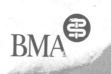

Textbook of
Clinical Occupational
and **Environmental Medicine**

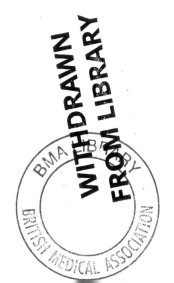

Commissioning Editor: Thomas H Moore
Project Development Manager: Hilary Hewitt
Project Manager: Susan Stuart
Designer: Andy Chapman
Illustration Manager: Mick Ruddy
Illustrators: Marion Tasker, Tim Loughhead

Textbook of
Clinical Occupational
and Environmental Medicine

Second Edition

Edited by

Linda Rosenstock MD MPH

Dean, School of Public Health
Professor of Medicine and Environmental Health Sciences
University of California, Los Angeles
Los Angeles, CA
USA

Mark R Cullen MD

Professor of Medicine and Public Health Director
Occupational and Environmental Medicine Program
Yale University School of Medicine
New Haven, CT
USA

Carl Andrew Brodkin MD MPH

Clinical Associate Professor of Medicine and
Environmental and Occupational Health Sciences
University of Washington
Seattle, WA
USA

Carrie A Redlich MD MPH

Professor of Medicine
Occupational and Environmental Medicine Program
and Pulmonary Critical Care Section
Yale University School of Medicine
New Haven, CT
USA

ELSEVIER
SAUNDERS

Philadelphia · Edinburgh · London · New York · St Louis · Sydney · Toronto 2005

ELSEVIER
SAUNDERS

© Harcourt Health Sciences Company 1994
© 2005, Elsevier Inc. All rights reserved.

First edition 1994
Second edition 2005

ISBN 0 7216 8974 4

British Library Cataloguing in Publication Data
A catalogue record for this book is available from the British Library

Library of Congress Cataloging in Publication Data
A catalog record for this book is available from the Library of Congress

---

Notice

Medical knowledge is constantly changing. Standard safety precautions must be followed, but as new research and clinical experience broaden our knowledge, changes in treatment and drug therapy may become necessary or appropriate. Readers are advised to check the most current product information provided by the manufacturer of each drug to be administered to verify the recommended dose, the method and duration of administration, and contraindications. It is the responsibility of the practitioner, relying on experience and knowledge of the patient, to determine dosages and the best treatment for each individual patient. Neither the Publisher nor the editors assume any liability for any injury and/or damage to persons or property arising from this publication.

The Publisher

Working together to grow
libraries in developing countries

www.elsevier.com | www.bookaid.org | www.sabre.org

ELSEVIER   BOOK AID International   Sabre Foundation

Printed in China

Last digit is the print number 9 8 7 6 5 4 3 2 1

Contents

Contributors

Michelle R Addorisio MD MPH
University of Connecticut Health
Center
Farmington, CT
USA

Bruce H Alexander PhD
Assistant Professor
Division of Environmental Health
Sciences
School of Public Health
University of Minnesota
Minneapolis, MN
USA

Thomas J Armstrong PhD
Professor, Industrial and Operations
Engineering
School of Public Health
The University of Michigan
Ann Arbor, MI
USA

Michael D Attfield PhD
Surveillance Branch Chief
Division of Respiratory Disease Studies
National Institure for Occupational
Safety and Health
Morgantown, WV
USA

Edward L Baker MD MPH
Professor and Director
North Carolina Institute for Public
Health
Chapel Hill, NC
USA

John R Balmes MD
Professor of Medicine
Division of Occupational and
Environmental Medicine
University of California
San Francisco, CA
Professor of Environmental Health
Sciences
University of California, Berkeley
San Francisco, CA
USA

Daniel E Banks MD
Professor of Medicine
Professor and Chair
Department of Internal Medicine
Louisiana State University Health
Sciences Center
Shreveport, LA
USA

Rebecca Bascom MD MPH
Professor of Medicine
Penn State College of Medicine
Milton S Hershey Medical Center
Hershey, PA
USA

Shirley Bassiri MD
Internal Medicine Residency Program
Department of Medicine
Columbia Presbyterian Medical
Center
New York, NY
USA

Alan R Berger MD
Professor of Neurology and Associate
Chairman
Department of Neurology
University of Florida
Jacksonville, FL
USA

Patricia Blackwell MD MPH
Medical Director
Occupational Health Clinic
Occupational Health and Prevention
Services
Centers for Disease Control and
Prevention
Atlanta, GA
USA

Paul Blanc MD MSPH
Professor of Medicine
Division of Occupational Medicine
University of California, San Francisco
San Francisco, CA
USA

Carl Andrew Brodkin MD MPH
Clinical Associate Professor of
Medicine and Environmental and
Occupational Health Sciences
University of Washington
Seattle, WA
USA

Sandy Bogucki MD PhD
Associate Professor
Section of Emergency Medicine
Yale University School of Medicine
New Haven, CT
USA

Chris Carlsten MD
Senior Fellow, Occupational and
Pulmonary Medicine
Occupational & Environmental
Medicine Program
University of Washington
Seattle, WA
USA

Tania Carreón MSc PhD
Associate Fellow
Division of Surveillance
Hazard Evaluations and Field Studies
National Institute for Occupational
Safety and Health,
Centers for Disease Control and
Prevention,
Assistant Professor
Department of Environmental
Health
University of Cincinnati Medical
Center
Cincinnati, OH
USA

Stephanie Carter MSPH CIH
Research Assistant and Doctoral
Candidate
Department of Environmental and
Occupational Health Sciences
University of Washington
Seattle, WA
USA

Moira Chan-Yeung MB FRCPC
FRCP
Professor of Medicine
Respiratory Division
Department of Medicine
University of British Columbia
Vancouver, BC
Canada

Harvey Checkoway PhD
Professor
Departments of Environmental and
Occupational Health Sciences and
Epidemiology
University of Washington
Seattle, WA
USA

Martin G Cherniack MD MPH
Professor of Medicine
Division of Occupational and
Environmental Medicine
University of Connecticut
Health Center,
Director
University of Connecticut
Ergonomics Technology Center
Farmington, CT
USA

H Gregg Claycamp MS PhD CHP
Director, Scientific Support Staff
Food and Drug Administration
Center for Veterinary Medicine
Rockville, MD
USA

David Eric Cohen MD
Director, Occupational and
Enviromental
Dermatology
Department of Dermatology
New York University Medical Centre
New York, NY
USA

Mark R Cullen MD
Professor of Medicine and Public
Health,
Director
Occupational and Environmental
Medicine Program
Yale University School of Medicine
New Haven, CT
USA

William E Daniell MD MPH
Associate Professor
Department of Environmental and
Occupational Health Sciences
University of Washington
Seattle, WA
USA

Paul S Darby MD PhD MPH CIME
Clinical Instructor
Department of Family Medicine
University of Washington
Seattle, WA
USA

John M Dement PhD CIH
Professor, Division of Occupational
and Environmental Medicine
Department of Community and
Family Medicine
Duke University Medical Center
Durham, NC
USA

Paul A Demers PhD
Associate Professor
School of Occupational and
Enviromental Hygiene
University of British Columbia
Vancouver, BC
Canada

Jeffrey Derr MD MPH
Occupational and Environmental
Medicine Residency Program
School of Public Health
University of Illinois at Chicago
Chicago, IL
USA

James R Donovan Jr MD MS
Professor
Department of Environmental Health
University of Cincinnati
Cincinnati, OH
USA

Alan M Ducatman MD MS
Professor and Chair
Department of Community Medicine
West Virginia University School of
Medicine
Morgantown, WV
USA

Derek E Dunn (deceased) PhD
National Institute for Occupational
Safety and Health, Centers for
Disease Control and Prevention
Cincinnati, OH
USA

David L Eaton PhD DABT FATS
Professor and Director
Center for Ecogenetics and
Environmental Health
University of Washington
Seattle, WA
USA

Ellen A Eisen ScD
Professor
Department of Health and
Environment
University of Massachusetts at Lowell
Lowell, MA
USA

Maadhava Ellaurie MBChB
Associate Professor of Medicine
Penn State College of Medicine
Milton S Hershey Medical Center
Hershey, PA
USA

Bradley A Evanoff MD MPH
Associate Professor of Medicine
Division of General Medical Sciences
Washington University School of
Medicine
St Louis, MO
USA

Peter S Evans PhD
Senior Research Scientist
Institute for Environmental
Health, Inc.
Seattle, WA
USA

Karin D E Everett PhD
Research Engineer Scientist
Department of Biology
University of Washington
Seattle, WA
USA

Nancy Fiedler PhD
Associate Professor
University of Medicine and Dentistry
of New Jersey
Robert Wood Johnson
Medical School
Environmental and Occupational
Health Sciences Institute
Piscataway, NJ
USA

Lawrence J Fine MD DrPH
Medical Advisor
Office of Behavioral and Social
Sciences Research
Office of the Director,
National Institutes of Health
Bethesda, MD
USA

Michael L Fischman MD MPH
Associate Clinical Professor and
Assistant Chief
Division of Occupational and
Environmental Medicine
Department of Medicine
University of California
San Francisco, CA
USA

Jordan A Firestone MD PhD MPH
Assistant Professor of Neurology,
University of Washington,
Staff, Harborview Medical Center
Seattle, WA
USA

Lora E Fleming MD PhD MPH MSc
Associate Professor
Department of Epidemiology and
Public Health and Division of Marine
Biology and Fisheries
School of Medicine and Rosenstiel
School of Marine and Atmospheric
Sciences
University of Miami
Miami, FL
USA

Brian G Forrester MD
Assistant Professor
University of Alabama School of
Medicine
Birmingham, AL
USA

Linda S Forst MD MPH MS
Associate Professor
University of Illinois at Chicago
School of Public Health
Environmental and Occupational
Health Sciences
Chicago, IL
USA

Susan H Forster MD
Associate Clinical Professor
Department of Ophthalmology and
Visual Science
Yale University School of Medicine,
Chief of Ophthalmology
Yale University Health Services
New Haven, CT
USA

Mark W Frampton MD
Professor of Medicine and
Environmental Medicine
University of Rochester School of
Medicine and Dentistry
Rochester, NY
USA

Alfred Franzblau MD
Professor of Occupational Medicine
University of Michigan
School of Public Health
Ann Arbor, MI
USA

Mary Carol Fromes (deceased) MD
MPH
University of Michigan School of
Public Health
Ann Arbor, MI
USA

Howard Frumkin MD MPH DrPH
FACP FACOEM
Professor and Chair
Department of Environmental and
Occupational Health
Rollins School of Public Health of
Emory University,
Professor of Medicine
Emory Medical School
Atlanta, GA
USA

David H Garabrant MD MPH
Professor of Occupational Medicine
and Epidemiology
University of Michigan
School of Public Health
Ann Arbor, MI
USA

Julie L Gerberding MD MPH
Director, Centers for Disease Control
and Prevention,
Administrator, Agency for Toxic
Substances and Disease Registry
Atlanta, GA
USA

Prajakta Ghatpande MSc MS
Research Scientist
Institute for Environmental
Health, Inc.
Seattle, WA
USA

Craig S Glazer MD
Assistant Professor
Department of Internal Medicine
University of Texas Southwestern
Medical Center at Dallas
Dallas, TX
USA

Michael Gochfeld MD PhD
Professor of Environmental and
Occupational Medicine
Enviromental and Occupational
Health Sciences Institute
University of Medicine and Dentistry
of New Jersey
Robert Wood Johnson Medical
School
Piscataway, NJ
USA

Bernard D Goldstein MD
Dean
Graduate School of Public Health
University of Pittsburgh
Pittsburgh, PA
USA

Daniel A Goldstein MD
Senior Science Fellow
Director of Medical Toxicology
Monsanto Company Regulatory
Affairs
St Louis, MO
USA

Audrey R Gotsch PH CHES
Interim Dean
University of Medicine and Dentistry
of New Jersey
School of Public Health
New Brunswick, NJ
USA

James W Grosch PhD
Research Psychologist
National Institute for Occupational
Safety and Health, Centers for
Disease Control and Prevention
Cincinnati, OH
USA

Mridu Gulati MD
Occupational and Environmental
Medicine and Pulmonary Clinical
Fellow
Department of Internal Medicine,
Yale University School of Medicine
New Haven, CT
USA

Mats Hagberg MD PhD
Professor and Director
Department of Occupational Medicine
Sahlgrenska Academy at Göteborg
University,
Chief Physician and Director
Department of Occupational and
Environmental Medicine
Sahlgrenska University Hospital
Göteborg
Sweden

William E Halperin MD DrPH
Professor and Chair
Department of Preventative
Medicine and Community Health
New Jersey Medical School
University of Medicine and Dentistry
of New Jersey
Newark, NJ
USA

Thomas E Hamilton MD PhD
MPH
Clinical Associate Professor of
Endocrinology and Metabolism
Division of Endocrinology and
Metabolism, University of
Washington Medical Center;
Fred Hutchinson Cancer Research
Center, Seattle, WA;
Private Practice, Endocrinology and
Metabolism
Bellevue, WA
USA

Philip Harber MD MPH
Professor of Family Medicine,
Chief, Division of Occupational and
Environmental Medicine
University of California, Los Angeles
Los Angeles, CA
USA

Amanda Hawes JD
Partner
Alexander, Hawes, and Audet
San Jose, CA
USA

Frank J Hearl BSChE SMChE PE
Senior Advisor
National Institute for Occupational
Safety and Health
Washington, DC
USA

Robin Herbert MD
Assistant Professor of Community
and Preventative Medicine
Mount Sinai Medical Center
New York, NY
USA

Christina A Herrick MD PhD
Assistant Professor of Dermatology
Yale University School of Medicine
New Haven, CT
USA

Robert F Herrick MS ScD
Senior Lecturer
Department of Environmental
Health
Harvard School of Public Health
Boston, MA
USA

Jessica Herzstein MD MPH
Global Medical Director
Air Products & Chemicals Inc.
Lexington, MA
USA

Michael J Hodgson MD MPH
Director
Occupational Safety and Health
Program
Department of Veterans Affairs
Office of Public Health and
Environmental Hazards
Washington, DC
USA

Christer Hogstedt MD PhD
Professor and Research Director
National Institute of Public Health
Stockholm
Sweden

Marilyn V Howarth MD
Assistant Professor of Occupational
and Emergency Medicine
University of Pennsylvania School of
Medicine,
Director of Occupational and
Environmental Consultation Services
Hospital of the University of
Pennsylvania
Philadelphia, PA
USA

Lea Hyvärinen MD PhD
Honorary Professor, Rehabilitation
Science, University of Dortmund
Dortmund, Germany,
Senior Lecturer, University of Oulu
and University of Tampere,
Helsinki
Finland

Louis F James MD MPH & TM
FACPM
Colonel, United States Air Force
(retired) Medical Corps Senior
Flight Surgeon,
Former Acting Director, Hyperbaric
Service, St Mary's Hospital
West Palm Beach, FL,
Former Co-Director, Hyperbaric
Service, Mariner's Hospital
Tavernier, FL
USA

Joel D Kaufman MD MPH
Associate Professor and Director
Occupational &
Environmental Medicine Program
Department of Occupational and
Environmental Health Sciences
University of Washington
Seattle, WA
USA

Matthew C Keifer MD MPH
Associate Professor
Departments of Environmental and
Occupational Health Sciences and
Medicine
University of Washington
Seattle, WA
USA

Karl T Kelsey MD MH
Professor of Cancer Biology and
Environmental Health
Harvard School of Public Health
Boston, MA
USA

Susan M Kennedy PhD
Professor, School of Occupational
and Environmental Hygiene,
Director, Centre for Health and
Environment Research
University of British Columbia
Vancouver, BC
Canada

Edwin M Kilbourne MD
Chief Medical Officer National
Center For Environmental Health/
Agency for Toxic Substances and
Disease Registry/United States
Department of Health and Human
Services/Office of the Director,
National Institutes of Health
Atlanta, GA
USA

Howard M Kipen MD MPH
Director and Professor of
Occupational Health
Environmental and Occupational
Health Sciences Institute
University of Medicine and Dentistry
of New Jersey
Robert Johnson Medical School
Piscataway, NJ
USA

Tord Kjellstrom BMed MEng PhD
(Medicine)
Professor of Public Health
National Institute of Public Health
Stockholm
Sweden

Jeffrey L Kohler PhD
Director, Pittsburgh Research
Laboratory
National Institute for Occupational
Safety and Health
Pittsburgh Research Laboratory
Pittsburgh, PA
USA

Anne Krantz MD MPH
Assistant Professor of Medicine, Rush
Medical College,
Chief, Section of Toxicology
Division of Occupational Medicine
John H Stroger Jr Hospital
of Cook County
Chicago, IL
USA

Kathleen Kreiss MD
Field Studies Branch Chief
Division of Respiratory Disease
Studies
National Institute for Occupational
Safety and Health
Morgantown, WV
USA

Anthony D LaMontagne ScD MA
MEd
Associate Professor
Centre for the Study of Health and
Society
The University of Melbourne
Parkville
Victoria
Australia

Philip J Landrigan MD MSc
Professor and Chairman
Department of Community and
Preventative Medicine
Mount Sinai School of Medicine
New York, NY
USA

Stan Lee MD
Senior Partner
The Polyclinic
Seattle, WA
USA

Carola Lidén MD
Professor of Occupational and
Environmental
Dermatology
Department of Medicine
Karolinska Institute
Stockholm
Sweden

James E Lockey MD MS
Professor and Director
Division of Occupational and
Environmental Medicine
University of Cincinnati
Cincinnati, OH
USA

William T Longstreth Jr MD MPH
Professor of Neurology
Harborview Medical Center
University of Washington
Seattle, WA
USA

Ulrike Luderer MD PhD MPH
Assistant Professor of Medicine
Center for Occupational &
Environmental Health
University of California, Irvine
Irvine, CA
USA

Ingvar Lundberg MD
Professor
National Institute for Working Life
and Department of Public Health
Sciences
Karolinska Institute
Stockholm
Sweden

Gregory J Ma MSPH SM(AAM)
Microbiology Supervisor
King County Environmental
Laboratory
Seattle, WA
USA

Steven Markowitz MD
Professor and Director
Center for the Biology of Natural
Systems
Queens College
City University of New York
New York, NY
USA

Carmen J Marsit PhD
Research Fellow
Harvard University School of Public
Health
Boston, MA
USA

Christopher J Martin MD MSc
Residency Director and Assistant
Professor
Institute of Occupational and
Environmental Health
Department of Community Medicine
West Virginia University School of
Medicine
Morgantown, WV
USA

Thomas P Matte MD MPH
Medical Epidemiologist
National Center for Environmental
Health
Centers for Disease Control and
Prevention
Atlanta, GA
USA

Donald R Mattison MD
Adjunct Professor
Department of Environmental
Health Sciences
Mailman School of Public Health
Columbia University
New York, NY
USA

Rob McConnell MD
Associate Professor of Preventative
Medicine, Keck School of Medicine
University of Southern California
Department of Preventative
Medicine
Los Angeles, CA
USA

James A Merchant MD PhD
Dean, College of Public Health
Professor of Occupational and
Environmental Health
University of Iowa College of Public
Health
Iowa City, IA
USA

Robert R Miksch PhD
Chief Research Scientist
Institute for Environmental
Health, Inc.
Seattle, WA
USA

Ben Hur P Mobo Jr MD MPH
Instructor of Medicine
Occupational and Environmental
Medicine Program
Yale University School of Medicine
New Haven, CT
USA

Sandra N Mohr MD MPH
Associate Medical Director
New York Life Insurance Company
New York, NY
USA

Jacqueline M Moline MD MSc
Assistant Professor
Community and Preventative
Medicine and Internal Medicine
Mount Sinai School of Medicine
New York, NY
USA

Gabrielle Morris MD
Diving Medicine Physician
Seattle and King County Department
of Health,
Occupational, Aviation and Diving
Medicine Physician, US
Healthworks, FAA Senior Aviation
Medical Examiner,
Seattle, WA
USA

Linda Rae Murray MD MPH
Chief Medical Officer – Primary Care
Ambulatory and Community Health
Network
Cook County Bureau of Health
Services
Chicago, IL
USA

James Nethercott MD (deceased)
University of Maryland,
Johns Hopkins Hospital
Baltimore, MD
USA

Gun Nise PhD
Assistant Professor and Senior
Occupational Hygienist
Department of Public Health
Sciences
Division of Occupational Medicine
Karolinska Institute
Stockholm
Sweden

Peter Orris MD MPH FACP
FACOEM
Professor and Director
Occupational Health Services
Institute
University of Illinois School
of Public Health,
Professor of Internal and
Preventative Medicine
Rush University School of Medicine
Cook County Hospital
Chicago, IL
USA

Adelisa L Panlilio MD MPH
Medical Epidemiologist
Centers for Disease Control and
Prevention
Atlanta, GA
USA

Edward L Petsonk MD
Senior Medical Officer
Division of Respiratory Disease
Studies
National Institute for Occupational
Safety and Health
Morgantown, WV
USA

Michael Pulley MD PhD
Assistant Professor of Neurology
Department of Neurology
University of Florida, Jacksonville
Jacksonville, FL
USA

Adrianna Quintero JD
Attorney
Environment and Health Outreach
Program
Director of Latino Outreach
Natural Resources Defense Council
San Francisco, CA
USA

Peter M Rabinowitz MD MPH
Assistant Professor of Medicine
Occupational and Environmental
Medicine Program
Yale University School of Medicine
New Haven, CT
USA

Carrie A Redlich MD MPH
Professor of Medicine
Occupational and Environmental
Medicine Program and Pulmonary
Critical Care Section
Yale University School of Medicine
New Haven, CT
USA

Thomas S Rees PhD
Associate Professor of
Otolaryngology – Head and Neck
Surgery
University of Washington,
Director of Audiology
Harborview Medical Center
Seattle, WA
USA

David M Rempel MD MPH
Professor of Medicine
University of California, San
Francisco
Richmond, CA
USA

Stephen J Reynolds PhD CIH
Professor of Industrial Hygiene
Department of Environmental and
Radiological Health Sciences
Colorado State University
Fort Collins, CO
USA

Caroline S Rhoads MD
Associate Professor of Medicine
Harborview Medical Center
University of Washington
Seattle, WA
USA

Frederick P Rivara MD MPH
The George Adkins Professor of
Pediatrics, Adjunct Professor of
Epidemiology
The Harborview Injury Prevention
and Research Center
University of Washington
Seattle, WA
USA

Mark G Robson BS MS PhD MPH
ATS
Chairman
Department of Environmental and
Occupational Health
University of Medicine and Dentistry
of New Jersey
School of Public Health
Piscataway, NJ
USA

Cecile S Rose MD MPH
Associate Professor of Medicine
Pulmonary and Occupational
Medicine
National Jewish Medical and
Research Center
Denver, CO
USA

Linda Rosenstock MD MPH
Dean, School of Public Health
Professor of Medicine and
Environmental Health Sciences
University of California, Los Angeles
Los Angeles, CA
USA

Mark A Rothstein JD
Professor, Director of the Institute for
Bioethics, Health Policy and Law,
Herbert F Boehl Chair of Law and
Medicine
Institute for Bioethics, Health Policy
and Law
University of Louisville
Louisville, KY
USA

Rachel Rubin MD MPH
Division Chair and Assistant
Professor of Medicine
Occupational and Environmental
Medicine
Rush Medical College
Stroger Hospital of Cook County
Chicago, IL
USA

Avima M Ruder PhD
Senior Research Epidemiologist
Division of Surveillance
Hazard Evaluations and Field Studies
National Institute for Occupational
Safety and Health, CDC
Cincinnati, OH
USA

Mark B Russi MD MPH
Associate Professor of Medicine and
Public Health, Yale University School
of Medicine,
Director, Occupational Health
Yale-New Haven Hospital
New Haven, CT
USA

Mansour Samadpour PhD
Director
Institute for Environmental
Health, Inc.
Seattle, WA
USA

Jonathan M Samet MD MS
Professor and Chair
Department of Epidemiology
Johns Hopkins Bloomberg School of
Public Health
Baltimore, MD
USA

Steven L Sauter PhD
Chief, Organizational Science and
Human Factors Branch
National Institute for Occupational
Safety and Health/Centers for
Disease Control and Prevention
Cincinnati, OH
USA

E Neil Schachter MD
Maurice Hexter Professor of
Medicine and Community Medicine,
Medical Director, Respiratory Care
Department
Mount Sinai Medical Center
New York, NY

Paul A Schulte PhD
Director
Education and Information Division
National Institute for Occupational
Safety and Health, Centers for
Disease Control and Prevention
Cincinnati, OH
USA

David A Schwartz MD MPH
Professor of Medicine and Genetics
Duke University Medical Center
Durham, NC
USA

Noah S Seixas PhD CIH
Professor
Department of Enviromental and
Occupational Health Sciences
University of Washington
Seattle, WA
USA

Stuart L Shalat BS BA ScM ScD
Associate Professor of Exposure
Epidemiology
Environmental and Occupational
Health Sciences Institute
Robert Wood Johnson Medical
School
Piscataway, NJ
USA

Elizabeth F Sherertz MD
Contact Dermatitis Specialist
The Skin Surgery Center
Winston-Salem, NC
USA

Gina Solomon MD MPH
Assistant Clinical Professor of
Medicine, University of California,
San Francisco,
Senior Scientist, Natural Resources
Defense Council
San Francisco, CA
USA

Akshay Sood MD MPH
Assistant Professor of Medicine
Division of Pulmonary and Critical
Care Medicine
Southern Illinois University School
of Medicine
Springfield, IL
USA

Nancy L Sprince MD MPH
Professor of Occupational and
Environmental Health and Internal
Medicine
Department of Occupational and
Environmental Health
University of Iowa College of Public
Health
Iowa City, IA
USA

Lawrence B Stein PhD
Psychologist
Private Practice
Red Bank, NJ
USA

Frances J Storrs MD
Professor Emerita
Department of Dermatology
Oregon Health and Science
University
Portland, OR
USA

Jaime Szeinuk MD
Assistant Professor of Community
and Preventative Medicine
Mount Sinai School of Medicine
New York, NY
USA

Oyebode A Taiwo MD MPH
Assistant Professor of Medicine
Occupational and Environmental
Medicine Program
Yale University School of Medicine,
New Haven, CT
USA

Tim K Takaro MD MPH MS
Clinical Assistant Professor
Department of Environmental and
Occupational Health Sciences
University of Washington
Seattle, WA
USA

Susan M Tarlo MBBS FRCP(C)
Professor of Medicine and Public
Health Sciences
University of Toronto
Toronto Western Hospital
Toronto, ON
Canada

Peter S Thorne MS PhD
Professor of Toxicology and
Environmental Health
Department of Occupational and
Environmental Health
The University of Iowa, The College
of Public Health
Iowa City, IA
USA

Mark J Utell MD
Professor of Medicine and
Environmental Medicine,
Director, Pulmonary/Critical Care
and Occupational Medicine Divisions
University of Rochester Medical
Center
Rochester, NY
USA

Gregory R Wagner MD
Director, Division of Repiratory
Disease Studies
National Institute for Occupational
Saftey and Health
Morgantown, WV
USA

Niel Wald AB MD
Professor of Environmental and
Occupational Health
Graduate School of Public Health
University of Pittsburgh
Pittsburgh, PA
USA

Elizabeth M Ward PhD
Director
Surveillance Research
Department of Epidemiology and
Surveillance Research
American Cancer Society
Atlanta, GA
USA

Daniel Wartenberg PhD
Professor
Department of Environmental and
Community Medicine
Environmental and Occupational
Health Sciences Institute
University of Medicine and Dentistry
of New Jersey
Robert Wood Johnson Medical
School
Piscataway, NJ
USA

Kalman L Watsky MD
Section Chief of Dermatology
Hospital of Saint Raphael,
Associate Clinical Professor of
Dermatology
Yale University School of Medicine
New Haven, CT
USA

Nargues A Weir MD FACCP
Attending Physician
Northern Virginia Pulmonary and
Critical Care Associates Inc.
Annandale, VA
USA

Laura S Welch MD
Medical Director
The Center to Protect Workers'
Rights
Silver Springs, MD
USA

Catharina Wesseling MD PhD
Coordinator, Health Section of
Central American Institute for
Studies on Toxic Substances
Universidad Nacional
Heredia
Costa Rica

Ellen Widess JD
Senior Program Officer
The Rosenberg Foundation
San Francisco, CA
USA

David A Youngblood MD MPH &
TM FACPM
Former Director
Hyperbaric Oxygen Department
Roper Hospital
Charleston, SC,
Haleiwa, HI
USA

Preface to the First Edition

The field of occupational and environmental disease is rapidly evolving. Questions and concerns about the health consequences of exposures to a seemingly endless array of potential hazards in the workplace and elsewhere in the environment are increasingly raised by clinicians themselves or brought to their attention by patients or other interested parties. Yet most practitioners find themselves ill-equipped to recognize, diagnose and treat occupational and environmental diseases. Further, textbooks in the field have not traditionally been dedicated to helping clinicians meet this challenge by presenting clinically relevant information that is both comprehensive yet practical and easily accessible.

The *Textbook of Clinical Occupational and Environmental Medicine* was conceived and written to address the needs of students, trainees, and clinicians who seek a resource to integrate occupational and environmental medicine into routine clinical practice. It evolved in part from our well-received, earlier effort—a concise and less encyclopedic text entitled *Clinical Occupational Medicine*. This textbook, although we hope it benefitted by our experiences with the first, is by intent and necessity markedly different in approach and scope. The role of workplace factors has been broadened to include environmental physical, chemical, and biologic agents that may have adverse effects on human health. Environmental diseases, although in general less well recognized and understood than those arising from the workplace, are integrated throughout the sections of the textbook.

The textbook is divided into four major sections. The first, Principles and Practice, provides a broad overview of the specialized skills central to the successful practice of occupational and environmental medicine, recognizing the strong interrelationship in the field between scientific and ethical, legal, economic, and social issues. The second section encompasses three core disciplines that are necessary complements to the diagnosis, treatment, and prevention of occupational and environmental diseases: toxicology, epidemiology and industrial hygiene. The third and longest section provides an organ system approach that enables the clinician to consider potential occupational and environmental diseases as they most commonly present in an individual patient. The last section, strongly cross-referenced to the third, enables the reader to consider specific toxins or hazards. Each chapter in this section is organized by exposure type (e.g., radiation, biologic factors, metals) and presented to provide an understanding of the environmental and occupational settings where specific agents are likely to be encountered, their acute and chronic health effects, and approaches to treatment and prevention of exposure to them.

The contributors to the textbook are well known and recognized experts from North America and Europe. The editors have worked closely with them to provide a consistent format throughout the textbook. We are extremely grateful for the spirit in which our contributors responded to this objective by accommodating to our evolving effort to achieve for the reader a coherent, comprehensive text. Long periods of silence on the part of some contributors were thankfully rewarded with remarkable chapters. One was preceded by a welcome fax from Greg Wagner, which—like a clear day in Seattle that may follow weeks of rain—served to brighten memories of the recent past. His doggerel is excerpted below

As midnight came
and the bell tolled
off the printer
the pages rolled

Now sitting with the rising sun
I know at least a draft is done!

The editors would also like to acknowledge the outstanding secretarial and editorial assistance provided by Paula Sandler, Rebecca Hubbard, Anne Gienapp, Lanita Stewart, and Marjorie E. Marenberg.

We also want to thank our colleagues at W.B. Saunders for encouraging us to proceed and at all turns strengthening the product, especially John Dyson, Ray Kersey, David Kilmer, Pat Morrison, and Carol DiBerardino.

And finally, we would like to acknowledge the influence of Bernadino Ramazzini, the Italian physician credited as the father of occupational medicine, who taught us many things, but in his extraordinary 1713 treatise, *Diseases of Workers,* understood very well the occupational hazards of authors. He wrote

The Author to His Book

Since you itch and are burning to be published,
First pay heed to an anxious father's warning,
Briefly here's what the fates have destined for you,
Since you bring them something novel,
All the learned at once will run to greet you.
Two short pages, I think are all they'll read through,
Then they'll fling you to factories or by-streets.
Where the poorest buy sausages and fish sauce.
Yes, you're fated to wrap up something greasy.
Still, cheer up, for the same thing often happens
Now to massive imposing legal Pandects.
All-receivers they are; they wrap up mackerel,
Or we screw them to hold the grocer's pennorth,
Pepper, maybe, or smelly seed of cumin.
You must know you were born in grimy workshops
Not in elegant mansions of our betters,
Not in glittering courts where chief physicians
Lay own laws for the cooks but sit down nowhere.
Trust me, then, you will suffer this more lightly
Than do books that can boast of prouder titles.
If they read you and straightway send you packing
Back to workshops, remember—you were born there.

From Diseases of Workers, *translated from the Latin text* De Morbis Artificium *of 1713 by Wilmer Care Wright Publishing Company, New York, New York 1964.*
LINDA ROSENSTOCK
MARK R. CULLEN

Preface to the Second Edition

The *Textbook of Clinical Occupational and Environmental Medicine* was originally conceived and written to address the needs of students, trainees and clinicians, as a resource to integrate occupational and environmental medicine into routine clinical practice. We found the response to the first edition extremely rewarding – the text was critically acclaimed and sustained broad national and international distribution. It enjoyed use by many working in different capacities in the occupational and environmental field, not merely clinicians.

In the decade since publication of the first edition, although many of the challenges in diagnosis, treatment and prevention remain, much in the world of occupational and environmental medicine has changed. Workers and others in the United States and abroad face new and emerging threats due to dramatic changes in globalization, technology and demographics. Even the merger of the two components, occupational and environmental – which a decade ago was still being questioned – is now all but taken for granted.

It is against this background that the editors of the first edition have drawn upon the prodigious efforts of two colleagues for this second edition. As with the first edition, we have worked closely with our distinguished contributors to provide a consistent format throughout the textbook and we are extremely grateful for the spirit in which our contributors responded to this objective. We have also undertaken some changes: chapters have been deleted, many more added, and all others significantly updated. In addition to reorganizing the initial four sections, a new section has been added to provide an overview of major workforce sectors, recognizing that an appreciation of the overall health risk in a given setting, such as mining, involves more than an isolated understanding of individual exposures.

Realignments in the publishing world, parallel to consolidations and acquisitions seen in other parts of the economy this past decade, brought us through a series of changes to our London-based publisher, Elsevier. We are grateful to our Elsevier colleagues, especially Rolla Couchman, Hilary Hewitt, Susan Stuart and Amy Head for facilitating this process, and for their support and constant professionalism. The editors would also like to acknowledge the outstanding support and editorial assistance provided by Linda Oliva and Gauri Balani.

As editors, we have in common wondrous appreciation for the support of family and friends – with special recognition by Linda (Lee, Adam and Matthew), Mark (Michele, Zoe and Esme), Drew (Kayla and Naomi), and Carrie (Mara, Joshua, Evelyn and Norman). We also share a deep and abiding respect for workers throughout the world, from whom we have learned so much and to whom we dedicate this book.

Linda Rosenstock
Mark R Cullen
Carl Andrew Brodkin
Carrie A Redlich

Section 1
Principles and Practice

Chapter 1
Introduction to Occupational and Environmental Medicine

Mark R Cullen, Linda Rosenstock, Edwin M Kilbourne

Work and economic development are fundamental to the human condition, and have contributed to enormous advancement in wellbeing and health over the centuries. Unfortunately, virtually every aspect of work entails risk of harm as well, both because of the physical nature of the activities involved and the intimate relationship in which workers are placed to natural and man-made hazards in the environment. Moreover, the activities of production themselves and the products generated by work have introduced into the broader environment innumerable hazards of everyday life: in the air we breathe, the food and water we consume, and the material goods we use and ultimately must dispose of. Occupational and environmental medicine (OEM) is an evolving medical specialty that seeks to identify and modify the adverse effects of these hazards on the health of individuals and larger populations.

The focus of OEM differs from many other specialties, which may encompass interest in particular agents (e.g., infectious disease), organ systems (e.g., pulmonary medicine), mechanisms of injury (e.g., immunology) or curative approaches (e.g., surgery). In these more traditional disciplines, the focus of attention is on factors that an individual patient or his/her clinician, or both, can modify to prevent, ameliorate or cure disease or the consequence of injury. In OEM practice, although individuals are of paramount importance, equally important are external factors beyond the direct control of individuals or physicians. The same external factors affecting one person often threaten the health of others. There is a natural tension between the clinical health issues relating to the individual patient and broader public health issues, which transcend the traditional doctor–patient relationship. These broader issues fall very centrally in the domain of OEM practice. The focus of this text, however, is the clinical side, placed in the context of these broader perspectives.

Historically the field of OEM has developed out of two formerly distinct disciplines: occupational medicine and environmental medicine. Though common clinical and public health perspectives, scientific underpinnings, training needs and practice approaches have fostered this 'merger' during the past several decades, there remain differences in the two components by dint of their distinct population foci, divergent societal approaches and distinctive histories. We shall begin here by describing the central principles of disease that irrevocably bind the two; in the sections that follow, unique issues relating to the scope and practice will be introduced.

PRINCIPLES OF OCCUPATIONAL AND ENVIRONMENTAL DISEASE

1. The clinical and pathologic expression of most environmentally caused diseases are indistinguishable from those of non-environmental origin

There is a widely held belief among medical practitioners outside of OEM that diseases of occupational or environmental origin are both rare and distinctive. In reality, diseases caused by work and ambient environment are neither rare nor often distinctive in their clinical presentations and laboratory findings. Most occupational diseases, such as occupational cancers, not only resemble diseases caused by other factors but are otherwise indistinguishable except by careful documentation of a history of a relevant exposure. Other occupational and environmental diseases, like asthma or dermatitis, may be distinguished clinically only through obtaining an exposure history, with or without specialized testing, which presupposes high suspicion for the diagnosis. Only a minority of occupational diseases, such as pesticide and heavy metal poisonings, are sufficiently distinctive that they are likely to be uniquely identified by routine laboratory testing procedures.

2. Many diseases of occupational or environmental origin are multifactorial, with non-environmental factors playing a contributory role

The majority of chronic diseases and even a fair number of acute ones are multifactorial in origin. Coronary artery disease, for example, cannot be simply attributed to hypertension alone in a patient who also smokes. In fact, the discovery of one cause not only does not preclude the possibility of a second, it often makes the effect of an environmental exposure more likely. For example, it has been well established that asbestos exposed workers who smoke have a far higher likelihood of lung cancer than individuals exposed to cigarettes or asbestos singly. Similarly, alcohol consumption is known to potentiate the effects of some environmental hepatotoxins by causing hepatocellular disease.

The most important consequence of this principle in practice is that the potential role of an environmental toxin is not reduced by the presence of another pathogenic factor; in fact, it may be increased. This holds true for common types of clinical complaints that result from exposure to the environment, such as irritation and sensitization of the skin and respiratory tract. Such problems are too often ascribed to causes such as smoking or viral infection, leaving remediable occupational and environmental causes undetected.

3. The effects of occupational and environmental exposures occur after a biologically predictable latent interval following exposure

Agents or chemicals capable of causing direct and acute injury to the body will typically exert their effects either immediately or soon after exposure. In these cases, because the onset of disease occurs early, possible causal connections are relatively easily identified. On the other hand, the effects of agents that act by sensitizing the immune system, such as those that cause dermatitis or asthma, more often are exhibited only after a period of months to years of exposure.

Other substances initiate insidious disease processes that may become clinically apparent only after a latent interval of many years. For example, carcinogens may not cause cancer until years after the individual's first exposure. Importantly, there is no uniform relation between these late outcomes and any early effects. For example, leukemia may occur in a person exposed to external ionizing radiation at levels far below that which would cause acute radiation sickness or other demonstrable health effect. Indeed, individuals unaffected by early effects may be at higher risk for later effects because they tolerate doses of higher intensity and duration than those who do suffer acute effects, and consequently remove themselves from further exposure, or are removed.

4. The dose of an exposure to a noxious agent is the strongest predictor of the likelihood and type of effect

Although this principle is elucidated in detail in Chapter 5, it is important to recognize that toxins, like drugs, have clear relationships between dose of exposure and subsequent effect, and proportion of exposed individuals affected. Although each host differs from others, knowledge of these relationships and estimation of the amount of each are key to diagnostic decision-making.

In general, higher exposures confer a higher likelihood of being affected (dose–response relationship) and of more serious effects (dose–effect relationship). As shown in Figure 1.1, three distinct patterns can be discerned. For direct acting toxins, such as heavy metals, organic solvents, or pesticides (Fig. 1.1a), there is for each individual a threshold dose below which there is no demonstrable effect. As the dose increases, the severity of effect increases up to a level that ultimately, at least theoretically, would be fatal. In addition, as the dose increases, the proportion of the exposed population adversely affected also increases.

Other harmful agents act by eliciting an immunologic or other hypersensitivity response (Fig. 1.1b). With these agents, such as those that cause asthma, dermatitis, and

allergic alveolitis, many persons experience no untoward effect regardless of dose, presumably based on genetic or other host factors. Increasing dose, however, increases the likelihood of sensitization in those who are susceptible. Once sensitization occurs, however, the severity of reactions is typically independent of subsequent exposure dose and may occur at a very low level.

Finally, there are agents that interact with genetic material to cause mutations or initiate cancers (Fig. 1.1c). With these agents, the administration of even the smallest dose confers a finite chance of a mutation. The risk of disease at the lowest end of the dose–response curve may be only theoretical or unmeasurable (e.g., the risk of lung cancer from smoking one cigarette). In this situation, as with agents inducing hypersensitivity, the dose does not affect the severity of disease once it is present; only the probability of disease increases as the dose of exposure increases.

Although these relationships are different, the importance of dose in arriving at a correct diagnosis, providing treatment, and preventing disease remains crucial in every case. As discussed more fully in Chapter 3, successful evaluation and management of the patient suspected of having a disorder of environmental origin or who has a risk for such a disorder depend on the clinician's ability to assess the patient's recent and past exposure dose, at least qualitatively. Primary prevention, on the other hand, depends on minimizing exposure dose in the first place.

5. People differ substantially in their responses to noxious exposures

Humans sometimes differ remarkably in their responses to environmental exposures. These differences may be due to a wide range of factors, including genetic differences in metabolism, age, gender or size, co-exposures to environmental substances that may interact with agents of interest, coexisting morbid conditions, or complex behavioral factors. The major principles that underlie this variability are discussed in Chapter 11. For present purposes, it is important to recognize such variability, which frequently obscures the relationship between environmental exposures and health effects. For example, a health problem in one among many individuals exposed to a harmful agent may suggest an alternative explanation for the effect when in reality only that single individual was susceptible to that dose of exposure. Similarly, the fact that many workers have functioned without adverse consequence around a chemical or process may wrongly suggest to an employer or susceptible coworker that the environment is equally safe for all. From the practitioner's perspective, it is important to recognize that although the pattern of occurrence of illness in a population may be a vital clue and should always be sought, the absence of an obvious pattern or a confusing pattern may be a function of host variability within the population.

OCCUPATIONAL MEDICINE

In developed countries the vast majority of adults – men and women – are active in the formal economy, inter-

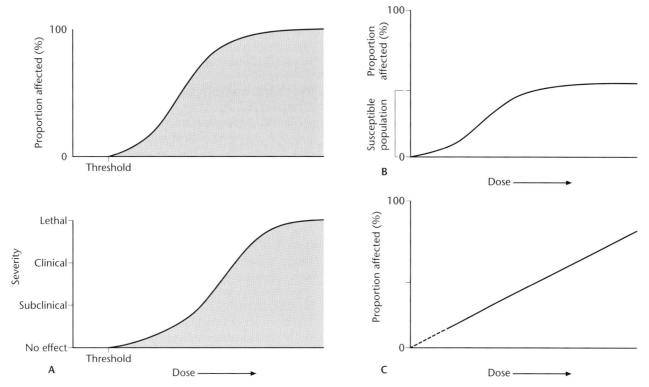

Figure 1.1: Schematic dose–response relations for environmental hazards. (a) For direct-acting agents, there is a threshold for each individual, followed by increasing severity with rising dose. Similarly, a rising fraction of the exposed population is affected as dose rises; eventually everyone is affected. (b) Indirect-acting toxins affect only susceptible individuals. The dose determines what proportion of these individuals are affected. Note that dose may not determine the severity of the reactions, which may be more related to host factors. (c) Carcinogens are believed to cause disease as a linear function of dose. The shape of the dose–response curve at very low doses (dotted line) is difficult to determine directly from studies; it is often assumed to be linear, but this assumption is controversial for some carcinogens.

rupted occasionally for reproduction, medical disabilities and economic dislocations such as layoffs. Virtually every form of work has attendant hazards – physical, chemical, biologic and social; these are discussed in Sections 2 and 4 of this text. Although some work environments are complex, involving many different hazards, and the potential human effects of many hazards remain incompletely studied, the range of possibilities is nonetheless circumscribed and, in theory at least, can be reconstructed and characterized – even quantified – in the effort to assess risk for injury and illness, and evaluate health problems that do arise. For complex historical and social reasons, however, attention to this relationship has been very limited until the past few decades, even in developed countries (Chapter 2). In developing countries, where far higher fractions of the adult population are either unemployed or engaged in informal work, characterization of the health effects of work is far less complete (Chapter 10).

Despite significant recent advances in worker health promotion, there remains as yet no reliable estimate of the magnitude of the medical and economic burden posed by occupational diseases and injuries. Efforts to determine the nature and extent of occupational diseases are more elusive than for injuries; the latter, in general, involving more physically apparent outcomes with more easily traced causes.

Chapter 31 provides an overview of data sources and information about the distribution of both fatal and non-fatal occupational injuries. In this section we review some of the problems defining the extent of occupational disease and injury in developed countries, focusing on what is known and not known in the United States. Readers can find more detailed information about the incidence and prevalence of specific disease entities in the organ system chapters of Section 3 of this text.

Two main factors contribute to the lack of reliable estimates about the extent of occupational diseases: clinical under-recognition that such diseases are in fact occupational and inadequacy of public surveillance systems to capture and summarize those that may be recognized clinically. Under-recognition, in turn, is based on a number of factors, including:

1. inadequate knowledge about the health effects of many hazards among employers, workers and health practitioners;
2. the absence of pathognomonic or even relatively specific findings for many occupational diseases;
3. latency between exposure and disease onset for most chronic conditions;
4. multifactorial causation for many occupational diseases, including those due to both occupational and

environmental factors and non-environmental ones; and

5. marked variations in individual susceptibility to most occupational hazards.

Compounding these complexities in disease recognition are the inadequate attention devoted to occupational diseases in medical education in the United States and the historical isolation that largely excluded attention to occupational factors and conditions from mainstream medical care. Beyond diagnostic difficulties lie fragmented and often biased reporting systems. Moreover, even if reporting systems functioned better, there are a number of significant disincentives for the physician to report an occupational disease. These include: burdensome paperwork and bureaucratic interactions; lack of payment, underpayment, and payment delays if cases are contested by employers; and the wish to avoid litigious involvement.

The burden of occupational injury and disease: sources and limitations of data

The following section provides a brief overview of some of the state and national data sources that have been used in deriving estimates of the nature and extent of the occupational disease burden in the United States. Although data systems in other developed countries differ, the fundamental limitations are common to all to varying degrees. The situation in developing economies is far more intractable, as discussed in Chapter 10.

Annual survey of occupational injuries and illnesses

In the United States the Bureau of Labor Statistics (BLS) program of OSHA, mandated by the 1970 OSH Act, maintains a national employer based system to monitor job-related illnesses and injuries and summarizes these data in annual surveys.[1] The BLS data are obtained by annual compilation of required injury and illness reporting logs from all eligible employers, with substantial penalties invoked for non-compliance. Many shortcomings of this reporting system limit its reliability and completeness including exclusion of many workers (the self-employed; small businesses and farms; and federal, state, and local agency employees); under-reporting of most occupational diseases (especially chronic, multifactorial and latent ones); and the disincentives inherent in any system linking reporting rates to regulatory priorities, however otherwise rational such links might appear. Needless to say, the quality of the aggregate data can be no better than the quality of the data input.

Nonetheless, the most recently available data do provide a broad and staggering picture of the magnitude of the occupational health problem in the US, limitations notwithstanding. In the year 2000 almost 5.3 million occupational injuries were self-reported at covered workplaces alone; 1.6 million of these resulted in lost work time. In addition, 362,000 occupational illnesses were reported, including over 200,000 cases of musculoskeletal disorders attributed by employers to work, over 40,000

skin conditions, and almost 80,000 respiratory cases, poisonings, etc – almost all acute in nature.[2] In a separate reporting function, 5,344 deaths were reported at work due to occupational causes.

Workers' compensation reports (see also Chapter 57.2)

Workers' compensation records, both state and federal, provide one of the most widely available sources of data about occupational diseases and injuries. There is ample support for the belief that these databases systematically underestimate the extent of occupational illnesses and distort the distribution of types.[3] For example, a recent study conducted in the northeastern United States found that as many as 90% of self-recognized musculoskeletal disorders had not been reported to the workers' compensation system.[4] Workers' compensation systems also vary as to their inclusiveness of coverage; agricultural workers, for example, are excluded from workers' compensation benefits in many states. In addition to problems of incomplete worker coverage and failures to report diseases – especially chronic diseases – to this system (whether because of patient or physician inclination not to do so), many of these systems report only those claims that are accepted; widespread experience suggests many are contested by insurance carriers in virtually every jurisdiction. The reverse also occurs: poorly documented claims are sometimes compensated. Nonetheless, some inferences can be derived from these data which form part of the incomplete whole picture.[3]

Morbidity and mortality from chronic conditions

In the United States, some states record the individual's usual occupation on death certificates; a smaller number of states include industry as well. These data and accompanying information about cause of death and contributory causes (so-called 'multiple causes of death') have proved useful in estimating excess mortality in different jobs and industries. Since the late 1960s, the National Center for Health Statistics (NCHS) has provided annual summaries of all conditions on death certificates from all states, including information about occupation and industry from the several states which code this; since 1989 more extensive information about industry and occupation has been coded.[5] These data allow exploration not only of the underlying cause of death but also about other conditions that may have contributed to death. Still, there are many limitations to using death certificates in general and multiple causes of death in particular, including: under-and over-reporting of causes by physicians unknowledgeable about occupational diseases; very limited and poor quality information about job and industry from which to infer exposures; and all those factors leading to under-recognition of occupational diseases alluded to earlier.

Nonetheless, manipulations with these data have led to various estimates of occupational disease mortality in the

US, ranging from 40,000 to 65,000 deaths from chronic occupational disease per year in the US.[6] Almost 10,000 of these are directly attributable to asbestos.[7] The majority of cases – cancers, and chronic disease of the respiratory tract, heart, liver and kidneys – have been imputed by comparing proportional death rates in various industries, adjusting as best possible for confounding factors such as tobacco and socioeconomic class. For this reason, caution is suggested in the interpretation of these data.

Canadian estimates of incidence and mortality, derived from similar databases, suggest comparable experience throughout North America, at least, adjusting for differences in the size of the workforces.[8]

National Hospital Discharge Survey

The National Hospital Discharge Survey (NHDS), conducted annually by the NCHS, provides data on hospital stays in non-governmental hospitals.[9] Information is provided regionally. Data on occupations and industries are not available, but the system does allow capture of diagnostic events that may be occupational in origin, e.g., carpal tunnel syndrome or asthma, or other so-called 'sentinel health events' – common disorders that have been linked to occupational causes in some significant fraction of all new cases.[10] These data, despite significant limitations, have been used in helping to derive estimates of the extent of certain occupational diseases in the United States, such as coal workers' pneumoconiosis, whose prevalence has

resulted in a drop from a peak of 24,000 hospitalizations in 1984 to 11,000 in 1996, and asbestosis, whose prevalence based on these data has increased during the same time period from 6000 a year to 13,000.[7]

Outpatient data

Occupational diagnostic referral clinics developed in the US in the 1970s and have become widespread in medical centers in the 1980s and 1990s.[11] These clinics have as their primary goal the identification and management of work-related diseases not readily handled by primary sources of worker care. Although workplace diversity and identified conditions of evaluated patients are limited by local or regional referral practices and patterns, and the availability of such clinics remains extremely limited, data from these clinics provide some insight into common diseases and exposures. Tables 1.1 and 1.2 give an overview of common diagnoses and exposures from 24 clinics, members of the Association of Occupational and Environmental Clinics (AOEC) who submitted case reports to the AOEC database describing patients with work-related diseases or injuries[12] who were diagnosed between January 1991 and December 2000. While not necessarily representative of all patients with work-related conditions, these case reports provide insight into the types of occupational conditions being treated by occupational medicine specialists, as well as into the types of exposures that are causing or exacerbating these diseases.

General diagnosis category	Specific diagnosis	# of cases	% of cases
Respiratory (5814 of 6021 diagnoses)*	Asbestosis/parenchymal disease only	3631	40.1
	Asthma (691 cases) and reactive airways dysfunction syndrome (156 cases)	847	9.4
	Asbestos-related pleural disease only	642	7.1
	Upper respiratory irritation, chronic or NOS	425	4.7
	Silicosis	155	1.7
	Parenchymal and pleural disease	114	1.3
Musculoskeletal (973 of 1755 diagnoses)	Carpal tunnel syndrome or median nerve neuropathy	318	3.5
	Tendinitis / tenosynovitis / bursitis of the forearm, wrist, hand, or fingers	192	2.1
	Epicondylitis	144	1.6
	Low back strain / sprain / tears	133	1.5
	Low back pain / radiculopathy / muscle spasm	98	1.1
	Upper extremity cumulative trauma disorder / musculoskeletal pain	88	1.0
Sensory organ disorders (909 of 965 diagnoses)	Noise-induced hearing loss	909	9.7
Symptom-defined and miscellaneous syndromes (443 of 626 diagnoses)	Multiple chemical sensitivity/acquired chemical intolerance	166	1.8
	Sick building syndrome	156	1.7
	Headache (chemical, migraine, tension, or NOS)	121	1.3
Chemical poisoning syndromes (313 of 458 diagnoses)	Toxic effect of lead	181	2.0
	Toxic effects of solvents	132	1.5
Skin (183 of 254 diagnoses)	Dermatitis, all	183	2.0
Psych/Neuro (165 of 395 diagnoses)	Toxic encephalopathy	165	1.8

*Numbers in parentheses represent number of cases with specific diagnoses listed in table, out of total number of diagnoses in category.
NOS = not otherwise specified.

Table 1.1 Diagnoses made in at least 1% of the occupational cases, 1991 to 2000 (*n* = 9044 cases; 10,882 diagnoses)

Exposure	Percent of 5641 occupational cases
Asbestos	49.9
Noise	16.0
Repetitive motion	8.3
Keyboard use	7.7
Indoor air pollutants	7.7
Solvents, NOS	4.8
Inorganic lead	3.3
Lifting	3.1
Crystalline silica	3.0
1,1,1-Trichloroethane	2.7
Tetrachloroethylene	2.5
Fall, NOS	2.5
Acute trauma, NOS	2.1
Dust, NOS	1.9
Smoke, NOS	1.6
Tuberculosis	1.5
Paint	1.4
Chemicals, NOS	1.4
Vibration, NOS	1.3
Isocyanates, NOS	1.3
Coal	1.2
Latex, natural rubber	1.2
Welding, NOS	1.1
Cutting oils	1.0
Formaldehyde	0.9
Ergonomic factors, NOS	0.9
Mold	0.9
Toluene	0.8
Hydrocarbons, NOS	0.7
Xylene	0.7
Pesticides, NOS	0.6
Ammonia solution	0.6
Glutaraldehyde	0.6
Epoxy resins	0.5
Methyl ethyl ketone	0.5
Struck by/against object	0.5

*Exposures contributing to at least 0.5% of the cases are included in table; some cases have more than one contributing exposure.
NOS = not otherwise specified

Table 1.2 Most frequent contributing exposures* associated with occupational conditions, AOEC cases, 1991–2000 ($n = 9044$ cases; 11,239 exposures)

Over a 10-year period, over 9000 patients were diagnosed with work-related diseases or injuries. The AOEC case report records up to three diagnoses and three exposures; therefore, the numbers of diagnoses and exposures exceed the number of patients. As seen from Table 1.1, asbestosis, diagnosed in 41% of all patients with work-related conditions, was by far the most common disease seen in these AOEC clinics; asbestos-related pleural disease was also common. This burden of disease from past asbestos exposures should diminish over time, as asbestos exposures are now well controlled in the US. Noise-induced hearing loss was seen in almost 10% of patients with occupational disease, almost all diagnosed within the patient subgroup with asbestos-related disorders. The AOEC clinics also treat numerous patients with diseases and injuries caused by more recent exposures. Chief among these are respiratory conditions and soft-tissue musculoskeletal disorders. Asthma or RADS (reactive airways dysfunction syndrome) was diagnosed in 9.4% of occupational cases, and upper respiratory irritation in 4.7%. Carpal tunnel syndrome, upper extremity tendinitis/

tenosynovitis/bursitis, epicondylitis, and low back problems together accounted for almost 10% of occupational cases. Table 1.1 also lists several other commonly diagnosed conditions, including dermatitis, lead poisoning, multiple chemical sensitivity, toxic encephalopathy, and sick building syndrome.

Table 1.2 details the occupational exposures most frequently related to patients' injuries or illnesses. Leading the list of associated exposures were: asbestos (49.9%); noise (16%); repetitive motion (8.3%); keyboard use (7.7%); and indoor air pollutants (7.7%). As can be seen from the remaining exposures on the list, occupational diseases and injuries are being caused by very diverse chemical, physical and biologic exposures.

Occupational disease surveillance systems

Both the federal government in the US and some states have developed surveillance systems to track incident cases of all occupational diseases or specific entities. Five states, for example, undertook reporting of occupational asthma under a program sponsored by the National Institute for Occupational Safety and Health: 1100 cases were reported between 1993 and 1995.[13] Twenty-eight states require reporting by laboratories of blood lead levels for adults as a way of tracking OSHA-mandated blood testing of exposed workers. Results suggest numbers of cases of lead poisoning still occur: Washington State reported almost 2800 levels greater than 25 micrograms/dL between 1993 and 2001;[14] Massachusetts reported 547 during a recent 5-year period.[15] Connecticut requires reporting of all work-related diseases, collecting between 1500 to 2000 reports per year since 1996, mostly musculoskeletal disorders, elevated lead levels, skin and lung conditions.[16]

Despite these and emerging efforts both nationally and regionally, it is noteworthy that no comprehensive system exists to capture occupational diseases and non-acute injuries, so all estimates of incidence and mortality must be viewed with caution as likely underestimates of the true burden.

Estimates of the prevalence of occupational conditions in the population

Because incidence data are limited, attempts have been made to estimate the prevalence of occupational effects in the population based on broader measures of the health of the population. The boldest attempt thus far was the Occupational Health Supplement to the National Health Information Survey (NHIS), a periodic populational sample survey conducted every several years by the National Center for Health Statistics.

Unfortunately the supplement has only been done once – in 1988 – limiting any inference about changes. Moreover, since the survey is self-administered, only conditions of which respondents may be aware, such as pain or skin rash, are amenable to study. Interpretation is further limited by potential bias in respondents' perceptions about what conditions are and are not related to their work.

Nonetheless, analyses of the 1988 survey have resulted in some evidence that the proportion of the population with work-related musculoskeletal disorders such as low back pain, carpal tunnel syndrome and dermatitis may dwarf estimates from BLS and the other sources described above,[17] with literally millions of workers affected by, and to a disturbing extent disabled by conditions perceived to have occurred on the job. While it would be presumptuous to apply these estimates as verified, the extent of positive responses regarding a small number of self-reported conditions further underscores both the large scope of the persisting occupational disease burden in our society, and ultimately the need for more valid, timely and longitudinal data to control it.

ENVIRONMENTAL MEDICINE

Since the birth of occupational medicine and continuing through very recent times, interest in the environmental determinants of non-infectious disease has centered overwhelmingly around the workplace. Substantial concern regarding the potential adverse effects on health of non-occupational environmental exposures has developed only relatively recently. The beginning of this trend is difficult to pinpoint, but in the United States, it has become particularly evident over the last three decades.

Today, the non-occupational environment rivals or exceeds the occupational environment as a source of health concerns among the public at large. Hardly a day goes by without news media coverage of one or more potential environmental health problems. At the national and international level, prominent environmental health issues currently include all of the following and more:

- increased cancer risk from radon in indoor air;
- neurologic dysfunction from exposure to lead in house dust and drinking water;
- respiratory and cardiovascular mortality from particulate and other ambient air pollutants;
- still-to-be-clarified consequences of the accumulation of measurable body burdens of biopersistent halogenated organic compounds (e.g., dioxins and polychlorinated biphenyls) in large segments of the population;
- possible neurotoxic, carcinogenic, and other effects of substances added to foods; and
- potentially devastating health consequences that may arise from global warming and depletion of stratospheric ozone.

Quantifying the precise levels of risk attributable to environmental exposures in a given population presents difficult methodologic problems. Nevertheless, in one major study, an estimated 75–80% of cancers in the United States were judged to be avoidable, and largely due to environmental factors.[18] Tobacco smoke, both actively and passively inhaled, may account for approximately 30% of all cancers in the United States. But other air pollutants are important as well. Over 1000 deaths per year occur in the United States as a result of unintentional exposure

to carbon monoxide, and the prevalence of asthmatic symptoms may double in children as a result of living close to a heavily polluting industrial facility. As many as 10,000 to 20,000 lung cancer deaths occur annually as a result of exposure to environmental radon.[19] A substantial proportion of preschool children in the United States, particularly those living in older housing, are at risk of developing measurable intellectual dysfunction owing to environmental lead.

At the local level, there is concern about the potential danger to people located close to hazardous waste sites and the possible effects of water or air pollution related to nearby industry. At the level of the individual, the practitioner may see patients whose illness or personal health concerns relate either to one of the major issues described earlier or to more unusual exposures or health problems that are specific to that individual.

Purview of environmental medicine

By comparison with occupational health, non-occupational environmental medicine presents both the researcher and the health practitioner with an unusually thorny set of issues and problems. Full consensus has yet to be reached even regarding the boundaries of the new medical discipline, but one could reasonably define non-occupational environmental medicine as that medical specialty involving the prevention, diagnosis, therapy, and study of disease and injury due to external influences but unrelated to the patient's workplace. Nevertheless, the potential problems accompanying such a broad definition of the field should be recognized. There is substantial overlap with extant and established specialties, such as infectious disease medicine and pulmonary medicine. Given the paucity of practitioners of this component until very recently, it would seem most appropriate for practitioners of non-occupational environmental medicine to concentrate both clinical and research activities on those problems and issues not already covered by other specialists.

Some might prefer a more limited (but potentially viable) definition that would exclude essentially all infectious agents from the purview of non-occupational environmental medicine. This limitation in scope would have the added benefit of focusing the specialty area on the effects and potential effects of chemical and physical environmental agents, which are not dealt with comprehensively in any other specialty area except occupational medicine. Whether certain chemical exposures related to lifestyle (e.g., tobacco smoking and ingestion of dietary lipids) should be excluded from the consideration as problems in non-occupational environmental medicine can also be debated. Despite potential overlap with the fields of allergy and clinical immunology, the potential contribution of the environmental medicine practitioner to the amelioration of health problems due to non-infectious biologic agents is large.

There is clearly some overlap between non-occupational environmental medicine and the developing specialty of clinical toxicology. However, clinical toxicologists tend to deal with sudden, generally well-characterized, chemical exposures for which the resulting clinical picture is often acute, rapidly terminating in death or resolution of clinical abnormalities. They deal less with chronic health effects related to cumulative exposure to relatively low doses of toxicants, whereas this area is a specific focus of environmental medicine. The practice of clinical toxicology is directed toward treating persons for clinical symptoms that are already apparent. Clinical toxicology is less oriented toward risk communication and counseling aimed at preventing adverse health outcomes over the long term. Finally, clinical toxicology does not deal with the physical environmental hazards that form an important focus of research and practice in environmental medicine.

Even if one defined the field in the most restrictive terms possible, the scope of environmental medicine would remain enormous. Potential chemical hazards are particularly numerous with potential human exposure outside of work to more than 50,000 registered with the US Environmental Protection Agency under the Toxic Substances Control Act (see Chapter 57.1) There are fewer physical than chemical environmental agents of concern. This set of etiologic agents requires very different and diverse bases of scientific knowledge to understand the processes involved in the etiology and pathogenesis of the documented and potential health effects produced by such diverse physical agents as ionizing radiation, electromagnetic fields, hot and cold temperatures, high and low atmospheric pressures, and mechanical force.

Differences from occupational medicine

Whereas occupational medicine is a well-established specialty, with a substantial (if still inadequate) number of practitioners focused on reasonably well-defined populations and hazards (earlier cautionary comments notwithstanding), there are relatively few physicians whose practices involve a substantial component of non-occupational environmental medicine. Moreover, many of those who do practice non-occupational environmental medicine do so only as part of a broader practice involving a recognized specialty or subspecialty (e.g., allergy/immunology, otolaryngology, neurology, or pulmonary medicine).

Information bases

For both the practitioner and the researcher, the non-occupational environment presents challenges, many of which are either absent from or present to a lesser extent in occupational medicine. Of these challenges, the frequent absence of quantitative and even certain qualitative information on exposure is particularly troublesome. The worker at a given site is subject to a particular set of exposures that are determined by the industrial process used there. If he or she becomes ill, a relatively rapid determination can, at least in theory, be made regarding whether a workplace exposure could plausibly account for the

illness. Such a determination could be based on the known adverse effects of the specific materials and processes used and the number, duration, and circumstances of contacts the patient has had with them. It is often possible (and always desirable) to conduct environmental measurements of exposures of concern in the workplace to provide quantitative data on both average and peak exposures (see later). Moreover, because a number of workers may share the same exposures, the presence of a pattern of symptoms among workers with common duties can alert one to the possibility that a workplace environmental exposure may be the cause. Workers themselves may have at least some familiarity with the potential adverse consequences of specific exposures in their industry, and, therefore, they may be more likely to report them to the physician.

By contrast, outside of the workplace, peoples' lifestyles and exposures are extremely varied. Patients rarely maintain an encyclopedic listing of the particular products they use or of other exposures that may be relevant to their complaints or illness. Often exposures affect only a single individual or family, substantially lessening the possibility that an association of a disease with a particular exposure could be identified by means of an analysis of the pattern of health effects seen among several persons. The patient may be unable to reproduce or even accurately report the typical pattern of use of potentially etiologic materials, substantially complicating any effort to quantify exposure. Moreover, particular activities (especially hobbies and avocations likely to involve repeated exposures) may or may not lead to exposures recognized by the patient as possibly relevant to symptoms or illness; the patient may fail to consider that his or her non-workplace exposures might be responsible for a health problem and, therefore, may fail to report them to the physician. A careful history that comprehensively reviews possible causative exposures is, thus, particularly important in non-occupational environmental medicine (see Chapter 3).

Comprehensive occupational medical coverage of employees often includes a program of medical surveillance of workers. Such programs are oriented toward the exposure(s) of particular concern in the industry that the program is designed to monitor. Biologic samples (e.g., urine or serum) may be tested periodically to determine whether or not any undue toxicant absorption has occurred. In addition, a worker may receive directed, periodic medical examinations, the purpose of which is the early detection of health effects from the particular substances or processes to which that worker is exposed, hopefully at a stage when those effects can be either mitigated or reversed. If the worker is seen because of a complaint or concern, the surveillance data serve as baseline information that facilitate the evaluation.

Conversely, physicians dealing with patients who are ill or fear they may be ill from environmental exposures incurred outside the workplace are unlikely to have data equivalent to the surveillance data to which occupational physicians may have access. Although testing of biologic specimens from the patient may still be informative, the perspective provided by prior baseline testing is almost always absent, as are data from previous examinations directed toward documenting information relevant to the particular environmental exposure(s) or health effect(s) of concern.

The practitioner of occupational medicine also may have the benefit of information from periodic environmental monitoring (e.g., air sampling) of substances that may threaten health, typically performed by industrial hygienists or other trained personnel. Such measurements may greatly aid in interpreting patients' complaints or the validity of their health concerns. Even if no measurements were taken before the fact, many industrial processes are performed under conditions that are sufficiently well characterized that they may be reproduced with reasonable precision at a time when the monitoring can be conducted. In contrast, it is rare for environmental measurements relevant to a specific individual to have been taken outside the workplace. Moreover, the patient with a non-occupational, environmental exposure is relatively unlikely to have maintained records on such items as the quantity of a potentially problematic substance used. As an individual, he or she is also much more likely to have varied his or her use of these substances over time in ways that are unlikely to be documented and about which the patient's own memory may be poor. These factors substantially limit the possibility of replicating the exact circumstances of exposure in order to make environmental measurements that may be ideal for clinical evaluation (see Chapter 3).

Scientific investigation of new problems

The complete spectrum of environmentally caused illnesses and their specific environmental antecedents has not yet been fully described. Thus, when one or more patients appear with symptoms that are either novel or unexpected for the set of environmental exposures experienced, it is reasonable to consider the possibility that the illness actually is caused by one or another of the exposures and that the particular disease–exposure link simply has not been described previously. This possibility may be easier to investigate in the workplace than outside it; reasons include specific awareness of the possibility of occupational disease in many populations of workers and the frequent occurrence in the workplace of qualitatively and quantitatively similar exposures among multiple, socioeconomically comparable but unrelated individuals, substantially increasing the statistical power of epidemiologic studies aimed at elucidating the cause of a new syndrome.

On the other hand, there may be situations in which investigations of both new and previously described environmental health effects are problematic in the workplace and more easily completed in the community at large. Such situations may arise, for example, when employees feel substantial pressure either not to report or to downplay their report of symptoms that could reflect negatively on the employer. Alternatively, there may be peer pressure or pressure from employee advocacy groups (e.g., unions)

to report symptoms that the employee might otherwise ignore. Either circumstance can complicate the conduct of an epidemiologic study.

Host populations

The special sensitivities of children and the elderly (i.e., those whose ages are outside the limits of those who typically make up the workforce) to certain environmental agents are more relevant to non-occupational than to occupational medicine (see Chapter 11). Thus, to a greater degree than the specialist in occupational medicine, the non-occupational environmental physician must take such potential differences in sensitivity into account.

Children appear more sensitive than adults to a wide variety of environmental exposures. For example, the developing nervous system of a child appears to be substantially more vulnerable to the toxic effects of lead than that of an adult. Babies tolerate excess nitrate in drinking water far less well than adults. Other potent neurotoxins, such as pesticides (organophosphates and organochlorines) and saxitoxins (the agents of paralytic shellfish poisoning), produce severe illness or death at lower doses in children than in adults. In addition, models for assessing cancer risk generally predict a quantitatively greater risk to children from a given level of exposure to a carcinogen than for adults.

Elderly persons also exhibit different responses to some environmental exposures than do younger adults. The elderly are far more likely to develop clinically apparent illness when exposed to extremely hot or cold conditions than are younger adults. Excretory functions involving renal and hepatic function may be diminished in the elderly, making them more likely to have adverse reactions to certain chemical exposures. In addition, chronic diseases and use of medicines for their treatment are more prevalent among the elderly than among other populations groups and may increase susceptibility to certain environmental exposures. Ambient air pollution, for example, results in excess respiratory and cardiovascular mortality, primarily among such persons. On the other hand, the importance of some environmental exposures may be diminished among the elderly. For example, assessment of exposures to certain carcinogens and counseling in this regard may not be as relevant to elderly persons, particularly if life expectancy is less than the anticipated latent period of the carcinogen. In addition, the adverse effects on reproduction of some environmental agents may be relatively unimportant to patients no longer in their reproductive years.

Thus, to an unusually large extent, physicians involved in non-occupational, environmental medicine must take basic differences in susceptibility into account in the assessment, counseling, and treatment of specific patients, and individual differences in susceptibility demand heavier emphasis in non-occupational, environmental medicine research. A corollary of this statement is that recommended limits for occupational exposure to chemical and physical environmental agents can by no means be automatically construed as appropriate or applicable to situations of exposure outside the workplace.

Social aspects (see also Chapter 9)

The administrative, regulatory, and economic contexts in which occupational medicine and non-occupational environmental medicine are practiced also create important differences between the two areas. Ethical issues similar to those related to potential conflicts of interest of occupational physicians employed by the same companies whose workers they care for are far less likely to arise among physicians dealing with environmental medicine outside the workplace. Moreover, non-occupational environmental specialists may escape much of the burden of the complex, time consuming, and red tape laden workers' compensation system.

Although they do not necessarily have to confront certain ethical dilemmas faced by occupational physicians, physicians involved in non-occupational environmental medicine – particularly consultants involved in epidemiologic evaluations – share with their colleagues in occupational medicine another set of complex social issues. Environmental physicians are frequently called on by the media – in public meetings, courts of law, or other public forums – to offer expert opinions regarding whether or not specific cases of disease or injury were caused by a specific environmental exposure. Often such opinions must be offered on the basis of few objective data or prior scientific studies and in the context of heated feelings and firmly established, preconceived notions on the part of those affected and their supporters. The expert may be confronted by equally daunting pressure from the party or parties responsible for the environmental exposure, who risk substantial economic losses from an expert opinion supporting a disease exposure link.

Established versus hypothetical hazards

Environmental medicine deals largely with questions of exposure and risk. In this regard it is useful to differentiate clear-cut hazards – those known to cause effects at occupational dose levels, from potential hazards – those known to cause human effects only at much higher dose levels, or those never demonstrated directly to cause harm in humans. Clear-cut environmental hazards can be designated as such on the basis of epidemiologic studies that show a cause-and-effect relationship between exposure to the hazard and the development of a particular illness or injury (usually, but not invariably, done in the occupational setting). For patients exposed to such environmental hazards, the physician's course of action is relatively clear. The exposed patient should be counseled regarding the nature of the risk, along with the likelihood – based on estimated dose and host factors – of possible health outcomes. When appropriate, the patient should be evaluated for the presence of the disease for which he or she may be at increased risk. If the disease is present, appropriate treatment should be instituted.

More problematically, much of the public's current concerns regarding the environment relate to exposures for which harmful effects in human populations have not yet been demonstrated. In general, such potential environmental hazards have been identified as possibly dangerous on the basis of their chemical or physical similarities to clear-cut hazards and/or their apparently harmful effects on animals or in in-vitro systems. Counseling patients about risk in such circumstances is substantially more complicated than for the former class, because the issue of whether or not the risk actually exists at all has to be considered. Quantitative estimates of the extent of possible risk may be lacking entirely. When such quantitative data exist at all, they are typically derived from animal studies or extrapolated from other data on similar (but not identical) compounds. Under these circumstances, some of the important caveats regarding the validity of risk assessment techniques (see Chapter 60) must be incorporated into the patient's counseling on risk related to the environmental exposure.

Data from community-based studies

Nowhere can the occupational roots of much of non-occupational environmental medicine be seen as clearly as in a review of currently recognized environmental hazards. Most such hazards have received their strongest and first scientific support for a causal relationship with human illness on the basis of studies performed on exposed workers. Well-known examples of exposures whose health effects were elucidated in this way include the linking of asbestos to asbestosis, mesothelioma, and carcinoma of the lung; vinyl chloride to angiosarcoma of the liver; and mercury exposure to adverse effects on the nervous system. It is primarily on the basis of these occupational epidemiologic data that practitioners of non-occupational, environmental medicine are aware of the potential risks such exposures pose to persons having non-workplace exposure.

Occupational studies are frequently more useful sources of data than studies of the same agents outside the workplace, because exposure in the workplace is often more intense, more prolonged, more regular, and more easily quantifiable than are comparable exposures outside the workplace. Thus, in a study population of a given size, the numbers of cases of the health outcome of interest are likely to be substantially greater in the occupational than in the non-occupational situation. Moreover, because exposure is generally more easily quantified in occupational studies, the extent of risk is more easily quantified, and the existence and shape of the dose–response curve can be estimated with greater precision.

Nevertheless, data from studies of environmental illness in non-occupational settings are important and continue to be needed to supply information that is missing or unobtainable from occupational studies alone. For example, occupational studies do little to address questions regarding the existence and extent of effects of specific environmental agents on children and others outside the range of demographic parameters in which workers usually fall. Moreover, what might happen in the home cannot easily be extrapolated from results of studies conducted under industrial conditions. For example, children's exposure to mercury (and consequent health effects) related to 'off-gassing' from household interior latex paint could not easily have been studied in the workplace. Diseases involving severe hypersensitivity to substances arising from industrial operations can sometimes be studied more satisfactorily outside than inside the workplace, because either the workers may be relatively few in comparison to the numbers of persons in nearby areas who are exposed to the substances emanating from the workplace or workers may systematically eliminate themselves from jobs involving contact with substances to which they are hypersensitive and that, therefore, cause them severe discomfort. Thus, non-occupational rather than occupational studies led to the discovery that severe (sometimes fatal) asthma attacks can be elicited in sensitized persons by soybean dust released during the course of industrial operations involving the bean.[20]

Risk assessment and environmental medicine (see also Chapter 59)

Here, the term risk assessment refers to the use of available data to develop a quantitative estimate of the probability that a given health outcome may result from a specific exposure experienced at a particular point in one's life, for a particular length of time, by a particular route, and at a particular dose level. Although risk assessments may be based on epidemiologic studies (i.e., those involving observation of human beings), they more frequently involve extrapolations based on data obtained from toxicity testing in animals.

Most often, the health outcome of concern is the development of malignant tumors. The test animals are almost always given far higher doses of the test compound than the dose levels for which one wishes to estimate risk, and the test generally lasts a period of about 2 years, the approximate lifespan of small rodents most often used as test animals. Malignant tumors or other health outcomes are assessed histopathologically or by other appropriate techniques. The data obtained from these studies are incorporated into mathematical models that attempt to estimate the maximum dose or concentration of the test chemical to which a human being could be exposed over the course of an approximately 70-year lifetime, while incurring an excess risk – i.e., incremental risk over background – of the health outcome of concern that is less than a particular fraction, frequently 1 per 1,000,000 or 1 per 100,000.

Despite widespread use in regulatory and public health decision making, full consensus has not been reached regarding many issues directly related to the validity of various risk assessment approaches. Some of the most problematic issues relate to:
- extrapolating findings from one species to another;
- adjusting incidence figures from relatively short-lived rodents to relatively long-lived human beings;
- calculating equivalent dosages across species;
- dealing with contradictory results obtained from studies of the effects of the same exposure on different animal species; and
- determining the proper mathematical function for extrapolating high-dose study exposures to the levels of exposure obtained from the environment, which are often several orders of magnitude lower.

Risk assessments based on human (epidemiologic) data are not limited by the problems of extrapolating data from animal models but do suffer from the other problems. Chief among these is quantification of dose. Many human studies of potential use in risk assessment involve retrospective examination of data collected over many years, often from times when the exposure of concern was not thought to be particularly harmful (which is logical, if one considers that large numbers of human beings would have been unlikely to have exposed themselves unnecessarily to a known substantial danger). The attention paid to documenting dose was, therefore, often correspondingly small, and the exposure data are, therefore, frequently imprecise. Human studies yielding positive results also may involve relatively high levels of exposure and, therefore, may suffer from the same problem as animal studies with regard to choice of an appropriate mathematical model for extrapolating data to dose levels more typical of home or community exposure.

All of the problems mentioned earlier lead to uncertainty in the risk estimate. Yet, the results of risk assessments are frequently presented as one or more specific numbers, with no mention of the underlying qualitative and quantitative uncertainties that must inevitably affect the interpretation of such estimates.

However they are derived and with whatever problems, the results of risk assessment are widely applied in formulating environmental regulations regarding the permissible levels of contaminating substances in air, water, soil, and food. The results of risk assessments also guide decisions on risk management made by environmental public health officials (e.g., in determining the extent to which spilled or unintentionally released chemicals must be removed or 'cleaned up' before usual activities in an area can be resumed).

Although the techniques of risk assessment play an important role in the approach to environmental regulation and environmental public health, their appropriate use in physicians' contacts with individual patients remains unclear. It may, in fact, be useful for a patient to be told that a particular exposure to which he or she may be subjected, when incurred constantly over the course of a lifetime, is estimated to lead to approximately a 1 in 10,000 lifetime additional risk of cancer. However, any counseling of the patient in this regard should be accompanied by full disclosure of the types of uncertainties mentioned earlier, all of which potentially affect the validity of the risk estimate. Moreover, to the greatest extent possible, any quantitative risk estimate used in counseling a patient should be set in the context of risks the patient faces frequently and, therefore, is likely to understand. For example, it may be useful to mention to the patient that 1 in 100 is the order of magnitude of risk for dying over a lifetime in a plane or car crash; by comparison, 1 in 1,000,000 approximates the lifetime risk of being killed by lightning.

Recommending behaviors for risk reduction is complicated by a number of factors, not the least of which is the varying tolerance of particular individuals for different levels of risk. In addition, the risk assessment information commonly available is based on assumptions of constant exposure over a lifetime. Comparable figures for acute exposures that may be of concern to individual patients may be lacking. Other specific features of individual patients' situations (e.g., very young or very advanced age) may result in substantially greater or less theoretical risk for a given patient than that indicated by the estimate used by public health personnel for protecting the general population's health. Currently, the health practitioner does not have easy access to individualized risk estimates fitting the individual circumstances of particular patients as are now readily available for other clinical risks such as cholesterol or body mass index. The best one can do is to emphasize the caveats associated with any quantitative estimate of risk given to a particular patient.

Clinical and public health practitioners and investigators

Close partnership between clinicians and public health practitioners is particularly important in the field of environmental medicine. The need for such collaboration arises, in part, from the fact that although a clinician may effectively treat the deleterious effects on health produced by an environmental exposure, he or she is rarely in a position to change the environmental factors that produced the illness, by contrast with occupational medicine where that relationship may be very much more tenable. For example, it would be senseless to provide chelation therapy for a child with lead toxicity and effectively reduce his or her lead level but then return the child to the same environment that caused the illness in the first place. In this situation, contact with the responsible public health authorities can lead to action that will be of immediate benefit to the patient.

Public health officials also may be a good source of data for health practitioners attempting to counsel patients in a reasonable way about recent highly publicized environmental health concerns. Such episodes of particular concern can be national (e.g., the escalating concern over radon accumulation in buildings and the episode of concern in 1989 regarding residues of daminozide [Alar] and its breakdown products in apples) or local (e.g., concerns of persons living near hazardous waste sites).

A close association with clinicians can provide important information to public health professionals as well. There is currently little formal surveillance for environmentally caused disease. Informal reports from clinicians can alert those working in public health to the presence of a problem that otherwise might have escaped notice

entirely or might have been recognized by them only much later on. In addition, because environmental medicine is a developing area in which previously unrecognized disease exposure associations may be anticipated from time to time, alert clinicians can play an important role in identifying new public health problems. In the early 1980s, clinicians in Barcelona, Spain, pointed out the sudden appearance of clusters of cases of exacerbation of asthma that, from time to time, flooded the city's emergency rooms. That report provided the stimulus for an investigation that eventually led to the discovery that dust arising from ships unloading soybeans in the nearby port was the instigating agent.[20] This discovery, in turn, allowed appropriate preventive measures to be taken. Similarly, the eosinophilia-myalgia syndrome was first reported to public health authorities by a group of clinicians who recognized a cluster of patients in New Mexico with similar, peculiar illnesses and a common history of ingestion of L-tryptophan. Subsequent investigation led to the discovery of over 1500 cases nationwide, a clear-cut association with L-tryptophan from a particular manufacturer, recall of implicated products, and an end to the epidemic.[21] Fostering recognition of such outbreaks is one of the greatest potential roles of practitioners in this emerging field.

References

1. The BLS website is: data.bls.gov.
2. Bureau of Labor Statistics. US Department of Labor News, December 18, 2001. USDOL-47. 2001.
3. Goldsmith DF. Uses of workers' compensation data in epidemiologic research. Occup Med State Art Revs 1998; 13:389–415.
4. Morse T, Dillon C, Warren N, Levenstein C, Warren A. The economic and social consequences of work-related musculoskeletal disorders: the Connecticut Upper Extremity Project (CUSP). Int J Eviron Health 1998; 4:209–16.
5. The website for these data is: www.cdc.gov/nchs/products/catalogues/subject/mortmed.html.
6. Herbert R, Landrigan PJ. Work-related death: a continuing epidemic. Am J Pub Health 2000; 90:541–5.
7. Division of Respiratory Disease Studies, NIOSH. Work-related Lung Disease Surveillance Report 1999. DHHS (NIOSH) Number 2000-105. Publications Dissemination, Cincinnati: NIOSH, 2000.
8. Krant A. Estimates of the extent of morbidity and mortality due to occupational diseases in Canada. Am J Ind Med 1994; 25:267–78.
9. The website for these data is: www.cdc.gov/nchc/about/major/hdasd/nhdsdes.html.
10. Rutstein DD, Mullan RJ. Sentinel health events (occupational): a basis for physician recognition and public health surveillance. Am J Pub Health 1983;73:1054-62
11. Rosenstock L, Daniell W, Barnhart S. The 10-year experience of an academically affiliated occupational and environmental medicine clinic. West J Med 1992; 157:425–9.
12. Data provided by Kathy Hunting, Association of Occupational and Environmental Clinics, June 2002.
13. NIOSH. Worker Health Chartbook 2000. DHHS (NIOSH) Number 2000-127. Publications Dissemination. Cincinnati: NIOSH, 2000.
14. Whittaker SG, Curwick CC. Surveillance for occupational lead poisoning, State of Washington 1993–2001: incorporating data from May 15 1993 through June 30, 2001. Technical Report 44-3-2001. Safety and Health Assessment and Research

for Prevention. Olympia, WA: Washington State Department of Labor and Industries 2001.

15. Tumpowski C, Rabin R, Davis L. Lead at Work. Elevated blood lead levels in Massachusetts workers. Occupational Health Surveillance Program. Massachusetts: Dept of Public Health, 1998.

16. Morse T. Occupational Disease in Connecticut 2001. Occupational Disease Surveillance Program. Connecticut: Department of Labor and Department of Health, 2001.

17. Lalich NR, Sestito JP. Occupational health surveillance contributions from the National Health Interview Survey. Am J Ind Med 1997; 31:1–3.

18. Doll R, Peto R. The causes of cancer: quantitative estimates of avoidable risks of cancer in the United States today. J Nat Cancer Inst 1981; 66:1191–308.

19. Darby S, Hill D, Doll R. Radon: a likely carcinogen at all exposures. Ann Oncol 2001; 12:1341–51.

20. Anto JM, Sunyer J, Rodriguez-Roisin R, Suarez-Cervera M, Vazquez L. Community outbreaks of asthma associated with inhalation of soybean dust. New Engl J Med 1989; 320:1097–102.

21. Varga J, Uitto J, Jimenez SA. The cause and pathogenesis of the eosinophilia-myalgia syndrome. Ann Intern Med 1992; 116:140–7.

Chapter 2
Occupational and Environmental Medicine: the Historical Perspective

Paul Blanc

The history of occupational and environmental medicine is composed of multiple threads continually interwoven over time into a single historical cord. One thread is formed by the key clinicians and researchers who have contributed to the development of this discipline. Most brief summaries of occupational and environmental medical history take this as their limited focus. Yet as important as these biographical elements are in the story of occupational and environmental medicine, other factors have come into play that make the evolution of this discipline distinct from that of other branches of medicine.

First, advances in technology have played a driving role in occupational and environmental medicine that is unparalleled in other fields of health. It is true that advances in diagnostic and therapeutic modalities, from the microscope to the laser, demonstrate the powerful impact that technologic innovation can have on medical practice as a whole. But despite the role that such inventions have played in clinical care, the underlying pathologic processes of concern to practitioners have not changed because of them. Simply put, the microscope did not create illnesses due to new strains of bacteria. In contrast, technologic change continually introduces new occupational and environmental hazards, leading to evolving patterns of established diseases as well as inducing entirely novel conditions never experienced before in human history. Radiation poisoning is an obvious example, but by no means an isolated one.

Second, the history of occupational and environment medicine reflects the impact of larger social movements outside the narrow confines of medicine. This is not to argue that other branches of medicine are immune to such forces. The course of modern medicine still reflects the impact of the French revolution, transmitted down through the influential work of French medical scientists working at the end of the 18th and in the first half of the 19th centuries.[1] So too, the Flexner Report and all that it brought with it for American medicine had a larger sociopolitical context.[2]

Nevertheless, occupational and environmental medicine, more than any other health discipline in the last 200 years, has tended to wax and wane as a consequence of societal forces. The hygienic movement of the 19th century (particularly in Great Britain), which was linked in turn to wider social reforms, is a case in point. The First World War marked another social–political confluence of forces distinctly impacting occupational and environmental medicine. More recently, the social movements of the late 1960s in the US coincided with the establishment of OSHA, NIOSH, and the EPA, all of which profoundly affected the field.

The goal of this chapter is to place the story of occupational and environmental medicine within the context of these three disparate, yet inter-related themes: the key historical figures that contributed to the development of the field, the technologic changes that have led to an ever-shifting burden of disease, and the sociopolitical forces that helped set the priorities of the discipline. An overview of this chronology is summarized in Table 2.1. Finally, key resources in occupational and environmental medical history will be summarized in order to direct interested readers further beyond the scope of this brief overview.

OCCUPATIONAL AND ENVIRONMENTAL MEDICINE IN THE ANCIENT WORLD

The remote history of occupational health is fragmentary and largely conjectural.[3–5] In terms of occupationally related illness and injury, as the medical historian Henry Sigerist many years ago pointed out eloquently, the most salient determinant of work-associated morbidity in the ancient world was the widespread use of slave labor.[5] In a 1936 address to the New York Academy of Medicine, Dr Sigerist remarked:

'Labor in ancient civilization was primarily slave labor. The pyramids were built by state slaves whose lives had no value whatever, whom every war would replace. We still can see the Egyptian workers laboring under the whip as represented on wall paintings and in reliefs. The lot of the city worker was hardly any better and we can still perceive their voice of rebellion . . . We admire the graceful Greek bronze statuettes that fill our museums but we do not think of the copper miners providing material for these works of art, or the coal miners digging for coal to make the bronze, working ten hours in narrow galleries suffocated by heat and smoke. They were prisoners of war or convicts as a rule.'[5]

As noted by Sigerist, the adverse occupational safety and health impacts of slave labor in the ancient world were most dramatic in mining operations. This industry was also one of the first to manifest the adverse impact on occupational safety and health of technologic advancements in

Historical period	Notable factors	Key documentation
Ancient–Classical	Slave labor Mining and metallurgy Agriculture and crafts	Scattered references in classical medical and non-medical writing
7th–17th Centuries	Early technological change Armaments and metallurgy Alchemical experiments	Ellenbog, Agricola, Paracelsus Chinese technological texts
1650–1800	Large-scale trades Renaissance technologies Coal fuel power pollution	Ramazzini and his translators Evelyn on air pollution
1800–1900	Industrial Revolution Novel exposures to toxins Germ theory predominates	Thackrah and Patissier Annales d'Hygiene Medicine Legale Hirt, Simon, Arlidge, Proust
1900–1950	The New Public Health First and Second World Wars Progressive movements Air pollution emergencies	Oliver, Hamilton, Legge Teleky, Underhill, Drinker Various governmental reports
1950–1970	Nuclear threats, Cold War Petrochemical industry OSHA, NIOSH, EPA	Carson, Brodeur, Berman, Sellars

Table 2.1 A brief chronology of occupational and environmental health

metallurgy[6] (which increased the demand for a variety of ores) and mining methods (especially pumping systems that allowed mining to delve deeper than ever before).[7] Such mining operations were important economic forces in Egypt and in Greece, but took place on a truly massive scale in the Roman Empire, particularly in the Iberian peninsula. Rosen's superb *History of Miner's Diseases* provides the most detailed history of this subject.[7]

Allusions by non-medical writers of the classical period to various labor hazards, including risks to miners, constitute some of the earliest written documentation of occupational safety and health problems. Many of these comments are terse references, such as those that have been noted in the epigrams of Martial or the satires of Juvenal.[3,4] One of the most notable references is the widely cited description of mining by Pliny the Elder (Natural History XXXIII, 40) in which he writes:

'Persons employed in the manufactories in preparing minium (red lead) protect the face with masks of loose bladder-skin, in order to avoid inhaling the dust, which is largely pernicious.'[5]

There are other occasional references to working conditions of artisans or laborers in ancient Western writings, including the Egyptian papyri Eber and Sallier.[4,5] Similar examples of fragmentary descriptions of working conditions and their inherent risks may also exist in the non-Western early written tradition (especially Chinese medical and technologic writing), but this literature, insofar as it might touch on occupational morbidity, has not been systematically reviewed in the English language.

The concept of 'environmental' health, in the modern sense of the term, is even more difficult to track in early history. A recent review of ancient Roman law makes it clear that statutory and other legal remedies for water and air pollution were indeed undertaken as early as the 1st century AD (for example, a legal opinion by the Roman

Aristo that a cheese maker should not emit smoke into the building above it).[8] Talmudic commentary provides further indication that legal concepts of environmental and even occupational protection have a surprisingly long history.[9]

Classical *medical* writing (as opposed to general works such as histories or satires) largely ignored occupation in relation to health. Certain vocations were addressed, for example, horseback riding (Hippocrates associated it with impotence and sterility; Aristotle with augmented sex drive).[3] This trend continued through Galen, although he may have been the first physician who recorded a personal brush with a significant occupational health hazard. According to one history of the subject:

'In the course of one of his numerous voyages, Galen spent some time on the Island of Cyprus. While there he had visited a mine where copper sulfate was recovered. Unaware of the danger, he himself was nearly overcome by the fumes in the mine. He records that the workmen who carried out a vitriolic liquid ran from the mine with all speed with each load to avoid perishing in the midst of the labors.'[3]

THE 7TH CENTURY THROUGH THE MID-17TH CENTURY

In the thousand years following the end of the Classical period, the foundations were set upon which modern Western medical science would later be built. Occupational health, as a medical concern, was marginal (at best) throughout most of this long period. Environmental health was given fairly short shrift too, being little discussed beyond a few generalities about climate and good air. This can be contrasted, by comparison, to the subject of diet and health, a topic addressed by many medical writers over these centuries.

During this time there were few, if any, social forces that would have worked to bring such concerns more to the forefront. There were, however, technologic innovations that began to have an impact through changing patterns of morbidity and mortality. These innovations, at first sporadic and isolated, became increasing important as the Middle Ages drew to a close.

One of the most straightforward examples is provided by technologic developments in armaments, especially the introduction of firearms. The traumatic risks of soldiering, essentially an occupational hazard, were well documented by the famous 16th century military surgeon Ambroise Pare, who gave special emphasis to the novel (at that time) phenomenon of gunshot wounds.[10] From the same period, the introduction of new sea-faring technologies (not only the sailing ships themselves, but as importantly, innovative navigational equipment) led to severe outbreaks of scurvy as an occupational disease of seamen.[11]

Even earlier than this, mining and metal working technologies became the engine driving the evolution of occupational health as a distinct medical issue.[7] As was noted previously, this was already true, although to a much lesser extent, in the Classical period. Lead was certainly very widely used during the Roman period and has even been the subject of speculation as to its potential role as a major environmental toxin in that time period.[12]

One of the first, clear-cut medical descriptions of lead colic was noted by the 7th century Byzantine physician Paul of Aegina.[13] In the Middle Ages, lead, arsenic, and mercury were all employed in the Western pharmacopeia and were the subject of study and misadventure by generations of alchemists. But above and beyond that, the appreciation of novel metals and alloys, and new ways of refining others, brought about the introduction of greater risks and even entirely new hazards to miners and metal workers.[7] The first publication devoted entirely to the subject of occupational health was Ullrich Ellenbog's fittingly titled, seven-page pamphlet, On the Poisonous Wicked Fumes and Smokes of Metals (*Von den gifftigen besen Tempffen und Reuchen der Metal*).[14] First printed in 1524, it was originally written in 1473 and warns the metal worker of the health hazards of metal, coal, and acid fumes.

Between 1500 and 1650, an increasing number of writers began to address the subject of miners' and metal workers' health. The first book-length treatment of the subject was that of Paracelsus (*Von der Bergsucht under anderen Bergkrankheiten*), written in 1533 but only first published posthumously in 1567.[15] Agricola's *De Re Metallica* (1556), although mainly devoted to the technology of mining and smelting, contains a notable section on occupational health in Book VI. Agricola writes:

'It remains for me to speak of the ailments and accidents of miners, and of the methods by which we can guard against these, for we should always devote more care to maintaining our health, that we may freely perform our bodily functions, than to making profits. Of the illnesses, some affect the joints, others attack the lungs, some the eyes, and finally some are fatal to men.'[16]

In addition to Paracelsus and Agricola, during this period authors of note on occupational exposures include Pansa, Ursinus, and Stockhausen.[7] Early technologic writing, for example, that of Ercker[17] or Birunguccio,[18] is also of interest in relation to likely occupational exposures. Some of the medical writing is straightforward, describing hazards, such as asphyxia, that are clear cut and readily discernible in modern occupational terms. Other writing is terribly obscure (especially Paracelsus).[15] Even Agricola, amidst his lucid descriptions of hazards such as stagnant air, falls from ladders, and cave-ins, warns that in some mines ('although in very few'), there are demons which can be put to flight by prayers and fasting.[16]

During this time, another technologic change in Europe that began to impact health was manifest in the environmental rather that the occupational arena. This was the introduction of fossil coal (as opposed to wood, peat, or charcoal) as a fuel.[19] At first, this practice was limited to Britain, with a particularly important industrial application in firing lime kilns. As early as the 13th century, a commission had been established in London to investigate the problem of pollution from coal burning. In 1306, a proclamation was issued banning the practice, albeit to little effect.[20] After a brief plateau, the coal market (and with it coal mining) increased logarithmically during the 16th and 17th centuries in Britain.[22]

Although fossil coal was employed in China for fuel long before its use in Europe, there has been no systematic review of the history of its use in China and its potential public health impact from an historical perspective. This parallels a general paucity of information on health impacts of early technologic innovations that originated in Asia, although the history of this technology as it pertains to chemistry and metal working is quite rich.[21–24]

1650 TO 1800

In 1700, after some years of preparatory work on the subject, Bernadino Ramazzini published the first edition of his landmark treatise, *De Morbis Artificum* ('The Diseases of Artificers', usually translated in modern terms as 'The Diseases of Workers').[25] This work is remarkable for its innovations. First, in simply approaching the subject matter as a topic worthy of a complete treatise, rather than by narrowly focusing on a single occupational group or exposure, Ramazzini fundamentally changed the way in which all medical writing would subsequently address occupational illness and injury. Second, and no less importantly, Ramazzini explicitly put occupational risk factors on the agenda in terms of the medical differential diagnosis. In the preface to *De Morbis Artificum*, Ramazzini directly addresses the reader with the following, often cited (deservedly so) admonition:

'The divine Hippocrates informs us, that when a physician visits a patient, he ought to inquire into many things, by putting questions to the patients and bystanders . . . to which I would presume to add one interrogation more; namely, what trade he is of. But I find it very seldom minded in the common course of practice, or if the physician knows it without asking he takes little notice of it. Though at the same time a just regard to that, would be of great service in facilitating a cure.'[26]

Ramazzini's text was divided into 42 chapters, although the number of occupations covered was even greater (for example, a single chapter covers oil pressers, tanners, lute-string makers, candle-makers and cheese-makers). Even this was not sufficiently comprehensive for the author. In 1713, he published a second edition of the work, adding to it a supplement of an additional 12 chapters to address occupations omitted from the original (including printers, carpenters, and sailors, among others).[27]

The work practices that Ramazzini documents provide a fairly exhaustive summary of manufacturing technology as it existed in Europe at the turn of the 17th to 18th centuries, just before the advent of the Industrial Revolution that would, by century's end, begin to fundamentally transform the workplace and the risks it entailed. Indeed, there is very little 'recent' technologic innovation driving Ramazzini's observations. Most of the occupations he describes, even those that entail metallurgy and mining, employed materials and methods well established for at least several generations. Other work practices described are virtually unchanged since Roman times, for example, the hazards of fullers (cleaners of cloth). Ironically, one of the few novel syndromes related to an emerging industry was that of nicotine toxicity among tobacco workers, especially for those involved in tobacco grinding.[27]

Although rapidly changing technology leading to novel illnesses is not a major factor in De Morbis Artificum, the work clearly reflects the impact on Ramazzini of the larger social, cultural, and political forces of his day. In broad historical terms, he was very much a product of the late Italian Renaissance. More specifically, he spent most of his career in Modena during the years leading up to the publication of the De Morbis Artificum under the patronage of the Ducal House of Este, one of the great liberal benefactors of the age.[27] This spirit imbues Ramazzini's work, which emphasizes the lot of the common worker with empathy and compassion on almost every page. Perhaps the most striking passage demonstrating Ramazzini's sociopolitical context is his chapter on the 'Diseases of Jews,' in which he ascribes these disease to the occupations into which the Jews were forced by the restrictions of the period. As odd as the chapter title strikes the modern reader, its actual content underscores Ramazzini's decidedly liberal approach to his subject.

It would be hard to overestimate the impact that Ramazzini's work had on the discipline of occupational medicine throughout the 18th century and well into the 19th. The work was translated from Latin into English within five years of its initial publication (1705); a new English edition in 1746 included the 1713 appendix.[26,27] More important were two other 18th century annotated translations with significant additions by the translators, one in French (1777)[28] and one in German (1780–83).[29] The latter is particularly noteworthy, more than doubling Ramazzini's original text. Beyond these translations, Ramazzini was widely cited by his contemporaries and

the generations that followed. His most famous student was the great pathologist Morgagni, whose classic text, The Seats and Causes of Diseases, is not only meticulous in documenting the occupations of many of its cases, but also directly discusses possible work-related contributions to the pathology that Morgagni observed in several instances.[30]

The key medical writers in the 18th century who addressed occupational subjects (although none with as all-encompassing a text) acknowledged their predecessor. One example is Tissot, whose text on the diseases of 'men of letters' was first published in 1768 and widely circulated.[31] Ramazzini's work on occupational diseases was even the subject of several 18th century doctoral theses,[32–34] the most well known of which was the work of a Swede, Nicholas Skragge.[35] Skragge wrote his thesis under the tutelage of Linneaus, whose lecture notes document that he gave considerable attention to Ramazzini.[36]

Ramazzini's presence within 18th century occupational and environmental medicine is so dominant that it obscures another pivotal contribution of this time, John Evelyn's Fumifugium; or, The inconvenience of the aer and smoak of London dissipated.[37] Initially published in 1661, it is the first tract (26 pages only) specifically focused on air pollution and its potential dangers. Although Evelyn's dates (1620–1706) overlap almost entirely with those of Ramazzini (1633–1714), the two could not be further apart. Evelyn, neither a medical practitioner nor a scientist, was a Royalist, a great diarist of the age (as was his contemporary, Pepys), and a colorful polemicist. In Fumifugium, railing against the coal smoke polluters of his day, he writes:

'Whilst these are belching forth their sooty jaws, the City of London resembles the face of Mount Aetna, the Court of Vulcan, Stromboli, or the Suburbs of Hell than an Assembly of Rationale Creatures . . .'[37]

Although it might be tempting to dismiss Evelyn as something of an Enlightenment crack-pot, Fumifugium is important in the history of air pollution specifically and environmental health generally. In this context, the unsigned, contemporary preface to a 1772 re-printing of the book is particularly relevant:

'Our Author [Evelyn] expresses himself with proper warmth and indignation against the absurd policy of allowing brewers, dyers, soap-boilers, and lime-burners to intermix their noisome works against the dwelling-houses in the city and suburbs; but since his time we have a great increase of glass-houses, foundries, and sugar-bakers, to add to the black catalogue; at the head of which must be placed the fire-engines of the water-works at London Bridge and York Buildings, which (while they are working) leave the astonished spectator at a loss to determine whether they do not tend to poison and destroy some of the inhabitants by their smoke and stanch than supply with their water.'[38]

At the beginning of the 18th century, Evelyn stood nearly alone in addressing air pollution in any modern sense of the word.[39] By century's end, a series of discoveries had led to an understanding of the precise chemical composition of air. This, in turn, provided a new scientific basis to consider how the contents of air, on a chemical basis, might act upon the body. The same chemical-analytic attention had not yet been given to water pollution, but was beginning to be applied to food contamination. For example, George Baker's classic ecologic analysis of the regional association between the practice of using lead in apple presses and the 'Devonshire colic' was combined with laboratory experiments demonstrating the lead content in various cider preparations.[6] Throughout the second half of the 18th century, the potential for systematic application of scientific discoveries to industrial manufacturing was gaining increasing attention. The Diderot's *Encyclopedia*, subtitled an 'Analytical Dictionary of the Science, Arts, and Trades', published its first volume in 1751.[41] The lavish illustrations of the *Encyclopedia*, detailing the mechanical state of the art in industry at the time, heralded the technologic transformations of manufacturing about to occur.

THE 19TH CENTURY

By 1800, 100 years after Ramazzini, the occupational and environmental health equation had been fundamentally altered. First, the Industrial Revolution was in full swing. Second, the French Revolution redefined the rights of the people, and, by extension, those of the worker. Third, medical research was beginning to link toxicology to pathophysiology in ways directly relevant to occupational and environmental as a scientific discipline.

Even after the first flush of the Industrial Revolution, technical innovation (chemical and mechanical) continued to remain a dominant force in occupational health and safety throughout the century. Far more than simply a series of manufacturing changes in the cotton textile industry,[42] it was introducing both entirely novel exposures as well as increasing old exposures to new levels of intensity.[43] Some key examples of novel exposures introduced in this period linked to outbreaks of entirely new syndromes include: chlorine gas inhalation,[44] work in high barometric pressure environments,[45] the introduction of white phosphorus ('lucifer') matches,[46] carbon disulfide-based rubber vulcanization,[47] aniline and other synthetics in textile dyeing,[48] and, just at the end of the century, ionizing radiation in medical radiography.[49]

One of the most important established exposures that was greatly magnified through new industrial processes was that of silica dust, especially through the introduction steam power-driven grinding wheels.[50,51] Lead is another prime example of a classic exposure with greatly increased exposure levels in the 19th century, particularly in the pottery, glass, and metal-working industries.[52] Even zinc oxide exposure, which was trivial in 18th century brass manufacturing, burst on the scene with new methods of making the alloy, and with that new technology a novel occupational syndrome – metal fume fever.[53]

During the 19th century, social forces came to bear on occupational health in important new ways. Despite the revolutionary tradition on the Continent (or perhaps in part because of it), occupational health had its clearest political manifestations in Great Britain, where it was part of a larger hygienic movement tied closely to a broad agenda of social reform. The key hygienic document of the first half of the 19th century is the famous Chadwick *Report on the Sanitary Condition of the Labouring Population*.[54] It addresses specific occupational exposures only briefly, although they are included. To a greater extent, the governmental sanitary reports of John Simon underscore the extent to which occupational safety and health was very much on the public health agenda.[55] Even Florence Nightingale's *Notes on Nursing*, which she intentionally adapted for working men and women, addresses occupational health hazards in general terms.[56]

The most important English language occupational text of the 19th century was that of Charles Thackrah, *The effects of the principal arts, trades, and professions, and of civic states and habits of living*. First published in 1831, Thackrah greatly expanded the work in a second edition in 1832.[57,58] He was planning a third edition when he died of tuberculosis (most likely occupationally acquired) in 1833.[59] It is the first text to address the myriad occupational health risks brought about by the new technologies of the Industrial Revolution, especially the health of textile workers. This was a subject of particular interest to Thackrah because he practiced in Leeds, a textile factory center. Thackrah's work had an immediate influence on other hygienists of the period, especially in Great Britain[60] and in the US.[61,62] It also had an impact on political reformers. Michael Sadler, rising to speak on pending social legislation in Parliament, is reported to have had a copy of Thackrah's book in his hand and to have quoted from it extensively.[59]

Invoking occupational health as a motivation for more broadly protective legislation was not without precedent: one of the first pieces of child labor legislation in Britain (1778) was for chimney sweeps[63] among whom scrotal cancer had been reported by Percival Pott in 1775.[64] British legislative reforms of working conditions were introduced in a series of landmark statutes promulgated in the second half of the 19th century. As a part of these enabling acts, governmental medical positions as 'factory inspectors' were established. These positions, in turn, provided the training ground for several generations of physicians specializing in occupational disease.[65,66]

In France, occupational medicine diverged from the discipline that was evolving in Great Britain. Industrial conditions differed between the two countries in significant ways. Although there were some relatively large manufacturing sectors (for example, textiles), production to a much greater degree than in Britain remained in smaller-scale workshops, especially in Paris.[67] Medicine in France was distinct as well, characterized by a greater emphasis on systematic analysis and characterization of pathophysiologic processes.[1] This was also manifest in occupational medicine.

Patissier in France played a role similar to Thackrah's in Britain. In 1822, Patissier wrote the first original French text on occupational medicine.[68] Often cited as an annotated translation of Ramazzini, it goes far beyond that. Patissier broke down occupational exposures into classes of risk, categorized hierarchically consistent with French regulations. Most of the later French writers on occupational health in the 19th century followed Patissier's somewhat didactic schema. Another major text of the early 19th century, Tanquerel des Planches' *Lead Poisoning,* demonstrates even more strikingly the emerging new 'science' of occupational medicine in France during this period.[69] In more than 1000 pages, it meticulously details over 1200 cases of lead poisoning at the famous Charite Hospital. It remains to this day the largest case series of its kind.

The emerging science of toxicology, dominated by researchers ranging from Orfila[70] to Bernard,[71] also had a major impact on occupational medicine in France. Indeed, the leading scientific journal of the 19th century for occupational medicine content was the toxicologically oriented *Annales d'Hygiene et de Medicine Legale.* Many of its key occupational articles were also reprinted as separate bound volumes, providing a major source of scholarship on the subject.

In the latter part of the 19th century, German occupational medicine became ascendant, particularly through a series of scientific and medical publications. Of these, the massive textbook of Hirt is the most noteworthy example.[72] At the same time, the first workers compensation insurance schemes were coming into being, starting with the German 'Accident Insurance Law or Trades and Industry' of 1884.[73]

Beyond Great Britain, France, and Germany, occupational medicine as a discipline had little presence in the 19th century. In the United States this was especially the case, although clinical reports and scholarly articles on the subject did appear sporadically.[74] Moreover, there was a subtle, but general decline in the field of occupational health as the century progressed, even in its former centers of strength in Great Britain and France. There were notable textbooks produced in this period, such as those by Aldridge[75] and by Proust (Marcel's father, who was one of the first to apply the term 'byssinosis' to illness in cotton textile workers),[76] but these are something of the exception proving the rule.

The explanation for this decline is not clear cut. Technologic innovation was still introducing new hazards and novel syndromes during this period (the association of aplastic anemia with benzene was first published in 1897, for example).[77] In part, the political climate may have been less conducive. Clearly, social reform was no longer at the forefront.

More importantly, however, occupational disease and, even more dramatically, 'environmental' illness were falling out of scientific favor among the very public health experts who had once touted these concepts. The reason may derive from germ theory and its role in preventive medicine. It became increasing clear that the major epidemic diseases (acute and indolent), especially those that attacked the poor and working classes, were infectious in nature and attributable to specific, transmissible microorganisms. With these insights came a major paradigm shift which became known as the 'new' public health.

Diffuse concerns over sanitary conditions were replaced with a focused emphasis on controlling contagion or on the innate resistance or vulnerability of the potential host.[39,78]

Although the discipline of occupational disease was overshadowed to the extent that it could not be illuminated by the new science of microbiology, environmental health concerns beyond bacterial pathogen and vector control were eclipsed almost entirely by the 19th century's end. Any discussion of air quality in terms of chemical or particulate pollution as a direct or proximate cause of disease was likely to be ignored as little more than miasmic superstition. So too, water- and food-borne illness prevention was approached as if wholly accounted for by microbiological factors.

1900–1970

The 20th century began with a few positive signs of renewed vigor in the discipline of occupational medicine. The first meeting of the International Association for Labor Legislation, the forerunner of the ILO, took place in 1901.[73] In the UK, a major multi-authored, state-of-the-art textbook appeared in 1902, edited by Thomas Oliver (later to be knighted for his work in the field).[79]

Workers' compensation legislation spread beyond Germany and Great Britain. During this time, agitation for worker protection and compensation for injury in the US was taking place within the context the larger progressive reform movement,[80–82] as well as in response to greater labor militancy, particularly among mine workers.[83–85] In 1909 the first state workers compensation law was passed in the United States.[73]

Even environmental health, from the standpoint of industrial point-source air and water pollution, began to receive some renewed attention, albeit sparingly. In Britain, alkali works were known to be a major producer of air contaminants since early in the 19th century. Various frustrated attempts at control finally culminated in the Alkali Works Regulation Acts in 1906.[73] In Britain and the US as well, smokestack control began to be evaluated, although negative impacts on property were often emphasized over adverse human health effects.[86,87]

Nonetheless, change was slow. Despite the modest advances noted above, occupational and environmental health was still dominated by the contagion-control agenda of the broader public health movement. In the US, the field was even further constrained by an emerging corporate influence, a history documented extensively in Christopher Sellers' scholarly work, *Hazards on the Job.*[88]

The First World War over-turned the status quo in occupational and environmental medicine. The industrial expansion of armaments production demanded by modern warfare, particularly in the manufacture of munitions and airplanes, led to outbreaks of chemically related illness for which contagion control had no role.[89,90] Governmental investigation and intervention led to revamping existing units or establishing new ones such as the US Public Health Service Bureau of Industrial Hygiene.[73,88] Research into the causes and prevention of 'industrial fatigue,' which was subsumed within the discipline of occupational health, was also born out of the same First World War driven needs.[91]

More dramatically, the introduction of chemical gas warfare on a mass scale put to rest completely any lingering dogmatic tenet that germs alone accounted for the only large-scale public health threat worth bothering with.[44,92,93] Ironically, it was research on mines and caissons that provided a key underpinning for the British war gas effort through the work of JS Haldane.[45]

In the years following the First World War, and particularly during the 1930s, renewed attention to occupational illness and injury was infused with a new political awareness. This coincided with the progressive labor movement of the period and drew from its growing strength. In the United States, the apotheosis of this revitalization was Alice Hamilton. Her work in occupational health began at Hull House and she continued to be socially and politically engaged throughout her long career.[89,94,95] As with past practitioners, Hamilton's occupational medicine concerns were driven both by old hazards made worse by new technology, such as silica spread by air-powered tools in quarries, and novel problems altogether, such as the outbreak of neurological disease among the workers in the new rayon industry (as with 19th century rubber workers, the disease was caused by carbon disulfide).[89]

Dr Hamilton stands out in this period as a great figure, but she was not alone. In Britain, Thomas Legge stepped down from governmental appointment as the Senior Medical Inspector of Factories in protest over Britain reneging on an international agreement to control lead and took a job as an advisor to the Trade Union Congress (an equivalent of the CIO).[90] In Spain, a young industrial surgeon named Josep Trueta developed a new system for treating open limb trauma with closed casts. He went on to become a leading Republican military physician in the Spanish Civil War; his closed-cast technique went on to become standard practice for the care of war wounds, saving many lives.[96]

The degree to which explicit occupational health concerns permeated the non-medical literature of the period is also indicative a wider recognition these problems. In the US, Theodore Dreiser's *Tragic America*, a non-fiction critique of the Depression era, specifically catalogues a number of occupational illnesses, including asbestos-related lung disease.[97] In fiction, one of the short stories that first brought success to Albert Maltz, later a major Hollywood screenwriter, was an eerie tale featuring a worker dying of acute silicosis.[98] This was one of the first print notices of the Gauley Bridge disaster, later also treated in a proletarian novel.[99,100]

Written in a slightly earlier period, but only published widely later, Franz Kafka's stories of the bureaucratic apparatus were imbued with the first-hand experiences that he gained as a successful operative of the Workmen's Accident Insurance Institute of the Kingdom of Bohemia.[101] In the UK, too, non-medical writing also turned to matters of workplace safety and health. The most remarkable novelis-

tic example may be the following, from A.J. Cronin's *The Citadel*:

'He went through the literature on the subject. Its paucity astounded him. Few investigators seemed to have concerned themselves greatly with the pulmonary occupational disease. Zenker had introduced the high-sounding term, pneumokoniosis, embracing three forms of fibrosis of the lung due to dust inhalation. Anthracosis, of course, the black infiltration of the lung met with in coal miners had long been known and was held by Goldman and Trotter in England to be harmless. There were a few treatises on the prevalence of lung trouble in makers of millstones, particularly the French millstones, and in knife and axe grinders ... "grinder's rot" ... and stone cutters. There was evidence, mostly conflicting, from South Africa upon ... gold miner's phthisis, which was undoubtedly due to dust inhalation. It was recorded also that workers in flax and in cotton and grain shovelers were subject to chronic changes in the lungs. But beyond that, nothing.' [102]

The Second World War and its immediate aftermath had an effect on occupational medicine, although not as transforming an event as the First World War. Certain sequelae are of note. Women entered the industrial workforce in large numbers, leading to renewed attention to their occupational health hazards[103] (although this subject had been of some concern since the 19th century).[104–106] The forced exile of large numbers of physicians and biomedical researchers, which crippled medicine in Germany and Austria generally,[107] had its impact on the disciplines of occupational medicine and toxicology as well. Ludwig Teleky, for example, one of the leading figures in German occupational medicine, was forced to flee to the US.[73] Industrial health-related medical research did not cease in Germany, however, particularly in aerospace medicine, where it was directly incorporated into the war effort. The German human research program on low barometric pressure environments, carried out on concentration camp victims, led to several Nuremberg indictments.[108]

As in the previous World War, chemical warfare research again was given high priority on both sides, driving toxicologic science to discoveries that would later be to the detriment of occupational health, most saliently through the development of organophosphates.[92] Paralleling the legacy of chemical warfare research, the birth of the nuclear weapons industry was also to have long lasting health consequences for a new workforce. It would be difficult to argue, however, that this created significant change within the discipline of occupational medicine, with much of the professional oversight of this issue divested to a new specialization of 'radiation safety.' Nonetheless, the threat of atomic warfare, and the reality of ongoing, aboveground testing of nuclear weapons, did mean that airborne pollution was once again destined to be on the public health agenda.

Even as the nuclear age was lending pressure to a reordering of public health priorities, other events supervened to accelerate this process. In Donora, Pennsylvania, from October 27th to 31st 1948, the US experienced its first air pollution disaster.[39,109,110] Four years later, from the

5th to 9th of December 1952, a larger and even more deadly episode occurred in England, the so-called 'killer-fog' of London.[111]

This was not the very first outbreak of such a crisis. In December of 1930, a similar event had taken place in the Meuse Valley in Belgium. The event was not ignored by scientists, on either side of the Atlantic.[112,113] Yet data from the event were limited and subject to conflicting interpretation. Moreover, there was a tendency to dismiss the episode as something of an anomaly. For example, Philip Drinker of Harvard, in one of the first scholarly reviews of air pollution in the US scientific literature, wrote in 1939 that:

'Naturally, we want to know whether such an accident could occur in industrial America. Our stacks emit the same gases as did the Belgian, but fortunately, so meteorologists tell us, we have no districts in which there is even a reasonable chance of such a catastrophe taking place.'[112]

In the US, Donora did more than simply prove the weather man wrong. It established air pollution control as a newly recognized and critical need.[39] Since there were no personnel trained specifically in this area, the early work in the field fell to the discipline of occupational health, largely to engineers in industrial hygiene. By 1957, the US Pubic Health Service had organized a separate Air Pollution Division, which began to develop criteria documents to address specific pollutants and their potential control.[110]

In this period there was no matching regulatory movement in occupational safety and health promotion in the US. Not only worker's compensation, but exposure standard-setting, too, was also a matter of state-by-state control. The only national guidelines available were the threshold limit values of a non-governmental organization, the American Conference of Governmental Industrial Hygienists.[84]

Nationally and internationally, this was a time of stagnation, if not retrenchment, in occupational medicine. The ILO, which had predated the League of Nations, joined with it, and then survived its demise, continued on with its work based in Geneva. The United Nations headquartered the World Health Organization there as well, but little effective collaboration emerged from this geographic proximity. In Great Britain, the long line of occupational medicine leaders stretching back to the 19th century hygienists and on down through Thomas Oliver and Thomas Legge appeared to have died off, although in 1955 Hunter did publish the first of what was to become many editions of a dominant text in the field.[114] On the Continent, the picture was even bleaker, with the sole exception of Italy. There, the major institute for occupational health research, the Milan University Clinica del Lavoro, had survived the fascist period remarkably intact and its director, Emilio Vigliani, took a leadership role in rebuilding the discipline.[115]

Cold War politics were not conducive to occupational safety and health promotion. In the United Sates certainly, in the aftermath of the McCarthy witch-hunts, any collaboration between academics and organized labor would have been suspect, at best. Outside of academic circles,

occupational medicine practice was corporate based and dominated by the Industrial Medical Association (IMA), whose membership between 1948 and 1959 more than doubled to 4000.[116] The IMA's presidents over this time included the medical directors of Caterpillar Tractor, Inland Steel, Ford Motor, and New England Telephone and Telegraph.[116] This period underscores, once again, the particular responsiveness of this discipline to larger political and cultural forces.

The first major sign of the ice breaking was not in occupational medicine, but rather in environmental health, in this instance primarily in relation to water and soil, rather than air pollution. Rachel Carson's seminal *Silent Spring*, was published in 1962.[117] Carson was explicitly concerned with emerging and novel manifestations of environmental damage resulting from a new technology: petrochemical synthetics, particularly chlorinated hydrocarbons. We look back on *Silent Spring* as a landmark publication, but its importance is not merely in retrospect. Immediately upon its release, its impact was widespread and powerful. Strong conservation organizations pre-dated *Silent Spring*, but their evolution into an environmental movement is difficult to imagine without it. The links between the environment, particularly non-human health effects, and traditional concerns of occupational disease were not straightforward to the general public, but were not lost on industry. Only recently has data emerged documenting the degree to which chemical manufacturers and their trade groups viewed with alarm the potential political and especially regulatory implications of Rachel Carson's work.[118]

The decade in the US that began with *Silent Spring* ended with the establishment of the Occupational Safety and Health Administration, the National Institute for Occupational Safety and Health, and the Environmental Protection Agency. These regulatory advances, made possible by series of enabling legislative acts, did not occur in a vacuum, culturally, politically, or scientifically.

RECENT HISTORY

As the preceding synopsis makes clear, the history of occupational and environmental medicine teaches us that this discipline has a long and complex past. Understanding that past, and the forces that have helped shape it, can better inform our understanding of the issues that face us going forward in an ever-changing world. It is not only convenient, but perhaps prudent as well, to use a cut-off of 1970 for an overview of the historical perspective in occupational and environmental medicine. Nonetheless, it is safe to assume that the interplay of technologic change and social forces continues to exert a substantial effect on the course of the discipline.

In the decades of the 1970s and 1980s, the United States assumed a critical leadership role internationally in key environmental areas such as removal of lead from gasoline, sulfur-containing coal emission reductions, and water pollution remediation. The regulatory evolution of occupational health protection in the US was less robust, although promulgation of a new OSHA lead standard in the 1970s did represent a major advance. Paralleling these trends, environmental medicine has grown to take on an increasingly prominent role within the discipline, particularly in the US.

Over the past 40 years, multiple exposure-related outbreaks of occupational or environmental disease have occurred worldwide. Some of the most notable episodes include vinyl chloride-caused angiosarcoma of the liver, kepone-induced neuropathy, methyl mercury-related teratogenesis (Minimata disease), and dibromodichlorpropane(DBCP)-induced male sterility. Although definitive historical assessments of these events have yet to be written, the importance of technologic and social factors is abundantly clear in the causes, identification, and struggle to control these outbreaks. The same confluence of forces is no less relevant to ongoing issues faced by occupational and environmental medicine.

ADDITIONAL RESOURCES

A complete history of occupational and environmental health is far beyond the limitations of a single chapter in a general text. There are, however, many additional resources that the interested reader can pursue in order to gain supplemental information.

In recent years, a number of excellent historical analyses addressing various aspects of occupational health have been published. These include *Hazards on the Job* (Sellers),[88] *Deadly Dust* (Rosner and Markowitz),[119] *Hawk's Nest Incident* (Cherniack),[99] *The Bends* (Phillips),[45] *Workers' Health, and Workers' Democracy: The Western Miners' Struggle, 1891–1925* (Derickson),[85] and *Occupation and Disease* (Denbe).[120] In addition to these works, there are noteworthy earlier histories. The two most important books that helped define the field of occupational health history are Rosen's *The History of Miners' Diseases* (1943)[7] and Teleky's *Factory and Mine Hygiene* (1948).[73] In the 1950s, the scholarly work of Meiklejohn was also groundbreaking.[59,66,121] From a somewhat later period, noteworthy works with considerable historical material include *Death on the Job* (Berman)[84] and *Expendable Americans* (Brodeur).[122]

In terms of 20th century memoirs by occupational medicine practitioners, the most important is Alice Hamilton's *Exploring the Dangerous Trades*[89] (and of related autobiographical interest, Sicherman's *Alice Hamilton: A Life in Letters*).[95] Another American occupational health memoir of the same period is that of McCord, *A Blind Hog's Acorns*.[123]

Some of the key library resources in occupational and environmental medicine also should be noted. The greatest single focused collection in the field of occupational medicine was undoubtedly that of Alfred Whittaker, which was later acquired by the Blocker History of Medicine Collections at the University of Texas, Galveston.[124] This collection includes the only extant copy of Ellenbog's *On the Poisonous Wicked Fumes and Smokes of Metals* (the earliest printed work in occupational medicine).[14] Another small, but important collection in the history of occupational medicine was donated by Robert Legge to the University of California San Francisco.

Occupational health titles are well represented in most of the great medical history collections, although some are particularly noteworthy in this regard, in particular that of the Wellcome Medical Trust (London). In addition to a large number of important printed items, it also holds other material, including the occupational medicine archives of Donald Hunter. The mining collection of Herbert Hoover, housed at Claremont College, contains a number of rare items especially relevant to mining safety and health.[125] A major resource on microfilm is available through the Goldsmiths'-Kress Library of Economic Literature, which reproduces a 60,000 document collection held at the University of London and Harvard University and includes many items relevant to occupational history prior to 1850.[126] Finally, the medical bibliography of Garrison and Morton provides an excellent citation listing of many of the key texts (including journal articles) that constitute landmarks in the history of the discipline.[127]

References

1. Foucault M. The birth of the clinic (translated by AH Sheridan Smith). New York: Vintage Books, 1973.
2. Starr P. The social transformation of American medicine. New York: Basic Books, 1982.
3. Goldwater LJ. From Hippocrates to Ramazzini: early history of industrial medicine. Ann Med History New Series 1936; 8:27–35.
4. Legge RT. The history of industrial medicine and occupational diseases. Ind Med 1936; 5:300–14.
5. Sigerist HE. The Wesley M. Carpenter Lecture. Historical background of industrial and occupational diseases. Bull New York Acad Med 1936; 12(11):597–609.
6. Humphrey JW, Oleson JP, Sherwood AN. Greek and Roman technology: a source book. London: Routledge, 1998.
7. Rosen G. The history of miners' diseases. New York: Schuman, 1943.
8. DiPorto A, Gagliardi L. Prohibitions concerning polluting discharges in Roman law. In: Grieco A, Iavicoli S, Berlinguer G, eds. Contributions to the history of occupational and environmental prevention. Amsterdam: Elsevier, 1999;211–21.
9. Chuwers P, Neumark Y. Worker health and environmental protection in Biblical and Talmudic sources. In: Grieco A, Iavicoli S, Berliguer G, eds. Proceedings, First International Conference on the History of Occupational and Environmental Protection. Rome: ISPESL, National Institute for Occupational Safety and Prevention, 1998;135.
10. Pare A. The apologie and treatise of Ambroise Pare containing the voyages made into divers places with many of his writings upon surgery. Edited with and introduction by Geoffrey Keynes, Chicago: University of Chicago Press, 1952.
11. McCord CP. Scurvy as an occupational disease: IV. Scurvy and the nations' men-of-war. J Occup Med 1971; 13:441–7.
12. Wedeen RP. Poison in the pot: the legacy of lead. Carbondale: Southern Illinois University Press, 1984.
13. Adams F. The medical works of Paulus Aegineta. Vol 1. London: J Welsh, 1834.
14. Ellenbog U. On the poisonous evil vapors. Lancet 1932; 1:230-1.
15. Sigerist HE, ed. Four treatises of Theophrastus von Hohenheim called Paracelsus. Baltimore: Johns Hopkins Press, 1941.
16. Agricola G. De re metallica. Translated by Herbert Clark Hoover and Lou Henry Hoover. New York: Dover, 1950.
17. Sisco AG, Smith CS. Lazarus Ercker's treatise on ores and assaying. Chicago: University of Chicago Press, 1951.

18. Birunguccio V. The pirotechnia. Sisco AG and Gnudi MT, translators. New York: American Institute of Mining and Metallurgical Engineers, 1942.

19. Nef JU. Coal mining and utilization. In: Singer C, Holymard EJ, Hall AR, Williams TI, eds. A history of technology. Vol III. New York: Oxford University Press, 1957;72–88.

20. Brimblecombe P. The big smoke. London: Methuen, 1987.

21. Li Ch'iao-p'ing. The chemical arts of old China. Easton Pennsylvania: Journal of Chemical Education, 1984.

22. Needham J. The development of iron and steel technology in China. London: Newcomen Society, 1958.

23. Singer C. East and west in retrospect. In: Singer C, Holymard EJ, Hall AR, Williams TI, eds. A history of technology. Vol II. New York: Oxford University Press, 1956;753–76.

24. Ying-Hsing S, T'ien-Kung K'ai-Wu. Chinese technology in the seventeenth century. University Park and London: The Pennsylvania State University Press, 1966.

25. Ramazzini B. De morbis artificum diatriba. Modena: Capponi, 1700.

26. Ramazzini B. Treatise on the diseases of tradesmen. London: Thomas Osborne, 1746.

27. Ramazzini B. De morbis artificum Bernardini Ramazzini diatriba. Disease of workers. The Latin text of 1713 revised, with translation and notes by Wilmer Cave Wright. Chicago: University of Chicago Press, 1940.

28. Ramazzini B. Essai sur maladies des artisans. M. Fourcroy, translator. Paris: Moutard, 1777.

29. Ramazzini B. Abhandlung von den krankheiten der kunstler un handweker neu bearbeit und vermehret von Johann Christian Gottlieb Ackermann. Stendal: D.C. Franzen und J.C. Gross, 1780, 1783.

30. Morgagni G. The seats and causes of diseases. Translated by Benjamin Alexander. (Facsimile of the 1769 edition). Birmingham: Classics of Medicine Library, 1983.

31. Tissot SA. An essay on the disorders of people of fashion; and a treatise on the diseases incident to literary and sedentary persons. Edinburgh: A Donaldson, 1772.

32. de Begontini A. Bernadino Ramazzini da morbis artificum prosequito. Vienna: Typis Geroldianis, 1778.

33. Giesl JF. Bernadino Ramazzini da morbis artificum prosequito. Vienna: Typis Geroldianis, 1778.

34. Tralles JW. De Praeservandis artificum et opificum morbis. Magdeberg: Johan Christian Hendel, 1745.

35. Skragge N. Disertationem medicam, qua morbi artificum leviter adumbrantur. Uppsala: Uppsala University, 1765.

36. Lindfors AO. Linnes dietetik. Uppsala: Akadmeiska Boktryckeriet, 1907;64–74.

37. Evelyn J. Fumifugium: or the inconvenience of the aer and smoake of London dissipated. Dorchester, Dorset and London: National Society for Clean Air, 1961.

38. Evelyn J. Fumifugium: or the inconvenience of the aer and smoake of London dissipated, 2nd edn. London: B White, 1772.

39. Blanc PD, Nadel JA. Clearing the air: the links between occupational and environmental air pollution control. Public Health Rev 1994; 22:251–270.

40. Baker G. An essay concerning the cause of the endemial colic of Devonshire, which was read in the theatre of the College of Physicians, in London, on the twenty-ninth day of June, 1767, 2nd edn. London: Payne and Foss, 1814.

41. Gillispie CC, ed. A Diderot pictorial encyclopedia of trades and industry. Manufacturing and the technical arts in plates selected from 'L'Encyclopedie, ou dictionnaire raisonne des sciences, des arts et des metiers' of Denis Diderot. New York: Dover Publications, 1987.

42. Baines E. History of the cotton manufacture in Great Britain. London: H Fisher, R Fisher, and P Jackson, 1835.

43. Clow A, Clow NL. The chemical industry: interaction with the industrial revolution. In: Singer C, Holmyard EJ, Hall AR, Williams TI, eds. A history of technology. Oxford: Clarendon Press, 1958; 230–56.

44. Underhill FP. The lethal war gases: physiology and experimental treatment. New Haven: Yale University Press, 1920.

45. Phillips JL. The bends. New Haven: Yale University Press, 1998.

46. Geist L. Die regeneration des unterkiefers nach totaler necrose durch phosphordampfe. Erlagen: Verlag von Ferdinand Enke, 1852.

47. Delpech A. Industrie au caoutchouc souffle. Researches sur l'intoxication speciale que determine le sulfure de carbone. Annales d' Hygiene Public et de Medicine Legale (Series 2) 1863; 19:65–183.

48. Richardson BW. Health and occupation. London: Society for Promoting Christian Knowledge, 1879.

49. Walsh D. Deep tissue traumatism from roentgen ray exposure. Br Med J 1897; ii:272.

50. Greenhow EH. On chronic bronchitis escpecially as connected with gout, emphysema and diseases of the heart, being clinical lectures delivered at Middlesex Hospital. London: Longmans, 1869.

51. Holland CG. Diseases of the lungs from mechanical causes. London: John Churchill, 1843.

52. Oliver T. Lead poisoning in its acute and chronic forms. The Goulstonian Lectures, delivered in the Royal College of Physicians, March, 1891. Edinburgh & London: Young J Pentland, 1891.

53. Blanc PD. Metal fume fever from a historical perspective. In: Grieco A, Iavicoli S, Berlinguer G, eds. Contributions to the history of occupational and environmental prevention. Amsterdam: Elsevier, 1999; 211–21.

54. Chadwick E. Report on the sanitary condition of the labouring population of Great Britain. London: W Clowes for HM Stationery Office, 1843.

55. Simon J. Public health reports (2 vols). London: The Sanitary Institute, 1887.

56. Nightingale F. Florence Nightingale's notes on nursing. Edited with an introduction, notes and guide to identification by Victor Skretkowicz. London: Scutari Press, 1992.

57. Thackrah CT. The effects of the principal arts, trades, and professions, and of civic states and habits of living. London: Longman, 1831.

58. Thackrah CT. The effects of arts, trades, and professions, and of civic states and habits of living, on health and longevity, 2nd edn. London: Longman, 1832.

59. Meiklejohn A. The life and times of Charles Turner Thackrah. Edinburgh: E & S Livingstone, 1957.

60. Noble D. Facts and observations relative to the influence of manufactures upon health and life. London: John Churchill, 1843.

61. Lee CA. On the effects of arts, trades, and professions, as well as habits of living, on health and longevity. Family Magazine (New York) 1840–41; 8:175–7,212–5,270–2,302–5.

62. McCready BW. On the influence of trades, professions and occupations in the United States in the production of disease – being the prize dissertation for 1837. Transactions of the Medical Society of the State of New York 1836–37; 3:91–150.

63. House of Commons, Great Britain. A copy of the report presented to the House of Commons by the committee appointed to examine the several petitions, which have been presented to the House, against the employment of boys in sweeping of chimneys. London: House of Commons, 1817.

64. Fleming LE, Ducatman AM, Shalat SL. Disease clusters: a central and ongoing role in occupational health. J Occup Med 1991; 33:818–25.

65. Holdsworth C. Dr. John Thomas Arlidge and Victorian occupational medicine. Med Hist 1998; 42:458–75.

66. Meiklejohn A. Industrial health – meeting the challenge. Br J Ind Med 1959; 16:1–10.

67. Chevalier L. Laboring classes and dangerous classes in Paris during the first half of the nineteenth century (translated by Frank Jellinek). New York: Howard Fertig, 1973.

68. Patissier P. Traite des maladies des artisans. Paris: Chez J.-B. Bailliers, 1822.

69. Tanquerel des Planches L. Traite des maladies de plomb ou saturnines. Paris: Ferra, 1839.

70. Orfila MP. Traite des poisons tires des regnes mineral, vegetal et animal, ou Toxicologie generale, consideree sous les rapports de la physiologie, de la pathologie et de la medecine legale, 2nd edn. Paris: Crochard, 1818.

71. Bernard C. Lecons sur les effets des substances toxiques. Paris: J.B. Baillier, 1857.

72. Hirt L. Die krankheiten der arbeiter. Breslau: F. Hirt, 1871–1878.

73. Teleky L. History of factory and mine hygiene. New York: Columbia University, 1948.

74. McCord CP. Occupational health publications in the United States prior to 1900. Ind Med Surg Med 1955; 24:363–8.

75. Arlidge JT. The hygiene, diseases, and mortality of occupations. London: Percival and Company, 1892.

76. Proust A. Traite d'hygiene publique et privee. Paris: G. Masson, 1877.

77. Santenson CG. Ueber chronische vergiftungen mit steinkohlentheerbenzin; vier todesfalle. Archiv fur Hygiene 1897; 31:336–76.

78. Sellers C. The Public Health Services Office of Industrial Hygiene and the transformation of industrial medicine. Bull Hist Med 1991; 65:42–73.

79. Oliver T, ed. Dangerous trades. The historical, social, and legal aspects of industrial occupations as affecting health, by a number of experts. London: John Murray, 1902.

80. Eastman E. Work accidents and the law. The Pittsburgh Survey. New York: Russell Sage Foundation (Charities Publishing Committee), 1910.

81. Kober GM. Industrial and personal hygiene. A report of the Commission on Social Betterment. Washington DC: The President's Homes Commission, 1908.

82. Overlock MG. The working people, their health and how to protect it. Boston: Health Book Publishing Co, 1911.

83. Andrews JB. Labor problems and labor legislation. New York: American Association for Labor Legislation, 1919;65–92.

84. Berman D. Death on the job. New York: Monthly Review Press, 1978.

85. Derickson A. Workers' health and workers' democracy: the western miners' struggle, 1891–1925. Ithaca, New York: Cornell University Press, 1988.

86. Haywood JK. Injury to vegetation and animal life by smelter wastes. U.S. Department of Agriculture Bulletin 113. Washington DC: US Government Printing Office, 1910.

87. Royal Sanitary Institute. Addresses, papers, and discussions at conference on smoke abatement, London, Dec. 12th–15th, 1905. London: Royal Sanitary Institute, 1906.

88. Sellers C. Hazards on the job: from industrial disease to environmental health science. Chapel Hill: University of North Carolina Press, 1997.

89. Hamilton A. Exploring the dangerous trades. Boston: Little, Brown, 1943.

90. Legge TM. Industrial maladies. London: Humphrey Milford Oxford Press (Oxford Medical Publications), 1934.

91. Brown AB. The machine and the worker. London: Ivor Nicholson and Watson Ltd, 1934.

92. Blanc PD. The legacy of war gas. Am J Med 1999; 106:689–90.

93. Fauntleroy AM. Report on the medico-military aspects of the European war. Washington DC: US Government Printing Office, 1915.

94. Grant MP. Alice Hamilton. Pioneer doctor in industrial America. London: Abelard-Schuman, 1967.

95. Sicherman B. Alice Hamilton, a life in letters. Cambridge: Harvard University Press, 1984.

96. Trueta J. Treatment of war wounds and fractures with special reference to the closed method as used in the war in Spain. London: Hamish Hamilton, 1939.

97. Dreiser T. Tragic America. New York: Horace Liveright, 1931;19,196.

98. Maltz A. The way things are. New York: International Publishers, 1938.

99. Cherniack M. The hawk's nest incident: America's worst industrial disaster. New Haven: Yale University Press, 1986.

100. Skidmore H. Hawk's nest. New York: Doubleday Doran and Co., 1941.

101. Pawel E. The nightmare of reason. A life of Franz Kafka. New York: Farrar Strauss Giroux, 1984;181–9.

102. Cronin AJ. The citadel. London: Victor Gollancz, 1937;209.

103. Mettert MT. The occurrence and prevention of occupational diseases among women. US Department of Labor, Bulletin of the Women's Bureau No. 184. Washington DC: US Government Printing Office, 1941.

104. Ames A. Sex in industry: a plea for the working girl. Boston: James R. Osgood and Company, 1875.

105. Hamilton A. Women workers and industrial poisons. Bulletin of the Women's Bureau No. 57. Washington DC: US Government Printing Office, 1926.

106. Hutchins G. Women who work. International Pamphlets No. 27. New York: International Publishers, 1932.

107. Ernst E. A leading medical school seriously damaged: Vienna 1938. Ann Intern Med 1995; 122:789–92.

108. West JB. Highlife: a history of high-altitude physiology and medicine. New York: Oxford University Press, 1998;246–53,427.

109. Schrenk HH. Causes, constituents and physical effects of smog involved in specific dramatic episodes. Arch Ind Hyg Occup Med 1950; 1:189-94.

110. Whittenberger JL. Health effects of air pollution: some historical notes. Environ Health Persp 1989; 81:129–30.

111. Logan WPD. Mortality in the London fog incident, 1952. Lancet 1953; 1:336–8.

112. Drinker P. Atmospheric pollution. Ind Engineer Chem 1939; 31(11):1316–20.

113. Roholm K. The fog disaster in the Meuse Valley, 1930: a fluorine intoxication. J Ind Hyg Toxicol 1937; 19:126–37.

114. Hunter D. The diseases of occupations. London: English Universities Press, 1955.

115. Grieco A, Chiappino G, Alessio L et al. La scomparsa del Prof. Encrio Vigliani. Med del Lavoro 1992; 83:4–17.

116. Selleck HB, Whittaker AH. Occupational health in America. Detroit: Wayne State University Press, 1962.

117. Carson RL. Silent spring. Cambridge: Houghton Mifflin, 1962.

118. Cushman JH Jr. After 'Silent Spring,' industry spin on all it brewed. New York Times, March 26, 2001;A14.

119. Rosner D, Markowitz G. Deadly dust: silicosis and the politics of occupational disease in twentieth-century America. Princeton, New Jersey: Princeton University Press, 1991.

120. Denbe A. Occupation and disease: how social factors affect the conception of work-related disorders. New Haven: Yale University Press, 1996.

121. Meiklejohn A. John Darwall, M.D. (1796–1833) and 'Diseases of Artisans'. Br J Ind Med 1956; 13:142–51.

122. Brouder P. Expendable Americans. New York: Viking Press, 1974.

123. McCord CP. A blind hog's acorns: vignettes of the maladies of workers. Chicago: Cloud Inc, 1945.

124. Moody Medical Library. The Truman G. Blocker, Jr. History of Medicine Collections: books and manuscripts. Galveston: University of Texas Medical Branch, 1986.

125. Claremont College. Hoover collection on mining and metallurgy. Claremont, California: Arcon Press, 1980.

126. Goldsmiths'-Kress Library. Goldmsiths'-Kress library of economic literature: a consolidated guide to segment I of the microfilm collection. (5 vol.). Woodbridge: Research Publications, Inc., 1976.

127. Morton L. Morton's medical bibliography: an annotated check-list of texts illustrating the history of medicine (Garrison and Morton), 5th edn. Brookfield: Gower, 1991.

Chapter 3
Approach to the Patient

Mark R Cullen, Linda Rosenstock

As noted in the Introduction, OEM includes both clinical and public health aspects. In this chapter, principles of clinical practice are explored that distinguish the field from the core disciplines of clinical medicine – internal medicine, orthopedics, dermatology, neurology, etc – with which the reader may be more familiar.

One very obvious distinction is that clinical OEM includes two very different components. The bread and butter of the field has come to be known as 'primary care' occupational medicine (there is no counterpart on the environmental side) and includes activities that have existed, primarily within heavy industry, long before they were glamorized by this designation or became the subject of scientific scrutiny. Primary care components include, among other things, the conduct of preplacement physical examinations; care of minor injuries and immediately recognized adverse effects of over-exposure in the workplace; return to work examinations and medical screening. Historically these services were deemed sufficiently straightforward that any practitioner of medicine would be qualified to perform them without additional or specific OEM training. Changes in public perception, regulations, rapidly advancing knowledge and legal/economic considerations have rendered each aspect worthy of formal training, now incorporated into the residency requirements for specialty training in OEM in the US.

PRIMARY CARE OCCUPATIONAL MEDICINE
Preplacement evaluation

Preplacement evaluation has superseded the previous construct of pre-employment examination because of societal discrimination concerns; in the US and many other countries, individuals may not be assessed medically prior to being offered provisional employment as a matter of law. Once a job offer has been made, an exam may be conducted – and for jobs entailing any substantial risks undoubtedly should – to determine that the employee is physically and mentally qualified to perform the essential functions of the job safely. The legal aspects of this are discussed in Chapter 57.3. From a medical perspective, the examination must be tailored to the specific physical requirements and hazards of the job; general considerations, such as pre-existing health conditions or disabilities, are irrelevant except insofar as they would interfere with the job. For this reason, primary care occupational medicine practice requires extensive knowledge about the work setting and job requirements for each position for which any exam may be performed. This knowledge must be sufficiently detailed to address any challenge that an employee has been discriminated against for any reason other than ability to perform the essentials of the job. While it is perfectly acceptable for the examiner – who does not enjoy a traditional doctor–patient relationship with such individuals – to inquire about or evaluate other health issues or behaviors (about which there may be concern from a preventive health perspective) he or she may do so only insofar as three things are borne in mind: such investigations must be voluntary, and the employee aware of that; the information must be maintained confidentially and not used to make employment decisions; and similar investigations must be requested of all new employees, irrespective of the positions for which they have been hired (including managers!).

Management of minor injuries and responses to work hazards

The routine management of minor injuries and acute responses to hazards at work falls into the purview of outpatient emergency medicine or surgery, and is beyond the scope of this text. However, as with preplacement, there are important occupational health components.

First, it is crucial that the underlying causes of the illness or injury be investigated in order to prevent further injuries from occurring. This may or may not be the responsibility of the primary care provider per se, but it is her or his obligation to make sure that all available information from the evaluation relevant to the event is provided to those at the workplace or company who are responsible.

Second, since most employers are now eager to limit lost work time and generally prefer early return to work, even if in restricted roles, the provider must be cognizant of the demands of the patient's job, to determine whether or not the injury or illness precludes it, unless there are overarching medical reasons for lost time such as the need for hospitalization, work-limiting medications or bedrest. Pressures from employee or his/her supervisor for premature or inappropriate return to work must be resisted, as must the temptation to prescribe time off for convenience or social reasons. Close communication with both the employee and the manager are essential in every case.

Evaluation for return to work

Evaluation for return to work is an extension of the above activities, and requires review of medical reports regarding any disabling illness – work related or otherwise – and then reiterating the preplacement approach in light of the new information. Even more crucially in this context, information without direct bearing on the patient's specific job is not relevant, and must not be communicated in any way to the employer.

Medical screening

Finally there is medical screening. This activity involves the collection of information from the patient – it may be a questionnaire, a hearing test, a blood test etc – to assess either level of exposure to a hazard or a possible preclinical health effect. The primary purpose is to protect the individual worker, although results are often scrutinized for other purposes, such as part of a surveillance program to prevent adverse workplace effects more generally (discussed more fully in Chapter 4.3). The first level of interpretation, however, pertains to the wellbeing of the individual tested. In this way, results may demonstrate an over-exposure or a work-connected effect. In either case the practitioner is obliged to inform the worker explicitly of that fact, and assure appropriate response such as reduction of exposure, removal, compensation and/or treatments as necessary. Often, however, abnormalities detected on screening exams are not job related in origin, nor directly affect the ability of someone already doing the job to continue doing it (although occasionally they might, and in that situation must be addressed). When non-work connected abnormalities are suspected, two things become essential: the provider must inform the employee of the abnormal finding and her/his opinion regarding its origins, and the provider must share responsibility that the findings are appropriately followed up.

TERTIARY CARE OCCUPATIONAL AND ENVIRONMENTAL MEDICINE

Unfortunately, despite all of the preventive aspects of those charged with making the workplace and outside environment free of excess hazard, some adverse consequences of exposure continue to occur; many more are suspected. Evaluation of such patients constitutes the 'tertiary' aspect of OEM practice, one that prior to a few decades ago could not be said to exist in organized form in the US or most other parts of the world. It is to that aspect that the rest of this chapter is devoted.

Patients, physicians, and third parties typically prompt diagnostic consultation with an OEM specialist for one of four reasons:

1. the patient (or referring party) suspects that symptoms, signs, or laboratory abnormalities may be due to some environmental or occupational factor;
2. a disorder has been diagnosed where the cause may not be evident: the question arises as to whether it may be due to an environmental or occupational factor;
3. exposure to a suspected harmful agent has raised concern that early manifestations of disease may be

present or that the patient may be at high risk for subsequent occurrence; and
4. assessment of disability and/or potential for work rehabilitation.

In the sections that follow we will concern ourselves with the first three scenarios; assessment of impairment and disability is the subject of Chapter 8.

CLINICAL EVALUATIONS IN OEM

In addition to the usual methods of clinical diagnosis, three tools are special to OEM practice: the occupational and environmental history, the environmental evaluation, and the use of specialized tests to establish causal associations. Despite variations in applicability, the principles are common to every case.

Occupational and environmental history and evaluation

The occupational health history is fundamental to the assessment of the work-relatedness of health problems; as such, even in abbreviated form it should become a routine component of every comprehensive health history, not exclusive to OEM referral care.[1,2] The environmental history complements the occupational health history by probing for the presence of non-occupational factors and their possible role in the disease process.

The occupational and environmental history has multiple purposes.

1. *To increase awareness of occupational and environmental factors.* It is more the exception than the rule that clues to the potential role of these factors emerge from the physical examination or routine laboratory testing. Unless this history is specifically elicited or otherwise offered by the patient, the opportunity will be lost to consider occupationally and environmentally related disease or risk.
2. *To make accurate medical diagnoses.* Failure to obtain the history in the setting where occupational and environmental factors have played a role inevitably results in at least a partial misdiagnosis. For example, if fatty liver disease is correctly diagnosed but is attributed to alcohol over-consumption when solvent exposures have also played a role, then the diagnosis of alcoholic fatty liver disease is not correct and important treatment interventions may be overlooked.
3. *To prevent the development of occupational and environmental disease.* By using the occupational and environmental health history as a screening tool, identification of exposures to potentially hazardous factors can result in the reduction or elimination of these exposures. This factor may be beneficial in the setting where exposures cause diseases of long latency, as well as those responsible for acute and recurrent conditions. Identifying past asbestos exposure, for example, may render counseling about smoking cessation more effective when this counseling is

provided in the setting of education about the synergistic effect of exposure to both carcinogens. In the case of exposures causing acute conditions – for example, pulmonary allergens – interventions to decrease exposure are likely to reduce the person's risk of subsequently developing hypersensitivity.

4. *To prevent the aggravation of underlying medical conditions by occupational and environmental factors*. The smoker with chronic bronchitis who is exposed to respiratory irritants in the workplace will, regardless of effectiveness of smoking cessation interventions, benefit by reducing his or her exposure to identified respiratory irritants. Similarly, in addition to optimizing glucose control in the individual with diabetes mellitus, avoidance of exposure to agents that may cause peripheral neuropathy is also an important intervention, because the individual predisposed to a peripheral neuropathy of any cause may be at increased risk for damage from environmental peripheral neurotoxins.

5. *To identify potential workplace hazards*. In addition to using the occupational and environmental history as a screening tool to identify and ameliorate the risk of exposure to hazards, the history can help identify factors that would otherwise not be suspected as injurious. For example, the worker who presents with a persistent nocturnal cough may have been exposed to an irritating or sensitizing agent, initiating bronchial hyper-responsiveness manifested as cough.

6. *To detect new associations between exposures and disease*. The field of occupational and environmental medicine is rapidly evolving. As more interest and attention are paid to environmentally induced illnesses, more is learned about the nature and extent of adverse effects of specific agents. Perhaps no other field offers the potential to uncover, through the evaluation of an individual patient, a previously unknown association between exposure and disease. Examples include adding to the list of now over 200 agents known to induce specific asthmatic responses, identifying new neurologic syndromes as chronic sequelae of past intoxications, and discovering new renal and hepatic toxins.

7. *To establish the basis of compensation for occupational and environmental disease*. Whether for workers' compensation for occupational disease or liability claims, the physician plays a key role in determining the likelihood that an environmental exposure has caused a given medical condition. The patient's history of exposure, its onset, intensity, and duration – sometimes alone or in conjunction with other available exposure information – is fundamental to this assessment.

8. *To establish rapport with patients*. This last benefit of the occupational and environmental health history in many ways is a secondary and unexpected bonus to the original objectives. In our experience, it is remarkable how often encouraging an otherwise taciturn person to describe the details of his or her job

facilitates a more relaxed and congenial medical evaluation. Demonstration of a physician's interest in activities fundamentally important to the patient can lessen anxieties attendant with first time physician–patient encounters.

Components of the occupational and environmental history

The occupational and environmental history can be obtained in several ways. One approach is to integrate a series of key questions directly into the routine health history. Another approach is to incorporate a screening history with all new visits, selectively updating this procedure as indicated. In either approach, however, the occupational and environmental history has two main components: the employment and exposure history and the occupationally and environmentally related health history. The first component contains information about current and past jobs as well as non-occupational environmental exposures. The health history component uses questions to elicit information about health problems and symptoms in relation to specific exposures and work settings, and about the existence of symptoms or illnesses in coworkers, household members, or community residents.

A sample history form that can be self-administered and maintained as part of the patient's database is shown in Figure 3.1. This form can serve as a screening tool; clinical judgment will determine when it is appropriate to take a more comprehensive history. Because in some clinical settings even this shortened form may not be readily administered, we are often asked what few questions should be asked of all new patients. A survey of members of the United States Association of Occupational and Environmental Medicine Clinics (AOEC) found the following three questions essential.

1. Please describe your job.
2. Have you ever worked with any health hazard, such as asbestos, chemicals, noise, or repetitive motion?
3. Do you have any health problems that you believe may be related to work?

The following section describes the elements of the two core components of the occupational and environmental health history in greater detail, as would be appropriate to OEM tertiary evaluation.

Work and exposure history

This component of the occupational and environmental health history extends beyond what might be routinely obtained in the clinical setting. Nonetheless, the objectives of the work history are similar to many other aspects of social history, particularly those that include identifying in an individual risk factors that indicate the need for prevention or intervention strategies.

The following discussion is relevant to information about the current or most recent job or, in some instances, a previous job of concern regarding the problem under evaluation. For example, if a patient is being evaluated for

---

I. Work and exposure history

A. *Current employment*

Questions 1–7 refer to your current or most recent job.

1. Job title _____

2. Type of industry _____

3. Name of employer _____

4. Year job began
   Still working?
   Yes _____ No _____ If no, year job ended

5. Briefly describe this job, noting any part that you feel may be hazardous to your health.

   _____
   _____

6. Do you wear protective equipment on this job?
   Yes _____ No _____ If yes, check equipment used:

   Gloves _____   Air supply respirator _____
   Mask respirator _____   Coveralls or aprons _____
   Hearing protection _____   Safety glasses _____

7. In this job, are you exposed to any of the following?
   If yes, mark those to which you are exposed:

   Fumes and dust _____   Elements and metals _____
   Solvents _____   Other chemicals _____
   Vibration _____   Excess heat/cold _____
   Emotional stress _____   Noise _____ Other _____

B. *Employment history*

It is important that we know all the jobs you have had. Job #1 is your current or most recent job. Beginning with the job before this one— Job #2—please fill in as much of the information requested as you can remember, and continue to do so until all previous jobs have been listed. Include any military service you have had. If you need additional space, use the back of this form.

	Years From To	Job title	Exposures
Job #2	_____	_____	_____
Job #3	_____	_____	_____
Job #4	_____	_____	_____
Job #5	_____	_____	_____
Job #6	_____	_____	_____
Job #7	_____	_____	_____
Job #8	_____	_____	_____
Wartime employment	_____	_____	_____

C. *Other exposures*

1. Does anyone in your household work at a job that you suspect involves exposures that may be brought home from work (e.g., asbestos fibers on clothes)? Yes _____ No _____

2. Are there any industries in the area in which you live that may pollute your environment? Yes _____ No _____

3. Do you have any hobbies that expose you to chemicals, metals, or other substances? Yes _____ No _____

4. Have you ever smoked cigarettes? ("No" means less than 20 packs of cigarettes in your entire life.) Yes _____ No _____

   If yes, please answer the following:

   a. Do you now smoke cigarettes (that is, as of 1 month ago)?
      Yes _____ No _____
   b. How many years have you smoked? _____
   c. Of the entire time you have smoked, about how many cigarettes per day do or did you smoke on the average? _____

II. General health history*

1. Is there any particular hazard or part of your job that you think relates to your problems? Yes _____ No _____

2. Do any of your coworkers have problems or complaints similar to yours? Yes _____ No _____

* For each positive response to review of systems, ask whether symptoms are better, worse, or no different in association with work

---

Figure 3.1: A sample of a screening occupational and environmental history form, which can be self-administered and serve as the basis for a more comprehensive history.

---

suspected occupational asthma, the key to a successful diagnosis is to focus on the job when the patient first began having symptoms. In addition to asking for the patient's job title (or occupation), it is important to ascertain the specific nature of the job. This information can be obtained by asking additional questions about the industry. For example, a painter in a shipyard is subject to different exposures from a painter in a residential setting. Hence, the key questions are: 'What product or service does your employer make or produce?' and 'What aspect do you do on your job?' If the job is already familiar to the physician, then the question may be modified; for example, one may ask 'Is there anything you do now that is different from past jobs where you've been an electrician?'

It may be helpful to ask the patient to describe a typical work day.

The screening history inquires about the use of personal protective equipment (PPE). Although the provision of good protective equipment should mitigate risks of exposure, it must be kept in mind that those who use protective equipment are often at increased risk for work-related illnesses. The protective equipment serves as a clue that hazardous materials are present, and exposure at least possible. For this reason a candid appraisal of the equipment's actual use is invaluable as well.

The patient should be asked directly about potentially hazardous exposures that are present at work, whether of biologic, chemical, physical, or psychologic origin. A checklist approach (as illustrated in Fig. 3.2) can be used to direct this inquiry. If a patient gives a positive response within any category, then further information can be obtained about specific exposures. For an overview of the patient's occupational and environmental history and for an evaluation of those conditions of long latency, such as cancer or pneumoconiosis, the history must include information about past jobs and exposures and potential important exposures in the non-work environment. An abbreviated history of all employment is provided in the sample history form (Fig. 3.1). Sometimes an individual omits information about employment during military service; therefore, this information, which may indicate that the individual was subject to other toxic exposures, should be specifically sought.

Many workers are well informed about specific exposures. In other instances, however, the exposure history requires further investigation to identify specific constituents of products and exposure levels. Consideration of the exposure dose is important in identifying, preventing, and managing occupational diseases; the history is an important first step in establishing the level of exposure. Although it is by no means precise, the patient's assessment of relative levels of exposure (i.e., low, medium, high) for specific agents can be valuable. One way of eliciting this information is shown in Figure 3.2, a portion of a comprehensive occupational and environmental history that can also be self-administered. Here, the patient is given an opportunity to report potential exposure to various widely prevailent hazards that appear or have appeared in the current or any past job. For physical

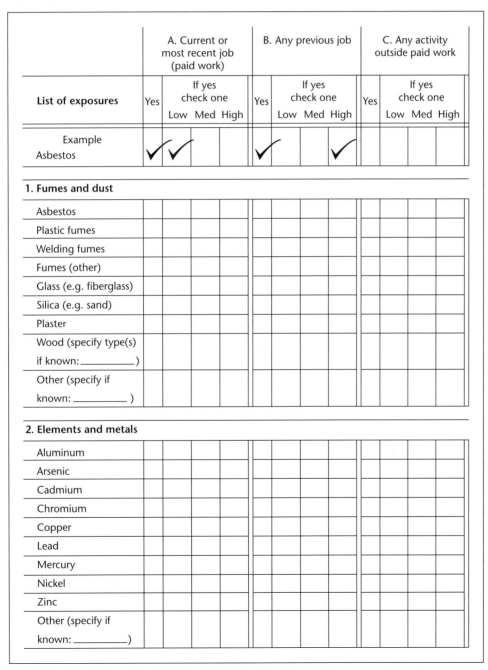

Figure 3.2: Sample of detailed self-report form for specific occupational and environmental exposures.

List of exposures	A. Current or most recent job (paid work)			B. Any previous job			C. Any activity outside paid work		
	Yes	If yes check one Low Med High		Yes	If yes check one Low Med High		Yes	If yes check one Low Med High	
3. Solvents									
Alcohols (e.g. methyl, wood)									
Benzene									
Toluene, xylene, naphtha									
Paint, varnish, degreasers									
Tri-, tetrachloroethylene									
Other (specify if known: _____)									
4. Other chemicals									
Acids									
Alkali (caustics)									
Ammonia									
Herbicides and pesticides									
Dyes									

Figure 3.2 (cont'd): Sample of detailed self-report form for specific occupational and environmental exposures.

hazards it is often best to have the patient compare levels to common comparisons, such as 'loud as a subway'. Sometimes acting out an activity or task may be useful for demonstrating potential risk, especially for musculoskeletal effects.

As noted, the nature and use of protective equipment may provide an additional clue about levels of exposure, as would information about the general cleanliness of the workplace and the adequacy of ventilation. Finally, for some exposures that have acute as well as chronic effects, such as organic solvents, the description of immediate symptoms in relation to exposure – e.g., acute intoxication or headache – may provide evidence that excessive exposure levels have been encountered; the absence of these symptoms would suggest more modest exposure levels.

Environmental history

The non-occupational environment, while generally less hazardous in terms of the number and dose of chemical, physical, and biologic hazards, is paradoxically more complex to query. Often the patient has a particular focus or concern, and detailed attention can be directed to that,

for example the consequence of a leaky furnace, or the installation of a new carpet in the home. However, in every OEM referral examination at least a survey of possible environmental contaminants should be made, covering at least a question about outdoor air, environment inside the home (e.g. heat sources, chemical use) hobbies and avocations, sources of toxic pollution in the community, drinking water and diet. Occasionally, patients are referred with cryptogenic signs or symptoms, such as recurrent hives or respiratory complaint, or an elevated body burden of some heavy metal, the source of which is obscure, rendering it necessary to probe all of these aspects in some detail.

The home is the source of most referrals and concerns. Wells may be contaminated with organic hydrocarbons, metals or pesticides. Exposure occurs during consumption or, in the case of volatile chemicals, from the air during bathing. Most people will be unaware of whether there are contaminants in their water, unless these have already been tested for a reason. From a history-taking perspective, the major issue is whether they use well or city water; if the former, whether there is reason to suspect contamination. Rarely the water will have an odor or abnormal appearance, but it's not a very discriminating question. An unrelated water concern is old plumbing, from which lead and copper may leech after water stands overnight.

Boilers, furnaces, fireplaces and stoves provide opportunities for carbon monoxide, gas, particles and fuel exhaust exposure if flues or other devices leak or are clogged. Carpets, a source of irritation when installed, harbor molds and mildew (as do ceiling and wall board) after exposure to moisture. Furnishings, computers, pets, cleaning materials or services and other merchandise may introduce chemical hazards, allergens or, occasionally, infectious risks. Radon gas occurs primarily in homes built on hard rock, but can only be evaluated by measurement – there are no other clues to be gleaned from the patient. Many, if not all of these hazards are enhanced by indoor tobacco use.

Questions about outdoor sources of contamination should focus on recognized point sources, since major air pollutants such as ozone and sulfate and oxides of nitrogen are more regionally distributed: the patient is unlikely to know what levels are, though these can be obtained from regulatory authorities. Of more usual concern are local polluters, which may include neighbors using chemicals on lawns and trees that patients find noxious or disconcerting.

Many people engage in hobbies or avocations at home or in their garage, involving hazardous risks. These should be specifically queried, since they may involve exposures to very dangerous materials at levels at or even above those seen in comparable occupations, usually without appropriate controls. Examples may include gardening, painting cars, sanding (leaded) paints from old furniture, building models with glues and solvents, home renovations or virtually anything which for another patient would be an occupation. Not rarely, people do at home something similar to their work, so that this line of questioning is crucial for screening all patients.

Finally, it is worth asking every patient at least briefly about their diet. The most important issues revolve around imported or unusual foods, a heavy portion of the diet coming from a single source (e.g. swordfish, an important source of environmental mercury exposure) or the use of non-commercially sold dietary supplements. Cookware of distant origin may also be a source of metal or other hazards. These factors are discussed at length in Chapter 53.

Health in relation to work and environment

The traditional part of the health history, including the chief complaint and review of systems, needs to be appropriately expanded to assess a possible relationship between occupational and environmental exposures and health problems. In each of the chapters in Section 3 of this text, specific questions pertinent to disorders under discussion are highlighted. But a few questions should be asked of all patients; others are specific to particular conditions. If nothing else, patients should be asked whether they feel their health problems are occupationally or environmentally related. In many instances, the first suspicion about an occupational or environmental disorder arises from the patient's concern about the effects of an exposure.

Although this suspicion may well prove to be unfounded, such concerns should always be taken seriously.

The presence of similar symptoms or complaints among coworkers or others exposed may be an important clue. Particularly for agents acting as direct toxins (see Chapters 1 and 5), the presence of symptoms among others similarly exposed may indicate that a common exposure is responsible and that the exposure levels are generally above typical 'thresholds'. Even for substances producing sensitization, such as chemical asthmagens, finding other persons in the workplace with similar symptoms may help identify the offending agent. The report of the presence or absence of symptoms in coworkers or others in an ostensibly contaminated environment should, however, be interpreted with caution. Sometimes an exposure affects only a single person, due to unique opportunities for exposure, an idiosyncratic reaction, or differing host susceptibilities. Conversely, 'epidemics' may seem to be occurring where common complaints are exhibited, whose causes turn out to be quite unrelated.

An important component of this part of the history, particularly for symptoms reflecting acute and recurrent conditions such as dermatitis or asthma, is the relationship between symptoms and time of work shifts or specific exposures. In the occupational setting, patients should be asked whether anything different at work preceded the onset of their symptoms, such as handling a new task, new product, or new job assignment. Patterns of symptoms in relation to time at work may provide helpful hints to both the diagnosis and the etiologic agent. Several patterns are described below; these patterns may occur alone or in combination in an individual patient. Inquiry about timing of symptoms in relation to non-workplace environmental exposure is essentially no different from inquiry about workplace exposures, and questioning should proceed along the general lines described below.

Change in symptoms during the work day

For a number of substances that induce their effect as direct acting toxins, such as solvents or non-specific dusts and respiratory irritants, the patient may arrive at work free of symptoms only to experience their onset in a predictable fashion after arriving at work. A person with building-related illness (Chapter 50), for example, may report the onset of headache and dizziness within 1 to 2 hours after arriving at work; abatement of these symptoms occurs within a few hours after leaving work. For agents causing immediate hypersensitization responses, such as flour in bakers sensitized to it, the patient often describes the onset of symptoms consistent with asthma (whether exhibited as cough, chest tightness, shortness of breath, or wheeze) within minutes of exposure. Common upper respiratory and mucosal symptoms, including coryza, eye discomfort, and itching, precede or occur concurrently.

Symptoms may not occur similarly on all work days, and they may vary depending on the level of exposure (e.g., when ventilation is on or off, climatic conditions, specific job responsibilities) and other host factors (e.g., extent of recent exposure, medication use).

Change in symptoms over the work week

For several agents, of which cotton dust exposure is the classic example, there may be a higher level of symptom intensity on first returning to work after several days away ('Monday morning fever'), although symptoms (and concomitant pulmonary function decline) may worsen gradually as the week passes. In some instances, symptoms may be apparent only at the beginning of the work week. In metal fume fever, for example, the symptoms of this flu-like illness are most likely to occur on a Monday or Tuesday, with the individual exhibiting loss of the tolerance acquired during the previous work week. On the other hand, workers exposed to nitrates may get headaches both in the beginning of the work week and on weekends. Weekend flare-ups are associated with a withdrawal syndrome from these potent vasodilators, with associated vasospastic coronary or cerebral events occurring most commonly on weekends.

Change in symptoms on weekends and on vacations

A number of work-related syndromes result from exposures that have immediate or early effects, such that associated symptoms resolve within hours or days and occasionally with longer periods away from work. The effects of overexposure to solvents are examples of this type of temporal change. Because some solvents have longer half-lives than others, it may take days for the acute effects of solvent intoxication (characterized by headaches, lightheadedness, dyspepsia, and irritability) to resolve. For individuals who are chronically exposed to these agents, these effects may persist longer but should gradually resolve unless permanent sequelae, such as chronic encephalopathy, have supervened.

Trials of removal of the individual to assess the effect of withdrawal from exposure have an important diagnostic role in OEM. Examples include: removing a worker because of exposure to potential hepatotoxins to determine whether or not several weeks or months away from work may result in resolution of dysfunction; removing a student with respiratory symptoms from a problem classroom; removing a worker with carpal tunnel syndrome from exposure to repetitive motion; and removal of the patient with contact dermatitis from consumption of suspect water. Occupation-related trials must be conducted in close cooperation with employers, to prevent unwanted economic sequelae or misunderstanding about the reason for work absence (see Chapter 9).

Onset of symptoms away from exposure

A few agents are known to have unique patterns of inducing effects in relation to time of exposure. Some occupational asthma-inducing agents, for example, cause as the most common pattern of sensitization a delayed reaction from 4 to 12 hours after exposure, often initially exhibited as nocturnal asthma. The diisocyanates (TDI, MDI, HDI)

and Western red cedar are two well-studied agents associated with this pattern, which is characteristic of exposure to low molecular weight compounds. Often, the patient presenting with new onset asthma from these causes describes first awareness of wheezing or cough on nights following days at work; over time, with the emergence of non-specific bronchial hyper-reactivity, this clear-cut association with time at work may be lost.

As mentioned earlier, some agents such as nitrates may not exert their effects until their levels are lowered, so that symptomatic vasoconstriction may occur on removal of the individual from exposure. Some solvents, notably trichloroethylene, may cause a reaction similar to that of the drug Antabuse; affected individuals experience a flushing response when consuming even modest amounts of ethanol, even hours after solvent exposure has ceased.

Other experiences with work-related events

The last component of the modified general health history is to inquire about previously diagnosed work-related injuries or environmental illnesses, including any experience with workers' compensation. In addition to completing the historical database, this information may be helpful in recognizing previous hazardous exposures and the patient's clinical and emotional response to these.

The validity of the occupational and environmental health history

As noted previously, the occupational and environmental health history can be obtained by using a self-reported questionnaire or by interview. In either case, the question of the accuracy of exposure information provided by the patient is often raised, particularly if the information is likely to be used in settings that may have adversarial connotations such as workers' compensation or litigation.

Several investigators have studied the reliability and validity of this part of the health history. In the occupational and environmental history, self-reported exposure information has been evaluated in comparison with other measures, including personnel records; outcome measures, such as vital status, chest x-ray studies, and cancer registries; and information obtained by interviews with individuals knowledgeable about workplace assessments. Studies have found varying degrees of association between self-reported information and data obtained from other sources.[3] Results are nonetheless reassuring when the occupational and environmental history is the main or only source of exposure data.

Wherever possible, however, self-reported exposures should be supplemented by other information, discussed in more detail in the next section. The need for additional data about the nature and extent of specific exposures varies on a case by case basis. In practice, the information obtained directly from the patient often is sufficient to raise suspicion, but adequate for diagnosis only when corroborating information cannot be obtained after appropriate effort.

Strategies for further evaluating occupational and environmental exposure

Unfortunately for the practitioner, for many reasons the history by itself is insufficient for an accurate diagnosis. These reasons include: lack of specificity about the identity of hazards; inadequate information about exposure levels; recall biases (greater attention to exposures that were at the time bothersome or otherwise perceived as being harmful); and other biases, e.g., patients fearful of possible job loss may under-report exposures, whereas litigants may exaggerate the intensities of exposures and purported effects. For these reasons, an essential component of the work-up is obtaining additional exposure information whenever possible. This additional information serves several purposes: to learn the specific identity of chemical or physical hazards to which the patient has been exposed; to establish information about dose; and to corroborate or modify the information that has been obtained directly from the patient. This includes both environmental and prior medical information that may clarify perceptions or reports of the relationship between the two.

The section that follows is a summary of avenues that may be used to obtain environmental and related health information. Strategies for obtaining this information are variable, and issues about confidentiality must always be considered (see Chapter 9). A further discussion of some of these sources is provided in Chapter 4.1.

Prior medical records

These records tend to be accessible and obtainable without risk of any disclosure for the patient. Although these records may not further etiologic assessment, they can confirm the patient's complaints on previous occasions and provide objective measures of his or her previous physiologic status. This information can help corroborate or modify the history and may be useful in applying one of the cardinal principles of occupational and environmental diseases: the biologic plausibility inherent in the time between exposure and effects (see below).

Exposure records from an employer

Under current regulations in the United States and most other developed countries, employers are obligated to maintain material safety data sheets (MSDS) for each potentially hazardous material with which employees may come in contact. The employer must make this information available to the employee or his or her physician in a timely fashion, together with any available information about exposure doses (e.g., air sampling information, blood tests). Despite this, there remain numerous problems. The MSDS themselves are often of limited quality. Much potentially useful information is lacking, such as information on minor ingredients that may be responsible for important health effects, especially allergic ones. In addition, the health information is often presented uncritically and without adequate discussion, much as the way adverse effects are uncritically listed in the Physician's

Desk Reference. In fact, for many of these MSDS, the most useful information is the telephone number listed to call for additional help. Employers or others working directly for them (e.g., physicians) may be able to provide more useful information, including the results of past workplace assessments, although other biases may be at play in such informational requests.

Health and regulatory agencies

Often, a workplace or environmental hazard has been inspected by an agency with regulatory authority. The results are generally available to physicians and, if so, may be an excellent source of information. Nonetheless, one limitation is that workplace inspections are generally conducted by industrial hygiene or safety personnel for the sole purpose of ascertaining whether or not there has been adherence to various regulations; the regulations may not reflect the possible harm that can occur at levels lower than the 'acceptable limits.'

Unions and community groups

Although they are not in the same position as current or past employers, who have direct access to exposure information, many such organizations take environmental health issues seriously and have substantial amounts of information, often of good quality, that is relevant to their members or residents of a community. On the other hand, the role of adversarial relations among parties may slant or bias information from these sources (see Chapter 9).

Direct site visit

When the issue is a current or recent exposure, there is perhaps no more satisfactory way to evaluate the environment than onsite inspection. This practice offers the advantages of contacting employees at the site, relating the history to observable facts, and directly assessing exposure and dose. The opportunity to correlate illness with the work environment is one of the special advantages of clinicians who are based at the workplace. Lack of this capability puts the diagnostician at a considerable disadvantage. Whether he or she is based inside or outside the plant, however, the clinician must recognize that the direct assessment of exposures is a highly complex and specialized process, requiring assistance of an industrial hygienist or a comparably trained professional (see Chapter 4); not every relevant exposure possibility may be evident to the untrained eye.

DIAGNOSTIC DECISION MAKING
Specialized use of the laboratory

Clinicians without experience in OEM diagnosis and practice may imagine that the laboratory could be used to compensate for the difficulties in obtaining reliable information about exposure or putative effects. This is not surprising, given the remarkable progress of clinical toxicologists in quantifying xenobiotics and the burgeoning array of technical capabilities that now allow measurement of many contaminants down to the level of parts per trillion in numerous body tissues. Unfortunately, at this time, the overall role of the laboratory in OEM remains limited. In this section, the role of the laboratory in tertiary OEM practice is described. Each of the organ system (Section 3) and exposure chapters (Section 4) in the text further details the role of the laboratory in the assessment of particular hazards and diseases.

Despite some overlap, laboratory tests can be conceptualized in one of three ways.

1. Tests that elucidate pathophysiology

These tests include almost all of the routine 'medical' tests, such as imaging studies, chemistry panels, and hemograms. Also included are tests that play more specific roles in OEM diagnosis, such as non-specific inhalational challenge tests (e.g., methacholine challenge test) or measurement of enzyme levels (e.g., cholinesterase or aminolevulinic acid dehydratase [ALA] test). The net effect of this kind of study is to clarify what is or is not wrong pathophysiologically with the patient. Some such studies, of course, may be invaluable for assessing causality, but the primary role is to evaluate effects, not exposures or causes.

2. Tests that elucidate or quantify exposures

Other tests may be performed to establish the presence of a suspected causal agent in an organ or body tissue. Such tests are often referred to as biologic monitoring because, in effect, they use the body as a sampling device to assess exposure. Examples include measurement of the whole blood lead level, which documents that lead at a given concentration is present in red cells, or polarizing light microscopy on a lung biopsy to quantify crystalline silica particles. These kinds of studies may lead to inferences about health effects, but they do not measure them, only exposures. Although there may be some rationale in using a measure of exposure as a surrogate for identifying 'cases' of disease (e.g., identifying an adult with a lead level over 40 g/dL as 'lead poisoned') for surveillance purposes, the identification of the toxin is not tantamount to demonstration of a causal health effect for clinical use.

3. Tests that directly assess the relationship between an exposure and an effect

A few tests are 'dynamic' in the sense that they inherently capture causal information. An example is determining the presence of a specific antibody to a sensitizing agent. The presence of the antibody in such a case confirms both that exposure has occurred and that it has generated an immunologic reaction (which may or may not prove to be related to a presenting symptom or sign!). Similarly, patch testing and specific inhalational challenge tests are types of tests that document that an exposure and sensitization have occurred and may even document the relation between the level of exposure and a specific health effect.

At times, a test of one of these three types may be used appropriately to establish information about another type. For example, zinc protoporphyrin (ZPP) in red cells, a measure of lead effect in the blockade of the enzyme heme synthetase, is a test commonly used as a surrogate measure of lead exposure because of its dose–response characteristics. Similarly, while measurement of urine cadmium level is a good index of recent absorption in workers exposed to the metal, in another setting – long after exposure has ceased – it may serve as a good measure of the renal effect of cadmium. In individuals who have not had recent cadmium exposure but who have suffered impaired renal function, the affected kidney leaks stored cadmium, whereas the intact kidney will not. In this case, an apparent measure of an exposure is used to measure an effect.

Even when the logic for ordering a laboratory test is clear to the clinician, there remain several problems with the application of results to diagnosis.

1. Limitations inherent in the laboratory itself

The clinician must always be alert to the factors that limit the quality of any data that are returned from the laboratory. These include (1) the ability of the laboratory to detect a substance or an effect, (2) the reliability of the laboratory at measuring such substances, (3) the validity of results, (4) the precision of the results, and (5) the standardization of the results. Notably, for example, the indiscriminant use of hair analysis to detect heavy metals has undergone scrutiny; in all but a small number of research labs, hair analysis has been found wanting in almost every one of these dimensions.[4]

2. Strategies for obtaining tests

Although many tests in clinical medicine do not vary significantly according to the time they are obtained (e.g., chest x-ray studies), others can be interpreted only on the basis of careful planning of how and when samples are obtained (e.g., plasma triglycerides). In many clinical situations in OEM, the strategy for sampling is crucial to interpretation of results. For tests of effects, the timing must be planned to avoid either missing the effect or confounding one effect with another. An example of the first situation is the use of spirometry to detect bronchospasm; even an individual with severe occupational asthma may have normal spirometry if the test is not timed to coincide with an expected effect. On the other hand, an audiogram performed within several hours of noise exposure is likely to document the temporary effects of noise but is incapable of establishing baseline hearing function.

Failure to consider testing strategy may also limit the interpretation of tests that directly assess the relationship between exposure and effect. For example, it is now well recognized that early in the course of occupational asthma, sensitization to agents such as isocyanates may rapidly reverse after removal of the individual from exposure. Therefore, even in a previously sensitized individual, a specific challenge with the agent may fail to produce bronchospasm if that person has been away from the exposure for a period of time before testing.

3. Interpretation of normal and abnormal results

Laboratories commonly supplement reports with statements as to whether or not a result is 'normal'. By convention, the term 'normal' usually means that a test result falls within the range of results for 95% of the healthy population. For a few tests, other guidelines are used by convention, such as within 20% of the mean result of a reference group. In OEM, unlike general medical practice, laboratory test results need to be placed in their appropriate context. For example, a young worker exposed to a known respiratory tract toxin may have 'normal' lung function on spirometry, yet comparison with a previous value from the same individual documents that loss in function has occurred. The laboratory's interpretation in this case is falsely reassuring. Conversely, a lead battery worker may be identified by the laboratory as having an 'abnormal' whole blood lead level of 20 µg/dL. Although this level is indeed higher than that found in any general population, it is unlikely to reflect significant lead toxicity, nor is it an unexpected value in a well-controlled battery plant. Recognition that this level of exposure is higher than that seen in other adults may have some utility, but cannot be used as the basis for the diagnosis of lead poisoning.

Further, as with all tests, the likelihood that an individual with an abnormal test in fact has the disease under evaluation (positive predictive value) is influenced not only by the test's sensitivity (that those with disease will test positive) and specificity (that those without disease will test negative) but also by the prevalence of the disease in the specific population from which the individual comes. For example, a minimal finding of interstitial fibrosis on a chest radiograph in an asbestos-exposed worker is, in itself, more predictive of disease than is the same finding in someone who has not been exposed to a fibrogenic material (see further, below).

The available databases for diagnostic inference

Having completed the basic evaluation, including the history, environmental exposure assessment, physical examination, and basic laboratory evaluation, the information needs to be integrated to answer three central questions.
1. Given everything already known about the patient, is it plausible that he or she has a disease or health effect related to environmental exposure?
2. If it is plausible, how likely is it, based on the exposure assessment and clinical pattern?
3. Given the exposure assessment and clinical setting, how should various laboratory tests be interpreted? What further studies or tests offer the possibility of substantially altering the likelihood that any clinical abnormality(ies) is (are) related to the environmental exposure?

In this section, we address the task of identifying existing sources of information and establishing how these sources can be used to assist in arriving at a working diagnosis.

Many different types of resources are available to address questions about disease plausibility and likelihood. Most, but not all, rely on a review and assessment of the scientific literature related to the exposures and the health effects in question. The most important are as follows.

1. Exposure assessment databases

For a variety of reasons, it is often not possible to confirm directly the occurrence of an exposure of interest or to obtain a reliable estimate of dose. Fortunately, there are many available resources for translating historic information into at least semi-quantitative estimates about exposure and likely dose. Texts, including this one, often summarize the hazards associated with particular kinds of activities and the range of doses to which such workers are potentially exposed. Large surveys, such as the ones performed periodically by the National Institute for Occupational Safety and Health (NIOSH), allow determination of the jobs and industries where certain hazards are likely to be found.[5] Scientific papers, often from the industrial hygiene literature, can frequently provide valuable summaries that may be relevant to a particular clinical problem. Such papers are easily searched using National Library of Medicine and related databases such as Medline or Toxline.

2. Epidemiologic databases

When there is some basis for estimating exposure and dose, epidemiologic studies often provide the most compelling data relating exposure to risk for disease Epidemiologic studies can provide direct evidence that an exposure causes an effect in humans. Moreover, such studies often establish certain limits for biologic plausibility of an association between exposure and disease, such as the timing between exposure and emergence of increased disease risk. These kinds of data are often helpful in the quantitative assessment of individual risk. If individuals who do precisely the same activity have been studied, quantitative determination of risk is relatively straightforward. Even if the patient's exposure setting differs from groups that have been reported, one can often learn enough about the patient's exposure to fit him or her into the range of exposures that have been studied.

Access to epidemiologic studies is readily achieved by using available texts and computerized literature searches. Unfortunately, occupational epidemiology studies vary dramatically in quality and applicability to the patient under evaluation. Issues related to the quality of epidemiologic studies are discussed in Chapter 6. The relevance of epidemiologic studies to the patient at hand is no less important.

First, the exposure dose in the patient should be reasonably similar to the exposure dose of at least a portion of the study population. Study findings can be extrapolated to results at higher and lower doses, but this approach is not always valid biologically and requires complex scientific judgements (see Chapter 5).

Second, the population under study ideally should resemble the patient's demographic characteristics, such as age and gender. Unfortunately, most studies historically have been limited to white males, so there is often little choice other than to use the data on white males and modify the interpretation as needed. Whether this is a meaningful limitation depends on the particular health effect and the likelihood that host susceptibility plays an important modifying role.

3. Toxicologic databases

Epidemiologic data are often inadequate alone for determining the likelihood that a patient's health problem can be related to an environmental exposure. Alone or in combination with epidemiologic data, the results of animal studies performed under experimental conditions may be helpful. One advantage of these studies is that they often provide very strong evidence of dose-related effects of hazards. Further, animal studies may provide information about certain laboratory findings, such as the presence of toxins in diseased organs, biochemical changes, and histopathology. Modern toxicologic studies of this kind are plentiful and are easily identified by computer searches of the scientific literature. Good summaries are often available as well in texts and in monographs such as the toxicologic profiles compiled by the United States Agency for Toxic Substances and Disease Registries located in Atlanta.[6]

Serious limitations of toxicologic studies include differences between species and routes of exposure. For example, gavage (tube feeding) differs greatly from the routes by which patients typically have been exposed. In addition, animal studies almost invariably depend on use of relatively high doses of single toxins, and invariably require extrapolation to be applicable to clinical situation. As with epidemiologic studies, such extrapolation sometimes requires complex scientific judgment. Additional limitations to the use of toxicologic studies for clinical purposes are identified in Chapter 5.

4. Clinical studies and case reports

Clinical reports and case studies, although of limited value for establishing cause and effect per se, often are exceptionally useful for clinicians in OEM. Compared with epidemiologic studies, very rich information is often provided regarding the actual characteristics of the patients being reported and the specific nature of their exposure and dose. Specific clinical information of importance may include the results of a wide array of tests and descriptions of the patterns of illness, clinical course, and responses to treatment. At their best, clinical case reports and studies may be sufficiently applicable to provide a rational basis for all subsequent steps in diagnosis and management. At their worst, clinical reports may create the illusion of a causal relationship between an exposure and an outcome that cannot be substantiated. Case reports relevant to an exposure, therefore, should be carefully reviewed, but strong weight should be given to them only if corroborating evidence (e.g., toxicologic or epidemiologic) is also available.

5. Clinical experience

Although direct clinical experience may create certain biases of perception because exposed individuals with problems are far more likely to have been seen than those without problems, relevant experience should be drawn upon whenever feasible. Specifically, when possible, physicians should consult those who may have previous experiences with patients like their own, such as physicians practicing in workplaces where relevant exposures are commonplace, or those caring for such workers. Such databases, while not 'scientific' in the usual sense of the term, have obvious relevance.

Quantitative clinical reasoning

Once the patient's health status has been evaluated, and the exposure history obtained and supplemented to the extent feasible, the task remains to establish a final diagnosis. In particular, it is necessary for the OEM practitioner to address the specific question regarding the suspect occupational and environmental cause. In most cases, despite every effort, this determination requires dealing with at least some uncertainty. Not only will the diagnosis often fail to be unequivocally established by information at hand, in many instances there is no single further test or source of information that could provide certainty even were patient safety, cost or practicality not at issue.

Going back to the principles outlined in Chapter 1, for many situations there are no discriminatory tests to resolve, for example, whether a bladder cancer was or was not caused by exposure to benzidine dye, or asthma by exposures in an aluminum potroom. For other situations, extensive quantitative data regarding former exposure might theoretically resolve the matter, or a test might in theory exist to assist, but the information or test cannot be obtained. Unfortunately, though in many domains of medicine such specific answers are not required – physicians treat such disease all the time without establishing their causes – this luxury does not extent to OEM where preventive and therapeutic efforts, as well as appropriate assignment of medicolegal benefits, require such a diagnosis. In this section we discuss the use of Bayesian reasoning to reach a diagnosis in the face of uncertainty. A fuller discussion of this subject can be found in various texts.[7,8]

Whether they do it explicitly or not, all clinicians rely on Bayesian reasoning in everyday practice, when deciding that a fever in a young adult is most likely mono, or a rash in an elderly patient most likely a reaction to a medication – and which medication is the most likely culprit. The theory, based on Bayes theorem, is straightforward: the probability of any diagnosis being correct is the mathematical product of two probabilities. The first probability is the 'risk' for the patient (given his/her age, race, gender, background, the season, etc) getting such a disorder, sight unseen. This is referred to as the 'prior' probability, and refers to the frequency with which such a diagnosis occurs in the population from which the patient comes.

For example, the prior risk of an adolescent getting mono in a given year is very high – perhaps as high as 1 per 100 – based on incidence in that age group. Likewise, the risk of an elderly patient on antibiotics getting a skin rash is also high, depending on the antibiotic. Contrarily, the risk of a young patient in otherwise good health getting tuberculosis in the US is very low – perhaps 1 per 100,000 – compared to the same person in South Africa, where the background rate is several orders of magnitude higher. Obviously, some knowledge of disease rates in the appropriate population is necessary for estimating this prior probability, but even in the absence of such detail, almost all practitioners should have enough experience to know what is common and what is rare. More detailed information comes from medical texts, periodicals like MMWR and descriptive epidemiologic studies. In occupational and environmental medicine practice, the sources may be the same, or knowledge is available from some of the sources of exposure information described earlier in this chapter.

The second factor in the calculation of the probability of each diagnostic consideration is the probability that some major finding – typically a physical sign or laboratory anomaly – would be expected in patients with that diagnosis. For example, 80–90% of all patients with mono have persistent fever. On the other hand, less than 1 in 10 with mono will be expected to be negative on the mono-spot test. Determining these 'posterior' probabilities depends on performing the most appropriate exams and/or tests for the major diagnostic possibilities dictated by knowledge of the patient's (prior) risks. The sources for this information, at least for diseases of OEM concern, are discussed in Section 3 of this text in relation to each of the major disorders.

Once these two probabilities are estimated for each major diagnostic possibility, comparison should yield either a clear 'winner' – the most likely – or leave a small number, usually two, about equally possible. In the former instance, the work-up is essentially complete, unless one of the more remote possibilities has health consequences that mandate exclusion. For example, even if metastatic cancer is a very unlikely possibility for a young coal miner with diffuse nodules on chest x-ray (unless he/she had a melanoma removed the year before!), consideration of cancer might dictate additional tests to further exclude this possibility if only because of the harm to the patient of overlooking it. More important is the use of additional tests when there remain competing probabilities, as the following case examples illustrate.

The first example is a 60-year-old African-American male, a foundry worker who has been a 'chipper-grinder' – a job entailing the grinding of sand off metal castings – for 35 years. He complains of cough and shortness of breath and has a symmetric reticulo-nodular infiltrate on his x-ray (Fig. 3.3). The ILO grade of the infiltrate is 2/2 (see Chapter 19.1 for a discussion of the ILO rating system for x-rays). The complaint and the x-ray are compatible with silicosis, but also with sarcoidosis, chronic beryllium disease, disseminated tuberculosis and other rarer diseases. Using the approach suggested above, it is first important to learn roughly how likely a chipper-grinder of this era (1968–2002) would be to get silicosis, i.e., the prior probability of that diagnosis.

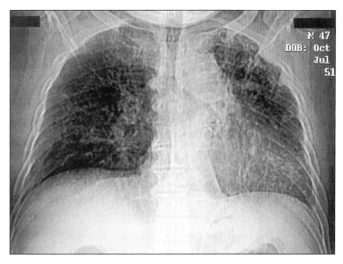

Figure 3.3: Abnormal chest x-ray for both hypothetical patients. The x-ray shows symmetric, bilateral reticulo-nodular opacities in the mid and upper lung zones, rated 2/2 by a B-reader using the ILO scale (see Chapter 19.1).

Based on review of the literature or, better yet, a call to the company or physicians caring for workers there, you learn that as many as 1 in 5 long-term workers have developed this common outcome of daily, historically uncontrolled exposure. Next, reviewing Chapter 19.9 of this text, you learn that his x-ray is typical of the disease, present in almost all cases, let's say 90% for the calculation purposes. Applying Bayes theorem, his likelihood of having silicosis is proportional to:

$$0.2 \text{ (prior)} \times 0.9 \text{ (posterior)} = 0.18.$$

The absolute number is unimportant, only its value compared to other possibilities. Compare it, for example, with his risk for sarcoid, the next most likely consideration from a clinical perspective. Sarcoid has a prevalence in this patient's ethnic group of about 1 per 1000. Even assuming the x-ray is seen in all such cases, the likelihood of sarcoid would be proportional to:

$$0.001 \text{ (prior)} \times 1.0 \text{ (posterior)} = 0.001.$$

Crudely estimating, silicosis is 180 times more likely than sarcoid in this case. For all of the other possibilities the prior would most likely be lower still, even though tuberculosis occurs more frequently in silica-exposed men than in the rest of the population. Although it makes sense to exclude tuberculosis because of the gravity if this were missed, the overwhelming likelihood is that this man has silicosis. Unless his illness takes an unexpected turn, no biopsy or further tests are easily justified, especially not for medicolegal reasons.

Now consider a second patient with the same complaint and the same x-ray from the same foundry. This second man, however, is only 35, and has worked in this environment only since 1995. For him, the prior probability of silicosis, by comparison to the previous case, is very low –

he has worked fewer years, all in the more modern period since environmental controls have been instituted (you learn using the approach above) and in a less exposed job category (other facts you could confirm). With silicosis far less likely a priori, his likelihood of having sarcoid, or even one of the rarer causes of this x-ray picture (Fig. 3.3) become greater by comparison. So likely, in fact, that additional tests, up to and including lung biopsy, would be justified to reach the correct answer, whereas in the first case the risk of such a test may exceed the risk of initially missing an alternative diagnosis (as might occur very rarely, of course).

Not every case is as clear as these, nor in every case is there an obvious test available to break 'ties'. Consider, for example, the elderly painter with heavy solvent exposure who develops depression, or mild dementia. There are numerous possibilities and no trivial test to distinguish chronic solvent intoxication. Another concern in many cases is the possibility of no disease at all. This must often be factored in as a possibility, when signs or laboratory findings are minimally deranged (not really a possibility in the previous examples). In such a case one calculates the probability of no disease in much the same way as a particular diagnosis, e.g., what is the (prior) probability that a 60-year-old foundryman is free of any respiratory disease? Having said that, and with full appreciation of the difficulty of providing estimates of many prior probabilities with great confidence, the overall approach is itself very robust, and OEM practitioners, whether in training or highly experienced, are well advised to make such estimates as explicitly as information allows, the more so the more complex and uncertain the case may be.

PATIENT MANAGEMENT

There are four conceptual stages in the management of patients suspected of occupational or environmental disease. Although actual treatment choices depend on the particular hazardous exposure, clinical disorder, and relevant social issues, the conceptual framework remains uniform.

The diagnostic period

In every case, there is a period of time from the first contact with the patient until the best possible working diagnosis can be achieved. Although this period may be as short as a single visit in cases of clear-cut exposure and a well-delineated physiologic response (or its absence), often this period spans days to weeks and occasionally even longer, during which relevant records of medical and exposure history are obtained, environments evaluated, and additional tests performed. Several important aspects of management should be kept in mind during this period.

1. Formulate the diagnostic plan at the outset. For reasons already given, it must be anticipated that many potentially knowable facts may remain unlearned. Therefore, at the outset, it is important to decide how the diagnostic process will proceed, whether or not one succeeds in obtaining desired information. This is another way of saying that the patient cannot be held hostage to impediments in getting access to information.

2. Use the diagnostic period to the fullest. An advantage of small delays in achieving best clinical diagnosis is that it facilitates ascertainment of various social issues, such as the agendas of all parties and likelihood of reactions if certain choices are proposed (see Chapter 9).

3. Do not initiate management decisions until a sound working diagnosis is achieved. Although a few occupational and environmental illnesses are true medical emergencies, the vast majority are not. In fact, many diagnostic issues, such as the temporal relationship between physiologic responses and exposures or the measurement of biologic exposure dose, are best studied while a patient remains in an exposed situation. Further, given the ramifications of certain courses of action, such as removal of a worker from a job or the designation of a particular health problem as occupational, it is important not to take such steps prematurely when there is a reasonable likelihood that subsequent facts may alter diagnostic thinking. Although further exposure may seem on the surface to place a patient at unnecessary additional risk, it is important to place that risk in the context of exposures that have already occurred and the very real risk of taking mis-steps that may be harmful in themselves, especially if they are premature and wrong.

4. In certain circumstances, diagnosis itself depends on the individual's response to a therapeutic trial, such as whether or not the symptoms abate on removal of the individual from an environment. Although such trials are sometimes necessary or desirable, they must be conducted as trials, with the explicit understanding that the goal is to establish a diagnosis and not misconstrued as treatment based on a putative or tentative diagnosis. Only in this way can future confusion be avoided and, with it, the attendant social costs to the patient.

Formulation of treatment plans

Once the diagnosis has become sufficiently clear, treatment plans can be developed. Sometimes the choice is strongly dictated by clinical circumstances, as in cases of disabling chronic diseases. More often, however, there are alternatives. Although one choice or another may seem preferable from a strictly medical perspective, it cannot be presumed that this choice satisfies the needs of the patient, or that it is included among the options offered by the employer or other relevant circumstances. Whenever feasible and safe, it is ideal to consider alternative possibilities for the management of every case. On other occasions, though, medical realities dictate clearly one course of action, such as discontinuing exposure of a patient with heavy metal or pesticide poisoning when the documentation is clear-cut.

Establishing and communicating the therapeutic plan

However limited or diverse the options considered, the actual choice of a treatment plan cannot be made without discussion with all parties who must participate, first and most importantly the patient. The benefits, costs, and health risks associated with each option must be identified so the patient can make an intelligent decision based on all the facts, including social factors (see Chapter 9). If necessary, he or she should be encouraged to include a spouse or other family member who may be affected by the choice. Advice from other advocates, such as a social worker, union representative, or advisor, may be invaluable – especially when one choice or another may disrupt the individual's normal life activities, work, or income.

Once the patient has agreed to a plan, it is reasonable to communicate that plan to the other parties who must cooperate, especially in the occupational setting. In every case, the patient should be aware of the planned communication and it should be limited to issues that are within the purview of the doctor's relationship with non-medical parties. Once an approach has been selected, it is important that results of the evaluation be put in writing for the patient, his or her personal physician, and others who need to have this information. Dissemination of this information can often be best accomplished by a single letter, which is sent to everyone. Although this method may limit communication of certain private issues and require use of language not technically ideal for every reader, the use of a single letter reduces the likelihood of anyone misunderstanding what has been found and recommended.

Therapeutic follow-up

Whatever plan is chosen, clinical and non-clinical consequences that arise during the initiation of the plan may lead to reconsideration by patient, physician, or both. For example, the impact of altered life circumstances, such as joblessness, or homelessness in environmental cases, may provoke re-evaluation of options, however strongly they are indicated from a clinical perspective.

By planning visits for no grander purpose than a progress update and plan re-evaluation, the physician offers the most flexible and supportive milieu in which the patient can accommodate to changes demanded in the management of occupational and environmental health problems.

Where does the physician's responsibility end?

One of the most inescapable realities of modern OEM practice in most parts of the world, including the United States, is that many hazardous situations will be recognized about which little can be done. Reasons include: limitations of resources available in the professional community, corporate sector, and governmental agencies; technical uncertainty about the solution; economic incentives to ignore or resist recognition of the problem or solution; inadequate regulatory, technical and administrative structures to resolve the matter; and last, but not least, widespread ignorance.

None of these factors should form the basis for physician apathy or reluctance to consider and act on the public health implications of a serious occupational or environmental disease or injury. At a minimum, the record should clearly indicate the physician's opinion that others may be at risk. The choice of strategy should be well documented in the patient's record. Finally, although various approaches may best be carried out verbally or informally, in the end it is important that the individuals who control the environment in question be formally notified that concern has been raised. This notification may come directly from the physician or, more often, indirectly through a government agency or their consultant. The physician's effort should be documented in writing, which is far more effective in motivating action than informal approaches.

Once these steps have been taken, the practitioner can and should return to the care and needs of the patient, whose OEM problems and their clinical and social sequelae may take months, often years, to resolve. This is the same timetable that public intervention may follow. Clinicians may choose early in the process of public health actions to turn responsibility over to others. Regardless, the often delayed but sometimes highly effective link between clinical evaluation and resultant greater public health good is one of the great satisfactions of OEM practice.

References

1. Frank AL. Occupational and environmental medicine: approach to the patient with an occupational or environmental illness. Primary Care Clin Office Pract 2000; 27:877–94.
2. Lax MB, Grant WD, Manetti FA, Klein R. Recognizing occupational disease – taking an effective occupational history. Am Fam Phys 1998; 58:935–44.
3. Rosenstock L, Logerfo J, Heyer N, Carter W. Development and validation of a self-administered Occupational Health History Questionnaire. J Occup Med 1984; 26(1):50–54.
4. ATSDR. Summary Report on Hair Analysis Panel Discussion, June 12–13, 2001. The website is: www.atsdr.cdc.gov/HAC/hair_analysis/index.html.
5. NIOSH. National Occupational Exposure Survey. The website is: www.cdc.gov/niosh/89-103.html.
6. ATSDR toxicologic profiles may be accessed at: www.atsdr.cdc.gov/toxfaq.html.
7. Albert DA. Reasoning in medicine: an introduction to clinical inference. Baltimore: Johns Hopkins Press, 1988.
8. Cutler P. Problem solving in clinical medicine: from data to diagnosis. Baltimore: Williams and Wilkins, 1998.

Chapter 4
Principles of Industrial Hygiene

4.1 Occupational Hygiene

Robert F Herrick, John M Dement

Occupational (industrial) hygiene is the health profession dedicated to the anticipation, recognition, evaluation and control of hazards in the workplace environment. The scope of interest includes chemical, physical and biologic hazards as well as ergonomic and human factors, that cause or contribute to impaired function, disease, disability, injury and discomfort resulting from work. As the profession grew up with the Industrial Revolution, it has been known as industrial hygiene, but the term occupational hygiene more accurately describes the field and the practitioner's range of activities. In fact, the term occupational hygiene is prevalent everywhere except in the United States. The term industrial/occupational hygiene is derived from the Greek Hygieia, the goddess of health and prevention, daughter of Asklepiose, god of medicine. Its roots trace back to Bernardino Ramazzini (1633–1714), considered the father of occupational medicine.

The modern history of occupational hygiene starts with the industrialization of the United States and western Europe. This process was chronicled by Theodore Hatch, who summarized the 'Major Accomplishments in Occupational Health in the Past Fifty Years' on the 50th anniversary of the Division of Occupational Health of the Public Health Service in 1964.[1] Hatch recounted that prior to the First World War (about 1914), societies were predominantly rural and based upon agriculture. Industrial processes were few, and conducted by manual labor. The only plastic available was celluloid, petroleum refining discarded most product as waste, and Henry Ford had just introduced the radical concept of a $5 daily wage. This was the industrial world Alice Hamilton found when she began to trace health problems among immigrant families back to the workplace. Pioneers like Hamilton and Hatch identified important problems, but they also had the vision to develop interdisciplinary approaches to solve them.

Occupational hygienists share responsibility with physicians and other occupational health practitioners and researchers in the identification of adverse health effects associated with the workplace environment. The occupational hygienist focuses upon the factors that are potential causes of work-related conditions, providing information on workplace processes, and exposures to physical, chemical and biologic agents that result from those workplace processes and conditions. The evaluation of those hazards frequently includes measurements to identify and quantitate contaminants in the workplace, as well as measurements of physical factors such as noise, radiation, heat and ergonomic conditions. In the practice of occupational hygiene, the evaluation of hazards leads to the selection and application of an appropriate exposure control strategy. These strategies include engineering controls, improvements in work practices and materials, and personal protective equipment to reduce workplace risks.

In addition to the occupational hygiene practice of hazard recognition, evaluation and control, research on exposures as potential causal factors for occupational disease advances the goal of promoting worker health and safety. Exposure assessment in epidemiologic research and hazard evaluation is a vital role for occupational hygienists. These assessments frequently involve current and past exposures, so occupational hygienists apply familiarity with workplace processes, controls, and exposure information in conjunction with the work histories of employees, to reconstruct exposures in retrospective epidemiologic studies and risk assessments.

Occupational hygienists integrate information and knowledge from disciplines including engineering, chemistry, physical science, toxicology and medicine. While occupational hygiene practitioners are usually trained in one of these disciplines, the majority have graduate degrees in occupational (industrial) hygiene, environmental health, or an allied field. There are programs for professional certification of occupational (industrial) hygienists in several countries, requiring demonstration of proficiency in the following technical areas: basic science; biohazards; biostatistics and epidemiology; engineering and other controls; ergonomics; ethics and management; analytical chemistry; sampling, monitoring and instrumentation; noise and vibration; ionizing radiation; nonionizing radiation; regulations, standards and guidelines; thermal and pressure stressors; toxicology; and general topics including community exposures, hazardous wastes, risk communication, indoor environmental quality, and others (unit operations, process safety, and confined spaces). Certification is achieved through a combination of work experience and a comprehensive written examination. In the United States, approximately 6500 industrial hygienists are certified by the American Board of Industrial Hygiene.

OCCUPATIONAL HYGIENE AND DISEASE PREVENTION

Prevention of environmental diseases may be thought of as a two-stage process involving primary prevention and secondary prevention.[2] The ultimate objectives are: (1) to avoid the establishment of disease, (2) to reduce the likelihood of disease recurrence or progression and (3) ameliorate the morbidity associated with the disease. Prevention of environmental diseases involves hazard recognition, hazard evaluation, and hazard control/intervention.

Hazard recognition: The hazard associated with a given exposure is a function of both the toxicity of a material and the extent of human exposure. Surveillance of both exposure and disease provides clues and hypotheses for further evaluation. Health data may be generated through environmental/occupational medicine and surveillance programs or through epidemiological studies. Toxicology often provides valuable information with regard to hazard recognition.

Hazard evaluation: Prevention strategies require knowledge of the effects caused by exposures as well as the dose levels where effects occur. These data allow development of risk assessment and strategies to reduce or eliminate significant human exposures. Toxicology, occupational medicine, and epidemiology provide the means for identifying chemical, physical, or biologic hazards. Toxicology testing in animals is an important component of early hazard recognition as well as hazard evaluation.

Hazard control/intervention: Primary prevention involves identification of environmental hazards which are factors or co-factors in disease development, followed by application of methods to reduce or eliminate human exposures. This represents the classical public health approach. Figure 4.1.1 depicts the components of the pathway from the source of a contaminant in the environment, through exposure, dose, and adverse health outcomes. The opportunities for intervention at various steps along the pathway are also shown. Principles and methods for controlling occupational hazards are discussed more fully later in this chapter.

RECOGNITION OF OCCUPATIONAL AND ENVIRONMENTAL HAZARDS
Classification of hazards

Workers may be exposed to contaminants by inhalation, absorption through the skin, ingestion, or injections (e.g., through accidental puncture wounds). Inhalation and skin absorption represent the predominant routes of exposure for most materials in the occupational environment. Ingestion may be an important source of exposure where poor hygiene practices, such as consumption of food and beverages in a contaminated work area, is allowed. Workers in healthcare facilities often are exposed to infectious agents through punctures with contaminated needles. Mucous membrane exposures to infectious agents from blood and body fluids may also be an important route of exposure in healthcare facilities.

Environmental agents are broadly classified by the Occupational Safety and Health Administration (OSHA) in the Hazard Communication Standard.[3] The following is a summary and elaboration of hazards listed in the OSHA standard.

Physical hazards

Materials such as explosives, flammable or combustible liquids, oxidizers, compressed gases, organic peroxides, pyrophoric materials, unstable (reactive) chemicals, or water reactive chemicals are regarded as physical hazards by OSHA. Other exposures in the workplace, such as excessive noise, ionizing and non-ionizing radiation, and temperature extremes are further examples of physical hazards.

Ergonomic hazards include repetitive and forceful movements, vibration, temperature extremes, and awkward postures that arise from improper work methods and improperly designed workstations, tools and equipment.

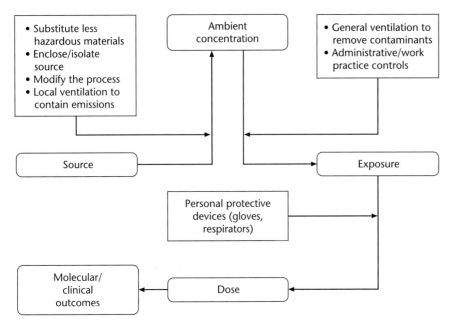

Figure 4.1.1: Hazard recognition, evaluation, control.

Ergonomic factors are increasingly important causes of injury in the workplace. Collectively, the term musculo-skeletal disorders (MSDs) refers to conditions that involve the nerves, tendons, muscles, and supporting structures of the body. Carpal tunnel syndrome is an example of a well-recognized work-related MSD of the wrist.

Chemical health hazards

Many chemicals are capable of producing adverse acute or chronic health effects. Chemical hazards include exposures to chemical mists, vapors, gases or particulates (dust and fumes) through inhalation or by absorption through the skin. OSHA defines hazardous chemicals to include carcinogens, reproductive toxins, irritants, corrosives, sensitizers, hepatoxins, nephrotoxins, agents which act on the hematopoietic system and agents which damage the lungs, skin, eyes or mucous membranes. Certain biologic materials are health hazards.

Biologic health hazards

Biologic hazards include bacteria, viruses, insects, plants, birds, animals and humans. Most biologic health hazards can be classified as infectious or immunologically active. As an example, accidental injection of blood-borne viruses is the major hazard of needlestick injuries, especially the viruses that cause AIDS (the HIV virus), hepatitis B, and hepatitis C. Anthrax is an example of a bacterium (*Bacillus anthracis*) that can affect the skin, the lungs, as well as the mouth, throat, and gastrointestinal tract. The infection sometimes can spread to other parts of the body, especially if treatment is not started early. The anthrax bacteria can form spores under certain conditions when, for example, body fluids infected with the bacteria are exposed to the air. The bacteria cannot live for long outside an animal; however, the spores can survive in soil and some other materials for decades.

Types of air-borne contaminants

Aerosols: Aerosols are composed of liquid droplets or solid particles fine enough to remain dispersed in air for a prolonged period of time. Aerosols may also be referred to as air-borne particulate matter with a wide range of particle size. Typical size ranges for aerosols are shown in Figure 4.1.2.

Dusts: Dusts are solid particles suspended in a gaseous medium. Dusts result from the mechanical disintegration of materials, such as grinding, with enough mechanical energy to propel particles into the air. Air-borne dust particles vary widely in size from approximately 50 μm to less than 1 μm. Only the larger particles may be seen without the use of a microscope. Most dusts produced from industrial operations as well as non-industrial operations such as construction or demolition consist of particles that vary widely in size, with the small particles greatly outnumbering the large ones. In general, when visible dust is noticeable in the air near a dust-producing operation, exposures to large numbers of smaller particles can be anticipated. The presence of a visible dust cloud, under typical indus-trial lighting conditions, may represent a serious overexposure condition for substances such as asbestos and silica.

Air-borne dusts show wide variability in particle shape. Figure 4.1.3 shows typical dusts from a rubber-processing operation using industrial talc. The particles vary from flat to rounded and compact. In comparison, Figure 4.1.4 shows a microscopic photograph of dusts from an industrial operation generating talc contaminated with asbestiform minerals. The photograph demonstrates greatly elongated asbestiform fibers, similar in appearance to fibers seen with commercial asbestos minerals.

Fumes: Fumes are formed when the material from a volatilized (evaporated or vaporized) solid condenses in cool air. The solid particles that are formed make up a fume that is extremely small, usually less than 1 μm in diameter. In most cases, the freshly generated fume reacts with the oxygen in the air to form an oxide. Welding, metalizing, and other operations involving heating of metals to high temperatures produce vapors from the molten metal which produce fumes. Arc welding volatilizes metal to form a vapor that condenses, usually as the metal or its oxide. Fumes, because they are extremely fine, are readily inhaled.

Smoke: Smoke is usually produced by the incomplete burning of carbonaceous materials such as coal and oil. The resulting aerosol consists of carbon or soot particles less than 0.1 μm in size. Smoke, such as tobacco smoke, generally contains droplets as well as dry particles.

Mists: Mists are finely divided liquid droplets which are air-borne. Mists may be generated by condensation of liquids from the vapor back to the liquid state, or by breaking up a liquid into a dispersed state, such as by splashing, foaming, or atomizing. In industrial operations, mists are produced during paint spraying, spray application of pesticides and herbicides, and during cutting and grinding operations. Acid mists are produced during metallurgical pickling operations and during electroplating.

Particle respiratory deposition

The hazard associated with air-borne particulate matter is a function of: (1) the biologic activity of the material, (2) concentration of the air-borne material, and (3) air-borne particle size. Particle size determines the site of deposition within the respiratory system. Many occupational diseases such as silicosis and asbestosis are associated with material deposited in particular regions of the respiratory tract. Criteria have been developed to define critical size-fractions most closely associated with various health effects.[4] The various critical fractions established by the American Conference of Governmental Industrial Hygienists (ACGIH) are shown in Figure 4.1.5 and are defined as follows.

Inhalable fraction: This is the fraction of air-borne particulate matter which can be hazardous when deposited anywhere in the upper or lower respiratory tract.

Thoracic fraction: Those particles which are hazardous when deposited anywhere within the pulmonary airways and the gas exchange region.

Respirable fraction: Those particles which are a hazard when deposited in the gas exchange region of the lungs.

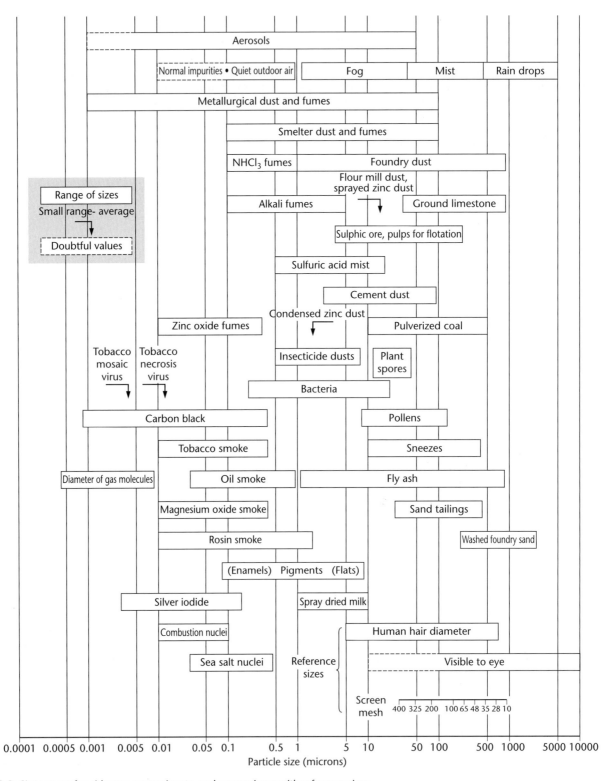

Figure 4.1.2: Size ranges for airborne contaminants, and comparisons with reference sizes.

Gases: Gases are formless fluids that expand to occupy the space or enclosure in which they are confined. The gaseous state is restricted to temperatures and pressures which would normally be present in the ambient or occupational environments.

Vapors: Vapors are the gaseous form of substances that are normally in the solid or liquid state at room temperature and pressure. Evaporation is the process by which a liquid is changed into the vapor state and mixed with the surrounding atmosphere. Many solvents will volatilize

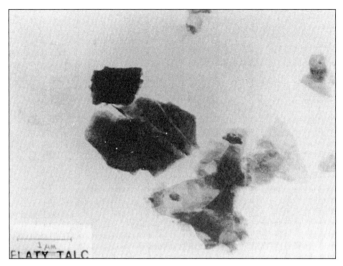

Figure 4.1.3: Electron microscope image of airborne particles from an industrial rubber operation using non-fibrous talc.

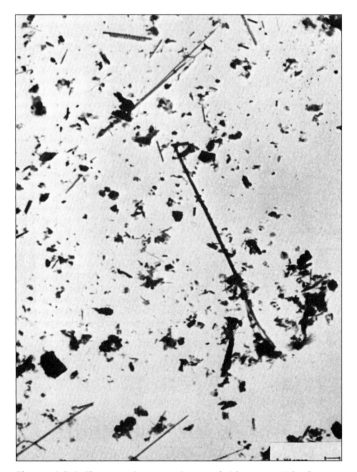

Figure 4.1.4: Electron microscope image of airborne particles from a talc mine and a mill processing talcs contaminated with asbestiform minerals (seen as long, thin fibers).

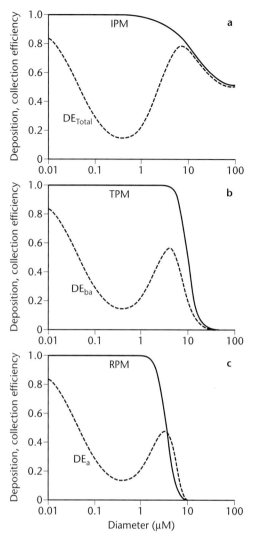

Figure 4.1.5: ACGIH reference curves for inspirable (a), thoracic (b), and respirable (c) fractions of airborne particulates. In (a), total inhalable fraction, or IPM, demonstrates that most particulates under 100 μm are *inhalable*. The DE_{total} curve reflects the fact that all but particles between 0.1 and 1.0 μm are well retained in the respiratory tract. In (b), it is apparent that particles under 10 μm are able to enter the bronchial tree and are called *thoracic*, or TPM. DE_{ba} shows the proportion of particles of each size deposited in the bronchoalveolar compartments. Particles of smaller size (<5 μm) are *respirable*, labeled RPM in (c). Alveolar deposition is indicated by the DE_a curve.

generation of elevated vapor concentrations near open sources or containers.

Fire and explosion hazards

Under appropriate conditions, gases, vapors and dusts present fire and explosion hazards. Fires and explosions account for a large majority of catastrophic industrial accidents resulting in injury and death. Health and safety personnel and workers must be trained to recognize fire and explosion hazards and their control. The following are key definitions and concepts.

Flash point: The flash point is the lowest temperature of the liquid at which the vapor/air mixture above the surface

to form vapors at normal temperatures and pressures. In addition, application of heat in many industrial operations produces more vapor. In general, the higher the vapor pressure of a liquid, the greater the potential for

will propagate (spread) a flame away from the source of ignition through the vapor/air mixture. A vapor/air mixture whose concentration is below the lower limit of flammability may burn in the zone immediately surrounding the source of ignition, without spreading away from the source ignition. The flash point is an important concept with regard to fire hazard recognition. If a liquid has no flash point, it is not flammable or combustible, and conversely the presence of a flash point indicates flammability or combustibility. In finely divided forms, such as mist or spray, liquids can be ignited at temperatures below their flash points.

Flammable (explosive) limits: Vapors of a flammable or combustible liquid must be mixed with air in the proper proportions, in the present of a source of ignition, for combustion or an explosion can occur. The proper mixture with air is called the flammable range and is also referred to as the explosive range. The flammable range includes all concentrations of flammable vapor or gas in air, in which a flash will occur or a flame will travel if the mixture is ignited. The minimum concentration of vapor or gas below which propagation of flame does not occur on contact with a source of ignition is called the lower flammable or explosive limit (LEL). Conversely, the maximum concentration of vapor above which propagation of flame does not occur is called the upper flammable or explosive limit (UEL). A vapor/air mixture below the lower flammable limit is too 'lean' to burn or explode, and a mixture above the upper flammable limit too 'rich' to burn or explode. As an example, the lower explosive limit of gasoline is 1.4% and the upper flammable limit or upper explosive limit is 7.6%.

Ignition temperature: The minimum temperature required to initiate or cause self-sustained combustion independent of the heating source is called the ignition temperature. Ignition temperatures may be changed substantially by a change of conditions, including composition of the vapor or gas–air mixture, shape and size of the space where the ignition occurs, rate and duration of heating, and temperature of the ignition source.

Autoignition or ignition temperature: The temperature at which a material self-ignites without any obvious sources of ignition, such as a spark or flame. Most common flammable and combustible liquids have autoignition temperatures in the range of 300°C (572°F) to 550°C (1022°F). Some have very low autoignition temperatures. For example, ethyl ether has an autoignition temperature of 160°C (356°F) and its vapors can be ignited by hot surfaces such as steam pipes.

Flammable liquids: The National Fire Protection Association, Flammable and Combustible Liquids Code, Standard No. 30,[5] defines a flammable liquid as any liquid having a flash point below 100°F (37.8°C), and having a vapor pressure not exceeding 40 psi at 100°F.

Combustible liquids: Combustible liquids are those with flash points at or above 100°F. Combustible liquids do not ignite as easily as flammable liquids, although they can be ignited under certain circumstances.

Explosive dusts: Many industrial dusts may be explosive when air-borne. Notable examples are finely divided particles of aluminum and magnesium. Many air-borne organic dusts are explosive. Fire and explosion hazards may be present in grain elevators, woodworking plants, feed, cereal, flour, and paper mills, and fertilizer plants. The particle size and the density of the dust cloud produced are factors which govern the potential fire and explosion hazards.

Many materials are themselves capable of detonation or of explosively decomposing, some may be sensitive to mechanical or local thermal shock, or react only at high temperatures. Some materials need only be slightly contaminated to produce a violent reaction. Materials such as peroxides, perchlorates, fluorine, and chlorine support combustion directly or by evolution of oxidizers.

Boiling point: The boiling point of a liquid is the temperature at which the liquid's vapor pressure is equal to the atmospheric pressure at its surface. The boiling point is highly dependent on the pressure of the liquid. Liquids such as solvents will evaporate to form vapor at lower temperatures. As the temperature of an organic liquid increases vapor formation will occur more rapidly. Liquids with low boiling points have relatively high vapor pressure at room temperature and will volatilize readily, whereas those with high boiling points will usually volatilize more slowly.

Vapor pressure: When a liquid of a substance is exposed to the atmosphere there is a continuous movement of molecules from the liquid into the atmosphere. The vapor pressure of a substance is the pressure at any given temperature at which equilibrium between the vapor phase and the liquid or solid form occurs. The vapor pressure of a solvent is an important parameter to be considered in predicting fire and inhalation hazards. The vapor pressure also determines the tendency of a substance to become air-borne and pose an inhalation hazard.

Organic liquids with high vapor pressures are potentially hazardous because they evaporate readily into the air to produce high vapor concentrations. The saturation vapor concentration (i.e., highest attainable) for a liquid at a given temperature and pressure can be calculated as follows:

$$ppm = \frac{p_v}{p_{atm}} \times 10^6$$

where: ppm = parts per million by volume, P_v = vapor pressure in mmHg, P_{atm} = atmospheric pressure in mmHg.

Measures of air-borne concentration

Air-borne concentrations of contaminants are expressed in several ways, depending on the form of the contaminant and the sampling and analytic method used to determine air-borne concentration. Terms used to describe degree of exposure are as follows.

Ppm: Parts of vapor or gases per million parts of contaminated air by volume at room temperature and pressure.

Mpp/cf: Millions of particles of a particulate per cubic foot of air. This concentration measure is used to express dust concentrations measured with an impinger.

Mg/m³: Milligrams of a substance per cubic meter of air. This measure can be used for gases and vapors as well as dusts. For gases and vapors, mg/m³ can be converted to ppm by volume using the following expression:

$$ppm = \frac{mg/m^3 \times 24.45}{m.w.}$$

where: ppm = parts per million by volume, mg/m³ = gravimetric concentration of the vapor, m.w. = molecular weight of contaminant.

Vapor %: Part of vapor or gas per 100 parts of contaminated air by volume at room temperature and pressure.

Fibers/cc: A measure of the numbers of fibers longer than 5 µm in length per cubic centimeter of air. This measure is used for asbestos and man-made fibers when concentrations are measured by the membrane filter sampling method, using phase contrast microscopy.

CFU/m³: A measure used to express the concentration of bacteria or fungi in an air-borne sample. The foci of growth of viable organisms on culture plates are counted and expressed as the number of *colony-forming units* (CFU).

PFU/m³: A measure used to express the concentration of viruses in an air-borne sample. Virus-infected cells in culture produce changes in appearance, or the cells may burst and produce *plaques*. The foci of virus-infected cells in cultures are counted and expressed as the number of *plaque-forming units* (PFU).

Occupational exposure standards and guidelines

REL: NIOSH recommended exposure limit. RELs are generally time-weighed average concentrations for up to a 10-hour workday during a 40-hour workweek.

STEL: Short-term exposure limit. A STEL is normally a 15-minute (or other specified time period) TWA that should not be exceeded during any time of the workday.

TWA: Time-weighted average. A method of calculating a daily or full-shift average exposure by weighting the different short-term average concentrations by exposure time:

$$TWA = \frac{C_1T_1 + C_1T_2 + \dots C_nT_n}{T_1 + T_2 + \dots T_n}$$

where: C_1 = concentration of contaminant measured during time period, T_1 = time for average concentration C.

PEL: OSHA permissible exposure limit. PELs are regulatory levels (usually TWAs) that must not be exceeded during any 8-hour work shift of a 40-hour workweek.

Ceiling Concentration: Maximum OSHA concentration which must not be exceeded during any part of the workday.

TLV: Non-regulatory exposure recommendations by the American Conference of Governmental Industrial Hygienists (ACGIH). There are TLVs for approximately 750 chemical compounds and materials. These are usually 8-hour TWA concentrations but STELS or ceiling values are recommended by the ACGIH for approximately 150 compounds.[6]

General principles of occupational hazard recognition

Hazard recognition involves a systematic review of a worker's occupational environment to identify exposures and potential exposures.[7] This review should provide the following types of information:

- Materials produced or stored and the process involved.
- Raw materials used or added to the process.
- By-products formed during the production process.
- Types of industrial equipment used.
- Cycle of operation and/or frequency of exposure, with attention to specific work tasks.
- Operational methods and work practices used.
- Health and safety controls in place.
- Use of personal protective equipment.
- Levels of exposure to harmful agents.
- Frequency and duration of worker exposure.
- Number of workers exposed.

Although the most useful data for hazard identification are the magnitude and frequency of exposure, such data are rarely available for all contaminants of interest. The health professional is then faced with estimating the *potential for exposure* using other surrogate data sources. Information concerning plant processes, hazardous raw materials and by-products, work practices, types of control measures, use of protective equipment and duration of exposure can often be obtained from plant personnel or through interviews with workers.

For many types of jobs, such as maintenance and construction work, worker exposures are often highly dependent on specific work tasks and related work practices. In evaluating worker exposure, it is important to recognize the wide variability in individual worker exposures, even when workers are doing the same or comparable jobs.

The OSHA hazard communication standard provides a valuable information resource for hazard identification.[3] This standard requires employers to:

1. develop a written hazard communication program
2. maintain a list of all hazardous chemicals in the workplace
3. make available to workers material safety data sheets (MSDS) for each hazardous chemical
4. place labels on containers as to the chemical identity and precautions in handling, and
5. provide workers with education and training in the handling of hazardous chemicals.

A material safety data sheet (MSDS) is a short document (several pages) which provides summary information concerning a hazardous material. The OSHA hazard communication standard does not require a standard format for MSDS; however, the types of information which must be provided are specified. Figure 4.1.6 is a non-mandatory MSDS format suggested by OSHA. The following is a summary of information to be provided by an MSDS.

Section I: Contains general information – (a) chemical identity, (b) manufacturer's name and address, and (c) emergency telephone numbers

Material Safety Data Sheet
May be used to comply with
OSHA's Hazard Communication Standard,
29 CFR 1910.1200. Standard must be
consulted for specific requirements

U.S. Department of Labor
Occupational Safety and Health Administration
(Non-Mandatory Form)
Form Approved
OMB No. 1218-0072

Identity (As used on label and list)

Note: Blank spaces are not permitted. If any item is not applicable, or no information is available, the space must be marked to indicate that.

Section I

Manufacturer's Name	Emergency Telephone number
Address *(Number, Street, City, State, and ZIP Code)*	Telephone Number for Information
	Date Prepared
	Signature of Preparer *(optional)*

Section II – Hazardous Ingredients/Identity Information

Hazardous Components (Specific Chemical Identity; Common Name(s))	OSHA PEL	ACGIH TLV	Other Limits Recommended	% (optional)

Section III – Physical/Chemical Characteristics

Boiling Point		Specific Gravity (H$_2$O = 1)	
Vapor Pressure (mmHg)		Melting Point	
Vapor Density (AIR = 1)		Evaporation Rate (Butyl Acetate = 1)	

Solubility in Water

Appearance and Odor

Section IV – Fire and Explosion Hazard Data

Flash Point (Method Used)	Flammable Limits	LEL	UEL

Extinguishing Media

Special Fire Fighting Procedures

Unusual Fire and Explosion Hazards

(Reproduce locally)

OSHA 174, Sept. 1985

Figure 4.1.6: OSHA-suggested format for material safety data sheet, or MSDS. Although required in the United States under the Hazard Communication Standard, many different formats are used by different companies.

Section V- Reactivity Data

Stability	Unstable		Conditions to Avoid
	Stable		

Incompatability *(Materials to Avoid)*

Hazardous Decomposition or By-Products

Hazardous Polymerization	May Occur		Conditions to Avoid
	Will Not Occur		

Section VI – Health Hazard Data

Route(s) of Entry:	Inhalation?	Skin?	Ingestion?

Health Hazards *(Acute and Chronic)*

Carcinogenicity:	NTP?	IARC Monographs?	OSHA Regulated?

Signs and Symptoms of Exposure

Medical Conditions
Generally Aggravated by Exposure

Emergency and First Aid Procedures

Section VII – Precautions for Safe Handling and Use

Steps to Be Taken in Case Material is Released or Spilled

Waste Disposal Method

Precautions to Be Taken in Handling and Storing

Other Precautions

Section VIII – Control Measures

Respiratory Protection *(Specify Type)*

Ventilation	Local Exhaust		Special
	Mechanical *(General)*		Other

Protective Gloves	Eye Protection

Other Protective Clothing or Equipment

Work/Hygienic Practices

Figure 4.1.6 (cont'd): OSHA-suggested format for material safety data sheet, or MSDS. Although required in the United States under the Hazard Communication Standard, many different formats are used by different companies.

Section II: Lists the hazardous ingredients and identification information. Includes any synonyms, TLVs or recommended occupational exposure limits.

Section III: Lists the physical/chemical characteristics that are applicable. Can include boiling point, vapor pressure, vapor density, specific gravity, melting, evaporation rate, and appearance and odor.

Section IV: Contains fire and explosion hazard data. This section includes flash point, flammable limits, extinguishing media, special fire fighting procedures, and any unusual hazards.

Section V: Provides data. States conditions of stability, any incompatibilities, hazardous decomposition products, and hazardous polymerization conditions.

Section VI: This section lists those health hazards which may arise from acute or chronic exposure, the route of entry, target organ, signs and symptoms of exposure, emergency first aid procedures, and whether the chemical is classified as a carcinogen.

Section VII: Lists the precautions for safe handling and use. Included are steps to be followed in case of a spill, waste disposal methods, and handling or storage precautions.

Section VIII: Contains control measures that are to be utilized when the chemical in question is used. This includes what type of respiratory protection is required, ventilation requirements, other personal protection devices/clothing, and specific work practices.

While MSDS are valuable for hazard identification, they must be used with a degree of caution for several reasons. Firstly, quality and completeness vary considerably between chemical producers. Secondly, the OSHA standard does not require chemical producers to conduct further toxicological studies to define the hazard of a chemical – the standard requires only the disclosure of a known hazard. Thus the quality of an MSDS is greatly dependent on published literature concerning the hazard of a substance.

In addition to information concerning raw materials used and by-products formed, information concerning the type of industrial process and jobs performed by workers is often helpful in hazard identification. In most industrial processes and occupational environments, several hazards will be present. Occupational hygienists have training and experience in identifying process and job specific hazards. Table 4.1.1 provides a brief summary of typical plant processes and the types of hazards that may be present. In considering possible exposures to workers, it is important to recognize exposures during non-routine tasks such as maintenance and cleaning. Maintenance workers may be exposed to most chemical hazards in the plant environment in addition to other materials such as asbestos, man-made mineral fibers from insulation materials, cutting oils, and lubricants. Cleaning operations, especially by dry sweeping, may re-suspend materials creating significant potential for particulate exposures.

The National Institute for Occupational Safety and Health (NIOSH) has conducted several national surveys to identify potential exposures and hazards by industry and job.[8] Data from these surveys are often helpful in identifying potential occupational exposures when a worker's job title and industry of employment are known. There are several sources of guidance which are very useful in the recognition and evaluation of workplace hazards.[1,9-24] These are included in the References, and should be consulted as sources of further information.

Occupational exposure limits and information sources

OSHA air contaminant standards

The goal of the US Occupational Safety and Health Act of 1970 is 'To assure safe and healthful working conditions for working men and women. . .'(Public Law 91-596). In order to achieve this goal, the Act authorizes the Secretary of Labor to issue occupational health and safety standards. In the case of air contaminants, the Act requires that these standards be set as exposure limits 'which most adequately assure(s), to the extent feasible, on the basis of the best available evidence, that no employee will suffer material impairment of health or functional capacity even if such employee has regular exposure to the hazard dealt with by such standard for the period of his working life. . . . .'. In accordance with this mandate, in 1971 OSHA promulgated approximately 425 permissible exposure limits (PELs) for air contaminants, derived principally from the American Conference of Governmental Industrial Hygienists Threshold Limit Values (ACGIH-TLVs) of 1968.

The Act also describes mechanisms for updating these standards, which include the requirements that OSHA must provide notice of proposed rulemaking, give interested parties an opportunity to comment, and hold a public hearing if requested. As of 2001, OSHA had issued 30 substance-specific and three 'generic' health standards under these provisions. In 1989 OSHA published a final rule for general industry, revising 212 existing exposure limits and establishing 164 new ones. However, in 1992 the 11th Circuit Court of Appeals ruled that OSHA did not sufficiently demonstrate that the new PELs were necessary or that they were feasible. The Court's decision to vacate the new limits forced the Agency to return to the original 1971 limits. While the updated standards were vacated, the substance-specific reviews do provide some additional guidance to health professionals. NIOSH scientific reviews in support of the PEL update project are available on the NIOSH Website.

OSHA may issue Emergency Temporary Standards under section 6(c) of the Act when it determines 'that employees are exposed to grave danger from exposure' to toxic substances. Once OSHA has published an emergency standard, proceedings must commence for issuance of a regular standard under section 6(b).

OSHA also has regulations on access to medical and exposure records. Under these regulations (29 CFR 1910.20), health professionals may obtain access to medical records, and exposure information from employers and former employers. Other OSHA generic health standards address

Process of operation	Nature and description of hazard
Abrasive blasting	Abrasive blasting equipment may be automatic or manually operated. Either type may use sand (free silica), steel shot or artificial abrasives. Excessive noise exposures may occur
Agricultural and food science technicians	Bioaerosols, caustics, acids and other agents causing contact dermatitis
Animal breeding/handling	Allergenic animal proteins, bioaerosols, dusts from bedding, grains, feeds, infection hazards Gases from fecal decomposition in animal confinement housing
Assembly operations	Improper positioning of equipment and handling of work parts present ergonomic hazards due to repeated awkward motion resulting in excessive stresses
Automotive repair/mechanics	Solvents and degreasers, asbestos and other fibers, automotive exhaust, lead, glues and sealants, benzene from solvents and automotive exhausts
Automotive body repair & painting	Paint aerosols, solvents, isocyanates, epoxy, dusts from body fillers, lead
Babbitting	Fumes and dusts of oxides of antimony, lead, tin and zinc
Bagging and handling	Conveying, sifting, sieving, screening, packaging, or bagging of any dry material may present a dust hazard. The transfer of dry, finely divided powder may result in the formation of considerable quantities of airborne dust. Inhalation and skin contact hazards may be present
Bakers	Flour dust, bioaerosols or biological enzymes
Cement cutting/grinding	Excessive dust, silica, and noise
Ceramic coating	Ceramic coating may present the hazard of airborne dispersion of toxic pigments and metal oxides plus hazards of heat stress from the furnaces and hot ware
Coal mining	Coal mine dust, silica, noise
Coal handling	Dusts and gases of carbon monoxide, coal, free silica, and sulfur dioxide
Coke handling	Coke and free silica dust
Coking	Contaminants encountered include ammonia, benzene, carbon disulfide, carbon monoxide, cyanamides, hydrogen sulfide, naphthalene and other polycyclics, phenols, pyridine, and sulfur dioxide
Dry grinding	Dry grinding operations may produce airborne dusts and ergonomic hazards
Dry mixing	Mixing of dry material may present a dust hazard
Earth moving, drilling, or boring	Elevated dusts exposures, potential high exposures to silica
Electro-tinning (alkaline and halogen)	Mists of caustics, chromates, fluorides, and sulfuric acid
Electron beam welding	Any process involving an electric discharge in a vacuum may be a source of ionizing radiation. Such processes include electron beam equipment and similar devices
Fabric and paper coating	The coating and impregnating of fabric and paper with plastic or rubber solutions may involve evaporation into the workroom air of large quantities of solvents
Farming & ranching	Pesticides, wood preservatives, bioaerosols and animal-derived proteins, grain dusts, hydrogen sulfide from manure pits and decaying organic matter, molds
Ferromanganese handling	Dust and gases of ferromanganese and hydrogen
Firefighting	Smoke, dusts, carbon monoxide, gases such as hydrogen chloride, from burning plastics
Forming and forging	Hot bending, forming, or cutting of metals or non-metals may have the hazards of lubricant mist, decomposition products of the lubricant, skin contact with the lubricant, heat stress (including radiant heat), noise, and dust
Furnace operations	Dusts, fumes, and gases of carbon monoxide, iron oxide, metal oxides, sulfur dioxide, and other combustion products
Galvanizing	Production of fumes, gases and mists of ammonium chloride, chromates, hydrochloric acid, hydrogen chloride, lead oxides, and zinc oxide
Gas furnace or oven heating	Products of combustion that may be released into the workroom atmosphere. Burner noise may be excessive
Grinding	Grinding, crushing, or comminuting of any material may present the hazard of contamination of workroom air due to the dust of the material being processed or of the grinding wheel
Healthcare workers	Blood-borne pathogens, tuberculosis, and other biological hazards, latex, drug exposures, chemotherapeutic agents, waste anesthetic gas, laser hazards, hazards associated with laboratories, radioactive material, ionizing radiation, formaldehyde, ethylene oxide and paracetic acid used for sterilization, patient lifting injuries, job stress, workplace violence
High temperatures	Any process or operation involving high ambient unlagged steam pipes, process temperatures (dry-bulb) temperature, radiant equipment, etc, heat load (globe temperature) or excessive humidity (wet-bulb temperature) may produce heat-related problems
Janitorial work/cleaning	Caustics, solvents and other agents causing contact dermatitis, dusts, bioaerosols from fleas, mites and rodents, asbestos from old insulation, potentially infected human wastes
Leaded steelmaking	Dusts and fumes of iron oxide and lead oxide
Industrial maintenance operations	Exposures to typical hazardous materials in the process plus asbestos, man-made mineral fibers, cutting oils and lubricants. Cutting and welding hazards and frequent solvent exposures
Materials handling, warehousing	Carbon monoxide and oxides of nitrogen arising from internal combustion engine fork-lift operations. Secondary spills from spills and re-suspended dusts

Table 4.1.1 Hazards associated with jobs, processes and tasks

Process of operation	Nature and description of hazard
Metalizing	A high-temperature coating of parts ('spraying') with molten metals presents hazards of dust and fumes of metals and their oxides, fluxes, carbon monoxide, in addition to heat and non-ionizing radiation
Microwave and radiofrequency	Microwave heating operations or induction heating may produce heating effects, electromagnetic field exposures and, in some cases, noise exposures
Molten metals	Melting and pouring of molten metals may produce toxic gas, metal fume or dust. Acrolein often is produced
Ore handling	Dusts of fluorides, free silica, and iron oxide. Some ores may contain other toxic metals as well as mineral fibers
Paint spraying	Paint spraying operations produce hazards from inhalation and skin contact with toxic and irritating solvents and inhalation of toxic pigments (cadmium, chromates and lead). The solvent vapor evaporating from the sprayed surface also may be source of hazard, because ventilation may be provided only for the paint spray booth
Pesticide application	Exposure to pesticides, herbicides, fungicides, or insecticides through sprays, dusts, vapors, soil incorporation or chemical application on trees, handling of agents causing allergic or contact dermatitis
Pickling (steel)	Gases and mists of hydrochloric acid, hydrogen chloride, hydrogen fluoride, oxide of nitrogen, and sulfuric acid
Plating	Electroplating processes involve risk of skin contact with strong chemicals and a respiratory hazard if mist or gases from the plating solutions are dispersed into the workroom air. Most commonly, these can be acids, alkalis, chromic acid mist, etc
Plumbers, pipefitters & steamfitters	Asbestos, man-made fibers, polyurethane, epoxy, styrene, glues, solvents, lead, coal tar, welding and soldering fumes
Punch press, press brake, drawing	Cold bending, forming, or cutting of metals or non-metals may involve hazards of contact with lubricant, inhalation of lubricant mist, and excessive noise
Refractory handling	Free silica dust as well as asbestos fibers
Sheet metal fabrication	Welding and cutting fumes and gases, glues, solvents, soldering fume, asbestos, man-made mineral fibers, urethane foam
Sintering	Dusts and gases of carbon monoxide, fluorides, free silica, iron oxides, and sulfur dioxide
Solvent degreasing	Vapors of perchloroethylene, trichloroethylene, vapor decomposition products (e.g., phosgene) and other solvents
Steelmaking (material handling)	Dusts of fluorspar, graphite, iron oxide, limestone, mill scale, and ore
Tandem rolling mills	Oil mist
Tool grinding, filing & sharpening	Tungsten-carbide, cobalt, beryllium alloys, abrasives containing silica, cleaning solvents
Vapor degreasing	The removal of oil and grease from metal products may present hazards
Veterinarians & technicians	Animal pathogens including hepatitis A from primates, animal proteins, therapeutic agents
Welding, gas or electric-arc ('brazing')	Processes involving the melting and joining of metal parts may produce exposures to fumes and gases. Oxides of cadmium, chromium, fluorides, iron, manganese, nickel, nitrogen, and vanadium may form, as well as pyrolysis by-products from fluxes and coatings. Welding on painted surfaces (e.g., lead-based paint) may produce a lead vapor hazard
Wet grinding	Wet grinding of any material may produce possibly hazards of mist, dust, and noise
Wet mixing	Mixing of wet materials may present possible hazards of solvent vapors, mist, and possible dust. Elevated noise levels also are possible
Woodworking/cabinet making	Hard and soft wood dusts, allergenic dusts such as Western red cedar, glues, epoxies, coatings, formaldehyde-resin adhesives, isocyanate

Table 4.1.1 (cont'd) Hazards associated with jobs, processes and tasks

blood-borne pathogens and occupational exposures to hazardous chemicals in laboratories.

Material safety data sheets (MSDS) are an important tool for communicating information about potentially hazardous chemicals in the workplace. The OSHA Hazard Communication Standard, 29 CFR 1910.1200,[3] mandates that employers inform employees of potentially hazardous materials. The regulation specifies requirements for the labeling, and communication of information on the hazardous properties of chemicals. It applies to chemical manufacturers, importers, and distributors. The standard includes a basic list of substances which must be treated as hazardous, and the term 'hazardous chemical' is defined as any chemical that is a physical hazard or a health hazard.

The OSHA hazard communication standard requires employers to: (1) develop a written hazard communication program, (2) maintain a list of all hazardous chemicals in the workplace, (3) make available to workers MSDS for each hazardous chemical, (4) place labels on chemical containers as to the chemical identity and precautions in handling, and (5) provide workers with education and training in the handling of hazardous chemicals.

OSHA also has issued a generic standard for respiratory protection (29 CFR 1910.134). OSHA's revised Respiratory Protection Standard became effective in 1998 and replaced the respiratory protection standards adopted by OSHA in 1971. The standard provides guidance for employers on how to establish and maintain a respiratory protection program to protect their respirator-wearing employees.

NIOSH recommendations

The NIOSH develops and recommends criteria for preventing disease and hazardous conditions in the workplace. These recommendations are issued in several forms, including exposure limits for physical and chemical hazards published as criteria documents and current intelligence bulletins. Information on recommended methods for prevention, including engineering controls, guidelines for selecting personal protective equipment such as respirators, and safe work practices are published in documents such as hazard alerts and occupational hazard assessments.

The NIOSH recommendations are not themselves legally enforceable; however, they are transmitted to OSHA and the Mine Safety and Health Administration (MSHA) for use in promulgating legal standards. NIOSH has recommended exposure limits for over 600 chemicals and compounds, as well as for physical hazards including hand-arm vibration, heat, noise, radon progeny, and ultraviolet radiation. Safety and health standards have also been recommended for industries, processes, and work environments including foundries, confined spaces, and logging operations.

Toxicological reviews

Reviews and evaluations of information on the toxicity of hazardous substances are prepared by several governmental and private organizations in the United States and internationally. The Agency for Toxic Substances and Disease Registries (ATSDR) (http://www.atsdr.cdc.gov/) of the US Department of Health and Human Services prepares toxicological profiles for compounds which are commonly found at hazardous waste sites, and may pose the most significant threat to human health. The profiles identify and review the key literature on each substance's toxicological properties. Each profile includes a public health statement which summarizes the compound's toxicological properties, a review of the information on human exposure, and known information on human health effects. The reviews are intended primarily for the use of health professionals, as well as private organizations and members of the public.

The National Institute of Environmental Health Sciences (NIEHS) of the US Department of Health and Human Services prepares an Annual Report on Carcinogens, which reviews and evaluates information on evidence of carcinogenicity. The report provides a listing of chemicals classified on the basis of the strength of the evidence of carcinogenic risk. Chemicals may be classified as 'known carcinogens' based upon sufficient evidence of a causal association between the chemical and cancer in humans. Chemicals for which less available evidence exists may be classified as compounds 'reasonably anticipated to be carcinogens'.

The American Conference of Governmental Industrial Hygienists (ACGIH) prepares a listing of Threshold Limit Values (TLVs) and Biologic Exposure Indices (BEIs) which is updated annually.[4] The TLVs are recommendations intended to be used as guidelines for limiting occupational exposures to more than 700 chemical and physical agents. They are prepared by technical committees of the ACGIH, which is an association of occupational and environmental professionals largely from academia and governmental agencies. In addition to the annual TLV listing, the ACGIH publishes a companion volume of documentation for the TLVs, which summarizes the pertinent scientific information and data that was used as the basis for the recommended exposure limits or indices.[6]

Several international organizations review scientific information for purposes of evaluating risks resulting from human exposure to chemicals. The International Agency for Research on Cancer (IARC) prepares a critical review of information on evidence of carcinogenicity for chemicals. The result of these reviews is a set of monographs which include several hundred chemicals, mixtures, processes and occupations.[25] The IARC classification of the evidence on carcinogenicity ranges from category 1 (carcinogenic to humans; sufficient evidence of carcinogenicity) to category 4 (probably not carcinogenic to humans). The International Programme on Chemical Safety (IPCS) is a joint venture of the United Nations Environment Program, the International Labor Organization, and the World Health Organization. This program develops Environmental Health Criteria Documents, which are summaries and evaluations of the information on toxic effects of specific chemicals and groups of chemicals. Over 200 chemicals have been reviewed, and are published in the criteria documents,[26] that summarize available information and include recommendations for further research.

Computerized databases and internet resources

Many excellent computerized databases and internet-based information sources are available. Only a few of the more important sources are highlighted in this section. These data sources are expanding rapidly. In addition to the primary information sites on the internet, links with other useful information sources are provided. As with all internet-based information, users should be careful to rely on information provided by reputable sites such as the various Federal and State agencies.

The National Library of Medicine (NLM) is an excellent starting point for research on agents and health effects (http://www.nlm.nih.gov/). The major bibliographic resource available through the NLM is MEDLINE/PubMed. MEDLINE/PubMed provides public access to over 12 million MEDLINE citations back to the mid-1960s and additional life science journals. PubMed includes links to many sites providing full text articles and other related resources.

In addition to bibliographic data resources, the NLM provides public access to a number of peer-reviewed databases concerned with chemical agents and health. These databases are briefly summarized below based on description provided by the NLM.

Hazardous Substances Data Bank (HSDB). HSDB is a toxicology data file that focuses on the toxicology of potentially hazardous chemicals. It is enhanced with information on human exposure, industrial hygiene, emergency handling procedures, environmental fate, regulatory requirements, and related areas. All data are referenced and derived from a core set of books, government documents, technical reports and selected primary journal literature. HSDB is peer reviewed by the Scientific Review Panel (SRP), a committee of experts in the major subject areas within the databank's scope. HSDB is organized into individual chemical records, and contains over 4500 such records.

Integrated Risk Information System (IRIS). IRIS is a toxicology data file that contains data in support of human health risk assessment. It is compiled by the US Environmental Protection Agency (EPA) and contains over 500 chemical records. IRIS data, focusing on hazard identification and dose–response assessment, is reviewed by working groups of EPA scientists and represents EPA consensus. Among the key data provided in IRIS are EPA carcinogen classifications, unit risks, slope factors, oral reference doses, and inhalation reference concentrations.

GENE-TOX. GENE-TOX is a toxicology data file created by the US Environmental Protection Agency (EPA) and contains genetic toxicology (mutagenicity) test data, developed from expert peer review of the scientific literature, on over 3000 chemicals. The GENE-TOX program was established to select assay systems for evaluation, review data in the scientific literature, and recommend proper testing protocols and evaluation procedures for these systems.

Chemical Carcinogenesis Research Information System (CCRIS). CCRIS is a scientifically evaluated and fully referenced databank, developed and maintained by the National Cancer Institute (NCI). It contains some 8000 chemical records with carcinogenicity, mutagenicity, tumor promotion, and tumor inhibition test results. Data are derived from studies cited in primary journals, current awareness tools, NCI reports, and other special sources. Test results have been reviewed by experts in carcinogenesis and mutagenesis.

TOXLINE. TOXLINE is the National Library of Medicine's extensive collection of online bibliographic information covering the biochemical, pharmacologic, physiologic, and toxicologic effects of drugs and other chemicals. It contains more than 3 million bibliographic citations, almost all with abstracts and/or indexing terms and CAS Registry Numbers. TOXLINE references are drawn from various sources grouped into two major parts – TOXLINE Core and TOXLINE Special – both of which operate under versatile search engines offering a variety of search and display capabilities.

Developmental and Reproductive Toxicology/Environmental Teratology Information Center (DART/ETIC) Database. DART/ETIC is a bibliographic database that covers teratology and other aspects of developmental and reproductive toxicology. It contains over 90,000 references

to literature published since 1965. DART/ETIC is funded by the US Environmental Protection Agency, the National Institute of Environmental Health Sciences (NIEHS), the National Center for Toxicological Research of the Food and Drug Administration, and the NLM.

EPA's Toxic Chemical Release Inventory (TRI). TRI is an annually compiled series of databases that constitute the toxic releases files on the National Library of Medicine's (NLM) Toxicology Data Network (TOXNET). This series, which includes 1995–1999 reporting years, contains information on the annual estimated releases of toxic chemicals to the environment and is based upon data collected by the Environmental Protection Agency (EPA). Mandated by the Superfund legislation, TRI's data cover air, water, land, and underground injection releases, as well as transfers to waste sites, and waste treatment methods and efficiency, as reported by industrial facilities around the United States. TRI also includes data related to source reduction and recyling.

ChemIDplus. ChemIDplus is a free, web-based search system that provides access to structure and nomenclature authority files used for the identification of chemical substances cited in National Library of Medicine (NLM) databases. ChemIDplus also provides structure searching and direct links to many biomedical resources at NLM and on the Internet for chemicals of interest. The database contains over 350,000 chemical records, of which over 114,000 include chemical structures, and is searchable by Name, Synonym, CAS Registry Number, Molecular Formula, Classification Code, Locator Code, and Structure.

All of the major Federal agencies concerned with occupational and environmental health, including NIOSH, OSHA, EPA, and NIEHS, provide excellent internet-based information resources. NIOSH (http://www.cdc.gov/niosh/homepage.html) provides many of their publications online as well as a number of useful data sources including:

NIOSH Certified Equipment List (CEL): A database of all certified respirators and coal mine dust personal sampler units.

NIOSH Manual of Analytical Methods: A collection of methods for sampling and analysis of contaminants in workplace air, and in the blood and urine of workers who are occupationally exposed.

NIOSH Pocket Guide: Provides a concise summary of physical and chemical properties of agents, health effects, exposure limits, recommended personal protective equipment including respirators, and sampling methods.

NIOSH has developed an electronic data source (NIOSHTIC-2) consisting of bibliographic databases of literature in the field of occupational safety and health. NIOSHTIC-2 is updated quarterly and is available online and on CD from several vendors. NIOSHTIC-2 covers the following subject areas: toxicology, occupational medicine, epidemiology, pathology, physiology, engineering, industrial hygiene, health physics, behavioral sciences, ergonomics, hazardous waste, chemistry, and control technology.

NIOSH also developed the Registry of Toxic Effects of Chemical Substances (RTECS) which is a compendium of data extracted from the open scientific literature concerning the toxicology of a chemical or chemical compound. RETECS is intended to be a comprehensive source of basic toxicity information for the assessment of hazards posed by exposure to chemical substances.

OSHA (http://www.osha.gov/) provides a comprehensive resource for standards, standard interpretations, and Electronic Products for Compliance Assistance on its internet site. This site also provides hundreds of links to other useful documents and technical resources. Medical Tests for OSHA Regulated Substances are included, providing specific information on medical tests published in the literature for OSHA regulated substances.

The Agency for Toxic Substances and Disease Registry (ATSDR) has developed the Medical Management Guidelines (MMGs) for Acute Chemical Exposures (http://www.atsdr.cdc.gov/mmg.html). These guidelines were developed by ATSDR to aid emergency department physicians and other emergency healthcare professionals who manage acute exposures resulting from chemical incidents. ATSDR also has developed ToxFAQs which serve as a quick and comprehensible guide regarding exposure to substances found around hazardous waste sites and the effects of exposure on human health.

EXTOXNET (http://ace.ace.orst.edu/info/extoxnet/pips/ghindex.html) is a cooperative effort of University of California-Davis, Oregon State University, Michigan State University, Cornell University, and the University of Idaho. EXTOXNET provides Pesticide Information Profiles (PIPs) which provide specific pesticide information relating to health and environmental effects. PIPs are not intended to be exhaustive literature reviews concerning a pesticide.

Resource hotlines

A number of emergency response services are in operation, some of which are primarily intended to provide information on environmental aspects of chemical hazards. These services are good sources of information on the toxicity and risk of exposure to a wide range of chemicals, regardless of whether exposure takes place in an environmental or an occupational setting. NIOSH operates a toll-free technical service to provide information on workplace hazards. The service is staffed by technical information specialists who can provide information on NIOSH activities, recommendations and services, or any aspect of occupational safety and health. The number is not a hotline for medical emergencies, but is a source of information and referrals on occupational hazards. The NIOSH toll-free number is 800-35- NIOSH (800-356-4674).

CHEMTREC (http://www.chemtrec.org/) is a 24-hour hotline to the Chemical Transportation Emergency Center operated by the Chemical Manufacturers Association (USA 800-424-9300; outside USA 703-527-3887). CHEMTREC assists in the identification of unknown chemicals, and provides advice on proper emergency response methods and procedures. It does not provide emergency treatment information other than basic first aid. CHEMTREC also facilitates contact with chemical manufacturers when further information is required.

The National Pesticides Information Center (http://npic.orst.edu/) is operated by Oregon State University and the US Environmental Protection Agency (800-858-7378). The hotline provides information on pesticide-related health effects, toxicity, and minor cleanup procedures to physicians, veterinarians, fire departments, first responders, and the general public. It is also a source of information on pesticide product formulations, basic safety practices, health and environmental effects, and cleanup and disposal procedures.

Several hotline and information lines are available for response to information requests on toxic materials and environmental issues. The US Environmental Protection Agency (USEPA) (http://www.epa.gov/) has several hotlines and information sources. The Center for Environmental Research Information is a central point for distribution of USEPA research results and reports (513-569-7562).

EPA also operates the Emergency Planning and Community Right-to-Know Act (EPCRA) hotline (800-424-9346) to provide information regulations and programs implemented for the Resource Conservation and Recovery Act (RCRA); the Comprehensive Environmental Response Compensation and Liability Act (CERCLA, or Superfund); and the Emergency Planning and Community Right-to-Know Act and the Toxic Substances Control Act. In addition, each of the ten USEPA Regional Offices has a hotline telephone number. ATSDR also operates an emergency response hotline manned 24 hours a day (404-498-0120). The ATSDR hotline staff is composed of toxicologists, physicians, and other scientists available to assist during an emergency involving hazardous substances in the environment.

EVALUATION OF HAZARDS

Occupational hygiene includes assessment of the nature and extent of human contact with biologic, chemical and physical hazards in the work environment. In the study of occupational disease, occupational hygiene techniques are applied to identify, evaluate and control the factors that cause work-related disease. While the techniques for evaluation are tailored to each type of hazard, the principles of evaluation can be generalized.

Over the range of types of air-borne exposures (e.g., gases and vapors, aerosols, biologic or physical agents), there are two general classes of measurement techniques. One class may be termed the extractive methods, in which the contaminants of interest are removed from the environment for laboratory analysis. With these methods, an air sampling device is used to collect the contaminants, usually from air in the vicinity of the worker's breathing zone. This sort of measurement of exposure is termed a personal sample, as it attempts to characterize the composition of the environment at the point the worker contacts it by inhalation. Most measurement methods assess air-borne contaminants due to the importance of inhalation exposures; however, methods to measure contamination of surfaces, as well as the exposure of the skin, are available.

The second general class of measurement techniques are those which determine the analyte directly in the atmosphere. These techniques are described as monitoring methods, and they are usually derived from instrumental methods first used in the laboratory. Devices which perform automated chemical analysis, or make measurements based upon chromatographic or spectrophotometric methods are common. These monitoring methods can measure continuously and report results immediately, which allows the examination of the pattern of exposure as it changes over time. This often represents substantial improvement over the information provided by extractive sampling methods, which accumulate material over the time of sampling, and give a result which is time integrated over that period.

Evaluating current hazards

Gases and vapors

Over the range of exposures which are found in the work environment, the greatest number are typically present in the form of a gas or vapor. Of the 567 chemicals and materials for which there are OSHA Permissible Exposure Limits (PELs), approximately 300 are usually found as gases or vapors in the workplace. As these materials pose a hazard primarily due to inhalation (although skin contact or ingestion may also be significant routes of exposure), exposure measurement methods typically involve the collection of air near the point of inhalation. These measurements are called personal breathing zone samples.

Most gas and vapor sampling is performed by using a sampling medium which removes the contaminants from air, and concentrates them for laboratory analysis. These sampling devices are small enough to be placed in the breathing zone of the person being sampled and they usually contain solid materials which adsorb the contaminants from air and retain them for analysis (materials such as activated charcoal, silica gel, and porous polymers are typically used). Other sampling devices contain liquids, which absorb contaminants based upon solubility or a reaction of the contaminant with the sampling solution. Air comes into contact with the collection media in these samplers either by active movement of air through the medium by a small portable pump, or by natural diffusion of the contaminants into the sampler to the collection medium. In both types of sampling devices, the total amount of contaminant collected during the sampling period is determined by removing the contaminant from the media (usually by chemical or thermal desorption), with analysis using a laboratory instrument such as a gas chromatograph, or a high performance liquid chromatograph. These devices may be coupled with a mass spectrometer to provide positive identification of contaminants.

An alternative method for air sampling is to collect a sample of air directly from the atmosphere using an evacuated container or a flexible bag. The composition of the air collected in this sample may be analyzed directly. Measurements made by these methods are described as grab samples. As the absolute quantity of material collected by these direct, or grab sampling techniques is small, these methods are generally limited to cases where very small amounts of contaminant can be accurately measured. Materials for which other methods are not applicable, such as highly reactive or unstable contaminants which cannot be preserved for later analysis, may be best measured by grab sampling.

Monitoring devices that can measure contaminants directly in the atmosphere are available for many gases and vapors. The simplest type of these are indicator or detector tubes, containing a chemically treated material that changes color in response to exposure to a contaminant. These devices are small and extremely simple to use, and can provide semiquantitative determination of a range of air-borne contaminants, such as carbon monoxide, mercury, and many organic solvents. At the next level of complexity are portable instruments that directly measure a single contaminant, such as oxygen, or provide a composite measurement of all combustible gases in an atmosphere. These latter two measurements are commonly made in the workplace to determine the safety of entering a confined space, such as a manhole or a storage tank.

The most sophisticated monitoring equipment is a set of instruments which are derived from devices previously used only in the laboratory. Instruments such as gas chromatographs with a range of detection systems, spectrophotometers, electrochemical monitors, and mass spectrometers have been miniaturized and made transportable for field use. These devices can provide the sort of detailed identification and analysis of air-borne contaminants which until recently has been only available by using extractive methods of sampling and analysis. Many of these devices are capable of providing continuous measurement of the concentration of air-borne contaminants, and displaying and recording results in real time. This capability allows observation of the change in level and composition of exposure through time, which is a powerful tool in the analysis of sources of exposures. This detailed information about the characteristics of exposure is also useful in the development of methods to control exposures.

Particulate material

A wide variety of solid and liquid materials suspended in air may be important as causes of occupational disease. These suspensions of particles in air can be collectively described as aerosols, a term which includes air containing solid particles (dusts), fine particles formed by condensation (fumes), and liquid particles (mists). The evaluation of exposure to these aerosols must consider the mass quantity and number of particles present in air (the concentration), as well as the size distribution, and chemical composition of the particles. As in the case of gases and vapors, exposure measures can be made by methods which remove the particulate materials from air for subsequent analysis, and by devices which measure the particulate content directly in air. Measurement methods which remove particulate material from air usually operate on the basis of the physical properties of the material, e.g., the particle size, mass, or electrostatic charge of the particles. Once the particles are removed from air, they can be subjected to a variety of chemical analyses to determine their composition, and they can be examined microscopically to evaluate their shape and size.

These methods for collecting particles for analysis operate in a fundamentally different manner from the techniques used to extract gases and vapors from air. Even the smallest particles in an aerosol are many times larger, and more massive than the molecules in the mixture of gases which comprise air. Particles which can be seen with an unaided eye are approximately 200 μm in diameter. (For comparison, a red blood cell is about 7.5 μm in diameter.) Particles large enough to be seen are generally too large to penetrate beyond the extreme upper oral and nasal passages, while most of the particles 100 times smaller (2 μm diameter) will enter, and be deposited in the respiratory tract. Even these 2 μm diameter particles, while far too small to be seen, are vastly larger and heavier than the gas molecules in air, which have an average diameter of 0.0004 μm. Most particulate sampling methods, therefore, utilize this difference in size and mass between aerosol particles and molecules in air to remove aerosol particles for analysis.

The method most commonly used for personal measurement of aerosol exposures is filtration. As is the case for gas and vapor sampling, small filters can be placed in the breathing zone, and the aerosol particles are collected from air approximately at the point of inhalation. Several types of filtering media are used, depending upon the type of analysis which will be performed, and the properties of the contaminant being measured. For example, the particulate material collected from air can be measured by chemical analysis for metals using a method such as atomic absorption spectrophotometry, or the organic fraction may be extracted from the filter and analyzed by a chromatographic method. Dusts such as those found in mining atmospheres may be analyzed for their mineralogic composition. Where the shape and size of the particle are important factors in evaluating the hazard, such as is the case for asbestos and other mineral fibers, the collected particulate material is analyzed by counting and sizing the individual particles using optical or electron microscopy.

The hazard from air-borne particulate material varies greatly, depending in large part on the site of deposition within the respiratory tract. The size of the particles, expressed as the aerodynamic diameter, is the major factor which determines the region of the respiratory tract where a particle may be deposited. Most aerosols found in the workplace contain mixtures of particles of widely varying sizes. It is not unusual, for example, to find particles ranging in size by a factor of 100 (i.e., an average diameter of 2 μm, but individual particles ranging from less than 1 to 100 μm) within an aerosol in a workplace such as a coal mine, a bakery, or a construction site.

When a worker is exposed to a mixture such as this, the inhaled particles are distributed throughout the respiratory tract on the basis of the particle aerodynamic diameter. Since the toxic effect of a particle may depend on the region of the respiratory tract in which it is deposited, exposure measurements are made using methods which classify aerosol particles on the basis of their size. There are many types of air sampling devices which are designed to separate particles into fractions that correspond to the region of the respiratory tract in which they are likely to be deposited. Particle size selective samplers include devices that are designed to effectively capture particles in several size ranges. Inhalable particle samplers efficiently collect particles up to 100 μm in aerodynamic diameter; which includes materials that are hazardous when deposited anywhere in the respiratory tract.

Samplers that are optimized to collect particles with aerodynamic diameters of 10 μm and smaller measure the thoracic particle mass fraction; these include particles that are hazardous when deposited in the pulmonary airways and the gas exchange region. Respirable particle samplers are optimized to efficiently collect particles with aerodynamic diameters of 4 μm and less; these particles are hazardous when deposited in the gas exchange region of the lung. This information about the size of the particles, along with the chemical analysis provides the data needed to fully evaluate the hazard which an aerosol exposure may present. For example, it has been shown that humans absorb lead differently depending on whether uptake is from inhalation or ingestion.

Depending upon the size of an inhaled aerosol particle, it may be deposited in the deep alveolar region of the lung, or it may be retained in the upper airways. The location of deposition is critical for a material such as lead, since virtually all the lead retained in the alveolar region is absorbed, while lead in the upper airways is cleared to the gastrointestinal tract where it is absorbed with an efficiency ranging from 10% to 30%.[9] The amount of lead contained in these small (less than 1 μm in aerodynamic diameter) aerosols may make a much greater relative contribution to the blood lead than larger particles which are deposited in the upper airways. Air sampling to assess a hazard such as this would be conducted using a device which separates the particles into two or more fractions based upon their aerodynamic diameter. Air samplers such as miniature cyclones, or impactors are used to separate aerosols in this way, so that the size fractions can be analyzed separately.

There are a variety of instruments which directly measure the atmospheric concentration of aerosols. These instruments depend upon the physical properties of the particles in air to provide the means of detecting and measuring aerosol concentration. For example, the tendency of particles to scatter light provides the basis for a family of instruments known as optical particle counters. In these devices, air is drawn into a chamber and a light source is focused on the air sample. Particles suspended in the air scatter a portion of the light, and this amount of light is proportional to the quantity of air-borne material in the sample. Instruments incorporating lasers as the light source are capable of directly measuring the size, as well as the concentration of the particles in an air sample.

Another type of direct reading instrument operates by subjecting the aerosol particles to electrical charges, and measuring their movement in a charged field. These instruments are also capable of directly measuring the mass of material present in air, and providing information about the size characteristics of the particles. A third type of instrument measures the mass of aerosol in a sample by collecting the particulate material on a surface which is placed between a source of beta radiation and a beta radiation counter. The attenuation of radiation is proportional to the mass of particulate material from the sample, allowing the direct measurement of aerosol mass concentration in air.

Biologic hazards in air

Methods for evaluating biologic materials in air are a specialized set of techniques derived from the methods for measuring air-borne particulate material. In terms of methods for air sampling, there are two general classes of biologic hazards: those considered viable, which pose a risk through their capacity to grow and multiply in an exposed host, and the non-viable particles, which are hazardous due to the ability to produce an allergic response, regardless of whether the exposure agent is viable. The methods for measuring exposure to these hazards tend to be specific to the agent being evaluated, and are not standardized to the degree of other aerosols. The importance of methods to measure biologic hazards is apparent in studies of indoor environments, particularly in buildings with outbreaks of respiratory complaints, and in healthcare facilities.[27]

Methods for measuring viable materials in air use equipment which is similar to that used for other air-borne particles, including filters, impactors, impingers, and open settling surfaces. The difference in these methods from the general aerosol sampling methods is in the need to preserve the viability of the collected material. The techniques for detecting and enumerating viable organisms require that conditions be suitable for the collected material to grow into observable colonies or plaques. The sampling devices therefore include a growth medium, in which the collected micro-organisms are retained, or can be preserved in a viable state so they can be transferred to a growth medium after sampling. Depending upon the purpose of the sampling, the growth medium can be tailored to support general growth, or it may be selective to favor the organisms of interest. In some investigations, the overall level of biologic contamination, measured in terms of total colony-forming units may be important.

Other investigations seek to address more specific concerns, such as the contamination originating from an air conditioning system in an office building. A study of this sort of problem would use selective media to evaluate particular types of micro-organisms. The range of collection and culturing techniques for air-borne micro-organisms, as well as the specialized nature of investigations of biologic hazards usually require expertise in microbiology for quantitative measurements and interpretation. Unlike other chemical and physical contaminants, there are no generally accepted standards for viable micro-organisms in air.

The second type of biologic hazard is an air-borne particle which produces an allergic response, regardless of whether the particle is viable. These particles are described as aeroallergens, and include pollens, some bacteria, fungal spores, and insect body parts. These materials are collected from air using techniques including filtration, impaction, and gravitational settling. The properties of the collected material may be determined by microscopic examination, culturing for the viable fraction, and immunoassay for the antigenic component of the air-borne material. These assay techniques are tailored to the property of interest, and investigations of air-borne allergens are usually designed to address specific exposures.

Measures of hazards in tissue or body fluids (biologic monitoring)

The use of exposure information in the investigation of occupational disease requires the assumption that exposure is a reasonable indicator or marker for the quantity of a toxic material which reaches a site in the body and elicits a response. Under some circumstances, this is a valid assumption, and useful exposure response associations can be observed. There are, however, many factors which can compromise the value of exposure measures as predictors of health effects. Exposure is a measure of the concentration of a contaminant in the environment external to the body. As was mentioned in the discussion of air sampling procedures, measurements can be made as close to the actual point of inhalation as possible (the breathing zone sample), but the air collected at this point is not identical to that which is inhaled. Once the air enters the respiratory tract, contaminants may be removed, distributed and metabolized by many possible mechanisms. There can be a great deal of variability in these mechanisms between individuals, resulting in very different quantities of an active material at sites where toxic effects occur, even though the individuals may have had the same measured level of external exposure.

Another factor which complicates the assessment of exposure is the ability of many toxic materials to enter the body by several routes. In addition to pulmonary absorption, materials may be cleared from the respiratory tract and swallowed, resulting in uptake from the gastrointestinal tract. Many industrial materials can also be absorbed directly through the skin. Measurement of contaminants in biologic media reflects the contributions from these multiple routes of exposure, as well as the variability in absorption, distribution, and metabolism between exposed individuals. Progress in biologic monitoring has been driven by the uncertainties in the relationship between measurement of contamination in the workplace environment, such as those made with conventional occupational hygiene air sampling methods, and the actual quantity of a toxic material which may be present in the body.

The measurement made in biologic media may be for a particular chemical itself, or its metabolites. A reversible biologic change which is characteristically induced by exposure to a chemical is another type of measurement used to evaluate workplace exposure. These measurements can be made in blood, urine, exhaled breath, or other media. Biologic monitoring methods are usually used to complement measurements of inhalation exposures, as they provide information on the total exposure from all sources (non-occupational and workplace), and by all routes, including skin and gastrointestinal absorption. The medium which is selected for sampling can be chosen to suit a particular purpose, as materials (e.g., organic solvents) may be eliminated by several pathways. In a study of workers exposed to n-hexane, for example, the solvent was rapidly cleared from the body in exhaled breath, with a biologic half-time of approximately 15 minutes. N-hexane vapor may be measured in exhaled air during the period of exposure, providing information about the level of exposure in the short time before sample collection. A n-hexane metabolite is also excreted in the urine, so end-of-shift urine samples could be collected from the same workers and analyzed for 2,6-hexanedione, providing a time integrated measure of daily exposure.

There are reference values for measurements made in biologic media.[4,6] The ACGIH has prepared these values, known as biologic exposure indices (BEIs), with documentation for their measurement and interpretation of results, for approximately 40 chemicals. In most cases, these values are chosen to represent the level of a determinant (the parent chemical, a metabolite, or a characteristic reversible biologic change) in biologic medium that would be observed in a healthy worker exposed by inhalation to the parent chemical at the level of the TLV. As such, the BEIs are not clear boundaries between safe and dangerous exposures; rather they are intended to be indirect reflections of dose, to be used in conjunction with environmental exposure measures.

Interpreting exposure measurement information

Information on exposure in the work environment is collected for a number of purposes. Exposure measurements may be compliance driven, that is, the measurements are made to determine the levels of workplace contaminants with reference to an exposure limit or guideline. There are several sources of exposure limits, as discussed earlier. Whilst the exposure limit values vary between sources, virtually all these limits are specific to the air-borne concentration of a single chemical, and the vast majority set a level which is not to be exceeded as a time integrated average over an 8–10-hour work shift. Exposure measurements made to determine compliance with these exposure limits, therefore, are usually made in a manner which allows direct comparison between a worker's exposure level and the limit, as measures of a single contaminant averaged over the full workshift.

Although these data help determine compliance with a limit, they may not be useful as a predictor of health risk or the relationship between exposure and health effects. Several factors must be considered in interpreting exposure information, including simultaneous exposure to mixtures of toxic agents, variability in the composition and levels of exposure over time, exposure by multiple routes, and unusual working conditions. In addition, a standard or limit may not be protective against a risk or health effect of interest. The interpretation of exposure measurements in comparison to a legally mandated exposure limit (such as the OSHA Permissible Exposure Limits) or a recommended value (such as the NIOSH Recommended Exposure Limits or the ACGIH Threshold Limit Values) must be done with caution. These limit values and exposure standards are not intended to be clear lines between safe and unsafe conditions, nor are they meant to be indices of relative toxicity between substances. The philosophy underlying these values is that they represent conditions under which it is believed that nearly all workers may be repeatedly exposed without adverse health effects. Variations in individual susceptibility, for example will result in some workers experiencing adverse health effects when exposed at or below the exposure limit value. It is not appropriate, therefore, to conclude that adverse health effects cannot be related to workplace exposures simply because exposure measurements do not exceed a limit value or exposure standard.

Evaluating mixed exposures

While most exposure limits are specific to a single agent, the work environment is likely to be composed of mixtures of potentially hazardous materials. Virtually all workers are exposed to environments containing more than one potentially hazardous agent, with work in agriculture, manufacturing, and construction commonly presenting combinations of chemical or physical agents. The evaluation of potential health risks posed by occupational exposures should also recognize the effects of non-work-related exposures, such as the consumption of alcohol, tobacco, or the use of insect repellants, cosmetics, or other chemicals that may act in concert with workplace exposures. The complexity of exposures and resulting biologic responses is illustrated by the synergisitic effect of exposures to noise and the solvent toluene, which results in a 2–3-times higher risk of hearing loss than exposure to either component alone.

Another example is exposure to carbon monoxide and methylene chloride, which both produce elevated levels of carboxyhemoglobin, reducing the blood's ability to carry oxygen. The combined effects of materials which act upon the same organ system are recognized in the ACGIH TLVs.[4] For example, an atmosphere containing a mixture of solvents, each of which may have neurotoxic effects, should be evaluated in consideration of the additive effect of the exposure. The TLVs provide guidelines for assessing the effect of exposures when the components of a mixture have similar toxicologic properties.

In epidemiologic investigations of exposure–response associations, the comprehensive assessment of exposure enhances the likelihood that a study will correctly identify and evaluate these relationships. Although these studies usually are conducted with some prior specification of the exposure(s) of interest, comprehensive exposure assessment is necessary to deal with confounding or effect modification by exposures which may not have been anticipated. Studies of the respiratory effects of sulfur dioxide (SO_2), for example, demonstrate the potentiating effect of inert aerosols such as sodium chloride when the two materials are present as combined inhalation exposures. Exposure to atmospheres containing both SO_2 and an aerosol results in a much greater restriction in pulmonary flow than is observed for SO_2 alone, while inhalation of sodium chloride aerosol alone has no effect on pulmonary flow.

One common pitfall of exposure assessment in these studies is discounting the possible role of an exposure as a causal agent because the association is not thought to biologically plausible. For example, the unexpected finding that carbon monoxide exposure (CO) potentiates noise-induced high frequency threshold shifts illustrates the importance of conducting comprehensive assessments of exposure, even in cases where a particular exposure is of primary interest.

Evaluating exposure variability

Exposure results from human contact with a contaminant in the environment. Regardless of the route (inhalation, dermal contact, or ingestion), exposure can be considered to be part of a pathway between the source of a contaminant in the environment, to a site in the body where it can cause molecular or cellular damage. Exposure is measured as a marker of human interaction with a contaminated environment. Since the nature of this interaction can vary, the characterization of exposure should consider exposure to be part of a dynamic process which changes through time, not as a fixed quantity.

The variability in exposure can be broken down into components. The characteristics (i.e., composition and intensity) of the contamination in the environment are described as the ambient concentration. The composition, e.g., the chemical makeup, or the distribution of particle sizes may change through time. The second characteristic is the intensity of exposure, expressed as its concentration, e.g., parts of benzene vapor per million parts of air, or number of asbestos fibers per cubic centimeter of air. In many occupational environments, these characteristics of exposure are highly variable over a workday, resulting in a constantly changing exposure. The third major component of exposure variability is introduced by the characteristics of the individuals in the exposure environment. Even among jobs at fixed workstations, where workers perform similar tasks, there can be substantial exposure differences between individuals because of personal work practices.

These sources of exposure variability should be considered in designing an exposure assessment strategy, and in the interpretation of exposure information. When exposure varies widely over time, the time course of exposure must be considered. Industrial hygiene sampling methods which collect air-borne contaminants for laboratory analysis provide a measurement which is integrated over the time of sampling. The temporal component of exposure variability is lost in such a measurement. For example, the atmosphere in a work environment could contain a steady state concentration of 1 ppm of a solvent, so the exposure of a worker spending a full shift in this area would be measured as 1 ppm as an 8-hour time-weighted average exposure. Another worker could spend a full shift in an environment in which the level of exposure to the same solvent varied widely, from periods of no detectable exposure, to very high but short-term peaks of exposure. If this second worker experienced a single, high peak exposure level of 48 ppm of the solvent for only 10 minutes a day, then spent the remainder of the shift in an unexposed area, this worker's 8-hour time-weighted average exposure would also be 1 ppm. Interpreting these two exposures to be equivalent, in terms of their likelihood of causing a toxic effect, could result in an erroneous conclusion. Without any further information about the actual time course of the exposure, however, these two workers could be classified as equally exposed.

Exposure limits and guidelines are set in a manner which attempts to recognize that the risk of health effects resulting from extremes of exposure over time. For rapidly acting chemicals which are known to cause toxic effects from brief exposures, exposure limits can be designated as short-term exposure limits (STELs). These values are intended to be levels measured over a short averaging period (usually 15 minutes), which should not be exceeded during any period, even if the 8-hour time-weighted average does not exceed the exposure limit. These STELs are set to prevent irritation, chronic or irreversible tissue damage, narcosis, or other impairment which would result in material risk. For some acutely toxic chemicals, the exposure limit is designated as a ceiling limit, which is a level not to be exceeded at any time. In practical terms, the duration of a ceiling exposure limit is defined by the shortest time period over which an exposure measurement can be made. Depending on the chemical of interest, and the availability of methods for measuring its concentration in air, this may be a virtually instantaneous measurement, or the limitations of the measurement method may extend it to a period of approximately 15 minutes.

Tasks as the basis for exposure assessment

The overall variability in exposure levels within a population can be very substantial. In some cases where workers have been grouped for air sampling and analysis on the basis of their job title (assembler, or chemical operator for example), exposure levels between individuals in the group have been found to vary by factors as great as 15-fold.[28] Repeated measures of exposure on individual workers made from day to day have shown that the level of exposure for the same worker can also be highly variable. The overall variability in exposure for individual members of a group can be partitioned into between-worker (differences between individual workers) and within-worker (day to day or variability over time for an individual worker) components. Environmental and production factors have been found to have a strong influence on the within-worker (day-to-day) variability, but not on the between-worker variability. Groups working outdoors and those working without local exhaust ventilation generally have greater day-to-day variability than groups working indoors and those working with local exhaust ventilation. Mobile workers, and workers involved in intermittent processes, also have great day-to-day variability in exposure.

The significance of this finding is that the title of a job may not be a good predictor of exposure, as workers with the same job title may have very different exposures. Sampling a subset of individuals in a group with the same job title, then applying these sampling results to the entire group, may severely misclassify individuals on the basis of their actual exposure. An alternative approach to exposure assessment is to use job task as the primary classifying variable, rather than job, group, or department title. The task-based approach identifies the characteristic work activities that influence exposure, then forms worker groups on the basis of similar activities.

A study of workers exposed to ethylene oxide in a hospital, for example, would seek to identify the primary work tasks and activities that may result in ethylene oxide exposure, then to characterize the exposure associated with each task. This exposure measurement approach has revealed that workers who load and unload the sterilizer, for example, have a very different level and pattern of ethylene oxide exposure than workers who sort the packages of sterilized materials for distribution throughout the hospital. While workers performing these different tasks may have the same department name (for example, Central Sterilization) and job title (for example, sterile area technician), those who load and unload the sterilizer may have much higher exposures than the other workers. Measuring the exposure associated with the work task therefore provides the information needed to correctly classify workers on the basis of exposure, and to target the workers at highest exposure risk and the specific work tasks that contribute to that risk. Tasks associated with high exposure can be prioritized for control measures.

When exposure is used as a risk factor in studies of exposure–response associations, unrecognized variability may occur, resulting in misclassification of exposure among the members of the study population, and obscuring actual exposure–response relationships.

In most studies, exposure is actually measured for a small sample of the population, and only for part of the period of interest. Based upon these measurements and other information which may influence exposure, such as production conditions, presence of ventilation, or use of protective devices, exposure values may be estimated and applied to entire groups of workers. The assumption underlying this approach is that it is possible to identify groups of similarly exposed workers to which a single exposure value may be correctly assigned. The extent to which this assumption can be validated should be considered in the interpretation of study results, particularly in studies which show no apparent association between exposure and response. This problem is especially serious in retrospective studies of diseases with long latency, as there is usually very limited historical information available on actual exposures. The likelihood of exposure misclassification, which is likely to obscure associations, should be considered carefully in interpreting the results of these studies.

Evaluating exposure by multiple routes

Exposure assessments typically focus on exposure by inhalation of gases, vapors and aerosols, but absorption through the skin can be another important route of exposure. This fact has been recognized in the case of exposures to pesticides, and dermal exposure has recently received more attention as a potential route of exposure for other chemicals. The OSHA permissible exposure limits, the ACGIH threshold limit values, and most other exposure guidelines include notations indicating cases in which skin contact may be a significant route of exposure. In the case of the TLVs, this notation appears for approximately 10% of the chemicals listed. The likelihood of dermal contact with potentially hazardous materials is great in some occupations and industries.

For example, dermal exposure to polycyclic aromatic hydrocarbons (PAH) among coke oven workers has been found to be as important as inhalation as a contributor to total exposure and absorbed dose.[29] When these workers implemented hygienic measures to reduce dermal absorption (including laundered work clothes and gloves before each shift), the weekly average excretion of a PAH metabolite (1-hydroxypyrene) was reduced by more than a third. This illustrates the importance of dermal exposure route in the classification of exposure when cumulative or average exposures are calculated, and in the development of control strategies to reduce exposure.

The uptake of chemicals through the skin depends on the molecular weight, lipid solubility, polarity, and state of ionization. There has been considerable effort to develop quantitative measurement methods for dermal absorption of chemicals. Methods of assessing dermal exposure have been classified into three general types: surrogate skin techniques which rely on a collection medium placed against the subject's skin; removal techniques where substances deposited on the skin are removed, generally by washing or wiping; and fluorescent tracer techniques that rely on the measurement of UV fluorescence from materials deposited and retained on the skin. An example of a surrogate skin technique is the use of cloth patches placed on the outside of workers' clothing and removed for analysis of chemical contamination as an estimate of the exposure of unprotected skin.

A similar method has been used with patches placed under the workers' clothing, to measure the quantity of a contaminant which penetrates protective clothing. Exposure to the surface of the hands has been estimated by providing workers with thin cotton inspector's gloves which are worn during tasks of interest. Analysis of the glove material then provides an estimate of the exposure of unprotected skin of the hands. This approach has also been used to evaluate the performance of protective gloves by wearing the cotton glove under the protective glove. The removal techniques include rinsing the hands, or both the inside surface of the protective gloves and the hands, after a worker has performed the task of interest. The volume of rinse solution is collected and analyzed for the contaminant.

The interpretation of information obtained by measuring dermal contact is complicated by the absence of guidelines or reference values. Measurement of skin contact does not necessarily provide a direct indication of the quantity of a chemical which may be absorbed, as the relationship between the material found on the skin and the absorbed amount depends on several factors. The physical and chemical properties of the material, the anatomical area of contact, the duration of contact, and the individual characteristics of the exposed individual can all influence the relationship between skin contact and dermal absorption. The importance of dermal exposure should not be underestimated, particularly in the case of pesticides that have been shown to enter the body primarily by dermal absorption.

Several techniques have been developed to measure contaminants on surfaces which may be sources of dermal exposure in the workplace. The measurement of surface contamination in a working environment can provide an indirect indication of dermal exposure. Techniques for wipe sampling have been developed to measure surface contamination. These methods have been widely used in industries where exposure may result from resuspension of settled aerosols. For example, surface sampling for lead in industries such as foundries and lead smelters have been extensively performed. In cases where exposure of interest is non-volatile, such as metals and polychlorinated biphenyls (PCBs), surface contamination is a useful measure of the risk of exposure from skin absorption, or ingestion resulting from eating or smoking with contaminated hands. There is a standardized surface wiping method specified by OSHA which describes techniques for collecting samples from contaminated surfaces (OSHA Technical Manual, Sampling for Surface Contamination).

Evaluating unusual working conditions

Information on exposure should be interpreted in view of the overall conditions in the working environment. Even the OSHA Permissible Exposure Limits, which are legally enforceable, are not intended to be used as specific lines to distinguish between safe and dangerous working conditions. When interpreting the results of exposure measurements, an environment should not be assumed to be free from risk when exposure levels do not exceed the limit value. In the case of individual workers in the environment, reported symptoms should not be dismissed as non-work-related because measured exposure levels are below a limit value. Any interpretation of exposure information should recognize that there is uncertainty associated with both measurement of exposure, as well as the limit value

to which it is compared. The extent of individual variability in response to workplace exposure may be considerable and a conservative approach to the interpretation of exposure is appropriate.

Among a number of factors which may influence the response to workplace exposures, the duration of exposure period is one which has been recognized in the OSHA permissible exposure limits. Exposure measurements are generally made with the expectation that the individuals are in the working environment for the 'normal' 8-hour day, and 40-hour work week. Many jobs, including a substantial portion of those in manufacturing, operate on a schedule which exceeds this. The potential effect of extended duration on occupational exposure may be recognized, but it is rarely quantified. Of the over 600 materials for which there are OSHA PELs, only the lead standard specifies that the maximum daily allowable exposure level be adjusted down in proportion to overtime activities exceeding 8 hours. Another factor which should be considered in the interpretation of exposure information is the time of day during which the exposure occurred. At least 20% of the workforce in manufacturing jobs work non-daytime shifts. Although limited information is currently available on the physical and psychological effects of shift work, overall job performance, as well as behavioral and psychological function, are diminished in night shift workers compared to day shift workers. The possibility of combined effects of exposure and the time of day during which it occurs should be considered in investigations where both could affect health outcomes.

Assessing previous work exposures

Many occupational and environmental exposures produce clinical disease years after the initial exposure. Past exposures are therefore important with regard to attribution of disease in an individual or establishing a causal association using epidemiologic data. In many instances, available data are sufficient for estimating past exposures only qualitatively; however, these estimates are often useful for establishing plausible ranges of exposure. Estimating past exposures requires a systematic approach to information gathering. First, an inventory of potentially toxic substances and exposures for various jobs, work locations, and work tasks must be developed. This effort requires detailed knowledge of industrial processes, work procedures, and materials, and familiarity with the toxic properties of the substances present in the workplace environment. In addition, the ever-changing character of work must be considered.

Use of past exposure measurement data
In ideal circumstances, quantified personal monitoring data, obtained from air sampling or other dosimetric methods (e.g., radiation film badges). However, in the more typical situation, quantified exposure data are sparse or non-existent. Even when data are available, they often represent special exposure situations that were measured in response to particular concerns about workers' health or because of

compliance enforcement requirements. Evaluations of sampling data are best determined when there is documentation of the circumstances under which exposure measurements were taken. Furthermore, occupational hygiene data tend to be most complete for recent years in which promulgated exposure guidelines and standards have required initial and periodic exposure monitoring.

For epidemiologic investigation, rather than for clinical evaluation, these limitations may be more significant. Industrial hygiene sampling data measuring individual exposures are by far the most useful for exposure classification. It is usually not feasible to measure all exposures for all individuals; therefore, samples are collected that are thought to be representative of employees doing the same or similar tasks. Typically in epidemiologic studies, attempts are made to assign workers to various exposure classifications, based on types of exposures and exposure levels. Occupational hygiene sampling data are useful for this purpose when sufficient descriptive data are recorded to allow identification of individual workers or specific jobs for which the exposure data pertain.

Because exposures can change qualitatively and quantitatively over time, it is important that these changes be taken into consideration. Changes in occupational hygiene and analytic laboratory techniques may diminish the validity of some past exposure monitoring data.

Special sampling studies are useful for correlating results from different measurement methods and for assessing the validity of the exposure rating scheme – at least in reference to current exposure levels. For example, exposure to asbestos containing dusts was formerly measured in units of millions of particles per cubic foot of air (all particles) using an impinger rather than fibers per cubic foot centimeter of air by the membrane filter method. Use of these old sampling data may require the investigator to estimate a conversion from the old impinger method to the membrane filter method. As no direct conversion is possible, statistical analyses of simultaneous sampling data using both methods can be used to arrive at an approximate conversion factor.

Estimates of exposure using surrogate data

In the absence of complete quantified exposure data, potential occupational exposures can be identified using an assessment of raw material, process, tasks, and control information. Jobs and work areas may be classified with respect to exposure levels and potential exposures. A 'job-exposure matrix' is frequently generated which links worker exposure histories with health outcomes for clinical and epidemiologic analysis.

The types of information that the occupational hygienist incorporates into the exposure rating scheme include data from the following: air sampling, physical agent exposures (e.g., noise dosimetry), biologic monitoring, materials usage records and purchase orders, plant production records, job and task descriptions, and documentation of engineering controls and use of protective equipment. Table 4.1.2 provides a summary of data useful for estimating exposures. The following are potential uses and limitations of various data source with respect to estimation of past exposure.

Company records
Process, descriptions, flow charts and plant layouts
Job and task descriptions
Raw materials and intermediates, by industrial process
Plant production records
Engineering control records
Industrial hygiene sampling records
Physical and biological agent measurements
Personal protective equipment availability and use
Inspection and accident reports
Biological monitoring results
Environmental discharge and incident reports
Medical records
Injury reports or workers' compensation records
Labor union records
Records of work locations
Injury/illness records
Government records
OSHA or State program inspections
NIOSH studies/Health Hazard Evaluation Reports
State OSHA or consultation reports
Workmen's Compensation Records
Insurance company records
Plant inspection/reports
Industrial hygiene studies

Table 4.1.2 Sources and types of information useful for evaluating past exposures

1. *Process descriptions, flow charts and plant layout.* Changing plant process and raw materials may significantly affect actual or potential occupational exposures. Process changes often result in new raw materials or intermediates of potential occupational health significance. Proximity of plant operations to each other also may be important. Ideally, plant records should be maintained in sufficient detail to permit identification of dates of process changes or major changes in plant layout or equipment.

2. *Job and task descriptions.* The most commonly used method for assigning employees to exposure categories in epidemiologic studies is the classification of job titles. In studies where only a few significant exposures are present, job titles generally allow suitable stratification into exposed and non-exposed populations. Changes in job titles over time should be recognized. While job titles are useful for exposure classification, additional information – such as specific tasks performed and plant location – may be needed to appropriately classify exposures. Assessment of task-specific exposures is very important for exposures experienced by maintenance and craft workers.

3. *Raw materials and intermediates by process.* Raw materials and intermediates should be recorded in sufficient detail to allow identification of processes or plant areas where raw materials are used and changes in the use of these over time. Because it is usually not possible to measure all exposures in a given process or area, it is important that the materials list be as complete as possible so that multiple potentially hazardous exposures may be evaluated in epidemiologic studies. Purchase records can be a valuable source of information on the types and quantities of materials used. Such data are particularly valuable for case-control studies that may be necessitated at some future time.

4. *Plant production records.* In addition to raw materials, plant production or output rate may affect exposures. In many instances changes in measured exposures without other apparent plant changes can be attributed to increased or decreased processing of the materials in question. Annual production volume by product is useful as a measure of change in potential exposures.

5. *Engineering control records.* Engineering controls are the preferred method for controlling occupational exposures and, typically, change significantly over time. Engineering records should be maintained in sufficient detail to identify controls by process or equipment over time. Both control system design and operational parameters are important. Special studies evaluating effectiveness of engineering control measures are especially useful as these may suggest important changes in employee exposures. Photographs can be valuable supplements to such record systems.

6. *Physical and biologic agents.* Plant raw materials lists are usually helpful in identifying potential chemical exposures; however, additional records are often necessary to characterize exposures to physical and biologic agents. Physical agents include ionizing and non-ionizing radiations, noise, and vibration; biologic agents include viruses, bacteria, fungi and other microbial antigenic material. Exposures to physical and biologic agents often are generated within the workplace, rather than resulting from the intended use of defined raw materials. The presence or absence of such exposures should be recorded as well as associated levels of exposure.

7. *Personal protective equipment.* Personal protective equipment – such as respirators, gloves, protective clothing and hearing protection – may affect actual worker exposures significantly. In addition to recording protective equipment in use during industrial monitoring studies, documents detailing protective equipment policies and procedures should be maintained. Specific processes or procedures requiring protective equipment should be identified in these records.

8. *Inspection and accident reports.* Accidental spills or leaks may represent significant exposures that must be considered when drawing conclusions from epidemiologic studies. Spills or accidents can result in greater potential for atypical routes of exposure, such as clothing contamination and skin contact. Failure to account for such exposures can lead to incorrect conclusions concerning health effects of apparently low exposures. Incidents such as major spills or leaks should be documented in sufficient detail to allow for estimation of the potential severity of intermittent excessive exposures, as well as identifying workers potentially exposed.

9. *Biologic monitoring results.* Although results of blood, urine, breath and other types of biologic monitoring usually are maintained in medical departments, they also are frequently used by industrial hygienists for exposure monitoring. These data are especially valuable when there are multiple routes of exposure entry, such as inhalation and absorption. The collection of these data and their integration with the environmental data should be made with proper and mandated safeguards for confidentiality.

10. *Environmental discharge and incident reports.* Health effects among residents of neighborhoods in close proximity to industrial plants may be of concern. Federal regulations require annual reports of environmental discharges for specified pollutants for certain manufacturing facilities.

11. *Employee surveys/interviews.* Surveys of long-term employees, wherein workers are asked to rate jobs according to perceived relative exposure intensities, provide ancillary information. Questionnaire survey results are most reliable when the variations in exposure levels of the agent of concern are readily apparent (e.g., dust, malodorous fumes, irritating gases). Validation of reporting with objective information (e.g., measurements) is desirable when available.

Historical reconstruction of workplace exposures is essential to the validity of occupational epidemiology, and for establishing a causal relationship between exposures and disease. When sufficient data exist that permit a quantitative exposure rating scale, it is possible to estimate, within reasonable limits, true relative exposure intensities. Estimates of potential exposures using production-related data are also useful for epidemiologic research and for relating workers symptoms and disease with potential occupational exposures.

While occupational exposure data vary substantially in both quality and quality within and across industries, there has been substantial progress toward a consensus set of standardized data elements to be captured with measurements and qualitative estimates of exposure to air-borne chemical hazards as well as noise. The Joint ACGIH/AIHA Task Group on Occupational Exposure Databases has developed consensus recommendations with the goal of harmonizing the collection of exposure data across different work sites, companies, agencies, and other institutions.[30] Occupational hygienists and other health professionals responsible for developing and maintaining exposure information should consult this document as well as similar guidelines developed in Europe, including the report of the Working Group on Exposure Registries in Europe and the information database (COLCHIC) developed by French insurance funds in collaboration with the French National Research and Safety Institute.[31]

Linkage of industrial hygiene and health outcome data

Strategies for evaluating occupational exposures may differ according to the population being studied and the available exposure data. Both quantitative and qualitative exposures are useful for purposes of disease surveillance as well as in etiologic research. For etiologic research, both the magnitude of the observed relative risk for disease in relation to exposure as well as trends in relative risks with increasing exposures are important considerations in establishing causal relationships. In industry-based studies, it is often possible to develop a more limited list of operations, jobs and tasks, and associated exposures. The process of retrospective exposure assessment is facilitated when at least some quantitative historical exposure data are available, and the number of possible exposures of concern is limited. Prospective studies of exposures and health conditions have the advantage of measuring both health outcomes and exposures simultaneously, thus the investigator has more control over the quality of exposure data, as well as their analyses and interpretation.

The link between occupational hygiene data and health outcome data, available from sources such as medical surveys, cancer registries, and death certificates, may be accomplished using employer personnel records or other records which characterize the study population. From such records, work histories, indexed by time interval at various exposure levels, can be constructed. Techniques for and difficulties associated with linking information on industrial work conditions with health data have been discussed by investigators active in this area (see Chapter 6). Studies such as the assessment of lung cancer among welders, and radon-related lung cancers among miners, provide excellent examples of linkage methods as well as associated strengths and limitations of these methods.

Direct exposure measurements from monitoring surveys that are specific for individual workers offer the best exposure data. More commonly, occupational epidemiology studies rely on exposure estimation where jobs and tasks within the industry are assigned exposure intensity levels. Creation of a job-exposure matrix that is specific for jobs, tasks and calendar years, and can be linked with employee personnel records, has become standard procedure in many epidemiologic studies. This approach allows for aggregation of jobs and tasks according to either exposure levels or similarity of tasks and materials handled, depending on the extent of available information.

A job-exposure matrix (JEM) is often used to define the presence or absence of specific exposures within a given industry or job title. In general, a JEM can be organized as an array of information which relates industry and/or job titles with occupational exposures. Each cell entry in the array then contains a measure of exposure for the job title/chemical pair. Entries can be quantitative when sufficient exposure measurement data are available, semi-quantitative (e.g., categories of exposure), or qualitative (e.g., exposed or unexposed). If exposures vary with time period, a third dimension can be added to the JEM to account for temporal variations. More elaborate JEMs can sometimes be developed if jobs are analyzed at the task level. Any given job may be further characterized as a specific number of tasks, each with an associated exposure level.

JEMs have been used effectively to combine observational or direct exposure measurements with past work histories, to derive a measure of overall exposure for both surveillance and etiologic research. JEMs provide a global evaluation of a job category which can be used, through data linkages, to estimate exposures of anyone who worked in that job, or task, with their cumulative exposures based on length of employment in that job. Clearly there is some loss of precision compared to direct expert assessment and personal exposure measurements, but there can be very significant cost savings thus making it possible to study larger groups of workers than would be

possible if individual longitudinal exposure assessments were needed. In addition to their value for etiologic research, JEMs provide a useful tool for surveillance where potential exposures to many substances or work circumstances can be evaluated.

JEMs have been developed using many different techniques and in varying degrees of detail. Population-based JEMs may use broad definitions of exposures based on industry SIC codes and occupational codes. Industry-specific JEMs can often provide a much greater degree of detail and precision in defining exposures. While JEMs have largely been used for studies of chemical or physical hazards, more recent efforts have extended the JEM concept to include a wider spectrum of hazards including physical, chemical, biologic, ergonomic, and psychosocial factors. In addition to new dimensions of the matrix allowing for factors other than chemicals, the conceptual model includes more extensive documentation concerning exposure definitions and reference data sources.

The types of data which can be used to develop a JEM for linking industrial hygiene and health data include the following: occupational hygiene survey data, job classifications and descriptions, personnel employment records of workers, information on work location within a plant for specific jobs, and where available, medical records. Medical records, although most valuable as a source for case finding for injuries, accidents, dermatitis and other non-disabling conditions, sometimes contain results of biologic monitoring that can be an ancillary source of exposure classification.

Existing occupational hygiene or health physics sampling data, which are of obvious research value, may need to be augmented by currently obtained measurements in cases where many jobs cannot be classified into exposure level categories. When major changes in sampling and quantification technology have occurred over time, it may be inappropriate to add the newly obtained data to the historical data. Instead, the new data can be incorporated to generate ordinal exposure scales for the various jobs in the plant, or to confirm judgments that certain work locations and jobs probably entail no or minimal exposure level.

Resources seldom permit extensive occupational hygiene surveys; thus, a selective approach is recommended in which special groups of workers or job types are targeted for monitoring. These groups can be workers for whom data have never been collected, or workers in jobs where previous research has indicated important disease risks. Maintenance, crafts, quality control and laboratory workers are groups that frequently go unmonitored. Periodic monitoring surveys of these workers, especially maintenance workers who represent sizable proportions of the workforce in many industries, would serve to rectify the common problem of unknown exposure profiles. Almost invariably there will be some jobs that cannot be classified according to exposure level, either because there is inadequate job description (e.g., the laborer designation) or because sampling cannot be performed. This circumstance will necessitate the creation of an unknown exposure category for some workers in the study. The health experience of such workers should be evaluated in a similar manner as that of workers with estimatable exposure profiles, although the results for the former will be less informative. Deletion of workers with unknown exposures would be wasteful of information and may introduce bias into the study.

The JEM that is generated should be documented carefully so as to indicate the basis for assignment of exposure levels. Thus, the occupational hygienist should maintain a file that indicates each job or task included in the analysis – the exposure value or rankings – by time period, and the data sources that were used to derive exposure estimates. The source information should indicate whether a given estimate was based on occupational hygiene sampling data, the nature of the sampling (e.g., area or personal, compliance or routine monitoring), the number of samples and the range of values, and whether the estimate was based on judgment. Documentation of sources of error and uncertainty as well as assumptions used in the exposure assessment process should be maintained.

PRINCIPLES AND LIMITATIONS OF CONTROLS

Hazard control in the working environment is one of the primary goals of occupational hygiene. The elimination, or reduction of hazards to the extent feasible is the primary means of prevention for occupational disease and injury. The strategy for effective hazard control is an ordered hierarchy, which NIOSH[32] has described as including three elements, in order of effectiveness:

1. first, prevent or contain hazardous workplace emissions at their source;
2. next, remove the emissions from the pathway between the source and the worker;
3. last, control the exposure of the worker with barriers between the worker and the hazardous work environment.

This strategy mandates the use of engineering control methods on the environment as the primary means of exposure prevention. These controls may be implemented in several forms, or in combinations as part of an overall prevention strategy. The methods include substitution of materials for less hazardous substances, modification of the working environment to contain the source of the hazard, isolation of the worker from the hazardous environment, removal of the hazardous substance by ventilation, modification of work practices to reduce exposure, and use of personal protective equipment to reduce exposure. Use of this protective equipment, including respirators, is intentionally mentioned last. Respiratory protective equipment should be considered the least preferable means of hazard control, implemented only when other means of control are not feasible or effective.

This hierarchical approach to exposure control has been recommended practice, but it is now specified in the regulatory language of the OSHA respiratory protection standard. OSHA has stated that 'In the control of those occupational diseases caused by breathing air contaminated with harmful dusts, fogs, fumes, mists, gases, smokes, sprays, or vapors, the primary objective shall be to prevent atmospheric contamination. This shall be accomplished as far as feasible by accepted engineering control measures (for example, enclosure or confinement of the operation, general and local ventilation, and substitution of less toxic materials). When effective engineering controls are not feasible, or while they are being instituted, appropriate respirators shall be used' (29 CFR 1910.134).

Material substitution

The preferred method of direct intervention to reduce workplace hazards is the removal of a toxic material and its replacement with a less toxic substitute. This practice is well established as a means of reducing risk in the workplace as well as in the general environment. Elimination or reduction of extremely toxic materials, such as asbestos as an insulating material, or benzene in solvents, adhesives, and gasoline illustrate the principle of substitution. These examples also demonstrate another factor which must be considered in substitution: the risk of replacing one hazard with another. Some of the materials used to replace asbestos as an insulating material, such as man-made mineral fibers and fibrous glass, may also have adverse respiratory effects, as more information is discovered about their toxicity. The replacement of benzene with another chemical with similar solvent properties, such as hexane, may reduce the risk of exposure to a carcinogen, but increase the hazard of exposure to a neurotoxin. Substitution is an important method of primary prevention of workplace exposures, but it should be practiced with a recognition of the effect the replacement material may have on the work environment. The result of substitution should not be the replacement of one hazard with another.

Process modification

The introduction of contaminants into the work environment may be prevented by changing the characteristics of the source. The application of engineering control technology in the design of industrial processes is a very effective method of intervention to reduce exposures. For example, the technology of spray painting has changed, substantially reducing solvent exposures by using airless atomization systems instead of compressed air spray guns. Many common industrial processes, such as material handling procedures can be redesigned to minimize the release of contaminants. At the design stage of a new industrial process, or in the modification of existing operations, exposure control should be included as a central design element. The anticipation and control of potential hazards at the design stage is more efficient than remediation of existing conditions.

Isolation

Isolation is an effective method of intervention to interrupt the pathway between the source of a hazard and the worker. The general approach of isolation can be implemented in two ways: (1) by enclosure to isolate a source from the working environment, or (2) by isolating the workers from a contaminated environment. Although a comprehensive exposure control strategy may include both approaches, containment of the source is generally preferable.

A common example of containment as a means of hazard control is the glove box used in handling infectious materials, extremely toxic chemicals, or radioactive materials. This approach is particularly well suited to control individual point sources of contaminants, or physical hazards such as noise. By preventing the release of a hazardous agent into the work environment, exposure is controlled at the source.

In cases where contaminants are released from multiple sources dispersed through the work environment, isolation of the workers from the contaminated environment may be preferable. While this approach does not prevent the release of the hazard into the environment, it is possible to control exposure by protecting workers through isolation. The use of clean-air-supplied control rooms in chemical production facilities is an example of isolation of workers from general environmental contamination.

Administrative and work practice controls

Measures can be taken to limit or restrict the opportunity for exposure through changes in the manner in which work is performed. These controls are a hybrid, incorporating some features of source control and some modifications of work practices. Administrative controls may be implemented to prevent release or contain hazardous emissions at their source. In the healthcare setting, for example, administrative controls such as rapid identification, early treatment, and isolation of potential tuberculosis transmitters, limiting worker access to acid-fast bacilli (AFB) isolation rooms and other administrative procedures could be implemented to reduce risk of exposure. Modification of procedures such as using portable x-ray units in the room of a confirmed or potential tuberculosis transmitter, rather than moving the infectious person to the central x-ray department, is another example of the use of administrative control to reduce the chance of exposure.

Work practice modifications also can be implemented to reduce exposures. For example, methods used for clean up of lead-containing dust at weapon firing ranges makes a significant difference in the general level of contamination and personal exposure. Instead of using brooms to sweep up dry dust, which generates large amounts of lead-containing aerosols, vacuuming with equipment incorporating high-efficiency particulate (HEPA) filters keeps lead dust from being suspended, significantly reducing exposures. Analysis of individual work tasks also can identify practices that contribute to exposure. Painters using spray guns in ventilated booths, for example, may unnecessarily increase their exposure to solvent vapors by moving into the booth when they paint the back of a large part, rather than turning the part so they can always spray paint into the booth. Changing work practices such as these can reduce exposure significantly, and they are most likely to be effective when they are developed through on-site evaluation, with full participation to the workers who are actually performing the job.

Ventilation

In the working environment, ventilation is a central component of hazard control. There are two general types of ventilation: (1) dilution ventilation (also known as general or comfort ventilation), and (2) local exhaust ventilation. Virtually any indoor space has some amount of dilution ventilation, even if it is only the natural infiltration of outside air. The control of contaminant sources in the workplace frequently requires additional ventilation, in the form of local exhaust to capture contaminants at or near their source, and remove them from the work environment. These two types of ventilation are very different in design and performance, and are discussed separately.

Dilution ventilation

Dilution ventilation operates on the principle of replacement of contaminated air with fresh air. The simplest form is the natural entry of outdoor air through drafts around windows, doors and other openings. Most buildings used as places of employment have at least some means of providing mechanical air movement to supplement the natural airflow. Mechanical roof ventilators or wall fans are common in buildings used as workplaces. In office buildings where there are no industrial processes which release contaminants, the human occupants may be the primary source of indoor pollution. General building air provided by a heating, ventilation, and air conditioning (HVAC) system may be the only means of controlling the carbon dioxide, water vapor, particulate material, and biologic aerosols which are the result of human occupancy. Ventilation guidelines for general dilution are provided by the American Society of Heating, Refrigerating and Air-Conditioning Engineers (ASHRAE)[33] to specify minimum ventilation rates and indoor air quality which provide an acceptable work environment to building occupants, and the quantity of ventilation needed '. . .to minimize the potential for adverse health effects.'

For workplaces where there are sources of contamination in addition to human occupancy, dilution ventilation is generally not as effective a control method. It may be applicable in a limited number of situations, only when several criteria are met. Typically, dilution ventilation may be adequate in workplaces where small amounts of contaminants are released at uniform rates. In these cases, a reasonable amount of air added to the work space may be sufficient to dilute the contaminants to a level at which they do not pose a hazard. This approach is limited, therefore, to contaminants with low toxicity, and environments in which workers do not have contact with the contaminant until after it has been diluted. The volume of air which is needed to dilute contaminants to acceptable levels is usually large, requiring large and expensive air-handling systems to move the air, as well as to heat and cool it. The lack of positive control over the sources of contaminants, as well as the high airflow requirements and operating costs, usually limit the usefulness of dilution ventilation systems as exposure control methods in the workplace. These systems may reduce the amount of contaminant present in the work environment, but they do not control its release.

Local exhaust ventilation

Local exhaust systems differ fundamentally from dilution systems. The operating principle of local exhaust ventilation is the capture of air contaminants at the source, preventing their dispersion in the environment. These local systems control emissions and prevent exposures, interrupting the pathway between the source of the contaminant and the worker. Local exhaust systems are usually tailored to the source they control. The components of the systems include the hood, which is the device to capture the air and facilitate its entry into the exhaust system; the fan which provides the force to move air into the system; and the duct work connecting the hood and the fan. Many systems also include an air cleaning device, such as a filter, to remove contaminants before the air is released to the environment. The hood, which is the collection point of the contaminated air, is typically designed in a manner which encloses the source to the extent possible. It may be designed to fit around the shape of existing machinery, or to receive material which is released from the source, such as the metal particles thrown from a grinding wheel, or the dust created by a circular saw (Fig. 4.1.7).

The design and testing of local exhaust systems is a specialized aspect of ventilation engineering. There are several sources of guidance which are very useful in the construction of systems which are effective in controlling exposures by local ventilation. These are included in the References, and should be consulted as sources of further information.

Personal protective equipment

A variety of devices are available to provide a barrier between a worker and a contaminated environment. These include equipment to protect the eyes, such as safety glasses, goggles, and face shields. There are many types of skin protection, including gloves, aprons, and full body suits made of materials which are impervious to chemicals. The selection and use of these devices is largely driven by the particular application, and there is a large number of choices of protective equipment available.

The choice of chemical protective clothing for the skin usually centers on gloves, although the principles guiding the selection can apply to equipment that protects part or all of the body. The selection of chemical-protective gloves should include analysis of both the job task and the exposure against which protection is needed. The job task analysis should also include ergonomic factors, such as the manual dexterity, grip, and tactility required by the task. Guidance in the selection of gloves is available from the American National Standard for Hand Protection Selection Criteria.[34] This document establishes performance classes for various types of protective gloves, and it includes rating scales for the following factors: permeation, penetration, degradation, cut, puncture, flame, abrasion, heat and cold. This information, along with the analysis of the exposure the glove will protect against, will guide the selection of a suitable glove for the situation. The MSDS for the materials in use may also be a good source of information to guide the selection of gloves, and specific recommendations are often included on the MSDS. This guidance should not be a substitute for a thoughtful analysis of each job-task exposure situation, however. The demands of each work environment and characteristics of the individual worker must be considered in the selection process.

Information on the properties and characteristics of gloves is available from a number of sources, including the glove manufacturers. Publications that summarize available guidance on the selection of gloves and other protective equipment are included in the references.[35-37]

Respiratory protective devices

Respiratory protective devices are used to provide protection from exposure by inhalation. There are several factors which must be considered in the use of respiratory protection beyond the general considerations for other protective devices. OSHA has a specific regulation for respirator use (29 CFR 1910.134). In addition, some OSHA standards for specific air contaminants such as asbestos and lead include requirements for respiratory protection programs. These legal requirements, as well as the importance of matching the choice of respiratory protection with both the hazard and the individual respirator user, make respirator selection and use more complex than other protective equipment. The correct choice of a respirator depends upon the identity of the particular contaminant, as well as the concentrations at which the contaminant is present in the workplace environment. The ability of the individual worker to wear the respirator in a manner that provides adequate protection also must be determined as part of a respirator selection and use program. The degree of protection that a respirator provides in the working environment

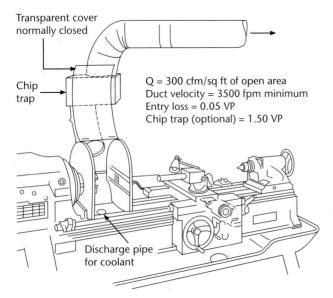

Transparent cover normally closed

Chip trap

Q = 300 cfm/sq ft of open area
Duct velocity = 3500 fpm minimum
Entry loss = 0.05 VP
Chip trap (optional) = 1.50 VP

Discharge pipe for coolant

Figure 4.1.7: An example of local exhaust ventilation, in this case used over a lathe-generated coolant mist and possible metal dusts.

varies widely between individual workers. Comprehensive respiratory protection programs must include respirator fit testing to ensure that each respirator performs effectively for the individual user.

NIOSH has exclusive authority over respirators, except for mine escape and rescue devices. Employers must select a respirator certified by NIOSH. There are two general types of respiratory protection. Respirators may remove contaminants from air by filtration, adsorption, or chemical reaction. Respirators which operate by this principle are described as air-purifying respirators. Respirators which supply air from a source other than the surrounding environment (such as from a cylinder of compressed air) are known as atmosphere-supplying respirators. Both types of respirators are tested and certified for use by NIOSH.

As a guide to the selection and use of respiratory protection, OSHA has prepared a respiratory protection advisor, which is based upon the requirements of the OSHA respiratory protection standard and the guidance of the NIOSH Respiratory Decision Logic. NIOSH has also incorporated information on respiratory protection in its Pocket Guide to Chemical Hazards. Both are sources of practical guidance on the selection of respiratory protection that is appropriate to the work situation for which respirator use is being considered. The OSHA advisor covers most elements of the respiratory protection program including selection criteria, medical evaluations, procedures for proper use, fit testing, and maintenance procedures. Proper selection and, if appropriate, fit testing of tight-fitting facepieces are necessary to assure that the respirator will provide adequate protection against the contaminants that affect use. Medical evaluations are necessary to determine whether the user is fit to wear a respirator without adverse health effects. Training on procedures for proper use and maintenance is needed so the wearer uses the respirator in a safe and healthful manner.

Some OSHA standards have specific respirator requirements when certain contaminants are present in the workplace, such as lead and asbestos. When these contaminants are present in the workplace, the substance-specific standard takes precedence over any recommendations provided by the respirator selection decision logic.

The OSHA respiratory protection advisor is designed to guide the user through the respirator selection process. The advisor asks if the atmosphere is oxygen deficient, that is if the oxygen content is less than 21%. For example, for work in an area with poor ventilation, or in a confined space, it is necessary to measure the oxygen level. If the atmosphere is oxygen deficient, then an atmosphere-supplying respirator is required. The user must be aware of the identity and approximate air-borne concentration of the contaminant the respirator will protect against. This requires an exposure assessment to determine the type and amount of hazardous exposure. The advisor asks the type of contaminant (particulate or gas) the respirator will protect against. It also asks whether the contaminant(s) is an eye irritant, or can cause eye damage at the exposure concentration. For gaseous contaminants, the maximum concentration of contaminants in the workplace must be known (in units of parts per million or milligrams per cubic meter). For respirators to protect against particles, the user is asked if there is oil present in the workplace air, the filter efficiency that is desired, and whether the filter will be used for more than 8 hours. The advisor also asks about the existence of special working conditions, such as welding in confined spaces and abrasive blasting.

This guidance is based upon the NIOSH Respirator Decision Logic and the OSHA Respirator Standard (29 CFR191 0.134). The actual choice of the appropriate respirator is made with consideration of the assigned protection factor for the respirator and the expected concentration of the contaminant(s) that are present in the working environment. The assigned protection factor (APF), which is the ratio of the concentration of the contaminant outside the mask to the concentration inside the mask, is the key to evaluating the respirator's efficiency at removing air-borne contaminants. For example, a single-use disposable dust mask may have an APF of 5, meaning there is a five to one ratio between the concentration of the contaminant in air outside the respirator to the concentration inside the respirator. Put another way, such a respirator would allow 20% penetration of the contaminant it is designed to protect against. A full facepiece respirator with an HEPA filter would have an APF of 50, allowing only 2% of the contaminant to penetrate.

In practice, the APF guides the selection of the respirator to the one that provides sufficient protection. To choose a respirator for a particular exposure situation, the expected concentration of the contaminant (either an 8-hour TWA, or a short-term concentration) is divided by the exposure limit for the contaminant (the OSHA PEL, the NIOSH REL, or some other exposure limit). The result of this division is the minimum respirator protection factor required. For example, suppose respirators were being considered to protect workers in a factory where exposure control measures such as ventilation were either not feasible or were in the process of implementation to reduce exposure to Portland cement dust. The OSHA and NIOSH exposure limit for total Portland cement dust is 10 mg/m^3. If the expected dust concentration in the workplace were approximately 20 mg/m^3, then the minimum respirator protection factor required would be 20 divided by 10, or 2. Using the tables of APFs for the various types of particulate respirators, as described in the respirator decision logic, a properly fitted single-use respirator (which has an APF of 5) would be appropriate. If the exposure agent were a material of greater toxicity, such as the pesticide Endrin, which has OSHA and NIOSH exposure limit of 0.1 mg/m^3, protection against an atmosphere containing 20 mg/m^3 of the contaminant would require a respirator with a minimum protection factor of 200, which would indicate that a positive-pressure supplied-air respirator is needed.

Respirators can provide effective personal protection only when they are properly selected and when they are used in the context of a comprehensive respiratory protection program. OSHA has specified the minimum requirements for an acceptable program (29 CFR 1910.134). In order for respirators to provide adequate worker protection, both the proper selection and the correct use of respirators are essential. Despite the apparent simplicity of respirator use, respirators can be unreliable if not selected and used in a comprehensive protection program and are cumbersome and uncomfortable when used for extended periods of time. Respirators are the least preferred method of protection from respiratory hazards, and they should be used only when engineering controls are not technically feasible, while controls are being installed or repaired, or in emergency and other temporary situations.

Education and training

Worker education and training are key components of effective primary prevention programs for workplace injuries and illnesses. Workers must understand the physical and chemical hazards associated with their work as well as methods for controlling these hazards. Worker training is defined as instruction in recognizing hazards, and in using available methods of worker protection, whereas worker education is defined as instruction in analyzing and responding to new circumstances and conditions.

OSHA substance-specific regulations such as asbestos, lead, arsenic, and cotton dust require worker education and training, although these regulations often lack detailed training specifications. Training requirements also are contained in several OSHA process specific standards such as the respiratory protection standard, the blood-borne pathogens standard and the standard concerning process safety management for highly hazardous materials. In addition, the OSHA Hazard Communication Standard which was promulgated in 1985 establishes generic training requirements for hazardous substances.

The OSHA Hazard Communication Standard requires chemical manufacturers and importers to provide hazard information to users of their products. Information must be provided in the form of MSDS and product labels. The standard requires that employees be provided with information and training on hazardous chemicals in the workplace. Training must include the following.

- Information concerning requirements of the OSHA standard.
- Identification of hazardous materials in the work area.
- Information on the company's written hazard communication standard.
- Methods for detecting presence or release of hazardous chemicals in the work area.
- Specific hazards of chemicals in the workplace.
- Measures to protect workers from exposure to hazardous chemicals.
- Details concerning the employer's hazard labeling system for chemicals in the workplace.

Quality worker education and training must consider special needs of the worker and appropriate means of training delivery. While OSHA standards require training, little specification is provided concerning training content, delivery or quality assurance. The National Institute of Environmental Health Sciences (NIEHS) was given major responsibility for initiating a training grants program under the Superfund Amendments and Reauthorization Act of 1986 (SARA). The primary objective of this program is to fund non-profit organizations, with a demonstrated track record of providing occupational safety and health education, to develop and deliver high-quality training to workers who are involved in handling hazardous waste or in responding to emergency releases of hazardous materials.

Since the initiation of the Hazardous Waste Worker Training Program in 1987, the NIEHS has developed a strong network of non-profit organizations that are committed to protecting workers and their communities by delivering high-quality, peer-reviewed safety and health curriculum to target populations of hazardous waste workers and emergency responders. A national clearinghouse for worker training has been established by NIEHS (http://www.wetp.org/). A consensus working group has developed minimum criteria recommendations for worker training quality assurance. The key components of these recommendations include: (1) experienced training program staff; (2) a well-defined training plan with tested curricula and materials; (3) students with prerequisite job skills; (4) adequate training facilities including provisions for hands-on training and demonstrations; and (5) quality control and evaluation plans including adequate peer review of the training program.

References

1. Hatch T. Major accomplishments in occupational health in the past 50 years. Ind Hyg J 1964; 25:108–13.
2. Harris RL, ed. Patty's industrial hygiene and toxicology, 5th edn. New York: John Wiley & Sons, 1999.
3. Occupational Safety and Health Administration. Hazard Communication Standard, 29 CFR 1910. 1200.
4. American Conference of Governmental Industrial Hygienists. Threshold limit values for chemical substances and physical agents & biologic exposure indices. Cincinnati: ACGIH, 2002.
5. NFPA. National Fire Protection Association, Flammable and Combustible Liquids Code, Standard No. 30.
6. American Conference of Governmental Industrial Hygienists. Documentation of threshold limit values and biologic exposure indices, 7th edn. Cincinnati: ACGIH, 2001.
7. Burgess WA. Recognition of health hazards in industry, 2nd edn. New York: John Wiley & Sons, 1995
8. National Institute for Occupational Safety and Health. National Occupational Exposure Survey, 1990. Cincinnati: NIOSH, 1990.
9. Bingham E, Cohrssen B, Powell CH, eds. Patty's toxicology, 5th edn. New York: John Wiley & Sons, 2001.
10. Berkow R, ed. The Merck manual, 16th edn. Rahway: Merck & Co., 1992.
11. Budavari S, O'Neil MJ, Smith A, Heckelman PE, eds. The Merck index, an encyclopedia of chemicals, drugs, and biologicals, 11th edn. Rahway: Merck & Co., 1989.
12. Chin J, ed. Control of communicable diseases manual, 17th edn. Washington DC: APHA, 2000.
13. Harber P, Schenker MB, Balmes JR, eds. Occupational and environmental respiratory diseases. St. Louis: Mosby, 1996
14. Hawley L. Hawley's condensed chemical dictionary, 12th edn. New York: Van Nostrand Reinhold, 1993.
15. LaDou J, ed. Occupational and environmental medicine, 2nd edn. Stamford: Appleton & Lange, 1997.
16. Levy BS, Wegman DH, eds. Occupational health: recognizing and preventing work-related disease, 3rd edn. Boston: Little, Brown and Company, 1995

17. Marks JG, DeLeo VA. Contact and occupational dermatology, 2nd edn. St. Louis: Mosby, 1997.
18. National Safety Council. Fundamentals of industrial hygiene, 4th edn. Chicago: National Safety Council, 1996.
19. Rom WN, ed. Environmental & occupational medicine, 3rd edn. Philadelphia: Lippincott-Raven, 1998.
20. Stellman JM, ed. ILO Encyclopaedia of occupational health and safety, 4th edn. Geneva: International Labour Organization, 1998.
21. Sullivan J, Krieger G, eds. Hazardous materials toxicology. Baltimore: Williams & Wilkins, 1992.
22. Ryan RP, Terry CE, eds. Toxicology desk reference: the toxic exposure and medical monitoring index, 4th edn. Washington DC: Taylor & Francis, 1997
23. Weeks JL, Levy BS, Wagner GR, eds. Preventing occupational disease and injury, Washington DC: APHA, 1991.
24. Zenz C, Dickerson BO, Horvath EP, eds. Occupational medicine, 3rd edn. St. Louis: Mosby, 1994.
25. International Agency for Research on Cancer, IARC Monographs Programme or the Evaluation of Carcinogenic Risks to Humans, IARC, Lyon CEDEX 08, France. http://www.iarc.fr
26. International Programme on Chemical Safety, Environmental Health Criteria Documents, http://www.who.int/pcs/
27. Macher J, ed. Bioaerosols: assessment and control. Cincinnati: ACGIH, 1999.
28. Kromhout H, Symanski E, Rappaport SM. A comprehensive evaluation of within and between-worker components of occupational exposure to chemical agents. Ann Occup Hyg 1993; 37:253–70.
29. VanRooij JG, Bodelier-Bade MM, Hopmans PM, Jongeneelen FJ. Reduction of urinary 1-hydroxypyrene excretion in coke-oven workers exposed to polycyclic aromatic hydrocarbons due to improved hygienic skin protective measures. Ann Occup Hyg 1994; 38:247–56.
30. ACGIH/AIHA. Joint ACGIH-AIHA task group on occupational exposure databases, data elements for occupational exposure databases: guidelines and recommendations for air-borne hazards and noise. Cincinnati: ACGIH, 1997
31. Working Group on Exposure Registries in Europe. European proposal for core information for the storage and exchange of workplace exposure measurements on chemical agents. Appl Occup Environ Hyg 197; 12:31–9.
32. National Institute for Occupational Safety and Health. The industrial environment – its evaluation and control. Cincinnati: NIOSH, 1973.
33. ASHRAE. American Society of Heating, Refrigerating and Air-Conditioning Engineers, Standard 6202001, Indoor Air Quality, 2001.
34. American National Standard for Hand Protection Selection Criteria. ANSI/ISEA 105.
35. Forsberg K, Keith LH. Chemical protective clothing: performance index, 2nd edn. Cincinnati: ACGIH, 1999.
36. National Institute for Occupational Safety and Health. A guide for evaluating the performance of chemical protective clothing. Cincinnati: NIOSH, 1990.
37. Schwope AD, Costas PP, Jackson JO, Weitzman DJ. Guidelines for selection of chemical protective clothing, 3rd edn. Cincinnati: ACGIH, 1987.

4.2 Occupational Health Surveillance
Edward L Baker, Thomas P Matte

GENERAL PRINCIPLES

Surveillance is the ongoing, systematic collection, analysis, and interpretation of health data essential to the planning, implementation, and evaluation of public health practice, which is closely integrated with the timely dissemination of these data to those who need to know.[1] To be effective, surveillance must be directly linked to preventive action.[2,3] In the case of occupational health, the actions prompted by the surveillance system should be directed not only at the individual case or the affected group, but also at the responsible workplace factors.[4] Surveillance programs (i.e., secondary prevention) should be designed to support programs intended to control workplace hazards (i.e., primary prevention). In occupational safety and health,[5,6] surveillance programs should:

- identify cases of occupational illness or injury; and/or
- monitor trends of occupational illness or injury.

Identifying cases

The purpose of case identification is to target an intervention of direct value to the affected individual and to others at risk of developing the same disorder.[7] Case identification is followed by attempts to identify other individuals at risk and to control environmental factors that are responsible for causing disease. Case identification is found in three types of surveillance programs:

- medical screening;
- healthcare provider reporting; and
- employer case reporting.

Monitoring trends

Surveillance programs in the workplace can also be used to monitor trends of illness, injury, or exposure to workplace hazards.[8] In such activity, surveillance data are developed to assess variations in rates between (1) different industrial groups, (2) different geographic areas, and (3) different time periods. From such comparisons, health officials can identify target industries or geographic areas requiring further investigation or intervention.

In this way, surveillance of health or exposure trends is used to evaluate the efficacy of programs designed to control occupational hazards. Surveillance of occupational disease and injury can involve monitoring of either health effects among the workforce, or hazards present in the workplace.[9] In many situations, surveillance of individual health effects or workplace hazards alone may be useful.[10] Linkage of the data derived from health effects with hazard surveillance for the same population is even more desirable.[11]

Health effects surveillance

In surveillance of health effects, a system may target the actual health event[12,13] (i.e., the occurrence of an occupational injury or the diagnosis of a case of an occupational illness) or a change in a biologic function[14,15] of an exposed individual (e.g., loss of pulmonary function or disruption of heme metabolism). For surveillance purposes, occupational illnesses can be divided into two groups:

- disorders caused primarily by a single occupational exposure or hazard (e.g., lead poisoning[16] or silicosis); and
- disorders of multifactorial etiology for which occupational factors may serve as one of several causal factors (e.g., lung cancer[17]).

Further, occupational hazards may exacerbate a pre-existing health condition.

Surveillance of disorders caused by a single exposure or hazard can be accomplished by specifically identifying the condition and developing an approach to evaluate the health status of the worker and the worker's exposure history. Such diseases caused primarily by a single occupational exposure or hazard are termed occupational diseases by the World Health Organization (WHO). Surveillance of multifactorial diseases for which occupational factors may play a contributing role is seldom useful. Surveillance is made difficult by problems in diagnosis of the condition or in ascertainment of the relative importance of non-occupational factors in disease etiology. Control of such conditions is best accomplished by relying on primary control of the offending hazard through environmental measures and through the performance of hazard surveillance to monitor the effectiveness of such controls.

Hazard surveillance

Hazard surveillance consists of the periodic characterization of chemical or physical hazards in the workplace.[11] Such characterization can be accomplished by direct measurement of air-borne contaminants, using industrial hygiene procedures, or by indirect approaches for assessment of the degree of hazard present in the work environment. Because many chemical, physical, and biologic agents have been found to present a significant hazard to the health of workers, surveillance of the occurrences of hazards provides very useful information, even in the absence of simultaneous health status assessment. In many industries, certain types of hazard surveillance (i.e., direct measurement of levels of air-borne contaminants or noise level) are used to direct strategies for primary prevention.[18]

CONDUCT OF SURVEILLANCE
Use of medical screening data

Medical screening is the administration of a medical test for the purpose of detecting organ dysfunction or disease before the person would normally seek medical care and at a time when intervention is beneficial.[19] Screening tests may indicate the presence of a disease or merely a higher probability of disease and the need for additional, confirmatory testing.

If it is performed correctly, conduct of an occupational health-screening program is one of the most complex processes in medical practice. In designing the program, the practitioner must be familiar with clinical medicine and toxicology, and understand the importance of a standardized approach to data collection.[20–22] In analyzing and interpreting the data, the practitioner must be familiar with epidemiology and clinical decision analysis, and understand the applicability of industrial hygiene exposure measurements. Finally, in making recommendations based on these interpretations, the practitioner must be cognisant of existing laws and regulations and act ethically in situations in which conflicts of interest often exist.[23,24]

Screening tests have certain operational characteristics that should be considered in designing and evaluating workplace medical programs.

- The *sensitivity* of a screening test is the probability that it will detect diseased individuals (i.e., recognize their disease).
- The *specificity* of a screening test is the probability that it will not label as diseased individuals who are free of the disease in question.
- The *predictive* value of a positive screening test (sometimes referred to as the positive predictive value) is the probability that a person with an abnormal test truly has the disease. Conversely, the predictive value of a negative screening test (sometimes referred to as the negative predictive value) is the probability that a person who has a normal test result is truly free of disease. The determination of 'true' disease status requires the administration of a definitive diagnostic test to a screened population. The predictive value depends not only on the sensitivity and specificity of the test used, but also on the proportion of truly diseased people in the population being screened.
- The *reliability* or *reproducibility* of a screening test is its ability to produce consistent test results on repeated administration to the same person (unless, of course, the person's disease status has changed).

Surveillance versus screening – terminology

As described in the definitions given earlier, the term surveillance encompasses a broad range of activities that includes monitoring the results of screening. The term medical surveillance in Occupational Safety and Health Administration (OSHA) Standards corresponds reasonably well in usage with the term screening.[19] The process of medical surveillance, or screening, involves direct medical evaluations of individuals at risk for the development of certain disorders. 'Surveillance' describes any use of health or exposure data to identify cases or monitor trends; screening is one source of health data.

Purpose of medical screening and biologic monitoring

The main focus of workplace medical examination programs should be screening to benefit individual workers. In the context of the workplace, screening tests are used to identify toxic health effects at an earlier stage than they would be identified without screening. Target conditions should be those for which interventions, such as reducing worker exposure to the offending agent and/or medical treatment, are more beneficial when applied early in the disease process. Thus, the principal objective of workplace medical screening is secondary prevention of disease in the people who are screened. Screening can also be used to establish the work-relatedness of a previously diagnosed condition and to generate data for use in the surveillance of groups of workers.

Biologic monitoring

Biologic monitoring is the measurement and assessment of workplace agents or their metabolites in biologic specimens (e.g., blood and urine), to evaluate exposure and absorption by all routes (i.e., inhalation, percutaneous, or ingestion). Biologic monitoring results, collected as part of a screening program, can be used to supplement the results of exposure monitoring.[19]

A general approach to the performance of screening programs

Design and conduct of a screening program should follow 13 steps[7] (Table 4.2.1). In addition to following these steps to screen individuals, the data collected can be aggregated for analysis of the health status of a group with similar risks.

Step 1: Hazard assessment

Exposure levels and routes of absorption of the substances in the work environment should be ascertained to assess individual worker risk. Situations in which exposure mixtures are seen and workload varies widely complicate the process of hazard assessment considerably.

1. Assessment of workplace hazards
2. Identification of target organ toxicities for each hazard
3. Selection of a test for each screenable health effect
4. Development of action criteria
5. Standardization of the testing process
6. Performance of testing
7. Interpretation of test results
8. Test confirmation
9. Determination of work status
10. Notification
11. Diagnostic evaluation
12. Evaluation and control of exposure
13. Record keeping

Table 4.2.1 Process of designing and implementing a screening program

Step 2: Identification of target organ toxicity

Potential toxicity for each significant workplace hazard can be identified in the toxicology, industrial hygiene, and medical literature.[25] Such information may be limited, particularly with respect to meaningful human dose–response data. Recommendations of the National Institute for Occupational Safety and Health (NIOSH) or regulations promulgated by OSHA are often based on data that are limited in this regard.

Step 3: Selection of tests

For a health effect to be identified through screening, a test must be available that can detect the toxic health effect before it would normally cause a worker to present for medical attention (i.e., during the preclinical phase), and at a time when intervention (reduction of exposure and/or medical treatment) is more beneficial than for more advanced disease. Generally, the preclinical phase of an effect must be of sufficient duration (at least weeks or months) to be detected by a screening test given at feasible intervals. Screening is of little help in preventing acute, severe health effects, such as cyanide poisoning, because the preclinical phase is too brief to be detected. Some acute, but intermittent, health effects, such as solvent intoxication,[26] may be amenable to screening by questionnaire, because workers may recall symptomatic episodes at screening examinations weeks or months after they occur. This information may be useful, because such episodes may precede the development of chronic central nervous system toxicity.

Test selection also should be governed by the considerations of sensitivity, specificity, predictive value, and reliability, as defined above.[27] Often, tests used in clinical practice are found to be inadequate if considered in this way.

Step 4: Development of action criteria

When medical evaluation of workers is undertaken, the health professional designing the program should have a plan for how medical data are to be interpreted and acted on.[28] This plan should include criteria to determine when action will be taken in response to medical test results. To assist in the interpretation of the results of some screening tests, guidelines have been developed by consensus groups. These guidelines exist primarily for biologic monitoring tests (e.g., the biologic exposure index [BEI] developed by the American Conference of Governmental Industrial Hygienists [ACGIH]). In certain OSHA Standards, guidelines are provided for the interpretation of such tests (e.g., blood lead levels). Guidance in the interpretation of the significance of other tests can also be found in selected OSHA Standards (e.g., pulmonary function testing in the Cotton Dust Standard). Unfortunately, guidance is limited and inconsistent. For this and other reasons, OSHA has proposed a generic approach to medical surveillance that would create a more comprehensive and uniform approach to this complex process.

Pending the development of more comprehensive guidance, practitioners should establish, for their programs, criteria for action that apply to each test. In developing these criteria, practitioners should evaluate testing data to determine action levels that are statistically appropriate and biologically meaningful.

Step 5: Standardization of testing process

Staff should be trained in the proper performance of tests so that the results are interpretable. If adequate systems of quality control do not exist, data integrity over time cannot be ensured. Therefore, use of quality control systems and standardized tests is essential for optimum reliability and comparability.

Step 6: Test performance

Testing should be performed on a voluntary basis. Employees should be given information regarding the risks and benefits of testing and provide written evidence of informed consent to testing. Confidentiality of records should be protected through development of a record access control system, which ensures that only those who need to know the results will have access to them.

Step 7: Interpretation of test results

Tests conducted as part of a screening program should be interpreted in two different ways. First, results are compared against the predetermined action criteria to establish whether or not any *individual* action (e.g., removal from an exposure, referral for further tests) needs to be taken. At the same time, results of tests should be analyzed in the aggregate to determine whether or not there is any pattern indicating even subthreshold dysfunction, which would point to a potential workplace problem.[29] Is there any relation between the test results and a specific exposure? Do workers in one job category or area show altered (although possibly still normal) function relative to others? This aggregate interpretation may be as important or more important than the individual interpretation for determining what actions should be taken with the work environment itself.

Step 8: Test confirmation

Abnormal test results should be confirmed immediately, before further action is taken. At the discretion of the responsible person directing the program, the employee may be removed from exposure, pending results of confirmatory testing.

Step 9: Determination of work fitness

The proper use of medical testing in determining whether or not a worker should be removed from a hazardous job has received considerable attention and is subject to a proportional amount of controversy. If continued work exposure may further compromise the health of the worker, the worker should be removed from exposure, pending resolution of the health problem or abatement of the offending hazard. Because retention of salary and benefits may not be guaranteed following such 'medical removal', the physician should stress the importance of these protections to management if workers are expected to comply. In the US, OSHA has legislated these guarantees in some situations, such as in cases of overexposure to lead.

Step 10: Notification

Frequently, employees do not receive notification of the results of medical screening tests. Such notification should be prompt and informative, and strict confidentiality procedures should be followed. The implications of the test results should be explained by a qualified health professional in a manner that is clearly understood by the employee.

Step 11: Diagnostic evaluation

Screening tests rarely, if ever, provide a definitive diagnosis, and abnormal results should be evaluated according to good medical practice.[30] In some instances, further investigation may be limited to a more detailed medical history to clarify symptoms reported on a questionnaire. In other cases, referral to a specialist may be required.[31] The action plan should include conditions under which such referrals are indicated.

Step 12: Evaluation and control of exposure

When a toxic effect is established or strongly suspected from medical test results, the most important action is to initiate a re-evaluation of the work environment of the affected employee and, if indicated, make modifications to reduce exposure to levels that are safe for the affected person.[32] In such instances, notification of the employer is necessary. However, employers should only be provided with information that is relevant and necessary for evaluation and modification of the work environment, and every effort should be made to keep medical data confidential to the greatest extent feasible.

Once an employer has been notified of a screening result requiring evaluation of the work environment, a sequence of measures should be followed until the problem is resolved. This sequence should include measurement of air-borne levels, assessment of engineering controls (e.g., ventilation systems) and personal protective equipment, modifications in control measures as appropriate, and assessment of the effectiveness of modifications.

Once environmental modifications have been effected, it is again necessary to determine whether the worker can safely return to or remain in the exposed job. When an affected person is returned to an exposed job, frequent, ongoing medical evaluation may be recommended. Whenever an examining physician recommends that an employee be removed from an exposed job, the employee should be informed of the basis for the recommendation (i.e., the risk and severity of an adverse outcome if the employee remains in the exposed job).

Step 13: Record keeping

Medical records should include examination results, interpretations, and documentation of employee and employer notifications. In addition, employers should keep records of notifications they have received of the adverse effects detected by screening and of exposure evaluations and modifications they have carried out in response to such notifications.

Interpretation and action based on group test results

Results from individuals with similar exposure situations can be pooled to evaluate group health status. Such an evaluation is useful in evaluating the efficacy of control measures. At times, group analyses may reveal important information not provided by individual analyses alone. For example, although all measured levels of a test in an exposed group may be within normal limits, there may be a shift in the distribution, suggesting an early group effect. Practitioners have a responsibility to perform group analyses of screening data, because such analyses can identify potential breakdowns in hazard control programs before they would be evident from individual data. Unfortunately, such population surveillance is frequently not performed.

POLICY ISSUES[33]
Responsibilities

Physician responsibilities

Screening programs should be designed by and administered under the direction of a licensed physician, preferably one with training in occupational medicine. The physician, or another appropriately licensed healthcare provider, has a responsibility both to the employee being screened and to the employer. If these responsibilities generate conflicting courses of action, the physician's responsibility to the employee takes precedence in determining the course of action.

Physicians should provide all medical test results to the employee, along with an interpretation of the abnormal tests. The physician also has a responsibility to ensure that appropriate medical follow-up of abnormal test results occurs. Further, the physician has a responsibility to the employee to ensure that if worksite exposures were responsible for abnormal test findings, these exposures are controlled to an acceptable level before the employee returns to work.

Finally, the physician should ascertain whether or not the employee's coworkers with similar exposures are at risk, and if so, the appropriate action that should be taken (e.g., screening). When a physician recommends an employee be removed from a particular job because of health risks from further exposure, he or she should inform the employee of the basis of the recommendation, including any uncertainty about the benefits of removal.

Physicians should only provide to the management of the company information that is needed to guide management actions. In situations in which the medical department is part of the company (i.e., in-house medical center), specific procedures should be developed to control access to medical information by personnel officers and by other company personnel. Medical results should be released by management if such knowledge would prompt action to protect the health of employees. In such situations, the employee should be informed that disclosure will take place.

Employer responsibilities

In addition to providing unrestricted access to medical screening for employees at risk, employers should provide information to the responsible physician and should act on the results of tests when a workplace factor is implicated. Exposure information (e.g., job history and results of environmental sampling) should be provided to the physician. Information about applicable standards, material safety data sheets, and the extent of use of personal protective equipment should also be provided. Finally, the employer has the primary responsibility for maintaining a safe and healthful workplace.

Employee responsibilities

As in any medical evaluation, employees are responsible for providing accurate information (e.g., medical history) and for cooperating with medical testing procedures (e.g., providing full effort on pulmonary function testing). In those instances in which individual behavior, either job practices or personal habits, contributes to the development of a health problem, the individual should assume personal responsibility for changing the behavior to reduce the risk.

OSHA requirements

In the US, under existing OSHA Standards, employers are required to provide employees with access to medical screening examination when the employees are exposed to certain hazards (Table 4.2.2). Specific requirements for

2-Acetylaminofluorene
Acrylonitrile
4-Aminodiphenyl
Inorganic arsenic
Asbestos
Benzene
Benzidine
Bischloromethyl ether
Cadmium
Coal tar pitch volatiles
Coke oven emissions
Cotton dust
Dibromochloropropane
3,3'-Dichlorobenzidine
4-Dimethylaminoazobenzene
Ethylene oxide
Ethylenimine
Formaldehyde
Hazardous waste
Lead
Methylchloromethyl ether
Alpha-naphthylamine
Beta-naphthylamine
4-Nitrobiphenyl
Nitrosodimethylamine
Noise
Beta-propiolactone

Table 4.2.2 Hazards requiring medical surveillance by OHSA Standards

OSHA mandated surveillance is provided in Chapter 59. In a few instances, decision models are provided (e.g., Lead and Cotton Dust Standards) that guide physicians in their evaluation of results and in their recommendations for action. In most instances, little or no guidance is provided in the interpretation of results. OSHA requires that records be maintained for the duration of employment plus 30 years, and that access of the employee to his or her personal records be provided on request.

Healthcare provider case reporting

Regulations have been developed in many cities, states, and countries that instruct healthcare providers to report suspected cases of occupational illness or injury to an office of government. In some cases, consultation services are made available to assist in the investigation and remediation of the suspected causes of a case report. Requirements for reporting vary widely, and are not well publicized within the medical community. Further, healthcare providers often fail to report problems because, at times, no action is taken in following up the report.

To develop a systematic approach to the use of reports received from healthcare providers in the US, NIOSH developed the Sentinel Event Notification System for Occupational Risks (SENSOR).[12] The system consists of a network of sentinel healthcare providers who are linked to the state health department. In addition to developing a network of providers, the health department determines which conditions should be reported.

For each condition, reporting guidelines were developed to facilitate recognition of the case by the provider. Once reports are received and confirmed by the health department's surveillance centers, an active response occurs. Three possible actions may take place:
• management of the individual case;
• screening of coworkers with similar job exposures; and
• investigation of the worksite.

Monitoring injury, illness, and exposure trends

General considerations

Surveillance systems designed to monitor trends for occupational disorders or exposure usually rely on existing records collected for purposes other than surveillance. These records are coded or modified in some way to make them suitable for analysis. Each data source has certain limitations and advantages that must be considered in assessing the usefulness of the data for surveillance purposes.

Pre-existing healthcare and vital records

Many types of health records contain diagnostic information on conditions appropriate for surveillance. Death certificates[34,35] (including those of fetal deaths), birth certificates, hospital discharge records, office records of healthcare providers, and insurance claim files represent potential data sources for surveillance activities. Limitations include:

- information on the occupation of the patient is often not in the record;
- physicians often fail to recognize disorders caused by occupational hazards;
- there may be misclassification or omission of conditions and occupations of interest.

Advantages include:

- records are available at modest cost;
- records are coded using generally accepted code schemes (e.g., International Classification of Diseases).

The process of using healthcare provider records in surveillance may serve to improve awareness among healthcare providers of the impact of work on health, particularly in light of the emergence of the electronic medical record.

In summary, healthcare records, if collected and coded, can be useful sources of surveillance data. Death certificates, which contain information on the occupation of the deceased person, may be particularly useful if the occupational disease leads to mortality, given the limitations noted above.

Employer case reporting

In the US, employers are required by OSHA to record occurrences of occupational illness and injury on a form maintained at the worksite (called the OSHA log). The responsibility for completing this record often falls to an individual who has had no medical training and guidance in determining what should be recorded. Studies have shown that many disorders, particularly occupational illness, are not reported in the OSHA log.

Each year, the Bureau of Labor Statistics of the US Department of Labor collects a sample of these records from a portion of employers; certain categories of the workforce are not included in the survey. This sample is used to generate national estimates for selected conditions.

Workers' compensation data

Each state in the US maintains a workers' compensation system that generates data that could be used in surveillance.[36] To be entered into the system, a worker must recognize his or her condition as work related and file a claim. To receive compensation, the worker must also satisfy state regulations for eligibility, and successfully win a decision by the workers' compensation board.

Limitations of workers' compensation data for surveillance follow.

- In view of reporting disincentives and inherent difficulties in recognizing occupational disorders, workers' compensation data consistently underestimate the true rate of occurrence of occupational disorders. Furthermore, the rate of underestimation varies among conditions, with greater under-reporting of diseases than for occupational injuries.
- Workers' compensation laws vary from state to state. Many workers' compensation systems have requirements that claims be filed within a brief time period (e.g., within 1 year) following the suspected exposure; this requirement may present substantial barriers to

filing claims for occupational diseases of long latency (e.g., cancer).

Nevertheless, significant advantages to the use of workers' compensation data include the following.

- All records in the data set relate to conditions of suspected occupational etiology.
- Information on the job and the industry for each claimant is contained in the record.
- The circumstances of the illness or injury are frequently described in a way that provides understanding of the cause of the condition.
- If case identification leads to improvement of workplace conditions, prevention of further claims should occur, thus benefiting both the employee and the employer.
- If these data are used for surveillance purposes, technical improvements in the data management system (e.g., better coding procedures or computer systems) could occur that would benefit the management of the workers' compensation insurance system itself.

In summary, workers' compensation data represent an important source of surveillance data that can be used to monitor trends in the occurrence of selected occupational disorders and to identify cases for follow-up action.[16]

Biologic monitoring data

In selected situations, employers and healthcare providers obtain samples for biologic monitoring (e.g., blood or urine) from workers exposed to toxic substances. Typically, analyses are performed by one or only a few laboratories in a state. Data from the laboratory can be collected by a government agency and analyzed to monitor trends in exposure to selected toxic substances. This approach has certain limitations.

- Biologic assays exist for only a few substances.
- Quality control programs for these analyses may be limited.
- Participation in biologic monitoring programs is often limited to larger workplaces in which hazards are well controlled.
- Within workplaces that participate in a biologic monitoring program, individual workers may choose not to be tested.

Nevertheless, there are advantages to this approach.

- Each test (e.g., blood lead concentration) is a specific index of exposure to the toxic substance of interest.
- In states where commercial laboratories are required to report results to the state agency, data can be obtained widely and at low additional cost.

In summary, for certain substances (blood lead testing is by far the best example), biologic monitoring test results can be a useful source of surveillance data.

National health surveys

Different countries maintain different health survey systems. Each year in the US, the National Center for Health Statistics (NCHS) performs surveys of statistical samples of the population. Within each sample, a subset of employed persons can be identified. In each survey, health status data and occupational listing information are collected. The US Health Interview Survey (HIS) is a questionnaire survey that currently contacts 50,000 households, with 130,000 individuals. The National Health and Nutrition Examination Survey (NHANES) uses both a questionnaire and detailed medical tests to obtain health status information on 30,000 to 40,000 individuals. NIOSH collaborated with NCHS researchers to include tests in the NHANES III protocol which evaluate selected occupational disorders, such as lung disorders and neurotoxicity.

Exposure surveillance systems

Exposure surveillance can be performed using existing data or through the performance of worksite surveys.[37] Existing environmental data are most commonly developed as part of compliance inspections performed by the US Department of Labor (either OSHA or the Mine Safety and Health Administration, MSHA). Direct surveys have been performed by NIOSH: the National Occupational Hazard Survey, the National Occupational Exposure Survey, and the National Mining Survey. Each approach has important advantages in describing trends in exposure to hazards in the workplace.

References

1. Langmuir AD. William Farr: founder of modern concepts of surveillance. Int J Epidemiol 1976; 5:13-18.
2. Foege WH, Hogan RC, Newton LH. Surveillance projects for selected diseases. Int J Epidemiol 1976; 5:29-37.
3. Halperin W, Baker EL, Monson RR. Public health surveillance. New York: Van Nostrand Reinhold; 1992.
4. Baker EL, ed. Surveillance in occupational safety and health. Am J Public Health 1989; 79:1-63.
5. Halperin WE, Schulte PA, Greathouse DG, eds. Conference on medical screening and biologic monitoring for the effects of exposure in the workplace, part I. J Occup Med 1986; 28:543-788.
6. Rempel D, ed. Medical surveillance in the workplace. Occup Med 1990; 5:435-652.
7. Matte TD, Fine LJ, Meinhardt TJ, Baker EL. Guidelines for medical screening in the workplace. Occup Med 1990; 5:439-56.
8. Mason TJ, Prorok PC, Costlow RD, eds. Conference on medical screening and biologic monitoring for the effects of exposure in the workplace, part II. J Occup Med 1986; 28:901-1126.
9. Fine LJ. Surveillance and occupational health. Int J Occup Environ Health 1999; 5:26-9.
10. Frye L. Occupational health surveillance. We're making progress, but is it enough? AAOHN J 1997; 45:184-7.
11. Kauppinen T, Toikkanen J. Health and hazard surveillance – needs and perspectives. Scand J Work Environ Health 1999; 25(Suppl 4):61-7.
12. Baker EL. Sentinel Event Notification System for Occupational Risks (SENSOR): the concept. Am J Public Health 1989; 79:18-20.
13. Matte TD, Baker EL, Honchar PA. The selection and definition of targeted work-related conditions for surveillance under SENSOR. Am J Public Health 1989; 79:21-5.
14. Ross DJ, Keynes HL, McDonald JC. SWORD '97: Surveillance of work-related and occupational respiratory disease in the UK. Occup Med (Lond) 1998; 48:481-5.
15. Attfield MD, Wagner GR. Chronic occupational respiratory disease. Occup Med 1996; 11:451-65.
16. Seligman PJ, Halperin WE, Mullan RJ, Frazier TM. Occupational lead poisoning in Ohio: surveillance using workers' compensation data. Am J Public Health 1986; 76:1299-302.
17. Merler E, Bulatti E, Vainio H. Surveillance and intervention studies on respiratory cancers in asbestos-exposed workers. Scand J Work Environ Health 1997; 23:83-92.
18. Stayner L, Kuempel E, Rice F, Prince M, Althouse R. Approaches for assessing the efficacy of occupational health and safety standards. Am J Ind Med 1996; 29:346-52.
19. Murthy LL, Halperin WE. Medical screening and biologic monitoring. A guide to the literature for physicians. J Occup Environ Med 1995; 37:170-84.
20. Amler RW, Anger WK, Sizemore OJ. Adult environmental neurobehavioral test battery. Atlanta, Georgia: DHHS, PHS, ATSDR; 1995.
21. Metcalf SW, Samet J, Hanrahan J, Schwartz D, Hunninghake G. A standardized test battery for lung and respiratory diseases for use in environmental health field studies. Atlanta, Georgia: DHHS, PHS, ATSDR; 1994.
22. Straight JM, Kipen HM, Vogt RJ Jr, Amler RW. Immune function test batteries for use in environmental health field studies. Atlanta, Georgia; DHHS, PHS, ATSDR; 1994.
23. Van Damme K, Casteleyn L, Heseltine E, et al. Individual susceptibility and prevention of occupational diseases; scientific and ethical issues. J Occup Environ Med 1995; 37:91-9.
24. Ashford N, Miller C, eds. Chemical exposures: low levels and high stakes, 2nd edn. New York: Van Nostrand Reinhold; 1998.
25. Baker EL. A review of recent research on health effects of human occupational exposure to organic solvents: a critical review. J Occup Med 1994; 36:1079-92.
26. Seward JP. Medical surveillance of allergy in laboratory animal handlers. ILAR J 2001; 42:47-54.
27. Saxton JM. A review of current literature on physiologic tests and soft tissue biomarkers applicable to work-related upper limb disorders. Occup Med (Lond) 2000; 50:121-30.
28. Welch L, Roto P. Medical surveillance programs for construction workers. Occup Med 1995; 10:421-33.
29. Eisen EA. Methodology for analyzing episodic events. Scand J Work Environ Health 1999; 25(Suppl 4):36-42.
30. Mani L, Gerr F. Work-related upper extremity musculoskeletal disorders. Prim Care 2000; 27:845-64.
31. Dedhia HV, Rando RJ, Banks DE. Can we protect workers from developing the adverse respiratory effects of isocyanate exposure? Occup Med 2000; 15:399-410.
32. Burdorf A, Van Der Beek A. Exposure assessment strategies for work-related risk factors for musculoskeletal disorders. Scand J Work Environ Health 1999; 25(Suppl 4):25-30.
33. Boden LL. Policy evaluation: better living through research. Am J Ind Med 1996; 29:346-52.
34. Herbert R, Landrigan PJ. Work-related death: a continuing epidemic. Am J Public Health 2000; 90:541-5.
35. National Institute for Occupational Safety and Health. National traumatic occupational fatalities: 1980-1985. Washington, DC: DHHS, PHS, CDC; 1989; DHHS publication no (NIOSH) 89-116.
36. Goldsmith DF. Use of workers' compensation data in epidemiology research. Occup Med 1998; 13:389-415.
37. Wagner GR. Asbestosis and silicosis. Lancet 1997; 349:1211-15.

Chapter 5
Toxicology

David L Eaton

INTRODUCTION

Toxicology has been defined as 'the study of the adverse effects of chemicals on living organisms, and the assessment of the probability of their occurrence' (Society of Toxicology). The discipline of toxicology has evolved over the past century from one that focused primarily on the acute adverse effects of therapeutic agents in patient populations (a subdiscipline within the field of pharmacology) to one that includes consideration of the adverse effects on both health and the environment of the much larger universe of industrial chemicals found in the occupational and general environment. There are a variety of identifiable subdisciplines within the field of toxicology, although there is extensive overlap and integration among these areas. For example, the subspecialty of environmental toxicology originally was developed to investigate the adverse effects of chemical pollutants in the environment on human health, but in the past decade it has been used frequently to describe environmental perturbations from chemicals in the environment (e.g., aquatic toxicology, wildlife toxicology, and ecosystems toxicology). Occupational toxicology (sometimes referred to as industrial toxicology) focuses principally on chemical hazards in the workplace and is closely aligned with the disciplines of industrial hygiene and occupational medicine. Many toxicologists employed in academia, industry, and government direct their research efforts on understanding the cellular, biochemical, and molecular mechanisms of the toxicity produced by chemicals.

The mechanistic information provided by research toxicologists often provides the scientific basis that supports many of the more applied areas of toxicology. Forensic toxicology is generally viewed as a subdiscipline of pathology that relates primarily to the resolution of medicolegal issues surrounding the causal connections between injury or death of an individual and specific chemical exposures. Forensic pathologists are generally physicians employed by medical examiner's offices or large hospitals. Clinical toxicology focuses primarily on the biologic basis for chemical-induced injury, and implications for diagnosis and treatment; historically focusing on drugs and natural products (e.g., poisonous plants and animals). Clinical toxicologists are usually physicians, most often employed by hospitals, laboratories, and poison control centers. Regulatory toxicology is perhaps the newest subdiscipline of toxicology, and relates primarily to the use of toxicologic principles and data to establish regulatory standards aimed at reducing the adverse impacts of chemicals on human health or the environment. Although the background and training of professionals involved in these subdisciplines of toxicology may vary widely, there is nonetheless a common body of knowledge shared by all, and integral to the practice of clinical occupational and environmental medicine, which will be the focus of the remainder of this chapter.

Historically, the heavy metals, most notably lead, mercury, and the metalloid arsenic, presaged the advent of occupational and environmental toxicology. Throughout recorded history outbreaks of poisonings were recorded based on interpretation of simple epidemiological observations. For example, the variety of symptoms attributable to lead were recognized and traced to such sources as plumbing systems, the glazing of pottery, and additives to wines to improve taste. With the advent of the industrial revolution, still other avenues for exposure to lead appeared, such as vaporization, with bioavailability to the respiratory tract during a variety of industrial operations. Mercury and arsenic have both plagued humankind as toxic substances, as well as being used in a variety of processes to improve our lifestyle. As an example, consider the remarkably widespread historic use of mercury in medicinal salves, ointments, oral diuretics, as well as in powders applied to the gums of infants to remedy the purported effects of teething. After the dire consequences of mercury were recognized in the middle of the 19th century, acrodynia, or pink disease, a unique hypersensitivity reaction to mercury in children, totally disappeared from clinical experience, only to re-emerge recently following exposure to mercury in latex paints.[1] Similarly, as these same metals were combined with organic chemicals, still new symptom complexes were recognized, such as the neurological toxicity of tetraethyl lead, and the teratologic consequences of exposure to methyl mercury. Although concerns about the toxic potential of modern organic pesticides may be justified, one need only remember that prior to the advent of synthetic organic pesticides, arsenic (often as lead arsenate) enjoyed widespread use in the world of agriculture, with significant detrimental effects on health.

By the turn of the century, with the emergence of the science of chemistry and its analytic techniques, a variety of new chemicals were synthesized and older forms and formulations were characterized. Much progress occurred in identifying 'toxidromes', combinations of clinical signs and symptoms that were associated with human and animal exposures. Initially, the focus was on acute exposure, but more than 100 years ago, the effects of chronic exposure to mercury in the felt-hat industry were delineated. Pressure to curtail mercury exposure culminated in Lewis Carroll's famous classic *Alice in Wonderland*, and parliamentary action in Britain led to the elimination of mercury by the mid-1860s. Comparable public health measures were not adopted in the USA until shortly after the beginning of the Second World War, emphasizing the constant conflict between the risks and benefits of chemical use and associated health consequences.

In recent years the emphasis in toxicology has shifted to understanding the molecular basis by which chemicals induce adverse effects. The new field of 'toxicogenomics' has evolved through coupling of traditional toxicology with the recent advances in molecular biology and genomics. Toxicogenomics holds the promise of providing simple genetic tests that will identify individuals who are highly sensitive to workplace and environmental exposures to toxic substances. However, with such capabilities come many important ethical, social and legal issues, that themselves have spawned a new field of 'public health genetics'.[2]

DOSE–RESPONSE RELATIONSHIPS

The principal paradigm of toxicology was framed more than four centuries ago by Paracelsus (1493-1531), who stated that 'All substances are poisons; there is none which is not. Only the dose differentiates a poison from a remedy.' Regardless of the source - toxic plants, industrial pollution, or therapeutic drugs - the responses of biologic organisms to toxic substances often follow a similar pattern, commonly referred to as the dose–response relationship. This intuitively obvious concept, that the magnitude of response increases with the dose, can be graphically depicted, as shown in Figure 5.1. In a given individual chemical (known as an intrinsic toxin), there exists some dose below which there is no evidence of adverse effects. The body has a limited capacity to handle a certain amount of chemical insult before biologic function is compromised. The amount of this 'functional reserve capacity' can vary among individuals, and specific chemicals may readily exceed this capacity for specific organ systems at relatively small doses, whereas for other chemicals, a very large amount may be required before the 'threshold of safety' is exceeded.

For some substances, such as vitamins and minerals, which are essential for life, the dose–response curve takes on a biphasic shape. An inverse dose–response relationship is evident at 'low doses,' e.g., during vitamin or mineral deficiencies. Increasing the dose of these essential nutrients brings one into the region of homeostasis; however, toxicity can occur if the dose is too great and the threshold for toxicity is exceeded. This threshold may vary greatly among individuals in the population, and is influenced by many intrinsic factors, such as age, gender, weight, and genetic makeup, as well as extrinsic factors, such as exposure to other chemicals, diet, or personal habits, such as smoking or drinking. Because of such variation in response to chemicals, there are always individuals who respond at doses much lower than those of the average person, and others who are more resistant to toxicity with observable effects at

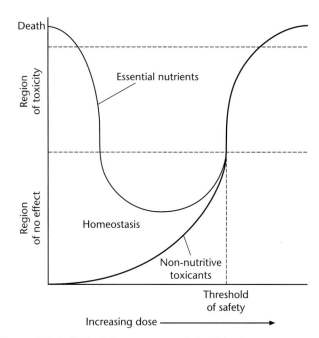

Figure 5.1: Individual dose–response relationship. dose–response curve for an individual exposed to either an essential substance or a non-nutritive substance. It is generally recognized that, for most intrinsic toxins, a threshold exists such that at doses below the threshold, no toxicity is evident. For essential substances, doses below the minimum daily requirement, as well as those above the threshold for safety, may be associated with toxic effects.

higher exposures. Today we recognize that many of such inter-individual differences are due to genetic factors.

The variation in population response to toxic chemicals often is presumed to follow a classic 'bell-shaped curve' (gaussian distribution, Fig. 5.2a), which is frequently depicted as a cumulative, quantal dose–response curve (Fig. 5.2b). These curves identify the response of a population to varying doses of a toxic chemical, with the midpoint of the curve representing the effective dose 50 or ED_{50}, that is, the dose at which 50% of the population responds. If the effect that is measured is death, then the ED_{50} is expressed as the lethal dose 50, or LD_{50}. For many years, the LD_{50} was used as the primary indicator of the relative toxicity of a chemical, and it can still be found as the principal measure of toxicity in many reference materials, such as material safety data sheets. It is important to recognize that the LD_{50} measures only the acute single-dose response to chemicals, and the only adverse response it reflects is mortality. It provides no meaningful insight into other types of non-lethal adverse responses, such as neurological effects, carcinogenic potential, teratogenic potential, reproductive effects, or other serious adverse effects that may occur at doses well below the LD_{50}. Furthermore, LD_{50} values are always based on laboratory animal data, and thus, they poorly reflect the diversity of human conditions and experiences that may drastically alter response to exposure. It is therefore never safe to assume that exposures far below the LD_{50} are harmless without much greater characterization of the types of effects a chemical may produce.

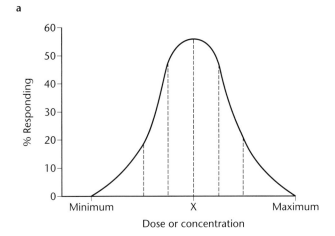

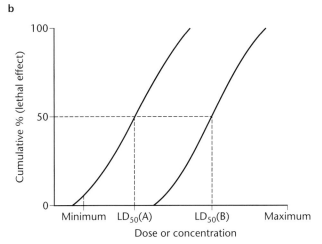

Figure 5.2: Frequency distribution and quantal dose–response relationship. Quantal dose–response curves for a population: a quantal (all or none) endpoint, such as death, is selected, and then the dose at which each individual in the population responds is determined. Curve (a) represents a frequency-response distribution curve for the quantal response of a 'normal,' or gaussian, distribution of responses among the population. Curve (b) plots the data for two different chemicals (A and B) as cumulative, quantal dose–response curves. The mid-point on the response curve represents the LD_{50} if the quantal response is death. (Adapted from Loomis TA. Essentials of toxicology, 3rd edn. Philadelphia: Lea & Febiger, 1978. © 1978, the Williams & Wilkins Co., Baltimore.)

TYPES AND NATURE OF ADVERSE RESPONSES
Acute and chronic toxicity

Humans generally respond to toxic chemicals in a manner similar to that of laboratory animals and usually in doses that are relatively similar on a body-weight basis (or, more accurately, on a dose per unit surface area basis). The variation of effects (e.g., hepatic necrosis, central nervous system depression, and renal damage) between different individuals, and between humans and laboratory animals, is generally predictable for a given chemical agent, although the doses necessary to produce characteristic symptoms may vary substantially. However, there are often individuals within a population who have some genetic variation that

causes them to respond at a dose far below the anticipated dose. This type of hyper-responsiveness is often referred to as an idiosyncratic response, and it is usually seen only in a small percentage of the population who are genetically predisposed to toxicity. Most chemical idiosyncratic responses that have been identified have been associated with administration of therapeutic drugs. For example, 3-5% of the population expresses a variant form of the gene that encodes for the enzyme protein pseudocholinesterase, which apparently plays little or no role in normal metabolism. However, when such individuals are administered the muscle-paralyzing drug succinylcholine for surgical procedures, they remain paralyzed for much longer periods of time (many hours) than does the average individual with adequate pseudocholinesterase levels (several minutes). This adverse response occurs because the pseudocholinesterase enzyme is primarily responsible for metabolizing succinylcholine; the genetic basis for poor metabolism has recently been characterized.[3]

Other common genetically determined drug idiosyncratic reactions include significant differences in the rates of acetylation (and thus deactivation) of certain amines and amides, such as phenytoin, isoniazid, and hydralazine, as well as deficiencies in glucose-6-phosphate dehydrogenase, which can result in a severe hemolytic response following exposure to a variety of oxidizing pharmaceuticals and non-pharmaceutical chemicals. Numerous other examples of genetically determined hypersusceptibility to the adverse effects of drugs and non-drug chemicals have been described, and may be important in determining susceptibility to cancer and birth defects.[4] Although such examples of idiosyncratic reactions are relatively rare for non-drug chemicals, it is certain that they do occur and one must always be alert to this possibility when a patient experiences symptoms of toxicity, even though others around him or her show no apparent effect.

Allergic reactions

In addition to the dose-related and idiosyncratic responses, some individuals may develop allergic reactions to chemicals. Although the incidence of this is usually small, for those substances capable of producing immunologic reactions, it can have important consequences. Unlike normal toxicologic responses, allergic reactions do not follow the classic population dose–response curve. In contrast, allergic individuals respond at doses far below those of non-allergic individuals; even within an allergic population, the magnitude of response is not always clearly dose-related. However, in a particular allergic individual, the development of an allergen response is usually related to the magnitude of exposure. In contrast to normal toxicological responses, individuals must first become sensitized, as the allergic response is dependent on the presence of specific antibodies that are directed against the chemical antigen (allergens). Many chemicals of environmental and occupational concern are not sufficiently large to stimulate the immune system directly, but must first combine with an endogenous protein. The chemical is then referred to as a

Classification	Examples	Mechanism
Type I anaphylaxis (immediate hypersensitivity)	Asthma, urticaria, rhinitis, atopic dermatitis	IgE bound to mast cell/basophil triggers release of soluble mediators (e.g., histamine)
Type II cytolytic	Hemolytic anemia, Goodpasture's syndrome	IgG and/or IgM binds to cells and results in destruction by complement, opsonization, or antibody-dependent cellular cytotoxicity
Type III Arthus	Systemic lupus erythematosus, glomerular nephritis, rheumatoid arthritis, serum sickness	Antigen-antibody complexes deposit in various tissues and may then fix complement
Type IV delayed-type hypersensitivity	Contact dermatitis, tuberculosis	Sensitized T lymphocytes induce a cell-mediated response

Adapted from Dean JH, Murray MJ. Toxic responses for the immune system. In Amdur MD, Doull J, Klaasen CD, eds. Casarett and Doull's Toxicology: the basic science of poisons, 4th edn. New York: Pergamon Press, 1991;282–333.

Table 5.1 Gell and Coombs classification scheme of allergy

hapten, and the chemical-protein complex becomes the antigen. After an antigen is formed, the production of antibodies requires several weeks following this first, or sensitizing, exposure. However, once antibodies have been formed, a subsequent exposure may result in a rapid and severe allergic response, involving one or more organ system's responses (Table 5.1).

A Type I, or immediate hypersensitivity, reaction is associated with the immunoglobulin (Ig)E-triggered release of endogenously active substances such as histamine from mast cells, most commonly presenting as rhinitis, asthma or atopic dermatitis. Far less commonly, it may result in angioedema or fatal anaphylactic shock. Occupational asthma from platinum salts and trimellitic anhydride are well-described Type I reactions but may also be associated with non-immunological responses. Other pulmonary irritants, such as formaldehyde, may produce asthmatic symptoms from a direct irritant effect on the airways, or non-IgE-related immune responses.[5] Other antibodies, such as IgG and IgM, when activated by an antigen, may interact with tissues to generate cytolytic processes (Type II reactions).

The major targets of Type II reactions are circulating cells, such as erythrocytes and white blood cells, but type II reactions may also occur in other tissues, such as lung and kidney. For example, Goodpasture's syndrome results from the development of cytolytic antibodies directed against basement membrane proteins in the kidney, and is generally thought to be an autoimmune condition,[6] although there is some suggestion that exposure to some solvents and other nephrotoxic agents can induce this response through cross-reactivity of the immune response with basement membranes.[7] Type III, or Arthus, reactions, are mediated by IgG, with resultant antigen-antibody-complement complexes being contained in the circulation, rather than fixed to tissues. The circulating immune complex becomes deposited in the vascular endothelium, producing a destructive inflammatory response. This type of reaction is most commonly associated with autoimmune diseases, such as systemic lupus erythematosus and rheumatoid arthritis, and is presumed to stem from endogenous antigens. However, this response can also result from exposure to exogenous antigens, especially

exogenous proteins (e.g., serum sickness produced by horse antiserum). Type IV, or delayed-type hypersensitivity, reactions, which are cell-mediated reactions, are relatively common with exposure to environmental and industrial chemicals, and may manifest as contact dermatitis. Type IV allergic reactions to latex rubber have become one of the most common occupational health complaints in the healthcare industry.[8,9]

Although allergic and idiosyncratic reactions occur in a relatively small percentage of the total population, they represent a significant portion of the adverse responses to chemicals found in selected workplaces with exposure to allergenic materials, as well as in workplaces with engineering controls limiting exposure to protect the majority of workers.

Carcinogenicity

The potential for the occupational environment to induce cancer has been recognized since Sir Percival Pott first identified scrotal cancer as an occupational disease among chimney sweeps in the 1700s. It was not until the early part of this century, however, that certain polyaromatic hydrocarbons (common chemical components of soots, tars, and oils) were identified as the probable carcinogenic agents in this industry. Since that time, there has been increasing concern regarding the potential carcinogenic effects of a variety of chemicals in the environment. The strong associations of asbestos with diffuse malignant mesothelioma and primary lung cancer, vinyl chloride with angiosarcoma of the liver, and certain aromatic amines with bladder cancer, stimulated the search for other possible associations between occupational and environmental chemical exposure and cancer.

There are numerous other chemicals for which substantial epidemiologic evidence exists to link occupational exposures with cancer. However, relative to the approximately 60,000 chemicals in commercial use in the United States, their number is currently small. The International Agency for Research on Cancer (IARC) has reviewed the literature on approximately 860 putative carcinogenic agents (chemicals, processes, infectious agents).[10] IARC currently lists 89 different chemicals, mixtures or chemical processes for which it judged there was adequate scientific evidence of carcinogenicity in humans (Group 1 carcinogens). Of these, 39 were occupationally related, 31 were pharmaceutical chemicals or radiation, 10 were infectious agents (e.g., hepatitis B, human papilloma virus), and nine were associated with diet or lifestyle (e.g., ethyl alcohol, aflatoxin and smoking). IARC identified another 64 chemicals for which the scientific data suggested probable, but not conclusive, evidence of carcinogenicity in humans (Group 2A), and another 236 chemicals that were possibly carcinogenic in humans, based primarily on laboratory animal studies (Group 2B). Nearly 500 chemicals or processes of industrial and pharmaceutical importance were identified by IARC for which there is some suspicion of carcinogenic potential, but for which the scientific evidence for carcinogenic potential remains inadequate (Group 3). Because exposure data are often inadequate, and limited to small numbers of cases (primarily because of the long latency period between exposure and development of cancers, requiring many years), it is extremely difficult to definitively characterize a specific chemical as a human carcinogen, against a high background incidence of cancer. Much of the data implicating chemicals as human carcinogens have been derived from laboratory animal studies, but some are a result of epidemiologic studies relating occupation to an increased risk of specific types of cancer. In some instances a process, rather than a specific chemical, has been linked to an increased incidence of cancer.

Although the precise biologic processes involved in the development of cancer are not fully understood, there is a consensus that chemical carcinogenesis is a multistep process.[11,12] The first step, referred to as initiation, involves the binding of the chemical to DNA (Fig. 5.3). Most chemicals lack the reactivity necessary to covalently bind to DNA, but in the process of biotransformation, reactive electrophilic intermediates may be formed that bind avidly to nucleophilic sites in DNA. Genetic differences in the ability to activate or detoxify chemical carcinogens are often considered one of the most likely reasons for inter-individual and inter-species differences in susceptibility to chemical carcinogens.[13] Most DNA damage is either inconsequential, lethal to the cell, or produces damage that is efficiently repaired by special DNA repair enzymes. However, some DNA adducts may escape repair, or be repaired incorrectly, and thus introduce a mutation into the cell. If this mutation is at a site important to the regulation of cellular replication, it may result in the loss of cellular growth regulation.

It is now recognized that there are certain genes present in all cells, called proto-oncogenes, which, when activated by mutation, transform a normal cell into a precancerous cell. Similarly, there are genes that act to suppress cell replication and, consequently, tumor growth, called tumor-suppressor genes. The mutation of tumor-suppressor genes appears to be a major factor in many types of malignancies. One particular gene, called p53, is mutated from the wild type in a high percentage of human malignancies.[14] The product of this gene appears to function as a check-point in the regulation of the cell cycle, ensuring adequate time for DNA damage to be repaired prior to cell division. In the absence of this regulation (e.g., mutated p53), cells can replicate before the DNA damage is repaired, passing on their mutations to daughter cells.

Precancerous, or latent, carcinoma cells may exist in a quiescent stage in tissues for many years. Many times, such transformed cells often express surface proteins that are recognized as abnormal to the immune system, and antibodies are generated that facilitate the destruction of these cells. However, if immune surveillance is ineffective or incomplete, these cells may begin to proliferate into tumors and eventually metastasize to distant sites. The multiple steps from initiation to early neoplastic foci and tumor development (promotion) to metastatic carcinomas (progression) are not well understood, although it is recognized that some chemicals can enhance the rate of these later processes. Chemicals that stimulate the development and growth of already initiated precancerous cells are often called promoters (Fig. 5.3). Promotion is often associated with stimuli that enhance the rate of cell division (e.g., mitogenic) and inflammatory responses. Thus, an increase in the rate of cell division and attendant DNA replication in a normally quiescent cell population greatly increases the chances of the fixation of mutations that arise continuously from natural processes and environmental mutagens. Therefore, drugs or other chemicals that enhance cell proliferation (the rate of cell division) may augment the expression of mutations accumulated over time, increasing the opportunity for mutated cells to expand in number and acquire additional mutations.[15]

Some chemicals may act as co-carcinogens, i.e., by themselves, they are incapable of inducing cancer but when given before or during exposure to initiators, they increase the potency or effectiveness of the carcinogen. Although promoters fit within this definition, the term co-carcinogen is usually reserved to describe chemicals that alter the effectiveness of protective pathways in the multistep process leading from initiation to tumor motion. For example, many chemicals can alter the relative fraction of procarcinogen that is activated to the ultimate carcinogenic form, by inducing competing inactivation pathways or inhibiting activation pathways. Likewise, chemicals that suppress immune function or alter the efficiency or accuracy of DNA repair processes, enhance the carcinogenic potency of other carcinogens and increase rate of tumor formation.

Chemicals that increase the incidence of cancer by promotional mechanisms are generally considered to respond in a threshold fashion; that is, they will not enhance tumor response at doses below that necessary to increase the rate of cell division. In contrast, chemicals that induce cancer through mutagenic processes (initiators) are often considered to act in a non-threshold fashion, that is, the incidence of cancer is directly proportional to the dose of carcinogen even at very low doses. Such a linear non-threshold model has important public health consequences, as there is theoretically no dose below which the probability of cancer becomes zero. The distinction

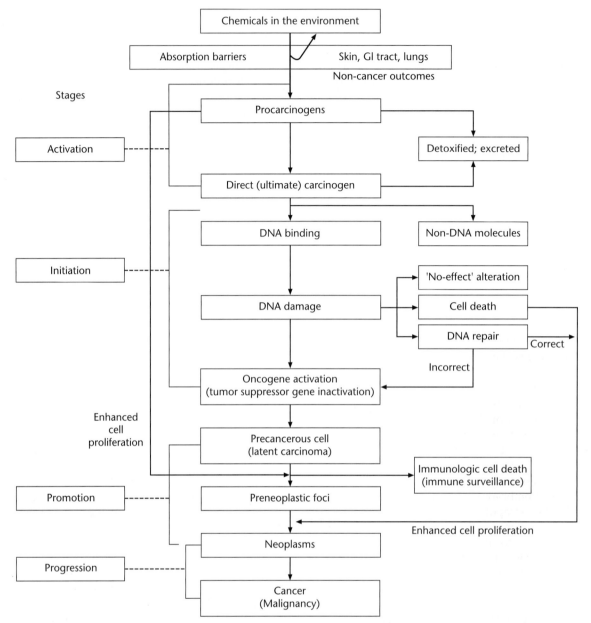

Figure 5.3: Process of chemical carcinogenesis. Carcinogenic chemicals must undergo a number of sequential events in order to produce tumors. Most chemicals require biotransformation to reactive intermediates (activation) before being able to induce somatic mutations. Mutation of a gene involved in cellular growth and differentiation (oncogene) often is referred to as initiation, whereas the stimulation of clonal expansion of the mutated cell to a colony of cells containing the mutated oncogene is referred to as promotion. Cells within this population may acquire additional mutations favoring growth, dedifferentiation, or both, ultimately leading to the development of cancers. This later stage is commonly referred to as tumor progression, and it may involve many successive changes in phenotype leading to increasing degrees of malignancy (e.g., benign to invasive to metastatic).

between chemicals that act by threshold processes (e.g., promoters) and chemicals that act through non-threshold mechanisms (e.g., initiators) also has potentially profound regulatory implications, as discussed later in this chapter.

Reproductive and developmental effects

With the increasing number of women of child-bearing age entering the industrial workforce, concern over the potential for occupational and/or environmental chemical exposures to produce reproductive disorders and birth defects has heightened during the last few decades. Because the developing embryo is often exquisitely sensitive to toxic substances, it is necessary to consider women of child-bearing age as being at particularly high risk for toxic chemical exposures, and efforts must be made to make the workplace safe for this important sector of the workforce. Many causes of birth defects, such as maternal malnutrition, medications, alcohol, genetic factors, and infectious agents, have been identified, but the etiology of 65-70% of all human birth defects remains unknown (Table 5.2; see Chapter 27.2).

Known genetic transmission	20%
Chromosomal aberration	3–5%
Environmental causes	
Radiation	<1%
– Therapeutic	
– Nuclear	
Infections	2–3%
– Rubella virus	
– Cytomegalovirus	
– Herpesvirus hominis	
– Toxoplasma	
– Syphilis	
Maternal metabolic imbalance	1–2%
– Endemic cretinism	
– Diabetes	
– Phenylketonuria	
– Virilizing tumors	
Drugs and environmental chemicals	7–10%
– Ethanol	
– Androgenic hormone	
– Folic antagonists	
– Thalidomide	
– Organic mercury	
– Some hypoglycemics	
– Some anticonvulsants	
Potentiative interactions	Unknown
Unknown	60–65%

Table 5.2 Known causes of developmental defects in humans

Literally hundreds of chemicals have been identified as having the ability to cause birth defects, usually at high doses in laboratory animals, but the list of documented human teratogens remains surprisingly small, of the order of 10-20, with many of these subject to debate. The large inter-species differences in sensitivity to some teratogens is of critical importance; moreover, the timing of the exposure and stage of embryonic development has made reliable, quantitative extrapolation of animal data to humans challenging. For example, the drug thalidomide, which was used in Europe to ameliorate nausea and vomiting during the early stages of pregnancy, was found to produce an extraordinarily high incidence of a rare birth defect, phocomelia (failure of limbs to develop) among the offspring of women who took this drug during a specific period early in their pregnancies. Only later was it found that humans are about 700 times more sensitive to the teratogenic effects of thalidomide than is the hamster, and 100 times more sensitive than the rat. Recently, thalidomide has resurfaced as a potentially valuable drug in the treatment of a variety of infectious and malignant conditions (e.g., thyroid cancer), although obviously great care must be taken to prevent its use in pregnant women.[16]

Even though inter-species differences complicate the interpretation of laboratory animal studies to predict human risks, there are some basic concepts regarding the teratogenic response that appears to be true in all animals, including humans. First, the age of development of the embryo at the time of exposure to the teratogen is very important. The period of greatest sensitivity to chemical teratogens is during the first trimester of pregnancy (Fig. 5.4), a time of maximal cell differentiation.

In humans, this highly sensitive period for teratogenic effects extends generally from about 2 weeks through 12 weeks gestation. Exposures to many toxic substances during the first 2 weeks of embryonic development are likely to result in the death of the embryo, and it is probable that the woman would not even be aware that she was pregnant due to early miscarriage. Exposure to teratogens occurring beyond the tenth to twelfth week of pregnancy are far less likely to result in physical or morphologic abnormalities because major morphologic characteristics (extremities, palate, ribs, and organs) have been formed. However, other developmental problems, particularly relating to the nervous system, may result from exposure during the later stages of fetal development, because the brain is not fully differentiated and developed until after birth. Methyl mercury, lead, and alcohol are all examples of chemicals that can affect the developing nervous system in utero during the later stages of pregnancy.

The second important factor relating chemical exposure to teratogenic responses is the dose of the teratogen.[17] Most, if not all, toxic substances can adversely affect the developing embryo and/or fetus, either directly, or indirectly if it produces a maternal toxic response. What generally defines whether a chemical is truly teratogenic is whether it affects embryonic and/or fetal development at a dose below that which produces maternal toxicity. As with other types of responses, teratogenicity follows the dose–response relationship for a population, although often the slope of this curve is exceedingly steep, e.g., the dose range is very small between no effect in the population and a very high percentage of the population responding. Although a steep dose–response curve argues for the concept of a threshold dose in experimental animals, it is very difficult to extrapolate such information to the human situation. Furthermore, because of the very wide genetic variability among individuals within the human population, relative to the highly inbred characteristics of laboratory animals, it is likely that the threshold for teratogenic response will

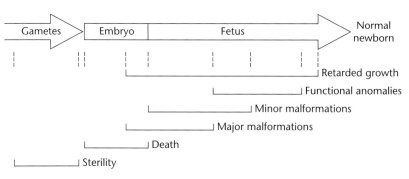

Figure 5.4: Sensitivity of the developing organism to birth defects. The period of development from fertilization to parturition is an important factor in reproductive toxicity. Damage to gametes usually results in infertility or early embryonic loss rather than frank birth defects. Exposure of the embryo during the early period of organogenesis may produce major malformations (teratogenic effects), whereas exposure during later periods of gestation more commonly produces functional anomalies and retarded growth.

vary more substantially among humans, making it more difficult to establish a safe level of exposure for everyone. Because of our relative ignorance about the causes of most birth defects and the likely high sensitivity of the developing fetus to some toxic chemicals, a high degree of caution in establishing so-called 'safe levels' of exposure for pregnant women is appropriate.

FACTORS THAT INFLUENCE TOXIC RESPONSES
Absorption

Although the terms exposure and dose are often used interchangeably, the two are substantially different. The term exposure has seldom been carefully defined, but generally, it connotes the amount or concentration of a pollutant present in air, water, soil, or other medium that potentially can be transferred to a subject. Dose, in contrast, generally refers to the quantity of material present in the medium of potential transfer that has actually passed from the medium into the organism. Different adjectives are sometimes provided to add more precision to these terms, such as exposed dose, administered dose, target dose, internal dose, and biologically available dose.[18] A term frequently used in pharmacokinetics to describe the variation in the amount of exposed dose that is actually absorbed into the bloodstream (e.g., becomes systemically available) is referred to as its bioavailability. Conceptually, bioavailability is simply the fraction of the exposed dose that is absorbed. Thus, for example, ingestion of 100 mg (0.1 g) of soil containing 10 ppm of cadmium (10 micrograms of Cd per gram of soil) would result in an exposure (exposed dose or administered dose) of 1 microgram of Cd. Because the bioavailability of Cd through the gastrointestinal tract is only about 5-8%,[19] the systemic or internal dose would only be 0.05-0.08 micrograms. The route of exposure (transdermal, gastrointestinal, or respiratory) is a critical determinant of the systemic dose, because some substances may be well absorbed by one route but poorly absorbed by another. For example, elemental mercury in its metallic form is extremely poorly absorbed following ingestion, yet inhalation of elemental mercury vapors results in rapid and nearly complete absorption by the respiratory tract.

There are several basic principles that dictate the extent of absorption of a substance at any given site of exposure. Because most toxic substances are absorbed by the process of simple diffusion, Fick's law of diffusion adequately describes the critical physicochemical parameters that influence absorption:

$$v_0 = dX/dt = \frac{PA}{d}(c_0 c_i)$$

where v_0 = the rate of flux of compound across the membrane, P = the permeability coefficient, A = the surface area available for diffusion, d = the diffusion distance (thickness of the diffusion barrier), and $(c_0 c_i)$ = the concentration gradient between the outside (c_0) and inside (c_i) of the compartment separated by the diffusion barrier.

Thus, for absorption of substances across the gastrointestinal, dermal, or pulmonary epithelium, where uptake occurs by simple diffusion, it is evident that the extent of absorption should be directly proportional to the surface area exposed, the concentration gradient, and the length of time over which exposure occurs, and inversely proportional to the thickness of the particular diffusion barrier. The permeability coefficient, P, is an arbitrary constant that is determined by both the physicochemical characteristics of the chemical and the particular diffusion barrier. Although small (molecular weight <100 Daltons) water-soluble molecules may pass with water directly through pores in biologic membranes, for the majority of toxic substances translocation across a biologic membrane occurs by diffusion through the lipid membrane. Because the diffusion barriers of skin, gastrointestinal, and pulmonary epithelium are principally lipid in nature, there tends to be a strong correlation between the permeability coefficient determined experimentally and the lipid solubility of the chemical. Lipid solubility, as determined by octanol/water partition coefficients (K_{ow}, unitless values that represent the ratio of a solute between two nonmiscible solvents, octanol and water, at equilibrium), frequently is used as a crude predictor of bioavailability for chemicals about which little experimental data are available. Chemicals that are highly lipid soluble are in general well absorbed, whereas highly water-soluble substances are generally poorly absorbed. However, the relationship between the partition coefficient (K_{ow}) and the permeability coefficient is most appropriately described as hyperbolic (Fig. 5.5).[20]

At low log K_{ow} values (e.g., low lipid solubility and high water solubility), chemicals cannot adequately diffuse through membranes. At log K_{ow} values between 1 and 10, substances are sufficiently water soluble to diffuse through the aqueous environment surrounding the cell barrier, yet

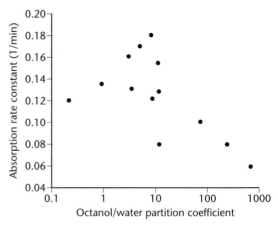

Figure 5.5: Relationship between partition coefficient (K_{ow}) and rate of absorption. Highly water-soluble chemicals (e.g., K_{ow}<0.01) are generally poorly absorbed across the intact epidermis. Chemicals that exhibit characteristics of both water and lipid solubility (e.g., K_{ow} between 0.1 and 10) tend to have the highest transdermal absorption rates, whereas highly lipid-soluble chemicals (e.g., K_{ow}>100) may partition into lipids in the epidermis and are only slowly absorbed into the systemic circulation.

they are also adequately lipid soluble to diffuse readily across the lipid membranes. Substances with very high log K_{ow} values may be unable to diffuse adequately through the aqueous unstirred layer that surrounds biologic membranes. Thus, organic chemicals that are highly lipid soluble but also sparingly soluble in water, such as some organophosphate insecticides, are generally well absorbed by either dermal or gastrointestinal routes and may have dermal LD_{50} values that are close to those of the oral route.

Because the permeability coefficient is closely correlated with lipid solubility, the absorption of weak organic acids and bases is greatly influenced by the pH at the site of absorption. The extent of ionization of a weak acid or base is a function of both the pH and the pKa for the chemical, as described by the Henderson-Hasselbalch equation:

$$\text{For weak acids, pKa - pH} = \log \frac{[\text{non-ionized}]}{[\text{ionized}]}$$

$$\text{For weak bases, pKa - pH} = \log \frac{[\text{ionized}]}{[\text{non-ionized}]}$$

Thus, weak organic acids, which generally have pKa values between 3 and 4, exist predominantly in the lipid-soluble, non-ionized form at pH values less than 3, whereas weak organic bases (pKa values usually between 6 and 8) are in the ionized, water-soluble form at low pH. From this, one might assume that weak organic acids would be primarily absorbed in the stomach, with a pH of 2 to 3, relative to the intestine with a pH of 6 to 7. Although the rate of absorption is higher in the stomach, the extent of absorption is often greater in the small intestine because both the time of contact and the total surface area are much greater in the intestine than in the stomach.

Because there are specific features of each common route of exposure, and an understanding of these differences can have important practical clinical implications in both the preventive measures used to reduce absorbed dose and in the management of poisoning, each route is discussed separately.

Absorption by the gastrointestinal tract

The gastrointestinal tract functions physiologically as an organ of absorption; therefore, it is not surprising that many chemicals are well absorbed when ingested. In contrast to drug intoxications and attempted suicides by poisoning, however, gastrointestinal absorption is not the most common route of exposure in the occupational environment. Nevertheless, secondary ingestion of toxic substances by hand-to-mouth contact or mucociliary clearance of contaminants collected in the upper respiratory tract can be a major route of exposure in the occupational environment. Ingestion of contaminated food and water also is a common route of exposure to environmental pollutants.

As noted, although the stomach can serve as a site of absorption for most chemicals, especially weak acids, the majority of absorption occurs in the small intestine.[21,22] In humans, the combined length of the duodenum, jejunum, and ileum is about 2.7 m. The inner surface of the intestine

pH
Acid and other secretory products (e.g., proteolytic enzymes, mucus, and lipases)
Gastric and intestinal contents
Gastric and intestinal motility
Bile salts and other constituents of bile
Bacterial flora

Table 5.3 Factors that influence gastrointestinal bioavailability

contains numerous villi of about 0.5 to 1 mm in length and 0.1 mm in diameter. There are approximately 25 villi per square millimeter of surface, and the villi are covered with a simple columnar epithelium. These cells, called enterocytes, make up 90% of the surface area of the small intestine and contain a brush border membrane of microvilli. The total absorptive surface area (villi and microvilli) of the small intestine in humans is thus about 200 m^2. The colon also is a site of absorption in humans, principally of water, sodium, and other minerals. The length of the human colon is about 1.1 m, and it does not contain villi, although transverse folds enhance the total surface area.

In addition to the large surface area and relatively thin diffusion distance (one cell layer) of the gastrointestinal tract, blood flow to the small intestine is relatively high, receiving about 6-7% of the cardiac output in usual circumstances. This increases substantially after a meal, with the increase in blood flow specifically directed to the mucosal area. The high rate of blood flow through the intestine quickly removes absorbed substances such that the concentration gradient from the intestinal lumen to the circulation is nearly maximal, enhancing the rate and extent of absorption.

There are numerous factors that can influence the extent of absorption of toxic substances in the gastrointestinal tract (Table 5.3). An important consideration for the absorption, and even toxic characteristics, of some chemicals is the presence of a high concentration of anaerobic bacteria in the colon. These bacteria may themselves metabolically alter drugs and chemicals, with consequent changes in both bioavailability and toxicity. For example, the presence of β-glucuronidase-containing bacteria in the gut can result in the hydrolysis of highly polar glucuronide conjugates of toxic substances excreted in the bile. Hydrolysis of the glucuronide conjugate returns the chemical to a lipid-soluble, bioavailable form where it can be reabsorbed.[23]

Early in life, the bacterial flora of the intestine is different in infants receiving only breast milk or formula, and is efficient at reducing inorganic nitrate to nitrite. In contrast, this bacteria-mediated reduction does not occur to any significant extent in adults. Thus, consumption of well water containing inorganic nitrate (e.g., 100 ppm) is of little consequence to the human adult but can result in serious or even fatal methemoglobinemia in infants.

Absorption of chemicals across the skin

In contrast to the gastrointestinal tract, the physiologic function of the skin is to act primarily as a barrier to the absorption of exogenous substances from the environment

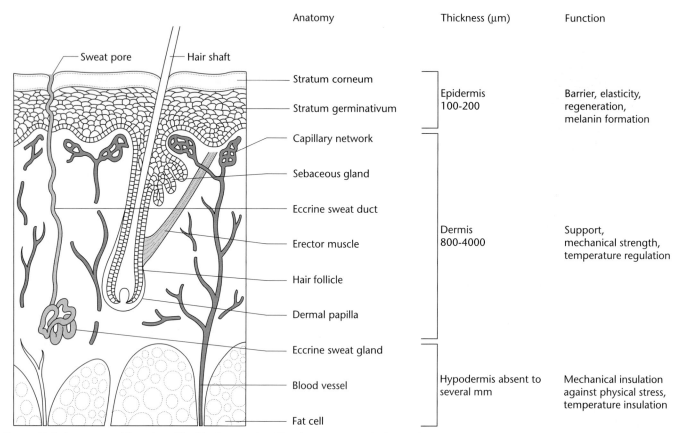

Anatomy   Thickness (µm)   Function

Anatomy	Thickness (µm)	Function
Epidermis	Epidermis 100-200	Barrier, elasticity, regeneration, melanin formation
Dermis	Dermis 800-4000	Support, mechanical strength, temperature regulation
Hypodermis	Hypodermis absent to several mm	Mechanical insulation against physical stress, temperature insulation

Figure 5.6: Anatomy and function of healthy human skin. The skin is composed of several layers (epidermis, dermis, and hypodermis) and contains a variety of appendages. The major barrier to absorption lies in the outermost layer of keratinous cells in the epidermis (stratum corneum). (From Ritschel WA, Hussain AS. The principles of permeation of substances across the skin. Methods Find Exp Clin Pharmacol 1988; **10**:39–56.)

and to prevent an excessive loss of water and electrolytes from the body.[24] The average adult has a skin surface area of approximately 1.8 m², which varies substantially among different anatomic areas in thickness and permeability to exogenous agents. The skin, as an organ, contains three anatomically distinct areas: the epidermis, the dermis, and the hypodermis (subcutaneous fat, Fig. 5.6). The protective function of the skin lies solely in the epidermis, which itself contains six identifiable layers (Fig. 5.7). The epidermis contains no blood vessels and varies in thickness from about 100 µm (eyelids and scrotum) to 800 µm (palms and soles). The outermost layer of the epidermis, the stratum corneum, consists of multiple layers of flattened, dead cells containing about 40% protein (primarily keratin), 40% water, and 15-20% lipids. This portion of the epidermis is between 10 and 50 µm in thickness, depending on the location and degree of hydration. The stratum corneum is continuously shed, with lost cells replaced by the migration of germinal cells toward the surface. The process of conversion of viable germinal cells to dead, keratin-filled cells in the outer layer of the stratum corneum takes approximately 5 days.

The dermis is about 20-30 µm in thickness and consists primarily of a gelatinous matrix of polysaccharides containing a fibrous protein structure of elastin, collagen, and reticulum. The dermis contains a rich blood supply, which traverses into the innermost layers of the epidermis (stratum malpighii) containing the germinal cells of the stratum corneum. Thus, the actual site of absorption into the systemic circulation occurs at the dermoepidermal interface.

The hypodermis, or subcutaneous fat layer, serves as a heat insulator and shock absorber and a source of energy. It varies in thickness from practically non-existent (eyelids) to several millimeters or more. Because of the high lipid content of this layer, it can potentially serve as a significant reservoir for the accumulation of highly lipid-soluble chemicals following extensive dermal contact.

Skin appendages include hair follicles, sebaceous glands, eccrine sweat glands, and apocrine sweat glands. Although such appendages provide a means of bypassing the stratum corneum, the total surface area covered by all skin appendages is less than 0.1% in most anatomic regions, and their contribution to total percutaneous absorption is considered negligible.[25]

The absorption of chemicals across the skin (percutaneous absorption) occurs exclusively by simple diffusion because no carrier-mediated transport systems or other means of translocation have been described. After a chemical has come into contact with the skin, it may enter the systemic circulation by either the transepidermal or transappendageal route (Fig. 5.8).[25]

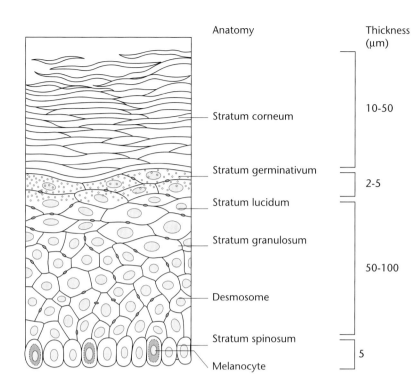

Anatomy | Thickness (μm)

Stratum corneum — 10-50

Stratum germinativum — 2-5

Stratum lucidum

Stratum granulosum

Desmosome — 50-100

Stratum spinosum

Melanocyte — 5

Figure 5.7: Anatomy of the human epidermis. The outermost layer of the epidermis, the stratum corneum, consists of multiple layers of dead, keratin-filled squamous cells, which serve as the principal barrier to dermal absorption of toxic substances. (From Ritschel WA, Hussain AS. The principles of permeation of substances across the skin. Methods Find Exp Clin Pharmacol 1988; **10**:39–56.)

As noted, the relative extent of absorption of chemicals across the skin that occurs by diffusion through the cells of the stratum corneum (intracellular) in contrast to between the cells (intercellular) has been the subject of debate. It has been postulated that the permeation of substances between cells may be a more important determinant of percutaneous absorption than either the thickness or number of cell layers. However, the diffusion distance postulated for intercellular absorption (359 μm) is nearly 15 times greater than the diffusion distance for intracellular absorption (25 μm), and the available surface area is 10 to 100 times less. Thus, the intercellular rate of diffusion would have to be several orders of magnitude greater than the intracellular rate if it were to contribute substantially to the total extent of percutaneous absorption. However, the dissolution of the extracellular lipids by repeated dermal contact with organic solvents, opening pores through the stratum corneum, may largely explain the large increase in percutaneous absorption that occurs following repeated dermal exposure to solvents.

The absorption of toxicants across the skin is a two-step process involving both (1) the diffusion of substances through the stratum corneum into the epidermis–dermis interface and (2) clearance of the diffused material from the dermis. Clearance depends on effective blood flow, interstitial fluid movement, and lymphatic vessels. Thus, depending on the relative rates of transepidermal diffusion and dermal blood flow, absorption may be either diffusion or flow limited. In places where the stratum corneum remains intact and blood flow is normal, diffusion is almost always the rate-limiting step. There is little question that the primary barrier to percutaneous absorption of chemicals is the stratum corneum. Removal of this horny layer of dead cells by repeated stripping with adhesive tape

Physiologic and pathologic factors
Condition of the skin
Skin diseases
Blood flow
Regional skin sites
Species variation
Biotransformation
Physicochemical factors
Hydration
Temperature
Chemical concentration
pH
Vehicle
Solubility characteristics
Molecular size
Presence of other substances (e.g., sorption promoters, surfactants, and barrier creams)

Table 5.4 Factors that influence percutaneous absorption

resulted in more than a 100-fold increase in uptake of several corticosteroids, demonstrating the importance of this outermost layer of skin.[25] On penetration of the stratum corneum, diffusion through the inner layers of the skin is extremely rapid for most substances. For example, the rate of diffusion of octanol through the lower viable epidermal cellular layers and dermis was approximately 500 times faster than the rate of diffusion through the outer stratum corneum.

Factors that influence percutaneous absorption. There are numerous factors that can influence both the rate and extent of absorption of chemicals across the skin (Table 5.4).[24] The single most important consideration is the integrity of the stratum corneum. Physical damage to this barrier results in greatly enhanced penetration, as does

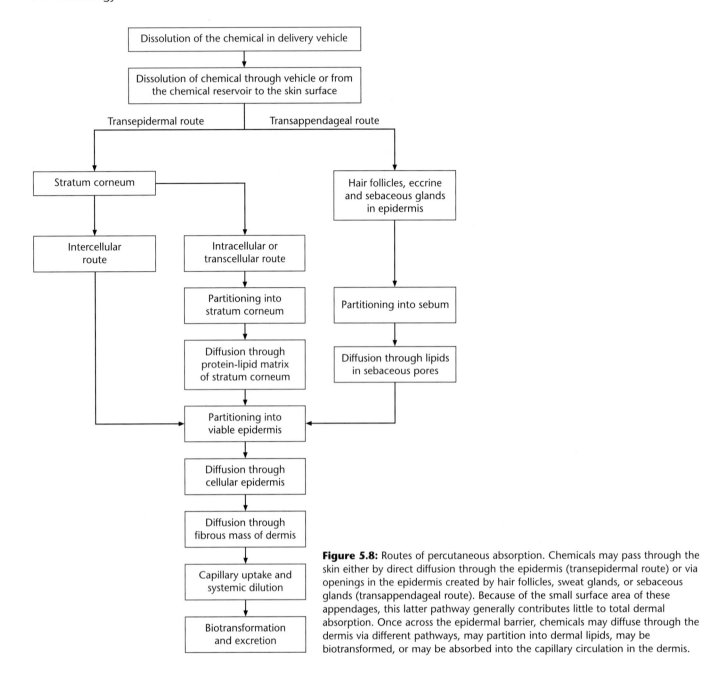

Figure 5.8: Routes of percutaneous absorption. Chemicals may pass through the skin either by direct diffusion through the epidermis (transepidermal route) or via openings in the epidermis created by hair follicles, sweat glands, or sebaceous glands (transappendageal route). Because of the small surface area of these appendages, this latter pathway generally contributes little to total dermal absorption. Once across the epidermal barrier, chemicals may diffuse through the dermis via different pathways, may partition into dermal lipids, may be biotransformed, or may be absorbed into the capillary circulation in the dermis.

irritation, inflammation, and other forms of injury. The age of the skin does appear to be important; children and elderly persons tend to have higher rates of percutaneous absorption than do young adults. The increased permeability of small children relative to adults may have to do with the increased degree of hydration, whereas the increase in percutaneous absorption in the elderly person is probably related to changes in skin structure caused by aging and cumulative solar damage. Skin diseases, such as eczema and psoriasis, also can alter the effectiveness of the stratum corneum barrier and increase the extent of blood flow to the dermis as a result of inflammatory processes. Enhanced blood flow facilitates the removal of diffused materials from the epidermal–dermal interface, which results in an enhanced concentration gradient from stratum corneum to dermis.

Regional differences in the absorption of chemicals across the skin have important implications for occupational and environmental exposures. There are relatively few studies that have carefully examined regional differences in absorption, and those that have are often contradictory. However, there is general agreement that the scrotum and posterior auricular skin are the sites of highest absorption, whereas plantar and palmar regions tend to be the least permeable. However, among different individuals, differences in the same region may be substantial. In general, the permeability across different areas of skin is inversely correlated with the thickness of stratum corneum. Penetration rates in cadaver skin increase in the following anatomic order: plantar, anterior forearm, instep, scalp and ventral thigh, scrotum and posterior auricular region.[24]

There are also wide differences in percutaneous absorption among different species.[20,24] The skin of rats, rabbits, and mice frequently have been used to examine the dermal bioavailability of drugs and chemicals, yet in the few studies in which comparisons have been made, the dermal permeability of most drugs and chemicals is greater in these animals compared with human skin. Although the relationship between species is not consistent for different substances, the permeability generally increases in the order monkey > dog > cat > rabbit > rat > guinea pig > mouse > forearm skin of humans.[20] The pig is often considered to be the best animal model for studies of transdermal penetration of drugs and chemicals.[26]

Although skin is generally not considered a major site of biotransformation of chemicals, biotransformation of some substances in the skin may be of critical toxicologic significance. The activity of most drug-metabolizing enzymes in the skin is low relative to the liver, but even low rates of metabolism for chemicals that are slowly absorbed or accumulate in the epidermis can be important in the ultimate disposition. The skin has the ability to perform a variety of oxidative biotransformations, including the oxidation of hydrocortisone, testosterone, aliphatic hydrocarbons, alicyclic hydrocarbons, and polyaromatic hydrocarbons. Indeed, the cytochrome P450-mediated oxidation of benzo[a]pyrene to the vicinal diol epoxide in the skin is thought to be essential to the ability of this compound to induce papillomas and carcinomas following repeated dermal application. Although the activity of aryl hydrocarbon hydroxylase in skin is only about 2% that of the liver, it is highly inducible following repeated dermal applications of polyaromatic hydrocarbons. The ability of the skin to perform a variety of other biotransformation reactions, including reduction reactions, hydrolysis of ethers, and glucuronide and sulfate conjugation, has been reported. Evidence for cutaneous first-pass metabolism of chemicals following dermal application has been demonstrated.

Among the various physicochemical factors that can influence percutaneous absorption, the extent of hydration is one of the more important. The permeability of skin has been shown to increase as much as 4-5-fold following hydration. The increase in penetration after hydration may result from an increase in the size of the pores in the stratum corneum. However, at high water concentrations, there are changes in both the diffusion and activity coefficients of the penetrating agent, in addition to physical changes in the stratum corneum. Dehydration also may enhance absorption by causing damage to the integrity of the stratum corneum. At water concentrations below 10%, the stratum corneum becomes brittle and loses its functional integrity.[20]

Occlusion of the skin is an especially effective means of enhancing percutaneous absorption; in one study, occlusion with an impermeable barrier resulted in a 50-fold increase in penetration compared with that of the same chemical in an identical formulation without occlusion. The significance of occlusion on skin permeability is especially noteworthy in the occupational setting. The use of gloves that serve as an incomplete barrier to chemicals may actually enhance percutaneous absorption by (1) increasing permeability by increased skin hydration and elevated temperature and (2) increasing the contact time and epidermal concentration, especially for volatile chemicals that would otherwise evaporate from the surface of the skin. Thus, it is imperative that gloves worn to protect against skin contact from chemicals be truly impermeable to the chemical of concern.

Occupational and environmental exposure to chemicals often occur in mixed media. For example, many pesticides are formulated in organic solvents. The nature of the vehicle that contains the solute may be of prime importance in determining dermal bioavailability. The rate and extent of penetration of a chemical is dependent on the relative partitioning of the substance between the vehicle and the epidermis. The use of barrier creams may reduce dermal absorption by preventing contact of the material with the dermis or by providing a 'skin-vehicle' partition coefficient that highly favors partitioning of the chemical into the vehicle. Conversely, chemicals that are only sparingly soluble in a solvent but are readily soluble in the lipid matrix of the epidermis may penetrate the skin much more rapidly than if they were applied directly or in a vehicle in which they are highly soluble. For example, when pure alcohols are applied to the skin, their rates of penetration are much lower than their corresponding rates in aqueous solutions. Some substances, such as dimethyl sulfoxide, dimethylformamide, and propylene glycol, can act as 'sorption enhancers', greatly increasing the permeation of other substances through the skin.[27] Percutaneous absorption of some substances has been increased 1000-fold by sorption promoters. Detergents and other surfactants also can alter the percutaneous absorption of other substances. Among the various types of surface-active agents, anionic surfactants are the most effective at enhancing percutaneous absorption, followed by non-ionic and cationic agents.

Classification of chemicals in terms of risk from dermal exposure. The American Conference of Governmental Industrial Hygienists (ACGIH) and a variety of occupational health regulatory agencies worldwide have identified compounds that are regarded as especially hazardous following dermal contact by use of the 'skin' denotation. The ACGIH lists 179 different compounds regarded as skin hazards. Although there is a large degree of inconsistency among the different lists that have been compiled, with nearly 400 chemicals appearing on at least one list, there is a smaller group of chemicals that are commonly identified as skin hazards (Table 5.5). Although the limitations of such lists have been discussed, they do provide a useful and quick reference for chemicals that may be especially problematic if they do come into contact with human skin. However, as noted by Granjean,[28] '. . . the lack of skin denotation for a particular substance does not necessarily exclude that hazardous quantities can be absorbed, provided that, e.g., the vehicle is right or the skin is occluded or damaged'. Finally, the contributions of dermal

Acrylamide	Epichlorohydrin	Nicotine
Acrylonitrile	EPN	Nitrobenzene
Aldrin	Ethylene chlorohydrin	Nitroglycerin
Alyl alcohol	Ethylene glycol dinitrate	Nitrotoluene
Aniline	Ethylene glycol monobutylether	o-Methylcyclohexanone
Benzene	Ethylene glycol monoethyl ether acetate	p-Nitrochlorobenzene
Carbon disulfide	Ethylene glycol monomethyl ether	p-Dioxane
Carbon tetrachloride	Ethylene glycol monomethyl ether acetate	p-Nitroaniline
Cellosolve (glycol ether)	Ethyleneimine	p-Phenylenediamine
Chlordane	Furfural	Parathion
Chlorinated naphthalenes	Heptachlor	Pentachlorophenol
Chloroprene	Hydrazine	Phenol
Cresol	Hydrogen cyanide	Phenylhydrazine
Demeton-methyl	Lindane	Picric acid
Diazinon	Malathion	Polychlorinated biphenyls
1,2-Dibromoethane	Mercury	Propargyl alcohol
2,2'-Dichlorodiethyl ether	Methyl acrylate	Sodium fluoroacetate
Dichlorvos	Methyl alcohol	1,1,2,2-Tetrachloroethane
Dieldrin	Methyl bromide	Tetraethyl lead
Diethylaminoethanol	Methyl sulfate	Tetryl
Dimethylacetamide	Mevinphos	Thallium
Dimethylaniline	Morpholine	Toluidine
1.1-Dimethylhydrazine*	n-Butylamine	Trinitrotoluene
Dinitrobenzene	n-Methylaniline	Xylene
Dinitro-o-cresol	N,N-Dimethylformamide	Xylidine
Endrin		

* Only 1,1-dimethylhydrazine does not have a 'skin' denotation on the ACGIH list.
Adapted from Granjean P, Berlin A, Gilbert M, et al. Preventing percutaneous absorption of industrial chemicals: the 'skin' denotation. Am J Ind Med 1988; 14:97-107. © 1988 John Wiley & Sons, Inc. Reprinted by permission of Wiley-Liss, Inc., a subsidiary of John Wiley & Sons, Inc.

Table 5.5 Chemicals commonly identified as hazardous by dermal exposure

absorption to overall exposure to toxic substances is often underestimated, especially for volatile chemicals. For example, using an experimentally determined dermal permeability value for benzene, the amount of benzene absorbed through the hands during long-term exposure to solvents contaminated with 0.1% benzene could increase the theoretical risk estimate for leukemia by 42%.[29]

Absorption of chemicals by inhalation exposure

The lung serves as an important site of contact with chemicals in the external environment. Such contact can result in direct damage to the respiratory epithelium or may lead to systemic toxicity following absorption into the blood stream. Like the gastrointestinal tract, the lung is designed for optimal absorption. It has a large total surface area (50-100 m^2) and a high blood flow (4 to 5 L/min) that is in intimate contact with the respiratory epithelium, which itself is of minimal thickness (10 μm diffusion distance).

Absorption of chemicals from inspired air can occur regardless of the physical form. For gases and fine vapors, absorption occurs by direct diffusion from alveolar air spaces across the epithelial cells, whereas for aerosols and other types of particles, deposition occurs along various aspects of the tracheobronchial tree, with the specific location depending on the size and density (mass median diameter). (See Roth[30] for a comprehensive review of toxicology of the respiratory system.)

Absorption of gases and vapors. The rate of absorption of gases and vapors by the lung is largely a function of the 'blood-gas partition coefficient'. Applying the principles of Henry's law to blood and alveolar gas, the concentration of a gas in the blood as it leaves the lungs is dependent on the solubility of the gas in blood, which is defined as the ratio of the concentration of the dissolved gas in the blood to the concentration in the gas phase at equilibrium.[31] Thus, chemicals with high blood-gas partition coefficients will have a high rate of uptake into the blood stream, relative to those chemicals with low blood-gas partition coefficients. For chemicals with a low solubility in blood, only a small fraction of the gas present in the alveolar space will be removed, and an increase in respiration will not enhance uptake. An increase in blood flow through the lung will greatly enhance uptake (perfusion limited). Conversely, an increase in respiration rate can significantly enhance the extent of absorption of gases that are readily soluble in blood because the delivery of gas to the blood, and not the dissolution into the blood, may be rate limiting in regard to uptake (ventilation limited). The solubility of a gas in the blood should not be equated to its solubility in water because components of blood other than water can greatly affect the solubility of some gases. For example, carbon monoxide, because of its high affinity for hemoglobin, has an extremely high apparent blood-gas partition coefficient even though it is only sparingly soluble in water.

The site of absorption of gases and vapors from the lungs is largely dependent on water solubility. Highly water-soluble gases present in low concentrations in inspired air, such as hydrochloric acid or sulfur dioxide, are usually removed in the upper respiratory tract, although higher concentrations and longer durations of exposure

Particle size (μm)

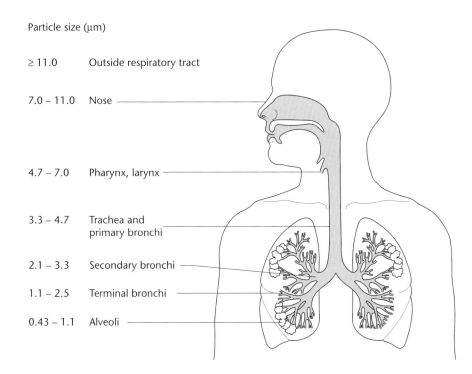

≥ 11.0	Outside respiratory tract
7.0 – 11.0	Nose
4.7 – 7.0	Pharynx, larynx
3.3 – 4.7	Trachea and primary bronchi
2.1 – 3.3	Secondary bronchi
1.1 – 2.5	Terminal bronchi
0.43 – 1.1	Alveoli

Figure 5.9: Particle deposition by size distribution in various regions of the lung. Particles deposit in different regions of the lung, based largely on the size of the particle. (From Kennedy GL. Inhalation toxicology. In Hayes AW, ed. Principles and methods in toxicology, 2nd edn. New York: Raven Press, 1989.)

allow bioavailability to the alveolar regions of the lung where they may cause serious pulmonary damage. Gases that are less soluble in water, such as nitrogen oxides and ozone, are not efficiently removed by the upper respiratory tract and tend to reach alveolar regions at relatively low concentrations. For those gases and vapors that impart their toxic properties systemically, the site of absorption is of far less concern than the rate and extent of absorption.

Deposition and clearance of particles from the lung. In contrast to gases, for which contact with the pulmonary epithelium occurs exclusively by diffusion, particles (aerosols) deposit on the pulmonary epithelium primarily through physical forces dictated by the particle size, shape, and mass. Inhaled aerosols are heterogeneous in size, and the size distribution usually follows a log-normal pattern. The geometric mean and geometric standard deviation of the particle size distribution is commonly obtained by plotting the cumulative percentage of particles less than a stated size increment against the log of the stated size on log probability paper. The 'mass median diameter' is a common means of characterizing aerosol size distribution because it considers not only the physical diameter of the particles, but also their density. For particles that are not spheric (e.g., asbestos fibers), a consideration of aerodynamic drag becomes important, and the determination of 'aerodynamic diameter' is most useful. This term describes the settling behavior of a non-spheric particle, whatever its size, shape, and density, in terms of a unit density sphere having the same settling velocity as the particle under study. The aerodynamic diameter of particles is a primary determinant of the site of deposition within the respiratory tract. Figure 5.9 shows the influence of particle size distribution on the regional deposition of an inhaled

aerosol. It is evident that aerosols with aerodynamic diameters greater than 10 μm are not capable of passing beyond the nasopharyngeal area.[32]

Particles may be deposited on the respiratory tract epithelium by three fundamental processes.

1. *Inertia.* Particles with sufficient mass will collide with the surface of the respiratory epithelium at points of branching and curvature. As the direction of air velocity changes, the inertial force of the particles will prevent them from changing directions at the same rate as that of the air flow. The greater the mass, the less the ability of the particles to change direction with air flow. Thus, deposition of particles occurs by impaction. For particles that are non-spheric (e.g., asbestos fibers), the term 'interception' is sometimes used to describe the deposition that results when an edge of the particle contacts the surface of the epithelium.

2. *Sedimentation.* Particles that are of sufficiently small size to escape deposition by inertia may deposit on the respiratory epithelium through sedimentation when the velocity of air flow becomes slow. Gravity is the predominant force behind sedimentation, and the rate of sedimentation is proportional to the density of the particle and the square of its diameter.

3. *Diffusion.* For extremely small particles, Brownian motion, in which suspended particles are bombarded by surrounding gaseous molecules, is the principal means of deposition. In contrast to both inertia and sedimentation, the rate of diffusion is not appreciably influenced by the particle density, but it is inversely proportional to the diameter.

Although particle size (i.e., aerodynamic diameter) is the principal determinant of deposition, other factors, such as breathing pattern, airway diameter, and the anatomy of the nasal, oral, and pharyngeal areas, are also important. Thus, pathologic or irritant conditions that result in narrowing or obstruction of airways, excessive bronchial secretions, or other conditions that alter the size and shape of the respiratory tract can alter the extent and pattern of particle deposition.

Clearance of particles from the lungs. Particles may be removed from the lungs by several mechanisms. Particles deposited in the upper nasopharyngeal area are cleared primarily by entrapment in the mucous lining and removal by reflex responses, such as sneezing or coughing, or through the continuous movement of mucus up the mucociliary escalator, where the entrapped particles are either swallowed or expectorated. The former is an important toxicologic consideration because it can result in significant ingestion of toxic materials even though exposure occurred by inhalation of particles. The mucociliary escalator is the primary means of clearance of particles in the tracheobronchial tree and functions down to the level of the terminal bronchioles. The clearance half-time by this process is between 12 and 24 hours.

Phagocytosis of particles by pulmonary macrophages is the principal route of elimination of particles that deposit in the alveoli and terminal bronchioles. Macrophage-containing particles may migrate to the ciliated epithelium of the terminal bronchioles and move up the mucociliary escalator, or they may enter the lymphatic vessels. This process takes from 2 to 6 weeks for effective elimination of particles. Some particles may actually be solubilized by body fluids and the constituents absorbed into the blood stream or lymph.

Obviously, any toxicologic response that reduces or eliminates particle clearance can result in more extensive accumulation of particles and potentially enhance the toxicity of the particles themselves or of toxic constituents that are slowly dissolved from the surface of the particles. Cigarette smoking has been demonstrated to reduce significantly the rate and efficiency of the mucociliary escalator. The inefficient removal of particles in heavy smokers may contribute, at least in part, to the well-described synergistic interaction in the lung cancer risk between asbestos and smoking.

DISTRIBUTION OF CHEMICALS IN THE BODY
First-pass effect

Because the critical dose parameter for any toxic effect relates to the concentration of a chemical at the biologic receptor site, the extent and nature of distribution of the absorbed chemical in the body can have a significant impact on the toxicity of that chemical. After a substance has entered the systemic circulation, it is potentially available to all tissues in the body. However, biologic activity at or near the site of absorption may drastically reduce the availability of the original chemical to distant sites, even

though absorption into the circulation is complete. This phenomenon, referred to as the 'first-pass effect,' is most often described in association with absorption of substances following ingestion.[33] Generally, the first-pass effect after oral absorption is the result of efficient extraction and metabolism of a chemical by the liver. The blood perfusing the gastrointestinal tract is collected in the portal vein, and thus, all substances absorbed from the gastrointestinal tract must pass through the liver prior to distribution to other organs. The liver maintains a high capacity for both extraction and biotransformation of exogenous substances, and can effectively prevent some chemicals from ever reaching the rest of the body. Although hepatic extraction is generally recognized as the most important site of removal for chemicals demonstrating a first-pass effect following oral administration, extraction and biotransformation by the gastrointestinal epithelium may also contribute.[34] The skin is also capable of first-pass metabolism of chemicals following dermal exposure, although the extent of this effect is generally far less important than that for oral exposure.

Binding and storage

Binding of chemicals to proteins can also have a dramatic effect on the toxicologic response to a given absorbed dose. Many chemicals bind to plasma proteins, especially albumin and globulins. Because only the concentration of 'free' (unbound) chemical is available for interaction with biologic receptors, extensive protein binding can greatly reduce the toxicity of a compound. For chemicals that are highly bound to plasma proteins, even a small shift in protein binding can have a large effect on their pharmacologic functions. For example, if the equilibrium binding of an absorbed chemical to plasma proteins is 98%, a change in binding status from 98% to 96% would result in a doubling of the concentration of free chemical and an attendant increase in its toxicity. This is especially a problem when multiple exposures occur to substances that share the same binding site, and it is a common mechanism of drug–drug or drug–chemical interactions.

If protein binding of toxic substances to intracellular proteins occurs, the tissue may serve as a 'sink' for accumulation of a chemical, prolonging the biologic half-life of the chemical. For example, Cd is a highly toxic element that binds avidly to intracellular binding proteins called metallothioneins. These low molecular weight proteins, which are inducible (their quantity increases) on repeated exposure to Cd and certain other metals, are present in relatively high concentrations in the liver and kidney. Following oral exposure to a dose of Cd, the majority of the absorbed dose (usually only a small percent of the exposed dose) is concentrated in the liver and bound largely to metallothioneins.[35] In this instance, the preferential binding serves as a protective mechanism against Cd-induced liver damage by preventing Cd from binding to essential cellular proteins. However, the Cd-metallothionein complex is slowly transported out of the liver to the kidney, where the complex is extracted by the proximal tubules. As the metallothioneins protein is degraded by normal catabolic processes, Cd is released and binds to either renal metallothioneins or other intracellular thiols, including critical proteins. The net effect of this is an extraordinarily long biologic half-life for Cd (up to 30 years), with the majority of the body burden eventually concentrated in the renal cortex. After the concentrations exceed the binding capacity of renal metallothionein, irreversible and potentially fatal kidney damage can result.

Lipid-soluble chemicals that are poorly metabolized will redistribute to poorly perfused fat depots following equilibration in the rapidly perfused tissues. Many lipid-soluble chemicals rapidly affect central nervous system function after exposure. A relatively high fraction of the absorbed dose enters the brain because of the high rate of perfusion of the brain and partitions into brain tissue because of the relatively high lipid content. The duration of action of this effect following an acute exposure is often short because the chemical quickly redistributes from the brain to the more slowly perfused peripheral fat stores, or to sites such as the liver where the chemical may be more rapidly metabolized to water-soluble forms and eliminated by urinary or biliary excretion.

Special barriers to distribution

The so-called 'blood–brain barrier' is an effective anatomic barrier to penetration of highly water-soluble chemicals into the brain.[36] This barrier is the result of several unusual anatomic characteristics, including the presence of tight junctions (desmosomes) between capillary endothelial cells, the presence of glial foot processes that effectively surround the capillary endothelium, a contiguous basement membrane, and a relatively low protein content in the interstitial fluid of the brain. The relative contribution of the last two elements to the barrier function is probably small compared with that of tight junctions and glial cells. Thus, in contrast to most other organ systems, where intercellular gaps in the capillary endothelium allow free access of chemical into parenchymal cells, in the brain a chemical must pass through several biologic membranes (capillary endothelial cells and glial cells) and interstitial fluid before coming into contact with neurons. This barrier is effective against most water-soluble chemicals, except very small substances that can diffuse with water through membrane pores, (e.g., lithium). However, it presents little impediment to the diffusion of lipid-soluble substances into the brain, and consequently, nearly all organic solvents can readily enter the brain and produce aberrant effects on central nervous system function.

A similar concept has been described for the testis. The 'blood–testis' barrier, like the blood–brain barrier, does limit the bioavailability of some water-soluble substances to germinal cells, but again, it provides little protection against lipid-soluble compounds.[37] Sertoli cells appear to be primarily responsible for the blood–testis barrier because adjacent Sertoli cells form occluding junctions between the germ cells in various stages of development.

The distribution of chemicals to different organs systems may also be affected by the presence of specific carrier-mediated transport processes. Such processes are most active in the liver, kidney, and intestine, although transport processes have been described in the choroid plexus and lung. The transport processes in the liver and kidney function primarily to aid in the uptake and elimination of foreign substances and metabolic byproducts from the blood, whereas those in the intestine function primarily to aid in the absorption of water-soluble nutrients that would otherwise not be absorbed. The physiologic functions of transport processes for organic substances identified in the lung are not known, but the presence of these transport systems can have important toxicologic consequences. For example, the herbicide paraquat is highly and specifically toxic to the lung, regardless of the route of administration, due in part to an active transport system that concentrates paraquat in type II pneumocytes.[38]

Biotransformation of chemicals

For many chemicals, the toxic effects are highly dependent on the metabolic fate of the chemical in the body. Because few xenobiotics are actually fully metabolized to carbon dioxide and water, the metabolic processes that change the structure and characteristics of a chemical are appropriately referred to as 'biotransformation' reactions. There are a multitude of enzymatic pathways capable of such reactions, and the quantitative and qualitative differences in the ability of different organs to conduct such processes is often responsible for the 'organotropic' (i.e., organ-specific) effects of many chemicals. For example, the liver is the most common site of toxicity for chloroform and carbon tetrachloride, largely because of the ability of this organ to biotransform these compounds rapidly into reactive free radical intermediates.[39]

Regardless of the specific pathways involved, conceptually the ultimate 'goal' of biotransformation reactions is to render potentially toxic chemicals less toxic. This is accomplished in two ways by: (1) the addition of polar groups to lipid-soluble chemicals, which decreases the ability of chemicals to penetrate cell membranes on the one hand and enhances the rate of elimination in urine or bile on the other, and (2) the alteration of chemical structure so that the chemical no longer 'fits' the specific biologic receptor (e.g., catalytic sites of enzymes or neurotransmitter receptors). However, it is now widely recognized that intermediates formed in the process may actually be of far greater toxicity than the 'parent' molecule, and thus, some biotransformation reactions may actually be deleterious 'activation reactions,' whereas others are considered 'detoxification' reactions.

Biotransformation reactions are commonly divided into two broad categories: phase I and phase II reactions.[40] Phase I reactions are so named because they are generally the first biotransformation step in what is often a multistep process leading to the eventual excretion of the biotransformed products. Phase II reactions are those enzymatic processes that use the products of phase I reactions to impart further structural changes, usually greatly increasing the water solubility. However, this classification can be confusing because some biotransformation enzymes may act as either phase I or phase II enzymes, depending on the substrate. For example, the hydrolysis of epoxides by the enzyme epoxide hydrolase could be considered a phase I reaction if it were the first enzyme to metabolize an exogenous epoxide, such as trichloropropene oxide or heptachlor epoxide, whereas it would be considered a phase II reaction if it were acting on an epoxide generated endogenously by an oxidative pathway. However, with numerous notable exceptions, oxidation, reduction, and hydrolytic pathways are generally considered phase I reactions, whereas conjugation reactions are usually classified as phase II reactions. Virtually all biotransformation reactions of toxicologic significance can be identified as proceeding by one of the following four basic categories of pathways: oxidation, reduction, hydrolysis, and conjugation.

Oxidation reactions

The majority of oxidative biotransformation reactions are mediated by the cytochrome P450-containing mixed-function mono-oxygenase system. However, there are other important oxidative pathways, and thus, oxidation reactions are most conveniently divided into 'cytochrome P450-mediated' and 'non-cytochrome P450-mediated' pathways.

Cytochrome P450-mediated oxidation reactions

Cytochrome P450 is a heme-containing, membrane-bound complex located in the smooth endoplasmic reticulum. For experimental purposes, this enzyme system is most easily studied in crude subcellular fractions of homogenized tissues. The subcellular fraction containing the smooth endoplasmic reticulum is referred to as the 'microsomal fraction,' and thus cytochrome P450-mediated reactions are often called microsomal oxidation reactions.[41] Microsomes are readily prepared by differential centrifugation of homogenized tissues. The cell membranes, nuclei, mitochondria, ribosomes, and most other intracellular organelles are pelleted after centrifugation at 9000-15,000 *g*. Because the fragments of the smooth endoplasmic reticulum are less dense than these other organelles, they remain suspended in the supernatant (sometimes referred to as the S9 fraction). The microsomes can be separated from the soluble fraction of the cell homogenate by centrifugation for 1 hour at 100,000 *g*. The microsomal pellet obtained by this process can then be resuspended and used for in-vitro studies. The 100,000 *g* supernatant contains only soluble enzymes, and it can also be used for studies of soluble biotransformation enzymes. It is important to recognize that, in addition to the cytochrome P450 system, microsomes contain many other important biotransformation enzymes, and thus, microsomal metabolism is not completely synonymous with cytochrome P450-mediated reactions.

There are actually numerous forms of cytochrome P450 enzymes (more than 30 distinct enzymes have been identified in the human liver), and the genetics of these enzymes is becoming well understood. Although there is generally a broad overlap in substrate specificity between individual enzymes, specific P450 enzymes play a major role in the biotransformation of specific xenobiotics, and genetic differences in the expression and activity of specific P450 enzymes can be of substantial toxicologic and pharmacologic significance (Fig. 5.10). Genetic polymorphisms in xenobiotic metabolism are discussed in detail subsequently.

The number of chemicals that can undergo oxidation by the cytochrome P450 complex is large, as is the variety

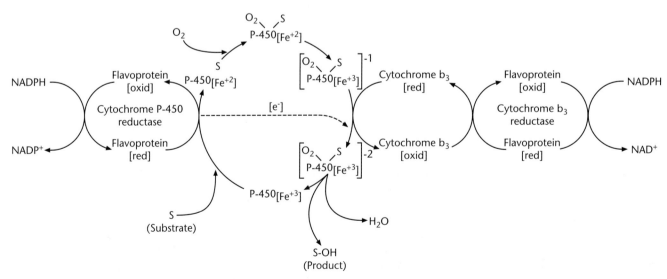

Figure 5.10: Catalytic cycle of the cytochrome P450-dependent, mixed-function mono-oxygenase system. The cytochrome P450-dependent, mixed-function mono-oxygenase system catalyzes the addition of atomic oxygen to lipophilic substrates such as hydrocarbons. The iron in the heme portion of the molecule undergoes oxidation and reduction, transferring electrons from an electron donor (NAD[P]H) to molecular oxygen (O_2) and the substrate (S). The net result is the insertion of one atom of molecular oxygen into the substrate, and the second atom combines with hydrogen ions to form water.

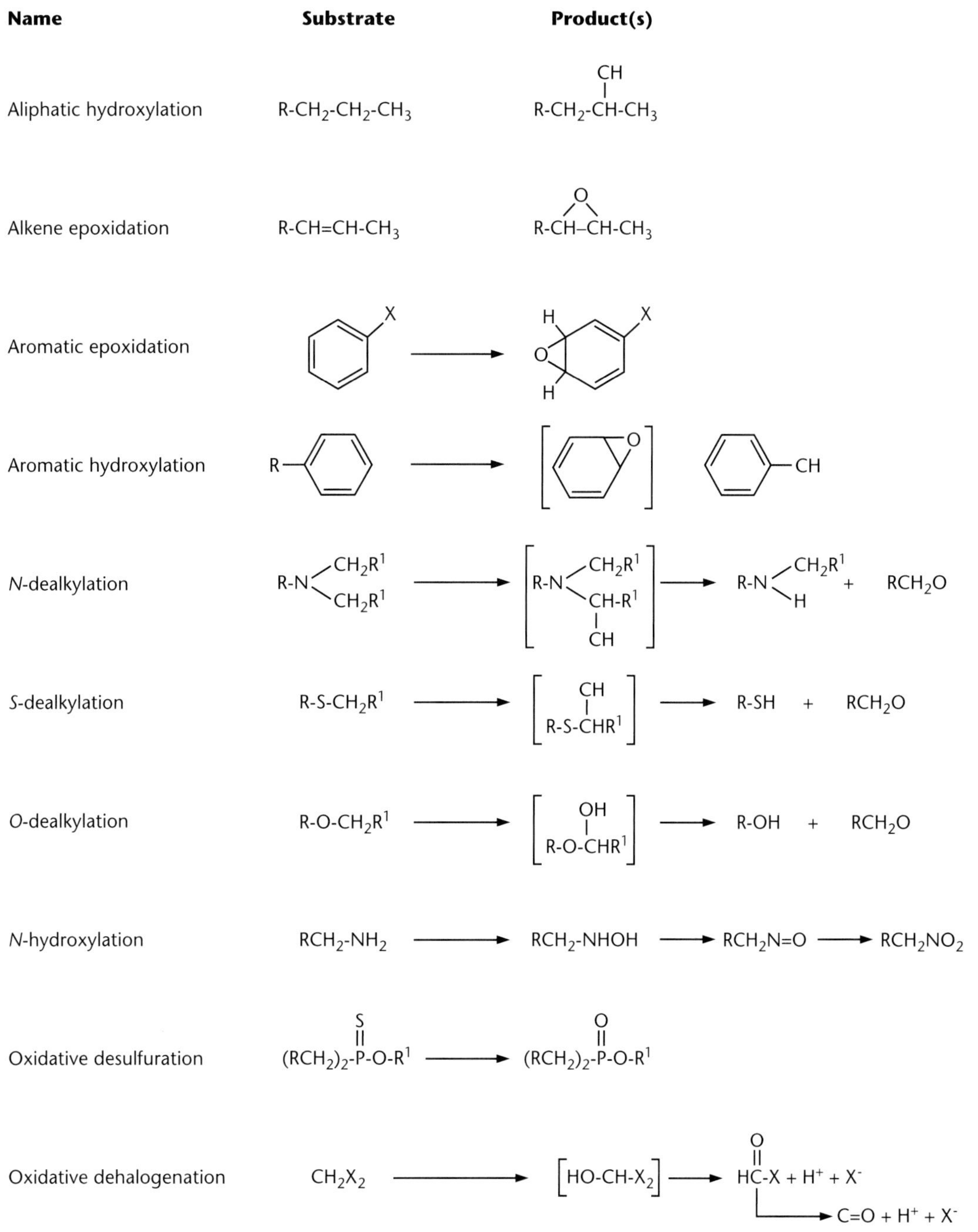

Name	Substrate	Product(s)
Aliphatic hydroxylation	R-CH$_2$-CH$_2$-CH$_3$	R-CH$_2$-CH-CH$_3$ with CH above
Alkene epoxidation	R-CH=CH-CH$_3$	R-CH–CH-CH$_3$ with O epoxide
Aromatic epoxidation		
Aromatic hydroxylation		
N-dealkylation		
S-dealkylation		
O-dealkylation		
N-hydroxylation	RCH$_2$-NH$_2$ → RCH$_2$-NHOH → RCH$_2$N=O → RCH$_2$NO$_2$	
Oxidative desulfuration	(RCH$_2$)$_2$-P-O-R^1 with S	(RCH$_2$)$_2$-P-O-R^1 with O
Oxidative dehalogenation	CH$_2$X$_2$ → [HO-CH-X$_2$] →	

Figure 5.11: Common oxidation reactions mediated via cytochromes P450. The cytochromes P450 system is capable of mediating the oxidation of a wide variety of drugs and other chemicals. See text for further discussion.

of biotransformed products that can result from a single substrate. However, it is possible to predict with some degree of confidence the possible array of metabolites that could result from cytochrome P450-mediated oxidation reactions by understanding the basic reactions that have been described. Cytochrome P450-oxidation reactions are commonly classified into ten different categories (Fig. 5.11).

The oxidation of aromatic and aliphatic hydrocarbons is one of the most common of the P450-mediated oxidations. The products of such reactions are generally hydroxylated metabolites. The hydroxyl group increases polarity and also provides a molecular site for conjugation with highly polar groups, such as glucuronic acid or sulfate, by phase II biotransformation pathways. However, oxidation of hydrocarbons can also lead to the formation of highly electrophilic epoxides or other reactive intermediates, which may bind to nucleophilic sites within the cell, disrupting cellular function. Two common nucleophilic sites within the cell are reduced thiols in proteins and certain bases in DNA. The binding of electrophilic intermediates to thiols or other nucleophilic sites in essential proteins may result in cell injury or death, with a resultant loss in organ function. The formation of reactive epoxide intermediates by cytochrome P450 oxidation is thought to be the initiating step in chemical carcinogenesis by a wide variety of chemicals, including polyaromatic hydrocarbons and the fungal toxin, aflatoxin B_1.

Oxidative dechlorination of carbon tetrachloride by cytochrome P450 is thought to be essential to the hepatotoxic effects of this chemical. Oxidative desulfuration by cytochrome P450 is essential to both the insecticidal activity and toxicity of many organophosphate insecticides because it is only the 'oxon' analogue that is capable of binding to and inhibiting acetylcholinesterase. Thus, although cytochrome P450-mediated oxidation reactions serve as a principal means of elimination of a wide variety of chemicals, this same pathway is also responsible for the activation of a variety of chemicals to more highly toxic and carcinogenic forms. Whether biotransformation through the P450 pathway results in net activation or detoxification is dependent on many other factors and is not always readily apparent. The kinetics of different cytochromes P450 enzymes toward the same substrate, relative to the kinetics of competing reactions, are critical to the ultimate outcome. For example, the widely used analgesic acetaminophen at normal therapeutic doses is largely metabolized by conjugation reactions (sulfation and glucuronidation), with only about 4% biotransformed by the cytochrome P450 system. Although one product of P450 biotransformation of acetaminophen is quite reactive, it is rapidly detoxified by intracellular reduced glutathione. However, at high doses, the ratio of biotransformation shifts more to the P450 system; with increasing doses, the tissue stores of glutathione become depleted, and the reactive intermediate then reacts with cellular thiols, binding to intracellular proteins and creating cellular damage, primarily in the liver where the majority of biotransformation of acetaminophen occurs.[42]

Induction of cytochrome P450. An interesting and clinically relevant phenomenon of most cytochrome P450 enzymes (and many other biotransformation pathways) is their ability to increase activity after repeated exposure to certain exogenous agents. Enzyme induction occurs by gene activation in which the rate of messenger RNA synthesis increases, with a concomitant increase in enzyme production and activity. A wide variety of chemicals have been identified as 'microsomal enzyme inducers', but the specific pattern of enzyme induction differs. The two most widely studied enzyme inducers are phenobarbital and 3-methylcholanthrene (3-MC). Phenobarbital induces a broad spectrum of P450 enzymes (P4502B, 2C, 3A, and several other important biotransformation enzymes, including some glutathione S-transferases and glucuronyl transferases). 3-MC, other polyaromatic hydrocarbons, and the controversial and potent toxicant 2,3,7,8-tetrachlorodibenzo-p-dioxin (dioxin) induce a much narrower spectrum of biotransformation enzymes, most notably the cytochrome P4501A family, via the aryl hydrocarbon hydroxylase receptor (AHH) complex.

Although the spectrum of enzymes induced via the AHH receptor complex is more limited, the extent of induction is often great, because constitutive (background) expression of the cytochrome P501A family of enzymes is very low. Thus, in the absence of exposure to AHH receptor agonists, enzyme activity is very low but increases dramatically on exposure. Because this enzyme system is principally responsible for the biotransformation of polyaromatic hydrocarbons, induction can be viewed as an attempt by the organism to respond to external stimuli by altering its capacity to deal with those stimuli. It is unclear whether induction of cytochrome P4501A enzymes is indeed beneficial to the organism because this enzyme system is responsible for the activation of polyaromatic hydrocarbons to carcinogenic intermediates, as well as formation of less toxic forms of the parent molecule.

Microsomal enzyme induction by phenobarbital-like inducers, which include many chemicals found in the workplace and general environment (e.g., some forms of polychlorinated biphenyls [PCBs] and organochlorine insecticides), can greatly accelerate the rate of biotransformation of numerous chemicals.[43] The significance of this effect is dependent on the relative toxicity of the products of biotransformation. Thus, induction with phenobarbital may decrease the toxicity of some compounds while enhancing the toxicity of others. Such chemical–chemical interactions are well described for therapeutic drugs, in which patients receiving chronic barbiturate therapy for epilepsy may require substantial dosage adjustment for other medications to be effective.

Non-cytochrome P450 oxidation reactions

Alcohol and aldehyde dehydrogenases. The pathways of oxidation of short-chain alcohols, such as methanol, ethanol, and isopropanol, are very important biotransformation routes because exposure to these substances is very common. Although cytochrome P450 2E1 enzymes are capable of oxidizing ethanol, the relative importance of this reaction to the overall metabolism of ethanol in humans is small. Primary oxidation of short-chain alcohols occurs by a two-step sequence involving alcohol dehydrogenase and aldehyde dehydrogenase.[44]

The relative rates of metabolism of these two enzymes are important to the toxicologic effects of various alcohols. In the case of ethanol, the oxidation to acetaldehyde proceeds relatively slowly and in a zero-order kinetic fashion at doses capable of inducing even mild inebriation. That is, the quantity of ethanol metabolized is a fixed amount, rather than a fixed percentage, of the available dose. Thus, with repeated consumption of alcohol, the fraction of the dose metabolized becomes less as the dose increases. Aldehyde dehydrogenase functions relatively more efficiently than does alcohol dehydrogenase, preventing any significant accumulation of acetaldehyde under normal circumstances. Acetaldehyde is toxic and causes numerous adverse effects (headache, nausea, vomiting, hypotension, and flushing), and thus, chemicals that inhibit aldehyde dehydrogenase may produce these effects when combined with relatively low doses of alcohol. Several drugs and a few non-drug chemicals are capable of this effect. Disulfiram has been used clinically for this purpose as a form of aversion therapy in the treatment of alcoholism.[45]

Methanol metabolism proceeds by the same pathway as that for ethanol, but at a rate about seven times slower than that of ethanol. However, the consequences of formation of the two sequential metabolites, formaldehyde and formic acid, are much more severe. Virtually all of the severe and potentially irreversible effects of methanol can be attributed to these two metabolites. Retinal damage and blindness is thought to result from the localized production of formaldehyde in the retina. Life-threatening metabolic acidosis results from the formation of formic acid by aldehyde dehydrogenase. Because ethanol is preferentially metabolized by alcohol dehydrogenase and methanol will be eliminated largely unchanged in the urine if given adequate time, the inhibition of methanol biotransformation by intravenous infusion of ethanol or administration of fomepizole, an inhibitor of alcohol dehydrogenase, is standard therapy for methanol poisoning.[46] If the amount of methanol ingested is large, pharmacologic treatment may be combined with extracorporeal hemodialysis to aid in the elimination of unchanged methanol. Alcohol and aldehyde dehydrogenases are also important in the biotransformation of various other alcohols, aldehydes, glycols, and glycol ethers and in the reduction of ketones to alcohols.

Flavin-dependent mono-oxygenases (FMOs). Oxidation of certain secondary amines, tertiary amines, imines, arylamines, and hydrazines, and many sulfur-containing chemicals proceeds by microsomal mono-oxygenases that are distinct from the cytochrome P450 enzyme family. This family of flavin-dependent mono-oxygenases appears particularly active in the human liver and competes with the cytochrome P450 system for the oxidation of nucleophilic nitrogen and sulfur atoms.[47] The primary function of FMOs is in the detoxification of xenobiotics, and is likely the major route of oxidation of nucleophilic nitrogen, sulfur, phosphorus and other heteroatom-containing chemicals, including several important pesticides. Like the cytochromes P450, the FMOs are a multi-gene family of enzymes, with five different genes identified in humans to date. Interestingly, a genetic variant in one of these genes, FMO3, is associated with a malodorous syndrome known as 'fish odor disease'. Individuals who inherit the variant form of FMO3 are unable to metabolize trimethylamine, a highly malodorous component of fish oil.[48] Lack of metabolic elimination results in secretion of the compound in skin. Although not physiologically detrimental, this condition may be associated with pyschosocial disorders.

Reduction reactions

Reduction reactions are relatively uncommon because cells function principally in an oxidizing environment. However, enzymatic reduction is important in the disposition of at least three general classes of chemicals: azo compounds, aromatic nitrates, and certain halogenated hydrocarbons. Surprisingly, these reactions are also mediated by the cytochrome P450 system, but the substrate, rather than molecular oxygen, accepts the electrons and is reduced.

Reduction reactions occur commonly in the gut flora and can be quite important in the disposition and toxicity of substances. As noted, the formation of nitrite from nitrate is a reduction reaction that can occur in the gut flora of infants, resulting in potentially severe methemoglobinemia. The reduction of azo dyes by the gut flora may alter the absorption and toxicity of these compounds. Complex azo dyes such as Direct Black 38 or Direct Blue 6 may release carcinogenic products, such as benzidine, after azo reduction, whereas the reduction of single azo compounds usually is a detoxification step.

NAD(P)H:quinone oxidoreductase (NQO1) is widely distributed in mammalian species and tissues, and is involved in the reductive activation and detoxification of a variety of chemicals that contain, or can form, quinones or their derivatives. NQO1 is thought to play an important role in protection against oxygen radical formation that can occur from redox cycling of quinones.[49] It also is involved in the metabolic activation of several widely used antitumor agents, including mitomycin C and streptonigrin.

Hydrolytic reactions

The hydrolysis of esters, amides, and epoxides is important in the disposition of a wide variety of drugs and chemicals. The products of the hydrolysis of esters are an organic acid and alcohol, whereas the products of amide hydrolysis are an organic acid and a primary or secondary amine. The hydrolysis of epoxides results in a dihydrodiol.

There are a variety of different esterase and amidase enzymes with broad and somewhat overlapping substrate specificities.[50] Arylesterases are principally active on aromatic esters, whereas carboxylesterases are active on aliphatic esters. One form of arylesterase, called paraoxonase, is active in the hydrolysis of parathion and a few other organophosphate insecticides and has a demonstrated polymorphic distribution in the human population.[51] Whether a genetic deficiency in paraoxonase activity places such individuals at increased risk for organophosphate insecticide poisoning is uncertain and the subject of current study. Genetic polymorphism in butyrylcholinesterase (pseudocholinesterase) is responsible for the prolonged muscular paralysis that occurs in 1-3% of the population following clinical use of succinylcholine. Cholinesterase is a more substrate-specific enzyme with important physiologic functions. A number of drugs and chemicals inhibit acetylcholinesterase activity, including all organophosphate insecticides. Esters may be hydrolyzed by plasma and hepatic esterases, whereas the metabolism of amides is more complicated, sometimes involving cytochrome P450-dependent N-dealkylation prior to amide hydrolysis. This is why amide-type local anesthetics (e.g., lidocaine) are generally longer acting that ester-type anesthetics (e.g., procaine).

The hydrolysis of epoxides by microsomal epoxide hydrolase is generally regarded as a detoxification pathway because the dihydrodiol product is far less reactive than the epoxides.[52] However, in some circumstances, such as in the biotransformation of polycyclic aromatic hydrocarbons, the hydrolysis of the first arene epoxide generated by cytochrome P450 oxidation is required for formation of the ultimate carcinogenic form, the 'diol-epoxide,' and thus, epoxide hydrolysis is considered part of the activation process.

Conjugation (Phase II) biotransformation reactions

Glucuronide conjugation

UDP-glucuronosyl transferases are a multigene family of microsomal enzymes that function to add a residue of glucuronic acid to a variety of xenobiotics.[53] Because these enzymes are not capable of adding glucuronic acid directly to hydrocarbons, functional groups such as alcohols (COH), carboxylic acids (CCOOH), amines (CNH_2), thiols (CSH), or sulfonamides are necessary. If such groups are present on the parent compound, conjugation can occur directly. However, for hydrocarbons or other chemicals that lack these sites, prior biotransformation to generate or 'expose' such functional groups is required.

The addition of the glucuronic acid moiety to the xenobiotic imparts a substantial degree of water solubility and generates a bulky addition that would likely interfere with any structure-specific receptor interaction. Glucuronic acid per se is not used in the reaction; rather, an activated form (UDPGA), in which glucuronic acid is linked to the terminal phosphate residue of uridine diphosphate (UDP), serves as the co-factor for the reaction. Typically, glucuronidation reactions have been viewed primarily as 'detoxification' events, although some glucuronidation reactions are considered 'activation' reactions.[54] Glucuronide conjugates are generally endproducts of biotransformation and are commonly found in both the urine and bile. Because bacterial flora contain the enzyme β-glucuronidase, which is capable of hydrolyzing the β-glycosidic linkage to re-establish the less polar substrate, glucuronide conjugates excreted in the bile may undergo extensive enterohepatic circulation if the degluconated molecule is sufficiently lipid soluble to be reabsorbed through the intestinal epithelium. β-glucuronidase activity has also been identified in the bladder epithelium and is thought to contribute to the etiology of bladder cancer for certain aromatic amines, which are conjugated with glucuronic acid, concentrated in the bladder, and then subsequently hydrolyzed by this enzyme to release a reactive, mutagenic form of the chemical.

Sulfate conjugation

The arylsulfotransferases are a multi-gene family of soluble enzymes present in the liver, kidney, and intestine that function to add inorganic sulfate to phenols, aliphatic alcohols and hydroxylamines.[55]

Sulfate is donated to the phenol or alcohol by 3'-phosphoadenosine-5'-phosphosulfate (PAPS), a molecule analogous to adenosine diphosphate, except that the terminal phosphate is a sulfate residue and the 3'-hydroxyl group is also phosphorylated. Because the products of this reaction are ionized regardless of pH, sulfate conjugates are rapidly excreted in urine. Although sulfate conjugation usually results in products that are less toxic than the substrate, sulfate conjugation of some hydroxylamines (R-NH-OH), such as the sulfate conjugate of N-hydroxy-2-acetylaminofluorene, can rearrange to form reactive electrophilic species capable of interacting with nucleophilic sites in DNA, and thus become potent mutagens and carcinogens.[56] The sulfate conjugation of phenol is a major metabolite of benzene, and the ratio of organic to inorganic sulfate in the urine was used at one time as a crude biologic indicator of benzene exposure in the occupational environment. However, much better biomarkers of benzene exposure are now available.[57]

Glutathione conjugation

Glutathione (γ-glutamylcysteinylglycine) is an intracellular tripeptide that provides a number of critical physiologic functions and is the most important intracellular antioxidant. In addition to its important physiologic functions, it serves as the co-factor for a multigene family of cytosolic enzymes, the glutathione S-transferases, which catalyze the conjugation of a variety of exogenous substances to glutathione.[58] The best studied, and perhaps toxicologically most important, of these reactions is the conjugation of aliphatic and aromatic epoxides.

Glutathione S-transferases can also catalyze the addition of glutathione directly across certain unsaturated aliphatic sites, such as with diethylmaleate, and can also facilitate substitution reactions on certain halogenated organic compounds, with replacement of one halogen atom with glutathione. Like the cytochrome P450 family of enzymes, the glutathione S-transferases contain a relatively large number of different enzyme forms that are the products of separate genes. There are at least 13 different isoenzymes that have been characterized in humans, with some forms exhibiting tissue-specific expression. The different enzymes have broad and overlapping substrate affinities but are readily classified into one of six families: alpha (hGSTA), mu (hGSTM), pi (hGSTP), theta (hGSTT), zeta (hGSTZ) and omega (hGSTO).[58] Glutathione S-transferase P1 is highly expressed in many neoplastic tissues, and its expression is frequently used as an early marker of neoplastic change in experimental carcinogenesis. There is also a microsomal form of glutathione S-transferase, but its function in the biotransformation of xenobiotics appears limited, relative to the various cytosolic forms.[59] Several GSTs are polymorphic in the human population, and have been the subject of considerable investigation as possible 'environmental susceptibility genes' due to their involvement in a wide variety of detoxification reactions.[60]

Glutathione conjugates are seldom excreted directly in the urine, although they may appear in the bile as intact glutathione conjugates. Most glutathione conjugates are sequentially metabolized by (1) γ-glutamyltranspeptidase (GGT), which removes the N-terminal glutamic acid residue from cysteine; (2) non-specific peptidases, which cleave the peptide bond between cysteine and the C-terminal glycine to generate a cysteine conjugate; and (3) N-acetylation of the cysteine conjugate to form the N-acetyl cysteine (mercapturic acid) conjugate. Mercapturic acid conjugates are then readily excreted in the urine.

Although glutathione conjugation is an important detoxification pathway, recent studies have demonstrated that certain haloalkanes, such as ethylene dibromide, when conjugated to glutathione, can rearrange to form highly reactive episulfonium ions.[61] Such glutathione metabolites may be at least partially responsible for the nephrotoxicity and carcinogenicity inherent in some of these compounds.

N-acetyl transferases (NATs)

Many aromatic amines are metabolized primarily by conjugation of the primary or secondary amine with an acetyl group.[62] Two different genes for NAT are commonly expressed in human tissues, referred to as NAT1 and NAT2. Because most primary aromatic amines are in the positively charged state at physiologic pH, this conjugation can actually result in products that are not appreciably more water soluble and, in some instances, may be less water soluble than the parent compound. Nevertheless, this pathway is a major route of biotransformation of many aromatic amines, such as hydralazine, isonicotinic acid hydrazide, aniline, 2,6-dinitrotoluene, and some sulfonamide drugs. Both NAT1 and NAT2 are polymorphic in the human population, and have been the subject of considerable study as potential determinants of adverse drug reactions and as environmental susceptibility genes.[63]

N-acetylation results in loss of pharmacologic activity of some widely used drugs and, as such, is a detoxification pathway. Occasionally, N-acetylated aromatic amines can undergo further metabolism by N-hydroxylation to yield the N-hydroxy-N-acetyl derivative. Both NAT1 and NAT2 are capable of catalyzing this 'activation' reaction. A different enzyme, called arylhydroxamic acid N,O-acyltransferase, catalyzes the transfer of the acetyl moiety from aromatic nitrogen to the hydroxyl group on the nitrogen, resulting in the formation of a highly unstable acyloxyarylamine that can react with DNA and proteins.[64] This complicated biotransformation pathway is implicated in the carcinogenesis of numerous aromatic amine compounds, including benzidine.[65]

Methyl transferases

The methylation of xenobiotics is not a frequent route of elimination. In contrast to most other biotransformation pathways, products of methylation are almost always less polar than the substrate. Thus, methylation reactions do little to enhance the elimination of non-polar compounds from the body. Methylation of endogenous proteins, nucleic acids, and catecholamines occurs frequently, and is an important biochemical process for the regulation of many intracellular functions. The methylation of xenobiotics thus occurs primarily in circumstances in which the xenobiotic mimics some endogenous substrate. Examples where this occurs are the methylation of pyridine and catechols. The co-factor for methyltransferase reactions is S-adenosylmethionine. A few examples where methylation of xenobiotics is important include the methylation of dopamine and related catechol drugs by catechol-O-methyl transferase (COMT) and the methylation of the chemotherapeutic agent, 6-mercaptopurine by thiopurine methyltransferase (TPMT).[66] The presence of a single nucleotide polymorphism in TPMT is an important consideration in treatment of leukemia patients with TPMT because those who are homozygous for the variant allele may suffer serious toxicity at standard therapeutic doses. Conversely, for those who are homozygous for the high activity allele, a standard dose may not be efficacious because of rapid systemic clearance of the drug.[67]

Amino acid conjugation

Organic cyclic carboxylic acids can undergo conjugation with several amino acids, including glycine, glutamine, and taurine.[68] For example, benzoic acid is rapidly conjugated with glycine to form hippuric acid. Because benzoic acid is the primary oxidative metabolite of toluene, hippuric acid is a primary urinary metabolite of toluene, and methylhippuric acids are primary urinary metabolites of xylenes. Both taurine and glycine are used biologically for the conjugation and biliary excretion of primary and secondary bile acids. Taurocholate, glycocholate, taurochenodeoxycholate, and glycochenodeoxycholate are the primary bile acids in human bile, and conjugation of newly synthesized bile acids in the liver is a prerequisite for biliary excretion.

Genetic polymorphisms in xenobiotic biotransformation

As noted throughout the previous discussion, several genetic polymorphisms in biotransformation pathways have been described. One of the best studied genetic polymorphisms is that associated with N-acetylation of various primary aromatic amines.[65] A bimodal distribution in N-acetylation activity has been described, with approximately 50-70% of caucasians having a slow acetylation phenotype, with only 10-15% of Japanese demonstrating this phenotype. The slow-acetylator phenotype has been associated with a high incidence of adverse drug reactions at normal therapeutic doses of isoniazid, hydralazine, procainamide, dapsone, and some sulfa drugs. In addition, a number of occupationally important arylamines, including naphthylamine, benzidine, 4-aminobiphenyl, and 4-nitrobiphenyl, are detoxified by N-acetylation. In occupations in which exposure to certain carcinogenic arylamines occurs (e.g., dyestuff workers), epidemiologic evidence has suggested that slow acetylators are at a slightly increased risk for bladder and perhaps a few other types of cancer.[69]

Genetic polymorphisms in several P450 cytochromes have been described in humans, and may have implications for individualized drug therapy.[70] For example, the alicyclic hydroxylation of the antihypertensive drug debrisoquin is mediated via human CYP2D6, which is polymorphically distributed, with 7-10% of the population characterized as extremely poor metabolizers. The differences in activity between poor metabolizers and the rest of the population are remarkable, with an approximately 20,000-fold difference in debrisoquin hydroxylation. This is a single-gene polymorphism, but the enzyme has broad substrate specificity and is important in the oxidation of a variety of other drugs and chemicals. Although several studies have evaluated whether the CYP2D6 'slow metabolizer' phenotype/genotype is associated with increased risk for certain cancers, no clear association has been found.[71] Thus, the importance of this genetic polymorphism in environmental and occupational toxicology remains to be established.

The cytochrome P450-mediated hydroxylation of polyaromatic hydrocarbons to mutagenic and carcinogenic intermediates is well established, although no clear polymorphic distribution in this activity has been identified in humans. However, some studies have suggested that high inducibility of aryl hydrocarbon hydroxylase activity may be associated with an increased risk of lung cancer in smokers.[72]

A genetic polymorphism in the M1 form of glutathione S-transferase (hGSTM1) has been extensively studied in human populations as a possible risk factor for cancer and other environmentally related diseases. Approximately 50-60% of the population are genetically deficient in hGSTM1, and this deficiency has been associated with a modest increase in the risk of lung[73] and bladder[74] cancer in numerous studies.

Much remains to be learned about the biochemical and molecular mechanisms that underlie important inter-individual differences in susceptibility to environmental and occupational pollutants. The study of the relationship between genetic factors and individual susceptibility to drugs and chemicals is the basis for the rapidly emerging field of ecogenetics.[75] Recent advances in molecular biology now provide the experimental tools necessary to identify important genetic differences in individuals, and the identification of variant alleles in the human population has grown at a remarkable rate.[76] Application of these tools to toxicology, epidemiology and other areas of public health will be critical to the rational evaluation of individual risk from chemicals in the workplace and general environment, but will also raise important ethical, legal and social issues that must be addressed in lockstep with the science.[77]

Excretory pathways

The ability of the body to rid itself of exogenous chemicals is largely dependent on the physicochemical characteristics of the chemical. Chemicals that have very low blood-gas partition coefficients (e.g., are poorly soluble in blood and have a high vapor pressure) may be effectively eliminated by exhalation, whereas chemicals that are highly water soluble will generally be eliminated by excretion into the urine or bile. Because many chemicals of occupational and environmental concern lack either of these characteristics, accumulation in the body is likely to occur unless biotransformation processes alter the chemical to a more readily excretable form. Thus, elimination of a chemical from the body occurs by two processes, direct excretion of the unchanged substance or biotransformation to a different chemical form that may then be excreted as a metabolite.

Urinary excretion

The kidney is highly efficient at removing many foreign substances from the blood. However, the extent and rate of urinary excretion are highly dependent on the water solubility of the substance. Most chemicals in the blood are readily filtered by glomeruli; the only exceptions are those chemicals that bind avidly to high molecular weight plasma proteins. The rate at which plasma is filtered through the glomeruli (glomerular filtration rate or GFR) is approximately 125 mL/min in normal adults, and the rate of urine production is less than 1% of this volume. As the volume of glomerular filtrate is reduced by reabsorption of electrolytes, nutrients, and water in the nephron, the filtered xenobiotics are concentrated in the remaining tubular fluid, generating a large driving force for diffusion of the xenobiotics from the tubular lumen to the interstitial space and blood stream.

Thus, relatively lipid-soluble chemicals are not effectively eliminated in the urine following glomerular filtration because they readily diffuse back out of the tubular fluid into the blood. However, water-soluble chemicals are incapable of diffusing across the tubular membrane, can thus be concentrated to a very high degree in tubular fluid, and eventually are eliminated in the urine. For weak organic acids and bases, the extent of urinary excretion can be greatly influenced by the pH of the urine. In contrast to blood, where the pH must be maintained in a narrow range, urinary pH can readily vary between 5 and 8, resulting in large potential differences in the fraction of chemical in the ionized form. This knowledge has been put to practical therapeutic use in the treatment of poisoning with several weak organic acids or bases. The renal elimination of a weak organic acid with a pKa in the range of normal urinary pH can potentially be increased by 4-6-fold by simply alkalinizing the urine with an intravenous infusion of sodium bicarbonate. The renal elimination of salicylates and barbiturates has also been enhanced by alkalinization of the urine.

For some organic acids and bases, urinary excretion occurs in part by the presence of specific carrier-mediated transport processes in the proximal tubules.[78,79] Such highly efficient active transport systems have been described for a number of weak organic acids and bases and are important in the elimination of certain drugs, such as penicillin, and a variety of glucuronide and sulfate conjugates. Because these carrier-mediated transport processes may be saturated at high doses or may be competitively inhibited by the presence of other substances, for the purposes of risk characterization, it is important to identify whether such processes are functional in the elimination of chemicals. For example, phenoxy acids and several other weak organic acid herbicides appear to be relatively more toxic to dogs than most other species, apparently because the renal organic anion transport system is saturated at relatively low doses, resulting in decreased elimination and somewhat greater rate of accumulation in dogs compared with other species given the same dose.[80] In humans, renal elimination of these weak organic acids can be enhanced by alkaline diuresis and/or hemoperfusion.[81]

For chemicals that enter the tubular lumen exclusively by glomerular filtration and are not reabsorbed across it, the rate of renal elimination from the blood stream equals that of the GFR. For chemicals that are partially reabsorbed or are incompletely filtered because of protein binding, the renal clearance rate may be much less than the GFR. Because the rate of renal plasma flow is about five times higher than the GFR (e.g., only 20% of total renal plasma flow passes through the glomeruli), chemicals that are cleared from the blood by active transport processes can have renal clearance rates much higher than the GFR.

Biliary excretion

In contrast to urine, bile is not an ultrafiltrate of plasma, and the biliary tree has very little direct contact with the vascular compartment. Therefore, all substances that enter the bile from the plasma must do so by passing first across the hepatic sinusoidal membrane and then from the hepatocyte across the canalicular membrane to the bile.[82] Bile flow is produced by the flux of water from the hepatocyte to the canalicular space in response to an osmotic gradient produced by active transport of bile acids and bicarbonate into the canalicular space. After chemicals enter the hepatocyte, they are generally biotransformed to polar metabolites, which may either re-enter the circulation for elimination in the urine or may be actively transported into the bile. As a general rule of thumb, polar chemicals with molecular weights in excess of about 325 to 350 Daltons will be secreted preferentially in the bile, whereas chemicals of lower molecular weights will be excreted primarily in the urine. The liver possesses several distinct active transport systems for endogenous and exogenous hydrophilic compounds. For example, biliary elimination of anionic compounds, including glutathione S-conjugates, is mediated by a transport protein known as MRP2, whereas bile salts are excreted by a bile salt export pump (BSEP); class I-P-glycoprotein (P-gp) is involved in the secretion of amphiphilic cationic drugs, whereas class II-P-gp is a phospholipid transporter.[83]

A widely used liver function test, based on the rate of plasma clearance of the blue dye sulfobromophthalein (BSP) or indocyanine green, is in fact a measure of the functional integrity of a hepatic organic anion transport system distinct from that which transports bile acids. Because the removal of these dyes from plasma occurs almost exclusively by hepatobiliary elimination, a decline in the rate of plasma clearance is a useful indicator of hepatic dysfunction. Bilirubin is also excreted in the bile (primarily as the diglucuronide conjugate), by active transport processes,

and a dysfunction in this system will result in elevated plasma bilirubin levels (jaundice; see Chapter 26.1). Indeed, genetic defects in biliary transport processes have led to new insights into how hepatobiliary transport processes function in humans.[84] Mutations in specific bile acid or lipid transporters have been identified within specific cholestatic disorders, and genetic polymorphisms have been established for specific diseases.[85]

Some metals are eliminated in the bile, albeit slowly, and this can be an important route of elimination. For example, methyl mercury is secreted in the bile, but it is largely reabsorbed in the intestinal tract. Interruption of this 'enterohepatic recirculation' by the administration of thiol-binding resins greatly reduces the half-life of methyl mercury and is a useful therapeutic approach to the treatment of methyl mercury poisoning.[86]

Some relatively non-polar compounds can also be excreted in the bile, probably by dissolution in biliary micelles. These are formed by the aggregation of bile acids and phospholipids, and are an important means of solubilizing the large quantity of cholesterol that is normally secreted in the bile. Too high a ratio of cholesterol to bile acids and phospholipids results in the precipitation of cholesterol as gallstones.[87] Because micelles are extremely effective at dissolving non-polar compounds, lipid-soluble xenobiotics can partition into the micelles from the hepatocyte. However, after biliary micelles reach the intestinal tract, the non-polar xenobiotics will be rapidly absorbed. Interruption of the enterohepatic circulation with the non-absorbable anion-exchange resin cholestyramine (used clinically to lower blood lipids) has been used successfully in humans to reduce the half-life and toxicity of the highly lipid-soluble pesticide kepone following very high occupational exposures.[88]

Hepatic dysfunction from disease or chemical toxicity can alter the kinetics of elimination and, thus, the toxicity of a wide variety of chemicals.[89] For example, the adverse effects of some digitalis glycosides can be enhanced in the presence of hepatic disease because hepatobiliary clearance is decreased, although this is a less common cause of digitalis sensitivity than other factors such as poor renal function, hypokalemia or hypothyroidism.[90] Some drugs that induce microsomal enzymes also enhance bile flow and may increase biliary excretion of other xenobiotics. Phenobarbital treatment increases bile flow and enhances the biliary elimination of methyl mercury. The potassium-sparing diuretic, spironolactone, has been shown experimentally to decrease the toxicity of several chemicals, including mercury and cardiac glycosides, by enhancing biliary excretion.

TOXICOKINETICS

The absorption, distribution, biotransformation, and excretion of xenobiotics in the body is a dynamic process. The concentration of toxicant at its receptor site is thus dependent on the various rates of reactions that affect absorption, distribution, biotransformation, and excretion. The field of pharmacokinetics developed largely out of a need to under-

a One-compartment open model

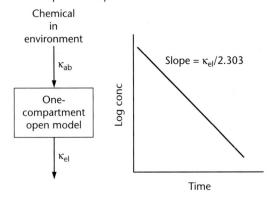

b Two-compartment open model

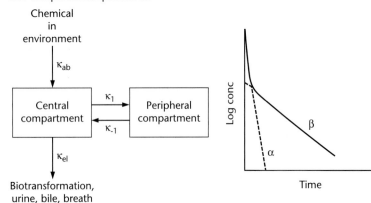

Figure 5.12: One- and two-compartment pharmacokinetic models. A one-compartment model (a) represents the simplest approach to understanding the distribution of chemicals in the body and assumes that the chemical is instantaneously distributed throughout the compartment (body) and that elimination from the compartment occurs by a first-order process (a constant per cent of remaining compound is eliminated per unit time). A two-compartment model (b) takes into account a slower, distribution phase between the central compartment (blood) and peripheral compartments (tissues). Elimination proceeds only from the central compartment, which is in dynamic equilibrium with the peripheral compartments. Absorption rate constants (k_{ab}), equilibrium rate constants (k_1, k_{-1}), and elimination rate constants (k_{el}) can be determined, which describe these processes under conditions of first-order kinetics.

stand the factors that dictate the determination of efficacious and non-toxic doses of pharmaceuticals. Essentially the same biologic factors also determine the biologic fate of non-drug chemicals in the body; therefore, toxicokinetics and pharmacokinetics are nearly identical disciplines, and toxicologists frequently use the terms interchangeably.

The mathematic modeling of the fate of chemicals in biologic systems commonly uses compartmental models and rate constants to reflect various physiologic functions.[91] A 'one-compartment open model' assumes that a chemical is instantaneously distributed equally throughout the body, and uses the concentration of a chemical in plasma as representative of the concentration throughout the compartment (Fig. 5.12a). For chemicals that more slowly redistribute from the vascular compartment to tissues, a two-compartment model is used (Fig. 5.12b). The central compartment conceptually represents the vascular space and rapidly perfused tissues, whereas the rest of the body represents the peripheral compartment. There is a rate constant for exchange between the two compartments, a rate constant for influx to the central compartment (where absorptive processes are involved), and a rate constant of elimination (k_{el}) from the central compartment. For chemicals that slowly redistribute to 'deep' compartments, such as fat and bone, a three-compartment model, with different rate constants between the central compartment and the two peripheral compartments, is sometimes used to explain the very long terminal half-life of some chemicals.

The volume in which a chemical is dispersed, of course, varies greatly, depending on its solubility in water and fat, whether it binds to proteins in the plasma, or whether it binds to intracellular sites. This so-called apparent volume of distribution is an important pharmacokinetic parameter and is essentially a constant that relates the concentration of a chemical in the plasma to the total amount of chemical in the body. Thus, for chemicals that are tightly bound to plasma proteins, the majority of the chemical is confined to the plasma (central compartment), and the apparent volume of distribution (Vd) is relatively small, perhaps on the order of 5-10 liters. In contrast, for chemicals that are highly lipid soluble or are sequestered in intracellular sites, the Vd may be very large, exceeding the 'true' volume of the body by many fold.

The apparent Vd is a necessary factor to estimate the 'body burden' or total amount of chemical in the body, at any point in time. Thus, the body burden is equal to the concentration of the chemical in the plasma times the Vd. 'Clearance' is a term that refers to the ability of the body to 'clear' a chemical from the blood and has units of flow rate (e.g., milliliters per minute). Thus, a chemical with a clearance of 50 mL/min is eliminated from 50 mL of blood in 1 minute. Clearance is thus a measure of the overall efficiency of the removal of a chemical from the body. Total body clearance (Cl_T) can be proportioned to specific pathways of elimination, such as the liver and kidney, such that:

$$Cl_T = Cl_H + Cl_R + \ldots ,$$

where Cl_H and Cl_R represent the rate of hepatic and renal removal, respectively. Clearance is thus related to the apparent Vd and a first-order elimination rate constant, k_{el}, according to the simple equation:

$$Cl_T = Vd\, k_{el}$$

Elimination of a chemical from the central compartment usually occurs exponentially by a first-order rate process, in which the fraction of chemical removed per unit time remains constant (a constant per cent of chemical is eliminated per unit time, e.g., 10% per minute). A plot of the log of the plasma concentration versus time will result in a straight line (Fig. 5.13). For first-order elimination rates, the plasma half-life (time required for the concentration of a chemical in plasma to decrease by 50%) is proportional to the elimination rate constant, k_{el}, by the following equation:

$$T_{1/2} = \frac{0.693}{k_{el}}$$

If elimination occurs by a process that is saturable (e.g., enzymatic metabolism or carrier-mediated transport), the rate of elimination will follow zero-order kinetics (a constant amount of chemical is eliminated per unit time, e.g., 10 mg/min), regardless of the concentration. The importance of enzyme saturation at high doses to toxicity is illustrated by the hypothetic situation shown in Figure 5.13b. This figure illustrates the hypothetical one-compartment elimination kinetics of two individuals given the same dose of a chemical, in which the elimination pathway in subject A is saturated at plasma concentrations above about 50 μg/mL, but saturation of the elimination pathway in subject B does not occur within the dose range shown. If toxic effects were evident at plasma concentrations above 10 μg/mL in both subjects, the period of time necessary for subject A to reduce the plasma concentrations to below the toxic level is over twice as long as that for subject B. The upper panel shows the plasma concentration versus time curve for the two subjects; the lower panel plots these same data as the log plasma concentration versus time. The linear response for subject B is typical of a first-order rate of elimination from a one-compartment model, with a half-life of 1 hour. The convex shape of the log-plasma concentration versus time curve in subject A is indicative of saturable metabolism or zero-order kinetics.

Toxicokinetic modeling of repeated exposure to chemicals in the workplace and/or environment requires the important additional consideration of the period between exposures, or the 'dosing interval'. If the dosing interval is longer than the elimination half-life, then accumulation of the chemical in the body will occur. Assuming a first-order rate of elimination at all concentrations, the amount eliminated between doses will eventually become equal to the amount taken in, and no further accumulation will occur. The point in time at which the amount of chemical eliminated equals the amount taken in during a dosing

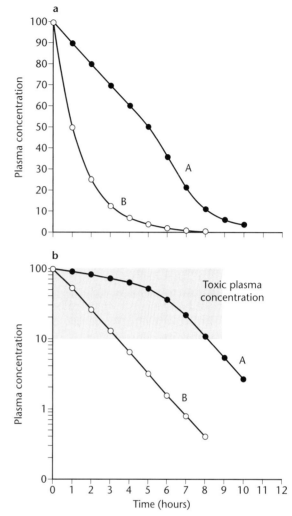

Figure 5.13 First-order and zero-order kinetics of elimination. When the plasma concentration of a chemical is plotted directly with time (a), a straight line is achieved only when elimination processes are saturated (A), and elimination from the plasma occurs via zero-order kinetics (a constant amount of chemical is removed per minute). However, elimination of most toxic substances occurs via first-order kinetics, in which a constant per cent (or fraction) of the dose is eliminated per unit time. When the log of the plasma concentrations is plotted against time (b), a straight line results when elimination is first order (B). Note how much longer chemical A remains in the region of toxic plasma concentration compared with chemical B, even though both have the same first-order elimination rates.

interval is called the 'steady state'. The average amount of chemical in the body (body burden) at the steady state is described by the following equation:

$$X_{ss} = \frac{(1.44)t_{1/2}D}{\tau}$$

where X_{ss} = the body burden at steady state, $t_{1/2}$ equals the elimination half-life, D = the amount of the dose at each dosing interval, and τ = the dosing interval (in the same time units as the $t_{1/2}$).

If the apparent Vd for the chemical is known, then the average plasma concentration at steady state can be obtained by simply dividing the body burden at steady state (X_{ss}) by Vd. From this relationship, it is evident that repeated daily exposure to a chemical with a half-life of 1 day would result in an accumulation of chemical in the body to an amount about 1.5 times greater than the amount of the daily exposure. For chemicals with very long half-lives, such as many chlorinated polyaromatic compounds (e.g., PCBs, DDT, and dioxins, which may have half-lives greater than several years) and some metals (e.g., Cd), accumulation may occur throughout a lifetime, potentially reaching toxic levels many years after the initial exposure. The relationship between toxicity and body burden is not always straightforward because accumulation may occur in body 'compartments', such as adipose tissue or bone, which may not be target organs for the toxicity of the chemical. As long as the chemical remains highly partitioned in non-target organ compartments, its presence may be of little toxicologic consequence. However, if for some reason this site of storage becomes mobilized (e.g., fasting in the case of fat storage of chlorinated hydrocarbons or osteolysis in the case of bone storage of lead), the subsequent release of stored chemical to the circulation and, thus, its redistribution to target organs could result in toxicity many years following the exposure.

Chemical–chemical interactions

The evaluation of toxicity for drugs and chemicals often assumes that the exposure to the suspect drug or chemical is isolated. However, this is seldom the case because simultaneous or sequential exposures to multiple drugs and chemicals are commonplace in our society. Interactions of prescription, over-the-counter, and/or recreational drugs with other such drugs, drugs with chemicals in the home or workplace, or with dietary factors can and do occur. There are many well-known adverse interactions, such as the interaction between monoamine oxidase inhibitors prescribed as antidepressants with other pressor drugs (sympathomimetics) and/or with tyramine, which occurs naturally in some foods (e.g., some types of wine and cheese). However, the number of chemicals for which specific interactions have been documented is likely to be only a small fraction of what really occurs. Of course, beneficial chemical–chemical interactions are the basis of antidotal therapy.

The number of potential drug–chemical combinations is, by definition, nearly infinite, and it would be impossible to study all such combinations systematically. Nevertheless, clinicians familiar with the basic mechanisms of action of drugs and chemicals can reasonably identify many potential interactions. Particularly because analytic techniques have emerged over the past few decades, the clinical problems seen as a consequence of such interactions have been recognized. Moreover, certain principles have been developed to estimate the likelihood of such problems, often in advance of their actual occurrence. These can be summarized as follows.

1. Interactions between two compounds prior to actual exposure by the host. For example, an acidic drug, when combined with an alkaline compound, may become insoluble and precipitate out of solution, thus becoming unavailable for absorption. Other examples include the high binding affinity of some drugs, such as cholestyramine, for other drugs, thus reducing their bioavailability.

2. Interactions that occur after ingestion but have an impact on the rate or the degree of absorption. Classic examples include antibiotics, such as penicillin, tetracyclines, many barbiturates, dicumarol, and a variety of hydroxide compounds. In these instances, multiple mechanisms may be involved so that the physician managing a given case will do well to consult the listing of such interactions. As a generalization, these types of interactions may serve to minimize therapeutic efficacy but seldom contribute to the enhancement of poisoning.

3. Drug interactions resulting from alterations in metabolism and/or disposition may lead to clinical problems.[92] For drugs that are largely bound to proteins, the displacement of as little as 1% or 2% from protein can greatly increase the biologically active compound. An example of this would be the interactions between various cardiac glycosides and dicumarol. Moreover, such displacement also alters the biologic half-life of the displaced drug. In other instances, concomitant administration of drugs, such as phenobarbital, with a wide variety of other drugs produces induction of enzyme systems (e.g., the cytochrome P450 series), with the result that the second drug will have enhanced elimination. In other instances, such as adding erythromycin to the regimen of a patient already taking theophylline, metabolism will be impaired such that the theophylline concentration may reach harmful levels.

4. 'Competition at the receptor site', the locus of pharmacologic activity, can occur. Classically, naloxone's ability to displace a variety of opioid entities is well known; other drugs, such as phenothiazines, tricyclic antidepressants, and antihistamines, exert comparable alterations at other receptor sites within the nervous system. With increasingly sophisticated analytic techniques, still more unanticipated interactions are being uncovered, although many have little or no clinical significance.

5. Alteration of pH of some body fluid and modifying the pharmacologic activity of a second compound. One example is the administration of sodium bicarbonate to treat an overdose of salicylate; the resultant alkalinization of the renal tubular fluid enhances the ionization of filtered salicylate, precludes its resorption, and significantly increases its excretion.

TOXICITY TESTING AND PREDICTIVE TOXICOLOGY

Although epidemiology can be an effective tool to identify and characterize chemical risks to humans, a major limitation of human epidemiologic studies is that the damage has been done by the time it is identified. Furthermore, the utility of epidemiology for purposes of 'predictive' toxicology is limited by a number of factors, including: (1) the presence of confounding, (2) difficulties in dose and exposure assessment, (3) difficulty in identifying suitable exposed populations, and (4) limited statistical power associated with many environmental and occupational epidemiologic studies.

Increased public awareness of chemical hazards, coupled with a few notable and highly publicized and potentially preventable chemical disasters, has stimulated the search for biologically meaningful and relevant tests to predict hazards from chemicals before human exposures occur. Most predictive toxicity tests rely on the use of common laboratory animals, such as rats, mice, and guinea pigs, although bacterial tests systems and cell and tissue cultures have gained widespread use in some types of toxicity testing, most notably mutagenicity. It is beyond the scope of this chapter to describe in detail the design and conduct of the multitude of toxicity tests that are currently available. However, a summary review of the nature and approaches used in toxicity assessment is given. (For a detailed description of these approaches and techniques, the reader is referred to the excellent reference text on this topic by Hayes.[93])

The fundamental principle that dictates the utility of animal models for predicting human response is that the adverse effects of a chemical on a test organism, when properly qualified, are applicable to humans; that is, laboratory animals are useful biologic surrogates for the human response to toxic substances. This premise underlies all experimental biology and medicine and is not unique to toxicology. The basic premise that laboratory animals are useful surrogates for human responses to toxic substances is well supported by a wealth of scientific data.[94] However, there are many circumstances in which the data obtained from animal models may differ from those in humans substantially, both quantitatively and qualitatively, because of mechanistic, pharmacokinetic, and/or pharmacodynamic properties. Thus, basic research into the biochemical and molecular modes of action and the biologic fate of chemicals in experimental animal and human tissues is a critical component of predictive toxicology.

Toxicity testing is generally divided into several major categories, based on the duration of exposure and/or the specific endpoint to be measured.

Acute toxicity testing

Acute toxicity studies involve the administration of a single dose of chemical to test animals. Acute toxicity tests can be conducted by a variety of routes of administration, including oral, dermal (percutaneous), inhalation, or parenteral (intravenous, intraperitoneal, or subcutaneous). A common measure of acute toxicity is the LD_{50}, although much additional useful information is generally obtained from acute toxicity studies. In addition to identifying the lethal and sublethal doses, acute toxicity tests provide information on target organs, mode of action, duration, and the reversibility of the non-lethal effects. In product safety evaluations, the acute toxicity test is used primarily to establish appropriate doses for subacute or subchronic studies, where repeated dosing occurs.

Subacute toxicity testing

For chemicals that are expected to accumulate in target organs or produce irreversible effects from individual doses, repeated administration of an agent over a period of 2-4 weeks is sometimes used to provide additional dose range information for the design of longer term studies. Additional information on target organs, pharmacokinetics, pharmacodynamics, and the mechanism of action is generated from such studies but does not generally fulfill regulatory requirements for the product safety evaluation of pesticides, food additives, and other chemicals for which routine exposures are likely to occur.

Subchronic toxicity testing

Routine toxicologic evaluation of a chemical for potential human health risks almost always requires the inclusion of studies in which the test chemical is administered daily for a period of 90 days.[95] Usually four to five doses are selected, the highest dose of which produces overt toxicity and limited mortality at the end of 90 days of dosing and the lowest dose selected approximates the maximum dose that would produce no observable adverse effects (NOAEL) even with 90 days of repeated dosing. For regulatory purposes, the objective of a subchronic bioassay is to identify the NOAEL. Because estimates of acceptable human doses are frequently derived from the animal NOAEL, the care and thoroughness of such studies can have a major impact on the regulatory standards for the workplace and environment. In general, most regulatory agencies establish acceptable levels of exposure by identifying the animal NOAEL (in units of milligrams of chemical per kilogram animal body weight per day), then dividing that value by an arbitrary 'safety' or uncertainty factor. Frequently a value of 100 or 1000 is used, depending on the degree of confidence the regulator has in the quality and relevance of the animal data to humans.

This approach assumes that a threshold exists in the dose–response relationship; that is, there is some dose below which no response will occur, regardless of the size of the population exposed. The animal NOAEL is an experimental estimate of the threshold dose in that strain of animal, and the safety factor is used to account for possible differences in species sensitivity, differences in response among various human individuals, and for 'scaling factor' differences (on a body weight basis, small animals generally require relatively larger doses than large animals to elicit the same response; the use of body surface area, rather than body weight, is often a better scaling factor). Because dose–response relationships for many toxic effects are steep, a 100-fold uncertainty factor in most circumstances may afford a large degree of protection. However, where there are significant differences in the mechanism of action, pharmacokinetics, or pharmacodynamics between the animal species used for estimation of the NOAEL and humans, the use of a 100-fold uncertainty factor may be significantly underprotective or overprotective. Thus, the establishment of relevant exposure standards for humans depends on a good understanding of the many factors that influence toxic responses, and how these factors may be similar or different between test animals and humans.

Chronic toxicity testing and carcinogenicity evaluation

In circumstances in which a chemical has a very long half-life, it causes irreversible effects at doses well below the lethal dose, and/or it is suspected of being potentially carcinogenic, a chronic bioassay may be warranted. These studies generally involve the administration of the test substance to animals for an entire lifetime, which for rodents is about 2 years. Generally, the route of administration is the one that is most relevant to human exposures. Administration of the test substance in the diet or drinking water is most common, although chronic bioassays using inhalation exposure are occasionally conducted. The latter are very expensive and, technically, much more difficult to conduct.

Although chronic bioassays may occasionally be conducted to assess endpoints other than cancer, by far the most frequent purpose for such studies is the assessment of oncogenic (carcinogenic) potential. Most chronic bioassays utilize both sexes of two species (almost always rats and mice), at least two exposure doses, and one unexposed control group, with approximately 40-50 animals per group. Dose selection is a major consideration in the design and conduct of a chronic bioassay, especially if the study is intended to evaluate the oncogenic potential of the chemical.[96]

For the purposes of quantitative cancer risk assessment, most regulatory agencies assume that all chemicals that increase tumor incidence do so in a non-threshold manner. Although studies in experimental animals have demonstrated that the extent of DNA damage is often proportional to dose at relatively low concentrations, experiments have not been, nor could they be, conducted at the very low lifetime doses that would be associated with cancer risks of less than about 0.1% (1 in 1000). The statistical power of studies that use even maximum experimentally manageable sample sizes (e.g., 50 animals per dose) is extremely limited. For example, consider a study that exposed 50 animals for a lifetime at dose x, with no tumors found in either the control or dose x group (Fig. 5.14). The most that could be said about such a negative experiment is that we would be 95% confident that, if a

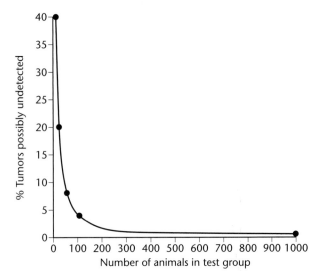

Figure 5.14: Statistical power of animal tests - power versus number. The statistical power of an animal test to determine a small positive response is highly dependent on the sample size. This curve tells us that we can be 95% confident that a chemical that tested negative in 100 animals will not produce more than about 4% incidence of tumors in a larger population. Thus, a negative test, even using 100 animals in a single dose, cannot be used to prove that a chemical is not capable of causing a significant incidence of cancer in a larger population exposed to the same dose.

human population equal in sensitivity to the test animals were exposed at dose x for a lifetime, the true incidence of cancer would not be greater than about 8%.

Obviously, it is experimentally impossible to demonstrate that a chemical poses no significant cancer risk using doses in the range of human exposures. For example, to detect a statistically significant ($P = 0.05$) tumor incidence of 1 in 1000 (0.1%), it would require the use of 460,000 animals in *each* dose group, plus control, assuming that the background incidence of tumors was near zero.[97] Thus, the only reasonable alternative is to assume that there is some describable dose–response relationship, test animals at doses high enough to give statistically measurable response levels (tumor incidence above about 5% to 10% in most instances), and then extrapolate the dose–response data down to the doses encountered by humans. Based on this logic, current carcinogenicity testing guidelines require that animal studies used for the quantitative risk assessment of potentially carcinogenic chemicals utilize the maximum tolerated dose (MTD) and some fraction (usually one half or one fourth) of the MTD to characterize tumor dose–response relationships and then extrapolate the dose–response data to the very low doses associated with 'acceptable' lifetime cancer incidence (e.g., one additional lifetime cancer per million exposed individuals). Thus, it is not uncommon to find that cancer risk estimates are based on extrapolation from animal studies with dose–response curves containing only two or three high-dose data points to doses four to six orders of magnitude below those in the measured response range. Figure 5.15 shows the process of extrapolation of observed animal data to the very low doses generally deemed necessary to

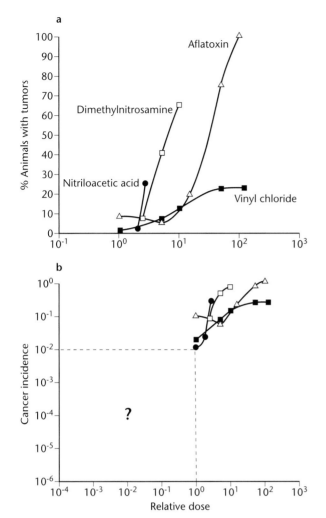

Figure 5.15: dose–response extrapolation to low doses. The upper panel represents the log-dose–response curve for four different chemical carcinogens. The lower panel represents the same data plotted on a log-log scale to demonstrate the extent of extrapolation typical of most quantitative risk assessments. The dose data for each carcinogen have been normalized by setting the lowest dose of each carcinogen that gave a positive result to 1, and subsequent doses as a multiplier of that dose. Actual dose ranges and routes of exposure for the four carcinogens were vinyl chloride, 50-6000 ppm (inhalation); aflatoxin, 1-100 ppb (diet); nitrilotriacetic acid, 7500-20,000 ppm (diet); dimethylnitrosamine, 5-20 ppm (diet). (From Amdur MO, Doull J, Klaassen CD. Casarett and Doull's Toxicology: the basic science of poisons, 4th edn. New York: Pergamon Press, 1991.)

protect public health. Regulatory agencies frequently use additional lifetime risk of 10^{-4}–10^{-6} (1 in 10,000 to 1 in million) as the level of socially acceptable risk.

Because of the uncertainty in the actual shape of the dose–response curve at very low doses, a great deal of potential error is introduced in modeling and extrapolation from the high-dose animal data to the low doses of environmental concern. This uncertainty is aggravated by the realization that high doses may produce tissue toxicity that does not occur at low doses, and that this toxicity in itself may produce a strong promotional effect by stimulating tissue repair and cell division.

The selection of a mathematic model to extrapolate the observed animal dose–response data to the very low dose levels encountered by humans can have a large effect on the projected acceptable risk level. Although numerous mathematic models have been proposed, there are few scientific data that would allow one to support the use of one model over another.

In addition to model selection, there are many other areas of uncertainty in the quantitative risk assessment process, such as the selection of animal data studies when more than one is available, the type of tumor responses to be used (e.g., total tumors or malignant tumors only), exposure assumptions, and human dose estimations. The current practice of making conservative assumptions (e.g., assumptions that tend to overestimate risk) when uncertainties exist is often justified as necessary to ensure that risks are not underestimated. Although the accuracy of risk projections based on these methods has limitations, and may overestimate risk, the process provides a useful means of comparing the relative magnitude of potential cancer risks posed by different chemicals, and is a useful addition to other scientific information necessary for the establishment of regulatory guidelines that are adequately protective of public health.

There is currently much controversy over the use of high-dose animal testing in cancer risk assessment. There is little question that the quantitative interpretation of the apparent magnitude of risk can be significantly altered by relatively small changes in the slope of the dose–response curve in the measured region, which can result from tissue damage and/or saturation of biotransformation pathways likely to occur at doses near the MTD. Consideration of the differences in pharmacokinetics and pharmacodynamics at high doses versus low doses will substantially enhance the reliability of predictive toxicology tests and represents a very active area of research in toxicology.[98]

Mutagenicity testing

There are numerous different tests commonly used to assess the mutagenic ability of chemicals.[99] There are two fundamentally important types of mutations, i.e., mutations in somatic cells and mutations in germinal cells. Mutations in somatic cells are not passed from generation to generation but may be associated with the development of cancer in the mutated somatic tissue. In contrast, germinal mutations may not express themselves as overt toxicity in the host but can be passed on to offspring in the form of a heritable genetic alteration.

Most chemicals encountered in the workplace and general environment are not sufficiently chemically reactive to interact directly with DNA, but they may be oxidized by enzymes in the liver and other tissues to highly electrophilic intermediates that covalently bind with nucleophilic sites in DNA. Because the interaction of electrophilic chemicals with nucleophilic sites in DNA is largely independent of the source and type of DNA, simple organisms such as bacteria, coupled with mammalian tissue fractions containing the enzymes necessary for activation, are commonly used. Thus, in contrast to most other predictive toxicity tests, mutagenicity assays most frequently utilize responses to bacteria or cells in culture.

The most widely used method for determining the mutagenic potential of a chemical is the Ames Salmonella mutagenicity assay. This test employs cultures of *S. typhimurium* bacteria that have been genetically altered from the wild type. These bacteria have a mutation in the gene that normally functions to synthesize the essential amino acid histidine. Because this gene is defective, the bacteria are unable to synthesize their own histidine (termed His⁻), and thus, they cannot grow in a histidine-deficient medium. However, the genetic alteration responsible for the histidine deficiency is readily altered back to the wild type (a 'reverse' mutation) in the presence of genotoxic chemicals. In addition to the His⁻ mutation, these strains of bacteria have additional mutations that enhance their responsiveness to mutagenic chemicals, such as genetic alterations that reduce the efficiency of DNA repair and increase the cell coat permeability to exogenous chemicals. Thus, one can plate millions of bacteria on a medium deficient in histidine, add a potentially mutagenic test chemical and the mammalian enzymes necessary for metabolic activation to the culture plates, and culture the bacteria for 48 hours. Readily visible bacterial colonies will form on the plate only where individual bacteria have been mutated back to the wild type.

The number of 'revertant' colonies formed per unit of mutagenic chemical is thus an index of the mutagenicity of the chemical. Generally, the 9000 *g* supernatant fraction (S9 fraction) of a rat liver homogenate is added to the culture plates as the source of the biotransformation enzymes. Because millions of bacteria can be used in a single plate, only a very small fraction of bacteria actually have to be mutated at the His⁻ locus to produce a readily measurable response. This simple and relatively inexpensive test has been used to screen thousands of different chemicals for mutagenic potential.

There are many other assays that employ other types of bacteria, yeast, and mammalian cells in culture to identify the mutagenic potential of chemicals.[99] The Ames test and other similar bacterial assays generally identify point mutations or 'microlesions', e.g., single base-pair substitutions or frame-shift mutations (deletions or additions).

There are also a number of in-vitro and in-vivo tests that have been developed to assess major alterations in DNA, sometimes referred to as 'macrolesions'. For example, incorporation of radiolabeled thymidine into high molecular weight DNA (unscheduled DNA synthesis) can be readily determined as a measure of DNA damage following exposure of normally quiescent mammalian cells in culture to a mutagenic chemical. Because the extent of DNA damage is reflected by the rate of DNA repair and thymidine incorporation, this test can be used to assess widespread but non-specific damage to DNA. Mammalian cells in culture are frequently used to identify chromosomal aberrations such as 'sister chromatid exchanges', chromosomal rearrangements or deletions, and micronuclei formation.[99] Increases in chromosomal aberrations in

circulating mononuclear leukocytes from occupationally exposed populations have been used as an in-vivo indicator of human exposure to mutagenic chemicals.[100] However, one should always insist on the use of appropriate controls because the association between exposure and effect can only be made when an appropriate non-exposed population is used for comparison.

Although short-term mutagenicity assays are extremely valuable in assessing the potential mutagenic activity of a chemical, the quantitative interpretation of such assays to human health risks has limitations. Generally, a chemical is tested in a variety of different mutagenicity test systems before qualitative judgments about the potential genotoxicity to humans are made. Chemicals that test positively in multiple different test systems are likely to be mutagenic and, thus, potentially carcinogenic in humans, whereas the mutagenicity of chemicals that test positively in only one or two assays but test negatively in several other tests may be of questionable relevance to humans.

Short-term mutagenicity assays are frequently used to assess carcinogenic risk. Although the qualitative relationship between mutagenicity and carcinogenicity is significant, it is not absolute. There are chemicals that may test positively in short-term mutagenicity assays that do not present a significant carcinogenic risk to humans (false-positive result relative to cancer risk) because of pharmacokinetic and/or pharmacodynamic factors. Similarly, there are chemicals that may pose a carcinogenic threat to humans that test negatively in short-term mutagenicity assays (false-negative result). For example, several inorganic substances, such as arsenic, chromium, and asbestos, test negative in the majority of mutagenicity assays, yet they are known human carcinogens. In general, all chemicals that modify the carcinogenic response by epigenetic mechanisms (e.g., promoters, co-carcinogens, and immune suppressants) may be important human carcinogens, even though they are not mutagenic. Conversely, the identification of chemicals that are mutagenic provides supportive, but not confirmatory, evidence of potential human carcinogenicity.

Reproductive and developmental toxicity tests

Well-defined experimental protocols have been developed for the assessment of the reproductive and developmental effects of chemicals in both male[101] and female[102] test animals. These tests often involve the exposure of laboratory animals throughout gestation, weaning, and early reproductive life. For example, a typical three-generation study (Fig. 5.16) to determine the effects of chemicals on reproductive capacity involves continuous exposure of both male and female animals (F₀, or Parental), generally by the diet or drinking water route, after weaning. Males are generally exposed for 8-11 weeks, and females for 2 weeks, prior to mating. The animals are then mated, reproductive success is evaluated, and the offspring (F₁A generation) are examined by autopsy at weaning for malformations. The parental generation (F₀) continues to

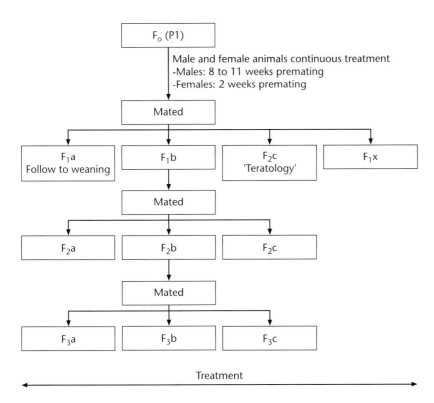

Figure 5.16: Three-generation reproduction study. Generations and time intervals involved in a three-generation study of effects on the reproduction process in rats. Adapted from Christian MS. Test methods for assessing female reproductive and developmental toxicology. In: Hayes AW, ed. Principles and methods of toxicology, 4th edn. Philadelphia: Taylor & Francis, 2001;1301–80.

be exposed and mated a second time after 1 to 2 weeks to produce the F_1B generation. These offspring are then continued on the study, receiving potential exposure by lactation from the exposed dams, and then are switched to the exposure diet at weaning.

Selected parents from this generation (F_1) are continued on the study and mated twice in the same manner, and the offspring (F_2A and F_2B) are treated as described previously, such that the cycle is repeated to a third generation (F_3A, F_3B). At one or more of the mating points in the three-generation study, one half of the pregnant female animals are killed and evaluated for the number and distribution of embryos, early implantation sites, and resorptions. These comprehensive studies provide useful information about the potential effects of the test chemical on male and female reproductive capacity and teratogenic effects. If abnormal responses are obtained in either category, more specialized tests can be performed to evaluate male and female reproductive effects individually and/or evaluate the teratogenic effects by limiting the exposure to specified portions of gestation at doses that are not associated with maternal toxicity.

Interpretation of reproductive and developmental tests must include an assessment of 0 relationships, the presence or absence of frank histopathologic damage to the reproductive organs, and evidence of maternal toxicity in which teratogenic effects have been identified. Because of the well-known occurrence of significant species differences in response to teratogenic agents, information on the mechanism of action, pharmacokinetics, and pharmacodynamics are again critical to the rational extrapolation of laboratory animal data to human health risks.

Specialized tests to assess other forms of toxicity

In addition to the basic toxicity testing discussed, numerous other special tests have been developed to assess ocular toxicity,[103] dermal toxicity,[104] neurobehavioral effects,[105] and immunologic alterations.[106] Ocular and dermal toxicity have classically been determined by direct application of the materials to the cornea or skin, usually using rabbits or guinea pigs as test animals. The 'Draize' test was originally developed in 1944 to identify human eye irritants using rabbits. Although this test is sometimes a regulatory requirement prior to manufacture of products that might result in eye contact, concerns over animal welfare have stimulated the search for better ways to assess the eye irritation potential of chemicals. Modifications of the procedure in recent years have reduced both the number of animals necessary and the level of discomfort, and new in-vitro procedures using corneal cells in culture and other similar approaches are now being used to screen for ocular irritancy potential.

The shaved surface of the guinea pig is frequently used to assess dermal irritation. A variety of protocols and methods of interpretation are available that attempt to quantify dermal irritation, delayed hypersensitivity, and other types of dermatoxicity. These tests generally involve the direct application of material to the shaved surface of the animal, followed by occlusion of the site with an impervious material for a defined period. A scoring system for erythema, eschar formation, and edema is then used to provide an overall score of dermal irritation. The assessment of allergic reactions, such as delayed hypersensitivity, usually involves the application of the test

Carcinogen	One-hit		Linearized multistage		Weibull		Multihit	
Vinyl chloride	1	(0.03)	1	(0.03)	1×10^{-7}	(0.56)	2×10^{-8}	(0.32)
Aflatoxin	1	(0.07)	20	(0.49)	1000	(0.64)	8000	(0.54)
Dimethylnitrosamine	1	(0.04)	600	(0.57)	600	(0.63)	200	(0.72)
Nitrilotriacetic acid	1	(<0.001)	10	(0.09)	30,000	(0.48)	40,000	(0.48)

* The numbers shown represent the difference in VSD estimates compared with those obtained from the one-hit model.
The values in parentheses represent the P value for goodness-of-fit of the data to the model.
Derived from Food Safety Council (1980), as adapted from Amdur MO, Doull J, Klaassen CD. Casarett and Doull's Toxicology: the basic science of poisons, 4th edn. New York: Pergamon Press, 1991.

Table 5.6 Differences in model-derived estimates of the virtually safe doses (VSD) at 10^6 risk level, relative to the one-hit model*

Motor system tests	Sensory system tests	Sensorimotor integration tests
Balancing rods	Startle response	Locomotor activity
Rotarod	Auditory discrimination	Circadian activity
Gait	Visual discrimination	Conditioned avoidance
Grip strength	Vibration sensitivity	
Cognitive tests: learning	**Social & emotional & memory behavior**	**Reproductive behavior**
Radial maze	Exploratory behavior	Female estrus behavior
Operant fixed interval	Aggressive behavior	Male mating behavior
Spatial discrimination	Social investigation	

Data from Norton S. Methods for behavioral toxicology. In: Hayes AW, ed. Principles and methods of toxicology, 2nd edn. New York: Raven Press, 1989;558–72.

Table 5.7 Methods for behavioral toxicity assessment

material and an adjuvant to facilitate the expression of dermal sensitization.

Experimental methods for the neurobehavioral assessment of chemicals have been developed and are finding increasing use in routine toxicity assessment.[105] Common tests in adult animals include the assessment of sensory and motor performance, sensorimotor integration, and the assessment of higher cognitive functions, such as learning, memory, and social, emotional, and reproductive behavior (Table 5.7).

In contrast to many other areas of predictive toxicology, routine protocols for neurobehavioral assessment have not been widely adopted by regulatory agencies, yet in recent years there has been increasing concern about the neurobehavioral toxicity that may result from environmental and occupational exposures. The standardization and widespread use of such tests are made difficult by the qualitative nature of the observations. Nevertheless, neurobehavioral assessment using experimental animals is an important area of toxicologic investigation, and refinements and broader applications of current methods should greatly enhance our abilities to identify, prior to distribution and widespread use, chemicals that may produce serious adverse neurobehavioral effects in humans.

References

1. Agocs MM, Etzel RA, Parrish RG et al. Mercury exposure from interior latex paint. N Engl J Med 1990; 323:1096–101.
2. Austin MA, Peyser PA, Khoury MJ. The interface of genetics and public health: research and educational challenges. Annu Rev Public Health 2000; 21:81–99.
3. Dey DC, Maekawa M, Sudo K, Kanno T. Butyrylcholinesterase genes in individuals with abnormal inhibition numbers and with trace activity: one common mutation and two novel silent genes. Ann Clin Biochem 1998; 35:302–10.
4. Kelada SN, Eaton DL, Wang SS et al. The role of genetic polymorphisms in environmental health. Environ Health Perspect 2003; 111: 1055–64.
5. Beach JR. Immunologic versus toxicologic mechanisms in airway responses. Occup Med 2000; 15:455–70.
6. Phelps RG, Rees AJ. The HLA complex in Goodpasture's disease: a model for analyzing susceptibility to autoimmunity. Kidney Int 1999; 56:1638–53.
7. Bombassei GJ, Kaplan AA. The association between hydrocarbon exposure and anti-glomerular basement membrane antibody-mediated disease (Goodpasture's syndrome). Am J Ind Med 1992; 21:141–53.
8. Yunginger JW. Latex allergy in the workplace: an overview of where we are. Ann Allergy Asthma Immunol 1999; 83:630–3.
9. Becker HS. An analysis of the epidemiology of latex allergy: implications for primary prevention. Medsurg Nurs 2000; 9:135–43.
10. International Agency for Research on Cancer (IARC), IARC Monongraphs Programme on the Evaluation of Carcinogenic Risks to Humans. http://monographs.iarc.fr.
11. Balmain A, Harris CC. Carcinogenesis in mouse and human cells: parallels and paradoxes, Carcinogenesis 2000; 2:371–7.
12. Hursting SD, Slaga TJ, Fischer SM, DiGiovanni J, Phang JM. Mechanism-based cancer prevention approaches: targets, examples, and the use of transgenic mice. J Natl Cancer Inst 1999; 91:215–25.
13. Lai C, Shields PG. The role of interindividual variation in human carcinogenesis. J Nutr 1999; 129(2S Suppl): 552S–555S.
14. Soussi T. The p53 tumor suppressor gene: from molecular biology to clinical investigation, Ann NY Acad Sci 2000; 910:121–39.
15. Cohen SM. Cell proliferation and carcinogenesis. Drug Metab Rev 1998; 30:339–57.
16. Calabrese L, Fleischer AB. Thalidomide: current and potential clinical applications, Am J Med 2000; 108:487–95.
17. Moore JA, Daston GP, Faustman E et al. An evaluative process for assessing human reproductive and developmental toxicity of agents. Reprod Toxicol 1995; 9:61–95.

18. Dahl AR. Toxicokinetics: concept of dose. In: Sipes IG, McQueen C, Gandolfi AJ, eds. Comprehensive toxicology, Vol. 1, General principles. New York: Elsevier Science, 1997;157–66.

19. Andersen O, Nielsen JB, Nordberg GF. Factors affecting the intestinal uptake of cadmium from the diet. IARC Sci Publ 1992;173–87.

20. Siddiqui O. Physicochemical, physiologic, and mathematical considerations in optimizing percutaneous absorption of drugs. Crit Rev Ther Drug Carrier Syst 1989; 6:1:1–38.

21. Walsh CT. Toxicokinetics: oral exposure and absorption of toxicants. In: Sipes IG, McQueen C, Gandolfi AJ, eds. Comprehensive toxicology, Vol. 1, General principles. New York: Elsevier Science, 1997;51–62.

22. Kararli TT. Gastrointestinal absorption of drugs. Crit Rev Ther Drug Carrier Syst 1989; 6:1:39–86.

23. Simon GL, Gorbach SL. Interactions of toxicants with gastrointestinal tract microbial flora, In: Sipes IG, McQueen C, Gandolfi AJ, eds. Comprehensive toxicology, Vol. 9, Hepatic and gastrointestinal toxicology. New York: Elsevier Science, 1997;589–604.

24. Ritschel WA, Hussain AS. Principles of permeation of substances across the skin. Meth Find Exptl Clin Pharmacol 1988; 10:39–56.

25. Feldman RJ, Maibach HI. Penetration of 14C hycrocortisone through normal skin: effect of stripping and occlusion. Arch Dermatol 1965; 91:661–6.

26. Simon GA, Maibach HI. The pig as an experimental animal model of percutaneous permeation in man: qualitative and quantitative observations – an overview. Skin Pharmacol Appl Skin Physiol 2000; 13:229–34.

27. Pannatier A, Jenner P, Testa B, Etter JC. The skin as a drug-metabolizing organ. Drug Metabol Rev 1978; 8:319–43.

28. Granjean P, Berlin A, Gilbert M, Penning W. Preventing percutaneous absorption of industrial chemicals: the 'skin' denotation. Am J Ind Med 1988; 14:97–107.

29. Kalnas J, Teitelbaum DT. Dermal absorption of benzene: implications for work practices and regulations. Int J Occup Environ Health 2000; 6:114–21.

30. Roth RA. Toxicology of the respiratory system. In: Sipes IG, McQueen CA, Gandolfi AJ, eds. Comprehensive toxicology, Vol. 8. New York: Elsevier Science, 1997.

31. Morgan MS, Frank R. Uptake of pollutant gases by the respiratory system. In: Brain JD, Proctor DF, Reid LM, eds. Respiratory defense mechanisms, Part. I. New York: Marcel Dekker, 1977;157–89.

32. Kennedy GL. Inhalation toxicology. In: Hayes AW, ed. Principles and methods in toxicology, 2nd edn. New York: Raven Press, 1989.

33. Rozman K, Klaassen CD. Absorption, distribution and excretion of toxicants. In: Klaassen CD, ed. Casarett & Doull's Toxicology: the basic science of poisons, 5th edn. New York: McGraw Hill, 1996;91–112.

34. Thummel, KE, Kunze KL, Shen DD. Metabolically-based drug-drug interactions: principles and mechanisms. In: Levy RH, Thummel KE, Trager WF, Hansten PD, Eichelbaum M, eds. Metabolic drug interactions. New York: Lippincott, Williams and Wilkins, 2000;3–20.

35. Klaassen CD, Liu J. Metallothionein transgenic and knock-out mouse models in the study of cadmium toxicity. J Toxicol Sci 1998; 2(Suppl):97–102.

36. Pardridge WM. Blood–brain barrier biology and methodology. J Neurovirol 1999; 5:556–69.

37. Pelletier RM, Byers SW. The blood–testis barrier and Sertoli cell junctions: structural considerations. Microsc Res Tech 1992; 20:3–33.

38. Smith LL, Lewis CP, Wyatt I, Cohen GM. The importance of epithelial uptake systems in lung toxicity. Environ Health Perspect 1990; 85:25–30.

39. Plaa GL. Chlorinated methanes and liver injury: highlights of the past 50 years. Annu Rev Pharmacol Toxicol 2000; 40:42–65.

40. Guengerich FP. Biotransformation. In: Sipes IG, McQueen CA, Gandolfi AJ, eds. Comprehensive toxicology, Vol. 3, Biotransformation. New York: Elsevier Science, 1997.

41. Guengerich FP. Cytochrome P450 enzymes. In: Sipes IG, McQueen CA, Gandolfi AJ, eds. Comprehensive toxicology, Vol. 3, Biotransformation. New York: Elsevier Science, 1997;37–68.

42. Cohen SD, Khairallah EA. Selective protein arylation and acetaminophen-induced hepatotoxicity. Drug Metab Rev 1997; 29:59–77.

43. Snyder R. Microsomal enzyme induction. Toxicol Sci 2000; 55:233–4.

44. Lieber CS. Microsomal ethanol-oxidizing system (MEOS): the first 30 years (1968–1998) – a review. Alcohol Clin Exp Res 1999; 23:991–1007.

45. Garbutt JC, West SL, Carey TS, Lohr KN, Crews FT. Pharmacological treatment of alcohol dependence: a review of the evidence. JAMA 1999; 281:1318–25.

46. Abramson S, Singh AK. Treatment of the alcohol intoxications: ethylene glycol, methanol and isopropanol. Curr Opin Nephrol Hypertens 2000; 9:695–701.

47. Cashman, J. Monoamine oxidase and flavin-containing monooxygenases. In: Sipes IG, McQueen CA, Gandolfi AJ, eds. Comprehensive toxicology, Vol. 3, Biotransformation. New York: Elsevier Science, 1997;69–96.

48. Akerman BR, Lemass H, Chow LM et al. Trimethylaminuria is caused by mutations of the FMO3 gene in a North American cohort. Mol Genet Metab 1999; 68 24–31.

49. Ross D, Kepa JK, Winski SL, Beall HD, Anwar A, Siegel D. NAD(P)H:quinone oxidoreductase 1 (NQO1): chemoprotection, bioactivation, gene regulation and genetic polymorphisms. Chem Biol Interact 2000; 129:77–97.

50. Sone T, Wang CY. Microsomal amidases and carboxylesterases. In: Sipes IG, McQueen CA, Gandolfi AJ, eds. Comprehensive toxicology, Vol. 3, Biotransformation. New York: Elsevier Science, 1997;265–81.

51. Costa LG, Li WF, Richter RJ, Shih DM, Lusis A, Furlong CE. The role of paraoxonase (PON1) in the detoxication of organophosphates and its human polymorphism. Chem Biol Interact 1999; 120:429–38.

52. Fretland AJ, Omiecinski CJ. Epoxide hydrolases: biochemistry and molecular biology. Chem Biol Interact 2000; 129:41–59.

53. Tukey RH, Strassburg CP. Human UDP-glucuronosyltransferases: metabolism, expression, and disease. Annu Rev Pharmacol Toxicol 2000; 40:581–616.

54. Ritter JK. Roles of glucuronidation and UDP-glucuronosyltransferases in xenobiotic bioactivation reactions. Chem Biol Interact 2000; 129:171–93.

55. Duffel MW. Sulfotransferases. In: Sipes IG, McQueen CA, Gandolfi AJ, eds. Comprehensive toxicology, Vol. 3, Biotransformation. New York: Elsevier Science, 1997;365–83.

56. Glatt H. Sulfotransferases in the bioactivation of xenobiotics. Chem Biol Interact 2000; 129:141–70.

57. Qu Q, Melikian AA, Li G et al. Validation of biomarkers in humans exposed to benzene: urine metabolites. Am J Ind Med 2000; 37:522–31.

58. Eaton DL, Bammler TK. Concise review of the glutathione S-transferases and their significance to toxicology. Toxicol Sci 1999; 49:156–64.

59. Estonius M, Forsberg L, Danielsson O, Weinander R, Kelner MJ, Morgenstern R. Distribution of microsomal glutathione transferase 1 in mammalian tissues. A predominant alternate first exon in human tissues. Eur J Biochem 1999; 260:409–13.

60. Hayes JD, Strange RC. Glutathione S-transferase polymor-phisms and their biologic consequences. Pharmacology 2000; 61:154–66.

61. Cmarik JL, Inskeep PB, Meredith MJ, Meyer DJ, Ketterer B, Guengerich FP. Selectivity of rat and human glutathione S-transferases in activation of ethylene dibromide by glutathione conjugation and DNA binding and induction of unscheduled DNA synthesis in human hepatocytes. Cancer Res 1990; 50:2747–52.

62. Cascorbi I, Brockmoller J, Mrozikiewicz PM, Muller A, Roots I. Arylamine N-acetyltransferase activity in man. Drug Metab Rev 1999; 31:489–502.

63. Grant DM, Goodfellow GH, Sugamori K, Durette K. Pharmacogenetics of the human arylamine N-acetyltransferases. Pharmacology 2000; 61:204–11.

64. Vatsis KP, Weber WW. Acetyltransferases. In: Sipes IG, McQueen CA, Gandolfi AJ, eds. Comprehensive toxicology, Vol. 3, Biotransformation. New York: Elsevier Science, 1997;385–400.

65. Zenser TV, Lakshmi VM, Rustan TD, Doll MA, Deitz AC, Davis BB, Hein DW. Human N-acetylation of benzidine: role of NAT1 and NAT2. Cancer Res 1996; 56:3941–7.

66. Lennard, L. Methyl transferases. In: Sipes IG, McQueen CA, Gandolfi AJ, eds. Comprehensive toxicology, Vol. 3, Biotransformation. New York: Elsevier Science, 1997;437–54.

67. Krynetski EY, Evans WE. Genetic polymorphism of thiopurine S-methyltransferase: molecular mechanisms and clinical importance. Pharmacology 2000; 61:136–46.

68. Vessey DA. Enzymes involved in the formation of amide bonds. In: Sipes IG, McQueen CA, Gandolfi AJ, eds. Comprehensive toxicology, Vol. 3, Biotransformation. New York: Elsevier Science, 1997;455–88.

69. Hein DW, Doll MA, Fretland AJ et al. Molecular genetics and epidemiology of the NAT1 and NAT2 acetylation polymorphisms. Cancer Epidemiol Biomarkers Prev 2000; 9:29–42.

70. Ingelman-Sundberg M, Oscarson M, McLellan RA. Polymorphic human cytochrome P450 enzymes: an opportunity for individualized drug treatment. Trends Pharmacol Sci 1999; 20:342–9.

71. Wolf CR, Smith G. Cytochrome P450 CYP2D6. Chapter 18. Geneva: IARC, 1999; 148:209–29.

72. Bartsch H, Nair U, Risch A, Rojas M, Wikman H, Alexandrov K. Genetic polymorphism of CYP genes, alone or in combination, as a risk modifier of tobacco-related cancers. Cancer Epidemiol Biomarkers Prev 2000; 9:3–28.

73. Houlston RS. Glutathione S-transferase M1 status and lung cancer risk: a meta-analysis. Cancer Epidemiol Biomarkers Prev 1999; 8:675–82.

74. Johns LE, Houlston RS. Glutathione S-transferase mu1 (GSTM1) status and bladder cancer risk: a meta-analysis. Mutagenesis 2000; 15:399–404.

75. Costa LG. The emerging field of ecogenetics. Neurotoxicology 2000; 21:85–9.

76. Nebert DW. Suggestions for the nomenclature of human alleles: relevance to ecogenetics, pharmacogenetics and molecular epidemiology. Pharmacogenetics 2000; 10:279–90.

77. Omenn GS. Public health genetics: an emerging interdisciplinary field for the post-genomic era. Annu Rev Public Health 2000; 21:1–13.

78. Berkhin EB, Humphreys MH. Regulation of renal tubular secretion of organic compounds. Kidney Int 2001; 59:17–30.

79. Inui KI, Masuda S, Saito H. Cellular and molecular aspects of drug transport in the kidney. Kidney Int 2000; 58:944–58.

80. Dickow LM, Podell M, Gerken DF. Clinical effects and plasma concentration determination after 2,4-dichlorophenoxyacetic acid 200 mg/kg administration in the dog. J Toxicol Clin Toxicol 2000; 38:747–53.

81. Bradberry SM, Watt BE, Proudfoot AT, Vale JA. Mechanisms of toxicity, clinical features, and management of acute chlorophenoxy herbicide poisoning: a review. J Toxicol Clin Toxicol 2000; 38:111–22.

82. McCusky RS, Sipes IG. Introduction to the liver and its response to toxicants. In: Sipes IG, McQueen CA, Gandolfi AJ, eds. Comprehensive toxicology, Vol. 9, Hepatic and gastrointestinal toxicology. New York: Elsevier Science, 1997;1–11.

83. Lecureur V, Courtois A, Payen L, Verhnet L, Guillouzo A, Fardel O. Expression and regulation of hepatic drug and bile acid transporters. Toxicology 2000; 153:203–19.

84. Kullak-Ublick GA, Beuers U, Paumgartner G. Hepatobiliary transport. J Hepatol 2000; 32(1 Suppl):3–18.

85. Bahar RJ, Stolz A. Bile acid transport. Gastroenterol Clin North Am 1999; 28:27–58.

86. Clarkson TW. Mercury: major issues in environmental health. Environ Health Perspect 1993; 100:31–8.

87. Dowling RH. Review: pathogenesis of gallstones. Aliment Pharmacol Ther 2000; 14 (Suppl 2):39–47.

88. Guzelian PS. New approaches for treatment of humans exposed to a slowly excreted environmental chemical (chlordecone). Z Gastroenterol 1984; 22:16–20.

89. Sauer JM, Stine ER, Gunawardhana L, Hill DA, Sipes IG. The liver as a target for chemical-chemical interactions. Adv Pharmacol 1997; 43:37–63.

90. Surawicz B. Factors affecting tolerance to digitalis. J Am Coll Cardiol 1985; 5(Suppl):69A–81A.

91. Johanson G. Toxicokinetics: modeling disposition, In: Sipes IG, McQueen C, Gandolfi AJ, eds. Comprehensive toxicology, Vol. 1, General principles. New York: Elsevier Science, 1997;167–88.

92. Levy RH, Thummel KE, Trager WF, Hansten PD, Eichelbaum M, eds. Metabolic drug interactions. Philadelphia: Lippincott, Williams & Wilkins, 2000.

93. Hayes AW, ed. Principles and methods of toxicology, 4th edn. Philadelphia: Taylor & Francis, 2001.

94. White WJ. The use of laboratory animals in toxicological research. In: Hayes AW, ed. Principles and methods of toxicology, 4th edn. Philadelphia: Taylor & Francis, 2001;773–818.

95. Wilson NH, Hardisty JF, Hayes JR. Short-term, subchronic and chronic toxicology studies. In: Hayes AW, ed. Principles and methods of toxicology, 4th edn. Philadelphia: Taylor & Francis, 2001;917–57.

96. Williams GM, Iatropoulos MJ. Principles of testing for carcinogenic activity, In: Hayes AW, ed. Principles and methods of toxicology, 4th edn. Philadelphia: Taylor & Francis, 2001;959–1000.

97. Gad SC. Statistics for toxicologists. In: Hayes AW, ed. Principles and methods of toxicology, 4th edn. Philadelphia: Taylor & Francis, 2001;285–364.

98. Foran J, ed. Principles for the selection of doses in chronic rodent bioassays. Washington DC: ILSI Press, 1997.

99. Brusick, D. Genetic toxicology. In: Hayes AW, ed. Principles and methods of toxicology, 4th edn. Philadelphia: Taylor & Francis, 2001;819–52.

100. Zhang L, Rothman N, Wang Y et al. Benzene increases aneuploidy in the lymphocytes of exposed workers: a comparison of data obtained by fluorescence in situ hybridization in interphase and metaphase cells. Environ Mol Mutagen 1999; 34:260–8.

101. Clegg ED, Perreault SD, Klinefelter GR. Assessment of male reproductive toxicity. In: Hayes AW, ed. Principles & methods of toxicology, 4th edn. Philadelphia: Taylor & Francis, 2001;1263–300.

102. Christian MS. Test methods for assessing female reproductive and developmental toxicology. In: Hayes AW, ed. Principles and methods of toxicology, 4th edn. Philadelphia: Taylor & Francis, 2001;1301–80.

103. DiPasquale LC, Hayes AW. Acute toxicity and eye irritancy. In: Hayes AW, ed. Principles and methods of toxicology, 4th edn. Philadelphia: Taylor & Francis, 2001;853–916.

104. Maibach, H, Patrick E. Dermatotoxicology. In: Hayes AW, ed. Principles and methods of toxicology, 4th edn. Philadelphia: Taylor & Francis, 2001;1039–78.

105. Weiss B, Cory-Slechta DA. Assessment of behavioral toxicity. In: Hayes AW, ed. Principles and methods of toxicology, 4th edn. Philadelphia: Taylor & Francis, 2001;1451–528.

106. Dean J, House RV, Luster MI. Immunotoxicology: effects of, and responses to, drugs and chemicals, In: Hayes AW, ed. Principles and methods of toxicology, 4th edn. Philadelphia: Taylor & Francis, 2001;1415–550.

Chapter 6
Epidemiology

Harvey Checkoway, Ellen A Eisen

Epidemiology is the systematic method of identifying occupational health hazards and quantifying the magnitude of risks. There is a long history of epidemiologic recognition of work-related risks, much of which was stimulated by clinical observations of seemingly unusual or unanticipated illnesses in workers. Respiratory diseases among underground metals miners in 16th century Germany and Czechoslovakia and scrotal cancer among London chimney sweeps in the 18th century are two prominent examples. Epidemiology has made significant contributions to occupational and environmental medicine, especially during the past 100 years. These contributions are directly related to advances in epidemiologic methods and to a growing appreciation by clinicians of the role of epidemiology in occupational and environmental hazard identification.

Although many important epidemiologic leads originate from clinical observations made on individual patients or small case series, the goal of formal epidemiologic research is to permit inferences about risks from exposures to populations. The at-risk populations typically studied initially are workers exposed to known or suspected toxic agents, and secondarily are community residents or consumers of industrial products exposed environmentally to the same agents. Ultimately, the findings from worker population studies can be used to evaluate risks to individual workers and other members of the population, thus contributing to the scientific bases of exposure guidelines for workplace and ambient exposures.

This chapter summarizes commonly used epidemiologic approaches to the study of occupational and environmental hazards. The intention is to provide an overview of study designs, including the relative advantages and limitations of each, a review of potential sources of bias that may undermine research findings, and a discussion of how clinicians and the public-at-large can interpret and make use of epidemiologic data. Most attention is focused on occupational exposures because risk factor identification is often more clearly derived from worker health studies due to generally higher and better assessed exposures in the workplace. Examples illustrating various research methods are drawn from the published occupational and environmental health literature. Readers seeking more in-depth treatment of epidemiologic methods are referred to texts devoted to this topic (see Further reading).

EPIDEMIOLOGY STUDY DESIGNS

Various approaches can be adopted for investigating relations between occupational or environmental exposures and disease risks. To a great extent, the design of a given study is governed by the types of exposures of concern, anticipated health outcomes, and feasibility. Epidemiologic investigations can range from case series reports of illness or injury to long-term follow-up studies of large occupational cohorts with well-characterized exposures. Typically, epidemiologists prefer relatively large studies of occupational populations, although size is by no means the sole determinant of the public health and scientific importance of a study. Other factors, especially the clarity of the research objectives, validity of exposure and health data, and the appropriateness of study design, are the distinguishing features of valuable epidemiologic research.

Case series and cluster investigations

As mentioned previously, case series reports provide insights into past or emerging occupational and environmental health problems. The recognition of cases of hepatic angiosarcoma at a polyvinylchloride manufacturing plant, and impaired fertility among male workers exposed to the pesticide dibromochloropropane (DBCP), are vivid occupational examples. Examples of adverse effects from secondary (indirect) exposures to workplace toxicants are reports of malignant mesothelioma, berylliosis, and lead poisoning among family members of workers exposed to the causative agents. In such instances, where the disease is rare and there are few if any other known causes, a case series is sufficient to trigger efforts to eliminate exposure.

More typical, however, are situations where there are reports of acute diseases or injuries among segments of a workforce or among individual workers from multiple workplaces with similar exposures. Case reports suggestive of environmental hazards also arise from the community-at-large. Noteworthy examples are reports of adverse reproductive outcomes and other morbidity among persons living near hazardous waste disposal sites or in communities exposed to polluted ambient air or water sources contaminated by industrial discharges. An epidemiologic study in many such situations may be unnecessary if the cause(s) can be determined (e.g., poor ventilation, contaminated water) and rectified.

Profound episodes of environmental pollution and subsequent illness can lead to epidemiologic follow-up studies of affected populations, particularly when the pollution source is readily identifiable and sequelae are severe. Two episodes of illness resulting from environmental water pollution in Japan, namely neurologic impairment in residents of Minimata Bay exposed to industrial mercury discharges, and bone and kidney disease ('itai-itai' disease) among Toyama Bay residents exposed to cadmium effluents from a mine, are well-known examples. In both instances, clinical recognition of unusual disease patterns prompted investigations into environmental causes and follow-up of cohorts of exposed populations for subsequent disease occurrence.

As with case series reports arising from the workplace, causal links with exposures in community case series are most convincing when the disease in question is either very rare or specific for the putative etiologic exposure. This was certainly true in the mercury and cadmium poisoning episodes in Japan. More generally, however, the consequences of environmental exposures are not clear-cut, as evidenced by findings from follow-up investigations of populations exposed to dioxins from a trichlorophenol factory explosion near Seveso, Italy, in 1976 and nuclear fallout from the 1986 Chernobyl disaster.

There are, however, numerous episodes of illness for which there are no obvious etiologic factors. The term 'disease cluster' has been used to describe such occurrences. Apparent clusters may simply be due to an especially intensive medical evaluation of workers or community residents in which previously unnoticed morbidity is reported. Alternatively, some clusters have been ascribed to heightened awareness or concern for potential health risks among workers or community residents. While such clusters may not represent exposure-related health effects, as a general rule, dismissing disease clusters as necessarily spurious without conducting some form of medical or epidemiologic inquiry, either by review of past data or by conducting a focused study of the problem, is unjustified both scientifically and from the perspective of protecting public health. Of course, the availability of resources to conduct an epidemiologic study will dictate its scope.

Case series reports or disease clusters should be appreciated for what they are: evidence of potential risks from exposure. There is no consensus among epidemiologists as to how one should address a disease cluster or what inferences can be drawn from case series reports. Initially, one would like to confirm that the cluster truly represents an excess. Data on disease incidence in relation to the timing of exposure is valuable in this regard. For example, either an increased incidence following the introduction of exposure or a decreased incidence after exposure reduction or removal would support a cause and effect association. Unfortunately, such unambiguous data are not readily available in many instances.

A second consideration in deciding whether a cluster warrants concern is the specificity of the reported health outcome. Case reports of homogeneous clinical entities, rather than a wide spectrum of adverse health outcomes, improves confidence that there has been an environmental factor contributing to risk. For example, a cluster of urinary bladder cancer cases in a workplace, as has been seen on numerous occasions among workers exposed to benzidine-based dyes, is more persuasive evidence of an occupational etiology than a cluster consisting of a mixture of various site-specific cancers. Also, conditions with relatively short latencies between exposure and case diagnosis or symptom reporting (e.g., reactive airway symptoms) are more readily assessed than conditions that typically have long induction and latency times (e.g., chronic bronchitis).

A reasonable approach for investigating a disease cluster might involve the following strategy. First and foremost, the priority assigned to investigating a cluster has to be determined by the medical significance of the problem. Importance of the problem to workers and management, in terms of psychological well being and workplace relationships, also deserves considerable weight. Next, the available resources to conduct a formal study need to be inventoried. For example, one case of acute myeloid leukemia in a small shop where solvents are used is a cause for genuine concern. However, if there were only a small number of exposed workers and no past exposure monitoring data, then a meaningful epidemiologic study would be unlikely. In such an instance, causality for the individual worker or recommendations for exposure control may have to be based on data from prior epidemiologic research.

Some have argued that, if an epidemiologic study is undertaken pursuant to a cluster, then one should delete the 'cluster cases' because their inclusion would bias the ultimate study findings. However, epidemiologic principles dictate that all relevant findings should be presented in a balanced manner. This means that the so-called 'cluster cases' are as valid as any other cases that might be detected on further inquiry. On the other hand, exclusion of some of the cluster cases would be justified when there is convincing evidence that case diagnoses or reports are biased, as might occur when aggressive case-finding efforts are made preferentially among persons exposed to presumed causal factors. A valid epidemiologic assessment requires that efforts should be made to expand the scope of the study to include events before and subsequent to the cluster occurrences, and that case identification should be performed in a uniform and unbiased manner.

Some researchers hold the opinion that cluster detection and follow-up are poor uses of resources; instead one should devote more attention to an understanding of basic disease mechanisms. This viewpoint certainly has some academic merit, but offers little guidance to practicing clinicians and epidemiologists. Epidemiologists generally prefer to conduct studies that examine well-formulated prior hypotheses, although there are situations where cluster recognition can offer valuable preliminary insights. Reaching conclusions about disease causation from cluster reports can be a vexing problem when they are the only available evidence. Statistical significance can be misleading because populations at risk and expected disease frequencies are seldom known when clusters are reported. Also, it should be appreciated that diseases in populations do not occur uniformly in time or place. Thus, some apparent clusters of disease are to be expected. (By analogy, inspection of a table of random digits will reveal clusters of repeated numbers in various places.) In general, the best evidence is obtained from formal epidemiologic studies. Determining whether an epidemiologic study should be mounted will always require clinical and epidemiologic judgment.

Cohort studies

Cohort studies involve the identification of an exposed worker population (cohort), follow-up over time, and determination of disease frequency in relation to exposure type and level. Among epidemiologic study designs, cohort studies are by far the best understood and recognized as scientifically valid because they mimic, at least in structure, an experimental approach. However, it should be appreciated that other designs, in particular case-control and cross-sectional, can also provide valid data, and are, in fact, more suitable than cohort studies in certain situations.

There are numerous types of cohorts that can be defined for study. The most typical is a population of workers from a single plant or industry. Other cohort definitions are workers from a trade or professional association, preferably with similar exposures, or persons with previously diagnosed occupational diseases, such as registered cases of pneumoconiosis. The choice of cohort depends on the goal of the study and availability of data necessary for cohort enumeration. If the research objective is to survey the exposure and health experience of workers in a particular industry, then a cohort defined as workers from plants in that industry will be most appropriate.

Trade union or professional association members might constitute the study population if plant- or industry-specific cohorts cannot be defined readily from existing data (e.g., construction painters), or if access to personnel and exposure records is denied. A cohort consisting of cases with certified or registered diseases customarily is followed to evaluate adverse sequelae related to those diseases, and for situations such as the pneumoconiosis or pesticide poisoning, to study workers assumed to have experienced the heaviest exposures to the causative agents.

Follow-up in a cohort study can be either prospective or historical. A prospective cohort study begins with a population of current workers and follows them into the future. Prospective cohort studies of diseases with long induction and latency intervals, such as most malignancies, are uncommon but not unprecedented in occupational epidemiology. The most efficient applications of the prospective cohort design are studies of common illnesses, injuries, or physiologic states that are observable within reasonably short time periods. Data from a prospective cohort study of longitudinal pulmonary function changes in cotton and silk textile workers in Shanghai[1] are shown

Cross-shift drop in FEV$_1$ at baseline	Annual change in FEV$_1$(mL)	
	Cotton workers*	Silk workers*
<5%	−35 (236)	−34 (243)
≥5%	−57 (73)	−36 (37)
* Number of workers in parentheses		

Table 6.1 Five-year mean annual change in forced expiratory volume in 1 second (FEV$_1$) among Shanghai cotton and silk textile workers in relation to cross-shift change at baseline

in Table 6.1. This study has features of both a short-term and longer-term prospective cohort study in that cross-shift FEV$_1$ measurements obtained at the baseline survey represent a follow-up of a single day, and the repeated FEV$_1$ measurement 5 years later is the longer-term component. In this study, although the differences between the cotton and silk workers, who were the non-exposed comparison (referent) group, were small, there was a detectable association of accelerated lung function decline among cotton textile workers who experienced the largest baseline cross-shift changes.

Historical cohort studies offer a more convenient and time-efficient method than prospective cohort studies for investigating chronic diseases. The principal limiting factors of most historical cohort studies are the availability of past data on employment, typically obtained from personnel records, and exposure, obtained from environmental monitoring data. The design and analysis of historical and prospective cohort studies are identical. The only distinction is the timing of when the studies are conducted relative to when exposures and disease have occurred. Thus, for example, a cohort may be followed from 1970 to 1999 for disease incidence. The study would be prospective if the investigators had enumerated the cohort in 1970 and followed it throughout the study interval. In contrast, the study would be historical if cohort enumeration and follow-up were conducted retrospectively after 1999.

As mentioned earlier, the identification of a case series of cancer among chimney sweeps was an important discovery in occupational medicine. A more modern investigation of this issue was addressed in a historical cohort study of Swedish chimney sweeps followed for 40 years[2] and is shown in Table 6.2. The cohort included 5542 chimney sweeps registered in a trade union that had been employed between 1918 and 1980. The cohort was traced for mortality outcomes during 1951–1990, and cause-specific mortality rates were compared with prevailing rates in Sweden. The chimney sweeps experienced mortality excesses for all causes combined, circulatory diseases, respiratory diseases, and various cancers. The two-fold elevated lung cancer risk was especially noteworthy because it was based on a reasonably large number of deaths and was consistent with the prior hypothesis regarding carcinogenic effects of inhaled soot particles. Additionally, data on cancer incidence were available from the Swedish National Cancer Registry for the years 1958–1987, and permitted contrasts with national rates for cancers with low mortality rates, such as bladder cancer. Analyses of cancer incidence according to duration employed as a chimney sweep revealed a trend indicative of a dose–response relation for lung cancer, although no such gradients were observed for cancer of the stomach and bladder (Table 6.3). The absence of gradients with duration for the latter cancers may reflect truly absent dose–response associations, although it is equally plausible that either employment duration is a poor surrogate for dose or that the actual dose–response relations are not continuously increasing.

Some special cohorts can be defined as workers who have experienced unusual exposure circumstances, such as

Cause of death	Observed	Expected*	Relative risk	(95% CI)+
All causes	919	680	1.35	(1.27–1.44)
Circulatory diseases	354	276	1.28	(1.15–1.42)
Respiratory diseases	44	27.8	1.59	(1.15–2.13)
Digestive diseases	39	20.1	1.30	(0.92–1.77)
All cancers	216	148	1.46	(1.27–1.67)
Esophageal cancer	12	3.1	3.86	(2.00–6.75)
Stomach cancer	20	16.6	1.21	(0.74–1.87)
Colon cancer	8	10.5	0.76	(0.33–1.50)
Liver cancer	11	3.3	3.31	(1.65–5.93)
Pancreatic cancer	10	10.0	1.00	(0.48–1.85)
Lung cancer	53	25.8	2.06	(1.54–2.69)
Prostate cancer	22	13.0	1.69	(1.06–2.56)
Bladder cancer	4	3.9	1.03	(0.28–2.64)
Kidney cancer	6	7.2	0.84	(0.31–1.82)

* Based on rates for Swedish males.
+ 95% confidence interval for relative risk.

Table 6.2 Mortality among Swedish male chimney sweeps 1951–1990

Employment duration (yr)	Lung cancer Observed	Lung cancer Relative risk*	Stomach cancer Observed	Stomach cancer Relative risk*	Bladder cancer Observed	Bladder cancer Relative risk*
1–9	4	0.88	4	1.58	10	3.34
10–19	16	2.17	5	1.12	13	2.91
20–29	15	2.70	5	1.29	7	2.12
≥30	15	2.34	9	1.58	7	1.82

* Relative to rates for Swedish males.

Table 6.3 Cancer incidence trends with duration of employment as a chimney sweep

	TCDD body burden (µg/kg body weight)					
	<0.1	(n = 108)	0.1–0.99	(n = 66)	≥1.0	(n = 69)
Cause of death	Obs	RR*	Obs	RR*	Obs	RR*
All causes	27	0.7	27	1.0	38	1.0
All cancers	8	0.8	8	1.2	15	1.6
Respiratory cancer	3	1.0	1	0.5	7	2.4
Digestive cancer	2	0.6	4	1.7	5	1.5
Leukemia, lymphoma	1	1.6	0	0	1	1.8
Circulatory diseases	13	0.8	11	1.0	13	0.8
Digestive diseases	0	0	1	0.5	4	1.6
Respiratory diseases	0	0	0	0	1	0.4

* Relative to rates in the former West Germany, 1953–1992.

Table 6.4 Mortality experience, 1953–1992, of 243 German workers exposed to dioxin (2,3,7,8-TCDD) following an industrial accident at a trichlorophenol plant

a chemical spill or explosion. An example is a 40-year mortality follow-up of 243 workers who were exposed to 2,3,7,8-tetrachlordibenzo-p-dioxin (TCDD) consequent to an accident at a trichlorophenol manufacturing plant.[3] Blood concentrations of TCDD measured periodically after the accident were incorporated into pharmacokinetic models to estimate cumulative dioxin doses, and permitted dose–response analyses (Table 6.4). Increasing gradients of relative risk for all cancers combined and for respiratory cancer, small numbers notwithstanding, support a carcinogenic potential for TCDD.

Special cohorts can be formed from workers with diagnosed disease. An example is a mortality follow-up study of a cohort of roughly 1500 workers, from numerous industries in Hong Kong, who were included in a silicosis registry organized largely for compensation purposes.[4] Compared to Hong Kong males, the cohort experienced a nearly two-fold increased risk of lung cancer, with a particularly accentuated risk gradient associated with the extent of large radiographic opacities (Table 6.5).

Studies in which workers are selected on the basis of health status frequently include cohorts whose source populations are less well characterized than conventional cohort studies of workers from particular plants or industries. The advantage of restricting cohorts in this manner is that this approach is efficient for estimating risks theoretically related to high dose levels. However, subtle selection biases may create confounded results. For example, if smoking-related morbidity increases the probability that a pneumoconiosis case will seek medical attention, and hence be more likely to

Group	No. workers	Observed	Expected*	Observed/ expected
All workers	1490	33	17.0	1.94
Small opacities				
1	316	6	3.44	1.74
2	588	13	7.61	1.71
3	102	2	1.03	1.94
Large opacities				
A	320	7	3.83	1.83
B	121	3	1.19	2.52
C	43	2	0.34	5.88

* Based on rates for Hong Kong males, 1981–1997.

Table 6.5 Lung cancer mortality among registered silicotics in Hong Kong by extent of silicosis 1981–1997

Cumulative exposure (mg/m³-yrs)	ILO radiographic category			
	< 1/0		≥1/0 or large opacity	
	Obs	RR*	Obs	RR*
<0.5	13	1.05	0	0
0.5–1.9	13	0.86	0	0
2.0–4.9	10	1.25	0	0
≥5.0	12	2.40	4	2.94

* Relative risk compared to rates for US males, 1942–1994.

Table 6.6 Lung cancer mortality among US diatomaceous earth workers classified by cumulative silica exposure and ILO radiographic category of silicosis 1942–1994

Occupational group	No. cases	Relative risk
Non-exposed	9	1.0
Exposed		
Coatings	17	2.2
Rubber	1	1.3
Chemical	7	3.6
Shoe	4	2.5
Other/mixed	9	2.5

Table 6.7 Leukemia incidence among Chinese workers exposed to benzene compared with non-exposed workers 1972–1987

Cumulative exposure (ppm-yrs)	No. cases	Relative risk
0	9	1.0
>0–<40	11	1.9
40–99	8	3.1
≥100	19	2.7

Table 6.8 Leukemia incidence according to cumulative exposure to benzene among Chinese workers

receive a definitive diagnosis and be awarded compensation, then a cohort study of subsequent lung cancer risk among compensated pneumoconiosis cases may overstate the effect of dust exposure. This problem may be overcome by including in the cohort exposed workers with and without the index condition. The data in Table 6.6 from a study of silica-exposed workers in the diatomaceous earth industry[5] illustrate this approach. An exposure–response lung cancer trend was evident among persons without radiographic evidence of silicosis (ILO category <1/0), suggesting that silica was an important contributor to risk that was independent of the presence of silicosis. Disentangling the carcinogenic effects to the lung of occupational dust exposures per se from effects secondary to fibrosis, which may be an intervening pathogenetic step, is a challenging epidemiologic problem with no simple solution.

There is a logical sequence to analyzing data from a cohort study. The first step is to examine the cohort's overall pattern of mortality and morbidity. This analysis identifies diseases that are occurring more or less commonly in the cohort than would be expected, based on rates in a reference population assumed not to be exposed to the agents of interest. The most commonly used measure of association in mortality studies is the standardized mortality ratio (SMR), which is the observed number of deaths from a particular disease divided by the number of deaths expected for that disease, based on reference rates, usually derived from the source national or regional population.

The standardized incidence ratio (SIR) is the analogue of the SMR in situations where comparative rates for disease incidence are available. The SMR (or SIR) provides an estimate of the relative risk among the cohort compared to expected in a non-exposed population, as was done in the study of Swedish chimney sweeps[2] (Table 6.2). Next, when there are sufficient job history or environmental data to classify workers according to exposure type or level, an analysis can be performed for subsets, or subcohorts, of the cohort. This approach is illustrated with data from study of leukemia incidence among Chinese workers from numerous factories exposed to benzene.[6] Workers from the same factories, but not exposed to benzene, provided the comparison group. Leukemia excesses were identified for exposed workers in all industries, with the largest excess seen in chemical manufacturing plants (Table 6.7).

The informativeness of an epidemiologic study is greatly enhanced when exposure data can be linked to employment for dose-response estimation. It was possible to reconstruct historical exposures to benzene in the study of Chinese workers[6] and to estimate a dose–response trend for leukemia with cumulative exposure (expressed in parts per million benzene × years, ppm-yrs) (Table 6.8). Unfortunately, quantitative data on exposure levels are often not available in historical cohort studies, or available data are incomplete. The reason is that, traditionally, exposure monitoring has not been performed for epidemiologic or medical surveillance research purposes, but rather to assess levels in relation to exposure standards, i.e., compliance testing. In the absence of representative and reliable quantitative exposure data, investigators are forced to rely on surrogates of dose, such as employment duration in various jobs ranked according to cumulative exposure level. This was the case in the Swedish chimney sweep study[2] where employment duration was the dose surrogate in the dose–response trends analyses (Table 6.3).

Many occupational cohort studies focus on fatal diseases because of their importance, and because of the relative ease of obtaining mortality data. Studies of cancer incidence also receive considerable attention, but require linkage to cancer diagnosis and reporting registration systems. Cancer incidence studies are facilitated when cohorts are located in population centers with cancer registries, such as the Surveillance, Epidemiology, and End Results (SEER) registries in the US, or the national population-based cancer registries maintained in some of the Scandinavian countries. The lack of national disease incidence registries in most countries (including the US) limits the ability to determine risks for workers who relocate after leaving employment. Some companies maintain their own disease registries as part of health surveillance programs, but this is not a widespread practice. Currently, most small industries are not likely to have adequate resources to maintain disease registries.

Cohort studies of health endpoints other than mortality or cancer incidence often require intensive questionnaire or clinical surveys of the workplace. An example is a historical cohort study of spontaneous abortion history among semiconductor fabrication workers.[7] In this study, self-reported reproductive histories were obtained from 506 active and 385 former workers who had been pregnant during 1986–1989. The cohort was identified from company records for more than 6000 women workers at 14 companies. Women were classified according to exposures to various chemicals that occurred at the estimated times of conception. As shown in Table 6.9, there were relatively strong associations for highest exposures to ethylene glycol ethers, xylene, and fluoride.

At times, the only available data for a worker cohort may be information on disease occurrence, generally death certificates. This situation occurs when the data necessary to assemble a cohort do not exist or cannot be obtained feasibly. Studies of union memberships sometimes encounter this problem when the membership represents workers from a large number of geographically scattered plants and companies. Data on disease frequency can be used to a limited extent by adopting a design known as a proportionate mortality or morbidity ratio (PMR) analysis. In a PMR study, the distribution of various diseases in the exposed group is compared with an expected distribution derived from the experience of a reference population. Thus, for example, if leukemia accounts for 10% of deaths for a group of workers exposed to solvents, but only 2% of deaths in the national population, then an estimate of the relative risk would be 5. Alternatively, one might compare the observed and expected proportions of death from a given cause in relation to a more specific encompassing category of diseases than all causes combined. Comparing observed and expected distributions of site-specific cancers as proportions of all cancers, rather than all deaths, is the most common application of this approach. For example, data from a proportionate mortality study of cancers among garment workers exposed to formaldehyde[8] suggest a relative excess of buccal cavity cancer, but not lung cancer (Table 6.10).

The main advantage of PMR studies is the relative speed with which they can be conducted, provided that a roster of deaths in the population of interest is available. A potential drawback of the PMR approach is that, without having followed a defined cohort, there is often no way of knowing whether the available deaths or cases constitute a biased sample, e.g., death certificates for cancer deaths may have been archived more completely than death certificates for other diseases. Another potential disadvantage is that, in a PMR analysis, excesses of certain diseases

Agent/level	Pregnancies	Spontaneous abortions	Rate	Relative risk
Ethylene glycol ether				
None	693	79	0.11	1.00
Low	135	23	0.17	1.50
Moderate	21	3	0.14	1.25
High	23	7	0.30	2.67
Xylene				
None	683	79	0.12	1.00
Low	117	14	0.12	1.04
Moderate	40	9	0.23	1.95
High	32	10	0.31	2.70
Fluoride				
None	652	70	0.11	1.00
Low	122	25	0.20	1.91
Moderate	85	14	0.16	1.53
High	13	3	0.23	2.15

Table 6.9 Spontaneous abortion history in semiconductor workers classified by exposure levels

Cause of death	Proportion of all deaths			Proportion of all cancer	
	Observed	Expected*	Observed/expected	Expected*	Observed/expected
Buccal cavity cancer	3	0.40	7.50	0.44	6.82
Colon cancer	8	7.32	1.09	8.61	0.93
Lung cancer	11	11.62	0.90	12.53	0.84

* Based on proportionate mortality distribution of US population.

Table 6.10 Proportionate mortality of garment industry workers exposed to formaldehyde

necessarily will be counterbalanced by deficits of the residual diseases. This occurs because the total number of deaths available for the study is fixed. Consequently, the investigator may not be able to determine which of the disease excesses and deficits are more valid findings. As a general rule, PMR studies serve best to give a general picture of disease experience, whereas follow-up studies of well-defined cohorts yield more complete and valid data.

One important aspect of cohort studies is that they are designed to assess multiple health outcomes, even in instances where a specific agent/disease association triggers the investigation. As a result, previously unanticipated associations may emerge and stimulate further research or interventions. As discussed earlier, prospective cohort studies of chronic diseases are seldom practical. Historical cohort studies are a convenient alternative, although a thorough analysis of disease risk in relation to complete occupational history can require several years of effort, even for relatively small cohorts. An alternative, more cost-efficient design is the case-control study which is considered next.

Case-control studies

In a case-control study, past exposure histories are compared between cases of index diseases and controls free of these conditions at the times when the cases are identified. Case-control studies were originally devised in the 1950s as a practical alternative to cohort studies. Some of the original case-control studies explored associations of lung cancer with cigarette smoking and cervical cancer with sexual history. Most of these studies were conducted in hospital settings. Early critics of the case-control design argued that an approach that begins with the outcome and works backward to its causes is inherently inferior to a cohort design that has the reverse, more intuitive, temporal sequence. This viewpoint, while not fully discarded, has in large measure been discounted following numerous theoretical and empirical demonstrations that, when conducted validly, cohort and case-control studies of the same research questions yield similar results. This has been amply demonstrated with smoking and lung cancer, for example.

There are two general types of case-control studies. The first are 'nested' case-control studies in which the cases and controls are both selected from within a defined occupational cohort. The other type are community-based case control studies in which study subjects typically are identified from hospitals, disease registries, or other sources of population-based data, rather than from enumerated industrial cohorts. The two types of case-control studies are considered in turn.

Nested case-control studies

Comparisons of disease rates can be made between subcohorts that comprise a defined occupational cohort. An example of this approach was given in Table 6.7. In many instances subcohort analyses of an entire cohort may not be practical, especially when an expensive and time-consuming exposure reconstruction effort is required. A more cost- and time-efficient alternative to a full subcohort analysis is to compare exposures of the cases with those of a sample of the non-cases, where both cases and controls are members of some defined occupational cohort. Typically, this involves identifying all or as many cases of the index disease(s) as can be ascertained from historical follow-up, and selecting a sample of other workers who were free of the index condition(s) at the times of the cases' diagnoses.

In a study of mortality outcomes, the date of death serves as the date of identification or diagnosis. The savings in time and cost for exposure assessment and data processing in a nested case-control study, relative to a subcohort analysis of an entire cohort, can be great. To illustrate, consider a cohort of 10,000 workers exposed to solvents from which 75 leukemia cases are identified during a 40-year historical follow-up. Exposure reconstruction for all 10,000 workers is an extremely labor-intensive effort, whereas exposure assessment and data processing for the 75 cases and 150 or 300 control workers can be accomplished much more efficiently. The savings becomes even more evident when there are multiple exposures of interest, which each engender detailed exposure assessments. In a study with a relatively small number of subjects, intensive efforts can be devoted to exposure reconstruction for each individual; this task can be unwieldy for a large cohort.

The diseases that are selected for nested case-control studies usually are those for which there are postulated a priori associations and those for which excesses are found from disease rate comparisons made between the cohort and an external reference population. Often in medical surveillance programs, apparent disease excesses emerge without prior evidence of toxicity, and these may prompt more in-depth analyses using the case-control design. As with disease cluster investigations, judgment concerning which diseases warrant further inquiry is needed to avoid unproductive expenditures of resources. In the absence of prior hypotheses or suspicions of toxicity associated with specific exposures, relatively stable, long-term trends of disease excess can serve as useful guides for decision-making.

The data in Table 6.11 are from a case-control study of fatal work-related injuries nested within a cohort of 22,000 Brazilian steel workers employed during 1977–1990.[9] The 37 cases who died from work-related injuries were compared with a sample of control steel workers; four controls were randomly selected for each case. Data on cases' and controls' demographic factors, history of injuries, physical disabilities (e.g., hearing loss), psychiatric disorders, and previous injuries at work and elsewhere were abstracted from plant personnel, occupational hygiene, and medical records. Occupational histories for study subjects were classified with respect to chemical and physical hazards. Prominent associations with fatal injuries were detected for employment in jobs classified as having moderate to high levels of noise, heat, and vibration; associations with dusts, fumes, gases and vapors were

Occupational hazard	Cases	Controls	OR*	(95% CI)
Noise				
None	4	50	1.00	–
Low	7	32	2.19	(0.60–8.04)
Moderate	16	27	5.72	(1.63–20.1)
High	10	31	3.05	(0.80–11.7)
Heat				
None	18	111	1.00	–
Low	1	10	0.45	(0.05–4.12)
Moderate	8	12	2.89	(0.92–9.07)
High	10	7	6.80	(2.13–21.7)
Vibration				
None	29	125	1.00	–
Low	3	11	1.01	(0.25–5.29)
Moderate	1	1	2.58	(0.15–49.8)
High	4	3	4.01	(0.81–19.8)
Dusts or fumes				
No	18	117	1.00	–
Yes	19	23	4.17	(1.87–9.31)
Gases or vapors				
No	24	124	1.00	–
Yes	13	16	3.85	(1.49–9.94)

* Odds ratio, adjusted for education.

Table 6.11 Nested case-control study of fatal work-related injuries in a cohort of 21,816 Brazilian steel workers

also identified (Table 6.11). This example clearly illustrates the chief advantage of the nested case-control design relative to a full cohort analysis: collection of occupational and non-occupational risk factor data was much more feasible than would have been the case had a similar effort been mounted for the entire cohort of 22,000 workers.

Case-control studies should yield estimates of exposure effects that are identical to those that would be obtained from a full exposure–response analysis of the base cohorts, provided that control sampling is performed in an unbiased manner. An absolute requirement for validity is that control selection should be made without respect to exposure status. Apart from this requirement, there is no one optimal method for control selection. It is generally sound practice to select controls such that they have similar distributions of age and gender as the cases. (The issue of confounding will be discussed in more depth later in this chapter.) In comparison with subcohort analyses, nested case-control studies may suffer from a loss of statistical precision by virtue of a reduced study size. However, statistical power can be increased by enlarging the study sample. This is usually accomplished by selecting more than one control per case, as the size of the case group is more likely to be fixed. Furthermore, the number of controls in the study may need to be enlarged if a goal of the study is to examine exposure effects in subgroups of the workforce (e.g., the effects of solvents on neurological disease risk separately for workers with and without metal exposures).

The foregoing discussion has emphasized the relative efficiency of the nested case-control design. This efficiency is realized when the time and cost required for exposure assessment and data management increase in proportion to the number of subjects in the analysis. However, there would be no need for a nested case-control study in situations where all of the pertinent work history and exposure data have already been compiled and assembled for analysis. Instead, a full cohort analysis would be preferred for reasons of statistical power and simplicity in explaining the results.

Community-based case-control studies

When it is not possible or convenient to enumerate and follow a defined occupational cohort, or when the disease of interest is especially rare so that only a prohibitively large cohort would be effective, community-based case-control studies provide a valuable alternative. For example, studies of soft tissue sarcoma among agricultural workers cannot be conducted easily in cohort studies because cohorts of such workers are usually difficult to enumerate, and the soft tissue sarcomas are very rare diseases. The frequency of exposure in the community is an important determinant of the success of the study, as some exposures may be too rare for evaluation. Consequently, the choice of study setting can be crucial. Thus, for example, towns in the Appalachian Mountains would be more suitable locations than large metropolitan areas in California for community-based studies of coal dust and non-malignant respiratory disease.

Community-based studies encompass research that is truly based in a community (i.e., surveys conducted among a defined population base), as well as studies that are conducted in hospital settings or other places where cases of disease are diagnosed and registered. Irrespective of the source of subjects, the design of community-based case-control studies is similar to that of nested case-control studies; exposure history profiles of index cases are compared with those of persons free of disease at the times when the cases' diagnoses are made. The difference between the two types of case-control studies is the source of subjects – persons identified from the population-at-large, or from disease registries in community-based studies.

Traditionally, most community-based studies have been conducted among hospital patients, which provided the source of both cases and controls. Controls may also be selected from the population-at-large, and are suitably compared with hospital cases when controls are sampled from the same population base that provides the hospital or clinic catchment area. As an illustration, Seidler et al.[10] conducted a case-control study of Parkinson's disease in Germany in which the exposures of cases identified from neurology clinics were compared with exposures of controls selected from the same regions where the clinics were located. Findings for pesticide exposures indicated associations with long-term use of herbicides and insecticides, including organochlorine compounds (Table 6.12).

Increasingly, there has been a trend toward using population-based disease registries to identify cases, and population rosters as sources of controls. Population-based disease registries greatly facilitate community-based case-control studies because they offer improved case ascertainment and diagnostic standardization over what are ordinarily available from studies relying on death certificates or hospital diagnosis logs for case accrual. National or provincial vital

Exposure/years	Cases	Controls	OR*
Herbicides			
0	238	287	1.0
1–40	59	44	1.7
41–80	34	15	3.0
>80	20	10	2.4
Insecticides			
0	213	258	1.0
1–40	70	55	1.8
41–80	46	25	2.5
>80	21	14	2.1
Organochlorines			
0	262	309	1.0
≥1	7	2	5.8

* Odds ratio, adjusted for smoking and education.

Table 6.12 Community-based case-control study of agricultural exposure and Parkinson's disease in Germany

	Blood lead concentration (µg/dL)			
	<15	15–24	25–39	≥40
Number of workers	32	46	29	12
Total sperm (million cells)*	186	153	137	89
Sperm concentration (million cells/mm³)*	79.1	56.5	62.7	44.4
Motile sperm (%)*	45.8	56.4	56.3	36.8
Abnormal morphology (%)*	17.7	18.4	17.3	16.2

* Geometric mean.

Table 6.13 Semen quality among Canadian lead smelter workers

statistics bureaus, which provide death certificate data, can also be regarded as special cases of disease registries. In some instances, exposure data can be inferred from occupations listed on death certificates, thus obviating the need for contacting next-of-kin.

A decided strength of community-based case-control studies is that they typically are designed to obtain data on a wide range of factors, including occupational and non-occupational exposures. Thus, it is often possible to obtain data on potentially confounding factors that are seldom accessible in industry-based studies, which ordinarily rely solely on personnel and exposure records. However, the principal disadvantage of many community-based studies is that exposure data are often determined from questionnaires administered to subjects or to proxy respondents, and thus may not offer quantified data on specific agents as can be obtained in most industry-based studies. This is especially true for studies in which occupational exposure information is inferred from occupations recorded on death certificates.

Cross-sectional studies

Epidemiologic studies of non-fatal outcomes frequently use a cross-sectional design in which health status is compared among worker groups classified with respect to exposure. Outcomes of interest can include overt clinical diseases, symptoms, or variations in physiologic measures. As the name implies, cross-sectional studies assess exposure/disease associations at a single point in time. As will be discussed below, exposure and health evaluations can be extended to multiple points in time, in which instance the study effectively assumes a cohort design.

An illustrative example of a typical cross-sectional design is a study of semen quality among Canadian lead smelters.[11] Total sperm count and sperm concentration were reduced markedly with increasing blood lead levels measured at the time of the study, although no consistent associations were observed for either sperm motility or morphology (Table 6.13). It is noteworthy that this cross-sectional study is conceptually similar to an exposure subgroup analysis that would be performed in a cohort study, except that there is no follow-up over time. In this

study, an effort was made to determine possible effects of chronic lead exposure by examining trends of semen quality parameters in relation to past lead exposures, but only among men whose most recent blood lead concentration was less than 40 µg/dL – similar associations were noted for chronic exposure as were observed for recent lead level.[11]

The lack of follow-up in a cross-sectional study can be a major hindrance to interpreting causal relations. Specifically, the concurrent measurement of exposure and health status can produce misleading results if changes in the latter influence exposure status. For example, a study of pulmonary function among workers exposed to metal-working fluids could show an inverse association with exposure if the appearance of respiratory symptoms causes workers either to leave employment altogether or to transfer to less heavily exposed jobs. Another significant limitation of many cross-sectional studies is that usually only currently employed workers are included; workers who previously had left employment, perhaps because of exposure-induced impaired health, may be the most relevant study subjects for detecting true exposure effects.

An improvement to the simple one-time cross-sectional study is a longitudinal follow-up with repeated measurements of exposure and health outcomes. The example of pulmonary function among Chinese cotton textile workers[1] partially fits this description (Table 6.1). Workers can be selected for repeated measures studies on the basis of past exposure, much in the same manner that cohorts of workers exposed to extraordinary exposure circumstances are assembled for cohort mortality studies (e.g., the dioxin-exposed workers in Table 6.4).

Repeated measures studies customarily involve assessments of physiologic function changes (e.g., lung function, nerve conduction velocity, semen quality), but may also include longitudinal evaluations of symptom prevalence. Such studies are more effectively conducted when there is a documented change of exposure in the workplace and the effect(s) of interest is thought to be reversible. A study from Sweden[12] took advantage of a 'natural experiment', caused by closure of a styrene-reinforced plastics plant, to examine post-exposure nervous system effects (Table 6.14). Questionnaires were administered one week and 7 months after exposure among workers with relatively low and high styrene exposures. The reductions over time in symptom prevalence in the heavily exposed workers suggest reversibility of effects.

Symptom	High exposure group (n = 9)		Low exposure group (n = 8)	
	1st exam*	2nd exam+	1st exam*	2nd exam+
Abnormal tiredness	9	0	5	0
Heart palpitations	4	0	2	1
Painful tingling	7	1	3	2
Unprovoked irritability	8	1	3	1
Depression	4	0	3	0
Problems concentrating	7	2	3	0
Short memory	9	2	8	2
Chest pain	6	0	1	1
Frequent headaches	8	1	3	1
Loss of libido	2	1	0	0

* One week post exposure.
+ Seven months post exposure.

Table 6.14 Nervous system symptoms among styrene-exposed workers following cessation of exposure

Attrition of the study population in a repeated measures survey, due to absenteeism, turnover of the workplace, or workers' refusals to continue participation, can pose a serious logistical problem. Losses or withdrawals of study subjects, per se, will not bias the study unless attrition is related both to health and exposure status. To illustrate, consider a hypothetical longitudinal study of pulmonary function in a dusty workplace in which subject attrition is proportionally greater among workers who have FEV_1 values less than 80% of predicted. If attrition among subjects with low FEV_1 values occurs equally across dust exposure levels, then the net effect will not be a bias, but rather a reduced statistical power to estimate a dose–response association because the study population will be over-represented with unaffected workers. On the other hand, the study would underestimate the effect of dust exposure on lung function if subject attrition were proportionally greatest among impaired workers in the highest exposure categories (i.e., biasing the study towards a negative result).

The likelihood of a successful longitudinal repeated measures study can be increased by attending to several practical considerations in the planning of the project. As a general guideline, the measurements should be relatively non-invasive and rapid. Blood, breath, or urine samples can be obtained readily on a routine basis, provided that workers understand the purposes of the tests, and the results are transmitted to workers within a reasonable period of time. Increasing application of molecular genetic markers in epidemiologic research to identify susceptible individuals in a population poses ethical concerns that need to be addressed and explained at the outset of research. Incorporating useful and interpretable clinical measurements, such as serum cholesterol, in a study involving more exotic tests can greatly improve worker interest in participating.

Long complicated test batteries, such as those used to measure neurobehavioral function, may be administered successfully on one occasion, but on repeated testing, participation will diminish in direct proportion to the time and effort required of subjects. One way to circumvent this problem is to obtain as much baseline data as necessary during the initial survey, but then to limit data collection for the repeat surveys to the minimally required informa-tion. Thus, the initial test battery results can serve as baseline data, and changes in the most relevant parameters can be assessed subsequently. So-called 'learning effects' whereby subjects improve their test performance due to increased familiarity can be mitigated by sufficient training at the baseline survey.

Repeated measures studies are most readily conducted as part of routine medical and exposure surveillance programs. Unfortunately, such programs are usually only affordable by large industries. Studying workers from work sites where exposures are frequently excessive and worker turnover tends to be high poses a more formidable, but important challenge.

TYPES AND SOURCES OF BIAS IN EPIDEMIOLOGIC RESEARCH

Virtually all occupational epidemiologic research studies are observational rather than experimental. Thus, epidemiologic studies are prone to a variety of potential biases that may undermine validity. It is convenient to classify epidemiologic biases into three broad types: selection bias, information bias, and confounding. The distinctions between these categories are not always sharp, as some biases have aspects of more than one type. Nonetheless, this taxonomy provides a useful framework for reviewing the topic of bias. Throughout this discussion, the term bias is used to denote distortion of study results such that observed associations are either spuriously over- or under-estimated.

Selection bias

Improper selection of study subjects can create bias in an epidemiologic study, irrespective of study design. However, in order to simplify the discussion, selection bias will be considered separately for cohort, case-control, and cross-sectional studies.

In cohort studies, selection bias is most commonly the result of inappropriate comparison groups. The most familiar form of such bias is known as the 'healthy worker effect'. In mortality studies, the healthy worker effect is recognizable as a lower mortality risk among the cohort compared to national or regional reference populations. Apparently reduced mortality rates from all causes combined, and more specifically from cardiovascular diseases, non-malignant respiratory diseases, diabetes, gastrointestinal diseases, and genitourinary diseases, are frequently observed among occupational cohorts. The explanation for this phenomenon is that industrial cohorts include workers who are healthy enough to gain and maintain employment, whereas national or regional (external) reference populations include persons unfit to work because of impaired health. In some industries, access to medical care is more readily obtainable than in the population-at-large, and this may account for some of the reduced mortality risk to the workforce. The healthy worker effect can be regarded as a form of selection bias because cohort members are selected preferentially on the basis of health status, either by themselves or as a result of job requirements.

An example of the healthy worker effect can be seen from a historical cohort mortality study of US electrical utility workers exposed to electromagnetic fields.[13] Reduced mortality, relative to national rates, was observed for all causes combined, heart diseases, non-malignant respiratory diseases, diabetes, all malignant neoplasms, and for the diseases of greatest a priori interest, leukemia and brain cancer (Table 6.15). Despite the absence of a deficit of brain cancer for the cohort as a whole, there was a trend of increasing risk related to cumulative EMF exposure in the 2–10-year period preceding death.[13]

The healthy worker effect does not necessarily occur in all cohort mortality studies. Obvious exceptions would be cohorts exposed to widely disseminated workplace hazards. Notably, occupational cohort studies of workers from large industries or trade unions from the developed countries have dominated the literature. A somewhat different picture would be anticipated for cohort studies of workers identified from small, non-unionized workplaces, or from developing countries.

The most suitable means of minimizing healthy worker effect bias is to substitute comparisons between worker cohorts and national or regional populations with comparisons among worker subgroups (i.e., internal comparisons). An internal reference group can be defined as workers with low or minimal exposures to toxic agents. This approach was used in the cohort study of Chinese factory workers

Cause of death	Observed	Relative risk*
All causes	20,733	0.77
Heart disease	7768	0.76
Stroke	1244	0.73
Respiratory diseases	1178	0.69
Diabetes mellitus	219	0.56
Malignant neoplasms	4833	0.86
Leukemia	164	0.76
Brain cancer	151	0.95

* Compared to rates for US males, 1950–1988.

Table 6.15 Cause-specific mortality among US electric utility workers 1950–1988

exposed to benzene.[6] However, care must be taken to avoid making inappropriate internal comparisons, as can occur when the least exposed workers are decidedly different in terms of lifestyle and sociodemographic factors than the more heavily exposed groups. An extreme case would be the inappropriate comparison of disease rates between office workers and heavily exposed production or maintenance workers. This problem can be mitigated somewhat by restricting comparisons to either 'blue collar' or 'white collar' groups, if such distinctions can be made.

However, difficulties can arise when internal comparisons are made. The most important is identification of a suitable reference group when exposures are relatively uniform across the cohort, or when the exposure data are too limited to permit meaningful exposure categorizations. A second difficulty is statistical in nature. The statistical precision of the outcome measure (e.g., relative risk) is dependent on the variability of the rates in the exposed and reference groups. Thus, disease rate comparisons made against a national population will have greater precision than comparisons made between subcohorts because the national rates are based on much larger numbers. This problem is an issue of statistical precision, rather than research validity. In fact, internal comparisons are generally more valid methods for assessing risk than external comparisons because the former minimize healthy worker effect bias and may reduce confounding from factors that differ between workers and the general population. In situations where there is a potential trade-off between validity and statistical precision (e.g., the choice between external and internal reference populations), validity concerns should take precedence.

An alternative approach to a strictly internal comparison analysis is to identify as a comparison group another occupational cohort not exposed to the agent(s) of concern or to agents that pose similar health risks, as was done in the study of Shanghai textile workers[1] (Table 6.1). This strategy has an intuitive appeal, although it is tantamount to conducting two studies, and hence the effort and resources required to enumerate and follow another cohort may at times be prohibitive. It may also prove difficult to identify a suitable occupational comparison group that is not exposed to hazardous agents for outcomes of interest.

The major issue relating to selection bias in case-control studies centers on the choice of controls. Certainly, controls in any case-control study should be selected 'blindly' without investigator knowledge of exposure history. The goal of a nested case-control study is to produce the same results (within sampling error) that would be obtained from a full cohort analysis. Accordingly, control selection should be made such that the nested case-control study mirrors the cohort design as closely as possible. Cohort studies measure temporal disease rate patterns in relation to exposure among an entire cohort. Therefore, case-control studies should be designed to evaluate a random sample of the cohort's experience, generally all of the cases and a sample of the remaining workers. This means that controls should be selected from among workers who do not have the index disease, but additional exclusions on the basis of other diseases should not be imposed.

To illustrate, consider a nested case-control study conducted among asbestos-exposed workers designed to evaluate exposure–response trends for stomach cancer. Given past knowledge of associations between asbestos and pulmonary fibrosis and lung cancer, it might be tempting to eliminate persons known to have developed the latter diseases from the pool of eligible control workers. This would introduce a bias into the study, in that it would artificially lower the likelihood of identifying heavily exposed controls. The extent of the bias will depend on the frequency of pulmonary fibrosis and lung cancer in the cohort, but the general principle of avoiding health-related control selection biases applies to any case-control study.

In hospital-based case-control studies, controls are typically hospitalized patients with conditions other than the index disease. Ideally, one would select controls with a condition that is unrelated, either positively or negatively, to exposure. Identifying suitable control conditions may not always be possible if the exposure under study is potentially associated with a range of health outcomes. In order to avoid introducing selection bias, it may be necessary to select control patients randomly from a variety of services rather than to choose controls with a particular condition.

Controls selected from the community should be representative of the base population insofar as there should not be any a priori reasons to suspect unusual exposure patterns among them. Excluding community controls with diseases known or presumed to be related to the index disease is generally not advisable for the same reason mentioned for control selection in nested case-control studies.

Selection bias in cross-sectional studies, and longitudinal repeat measures studies, are the same as those discussed above. A variant of the healthy worker effect bias is particularly prominent in some cross-sectional studies, where the only workers available for study may include a disproportionate number of persons who are resistant to the effects of exposure. This is often found in studies of acute toxicity where the most responsive or sensitive workers are 'selected out' of exposure. One should attempt to obtain data on subjects' entire work histories, although this may be impractical in many instances. Recruitment of volunteer subjects in cross-sectional studies may be a source of selection bias, although bias will only occur when subject participation is related both to exposure and health status. This can usually be accomplished by explaining to workers that the purpose of the study is not necessarily to screen for disease, and that the validity of the findings depends on inclusion of workers with varying exposure and health status. By way of illustration, in the study of semen quality among lead smelter workers,[11] only 119 workers out of 2469 active and retired workers whose participation was invited donated semen samples. While this raises the possibility of selection (participation) bias it is reassuring that there were no systematic differences between semen donors and non-participants with respect to age, blood lead level, work assignment, or history of having sought fertility consultation.[11]

Information bias

The main form of information bias is misclassification of either health or exposure status. Information bias can be considered to be either differential or non-differential. For example, exposure misclassification should be regarded as non-differential if the exposure classification error is similar for persons with and without disease. Likewise, misclassification of health status would be non-differential if the sensitivity and specificity of diagnoses were the same across exposure categories. The effect of non-differential misclassification of either exposure or health status is that relations between exposure and disease are usually underestimated. Thus, for example, the failure to detect a true contact dermatitis case due to beryllium in a study where exposure classification is equally erroneous for affected and unaffected workers is a case of 'noise in the system obscuring the signal'. On the other hand, misclassification that is differential can produce bias in either direction – toward over- or under-estimating effects. Thus, for example, in a study of mercury-related neurotoxicity, a more accurate exposure classification among affected than unaffected workers would produce an over-estimate of effect. In practice, one can seldom determine with any confidence whether misclassification is non-differential or differential. Generally, unless there is evidence to the contrary, it is most justifiable to assume that misclassification is non-differential because it is more likely that errors occur uniformly than in a systematic manner.

Health status classification is determined by diagnostic accuracy. Biases caused by differences in the quality of diagnoses can arise in cohort studies when the cohort has undergone more intensive medical scrutiny than an external comparison population. Diagnostic bias may also arise within a cohort if the most heavily exposed workers undergo more thorough medical evaluations than other workers. In general, however, differences in diagnostic accuracy between subgroups of a cohort, and hence biases, are less likely to occur in studies involving internal comparisons than those relying on external comparisons.

Misclassification of exposure is a pervasive concern in occupational epidemiology. The primary cause of exposure misclassification is inadequate or incomplete data on job histories or environmental exposure levels. Missing information includes not only data that cannot be retrieved or are truly absent (e.g., no monitoring had ever been performed), but also incomplete data on factors that affect exposure levels, such as changes in control measures and the use of personal protective equipment. This generalization applies to any industry- or community-based epidemiologic study. As mentioned earlier, exposure misclassification is generally non-differential with respect to health status. Thus, most observed associations will be biased toward observing no effect. It is possible to 'correct' observed associations statistically so as to take into account exposure misclassification by making assumptions about the sensitivity and specificity of exposure classification, and re-computing effect estimates. However, results that are corrected or adjusted for misclassification should be reported along with, rather than instead of, the observed data, because the assumptions underlying the adjustments are only approximations of reality.

Inaccurate reporting of data by study subjects is another potential source of information bias. This is seldom an issue in cohort mortality or nested case-control studies because most or all of the data are obtained from recorded information rather than from subject interviews. On the other hand, health and exposure data are frequently obtained from subject interview in community-based case-control studies and cross-sectional studies. Faulty recall of exposures that is non-differential for diseased and healthy subjects (e.g., cases and controls) will tend to mask true associations, as discussed above. There are instances, however, when recall may be differential and the resulting biases will cause over-estimation of associations.

For example, it is possible that affected cases may have more reason to remember past exposures than healthy controls, in which case exposure classification would not be equivalent for the two groups. There is no one effective safeguard against reporting bias. Instead, investigators have tried a variety of approaches, including selecting as controls persons with other diseases presumed to be unrelated to the exposures of concern, asking unrelated questions to elicit patterns of over- or under-reporting, and, where possible, verifying self-reported health or exposure information against objective sources, such as employment personnel and medical records. Studies of diseases with cognitive impairment, of which Alzheimer's disease would be a prototype, pose challenges of obtaining valid interview data. Interviewing proxy respondents, typically spouses or offspring, may be required; in case-control studies, interviews of proxy respondents for controls, even when they have full cognitive capacity, is advisable in order to balance interview data quality.

Although subject interviews may be a source of bias in some instances, they are also one of the most valuable sources of direct information about exposure conditions and confounding factors. Workers can often provide much better insights into past working conditions than what can be gleaned from reviews of industrial hygiene and production records. In fact, information on the use of protective equipment is usually better determined from workers' self-reports than from other sources. The opportunity to collect data on lifestyle factors, one that seldom exists in strictly record-based investigations, is another decided advantage to worker interviews. The use of in-person interviews to obtain morbidity information has obvious clinical advantages.

Confounding

Biased results can be observed when the effects of the exposures under investigation cannot be disentangled from the effects of other, unmeasured variables. Confounding is thus defined as a mixing of effects of exposure with the effects of extraneous factors. Differences between exposed and comparisons groups in the distributions of age, gender, race, and socioeconomic status may cause confounded results because these attributes are frequently related both to exposure and disease. The importance of these factors is widely acknowledged, and most epidemiologic studies include attempts to control confounding, in either the design or analysis phases.

In order for an extraneous factor to be a confounder, it must be associated with exposure and must be a risk factor for the disease under study. The second criterion implies that the confounder must be capable of inducing or contributing to disease etiology in the absence of the occupational exposure of concern. For example, cigarette smoke can cause lung cancer in the absence of asbestos, radon, or any other environmental lung carcinogen. A final requirement for confounding is that the suspected confounder should not be an intermediate step in the causal pathway of exposure leading to disease. Thus, for example, it would be inappropriate to consider impaired ventilatory capacity as a confounder in a study of coal dust and pulmonary disability.

There are several epidemiologic approaches to control (eliminate or minimize) confounding. It is always valuable to examine associations between the potential confounder(s) and the exposure(s) of interest. Weak or absent correlations of confounders and study exposures offer reassurance that confounding is likely to be minimal. In the semen quality study of lead smelter workers,[11] the distribution of age, smoking, alcohol use, and histories of delayed fertility and fertility consultation among subgroups of workers stratified by blood level was compared. Age was unrelated to exposure, whereas the other factors were either positively or negatively associated with exposure (Table 6.16). Subsequent analyses took these factors into account in the analysis. In addition, blood measurements of metals other than lead, such as zinc, cadmium, and thallium, enabled control in the analysis.[11]

Control of confounding may be accomplished by limiting study subjects to persons who have identical histories of exposure to the putative confounder. For example, studies of indoor radon and environmental tobacco smoke have intentionally focused on persons who were never active cigarette smokers. However, restrictions of this type will preclude opportunities to examine interactions among causal factors, e.g., active smoking and radon on lung cancer risks. Often, control of confounding is attempted

	Blood lead concentration (µg/dL)			
	<15	15–24	25–39	≥40
No. workers	32	46	29	12
Age (mean)	41.4	38.2	40.7	41.8
Smokers (%)	12.5	13.0	6.9	33.3
≥10 Alcoholic beverages per week (%)	15.6	10.9	24.1	33.3
Delayed pregnancy (%)	18.5	18.6	15.4	8.3
Sought fertility consultation (%)	14.8	9.3	7.7	8.3

* Unable to achieve pregnancy with partner after trying ≥1 year.

Table 6.16 Characteristics of Canadian lead smelter workers who provided semen samples, by blood lead level

by statistical correction of the observed results, with corrections made for imbalances in the distributions of the confounder between study and comparison groups. Age adjustment is a well-known approach to correct results for age differences among exposure levels. This type of direct statistical adjustment requires that data on the confounder are available in sufficient detail for use in the analysis. By way of illustration, consider the data in Table 6.17 from a community-based case-control study of lung cancer and occupation in Germany.[14] Relative risks for both unadjusted (crude) and adjusted smoking and asbestos exposure were computed for various occupational groupings. Fairly small differences between the two sets of results indicate that smoking and asbestos were not serious confounders in this study.

When there are no available data on smoking or other potential confounders, as is typically the case in many industry-based studies, then indirect methods of control can be used. The most commonly used technique is to estimate the extent of confounding that would be required for the observed effects to be attributable solely to confounding. This requires assuming a level of risk associated with the confounder, in the absence of the exposure of interest, and computing hypothetical values of effect estimates for a range of distributions of the confounder across exposure categories. The data in Table 6.18 illustrate this method.[15] In this hypothetical example, lung cancer incidence is compared between an occupational cohort and a national reference population. The prevalence of smoking in the reference population is given as 50% non-smokers, 40%

moderate smokers, and 10% heavy smokers, and the corresponding relative risk are, respectively 1, 10, and 20. There will be no spurious excess or deficit in the observed relative risk among the cohort when it has the same smoking distribution as the reference population, whereas departures from this distribution will create biased relative risk estimates.

It is worth noting that a very skewed distribution of smoking, weighted toward more heavy smokers in the cohort than the reference population, is required to produce a relative risk as high as 2, which is merely an artifact of confounding. This approach is considered an indirect method of control of confounding because, unlike explicit adjustment procedures that make use of available data, this method is based on assumed associations of the confounder with exposure and disease risk. Ordinarily, direct adjustment is preferable to an indirect assessment of confounding, provided that the data on the confounder(s) are sufficiently complete and valid. The indirect method offers a convenient alternative when data quality is inadequate, to assess the potential impact of bias.

In some studies, factors other than age, gender, race or smoking can be considered as potential confounders, and their control can be accomplished with the same methods outlined above. Previous employment in hazardous industries and occupations, like smoking, is often of concern in industry-based studies. Additionally, one may want to isolate the hazardous effects of a single agent in a multi-exposure environment, in which case each exposure is considered in turn while treating the other exposures as confounders. For example, one might try to control for the effects of xylene when examining the neurotoxic effects of toluene in a study of painters. Although in principle, control of confounding from concurrent workplace exposures should be as attainable as control of lifestyle confounding, strong and sometimes complex correlations among many chemicals will complicate the process. Thus, for example, exposures to multiple chemicals may be so highly inter-correlated in an industry that control of mutual confounding may be impossible. In such instances, the best that can be done is to determine the crude (potentially confounded) effects of each exposure, and to make qualitative judgments as to which associations are most meaningful.

Occupational group	Relative risk	
	Crude	Adjusted*
Farmer, agricultural worker	1.26	1.31
Miner, quarryman	1.92	1.65
Bricklayer, carpenter	1.65	1.33
Unskilled worker	1.60	1.36
Stationary engine, heavy equipment operator	2.35	1.78
Administrative, clerical work	0.58	0.65
Medical, dental, veterinary	0.50	0.60

* Adjusted for smoking and asbestos exposure.

Table 6.17 Crude and adjusted relative risks from a community-based case-control study of lung cancer and occupations in Germany

ANALYZING EPIDEMIOLOGIC DATA

In occupational and environmental epidemiology, we are interested in the effects of exposures on the probability of the outcome, (e.g., the dose–response association). In this section, we briefly describe some general principles of data analysis. A more thorough treatment of statistical analysis methods can be found in other texts, such as Rothman and Greenland.[16]

Statistical methods are used to make inferences, based on a sample of subjects, about the magnitude of the true association between an exposure and a health outcome. All statistical methods, from the simple comparison of means to multivariate modeling, are based on probability

	Population fraction (%)			
Non-smokers	Moderate smokers*	Heavy smokers+	Bias in relative risk
60	35	5	0.78
50	40	10	1.00
40	45	15	1.22
30	50	20	1.43
0	65	35	2.08

* Assumed relative risk of 10 for moderate smokers.
+ Assumed relative risk of 20 for heavy smokers.

Table 6.18 Indirect estimation of confounding from smoking in a cohort study of lung cancer

models. These models describe the probability of observing a particular health event or a particular value of a physiologic measurement. When the outcome is a health event, such as disease diagnosis, the exposure effect is usually expressed as a ratio of risks or rates, and is referred to as a relative risk. When the outcome is a physiologic measurement, such as pulmonary function or nerve conduction velocity, the effect of exposure is typically measured by the change in response per unit change in exposure.

Estimating relative risks and confidence levels

There are several reasons why the relative risk or the slope of a dose–response curve computed from the analysis of observed data may not be equal to the true underlying risk. We have discussed how confounding and other forms of bias can distort epidemiologic data so that the observed relative risk is misleading. However, even in the absence of confounding or other bias, risk may be imprecisely estimated because of statistical error. Two primary sources contribute to statistical error: errors in the measurement of study variables and sampling variability.

Sampling variability measures the spread of results derived from hypothetical repetitions of a study, each based on a random sample of the same size, from the same population (workforce or community), under identical conditions. The larger the sample size of the study, the less variability there will be among replicate samples. Sampling variability is reflected in the width of the confidence interval around the relative risk. The larger the study, the smaller the sampling variability, and the narrower the confidence intervals. As described further below, evaluating sampling variability is important in interpreting the results of an epidemiologic study. To attribute the findings of a small study to chance raises concerns about large sampling variability.

Hypothesis testing and study power

Inference is a procedure by which observed data from a sample are used to estimate a population parameter or to test a formal hypothesis about the value of that parameter. Hypothesis testing relies on a rigorous algorithm for deciding whether to reject the null hypothesis in favor of a specified alternative. The algorithm involves the calculation of a test statistic based on the data and a probability value (*P*-value) derived from the assumed probability distribution of the test statistic. The *P*-value is the probability of observing data as far from the null as was actually observed, given that the null hypothesis is true.

For example, a null hypothesis is typically stated as: there is no association between the exposure and the health outcome, i.e., the relative risk is 1.0. The analysis of epidemiologic data will result in an estimate of the relative risk and a *P*-value. If the data are inconsistent with the null hypothesis, the estimated relative risk will be different from the null value, the *P*-value will be small, and one will be inclined to reject the null hypothesis; an association

between exposure and outcome is therefore inferred. Although rigid rules for rejecting a null hypothesis, such as *P*<0.05, are ill-advised, the *P*-value does provide a measure of the robustness of the inference. *P*-values are closely related to confidence intervals but are not entirely redundant. A *P*-value less than 0.05 is equivalent to a 95% confidence interval that excludes the value of relative risk under the null hypothesis (typically 1.0). Thus, one can formally test a hypothesis on the basis of a confidence interval. One cannot, however, distinguish a *P*-value of 0.10 (indicating data fairly consistent with the null) from a *P*-value of 0.30 (data more consistent with the null) based on a confidence interval alone.

The statistical power of a study is also related to the concept of a power. Power is the probability of rejecting the null hypothesis when it is false. In a small study, the estimated relative risk would need to be quite far from 1.0 in order to result in a *P*-value small enough to reject the null. Conversely, in a large study, the difference between the estimate and the null could be trivial and still result in a 'statistically significant' difference. The larger the sample size, the greater the statistical power. Of course, statistical significance is not necessarily synonymous with clinical or public health significance.

Building regression models

The estimation of an exposure effect often involves consideration of several extraneous risk factors that my be acting as confounders. For example, in the German community-based case-control study of occupations and lung cancer[14] (Table 6.17), relative risk estimates were presented with and without adjustment for smoking and asbestos exposure. One way to control confounding in the analysis is to perform a separate exposure/outcome analysis for each level of the confounder (e.g., by age category). However, stratified analysis becomes a less effective way to address confounding as the number of confounders increases because the size of each stratum decreases. The decrease in sample size of each stratum increases sampling variability, and thus reduces the statistical power to identify underlying risk.

To address the problem of sparse data created by multiple confounders, epidemiologic studies commonly use multiple regression models to derive adjusted risk estimates. Regression models smooth across sparse strata by making statistical assumptions about the probability distribution of the outcome and the generic shape of the exposure–response curve.

A regression model is a function of the health outcome, Y, on a set of variables, X_i, that includes the primary exposure and potential confounders. For an outcome measured as a continuous variable, like pulmonary function, a linear regression model has the following general form:

$$E(Y) = \beta_0 + \beta_1 X_1 + \beta_2 X_2 + \ldots + \beta_k X_k$$

where E(Y) is the expected value, or mean value, of the outcome Y for every combination of specific values of the X variables. E(Y) can also be written as E(Y|X) to reflect the fact that the value of E(Y) is dependent on the values of X. When the outcome of an epidemiologic model is risk of a binary event, such as disease or cause of death, E(Y) can be replaced by R(x), or average risk. Analogous regression models can also be defined for modeling incidence rates.

The β coefficients of the X values are the regression parameters that specify the particular exposure–response curves that define the relationships. Each β can be interpreted as a slope, i.e., the change in Y, or change in risk or rate, associated with a unit change in a particular X variable. The β coefficient of the exposure of interest, is the primary exposure–response parameter. Because confounders are also present in the model, the estimate of the exposure effect has been adjusted for confounding.

Model specification concerns the generic shape of the curve defined by the form of the regression model. The most common forms of epidemiologic risk models are linear and exponential. The exponential risk model is linear on the logarithmic scale, and can be written either by taking an exponential function of the right-hand side of the model as follows:

$$R(x) = \exp(\beta_0 + \beta_1 X_1 + \beta_2 X_2 + ... + \beta_k X_k)$$

or equivalently as:

$$\text{Log }(R(x)) = \beta_0 + \beta_1 X_1 + \beta_2 X_2 + ... + \beta_k X_k$$

Once the form of the model has been selected, the model is 'fit' to the data and the parameters are estimated. Model fitting includes decisions about which variables need to be included in the model, as well as the calculation of the parameter estimates and their confidence intervals. The statistical method used to estimate regression parameters is called maximum likelihood. This method is based on the concept that the best estimates of the β parameters are those values that make the observed data most likely to have occurred under the structural constraints of the model.

Fitting models requires judgments about what variables to include. These judgments will affect the findings of a study because parameter estimates can change when other variables are added to or removed from the model. In fact, the presence of confounding is generally evaluated by comparing the β coefficient for exposure between models with and without the potential confounder included. A change in the magnitude of the exposure–response parameter estimate in the presence of an extraneous variable is evidence that confounding exists and needs to be controlled.

INTERPRETING EPIDEMIOLOGIC DATA

In one form or another, two related questions emerge from a review of epidemiologic findings. (1) Is the agent(s) hazardous? (2) If so, is there a safe level of exposure below which impaired health is unlikely to occur? These questions, or variations thereof, will inevitably be asked by workers, employers, epidemiologists, clinicians, exposure assessment professionals, policy makers, lawyers, and the general public. Answers to these questions cannot usually be obtained from the results of a single study, as most studies can only add evidence to a body of information. Although there are some dramatic examples where causality is unambiguous, most studies fall far short of providing definitive data on disease risk or safe exposure levels. Therefore, the reviewer's task in making sense of data is to evaluate the results from a single study, and to place them in context with findings from other epidemiologic, and at times, toxicologic studies of the same or related issues.

Some general guidelines for interpreting data and assessing causality can be stated, although these are by no means formal rules nor are they offered as a comprehensive list. Standard criteria for assessing causal associations in epidemiology include some necessary as well as some merely desirable conditions that, when met, improve confidence in interpreting data. One necessary condition is that exposure precedes disease. Desirable, although not always demonstrable, conditions are the strength and specificity of the association, evidence for a dose–response relation, biologic plausibility, absence of bias, internal consistency of the study findings, and consistency of results with prior epidemiologic and toxicologic research. Statistical significance (P-values) can aid interpretation, as discussed earlier. However, statistical significance can be a misleading concept in non-experimental research, and some have argued that there is no place for 'P-value testing' in epidemiology. Too often, there has been a failure to appreciate that the nominal level of 'significance' (customarily, $P<0.05$) is an arbitrary numerical boundary. Most epidemiologic studies generate large data sets, and hence large numbers of statistical evaluations. Cohort studies may typically involve assessments of risks for some 30 to 60 diseases. Likewise, case-control studies often include examinations of the effects of numerous exposures.

The number of statistical evaluations will also increase with data stratification, such that a given study may engender literally hundreds of comparisons. In such instances, the chance of detecting statistically significant results will increase with the number of statistical associations evaluated. Corrections of P-values for multiple tests have been proposed by some authors, although it is never clear just how many hypotheses are actually tested in a given study, or whether all tests of hypotheses should be treated equivalently. For example, in a study of risks related to asbestos, statistical testing (by P-value estimation or calculation of confidence intervals) may be conducted for established associations, such as with lung cancer, as well as for relations that have less support, such as for athero-sclerotic vascular disease. The prior expectations for these two outcomes would be clearly different: a much smaller P-value for the lung cancer relative risk would be anticipated.

For these reasons, corrections for multiple testing have gone out of favor in observational epidemiology research. In general, statistical significance testing alone provides little guidance in discriminating between true and spurious associations. Similar cautions can be invoked for interpreting confidence intervals. Like the nominal level of statistical significance, the choice of confidence interval width (90%, 95%, etc.) as a benchmark is arbitrary. Correcting confidence interval widths for multiple effect estimation would suffer the same ambiguities as correcting P-values for multiple testing. Thus, decision making regarding causation should emphasize other considerations, especially consistency with prior epidemiologic and experimental research, biologic coherence, and clinical interpretability.

Detecting the effects, presumably beneficial, of interventions, such as a reduction of exposure levels on disease and injury risks, can seldom be done in any one epidemiologic study, unless the study spans a very long time period. In contrast, the effects of interventions imposed to reduce the incidence or severity of acute health effects are usually more readily demonstrable. However, even when an apparent reduction in risk has been observed, alternative explanations, such as susceptible individuals leaving the workforce, should be considered before accepting the results at face value.

An example where there would be little doubt concerning a causal association is the cohort study of bone sarcoma among female radium dial painters[17] summarized in Table 6.19. The rarity of the disease, the biologic plausibility of the association between a radioactive bone-seeking compound and bone malignancy, and obvious antecedent/consequent relation between the practice of ingesting radium and the occurrence of bone sarcoma, the strong dose–response trend, and the small chance that bias, especially confounding, distorted the findings, all argue in favor of causation.

Most epidemiologic studies, however, do not reach such clear-cut conclusions as the radium dial painters study. The following examples illustrate some of the complexities that arise when interpreting epidemiologic findings. Consider the data on leukemia and multiple myeloma in Table 6.20 derived from a historical cohort mortality study

Dose (μCi)	Cases	Person-yrs	Rate per 1000 person-yrs
0–99	0	29,936	0
100–249	2	1164	1.72
250–499	9	1249	7.21
500–999	8	610	13.1
1000–2499	15	419	36.8
≥2500	4	219	18.3

Table 6.19 Incidence of bone sarcoma among female radium dial painters according to radium (^{226}Ra + ^{228}Ra) dose

	Test participants		Other military personnel	
Cause of death	Obs	RR*	Obs	RR*
Leukemia	29	1.00	17	0.56
Multiple myeloma	8	0.72	6	0.51

* Relative risk compared with rates of UK men.

Table 6.20 Leukemia and multiple myeloma mortality among UK atomic weapons testing and other military personnel

of cancer among UK military personnel exposed to atomic weapons testing.[18] Two cohorts were identified: the exposed group consisted of approximately 22,000 males who had participated in testing activities, and a comparison group including an equal number of military personnel in service at the same times as the exposed cohort, but not assigned to atomic weapons test areas. The two groups were matched according to gender, age, branch of armed service, and military rank. Mortality in both groups was compared against prevailing rates for UK males.

Two conflicting interpretations can be drawn from these data. Based strictly on comparisons with mortality rates for UK males, it would appear that there were no excesses of leukemia and multiple myeloma in the exposed group. However, direct comparisons between the two groups would support a conclusion of increased risks for both diseases (nearly two-fold for leukemia) in the exposed military personnel. The interpretation of the data depends principally on what is regarded as the more suitable reference population, the UK general population or the non-exposed military personnel. Insofar as the latter were probably more similar to the exposed group in regard to socioeconomic factors, access to medical care, and hence diagnostic certainty, comparisons with the non-exposed cohort should be more valid than general population comparisons. As such, the data are consistent with associations between leukemia and multiple myeloma and exposure to atmospheric nuclear tests, although other explanations, including chance and an unexplained deficit of hematologic malignancies in the non-exposed military personnel, could still be considered.

Reducing bias from confounding is necessary to ensure valid findings. Accordingly, epidemiologists pay substantial attention to minimizing confounding. Studies that do not take into account potential confounding factors in the design or analysis may be viewed with some degree of skepticism, although it is important to realize that very strong associations (e.g., relative risks of 2 and greater) that are based on reasonably stable statistical estimates are very unlikely to be spurious. This point should be evident by referring to Table 6.18, which shows that even a very potent extraneous risk factor (smoking in the case of lung cancer) would have to be highly related to the exposure under study in order to create a severe confounding bias. On the other hand, control of confounding becomes a substantially more important issue when there are relatively weak associations (relative risks of 1.5 and less) or the observed effects, irrespective of magnitude, are based on small numbers.

Factors that may be confounders should also be considered as possible modifiers of the hazards of occupational and environmental exposures. Thus, there may be synergistic (or in some cases, antagonistic) effects between various occupational or environmental exposures and host factors, including confounders, on disease risk. An illustration is provided from a case-control study of lung cancer and sugar cane farming in India.[19] As shown in Table 6.21, the trend of lung cancer risk with cigarette smoking was considerably stronger among persons with a history of

Pack-years of cigarette smoking	Never farmed sugar cane OR	Farmed sugar cane OR
0	1.00*	1.10
1–225	1.45	2.70
225	1.41	5.89

* Reference category.

Table 6.21 Case-control study of lung cancer and sugar cane farming

Control group	Males OR	Females OR
Stomach cancer	0.7	3.2
Myocardial infarction	0.6	3.7

Table 6.22 Case-control study of liver cancer and solvent exposures

sugar cane farming, and there was a nearly six-fold elevated risk in persons who farmed sugar cane and had the largest pack-years of smoking compared with non-farmers who never smoked. However, interactions among workplace exposures on disease and injury risks can be difficult to detect in many instances, particularly when exposures are strongly intercorrelated.

Consistency of an association can be an elusive concept in epidemiologic studies. Consistency can be considered as internal to a particular study, or in reference to external information, such as data from prior research. Internal consistency would be indicated when exposure is equally potent, or at least qualitatively similar in effect, for various members of the study population (e.g., for males and females). Of course, departure from homogeneity of effect may be related to dose–effect relations, in which case an argument for causation is strengthened. Alternatively, differences in effect that are not dose-dependent may have some other plausible explanation, such as the requirement for a potentiating factor (e.g., alcohol consumption and hepatoxicity).

However, there are no ready explanations for heterogeneity of effect in many instances. As an illustration, consider the data in Table 6.22 from a community-based case-control study of primary liver cancer. The data are both internally consistent and inconsistent; the results do not vary depending on the control group considered, stomach cancer or myocardial infarction cases, yet the effects for males and females are in opposite directions. There are numerous possible speculative explanations for the data, many of which were considered by the investigators. These include unmeasured confounding (e.g., hepatitis B or C infection), differential exposure misclassification, or true gender differences in susceptibility. The possibility of different types of solvent exposures among men and women, namely a higher prevalence of chlorinated solvent exposures (e.g., perchloroethylene) among women than men, is also a candidate explanation. This illustrates the importance of seeking exposure information for specific substances. Regrettably, limited exposure data in many epidemiologic studies only permit insights into patterns of associations with broad categories or agents, rather than with specific substances.

Consistency of findings across studies is also an important criterion for assessing causation. In deciding whether or not an association exists between an occupational exposure and a particular health outcome, one ultimately synthesizes information form the available literature. This can be a informal process, in which the reviewer determines which evidence is most suitable for the question at hand. A more formal approach, known as 'meta-analysis,' involves weighting the data from multiple studies to derive a single best estimate of the strength of association. Approaches for 'meta-analysis' have been developed for this purpose.[20]

Epidemiologic data generally refer to groups, but can also contribute significantly to clinical determinations of risks and causal attribution for individuals, provided that the strengths and limitations of the research that generates the data are appreciated. Mutually reinforcing substantive and technical advances in epidemiology and clinical medicine should continue to facilitate the integration and interaction between both disciplines.

References

1. Christiani DC, Ye T-T, Wegman DH et al. Cotton dust exposure across-shift drop in FEV1, and five-year change in lung function. Am J Respir Crit Care Med 1994; 150:1250–5.
2. Evanoff BA, Gustavsson P, Hogstedt C. Mortality and incidence of cancer in a cohort of Swedish chimney sweeps: an extended follow-up study. Br J Ind Med 1993; 50:450–9.
3. Ott MG, Zober A. Cause-specific mortality and cancer incidence among employees exposed to 2,3,7,8-TCDD after a 1953 reactor accident. Occup Environ Med 1996; 53:606–12.
4. Chan CK, Leung CC, Tam CM, Yu TS, Wong TW. Lung cancer mortality among a cohort of men in a silicotic register. J Occup Environ Med 2000; 42:69–75.
5. Checkoway H, Hughes JM, Weill H, Seixas NS, Demers PA. Crystalline silica exposure, radiological silicosis, and lung cancer mortality in diatomaceous earth industry workers. Thorax 1999; 54:56–9.
6. Hayes RB, Yin S-N, Dosemeci M et al. Benzene and the dose-related incidence of hematologic neoplasms in China. J Natl Cancer Inst 1997; 89:1065–71.
7. Swan SH, Beaumont JJ, Hammond SK et al. Historical cohort study of spontaneous abortion among fabrication workers in the Semiconductor Health Study: agent-level analysis. Am J Ind Med 1995; 28:751–68.
8. Stayner L, Smith AB, Reeve G et al. Proportionate mortality study of workers in the garment industry exposed to formaldehyde. Am J Ind Med 1985; 7:229–40.
9. Barreto SM, Swerdlow AJ, Smith PG, Higgins CD. A nested case-control study of fatal work related injuries among Brazilian steel workers. Occup Environ Med 1997; 54:599–604.
10. Seidler A, Hellenbrand W, Robra B-P et al. Possible environmental, occupational, and other etiologic factors for Parkinson's disease: a case-control study in Germany. Neurology 1996; 46:1275–84.
11. Alexander BH, Checkoway H, van Netten C et al. Semen quality of men employed at a lead smelter. Occup Environ Med 1996; 53:411–6.
12. Flodin U, Ekberg K, Andersson L. Neuropsychiatric effects of low exposure to styrene. Br J Ind Med 1989; 46:805–8.
13. Savitz DA, Loomis DP. Magnetic field exposure in relation to leukemia and brain cancer mortality among electric utility workers. Am J Epidemiol 1995; 141:123–34.

14. Bruske-Hohfeld I, Mohner M, Pohlabeln H et al. Occupational lung cancer risk for men in Germany: results from a pooled case-control study. Am J Epidemiol 2000; 151:384–95.
15. Axelson O. Aspects on confounding in occupational health epidemiology. Scand J Work Environ Hlth 1978; 4:85–9.
16. Rothman KJ, Greenland S. Modern epidemiology, 2nd edn. Philadelphia: Lippincott-Raven, 1998.
17. Rowland HE, Stehney AF, Lucas HF. Dose–response relationships for female radium dial workers. Radiat Res 1978; 76:368–83.
18. Darby SC, Kendall GM, Fell TP et al. Further follow-up of mortality and incidence of cancer in men from the United Kingdom who participated in the United Kingdom's atmospheric nuclear weapon tests and experimental programmes. Br Med J 1993; 307:153–5.
19. Amre DK, Infante-Rivard C, Dufresne A, Durgawale PM, Ernst P. Case-control study of lung cancer among sugar cane farmers in India. Occup Environ Med 1999; 56:548–52.
20. Greenland S. Meta-analysis. In: Rothman KJ, Greenland S, eds. Modern epidemiology, 2nd edn. Philadelphia: Lippincott-Raven, 1998;643–73.

Further reading

Checkoway H, Pearce N, Kriebel D. Research methods in occupational epidemiology. New York: Oxford University Press, 1989.
Hernberg S. Introduction to occupational epidemiology. Chelsea: Lewis Publishers, 1992.
Monson RR. Occupational epidemiology, 2nd edn. Boca Raton: CRC Press, 1990.

Chapter 7

Biologic Markers in Occupational and Environmental Medicine

Carmen J Marsit, Anthony D LaMontagne, Karl T Kelsey

INTRODUCTION

A biologic marker, or biomarker, is any substance, structure, or process that can be measured in the human body or human body products, and that may influence or predict disease.[1] Traditionally, in occupational medicine, biomarkers of exposure – or internal dose – have been used most frequently (e.g., lead in blood, cadmium in urine). Personal exposure to over 100 different chemicals in the workplace can be assessed in biologic media.[2] In addition to exposure or dose, biomarkers can also be used to assess biologic effects or to identify susceptibilities to the effects of specific exposures. Markers of susceptibility are the newest and most rapidly expanding class of biomarkers in occupational medicine, and in contrast to most biomarkers of exposure and effect, these are typically inherited or acquired genetic properties of a given individual.[3]

In occupational and environmental medical practice, biomarkers of exposure and effect related to hazardous substance exposures are most widely used, though biomarkers of dietary intake, tobacco smoke exposure, biologic agents, and a wide range of other agents are also important. Biomarkers of susceptibility, though the most active area of biomarker research currently, are rarely used in medical practice due to low or unknown predictive value of actual disease risk under common exposure conditions, as well as social and ethical problems raised by their use.[4]

This chapter will focus on biomarkers relevant to hazardous exposures and consequent risks and their use in occupational and environmental medicine. Interested readers are referred to other monographs on the rapidly evolving application of biomarkers in cancer and other chronic disease epidemiology contexts.[1,5] However they are used, it is critical to understand the methodology behind the sample collection and the methods involved in generation of the values reported as well as the methods used for determination of the reference values.

Environmental vs biologic monitoring

Used in conjunction with environmental monitoring, biologic monitoring can help to more accurately determine individual levels of exposure. Environmental monitoring measures the ambient exposure of a chemical through sampling of the air or surfaces at the workplace. This ambient monitoring has been used for many years and therefore accurate methods of sampling and detection exist for numerous exposures (see Chapter 4.1). Environmental monitoring can be useful to detect acute exposures to dangerous chemicals, to identify emission sources, to evaluate engineering control measures, to prevent overexposure, and to provide a more accurate monitoring of chemicals that demonstrate their effect at the site of contact such as skin, eye, or respiratory tract irritants. Exposure limits used in environmental monitoring have been established for approximately 700 potentially hazardous chemicals.

Interestingly, biologic levels of exposure predicted by modeling from environmental exposure levels often vary greatly from actual biomarker values reported upon testing markers. Such variability can be accounted for by the biologic and work practice variations between individuals. Table 7.1 summarizes the principal sources of this variability. All of these factors can greatly affect the biologic levels of a given chemical in individuals working in an environment with a single environmental exposure level.

Also important to keep in mind is the fact that use of biomarkers will include measurements that reflect all sources of exposure, including occupational as well as background exposure from dietary habits, residence, and other lifestyle factors.

Due to the limitations as well as the strengths of both environmental and biologic monitoring, it is important that these two approaches be considered complementary and both important parts of a total occupational health program.

Biologic monitoring program

Biologic monitoring poses many challenges as well as advantages. The media being tested – blood, urine, or exhaled air – are complex mixtures that require powerful analytical tools to separate and quantitate the various biomarkers in question. Timing of sampling is also critical, as some chemicals may be quickly metabolized or excreted from the body, while others may be present for longer periods. Selection of the appropriate biomarker is also a key issue, as it must be specific to the chemical exposure and serve as an accurate measure of the exposure.

Point of variability	Potential mechanism
Route of exposure	Differences in uptake between respiratory and skin routes and differences in exposure routes between individuals
Respiration rate	Increased respiratory rate can significantly affect absorption
Metabolic and excretion rate	Normal variation in hepatic and renal function can account for individual variation
Genetic	Polymorphisms in metabolic enzymes may change their level of function
Adipose tissue level	Increased adipose tissue levels may allow greater accumulation of lipid-soluble compounds

Table 7.1 Sources of biologic variability in biomarker assessment

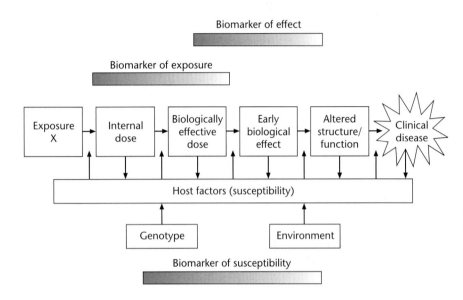

Figure 7.1: Various interactions involved as an exposure progresses to clinical manifestation of disease. Adapted from Van Damme K, Casteleyn L, Heseltine E et al. Individual susceptibility and prevention of occupational disease: scientific and ethical issues. J Occup Environ Med 1995;37:91–9.

Biomarkers

Selection of an appropriate biomarker depends on many variables, including those referred to in Table 7.1. In assessing the biologic level of a chemical in the human body, there needs to be a thorough understanding of the route and level of absorption of the chemical, of the chemical properties of the substance, which can account for differences in the absorption and distribution (i.e. a lipophilic chemical is more likely to deposit in high lipid regions of the body such as fat or nerve tissue, while hydrophilic chemicals remain in the blood stream and visceral organs), as well as of the metabolism of the chemical and its excretion. Figure 7.1 schematically represents the various interactions involved as an exposure progresses to clinical manifestation of disease. Biomarkers have been classified into biomarkers of exposure, of effect, and of susceptibility, but, due to the complex interactions and biology of the progression from exposure to disease, the lines are somewhat blurred. A thorough knowledge of the agent in question can help to determine which type of biomarker, or combination of biomarkers, is most appropriate for the environment in question.

Biomarkers of exposure

A biomarker of exposure measures the exposure to a chemical independent of route of exposure. Table 7.2 discusses the important characteristics that define a useful biomarker of exposure. This type of biomarker can be further subdi-

vided into a biomarker of internal dose or a biomarker of effective dose.

The biomarker of internal dose reflects the amount of the chemical in question or its metabolite present in the biologic sample. These levels can be measured directly through analytical methods from urine, blood, exhaled air, feces, hair, nails, saliva, or breast milk. An example would be a measurement of S-phenylmercapuric acid or t,t-muconic acid levels in urine to assess benzene exposure.[6] New developments now allow for assessment of organ or body exposure in vivo directly at the site of accumulation for selected agents. These methods utilize imaging techniques such as neutron activation that can identify cadmium burden of the kidney and x-ray fluorescence, which can evaluate lead content in bones. The biomarker of effective dose is used to directly estimate the exposure to the chemical in question through its interaction with the target site.[7] Such a biomarker is the measurement of carboxyhemoglobin used to assess carbon monoxide exposure.

For the practicing occupational health and safety person on the shop floor (e.g., industrial hygienist or safety officer), air monitoring would be preferred if the goal is representative exposure assessment and exposure control with limited expense (preventative, group-level perspective). On the other hand, for the occupational medicine provider (e.g., occupational health nurse or physician), the ability to establish exposure or biologic effects for an individual, even in the absence of environmental monitoring data, is invaluable. To date relatively few

Characteristic	Notes
Correlation with exposure	Limits of quantitation and correlation must exist at exposure levels in industrial setting[22]
Correlation with target tissue dose	Sampled media must reflect target tissue exposure, as target tissue itself often cannot be sampled[22–25]
Appearance is reversible	Helps to distinguish industrial exposure from background exposures. Also demonstrates effectiveness of exposure control methods.[22,23,26,31]
Influence of confounding and modifying factors is well characterized	Thorough knowledge of the physical, chemical, and metabolic properties of the chemicals and host factors response is needed for an accurate analysis[25]
Suitable for application in the workplace	Sampling methods should be minimally invasive, pose minimal risk, and be as convenient to workers as possible[28–29]

Table 7.2 Characteristics of useful biomarkers of exposure[12]

biomarkers of exposure, such as blood lead levels or urinary excretion of certain metals, are routinely used in clinical practice.

Biomarkers of effect

These biomarkers measure reversible biochemical changes that occur after receipt of an internal dose. Although these are effects of exposure, they are less than the degree of change associated with injury or irreversible pathological effect and should not be considered health effects per se. In other words, these markers may predict adverse effects, yet they must be distinguished from tests that monitor true pathological effects. Some examples include the inhibition of specific enzymes by various chemicals (e.g., δ-aminolavulinic acid dehydratase which is inhibited by lead), or the production of antibodies to low molecular weight molecules. The measurement of protein or DNA adduct burden which can be correlated to aromatic amine or polycyclic aromatic hydrocarbon (PAH) levels in the blood and can reflect intensity of exposure as well as effective dose. Studies continue to provide new markers, such as presence of various proteins and enzymes in urine due to nephrotoxic chemicals, but the debate continues as to whether or not such markers should be considered adverse effects or rather markers of developing health consequences (thus questioning their role in workplace monitoring).

Biomarkers of susceptibility

Biomarkers of susceptibility provide an indication of an inherent or acquired ability of an organism to respond to the challenge of exposure to a specific xenobiotic substance.[8] In other words, these biomarkers demonstrate the possible differences between individuals in metabolism, DNA repair mechanisms, immune responsiveness, or alterations of oncogenes' and tumor suppressor genes' activities, thereby providing an idea of how an individual will respond when confronted with an exposure. Such bio-markers may be able to identify 'susceptible' individuals who, through impaired or altered enzymatic functioning, may react adversely at low exposures to effective doses.[9]

Biomarkers that reflect differences in metabolism can be measured by administration of a test drug and observation of its clearance from the body. Alternatively, the genotype of an individual can be determined using DNA collected from circulating lymphocytes in a blood sample. Using modern molecular biologic techniques, including the polymerase chain reaction (PCR), the polymorphisms, or genetic differences, of an individual, can be determined for various enzymes known to metabolize specific chemicals. Theoretically that individual's genotype could then be compared to a database of known polymorphisms to determine to what extent he or she can metabolize certain chemicals, thereby potentially determining how susceptible the individual is to an exposure and to what level he or she can be safely exposed.

Ideally, this type of biomarker could be used preventatively to assess possible risk. However, in reality most diseases are the result of multigenetic processes and thus risk of disease is likely related to complex interaction between exposure and multiple genetic markers. The genes encoding enzymes of the cytochrome P450 family, the glutathione S-transferases, and the N-acetyltransferases are some of the most widely studied and best documented polymorphic biomarkers, as these enzymes are involved in the early metabolic stages of various chemicals. They have also been shown to have polymorphisms, which lead to decreased activity and thus altered susceptibility to pathological disease.

Perhaps the most illustrative example of biomarkers of susceptibility involves the use of genetic testing for susceptibility to beryllium exposure. Particular HLA types may be important for an individual to mount an immunologic response to beryllium exposure.[10,11] Workers who have a particular HLA subtype have been shown to be more susceptible to the adverse effects of beryllium exposure. However, the allele specific risks and positive and negative predictive values of these tests remain unclear. Thus genetic testing currently is not recommended as part of a preplacement exam for workers exposed to beryllium. Genetic testing does not substitute for the mandate that exposures should be minimized such that all workers be protected from exposure-related harm.

INSTITUTING A BIOLOGIC MONITORING PROGRAM

Several key issues need to be addressed when instituting a biologic monitoring program, as such a program needs

1. Determinate must be present in an available biologic medium and should be suitable for sampling
2. The sampling method must be convenient and acceptable to the population being tested
3. The sampling method must produce representative and useful samples for analysis
4. A method of analysis of the biomarker must exist that is practical, accurate, and reproducible
5. A plan of action should be established for responding to aberrant results

Table 7.3 Criteria for choosing and implementing a biomarker

to produce meaningful results that can impact the safety of the working environment but be implemented in a convenient and cost-effective manner.[12] Table 7.3 lists conditions to be considered in choosing a biomarker and instituting its use in biologic monitoring. Considering these conditions can lead to the appropriate sampling and analysis conditions.

Sampling

In order to obtain accurate monitoring of exposures, the timing and appropriateness of sampling must be considered for each type of exposure. Chemicals that are rapidly cleared from the body may require more immediate sampling such as sampling during or at the end of a working shift, while those with longer residence times can be sampled more randomly.

The collection method may also play a key role in the accurate analysis of a biomarker. It is advisable to consult with the lab performing the analysis to determine appropriate sampling and storage conditions of samples. Inappropriate sampling containers may contaminate the sample or adsorb the sample, and improper storage can lead to deterioration of the analyte. Also, the appropriate preservatives (in urine or blood sampling) or anticoagulants (blood sampling) need to be added as directed by the analyzing lab.[13]

In some cases, specifically for chemicals that can accumulate in the body or for which there is substantial interindividual variability, baseline testing may need to be performed. Examples of such exposures include cadmium, polychlorinated biphenyls (PCBs), and lead, which show bioaccumulation and pseudocholinesterase in plasma, which is highly variable between individuals.[13]

Most commonly, blood, urine, and exhaled air are used as the media for analysis. Hair and fingernails have also been used, but their utility is somewhat limited, while the use of adipose tissue has proven difficult for sample collection outside a clinical setting.

Blood

Blood serves as the transportation route for chemicals and their metabolites throughout the body, and therefore is often the most accurate medium for biomarker sampling. On the other hand, volatile compounds and substances with short half-times should not be determined with blood sampling. One advantage of blood monitoring is that the composition of blood varies little between individuals and thus correction for individual differences is not usually necessary. Also, obtaining specimens is relatively straightforward and can be accomplished with little risk of contamination, but must only be done by trained individuals, as it is an invasive procedure. The dynamic equilibrium of the analyte within various parts of the body must also be considered, as the concentration of the chemical can vary depending on route of exposure, metabolism timing and efficiency, and excretion.[14]

Urine

Urine sampling can be the easiest method of body fluid sampling, and can be used for detection of various hydrophilic chemicals, metals, and metabolites. A 24-hour urine collection provides the most accurate assessment, as this will eliminate error based on urine output and concentration. If 24-hour screens are impractical and spot checks are to be used, corrections must be made dependent on the concentration, which can be done by adjusting levels to a standardized specific gravity or urine creatinine level. Urine levels of chemicals that are targeted to the kidney (such as cadmium) may not reflect an accurate level of exposure, and urine sampling would be inappropriate for workers with advanced renal disease.[15]

Exhaled air

Exhaled air monitoring has limited use for determining levels of volatile chemicals. The sampling involves breathing into a plastic bag, which is then exhausted through a charcoal filter onto which the analyte is adsorbed and can then be analyzed. This approach is not useful for aerosols, or for gases or vapors that decompose upon contact with body tissues or that are highly water soluble (such as alcohols). Workers with emphysema should not be monitored with exhaled air sampling.[16]

Analysis

The analysis of the biomarker in the sample media needs to be performed by a qualified laboratory. Table 7.4 lists some criteria to be considered when choosing the laboratory for analysis. National and international certification and quality assurance programs continue to be sponsored by the United States government as well as the World Health Organization. In 1992, the Clinical Laboratory Improvement Amendments (CLIA) guidelines were introduced and apply to biologic monitoring data. These guidelines include strict management of sampling, transportation, handling, storage, and evaluation of specimens including accurate analytical quality assurance and method verification.

The laboratory should provide all information on the sample collection method, containers, and sources of contamination. They may also be able to offer 'background' and 'normal' levels which they have gathered from unexposed populations, although it is important to the laboratory's definition of 'normal' (i.e. is it a normal level for workers or for non-occupational exposures?). Some laboratories may provide sample collection equipment and service and may deliver and pick up samples. These types of considerations may affect the convenience and cost of instituting a biologic monitoring program.

Interpretation

The analytical result obtained from the biologic monitoring program indicated the level of a biomarker in the given biologic media at the time of sampling. Again, thorough understanding of the biologic response of the human body to the agent is necessary to extrapolate these data to understand exposure. Further, the sensitivity and

Analytical accuracy	Must be assessed through intra- and inter-laboratory QA
Convenience	Processing methods should rely on convenient sampling and sample preparations on site
Turnaround time	Timely indications of possible exposures so that corrective actions can be quickly undertaken
Cost	Cannot be prohibitive

Table 7.4 Characteristics of analysis lab

specificity of the biomarker should be well established. Moreover, use of the biomarker assumes that there is a quantitative relationship between biomarker level and exposure, or at least that presence of a biomarker above its background level indicates an exposure.[17]

In order for judgments to be made about the exposure levels indicated through biologic monitoring, a series of reference values must be utilized. These values can help an environmental health clinician in consultation with industrial hygienists to determine whether or not action needs to be taken because of biologic exposure levels being reported in the workplace population. Various values have been reported due to a variety of methods used to derive these values. Table 7.5 discusses the various biologic exposure indices as well as their derivation and possible usage. A thorough understanding of these values and their derivations is necessary for their correct interpretation. Generally, the Biologischer Arbeitsstoff-Toleranz-Wert (BAT) and exposure equivalents for carcinogenic materials (EKA) values are based on health consequences and are generally used by physicians while the biologic exposure indices (BEI) as well as the biomonitoring action level (BAL) are based on external exposure and are considered tools of industrial hygiene.[18] Therefore, if a worker's biologic exposure persistently exceeds the BEI value, this may not indicate potential health consequences, but if exposure results from a group of workers consistently exceed the BEI, further investigation and possible corrective action may be needed.[19]

Values index	Organization	Derivation	Usage
Biologic exposure indices (BEI)	American Conference of Governmental Hygienists (ACGIH)	Internal dose arising from inhalation exposure at the TLV concentration* [30]	Represents the highest acceptable internal dose that will not typically result in future health consequences
Biologischer Arbeitsstoff-Toleranz-Wert (BAT)	German independent scientists of various disciplines	Maximal permissible quantity of a chemical compound, its metabolites, or any deviation from the norm of biological parameters induced by these substances based on exposed human beings[27]	Provides an absolute ceiling value for healthy individuals not to be exceeded[†]
Exposure equivalents for carcinogenic materials (EKA)	German independent scientists of various disciplines	Internal dose arising from inhalation exposure alone for carcinogenic materials without BAT value[6]	Relates external exposure to internal dose, but does not imply any safe limit
Biomonitoring action level (BAL)	Finnish Institute of Occupational Health (FIOH)	Some based on health outcomes. Others extrapolated from external exposure limits or based on good working habits[31]	Provide levels that even if at or below for an entire lifetime, no negative health consequences would be expected
Human biologic monitoring (HBM) values	Commission on Human Biological Monitoring (Germany)	Based on human toxicologic and epidemiologic evidence[20]	HBM I – level at or below which there is no adverse effect. HBM II – level at or above for which there is increased risk for adverse health effects in susceptible individuals[‡]

* A small number of these values do not reflect this derivation and are derived based on levels which result in prevention of systemic health risk.
† No BAT value is given for carcinogenic substances as no value can be considered harmless.
‡ Reference values also exist which demonstrate the upper margin of the current background exposure level in a given population and can identify subjects at risk.

Table 7.5 Monitoring reference values for exposure biomarkers

Also important for consideration in interpretation of biologic monitoring data is the significance of background levels of exposure and the ability to distinguish this exposure from that associated with occupational exposure. Individuals can be exposed to a variety of chemicals depending on their residence, air quality in the home or work community, dietary habits, hobbies, and most importantly smoking habits, these exposures can affect the biologic levels observed in the tested population. Finally, it is important to note that the reference values, including the BEI and BAT, are for occupational exposure based on an average workday of exposure, and therefore do not apply to residential or other non-occupational sources of exposure.[6] On the other hand, the HBM reference values can be utilized as warnings for increased exposure and for the potential of negative health consequences in susceptible populations who may require medical action to abrogate the exposure. These values vary depending on the age group and sex of the population being tested and are meant to reflect the exposure outside of occupational exposure and therefore can be applied to background and environmental exposure situations.[20]

SOCIAL AND ETHICAL ISSUES

Biomarker use must be carefully considered, specifically incorporating safeguards essential for insuring that they are used ethically and in a socially responsible manner. The most obvious potential problem is presented by the use of genetic markers. The US Office of Technology Assessment determined in the 1980s that there was relatively sparse use of genetic testing in the workplace.[4] This seems wise, given the still investigative nature of most markers. Where genetic testing is used, there are also important questions that are related to the Americans with Disabilities Act of 1990. This legislative act highlights the primacy of exposure control in the workplace. Regardless of technical advances in terms of predictive value, social advances will be required in areas such as privacy protection, rate retention for workers with identified susceptibilities (analogous to OSHA's medical removal protections for high blood lead levels), and accommodations made for identified susceptibilities in order to facilitate the use of susceptibility markers in the future.[4] The strategy for reducing occupational disease should continue to be through modification of the workplace and not modification of the workforce.[21]

References

1. Toniolo P, Bofetta P, Shuker DEG, Rothman N, Hulka B, Pearce N, eds. Application of biomarkers in cancer epidemiology. IARC Scientific Publications No. 142. Lyon, France: IARC, 1997.
2. Rosenberg J, Harrison RJ. Biologic monitoring. In: LaDou J, ed. Occupational and environmental medicine. Stamford: Appleton and Lange, 1997.
3. Berlin A, Yodaiken RR, Henman BA. Assessment of toxic agents at the workplace. Roles of ambient and biologic monitoring. Boston, The Hague: Nijhoft, 1984.
4. Gochfeld M. Susceptibility biomarkers in the workplace: historical perspective. In: Mendelsohn ML, Mohr LC, Peeters JP, eds. Biomarkers: medical and workplace applications. Washington DC: Joseph Henry Press, 1998;3–22.
5. Schulte PA, Perera FP, eds. Molecular epidemiology: principles and practices. San Diego: Academic Press, 1993.
6. Morgan MS, Schaller K-H. An analysis of criteria for biologic limit values developed in Germany and the United States. Int Arch Occup Environ Health 1999; 72:195–204.
7. Hoet P, Haufroid V. Biologic monitoring: state of the art. Occup Environ Med 1997; 54:361–6.
8. World Health Organization. Biomarkers and risk assessment: concepts and principles. International programme on chemical safety. Geneva: WHO, 1993.
9. Mutti A. Biologic monitoring in occupational and environmental toxicology. Toxicol Lett 1999; 108:77–89.
10. Richeldi L, Sorrentino R, Saltini C. HLA-DPB1 Glutamate 69: a genetic marker of beryllium disease. Science 1993; 262:242–4.
11. Richeldi L, Kreiss K, Mroz MM, Shen B, Tartone P, Saltini C. Interaction of genetic and exposure factors in the prevalence of berylliosis. Am J Ind Med 1997; 34:337–40.
12. Morgan M. The biologic exposure indices: a key component in protecting workers from toxic chemicals. Environ Health Perspect 1995; 105 (suppl 1):105–15.
13. Lauwerys RR, Hoet P. Industrial chemical exposure. Guidelines for biologic monitoring. Ann Arbor: Lewis Publishers, 1993.
14. Lowry LK, Rosenberg J, Fiserova-Bergerova TV. Biologic monitoring III: measurements in blood. Appl Indust Hyg 1989; 4(3):F-11.
15. Rosenberg J, Fiserova-Bergerova TV, Lowry LK. Biologic monitoring IV: measurements in urine. Appl Indust Hyg 1989; 4(4):F-16.
16. Fiserova-Bergerova TV, Lowry LK, Rosenberg J. Biologic monitoring II: measurements in exhaled air. Appl Indust Hyg 1989; 4(2):F-10.
17. Teass AW, Biagini RE, DeBord DG, Hull RD. Application of biologic monitoring methods. NIOSH/DBBS NIOSH/DSHEFS
18. Bolt HM, Rutenfranz J. The impact of time and duration of exposure on toxicokinetics and toxicodynamics of workplace chemicals. In: Notten WRF et al, eds. Health surveillance of individual workers exposed to chemicals. Berlin, Heidelberg, New York: Springer, 1986;91–5.
19. Rosenberg J, Rempel D. Biologic monitoring. Occup Med State-of-the-Art Rev 1990; 5:491–8.
20. Ewers U, Krause C, Schulz C, Wilhelm M. Reference values and human biologic monitoring values for environmental toxins. Int Arch Occup Environ Health 1999; 72:255–60.
21. Rawbone RG. Future impact of genetic screening in occupational and environmental medicine. Occup Environ Med 1999;56:721–4.
22. Aitio A. Biologic monitoring at the Institute of Occupational Health. Scand J Work Environ Health 1992; 18(suppl 2):69–71.
23. Bernard A, Lauwerys R. Present status and trends in the biologic monitoring of exposure to industrial chemicals. J Occup Med 1992; 28:558–63.
24. Greim H, Csanady G, Filser J et al. Biomarkers as tools in human health risk assessment. Clin Chem 1995; 41:1804–8.
25. Vainio H. Current trends in the biologic monitoring of exposure to carcinogens. Scand J Work Environ Health 1985; 11:1–6.
26. Aitio A. Biologic monitoring today and tomorrow. Scand J Work Environ Health 1994; 20(special issue):46–58.
27. Lehnert G, Schaller K-H. Strategy of biologic monitoring and setting of biologic threshold limits (BAT values) in Germany. Isr J Med Sci 1995; 9:549–57.
28. Friberg L, Elinder C-G. Biologic monitoring of toxic metals. Scand J Work Environ Health 1993; 19(suppl 1):7–13.
29. Greim H, Lehnert G, eds. Biologic exposure values for occupational toxicants and carcinogens, Vol. 2. Weinheim, Germany: VCH Verlagsgesellschaft, 1995.

30. ACGIH. Threshold limit values (TLVs) for chemical substances and physical agents and biologic exposure indices (BEIs). Cincinnati: American Conference of Governmental Industrial Hygienists, 1996.

31. Kiilunen M. Biomonitoring action levels in Finland. Int Arch Occup Environ Health 1999; 72:261–7.

Chapter 8
Impairment and Disability

Philip Harber

Evaluating work ability and disability requires both clinical and environmental expertise. Disability and impairment are not static; rather, they are subject to intervention. The extent of disability is determined by several factors: severity of the impairment itself, concurrent impairments in other systems, efficacy of medical care, job demand, ability to adjust job demands as needed, attitude of the worker, policies of the employer, and social context.

Evaluating the match between a person and the job requires understanding of both the individual's clinical condition and the stressors imposed by work. Five general questions may be asked in assessing occupational disability. These questions are summarized in Table 8.1. Certain jobs are sufficiently arduous or have sufficiently frequent risk that they are inappropriate for nearly all workers. This chapter, however, focuses on evaluation of the individual for jobs that are not inherently unacceptably dangerous.

GENERAL CONCEPTS

Several general concepts are involved in the evaluation of an individual's ability/disability. This section will define basic terms.

An *impairment* is the loss of physiologic function or anatomic structure, such as decreased maximal strength or loss of a hand. Traditionally, physicians have emphasized assessment of impairment.

A *handicap* is the specific activity that may not be performed (e.g., the person cannot walk one flight of stairs, cannot use a respirator, cannot calculate change). In the United States, the term 'handicap' is used less frequently, and the distinction between disability and handicap is less clear.

A *disability* is the impact of the impairment or handicap on the person's life. Disability may be assessed in several spheres. *Job-specific disability* describes the inability of a person to do a specific job, typically his or her current or most recent job. *General occupational disability* relates to the inability to do most jobs in the economy. Disability may also be described in terms of the activities of daily living (ADL) without reference to a specific occupation. For example, can the person live independently? As discussed below, the extent of disability depends on many factors besides the actual impairment, and it is common that two individuals may have similar impairments but different consequent disabilities.

A disability may be characterized as either *permanent* or *temporary,* depending on anticipated healing or response to treatment. Furthermore, a disability may be characterized as partial or total. *Total disability* usually implies that the individual is unable to do any substantial work. *Diagnosis* usually refers to a description of the underlying etiology (the traditional medical diagnosis). Unfortunately, many physicians limit their evaluation to establishment of the diagnosis rather than considering its functional impact. *Accommodation* is the process of making workplace adjustments to permit a person with impairment to continue working. Even when impairment cannot be eliminated by medical treatment following an injury or an illness, a physician may serve as a member of an interdisciplinary team to significantly diminish the consequent disability.

Whole-person impairment considers the impact of combined impairments from several organ systems on the total person. In some instances, two non-total impairments may combine to become completely impairing. For example, the patient with an otherwise compensated psychiatric impairment may become totally impaired if a back injury occurs.

There also are several concepts that relate to the administrative and legal aspects of evaluation. Several administrative/legal systems require reducing complex patient and worksite factors into a single number upon which to determine the size of an award of benefits. *Percent disability* is a legal concept, not a medical reality. It applies a single number to the individual; this number is commonly used by agencies to determine directly the amount of financial award. The specific method for calculating this award varies. Some systems base this award on impairment (physiologic and anatomic loss), whereas others are truly disability based, such as an estimation of the loss of wage-earning capacity. Another administrative term is *apportionment*, in which the patient's impairment or disability is ascribed in a quantitative fashion to different causes. Ascribing a certain degree of the current impairment or disability to a job as a welder and the remainder to smoking is an example. A *preclusion* represents an activity or exposure that is not recommended for the individual. Such preclusions may be for chemical exposures, physical job demands, or even workplace emotional stressors, that result in work restrictions.

Clinical evaluation of disability requires an assessment of five basic factors, outlined in Table 8.1 and discussed in detail below.

A. Can the worker do the job?

Determination of whether or not a worker is currently capable of performing a particular job necessitates evaluation of both the worker and the job characteristics. Only after both the worker and the job have been carefully assessed is it

1. *Can* the worker do the job?
2. *Should* the worker do the job (i.e., what is his or her risk of future illness)?
3. What is the extent of deviation from normality (impairment)?
4. How can the job be modified to accommodate the worker?
5. Can the worker's health be modified to meet job requirements?

Table 8.1 Basic questions

possible to comment specifically on the match between the two. If the clinician has sufficient understanding of the job demands he/she may comment upon ability to do the specific job.

Evaluation of a person's current capability to do a job are commonly performed in three contexts: (1) preplacement examination, in which a potential worker is evaluated prospectively to determine whether or not he or she can do a job; (2) fitness-for-duty evaluation, in which a worker who is currently employed in a job is evaluated to determine whether or not he or she should remain in the job; and (3) disability compensation evaluation, in which job-related disability is determined to guide a legal decision about financial payment. Although the contexts differ, the same scientific principles apply.

Characterizing the individual

In evaluating whether or not someone can do a job, each individual must be assessed *individually*. Information about classes of workers should not be applied to evaluating a particular worker–job match. For example, although women may on *average* be able to supply less muscular force for lifting than men, it is inappropriate to exclude a woman from a job requiring heavy lifting without carefully evaluating her specific strength. Similar comments apply to the aging worker and individuals who have known impairments.

Preplacement medical assessment determines whether or not an individual can meet the basic job requirements; the medical evaluation is not aimed at selecting the best worker (this is a personnel decision).[1,2] In the United States, the Americans with Disabilities Act (ADA) defines the information that may be collected and how it should be used. Information that is collected should be relevant to the job. If additional medical information is collected (as part of a baseline evaluation or for general health purposes), the clinician must not allow irrelevant information to affect the placement recommendation.

The information to be collected must be carefully selected based on knowledge of the job rather than relying on a generic preplacement examination. Each worker's specific medical history may lead to individualization of testing. In the United States, several Occupational Safety and Health Administration (OSHA) regulations require specified examinations soon after placement, and many incorporate these specified examinations into the general preplacement examination. In addition, different situations warrant different clinical emphases. For example, lower extremity sensation and reflexes warrant special attention for baseline documentation for jobs stressing the low back,

whereas testing for Phalen's and Tinel's signs is warranted when there is likely to be repetitive wrist motion.

Considerations for compensation disability evaluation are similar, but the examiner is generally afforded more leeway in choosing tests.

Characterizing the job

The job must be described adequately to determine whether or not the worker can do it. Assessment of disability must include evaluation of the job in addition to examination of the individual.[3] In those instances in which a global rather than job-specific disability assessment is performed, the examiner must have a clear concept of the average and the minimal demand jobs in the economy.

Job-specific work characterization information can be obtained from many sources. For example, the worker may provide descriptions when seeking information supplied by the employer. Other methods include a worksite visit, discussions with coworkers, or viewing of videotapes about the job. Review of industrial hygiene data is useful for evaluating the chemical environment. Finally, occupational medicine textbooks and industrial process books include useful information.

When the physician does not have sufficient work characterization information on which to base a *disability* recommendation, the report should be explicitly limited to a description of *impairment, handicap, or work ability* with the clear understanding that translation to disability is to be done by others. For example, a clinician may express ability (e.g., 'can lift 20 pounds 5 times an hour') or handicap ('cannot lift more than 20 pounds') rather than job-specific ability ('cannot work at a specific position at a specific company').

B. Should the worker take the job? (Future risk assessment)

While the previous section addressed whether or not an individual can do a job *at the current time,* this section deals with the more difficult question of assessing future risk. The clinician's role is to make an assessment and provide advice; the worker and the employer have the ultimate responsibility for actually making the decision about whether or not the estimated risk is acceptable. This decision is affected by non-medical considerations, including the availability of alternative work or alternative workers with lower risk, and the potential benefits of the work. Also, there is a societal acceptance of differential risk for various occupations; for example, a higher risk is thought to be more acceptable for astronauts, US presidents, and soldiers than for schoolteachers and physicians. Assessment of the significance of future risk is guided by several principles: (1) likelihood that an adverse event will occur; (2) severity of the effect; (3) temporality regarding how soon the event will occur; and (4) public impact or the extent to which the public would be placed at risk if an event occurs. Thus, a police officer with angina and a high likelihood of developing a myocardial infarction in the near future while chasing a felon would carry far more weight than an unlikely skin irritation developing in the far future.

Certain risk estimates are generic for the job or industry, but characteristics of a specific worker may significantly modify the generic risk associated with a job. These individual risk modifications arise in the following ways.

1. Sensitization to a specific agent

An allergic, chemical or biologic agent-specific sensitization generally precludes a worker from a job with a high probability of exposure to that particular agent. Even if the worker has no current impairment, disability for specific jobs may exist because of the necessity to avoid certain chemicals. Such allergic sensitization may be manifested by asthma, allergic rhinitis, or contact dermatitis. Once sensitized, low levels of exposure may produce active disease, and typical regulatory standards cannot be relied on for protection.

2. High risk of recurrence of a previous injury or illness

Often, a worker who has had previous injury is more likely to have a recurrence than are his or her coworkers. Each situation must be individually evaluated to assess specific risk rather than simply assuming that previous illness predicts future illness. One should determine whether the original injury indicated a particular individual susceptibility, or occurred purely by chance. Furthermore, one must determine whether the individual risk factor leading to the original illness or injury still exists, has been corrected, or is subject to modification. For example, inadequate strength for a job can lead to back injuries; however, strength may be improved by training, and therefore, an injury that occurred in an untrained individual does not indicate that the risk persists. In addition, the previous injury may have been due to unusually adverse working conditions that are unlikely to be found in any other situation on the job.

3. High risk of total disability in the event of a second injury

An existing impairment, whether due to occupational or non-occupational factors, may sufficiently limit the person's physiologic reserve that any additional loss, even one that is transient, would be unacceptable. This concept applies to traumatic loss (e.g., a worker with only one hand is at very high risk for incapacitation should any injury occur to the remaining hand), physiologic loss (destruction of lung tissue by asbestosis or emphysema markedly exaggerates the effect of any subsequent fibrosis), or psychiatric loss (a usually minor workplace psychosocial stressor may completely disable an otherwise compensated individual). Assessments, therefore, require evaluation of the potential for subsequent injury.

Many states have second injury laws to protect employers against large expenses incurred by employing partially disabled workers. In the absence of such laws, however, there is strong incentive to discriminate against the partially impaired worker at the time of hiring and placement.

4. High risk of developing an unrelated problem

A previous injury or illness may increase the risk of developing a new, unrelated problem at work. For example, occupational hearing loss may increase the risk of subsequent bodily injury if it interferes with a worker's ability to hear warnings or oncoming traffic. Similarly, reactive airways dysfunction syndrome (RADS), which was induced by a single high-level exposure to a specific agent such as sulfur dioxide, may leave a worker more susceptible to a variety of non-specific respiratory irritants.

5. Difficulty in discerning job-related health effects in cases of pre-existing impairment

A pre-existing impairment may interfere with the ability to screen for health effects. For instance, approximately 5% of workers exposed to certain isocyanates become sensitized and develop asthma. A worker in an isocyanate facility who develops even mild wheezing will likely be detectable by spirometry surveillance programs or by symptom reporting, whereas occupational sensitization would be much more difficult to detect in the worker with pre-existing wheezing. Similarly, the increasing reliance on early symptom reporting for secondary prevention of cumulative trauma disorders is complicated by the presence of pre-existing symptoms. In such instances, it is difficult to determine whether a symptom is new or simply a manifestation of existing dysfunction. These limitations may be minimized by obtaining appropriate baseline clinical information.

6. Psychologic sensitization

Individuals may encounter considerable difficulty in returning to former work because of significant fear of a recurrent episode after recovering from the effects of one earlier accident. For example, a worker who sustained major burns (from which he or she has fully recovered) following rupture of a steam line may have sufficient fear to preclude him or her from working in a power or steam plant. Similarly, a worker who has experienced high-level exposure to a toxic material with a strong odor may subsequently feel anxiety in the presence of non-specific odors, having learned to associate odor with danger.[4]

7. Increased risk to coworkers or the general public

A previous impairment or injury may increase the future risk to coworkers or the general public without necessarily increasing the risk to the worker personally. The important distinction between future risk to self versus others has been made by the ADA, which differentially emphasizes risk to others. For example, a schoolteacher with paranoia or a narcoleptic police dispatcher represents future risk not to himself (or herself) but to others.

Because preplacement evaluation and job-specific disability assessment are fundamentally the same, the same principles guide both. Preclusions frequently are specified in the course of a disability evaluation and are based on the evaluator's opinion about future risk. As such, they are frequently called 'prophylactic preclusions'. These preclusions are used as the basis for determining monetary awards in several disability compensations systems.

In describing a work limitation, the evaluator should clearly differentiate a prophylactic preclusion, based on an estimate of future risk, from the determination that the worker is currently incapable of performing the job tasks. The evaluator also should describe the rationale for such recommended preclusions as well as the estimated probability of an adverse effect if the preclusion is not followed. Furthermore, to the greatest extent possible, the recommended preclusions should be carefully described. A frequently used phrase, such as 'precluded from exposure to gases, mists, and fumes', would effectively preclude the individual from life on earth, since air is a gas. Similarly, 'precluded from moderate lifting' is far too vague to be helpful. In addition to specifying a recommended weight limitation for lifting, the evaluator also should comment on frequency; for example, 'Lifting 25 pounds once a shift is not likely to produce recurrent injury and is thus acceptable, but lifting 25 pounds 100 times per hour is risky'.

C. Quantifying impairment: how much function has the patient lost?

Here, the emphasis is on the decrement rather than on the residual abilities or future risk. Therefore, in answering this question as part of a disability evaluation, it is necessary to provide an assessment of the functional ability at two times: prior to the injury and currently. Some disability evaluation systems, such as the United States Social Security Disability Insurance System, are based solely on the individual's current functional ability, whereas most workers' compensation systems are concerned with the *loss* of function *due to work*. Simply subtracting current function from pre-hire function often does not adequately evaluate the functional loss due to work, because aging and other unrelated factors also might produce loss. These factors should be delineated as carefully as possible. Even though factors other than work may have caused some decrement in function, an additional impairment component due to work may represent the proximate cause, or the proverbial 'straw that broke the camel's back' and create disability for a job.

Retrospective evaluation of preinjury status with precision is often difficult. Several approaches may be used to estimate the individual's preinjury function; these approaches are summarized in Table 8.2 and include the following.

1. Available preinjury objective data
Where available, such objective information is particularly useful. For example, the worker may have participated

in an annual medical surveillance program involving pulmonary function testing, thereby providing objective information about his or her preinjury status. The results of periodic medical examinations or preplacement examinations may be similarly useful. Medical testing performed outside the occupational setting by the personal physician or as part of insurance or military service examinations also may be available.

2. Objective evidence of prior activities indicating a high functional level
Life activities prior to the injury may imply a specific level of functioning. For example, having worked successfully in a heavy manual materials handling job suggests the absence of pre-existing back impairment and may imply a preinjury strength that is greater than average. Similarly, marathon running suggests high cardiopulmonary fitness. Evaluation of loss of cognitive function is more challenging; given the wide range of cognitive ability (e.g., as measured by IQ testing) in a population, it is difficult to determine whether someone who has low-normal function always functioned at that level or has had a significant loss. Educational attainment and occupational achievement may provide insight into preillness capability. However, before concluding that poor prior educational/vocational attainment indicates a low premorbid cognitive ability, one must consider if opportunity and cultural barriers, rather than low ability, account for the low attainment.

3. Intraindividual comparison
For certain functions, the person may serve as an internal reference (e.g., the general symmetry of muscle bulk and strength allows comparison of one side to another). Range of motion evaluations should compare the affected side to the contralateral side. Comparisons of the left and right sides should be made soon after onset of the impairment. A delay of many years may lead to secondary disuse or overuse of the unaffected side.

4. Comparison to population norms
Statistical description of the distribution of many specific functional characteristics is available. When there are no data about the individual's preinjury functional status, one may compare the patient's current result with the relevant population average and make the assumption that prior to injury, he or she was 'average'. Such general comparisons must be interpreted with caution. Working populations should not be assumed to be 'average'. Unhealthy individuals are often less likely to apply for or be placed in jobs than healthy applicants ('healthy worker effect') or to remain in a demanding job ('survivor effect'). For example, individuals with naturally low lung function may tend to leave jobs requiring heavy exertion, and individuals with airway hyper-responsiveness will leave jobs entailing exposures that produce bronchospasm (e.g., grain dust exposure), thereby leaving working populations that have higher-than-average functional availability for the given job.

Conversely, the reference values may have been derived from subjects selected for above-average health. To under-

Preinjury objective data
Prior activities
Intraindividual comparisons (e.g. right vs. left)
Population norms
Self-reported status

Table 8.2 Methods of estimating preinjury functional status

stand the limitations of this approach, consider the following example. There are predicted values for pulmonary function tests such as spirometry. These predictions are often based on regression equations derived from empiric testing of carefully selected 'normal' individuals. Cigarette smokers, persons with asthma or other respiratory symptoms, and those who perform suboptimally on the tests were excluded. Therefore, the predicted values do not reflect average results for a typical community population, because those with naturally occurring disease and smokers were excluded. Therefore, an unselected community population should not automatically be expected to have average values equal to those that are predicted.

Thus, the source of the reference population and factors affecting selection of workers must be considered. Reference values based on atypically fit subjects may overestimate expected values; similarly the 'healthy worker' and 'survivor' effects may increase expected values for some worker groups above usual reference values.[5-7] Furthermore, there is considerable interpersonal variation in ability even among the carefully selected study population, requiring that a *range* of normality, rather than a single value, be defined. For arbitrary reasons, this has traditionally been set at a value that creates a 5% false-positive rate for each test (i.e., 5% of the carefully selected normal population would still have values outside this range). Population norms of muscle strength are even more complex because the job itself may have a significant training effect, leading to increased muscle strength in comparison to overall population averages. For these reasons, population averages as the estimate of preinjury functional status must be used cautiously, and clinical judgment must be employed to make necessary adjustments.

5. Self-reported status

Subjective information collected from the worker also facilitates evaluating prior function. Clinical assessments of function loss using self-reported status should be conducted where possible. Family and friends also may provide significantly useful subjective data. This information is especially helpful when changes in central nervous system functional status are evaluated.

The loss should be carefully described. However, unlike the preplacement testing situation, more detailed, individualized testing is traditionally acceptable for impairment assessment when the assessment is part of a compensation disability evaluation. Testing should be as objective as possible, and optimal patient cooperation must be obtained. When appropriate, physicians should state in a written report that adequate testing could not be performed for technical reasons or due to lack of full cooperation. Whenever possible, clinical evaluation and testing results should be recorded in a way that permits external validation and review. For example, spirometry tracings should be incorporated in reports; raw psychometric data, rather than just a final interpretation of results, also should be available for review.

In addition to simply listing results of current function evaluation and estimated prior function, physicians should describe which findings are the most important. For example, loss of FEV_1 is more significant than loss of $FEF_{25-75\%}$, and loss of dominant hand function is more important than loss of function of the non-dominant hand.

For occupational disease and cumulative trauma disorders, functional loss is frequently multifactorial and the clinician is asked to apportion the functional loss to multiple causes. For example, aging and cigarette smoking cause decline in lung function and may confuse the evaluation of loss of lung function due to cotton dust exposure (chronic byssinosis). Unfortunately, there is difficulty in simply applying the average excess decline in lung function found in cigarette smokers and assuming that any loss above this level is due to the occupational exposure. Only a minority of smokers develop high rates of decline of lung function; therefore, applying the average annual excess decline among smokers would underestimate the effects of byssinosis in some and overestimate it in other cotton dust-exposed workers. Unlike smoking, aging significantly affects all individuals and should be accounted for using standard reference equations provide an age adjustment.

When attempting to ascribe functional loss to certain jobs, estimates of the level of risk associated with each job must be evaluated. For illness related to chemical exposure, one must consider dose, exposure levels, frequency, mitigating factors (personal protective equipment such as respirators), and the time course of exposure relative to the onset of disease. In essence, one must apply epidemiologic and toxicologic approaches to the individual rather than to populations or laboratory animals.

D. Accommodation: how can the job be modified to decrease the worker's disability?

Modification of a job may significantly decrease the extent of occupational disability. Such possibilities should be considered in most occupational disability evaluations. Modifications such as creating a flexible work pace or work schedule may convert a disabled worker to an able worker. Providing mechanical assist devices may permit a worker to use any residual abilities; similarly, coworkers may be assigned a small number of relatively heavy tasks to permit a partially impaired individual to remain in the workforce. Modification of chemical exposures also may be accomplished; for example, a worker may be transferred to another department that does not deal with a specific chemical agent or process.

The psychosocial and organizational structure of the worksite also may be improved to decrease occupational disability. For example, education of the immediate supervisor about the worker's specific limitations and residual abilities can facilitate the worker's re-entry to the workforce. Upper management (and often union) support may be needed to encourage the immediate line supervisor to become an ally in returning someone to modified work.

E. Can the worker's condition be modified to decrease occupational disability?

There are four ways in which changes to the worker can affect the degree of disability. The first two apply directly to the injury- or illness-related impairment, the third applies to the individual's psychologic response to the injury, and the fourth applies to the occupational disability per se.

1. Natural course of the illness

Many illnesses and injuries are not static but change over time. For example, certain diseases, such as progressive massive fibrosis or severe asbestosis, may progress even after exposure ceases, whereas many others, such as post-irritant tracheobronchitis, may improve with time. Most musculoskeletal strains and sprains also improve with time. Therefore, one must carefully consider the point in the natural history of the illness at which the evaluation is being performed.

2. Medical treatment

Proper medical treatment may modify the level of impairment and, consequently, the disability. Therefore, in addition to assessing current functional status, physicians should consider the extent to which improved treatment would modify the functional condition. In some instances, treatment may be directed at the injury itself (operative repair of a fracture, bronchodilator therapy); in other situations, the individual may require medical rehabilitation (physiatry, physical therapy). Treatment of coexisting conditions also may decrease the disability consequent to the occupationally related problem.

Hence, impairment should be assessed in its current state as well as on the assumption that the patient will receive optimal medical treatment. Some residual uncertainty about future impairment always exists, because an individual's response to therapy is often variable. The clinician should indicate if the worker has obtained 'maximal medical improvement'. For these reasons, the evaluating physician should consider whether the patient is in a 'permanent and stationary' status. If so, then a 'permanent disability/impairment' may be described.

3. Improvement of psychologic effects

Occupational illnesses or injuries may lead to secondary psychiatric or psychologic effects. For example, the inability to go to work may significantly affect an individual's self-image, or fear of subsequent workplace events may lead to inability to work even if the primary illness has ameliorated. These psychologic effects are not permanent in most instances and can be managed with appropriate treatment. The management includes both medical and psychologic treatment, as well as altering attitudes at the workplace and managing physical factors, as described earlier.

4. Vocational training

Often, a worker who has received maximal medical treatment may still improve his or her disability status through vocational rehabilitation. The individual's remaining skills and abilities may often be redirected into other productive areas. Vocational rehabilitation is best begun as soon as it is clear that a worker will not be capable of returning to the former job and that he or she is not totally disabled for all work.

INTEGRATED DISABILITY PREVENTION

Worker productivity is reduced by injuries and illnesses, whether or not caused by work exposures. The indirect costs of worker disability include reduced productivity, necessity to hire and train new employees, and reduced morale. Therefore, there is increasing recognition of the value of efforts to reduce disability, whether or not consequent to work itself. Integrated disability management programs do not distinguish between workers compensation and group health, but apply similar approaches to optimize worker functional status.

Disability is the end result of many factors. Figure 8.1 demonstrates schematically the factors that affect disability. Exposure to workplace hazards or personal health conditions can gradually or acutely produce pathophysiologic effects (injury), which lead to a clinically diagnosable condition (e.g., asthma, low back strain) and its consequent impairment. The latter may resolve or leave some degree of permanent impairment. This in turn interferes with the ability to do certain tasks, such as lifting specific poundage (the handicap). This produces work disability if the job cannot be done without the task. In considering disability, clinicians should recognize the critical importance of functional assessment, rather than the medical diagnosis per se.

The likelihood and extent of permanent disability are significantly modified by factors external to this direct sequence from injury to disability. The dashed boxes in Figure 8.1 show these factors. Each is a potential site for preventive intervention.

As shown in Figure 8.1, most of the aspects influencing disability are the same whether the medical problem is of occupational or non-occupational origin. Regrettably, some compensation systems penalize workers for any contribution not due to a work hazard and therefore discourage attention to many relevant issues.

Efforts to prevent occupational disability may be directed at various points. Effective approaches towards prevention of occupational injury/illness are discussed throughout this book. Although the term 'disability management' is popular, 'disability prevention' is more consistent with primary, secondary, and tertiary prevention approaches for most occupational problems. Some methods are directed at individual workers/patients, whereas others focus upon the work environment or policies. Disability prevention approaches should be considered soon after an injury has occurred; once a pattern of disability has been established, it is difficult to change.

By appropriate early interventions, secondary prevention limits the extent of disability following an injury.

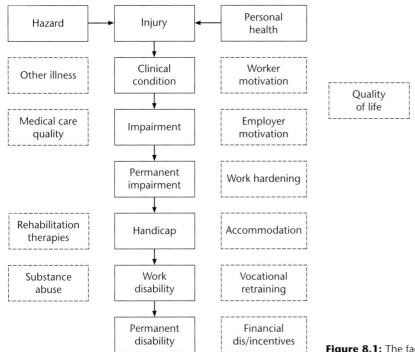

Figure 8.1: The factors that affect disability.

Reducing impairment by good medical care (e.g., optimizing medications for reactive airways disease syndrome) and avoiding unnecessary surgery (e.g., inappropriate lumbar fusions) will reduce the consequent disability.[10,11] Methods as simple as occasional telephone calls from coworkers and supervisors increase the likelihood of effective return to work after a back injury.

Secondary prevention efforts include establishing policies which encourage job accommodation and availability of limited duty. They also include programs addressing factors such as drug/alcohol abuse that tend to prolong disability. The quality of work life affects both employer and patient motivation to return to work. For example, worker assessment of the quality of work life was a major determinant of disability due to back pain.[8,9]

Identifying social factors, whether at home or work, which tend to prolong the period of disability may lead to effective secondary prevention efforts. Numerous studies have shown that perception of work stress affects extent of disability after reporting a back injury.[12-14] For example, this may involve remediation of worksite stressors such as lack of respect for workers, inconsistent management, lack of autonomy, or conflicts with specific supervisors or coworkers. Personal stressors, such as alcohol abuse or a dysfunctional family situation, are also subject to intervention. When the period of disability seems inappropriately long, clinicians must consider the possibility of 'medicalization' of personnel issues, a situation in which managers or workers camouflage personnel issues as clinical issues.

Traditional functionally oriented therapies (such as physical and occupational therapy) may be supplemented by job task-specific rehabilitation.[15] Such 'work hardening' should be based upon understanding the specific types of job demands and emphasize strengthening the most relevant functions. Work hardening may be helpful even for physical aspects not involved in the injury itself, if deconditioning has occurred while the affected anatomic area heals.

Tertiary disability prevention methods include vocational rehabilitation such as training for a new occupation. Modification of the job (accommodation) by reassigning or modifying the tasks leading to disability can be effective. Eliminating employer and employee disincentives to work (e.g., by 'second injury laws') reduce disability.

Policies that affect disability must be carefully formulated. The 'indirect' cost of occupational injury/illness (e.g., reduced productivity) often exceeds the cost of direct medical care and workers compensation payments; 'cost containment' efforts which delay care may therefore actually increase the total cost of an injury. Rigid work rules, which assign lighter jobs solely on seniority, may reduce the flexibility necessary for accommodation.

EXAMPLES: IMPAIRMENT AND DISABILITY RELATED TO LOW BACK, PULMONARY DISORDERS AND PAIN

The earlier sections outlined general principles underlying disability assessment. Specific methods are appropriate for evaluation of each organ system, and several examples are presented here. Nevertheless, the impairment and disability evaluator must recognize the person as a whole rather than simply as a collection of individual systems. An approach to impairment assessment is provided, using back disability as a prototype. Evaluation of low back impairment, despite a plethora of physical examinations and laboratory tests, still relies heavily on subjective factors from both the patient's and the examiners' standpoint.

Low back

Acute and cumulative trauma injury to the low back is the most costly occupational health problem in industry in the United States (see Chapter 23.4). It occurs both as a consequence of single specifically identifiable events as well as from repetitive strain. Most low back problems are relatively limited in their impact, with return to work occurring in less than 2 weeks. However, a small proportion of workers with low back injuries have prolonged or even permanent total inability to work. Many such injuries affect manual materials handling workers with limited alternative skills. However, trained service sector professionals, such as nurses, also have very high rates of low back injury.

Early workers' compensations systems were oriented toward acute traumatic loss (e.g., amputation) and did not address anything as subjective as low back pain. Therefore, the discovery of the entity of herniated nucleus pulposus (HNP) in the early part of the century provided the rationale for including this large group of occupational problems. Occupational back pain was believed to be the consequence of an acute rupture of the annulus, with herniation of the disc and compression of neural structures. To be considered work related and compensable, the pain had to begin following a specific identifiable incident, in which the annulus was acutely torn. In this theory the disc herniation was believed to be both necessary and sufficient to diagnose and explain the impairment. Workers with gradual onset of pain or those without a disc herniation on myelography were believed not to have demonstrable impairment. Unfortunately, this attractively simple scheme is incorrect. Repetitive overuse can contribute significantly to occupational low back pain without a single severe incident.

Current disability

The best way to determine whether or not an individual currently is capable of doing a job with demands on low back function is to have the individual attempt the work. If this approach is not feasible, work simulation also may be conducted, often in a clinical setting. In many cases, work limitation due to back pain is related to decreased lifting ability and, therefore, evaluation tends to focus on this area. The type of lifting associated with a particular job may be characterized by several parameters; these are shown in Table 8.3. These lifting parameters are very

Weight lifted
Frequency of lift
Starting position for lift
Vertical travel
Body position relative to starting and final positions
Load factors (size, shape, handles, footing)

Table 8.3 Parameters describing lifting jobs

comparable to those recommended in the National Institute for Occupational Safety and Health (NIOSH) manual materials handling guides. However, they must be supplemented by information about whether the lift is typically one-handed or two-handed, or in the sagittal plane or asymmetrical.

Most jobs involve heterogeneity of lifting tasks. In some instances, the current ability of an individual to do a particular job is determined by the most arduous of the tasks, even if this task is performed only once or twice a day. In other circumstances, typical work is performed at high repetition rates throughout the day. In the latter case, the work simulation test, which is used to determine whether or not a worker is able to do a particular job, must not be based on the ability to generate a single forceful lift.

Unfortunately, work simulation is generally impractical. The evaluator frequently does not have adequate information about the job. Furthermore, there is considerable concern about performing significant lifting tasks as part of the disability evaluation. Clinicians may be appropriately concerned about the possibility of further exacerbation of injury as a consequence of the testing. Moreover, this testing is subject to motivational factors. A worker who strongly desires a particular job placement may tolerate an otherwise unacceptable level of discomfort during the preplacement simulation test, and conversely, a worker who seeks compensation may have a subtle bias in the opposite direction. Therefore, rather than relying on direct workplace or workplace simulation testing, more indirect methods are commonly used.

An intermediate approach is to determine whether or not the worker has strength and endurance comparable to typical workers who are currently successfully performing the work. Specific methods for determining strength are described in more detail later. Although strength often may be measured conveniently in a clinical setting, it is more difficult to evaluate the strength of workers in a particular job for comparison purposes. Nevertheless, there are published data about the typical strength of certain working populations. In addition, the strength data are incorporated in several commercially available computer programs for easy use.

Relative perceived exertion (RPE) techniques also may be applicable in the absence of concern about secondary gain.[16] Workers are remarkably good at describing the work demands, and a series of formal scales (RPE) can be used for this purpose. Instead of measuring strength, a worker may be evaluated by performing several typical tasks in the clinical setting and being asked how the tasks compare with the worker's perception of his or her former job.

In actual practice, clinical judgment by clinicians without direct knowledge of the workplace often is the basis for determining whether or not impairment leads to current disability. To improve the usual situation, in which the clinician has neither the time nor the training to conduct a worksite survey to determine the specific lifting requirements, as much useful information as possible should be provided. There is a tradition that requires physicians to 'pigeonhole' disability evaluees into vaguely characterized categories such as 'capable of light lifting' or 'capable of very heavy lifting'. Even specifying the duration in hours per day is inadequate unless the frequency per hour is also described. Positional terms such as kneeling, stooping, and bending also require quantitation to be of any use to the clinical evaluator.

Future risk

Assessment of future risk and recommendation of consequent preclusions are more difficult than description of current disability. Previous episodes of severe impairment are a significant predictor of future risk. Certain clinical diagnoses imply a high degree of instability and consequent elevated risk. For example, an untreated large herniated disc that is beginning to impinge on the spinal canal or neural foramina warrants particular caution.

Current muscle strength is believed by many to be a modifier of future risk and is recommended by NIOSH for preplacement testing in manual materials handling tests. There is at least one study that has shown validity of the concept that a worker's strength in relation to the job requirement is a major predictor of future risk.[17] Although this study has not been specifically validated for workers with existing impairment, it is reasonable to assume that strength testing will play an increasingly important role in assessing disability due to low back disorders.

Extent of loss

Several approaches are available to estimate the loss of function (impairment) due to low back problems. As discussed previously, antecedent (preinjury) status may be assessed by several methods. In some instances, previous medical data such as strength testing and preplacement physical examination data, or both, may be available for comparison. The ability of the individual to have conducted heavy work prior to the illness is frequently the best indicator of a high functional status. Moreover, there are population norms available for specific measures of strength and range of motion.

Evaluation of current functional status has several functional components: subjective statements made by the patient, medical diagnoses, range of motion testing, and performance testing. Each of these components can and should be used in effectively comparing current function with previous function. There are two commonly used methods for summarizing and rating impairment related to back disorders – range of motion (ROM) and diagnosis related estimated (DRE). The former approach (ROM) has been traditionally used and is based largely upon reduction in the measured range of motion of the spine also considering associated neurologic deficits. Measurement of range of motion requires attention to detail and it is dependent upon adequate cooperation of the patient. Many feel that accuracy is enhanced by use of an inclinometer rather than by visual estimation or use of a goniometer. An inclinometer measures deviation from the vertical plane and is similar to levels used by carpenters. Spinal motion is measured in three planes: extension–flexion; axial rotation, and frontal motion. The

measurement should be repeated several times to estimate consistency.

The other method, DRE, depends upon assigning diagnostic categories. According to the AMA Guidelines, the following factors are considered: muscle spasm, muscle guarding, spinal motion asymmetry, radicular pain, reflex abnormality, weakness, hyperesthesia, atrophy, electrodiagnostic abnormality, motion segment integrity loss, cauda equina syndrome, urodynamic abnormalities. The DRE method is particularly useful when there has been a specific, well-defined injury. Conversely, the ROM approach is preferable when it is not possible to delineate a specific diagnosis or injury. Increasingly, the DRE method is preferred. The medical evaluation also helps determine if impairment is likely to be permanent. Some disorders may be expected to improve with treatment, whereas others, even if less severe, may not (e.g., nerve root impingement versus chronic musculoligamentous strain without specific remediable lesion).

Strength measurements are also employed to assess functional status and impairment performance. Relatively simple equipment can often give very useful information. By the same token, expensive, computerized equipment may give misleading results unless carefully calibrated and maintained and unless the clinician interpreting the results fully understands the basis for the printed results. Strength testing techniques fall into three general categories: static, performance, and dynamic. In a static strength test, the subject exerts force against a non-moving object (typically a grab bar) that is attached to a force transducer.[18,19] Performance-based strength measurements are similar to work simulation methods described earlier. However, for this type of testing, the subject modifies the load to be lifted. For example, the subject may be asked to place unmarked lead weights into a tote box, modifying the number of weights upward or downward until the lift can be comfortably accomplished. Dynamic testing measures strength while the region is in motion. Equipment for this method typically is expensive and provides a large number of graphs and data points. For dynamic testing, the subject is directly linked to the measurement apparatus that controls the motion. Dynamic testing has the advantage of measuring strength throughout the range of lumbosacral spine motion rather than only in one or two positions. While these techniques produce many graphic displays, that may seem impressive, they have not been as widely validated as the isometric methods.

Certain caveats apply to ROM testing and strength testing. The subject must be motivated, and instructions must be clear. The subject should be instructed to produce good efforts but not to risk injury. Repeatability must be determined. In the absence of specific coaching, it is very difficult for a malingerer to exert consistently only 75% of his or her true capability.

Possibility of accommodation

Modification of the job to accommodate workers with low back impairments may often be accomplished. This modification may range from transferring the individual to lighter work or providing mechanical assist devices. Permitting self-pacing also is very useful. In some situations, such as nursing, having a second person available when lifting also may be useful. In assessing possible jobsite modifications, the full cooperation of the patient must be enlisted in order to avoid the opposing dangers of lack of motivation due to fear of re-injury and risk of injury due to overzealous return to work.

Worker treatment also plays a very important role. In addition to specific medical treatment for the underlying back disorder, there has been considerable interest in worker training for impaired workers. Various programs, commonly called 'work hardening' or 'back' schools, have been widely used. Limited outcome data, rather than randomized clinical trials to assess their efficacy, suggest they are useful in some cases. In general, such programs incorporate a combination of physical training, worker education, and psychologic motivation. The truly effective programs typically include specific knowledge of the worksite for which the subject is being rehabilitated rather than applying broad generic methods. For instance, the stressors and techniques for a railroad crew worker are quite different from those for a back-impaired office worker.

Subjective aspects

Despite the existence of many objective physical examinations and laboratory tests, evaluation of low back disorders still must consider the subjective reports of the patient about his or her pain. Pain may be described in terms of its severity, frequency, precipitating events, and impact. The severity description should include the patient's own words as well as traditional qualifiers such as 'mild' or 'severe'. The quality of the pain should also be described, using the patient's own words. There are formal pain scales that, when integrated with a clinical interview, have some value for workers who are socioculturally comparable to the population for whom the scales were developed. The frequency of pain also should be described. This description should include discussion of typical number of days per week during which it occurs, as well as the number of episodes per day.

The duration of pain for average episodes and for more severe episodes also should be reported. In addition, the clinician should query whether or not the onset is predictable. Precipitating factors should be evaluated. Is the pain brought on by simply tying shoes or does it require carrying a 20-pound grocery sack? Does it occur with short duration of exertion or only with prolonged, repetitive exertion? Are there certain positions that precipitate the pain? Does sitting for prolonged periods induce it? To what extent does anxiety or stress bring out the pain?

Establishment of a medical diagnosis also is important.[20] Low back disorders actually represent a very heterogeneous group of underlying pathophysiologic sequences (see Chapter 23.4). In addition to regional disorders causing back pain, the pain may be a manifestation of a significant underlying disease unrelated to the low back. The disability evaluation may be the only opportunity for a second opinion or, in some instances, may be the only chance for a specialty evaluation.

History of injury
Distribution of pain in a dermatomal pattern
Muscle spasm
Specific signs on examination
Limitation of range of motion
Observation in a structured setting
Reflex asymmetry
Muscle weakness or atrophy
Thermography
Chiropractic evaluation
Discography
Magnetic resonance imaging
CAT scanning
Electromyography
Nerve conduction studies
Lumbar spine radiographs

Table 8.4 Historical list of objective methods of evaluation of low back pain

Many methods have been proposed for 'objective' evaluation of low back pain. Some of these methods are listed in Table 8.4. Unfortunately, many of these methods have not been well validated. In addition, the most objective of these methods primarily apply to low back disorders that involve neural damage (either to the spinal cord or peripheral nerves at the root). The majority of patients with low back disorders do not have demonstrable abnormalities of spinal canal or foraminal encroachment.

Assessment of pulmonary impairment and disability

The pulmonary system may be objectively assessed by numerous functional tests as well as imaging studies. However, even though current functional status may generally be objectively and reasonably precisely measured, determination of impairment (functional loss) and disability/work ability are still somewhat imprecise.[21-23]

Spirometry, static lung volume, diffusing capacity of the lung for carbon monoxide, methacholine challenge testing, and cardiopulmonary exercise testing allow characterization of the physiologic status. These methods are discussed elsewhere (see Chapter 19.1). These tests are not necessary in every case and should be used selectively.[24] For example, exercise testing is necessary only when the pulmonary function testing is equivocal. If spirometry and diffusing capacity are both strikingly abnormal, exercise testing is unlikely to yield additional information for assessing impairment.[25] Methacholine challenge testing is particularly useful for determining the extent of impairment in individuals with asthma.

In general, a careful history and physical examination should be supplemented with determination of ventilatory (spirometry) and diffusing capacity in nearly all cases. If asthma is a concern, yet spirometry is normal, methacholine challenge may be performed. Similarly, if the basic tests are equivocal or the extent of dyspnea is markedly greater than the degree of abnormality of the basic tests, exercise testing may be useful. There are several well-accepted guidelines for test performance and interpretation.

Determining impairment requires comparing current physiologic status with the condition which would have been present in the absence of respiratory disease/injury. In some instances, the patient had spirometry or other lung function tests performed prior to a specific injury. In many situations, however, the current results must be compared to population norms rather than results for the specific individual. Because the range of 'normal' is large, this introduces some uncertainty; this is particularly true with highly variable tests such as the forced expiratory flow over the mid vital capacity range ($FEF_{25-75\%}$).

Translating clinical pulmonary function tests into work ability/disability determinations requires understanding of the job. Both the typical and the maximal exertion levels must be considered. Most persons can maintain approximately 50% of the maximal attainable oxygen consumption for prolonged time periods but can perform work at higher levels of exertion for briefer episodes.[21,23] Individuals with asthma are more sensitive than others to workplace irritants. Although they may have nearly normal spirometry on the date of clinical testing, workplace conditions may cause reduction in lung function.

Occupational asthma due to allergic sensitization to workplace chemical or biologic agents generally precludes any continued exposure.[26] Once sensitized, even low-level exposure can be adverse. Thus, an individual may be disabled for his/her usual job even though lung function testing performed when non-exposed may be normal. For this reason, clear diagnostic distinction between occupational asthma due to allergic sensitization and occupational asthma due to high levels of irritants (such as reactive airways dysfunction syndrome or asthma without latency) is essential. The former situation usually precludes continued work in the specific job, but the latter situation may permit work if irritant levels are controlled to acceptable levels.

Occupational asthma also illustrates the importance of considering adequacy of medical therapy. A person with asthma who is receiving inadequate treatment cannot be evaluated for permanent impairment until appropriate therapy is characterized.

Respiratory disorders, therefore, illustrate the importance of considering workplace as well as clinical factors in assessing impairment. Despite objective testing of function, characterization of the workplace is also important.

Pain

Assessment of pain in the absence of definite objective abnormalities may be complex. The basis of pain itself is poorly understood and probably depends upon a combination of physical and psychologic factors. Pain-related behavior reflects the impact of pain on an individual's life; in some instances, pain becomes chronic as the person's life is organized around this central aspect. It is not surprising that there are frequent differences of opinion in the assessment of impairment in disability related to pain per se. Some syndromes such as the chronic regional pain syndromes (e.g. reflex sympathetic dystrophy) are controversial and depend very heavily on subjective findings. To the extent possible, evaluating physicians should be as objective as possible, describing the areas of pain and the impact on life, and avoiding advocacy for or against the 'validity' of symptoms.

While malingering (intentional deception, often for the purpose of financial gain) occurs, it is present in a small minority of individuals claiming disability. Although estimates of the proportion of malingerers among chronic pain subjects have ranged from 1% to 10%, the data supporting this are weak.[27] Although not foolproof, several clinical signs (commonly called the Waddell signs) are suggestive that an organic basis is absent.[28] For example, compression of the head while standing is unlikely to produce back pain in most cases on a purely organic basis.

GENERAL APPROACH TO EVALUATION

The principles outlined in the first section and the specific organ system examples discussed subsequently illustrate the breadth of approaches that are necessary for impairment and disability assessment. Such an evaluation must be performed as objectively as possible. In theory, since the underlying principles are the same, a clinician should reach the same conclusions about the impairment and disability of a specific patient whether the patient is being seen for a preplacement evaluation or a disability evaluation.

Impairment and disability evaluations are frequently performed in the context of an administrative, regulatory, or legal procedure. Therefore, the examiner should define the specific needs of the overall system of which the evaluation is part. Table 8.5 lists several questions about the role of the particular evaluation to guide report prepara-

1. Why was I selected as examiner?
2. To whom does the report go? Will it be used as a medicolegal document?
3. How 'technical' should the report be? Will it be read by a physician, or is it primarily for non-clinicians?
4. Who is paying for the evaluation? Will they fund extensive documentation?
5. What is the scope of the report (whole person or simply one organ system or one injury)?
6. Is impairment alone the concern, or is disability also to be discussed?
7. Should ability to do a specific job (e.g., most recent) be discussed or is evaluation more generic?
8. Must non-occupational and occupationally caused illness be differentiated?
9. Should my opinions about causation be stated?
10. Will there be another opportunity to evaluate the patient again, or must this truly be a *final* report?
11. Are there particular 'rating terms' that I must use in specific senses? If so, were these terms defined in writing for me?
12. If the problem is occupational, must I prepare a separate report to public health authorities?
13. What specific documentation must be included (e.g., hard copies of spirometry, specific statement listing each staff member who spoke with patient)?
14. How shall the results be communicated to the patient?
15. Am I allowed to treat the patient now or in the future?

Table 8.5 Questions for perspective on preparing reports

tion. Because the medical role is only part of the disability assessment process, effective communication is essential, and the written report should be carefully prepared and reviewed prior to submission; it should not be dashed off as an afterthought following the examination.

Answering the specific questions posed at the time of referral is important. The evaluator should determine whether impairment, disability, or handicap should be addressed. There should be clear separation of subjective and objective data. The rationale for conclusions reached should be stated. When there is some residual uncertainty, this factor also should be identified. In some instances, the physician is simply an information transducer (e.g., reporting the FEV_1 or the ROM of the left elbow) and no conclusions are requested. Other systems request the physician's opinion as well as objective fact. In these circumstances, the physician's opinion should be identified as such. Furthermore, when issues of causation are involved, clinicians should feel comfortable in carefully delineating their area of expertise and commenting only within that area. For example, many cardiologists can very effectively describe the functional impact of a cardiomyopathy but have not had sufficient training in epidemiology, toxicology, or industrial hygiene to discuss whether or not a putative cobalt exposure at work produced a cardiomyopathy.

Finally, certain terms have very specific meanings in many administrative systems. The written reports of physicians are often interpreted extremely literally by individuals who seek to translate specific terms into administrative action or compensation. Therefore, the report should be carefully composed and specific words should be used with appropriate clarification. For example, in many of the workers' compensation systems in the United States, the choice between the adverbs 'probably' and 'possibly' describing causation may determine if a compensatory award is made. Similarly, in some systems, ordered terms such as 'slight,' 'moderate' and 'severe' have very specific meanings and should be used in the context of the system. When uncertain of the specific meaning of one of these terms, the examiner may append a phrase illustrating his or her meaning, such as, 'He has *moderate* pain in the knee, such that he walks more slowly but does not have to remain in a chair'. Amplifying terms in this fashion defers the responsibility for assigning specific ratings to the program administrators.

Role of guidelines and standards

Guidelines and formal standards are used in several ways as summarized in Table 8.6. They may be purely advisory, offering educational suggestions, or they may be mandatory, defining precisely how the clinician must proceed. Some are translational, providing tables to inter-convert clinical and administrative systems or impairment and disability. They may also serve legal purposes. Even if somewhat arbitrary, the presence of standards fosters consistency (and hence fairness) among individuals.

There are many published sets of guidelines for assessment and rating. The most comprehensive and influential

Education of clinicians
Suggestions to clinicians
Default procedures and rating scheme
Used unless clinician has a rationale for alternative
Quality assurance: defines minimum data requirements
Prescriptive
Mandatory without major rebuttal effort
Regulatory
Arbitrary but consistent
Translational
Converts impairment into disability by formula

Table 8.6 Utilization of guidelines and standards for assessing impairment and disability

set is the Guidelines to the Evaluation of Permanent Impairment of the American Medical Association (the 'AMA Guidelines'). The fifth edition was published in 2001. This work is comprehensive and includes sections for most organ systems (including mental). It represents the opinion of a series of expert committees appointed by the AMA. Prior to release, the AMA sent the Guidelines for external review. The AMA Guidelines offer a practically oriented approach to defining clinical data to be collected (history, exam, tests). They also contain numerous tables for converting clinical data into numerical summary indexes. For example, tables suggest using lung function tests to categorize patients into one of four classes of impairment. In addition, the Guidelines seek to provide a common scale across different body parts. The AMA Guidelines are widely accepted.[29]

Several state workers' compensations systems and non-US entities also have produced rating guidelines. Unlike the AMA, some were produced by governmental agencies and carry regulatory force. In addition, professional organizations have produced organ system-specific guidelines for impairment and/or work ability/disability.[30]

Although many of the sets of guidelines contain basic tables, they generally are not meant to be fully prescriptive. Rather, they permit (and encourage) clinicians to use good judgment and to consider additional relevant information. However, in some settings, their use is mandatory and fully prescriptive. This creates a problem when the Guidelines are updated.

The AMA Guidelines and many others explicitly are limited to translating clinical findings into rating of impairment per se rather than disability. The AMA Guidelines explicitly state that the rating scheme is for 'activities of daily living, excluding work'. The Guidelines state, 'impairment ratings are not intended for use as directed determinants of work disability'. Therefore, the percentage ratings and class system should not be directly translated into work disability assessments: 'Impairment percentages derived from the Guides should not be used as direct estimates of disability.' Thus, the impairment percentage ratings are not related to income loss or other measures of disability.

By contrast, several systems directly relate clinical findings into disability terms. The US Social Security Disability Insurance system uses tables of clinical test and examination results to discern applicants who are disabled for substantial gainful employment. Certain state workers' compensation systems also seek to directly interrelate clinical findings into disability and consequent monetary awards. Others, such as California, allow clinicians or 'rating bureaus' to indicate the work loss due to the impairment.

Rating schemes: principles and validity

In a preplacement or fitness for duty evaluation, the clinician's focus is upon a specific individual, as is the case with most diagnostic and therapeutic considerations. However, often in assessing disability for compensation purposes, the clinician's role is not primarily as a patient advocate, but to document objectively and without bias. Generally, there is a non-clinical context for selecting the amount of awards (e.g., rating tables). The system seeks a fair balance among the rights of worker applicants, employers, and governments. There are often very disparate awards for the same impairment depending upon the social context. Workers' compensation benefits vary considerably among states. Where work causation is an issue, the standard of proof varies considerably, as does the underlying logic employed.[31] In comparison to workers' compensation, tort awards often are larger but require a higher standard of proof.

The validity of assessment systems has received only limited attention.[3] Most often, schemes are derived from consensus of expert opinion or political compromise rather than empiric data. However, some have provided limited evaluation by showing that there is a demonstrated correlation between adverse health impact associated with award or diagnosis.[32-34] For instance, mortality is higher among applicants who receive awards than among those who do not.[35] In addition, the economic impact of a diagnosed disease has been evaluated in several studies by follow-up of cohorts of applicants.[36]

References

1. Blanck PD, Pransky G. Workers with disabilities. Occup Med 1999; 14:581–93.
2. Himmelstein JS. Worker fitness and risk evaluations in context. Occup Med 1988; 3:169–78.
3. Harber P, Hsu P, Chen W. An 'atomic' approach to dis/ability assessment. J Occup Environ Med 1996; 38:359–66.
4. Shusterman DJ, Dager SR. Prevention of psychological disability after occupational exposures. Occup Med 1991; 6:11–27.
5. Knudson RJ, Slatin RC, Lebowitz MD, Burrows B. The maximal expiratory flow-volume curve. Normal standards, and effects of age. Am Rev Respir Dis 1976; 113:587–600.
6. Petersen M, Hankinson J. Spirometry reference values for nonexposed blue-collar workers. J Occup Med 1985; 27:644–50.
7. Miller A, Thornton JC, Warshaw R, Bernstein J, Selikoff IJ, Teirstein AS. Mean and instantaneous expiratory flows, FVC and FEV1: prediction equations from a probability sample of Michigan. Bull Eur Physiopathol Respir 1986; 22:589–9.
8. Bigos SJ, Battie MC, Spengler DM et al. A longitudinal, prospective study of industrial back injury reporting. Clin Orthop 1992; 21–34.
9. Bigos SJ, Battie MC, Spengler DM et al. A prospective study of work perceptions and psychosocial factors affecting the report

of back injury [published erratum appears in Spine 1991; 16:688]. Spine 1991; 16:1–6.
10. Elam K, Taylor V, Ciol MA, Franklin GM, Deyo RA. Impact of a worker's compensation practice guideline on lumbar fusion in Washington State. Med Care 1997; 35:417–24.
11. Feuerstein M, Berkowitz SM, Huang GD. Predictors of occupational low back disability: implications for secondary prevention. J Occup Environ Med 1999; 41:1024–31.
12. Krause N, Lynch J, Kaplan GA, Cohen RD, Goldberg DE, Salonen JT. Predictors of disability retirement. Scand J Work Environ Health 1997; 23:403–13.
13. Turner JA, Franklin G, Turk DC. Predictors of chronic disability in injured workers: a systematic literature synthesis. Am J Ind Med 2000; 38:707–22.
14. Oleske DM, Andersson GB, Lavender SA, Hahn JJ. Association between recovery outcomes for work-related low back and personal, family, and work factors. Spine 2000; 25:1259–65.
15. Colledge AL, Johns RE, Jr, Thomas MH. Functional ability assessment: guidelines for the workplace. J Occup Environ Med 1999; 41:172–80.
16. Asfour SS, Ayoub MM, Mital A, Bethea NJ. Perceived exertion of physical effort for various manual handling. Am Ind Hyg Assoc J 1983; 44:223–8.
17. Keyserling WM, Herrin GD, Chaffin DB. Isometric strength testing as a means of controlling medical strenuous jobs. J Occup Med 1980; 22:332–6.
18. Chaffin DB, Herrin GD, Keyserling WM, Garg A. A method for evaluating the biomechanical stresses resulting from materials handling jobs. Am Ind Hyg Assoc J 1977; 38:662–75.
19. Keyserling WM, Herrin GD, Chaffin DB, Armstrong TJ, Foss ML. Establishing an industrial strength testing program. Am Ind Hyg Assoc J 1980; 41:730–6.
20. Johanning E. Evaluation and management of occupational low back disorders. Am J Ind Med 2000; 37:94–111.
21. Armstrong BW, Workman JM, Hurt HH Jr, Roemich WR. Clinico-physiologic evaluation of physical working capacity in with pulmonary disease. Rationale and application of a method estimating maximal oxygen-consuming capacity from MBC and O2ve. Am Rev Respir Dis 1966; 93:223–33.
22. Harber P. The evaluation of pulmonary fitness and risk. Occup Med 1988; 3:285–98.
23. Roemmich W, Blumenfeld HL, Moritz H. Evaluating remaining capacity to work in miner applicants with pneumoconiosis under 65 years of age under Title IV of Public Law. Ann NY Acad Sci 1972; 200:608–16.
24. Harber P, Discher D. Occupational respiratory function testing – an algorithm. Occup Med 1997; 12:485–512.
25. Cotes JE, Zejda J, King B. Lung function impairment as a guide to exercise limitation in lung disorders. Am Rev Respir Dis 1988; 137:1089–93.
26. American Thoracic Society. Guidelines for the evaluation of impairment/disability in asthma. Am Rev Respir Dis 1993; 147:1056–61.
27. Fishbain DA, Cutler R, Rosomoff HL, Rosomoff RS. Chronic pain disability exaggeration/malingering and submaximal research. Clin J Pain 1999; 15:244–74.
28. Waddell G, McCulloch JA, Kummel E, Venner RM. Nonorganic physical signs in low-back pain. Spine 1989; 5:117–25.
29. Cocchiarella L, Turk MA, Andersson G. Improving the evaluation of permanent impairment. JAMA 2000; 283:532–3.
30. American Thoracic Society. Evaluation of impairment/disability secondary to respiratory disorders. Am Rev Respir Dis 1986; 133:1205–9.
31. Harber P, Shusterman D. Medical causation analysis heuristics. J Occup Environ Med 1996; 38:577–86.
32. Liss GM, Tarlo SM, Banks D, Yeung KS, Schweigert M. Preliminary report of mortality among workers compensated for asthma. Am J Ind Med 1999; 35:465–71.
33. Liss GM, Tarlo SM, Macfarlane Y, Yeung KS. Hospitalization among workers compensated for occupational injury. Am J Respir Crit Care Med 2000; 162:112–8.

34. Rosenman KD, Stanbury MJ, Reilly MJ. Mortality among persons with silicosis reported to disease systems in Michigan and New Jersey in the United States. Scand J Work Environ Health 1995; 21:73–6.

35. Coutts II, Gilson JC, Kerr IH, Parkes WR, Turner-Warwick M. Mortality in cases of asbestosis diagnosed by a pneumoconiosis panel. Thorax 1987; 42:111–6.

36. Ameille J, Pairon JC, Bayeux MC et al. Consequences of occupational asthma on employment and financial follow-up study. Eur Respir J 1997; 10: 55–8.

Chapter 9
Social Issues in the Practice of Occupational and Environmental Medicine

Mark R Cullen, Linda Rosenstock

Individuals seek the services of an OEM practitioner for a broad array of reasons. In workplaces with in-house or contractual medical services, patient choice is limited to either utilizing these or seeking care elsewhere; in emergencies there is no option. For practitioners outside this setting, sources of referral include primary practitioners and other medical specialists, as well as such diverse parties as employers, lawyers, unions, insurance companies, and government agencies. Sometimes it is the patient who encourages the referral or who directly refers him- or herself.

The referral source may influence the context and basis for the evaluation. Patient expectations also have important ramifications, both during the diagnostic evaluation and after. Understanding the expectations of the patient and referring party early in the evaluation process is a central tenet of OEM practice.

In this chapter, we shall explore the major *non-biologic* issues – social, economic and legal – that arise in practice, and introduce the ethical responsibilities that accrue in this practice domain.

THE AGENDA OF PATIENTS AND THIRD PARTIES
The patient's agenda

There are three areas of relevant inquiry into understanding the patient's perception of and interest in an OEM examination: health perception and concern, job situation, and life situation.

Health perception
Individuals seek medical care generally because they have been injured, are experiencing symptoms or are concerned about future health risks. These are the most common reasons to seek OEM evaluation as well, whether the visit is mandated or voluntary. Changes in the societal view about chemicals and other hazards, notification requirements of new laws, wide public attention to certain hazards and extensive information available over the internet – of variable quality – have created more awareness about risk and, to some extent also, confusion. Individuals generally have too little knowledge to apply probabilistic reasoning and are often unsophisticated about the influence of dose on risk (see Chapters 1 and 5). At one end of the spectrum, patients may have been led to believe that a minor exposure has conferred an imminent risk of serious disease. At

the other end are disbelievers who deny or underestimate risks and fail to act appropriately, either in terms of limiting their exposures or undertaking recommended surveillance examinations.

Distorted perceptions of risk and harm may be closely linked to social issues, such as a community's fight against a toxic waste site or a union's struggle for a new contract. Misleading information may have come as well from a highly respected source within the patient's circle – including poorly informed physicians or other health professionals, however well intended. Moreover, correct information may sound disturbingly like information provided by an employer, a suspect polluter or the government, agents the patient may have come to mistrust.

For these reasons and more, it is important to know not only what the patient believes might be going on but the basis for that belief. Responses to this line of inquiry, ideally early in the evaluation process, often disclose the reason(s) for the visit and better define the context in which the clinician can perform most effectively.

Exploring the current job situation
In addition to being a potential source of health risk, work is also a central and crucial component of life for most adults, encompassing both positive and negative aspects. On the positive side, work provides a basis for identity and self-worth, an organizing principle for time, the primary source of income, and a series of relationships, including those with superiors, colleagues, and those supervised. On the negative side, work also provides one of the most enduring of life's stresses, a distraction from family and friends and a source of alienation and self-doubt.

Moreover, work is not necessarily constant in any of these features. Tasks and personnel fluctuate, responsibilities grow or diminish, and the economic picture is always subject to change, sometimes with minimal warning. Given this spectrum of roles that work may fulfill and its inherent variability, it is not surprising that social and personal factors related to work may impact patient management to a larger degree in OEM practice than in other specialties. For the clinician, the following two important questions should always be answered.

1. To what extent are these work factors (above and beyond specific environmental health risks per se) responsible for the timing and presentation of illness?

This question is central in several settings. An example is seen in the older worker who presents with a chronic or slowly progressive disorder, such as mild central nervous system, musculoskeletal, or respiratory dysfunction. While these problems typically evolve over years, the timing of presentation often coincides with other disturbances or changes at work, such as increasing difficulty accomplishing former tasks (often with some attendant rebuke or discipline), threat of job security from younger workers, perceived obsolescence of the job itself, or the possibility of a plant closing or lay-off. Deeper concerns about the work situation also afflict displaced workers who have moved into unaccustomed jobs, as well as formerly unemployed persons who have been pressed into the job market unexpectedly by economic needs, such as former welfare recipients or 'housewives'.

Whatever the setting, correct diagnosis and treatment require that the clinician understand the patient's conscious or not so conscious agenda for seeking attention at the time they do. For older workers who are failing at their jobs, aggressive approaches at rehabilitation based solely on health considerations are doomed to fail. Assistance with the often traumatic but appropriate transition to the next phase of life is probably more likely to meet the needs of patient and employer alike. For younger or transitional workers, early health concerns may be important signs of a constitutional mismatch between worker and job. In these instances, blind focus on treatment and return to work without consideration of larger issues may lead to costly and ineffective treatment options.

2. To what extent will work factors limit the range of options available for managing a work-related – or non-work related – health problem?

The willingness and ability of patient and employer to accept medical recommendations that dictate any but the most temporary or trivial change in work depend on many factors unrelated to health. Often, the patient is well aware of these constraints and will explicitly discuss them with the physician. Sometimes, however, they are couched in terms of health, leading to denial or exaggeration of certain complaints based on how the patient perceives they might translate into treatment recommendations. For example, if a patient is struggling with a particular supervisor, factors attributed to that supervisor or work area may be accentuated to the exclusion of other important environmental issues at the workplace. Likewise, a task that is frustrating or onerous might be presented as painful or dangerous. The best approach for the clinician to take is to attempt to elicit these non-health-related factors about the patient's job as early and as explicitly as possible. Such knowledge offers the best way to avoid confounding diagnostic issues by social factors and to focus clinical choices.

Exploring the home and family situation

Although knowledge of family is crucial in the practice of medicine generally and is a usual part of every clinical history, home and family considerations have special importance in the practice of OEM. Work may be a major family stressor because the demands of the individual's job compete against those of his or her family for time and energy. In some cases the earliest effects of work-related illnesses, such as noise-induced hearing loss or central nervous system dysfunction due to metals, solvents, or pesticides, may be first recognized because of their impact on family functioning rather than work functioning. Conversely, stresses within the family may result in changes in work performance, which, in turn, may enhance stresses on the job. Further, perception of risk may differ between those in the work environment, where certain hazards are seemingly accepted, and the family setting, where the possibility of illness or injury is deemed threatening or even unacceptable.

A special consideration in occupational practice is the impact occupational injury or disease may have on family dynamic. A spouse, currently not working or underemployed, may find him- or herself pressed into the role of primary household provider. With family roles other dynamics may also change, stressing primary dependency needs or other dysfunctional responses. These pressures can enormously impact the perception of the patient about what is going on, and the range of options perceived by the patient and family as acceptable. Such stressors may also serve to delay recovery (in patients prone to dependency) or lead to inappropriate risk taking before full recovery (in patients averse to being dependent).

In environmental health outside the workplace, the family takes on a whole new dimension. Here, the home itself may be the focus of concern, because of a hazardous substance perceived to be in the air, walls and furnishings, or water supply. This threat to family health may have symbolic importance that in some cases exceeds health risk or impact. Not only is the home important symbolically, it is often the foundation of the family's economic and social security. People are not easily moved from their homes, even under the direst environmental threats. The prospect of reduced property values based on environmental risk also sharply heightens the sense of threat. The fact that levels of harm or risk from contaminants in or near the home often are modest compared with those in the industrial workplace must never translate into a lesser level of concern or attention paid by clinicians.

Environmental concerns in and around the home also severely stress family dynamics and roles. Often there are issues of blame and responsibility for contamination lurking below the surface, e.g., 'it was *your* idea to build that', or 'it was *you* who wanted to move here', etc. Moreover, the house may have different meanings or value to different family members, whose differing responses to the threat may prove dysfunctional or problematic as therapeutic choices are considered. As in the occupational situation, the most important ramification for practice is to explore these issues in every case, and deeply in circumstances where evident issues surface.

The agenda of third parties

As noted above, OEM is unique among medical specialties in the high fraction of patient referrals initiated by non-physicians, such as employers, insurance companies, and lawyers. Even when patients are referred by physicians, the underlying agendas of outside parties often account for the referrals. Of course the interests of these parties, like the special interests of the patient and family addressed above, do not alter the actual diagnosis or risk. However, like the agendas of the patient, the interests of these parties may serve to distort reality or limit access to information and could, unless recognized, interfere with the clinician's ability to make a correct diagnosis or risk assessment.

Beyond the diagnostic stage, the interests of outside parties have an impact on the range of therapeutic choices, whatever the correct diagnosis. For example, a lawyer or outside advisor might be advising the patient that return to modified work would result in diminished worker compensation payments in the future, resulting in patient resistance to this option. For all these reasons, the current or potential interest or perceptions of each of the major third parties, including employers, lawyers, and insurance carriers, must always be assessed as part of the evaluation of any significant occupational or environmental medical problem.

THE ETHICS OF OCCUPATIONAL AND ENVIRONMENTAL MEDICINE PRACTICE

Relatively little attention has been given to ethical issues faced by physicians who provide healthcare to workers or to those with other environmental concerns or risks. Until now, the focus of the limited ethical debate has largely centered on occupational physicians employed by industry. This focus has neglected the important role of primary care physicians, who frequently face the same ethical dilemmas and are often the point of first contact with the patient. The following discussion identifies ethical issues to be considered by providers regardless of practice setting, recognizing that the dynamic legal and regulatory environment surrounding OEM practice may introduce further complexities.

Ethical problems arise often for physicians who provide health services to workers, although many would argue that it is the frequency rather than the nature of the issues that distinguishes the practice of OEM from other specialties. In fact, the ethical principles universal to all clinical medicine can be applied reasonably to the circumstances of providing healthcare to individuals with known or suspected occupational and environmental conditions. All of these issues, as well as special issues in OEM, such as preplacement or independent medical examinations, are discussed in greater detail in Chapter 55. The following section provides an overview of the principles as applied to six aspects of OEM practice.

Awareness of occupational and environmental health

Physicians are understandably challenged and even intimidated when considering the rapidly changing and growing field of occupational and environmental medicine, and discerning strategies to incorporate relevant material into traditional clinical practice. Increasingly, the patient brings questions of environmental concern to the physician's attention. And physicians, although seen as trusted sources of information, have become identified by patients as generally not well informed about these matters. Many factors have been identified as contributing to physicians' inadequate knowledge about and underinvolvement in the occupational and environmental health arena, including: insufficient medical education; isolation of many of these services and reimbursement from mainstream medical practice; and the increasingly complex array of potential exposures and known, let alone suspected, health effects arising from them.

Nonetheless, the physician in OEM, as in other areas of medicine, has an ethical obligation to be as informed as possible and, perhaps most importantly, to recognize when his or her own knowledge or experience is insufficient to resolve the problem and consultation is needed. In much the same way that a generalist might ask a cardiologist for assistance with a case, physicians faced with potential occupational and environmental health problems that are beyond their own capabilities or resources should seek professionals with appropriate expertise. This minimum standard, maintaining awareness about occupational and environmental health risks or conditions, is a fundamental ethical principle and one that, at least in the United States, is likely to be accompanied by legal responsibility as well. Judicial opinion has held that the physician exploring a health problem that may have an occupational basis bears a responsibility to inquire fully into the work history of a patient.

The physician–patient relationship

The physician–patient relationship is the foundation on which virtually all activities in clinical medicine rest. This relationship is frequently challenged in occupational and environmental medicine practice, but ethical and legal considerations common to general medical practice can be applied even to situations seemingly unique to this field.

Loyalty
Long a basic tenet of medical ethics in general, the primary loyalty of a physician is to his/her patient. Although there is evidence to substantiate the concern among workers that physicians employed by industry have not always followed this dictum, the issue of loyalty is by no means confined to the company physician. Physicians in all aspects of clinical practice may face the challenge of having payment and referral sources shape the nature of their interaction with the patient; pressure to respond to competing needs is sometimes explicit and often implicit. Whether the pressure arises from the direct financial interest of an employer or cost containment effort of an insurance carrier or preferred provider organization, the response to it may not always serve the patient's best interests.

Physicians providing occupational and, to a lesser extent, environmental health services must appreciate that although ideally both the patient's and any third party's interests are best served by the same good medical practice and preventive interventions, these ends can and do at times come in conflict. In these challenging but not infrequent situations, the physician must rely on the primary ethical responsibility to serve the patient's needs first. This mandate is derived from the larger context of the physician–patient relationship, although a possible exception is the setting of preplacement examinations, which is discussed later in this section.

Confidentiality

The patient's right to confidentiality in all aspects of the physician–patient relationship is another basic principle of medical care. Perhaps more than in most areas of specialization, the disclosure of information about evaluation and treatment of known or suspected occupational or environmental conditions has the potential to cause serious harm to the individual and may affect the individual's employment security. Although recent regulatory efforts in the United States and elsewhere have tried to ensure that information obtained from medical records cannot be used to block hiring or continued employment, the information can still be seriously damaging. In caring for individuals with occupational and environmental conditions, once a doctor–patient relationship is formed, the usual rules of confidentiality should apply.

Confidentiality refers to both the written and verbal release of information. Medical records should be maintained to optimize protection; patients should sign a release form for any information that is to be disclosed to a third party (and he or she should have a reasonable understanding of the implications of doing so), and no record should be released to a third party unless the patient has signed a release form. Just as important, patients must be informed of the special circumstances in which confidentiality cannot be protected. For example, once a workers' compensation claim is filed, confidentiality can no longer be protected in reference to information relating to that claim because the employer and appropriate agencies have legal access to it. Medical records can be subpoenaed, as will often happen if the patient becomes involved in litigation such as third-party liability. Mandatory reporting of occupational diseases in many countries and jurisdictions contributes another breach of the usual confidence; the patient should be so advised.

The over-riding ethical obligation to maintain patient confidentiality is not absolute, and there are situations other than those legally mandated in which it may be more appropriate to reveal than withhold information that the patient wishes to be kept confidential. Such decisions to violate confidentiality undoubtedly should be rare and need serious consideration on a case-by-case basis. In addition, the circumstances in which they may arise are not unique to OEM. They fall in two general categories: either in the patient's best interests or because of an over-riding duty to protect the public health (such as notification of contacts in venereal disease cases). What arises more commonly in OEM practice than in virtually all other fields is that the detection of disease or hazardous exposures in one person may point to the probability that the same problem may arise with other coworkers, household members, and community residents. In instances in which concern about others is sufficiently high, consideration must be given to the serious step of breaching confidentiality.

Patient advocacy and conflicts of interest

Practitioners who provide occupational or environmental medicine services, particularly those who do so in the context of a broader general practice, may face the challenge of making objective decisions about patient illnesses and employability when they have a personal, emotional, or financial interest in these patients and their families. This potential conflict, of course, is not unique to the occupational or environmental health arena; society relies on physicians to undertake a number of activities that are aimed primarily at societal welfare rather than the benefit of individual patients or their families.

Included in these are physical examinations for insurance, participation in sports, or disability purposes. Here, it is either the public at large or some subset, including special interest groups, who ask the physician to make judgments that may differ from an individual patient's desires or interests. The physician often can decline to perform such evaluations; however, this approach is not always possible and, even when it is, does not necessarily result in an equitable solution. The best approach to use in cases in which patient advocacy may conflict with the physician's objectively performing an appropriate and reasonably requested social function is to apply ethical principles of loyalty and confidentiality and to inform the patient fully of explicit and implicit uses of such information. The specific circumstance of medical screening that may stress the physician–patient relationship either for or against advocacy is discussed in Chapter 3.

Disclosure to patients

Another fundamental aspect of the physician–patient relationship is informing patients fully about their conditions, including reasons for and against various diagnostic and therapeutic strategies. In conditions related to occupational or environmental factors, this requires full discussion about the implications of undertaking evaluations, including legal or other constraints on protecting confidentiality, and the implications of treatment interventions. The last-mentioned issue is particularly important given the major impact of therapeutic choices that may include job or home modification or relocation so that the individual can avoid continued hazardous exposure. The physician has a responsibility to discuss the range of reasonable choices, acknowledging that sometimes the optimal medical choice may be forsaken for one less ideal because of the social, economic, or legal ramifications. Included in the ethical responsibilities of disclosure are providing information and participating as dictated by local custom and regulations in the workers' compensation process, however irksome.

Reporting to third parties

In addition to disclosing information about environmental risks to the patient, the physician has an ethical and occasionally legally mandated responsibility to notify third parties (e.g., employers, agencies, insurance carriers) who would benefit from information derived from the physician–patient relationship. The potential to instigate meaningful preventive activities by undertaking this follow-up of suspected or known occupational or environmental diseases or risks is one of the most satisfying aspects of clinical practice in OEM. In the United States, legal responsibilities to report these conditions vary considerably from state to state; however, independent from legal mandates, physicians should identify the most appropriate means to report these risks or conditions.

Examples of reporting include: notifying local or state health departments, regulatory agencies, employers, and unions; publishing in scientific journals; and, in certain instances, informing the public through the media. Which, if any, of these avenues should be pursued depends on numerous factors, including the seriousness of the risk and the likelihood of occurrence in others. Unless there are extraordinary reasons to do otherwise, all actions should be taken with full respect for the promise of confidentiality inherent in the physician–patient relationship. The following sections are a brief overview of those parties the physician should consider contacting in dealing with cases of known or suspected occupational and environmental diseases or hazards.

Employers

After a thorough discussion with the patient about the implications of doing so, the employer, whenever feasible, should be informed about workplace hazards or conditions. The employer is in the best position to undertake preventive action and further environmental or medical assessment as needed. In addition, the employer may be able to provide the physician with additional data on the nature and intensity of exposures that will enhance clinical evaluation of the patient.

Labor unions

In occupational health practice many patients will be members of labor unions. Unions vary in the extent to which they become involved in workplace health and safety issues. In some instances the union may be able to provide valuable exposure information and may directly or indirectly identify other coworkers at risk. They also may be well positioned to optimize the likelihood of appropriate interventions. As with other third parties, the patient must first consent before anything is reported to a union.

Health agencies and referral centers

Local, regional, and national health agencies play variable roles in occupational or environmental health issues. In some settings, the health agency may be the best place to report initially a known or suspected hazard, with subsequent appropriate follow-up delegated to the agency. In other instances, specialty referral centers, such as those affiliated with academic medical centers and hospitals, are best equipped to follow up the results of an individual evaluation. In the United States, the National Institute for Occupational Safety and Health (NIOSH), in addition to its training and research functions, provides consultation services about hazardous workplaces, a function also provided by some state and local health departments.

Regulatory agencies

A number of regulatory agencies, such as the Occupational Safety and Health Administration (OSHA) in the United States, can provide assistance to the physician and respond to reports of occupational hazards or unsafe conditions. In some situations OSHA or its equivalent may be able to provide, on employer request, consultation about workplace hazards without threat of reprisal for violations of the law or best practice. On the other hand, if circumstances warrant and after confidentiality considerations have been reviewed, a physician may file a complaint about a workplace hazard, which, in turn, should generate a regulatory inspection. Although such complaints can be made anonymously, the physician should appreciate and advise the patient that the nature of the complaint may nonetheless result in their identification and possible subsequent harm.

Similarly, agencies that are involved in control of the non-workplace environment, such as the federal Environmental Protection Agency (EPA) and related state and local agencies in the United States, may be contacted. In both occupational or other environmental settings, these agencies may also have valuable information about exposures and results of past investigations or monitoring that may aid the physician in the clinical assessment.

News media

Often parties impacted by environmental or occupational hazards, or their health providers, may perceive the news media as a particularly rapid and effective means of disseminating information. While this is undoubtedly true, it must be borne in mind that that such media are neither peer reviewed nor without their own strong agendas – for drama, conflict, human interest and polarization. While this may make good copy, it often serves to confuse issues and inflame already complex health situations. In general, practitioners should resort to this pathway only as a very last resort. Even when reporters directly approach the practitioner for information, extreme discretion is advised: what a clinician believes he or she has said may or may not be what a reporter has heard, or what his/her editor chooses to print or show on television as a soundbite. These issues are further discussed in Chapter 60.

Litigation

Hanging over many occupational and environmental health situations is litigation – actual, threatened or feared. Other than workers' compensation, a no-fault insurance scheme, the demands of litigation often lead to hyperpolarization and extreme responses, severely limiting clinical options. These issues are discussed in detail in Chapters 56 and 57. For present purposes, suffice it to say that practitioners should always assess whether legal action is pending or anticipated, and appreciate the possible role(s) it may play in delimiting the behaviors of patient and third parties alike.

Chapter 10
Susceptible Populations

Jessica Herzstein

Our society has become increasingly concerned about the health consequences of exposure to chemical and physical agents in outdoor and indoor environments. As we acquire more knowledge regarding the basic adverse health effects of the spectrum of environmental exposures, it is becoming clear that certain groups are more susceptible to the toxicity of specific environmental exposures than is the general population. These susceptible groups may experience exposure-related health problems that others do not have at all, or the health effects may be more severe or occur earlier in time or at a lower exposure levels than is seen in the general population.

Public policy is beginning to reflect the need to consider differences in vulnerability among subpopulations. For example, USEPA cancer guidelines promote the incorporation of information on susceptibility.[1] The Presidential Commission on Risk Assessment and Risk Management has recommended that the USEPA use accurate data on susceptible populations, including molecular epidemiology and other population-based information, to determine the magnitude of variability in disease risk. Human risk assessment methodology in current use does not usually include measures of susceptibility.[2] Another example of public policy responding to the potential for health effects in a vulnerable population is the agreement by USEPA and manufacturers to eliminate the application of the insecticide chlorpyrifos in places where children could be exposed (homes, schools, day-care centers, stores, etc.). The 1996 Food Quality Protection Act requires EPA to review pesticides to ensure they meet new standards specifically designed to protect children.[3] The review of chlorpyrifos is part of that process.

Strategies to improve environmental health have focused on reduction of exposure in the workplace and in the indoor and outdoor environment. Societal interventions to lower risk have addressed the population as a whole (e.g., all persons with exposure above the maximum contaminant level (MCL) to arsenic or trichloroethylene (TCE)) and have not focused on genetic and acquired differences among individuals, which may allow development of more effective policies. Assuming similar biologic responses from all persons for a specified dose of a toxic agent may not offer sufficient protection for certain subgroups.[4] Default safety factors used in human risk assessment are controversial and may be overprotective or underprotective of certain segments of the population. Developing standards for environmental quality that protect the average person has been criticized for overlooking vulnerable groups who may suffer significant harm

from low-level exposures. Principles for applying greater precaution to children's environmental health policy have been proposed.[5] More mechanistic information is needed in order to understand how genetics, behavior, and age influence an individual's response to an environmental agent.

The goal of this chapter is to review major subgroups within the larger population who may be particularly susceptible to environmental exposures. Existing data on common exposures that may cause increased toxicity for certain groups are summarized, emphasizing those populations at risk and exposures on which some empiric information is currently available or on which a risk-exposure relationship is anticipated on theoretical grounds. For most environmental chemicals, data on susceptible subgroups have not been collected. Most of the existing data are controversial or preliminary. Research focusing on identification of markers for host susceptibility has identified promising areas but also significant limitations. To date, markers for host susceptibility have minimal clinical applications.[6]

As a caveat, it must be emphasized at the outset that host-response differences are highly complex. In many areas, only one aspect of an obviously multifaceted problem has been studied. In turn, studies have conspicuous methodological flaws. Issues such as dose and duration of exposure, documentation of exposure, and presence of confounding factors arise with most of the populations and hazards studied. Therefore, no attempt is made to offer definitive answers to these important questions, nor should any of the following information be applied dogmatically in practice. Although clinicians need to know how these adverse effects can be recognized early, treated, and prevented - and policy makers need to ensure protection from environmental hazards for some sensitive populations - the main objective here is to define the scientific basis for the role host factors play in response to specific environmental agents.

A person's response to environmental agents is affected by physiologic variables including exposure routes and absorption (respiratory minute ventilation, dermal penetration, etc.), pharmacokinetics (distribution, metabolism, excretion) and pharmacodynamics (receptor density and specificity, target organ). These variables are each significantly affected by constitutive factors (genetics, age, gender, ethnicity) and acquired factors (altered health state, effects of previous or concurrent exposures, diet, exercise, and stress). To simplify these complex sets of possibilities, three main groups of host factors are presented:

Behavioral, genetic, and lifestyle factors
    Genetic factors
    Tobacco smoking
    Ethanol intake
    Stress
    Dietary intake
Age-defined populations
    Fetus and child
        Air pollution
        Indoor air pollution
        Carcinogens
        Neurotoxins
    The elderly
        Neurotoxicants
        Air pollution
        Carcinogen exposure
Risks associated with pre-existing conditions
    Chronic lung disease
        Asthma
        COPD
    Heart disease
    Diabetes
    Obesity

Table 10.1 Host factors modifying environmental susceptibility

personal (lifestyle, genetic, behavioral), age related, and underlying disease related. These factors are summarized in Table 10.1.

GENETIC, BEHAVIORAL, AND LIFESTYLE FACTORS
Genetic factors

In contrast to the increasing amount of data about the effect of biologic phenotypes on risk of environmental susceptibility, scant empiric data exist regarding the relationship between genotype and disease susceptibility. It is widely recognized by experimentalists and epidemiologists that hosts vary enormously in their response to comparable doses of environmental agents. However, the number of genetic polymorphisms or identifiable genetic differences that have been pinpointed to explain such differences are few. Susceptibility occurring on the basis of genetic variation is likely to play an increasingly important role in risk assessment. Genetic modulation of exposure risk incorporates the concept that following exposure at low levels, disease can be detected only among sensitive genotypes. These genotypic subgroups may herald risks for the greater population.

A great deal of research now focuses on genetic polymorphisms impacting the risk of cancer. The polymorphisms involving metabolic enzyme genes, cell cycle control genes and DNA repair have complex effects and their specific roles in different cancers are unclear. Areas of promising work in polymorphisms affecting lung cancer include the following: myeloperoxidase-induced metabolism of benzo[a]pyrene which results in DNA adducts and mutation; glutathione S-transferase which activates and deactivates carcinogens and can promote elimination of anticarcinogens such as isothiocyanates; and DNA repair genes. Understanding which are the common genes impacting cancer risk has been a slow process involving a few genes at a time in case control studies. Future work will likely benefit from advances such as nested cohorts, non-invasive specimen collection, and rapid genotyping.

Susceptibility genes, defined as common polymorphic genes found in over 1% of the population, affect activation and detoxification of environmental agents. Specific environmental exposures are required to induce disease associated with susceptibility genes. Although only a modest risk of disease is associated with carrying these genes, they pose an important public health problem because large numbers of people can be affected. An overview of common polymorphisms that interact with environmental agents to cause cancer and other diseases is presented in Table 10.2.[7-9] Differences in the expression of these enzymes are likely to yield differences in susceptibility to both carcinogenic and non-carcinogenic exposures. The onset and the severity of the resulting disease are determined by the combination of genetic and environmental factors.

Epidemiologic studies of polymorphic metabolic genes have concentrated on cancer. Less than 20% of long-term smokers develop lung cancer in their lifetime. Genetically determined factors that negate the effects of environmental carcinogens may explain differences in susceptibility. Lung cancer risk is dependent on the dose of tobacco carcinogens. This dose is modulated by genetic polymorphisms in the enzymes that activate and detoxify these carcinogens, as well as by the efficiency of host cells in

Cancer: metabolic (activation and inactivation)	Cancer: DNA repair	Non-cancer
cyt P450 (CYP)-dependent oxygenase systems (PAHs and lung cancer)	DNA repair capability measured as mutagen sensitivity (e.g. to bleomycin) (Ataxia telangiectasis, Fanconi's anemia, xeroderma pigmentosum)	Paraoxonase: inactivation of toxic metabolite (paraoxon) of organophosphate & carbamate pesticides (neurologic disease)
Glutathione S-transferase (GST) (a) metabolize mutagenic intermediates of CYP-mediated oxygenation reactions (b) metabolize PAH constituents of tobacco smoke (lung cancer and bladder cancer)		Alpha antitrypsin (emphysema) HLA alleles (may be associated by beryllium oxide-induced lung disease and acid anhydride-induced asthma) Aminolevulinate dehydrase (lead retention)

Table 10.2 Genetic polymorphisms associated with environmentally related disease

monitoring and repairing DNA damage caused by tobacco carcinogen. Recent research has shown that individuals with susceptible genotypes tend to develop lung cancer at earlier ages and with lower levels of tobacco exposure than do individuals with non-susceptible genotypes.[10] Forthcoming technology will enable the performance of large-scale and low-cost genotyping of nested cohorts and will allow the identification of smokers with the highest risk of developing cancer. These individuals would be candidates for the most intensive preventive interventions.

The metabolism of xenobiotics involves hydrolysis, oxidation and other reactions that lead to the formation of compounds that are more hydrophilic. The enzymes involved in the biotransformation reactions include cytochrome P450 (CYP), alcohol dehydrogenase, aldehyde dehydrogenase and glutathione S-transferase (GST). Bladder cancer and lung cancer occur at a higher frequency among persons with defective GST genes. Fifty to sixty percent of Caucasians and 30% of African-Americans are homozygous for the null allele of GSTM1; this is associated with a higher risk for lung and bladder cancer and possibly skin and colon cancer. The elevated cancer risk requires gene–environment interaction; non-smokers with GSTM1 null phenotype do not show elevated risk, whereas smokers with the phenotype have a 2–6 times higher cancer risk. GSTM1 homozygous null phenotype has also been associated with a statistically significant lung cancer risk in never-smoking women exposed to high levels of environmental tobacco smoke (ETS).[11]

The CYP family of enzymes includes many genetic variants and a wide spectrum of interindividual variability exists in humans, resulting in up to a 10-fold difference in metabolic activity by CYP. Smoking-induced lung cancer has been associated with altered genotypes in several CYP450 enzymes.[12] CYP2E1 metabolizes over 80 xenobiotic substances, including nitrosamines and chlorinated solvents. A wide range of interindividual variability (10–50-fold) as well as inter-racial variability has been observed with CYP2E1 activity. Molecular markers have documented differences in these metabolic genes among certain populations. Lacking data relating polymorphisms directly to enzymatic activity, the markers are not currently useful clinically for predicting disease risk.

An individual's genetic make-up also plays an important role in determining his or her susceptibility to environmentally related illness other than cancer. For example, the increased sensitivity of some persons to the effects of lead may be due to the existence of genetic polymorphisms in delta-aminolevulinic acid dehydratase (ALAD). Individuals with ALAD1 allele are more likely to experience toxicity with lead exposure. Notably, lead workers have a higher prevalence of the ALAD2 allele.[8] Occasionally, a genetic predisposition may require an environmental exposure for expression of disease. For example, multiple sclerosis appears to require the combination of a specific genetic factor and exposure to an unidentified environmental factor prior to adulthood. Also, males with the X-linked glucose-6-phosphate dehydrogenase deficiency are predisposed to hemolytic crises from a number of oxidizing

drugs, naphthalene, and fava beans. Such individuals are more likely than others to develop hemolysis following exposure to oxidizing chemicals in the workplace (documented with trinitrotoluene).

Inherited homozygous alpha$_1$-antitrypsin deficiency is associated with a markedly increased risk of pulmonary emphysema. Persons with the heterozygous carrier state may be at increased risk of obstructive lung disease if they are tobacco smokers. Tobacco smoke has been shown to decrease the lung's capacity to inhibit proteolytic enzyme action. There is evidence to support the hypothesis that amyotrophic lateral sclerosis, a degenerative neurological disease of unknown etiology, involves genetically determined metabolic pathways that increase susceptibility to one or more environmental toxins. Genetic susceptibility, in combination with environmental exposures, may play a role in many common diseases, such as coronary artery disease, diabetes, asthma, peptic ulcer disease, and breast, colon, and lung cancers.

The N-acetyltransferase phenotype is another example of the potential effect of genetic differences in toxin metabolism on carcinogenesis. Arylamines, a class of potent bladder carcinogens, are detoxified by N-acetylation. Persons with bladder cancer have been shown to have an increased prevalence of the slow acetylator phenotype. Thus, in this case, genetic control of the rate of metabolism of xenobiotics may affect the risk of carcinogenesis. The acetylator phenotype is known to play an important role in drug–drug interactions and is likely to be important in interactions between chemicals in the environment and in drug–chemical interactions. The metabolism of tobacco and alcohol-derived carcinogens may also be genetically determined. Large interindividual differences have been found in both the activity and DNA binding of benzo[a]pyrene, a potent carcinogen in cigarette smoke, likely due to inherited differences in the P450 enzyme system responsible for its metabolism.

Another important process in carcinogenesis, the ability of cells to repair DNA damage, may also be affected by environmental exposures. The best-studied example of a heritable genetic abnormality associated with a markedly increased susceptibility to environmentally induced cancer is the autosomal recessive disease xeroderma pigmentosum. Persons with this disease develop multiple skin cancers in sunlight-exposed areas of the body, often within the first few years of life. The somatic cells from these patients have a defect in the repair process for DNA base-pair damage induced by ultraviolet light. The cells are highly sensitive to a variety of carcinogenic chemicals and ultraviolet light.

Behavioral and lifestyle factors

Tobacco

Tobacco use, alone or in combination with alcohol, is the most important cause of cancer in developed countries. Active smoking or direct exposure to other tobacco products accounts for almost all cases of tobacco-related cancer. However, non-smokers who are exposed to sidestream smoke from burning tobacco and to mainstream smoke exhaled by smokers appear to have a small increase in risk of lung cancer and perhaps other cancers.

Active smoking is associated with the development of chronic obstructive lung disease and cardiovascular disease. There also is evidence that tobacco smoking increases a person's risk of chronic lung disease associated with other air-borne exposures. A number of possible mechanisms for interactions between tobacco smoke and other environmental pollutants have been theorized. Cigarette smoke can increase exposure to other inhaled carcinogens by altering the normal mechanism of absorption, distribution, and clearance. The irritants in cigarette smoke – including hydrogen cyanide, acrolein, formaldehyde, and nitrogen oxides – induce ciliostasis, thereby impairing clearance and permitting larger doses of pollutants access to the lungs. In addition, aerosols are deposited differently in the lungs of smokers than in the lungs of non-smokers. Tobacco aerosols enhance particle deposition in the central regions of the lungs. Lung clearance mechanisms are less efficient here than in the upper respiratory tract. Smokers, for example, have dramatically increased long-term retention of some dusts in the lung compared with non-smokers.

There is evidence that lung cancer occurs at a higher frequency in a susceptible subgroup of smokers and former smokers. Current research aims to identify who is susceptible (e.g., testing for genetic polymorphisms and in-vitro assays for mutagen sensitivity) and then focus on behavioral change, chemoprevention and other primary and secondary prevention methods in this high-risk population.

The cigarette smoker is considered to be susceptible to an environmental exposure if there is an additive effect or greater-than-additive effect (synergism) between smoking and the exposure. Such synergism has been documented for a wide range of respiratory toxins. Grain dust and cotton dust act synergistically with smoking to increase coughing and phlegm production. Additive effects have been observed with smoking and the development of symptoms and decrements in lung function with exposure to grain dust, coal dust, and other agents. Less-than-additive effects also may exist; tobacco smoking may reduce the risk of the non-malignant effects of silica exposure.

In occupational settings with heavy long-term exposures to asbestos, tobacco and asbestos have been shown to act synergistically to cause an increase in lung cancer rates. Among insulators, for example, the risk of lung cancer increases 10-fold with tobacco smoking, 5-fold with occupational asbestos exposure, and 50-fold with both exposures. Asbestos is present in the ambient environment and in many buildings. The cancer risk associated with low-level ambient asbestos exposure superimposed on tobacco smoking has not been well defined.

The relative excess of proteases over antiproteases in the lung in smokers has been associated with the development of emphysema and chronic airflow obstruction. One theory is that exposure to environmental agents other than tobacco may increase the relative excess of proteolytic enzymes in the lung parenchyma and, thus, increase the risk of emphysema in smokers who already have an excess of proteases. Environmental agents also could interact with the effects of smoking to cause a deterioration in the level of chronic airflow obstruction by contributing to airway pathology. A wide range of agents can exacerbate airways disease, including respiratory irritants such as oxides of nitrogen, ozone, chlorine, and sulfur dioxide (SO_2).

Smoking may enhance systemic effects of toxins as well. The cigarette, or its smoke, may interact with physical or chemical agents, causing new adverse effects. For example, polymer fume fever, which develops in some Teflon manufacturing workers, is caused by the transformation of inert fluorocarbon polymers into toxic decomposition (pyrolysis) products by the heat of burning cigarettes (see also Chapter 41). Tobacco can serve as a vector for entry of chemicals into the body by inhalation or by ingestion. Smokers exposed to agents such as lead, mercury, carbonyl, organotin, inorganic fluoride, methyl parathion, boron trifluoride, and formaldehyde have developed more systemic effects than similarly exposed non-smokers. Tobacco smoke has been reported to increase the risk of development of sensitization by inhaled occupational asthmagens. Smokers also may be more susceptible to infectious agents in the environment. Studies of smokers reveal an increase in incidence of respiratory infections as well as impairment of bactericidal activity such as macrophage phagocytosis.

Alcohol consumption

Alcohol consumption is now known to be a major factor affecting human susceptibility to a broad spectrum of environmental and industrial contaminants. The health of persons who are not heavy drinkers may be affected by the interaction of ethanol with pollutants and drugs. For example, beer may modify the metabolism of nitrosamines and theoretically increase cancer risk. The interactions of alcohol with inorganic agents and with a wide variety of organic drugs, industrial chemicals, and pollutants have been reviewed in depth.[13] The interaction of alcohol with a few important environmental agents affecting the liver, kidneys, heart, and carcinogenesis is presented here.

Ethanol can enhance the hepatotoxic effects of some chemicals. Ethanol potentiates the toxicity of carbon tetrachloride in humans and animals. Administration of ethanol concomitant with carbon tetrachloride has been shown to increase the toxicity of the latter, probably through induction of the mixed function oxidase (P450) system. It is likely that a similar toxicity pattern exists for ethanol combined with other hepatotoxic agents, especially those that require bioactivation in the liver (such as the solvent trichloroethylene, TCE).

Alcohol consumption (or exposure to alcohols in industry) can potentiate the toxic effects of chemicals on organs other than the liver. For example, induction of the mixed function oxidase system by alcohol may enhance the bioactivation of carbon disulfide, resulting in increased neurotoxicity and hepatotoxicity. Acute ethanol consumption also magnifies the central nervous system effects of TCE.[14]

Ethanol may act to enhance the potency of a number of different chemical carcinogens. Animal studies suggest that the increased incidence of cancer among alcoholics may be attributed partially to the enhanced ability of these individuals to bioactivate procarcinogens (such as benzo[a]pyrene and dimethylnitrosamine) in the intestines. Investigators using animal models have concluded that ethanol can increase the rate of formation of toxic metabolites from benzene. Animal data suggest that ingestion of ethanol enhances the hematotoxicity of inhaled benzene. Extensive studies have shown that alcohol also may directly affect carcinogenesis at different stages of initiation and promotion. Chronic ethanol exposure results in an up to 10-fold induction of CYP2E1 activity. This has the potential to increase the formation and elimination of toxic metabolites. Some authors have recommended that physicians warn heavy alcohol users regarding a potential increase in adverse health effects from environmental chemicals.[15]

AGE-DEFINED POPULATIONS

The extent to which those at the extremes of age (the young and the elderly) may be more susceptible to certain toxins and why is addressed in this section. Because these subpopulations include a high proportion of the total population, a very large sector of society may be placed at risk when exposures occur. The United States government has generally taken into account the susceptibilities of the very young in establishing national exposure standards. For example, the Environmental Protection Agency (EPA) has set a drinking standard for nitrate that minimizes the risk of nitrite-induced methemoglobinemia in infants, the most susceptible group. The EPA, the Food and Drug Administration (FDA), and the Consumer Product Safety Commission have attempted to reduce exposure to lead in drinking water, food, ambient air, and paints in order to protect children from irreversible neurological damage.. Although in theory the elderly may be more susceptible to environmental exposures for a number of reasons[16] there is a paucity of research in this area and, therefore, very little regulatory policy.

The fetus and child

Exposures during the prenatal and childhood periods may result in more frequent or severe adverse health effects, or both, than do exposures of adults. The current areas of concern regarding the susceptibility of children include (1) respiratory effects of outdoor and indoor air pollutant exposure, (2) cancer caused by environmental exposures, and (3) the neuropsychologic effects of metals such as lead. The potential for increased sensitivity of the fetus, infant, and child to adverse effects from environmental exposures may be attributed to several mechanisms (see Table 10.3). These critical periods of developmental vulnerability deserve particular attention, given the potential risk to the entire population.

Recently, risk exposure experts and other scientists have challenged the assumption that children are more susceptible to environmental toxins than adults.[17,18] Sensitivity

Mechanism	Example
High number of rapidly dividing cells (fetus)	Radiation injury
Immaturity of enzyme activity (infant), e.g. superoxide dismutase, methemoglobin	Oxidant injury
Increased absorption (GI, dermal, inhalation) per unit weight	Lead absorption
Immature blood–brain barrier (developing endothelial capillaries)	Lead-induced CNS injury
Immature immune system (infants)	Deficient antibody response
Increased exposure	Environmental exposure Indoor air pollution Lead dust and paint chips

Reference: Calabrese 1986,[31] Kane 1985[44]

Table 10.3 Enhanced susceptibility of the young

to a risk is a function of exposure and susceptibility. The following issues have been raised: (1) young animals are not always more sensitive to chemical-induced carcinogenesis, (2) rates of metabolism and clearance (e.g., of xenobiotics) are generally faster in children than in adults, (3) knowledge of dose–response relationships is too limited to predict whether stricter regulations improve children's health (current exposure levels may be below a threshold for effect), (4) data on children's actual exposures are inadequate to assess risk and therefore default assumptions are utilized. Agreement exists that additional research data are needed to accurately assess both the exposure and the inherent susceptibility of children.

The report *Pesticides in the diets of infants and children* written by the National Research Council in 1993[19] brought international attention to the susceptibility of children and the lack of scientific research and data in this area. In 1996, the EPA developed the National Agenda to Protect Children's Health from Environmental Threats. The National Agenda mandates that the EPA ensure that its standards protect children, and instructs the agency to broaden research, policies and education in this area. The Food Quality Protection Act (1996) is the first environmental law to require explicit analysis of risk to children in establishing standards for pesticide residues in food.[3] The 1997 Presidential Executive Order 13045 on Children's Environmental Health (1997) requires federal agencies to consider 'disproportionate risks' to children related to environmental health or safety in their programs and policies.[20]

In-utero exposures

The fetus is particularly susceptible to a number of environmental toxins. The precise point of fetal development may determine the degree of risk (see also Chapter 27.2). Toxic agents usually exert the greatest risk for injury and malformations if exposure occurs during the embryonic period, when organogenesis is taking place. For most organs, this period occurs between the third and ninth weeks of gestation. The main development of the brain occurs later, between the eighth and fifteenth weeks of gestation. Earlier exposures may increase the risk for spontaneous abortion, whereas later exposures may affect growth and development.

Intrauterine lead exposure causes greater chronic and irreversible neurotoxicity at lower levels than occurs in late childhood or adulthood (see Chapter 39.8). The greatest risk to humans from ionizing radiation occurs during the in-utero period. Studies of persons exposed in the atomic bombings of Hiroshima and Nagasaki have documented that the brain is most susceptible to radiation injury during fetal development. Exposure to radiation during this period increases the risk of mental retardation, small head size, seizure disorder, and poor performance on standardized tests of intelligence.

All forms of mercury can cross the placenta, with bioavailability to the fetus. The major concern rests with organic forms of mercury (e.g. alkyl mercury) the critical target organ of which is the brain. In-utero exposures can cause abnormal neuronal migration and disordered neuronal organization; psychomotor retardation may result. The threshold for neurological adverse effects is lower for prenatal than for adult exposure. Rates of neonatal exposure can also be significantly increased by nursing. The resulting neurotoxicity is usually irreversible.

Exposure to solvents in drinking water has been variably reported to increase the rates of spontaneous abortion and congenital anomalies by unknown mechanisms. Similar findings have been observed in studies of pregnant women occupationally exposed to solvents. In animal studies, there is evidence that solvents can be fetotoxic, although they usually are not teratogenic. Ethylene glycol ethers in particular have documented reproductive toxicity.

The fetus is particularly susceptible to acute toxicity from carbon monoxide (CO). CO readily crosses the placenta from the maternal bloodstream to the uterine bloodstream. The fetus is highly sensitive to CO-induced hypoxia. Low levels of CO (resulting in carboxyhemoglobin levels of 4% and greater) appear to be associated with deficits in cognitive and motor functions; such concentrations are without apparent effects in healthy children and adults. Neurologic sequelae reported include mental retardation, microcephaly, and cerebral atrophy.

The rapidly dividing cells of the fetus may increase its susceptibility to carcinogens. The fetus appears highly sensitive to direct-acting alkylating agents, for example. However, fetuses may have lower levels of enzymes that activate procarcinogens and, therefore, may be more resistant to certain carcinogens. Other variables also affect fetal susceptibility to carcinogens. These variables include the differential transport of active metabolites from mother to fetus across the placenta, the status of cell differentiation in various tissues, and the capacity for immunosurveillance. In general, the fetal and infant stages of development should be considered highly susceptible to carcinogens until there is greater understanding of the fetal response to specific carcinogens.

Inhaled toxins

There is growing evidence that air pollutants may have a special impact on children's health. Of particular concern is the accumulating scientific data suggesting that (1) respiratory illness in childhood is a risk factor for the subsequent development of respiratory illness in adulthood and (2) lower respiratory tract illness in children may be a risk factor for chronic airways obstruction. The latter hypothesis holds that airway damage occurs during a vulnerable developmental stage and is followed by an excessive rate of decline in FEV_1 over many years, resulting in fixed airways disease.

The effects of air pollution on healthy children have been researched at length during the past four decades and have been reviewed by Angle[21] and Balmes[22] and summarized by the World Health Organization.[23] Issues of particular interest have been the incidence and severity of respiratory symptoms, the reversibility of symptoms, the magnitude and duration of pulmonary function decrements, and the effect on the lungs' growth and development. The data concerning these potential health risks and how they relate to some common air contaminants are summarized in Table 10.4.

The impact of air pollution on the developing lungs of children has been partially substantiated by animal studies demonstrating effects on growth and airway function; human data are consistent with these animal studies. The Six Cities Study of Air Pollution and Health is an ongoing prospective epidemiologic study that began in 1974, which compares the health of populations living in cities with high pollutant levels with those living in less polluted areas.

Population at risk	Exposure	Effect
Children and infants	SO_2 particulates, suspended sulfates, low-level air pollution	Increased rate of respiratory illness (Ware et al,[45] Jaakkol et al[46])
Children and infants	Acute pollution episodes with SO_2 and total suspended particulate	Acute decrements in pulmonary function (Dockery et al,[47] Dassen et al[48])
Preadolescent children	Particulate pollution	Increase in chronic cough and chest illness (Speizer,[49] Dockery et al[50])
	Fine particles	Acute respiratory symptoms (Schwartz J[51])
	SO_2	Persistent cough (Chapman et al,[52] Dodge et al[53])
Children and adolescents	O_3	Reduction in lung function (Spektor et al,[54] Castillejos et al,[55] Kinney,[56] Braun-Fahrlander[57])
Children	Air pollution	Reduction in single breath nitrogen test (Detels et al[58])

Table 10.4 Effects of outdoor air pollution on normal children

The study has documented a strong association between rates of chronic cough, bronchitis, and chest illness in preadolescent children and measurements of pollution, including acid aerosols, SO_2 and NO_2. Asthma, persistent wheeze, hay fever and measurements of pulmonary function were not associated with any pollutant concentrations. Other studies also have documented an association between SO_2 exposures and persistent cough in children.

Studies assessing the impact of ambient NO_2 exposures on health have suggested an increase in respiratory symptoms in children, but these results have been controversial owing to simultaneous exposures to other pollutants and unreliability of the method for monitoring NO_2. Data from several epidemiologic studies of school-aged children suggest that low-concentration ozone exposure is associated with small short-term, reversible decrements in lung function and also may affect the rate of lung growth in children.

Fine particulates (e.g., particulate matter less than 10 μm in diameter, termed PM 10) are increasingly recognized as a potential source of serious adverse health effects, both systemically and in the respiratory tract. They constitute a diverse mixture of pollutants, including arsenic, lead, sulfates, and carcinogens, not yet covered by federal standards for ambient air quality. Suspended sulfates, a major component of acid aerosols, have been related to respiratory tract infections and decreased lung function in children. Unlike the larger particles, fine particulates are frequently deposited in the alveoli and they may be carriers of toxic and carcinogenic vapors, even if the particulates themselves are inert. The particulates also interfere with the ciliary-mucosal filter system in the bronchial airways, thus promoting the potential toxicity of other inhaled toxins. The lung clearance mechanisms in small airways, which protect airways in adults, function less effectively in the early years of life.

An ongoing prospective study[24] in 12 California communities is assessing children's respiratory health following chronic exposure to respirable particles (PM10 and PM2.5), O_3 and NO_2. Results after 4 years show a decrease in lung function growth among children living in polluted areas as compared with children who breathe cleaner air, and the effects are more pronounced in areas with higher pollutant levels. Children with decrements in lung function may be more susceptible to respiratory disease and may be more likely to develop respiratory conditions as adults.

Indoor air pollution (see also Chapter 50) is of particular concern for children because children spend a large percentage of time in the home during the first 5 years. The home environment contains many potential sources of air pollution. CO, NO_2, and other particulates are produced by cigarette smoke. Similar compounds and SO_2 are produced by combustion of biomass fuels and accumulate, for example, with the use of improperly vented wood or coal fireplaces or stoves, gas cooking stoves, kerosene heaters, or malfunctioning furnaces. Volatile organic compounds, asbestos fibers, radon gas, and aeroallergens also may be present in indoor air.

Children have been found to be susceptible to a number of health effects attributable at least in part to indoor air pollutants. Some of the major exposures and associated health effects are summarized in Table 10.5. It is important to keep in mind that conflicting data exist on most of these exposure–effect associations. Three products of incomplete combustion (NO_2, CO, and SO_2) are important contaminants of indoor air. CO can be measured in almost all indoor environments, especially in winter, and may on occasion exceed the National Ambient Air Quality Standards set by the EPA. Overt CO poisoning of pregnant

Population at risk	Exposure	Effect	Citation
Fetus and young children	Ambient CO	Reduced birth weight Delayed postnatal growth SIDS	Angle 1988[21]
Infants and children	Formaldehyde (UFFI)	Mucous membrane and upper airway irritation SIDS Chronic respiratory symptoms Decrements in lung function	Woodbury and Zenz[59]
Children	Environmental tobacco smoke (ETS)	Asthma: increased prevalence and severity Respiratory illnesses Lower respiratory infections Decreased lung function (exposed in utero) and decreased lung function growth Possibly increased risk for COPD Chronic ear infections, middle ear effusions Increase in tonsillectomy and adenoidectomy Abnormal child behaviour including hyperactivity (fetal and child exposure)	Weitzman et al 1990,[27] Chilmonczyk 1993[28] Samet[29] Tager[60] Tager et al,[61] Tager[60] Samet[29] Angle 1988[21] American Thoracic Society[62] Eskenazi[63]
Children	Aeroallergens, e.g., house-dust mite, cockroach allergen	Asthma and atopic sensitization	Litonjua[64]

Table 10.5 Effects of indoor air pollution on normal children

women causes severe adverse effects on the fetus. Ambient exposure to CO is thought to cause the reduced birth weight of infants that is seen following exposure to environmental tobacco smoke (ETS); sensitivity to CO after birth has not been established.

NO_2 levels are frequently higher in the home than outdoors owing to cigarette smoking and the use of gas stoves. Whether or not children who live in homes with gas stoves have altered lung function or an increased incidence of respiratory illness is controversial, although a number of epidemiologic studies have addressed this issue. There is evidence that school children may develop increased respiratory symptoms and, in some studies, decreased pulmonary function in atmospheres with mildly elevated concentrations of SO_2 and particulates.

Volatile organic compounds are common constituents of indoor air. Formaldehyde has been associated with an increased risk of the development of chronic respiratory symptoms and transient decrements in lung function. Infants have been reported to develop restlessness, red eyes, diarrhea, vomiting, rhinorrhea, and cough in homes with elevated levels of volatile organic compounds in the air. Apnea has been documented following exposure of animals to chemical irritants. Knowledge of these factors has raised the possibility that home air contaminants may contribute to the sudden infant death syndrome.

Exposure of children to aeroallergens such as house-dust mite allergens is increasingly recognized to be an important determinant of the subsequent development of asthma and atopic sensitization. The expression of genetic factors such as atopy and allergic disease may require environmental triggers in childhood in order to induce allergic responses.

Environmental tobacco smoke (ETS) poses a health risk for infants and children (see Table 10.5). National data estimate that approximately 50% of children aged 5 years and under are exposed to environmental tobacco smoke in their homes.[25] Studies have examined prenatal exposure, acute respiratory illness morbidity, chronic respiratory symptoms, asthma and bronchial responsiveness, and pulmonary function of children in relation to ETS exposures. ETS exposure of young children increases the symptoms of respiratory disease.[26] Maternal smoking during pregnancy has been associated with an increased risk for childhood asthma. ETS exposure among children is associated with an increased prevalence and severity of asthma.[27,28] ETS exposure appears to increase the severity of asthma in those with pre-existing airways disease.

A reduction in lung growth during childhood may be a risk factor for chronic obstructive lung diseases. This predisposition may occur as a result of reduced peak lung volumes or accelerated ventilatory loss. The infants of smoking parents have increased rates of lower respiratory infections. It has been hypothesized that the altered pulmonary function in smoke-exposed children may result from these recurrent infections.

Children exposed to tobacco smoke in the home have increased rates of chronic ear infections and middle ear effusions. Persistent ear infections may be more likely to develop in children with nasal allergies and recurrent otitis media who are exposed to ETS. Increased frequency of tonsillectomy and adenoidectomy has been identified in children exposed to ETS.

Parental smoking, including maternal smoking during pregnancy, has been associated with changes in neurodevelopment and child behavior, particularly hyperactivity, in a number of studies.[29] The many unexplored social, demographic, and psychologic confounding variables preclude any conclusion about a causal relationship.

Carcinogens

The young are at increased risk of tumor development following exposure to certain carcinogens. Elevated relative risks have been reported for radiation-induced thyroid tumors, skin cancer, adult-onset leukemia, and vinyl chloride-induced angiosarcoma.

Prenatally exposed survivors of the atomic bombings in Japan appear to be more susceptible to radiation-induced cancer than those who were exposed after birth. Controversy remains over whether or not preconception exposure (maternal or paternal) to ionizing radiation can cause genetic mutations or heritable effects. Epidemiologic studies have failed to document a relationship between low-frequency magnetic fields in the home and outdoors with childhood cancer.

Transplacental carcinogenesis has occurred with diethylstilbestrol and could theoretically occur with other environmental exposures. In addition to chemicals and ionizing radiation, children may be at increased risk of developing cancer compared with adults following exposure to sunlight. Analyses of the relationship between ultraviolet light and melanoma suggest that childhood exposures may be disproportionately important. Children also may be particularly susceptible to carcinogens, such as aflatoxins and nitrites, found in food. Despite these several associations and theoretical reasons for suspecting that children are at greater risk from carcinogen exposure, empiric data for excess risk do not exist for most carcinogens.

Interindividual differences are known to play a role in susceptibility to environmental insults that increase cancer risk (e.g., asbestos, alcohol, and tobacco). Heritable differences in susceptibility have been identified at almost every stage of carcinogenesis, including metabolism of carcinogens, DNA repair, and proto-oncogene and tumor suppressor gene expression[9] (see Table 10.3).

Neurotoxins

There is growing evidence that the young are more susceptible than adults to the neurotoxic effects of a variety of agents including lead, mercury, organophosphate insecticides, and anesthetics and analgesics. A number of factors may explain this increased susceptibility. Children absorb a larger dose per unit of body weight of toxins through the gastrointestinal and respiratory tracts than adults do. Examples include increased absorption of lead and retention of larger amounts of mercury in the brain. The extended period of central nervous system development, beginning in the ninth week of gestation and extending into the early school years, results in a long 'window' of susceptibility.

The developing fetus has even greater sensitivity to lead exposure than do other age groups. There is no impediment to the transplacental transport of lead; umbilical cord blood lead levels are equal to those in maternal blood. There is evidence that the fetal brain is more sensitive than the mature brain to the effects of lead. Lead can more easily penetrate the developing endothelial cells of the capillaries and reach the brain's neurons and astrocytes. In addition, the immature blood–brain barrier may allow greater access of lead to the central nervous system. Most importantly, most of the neuropsychologic damage that infants and children may suffer when they are exposed to lead is irreversible (see Chapter 39.8).

At present, there are few additional empiric data on the differential effects of neurotoxins in the young. However, it remains prudent public policy to presume that children are particularly susceptible, based on the experience with lead and the compelling theoretical concerns.

The elderly

The proportion of persons in developed countries who are aged 65 or older is growing at a rapid rate. According to census projections, this proportion will increase in the United States from 12% in 1986 to 22% in 2050. The elderly are known to be more vulnerable than the rest of the population to a number of factors, including adverse side effects of drugs, thermal stress, and infections. However, very little scientific information exists concerning how or the extent to which an elderly person is more susceptible to adverse effects from a potentially hazardous environmental exposure. It is clear that the susceptibility of the human body to disease changes throughout the lifespan, but our knowledge of the underlying mechanisms is limited.

It has been suggested that because the elderly develop toxicity from drugs at lower doses than younger adults, they may be more susceptible to toxic chemicals present in home, work, and outdoor environments.[30,31] Environmental agents (termed gerontogens) also may be capable of accelerating the onset or rate, or both, of progression of certain aging processes.

The elderly person may be at increased risk for adverse effects following an environmental exposure for a number of reasons. Some proposed mechanisms underlying this susceptibility of the aged are listed in Table 10.6. For example, the cellular and biochemical responses of lung epithelium to oxidant damage are age dependent. Older animals are less protected from oxidant injury to the lung than are younger animals. One hypothesis is that older cells have higher basal levels of peroxidation of lipid membranes than younger cells. Decreased tissue dietary antioxidants such as vitamin E also may contribute to the increased susceptibility of older animals to lung injury.

Mechanism	Outcome
Changes in physiologic, biochemical, immune, homeostatic parameters	Diminished inherent protective mechanisms; immunosenescence Aging cells have an intrinsic sensitivity to certain toxins
Long exposure period to toxin (increasing lifespan)	High total exposure dose
Survival of years or decades since exposure began	Latency period exceeded and toxic effect is manifest Effects of complex chemical interactions become manifest
Diminished functional reserve	Acute exposure is more likely to cause adverse effects
Decreased xenobiotic metabolism, increased production of toxic metabolites, reduced successful chromosome repair	Potentiation of the toxin's effects

Table 10.6 Enhanced susceptibility of the elderly

Sensitivity to free radicals also appears to be age related. Free radical stress may be more prevalent in aged animals, and the aging process may allow the unrepaired damage caused by free radicals to accumulate. The elderly have lower levels of superoxide dismutase, an important enzyme in antioxidant defense. These low levels may be a risk factor for oxidant pollutant toxicity; there is evidence that ozone and NO_2 cause pulmonary toxicity via free radicals. Xenobiotic-related effects, such as carcinogenicity (e.g., carbon tetrachloride), hepatotoxicity (e.g., carbon tetrachloride and ethanol), nephrotoxicity (e.g., gentamicin), pulmonary fibrosis (e.g., bleomycin), and cardiotoxicity (e.g., adriamycin), are all age related, and available evidence supports free radical mechanisms.

Despite the difficulty of assessing the potential for increased susceptibility of the elderly to xenobiotics, a number of agents have been identified that are more likely to cause adverse effects in older adults and the elderly, based on animal models. Various studies show higher rates of acute respiratory and neurological toxicities, cancer, and other health effects in older animals compared with younger animals following exposure to a variety of chemicals.

Neurotoxicants

The elderly are more susceptible to some neurotoxic effects of pharmaceuticals than are young individuals. Examples include elderly people's increased sensitivity to tardive dyskinesia after neuroleptic use and to neuroleptic malignant syndrome following the administration of dopamine antagonists. There is evidence that senescent loss in neurons causes increased vulnerability to neurotoxicants. The age-related cell attrition causes reduced structural redundancy and reserve in the nervous system. Thus, subclinical injury can occur without apparent associated impairment until the finite reserve is depleted, at which point subsequent neurotoxin exposure or further age-related neuronal loss causes more profound disturbances of longer duration than those seen in younger individuals.

Aging can cause metabolic alterations, as well as changes in cell number, which may compound the neurotoxic effects of exposures. Carbon disulfide, acrylamide, lead, and the pesticides chlordecone, methylbromide, and DDT appear likely to potentiate neurotoxicity in the elderly because they affect the catecholamine/indolamine balance that is already perturbed by aging. In addition, aging can result in reduced metabolism of toxic compounds and increased production of toxic metabolites.

Inhaled toxins/air pollution

Age is a factor affecting the susceptibility of the lung to diseases and its vulnerability to inhaled toxic materials. Our understanding of the functional and structural mechanisms underlying the susceptibility of the aged lung is limited. Differentiating between 'true' aging effects and changes caused by the damaging effects of repeated exposures to inhaled contaminants is extremely difficult. Age-related changes in the human respiratory system, including tissue structure and respiratory function, have been described in some detail.[32] A decline occurs in elastic recoil of the lung and the decline is greater in smokers and in those who are susceptible to ETS. Multiple parameters decline with age, including resting arterial tension, diffusion capacity for carbon monoxide, maximum aerobic capacity with exercise and respiratory muscle strength.

In addition, immunosenescence causes an age-related decline in protective immunity against various infections as well as a less robust response to vaccinations. The impact of these parameters on susceptibility to environmental agents is not known. Age-related changes in aerosol deposition are not well understood. Animal models have been developed to define aerosol deposition as a function of age, though interindividual variability is known to be high.

The aging process is an important variable in exposure to environmental toxins and the susceptibility to lung disease. Age-related decreases in pulmonary function, cough efficiency, mucociliary transport, and cell-mediated immunity are some changes that may affect susceptibility and certain types of lung injury. The association between exposure to ambient concentrations of air pollutants and a decline in lung function with age is controversial. Animal studies have shown an age-related sensitivity to the pulmonary toxicity of ozone and NO_2, as noted earlier. In addition, non-specific airway hyper-responsiveness increases with age and, therefore, the elderly are potentially at increased risk for irritant and bronchospastic effects of inhaled pollutants. In acute air pollution episodes such as those in Donora, Pennsylvania (1948), and in London (1952), the elderly had higher rates of illness and death. However, many of the affected elderly had pre-existing diseases.

Although the risks of particulate matter (PM) or PM combined with other air pollutants have been discussed as a predictor of asthma in children, there are other subpopulation effects (see Table 10.7). One of the most challenging debates has been to explain the 0.5% increase in death rates related to days where PM10 levels increase by 10 ppm. This finding is reproduced in epidemiologic studies[33-35] yet challenged by occupational studies of 'dusty' trades such as coal miners where this effect is not apparent. It has been hypothesized that the increased

Exposure	Outcome
Adults:	
Particulates	Increase in death rates and emergency room admissions
	Exacerbation of asthma
	Exacerbation of pneumonia
	Increased cardiovascular effects
NO_2	Increased airway responsiveness (controversial)
O_3	Increased inhaled antigen sensitivity
Polluted ambient air (low O_3)	No change in lung function and symptoms
Polluted ambient air (O_3 and particulates)	Decline in lung function in asthmatics and controls
SO_2 (controlled exposure)	Small decline in lung function (versus purified air exposure): wheezing
	Increased airway responsiveness in asthmatics compared with non-asthmatics and atopics
	Increased bronchoconstriction with exercise
Sulfate aerosols (controlled exposure)	Decrease in lung function, no change in respiratory symptoms, increased airway responsiveness
	Increased respiratory symptoms, correlation with sulfate levels
Children:	
Particulates (epidemiologic studies)	Exacerbation of respiratory symptoms
	Change in pulmonary function
	Decrease in lung function growth
Adolescents:	
SO_2 aerosols (controlled exposure)	Reversible decrements in lung function
O_3 and SO_2 in sequence	Decreased pulmonary function
O_3 and NO_2	No significant differences in pulmonary function change between asthmatics and healthy persons

References: Balmes 1996,[4] Gauderman 2000,[24] Samet 2000,[33] Speizer 1990,[65] Zanobetti 2000[42]

Table 10.7 Responses to air pollutants in individuals with asthma

death (and emergency room admission) rates are in the elderly who are already debilitated, particularly with cardiovascular and respiratory diseases. Studies are currently underway to determine if such a susceptible subpopulation exists and if it may account for the increased morbidity and mortality seen on days with high ambient fine PM levels.

Carcinogens

The incidence of cancer increases markedly with age. This increased incidence can be partially attributed to the fact that cumulative exposure to toxins is related to the development of cancer. The longer duration of exposure accounts for the age-related increase in lung cancer in smokers. However, studies of people exposed to radiation from the bombs at Hiroshima and Nagasaki and from a single course of radiotherapy for ankylosing spondylitis reveal that the incidence of certain types of cancer (acute leukemia and lung cancer) was substantially higher in persons older than 50 years of age at the time of exposure, given the same exposure dose.

The age-dependent susceptibility to carcinogens and other environmental toxins is not universal. Animal studies suggest that this susceptibility is dependent on the chemical and the target organ; human data are sparse except for those on ionizing radiation.

POPULATIONS WITH PRE-EXISTING CONDITIONS

The healthiest workers have historically been selected for jobs with physical and/or chemical stressors. However, over time, many workers develop various chronic health problems related to work or other factors, bringing diseased individuals into contact with environmental risk factors. Legislation in the United States (the Americans with Disability Act) to protect the right to work of individuals with pre-existing diseases may further accentuate the potential for exacerbation of underlying disease in certain situations.

Unfortunately, at present, knowledge of the special risks from environmental exposures for those with specific diseases is very limited. This will severely hamper rational preventive practice, especially when the law requires that a worker be allowed to work unless good information is available to recommend otherwise. Such limitations in available data also interfere with providing effective advice to clinicians who must advise their patients with various ills how to cope with environmental stressors.

The remainder of this chapter reviews basic data regarding common medical problems whose interaction with environmental factors has been explored. For many others, including such common conditions as chronic renal and liver disease, specific data are totally lacking and the practitioner is forced to make judgments using conservative theory, based on knowledge of how each toxin is absorbed, metabolized, and excreted, and its target organs and effects at potentially excessive doses of exposure.

Chronic lung disease

Asthma

The prevalence of asthma is dramatically increasing in the western world. Scientists are focusing on identifying what risk factors account for this. The widening disparity in asthma prevalence between western industrialized countries and China, for example, has been explained as an interaction between susceptibility genes and new environmental exposures. Research suggests that environmental risk factors for disease may (1) exacerbate the effect of a genotype, (2) work with the genotype to increase risk, or (3) be acted upon (via increased gene expression or increased effect) by the genotype. Recent data[36] implicate obesity in the western world as an important risk factor for asthma. Differences in antibiotic use, diet, immunizations, parasite exposure, endotoxin exposure, host resistance, particulate air pollution, breast feeding, and sedentary lifestyle are also under investigation as possible factors contributing to the asthma epidemic.[37,38] At this time we have too few data to draw definitive conclusions about which groups of children and adults are more likely to develop airways disease and why.

Persons with asthma and airway hyper-reactivity, as well as atopic and allergic persons, may develop bronchoconstriction following exposure to certain air pollutants, which are summarized in Table 10.7. Several types of investigation support this generalization. Controlled human exposure studies with low concentrations of SO_2 have demonstrated that asthmatics experience bronchoconstriction at significantly lower concentrations than do non-asthmatics. As has been documented by asthma outbreaks in cities, asthmatics are more sensitive than the general population to acute increases in air pollution. In Donora, Pennsylvania, in 1948, a thermal inversion layer trapped high levels of SO_2 and particulates and 80% of persons with asthma experienced exacerbations. Animal models have demonstrated that inhaled pollutants such as ozone, SO_2, and NO_2 can enhance IgE production and airway reactivity. Immunologically mediated responses, especially IgE-dependent mechanisms, are an integral component in the development of airway inflammation and therefore the onset, severity and persistence of asthma.[39]

A spectrum of irritant gases, fumes, and particulates may precipitate respiratory symptoms in persons with asthma through a non-immunologic mechanism. Vapors of volatile organic compounds, including common solvents such as toluene and formaldehyde, are often found in indoor air. Acute exposure of asthmatics to these irritant compounds may result in mild decrements in lung function and bronchial irritation. ETS is an irritant that increases non-specific bronchial reactivity in asthmatics. Low concentrations of irritants (such as SO_2) may cause bronchoconstriction in exercising asthmatics. Persons with atopy or allergy are more sensitive to the effects of some irritant inhaled pollutants (e.g., ozone), even if the allergic individuals are asymptomatic (see Table 10.7).

Another major mechanism of asthmatic responses to environmental exposures involves sensitization to a specific agent through synthesis of IgE (or gamma G immunoglobulin, IgG) antibodies. Occupational asthma caused by animal proteins or bacterial enzymes in the detergent industry is an example of IgE-mediated asthma. Atopic individuals are more likely than non-allergic persons to become sensitized to these high-molecular-weight substances. However, in other exposure settings (for example, with polyurethane precursors or wood dust), there is no relationship between atopic status and the risk of hyper-sensitivity reactions (see Chapter 19.2).

Once an individual becomes asthmatic as a result of an environmental exposure, bronchospasm usually can be triggered by a variety of non-specific stimuli in the environment. A proportion of persons with new environmentally triggered asthma will have persistent airway hyper-reactivity and respiratory symptoms indefinitely after removal from the environment containing the sensitizing agent.

Table 10.7 reviews selected studies on the response of atopics and asthmatics to common air pollutants. Exposure to O_3, a potent oxidant and cause of airway inflammation, has resulted in exacerbation of asthma in epidemiological studies, although sensitivity to O_3 is not seen in chamber studies of asthmatics. Chronic exposure to O_3 may cause a decrease in flow rates.[40,41] Epidemiological studies have documented decrements in peak expiratory flow and lower respiratory symptoms associated with NO_2 exposure. Data from controlled exposures are not consistent. An increased bronchoconstriction response to allergen is seen with NO_2, similar to O_3.

Young asthmatics may be particularly susceptible to inhaled environmental exposures. Data from a 12-year follow-up in the Six City Study of air pollution have shown that exacerbations of symptoms in asthmatic children (but not a decrease in pulmonary function levels) are associated with levels of exposure to particulates at or below the current United States ambient standards. The occurrence of new cases of asthma did not appear to be related to ambient levels of pollutants. In contrast, as a group, children do not have increased respiratory symptoms as pollutant exposures increase. The long-term consequences of modestly elevated ambient pollutant levels and increased symptom burden on asthmatic children are unknown at present.

Controlled exposure studies of adolescent asthmatics have shown increased sensitivity to inhaled sulfuric acid, a common atmospheric transformation product of SO_2. Asthmatics are more sensitive to SO_2 and may experience exacerbations caused by brief exposures allowable under the National Ambient Air Quality Standards. The interactive effects of air pollutants may cause pulmonary toxicity that is not detected in single-exposure challenges. Very few studies have investigated the combined effects of pollutant exposures. There are no controlled human exposure studies evaluating the impact of PM on airways disease. There is some evidence in animals and humans that diesel exhaust increases local airways allergic responsiveness. PM

and diesel exhaust are currently intense areas of research in pollution health effects.

Overall, there are data to suggest that a number of inhaled pollutants may affect pulmonary function or respiratory symptoms, or both, of asthmatic children and adults.

Chronic obstructive pulmonary disease

Historical episodes of uncontrolled air pollution have demonstrated serious adverse health effects, particularly among those with pre-existing respiratory diseases. In the London fog incident of 1952, the maximal 24-hour concentration of SO_2 soared to levels estimated at 10 times the current maximum permissible level. Among the 4000 excess deaths attributed to pollution, the majority were ascribed to bronchitis, pneumonia, tuberculosis, and other respiratory diseases.

Chronic obstructive pulmonary disease (COPD) alters the structure and physiologic functioning of the lung, causing a loss of elastic recoil and a decrease in airway caliber, with a resulting increase in resistance to flow. These changes affect both the deposition and clearance of inhaled particles. Particle deposition occurs more centrally because terminal air units are not accessible. More particles are deposited at sites of obstruction. Thus, in diseased lungs, inhaled toxins may exert more pronounced and varied effects compared with healthy lungs. For example, there are some data to suggest that persons with COPD (and not normal elderly persons) experience considerable decrements in pulmonary function following acute NO_2 exposure. Persons with COPD, particularly those with increased bronchial reactivity, are probably also at greater risk of developing symptoms (and possibly deteriorating lung function) from inhaled toxins than are persons without lung disease. Persons with COPD have increased symptoms on days with high PM10 levels in ambient air.[42] Insufficient data preclude more specific conclusions about the risk of exacerbation or the effect on overall prognosis of various environmental exposures among persons with COPD.

Heart disease

Although there is epidemiologic evidence that patients with heart disease have increased susceptibility to inhaled pollutants, there are no controlled laboratory studies of exposure. In a small exercise study, patients with coronary artery disease were exposed to high ambient ozone concentrations; no changes in pulmonary or cardiovascular function were detected. However, the authors caution that the limited exercise tolerance of these patients may have resulted in inhalation of low concentrations of ozone. Persons with cardiorespiratory disease, which limits exercise performance, thus may have a protective mechanism restricting their total dose of inhaled pollutants.

Individuals with cardiovascular disease are considered to be at greatest risk for adverse effects from CO exposure. Low levels of CO can exacerbate myocardial ischemia during exercise. This was confirmed in a multicenter study of patients with coronary artery disease. Even small decreases in the oxygen-carrying capacity of blood in persons with coronary artery disease can produce myocardial ischemia because coronary blood flow cannot be augmented appropriately.

There is some laboratory and anecdotal evidence to suggest that patients with cardiomyopathies and ventricular rhythm disorders may be at risk for dysrhythmia from exposure to organic solvents, especially fluorinated ones. This is discussed more fully in Chapter 24.

Diabetes

Diabetes mellitus is frequently complicated by symptoms and signs of peripheral neuropathy. A number of chemicals, including certain metals, solvents, gases, pesticides, and substances used in plastics, are known to be peripheral nervous system toxins. In theory, there is reason to suspect that additive or perhaps synergistic toxicity could result when a diabetic is exposed to these toxins. Thus, a diabetic theoretically may be more likely to develop peripheral neurotoxicity and the disease may be more extensive or produce more severe symptoms than in a non-diabetic following exposure to a neurotoxin. However, there are no empiric data nor a convincing laboratory model for any toxin to confirm this theoretical possibility.

Obesity

Extreme obesity is associated with a reduction in lung volumes. The clinical picture of restrictive lung disease can be found in very obese persons without intrinsic lung pathology.[43] Because baseline pulmonary function is altered, obese persons may be at greater risk for the development of further respiratory impairment following exposure to respiratory toxins such as tobacco smoking and pulmonary infections. However, this possibility has not been confirmed in human epidemiologic studies.

In addition, obese persons may be at risk for sudden increases in the concentration of lipophilic chemicals in the blood because these chemicals are stored mostly in adipose tissue. Examples include organochlorine pesticides and dioxins. Higher amounts of lipophilic toxins accumulate in fat in an obese person than in a lean, athletic individual. The concentration of the toxin in the target organ may be lowered by such storage, and thus, this toxin may produce less toxicity in an obese individual than in a lean individual. However, when rapid mobilization of fat occurs, an obese person may have a greater increase in the concentration of the lipophilic chemical in the blood and, therefore, suffer acute toxic effects. This hypothesis has been studied and confirmed in animals exposed to organochlorine insecticides followed by starvation periods. Clinical toxicity in this setting has not been proved in humans.

Prospective studies have found a strong association between body mass index (BMI) and the risk of adult-onset asthma. Asthma severity may also be related to BMI.[43] Inner city asthmatic obese children show evidence of more severe asthma than those who are not obese. This effect is independent of age, gender, family income, allergy or mental health. The dramatic increase in asthma prevalence rates in the US may be related to obesity and western lifestyle and diet changes.[36]

SUMMARY

In order to better protect vulnerable groups and the population as a whole, accurate data on susceptibility are needed and should be incorporated into risk assessment to improve health-based policy development. Research and public policy are intensely focused on understanding and reducing risks among susceptible populations, particularly children. More mechanistic information is needed to increase understanding of how different factors impact toxicity and how these factors vary with genetic profile, behavior and age. Estimation of risk is becoming increasingly sophisticated. A new layer of complexity has been added to our understanding of disease causation with evidence that host factors may determine the impact of exposure to a carcinogen or other toxin.

Host factors may play a particularly important role in outcomes with low-level exposures. The challenge for risk assessment is to account for the wide interindividual variation in susceptibility to environmental agents, including for example the spectrum of interaction between environmental carcinogens and host factors. Public policy is creating the need for rapid advancement of scientific knowledge in human susceptibility to disease impacted by environmental exposures.

References

1. USEP. Proposed guidelines for carcinogen risk assessment. EPA/600/P-92/003C. Washington DC: US Environmental Protection Agency, 1996.
2. Presidential/Congressional Commission on Risk Assessment and Risk Management. Risk assessment and risk management in regulatory decision making. Final report, Vol 2. 519348/900115. Washington: US Government Printing Office, 1997.
3. Food Quality Protection Act, August 3, 1996, Title 7 US Code at Section 1261, as amended.
4. Balmes JR. Outdoor air pollution. In: Harber P, Schenker M, Balmes J, eds. Occupational and environmental respiratory disease. St. Louis: Mosby, 1996.
5. Tickner JA, Hoppin P. Children's environmental health: a case study in implementing the precautionary principle. Int J Occup Environ Health 2000; 6:28.
6. Cullen MR, Redlich CA. Significance of individual sensitivity to chemicals: elucidation of host susceptibility by use of biomarkers in environmental health research. Clin Chem 1995; 41:1809.
7. Eaton DL, Farin FM, Omiecinski CJ, et al. Genetic susceptibility. In: Rom WN, ed. Environmental and occupational medicine, 3rd edn. Philadelphia: Lippincott-Raven, 1998;209.
8. Schwartz BS, Lee Byung-kook, Lee Gap-soo, et al. Associations of blood lead dimercaptosuccinic acid-chelatable lead and tibia lead with polymorphisms in the vitamin D receptor and delta aminolevulinic acid dehydratase genes. Environ Health Perspect 2000; 108(10):949.
9. Spitz MR. Risk factors and genetic susceptibility. In: Hong WK, Weber RS, eds. Head and neck cancer. New York: Kluwer Academic Publishers, 1995.

10. Wei Q, Spitz MR. The role of DNA repair capacity in susceptibility to lung cancer: a review. Cancer Metastasis Rev 1997; 16: 295.

11. Bennett WP, Alavanja MCR, Blomeke B, et al. Environmental tobacco smoke genetic susceptibility and risk of lung cancer in never-smoking women. JNCI 1999; 91: 2009.

12. Wrighton SA, Stevens JC. The human hepatic cytochromes P450 involved in drug metabolism. Crit Rev Toxicol 1992; 22:1.

13. Calabrese EJ. Alcohol interactions with drugs and chemicals. Chelsea, MI: Lewis Publishers, 1991.

14. Barret L, Faure J, Guilland B, Chomat D, Didier B, Debru JL. Trichlorethylene occupational exposure: elements for better prevention. Int Arch Occup Environ Health 1984; 53:283.

15. Pastino GM, Yap WY, Carraquino M. Human variability and susceptibility to trichlorethylene. Environ Health Perspect 2000; 1008(suppl 2):201.

16. Snodgrass WR. Physiologic and biochemical differences between children and adults as determinants of toxic response to environmental pollutants. In: Guzelian PS, Henry CJ, Olin SS, eds. Similarities and differences between children and adults: implications for risk assessment. Washington DC: ILSI Press, 1992;35.

17. Charnley G, Putzrath RM. Children's health, susceptibility, and regulatory approaches to reducing risks from chemical carcinogens. Environ Health Perspec 2001; 109:187.

18. Cohen Hubal EA, Sheldon LS, Burke JM, et al. Children's exposure assessment: a review of factors influencing children's exposure, and the data available to characterize and assess that exposure. Environ Health Perspect 2000; 108:475.

19. National Research Council. Pesticides in the diets of infants and children. Washington DC: National Academy Press, 1993.

20. Protection of children from environmental health risks and safety risks. Executive Order 13045. Fed Reg 62: 19885, 1997.

21. Angle CR. Indoor air pollutants. Adv Pediatr 1988; 35:239.

22. Balmes JR. Emerging issues in ambient air quality and respiratory health. Probl Respir Care 1990; 3:163.

23. World Health Organization. Air Quality Guidelines, 1999 (chapter 3) www.who.int/environmental-information/air/guidelines

24. Gauderman JW, McConnell R, Gilliland F, et al. Association between air pollution and lung function growth in southern California children. Am J Respir Crit Care Med 2000; 162(4pt1):1383.

25. Overpeck MD, Moss AJ. Children's exposure to environmental cigarette smoke before and after birth. Health of our Nation's Children, United States, 1988. Adv. Date, 1991, p.1.

26. Gergen PJ, Fowler JA, Maurer KR, Davis WW, Overpeck MD. The burden of environmental tobacco smoke exposure on the respiratory health of children 2 months through 5 years of age in the United States: third national health and nutrition examination survey, 1988–1994. Pediatrics 1998; 101:e8.

27. Weitzman M, Gortmaker S, Walker DK, Sobol MA. Maternal smoking and childhood asthma. Pediatrics 1990; 85:505.

28. Chilmonczyk BA, Salmun LM, Megathlin KN, et al. Association between exposure to environmental tobacco smoke and exacerbations of asthma in children. N Engl J Med 1993; 3218:1665.

29. Samet JM. The relationship between respiratory illness in childhood and chronic air-flow obstruction in adulthood. Am Rev Respir Dis 1983; 127:508.

30. Cooper RL, Goldman JM, Harbin TJ, eds. Aging and environmental toxicology. Baltimore: The Johns Hopkins University Press, 1991.

31. Calabrese EJ. Age and susceptibility to toxic substances. New York: John Wiley and Sons, 1986.

32. Crystal RG, West JB, Barnes PJ, Weibel ER, eds. The lung: scientific foundations, vols I and II, 2nd edn. Philadelphia: Lippincott-Raven, 1997.

33. Samet JM, Dominici F, Curriero FC, Coursac I, Zeger SL. Fine particulate air pollution and mortality in 20 US cities, 1987–1994. N Engl J Med 2000; 343:1742.

34. Pope CA, Thun MJ, Namboodiri MM, et al. Particulate air pollution as a predictor of mortality in a prospective study of US adults, Am J Respir Crit Care Med 1995; 151:669.

35. Dockery DW, Pope CA, Xu X, et al. An association between air pollution and mortality in six US cities. N Engl J Med 1993; 329:1753.

36. Camargo CA, Weiss St, Zhang S, Willett WC, Speizer FE. Prospective study of body mass index, weight change, and risk of adult onset asthma in women. Arch Intern Med 1999; 159:2582.

37. Platts-Mills T, Woodfolk JA, Chapman MD, Heymann PW. Changing concepts of allergic disease: the attempt to keep up with real changes in lifestyles. J Allergy Clin Immunol 1996; 98:297.

38. Gern JE, Weiss ST. Protection against atopic diseases by measles – a rash conclusion? JAMA 2001; 283:394.

39. Busse W, Lemanske RF. Asthma. N Engl J Med 2001; 344:250.

40. Kunzli N, Lurmann F, Segal M, et al. Association between lifetime ambient ozone exposure and pulmonary for a college freshman – results of a pilot study. Environ Res 1997; 72(1):8.

41. Galizia A, Kinney PL. Long-term residence in areas of high ozone: association with respiratory health in a nationwide sample of nonsmoking young adults. Environ Health Perspect 1999; 107:657.

42. Zanobetti, A, Schwartz J, Gold D. Are there sensitive subgroups for the effects of air-borne particles? Environ Health Perspect 2000; 108(9):841.

43. Luder E, Melnik TA, Dimaio M. Association of being overweight with greater asthma symptoms in inner-city black and Hispanic children. J Pediatr 1998; 132:699.

44. Kane DN. Environmental hazards to young children. Phoenix: The Oryx Press, 1985.

45. Ware JH, Ferris BG, Dockery DW, et al. Effects of ambient sulfur oxides and suspended particles on respiratory health of preadolescent children. Am Rev Respir Dis 1986; 133: 834-42.

46. Jaakkola JJK, Paunio M, Virtanon M, et al. Low-level air pollution and upper respiratory infections in children. Am J Public Health 1991.

47. Dockery DW, Ware JH, Ferris BG Jr, et al. Change in pulmonary function in children associated with air pollution episodes. J Air Pollut Control Assoc 1982; 32:937-42

48. Dassen W, Brunekreef B, Hoek G, et al. Decline in children's pulmonary function during an air pollution episode. J Air Pollut Control Assoc 1986; 36:1223-7.

49. Speizer FE, Ferris B Jr, Bishop YM, et al. Respiratory disease rates and pulmonary function in children associated with NO$_2$ exposure. Am Rev Respir Dis 1980; 121: 3-10.

50. Dockery DW, Speizer F, Stram D. Effects of inhalable particles on respiratory health of children. Am Rev Respir Dis 1989; 139: 587-94.

51. Schwartz J, Neas LM. Fine particles are more strongly associated than coarse particles with acute respiratory effects in schoolchildren. Epidemiology 2000; 11: 6-10.

52. Chapman RS, Calafiore DC, Hasselblad V. Prevalence of persistent cough and phlegm in young adults in relation to long-term ambient sulfur oxide exposure. Am Rev Respir Dis 1985; 132: 261-7.

53. Dodge R, Solomon P, Moyers J, et al. A longitudinal study of children exposed to sulfur oxides. Am J Epidemiol 1985; 121:720-36.

54. Spektor DM, Lippmann M, Lioy PJ, et al. Effects of ambient ozone on respiratory function in active, normal children. Am Rev Respir Dis 1988; 137: 313-20.

55. Castillejos M, Gold DR, Dockery D, et al. Effects of ambient ozone on respiratory function and symptoms in Mexico City schoolchildren. Am Rev Respir Dis 1992; 145:276-82.

56. Kinney PL, Ware JH, Spengler JD, et al. Short-term pulmonary function change in association with ozone levels. Am Rev Respir Dis 1989; 139:56–61.

57. Braun-Fahrlander C, Kunzli N, Domenighetti G, et al. Acute effects of ambient ozone on respiratory function of Swiss schoolchildren after a 10-minute heavy exercise. Pediatr Pulmonol 1994; 17:169–77.

58. Detels R, Tashkin DP, Sayre JW, et al. The UCLA population studies of CORD: X. A cohort study of changes in respiratory function associated with chronic exposure to SOx, NOx, and hydrocarbons. Am J Public Health 1991; 81:350–9.

59. Woodbury MA, Zenz C. Formaldehyde in the home environment: prenatal and infant exposures. In: Gibson JE, ed. Formaldehyde toxicity. New York: Hemisphere Publishing Corporation, 1983.

60. Tager IB, Hanrahan JP, Tosteson TD, et al. Lung function, pre- and post-natal smoke exposure, and wheezing in the first year of life. Am Rev Respir Dis 1993;147:811–7.

61. Tager IB, Weiss ST, Munoz A, et al. Longitudinal study of the effects of material smoking on pulmonary function in children. N Engl J Med 1983; 309:699–703.

62. American Thoracic Society. Environmental controls and lung disease. Am Rev Respir Dis 1990; 142:915–39.

63. Eskenazi B, Castorina R. Association of prenatal maternal or postnatal child environmental tobacco smoke exposure and neurodevelopmental and behavioral problems in children. Environ Health Perspect 1999; 107:991–1000.

64. Litonjua AA, Carey VJ, Burge HA, et al. Exposure to cockroach allergen in the home is associated with incident doctor-diagnosed asthma and recurrent wheezing. J Allergy Clin Immunol 2001; 107:41–7.

65. Speizer FE. Asthma and persistent wheeze in the Harvard Six Cities Study. Chest 1990; 98:191–5.

Chapter 11
Occupational and Environmental Health and Safety in Developing Countries

Mark R Cullen, Linda Rosenstock, Tord Kjellstrom

Although there are substantive differences in occupational and environmental health practice among the developed countries because of differences in history, culture, political system, and professional practice, the principles of clinical practice described throughout this text are generally applicable in all. On the other hand, about 80% of the world's population lives in areas that are defined under the label 'developing countries'. In some, such as Mexico, Brazil, and most of Southeast Asia, transformation to patterns of health more typical of developed societies has occurred, but other features of underdevelopment, such as high rates of poverty and low educational attainment, persist. In others, such as most of those in sub-Sahara Africa, Central America, and many of the world's island nations, the major determinants of health remain poverty, poor sanitation, and malnutrition. There is compelling evidence that a disproportionate amount of the world's occupational and environmental injuries and disease occur in these societies as well. The clinical effects of the major environmental and occupational hazards may occur anywhere, but the likelihood is higher, the consequences often more profound, and the strategies for prevention and treatment more problematic in poor nations than rich. Some of the classic occupational diseases, such as silicosis, lead poisoning, and benzene poisoning, that have been virtually eradicated in most developed countries remain endemic in many developing countries.[1-3] Lack of foresight, lack of interest, and lack of resources combine to create health risks, which could be avoided, sometimes at very limited cost.

What happens now in many industries in poor countries is a replay of what occurred in the affluent countries 30 to 50 years ago. The difference is that then most practitioners, industrialists, and decision-makers were genuinely ignorant about the attendant health risks. Control technologies and access to information were far more limited than they are now. In the 21st century, information systems and the communication infrastructure are so well developed that ignorance is no excuse for inaction anywhere in the world. The workers of the developing countries deserve a better fate than those who were the guinea pigs of seminal epidemiologic studies in developed countries. However, experience shows that the demonstration of significant exposures and sentinel cases of health effects are not enough in themselves to trigger preventive action. Just as in developed countries, pressure from government, worker organizations, and the community

advocacy groups, in combination with locally conducted studies, are often necessary to initiate such action.

The continued industrialization of many developing countries without sufficient attention to occupational health and safety presents an increasing public health problem, despite the availability of preventive interventions. In the sections that follow, we estimate the magnitude of the problem, then review the major, generic factors that distinguish occupational and environmental medicine (OEM) practices in developing countries from those with which the reader is likely more familiar. These are summarized in Table 11.1, and reviewed in more detail later in the chapter. While there are myriad issues specific to each country, different regions within the same country, and even different workplaces or environmental settings within the same region, these factors are almost universally important and should serve as an overview to practice issues in the developing context.

THE MAGNITUDE OF THE PROBLEM

The overall picture that emerges from all parts of the developing world is one of increased health and safety risks in all occupations for which data are available. Similarly, in most of the developing world, attention to environmental hazards is a low, often non-existent priority, with the individual and community being vulnerable to increased levels of exposure to both workplace and non-workplace factors. Because of inadequate data and reporting systems, capturing the impact of this increased risk is daunting. Nonetheless, several recent efforts by international bodies have shed some light on the staggering burden although, in general, attempts to derive evidence-based estimates are likely to systematically and significantly under-represent the extent of the problem.

Worldwide, it is estimated that there are at least two million deaths per year due to occupational diseases and injuries.[4] The World Health Organization (WHO) recently evaluated the contribution of five select occupational factors in relation to the overall burden of disease.[5] These data provide a more in-depth yet still incomplete picture of the overall problem. Nonetheless, a picture emerges of the significant impact of largely preventable conditions associated with these factors, as described below.

Condition	Implication
Distribution of economic activity	High proportion of workers in high-risk occupations
Susceptibility of the populations	Greater co-morbidity Multiple hazards
Proximity of workplaces to residential communities	Additive exposures Risk of catastrophic accident Risk to family/children
Demographics of population	Risk to children High job turnover
Climactic factors	Problems with PPE* Interference with sampling New hazards, i.e. parasites and animals
Inadequate regulations and enforcement	Poorly controlled exposures Importation of hazardous materials, equipment and waste
Low educational level of managers/OEM professionals	Poor supervision Limited professional guidance
Low educational level of population	Training difficulty
Higher proportion of migrant work	Social instability STD risk
Extent of informal sector work	Undocumented, unregulated work
Resource limitations	Low investment in public and private sectors Substandard equipment, PPE,* source materials

* Personal protective equipment

Table 11.1 Work conditions differentiating developed and developing countries, and potential impacts on occupational health practice

WHO found that occupational injuries result in more than 300,000 deaths per year. Contrast this to the approximately 6000 lives lost each year in the US due to occupational injuries. As in the developed world, high injury fatality rates in the developing world are clustered in certain sectors, including agriculture, construction, and mining. Understanding the role of occupational injuries in relation to quality of life is accomplished by use of the 'common currency' called DALYs (disability-adjusted life years, with one DALY being equal to the loss of one healthy life year). Occupational injuries account for nearly 1% of all DALYs and 16% of the unintentional injuries in the working population aged 15 to 69 years.

The second occupational factor analyzed by WHO was the effect of exposure to workplace carcinogens. Estimating that globally about 20–30% of men and 5–20% of women of working age (15–64 years) are exposed to occupational lung carcinogens (such as asbestos, diesel exhaust, and silica), WHO concluded that these exposures account for about 10% of all cancers of the lung, trachea, and bronchus. They also attributed about 2.4% of all leukemia to occupational exposures. Overall, the worldwide burden of occupational cancers was estimated at 146,000 deaths per year (0.3% of all) and 1.4 million (0.1%) DALYs.

Estimates of the global burden of chronic lung disease demonstrate the significant contribution of occupational exposures, which account for about 15% of all chronic obstructive pulmonary disease (COPD). In total, WHO found the annual worldwide burden of work-related COPD to be 243,000 deaths (0.4% of all) and 3 million (0.2%) DALYs.

WHO found that 37% of all back pain worldwide is attributable to work, resulting in an estimated 0.8 million DALYs, significant loss of time from work, and high economic loss. Worldwide, 16% of all hearing loss is attributable to workplace exposures, resulting in 4.2 million (0.3%) DALYs.

The WHO analyses also provide some important insights into the global burden of select environmental risks. Again, as in the case of occupational conditions, WHO estimates, because they assess only a limited range of factors and because of under-reporting and inadequate or non-existent data, are thought to under-represent the overall burden. Beyond the workplace, unsafe water, sanitation, and hygiene were found to account for 3.1% of deaths (1.7 million) and 3.7% of DALYs (54.2 million). Urban air pollution was attributed as causal in 5% of trachea, bronchus, and lung cancer cases, 2% of cardiorespiratory mortality and 1% of respiratory infections mortality, amounting worldwide each year to 0.8 million deaths (1.4%) and 7.9 million (0.8%) DALYs. Indoor smoke from solid fuels, a source of heat for cooking for half the world, is associated with respiratory infection and lung cancer, and accounts for 2.7% of DALYs worldwide. Lead exposure accounts for 234,000 deaths per year worldwide (0.4%) and 12.9 million (0.9%) DALYs. Climate change was considered by the WHO to account for increased risk for diarrhea, malaria, and dengue fever, with an attributable mortality of 154,000 (0.3%) and attributable burden of 5.5 million (0.4%) DALYs.

Despite the importance of using systematic and transparent methods to better grasp the global burden of select factors, these new analyses fail to capture a broad range of significant workplace and environmental exposures, likely under-representing even further the burden that falls on the developing world. For example, pesticide exposures (both intentional and unintentional) cause a disproportionately high global burden of mortality and morbidity in the developing world (see Chapter 48). In addition, the many millions of workers in developing countries are exposed to a combination of health hazards both in the workplace and outside that lead to poor health status overall. Estimates of adult (age 15 to 59 years) mortality have shown that in a highly developed country, about 10% of 15-year-old persons will die before age 60, whereas in a country such as Egypt, about 30% will die, and in rural India, about 50%. How much of this preventable mortality rate is related to occupational hazards or other environmental hazards is not known.

DISTRIBUTION OF ECONOMIC ACTIVITY

One important reason for differences in occupational and environmental health priorities between developed and developing countries is the difference in the relative types of occupations and differences in the major sources of pollutants. The majority of people in the poorest developing countries (including India and China) work in subsistence agriculture. Health in the workplace is integrated into all aspects of daily life because the distinction between time at work and time at home is often blurred (see below). In societies where women work predominantly in the home, tasks such as cooking, gardening, water collection, firewood collection, and other chores may engender major risks, as has been established in relation to cooking and heating with biomass fuels (see Chapter 50). Beyond subsistence farming, formal sector agriculture is one of the largest occupational groups in many developing countries, entailing exposures to the entire spectrum of physical, biologic, and chemical hazards seen in developed countries (see Chapter 12) but often with exposures far less well controlled. In developed countries, by contrast, the proportion of the population involved in agriculture is rapidly dwindling, less than 2% currently in the US. Moreover, farm laboring is often a family affair in developing countries, with children exposed as well as pregnant women and the elderly.

One specific type of agriculture that is on an industrial scale is forestry, which has become a very important contributor to the economy of developing countries with rain forests. The destruction of the world's rain forests is, in itself, a well-known hazard to the global environment. Less well recognized is the high injury rate among forestry workers. Problems are similar in planted forests, and although there is better control of the environment in such forests, these workers often have to reside in poorly designed camps far from their families and the community support of village life, engendering an additional set of health risks (see below).

Another primary industry of greater importance in many developing countries is mining. Extraction of ore (or coal) for direct export is widespread, and refining of the ores is increasingly carried out in the country of origin. Mining in these settings often involves greater risks for injuries from falls, slips, and unexpected movements of ore or rocks than in more highly regulated settings (see Chapter 13). Mining still involves high risk of silicosis or coal-workers' pneumoconiosis (anthracosis and anthracosilicosis) in many countries.[1,6] Coal mines are also prone to explosions and fires, which can trap workers and lead to multiple fatalities.

Closely linked to the mining industry is the metal refining industry, which also is of major importance in developing countries. The occupational hazards in this field depend on the product. Limestone and quarrying industries create risks of silicosis. A special case is the mining (quarrying) of asbestos or other asbestos fiber-containing minerals, which can give rise to asbestosis, lung cancer, and mesothelioma. Non-ferrous metal refining involves risks of poisoning by a number of agents, including lead, cadmium, arsenic, and sulfur dioxide (SO_2).

As part of the development process itself, employment in construction and transport industries increases.

Generally, developed countries have a larger proportion of such workers than developing countries. Although in many countries sophisticated and modern buildings are going up rapidly, construction is often accomplished without the benefit of comparably sophisticated safety programs; risk of falls and fatalities is very high. In Singapore, for example, there was a dramatic increase in the number of serious injuries reported in the construction industry during the transformation of the municipality in the 1970s. A report from China in the last decade underscores the seriousness of this pattern.[7]

The transport system and the hazards in the transport industry depend on geographic factors, with increased risks of injuries in traffic accidents among drivers in countries with difficult terrain and bad roads. Vehicles are frequently substandard, often lacking mirrors, seatbelts and other modern safety devices, and open vans and lorries are widely used to transport workers. Increasing motor traffic also leads to an increase in non-occupational traffic accident injuries, with young and elderly pedestrians at the highest risk. In many countries, the per capita rate of occupational and non-occupational fatalities exceeds levels in the US and Europe by 10-fold or more.[8]

Light industry emerges in developing countries at early stages of development. The textile industry, assembly and repair industry for imported machinery, and small chemical formulation (mixing) factories may be the first to appear. To support an increasing use of cars, lead battery factories often are established early and are found in almost every developing country. The hazards in these industries are well known; however, protection for the workers is typically insufficient. High prevalence rates of systemic poisonings, hearing loss, respiratory conditions such as byssinosis, and other occupational diseases largely eradicated in western industry have been reported. Moreover, as is true with a number of other manufacturing processes at early stages of development, lead battery re-smelting is often performed as a cottage industry to extract the lead for paints and glazes. These conditions create not only the occupational health risks but also health risks to the family and the community.[2] These small-scale enterprises, which often fall outside government administrative control, play an important role in grass roots industrial development, but the lack of local knowledge about health hazards and the varying involvement of family members and neighbors as workers make them very difficult to track for health consequences. The special problem of so-called informal sector work, the most primitive of these, is discussed further below.

SUSCEPTIBILITY OF THE POPULATION

Many of the occupational and environmental health hazards that occur in developing countries are similar to those in developed countries, albeit more frequent and often more severe. But others are features of poverty and early development that are scarcely, if ever, seen nowadays in developed countries. For example, not only are injuries more common, but poor sanitation and inadequate surgical care and public health infrastructure result in far poorer outcomes and, sometimes, unheard-of complications such as tetanus. In the poorest countries, this totally preventable complication still ranks as an important cause of death; it has been estimated that a high proportion of tetanus cases in adults are caused by agricultural injuries.[9]

Poor sanitary conditions mean that for many workers in developing countries, the health problems of poverty overshadow the specific health effects of occupational hazards. Malaria and other tropical diseases, tuberculosis, diarrheal diseases, and other infectious diseases take a heavy toll not only among children, but also among people in the working age group. Such risks are often exacerbated by conditions of work – e.g., exposures in the field – as well as by associated living conditions such as overcrowding, inadequate potable water, and contamination of living space by chemicals and pollutants from the workplace.

Some occupational hazards combine with the diseases of poverty and make the exposed person more vulnerable. For instance, the problem of silicosis in Chinese mines is made worse by the relatively high incidence of tuberculosis, leading to silico-tuberculosis. In South Africa, miners face not only the same high risk of tuberculosis, but also the risk of HIV, to make all too common the devastating triad of AIDS, silicosis, and tuberculosis.[10] Anemia is a common condition among workers in developing countries due to poor nutrition and parasite infections. Both the degree of anemia and the symptoms of such can be exacerbated in workers exposed to, for instance, arsenic, nitrites, lead or carbon monoxide. Child labor (see below) adds another dimension to these problems of vulnerability. Although data are still limited in this regard, it is widely believed that risk for many, if not all, occupational and environmental diseases may be enhanced by co-morbidity, poor nutrition, and the coexistence of multiple health risk factors.

PROXIMITY OF THE WORKPLACE TO PLACES OF RESIDENCE

Because arable land, mines, and other large manufacturing complexes are most typically situated remote from sources of labor, the provision of residential housing at the worksite is commonplace throughout the developing world. Often, whole cities have sprung up, sometimes shockingly close to sources of pollution and dangerous activities, creating three major concerns. First is the blurring of the exposure context of work: workers are exposed to many of the same hazards on and off the job. Second, fires, explosions and toxic discharges may pose a direct threat to large populations. Third, industrial levels of exposure are often conferred on spouses, children, and other family members living in this often intrinsically overcrowded and undesirable housing stock. Contamination of residential air, water, food, and soil from this source is commonplace. A particularly gruesome and everyday example is the domestic use

of the large drums in which agricultural chemicals are typically supplied. Residues from these are sufficiently lethal to result in hundreds of thousands of cases of pesticide poisoning per year, inadvertent or intentional. This source likely exceeds the already vast toll in human health taken by occupational application of the chemicals. The special health problems of migrant workforces, where housing is typically provided for workers but not for their families, will be discussed further below.

The smelter town of La Oroya, Peru, illustrates the first concern. Rows of workers' huts line up in front of the main entrance to the smelter, which is situated in a narrow valley at an altitude of 3600 m (about 12,000 ft). The emissions of SO_2, lead, cadmium, arsenic, and other toxic metals create high concentrations in the air and contaminate house dust, leaving workers and their families exposed for essentially 24 hours each day.

Living close to the workplace was the major reason for the disaster in Bhopal, India. A cloud of methyl-isocyanate was released from a storage tank during a night in December 1984, owing to erroneous procedures, faulty equipment, and other factors. The highly toxic gas was heavier than air and spread throughout the densely populated neighborhood of the factory. An estimated 2000 persons died and as many as 250,000 were affected, mainly by lung and eye damage. In many, the effects have persisted for years in spite of the fact that the exposure lasted only a few hours.[11]

DEMOGRAPHIC FACTORS

In addition to the blurring of the work and domestic environment, demographics in many developing countries strongly favor risk for children. In part this is due to the economic advantage for women in subsistence farming, cottage industries, and other activities paid by the 'piece' to bring young children to the workplace, often to work. Child labor laws are often either non-existent or unenforced. The complementary problem is the contamination of the home for the reasons discussed above, and because little attention is given to accidental transportation of work materials into the home.

Another demographic factor of importance to practice is the reality of an unskilled labor force that vastly exceeds the size of the formal workforce in most developing countries, resulting in wide-scale unemployment. Up to 70% of the population in the poorest nations exist outside the formal economic sector. The consequences are manifold, above and beyond the obvious issue of poverty. The replacement cost for sick and injured unskilled workers is effectively zero, sharply reducing economic incentives to prevent such turnover. For these workers, low job security results in a willingness to work in undesirable conditions, to continue working despite illness, to under-report injury for fear of job loss, and the like. Even multinational corporations, which in their home countries may adopt a cradle-to-grave ethic towards workers who typically devote careers to that single employer, may behave very differently in such divergent economic circumstances.

CLIMATE

Most, but by no means all, of the developing countries have climates very different from the developed countries of the temperate zones. In addition to the obvious issues of heat stress, there are a host of unexpected consequences. First, many extreme climates introduce a multitude of new hazards, including insects, reptiles, wild animals and hazardous terrain. Second, the chemistry of many commercial operations may be quite different in tropical climates, such that contaminants may evolve that are not a problem, or far less of one, in temperate climates. Volatile chemicals, or those reactive with water in densely saturated air, are the most obvious examples. Sampling equipment may function poorly in these climates, or give results divergent from the same operation sampled in a cooler climate. Personal protective equipment, often designed for ambient conditions in developed countries, may also fail more readily or may simply not be tolerated in warm climates.

INADEQUATE REGULATION AND ENFORCEMENT

There is reasonable evidence to support the proposition that for the largest employers in developed countries, social, legal, and public relations considerations may outweigh the importance of regulation as the primary driver to minimize occupational and environmental health risks. But the same cannot be readily said of smaller employers, for whom the regulatory framework and its enforcement provide incentives without which behavior would likely revert to what it was before the modern regulatory era. Unfortunately, in most developing countries, regulations are inadequate or inadequately enforced or both. There are many reasons for this, including lack of political will, compromises against the perceived need for rapid economic expansion, inadequate resources, few professionals to fill key technical responsibilities, corruption, etc. Whatever the reasons, lack of strong regulations for workplace and environmental standards, or poor enforcement of those standards that exist, results in greatly increased risk of injury or disease from environmental contaminants and work.

The consequences of a voluntary approach to occupational and environmental risk reduction, in the context of the other issues listed in Table 11.1, are not hard to imagine. Two are of the greatest overall importance. First is the export of hazardous industries and materials from developed to developing countries for the purpose of escaping strict health and safety regulations.[12] This is becoming increasingly attractive to some industrial sectors, for whom restrictions on the sale or requirements to divulge contents effectively preclude economic utility. For some materials, pressure builds to find a place to 'dump' it, as is the case with asbestos, which has limited marketability in the developed world. Likewise, older technologies, such as machines without baffling (to prevent noise) or guards (to prevent injury), may find second homes in workplaces where such technical advances are not requisite. In other situations, products, although deemed harmful in some or all developed countries, are so cheaply produced relative to their value that companies are reluctant to dispense with them, and there is pressure for entrepreneurs in less regulated areas to adopt them. Export of hazardous waste, which can be very costly to dispose of in regulated environments, is a related practice. It leads to a few jobs, but brings health risks that may be almost impossible to predict or prevent. International agencies have managed, albeit slowly and incompletely, to induce agreements between governments in developed and developing countries which explicitly forbid the trans-boundary transport of hazardous waste and hazardous technologies without information about the hazards involved, which at least gives the recipient country an opportunity to take action. In an economic climate where developing countries are desperate for income, there is still a risk that hazardous technologies and materials end up where they are most difficult to control.

Far and away the most common consequence of inadequate regulation is uncontrolled exposure, widespread contamination, and poor preventive practice. Numerous investigations have documented very high exposures to hazards well controlled in the US and Europe, such as lead, silica, and benzene. Not surprisingly, higher prevalence of effects in developing countries is the rule.

The often inadequately controlled workplace environment is further worsened when coupled with an especially unregulated non-work environment. To individual and community, the result is quite simply greater exposure, whether to lead, diesel or injury risk.

LOW EDUCATIONAL LEVEL OF MANAGERS AND OEM PROFESSIONALS

Most developing countries have few OEM-trained physicians and industrial hygienists to provide expert guidance and policy for government, or to support practice by employers. In general, reliance is placed on physicians and engineers trained in other disciplines, with predictable suboptimal results. Sadly, for those who receive training – usually in developed countries – demand and opportunities for advancement are often greater in the developed context, resulting in a drain of these crucial resources from the societies that need them most. Even employers with the most extensive resources and motivation may be unable to develop optimal programs because of these manpower limitations.

Equally problematic is the low level of training and knowledge regarding occupational and environmental health and safety among managers and the personnel in the workplace charged with day-to-day protection of workers and the environment. Although the dearth of such training may be in part attributable to the lack of regulations mandating it, much is attributable to the historic inattention to such issues in all aspects of the educational system in many parts of the world. In addition to the traditional occupational diseases and injuries referred to above, industrialization leads to an increased risk of major hazard incidents caused by mismanagement of modern technologies, as occurred at Bhopal and other sites of industrial disaster.

LOW EDUCATIONAL LEVEL OF WORKERS AND THE POPULATION

Although training in occupational and environmental safety and health has not been widely adopted as part of public or technical education in most developed countries, there is nonetheless widespread public awareness of these issues, reinforced by media and employer efforts, in the US and Europe. An obvious example is the use of seatbelts in motor vehicles, in which the disparity between developed and developing countries is huge. Comparable societal awareness is not evident in many regions of the world – one of the factors underlying inappropriate exposure of children to industrial risks and chemicals, expropriation of industrial materials for domestic purposes, and failure to apply even 'lay' precautions such as natural ventilation or protective clothing. This puts a higher burden on employers to engineer out risk to the extent possible, and to train workers in matters including those of hygiene and safety that might otherwise be considered 'common sense' in developed countries.

MIGRANT WORKERS

As noted above, mining, agriculture, and many industrial activities in developing countries rely on large migrant workforces, in which workers typically live in provided housing separate from the family home for large portions of the year. Beyond the issues of poor living and working conditions, job insecurity, and the effects of low-wage, dangerous work, migrancy creates other serious concerns. First, the cultures that develop around migrant workforces may be extremely unhealthful, with prostitution, alcohol abuse, and violence commonplace. In many parts of the world, these are important sources of HIV spread, as they are to a far smaller extent in truck drivers and transportation workers in developed countries. A second consequence is lack of health services. Workers may be dependent on employer-provided service since community resources are typically not available in these remote regions. Finally, because the employment relationship is even more transitory in this setting than in high-turnover non-migrant workplaces, incentives for employers to provide training, health services and prevention may be weak or non-existent.

INFORMAL SECTOR WORK

In every society there are some economic activities which are 'informal', i.e., not documented through tax or other systems that, in theory, provide government with some knowledge and control of conditions. For the most part in developed countries these are limited to less than 10% of the workforce and involve mobile selling of goods, illicit activities such as prostitution and drug trade, and domestic labor, including day care. In many developing countries, however, a far higher (upwards of 70%) and more diverse cross-section of economic activities are informal, including subsistence farming, transportation work, construction, vending and commerce, and even light manufacturing. Not only are these enterprises and the people they affect usually well outside the scope of possible government regulation or surveillance, but employers have little reason not to discharge anyone sick or injured as expeditiously as possible. Since so much of the workforce may be engaged in just such work in many developing countries, these enterprises form a particularly intractable problem for control of occupational and environmental health and safety risks.

RESOURCE LIMITATIONS

Although many of the issues raised above are themselves amenable to intervention, the absolute limitations on financial and technical resources cannot be underestimated. In many parts of the world, per capita expenditures for all health are less than a US employer spends for each employee for occupational and environmental services alone. Machinery and technologies proven to reduce exposures or safety risk are often unfeasible economically, as are substitutions from dangerous to safer chemicals. The cost of appropriate safety equipment may be prohibitive, as may be even its availability, for example in countries with limited foreign exchange capacity. At the government level, expenditures on environmental health and safety must be balanced against other health priorities, such as care for AIDS, or provision of community health services. In this context, locally performed studies documenting the extent of risk and cost to employers may be extremely important in driving resource allocation. Programs oriented towards outcomes with proven economic advantage are most likely to be implemented – for example, those that reduce neuro-intoxication or musculoskeletal injuries, whose impact on productivity can be demonstrated. One of the most valuable services highly trained OEM professionals can offer is demonstration of such links, to encourage investments that might otherwise be deemed as economically impossible or undesirable, whether for government or employers.

POTENTIAL SOLUTIONS

A rather bleak picture of the occupational health and safety situation in developing countries has been painted in the previous sections. The lack of published data makes it difficult to assess accurately whether the situation is getting worse or better. Based on the overall increase in the number of workers and the changes in occupational structure over time, increasing occupational health and safety problems can be expected; however, in some developing countries, concerted efforts are being made to introduce effective prevention programs and some reports show that improvements are taking place.

In some ways, the increasing dependency of developing countries on foreign capital for investment in industry is an opportunity to introduce enlightened occupational health and safety practices into countries where legislation and practices lag behind. The World Bank, for example, has prepared guidelines for environmental and occupational health issues that should be taken into account when new investments are made.[13] Such guidelines can be used by government agencies and community groups as a pointer to practices that should be adopted.

Recent environmental protection agreements at an international level will also provide opportunities to protect worker health and safety; for example, the Basel Convention on Export of Hazardous Waste, initiated by the United Nations Environment Program (UNEP). This convention aims at reducing the uncontrolled dumping of hazardous waste in countries that are not prepared to deal with the hazards. Another example is the voluntary code of practice between the pesticide-producing industries and the Food and Agriculture Organization of the United Nations (FAO) concerning the export to and use of pesticides in developing countries. This code of practice gives guidelines for information supply, labeling, training, and other preventive methods. These guidelines provide a means for local users of pesticides, local inspectors, and community groups to implement appropriate practices of import and use of pesticides.

There is no lack of information on occupational health and safety in the international arena. Several publications from WHO and the International Labour Organization (ILO) are identified in the reference section.[4,5,14] A large amount of material on individual hazards is available, e.g., the Environmental Health Criteria, the Health and Safety Guides and the International Chemical Safety Cards from the WHO/ILO/UNEP International Program on Chemical Safety. Other international organizations, such as the international trade unions (e.g., the International Chemical and Energy Workers' Federation [ICEF] and the International Metal Workers' Federation [IMF]) and the international industry groups (e.g., Groupement International des Associations Nationales de Fabricants de Produit Agrochimiques [GIFAP] and the International Lead Zinc Research Organization [ILZRO]), produce review reports and information material on occupational health and safety hazards. National agencies in many developed countries also produce material that could be used in developing countries to attain local solutions.

The challenge lies in making all this information and knowledge available in developing countries and in translating the knowledge into practical actions in the workplace. Occupational health and safety professionals, government agencies, industry, trade unions, and community groups in developed countries can provide support, by advising and assisting specific projects at a bilateral level or by contributing to broader growth of technical cooperation. WHO has developed an infrastructure for such activities via the collaborating centers in occupational health.

Experience shows that it is seldom enough to identify potential health risks from known occupational health and safety hazards. Local health effect studies can be powerful tools in bringing a sense of urgency into prevention work. Clearly, the results of health effect studies have to be interpreted in the context of other health risks in the country. The challenge for occupational health and safety professionals in all countries is to unite in an effort to rapidly reduce all the unnecessary suffering and death that uncontrolled occupational health hazards in developing countries are causing. More and better epidemiologic information is required, as well as improved access to information in the field. Clean technology and better control technology need to be used when industry is established. Local initiatives for self-reliance need support. We can all contribute in one way or another.

References

1. Chien VC, Chai SK, Hai DN, et al. Pneumoconiosis among workers in a Vietnamese refractory brick facility. Am J Ind Med 2002; 42:397-402.
2. Harari R, Cullen MR. Childhood lead intoxication associated with manufacture of roof tiles and ceramics in the Ecuadorian Andes. Arch Environ Health 1995; 50:393.
3. Yin S-N, Li Q, Liu T, et al. Occupational exposure to benzene in China. Br J Ind Med 1987; 44:192-5.
4. International Labour Organization. Global estimates of occupational accidents and work-related diseases. Geneva: International Labour Organization; 2002. www.ilo.org/safework
5. World Health Organization. The World Health Report 2002: reducing risks, promoting healthy life. Geneva: WHO; 2002.
6. Cullen MR, Baloyi RS. Prevalence of pneumoconiosis among coal and heavy metal miners in Zimbabwe. Am J Ind Med 1990; 17:321-6.
7. Xia ZL, Courtney TK, Sorock GS, et al. Fatal occupational injuries in a new development area in the People's Republic of China. J Occup Environ Med 2000; 42:917-22.
8. Schoemaker MJ, Barreto SM, Swerdlow AJ, Higgins CD, Carpenter RG. Non-fatal work related injuries in a cohort of Brazilian steelworkers. Occup Environ Med 2000; 57:555-62.
9. Kanchanapongkul J. Tetanus in adults: a review of 85 cases at Chon Buri Hospital. J Med Assoc Thailand 2001; 84:494-9.
10. Corbett EL, Churchyard GJ, Clayton TC, et al. HIV infection and silicosis: the impact of two potent risk factors on the incidence of mycobacterial disease in South African miners. AIDS 2000; 14:2759-68.
11. Gupta BN, Rastogi SK, Chandra H, et al. Effect of exposure to toxic gas on the population of Bhopal, India. Indian J Exp Biol 1988; 26:149-160.
12. LaDou J. Deadly migration: hazardous industries' flight to the third world. Technol Rev 1991; July:46-53.
13. Feachem RGA, Kjellstrom T, Murray CFL, et al. The health of adults in the developing world. Washington, DC: The World Bank; 1992.
14. Kogi K, Phoon W-O, Thurman JE. Low-cost ways of improving working conditions: 100 examples from Asia. Geneva: International Labour Organization; 1989.

Section 2
Work Sectors and Special Populations

Chapter 12
Agricultural Workers

Stuart L Shalat, Mark G Robson, Sandra N Mohr

INTRODUCTION

Agricultural workers consist of individuals that range from owners of family farms to employees of large corporate enterprises. They may be full-time permanent employees of a single farm or they may be migrant or seasonal farm workers. The term farming includes a variety of enterprises encompassing the cultivation of row crops, fruit orchards, dairy farms and the raising of livestock and poultry. In the United States, the number of family farms has steadily decreased since the Second World War from 9 to 2.2 million in the period between 1940 and 1999.[1] The size of the average farm between 1953 and 1993 has almost doubled from 242 to 474 acres, reflecting the switch from small family to large corporate farms. In general these corporate enterprises are not only far larger in acreage, but employ more workers and are more highly mechanized.

Row crops

For those unfamiliar with farming in general, it is useful to consider the activities involved in each type of farming as a framework to understanding how health and safety problems arise in each category of farming. What most people think of in terms of farming is most likely to be the cultivation of row crops. These include the raising of grains (i.e., wheat, oats, rye, sorghum) and vegetables (i.e., carrots, corn, broccoli, peppers) to name just a few. It also can be used to describe vineyards, although these crops require different and unique activities and have occupational hazards of their own. The cultivation of row crops routinely employs the use of numerous farm chemicals including fertilizers, insecticides, herbicides, and fungicides. Additionally, row crops are highly amenable to mechanization in all stages of cultivation including tilling, irrigation, fertilizer and pesticide application, and harvesting. The cultivation of row crops employs the use of chemicals in a cyclical manner. Prior to planting, fertilizer and pre-emergent chemicals (herbicides and insecticides) are applied. This is followed by periodic re-applications during the growing season. Pesticides may be applied from once to several times as the crops mature. While in some climates there is only one growing season, others may be capable of two or more growing seasons.

Often different crops may be cultivated in the same field in different seasons. In the US, excellent sources of information of the types of crops grown locally and the types and quantities of pesticides employed can be obtained from county agricultural extension offices and extension specialists at the state land grant colleges and univer-sities and state departments of agriculture. This is important in that pesticides are employed and applied in highly specific patterns dependent on the crop and the region. The county extension office is the primary source of information for the agricultural community and the main source of training for new application techniques, safety equipment, new chemicals and changes in state and federal regulations.

In terms of health and safety issues in the cultivation of row crops, two of the major acute sources of health problems arise from worker exposure to agricultural chemicals and heat stress. In warmer climates, these may be highly correlated, because the use of personnel protection equipment (PPE) may exacerbate the potential for heat exhaustion. Injuries can arise from the mechanized equipment employed or from the moving of irrigation equipment. Because of the widespread use of mechanized equipment in the US, the greatest risk of death in a farm setting is from trauma associated with farm equipment and in particular from tractor accidents. Farm vehicles account for approximately half of all fatal farm accidents, and the majority of these deaths are due to tractors. Farm equipment, and specifically tractors, are also the predominant cause of fatal injuries to children in agricultural settings. Deaths of children due to machinery are 80 times more likely to occur in a farm setting.[2] Pesticides may be applied on row crops by a variety of mechanized techniques including towed spray rigs as well as from aerial application. While most row crops in the US are amenable to mechanical harvesting, some – including celery, onions and strawberries (among others) – are still harvested by hand (Fig. 12.1). During the harvest, health concerns arise from the use of pre-harvesting pesticides (in particular insecticides and fungicides) and the resultant potential worker exposure.

Orchards

Orchards involve the year-round growing and maintenance of fruit and nut trees. By their very nature, orchards require a higher degree of manual labor and less mechanization. They require very different types of equipment and periodic maintenance of the trees, including pruning. This usually requires the use of ladders or mobile 'cherry picker' cranes, which introduce the potential for falls. As in row crops, the use of agricultural chemicals is highly crop and region specific. Depending upon the crop, the harvesting may also be highly labor intensive and utilize migrant and seasonal farm workers. Pesticide application is often mechanized, but may also be by hand, using backpack spray rigs. These can

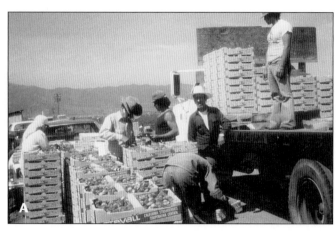
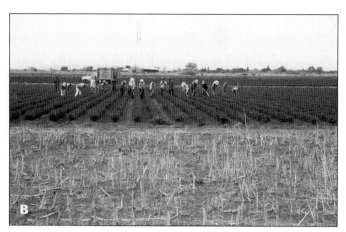

Figure 12.1: (a) and (b) Workers harvesting fresh strawberries. Workers are in the fields 8–12 hours per day harvesting crops. Note that crops are also sorted and stacked by workers in the field.

pose particular problems from leakage and spillage on the worker. One unique method of pesticide application is employed in the growing of bananas. This method makes use of pesticide-impregnated polyethylene bags. These bags, which contain a small quantity of organophosphate pesticides, are placed over bunches of bananas as they grow on the tree. This method results in lower exposures to workers, compared to manual spraying of the bananas, but may transfer the hazard to the workers involved in the manufacturing and preparation of the bags.

Livestock and poultry

The raising of livestock and poultry, as well as dairy farming, is very different in nature from the previously described types of farming activities and thus very different in the types of hazards to workers. This type of farming involves the breeding and care of farm animals ranging from chickens and turkeys to pigs, sheep, and cattle. It may include large indoor facilities and/or outdoor holding pens and feed lots. Typically, the raising of poultry for either egg production or meat usually occurs indoors. Cattle, with the exception of veal and dairy cattle, typically spend all their time outdoors. Pigs and sheep may be raised either indoors or out. While a large variety of insecticides and herbicides are used in the cultivation of row crops and fruits, a relatively limited number of insecticides and biocides are usually employed in the raising of livestock and poultry. These chemicals are applied for insect pests on the animals, or biocides for disinfections. This is often performed by workers using either hand spray or dips. While crushing injuries are possible in the handling of large animals, greater risks may be present from infectious agents (zoonoses) and from the handling of silage and grains and the inherent confined spaces and explosion hazards in storage facilities (i.e. silos, grain elevators).

Occupational hazards

Occupational hazards in farm settings may arise from several different factors including physical, chemical, and biologic factors, as well as structural and engineering practices. Physical hazards arise from lifting, climbing, heat and sunlight (ultraviolet radiation), and farm equipment (trauma). Lifting hazards can result from such diverse activities as lifting or handling irrigation pipes and equipment, and moving boxes of produce or bales of hay. While most people think of hay as something that is light, a bale of hay (depending upon type of equipment employed and moisture content) can weigh up to several hundred pounds.

Heat exhaustion can be a major problem in farming that employs manual and stoop labor for harvesting of crops, particularly in warmer climates. These workers are often paid by the quantity picked, so that workers may go from sunup to sunset with few to no work breaks. In addition, despite field sanitation laws, access to potable water may be limited. This may be compounded by requirements for the use of personal protective equipment (PPE) in the handling of pesticides (see appropriate sections below). In extreme heat, such as occurs in the southern US during the summer, as well as numerous tropical climates, the use of full PPE may be contraindicated by concerns for heat stress. In as little as 15 to 20 minutes, workers' lives can be endangered by respirators and impermeable jump suits.

Chemical hazards

In the agricultural setting, by far the most common method used to minimize dermal and/or respiratory exposures to farm chemicals is personal protective equipment (PPE). PPE may range from gloves and half-face respirators to full protective plastic suits and full-face respirators (Fig. 12.2). While PPE in agricultural settings is most commonly thought of in terms the handling of pesticides, other chemicals used on the farm can require protection of the workers as well. For example the use of anhydrous ammonia as a farm fertilizer, requires PPE for both dermal and respiratory protection. The use of PPE in particular applies to pesticide mixers, loaders, sprayers, and flaggers. It is important to consider that mixers and loaders may

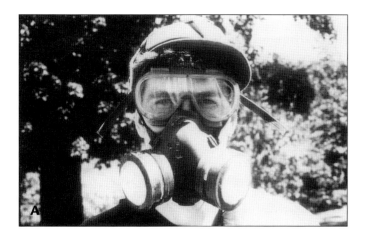

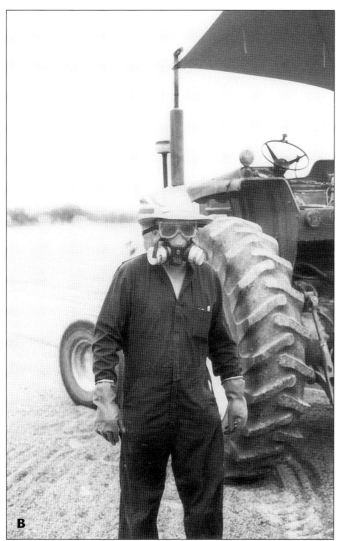

Figure 12.2: (a) and (b) A farmer wearing personal protective equipment (PPE) during a planting operation. Treated seed and granular insecticide are applied during the planting operation. Typical protection includes a respirator, gloves, goggles, and coveralls.

not even work on a farm, but rather may be employed at a small airfield where aircraft utilized for aerial spraying of pesticides and herbicides are maintained and serviced.

Mixers are involved in the preparation of the pesticide by mixing pesticides either in powder or liquid form from diluents. Diluents may be either water or organic solvents including kerosene. Additionally, surfactants such as nonyl-phenol may be added to improve the adherence of pesticides to the plants. Compounds such as nonyl-phenol and many others are viewed as 'inerts' in the technical terminology of pesticide formulation. This should not be construed to mean that these compounds may not also present some hazard. For example, in several studies nonyl-phenol has been found to be an estrogen disruptor.[3,4]

Loaders are involved in transferring the mixed pesticide to containers for application. Particular hazards may arise during pouring of solutions. Fatalities have been documented when loaders have spilled organophosphate pesticide mixtures into boots which they then failed to remove, and subsequently failed to wash the affected area promptly. The US Environmental Protection Agency estimates that farm workers experience approximately 300,000 acute illnesses and injuries each year related to pesticides. This is likely to be an underestimate of the true number as adequate clinical tests for pesticide poisonings only exist for organophosphates. There are very few states that require mandatory reporting of pesticide illnesses. In California in 1990, almost 2000 pesticide-related illnesses caused by occupational exposure were reported. More than half of these involved exposure during mixing and loading and an additional one-quarter involved exposure of workers to residues on crops.[2] Sprayers may be involved in manual spraying of crops or the operation of spray rigs. Hand spraying may involve either hand-carried tanks or spray backpacks (Fig. 12.3).

A major hazard may arise when tanks are filled while the worker is wearing these backpacks, as spillage onto the worker often occurs. Again, as with loaders, particular problems can arise from spillage into gloves or boots. Failure to remove them and wash promptly may result in acute poisoning episodes or even death. The availability of water for washing of workers who accidentally come in direct dermal contact with pesticides is another reason that field sanitation rules are important to worker health and safety. Flagging involves the use of workers on the ground, to mark areas to be treated by aerial spraying. These workers are at risk of over flight by the aircraft applying the chemicals. For this reason, the use of PPE by these workers is also important.

Once the pesticides have been applied, it is important that workers are not allowed into the field for a prescribed amount of time, termed the 're-entry' period. This is particularly important prior to harvest as a large number of workers, far more than are usually involved in the pesticide application itself, may be exposed. Re-entry periods are well established for all pesticides utilized in the US. However, re-entry time may be modified by weather, as temperature and humidity can effect how long the pesticide may remain wet and thus more readily transferable to workers. Some of the largest pesticide poisoning episodes have been associated with premature re-entry to fields following the application of organophosphate pesticides.

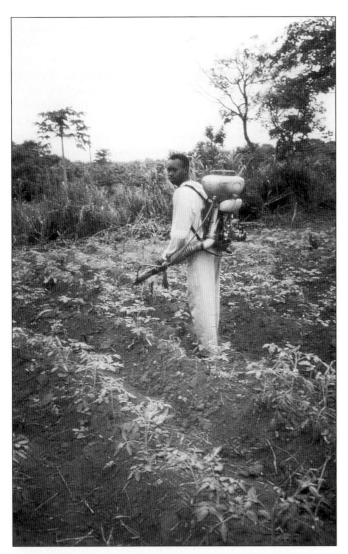

Figure 12.3: A worker applying pesticide using a backpack, mist blower sprayer. This application is taking place in West Africa; the worker is applying an organophosphate insecticide. He is not using any personal protective equipment (PPE).

Another factor that is often not considered is the potential for exposure of families of pesticide mixers, loaders, flaggers and applicators. This can result from several factors: (1) proximity of the family residence to mixing areas, (2) storage of pesticides in homes, (3) and washing of work clothes with the family laundry.[5] Workers may also reuse containers that previously held pesticides and employ these for carrying potable water. This practice has resulted in numerous poisonings and even fatalities. It is therefore important for the clinician not just to consider the potential for the exposure of pesticide workers, but the potential for exposure to their families as well.

Zoonoses

While hazards from zoonoses may most readily come to mind in the case of farms which raise livestock and poultry, they are certainly possible in other farm settings as a result of insect and arachnid bites arising from the handling of

fruits and vegetables. In the latter category, the rickettsials and arboviruses may be of concern. In addition, in the Southwestern part of the US storage of grains may lead to infestations of rodents, which may harbor fleas that carry Hanta virus. The focus of the clinician should be such that where locales are known to have problems with insect-borne viruses, zoonoses should certainly be part of the differential diagnosis and the determination of treatment of farm workers. With respect to zoonoses, animal handlers are clearly at a higher risk. With more and more farmers raising exotic livestock (i.e., alligators, llamas, emus, ostriches, etc), the possibility of non-traditional farm zoonoses must also be considered. The astute clinician needs to bear in mind these possibilities in the evaluation of infectious diseases in these workers. Despite recent concerns in Europe regarding bovine spongiform encephalopathy ('mad cow disease'), there is little evidence to suggest that farm workers are at specific risk from this agent.

Confined spaces

Though more common in grain elevators than farm silos, the hazards of confined space accidents and fatalities represent a small, but real health and safety factor on some farms. Workers who are employed at farms that store grain (either awaiting sale or for feed) are at particular risk. The hazards involved are three-fold: (1) oxygen-deficient atmospheres; (2) explosive dusts; (3) pneumoconiosis. Workers should be cautioned regarding these hazards. The hazards can be minimized either by the use of PPE or through ventilation of the spaces and testing of the atmosphere prior to entry.

Sunlight (ultraviolet radiation)

Separate from the health risks posed by heat from working in the hot sun are the risks from exposure to ultraviolet radiation during long days spent outdoors. Both acute problems such as severe sunburns, as well as chronic risks of skin cancer are associated with repeated long-term exposure to sunlight. Even though this might be perceived as being of greater concern in the warmer climates or high altitudes, these risks are quite real regardless of the locale. The preventive measures are relatively simple and include the use of sun blocks, long-sleeved shirts, and hats.

HEALTH AND SAFETY PRECAUTIONS
Personal protective equipment

The nature of farm work presents several health and safety hazards, which can be minimized by the use of proper personal protective equipment (PPE), as well as by proper engineering. Both of these methods may be employed with respect to workers' exposure to agricultural chemicals. As previously pointed out, while usually thought of in terms of pesticide application, other farm chemicals may also require PPE. The use of the correct and adequate PPE is a common problem on the farm. Farmers and farm workers often perceive pesticides as beneficial substances. Among Mexican-American farm workers, insecticides and herbicides are commonly referred to as *medicinas*, medicines for the plants. What is not obvious is that these chemicals can present both acute and chronic health risks to workers. The level of risk these chemicals may represent to human health is often not apparent to the farmers and farm workers, because technical language warning labels are frequently difficult to understand. This can be further confounded by language problems, as many farm workers in the US are illiterate in English. These workers may also be at the greatest risk for not having access to proper equipment or adequate training in its proper use. Compounded by the fact that a large proportion of farm work is done during the warm growing season, it is not surprising that PPE is underutilized on farms. Detailed studies by Fenske et al. have demonstrated that limitations of the use of some types of personal protective equipment on farms is a significant and important source of excessive exposure of workers to agricultural chemicals.[6]

The appropriate PPE for mixing, loading, and spraying of pesticides varies between specific compounds; however, in general the hazard is greatest for those involved in mixing, since they handle the most concentrated form of the chemical. PPE for agricultural workers may include either half- or full-face respirator, rubber gloves, and either a protective suit or chemical-resistant apron. In addition to inhalation as a route of exposure, some compounds can be absorbed through intact skin. The soles of the feet can be a major area of concern from accidental chemical spills in rubber protective boots. One of the difficulties in minimizing dermal exposure is to convince workers of the necessity for protective clothing. The other problem is the previously mentioned issue of balancing the chemical hazards against the heat stress that wearing PPE may entail. Since most small farming operations lack the resources and ability to train workers, problems of excessive exposure and poisoning of farm workers will unfortunately continue. For this reason clinicians, and particularly emergency room workers, need to be familiar with the recognition and treatment of acute organophosphate poisoning.

Controlled-environment cabs

Due to the increased mechanization of the application of agricultural chemicals, the use and desirability of controlled-environment cabs has increased in farm equipment. While the move to controlled-environment cabs has been driven by driver comfort (air conditioning), these cabins are increasingly being engineered into farm equipment for the increased protection they offer operators to inhalation exposure to agricultural chemicals. These systems may include the use of both high efficiency particulate filters (HEPA), as well as those for organic vapors. There may also be pre-filters to trap large dust particles. If manufacturer's recommendations are followed including appropriate routine replacement of filters; these cabs can reduce or eliminate major sources of worker exposure to agricultural chemicals. This has a two-fold benefit in eliminating the direct health effects of the exposure to the worker, as well as the additional protection from the potential of some chemicals to impair the ability of the operator to safely operate farm equipment.

Rollover protection

Injury data on farm accidents that result in serious injuries or death indicate that single greatest risk for farmers and farm workers results from rollover accidents of tractors and farm equipment. Tractor accidents account for an estimated 600 fatalities per year. Rollovers account for more than half of these deaths. Tractors made more than 40 years ago are still in operation today. It is estimated that fewer than one-third of the 4.4 million tractors used for agricultural purposes have rollover protection. Older tractors often are used in situations typically associated with tractor rollover accidents, such as mowing the road ditch area, using a front-end loader, and hauling fallen trees.[7,8] Because many tractors are based on a tripod like structure with two closely spaced wheels in the front (Fig. 12.4), they are prone to tip and roll over. While some tractors have adopted a wider spacing of the front wheels (Fig. 12.5) to decrease the risk of rollover, this does not totally eliminate the problem. In the US, tractors have been required to be fitted with seat belts and rollover protection since 1976. When used properly, this combination has been shown to significantly reduce the risk of injury from tractor rollover accidents.[7] Unfortunately, many older tractors still in use do not have these safety devices; however, retrofitting kits are available at reasonable costs. Given the high rate of injuries from tractors without rollover protection and seatbelts, the cost/risk benefit for these devices cannot be overstated.

Equipment guards

Another significant source of farm-related injuries is limb crushing and amputations from power take-off attach-

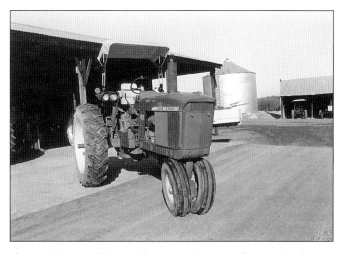

Figure 12.4: An older model tractor with narrow front end and no rollover protection system (ROPS), with only a shade used to reduce exposure to the sun.

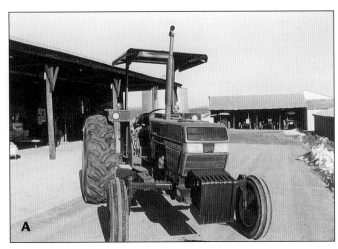
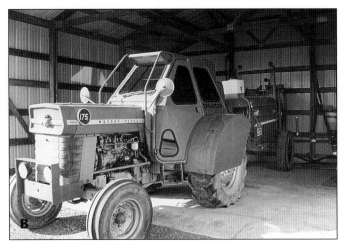

Figure 12.5: (a) and (b) Modern tractors with rollover protection system (ROPS). Note the tractors have a wide front end and front-end weights to counterbalance any equipment attached to the drawbar at the rear.

ments to farm equipment. While most modern farm equipment includes appropriate guards for pulleys and power take-offs, this equipment may be removed or not properly re-installed when the equipment undergoes repair or maintenance. It is important that farmers and farm workers appreciate the severity of injuries that may result from failure to employ these important safety devices.

CHRONIC DISEASE AND INJURY
Cancer

Numerous studies of farmers and farm workers have observed an increased risk of cancer. In particular, studies have found elevated risks for the development of hematopoietic malignancies including leukemias and non-Hodgkin's lymphomas.[9] These studies examined a broad range of farm activities as potential risk factors, including a variety of agricultural chemicals and possible zoonoses associated with livestock and poultry production. Most of the studies have focused on specific herbicides and pesticides used on farms. This has proven to be a difficult task for several reasons. First, a large variety of pesticides are applied on many farms. Second, changes have taken place both in the types of pesticides applied, as well as the method of application. Finally, a large group of agricultural workers, who are employed as migrant and seasonal employees, have been difficult to track with respect to health endpoints. However, despite these limitations, several chemicals have been implicated in epidemiologic studies including 2,4-D (2,4-dichlorophenoxyacetic acid). While no firm conclusions have been reached with respect to these pesticides and the apparent increased risks of cancer, it would appear to be prudent for farmers and farm workers to minimize their exposure to farm chemicals.

Clearly it is important for farmers and farm workers to make use of protective measures (as previously described) in handling farm chemicals. In addition, it is important for them to follow manufacturer's guidelines with respect

to proper use of PPE for mixing, application, and field re-entry. By following these procedures exposure and cancer risks should be minimized.

Even though the source of the increased risk of hematopoietic cancers in agricultural workers is not fully understood, one well-understood cancer risk is ultraviolet radiation from sunlight. Agricultural workers are thus at increased risk for skin cancers including squamous and basal cell carcinomas and malignant melanoma. While skin pigment (level of melanin) is important in the actual level of risk, even dark-complexioned farm workers are at elevated risk. As was previously discussed, the use of sun block, hats and long-sleeved shirts can help minimize these risks.

Dermatologic conditions

Besides the risk of skin cancer, other dermatologic conditions are also associated with work on farms. These may arise from a variety of different types of exposures. These include, but are not limited to, the maintenance of farm equipment, handling of farm chemicals and certain farm produce. Irritant contact dermatitis from the maintenance of farm equipment results from the handling of gasoline, diesel, and oil. Allergic contact dermatitis may also result from handling the crops or livestock. Skin problems associated with insecticides and herbicides can arise from the use of organic solvent diluents acting as defatting agents, as well as from the chemicals themselves. Some of the earliest dermatologic problems documented in the medical literature, pertaining to agricultural workers, were keratoses associated with the use of arsenical compounds in vintners.[10]

Clearly those individuals who are involved in mixing of pesticides may be at greatest risk due to their handling of the concentrated chemicals. It is also important to point out that the risk of dermatitis may not just arise from the handling of chemicals, but also from improper hygiene in the use of rubber gloves. If the protective rubber gloves are not thoroughly cleaned and dried inside and out, bacterial growth can lead to secondary infection, e.g. cellulitis. Therefore the availability and use of clean, dry gloves for PPE is essential. This can be aided by the use of disposable cotton liners for rubber gloves.

Musculoskeletal disorders

Musculoskeletal problems on the farm arise at least to some extent from the combination of light activities such as running farm equipment, in conjunction with other tasks requiring heavy lifting. Even though increased mechanization has made many tasks easier, lifting is still required for numerous farming activities. Lifting tasks on farms can range from replacement of tires on farm equipment to lifting bales of hay or boxes of produce. In addition, repetitive trauma to the wrist and elbow joints may arise from activities relating to hand picking of crops and/or trimming of vines. Migrant or seasonal farm workers are at particular risk for this type of injury. While the repetitive nature of hand milking has mostly disappeared from dairy farms in the US, musculoskeletal problems are still present from the bending and/or kneeling involved in attaching the automatic milking equipment in some dairy farm settings. This can be minimized by ergonomic design of the milking area, including the use of different elevations that allow workers to attach the equipment while in a standing position. There are also risks to workers of being stepped on or kicked, resulting in either crushing injuries or fractures in the handling of large animals.

Neurologic disorders

The use of pesticides, in particular organophosphates (OPs) and carbamates, has long been associated with acute neurologic conditions (see Chapters 28.1 and 48) but relatively little research has been conducted on possible chronic health effects of these compounds. Many of the older OPs were highly lipophilic and so long-term effects are possible. Future research is clearly called for in this area.

Reproductive disorders

Another area which has been of concern with respect to agricultural workers is the possibility of adverse reproductive effects. Areas that have been studied include both effects to males (i.e. azoospermia, oligospermia), female infertility and effects to the developing fetus (i.e. spontaneous abortion, low birth weight, stillbirth, and congenital malformations).[11-19] An increasing number of human epidemiologic studies have examined this issue. Clearly the majority of studies have examined the potential for health effects to the fetus (see Endocrine & Reproductive Disorder).[11-17] The evidence for significant adverse health effects to the fetus from pesticides and herbicides used on farms is increasing. In comparison to the volume of work on direct effects to the fetus, relatively little is know about effects on male gamete production (i.e. sperm abnormalities, oligospermia, azoospermia).

Perhaps the best documented effects on males involved farm workers using the pesticide dibromo-chloropropane (DBCP) in Rio Frio, Costa Rica.[18] In this study, male workers who were exposed to DBCP experienced sharp reductions in sperm production. While in most individuals this was found to be reversible, some men experienced permanent azoospermia. Arsenical compounds have been utilized both as pesticides and as defoliants on cotton. Based primarily upon a large number of animal studies, but also on studies of workers in production facilities, concern has been raised about arsenic compounds and a variety of reproductive endpoints.[17] These include increased rates of spontaneous abortion, stillbirths, and congenital malformations. Unfortunately, for many agricultural chemicals the issue of reproductive toxicity has been largely overlooked.

Respiratory diseases

Upper and lower respiratory symptoms among farm workers can result from non-specific mucous membrane irritation due to the fumes and dusts associated with crops, animal waste, and farm chemicals. Asthma and allergies are common from exposure and sensitivity to plant and animal allergens. 'Farmer's lung' is an illustrative term used to describe hypersensitivity pneumonitis among farmers. Although historically described as due to thermophilic actinomycetes contamination of hay, sugar cane, and mushrooms, hypersensitivity pneumonitis has now been ascribed to numerous bacterial, mold, and animal antigens found in various farming processes. In its acute form, hypersensitivity pneumonitis may mimic influenza, presenting with fever, chills, malaise, cough and shortness of breath, which usually resolves within a few days after removal from exposure. Chronic hypersensitivity pneumonitis may develop after repeated acute episodes and continued antigen exposure or rarely after a single severe attack. This can lead to irreversible progressive airflow limitation and parenchymal changes (see Chapter 19.6). While corticosteroids may be used to treat acute episodes, prevention either by removal of the exposure or avoidance of the exposure by the affected worker remains the mainstay of treatment.

CHILD LABOR

Perhaps no area is of greater concern with regard to the health and safety of agricultural workers than the plight of children as farm workers. This takes two forms: first, children who work on the family farm, and second, those children whose families are employed as migrant and seasonal farm workers. With regard to the former group, the major concern is the operation of farm equipment, where a disproportional number of tractor accidents involve young drivers. In respect to the latter group, the effect may be far less obvious, but no less serious. These children, some less than one year of age, are exposed to long days in the field. Those only slightly older (age 3) may be actively involved in the harvesting of row crops. This brings up not just the issue of repetitive trauma, but possible health effects of pesticides on infants and young children.

Unfortunately, little research has been conducted to determine the full range of health hazards these chemicals may represent to young children. It is also essential to keep in mind that personal hygiene is usually poorer in young children and infants. This, coupled with the high frequency of hand/mouth and object/mouth activities, results in a high risk for pesticide ingestion. For these reasons, it should be clear these children represent a high-risk population. Unfortunately, neither state nor federal laws in the US appear to adequately address this problem. Pediatricians in agricultural communities need to be cognizant of pesticide-related health effects and well educated in recognition and treatment of acute poisoning.

While many people view the farm environment as a safe place for children, the truth is that many children who work on farms suffer serious injuries and death. The National Agricultural Worker's Survey indicated that between 1993 and 1996 there were approximately 128,000 farm workers aged 14 to 17.[20] In the US in 1998, approximately 33,000 agricultural injuries occurred to children or adolescents under the age of 20. Injuries occur annually at a rate of 17 per 1000 farms. Boys were almost four times as likely as girls to suffer an injury. Approximately a third of all youth injuries occurred in children age 10 to 15, resulting in almost 300 deaths per year. Sixty-four percent of the work-related fatalities in children under age 16 occur on family-owned farms. Farm machinery, in particular tractors, is the leading cause of fatal farm accidents, accounting for 36% of deaths in workers under the age of 20. Perhaps most tragically, 30% of farm equipment accidents take the life of children under the age of 5. This same age group also falls victim to drowning, which is the second leading cause of farm deaths.[21]

References

1. United States Department of Agriculture, National Agricultural Statistics Service. 1997 Census of Agriculture: Geographic Area Series, Volume 1. Washington DC: The National Agricultural Statistical Service, 1999.
2. California Environmental Protection Agency, Department of Pesticide Regulation. Summary of illness and injuries reported by California physicians as potentially related to pesticides in 1990. Sacramento, CA: HS-1666, March 1, 1993.
3. Odum J, Lefevre PA, Tittensor S et al. The rodent uterotrophic assay: critical protocol features, studies with nonyl-phenols, and comparison with a yeast estrogenicity assay. Reg Toxicol Pharmacol 1997; 25:176.
4. Clement B, Donnelly KC, Ake CL et al. Chemical and bioassay analysis of water and soil extracts from south Texas. Organohal Comp 1997; 32:216.
5. Gladen BC, Sandler DP, Zahm SH et al. Exposure opportunities of families of farmer pesticide applicators. Am J Ind Med 1998; 34:581.
6. Fenske R. Visual scoring system for fluorescence tracer evaluation of dermal exposures to pesticides. Bull Environ Contam Tox 1988; 41:727.
7. Kelsey T, Jenkins P. Farm tractors and mandatory roll-over protection retrofits: potential cost of the policy in New York. Am J Public Health 1991; 81:921.
8. Schwab C, Hanna M, Miller L. Use tractors with ROPS to save lives. Fact Sheet PM 1265. Ames, IA: Iowa State University, 1992.
9. Keller-Byrne J, Khuder S, Schaub E, McAfee O. A meta-analysis of non-Hodgkin's lymphoma among farmers in the Central United States. Am J Ind Med 1997; 31:442.
10. International Agency for Research on Cancer (IARC). Some inorganic and organometallic compounds, Vol. 2. Lyon, France: International Agency for Research on Cancer, 1973.
11. Garcia AM. Occupational exposure to pesticides and congenital malformations: a review of mechanisms, methods and results. Am J Ind Med 1998; 33:232.
12. Garcia AM, Benavides FG, Fletcher T, Orts E. Paternal exposure to pesticides and congenital malformations. Scand J Work Environ Health 1998; 24:473.
13. Ihrig MM, Shalat SL, Baynes C. A hospital-based case-control study of stillbirths and environmental exposure to arsenic using an atmospheric dispersion model linked to a geographical information system. Epidemiology 1998; 9:290-294.
14. Arbuckle TE, Sever LE. Pesticide exposures and fetal death: a review of the epidemiologic literature. Crit Rev Toxicol 1998; 28:229.
15. Kristensen P, Irgens LM, Andersen A, et al. Gestational age, birth weight, and perinatal death among births in Norwegian farmers, 1967–1991. Am J Epidemiol 1997; 15:329.
16. Shaw GM, Wasserman CR, O'Malley CD, et al. Maternal pesticide exposure from multiple sources and selected congenital anomalies. Epidemiology 1999; 10:60.
17. Shalat SL, Walker DB, Finnell RH. The role of arsenic as a reproductive toxin with particular attention to neural tube defects. J Toxicol Environ Health 1996; 48:101.
18. Fuortes L, Clark M, Kirchner H, Smith E. Association between female infertility and agricultural work history. Am J Ind Med 1997; 31:445.
19. Thrupp LA. Sterilization of workers from pesticide exposure: the causes and consequences of DBCP-induced damage in Costa Rica and beyond. Int J Health Serv 1991; 21:731.
20. A profile of US farm workers. Demographics, household composition, income and use of services. Based on the data from the National Agricultural Workers Survey. Washington DC: US Department of Labor, 1997.
21. National Children's Center for Rural and Agricultural Health and Safety. Fact sheet – agricultural safety and children. Marshfield, WI: Marshfield Clinic National Farm Medicine Center, 2000.

Chapter 13
Mining

Jeffrey L Kohler

INTRODUCTION

Mining is a basic industry, providing modern society with the energy and material resources required for everyday life as we have come to enjoy it. The role of our mineral wealth is apparent when we see copper plumbing, a concrete sidewalk, or a piece of gold jewelry. Although the use of electricity is ubiquitous, many are unaware that over 50% of it is generated in coal-fired plants. Even less obvious dependencies include carpets (whose components include five mined products), plastic pipe (with a pulverized stone content of 50%), computers that contain more than 30 mined products, and paint and many medicines that depend upon mined constituents for their prized properties, to name but a few. Agriculture is heavily dependent on mined products in the form of fertilizers, and other industries utilize mined products even when those mineral commodities do not show up in the manufactured article. Indeed, it is difficult to find any corner of the economy that is not tied to the availability of quality minerals or mineral resources.

Mineral resources come from the Earth's crust, and their extraction is seldom easy. Even after extraction, considerable effort may be expended to separate, refine, and concentrate the valuable minerals that are often mixed or bound with waste materials. Minerals production can be divided into two general phases: the *extraction phase* is concerned with removing the material from the Earth; the *processing phase* separates the valuable component from the less valuable or waste material. In practice the distinction between the two phases is often blurred. Commonly, the term mining is used to describe the extraction phase, while processing is used to describe the phase of preparing the product for human use. Usually, the people involved in both are called miners or mineworkers, although in some quarters other terms are used.

In its simplest definition, mining includes all of the job processes required to produce a mineral commodity in saleable form. A simple example would be the mining of a limestone deposit and the subsequent processing to a crushed stone for sale to a concrete producer. A more complex example would be the mining of an iron ore deposit and the subsequent processing to concentrated taconite pellets for sale to a smelter. An increasing number of mining operations are becoming vertically integrated – that is, an end product for direct sale to the consumer is produced and processed on the mine site.

Economics and globalization of mining

Mining occurs where the deposit is found, of course, and where the mined commodity can be converted economically to the desired product. Transportation costs are often a limiting factor, and accordingly coal will be mined for the use of a nearby power plant or perhaps a plant that is hundreds of miles away but readily served by rail. Stone, on the other hand, has a lower value with respect to its transportation cost, so a stone mine will typically serve customers within only several miles. The transportation factor and the geographic linkage between mining and manufacturing have become more evident in recent years as metal mines employing hundreds of workers (e.g., copper mines) have closed and moved operations to other countries. Shortly thereafter, the associated manufacturing plants (e.g., copper rod and wire), also employing several hundred workers, close and move operations nearer to other mines. Of course, certain rare and precious commodities are completely decoupled from the transportation cost constraint – e.g., gold and diamonds.

Mined products had a value of 60 billion dollars in 2002, and added nearly one-half trillion dollars in value to the US economy. Approximately 300,000 people were directly involved in mining, and another 3 million people were employed downstream in the support, processing, and conversion of these mineral resources. Figure 13.1 illustrates the location of mines, by sector, within the United States – as the data reveal, mining occurs in almost every part of the country. (The sectors in common use are coal, metal, stone, and non-metal. Non-metal includes such commodities as boron, potash, sulfur, salt, and vermiculite. The US Geological Survey[1] provides an excellent discussion of all US mineral commodities.)

Mining has always been a global endeavor, but over the past decade the globalization of the industry has accelerated. Large multinational corporations now conduct extensive metal, non-metal, and coal mining in the United States and in South America, Africa, Europe, Asia, and Australia. Mining methods and equipment have become similar throughout much of the developed world, as have occupational health and safety hazards to which mineworkers are exposed. At the same time, this globalization has presented significant parallel opportunities to improve conditions on a global basis. For example, successful health and safety interventions are developed in one country and then applied to similar mines throughout the world. While many of the examples used in this chapter are drawn from

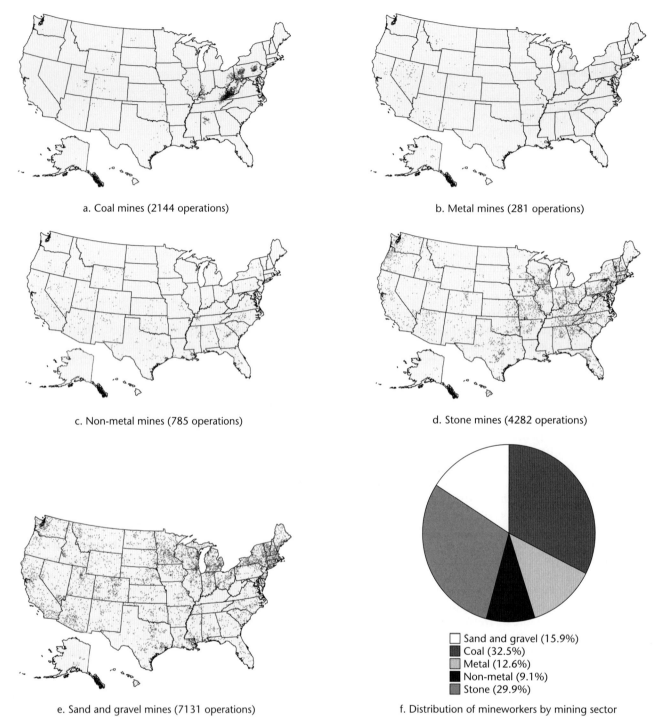

a. Coal mines (2144 operations)

b. Metal mines (281 operations)

c. Non-metal mines (785 operations)

d. Stone mines (4282 operations)

e. Sand and gravel mines (7131 operations)

f. Distribution of mineworkers by mining sector

☐ Sand and gravel (15.9%)
■ Coal (32.5%)
☐ Metal (12.6%)
■ Non-metal (9.1%)
■ Stone (29.9%)

Figure 13.1: Location of mines and distribution of mineworker employees by mining sector in the Unites States. Parts (a)–(e) from MSHA 2001,[21] part (f) from NIOSH 2003.[22]

the US mining industry, the mining methods, descriptions and associated health and safety issues apply to mining throughout most of the world.

Human costs of mining

In the course of meeting society's direct and multifaceted needs for mineral commodities, mineworkers have been killed, others have suffered lost-time injuries, and still others have endured the silent progression of occupational illnesses brought on by excess exposures to noise, dust, or other potentially harmful substances. Similar injuries and illnesses occur throughout the mining industry. At the most severe levels are traumatic injuries, cumulative trauma disorders, respiratory diseases, and hearing impairment or loss. Certain injuries and illnesses are far worse for certain commodities or mining methods, and a few are particular to a specific commodity or method.

Mines are 'built' directly within the crust of the Earth and therefore are made of whatever geologic materials exist at the site. Thus, the geologic setting can be inhospitable, containing dangerous gases, and the associated rock can be weak and prone to failure. This creates special health and safety challenges well beyond those of a factory setting, where the construction is entirely man-made materials and the factory operations are comparatively routine and predictable. Moreover, the dimensions of the working spaces within the mine are generally limited by the deposit dimensions, and in many cases this results in confined space working conditions.

A more detailed discussion of health and safety issues is presented later in the chapter.

MINING METHODS

The classification of mining methods for engineering purposes is complex, with many individual methods and sub-methods in use. However, in the interest of focusing on health and safety issues, a number of simplifications can be made. First, all mines can be classified as one of three types: *surface*, *underground*, or *solution*. Deposits that are close to the surface can be accessed by removing the relatively shallow cover or overburden materials, thereby exposing the deposit that can then be recovered. Copper, coal, and stone are examples of materials that are commonly mined by surface mining methods. Deposits buried deeper within the Earth's crust cannot be accessed simply by removing the overlying materials, so access to the deposit is gained by sinking shafts or driving other openings from the surface down one hundred to a few thousand meters deep to the deposit. Then an extensive network of 'tunnels' is driven into the deposit itself and/or within the host rock surrounding the deposit. This network of openings both facilitates the extraction of the ore and provides a way for the services infrastructure to get the ore from the solid ore body to the surface. Underground mining is much more difficult, expensive, and dangerous than surface mining, so it is primarily used for commodities that are otherwise unavailable from surface mines. Examples of underground mines include coal, gold, salt, and stone.

Occasionally a deep deposit can be mined with a solution method, in which 'wells' are drilled into the deposit, a dissolution agent is pumped down the well, and the solution is pumped back out for removal of the desired metal or mineral. This type of mining is used for commodities such as sulfur, trona, salt, and uranium, and is sometimes known as borehole mining. A modification of this is heap leaching, in which low-grade ores are mined, typically by surface methods, and placed into engineered piles where the lixiviant percolates through the pile. The resulting solution is then treated to recover the mineral product of interest. Heap leaching remains an important method for recovering gold.

The mining engineer chooses the mining method based on several technical and market factors. While it may be significantly cheaper to surface mine 100-foot-thick coal seams in Wyoming than to underground mine five-foot-thick seams in West Virginia, the cost of transporting the Powder River Basin coal to the East Coast tips the balance in favor of the more expensively mined coal in West Virginia.

Mine type	Class	Method	Commodities
Surface	–	Strip (open cast)	Coal
		Quarry	Stone
		Open pit	Metal
		Dredging	Metal, non-metal
Underground	Stoping	Room and pillar mining	Coal, non-metal
		Stope and pillar mining	Metal, non-metal
		Sublevel stoping	Metal, non-metal
		Cut and fill stoping	Metal
	Caving	Longwall mining	Coal
		Block caving	Metal
Solution	–	Leaching	Metal
		Borehole	Non-metal

Table 13.1 Important methods used to mine coal, metal, and non-metal commodities

Another example described earlier is stone. As a very low-cost commodity, it would appear that surface mining would be the only economic choice. However, some limestones are of very high purity, often called 'pharmaceutical grade', and because of this they fetch higher prices.

Major mining methods are summarized in Table 13.1. These methods will be described in more detail for each of the major mining sectors of coal, metal, and non-metal. For each sector the more important underground and surface methods will be summarized. The presentation of the mining methods is then followed with an overview of mineral processing operations. A complete treatment of mining methods is given by Hartman and Mutmansky.[2]

Underground coal mining

Deep coal deposits are tabular in nature (i.e., they lie in horizontal layers), and those being mined range from under a meter to several meters in thickness, with a thickness of a few meters accounting for the majority of underground mines. Within the coal seam, rooms are mined and pillars are left behind to support the overlying strata or roof of the mine. This is known as room and pillar mining, and is conducted usually with continuous mining equipment, and rarely today with the older conventional mining equipment. Continuous mining involves equipment that both cuts and removes material without the more conventional use of drills or explosives.

As the rooms are mined a vast network of 'tunnels' is created, stretching for many miles in larger mines. These mined openings are known as 'entries' and 'cross-cuts'. As these are developed they serve as conduits for ventilating air, travel and haulage ways for people, machines, conveyor belts, and even a mine-size railway system. Indeed, the underground mine is like a small city, complete with an electricity distribution system, as well as fresh and contaminated water distribution systems. While it is protected from the weather by virtue of being underground, parts of the mine closer to the intake air portals reflect the outside air temperature due to the high volumes of air drawn into the mine, whereas parts more distant from the fresh air

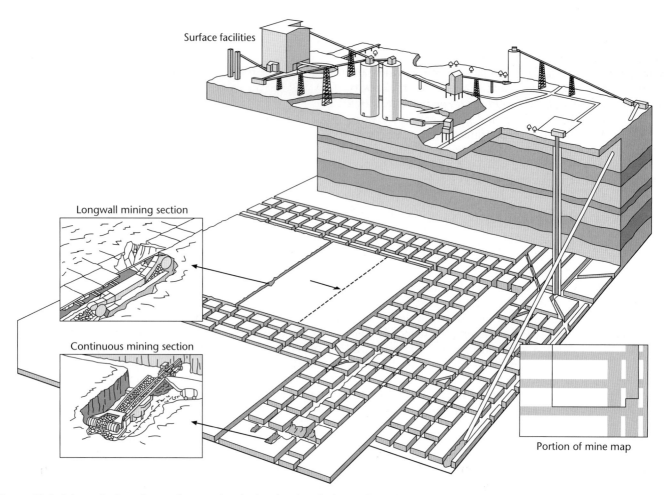

Surface facilities

Longwall mining section

Continuous mining section

Portion of mine map

Figure 13.2: Schematic view of an underground coal mine showing the longwall panel and the 'rooms and pillars' comprising the network of underground openings.

intakes more closely reflect the temperature of the deposit. During the winter, for example, the temperature of the intake air may be well below freezing and remain near freezing through much of the main entryways of the mine, although it would be warmed by the underground rock, which may be close to 15 degrees C. By the time this air reaches the working face, the air temperature may approach 25 degrees C. Such significant temperature differentials are not uncommon in other locations and mining types. The air in some parts is further warmed by the equipment, but throughout the mine the air tends to be very humid. Some mine operations cut through or break into the water table, and in these situations it may even seem to be raining in parts of the mine with generally wet conditions throughout.

Room and pillar mining is practiced by itself in smaller mines, whereas in larger mines room and pillar mining is used to facilitate a more productive method known as longwall mining. In this method, room and pillar mining is used to create the main infrastructure – in a sense the major highways and secondary roadways of the mine 'city' – and to delineate large blocks of coal. These large blocks

are then longwall mined at great efficiency and with additional safety over the room and pillar method. A brief overview of continuous and conventional mining methods is presented in Chapter 19.10. Figure 13.2 illustrates an underground coal mine with room and pillar workings and longwall panels. A longwall face is shown in Figure 13.3.

The primary hazards of underground coal mining fall into four general categories, each of which is discussed in greater detail below and in subsequent chapters:

* *traumatic injuries* – these are caused by rock falls or the consequence of large machines and people working in close proximity in a confined space;
* *cumulative stress disorders* – these disorders arise from working in a confined space in which the distance between the floor and roof may be well under a meter, necessitating extensive crawling, kneeling, and 'duck walking,' or from operating equipment mechanisms, such as remote control consoles that require repetitive motions;
* *respiratory disease* – respirable coal dust is liberated during the mining process, and silica dust is generated during different phases of mining, especially during drilling to

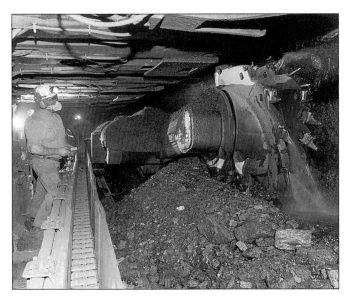

Figure 13.3: Coal mine longwall face, showing the shearer operator with the remote control pendant for the shearer. An important engineering control, the dust suppression water sprays, is visible, as is the personal protective equipment used by the operator. Note the confined conditions under which the operator performs the job over a period of 8–12 hours. (Photograph courtesy of Joy Mining Machinery, 2003.)

install roof bolts and from the action of longwall shields;
- *hearing loss* – the act of ripping tons of rock per minute from the deposit, rock drilling, and the many associated operations are inherently noisy, and harmful noise levels may result.

Surface coal mining

When the deposit lies close enough to the surface, it may be economically feasible to remove all of the overlying materials to expose and then mine the coal. Various methods used to do this make up surface mining, also known as open cast mining. Regardless of the specific method employed, surface coal mines follow a typical sequence of operations.
1. Vegetation is removed and soil layers are removed and stored for subsequent use.
2. The rock layers overlying the coal seam – referred to as 'overburden' – are removed and stored. Generally this overburden removal involves the drilling of holes for explosives, then blasting, loading, and hauling the overburden.
3. The exposed coal seam is mined, which may involve some additional drilling and blasting prior to loading and hauling.
4. After the coal has been harvested, the overlying materials are then returned in an exact sequence, which may involve the addition of materials such as stone or lime to neutralize acid-bearing layers and to facilitate the reclamation of the disturbed area.

Often the terrain overlying the coal is not flat but mounainous, and as mining advances the depth of the overburden will increase until it is no longer economically wise to remove it. At this point, surface mining stops, leaving an exposed highwall. Sometimes an underground coal mine will be developed, gaining access through the exposed coal seam in the highwall, and other times mining is terminated. An alternative to both of these is to engage in some form of highwall mining, in which a mining machine, such as a thin seam miner or an auger, is set up and operated on the bench – a horizontal working surface created during mining – at the highwall face. This allows some coal to be retrieved at a low cost without the expense or risk of developing an underground mine. The distance to which these machines can 'burrow' under the mountain top is of the order of 300 meters or less. While the mining operations are obviously vastly different for the surface mining of a 30-meter-thick seam in the wide open spaces of Wyoming versus a 1-meter-thick seam on a mountainside of West Virginia, similar health and safety issues exist for both.

By definition, the health and safety hazards are somewhat less in surface than underground mining. Many of the confined space issues of underground mining disappear, as do many of the respiratory hazards. The open spaces of surface mining also permit the use of cabs on equipment to protect workers from excessive noise levels, which cannot be done as practically in an underground mine. Generally, all of these facts are also reflected in surveillance data. Nevertheless, some surface coal mineworkers are exposed to hazardous levels of respirable coal dust, and drillers have the potential to be exposed to silica dust when the overburden contains crystalline quartz. Traumatic injuries still occur, and cumulative stress disorders are as prevalent as in underground mining, although slightly different in cause.

Underground metal mining

Underground mining of deposits containing metal – called 'metaliferous' – is dramatically declining in the United States, due to the high cost of recovering relatively low-grade ores, although many new metal mines are being developed in South America, Australia, and Asia. Within the US, there are some remaining underground mines, primarily in the western part of the country, principally for mining gold, silver, lead, zinc, molybdenum, and platinum. Of course, if a high-grade deposit were discovered, it is likely that new operations would open. Metaliferous deposits tend to be complex in shape when compared to the relatively tabular coal deposits, and accordingly, the mines tend to be more complex as their workings access different parts of the deposit. These mines are typically developed at many different depths or levels, and there may be extensive development within the host rock as well as in the ore body itself.

Access into the mine is usually by way of a vertical or inclined shaft (called a 'winze'), although ramps may wind between levels as well. Various openings are mined to access the ore body, and various levels are interconnected by raises and winzes. The term 'stopes' refers to working areas where ore is being removed. Depending on the method, openings are mined to provide chutes and funneling channels to drawpoints, where the broken material is concentrated and removed. Given the complex three-dimensional nature of the mine and the varying combination of properties between the deposit and surrounding rock, a variety of caving and stoping methods have evolved. In the *caving method*, the relatively weak ore is undercut in some fashion, and the ore then 'caves' under its own weight, with or without some blasting, into areas from which it will be loaded and removed. In the *stoping method*, openings are driven into the ore body and the material is drilled, blasted, loaded, and removed. As caving methods are less costly than stoping, they can be used to recover lower-grade ores economically. As with the underground coal mine, underground metal mines usually have a significant infrastructure of utilities and materials handling systems. From an occupational health and safety perspective, however, the complex mining nuances are less important than the commonalities of health and safety risks inherent in all mining processes.

Drilling and blasting

Drilling – which utilizes large rubber-tired equipment such as jumbo drills or portable drills such as drifters or stoppers – is a major unit operation in underground metal mining. This drilling is done to provide a cavity to accept explosives and the holes are drilled to exact, calculated depths and in carefully controlled patterns. Care is taken to ensure safe and efficient rock breakage without undue overbreakage of the surrounding rock, proper size distribution of the fragments, and appropriate positioning of the blasted material. In any drilling operation, respiratory hazards are associated with generated dust and air-borne lubricants in the drill exhaust. Repetitive stress trauma and noise exposure are also common health issues associated with drilling. Cumulative stress and vibration problems are especially worrisome with portable drills.

Established blasting practices ensure that the substantial hazards of handling explosives result in very few injuries. As personnel are evacuated prior to blasting, the potential hazards of toxic fumes, dust, and noise are drastically reduced. However, it is possible for fumes to remain in a pile of blasted rock until the pile is disturbed by loading operations, with the fumes then liberated. A more common worry is the possibility of a 'bootleg' hole that failed to 'fire', leaving open the possibility of an inadvertent explosive discharge during loading with potentially serious consequences to workers in the area.

Loading and haulage

Loading of the ore, or waste rock, is likely to be done using diesel-powered vehicles in the form of separate loaders and trucks, or using a hybrid vehicle known as a load-haul-dump (LHD). The hazards associated with loading include excessive noise, diesel exhaust, and repetitive stress trauma. In some operations, electrically powered trucks may be used with a significant reduction in the respiratory hazards to the miner. Electrically powered slushers – machines that employ scraper blades to move material – are still used in some mining methods to move the ore from a drawpoint

to a point where it is either loaded or flows by gravity to a collection point.

Mining support workers

In all types of mining, a large number of workers who are not involved directly in the extraction or processing nevertheless perform essential support services. Ground control, ventilation, electrical power, compressed air, and materials handling are but a few examples. In addition to being at risk for traumatic injuries, these workers also undergo health and safety risks due to their exposure to high-noise environments and from repetitive stress trauma. A significant health hazard present in many underground metal mines, but absent from most coal mines, is heat stress. Often there are significant geothermal gradients in proximity to the metaliferous deposits, and it is not unusual for the wall rock to exceed temperatures of 35 degrees C.

Surface metal mines

Open pit mining is a common method used to extract metaliferous ore bodies lying close to the surface. Unlike coal deposits, these can be a thousand meters or more in thickness, and as a result mining develops and continues downward until an economic limit is reached. In the case of an especially large deposit, this can take many years or several decades. The need to gradually spiral down through the deposit – and to facilitate the movement of equipment and ore in and out of the pit – gives rise to the characteristic shape of open pit mines. The 'steps' or benches are built to provide a working surface, and the combination of benches reduces the chance of a slope failure – when sections of the pit walls break free and fall downward with potentially disastrous results for workers below.

The general sequence of mining in open pit operations is as follows. Large drills are used to drill blastholes, which are then filled with explosives. Periodically these explosives are 'shot', resulting in a large pile of broken material, which is then loaded using front end loaders, shovels, or hydraulic excavators, and finally placed in large haul trucks. The trucks then travel out of the pit to a dump where the ore is often crushed and transported by belt to a plant for processing. Sometimes the trucks only travel part-way out of the pit and then dump onto an in-pit crusher. This crusher feeds a conveyor belt that transports the ore more economically out of the pit and directly to the nearby processing plant.

The health and safety hazards are again less in surface metal mines as compared to underground mines, but still include traumatic injury, repetitive stress trauma, noise exposure, and dust. Drillers and blasters have the greatest exposure to dust and noise, and jarring and jolting can be particularly problematic for truck drivers.

Underground non-metal mining

The primary non-metallic materials mined underground include salt, trona (a mineral used as a source of sodium carbonate), and stone. Trona mining is concentrated in Wyoming, while underground salt mines are dotted in a few locations of the East and Midwest. Underground stone mines are primarily located in the East, and their numbers are increasing. Methods similar to the room and pillar used in coal mining are frequently used in these tabular stone deposits, although a more irregular spacing of the pillars is necessary in both salt and stone, and thus the method is often termed stope and pillar rather than room and pillar mining.

Trona mines utilize mining machinery similar to coal mines, whereas salt and stone mines utilize equipment more characteristic of underground metal mining. Thus continuous mining machines, full-face boring machines, and roadheaders (boom-type tunneling machines) are found in underground non-metal operations such as trona, while diesel-powered drills, front end loaders, and haul trucks are found in stone and salt mines.

Surface non-metal mining

The surface mining of non-metallics ranges over several important materials, but such mining constitutes a small portion of overall mining activity with the exception of aggregates – the mineral materials used in making concrete – including stone, sand, gravel, and dimension stone. Aggregate operations occur in large numbers throughout the country. Dimension stone is a localized but important industry in certain parts of the country, where granite, marble, and slate are carefully mined for a variety of architectural uses.

The surface mining of stone is known as quarrying, and the open pit mine is called a quarry. The unit operations and sequence of quarrying are nearly identical to those of open pit metal mining – i.e., drilling, blasting, loading, and hauling – as are the health and safety hazards.

A few different methods are used to surface mine sand and gravel. Sometimes a pit is created and the material is simply dug out with an excavator. Other times the pit is flooded and a dredge is used to recover the material. Occasionally water cannons, which generate high-powered water-jet impulses, or hydraulic monitors, devices that employ large flows of water under high pressure, are used to break the material away from a bank where it is then recovered, although this is more likely to be used in placer deposits to access precious metals. Dredging is often utilized on lakes, rivers, and harbors to recover gravel. The primary risks with sand and gravel operations are traumatic injury and noise exposure.

Dimension stone mines have remained relatively unchanged over the years. Everything in these operations centers on cutting large blocks of material, such as granite or marble, from the solid deposit, with minimal damage to either the cut block or the remaining material. Blocks of material are removed by the careful use of explosives or a high-powered mechanical saw, and then they are hoisted intact or toppled and broken into smaller blocks. The use of ever larger and more powerful mining machines has no place here. Consequently, it is still a difficult and tedious process to carefully cut sections off the solid. Many of the cutting operations are deafeningly loud, and noise exposure is a high risk. Repetitive stress trauma is also a risk, and at a lower level, so is traumatic injury. Respirable dust risks have not appeared as a significant problem in this setting.

Solution mining

Solution mining methods are limited in application, but are becoming increasingly important especially for certain commodities. Consider, for example, that approximately 35% of gold, 50% of common salt, and 100% of lithium are derived from one of the solution mining methods. Sulfur is recovered using a solution mining process known as the Frasch method, in which superheated water is pumped down holes that have been drilled into the sulfur dome to melt the sulfur. The molten mixture is then recovered through other holes, or parts of the same borehole, and the sulfur is separated from the water and other impurities. The solution mining of uranium in particular offers a much safer method than the underground room and pillar method once used in uranium mines in the US, and like the solution mining of other commodities, it offers improved health and safety benefits as well as economic ones.

A modification of the solution mining method is heap leaching, discussed earlier in 'Mining methods'. Heap leaching remains an important method for recovering gold from low-grade deposits because it is unprofitable to run the low-grade ore through the traditional circuit of a mineral processing plant. Another similar application is the leaching of copper from waste piles created from material too low in grade to be sent to the mill, or from mill tailings that may still contain small percentages of copper. Vat leaching is a similar process that is conducted in large vats rather than heaps. Evaporation operations are an important method of solution mining, in which the liquid part of the solution is evaporated, typically with solar energy, leaving the desired component.

There are no documented health problems associated with solution mining, although the hazards associated with the use of solvents containing cyanide and acids, among other chemicals, are clear. In the past, some leaching sites have created serious environmental contamination, but modern environmental regulations and engineering practices are believed to be adequate to prevent future contamination of the environment from solution mining.

Mineral processing

Mineral processing plants are part of most mining operations. Their purpose is to convert the mined ore into a product for sale or subsequent use. A sand and gravel operation typically has a plant to wash the product and separate it by size. A stone plant typically includes several circuits to crush and separate the rock into a variety of sizes. In some cases this crushing includes pulverizing the stone down to micron sizes.

Coal preparation plants are somewhat more complex. While some crushing and sizing occur to meet customer requirements, most of the processing is concerned with separating the coal from impurities to reduce the ash and sulfur content. Thus, in addition to screen sizing, gravity separations are usually performed – where specialized machinery uses gravity to separate heavier and lighter materials. Moreover, as more sulfur can be released through crushing coal to increasingly smaller sizes, there is a significant fine coal component that must be recovered through sink-float processes that are heavily dependent upon organic chemicals. The plants associated with metal mines can be the most complex, with crushing and screening circuits and significant chemical circuits to isolate and concentrate the desired and undesirable constituents. These plants may include circuits for the beneficiation of metals associated with the primary metal, e.g., bismuth from a gold operation.

The health and safety hazards related to processing depend to some extent on the type of plant. Most plants have large machinery and are multileveled with numerous potential slipping hazards, and the processes are intrinsically noisy. Respirable dust can be a problem in certain locations of these plants, particularly near crushers. Traumatic injury problems and the problems associated with excess levels of noise or respirable dust are well known and well understood in mineral processing plants. The use of toxic chemicals such as cyanide has been studied extensively, whereas the risks associated with the use of neurotoxic chemicals in coal preparation plants, for example, is understood less well. Acids and other caustic materials used in these plants present safety hazards, if proper precautions are not applied.

MINING SAFETY AND HEALTH PROBLEMS

At the end of the 19th century, mining fatalities within the US numbered greater than 2000 a year; today the figure is less than 100 per year. Similar reductions have occurred for many injury classes and occupational illnesses. In some parts of the world these metrics are slightly better than in the US and in other parts are far worse. Efforts within the US by organized labor and progressive companies, research in university and government labs, and increasingly stringent regulations by state and federal agencies have all had a positive impact on mineworkers. Nonetheless, mining occurs under extremely difficult, and sometimes unpredictable, physical and environmental conditions. The Mine Safety and Health Administration (MSHA) has a mandatory reporting system for mine injuries and fatalities, and therefore good data are available to study the number and type of fatalities and injuries by commodity, work location, geographic region, and other variables.

Occupational illnesses in mining do not occur as discrete events, and as a result they are not reported with the same degree of certainty as fatalities or lost-time injuries. In fact, it is commonly believed that occupational illnesses among mineworkers are grossly under-reported, although this has not been substantiated through study.

Non-fatal lost-time injuries

Lost-workday injuries have declined over the past decade for mine operators in all commodities. Still, the rate in 2001 was 4.4 cases per 100 full-time coal mineworkers, as compared to a rate of 2.6 for general industry. Table 13.2 summarizes the number and annual average rate of lost-workday cases associated with various types of employers and commodities by work location. Note that the order and approximate magnitude of the injuries have changed little over the past few decades. During the period 1988 to 1997, for example, the five leading types of injuries were associated with materials handling (34%), slips or falls (21%), powered haulage (11%), machinery (11%), and hand tools (9.5%). The five most severe injuries, as reflected in the median number of days lost per injury between 1996 and 2000, were falling or caving rock (20 days for underground mining and 21 days for surface mining), slips or falls (25 days for underground and 17 days for surface), powered haulage (23 days for underground and 16 days for surface), stepping/kneeling on an object (22.5 days for underground and 9 days for surface), and materials handling (19 days for underground and 12 days for surface). Sprains to the back region due to overexertion accounted for the largest proportion of lost workdays. On a positive note, the number of back injuries has decreased over the years from nearly 5500 in 1992 to approximately 3500 in 2001.[3]

Many of these injuries are attributable to the natural conditions under which mining is conducted. Small slabs of rock may peel off the roof or back of the underground mine, striking a worker and causing a serious non-fatal injury. The presence of water and clay materials in the floor can cause a dangerously slippery condition. The close proximity of large machines and workers is always hazardous, but even more so in the confined spaces of underground mines. Visibility is often limited, further exacerbating the confined space hazard.

Despite extensive research over the years, significant improvements can still be made to reduce injuries resulting from these factors. Slips and falls have been a particularly difficult injury to reduce, because they occur in diverse settings and from many causes. Materials handling injuries have been reduced through improved workplace design. The increasing practice of palletizing supplies and providing vehicles with lifting forks has dramatically reduced the lifting and manual handling of supplies and materials that must be done each day in the mine. The development of stronger yet lighter materials for roof supports and stoppings has led to a reduction in materials handling injuries. A few mines have even installed exercise facilities at the mine site and encouraged employee fitness programs, and they report anecdotal evidence of reduced back injuries.

Work-related musculoskeletal disorders (WMSDs)

The leading illnesses among mine workers reported to MSHA in 2001 (excluding hearing loss) were repetitive trauma, accounting for 45.7% of illnesses. Numerous tasks

	All		Underground		Surface areas		Strip/open pit/quarry		Dredge		Other surface operations†		Mills/plants	
Type of employer and commodity	Number	Rate	Number	Rate	Number	Rate	Number	Rate	Number	Rate	Number	Rate	Number	Rate
All	170,635	5.5	74,264	10.9	6272	5.7	46,396	3.6	2270	4.1	1250	4.7	40,183	4.3
Mine operator:														
Coal	89,895	7.9	65,668	11.9	4348	8.0	12,453	3.2	9	1.7	848	5.4	6569	5.0
Metal	17,622	3.9	4534	7.2	641	3.9	5152	3.1	193	4.5	214	3.3	6888	3.5
Non-metal	9855	3.7	1528	4.4	308	5.0	1623	2.7	31	5.6	NA‡	NA	6365	3.8
Stone	31,642	4.7	748	4.7	270	6.9	13,426	4.8	66	5.6	82	3.3	17,00	4.7
Sand and gravel	12,059	4.1	NA	NA	NA	NA	10,106	4.1	1953	4.2	NA	NA	NR§	NR
Independent contractor:														
Coal	4363	3.4	1367	12.1	499	2.2	1385	2.2	2	1.0	96	4.9	1014	3.8
Metal and non-metal**	5199	3.3	419	7.1	206	3.4	2251	2.4	16	1.5	10	2.3	2297	4.6

Source: MSHA 1999[23]
* Computed per 100 full-time workers or 200,000 employee hours.
† Includes culm banks, auger mining, independent shops and yards, and surface mining n.e.c.
‡ NA = Not applicable for this commodity.
§ NR = Not reported separately. Sand and gravel operators report mill employment under strip or dredge operations.
** Includes metal, non-metal, stone, and sand and gravel.

Table 13.2 Number and annual average rate* of lost-workday cases associated with various types of employers and commodities by work location, 1988–1997[3]

within mining require repetitive actions, and many of these are physically demanding. Often, especially in underground mining, these actions must be performed in awkward postures. Many underground coal miners perform tasks where the total vertical clearance available to them is less than their body height. Over the past two decades, more attention, primarily through research, has been focused on WMSDs, and on the design of mining equipment, supplies, and processes (see Chapter 23). However, during this same time, equipment innovations to achieve higher levels of efficiency and productivity have at times placed even more demands on the human body. A comprehensive treatment of ergonomic issues in mining is presented by Gallagher.[4]

Lower back problems make up a significant proportion of the WMSDs in mining. Upper body problems of the shoulder and hands are not as severe, and carpal tunnel syndrome is relatively rare in mining.[5] The increased use of remote controls, as well as other changes to mining machinery, may contribute to an increase in upper-body WMSDs.

A final WMSD of note is miner's knee. This problem occurs in workers mining in thin seams, which requires extensive walking on the hands and knees. The resulting constant pressure leads to bursitis in the knee. The combination of pressure and frequently wet conditions also leads to infected hair follicles and thickened macerating skin that is easily infected. Miner's knee is confined primarily to the low coal fields, and in the United States, predominantly appears in mineworkers from Pennsylvania, West Virginia, and Virginia. Knee pads are provided to workers, but in many cases the design of the knee pads may worsen the problem by trapping moisture under the pad, or concentrating stresses behind the knee.[6]

Hearing loss

Unlike many occupational illnesses in mining, noise-induced hearing loss (NIHL) is of epidemic proportion. NIHL and noise exposures are discussed in Chapters 20.2 and 35 respectively. Despite 30 years of regulation, research, and intervention, 91% of coal miners and 64% of metal/non-metal miners have a hearing impairment greater than 25 dB by age 50, as compared to 9% of non-exposed males of the same age.[7,8] The resulting problems of hearing-impaired mineworkers go beyond quality of life issues, and include difficulties in communication or understanding speech, along with an increased accident risk on the job when normal safety cues cannot be discerned. MSHA's enactment of more protective rules combined with significant research efforts should help stem the tide of new cases in the future. However, mining is an inherently noisy endeavor, and even if engineering controls were 100% effective and applied diligently throughout the industry, it is estimated that only 20% of future cases would be prevented. Reduction of the remaining cases will depend heavily on the use of recommended hearing protectors. While engineering or administrative controls are the preferred approach, the proper use of individual hearing protective devices must be part of the solution to address the problem effectively.

Mineworkers, like those in other occupations, do not fully appreciate the risks to their hearing, nor do they fully understand the consequences of noise-induced hearing loss. For example, a common belief is that it will simply become quieter as hearing is lost – miners are often completely unaware of tinnitus and the fact that it often accompanies NIHL. Mineworker understanding of the risks posed by excessive noise levels is essential to gaining their co-operation in maintaining noise controls, as well as getting them to take steps to protect their hearing, such as wearing hearing protectors. New training approaches are being explored to more effectively educate miners on the causes of NIHL and the actions they can take to prevent it. Low-cost personal dosimeters have been developed to empower individual mineworkers to measure their noise exposure and take protective actions as their dose accumulates during the shift.

Most noise sources found in mining cause a temporary threshold shift, and given sufficient exposures over time, the temporary shifts will become permanent. There are a few noise sources, however, which are loud enough to cause damage over relatively short time periods, so-called "impulse" noise. These include air arc welding, channel jet drilling, and the impulse noise from the detonation of some explosives. For workers exposed to these tasks in particular, it is imperative that adequate hearing protection be worn and that exposure to these sources is limited.

Work-related lung diseases

Coal worker pneumoconiosis (CWP) and silicosis are the two lung diseases most relevant to mining, discussed in greater detail in Chapters 19.10 and 19.9, respectively. CWP is more commonly referred to as black lung. CWP primarily affects underground coal workers, although cases in surface mine and coal preparation plant workers do occur infrequently. Silicosis, while affecting fewer miners, occurs across all sectors. Among the illnesses reported to MSHA in 2001, dust-related diseases made up 13.4%. Fiber-related dust diseases associated with the mining and processing of asbestos or vermiculite are rare among US mineworkers, but might be seen in areas where these commodities are actively mined.

Coal worker pneumoconiosis

Over the past three decades, average shift production levels have increased by an order of magnitude while respirable coal dust concentrations have been cut nearly in half. This is a remarkable testament to the development and application of engineering controls during this period. Despite these gains, however, CWP remains a large problem of the coal mining industry, and while there has been a steady decline in the number of cases reported per year, there is still a significant problem.

Respirable coal dust generation is largely a function of cutting rates, and therefore respirable dust increases with production. Longwall mining is the most productive coal mining method, and it is not surprising that the two highest exposure occupations are stationed at the longwall. Advances in control technology in recent years have just been able to keep up with the increasing production levels. Of course, there is less margin of error as well. If one of several control parameters is set incorrectly or a part of the

dust control system malfunctions even briefly, significant concentrations of respirable dust can become air-borne. The coursing of ventilating air throughout the working face is a primary means of diluting and carrying away excess dust. However, in many cases limiting factors that could negatively affect mineworkers prevent further increases in this quantity of ventilating air.[9]

Full-shift sampling using the traditional gravimetric sampler – which employs quartz filters to collect particulate matter – captures the mineworker's exposure, but this information is not available until the sample has been weighed at the MSHA lab and the results are reported back to the mine – a process that takes weeks. Thus, the use of a real-time dust dosimeter is a crucial step towards the elimination of black lung. After years of development, prototypes of a new personal dust monitor (PDM) have been successfully tested in underground coal mines, and they are expected to be commercially available in 2005. These devices will allow mineworkers to make nearreal-time changes to the dust control system to reduce respirable dust levels. MSHA is also developing more stringent regulations, which include provisions requiring operators to utilize the PDM, to aid in the fight against CWP.

Silicosis

A chronic overexposure to respirable crystalline silica causes the progressive lung disease known as silicosis (see Chapter 19.9). The respirable crystalline silica is released by silica-bearing minerals as they are fragmented during mining processes. The strata surrounding many coal seams contain these quartz minerals. Three common sources of silica exposures in underground coal mines are:
1. cutting by the continuous miner into the roof for additional clearance or to construct overcasts;
2. drilling by the roof bolter into the roof to install bolts;
3. advancing longwall shields, which crush the immediate roof and distribute this dust as the shields move forward.

Dust exposure in coal mines
Water sprays and fan-powered dust collectors are commonly used on continuous miners to limit respirable coal dust, and are effective for reducing silica. The dry dust collection systems on roof bolters also capture much of the generated silica. A water misting system to reduce noise levels during the drilling cycle of roof bolting is undergoing field trials, and air-borne silica reduction may be an important side benefit from this noise control technology.

Despite these engineering controls, roof bolter operators are often careless when they empty and dispose of dust from the dust collection system, spilling the contents. In addition to the immediate air-borne exposure they suffer, significant amounts of respirable silica dust remain on the miner's clothes, which become a source of additional exposure for the remainder of the shift. Although this is smaller than the exposure from the actual drilling, it is not insignificant.

Dust exposure during surface coal mining occurs primarily during the drilling or handling of the silica-bearing overburden materials. Blasthole drillers can be exposed, particularly if the dust collection system around the drill-hole collar is functioning poorly, which many do. Dozer operators can have a significant exposure as they move and further break silica-bearing overburden. Front end loader operators can be overexposed as they handle these materials. Workers in the vicinity of drilling and materials handling operations can receive an overexposure as well.

To address these issues, better dust collection technology is needed for surface drills, and existing systems need to be better maintained. Part of the problem is that workers underestimate the hazard, so better worker training is needed. The widespread adoption of environmentally controlled cabs has been a boon to reducing dust as well as noise exposures, and fortunately most equipment in the surface mining industry now has cabs. Surprisingly, respirable dust concentrations within these cabs can be high. The obvious case occurs with older equipment in which cabs have holes and are poorly sealed to the outside. Many of these older cabs have poor air-conditioning systems that are unable to filter out much of the dust. These deficiencies are being addressed through the development of retrofit kits and training materials on cab sealing.

An unexpected but significant source of respirable silica is tracked into the cab on the operator's boots, and then re-circulated within the cab. Some effective means of reducing this hazard are operator training, the sprinkling of a natural canola oil-base sweeping compound onto the cab floor, and improvements to the cab filtration system.[10]

Dust exposure in other mines

The generation and exposure mechanisms in metal/non-metal surface and underground mining are similar to those described for coal. In underground mining, exposure occurs primarily from drilling operations and materials handling by loaders, load-haul-dump vehicles, trucks, and slushers. Surface mining exposures come from drills, dozers, and loaders. One important difference, however, is that the crystalline silica is part of the ore itself, rather than only being present in the surrounding rock, as is the case for coal. Accordingly, a significant dust source in metal/non-metal mining occurs around crushers. For underground crushers, the problem is amplified because of the confined space and the limited ventilation. For surface crushers, dust generation is generally less of a problem because of the open-air nature of the application. Sometimes an operator is stationed at the primary crusher, but is normally inside an environmentally controlled booth and well protected from the noise and dust of the crushing operation. If the crusher is fed by trucks dumping into it, the truck driver can be overexposed depending on the site arrangements.[11]

Air quality regulations by the Environmental Protection Agency to control visible or fugitive dust help reduce the respirable dust concentrations in the vicinity of the crusher. Dust reduction in surface plants – e.g., at transfer points and stock piles – is accomplished through the use of water sprays and to a lesser extent shrouds and mechanical efforts to limit dust generation. As with coal, training of metal/non-metal mineworkers is important to ensure that available control technologies are maintained and used effectively.

Many of the silica hazards present in mining also occur in other industries where surface drilling is an integral activity. Two large populations are water well drillers and heavy construction workers. Efforts are under way to apply the lessons learned in mining to these workers as well.

Heat stress

Heat stress can occur from mining in hot environments, further discussed in Chapter 34. The temperature of virgin rock in a mine is dependent on several factors including the depth of the deposit, the proximity to geothermal gradients, and the thermal conductivity of rock overlying the deposit. As an example, the temperature may be 25 degrees C at 250 m of depth and rise to 45 degrees C at 2000 m. Heat is released into the mine environment as mining progresses, and then ventilating air passing over the hot rock is warmed, increasing the ambient air temperature. The common use of water to control dust contributes to very high humidity levels in addition to elevated temperatures. The high temperature alone, and especially in combination with the additional high wet bulb temperature, creates significant health hazards to miners. Chilling of the air used to ventilate the mine can reduce the temperature and humidity levels to uncomfortable but safe values. Heat acclimatization regimens have been developed and have been shown to reduce heat stroke among miners.[12]

The problems of mining in hot environments have not been as severe in the US as in some other mining countries, due to the nature of the deposits. This may change as deeper deposits are mined in the future. Two fatalities from heat stroke occurred in the Nevada gold mines in 2003, after several years with none reported. In addition to adverse health effects of heat stress, the adverse impact on safety is also well documented. Accident rates are decidedly higher for persons working in hot humid conditions,[13] likely due to the resulting fatigue.

Toxic fumes from blasting

Gases, including some that are toxic, are produced during the chemical reaction process of explosive detonation and deflagration. Generally these are well understood, and proper material selection and blasting techniques are used to minimize any risk to workers. A relatively new problem has shown up with increasing frequency over the past several years, and that is carbon monoxide poisoning in structures and manholes at some distance form the blast site. The problem has been observed in trench blasting for construction purposes – e.g., municipal sewer projects – and in surface coal mining. Significant quantities of CO are produced during a normal blast, but this and other gases may not be vented to the atmosphere; rather the gas is confined beneath the surface, where it then travels along a path of least resistance. This path may be fractures in the bedrock, a gas or water line path into a residential basement, and so forth.

CO is a very stable gas and may persist for days. CO poisonings (discussed further in Chapters 19.5 and 47) have been documented in both the US and Canada. Ironically, practices designed to minimize ground vibration and flyrock (rocks being propelled from the blast area), both of which are undesirable at blast sites near population centers, may contribute to excess entrapment of gas. Techniques to minimize the presence of gas and to provide relief to the atmosphere are under investigation. Until they are in practice, however, blasters are being encouraged to deploy CO detectors in nearby buildings and to recommend CO checks before workers enter any confined space, such as a manhole, near a blast site.[14,15]

Other toxic substances

A variety of toxic or potentially toxic substances are used or encountered in mining, and they range from chemicals used in mineral processing to the byproducts of operations. There are no proven adverse effects from the presence of these agents in the mining workplace. However, studies that would detect adverse health effects have not been conducted for many of these substances, or in some cases studies have been conducted but were inconclusive. Four such agents of note are diesel particulate matter, froth flotation chemicals (where chemicals are used to separate minerals from one another), solcenic (a hydraulic fluid similar in formulation to emulsifiable metalworking fluids), and molds.

Diesel particulate matter (DPM) in diesel exhaust is considered carcinogenic and DPM levels are regulated in mining (see Chapter 44). DPM emissions into the mine environment can be reduced by fuel selection, through the use of filters and catalytic converters, or with newer engine designs. However, there are significant gaps in the current understanding of these control technologies. For example, the reduction of DPM by certain converters can result in dangerously elevated levels of nitrogen oxide or the release of potentially harmful heavy metals in respirable particles.[16]

Direct worker exposure to chemicals used in modern coal preparation plants has been reduced through changes to the delivery, mixing, and application phases. Nonetheless, some exposure during maintenance and operation does occur. A link between Parkinson's disease and exposure to neurotoxic chemicals used in coal preparation has been postulated, but remains unproven.[17]

Solcenic, a non-flammable hydraulic fluid commonly used in underground coal mining, was suspected of causing respiratory disorders, work-related asthma, and allergic and irritant skin disorders among longwall coal miners, but studies have failed to establish any relationship.[18] Reasonable precautions to minimize exposure, for example from leaks in the hydraulic lines, will prevent adverse effects in susceptible individuals. Large spills may result in atmospheric formaldehyde concentrations at or above the NIOSH-recommended REL, and precautions should be taken during these atypical events to protect workers. Notwithstanding, chemical exposures in the mining industry are poorly understood, and any unexplained symptoms presented in mineworkers should be investigated with chemical exposure in mind.

Humidity and temperature conditions in mines are particularly well suited to the growth of molds. There has been increasing interest in the health effects of these molds, but no investigations have been performed to date. Special precautions are necessary for underground lead miners to ensure that lead ore is not ingested or tracked out of the workplace. Strict rules regarding showering and changing clothes before eating or leaving the mine site, among others, are successfully applied.

Work-related stress and fatigue

Work schedules in mining have changed over the years. Work-related stress and fatigue (see Chapter 28.3) are increasingly being recognized in the mining industry. Many modern operations are in production 24 hours per day or in some combination of maintenance and production round the clock. Some operations stay open on the weekends, and some work almost every day of the year. Thus, workforce scheduling is obviously a challenge in these operations, and has resulted in various shift schedules in relation to consecutive days of work, i.e., a worker might be on the job 10 consecutive days, followed by a smaller block of days off, e.g., 4. Sometimes a more extended off-period is given after several of these cycles to help reduce work-related stress and fatigue.

Rotations from first to second and then to third shift still occur, but are not as common as they once were. Mining has become increasingly capital intensive, and as such, idle time of the expensive equipment involved is less acceptable. In underground coal mining, for example, it used to be common for one crew to leave the working face and travel to the outside portal for arrival at the end of the 8-hour shift. Then the next crew departed from the portal and traveled to the working face, where it restarted the production cycle. Travel times of 30 minutes or more on each end of the shift, along with the lost-time of cycling down and then restarting production, meant that less than 60% of the total shift time was spent in production. As mining became more competitive, the practice of changing crews directly at the working face, sometimes called a hot-seat change at the face, became common. This significantly improved productivity and effectively increased the shift length by as much as 2 hours because a full 8 hours of production time per crew was established. Two 10-hour production shifts with a 4-hour maintenance period evolved as one popular schedule. Some companies even went to 12-hour shifts.

Studies have been conducted primarily on the effect of these work schedules on safety, and as expected worker fatigue and disorientation from shift rotations is a factor in accidents, although the findings are not as dramatic or definitive as might be expected. Long-term health effects on workers are less understood, although significant interest in examining stress-related health effects on cardiovascular disease and worker depression is developing in the research community, and work schedules would likely be an important focus.[19]

There was significant research interest in the effects of work organization in mining several years ago, as the changes described previously began to evolve. More recently, a new complication has developed. Deposits located far from established communities are being mined. In the US, workers are now being transported by bus for up to 2 hours each way, each day, to work a 10- or 12-hour shift as part of an extended workweek schedule. This is common in the coal fields of the Powder River Basin in Wyoming and the gold fields of Nevada, and less common elsewhere. In Australia, even more remote locations are being mined, and workers are flown in, stay for several weeks, and are then flown back out. Concern over the health effects of these practices on workers in Australia has spawned several research studies, which are now in progress.[20]

Informational resources on mining health and safety

The understanding of mining safety and health problems is increasing, as are prevention and intervention measures. The clinician is ideally positioned to detect heretofore unknown adverse health effects from occupational exposures. A detailed occupational history of the patient may provide key clues, and unexplained or otherwise worrisome relationships should be reported. NIOSH scientists can conduct targeted health hazard evaluations to investigate such concerns.

Several sources can provide timely information to supplement the technical literature. The NIOSH and MSHA websites (http://www.cdc.gov/niosh/homepage.html and http://www.msha.gov/) are good places to start. Labor unions such as the United Mineworkers of America (coal), the United Steelworkers of America (metal), and the International Union of Operating Engineers (stone) have active health and safety departments. Finally, trade associations such as the Bituminous Coal Operators' Association (coal), the National Mining Association (metal/non-metal and coal), and the National Stone, Sand, and Gravel Association also aggressively promote health and safety for mineworkers. Labor and trade organizations have partnered to solve a number of important health and safety problems, and they provide a valuable source of information and training materials, in addition to the government agencies. States with significant mining interests often have their own mining agencies as well, which provide yet another source of information.

References

1. Geological Survey. Minerals Yearbook, Volume I, Metals and Minerals. Reston, VA: US Geological Survey, 2001.
2. Hartman, HL, Mutmansky JM. Introductory mining engineering, 2nd edn. Hoboken, NJ: John Wiley & Sons, Inc., 2002.
3. National Institute for Occupational Safety and Health. Worker health chartbook, 2000, focus on mining. DHHS (NIOSH) Publication No. 2002-121. Pittsburgh, PA: US Department of Health and Human Services, Public Health Service, Centers for Disease Control and Prevention, National Institute for Occupational Safety and Health, 2002.
4. Gallagher S. Ergonomics issues in mining. In: Marras WS, Karnowski W, eds. Occupational ergonomics handbook. Boca Raton, FL: CRC Press, 1999;1893–915.
5. Hudock SD, Keran CM. Risk profile of cumulative trauma disorders of the arm and hand in the US mining industry. Information Circular 9319. Minneapolis, MN: US Bureau of Mines, 1992;1–5.
6. Sanders MS. Personal equipment for low seam coal miners: VII improved knee pads. US Bureau of Mines Contract Report JO387213. Westlake Village, CA: Canyon Research Group Inc., 1982.
7. Franks JR. Analysis of audiograms for a large cohort of noise-exposed miners (and cover letter to Davitt McAteer from Linda Rosenstock, August 6, 1996). Pittsburgh, PA: US Department of Health and Human Services, Public Health Service, Centers for Disease Control and Prevention, National Institute for Occupational Safety and Health, 1996;1–7.
8. Franks JR. Prevalence of hearing loss for noise-exposed metal/nonmetal miners (and cover letter to Andrea Hricko from Gregory Wagner, October 7, 1997). Pittsburgh, PA: US Department of Health and Human Services, Public Health Service, Centers for Disease Control and Prevention, National Institute for Occupational Safety and Health, 1997;1–5
9. Rider JP, Colinet JF, Prokop AE. Impact of control parameters on shearer-generated dust levels. Transactions 2002, vol. 312. Littleton, CO: Society for Mining, Metallurgy, and Exploration, Inc., 2002;28–34.
10. National Institute for Occupational Safety and Health. Technology news 487: sweeping compound application reduces dust from soiled floors within enclosed operator cabs. Pittsburgh, PA: US Department of Health and Human Services, Public Health Service, Centers for Disease Control and Prevention, National Institute for Occupational Safety and Health, 2001.
11. Chekan GJ, Colinet JF, Grau RH III. Silica dust sources in underground metal/nonmetal mines: two case studies. Transactions 2002, vol. 312. Littleton, CO: Society for Mining, Metallurgy, and Exploration, Inc., 2002;187–93.
12. Wyndham CH. The physiologic and psychological effects of heat. In: The ventilation of South African gold mines. Yeoville, South Africa: Mine Ventilation Society of South Africa, 1974;95–100.
13. Hartman HL, Mutmansky JM, Ramani RV, Wang YJ. Mine ventilation and air conditioning. New York, NY: John Wiley & Sons, Inc., 1997.
14. Decker JA, Deitchman S, Santis L. Hazard evaluation and technical assistance report: carbon monoxide intoxication and death in a newly constructed sewer manhole, NIOSH HETA 98-0020. Pittsburgh, PA: US Department of Health and Human Services, Public Health Service, Centers for Disease Control and Prevention, National Institute for Occupational Safety and Health, 1998.
15. Sapko M, Mainiero R, Rowland J, Zlochower I. Chemical and physical factors that influence NOx production during blasting – exploratory study. Proceedings of the 28th Annual Conference on Explosives and Blasting Technique. Cleveland, OH: International Society of Explosives Engineers, 2002;317–30.
16. Schnakenberg GH, Bugarski A. Review of technology available to the underground mining industry for control of diesel emissions. DHHS (NIOSH) Publication NO. 2002-154, IC 9462. Pittsburgh, PA: US Department of Health and Human Services, Public Health Service, Centers for Disease Control and Prevention, National Institute for Occupational Safety and Health, 2002.
17. Mulloy KB. Two case reports of neurological disease in coal mine preparation plant workers. Am J Ind Med 1996; 30:56–61.

18. Cocalis JC, Rao CY, Kestenberg KA, Martin JE. Hazard evaluation and technical assistance report: Robinson Run Mine, Shinnston, WV. NIOSH Report No. HETA 2000-0098-2862. Morgantown, WV: US Department of Health and Human Services, Public Health Service, Centers for Disease Control and Prevention, National Institute for Occupational Safety and Health, 2000.

19. Duchon JC, Smith TJ. Extended workdays in mining and other industries: a review of the literature. US Bureau of Mines Information Circular No. 9378. Minneapolis, MN: US Bureau of Mines, 1994.

20. Leary C, Cliff D. A study of the health and safety aspects of shiftwork and rosters at the PCML. Conference Record of the Queensland Mining Industry Health and Safety Conference, August, 2003. Brisbane: Queensland Resources Council, 2003.

21. MSHA. Quarterly employment and coal production: accidents/injuries/illnesses reported to MSHA under 30 CFR Part 50, 2001. Denver, CO: US Department of Labor, Mine Safety and Health Administration, Office of Injury and Employment Information, 2001.

22. NIOSH. NIOSH Mining Internet site, Mine Employees, 2003. http://pit/prl/surveillance/Employees.htm

23. MSHA. Quarterly employment and coal production: accidents/injuries/illnesses reported to MSHA under 30 CFR Part 50, 1986–1997. Denver, CO: US Department of Labor, Mine Safety and Health Administration, Office of Injury and Employment Information, 1999.

Chapter 14
Construction Industry Hazards

Laura S Welch

INTRODUCTION

Construction workers build, repair, renovate, modify, and demolish structures: houses, office buildings, temples, factories, hospitals, roads, bridges, tunnels, stadiums, docks, airports, and more. In industrialized nations, construction is consistently ranked among the most dangerous occupations. In the United States, 19% of all fatal on-the-job injuries occur in construction, about three times its 6% share of the total employment;[1] half of all fatal falls occur in construction. High fatality rates occur around the globe as well.[2] Construction also has a high rate of non-fatal injuries. In 2000 there were four lost workday cases per 100 full-time equivalent construction workers compared to a rate of 3/100 full-time equivalent workers in all private industry; the rate in construction exceeded all other sectors.[3]

Construction work is composed of many different tasks undertaken by many different trades. To understand the risk for injury and illness, one must understand the work of specific trades and their characteristic tasks. In the United States, the unionized industry consists of 15 distinct trades, with specific tasks defined by the jurisdiction of each trade. In other countries, and on non-union job sites in the United States, the tasks of these trades may vary. A description of the work of each trade as defined by the US Bureau of Labor Statistics (BLS) is helpful in describing the variety of work in construction (Table 14.1).

Occupational diseases are also an important cause of morbidity in construction workers. Table 14.2 summarizes sentinel health events that may occur in construction workers and specific exposures that can lead to these diseases. This list was developed to identify diseases that, if they occur, point to an opportunity for intervention and prevention of future cases. These diseases do not represent an exhaustive list of occupational disease in construction, but illustrate the extent of the possible problem.

The costs of injuries in the construction trades are substantial. Estimates in the US range from $10 billion to $40 billion annually.[4] Assuming a cost of $20 billion, the cost per construction worker would be $3500 yearly. One cost indicator, worker's compensation premiums for three trades (carpenters, masons, and structural iron workers), averaged 28.6% of payroll. In addition to worker's compensation, there are liability insurance premiums and other indirect costs, including reduced work crew efficiency, clean-up (from a cave-in or collapse, for instance), or overtime necessitated by an injury. These indirect costs can exceed the worker's compensation claim for an injury by several multiples.

Construction work entails a number of physical hazards and psychophysiologic stressors, including extreme temperatures, shift work, and unpredictable work (discussed in Chapters 34, 38). Construction often must be done in extreme heat or cold, in windy, rainy, snowy, or foggy weather. Night-shift work is common in highway and bridge construction. On-again, off-again work adds to the health risks, including the emotional toll of uncertainty regarding job security and seasonal work.[5] In the US, where there is no universal health insurance, intermittent employment and the high cost of health insurance can leave construction workers and their families without healthcare coverage. Even when construction workers work the 30 or 60 days frequently needed to qualify for insurance coverage on a job (if coverage is available), they often cannot afford to maintain coverage between jobs.

For workers who do have healthcare coverage, episodic employment, frequent changes of employer, and continuous changes in worksite exposures and ambient conditions limit the clinician's or the researcher's ability to trace the individual's work history or exposures to hazards. Because of these factors, many of which are unique to construction, data on the extent or effect of toxic exposures in the construction industry are limited.

Construction work is demanding, both physically and socially. Data from the United States suggest that construction workers retire at an earlier age than does the average US worker. Construction workers who work in production jobs, as contrasted with management jobs, retire earlier than the general workforce; the average of age retirement is 54 for production jobs in construction, and 56 for the general workforce.[6] Tuomi characterized risk factors for early retirement or disability retirement in a follow-up study of over 6000 Finnish workers aged 45–58.[7] Specific aspects of the job that increased the likelihood of disability included static muscular work, diminished muscular strength, lifting and carrying, sudden peak loads, repetitive movement, and simultaneously bent and twisted work postures.

Most of these risk factors for early retirement are common in construction work. A study in Ireland found that 30% of construction workers who retired early because of a medical problem retired because of a musculoskeletal condition.[8] Arthritis was responsible for 70% of these musculoskeletal conditions, and degenerative disk disease for another 20%. An analysis of the medical conditions leading to retirement among unionized sheet metal workers in the United States reported that musculoskeletal conditions made up 70%.

Boilermakers
Construct, assemble, maintain, and repair stationary steam boilers and boiler house auxiliaries. Work involves use of hand and power tools, plumb bobs, levels, wedges, dogs, or turnbuckles. Assist in testing assembled vessels. Direct cleaning of boilers and boiler furnaces. Inspect and repair boiler fittings, such as safety valves, regulators, automatic-control mechanisms, water columns, and auxiliary machines.

Brick masons
Lay and bind building materials, such as brick, structural tile, concrete block, cinder block, glass block, and terracotta block, with mortar and other substances to construct or repair walls, partitions, arches, sewers, and other structures.

Carpenters
Construct, erect, install, or repair structures and fixtures made of wood, such as concrete forms; building frameworks, including partitions, joists, studding, and rafters; wood stairways, window and door frames, and hardwood floors. May also install cabinets, siding, drywall and batt or roll insulation.

Carpet installers
Lay and install carpet from rolls or blocks on floors. Install padding and trim flooring materials.

Cement masons and concrete finishers
Smooth and finish surfaces of poured concrete, such as floors, walks, sidewalks, roads, or curbs using a variety of hand and power tools. Align forms for sidewalks, curbs, or gutters; patch voids; use saws to cut expansion joints.

Construction laborers
Perform tasks involving physical labor at building, highway, and heavy construction projects, tunnel and shaft excavations, and demolition sites. May operate hand and power tools of all types: air hammers, earth tampers, cement mixers, small mechanical hoists, surveying and measuring equipment, and a variety of other equipment and instruments. May clean and prepare sites, dig trenches, set braces to support the sides of excavations, erect scaffolding, clean up rubble and debris, and remove asbestos, lead, and other hazardous waste materials.

Drywall and ceiling tile installers
Apply plasterboard or other wallboard to ceilings or interior walls of buildings. Apply or mount acoustical tiles or blocks, strips, or sheets of shock-absorbing materials to ceilings and walls of buildings to reduce or reflect sound. Materials may be of decorative quality. Include lathers who fasten wooden, metal, or rockboard lath to walls, ceilings or partitions of buildings to provide support base for plaster, fire-proofing, or acoustical material.

Electricians
Install, maintain, and repair electrical wiring, equipment, and fixtures. Ensure that work is in accordance with relevant codes. May install or service street lights, intercom systems, or electrical control systems.

Insulation workers
Apply insulating materials to pipes or ductwork, or other mechanical systems in order to help control and maintain temperature. Also line and cover structures with insulating materials. May work with batt, roll, or blown insulation materials.

Operating engineers
Operate one or several types of power construction equipment, such as motor graders, bulldozers, scrapers, compressors, pumps, derricks, shovels, tractors, or front-end loaders to excavate, move, and grade earth, erect structures, or pour concrete or other hard surface pavement. May repair and maintain equipment in addition to other duties.

Painters
Paint walls, equipment, buildings, bridges, and other structural surfaces, using brushes, rollers, and spray guns. May remove old paint to prepare surface prior to painting. May mix colors or oils to obtain desired color or consistency.

Paperhangers
Cover interior walls and ceilings of rooms with decorative wallpaper or fabric, or attach advertising posters on surfaces, such as walls and billboards. Duties include removing old materials from surface to be papered.

Plumbers, pipefitters, and steamfitters
Assemble, install, alter, and repair pipelines or pipe systems that carry water, steam, air, or other liquids or gases. May install heating and cooling equipment and mechanical control systems

Plasterers and stucco masons
Apply interior or exterior plaster, cement, stucco, or similar materials. May also set ornamental plaster.

Reinforcing iron and rebar workers
Position and secure steel bars or mesh in concrete forms in order to reinforce concrete. Use a variety of fasteners, rod-bending machines, blowtorches, and hand tools. Include rod busters.

Roofers
Cover roofs of structures with shingles, slate, asphalt, aluminum, wood, and related materials. May spray roofs, sidings, and walls with material to bind, seal, insulate, or soundproof sections of structures.

Sheet-metal workers
Fabricate, assemble, install, and repair sheet-metal products and equipment, such as ducts, control boxes, drainpipes, and furnace casings. Work may involve any of the following: setting up and operating fabricating machines to cut, bend, and straighten sheet metal; shaping metal over anvils, blocks, or forms using hammer; operating soldering and welding equipment to join sheet-metal parts; inspecting, assembling, and smoothing seams and joints of burred surfaces. Include sheet-metal duct installers who install prefabricated sheet-metal ducts used for heating, air conditioning, or other purposes.

Stonemasons
Build stone structures, such as piers, walls, and abutments. Lay walks, curbstones, or special types of masonry for vats, tanks, and floors.

Structural iron and steel workers
Raise, place, and unite iron or steel girders, columns, and other structural members to form completed structures or structural frameworks. May erect metal storage tanks and assemble prefabricated metal buildings.

Terrazzo workers and finishers
Apply a mixture of cement, sand, pigment, or marble chips to floors, stairways, and cabinet fixtures to fashion durable and decorative surfaces.

Tile and marble setters
Apply hard tile, marble, and wood tile to walls, floors, ceilings, and roof decks.

From Bureau of Labor Statistics, Standard Occupational Classification Manual, 1998 revision. http://stats.bls.gov/soc/socguide.htm

Table 14.1 Construction occupations

The remainder of this chapter will highlight exposures and occupational diseases that are prevalent in construction, or those for which unique characteristics of the construction industry warrant attention. More extensive discussion of specific occupational disorders or exposures can be found in subsequent chapters.

WORK-RELATED MUSCULOSKELETAL DISORDERS

Musculoskeletal injuries make up a high proportion of all work-related injuries in construction. Key musculoskeletal disorders and associated construction trade or risk factors

Condition	Industry/process/occupation	Agent
Asbestosis	Asbestos industries and utilizers	Asbestos
Bronchitis (acute), pneumonitis, and pulmonary edema due to fumes and vapors	Arc welders, boilermakers	Nitrogen oxides
Chronic or acute renal failure	Plumbers	Inorganic lead*
Contact and allergic dermatitis	Cement masons and finishers, carpenters, floorlayers†	Adhesives and sealants, irritants (e.g., cutting oils, phenol, solvents, acids, alkalis, detergents); allergens (e.g., nickel, chromates, formaldehyde, dyes, rubber products)
Extrinsic asthma	Wood workers, furniture makers	Red cedar (plicatic acid) and other wood dusts
Histoplasmosis	Bridge maintenance workers	*Histoplasma capsulatum*
Inflammatory and toxic neuropathy	Furniture refinishers, degreasing operations	Hexane
Malignant neoplasm of scrotum	Chimney sweeps	Mineral oil, pitch, tar
Malignant neoplasm of nasal cavities	Wood workers, cabinet and furniture makers, carpenters	Hardwood and softwood† dusts Chlorophenols
Malignant neoplasm of trachea, bronchus, and lung	Asbestos industries and utilizers	Asbestos
Malignant neoplasm of nasopharynx	Carpenter, cabinet maker	Asbestos
Malignant neoplasm of larynx	Asbestos industries and utilizers	Asbestos
Mesothelioma (malignancy of peritoneum and pleura)	Asbestos industries and utilizers	Asbestos
Noise effects on inner ear	Occupations with exposure to excessive noise	Excessive noise
Raynaud's phenomenon (secondary)	Jackhammer operator, riveter	Whole body or segmental vibration
Sequoiosis	Red cedar mill workers, wood workers	Redwood sawdust
Silicosis	Sandblasters	Silica
Silicotuberculosis	Sandblasters	Silica + *Mycobacterium tuberculosis*
Toxic encephalitis	Lead paint removal	Lead
Toxic hepatitis	Fumigators	Methyl bromide

*Lead exposure occurs in at least 23 construction-related industrial/occupational groups; including painting contractors, bridge and highway construction, and demolition work. Extremely high levels of lead exposure have been documented for workers in these groups.
†Not included in original 1991 table.
Adapted from Mullan R, Murthy L. Occupational sentinel health events: an updated list for physician recognition and public health surveillance. Am J Ind Med 1991; 19:775-99. © 1991 John Wiley & Sons, Inc. Reprinted by permission of Wiley-Liss, Inc., a subsidiary of John Wiley & Sons, Inc. Reprinted from Sullivan P, Moon Bank K, Hearl F and Wagner G: Respiratory risk in the construction industry. In: Ringen K. Englund A, Welch LS, Weeks JL and Seegal J (eds). Health and Safety in Construction: State of the Art Reviews in Occupational Medicine, Hanley and Belfus Philadelphia PA 10:2 269–284, 1995

Table 14.2 Sentinel health events in construction

are shown in Table 14.3. Strains and sprains were second in frequency only to lacerations among construction workers treated in a large emergency department.[9,10] Data from workers' compensation claims indicate that strains and sprains are the leading compensable injury for construction workers. In a study of carpenters,[11] 45% of all compensation claims were for musculoskeletal injuries and disorders. Cross-sectional studies also reveal a high prevalence of chronic musculoskeletal complaints (pain, ache, and discomfort) among construction workers.[12]

A survey of electricians showed that 51% had back symptoms, and 47% had hand or wrist symptoms;[13] 82% had symptoms to at least one body location in the prior year that lasted more than a week or recurred at least three times, while 63% reported symptoms to two or more locations. In a Swedish study, early retirements due to these disorders were more common among construction workers than other men. During 1988-1989, 72% of all sick leaves longer than 4 weeks in the construction industry in Sweden were due to musculoskeletal disorders.[12]

In the United States 33% of all worker compensation costs were due to low back pain, based on an analysis from a large workers' compensation insurance carrier.[14] The median cost of a low back claim in construction was 150% that of the reference group, and the cost of the 90th percentile cases was over 200% of the reference group. Clearly musculoskeletal problems in construction are frequent and more severe than in other industrial sectors.

Epidemiological studies of construction workers have found an increased risk of various musculoskeletal disorders, summarized in Table 14.3. Interview surveys in Finland and Sweden studied the relationship between work and musculoskeletal disorders in construction workers. Carpenters, bricklayers, concrete workers, plumbers, and machine and crane operators had a significantly increased standardized morbidity ratio for musculoskeletal diseases compared with Swedish men.[15] In Finland neck and shoulder symptoms, low back pain, and sciatica were more prevalent among machine operators and carpenters than sedentary workers,[16,17] indicating that construction work is a risk factor.

Several studies have looked at the occurrence of specific medical disorders of the knee, back and shoulders in construction workers (Table 14.3). A Finnish work analysis of carpet and floor laying and painting showed that carpet and floor layers kneeled, on average, 42% of the time in the observed work tasks. Among painters, kneeling was rare.[18] Bursitis in the front of the knee was more frequent among carpet and floor layers than painters,[18-20] suggesting kneeling and squatting as contributory factors. Ultrasonography

Disorder	Work posture, psychosocial factor, or trade	Reference
Neck, shoulder symptoms	Machine operators, carpenters	Tola 1988[16]
Neck, shoulder pain	Hand-held machines, hands above shoulder level, reported high psychological stress	Homstrom 1992[12]
Shoulder tendinitis	Rockblaster	Stenlund 1993[21]
Rotator cuff disorders	Sheet metal workers	Welch 1995[99]
Acromioclavicular joint osteoarthritis	Heavy manual work, vibration exposure Bricklayers, rockblasters	Stenlund 1992[100]
Elbow and wrist osteoarthritis	Using pneumatic, percussive tools (chipping hammers, scalers)	Gemme 1987[101]
Carpal tunnel syndrome	Repetitive, forceful work	Stock 1995[102]
	Sheet metal worker	Welch 1995[99] Rosencrance 2002[103]
Disk degeneration	Heavy manual work	Anderson 1981[104] Riihimaki 1990[105] Wickstrom 1978[106]
Herniated disk	Heavy manual work, motor vehicle drivers	Heliovaara 1987[107] Luoma 1998[108]
	Carpenters	Kelsey 1975[109] Budorf 1991[110]
	Construction workers, not further specified	
Low back pain	Concrete workers, roofers, carpet layers, scaffold erectors	Budorf 1991[110]
	Bricklayers, carpenters	Latza 2000[111] Arndt 1996[112]
	Construction workers, not further specified	Arndt 1996[112]
Sciatica	Concrete reinforcement workers	Riihimaki 1989[17]
	Carpenters, bricklayers	Nurminen 1997[113] Latza 2000[111]
Hip (coxarthrosis)	Heavy manual work	Lindberg 1984[114]
Knee, hip osteoarthritis	All construction	Vingard 1991[115]
Knee osteoarthritis	Heavy shipyard industry (laborers)	Lindberg 1987[116]
	Heavy manual labor	Kohatsu 1990[117]
	All construction workers	Lindberg 1987[116] Sandmark 2000[118]
	Floor layers and carpenters	Jensen 2000[119,120]
Knee symptoms	Carpet and floor layers	Kivimaki 1992[18,19] Thun 1987[20] Jensen 2000[119]
Thickening of prepatellar or superficial infrapatellar bursa	Carpet and floor layers	Kivimaki 1992[18,19]
Bursitis of knee	Carpet and floor layers	Kivimaki 1992[18,19] Thun 1987[20]

Table 14.3 Key disorders and associated work postures, psychosocial factors, or trades

showed thickening of the prepatellar or superficial infrapatellar bursa in 49% of the carpet and floor layers and in 7% of the painters. In addition, radiographic changes of the patella were more common among carpet and floor layers than among painters.

A study of bricklayers and rock blasters found that physical workload contributed to the development of radiographic osteoarthritis of the acromioclavicular joint, and exposure to vibration contributed to the development of shoulder tendonitis.[21] An association between severe low back disorders such as sciatica and herniated disk and heavy work has been shown in prospective studies, where heavy work was defined as construction work of some kind. An association between less severe non-specific back pain and workload is less well established in construction workers.[17,22]

NOISE-INDUCED HEARING LOSS AND OTHER PHYSICAL HAZARDS

Excess noise exposures among construction workers and high rates of noise-induced hearing loss among these workers are well documented.[23,24] More than 500,000 construction workers are exposed to potentially hazardous levels of noise. The United States has separate noise regulations for construction and general industry; in the construction standard there is no action level above which a hearing conservation program is required, and no detailed requirements for training or recordkeeping. Yet the work is very noisy. For example, a laborer using a heavy duty bulldozer is exposed to 91–107 dBA, with a mean of 99 dBA. Exposure from other heavy equipment ranges from a mean of 81 dBA in a crane with an insulated cab to 97 dBA without insulation. Studies of hearing thresholds show damage from these exposures. The Workers' Compensation Board in British Columbia has developed a successful program to prevent hearing loss in construction workers, and the 'Blue Angel' program in Germany can also be a model for the future. The article by Suter[23] provides an excellent review of noise control programs for construction.

HAZARDOUS MATERIALS IN CONSTRUCTION

Construction workers use a wide range of hazardous materials. Carcinogens that may be found on construction sites are shown in Table 14.4. Selected dermally absorbed and sensitizing agents found in the industry[25,26] are listed in Table 14.5. Construction exposures that can result in nonmalignant respiratory effects are listed in Table 14.6. Effects

	Uses or where encountered
C1: Established human carcinogens	
Beech wood dust	Joinery, circular saw on building sites
Benzene	Gasoline
Nickel compounds	Welding electrode
Oak wood dust	Joinery, circular saw on building sites
Tar, pitch	Road works
Zinc chromates	Old coatings
C2: Probable human carcinogens	
Benzo[a]pyrene	Road works, diesel engine emission, chimney sweeping
Cadmium compounds	Old coatings
Chromium(VI) compounds	Wood protection
Diesel engine emissions	Diesel engines
Hydrazine	Water treatment
C3: Suspected human carcinogens	
Dichloromethane	Stripper, solvent
Diphenylmethane-4'4 diisocyanate	Polyurethane
Formaldehyde	Conservation of dispersion products
Lead chromate	Old coatings
Wood dust (besides beech wood and oak wood dust)	Joinery, circular saw on building sites

From: Ruhl R, Kluger N. Hazardous materials in construction. In: Ringen K, Englund A, Welch LS, Weeks JL, Seegal J, eds. Health and safety in construction: state of the art reviews in occupational medicine, vol. 10. Philadelphia: Hanley and Belfus, 1995;335–52.

Table 14.4 Carcinogens relevant to construction

Substance	Transdermal (T) or sensitizing (S)	Areas of use
Benzene	T	Gasoline
Carbon tetrachloride	S	Solvent
Diphenylmethane-4,4'diisocyanate	S	Polyurethane
2-Ethoxyethanol	T	Solvent
Ethylbenzene	T	Solvent
Formaldehyde	S	Cleaning, disinfection
Hexamethylene diisocyanate	S	Polyurethane
Hydrazine	T,S	Water treatment
Isophorone diisocyanate	S	Polyurethane
Methanol	T	Solvent
2-Methoxyethanol	T	Solvent
Methyl methacrylate	S	Coating
Nickel	S	Welding electrode
Oil of turpentine	S	Solvent
Phenol	T	Solvent
Tin compounds	T	Wood protection
Toluene diisocyanate	S	Polyurethane
Wood dust	S	Joinery
Xylene	T	Solvent

From: Ruhl R, Kluger N. Hazardous materials in construction. In: Ringen K, Englund A, Welch LS, Weeks JL, Seegal J, eds. Health and safety in construction: state of the art reviews in occupational medicine, vol. 10. Philadelphia: Hanley and Belfus, 1995;335–52.

Table 14.5 Areas of use of transdermal and sensitizing materials in construction

of these exposures on respiratory health are summarized below. More detailed descriptions of the health effects of specific compounds can be found in subsequent chapters.

Lead (see Chapter 39.8)

Lead exposure and lead toxicity are particularly important problems in the construction industry. Nearly 1 million US construction workers are exposed to lead on the job;[27] more than 80% of these workers are involved in commercial or residential remodeling. Despite this risk in construction, the OSHA lead standard applied only to general industry before 1993. In 1992, NIOSH published an alert

for preventing lead poisoning in construction workers and reported on blood lead levels in bridge construction workers; levels ranged from 51 to 160 µg/dL whole blood with 62% of elevated blood lead levels involving work in a containment structure.[28,29] This publication identified high-risk activities associated with lead dust and fumes among bridge and structural steel workers including: abrasive blasting, sanding, burning, cutting or welding on steel structures coated with lead paint, and the use of containment enclosures. In 1993 OSHA promulgated a lead standard for construction.

In addition to setting a Permissible Exposure Level (PEL) for lead, the standard incorporates a presumption of expo-

Lung cancer	
Arsenic, inorganic (measured as AS)	Coal tar pitch volatiles
Asbestos	Formaldehyde
Beryllium	Zinc chromates
Chromic acid and chromates	
Non-malignant respiratory effects	
Aluminum	Mica, respirable dust
(pyro powders)	containing <1% quartz
Asphalt fumes	Mineral wool fiber
Bismuth telluride (Se-doped)	Nickel (soluble compounds)
Carbon black	Nitrogen oxide
Chlorine dioxide	Oxygen difluoride
Chromium (II) compounds (as Cr)	Ozone
Chromium metal (as Cr)	Paraquat, respirable dust
Coal dust	Silica
Cotton dust	Soapstone
Ethyl acrylate	Sulfur dioxide
Ferrovanadium dust	Sulfur tetrafluoride
Fibrous glass	Talc (containing no
Grain dust (oat, wheat, barley)	asbestos)
Graphite, natural, respirable	Tin oxide
<1% quartz	Trimelitic anhydride
Indium and compounds	Wood dust
Iron oxide (dust and fumes)	Yttrium
Methylene bis	
(4-cyclohexylisocyanate)	

Reprinted with permission from: Sullivan P, Moon Bank K, Hearl F, Wagner G: Respiratory risk in the construction industry. In: Ringen K, Englund A, Welch LS, Weeks JL, Seegal J, eds. Health and safety in construction: state of the art reviews in occupational medicine, vol. 10. Philadelphia: Hanley and Belfus, 1995; 269–84.

Table 14.6 Construction exposures identified by OSHA as potentially resulting in respiratory effects

sure during specific high-risk tasks, and requires specific protections during these tasks, unless air monitoring demonstrates exposure below the PEL. Levin demonstrated that implementation of the standard can reduce blood lead levels in construction workers.[30,31] However, the OSHA standard may not fully protect construction workers from lead toxicity.[31] Although the OSHA standard requires monitoring every 2 months, some tasks such as burning lead-coated steel can cause a rapid rise in lead levels in the blood. Thus more frequent monitoring and a lower threshold for industrial hygiene inspection or medical removal have been recommended in some circumstances.

Occupational lung diseases

Construction workers are exposed to a variety of hazardous agents that may pose risks to the respiratory system, including asbestos, silica, dust, synthetic vitreous fibers, cadmium, chromates, formaldehyde, resin adhesives, cobalt, metal fumes, creosote, gasoline, oils, diesel fumes, paint fumes and dusts, pitch, sealers, solvents, wood dusts and wood preservatives, and excessive cold. Selected construction exposures that can cause chronic non-malignant respiratory effects are shown in Table 14.6. Potential lung carcinogens are also included in Table 14.6

Lung cancer (see Chapter 30.1)
Studies from several countries, using a variety of study designs, have documented an increased risk of lung cancer among construction workers,[32] even after controlling for smoking.[33-38] Studies of specific construction trades have also shown an increased risk of lung cancer. Painters and plasterers appear to be at increased risk of lung cancer.[39-41] One factor may be cadmium, used as a pigment in paint. NIOSH has also documented an excess risk of lung cancer associated with cadmium exposure and identified the construction industry as an area where OSHA standards are needed to better protect workers.

High exposures may occur during unventilated renovation work. In addition, painters and plasterers may be exposed to acetone, acids, alkalis, benzene, chlorinated hydrocarbons, chromates, drying agents, paint strippers, oil base and resin paints, pigments, silica, solvents, thinners, and turpentine, as well as asbestos from spackling compounds and building restoration. Selikoff and Seidman documented a significant increase in lung cancer mortality among 17,800 asbestos insulation workers in the United States and Canada.[42] Finkelstein also documented an increased risk of lung cancer among insulators.[43] Sheet metal workers, who may be exposed to asbestos when working near insulators, are at increased risk of lung cancer.[44]

Construction welders may be exposed to filler metals containing cadmium, fluxes containing fluorine compounds, and metal fumes including nickel and chromium. Several studies have found increased risk of lung cancer among welders in a variety of work settings.[45-47] Masons have an excess of lung cancer[48,49] and are exposed to lung carcinogens such as asbestos, silica,[50] nickel, and hexavalent chromium. Other construction trades in which increased risk of lung cancer has been observed include electricians,[51-53] carpenters and woodworkers,[54] plumbers and pipefitters,[53,57-58] and roofers and mastic asphalt workers.[59,60] Roofers are exposed to volatile materials vaporizing from heated asphalt, including polycyclic aromatic hydrocarbons from coal tar pitch and bitumen fumes.

Nasal cancer (see Chapter 30.1)
Woodworkers, cabinetmakers, and furniture makers have an increased risk of nasal cancer.[61-63] Carpenters and joiners also appear to be at increased risk of developing nasal cancer.[64,65] Carpenters and cabinetmakers may be exposed to wood dust, formaldehyde, solvents, toluene, wood preservative, shellac, stains, bleaches, resin and casein glues, oils, polishes, and insulation agents including asbestos. Given the rarity of nasal cancer, the evidence for a relationship between nasal cancer and occupational exposure to wood dust is compelling. Several studies have also found an increased risk of nasal cancer among general construction workers.[33,62,65-67]

Mesothelioma (see Chapter 30.1)
Reports of mesothelioma among construction workers come from several countries.[34,44,66,69,70] Mesothelioma has been observed among construction workers who worked as insulators,[42,71] shipyard construction workers,[70-72] carpenters,[73] sheet-metal workers,[44] construction/maintenance workers,[71] and electricians.[72]

Respiratory condition	Prevalence rate per 1000 workers	Rate ratio
Lung cancer	1.7	1.31
Asbestosis	2.8	2.15
Asthma	19.6	0.82
Emphysema	25.8	1.34
Chronic bronchitis	24.1	1.30

Note: The rate ratio is the ratio of the rate in construction workers compared to the rate among other workers who participated in the survey. Reprinted with permission from: Sullivan P, Moon Bank K, Hearl F, Wagner G. Respiratory risk in the construction industry. In: Ringen K, Englund A, Welch LS, Weeks JL, Seegal J, eds. Health and safety in construction: state of the art reviews in occupational medicine, vol. 10. Philadelphia: Hanley and Belfus, 1995; 269–84.

Table 14.7 Prevalence rate and rate ratio of self-reported respiratory conditions among 1785 white male construction workers age 15 and older

Respiratory morbidity

Surveillance data on respiratory disease incidence or prevalence among construction workers are limited. Respiratory conditions accounted for 14.3% of approximately 7000 reported occupational illness cases among construction workers, based on the US BLS. NIOSH estimated the prevalence rate of reported respiratory conditions based on a national probability sample of construction workers. Prevalence rates ranged from 1.7 to 25.8 per 1000 white male construction workers for lung cancer and emphysema, respectively (Table 14.7). Construction workers reported asthma less frequently than in the general population, but since sensitized individuals may voluntarily leave the construction workforce, the reported prevalence may be low due to a healthy worker effect. Table 14.8 shows proposed exposure limits based on avoidance of respiratory effects for substances common in construction.

Asbestosis (see Chapter 19.8)

Asbestos has been recognized as a respiratory health risk for a number of construction trades.[75,76] Occupational exposure to asbestos, and a diagnosis of asbestosis, can occur in many construction trades, particularly among those working as insulators, plumbers and pipefitters,[76] electricians and sheet-metal workers,[77] and several studies have suggested that all construction workers may be at risk for asbestos-induced disease resulting from exposure associated with working adjacent to insulation workers.[77,78] Although asbestos is no longer used in new residential or heavy construction, workers may continue to be exposed to previously installed asbestos material during maintenance, renovation, addition, or demolition activities. For example, asbestos-containing fireproofing was sprayed on structural steel and other components of many US high-rise buildings before it was banned in 1973.

Silicosis (see Chapter 19.9)

Occupational exposure to silica can occur among various types of construction workers including those employed in concrete removal and demolition work, bridge and road construction, tunnel construction, and concrete or granite cutting, sanding, and grinding.[79,80] Sandblasters are at increased risk from exposure to crystalline silica. Those working nearby on the same construction site may also be at risk from silica-related disease. In the United States, sand containing crystalline silica is still used in abrasive blasting operations for maintenance of structures, preparing surfaces for painting, and in forming decorative patterns during installation of building materials. OSHA compliance monitoring data suggest that silica exposures within the construction industry continue to exceed recommended limits, and data in the US and in other countries show evidence of silicosis risk among construction workers.[50,80,81]

Bronchitis and chronic obstructive pulmonary disease (see Chapter 19.4)

Bronchitis has been reported among construction workers exposed to asbestos[82] and man-made mineral fibers,[83,84] spray painters,[85] and arc welders.[86] COPD has been reported among tunnel construction workers, construction painters,[85,87] sheet-metal workers,[84] and construction arc welders.[88] Chronic non-specific lung disease symptoms have been found among construction workers, wood workers, and painters,[89] even after adjusting for smoking and age. Specific exposures associated with excess risk of chronic non-specific lung disease included heavy metals, mineral dust, and adhesives.[90]

Occupational asthma (see Chapter 19.2)

Construction workers can be exposed to a number of agents that can cause asthma or exacerbate underlying asthma. Chan-Yeung reviewed agents and trades at risk for occupational asthma, including construction.[91] Possible causal exposures include wood dust and welding flux. Welders are at increased risk of occupational asthma; Kilburn and Warshaw found that 11% of male arc welders who had worked at construction sites reported a history of asthma.[86] Karjalainen confirmed the risk among welders, but also found an increased risk for asthma in almost all construction occupations.[92] Numerous exposures common among construction workers can exacerbate underlying asthma including exposure to cold, various particulates, dusts, fumes, and irritants.

Respiratory irritation (see Chapter 19.5)

Such exposures can also cause respiratory tract irritation in various construction workers. Painters may experience irritation of the respiratory system following exposure to solvents such as acetone, methyl ethyl ketone, and n-butyl lactate used in paints, varnishes, or lacquers.[93] Cement workers are at risk of respiratory irritation from components of cement, including amyl acetate and methyl ethyl ketone. Welders are exposed to several respiratory irritants, including ammonium chloride and boron trifluoride in soldering flux. Metal fume fever has been reported with exposure to nickel, chromates, copper, beryllium, cadmium, and other metal fumes which may be present during welding operations.

Chemical name	NIOSH recommended exposure limits*	OSHA permissible exposure limits	1994–95 ACGIH threshold limit values	Species	Comments
Asphalt fumes	5 mg/m³ ceiling (15-min) (total particulate)		5 mg/m³ TWA*		
Chromium (II) compounds (as Cr)	0.5 mg/m³ TWA	0.5 mg/m³ TWA	0.5 mg/m³ TWA		
Chromium (III) compounds (as Cr)	0.5 mg/m³ TWA	0.5 mg/m³ TWA	0.5 mg/m³ TWA		
Chromium metal (as Cr)	0.5 mg/m³ TWA	1 mg/m³ TWA	0.5 mg/m³ TWA		
Fibrous glass	5 mg/m³ TWA total fibrous glass		10 mg/m³ TWA		
Graphite, natural, respirable <1% quartz	15 mppcf TWA	2 mg/m³ TWA		Humans	Anthracosilicosis, similar to that seen in coal miners
Iron oxide (dust and fumes)		10 mg/m³ TWA	5 mg/m³ TWA		
Methylene bis(4-cyclohexylisocyanate)			0.005 ppm TWA		
Mica, respirable dust containing <1% quartz		20 mppcf TWA	3 mg/m³ TWA	Humans	Signs and symptoms resembling silicosis and pneumoconiosis in 8 of 57 workers
Mineral wool fiber			10 mg/m³ TWA		
Nickel (soluble) compounds	0.015 mg/m³ TWA (inorganic compounds)	1 mg/m³ TWA	0.1 mg/m³ TWA		
Nitrogen dioxide	1 ppm ceiling (15-min)	5 ppm ceiling	3 ppm TWA, 5 ppm STEL	Humans	Generated by welding Fatal pulmonary edema
Ozone		0.1 ppm TWA	0.1 ppm ceiling	Humans	Generated by welding Significant reduction in pulmonary vital capacity
Silica C amorphous, diatomaceous earth		20 mppcf	10 mg/m³ TWA	Mice	Damage to alveolar tissue
Silica C amorphous, precipitate, and gel			10 mg/m³ TWA		
Silica C crystalline cristobalite	50 g/m³ TWA	250/% SiO₂ +5 (as mppcf)	0.05 mg/m³ TWA	Dogs	Cellular infiltration of lung and fibrotic nodules in pulmonary lymph nodes
Silica C crystalline quartz, respirable	50 g/m³ TWA	250/% SiO₂ +5 (as mppcf)	0.1 mg/m³ TWA	Humans	Accelerated loss of pulmonary function beyond effects of aging alone
Silica C crystalline tridymite (as respirable quartz dust)	50 g/m³ TWA	250/% SiO₂ +5 (as mppcf)	0.05 mg/m³ TWA	Rats	Most active form of free silica when administered by intratracheal injection
Silica C crystalline tripoli (as respirable quartz dust)	50 g/m³ TWA	250/% SiO₂ +5 (as mppcf)	0.1 mg/m³ TWA	Lab animals	Progressive nodular fibrosis
Silica, fused	50 g/m³ TWA	250/% SiO₂ +5 +5 (as mppcf) 20 mppcf TWA	0.1 mg/m³ TWA (respirable dust)		
Soapstone C total dust			6 mg/m³ TWA		
Soapstone C respirable dust			3 mg/m³ TWA		
Sulfur dioxide	0.5 ppm TWA	5 ppm TWA	2 ppm TWA, 5 ppm STEL	Humans	Accelerated loss of pulmonary function
Sulfur tetrafluoride			0.1 ppm ceiling	Rats 4 hrs/day/10 days	Emphysema, marked clinical signs of respiratory impairment

Table 14.8 Substances common in construction for which proposed limits are based on avoidance of respiratory effects

Chemical name	NIOSH recommended exposure limits*	OSHA permissible exposure limits	1994–95 ACGIH threshold limit values	Species	Comments
Talc (containing no asbestos)		20 mppcf TWA	2 mg/m³ TWA (respirable dust)		
Tin oxide			2 mg/m³ TWA		
Trimelitic anhydride			0.04 mg/m³ ceiling	Rats	Intra-alveolar hemorrhage (no exposure duration indicated)
Wood dust, hard			1 mg/m³ TWA		
Wood dust, soft			5 mg/m³ TWA 10 mg/m³	STEL	

*NIOSH time-weighted-average (TWA) limits are for 10 hour/day, 40 hour/week exposures unless otherwise specified, and its ceilings are peaks not to be exceeded for any period of time unless a duration is specified in parentheses; OSHA's TWA are for 8-hour exposures; its short-term exposure limits (STELs) are for 15 minutes, unless otherwise specified, and its ceilings are peaks not to be exceeded for any period of time. The American Conference of Government Industrial Hygienists (ACGIH) sets threshold limit values (TLVs). The TLV-TWA is for an 8-hour exposure; the 'ceilings' are peaks not to be exceeded for any period of time during a working shift.

Reprinted with permission from: Sullivan P, Moon Bank K, Hearl F, Wagner G. Respiratory risk in the construction industry. In: Ringen K, Englund A, Welch LS, Weeks JL, Seegal J, eds. Health and safety in construction: state of the art reviews in occupational medicine, vol. 10. Philadelphia: Hanley and Belfus, 1995; 269–84.

Table 14.8 (Cont'd) Substances common in construction for which proposed limits are based on avoidance of respiratory effects

Respiratory infection (see Chapter 22)

Construction workers can be at increased risk of several infectious processes. For example, workers involved in excavation in tropical or subtropical areas may be at risk for nocardiosis, especially if they have another risk factor for the disease (such as lymphoma or deficient cell-mediated immunity). Road and bridge work and other construction activities which involve clearing of bird and bat roosts in river valleys in the eastern and central US can result in histoplasmosis, a pneumonitis caused by respiratory infection occurring after inhalation of air-borne fungal spores. The disease may be acute, inactive, or chronic, and can result in disability and death if untreated.[94-97] Elevated tuberculosis risk is found among silicotics. Legionnaire's disease has occasionally been reported in construction activities involving excavation or in the vicinity of cooling towers.[98]

Construction is a complex industry, involving many trades and employers on any single project. Because of that complexity, research and prevention activities have targeted construction less frequently than general industry, even though the need is great. These circumstances leave the industry with much room for improvement. The next decade should bring great improvement in health and safety in this industry.

References

1. US Department of Labor and Bureau of Labor Statistics. Fatal Occupational Injuries (1992–most current) www.bls.gov/iif/home.html. 2002.
2. Engholm G, Englund E. Morbidity and mortality patterns among construction workers in Sweden. In: Ringen K, Englund A, Welch LS, Weeks JL, Seegal J, eds. Health and safety in construction: state of the art reviews in occupational medicine, vol 10. Philadelphia: Hanley and Belfus, 1995;261–8.
3. US Department of Labor and Bureau of Labor Statistics 1989–current. Occupational injuries and illnesses: industry data. www.bls.gov/iif/home.html. 2002.
4. Meridian Research. Worker protection programs in construction. (OSHA Contract J-9-F-1-0019). Silver Spring, MD: Meridian Research, 1994.
5. Ringen K, Englund A, Welch LS, Weeks JL, Seegal J. Why construction is different. In: Ringen K, Englund A, Welch LS, Weeks JL, Seegal J, eds. Health and safety in construction: state of the art reviews in occupational medicine, vol 10. Philadelphia: Hanley and Belfus, 1995;255–60.
6. Construction chart book, 2nd edn. Silver Spring, MD: Center to Protect Workers Rights.
7. Tuomi K, Ilmarinen J, Klockars M, et al. Finnish research project on aging workers in 1981–1992. Scand J Work Environ Health 1997; 23:Suppl 1:7–11.
8. Brenner H, Ahern W. Sickness absence and early retirement on health grounds in the construction industry in Ireland. Occup Environ Med 2000; 57:615–20.
9. Hunting KH, Nessel-Stephens L, Sanford SM, Shesser R, Welch LS. Surveillance of construction worker injuries through an urban emergency department. J Occup Med 1994; 36:356–64.
10. Hunting KL, Welch LS, Nessel-Stephens L, Anderson J, Mawadeku A. Surveillance of construction worker injuries: utility of trade specific analysis. Applied Occup Environ Hyg 1999; 14:458–69.
11. Lipscomb HJ, Dement JM, Loomis DP, Silverstein B, Kalat J. Surveillance of work-related musculoskeletal injuries among union carpenters. Am J Ind Med 1997; 32:629–40.
12. Holmstrom E, Lindell J, Moritz U. Low back and neck/shoulder pain in construction workers; physical and psychosocial risk factors. Part 2: Relationship to neck/shoulder pain. Spine 1992; 17:672–7.
13. Hunting KL, Welch LS, Cuccherini BA, Seiger LS. Musculoskeletal symptoms among electricians. Am J Ind Med 1994; 25:149–63.
14. Webster BS, Snook SH. The cost of 1989 workers' compensation low back pain claims. Spine 1994; 19:1111–5.
15. Holmstrom, E, Moritz U, Engholm G. Musculoskeletal disorders in construction workers. In: Ringen K, Englund A, Welch LS, Weeks JL, Seegal J, eds. Health and safety in construction: state of the art reviews in occupational medicine, vol 10. Philadelphia: Hanley and Belfus, 1995;29–311.
16. Tola S, Riihimaki H, Videman T, et al. Neck and shoulder symptoms among men in machine operating, dynamic physical work and sedentary work. Scand J Work Environ Health 1988; 14:299–305.
17. Riihimaki H, Tola S, Videman T, Hanninen K. Low-back pain and occupation. A cross-sectional questionnaire study of men in machine operating, dynamic physical work and sedentary work. Spine 1989; 14:204–9.
18. Kivimaki J, Riihimaki H, Hanninen K. Knee disorders in carpet and floor layers and painters. Scand J Work Environ Health 1992; 18:310–6.
19. Kivimaki J. Occupationally related ultrasonic findings in carpet and floor layers' knees. Scand J Work Environ Health 1992; 18:400–2.
20. Thun M, Tanka S, Smith SB. Morbidity from repeated knee trauma in carpet and floor layers. Br J Ind Med 1987; 44:611–20.
21. Stenlund B, Goldie I, Hagberg M, Hogstedt C. Shoulder tendinitis and the relation to heavy manual work and exposure to vibration. Scand J Work Environ Health 1993; 19:43–9.
22. Heliovaara M. Occupation and risk of herniated lumbar intervertebral disc or sciatica leading to hospitalization. J Chron Dis 1987; 40:259–64.
23. Suter AH. Construction noise: exposure, effects, and the potential for remediation; a review and analysis. AIHA J 2002; 63:768–89.
24. Kerr MJ, Brosseau L, Johnson CS. Noise levels of selected construction tasks. AIHA J 2002; 63:334–9.
25. Jolaniki R, Kanverva L, Estlander T, et al. Occupational dermatoses from epoxy resin compounds. Contact Derm 1990; 172–83.
26. Ruhl R. GISBAU-Hazardous Substances Information System for the Contruction Sector. International Section of the ISSA for the Prevention of Occupational Risks in the construction Industry, XIII. Brussels: International Colloqium, September 1991.
27. Levin SM, Goldberg M. Clinical evaluation and management of lead-exposed construction workers. Am J Ind Med 2000; 37:23–43.
28. National Institute for Occupational Safety and Health. NIOSH Alert: Request for assistance in preventing lead poisoning in construction workers. NIOSH Publication 91–116a. Cincinnati, OH: NIOSH, 1992.
29. Waller K, Osorio AM, Maizlish N, Royce S. Lead exposure in the construction industry: Results from the California Occupational Lead Registry, 1987 through 1989. Am J Public Health 1992; 82:1669–71.
30. Levin SM, Goldberg M, Doucette JT. The effect of the OSHA lead exposure in construction standard on blood lead levels among iron workers employed in bridge rehabilitation. Am J Ind Med 1997; 31:303–9.
31. Vork KL, Hammond SK, Sparer J, Cullen MR. Prevention of lead poisoning in construction workers: a new public health approach. Am J Ind Med 2001; 39:243–53.

32. Sullivan P, Moon Bank K, Hearl F, Wagner G. Respiratory risk in the construction industry, In: Ringen K, Englund A, Welch LS, Weeks JL, Seegal J, eds. Health and safety in construction: state of the art reviews in occupational medicine, vol 10. Philadelphia: Hanley and Belfus, 1995; 269–84.

33. Neuberger M, Kundi M. Occupational dust exposure and cancer mortality: results of a prospective cohort study. In: Simonato L, Fletcher AC, Saracci R, Thomas TL, eds. Occupational exposure to silica and cancer risk. IARC Sci Publ 1990; 97:65–73.

34. Koskinen K, Pukkala E, Reijula K, Karjalainen A.Incidence of cancer among the participants of the Finnish Asbestos Screening Campaign. Scand J Work Environ Health. 2003; 29:64–70.

35. Robinson C, Stern F, Halperin W, et al. Assessment of mortality in the construction industry in the United States, 1984–1986. Am J Ind Med 1995; 28:49–70.

36. Boffetta P, Burstyn I, Partanen T, et al. Cancer mortality among European asphalt workers: an international epidemiological study. I. Results of the analysis based on job titles. Am J Ind Med 2003; 43:18–27.

37. Meyer JD, Holt DL, Chen Y, Cherry NM, McDonald JC. SWORD '99: surveillance of work-related and occupational respiratory disease in the UK. Occup Med (Lond) 2001; 51:204–8.

38. Hooiveld M, Spee T, Burstyn I, Kromhout H, Heederik D. Lung cancer mortality in a Dutch cohort of asphalt workers: evaluation of possible confounding by smoking. Am J Ind Med 2003; 43:79–87.

39. Brown LM, Moradi T, Gridley G, Plato N, Dosemeci M, Fraumeni JF Jr. Exposures in the painting trades and paint manufacturing industry and risk of cancer among men and women in Sweden. J Occup Environ Med 2002; 44:258–6.

40. Steenland K, Palu S. Cohort mortality study of 57,000 painters and other union members: a 15 year update. Occup Environ Med 1999; 56:315–21.

41. Wang E, Dement JM, Lipscomb H. Mortality among North Carolina construction workers, 1988–1994. Appl Occup Environ Hyg 1999; 14:45–58.

42. Selikoff IJ, Seidman H. Asbestos-associated deaths among insulation workers in the United States and Canada, 1967–1987. Ann NY Acad Sci 1991; 643:1–14.

43. Finkelstein MM. Analysis of mortality patterns and workers' compensation awards among asbestos insulation workers in Ontario. Am J Ind Med 1989; 16:523–8.

44. Zoloth S, Michaels D. Asbestos disease in sheet metal workers: the results of a proportional mortality analysis. Am J Ind Med 1985; 7:315–21.

45. Steenland K. Ten-year update on mortality among mild-steel welders. Scand J Work Environ Health 2002; 28:163–7.

46. Becker N. Cancer mortality among arc welders exposed to fumes containing chromium and nickel. Results of a third follow-up: 1989–1995. J Occup Environ Med 1999; 41:294–303.

47. Moulin JJ. A meta-analysis of epidemiologic studies of lung cancer in welders. Scand J Work Environ Health 1997; 23:104–13.

48. Rafnsson V, Gunnarsdottir H, Kiilunen M. Risk of lung cancer among masons in Iceland. Occup Environ Med 1997; 54:184–8.

49. Stern F, Lehman E, Ruder A. Mortality among unionized construction plasterers and cement masons. Am J Ind Med 2001; 39:373–88.

50. Flynn MR, Susi P. Engineering controls for selected silica and dust exposures in the construction industry – a review. Appl Occup Environ Hyg 2003; 18:268–77.

51. Milne KL, Sandler DP, Everson RB, Brown SM. Lung cancer and occupation in Alameda County: a death certificate case-control study. Am J Ind Med 1983; 4:565–75.

52. Ronco G, Ciccone G, Mirabelli D, et al. Occupation and lung cancer in two industrialized areas of Northern Italy. Int J Cancer 1988; 41:354–8.

53. Menck HR, Henderson BE. Occupational differences in rates of lung cancer. J Occup Med 1976; 18:797–801.

54. Pukkala E, Teppo L, Hakulinen T, Rimpela M. Occupation and smoking as risk determinants of lung cancer. Int J Epidemiol 1983; 12:290–6.

55. Ng TP. Occupational mortality in Hong Kong, 1979–1983. Int J Epidemiol 1988; 17:105–10.

56. National Institute for Occupational Safety and Health. Occupational characteristics of white cancer victims in Massachusetts, 1971–1973. (NIOSH) Publication No. 84-109. Cincinnati, OH: NIOSH, 1984.

57. Kaminski R, Geissert KS, Dacey E. Mortality analysis of plumbers and pipefitters. Cincinnati, OH: NIOSH, 1979.

58. Lynge E, Thygesen L. Occupational cancer in Denmark. Cancer incidence in the 1970 Census population. Scand J Work Environ Health 1990; 16(suppl 2):1–35.

59. Melius J. Asphalt – a continuing challenge. Am J Ind Med 2003; 43:235–6.

60. Boffetta P, Burstyn I, Partanen T, et al. Cancer mortality among European asphalt workers: an international epidemiological study. I. Results of the analysis based on job titles. Am J Ind Med 2003; 43:18–27.

61. Imbus HR, Dyson WL. A review of nasal cancer in furniture manufacturing and woodworking in North Carolina, the United States, and other countries. J Occup Med 1987; 29:734–40.

62. Luce D, Leclerc A, Morcet JF, et al. Occupational risk factors for sinonasal cancer: a case-control study in France. Am J Ind Med 1992; 21:163–75.

63. Mohtashamipur E, Norpoth K, Luhmann F. Cancer epidemiology of woodworking. J Cancer Res Clin Oncol 1989; 115:503–15.

64. Vaughan TL. Occupation and squamous cell cancers of the pharynx and sinonasal cavity. Am J Ind Med 1989; 16:493–510.

65. Comba P, Battista G, Belli S, et al. A case-control study of cancer of the nose and paranasal sinuses and occupational exposures. Am J Ind Med 1992; 22:511–20.

66. Hall NEL, Rosenman KD. Cancer by industry: analysis of a population-based cancer registry with an emphasis on blue-collar workers. Am J Ind Med 1991; 19:145–59.

67. Roush GC, Meigs JW, Kelly J, et al. Sinonasal cancer and occupation: a case-control study. Am J Epidemiol 1980; 111:183–93.

68. Begin R, Gauthier JJ, Desmeules M, Ostiguy G. Work-related mesothelioma in Quebec, 1967–1990. Am J Ind Med 1992; 22:531–42.

69. Chellini E, Fornaciai G, Merler E, et al. Pleural malignant mesothelioma in Tuscany, Italy (1970–1988): II. Identification of occupational exposure to asbestos. Am J Ind Med 1992; 21:577–85.

70. Mowe G, Andersen A, Osvoll P. Trends in mesothelioma incidence in Norway. Ann NY Acad Sci 1991; 643:449–53.

71. Muscat JE, Wynder EL. Cigarette smoking, asbestos exposure, and malignant mesothelioma. Cancer Res 1991; 51:2263–7.

72. Tagnon I, Blot WJ, Stroube RB, et al. Mesothelioma associated with the shipbuilding industry in coastal Virginia. Cancer Res 1980; 40:3875–9.

73. Milham S. Mortality Experience of the AFL-CIO United Brotherhood of Carpenters and Joiners of America, 1969–1970 and 1972–1973. NIOSH Publication Number 78-152. Washington DC: USGPO, 1978.

74. Cogan D, Pannett B, Osmond C, Acheson ED. A survey of cancer and occupation in young and middle aged men. I. Cancers of the respiratory tract. Br J Ind Med 1986; 43:332–8.

75. Baker EL, Dagg T, Greene RE. Respiratory illness in the construction trades. I. The significance of asbestos-associated pleural disease among sheet metal workers. J Occup Med 1985; 27:483–9.

76. Sprince NL, Oliver LC, McLoud TC. Asbestos-related disease in plumbers and pipefitters employed in building construction. J Occup Med 1985; 27:771–5.

77. Welch LS, Michaels D, Zoloth S. Asbestos-related disease among sheet-metal workers. Preliminary results of the National Sheet Metal Worker Asbestos Disease Screening Program. Ann NY Acad Sci 1991; 643:287–95.

78. Kilburn KH, Warshaw RH. Asbestos disease in construction, refinery, and shipyard workers. Ann NY Acad Sci 1991; 643:301–12.

79. National Institute for Occupational Safety and Health. ALERT - request for assistance in preventing silicosis and deaths in rock drillers. DHHS (NIOSH) Publication No. 92-107. Cincinnati, OH: NIOSH, 1992.

80. Tjoe Nij E, Burdorf A, Parker J, Attfield M, van Duivenbooden C, Heederik D. Radiographic abnormalities among construction workers exposed to quartz containing dust. Occup Environ Med 2003;60:410–7.

81. Ng TP, Yeung KH, O'Kelly FJ. Silica hazard of caisson construction in Hong Kong. J Soc Occ Med 1987; 37:62–5.

82. Hedenstierna G, Alexandersson R, Kolmodin-Hedman B, et al. Pleural plaques and lung function in construction workers exposed to asbestos. Eur J Respir Dis 1981; 62:111–22.

83. Engholm G, von Schmalensee G. Bronchitis and exposure to man-made mineral fibres in non-smoking construction workers. Eur J Respir Dis 1982; 63(Suppl 118):73–8.

84. Hunting KL, Welch LS. Occupational exposure to dust and lung disease among sheet metal workers. Br J Ind Med 1993; 50:432–42.

85. White MC, Baker EL. Measurements of respiratory illness among construction painters. Br J Ind Med 1988; 45:523–31.

86. Kilburn KH, Warshaw RH. Pulmonary functional impairment from years of arc welding. In: Proceedings of the VIIth International Pneumoconiosis Conference, Part II. Pittsburgh, Pennsylvania, August 23–26, 1988. NIOSH Publication No. 90-108. Cincinnati, OH: NIOSH, 1990;1264–8.

87. Schwartz DA, Baker EL. Respiratory illness in the construction industry: airflow obstruction among painters. Chest 1988; 93:134–7.

88. Kilburn KH, Warshaw RH. Pulmonary functional impairment from years of arc welding. Am J Ind Med 1989; 87:62–9.

89. Heederik D, Kromhout H, Kromhout D, et al. Relations between occupation, smoking, lung function, and incidence and mortality of chronic non-specific lung disease: the Zutphen Study. Br J Ind Med 1992; 49:299–308.

90. Heederik D, Kromhout H, Burema J, et al. Occupational exposure and 25-year incidence rate of non-specific lung disease: the Zutphen Study. Int Epidemiol 1990; 19:945–52.

91. Chan-Yeung M. Occupational asthma. Chest 1990; 98:148S–61S.

92. Karjalainen A, Martikainen R, Oksa P, Saarinen K, Uitti J. Incidence of asthma among Finnish construction workers. J Occup Environ Med 2002; 44:752 7.

93. Occupational Safety and Health Administration 29 CFR paragraph 1910. Air Contaminants: Proposed Rule. Fed Reg 57:26002–26601, 1992.

94. Bertolini R. Histoplasmosis – a summary of the occupational health concern. Report No. P88-8E. Hamilton, Ontario: Canadian Centre for Occupational Health and Safety, 1988.

95. George RB, Penn RL. Histoplasmosis. In: Sarosi GA, Davies SF, eds. Fungal diseases of the lung. Orlando, FL: Grune and Stratton Inc., 1986;69–85.

96. Powell KE, Hammerman KJ, Dahl BA, Tosh FE. Acute reinfection pulmonary histoplasmosis. Am Rev Respir Dis 1973; 107:374–8.

97. Sorley DL, Levin ML, Pukkala E, Teppo L, Hakulinen T, Rimpela M. Occupation and smoking as risk determinants of lung cancer. Int J Epidemiol 1983; 12:290–2.

98. Morton S, Bartlett CLR, Bibby LF, et al. Outbreak of legionnaires' disease from a cooling water system in a power station. Br J Ind Med 1986; 43:630–5.

99. Welch LS, Hunting KL, Kellogg, J. Work-related musculoskeletal symptoms among sheet metal workers. Am J Ind Med 1995; 27:783–91.

100. Stenlund B, Goldie I, Hagberg M, et al. Radiographic osteoarthrosis in the acromioclavicular joint resulting from manual work or exposure to vibration. Br J Ind Med 1992; 49:588–93.

101. Gemne G, Saraste H. Bone and joint pathology in workers using hand-held vibrating tools. Scand J Work Environ Health 1987; 13:290–300.

102. Stock S. Workplace ergonomic factors and the development of musculoskeletal disorders of the neck and upper limbs: a meta-analysis. Am J Ind Med 1991; 19:87–107.

103. Rosecrance JC, Cook TM, Anton DC, Merlino LA.Carpal tunnel syndrome among apprentice construction workers. Am J Ind Med 2002; 42:107–16.

104. Andersson GBJ. Epidemiologic aspects on low-back pain in industry. Spine 1981; 6:53–60.

105. Riihimaki H. Radiographically detectable degenerative changes of the lumbar spine among concrete reinforcement workers and house painters. Spine 1990; 15:114–9.

106. Wickstrom G. Effects of work on degenerative back disease. Scand J Work Environ Health 1978; 4(suppl 1):1–12.

107. Heliovaara M. Occupation and risk of herniated lumbar intervertebral disc or sciatica leading to hospitalization. J Chron Dis 1987; 40:259–64.

108. Luoma K, Riihimaki H, Raininko R, et al. Lumbar disc degeneration in relation to occupation. Scand J Work Environ Health 1998; 24:358–66.

109. Kelsey JL. An epidemiological study of the relationship between occupations and acute herniated lumbar intervenebral discs. Int J Epidemiol 1975; 4:197–205.

110. Budorf A, Govaert G, Elders L. Postural load and back pain of workers in the manufacturing of prefabricated concrete elements. Ergonomics 1991; 34:909–18.

111. Latza U, Karmaus W, Sturmer T, Steiner M, Neth A, Rehder U. Cohort study of occupational risk factors of low back pain in construction workers. Occup Environ Med 2000; 57:28–34.

112. Arndt V, Rothenbacher D, Brenner H, et al. Older workers in the construction industry: results of a routine health examination and a five-year follow-up. Occup Environ Med 1996; 53:686–91.

113. Nurminen M. Reanalysis of the occurrence of back pain among construction workers: modelling for the interdependent effects of heavy physical work, earlier back accidents, and aging. Occup Environ Med 1997; 54:807–11.

114. Lindberg H, Danielsson LG. The relation between labor and coxanhrosis. Clin Orthop 1984; 191:159–61.

115. Vingard E, Alfredsson L, Goldie I, Hogstedt C. Occupation and osteoarthrosis of the hip and knee: a register based cohort study. Int J Epidemiol 1991; 20:1025–31.

116. Lindberg H, Montgomery F. Heavy labor and the occurrence of gonarthrosis. Clin Orthop 1987; 214:235–6.

117. Kohatsu ND, Schurman DJ. Risk factors for the development of osteoarthrosis of the knee. Clin Orthop 1990; 261:242–6.

118. Sandmark H, Hogstedt C, Vingard E. Primary osteoarthrosis of the knee in men and women as a result of lifelong physical load from work. Scand J Work Environ Health 2000; 26:20–5.

119. Jensen LK, Mikkelsen S, Loft IP, Eenberg W. Work-related knee disorders in floor layers and carpenters. J Occup Environ Med 2000; 42:835–42.

120. Jensen LK, Kofoed LB. Musculoskeletal disorders among floor layers: is prevention possible? Appl Occup Environ Hyg 2002; 17:797–806.

Chapter 15
Office and Service Workers

Sandra N Mohr, Stuart L Shalat

INTRODUCTION

Office workers employed in traditional 'white collar' jobs are found in almost every industry. While some segments of industry employ office workers almost exclusively (e.g. insurance and finance), others such as manufacturing, construction, and transportation have some clerical, bookkeeping, personnel management, and other work performed in an office setting. Service work refers to activities that provide ancillary support to individuals, businesses, or industrial processes. Service work typically addresses needs other than manufacturing or fabrication. Examples include transportation, computer, hotel, personal service work (i.e. laundry, dry cleaning, barbers and beauticians, etc), business, entertainment, legal, social, and other services.

Historically, clinical and research aspects relating to occupational illness and injury have focused primarily on workers in the manufacturing and industrial sector. As job growth in the US migrated from manufacturing to office and service work, the nature of occupational health problems in this sector has become more important. Currently over 50 million workers are employed in service and office work in the US. The Bureau of Labor Statistics projects that service-related jobs will represent 95% of the total employment growth in the US over the next decade, with growth approaching 20%.[1] The development of the non-manufacturing workforce presents challenges to occupational medicine, with unique health issues not encountered in the traditional industrial sector.

The nature of the workplace environment has changed dramatically over the last 40 years, including workplace equipment, and office buildings themselves. Office workers may work in large buildings, with closed ventilation systems, or with limited make-up air. Ubiquitous use of computers has resulted in office workers spending longer periods of time in static postures at their workstation, at risk for repetitive motion from keying activities and challenges with ambient lighting, as well as video displays. Currently it is estimated that there are over 100 million computers in workplaces in the US.

As in other types of work, it is important to understand the nature of the workplace and the activities these tasks involve. Service jobs cover a broad range of occupational requirements ranging from sedentary activities at office workstations to physically demanding jobs such as postal carriers, and sales clerks standing all day in retail stores.

THE NEW WORKPLACE

Over the last 20 years, the number of individuals employed at computer-related occupations has grown exponentially. A broad array of occupations were created, and many that had previously existed have been significantly modified by an ever-increasing reliance on technology. The ergonomic problems associated with secretarial office work have expanded with the use of computers to involve numerous occupations and professions. While the computer keyboard is similar to that of a typewriter, several factors distinguish the computer operator. First, the worker at a computer faces a keyboard with more variable wrist postures and use of a mouse. Second, the nature of the work is often more continuous. For example, former use of typewriters would allow workers to replace paper at every page. The advent of the computer terminal meant that a worker could literally spend hour after hour performing the same repetitive task. Finally, in addition to working on the keyboard, the individual faces a computer screen with many of its own unique postural and ocular problems, as well as substantial productivity demands.

Service work in many different industries also makes broad use of computers. Workers may be located in large telephone and computer banks, consisting of many small cubicles. This type of organization is found in catalog and online retail sales, the insurance industry, transportation (reservations and dispatchers), and a variety of companies serving businesses. The common factor is the repetitive and sedentary nature of the workplace, with workers often at their workstation for long durations.

Office workers and ergonomics

The Occupational Safety and Health Administration has been attempting to improve ergonomic conditions in the workplace. While this resulted in the OSHA Ergonomics Program Standard in November 2000, this was overturned by Congress in the winter of 2001. In April of 2002, OSHA announced its Comprehensive Plan on Ergonomics to address musculoskeletal disorders in the workplace, in an ongoing effort to reduce illness and injury rates that will directly impact on office workers.

In the last two decades, ergonomics has risen to become one of the most critical factors in workplace injuries. Poor ergonomic design of the workplace is a major cause of musculoskeletal problems. Despite numerous studies that have examined workplace injuries that result from poorly designed workstations, many office design issues that contribute to worker health problems continue.[2-5] Common clinical syndromes among office workers include neck and back pain from poor postural position at the workstation, upper extremity problems from keying motion and improper positioning of keyboards, chairs, and arm supports.[6] In addition, many also complain of eye strain which can result from video display use.

Neck and back symptoms are among the most common experienced by office workers.[4] In many offices, desks without any provision for keyboard adjustment are still employed. The worker is therefore left with the choice between raising their arms to an uncomfortable height, or having their chair so high that their legs may be left dangling with no proper support. The use of adjustable keyboards and footrests can alleviate many of these problems. Customer service workers required to talk on the telephone and operate a computer simultaneously will often cradle the telephone receiver between their head and shoulders, leading to neck and shoulder strain. The use of headsets can alleviate this problem, as well as rotating tasks.

However, in many jobs in the service sector, such as phone bank workers or other telephone-based sales or customer assistance workers, there is likely to be little diversity in task. Constant repetition of tasks may also be exacerbated by productivity quotas, involving direct monitoring or surveillance of individual workers. Increasing task speed may increase short-term productivity, but may result in increased illness and injury rates. While having workers maintain high productivity is one measure of efficiency, it must be emphasized that a work force with fewer health complaints results in decreased lost time, as well as lower worker turnover. Research has suggested that frequent short rest breaks from computer work can have beneficial effects on workers' health and productivity.[7]

Prospective studies have been carried out to examine the role of workplace modifications in ameliorating musculoskeletal problems associated with visual display units (VDU). Key factors include the height of the display in relation to the operator, lighting of the room, and the adjustability of the keyboard and the operator's chair. Assessment of mechanical stressors in the office is reviewed in Chapter 32.

The development of functionally designed workstations for computers has helped to remedy some, but not all, problems associated with computer usage. The use of adjustable height and angle keyboards has significantly improved posture.[2] The use of footrests may assist in lower back problems. Chairs that tilt have been suggested to improve discomfort and lower extremity circulation.[8] The ability to adjust VDUs for height as well as angle has also proven useful.[9,10] Another ergonomic device that appears to be beneficial in reducing shoulder, neck, and back pain is the lower arm support on computer keyboards.[11]

Workers with upper extremity problems associated with keyboard use have shown clinical response to multidisciplinary therapeutic approaches.[12] In a retrospective study, 25% of patients who presented with bilateral hand and forearm pain achieved complete resolution of most symptoms, with an additional 54% reporting moderate improvement. Treatment consisted of medical management with pharmacologic interventions, occupational therapy, job-site evaluations, and psychological support with pain management and biofeedback training.

The efficacy of engineering modifications in computer keyboard and mouse shape and function, as well as wireless keyboards and mice, has not been well investigated. To the extent that these make an individual more comfortable, they may decrease the likelihood of injury and strain.

One workplace factor that has not been adequately studied is the recent introduction of the flat panel monitor into the workplace. The two primary types of flat panel monitors are light-emitting diode (LED) and plasma monitors. There are two factors in the design of these types of monitors which may make them more desirable for VDU operators. First, because they are truly flat, they are less likely to pick up reflections and create glare, as occurs with cathode ray tube (CRT) displays. Additionally, LED panels have a textured surface, which minimizes light reflection. Second, flicker rate has been blamed for many eye strain complaints associated with computer use in office spaces and fluorescent lighting. While the cost of plasma screens has limited their availability, the decreasing cost differential between CRTs and LED type displays make the latter an obvious choice for reducing visual fatigue.

A related issue in the use of VDU is eye strain that results when individuals change their plane of focus from computer display to paper copy. This is common both among office workers who are transcribing text from paper, and individuals reading from printed lists. The problem may also be exacerbated in older workers who require vision correction for presbyopia. If the distance from an operator's eyes to the VDU and to the paper copy is significantly different, it becomes difficult to maintain focus. It may therefore be useful to make use of copy holders that can be placed adjacent to display text at the same distance from the operator as the VDU.

Workplace lighting is another key factor in avoiding eye strain. Most office lighting is designed around standards that date back to the pre-Second World War era, for offices that used typewriters, not computers. The illuminated nature of the VDU screen and the potential for reflections from CRTs are a recognized problem for many VDU users. The use of glare-reducing screens can be of significant benefit, as can the use of light diffusers to soften lighting in offices. Many offices remain over-lit for current office needs. A re-evaluation of office lighting may have the dual benefit of reducing both eye strain and electricity costs.

Another area in which light is a problem is in electrostatic or dry copying. Workers who make copies, in particular when the document cannot be fed through a sheet feeder, often complain of the blinding light from the xenon flash tubes employed in many copiers. The primary recommendation for minimizing bright flashes from copier operation is use of engineering controls (i.e. covers).

Retail workers

One area of employment that is often overlooked in terms of occupational health problems is retail store clerks and sales assistants. Tendonitis, tenosynovitis, and carpal tunnel syndrome are common complaints. While this was initially thought to be related to the use of cash registers, electronic price scanners continue to cause problems.[13-15] Another problem in clothing sales is related to the folding of garments on display, and stacking activities. Complaints of carpal tunnel syndrom from this type of repetitive motion have been reported, that may be ameliorated by the use of folding templates.

Lifting during stocking and inventory activities results in risk for musculoskeletal injuries. Bulk packaging containers can be heavy, and when combined with twisting motions to place merchandise on display, may result in lower back injuries. Concern for low back injury in many retail businesses can be seen in frequent requirements to wear back braces. Unfortunately, numerous studies have not established the efficacy of these devices.[16-18]

INDOOR AIR QUALITY

One area frequently cited for health concerns among office workers is indoor air quality. Energy conservation measures since the 1970s have resulted in central heating, ventilation and air conditioning systems (HVAC) with closed windows, substantially reducing the amount of make-up air allowed into buildings. This overall decrease in air turnover rate means that any air pollutants within the workplace tend to remain in the ambient indoor environment. While the sources of air contaminants are not as obvious as those that may occur in manufacturing settings, there are a number of air contaminants that may affect workers' health.

Second-hand smoke

Among the most noxious indoor air pollutants, and the most likely to lead to long-term health effects, is second-hand (sidestream) tobacco smoke, also termed environmental tobacco smoke (ETS). Service workers in restaurants and bars in particular have health concerns associated with their exposure to second-hand tobacco smoke.[19] Other studies have examined airline flight crews, concluding that they are exposed to a variety of air contaminants.[20-23] Concern for cancer risk arises since flight attendants dating back to the 1950s were exposed to cigarette smoke for long periods of time in the close confines of the passenger cabins. Just as buildings have decreased make-up air to conserve heating and cooling costs, so airplanes have reduced make-up air to minimize jet fuel costs. Since the jet engines provide the energy for heating and cooling cabin air, decreasing the utilization of air handling units (termed 'packs') can lead to significant fuel savings. Studies have shown that such practices increase the levels of air contaminants including CO_2, and tobacco smoke in the cabin air.[22]

Despite the banning of smoking on domestic flights within the US, smoking continues on many international flights by non-US flag carriers, and so remains a continuing problem for some flight attendants. Bartenders, waiters, and waitresses continue to be at risk for smoking-related illnesses due to environmental tobacco smoke in their workplace. It must be emphasized that any service or office worker who is employed in a non-smoke-free workplace is placed at risk for complications of second-hand smoking.

Chemical contaminants

Other indoor air pollutants in the workplace may result from office equipment or furnishings. Copy machines and laser printers are often cited as sources; formaldehyde from composite wood products also causes respiratory effects.[24] Copy machines and laser printers rely on high voltage to generate an electrostatic charge, producing carbon black deposits on paper, as well as high-voltage xenon flash tubes. The paper then passes through a heating process to fix the pigment. This process results in two separate air pollutant streams, namely ozone, a well-recognized respiratory irritant, and vaporization of fuser oil. Workers may experience both eye irritation and respiratory symptoms from these exposures. Local ventilation with exhaust engineering can often eliminate these problems.

Office furnishings can contribute significantly to indoor air pollution. These can derive from carpets and carpet padding, as well as adhesives used to secure carpet and tiles to the floor.[25] While off-gassing from glues usually dissipates in a relatively short period of time after the carpet is put down, the carpet and padding may continue to off-gas formaldehyde for weeks or months after it has been laid. Similarly, office furniture, including fabric-covered office dividers, chairs, and wood furniture made of wood composites, can off-gas formaldehyde for long periods of time. In combination with the decreased make-up air in many office places, these contaminants can linger in office air for long periods of time.

The lack of make-up air from outdoors can often affect levels of air contaminants in buildings, contributing to mucous membrane and respiratory irritant effects and neurocognitive symptoms termed sick building syndrome (SBS).[26] Poor maintenance and under-utilization of air exchange from HVAC systems can further exacerbate indoor pollution problems. An example of problems in HVAC installations can be seen in the following case. Workers at a Federal Air Traffic Control facility experienced severe eye irritation and fatigue. Many of the workers smoked cigarettes on the job. The nature of the work required hyper-vigilance utilizing computers for hours at a time. Management thought these two factors might have been the primary source of the health complaints. However, an industrial hygiene inspection of the HVAC system determined that a recently installed HVAC system had never had the shipping blank plate removed from the make-up air inlet. This resulted in build-up in the indoor air of tobacco smoke and volatile compounds from electronic equipment components.

Certain service occupations have specific chemical exposures. Two examples are individuals who are employed in the dry cleaning industry and those involved in personal care, including hair and nail stylists. Concerns in the dry-cleaning industry have focused primarily on the use of perchloroethylene, a chlorinated solvent with neurotoxicity, hepatotoxicity, and potential carcinogity.[27-29] Inhalation is the primary route of exposure for most workers, although operators who remove the clothing from the washers (wet transfer processes) may have dermal exposure. While a variety of dermatologic problems exist, even greater health concerns have focused on inhalation exposures.[30] It is important to note that exposures are not limited to operators, but involve other dry-cleaning personnel (e.g. pressers, counter workers). Perchloroethylene may continue to off-gas from clothing for significant periods after cleaning.

In the case of hair and nail stylists, exposures include a variety of chemicals used for hair coloring, conditioning, and curling. Some of these chemicals can be highly irritating or sensitizing, resulting in contact dermatitis. Inhalation exposures to hair care products by stylists, and bonded acrylic nail components by manicurists, can lead to respiratory illness. While in the past most exposures were related to ketone mixtures, the advent of acrylic nail applications has resulted in an increase in exposure to a variety of epoxy glues and organic solvent systems. These include heat application processes resulting in increased volatilization. Hairdressers and manicurists often work from home or in small shops with inadequate ventilation, resulting in exposures above permissible short-term exposure limits (STEL). A number of studies have examined health issues in this population, which include dermatologic, respiratory, and neurologic problems, as well as increased risk of miscarriage.[31-36] Since these are small workplaces with small workforces, it is extremely difficult to fully examine less common outcomes such as cancer.[37]

The problem of infectious agents in office and service workplaces has been recognized for over a quarter of a century. Since the well-publicized outbreak at an American Legion Convention at a hotel in Philadelphia, Pennsylvania, in the 1970s, the importance of design and maintenance of HVAC systems has been established as an important factor in controlling *Legionella pneumophila*. Over 15,000 cases of *Legionella* are estimated to occur in the US each year. This bacterium is known to grow in cooling towers which are part of many HVAC systems. When systems are designed so that intake air for the HVAC system can become entrained in cooling towers, a problem potentially exists. Periodic maintenance and use of biocides in cooling towers are methods that have been utilized to control this problem. However, some controversy exists over the effectiveness of chlorination, copper-silver ionization, monochloramine, and heat in controlling the bacterium.

Molds and mycotoxins

In recent years there has been increasing concern over health risks associated with mold in indoor air.[38,39] The ability of various molds to trigger allergic and asthmatic responses in atopic individuals is well established.

Stachybotrys chartarum is a fastidious-growing mold associated with more severe mold contamination, and has generated substantial health concerns.[40-42] A wide range of symptoms including, but not limited to, respiratory difficulties, headache, body aches, fatigue, and neurocognitive symptoms have all been reported in association with *Stachybotrys*. In part, the origin of this concern centers on two reports of clusters of acute pulmonary hemorrhage in infants published by the CDC in 1994 and 1997. Even though the CDC later concluded that insufficient evidence existed to definitively link *Stachybotrys* to these serious respiratory problems, concern has continued. Clearly when dampness is present in office buildings, mold growth is possible, with potential allergenic or irritant responses in workers. The role of *Stachybotrys* in particular continues to be a source of concern and controversy.

VIOLENCE AND SERVICE WORKERS

An area of increasing concern in many workplaces is escalating violence in the workplace. In particular, service workers have become the target of violence with increasing frequency.[43] Police statistics have shown that personal assaults, including rape, serious injury, and death, represent the most serious acute health threat to service workers.[44,45] The rate of assaults on employees of convenience stores is particularly high. In the year 2000 there were a total of 674 homicides committed in the workplace; over 65% of these occurred among service workers. Studies have shown that a disproportionate number of these crimes occur during evening and night-time work. Since these jobs are often held by young people and individuals of color, they experience a disproportionate burden as victims of crime in the workplace.[46] In addition, women are frequently victims of domestic violence, including homicide, in the workplace. The need for workplace security to prevent such violence represents an important public health concern.

STRESS

An area of increasing concern both to workers and employers is stress in the workplace. Stress has been shown to affect workers' performance and overall health.[2,47] Although it is beyond the scope of this chapter to review all causes and implications of stress in service and office workers, several risk factors are notable in causing work-related stress among service and office workers.

Research has suggested that the amount of stress an individual experiences in the workplace is directly associated with the physical demands of their jobs and inversely associated with the amount of control a worker has over their daily tasks.[47] Since many service workers have relatively little control over their jobs, they may be at increased risk for stress. One aspect that may contribute to stress is electronic surveillance of productivity. This can take various forms, ranging from evaluation of the number of customers served, to direct video surveillance of workers. Such surveillance impacts workers' sense of control and security and may be associated with stress.

The result of stress in the workplace may not be limited to psychologic symptoms, but may be manifest in an increase in physical symptoms. For example, a worker with musculoskeletal symptoms may experience greater severity or greater frequency of these symptoms due to stress.

Assisting workers in coping with stress in the workplace can be advantageous to both workers and employers, as a sense of job satisfaction and security is likely to result in lower rates of job turnover. There is also the potential for greater productivity with a more contented workforce. Such methods as worker empowerment, including quality control networks and workplace discussion groups, can provide workers with a greater sense of control, as well as providing management feedback on improvements that may increase productivity.

The attacks on the Alfred P. Murrah Building on April 19 1995 in Oklahoma City, and on the World Trade Center towers and Pentagon on September 11 2001 have resulted in heightened concern for terrorism in the workplace. It should be noted that most of the victims of these attacks were service and office workers. Anecdotal reports exist for employees working in high-rise buildings, as well as airline transportation workers, who have expressed concern for their safety following these incidents. These concerns may lead some employees to experience stress, with the potential for anxiety or depression.

Once thought to be a problem limited to healthcare, manufacturing, and transportation industries, shift work has become more prevalent in retail, food service, and customer service sectors moving towards a 24-hour economy. In numerous industrial settings, it has been demonstrated that workers on rotating shift work exhibit disrupted sleep patterns on both day and night shifts.[48] Shift work is also associated with gastrointestinal and cardiovascular diseases.[49] Studies on age and shift work seem to show an interactive effect[50,51] and it is likely that office and service workers will experience a similar response.[52]

Unlike shift work, there are very limited data on the health consequences of overtime in either voluntary or mandatory settings. Several studies have demonstrated psychological, cardiovascular and reproductive effects as well as impact on workplace performance.

CHILDREN IN SERVICE INDUSTRIES

The use of children and adolescents in service industries raises a variety of health and safety issues.[53] In addition to the traditional employment of children and adolescents in agriculture, the most common areas of employment are in the food service industry. In particular, the fast food industry in the US frequently relies on entry level workers. While not always apparent, a variety of health issues are present in these workplaces, including burns from stove top grills and open fry vats. The need for speed in food preparation and service of customers can result in slips and falls, resulting in significant injury. In addition to illness and injury, the social impact of child labor includes potential adverse effects on school work due to fatigue and lack of study time.

References

1. Bureau of Labor Statistics, US. Washington DC: Department of Labor, Bureau of Labor Statistics, 2002.
2. Aras A, Horgen G, Bjorset HH, Ro O, Walsoe H. Musculoskeletal, visual and psychosocial stress in VDU operators before and after multidisciplinary ergonomic interventions. A 6-year prospective study-Part H. Appl Ergon 2001; 32:559–71.
3. Berqvist V, Wolgast E, Nilsson B, Voss M. Musculoskeletal disorders among visual display terminal workers: individual ergonomics and work organization factors. Ergonomics 1995; 38:763–76.
4. Ong CN, Chia SE, Jeyaratnam J, Tan KC. Musculoskeletal disorders among operators of visual display terminals. Scand J Work Environ Health 1995; 21:60–4.
5. Sauter SL, Schleifer LM, Knutson SJ. Work posture, workstation design and musculoskeletal discomfort in a VDT data entry task. Hum Factors 1991; 33:151–67.
6. Marcus M, Gerr F. Upper extremity musculoskeletal symptoms among female office workers: associations with video display terminal use and occupational psychosocial stressors. Am J Ind Med 1996; 29:161–70.
7. Henning RA, Jacques P, Kissel GV, Sullivan AB, Alteras-Webb SM. Frequent short rest breaks from computer work: effects on productivity and well-being at two field sites. Ergonomics 1997; 40:78–91.
8. Stranden E. Dynamic leg volume changes when sitting in a locked and free floating tilt office chair. Ergonomics 2000; 43:421–33.
9. Jaschinski W, Heuer H, Kylian H. Preferred position of visual displays relative to the eyes: a field study of visual strain and individual differences. Ergonomics 1998; 41:1034–49.
10. Svensson F, Svensson OK. The influence of the viewing angle on neck-load during work with video display units. J Rehabil Med 2001; 33:133–6.
11. Lintula M, Nevala-Puranen N, Louhevaara V. Effects of Ergorest arm supports on muscle strain and wrist positions during the use of the mouse and keyboard in work with visual display units: a work site intervention. Int J Occup Saf Ergon 2001; 7:103–16.
12. Barthel JR, Miller LS, Deardorff WW, Portenier R. Presentation and response of patients with upper extremity repetitive use syndrome to a multidisciplinary rehabilitation program: a retrospective review of 24 cases. J Hand Ther 1998; 11:191–199.
13. Hinnen D, Laubil T, Guggenbuhl D, Krueger H. Design of check-out systems including laser scanners for sitting work posture. Scand J Work Environ Health 1992; 18:186–94.
14. Lannersten L, Harms-Ringdahl K. Neck and shoulder muscle activity during work with different cash register systems. Ergonomics 1990; 33:49–65.
15. Lehman KR, Psihogios JP, Meulenbroek RG. Effects of sitting versus standing and scanner type cashiers. Ergonomics 2001; 44:719–38.
16. Genaidy AM, Simmons RJ, Christensen DM. Can back supports relieve the load on the lumbar spine for employees engaged in industrial operations? Ergonomics 1995; 38:996–1010.
17. Krauss JF, McArthur DL. Back supports and back injuries: a second visit with the Home Depot cohort study data on low-back injuries. Int J Occup Environ Health 1999; 5:9–13.
18. Krauss JF, Brown KA, McArthur DL, Peek-As AC, Samaniego L, Kraus C. Reduction of acute low back injuries by use of back supports. Int J Occup Environ Health 1996; 2:264–73.

19. Jones S, Love C, Thomson G, Green R, Howden-Chapman P. Second-hand smoke at work: the exposure, perceptions and attitudes of bar and restaurant workers to environmental tobacco smoke. Aust NZ J Public Health 2001; 25:90–3.

20. Dechow M, Sohn H, Steinhanses I. Concentrations of selected contaminants in cabin air of airbus aircrafts. Chemosphere 1997; 35:21–31.

21. Lindgren T, Norback D, Andersson K, Dammstrom BG. Cabin environment and perception of cabin air quality among commercial aircrew. Aviat Space Environ Med 2000; 7:774–82.

22. Mattson ME, Boyd G, Byar D, et al. Passive smoking on commercial airlines flights. JAMA 1989; 261:867–72.

23. Wieslander G, Lindgren T, Norback D, Venge P. Changes in the ocular and nasal signs and symptoms of aircrews in relation to the ban on smoking on intercontinental flights. Scand J Work Environ Health 2000; 26:514–22.

24. Malaka T, Kodama AM. Respiratory health of plywood workers occupationally exposed to formaldehyde. Arch Environ Health 1990; 45:288–94.

25. Hodgson AT, Rudd AF, Beal D, Chandra S. Volatile organic compound concentrations and emission rates in new manufactured and site-built homes. Indoor Air 2000; 10:178–92.

26. Wargocki P, Wyon DP, Sundell J, Clausen G, Fanger PO. The effects of outdoor air supply rate in an office on perceived air quality, sick building syndrome (SBS) symptoms and productivity. Indoor Air 2000; 10:222–36.

27. Vaughan TL, Stewart PA, Davis S, Thomas DB. Work in dry cleaning and the incidence of cancer of the oral cavity, larynx, and oesophagus. Occup Environ Med 1997; 54:692–5.

28. Ruder AM, Ward EM, Brown DP. Mortality in dry-cleaning workers: an update. Am J Ind Med 2001; 39:121–32.

29. Lynge E, Anttila A, Hemminki K. Organic solvents and cancer. Cancer Causes Control 1997; 8:406–419.

30. Redmond SF, Schappert KR. Occupational dermatitis associated with garments. J Occup Med 1987; 29:243–4.

31. Belsito DV. Contact dermatitis to ethyl-cyanoacrylate-containing glue. Contact Derm 1987; 17:234–6.

32. Hilpakka D, Samimi B. Exposure of acrylic fingernail sculptors to organic vapors and methacrylate dusts. Am Ind Hyg Assoc J 1987; 48:230–7.

33. John EM, Savitz DA, Shy CM. Spontaneous abortions among cosmetologists. Epidemiology 1994; 5:147–155.

34. LoSasso GL, Rapport LJ, Axelrod BN, Whitman RD. Neurocognitive sequelae of exposure to organic solvents and (meth)acrylates among nail-studio technicians. Neuropsychiat Neuropsychol Behav Neurol 2002; 15:44–55.

35. LoSasso GL, Rapport LJ, Axelrod BN. Neuropsychological symptoms associated with low-level exposure to solvents and (meth)acrylates among nail technicians. Neuropsychiat Neuropsychol Behav Neurol 2001; 14:183–9.

36. Lundberg I, Alfredson L, Plato N, Sverdrup B, Klareskog L. Occupation, occupational exposure to chemicals and rheumatological disease. A register based cohort study. Scand J Rheumatol 1994; 23:305–10.

37. Pukkala E, Nokso-Koivisto P, Roponen P. Changing cancer risk pattern among Finnish hairdressers. Int Arch Occup Environ Health 1992; 64:39–42.

38. Burr ML. Health effects of indoor molds. Rev Environ Health 2001; 16:97–103.

39. Page E, Trout D. Mycotoxins and building-related illness. J Occup Environ Med 1998; 40:761–4.

40. Etzel RA, Montana E, Sorenson WG, et al. Acute pulmonary hemorrhage in infants associated with exposure to *Stachybotrys atra* and other fungi. Arch Pediatr Adolesc Med 1998; 152:757–62.

41. Hodgson MJ, Morey P, Leung WY, et al. Building-associated pulmonary disease from exposure to *Stachybotrys chartarum* and *Asperigillus versicolor*. J Occup Environ Med 1998; 40:241–9.

42. Mahmoudi M, Gershwin ME. Sick building syndrome, III. *Stachybotrys chartarum*. J Asthma 2000; 37:191–8.

43. Nelson NA, Kaufman JD. Fatal and nonfatal injuries related to violence in Washington workplaces, 1992. Am J Ind Med 1996; 30:438–46.

44. Peek-Asa C, Runyan CW, Zwerling C. The role of surveillance and evaluation research in the reduction of violence against workers. Am J Prev Med 2001; 20:141–8.

45. Peek-Asa C, Erickson R, Kraus JF. Traumatic occupational fatalities in the retail industry, United States 1992-1996. Am J Ind Med 1999; 35:186–91.

46. Hammermesh DS. Changing inequality in work injuries and work timing. Monthly Labor Rev October, 1999.

47. MacDonald LA, Karasek RA, Punnett L, Scharf T. Covariation between workplace physical and psychosocial stressors: evidence and implications for occupational health research and prevention. Ergonomics 2001; 10:696–718.

48. Budnick LD, Lerman SE, Baker TL, Jones H, Czeisler CA. Sleep and alertness in a 12-hour rotating shift work environment. J Occup Med 1994; 36:1295–300.

49. Koller M. Health risks related to shift work. An example of time-contingent effects of long-term stress. Int Arch Occup Environ Health 1983; 53:59–75.

50. Brugere D, Barrit J, Butat C, Cosset M, Volkoff S. Shiftwork, age and health: an epidemiologic investigation. Int J Occup Environ Health 1997; 3(Supplement 2):S15–S19.

51. Harma MI, Ilmarinen JE. Towards the 24-hour society – new approaches for aging shift workers? Scand J Work Environ Health 1999; 25:610–5.

52. Spurgeon A, Harrington JM, Cooper CL. Health and safety problems associated with long working hours: a review of the current position. Occup Environ Med 1997; 54:367–75.

53. Kinney JA. Health hazards to children in the service industries. Am J Ind Med 1993; 24:291–300.

Chapter 16
Manufacturing Sector

Tim K Takaro

INTRODUCTION

In characterizing the manufacturing sector, it is useful to consider the US Bureau of Labor Statistics definition for manufacturing, namely, any mechanical or chemical transformation of materials into new products. Manufacturing establishments are generally described as plants, factories, or mills where production may include fabrication, assembly, or blending of materials as finished products, or as raw material for subsequent manufacture. Manufacturing does not include facilities where the product is a structure or similar fixed improvement.

The products of the manufacturing sector are usually produced for the wholesale market, and are limited to orders for industrial uses as opposed to retail sale to the consumer. For example, food and associated products industries supply grocery stores, which are considered within the trade sector. The nature of manufacturing, requiring the mechanical transformation of materials into new products, presents numerous risk factors for illness and injury to workers.

Table 16.1 provides some examples of manufacturing establishments, along with average annual employment and injury and illness rates in 1994 and 1999 for the industries with the highest morbidity. Industry groups which are not on this list and have lower injury and illness rates include durable goods, electrical and other equipment and instruments; and non-durable goods such as tobacco, textile mill products, apparel, paper and allied products, printing and publishing, chemicals and allied products, and petroleum and coal products. Because the manufacturing sector is so large, diverse and complex, this chapter will focus mainly on the ten industries within the sector with the highest incidence of illness and injury in the United States.

The principal hazards associated with the manufacturing sector will be defined and the primary associated health outcomes described, according to the most recent statistics from the United States Bureau of Labor and Statistics. In a few cases, a major industry has some industrial subgroupings with a higher injury and illness rate than the more general description provided in Table 16.1 (representing a two digit Standard Industrial Classification (SIC)). For example, household appliances (three digit SIC) and electron tubes (four digit SIC) within electronic industries, and coated fabrics and tire cord (four digit SIC) within the textile industry, have rates comparable to those higher risk industries described in Table 16.1. The reader must bear in the mind the specificity of the industrial classification when interpreting the data described.

Other chapters in this book will provide details regarding treatment and management of specific conditions associated with the hazards of the manufacturing sector such as musculoskeletal disorders (Chapter 23), diseases of the lung and pleura (Chapter 19), and dermatologic disease (Chapter 29). Specific hazards relevant to this industrial sector are described in detail in Section 4 of the text.

Manufacturing is the hallmark of the industrial era beginning in the 19th century. In most of the developed world, it is still the largest sector of employment in production. Factories employ more workers on average than non-manufacturing businesses. For example, in the United States, factories account for just over one-third of industrial establishments, but manufacturing employees outnumber workers in the next largest production sectors, construction and mining, by three to one.[1] In the US in 2000, the manufacturing employment level was 18.5 million, decreasing from 18.8 million in 1998, following a market-driven cyclical trough in the early 1990s (Fig. 16.1). Despite the shift of manufacturing jobs in the US and other developed nations to countries with lower wage rates, such as the emerging

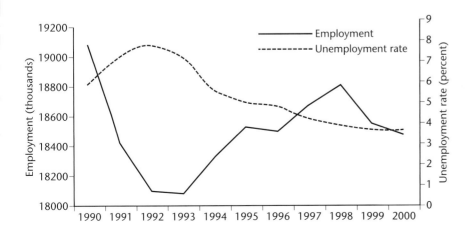

Figure 16.1: The figures for employment and unemployment in the US manufacturing sector have converged in recent years as the number of US manufacturing jobs declined since 1998, concomitant with a national decline in unemployment. US manufacturing jobs are expected to further decline.

	Annual average employment 1999	Total injury and illness incidence 1999	Total injury and illness incidence 1994	Total illness incidence 1999	Skin diseases or disorders	Dust disease of the lungs	Respiratory condition due to toxicant	Poisoning	Disorder due to physical agent	Repetitive trauma disorder	All other occupational illnesses
Lumber and wood products	831,900	1300	1570	56.2	4.0	0.3	0.6	0.2	2.9	44.9	3.40
Furniture and fixtures	547,000	1150	1500	120.8	6.7	0.2	1.5	0.1	4.6	99.3	6.00
Stone, clay, and glass	566,666	1070	1320	60.4	9.6	0.4	1.4	2.2	3.9	37.5	5.40
Primary metal industries	698,800	1290	1680	108.8	8.9	3.2	4.7	5.1	10.0	69.9	7.0
Fabricated metal products	1,521,900	1260	1640	99.0	15.1	0.1	3.2	0.9	5.9	67.6	6.3
Industrial machinery and equipment	2,132,800	850	1160	72.5	11.8	0.1	2.6	0.6	2.7	50.5	4.1
Transportation equipment	1,891,800	1370	1960	326.6	24.3	1.0	8.7	3.1	13.9	258.5	17.0
Food and kindred products	1,686,200	1270	1710	225.7	17.4	0.2	5.8	0.6	5.3	189.5	7.0
Rubber and misc. plastics	1,008,600	1010	1400	84.2	10.3	0.5	4.2	0.1	1.8	59.0	8.2
Leather	76,900	1030	1200	277.4	29.1	1.2	1.0	0.5	1.0	228.9	15.8

Table 16.1 Occupational illness incidence for top ten manufacturing industries in 1999 per 10,000 FTEs

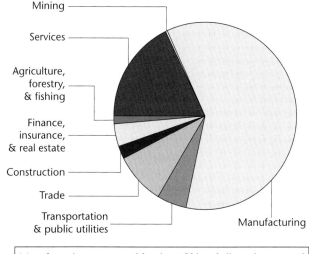

Mining

Services

Agriculture, forestry, & fishing

Finance, insurance, & real estate

Construction

Trade

Transportation & public utilities

Manufacturing

Manufacturing accounted for three-fifths of all newly reported occupational illnesses for private industry in 1999

Figure 16.2: Non-fatal workplace illnesses by industry division, 1999. Manufacturing is defined as those establishments which are engaged in the mechanical transformation of materials into new products. This sector of the US economy accounted for three-fifths of all newly reported occupational illnesses for private industry in 1999. Source: Bureau of Labor Statistics, US Department of Labor, December 2000.

manufacturing sectors such as the maquiladoras sector. These international manufacturing sectors are expected to cause a decline in employment in the United States manufacturing in the near future. Mining is the only other industrial sector expected to decline during this period.[1]

According to the US Bureau of Labor Statistics (BLS) the manufacturing sector accounts for more illness and injury than any other sector of the US economy, with 9.5 cases of illness or injury per 100 workers in 1999. Despite a decline in this rate during the past 5 years in most industries (Table 16.1) this sector accounted for three-fifths of all newly reported occupational illnesses for private industry in 1999 (Fig. 16.2). The sector's distinction in this regard has been consistent throughout the past decade in the US. Since 1993, manufacturing has surpassed the construction industry in total injury and illness rates, though the construction trades' annual rates remain nearly as high during the past decade with 8.8 cases per 100 workers per year, and exceed manufacturing in days lost from work. As demonstrated in Figure 16.3, the manufacturing industries with the top ten injury and illness rates are all well above the manufacturing sector's average incidence of illness and injury of 125.5 per 10,000 full-time employees.

Manufacturing accounted for 11.3% of all work-related fatalities in the US in 2000. The manufacturing industries with the top ten injury and illness rates accounted for 80% of all the fatalities in this sector. Lumber and wood products had more than twice as many fatalities as any other industry group, with logging accounting for the vast majority of these (122 fatalities in 2000). Most of the industries have had a slow rate of decline in fatalities over the past decade, except for the industrial machinery and equipment sector, which has increased by 1% over the past five years.[1] The distribution of the 668 fatalities in the manufacturing sector is shown in Figure 16.4.

Data sources

Much of the current data for health and safety in the manufacturing sector comes from the Survey of Occupational Injuries and Illness of the United States BLS.

economies in Asia and Mexico, the unemployment rate in manufacturing dropped in the late 1990s in the US to 3.6% in 1998 and 1995, though this has increased during the recent recessionary cycle.[1]

The fastest growing manufacturing zone in North America is in the US–Mexican border region, including foreign-owned factories with special tax status known as maquiladoras. Once assembly spots for multinational corporations, the maquiladoras have flourished and are now a manufacturing sector in their own right. Over 4000 maquiladora plants produce durable goods, including electronic equipment, household appliances, batteries, garments, furniture, and miscellaneous consumer products.[2,3]

Chapter 10 in this book addresses some of the challenges of worker health and safety in the emerging economy and

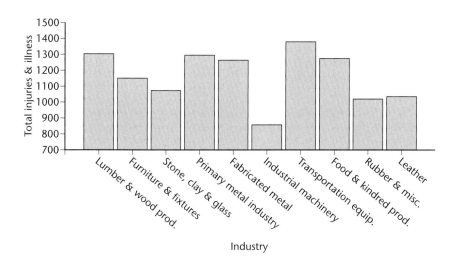

Figure 16.3: The top ten major US industries by injury and illness rate in 1999. These injury and illness rates are all well above the manufacturing division average incidence of illness and injury of 125.5 per 10,000 full-time workers.

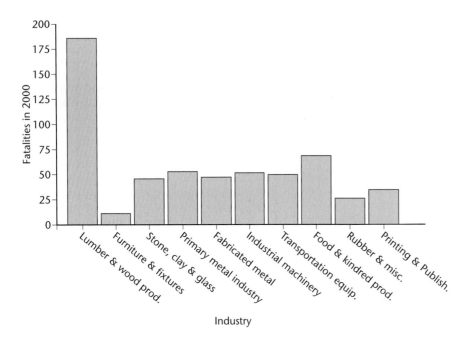

Figure 16.4: Manufacturing accounted for 11.3% of all work-related fatalities in the US in 2000, with these industries in the top decile in 1999. Most of the industries have had a slow rate of decline in fatalities over the past decade except for the Industrial Machinery and Equipment, sector which has increased by 1% over the past five years.

This survey is collected annually on a state-by-state basis, from approximately 169,000 private industrial establishments. The survey measures non-fatal injuries and illnesses in private industry, with the exception of self-employed firms and those with fewer than 11 employees, private households, government agencies, or state and local governments. The survey is based upon logs kept by individual employees, which are subject to various incentives that may result in substantial under-reporting or over-reporting.

The survey probably underestimates the true occupational illness and injury rates. For example, in Washington State in 1997, the BLS indicated 4.4 cases of carpal tunnel syndrome per 10,000 full-time employees (FTEs) resulting in time loss. The rate for claims that were accepted for compensation through the state's workers' compensation program for this illness was 16.6 per 10,000 FTEs during the same period.[4] The survey also likely under-measures long term chronic or latent illnesses.[1,5] This latter deficiency is particularly important for cancers secondary to chemical exposures.

The estimates of occupational injury and illness are based upon a probability sample, with a standard error calculated around the estimate. For example, the 1998 incidence rate for all occupational illnesses of 6.7 per 100 full-time workers in the private industrial sector has an estimated relative standard error of 0.9%. Data are also subject to non-sampling error such as mistakes in recording and counting, misclassification due to imprecise definitions, which may not accurately describe the industry, and the inability to obtain information about all cases. These errors are not measured directly, though procedures have been implemented by the BLS to minimize non-sampling error. Industries are classified by the 1987 Standard Industrial Classification (SIC) Manual established by the Office of Management and Budget. This classification system will be replaced by the North American

Industrial Classification System beginning December 2004 in order to better represent new industries across North America.

Since the 1990s, restricted work activity, as opposed to days away from work, has become a much more common response by employers to workplace injury and illness. While the total number of injuries and illnesses requiring days away from work has continuously declined since 1992, the number of injuries and illnesses requiring work restriction has increased by over 70% during this same period.[6] This trend is especially apparent in the manufacturing sector, where the rate of injury or illness requiring restricted work has been increasing since 1986.[5] For injury or illness requiring restricted work, the manufacturing sector is 50% higher over the past decade than the next highest sectors, agriculture and transportation. This trend seems to indicate an effort on the part of employers to maintain employee productivity by restricting duty to accommodate an injury or illness. However, the trend also demands more scrutiny of the BLS data to include tracking of the outcomes of work restriction (follow-back analysis). Without such effort, the information needed for the design of future illness and injury prevention intervention strategies will be lacking.

In 1999, 76% of injuries and illness in the manufacturing sector could be attributed to the ten industrial groups with data shown in Table 16.1 (classified by two digit SIC code): Durable Goods: Lumber and Wood Products (24), Furniture and Fixtures (25), Stone, Clay and Glass Products (32), Primary Metal Industries (33), Fabricated Metal Products (34), Industrial Machinery Production (35), Transportation Equipment (37); and the Non-durable Goods: Food and Kindred Products (20), Rubber and Miscellaneous Plastics (30), and Leather Industries (31). In the US these industries all had rates of illness and injury greater than 850 per 10,000 workers in 1999, and have been the sector leaders for the past five years. Miscellaneous Manufacturing

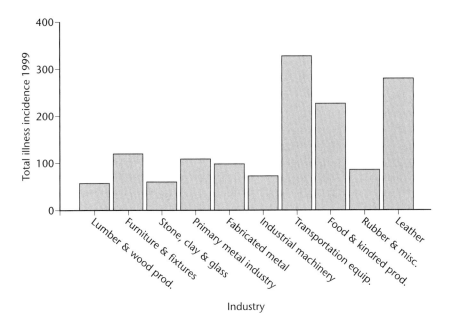

Figure 16.5: The top ten major US industries by illness rates per 10,000 FTE in 1999. Though occupational illnesses are often more difficult to associate directly with work practices, they are particularly important in this industrial sector.

Industries (SIC code 39) has a comparable incidence of illness and injury, but is not addressed in the chapter due to the difficulty in defining specific industries and exposures of interest.

Disease outcomes associated with manufacturing

In 1999 (Figs. 16.2 and 16.5) it is important to note that the manufacturing sector accounted for fully three-fifths of all occupational illnesses reported by private industry. Although injuries account for more total cases and lost work days than illness in all manufacturing categories, they are more readily linked to work practice. Their prevention can thus be effectively addressed by standard industrial safety measures (described in Chapters 31 and 32). In contrast, illnesses are often more difficult to associate directly with work practices, and because of their importance in this industrial sector, this chapter will give special attention to these outcomes.

Common conditions experienced among manufacturing workers

Manufacturing accounts for over 70% of all repetitive trauma disorders in the US workforce,[5] with industry specific rates described in Table 16.1. The proportions of illness due to repetitive trauma in each industrial group are similar to the total injury and illness rate proportions, except for textile mill production and apparel production, which have relatively low injury rates and high illness rates (69.2 cases per 10,000 full-time workers and 121.6 cases per 10,000 full-time workers, respectively) in 1999. For each of these industrial groups, repetitive trauma disorders are by far the largest contributor, frequently by an order of magnitude. The transportation equipment industries (e.g. autoworkers), food and associated products sectors, and leather workers have nearly three times the incidence

of repetitive strain injury than others in the manufacturing sector. This high incidence might be expected, based upon the repetitive job tasks of these workers, though the magnitude of difference is striking. Details of the hazardous exposures that are associated with musculoskeletal disorders, and the diagnosis and treatment of the associated disorders are described in Chapters 23 and 32.

Skin diseases are the next most common illness and are most prevalent in the transportation equipment sector, probably due to the heavy use of cutting fluids and other irritating lubricants.[7] In 1998, the manufacturing sector accounted for more than half of the total number of permanent hearing loss cases reported by clinicians to the NIOSH Sentinel Event Notification System for Occupational Risks (SENSOR) program for hearing loss.[5] Table 16.1 classifies this illness under Disorders due to Physical Agents. The NIOSH SENSOR program for silicosis, which covered seven states between 1993 and 1995, found that 75% of cases were from the manufacturing sector compared with 7% for mining and 9% for construction.[5]

INDUSTRY-SPECIFIC HEALTH CONCERNS IN THE MANUFACTURING SECTOR
Lumber and wood products

This industrial group includes the following industries: logging, saw and planing mills; fabricated wood products, ranging from cabinetry to prefabricated buildings, and wood composite manufacturing, representing in aggregate approximately 831,900 workers in the US in 1999. By far the largest fatality rate in this group is associated with logging, with 122 deaths in 2000 (65.6% of all deaths in this group). However, the illness and injury rates for workers manufacturing prefabricated buildings and wooden containers is much greater than that of loggers

(487.1 lost-work days per 10,000 full-time logging workers compared with 612.7 for prefabricated buildings and 661.7 for wooden containers, respectively in 1999).

Illnesses in lumber and wood products manufacturing are most common in mills and specialized production such as bowls, masts, poles and toothpicks. This latter category has the highest illness rate at 112.7 cases per 10,000 full-time workers. Ninety-six of these are associated with repetitive trauma, while the next highest illness in this category is dermatitis at 7.1 cases per 10,000 full-time workers. This relative proportion of repetitive trauma and dermatitis is seen throughout this group, and is consistent with the manual job tasks, exposures to irritants and allergens (such as allergenic wood dusts, preservatives, adhesives, lacquers and paints). The highest respiratory disease rate is seen in the hardwood and veneer industry, at 3.9 cases per 10,000 full-time workers. This rate is consistent with epidemiologic studies in wood workers that show symptoms of airway obstruction and decreases in lung function (FEV_1 and FVC),[8,9] also consistent with a combination of irritant and allergic effects. Several hundred species of trees have been associated with dermatitis and some specifically with asthma (e.g., Western red cedar, mahogany, and rosewood).[10-12]

Carcinoma is also a significant problem for wood workers. Nasal cancers are clearly associated with wood dust exposures from various species, although the mechanism has not been well characterized.[13,14] Leukemia and non-Hodgkin's lymphoma have also been elevated in mortality studies of wood workers,[15,16] as has colon cancer, most frequently reported in wood pattern makers, though this risk has diminished substantially as car design has evolved to other methods.[17,18] Elevations in lung cancer and pleural mesothelioma have been reported, though the data for these latter two cancer types are likely due to exposures to asbestos and other carcinogens found in the industry, rather than wood dust.[19,20]

Furniture and fixtures

This industrial group includes the production of wood, metal, plastic and composite fabricated furniture, partitions, fixtures, drapery and blinds. This group employed approximately 547,000 workers in the US in 1999.[1] Some of the same hazards as seen in wood products, e.g. laceration, crush, and repetitive strain injury, as well as exposure to wood dust, paints, lacquers, and solvents are found in this group. The injury rate is comparable at 1030 per 10,000 full-time workers per year; however, the illness rate is more than double that of lumber and wood products (Table 16.1). The illness distribution is similar to lumber and wood products, with repetitive trauma and dermatitis accounting for nearly 90% of the reported US cases in 1999.

The subgroup of workers engaged in fabrication of seating and fixtures for public buildings (SIC 253) stand out in the furniture and fixtures group, with an illness rate of 301.1 per 10,000 full-time workers compared with the group average of 120.8 per 10,000 full-time workers annu-

ally. Eight-five percent of this illness is due to repetitive trauma and 9% due to dermatitis. It is not clear what hazards separate this group from workers in related industries such as office furniture workers (annual illness rate of 154.9 per 10,000 full-time workers), but it may be due to the increased exposures to metals and plastics used in furniture for public buildings, since the only comparable rate in this group is in the category of non-wood office furniture, with an illness rate of 191.5 per 10,000 full-time workers per year.

Respiratory effects are also more common in this subgroup, with an illness rate of 3.2 per 10,000 full-time workers per year. An analysis of Italian furniture workers showed that spray painters were more likely to have asthma-like symptoms (though not positive methacholine challenge) than assemblers or wood workers from the same factories.[21] Isocyanate-containing paints are implicated as the etiologic agent in this study. The cancer epidemiology in the furniture and fixtures group is similar to that seen in the wood products industries, except for an additional increase in stomach cancer observed in white males working in metal furniture.[16] This finding is consistent with other studies in metal workers.[22]

Stone, clay, and glass products

This industrial group includes workers engaged in the manufacture of flat glass and other glass products, cement, concrete and gypsum products, pottery, cut stone, abrasives and some asbestos products. This group employed approximately 566,600 workers in the US in 1999.[1] The injury rate was 1010 full-time workers for 1999, with 60.4 illnesses per 10,000 full-time workers. While repetitive trauma accounts for 62% of this rate, the incidence of dermatitis is also relatively high at 16%. Dermatitis in porcelain workers is particularly high at 32.4 cases per 10,000 full-time workers per year, followed by concrete block and brick production at 25.9 per 10,000 full-time workers per year. Disorders associated with repetitive trauma were most problematic for china table and kitchenware workers, with 233.5 episodes per 10,000 full-time workers in 1999. Respiratory conditions are also high in this group at 6.0 per 10,000 full-time workers, though not as high as in abrasive products at 10.9 per 10,000 full-time workers per year. Abrasive products workers also show high levels of dermatitis, with 33.9 cases per 10,000 full-time workers.

Exposure hazards in this group are both physical (heat and infrared radiation) and chemical agents (silica, metal fumes, and vapors often found in colorants, hydrogen fluoride in etching processes, epoxies and polymer-based binders, noise, nitrogen oxide, other combustion products, and dusts). These hazards help explain the profile of illness in stone, clay, and glass products workers described above, since many of these agents can cause respiratory disease and/or dermatitis from either irritant (e.g. etching agents for glass) or allergic (e.g. chromates in cement) mechanisms. Pneumoconiosis remains a significant respiratory problem for this group (as shown for silicosis in Table 16.2).[23] The proportionate mortality ratios in stone, clay, and glass

Industry	Deaths	PMR	95% CI
Metal mining	105	81.30	66.10–98.91
Misc. non-metallic mineral and stone products	65	60.58	46.24–98.91
Non-metallic mining and quarrying	59	55.05	40.78–72.63
Iron and steel foundries	53	35.31	26.16–46.58
Pottery and related products	22	31.12	19.45–47.15
Structural clay products	22	30.15	18.84–45.68
Coal mining	68	9.41	7.18–12.11
Misc. fabricated metal products	21	7.93	4.90–12.13
Blast furnaces, steelworks, mills	68	6.29	4.80–8.10
Other primary metal industries	11	5.82	2.91–10.41
Cement, concrete, gypsum and plasters	6	4.63	1.70–10.09
Glass and glass products	10	3.54	1.70–6.51
Construction	114	1.86	1.51–2.26

Table 16.2 Proportionate mortality ratio for silicosis 1987–1996 in selected US states (adapted from Lewis[40])

products workers are comparable to those found in the mining industry, and represent an excellent opportunity for prevention of this potentially fatal lung condition.

Work in some sectors of this group have been associated with cancer, particularly lung cancer and to a lesser extent gastric cancer (IARC class 2A). Because flat glass manufacturing is largely automated, thereby reducing exposures in this subgroup, the main cancer risk in glass manufacturing currently is found in pressed glassware, art glass, and glass containers.[24]

Primary metal industries

This group is composed of workers engaged in the smelting and refining of ferrous and non-ferrous metals from ore, pig iron, or scrap. Associated mills are involved in rolling, drawing, and alloying metals; in manufacturing castings and other basic metal products including nails, spikes, manufacturing of insulated wire and cable, and production of coke. In 1999, approximately 698,800 workers were engaged in these industries in the US. That year there were 1190 injuries per 10,000 full-time workers and 108.8 illnesses per 10,000 full-time workers.

Foundry workers have the highest illness rates in this group, with 183.5 cases per 10,000 full-time workers overall. These workers primarily fabricate castings, such as fittings, manhole covers, and railroad wheels. The illnesses are due to repetitive trauma (78%), dermatitis (6%), and physical agents such as heat and noise (5%). Aluminum foundry workers had the most cases of dermatitis, with 31.2 per 10,000 full-time workers per year. This accounted for 22% of all occupational illness in this group in 1999, and was twice the rate seen in 1998. Dermatitis is due in part to the heavy use of caustics (particularly with the Bayer process) and production of sulphuric acid during smelting, producing irritant skin effects and in some cases sensitization to alloys in metals such as nickel, chromium and zirconium. Chronic respiratory diseases including asthma, emphysema, and chronic bronchitis are also seen in aluminum and other foundry workers.[25] Respirating hazards specific to manufacturing of alloys include fluorides (aluminum), nickel carbonyl (nickel), arsenic (copper and lead), mercury and cyanide (gold). Some metals are directly toxic and are produced in pure forms (e.g. lead). Silica is also a significant

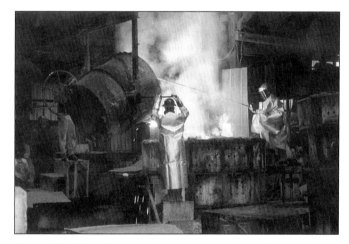

Figure 16.6: Foundry workers performing metal pour into a sand-filled form for steel manufacture. The worker on the left is controlling the rate of the pour by controlling the angle of dip of the crucible. The worker on the right uses the long pole with bar to prevent floating slag (waste products generated during the melting process) from getting into the form. There are several unsatisfactory safety practices that are occurring simultaneously during this pour, which include the absence of respiratory and hearing protection, face and body shielding, or proper elevation equipment for all workers present. Courtesy of Susan Swan.

hazard in the industry, as shown in Table 16.2. This exposure, along with coke oven and other furnace emissions, accounts for much of the relatively high respiratory disease rates seen in this group (Fig. 16.6).

A large prospective study of Finnish foundry workers from 1950 to 1987 found excess all-cause mortality (SMR 135 (95% CI 128–142)) and disease-specific mortality, including respiratory disease (SMR 153 (120–192)), lung cancer (SMR 143 (117–174)) and digestive organ cancers (SMR 150 (114–194)).[26] Polyaromatic hydrocarbon exposures are a significant hazard in the industry both for ferrous and non-ferrous metals utilizing coke, coal tar pitch, and related compounds, likely accounting for much of this increased risk.

Fabricated metal products

This manufacturing group covers the fabrication of metal products, such as cans, tinware, hand tools, cutlery, radiators, fabricated structural metal products, hardware, stamped and forged metal, small ordnance, and a variety of metal and wire products. Machinery, precision scientific equipment, jewelry, silverware, and transportation equipment are classified in other SIC groups. In 1999, approximately 1,521,900 workers were employed in these industries. The injury rate is similar to the primary metal industries at 1260 per 10,000 full-time workers, and the illness rates are comparable at the general level described in Table 16.1 for 1999 (99.0 cases per 10,000 full-time workers compared with 108.8 for the primary metal industries). Repetitive trauma disorders are similar in each group. Dermatitis is a significantly greater problem for this group than primary metal industries, while lung disease is a greater problem for the latter group, due in part to the silica exposures noted above.

Fabricated metal products workers are often exposed to cutting oils, hard metal, and other particles from cutting, grinding, and polishing. The hazards of cutting fluids are described in detail in Chapter 43 and include a significant risk of irritant and allergic dermatitis, folliculitis, as well as acute and subacute respiratory effects.[27,28] Particularly high rates of dermatitis are noted in the subgroup involved in metal forging and stamping (27.4 cases per 10,000 full-time workers) and other fabricated metal products (37.7 cases per 10,000 full-time workers). This latter subgroup also has a high rate of respiratory illness with 33.3 cases per 10,000 full-time workers in 1999, twice the group average in 1998 at 6.5 cases per 10,000 full-time workers.

Elevated cancer rates are reported in this group of industries. Cancer of the stomach, pancreas, larynx, and rectum were associated with metal-working fluids in a review by NIOSH in 1996.[29] Excesses in cancer of the digestive tract were also found in Finnish metal products workers in the large prospective study noted in the previous section,[26] and in several studies of workers involved in machining and grinding metals.[30-32]

Industrial machinery production

This group consists of workers manufacturing industrial and commercial machinery and equipment, including computers. Manufacture of engines and turbines; farm and garden machinery; construction, mining and oil field machinery; elevators and conveying equipment; hoists, cranes, monorails; industrial trucks and tractors; metal-working and other industrial machinery; power tools; computer and office equipment, and refrigeration and service industry machinery are included in this group. Machines powered by built-in or detachable motors ordinarily are included in this major group, with the exception of electrical household appliances. Workers who manufacture electrical equipment are classified elsewhere. This is the largest manufacturing group in the US, employing 2,207,800 full time workers in 1999. In that year there were 870 injuries per 10,000 full-time workers and 72.5 illnesses according to the BLS.[1] Disorders associated with repetitive trauma accounted for 50.5 cases per 10,000 full-

time workers, and dermatitis 11.8 per 10,000 full-time workers.

The highest repetitive trauma rates were found in the subgroups of carburettors, pistons, rings, and valves machining with 141.9 cases per 10,000 full-time workers (105.6 in 1998), lawn and garden equipment with 135.8 cases per 10,000 full-time workers (200.0 in 1998), and refrigeration equipment with 116.3 cases per 10,000 full-time workers (129.7 in 1998). Workers manufacturing carburettors, pistons, rings, and valves also have the highest subgroup rates of dermatitis, and their rate competes with pumps and pumping equipment (24.1 cases per 10,000 full-time workers) and industrial furnaces and ovens (12.5 cases per 10,000 full-time workers) for the highest respiratory disease rates due to toxic agents in 1999. While these other groups have lower rates of illness in 1998, workers manufacturing carburettors, pistons, rings, and valves had consistently elevated rates of respiratory illness. This is possibly related to the use of cutting fluids contributing both to acute and subacute respiratory illness.

The semiconductor industry is not encompassed by this group, though computer assembly is. The total injury and illness rate for computer and office equipment at 270 cases per 10,000 full-time workers per year is well below the group average of 850 cases per 10,000 full-time workers and consists primarily of injuries (210 cases per 10,000 full-time workers) and repetitive trauma (56.8 cases per 10,000 full-time workers).

Transportation equipment

This group includes workers engaged in manufacturing motor vehicles, aircraft, guided missiles and space vehicles, ships, boats, railroad equipment, motorcycles, bicycles, and snowmobiles. It does not include mobile home fabrication (see lumber and wood products above), or most off-highway farm, construction, or mining equipment (see Industrial machinery production, above). In 1999, 1,891,800 full-time workers were employed in the US in this group.[1]

Transportation equipment manufacturing has the highest rate of injury and illness in the manufacturing sector. With 1370 cases per 10,000 full-time workers in 1999, it surpassed all other industrial groups in the US according to BLS statistics. This group's injury rate of 1050 cases per 10,000 full-time workers is also consistently higher than the manufacturing sector average of 800 cases per 10,000 full-time workers for 1999. The very high rate of illness in this group is of considerable public health concern. The illness rate of 326.6 cases per 10,000 full-time workers (343.3 in 1998) is considerably higher than any other group in the manufacturing division. The rate is contributed to primarily by the motor vehicles and car bodies subgroup with 789.7 cases per 10,000 full-time workers (818.2 in 1998). This group has a high rate of repetitive trauma disorders at 685.5 cases per 10,000 full-time workers, and also the highest rates of dermatitis (34.7 cases per 10,000 full-time workers), high respiratory disease due to toxic agents (12.4 cases per 10,000 full-time workers), poisonings and disorders due to physical agents, particularly noise. The rate of carpal tunnel syndrome and tendonitis is 15.9 per 10,000 full-time workers per year.

In addition to the hazards and associated health effects described above for fabricated metal workers utilizing cutting fluids, occupational asthma and hypersensitivity pneumonitis (HP) has been associated with cutting fluid use in this industry.[33-35] Although chemical constituents in fluids and their associated biocides and preservatives have been suggested as a cause for the immunologically mediated lung disease HP, a 1996 NIOSH workshop on the subject considered microbiological contaminants, including several disinfectant-resistant *Mycobacterium* species to be a more likely cause.[36] Endotoxin is often found in association with Gram-negative bacterial growth in these fluids, particularly when the reservoirs are not well maintained. This exposure may contribute to both HP and asthma in this group. In the case of HP, endotoxin is a proposed adjuvant to the antigenic response.[37] Elevated cancer rates for stomach, pancreas, lung, and bladder have all been associated with machining fluid use in this industry.[38,39]

Food and associated products

The food and kindred products industrial group consists of food and beverage processing plants, including manufactured ice, chewing gum, vegetable and animal fats and oils, and prepared animal feeds. In 1999, 1,686,200 workers were employed in these industries in the US.[1] The injury and illness rate was 1270 total cases per 10,000 full-time workers per year. Eighty-two percent of these injuries were related to sprains and strains, often due to slips on wet surfaces (40%).[1] This mechanism of injury was highest in the dairy industry subgroup at 228.2 total cases per 10,000 full-time workers. Meat packers had the highest injury and illness rates of any subgroup with 2670 total cases per 10,000 full-time workers per year. In addition to sprains and strains, this group has the highest rates of lacerations and punctures, with 56.3 cases per 10,000 full-time workers per year.

As one might expect from the frequent repetitive motions performed by food preparation workers, illness from repetitive trauma is very common, with an overall rate of 189.5 cases per 10,000 full-time workers in 1999. With a rate of repetitive trauma disorder of 912.5 cases per 10,000 full-time workers, meat packers remain a group at risk for increased morbidity, with more than four times that of the next highest subgroup of workers, in cookies and cracker products (213.7 cases per 10,000 full-time workers). Tendonitis accounted for 15.0 cases per 10,000 full-time meat packers, and carpal tunnel 12.0 cases per 10,000 full-time workers in that year, with back pain the next highest category.

Dermatitis is another significant source of illness in this industrial group, with 17.4 cases per 10,000 full-time workers per year. Meat packers have the highest rates at 85.6 cases per 10,000 full-time workers, more than twice that of chewing gum processing, the next highest subgroup. Respiratory conditions are also a problem with this group, particularly for cheese processing workers, with 29.5 cases per 10,000 full-time workers.

Rubber and plastics

This manufacturing group includes the production of products from plastics, resins, and from natural or reclaimed rubber. It includes tire manufacture, but not recapping. Some products made from these materials are included in other major groups, such as boats, toys, buckles, and buttons. Establishments primarily engaged in manufacturing synthetic rubber are classified within the group Chemicals and Allied Products. The US employed an estimated 1,008,600 workers in the rubber and plastics industries in 1999, with over 73% in plastics, 8% in tires and inner tubes, and the remainder in hose gasket and seal production.[1] The group's overall injury and illness rate was 1010 total cases per 10,000 full-time workers. Over 92% of this total is due to injuries, primarily sprains and strains (43%), lacerations and punctures (10%), and bruises (9%). Occupational illness rates for this group in 1999 were 84.2 cases per 10,000 full-time workers, with 70% of the illness attributable to repetitive trauma, 12% to dermatitis, and 5% due to respiratory conditions caused by toxic agents. The dermatitis is due to both irritant and allergic mechanisms. Many skin sensitizers exist in the industry, including latex, isocyanates, thirams, amines, and mercaptobenzothiol. In addition to allergic contact dermatitis, many of these agents have also been implicated in asthma and reactive airways dysfunction syndrome (RADS), particularly in workers exposed to curing fumes and epoxies.[40]

Several carcinogenic hazards exist in the industry. These include benzene, 1,3-butadiene, and other polyaromatic hydrocarbons, nitros and aromatic amines, and asbestos. Elevations in standard mortality ratios have been described in several large studies of the industry and are reviewed by Roth.[41] The most consistent findings are for leukemia, bladder, stomach, throat, lung, and pleura (mesothelioma). Several of these studies are limited due to the absence of control for the confounding effects of smoking, though the relationship to mesothelioma is not affected by this confounding exposure. The relationship between benzene and butadiene with leukemia is strong, with a consistent dose–response relationship shown.[42] Benzene was the first chemical classified as a definite carcinogen by IARC (1A), and 1,3-butadiene is classified as a probable human carcinogen (2A).[43,44]

Leather industries

These manufacturing industries are composed primarily of workers who are engaged in tanning, curing, and finishing hides, skins, leather converters, and artificial leather products, and other related products. The US employed 76,900 workers in this industry in 1999. The total injury and illness rate for that year was 1030 cases per 10,000 full-time workers. Injuries accounted for 73% of these cases in 1999.

Most notable is the leather industry illness rate, which is the second highest in the manufacturing division, with 277.4 cases per 10,000 full-time workers per year, which has been stable for several years.[1] Repetitive trauma disorders are common in this industry, with 228.9 cases per 10,000 full-time workers per year. The industry has the highest rates of dermatitis found in the manufacturing division, with a rate of 29.1 cases per 10,000 full-time workers in 1999. Tanning is particularly hazardous in this regard, with 75.3 cases of dermatitis per 10,000 full-time workers. The likely sources of these dermatalogic findings are trivalent chromium, potassium dichromate, glutaraldehyde, and formaldehyde. These agents are toxic by both allergic and irritant mechanisms.[45,46] Many of these agents are also implicated in asthma, as demonstrated in a recent community-based survey in Spain among workers in the leather industry.[47] Another recent study from Spain utilizing a case-control design found an increase in oral cleft defects in children of mothers who worked in the leather industry (OR 6.18, 95% CI 1.48–25.69).[48] Other relationships to congenital malformations were also suggested by the data, but did not reach statistical significance.

SUMMARY

Manufacturing is the largest and most diverse sector of the goods producing economy of most developed countries. It employs over 18 million workers in the US, and accounts for the largest burden of illness and injury of any sector in the US economy, both in absolute terms as well as incidence. These incidence rates have steadily declined from 1994 to 1999, from an average of 1220 cases per 10,000 full-time workers to 920 cases per 10,000 full-time workers per year, but a significant opportunity for disease and injury prevention remains. An important decade-long trend which deserves scrutiny is the increasing rate of days with work restrictions, as opposed to lost work days, which have been in decline. Follow-back evaluations of specific manufacturing industries could provide valuable insights for illness and injury preventive strategies within these industries.

In the year 2000, manufacturing accounted for 11.3% of all worker fatalities, with nearly 20% of these related to logging. Although likely an underestimate, this sector accounts for over 60% of all occupational injury and illness among private industry in the US, with 8800 cases per 10,000 full-time workers per year. Injury, particularly sprains and strains, is the cause of most of this morbidity, but at least 10% is due to preventable occupational disease. The production of transportation equipment, processed foods, and leather goods are associated with the highest illness rates, more than twice that of other manufacturing subgroups. On average, repetitive trauma disorders account for approximately 80% of illnesses, with occupational dermatitis and lung disease the next most commonly diagnosed conditions. Repetitive motions, vibration, cutting fluids, metals, and dusts are common hazards in these sectors. Control of these exposures offers an excellent opportunity for preventive intervention.

Acknowledgment

Michael Silverstein MD MPH provided important guidance and reviews of this chapter.

References

1. Bureau of Labor Statistics, United States Department of Labor. Workplace injuries and illnesses in 1999. http://stats.bls.gov/oshhome/htm.
2. Moure-Eraso R, Wilcox M, Punnett L, MacDonald L, Levenstein C. Back to the future: sweatshop conditions on the Mexico–US border. II. Occupational health impact of maquiladora industrial activity. Am J Ind Med 1997; 31:587–99.
3. Takaro TK, Arroyo MG, Brown GD, Brumis SG, Knight EB. Community-based survey of maquiladora workers in Tijuana and Tecate, Mexico. Int J Occup Environ Health 1999; 5:513–5.
4. Silverstein B, Viikari-Juntura E, Kalat I. Work-related musculoskeletal disorders of the neck, back, and upper extremity in Washington State, 1990–1998. Safety and Health Assessment and Research for Prevention. Technical Report Number 40-4a-2000. Washington DC: Washington State Department of Labor and Industries.
5. National Institute for Occupational Safety and Health. Worker Health Chartbook, 2000. Publication Number 2000-127. Cincinnati: NIOSH, 2000.
6. Bureau of Labor Statistics, United States Department of Labor. Lost-worktime injuries and illnesses: characteristics and resulting time away from work, 1998. http://stats.bls.gov/oshhome/htm.
7. Alomar A. Occupational skin disease from cutting fluids. Dermatol Clin 1994; 12:537–46.
8. Goldsmith DF, Shy CM. Respiratory health effects from occupational exposure to wood dusts. Scand J Work Environ Health 1988;14:1–15.
9. Hessel PA, Herbert FA, Melenka LS, Yoshida K, Michaelchuk D, Nakaza M. Lung health in sawmill workers exposed to pine and spruce. Chest 1995; 108:642–6.
10. Chan-Yeung M, Abboud R. Occupational asthma due to California redwood (Sequoia sempervirens) dusts. Am Rev Respir Dis 1976; 114:1027–31.
11. Chan-Yeung M, Barton GM, MacLean L, Grzybowski S. Bronchial reactions to western red cedar (Thuja plicata). Can Med Assoc J 1971; 104:56–8,61.
12. Warsaw L. In: Stellman JM, ed. Encyclopaedia of occupational health and safety, 4th edn. Vol III. Geneva: International Labour Organization, 1998;86.13–86.19.
13. Demers PA, Kogevinas M, Boffetta P et al. Wood dust and sino-nasal cancer: pooled re-analysis of twelve case-control studies. Am J Ind Med 1995; 28:151–66.
14. Imbus H. Wood dust. In: Wald PH, Stave GM, eds. Physical and biologic hazards in the workplace. New York: Van Nostrand Reinhold, 1994.
15. Miller BA, Blair AE, Raynor HL, Stewart PA, Hoar ZS, Fraumeni JF. Cancer and other mortality patterns among United States furniture workers. Br J Ind Med 1989; 46:508–15.
16. Miller BA, Blair A, Reed E. Extended mortality follow-up among men and women in a US furniture workers union. Am J Ind Med 1994; 25:537–49.
17. Hoar SK, Bang KM, Tillett S, Rodriguez M, Cantor KP, Blair A. Screening for colorectal cancers and polyps among pattern makers. J Occup Med 1986; 28:704–8.
18. Tilley BC, Johnson CC, Schultz LR, Buffler PA, Joseph CLM. Risk of colorectal cancer among automotive pattern and model makers. J Occup Med 1990; 32:541–6.

19. Minder CE, Vader J-P. Malignant pleural mesothelioma among Swiss furniture workers: a new high-risk group. Scand J Work Environ Health 1988; 14:252–6.
20. Stellman SD, Demers PA, Colin D, Boffetta P. Cancer mortality and wood dust exposure among CPS-II participants. Am J Ind Med 1998; 34:229–37.
21. Talini D, Monteverdi A, Benvenuti A et al. Asthma-like symptoms, atopy, and bronchial responsiveness in furniture workers. Occup Environ Med 1998; 55:786–91.
22. Dubrow R, Wegman DH. Cancer and occupation in Massachusetts: a death certificate study. Am J Ind Med 1984; 6:207–30.
23. National Institute for Occupational Safety and Health. Work-related lung disease surveillance report. Cincinnati: NIOSH, 1999.
24. International Agency on Research in Cancer. Meeting of the IARC working group on beryllium, cadmium, mercury, and exposures in the glass manufacturing industry. Scand J Work Environ Health 1993; 19:360–3.
25. Romundstad P, Anderson A, Haldorsen T. Nonmalignant mortality among workers in six Norwegian aluminum works. Scand J Work Environ Health 2000; 26:470–5.
26. Koskela RS. Mortality, morbidity and health selection among metal workers. Scand J Work Environ Health 1997; 23(suppl2):80.
27. Kriebel D, Sama SR, Woskie S et al. A field investigation of the acute respiratory effects of metal working fluids. I. Effects of aerosol exposures. Am J Ind Med 1997; 31:756–66.
28. Park RM, Mirer FE. A survey of mortality at two automotive engine manufacturing plants. Am J Ind Med 1996; 30:664–73.
29. National Institute for Occupational Safety and Health. Criteria for recommended standard occupational exposures to metalworking fluids. Cincinnati: NIOSH, 1996.
30. Acquavella I, Leet T, Johnson G. Occupational experience and mortality among a cohort of metal components manufacturing workers. Epidemiology 1993; 4:428–34.
31. Eisen EA, Tolbert PE, Monson RR, Smith TJ. Mortality studies of machining fluid exposure in the automobile industry. I: a standardized mortality ratio analysis. Am J Ind Med 1992; 22:809–24.
32. Silverstein MA, Park RM, Marmor M, Maizlish N, Mirer F. Mortality among bearing plant workers exposed to metal-working fluids and abrasives. J Occup Med 1988; 30:706–14.
33. Bernstein DI, Lummus ZL, Santilli G, Siskosky I, Bernstein LL. A hypersensitivity pneumonitis disorder associated with exposure to metalworking fluid aerosols. Chest 1995; 108:636–41.
34. Eisen EA, Holcroft CA, Greaves IA, Wegman DH, Woskie SR, Monson RR. A strategy to reduce healthy worker effect in a cross-sectional of asthma and metalworking fluids. Am J Ind Med 1997; 31:671–7.
35. Greaves IA, Eisen EA, Smith TJ et al. Respiratory health of automobile workers exposed to metal-working fluid aerosols: respiratory symptoms. Am J Ind Med 1997; 32:450–9.
36. Kreiss K, Cox-Ganser I. Metalworking fluid-associated hypersensitivity pneumonitis: a workshop summary. Am J Ind Med 1997; 32:423–32.
37. Rylander R. Evaluation of the risks of endotoxin exposures. In: Rylander R, ed. Endotoxins in the environment: a criteria document. Int J Occup Env Health 3:S32–S36.
38. Mirer FE, Silverstein MA, Park R, Maizlish N. Occupational cancer in metalworking and transportation equipment industries. Ann NY Acad Sci 1988; 534:387–93.
39. Parks RM. Medical insurance claims and surveillance for occupational disease: analysis of respiratory, cardiac, and cancer outcomes in auto industry tool grinding operations. J Occup Environ Med 2001; 43.
40. Lewis R. Overview of the rubber industry and tire manufacturing. In: Health issues in the plastics and rubber industries, vol. 14. Philadelphia: Hanley & Belfus, Inc., 1999;707–18.
41. Roth VS. Rubber industry epidemiology. In: Occupational medicine: state of the art reviews. Philadelphia: Hanley & Belfus, Inc., 1999;849–56.
42. Macaluso M, Larson R, Delzell E et al. Leukemia and cumulative exposure to butadiene, styrene, and benzene among workers in the synthetic rubber industry. Toxicology 1996; 113:190–202.
43. National Institute for Occupational Safety and Health. Special NIOSH hazard review: rubber products manufacturing industry. Publication number 93-106. Cincinnati: NIOSH, 1994.
44. Rice JM, Boffetta P. 1,3-Butadiene, isoprene and chloroprene: reviews by the IAR monographs programme, outstanding issues, and research priorities in epidemiology. Chem Biol Interact 2001; 135–136:11–26.
45. Estlander T, Iolanki R, Kanerva L. Occupational allergic contact dermatitis from trivalent chromium in leather tanning. Contact Derm 2000; 43:114.
46. Mancuso G, Reggiani M, Berdondini RM. Occupational dermatitis in shoemakers. Contact Derm 1996; 34:17–22.
47. Monso E, Munoz-Rino F, Izquierdo J et al. Occupational asthma in the community: risk factors in a western Mediterranean population. Arch Environ Health 1998; 53:93–8.
48. Garcia AM, Fletcher T. Maternal occupation in the leather industry and selected congenital malformations. Occup Environ Med 1998; 55:284–6.

Chapter 17
Occupational Medicine in the Healthcare Industry

Mark B Russi, Marilyn V Howarth

The healthcare industry employs over 10 million workers in the US and encompasses an unusually broad spectrum of occupations and exposures. Job categories include physicians, non-MD clinicians, dentists, pharmacists, a range of clinical technicians, nurses, nurses' aides, housekeeping and maintenance personnel, engineers, security personnel, laboratory technicians, office and administrative personnel, and food service workers (Table 17.1). Work settings include hospitals, long-term care facilities, freestanding clinics, laboratories, and home care settings. Depending upon the specific work environment, healthcare industry personnel are at risk for exposure to hazardous biologic, chemical and physical agents, as well as to repetitive strain, violence, and fatigue.

Biologic exposures include blood-borne pathogens, principally HIV, hepatitis B and hepatitis C; and air-borne pathogens such as tuberculosis and a wide variety of respiratory viruses. Many medical centers also contain animal laboratories which may expose personnel to animal allergens and zoonotic illnesses. Chemical exposures include antineoplastic drugs, anesthetic agents, sterilants and disinfectants, latex, and a variety of laboratory reagents and cleaning chemicals. Physical agents include radiation from external beams or radionuclides, lasers, and the substantial physical stresses entailed in patient care. This chapter considers the principal occupational exposures of

Clinical	Physicians
	Dentists
	Physician assistants
	Podiatrists
	Physical and occupational therapists
Nursing	Nurse practitioners
	Medical/surgical/pediatric nurses
	Nurses' aides
Clinical support	Pharmacists
	Laboratory technicians
	Diagnostic imaging technicians
	Operating room technicians
Facility support	Police/security personnel
	Engineering personnel
	Building maintenance staff
	Housekeeping staff
	Food services staff
Office based	Administrators
	Clerical support personnel

Table 17.1 Categories of healthcare workers

healthcare workers, addressing health effects, methods of exposure reduction, and applicable laws and guidelines.

BIOLOGIC HAZARDS
Blood-borne pathogens

A broad range of blood-borne infections can be transmitted to healthcare workers via needlesticks, splashes onto mucous membranes of the mouth, eyes, and nose or exposures to abraded skin. While an exact tally of such exposures is not at hand – due in part to the practical challenges of active surveillance – it has been estimated that well over 500,000 needlesticks occur annually in the US, of which at least 5000 involve HIV-contaminated blood.[1] Despite the hazard of percutaneous and mucocutaneous blood or body fluid exposures, a number of studies document substantial under-reporting of blood and body fluid contacts among healthcare workers, particularly in the operating room setting, where it is estimated that in as many as 15% of all procedures at least one person at the surgical table sustains a needlestick, and where blood contact may occur in as many as 50% of all surgical procedures.[2,3] A study comparing incident reports of blood exposures with the actual frequency of such exposures observed at the operating table demonstrated that only approximately 2–11% were reported.[4] Studies of percutaneous exposures with hollow-bore needles have also demonstrated significant differences between the frequency of needlesticks reported and that estimated through retrospective questionnaires. Since early prophylactic therapy is now indicated for exposures to HIV-infected blood or body fluids, under-reporting may place healthcare workers at unnecessary risk of infection.

Exposure prevention
A number of guidelines and regulations have been designed to reduce blood-borne exposures among healthcare workers. Universal Precautions, developed by the Centers for Disease Control (CDC) in 1987, were incorporated into the OSHA Blood-borne Pathogen Standard of 1991, along with a requirement for annual training, exposure reduction plans, engineering controls, and provision of hepatitis B vaccine to potentially exposed healthcare workers. In 1995, Standard Precautions were introduced, combining Universal Precautions with body substance isolation, to establish a single set of procedures for patient

care and handling of blood and potentially infectious body fluids. Standard Precautions include use of barrier protections, such as gloves, gowns, and facial protection, where exposures to blood or body fluids may occur. They also include basic elements of infection control, such as handwashing and proper sharps disposal. Fundamental to the concept of Standard Precautions is the assumption that all blood and body fluids, except sweat, are potentially infectious, regardless of the infectious status of the patient.

Substantial evidence has accumulated that needlestick injuries can be reduced through educational programs and replacement of standard instruments with safer devices. Significant reductions in injury rates have been demonstrated for phlebotomy devices with engineered safety features and for needleless intravenous delivery systems.[5-8] Reductions in the rates of percutaneous injury among operating room staff following implementation of blunt needles for certain procedures have also been documented.[2,9] Several studies show the value of educational programs addressing needle safety.[11-16] Based on the potential for safer devices to reduce blood-borne pathogen exposures among healthcare workers, the OSHA Blood-borne Pathogens Standard was amended in 2001 to require that employers document consideration and implementation of appropriate commercially available and effective safer medical devices designed to eliminate or minimize occupational exposure. Employers are also required to maintain a sharps injury log containing information regarding the type and brand of device involved in an exposure incident, and an explanation of how and where the incident occurred.[17]

Although a broad range of infections can be transmitted percutaneously or mucocutaneously, the blood-borne pathogens of greatest significance for healthcare workers are human immunodeficiency virus (HIV), hepatitis B virus (HBV) and hepatitis C virus (HCV).

HIV

In the US approximately 5% of individuals with AIDS for whom occupational information is known have been employed in healthcare. A very small number (<0.3%) of those healthcare workers were documented to have become HIV positive following occupational exposure, of whom most are nurses and laboratory workers. Among healthcare workers infected on the job, the majority suffered percutaneous exposure, and a few became infected following mucocutaneous exposure. Nearly all transmissions have been due to exposures to HIV-infected blood.

A 0.3% risk of HIV infection following needlestick exposures is commonly quoted. Characteristics which may be associated with higher risk of seroconversion include deep injury, visible contamination of the device with blood, needle placement directly into an artery or vein, or exposure to an individual with elevated viral titers.[18] Risk of seroconversion following mucous membrane exposure has been estimated at 0.09%.[1] The risk of seroconversion following isolated skin exposure has not been quantified, but is likely to be of extremely low magnitude.

When percutaneous or mucocutaneous exposures to HIV-contaminated blood or body fluids occur, current US Public Health Service recommendations call for prophylactic treatment of exposed individuals with antiretroviral medications.[19] Several lines of evidence support use of prophylaxis. A case-control study has assessed risk factors for seroconversion in healthcare workers (HCWs) who became HIV positive following blood-borne occupational exposure to HIV.[18,20] Compared to a control group who did not seroconvert, cases were significantly less likely to have used antiretroviral prophylactic medication (zidovudine) when adjusted for other HIV transmission risk factors. A study of HIV-positive pregnant women demonstrated that administration of zidovudine during pregnancy markedly lowered transmission of HIV to the fetus. Viral load testing revealed that a relatively small proportion of the difference could be attributed to reduction in maternal viral load, suggesting that zidovudine may have acted prophylactically in the fetus.[21-23] Subsequent studies utilizing alternate dosing regimens or other antiretrovirals have yielded similar results. Animal studies have shown mixed results, but demonstrate decreased drug efficacy if treatment is not begun until 48 or 72 hours following exposure, or if animals are treated for only 3 or 10 days.[24-26]

Despite convincing evidence that prophylaxis can prevent HIV infection, it clearly is not always effective. Several seroconversions have occurred despite prophylaxis with one or more antiretroviral medications, likely due to viral resistance, late initiation of therapy, inadequate length of therapy, or an overwhelming inoculum of virus. Clinicians prescribing combination antiretroviral therapy to exposed HCWs should consider probable patterns of viral resistance based on knowledge of source patient medication history. Drug toxicities also should be monitored closely in HCWs receiving prophylaxis. A broad range of side effects have been reported, including an individual who suffered fulminant hepatic failure following prophylactic treatment with a nevirapine-containing regimen.[27-29]

For HCWs exposed to HIV-infected blood or body fluids, mechanisms should be put into place to begin prophylaxis as soon as possible following exposure, to ascertain source patient infectious status, and to monitor side effects and serological results in the exposed. Mechanisms should also be put into place to provide prophylactic medications to HCWs working in HIV-endemic areas of the world where such medications may not be readily available.[30]

Hepatitis B

The incidence of hepatitis B infection among HCWs in the US has declined dramatically since the 1980s to a rate below the current US population incidence. Although new infections among healthcare workers have fallen sharply in recent years due to widespread implementation of Standard Precautions and hepatitis B vaccine, prevalence figures among surgeons of 13–18% attest to the high risk of hepatitis B transmission in the past.[31] Not surprisingly, hepatitis B prevalence rates are higher among physicians with frequent blood contact than among those who rarely performed invasive procedures.

Risk of HBV infection following exposure is dependent upon exposure characteristics, body fluid to which the

HCW is exposed, and whether or not the source patient has e-antigenemia. Percutaneous exposure to HBV-infected blood is associated with a risk of 1–6% if the source patient is e-antigen negative, but 22–31% if the source patient is e-antigen positive.[19] The difference in risk results from higher rates of viral replication among e-antigen positive individuals. Viral titers may vary considerably, and may be as high as 1 billion virions per mL of blood or serous fluid. Titers are generally several orders of magnitude lower in saliva, semen, and vaginal secretions. In contrast to HIV and HCV, HBV is resistant to drying, ambient temperatures, simple detergents, and alcohol, and may survive on environmental surfaces for up to one week.[32] Hence, contaminated sharp objects may pose a threat to HCWs for several days following last contact with a source patient.

The incubation period of the virus ranges from 7 to 23 weeks, and less than half of individuals who become infected with hepatitis B manifest acute symptoms. Acute illness generally consists of several weeks of malaise, jaundice, and anorexia, but fulminant hepatitis may develop in approximately 1% of patients. Chronic infection develops in approximately 5% of patients and is generally accompanied by persistent hepatitis B surface antigenemia. In individuals whose infections do not become chronic, hepatitis B surface antibody develops as surface antigen levels fall. IgM antibodies to hepatitis B core antigen indicate current infection, while IgG core antibodies are a marker of past infection. The core antigen itself is not found in blood, but e-antigen, which is separated from core antigen during intracellular processing, is a marker of core antigen production and viral replication. It has been estimated that cirrhosis develops in approximately 20–35% of individuals with chronic hepatitis B, 20% of whom will develop hepatocellular carcinoma.[33]

Administration of hepatitis B vaccine, which contains recombinantly produced surface antigen, generates immunity in greater than 90% of individuals who receive three vaccine doses. Immunity lasts for at least 12 years following immunization, even if surface antibody titers fall or become undetectable, and there is currently no recommendation for periodic booster doses. Individuals who do not produce surface antibody following vaccination should have the three-vaccine series repeated. Those who do not mount a surface antibody response to the vaccine following repetition of the series should be counseled regarding their susceptibility to hepatitis B and should receive hepatitis B immune globulin and possibly additional vaccine if exposed percutaneously or mucocutaneously to hepatitis B-contaminated blood or body fluids. Hepatitis B immune globulin, which should be administered as soon as possible but which may be effective when administered as late as 7 days following exposure, is approximately 75% effective in preventing HBV infection in those without vaccine-induced protection.[34]

The single most effective step to prevent hepatitis B infection among healthcare workers is vaccination. Despite an OSHA requirement that employers provide vaccine free of charge to healthcare workers, a surprising number of workers remain at risk. A survey of more than 100 hospitals revealed that approximately two-thirds of employees had completed the vaccine series.[35]

Hepatitis C

An estimated 1.8% of the general US population is infected with hepatitis C virus.[36] Primary risk factors for the disease in the general population are intravenous drug abuse and receipt of contaminated blood transfusions. Among healthcare workers, several surveys show hepatitis C prevalence to be approximately equivalent to that of the general population. Needlestick exposures are independently associated with increased risk.

Following percutaneous exposure to infected blood, risk of hepatitis C seroconversion among exposed healthcare workers ranges from 0% to 10%, with an average risk of 1.8%.[37,38] Infection following mucocutaneous exposure appears to be less common, though several case reports document its occurrence. HCV viral titers are low compared to HBV, and virus is generally not detected in urine, feces, or vaginal fluids.

Incubation period for hepatitis C varies from 2 to 24 weeks, and averages 6–7 weeks.[32] Antibodies to HCV may be detected within 5–6 weeks of infection, and may persist regardless of whether virus is actively replicating. The vast majority of those who become infected with hepatitis C have no acute symptoms, and chronic hepatitis develops in approximately 85%.

There is no known neutralizing antibody to HCV, and no vaccine is available. Administration of immune globulin has not been shown to be effective and is not recommended following exposure. Several studies have demonstrated the efficacy of interferon alfa-2b as an effective treatment of chronic hepatitis C, and treatment early in the course of chronic disease may be associated with higher cure rates.[39-41] To date, treatment efficacy has been demonstrated in individuals with liver enzyme elevations, but it is not known whether there is an advantage to treating prior to any liver enzyme elevation, or whether treating acute illness begets a more favorable prognosis than treating early chronic disease.[32] One report has demonstrated high cure rates when interferon alfa-2b was begun during acute disease at an average of 90 days following infection.[42]

Healthcare workers exposed percutaneously or mucocutaneously to hepatitis C-infected blood or body fluids should have hepatitis C antibody checked at baseline, and at 6, 12, and 24 weeks. Individuals who seroconvert should undergo PCR testing to detect viral replication, and should be referred to a liver specialist for consideration of early treatment with interferon and ribavirin.

Infected healthcare workers

Since the onset of the AIDS epidemic there have been two reported instances in which healthcare workers transmitted HIV to patients. The first was a case in which a dentist transmitted HIV to six patients in his practice.[43-47] More recently, a French orthopedic surgeon transmitted HIV to a patient on whom he performed a 10-hour surgical procedure.[48] Of 982 other patients who underwent procedures with the same surgeon, serological testing revealed no other transmissions.[49] Numerous serological surveys of patients treated by other HIV-positive healthcare workers, including dentists, surgeons, obstetricians, and other physicians, have revealed no other transmissions of HIV from healthcare workers to patients. Infection with hepatitis B following procedures by hepatitis B-infected healthcare workers is more common.[50,51] Transmissions have taken place during dental procedures prior to widespread use of examining gloves, and during vaginal hysterectomies, major pelvic surgeries, and cardiac surgeries, and nearly all transmissions were linked to hepatitis B e-antigen-positive healthcare providers. Clusters in which hepatitis C was transmitted from healthcare providers to patients have been recently reported.[52,53] The CDC has estimated that the risk for transmission of HIV or hepatitis B lies between 1/42,000 and 1/420,000.[54]

On July 12 1991, the CDC issued guidelines addressing HIV and hepatitis B infection of healthcare workers, particularly among those who performed certain 'exposure-prone' procedures.[55] The guidelines stated that infected healthcare workers who adhere to universal precautions and who do not perform invasive procedures pose no risk for transmitting HIV or hepatitis B to patients, but that those who perform certain exposure prone procedures pose a small risk for transmitting hepatitis B or HIV. Exposure-prone procedures were characterized as those in which a needle tip was digitally palpated in a body cavity, or those in which a healthcare worker's fingers and a needle or other sharp instrument or object are simultaneously present in a poorly visualized or highly confined anatomic site.

The guidelines stated further that healthcare workers performing exposure-prone procedures should know their HIV antibody status, and if non-immune to hepatitis B, their hepatitis B surface antigen and hepatitis B e-antigen status. Healthcare workers infected with HIV or hepatitis B (and e-antigen positive) were further instructed not to perform exposure-prone procedures unless they had sought counsel from an expert review panel and been advised under what circumstances, if any, they might continue to perform these procedures. Such circumstances would include notifying prospective patients of the healthcare worker's seropositivity before they underwent exposure-prone invasive procedures. Mandatory testing of healthcare workers for HIV antibody, hepatitis B surface antigen or hepatitis B e-antigen was not recommended.

Several court decisions have rejected healthcare workers' discrimination claims regarding forced alterations of medical practice.[56] In contrast, a number of professional organizations including the Society for Healthcare Epidemiology of America have affirmed the ability of most physicians to continue to perform invasive procedures. This society also stated that patients should not be informed of a surgeon's serological status unless a clear exposure had taken place.[57] The American College of Physicians and the Infectious Disease Society of America generally reflected the CDC guidelines, but stressed the need for case-by-case evaluations of practice restrictions and the ethical obligations of individual physicians.[58] The

American College of Occupational and Environmental Medicine similarly reflected the guidelines, but stated that based on accumulated evidence, no invasive procedure had distinguished itself as 'exposure prone' with respect to transmission of HIV, and that HIV-positive healthcare workers performing invasive procedures with proper precautions, including double gloving, should not be otherwise restricted.[59]

The American College of Surgeons distinguished between HIV and hepatitis B, stating that HIV-infected surgeons should be allowed to continue to practice and perform invasive procedures unless there were clear evidence that a significant risk of transmission existed, but that surgeons who were hepatitis B e-antigen positive should seek counsel from an unbiased expert review panel.[60,61] In contrast, the American Academy of Orthopedic Surgeons stated that HIV-infected orthopedic surgeons should not perform invasive surgical procedures where there is substantial risk that the patient will come into contact with the surgeon's blood. The American Hospital Association stated that if an expert panel has already made a determination that a healthcare worker poses no reasonable risk to a patient, disclosure of the healthcare worker's infection status unnecessarily invades the healthcare worker's privacy. They stated further that providing patients with the HIV status of their caregivers is unacceptable.[62]

Decisions regarding a healthcare worker's continued ability to perform invasive procedures should take into account the surgeon's adherence to appropriate precautions and nature of the specific invasive procedures performed. The higher frequency of transmission from hepatitis B e-antigen-positive surgeons, compared with the very low chance of transmission from HIV-positive or hepatitis C-positive surgeons should also be considered. While the accumulated evidence provides very little support for restricting surgical privileges among HIV-positive or hepatitis C-positive surgeons, greater hazard may exist among hepatitis B-infected surgeons with e-antigenemia. Suppression of hepatitis B viral replication with antiviral medications may influence transmission potential, and could play a role in future decision making for such cases.

Tuberculosis

Following an alarming rise in US incidence of tuberculosis (TB) through the 1980s and early 1990s, the incidence of TB in the United States has fallen in recent years. In 2000, 5.8 cases of TB were reported per 100,000 US population compared with 12.25 in 1980.[63,64] Risk to healthcare workers increased substantially in the 1980s due to the emergence of multidrug-resistant TB and the need to hospitalize patients not responding to traditional outpatient antibiotic regimens. More recently, multidrug-resistant TB has also fallen, with approximately 1% of isolates collected during 2000 resistant to at least isoniazid and rifampin. Despite a currently decreasing population incidence, healthcare workers remain at risk without careful adherence to engineering and administrative controls.

The CDC has issued guidelines recommending that healthcare facilities at high risk for TB transmission develop and implement programs to prevent occupational exposure to TB.[65] The guidelines address early identification of potentially infectious patients, engineering controls to minimize spread of TB bacilli within a medical center, use of personal protective equipment, and medical surveillance among healthcare workers.

Strategies to identify potentially infectiozus patients before they expose healthcare workers in large numbers are integral to a successful tuberculosis prevention program. Tuberculosis is more prevalent among those infected with HIV, the homeless, prison inmates, persons from countries with high rates of TB, residents of long-term care facilities, and intravenous drug users. Use of epidemiologic indicators in addition to signs and symptoms of disease enhance early identification of potentially infectious patients. Once such patients are identified and isolated, the effectiveness of engineering controls is enhanced by keeping doors and windows closed, ensuring that room pressure is set properly, and performing regularly scheduled testing such as smoke-trail visualization.[66]

Laboratory healthcare workers may also be exposed when clinical specimens are manipulated in a manner that generates respirable aerosols. Engineering controls in mycobacteriology laboratories include the use of class I or II biologic safety cabinets. Routine maintenance and effectiveness testing are essential and have been well described.[67]

For the potentially infectious patient placed in negative pressure isolation, work practice controls include respiratory isolation signage, appropriate personal protective equipment, and restriction of diagnostic and therapeutic procedures to negative pressure isolation settings. Appropriate personal protective equipment, such as an N95 respirator, should be used by all individuals entering the isolation room of a patient with known or suspected TB, and while performing procedures with risk of aerosol production. OSHA requires that employers institute a respiratory protection program whenever respirators are in use. NIOSH has published guidelines to assist healthcare facilities implement respiratory protection programs for TB.[68] Appendices of the document include names and addresses of respirator manufacturers, respirator fit testing procedures, and checklists useful for program evaluation.

Medical surveillance of healthcare workers with tuberculin skin testing and symptom questionnaires may lead to the early detection of exposure and infection. Healthcare workers with negative tuberculin tests should be tested at time of hire. Those in whom testing has not been carried out within the preceding year should receive a two-step test to ensure adequate test sensitivity, as the tuberculin reaction may wane among infrequently tested individuals. Recommended frequency of ongoing testing is based on a risk assessment which considers community TB prevalence and frequency of inpatient TB admissions. Individuals with documented positive tuberculin tests should not be retested, and require only regular monitoring of symptoms suggestive of active TB. Several investigators have shown that skin test conversion rates may be more substantially influenced by community tuberculosis prevalence and workforce demographic factors than by frequency of clinical exposure. Others have demonstrated elevated skin test conversion rates among highly exposed healthcare workers, such as emergency medicine residents and respiratory therapists.[69,70] High rates of skin test conversion, as well as early progression to active disease, have also been demonstrated in hospital outbreak settings.

The Occupational Safety and Health Administration has made the decision not to proceed with a standard for TB, despite publishing a proposed standard in 1997.[71] OSHA has used the CDC guidelines in issuing compliance directives and has cited hospitals based on such directives.

Infection control and immunizations

An effective infection control program is essential to minimize infectious disease spread within a medical center setting. Patients are at risk from infectious healthcare workers just as healthcare workers may be at risk for transmission from patients. Prompt assessments of patients and healthcare workers for signs or symptoms of infectious disease are necessary to ensure proper disease containment or use of personal protective equipment. Medical center facility design has also been shown to directly affect spread of infection. Primary design and renovation of medical centers should include consideration of modern techniques of engineering control (i.e., ventilation, selection of finishes for surfaces, flooring, privacy curtains, disposable versus re-usable medical equipment).[66,72]

The Advisory Committee on Immunization Practice strongly recommends the following vaccines for healthcare workers who have not already received them or who can not document natural immunity: hepatitis B, influenza, measles, mumps, rubella, varicella, and tetanus.[73] Other pathogens commonly found in the hospital setting for which no vaccines are currently available include enteric pathogens, *Staphylococcus aureus*, CMV, cryptosporidium, scabies, and herpes simplex. Hepatitis A is a vaccine-preventable illnesses to which exposure may occur in medical centers, though hepatitis A vaccine is not currently recommended for healthcare workers.

Infection by varicella, CMV, and rubella can present teratogenic risk for pregnant medical center employees. Immunization for varicella and rubella prior to pregnancy reduces this risk. Though it was previously recommended that women refrain from becoming pregnant for 3 months after receiving live vaccines (i.e. rubeola, mumps, and rubella), recent recommendations have shortened the waiting period for rubella to 28 days.

Occupational health clinicians play an important role in the restriction of healthcare workers exposed to or infected with infectious diseases. State and local regulations may also restrict healthcare workers with infectious diseases. Table 17.2 lists work restrictions for healthcare workers with infectious diseases.[74]

Diseases requiring no patient contact	Work restriction
Infectious conjunctivitis	Until the discharge ceases
Acute diarrhea with symptoms* (i.e. fever, cramps, bloody stools)	Until symptoms resolve and infection with salmonella is ruled out, or if caused by salmonella (non-typhoidal), until stool is free of salmonella on 2 consecutive cultures not less than 24 hours apart
Group A streptococcal disease	Until 24 hours after adequate treatment begun
Hepatitis A*	Until 7 days after onset of jaundice
Herpes simplex infection on the hands	Until lesions heal
Active measles infection	Until 7 days after the rash appears
Post-exposure to measles	Susceptible personnel should remain out of the workplace from days 5–21 after exposure, and/or 7 days after rash appears
Active mumps	Until 9 days after onset of parotitis
Post-exposure to mumps	Susceptible personnel should remain out of the workplace from days 12–26 after exposure, and/or 9 days after onset of parotitis
Active pertussis	From beginning of catarrhal stage through the 3rd week after onset of paroxysms or until 7 days after start of effective therapy
Active rubella	Until 5 days after rash appears
Post-exposure to rubella	Susceptible personnel should remain out of the workplace from days 7–21 after exposure and/or 5 days after rash appears
Scabies	Until treated
Staphylococcus aureus infection of skin	Until lesions have resolved
Group A streptococcal infection*	Until 24 hours after starting adequate therapy
Active tuberculosis	Until proven non-infectious
Active varicella (chicken pox)	Until all lesions dry and crust
Post-exposure to varicella (chicken pox or shingles)	Susceptible personnel should remain out of the workplace for days 10–21 after exposure and/or until all lesions dry and crust
Diseases requiring partial work restrictions	**Work restriction**
Acute febrile viral respiratory infection	During community outbreaks of influenza and respiratory syncitial virus consider excluding symptomatic personnel from caring for high-risk patients
Diarrhea caused by enteroviral Infection	Personnel should not take care of infants and newborns until symptoms resolve
Hepatitis B – e-antigen positive	Personnel should be excluded from invasive procedures until recommendations from an expert review panel are made based on the specific job tasks and their risk for exposing patients
Orofacial herpes simplex	Personnel should not take care of high-risk patients until lesions heal
Human immunodeficiency virus	Personnel should be excluded from invasive procedures until recommendations from an expert review panel are made based on the specific job tasks and their risk for exposing patients
Staphylococcus aureus respiratory infections	Personnel should not take care of high-risk patients until acute symptoms resolve
Active varicella zoster	Personnel should keep lesions covered and should not take care of high-risk patients until lesions dry and crust
Diseases not requiring work restriction	
Cytomegalovirus infection	
Mild diarrhea lasting less than 24 hours without other symptoms	
Hepatitis B – acute or chronic antigenemia: personnel who do not perform exposure-prone procedures should follow standard precautions	
Hepatitis C	
Genital herpes simplex	
Post-exposure pertussis (asymptomatic personnel)	

* Food handlers should also remain out of work with these infections
Table based on: Bolyard EA, Tablan OC, Williams WM, Pearson ML, Shapiro CN, Deitchman SD and the Hospital Infection Control Practices Advisory Committee. Guideline for infection control in healthcare personnel, 1998. Am J Infect Control 1998;26:289–354, with permission from the American Academy of Dermatology.

Table 17.2 Work restrictions for healthcare workers with infectious diseases

CHEMICAL HAZARDS
Anesthetic gases

Healthcare personnel working in operating rooms, labor and delivery areas, postanesthesia recovery units, and certain ambulatory settings are at risk for exposure to anesthetic gases. Exposure may occur to nitrous oxide alone, or nitrous oxide in combination with halogenated agents such as fluoroxene, methoxyflurane, enflurane, halothane, isoflurane, desflurane, or sevoflurane. Scavenging devices are capable of reducing exposures to below 25 ppm for nitrous oxide and below 0.5 ppm for halogenated agents, but may allow levels well in excess of this if functioning improperly. Nitrous oxide levels as high as 300 ppm in hospital operating rooms and 1000 ppm in dental operatories using scavenging equipment have been documented.[75] Personnel working in postanesthesia care units may also be highly exposed to anesthetic gases due to exhalation by surgical patients of absorbed agents. Specific concern has been raised regarding exposures to desflurane and sevoflurane, due to the higher concentrations at which these two anesthetic agents are typically administered.[76] During inhaled induction with a rebreathing bag or a circle circuit system, sevoflurane concentrations as high as 20 ppm have been demonstrated, with nitrous oxide concentrations of approximately 100 ppm.[77]

A number of epidemiologic studies have evaluated an association between anesthetic gas exposure and adverse reproductive outcomes (see Chapter 27.2). Although methodological flaws undermine the reliability of many studies, the data suggest an elevated spontaneous abortion rate among highly exposed women. Animal studies also suggest adverse reproductive effects. It is uncertain whether current reduced levels of anesthetic gas exposure in operating rooms using adequately maintained gas scavenging systems remain a source of excess risk. A recent meta-analysis revealed an overall relative risk for spontaneous abortion of 1.48 (95% CI 1.4–1.58).[78] However, nearly all data were collected prior to widespread use of gas scavenging systems.

Infertility has also been evaluated in a study of female dental assistants. Women with five or more hours of exposure to unscavenged nitrous oxide were 41% (95% CI 23–74%, P<0.003) as likely as unexposed women to conceive during each menstrual cycle, adjusted for age, race, smoking habits, and reproductive/gynecologic history.[79] Among those exposed to scavenged nitrous oxide, there was no relation between the number of hours of exposure and fertility.

Elevated rates of congenital anomalies have been reported in women occupationally exposed to anesthetic gases. One survey found rates of congenital anomalies to be 25–50% higher among exposed women compared to unexposed controls, though no specific type of abnormality was predominant.[80] Another survey suggested elevated rates of musculoskeletal anomalies among children born to exposed dental assistants, while a third demonstrated increased anomalies when all defects were analyzed jointly, including minor malformations such as birth marks and nevi.[81,82] It is uncertain how applicable the findings of these studies are to current operating room exposures, since the questionnaire-based data were collected prior to widespread use of gas scavenging systems.

Evidence for an elevated risk of cancer among healthcare workers exposed to anesthetic gases is limited, and pertinent studies, which were carried out prior to widespread use of scavenging equipment, suffer from selection biases, lack of information regarding confounders, and near absence of dose information. A large American Dental Association survey revealed no statistically significant increases in cancer risk among exposed men or women with the exception of highly exposed female chairside assistants, who had higher rates of cervical cancer.[83] A large survey of US operating room personnel was suggestive of increased leukemia and lymphoma risk among female but not male study participants. A survey of cancer mortality among physicians revealed no increase among anesthetists.[84]

Although human epidemiological data do not exist to evaluate whether current exposure levels are associated with an excess risk of cancer, mutagenic activity has been associated with trace levels of anesthetic gases. Sister chromatid exchanges and micronuclei in peripheral blood lymphocytes of operating room personnel were shown to be elevated in personnel exposed to nitrous oxide and isoflurane.[85,86] In contrast, an earlier study among dental personnel exposed to nitrous oxide in excess of 100 ppm did not reveal elevated rates of sister chromatid exchange.[87]

There is no OSHA standard for waste anesthetic gases in general or for specific agents in use today. The NIOSH recommended exposure limit (REL) is 25 ppm time-weighted (over the time of exposure) average. The REL for halogenated anesthetics is a ceiling level of 2 ppm. The ACGIH has set TLVs for nitrous oxide, halothane, and enflurane but not for other halogenated anesthetic gases.

Reduction of exposures is best accomplished through a multidisciplinary effort including regular maintenance and inspections of anesthesia delivery equipment and scavenging systems, maintenance of room ventilation rates, provision of training to staff members, and regular (at least every 3 months) measurement of nitrous oxide levels. In most situations, control of nitrous oxide to a time-weighted average concentration of 25 ppm during anesthetic administration will result in levels of approximately 0.5 ppm of the halogenated agent.[88]

Hazardous drugs

The principal hazardous drugs of concern in medical centers are antineoplastic agents. Exposure to antineoplastic drugs may occur in a wide range of occupations. Pharmacists may be exposed if drugs are mixed outside a biologic safety cabinet, if inadequate personal protective equipment is used, or if a spill occurs. Personnel who transport medications are also at risk for exposure from spills. Oncology nurses and other nursing and medical personnel who administer medications are at risk if medication vials are opened at the bedside, if trapped air is emptied from a syringe, if skin contact with drug or a patient's urine occurs, or if soiled linens from a patient administered hazardous drugs are improperly disposed. Housekeeping and maintenance personnel who clean linens and patient rooms similarly have potential for exposure to excreta containing hazardous medication or hazardous medication metabolites. A recent survey of cancer treatment centers in the United States and Canada found surface contamination with antineoplastic agents in 75% of pharmacy preparation areas and in 65% of oncology drug administration areas.[89]

Human epidemiologic studies over the past 15 years have evaluated risk of spontaneous abortion, infertility, ectopic pregnancy, stillbirth, low birth weight or preterm delivery, and congenital anomalies (see Chapter 27.2). Data for many studies were gathered prior to widespread implementation of safety precautions designed to minimize exposures among pharmacy and nursing personnel.

Several studies suggest that spontaneous abortion may occur more frequently among personnel exposed to antineoplastic agents in hospital environments where adequate exposure controls are absent. Two studies which revealed relative risks for miscarriage of 2.3 (95% CI 1.20–4.39) and 1.7 (95% CI 1.0–2.8) respectively were carried out among personnel who were more likely to have had higher exposures based on job descriptions and work practices.[90,91] A more recently published positive study, which revealed an odds ratio of 1.5 (95% CI 1.2–1.8) associated with antineoplastic drug exposure, examined pregnancies which occurred primarily before 1986, when OSHA guidelines were issued regarding the safe handling of hazardous drugs. Spontaneous abortion and stillbirth combined was also significantly associated with antineoplastic drug exposure, but stillbirth alone was not.[92] Studies carried out in work settings where exposures to chemotherapeutics were well controlled generally have not revealed excess rates of spontaneous abortion.[93,94] Limited studies have suggested that exposure to chemotherapeutic agents is associated with an increase in infertility,[95] ectopic pregnancy,[96] and congenital anomalies,[93,97] while other studies reveal no increased risk.

Several antineoplastic agents are listed as known carcinogens by the International Agency for Research on Cancer (IARC).[98-100] Elevated risk of secondary tumors, particularly leukemias and lymphomas, in chemotherapy recipients is also well documented. Among healthcare workers with occupational exposures to antineoplastic drugs, however, there are almost no data regarding increased risk of malignancy. One study, primarily designed to assess reproductive outcomes among Danish nurses handling antineoplastic drugs, reported an elevated risk of leukemia (relative risk 10.65, 95% CI 1.29–38.5), based on only two cases.[94]

A number of studies have addressed indices of mutagenic activity among healthcare personnel exposed to chemotherapeutic agents. Investigators have utilized sister chromatid exchange assays in peripheral lymphocytes, micronuclei, chromosomal aberrations, DNA single-strand breaks, urine mutagenicity, and other test methods. No clear consensus regarding dose–response, correlation with measured workplace levels, utility of the testing methods for screening programs, nor association with any increased risk of malignancy has emerged.

Adverse health effects have also been reported among healthcare workers exposed to hazardous drugs other than antineoplastic agents. Upper respiratory symptoms, bronchospasm, and pulmonary function abnormalities have been observed in personnel administering aerosolized pentamidine.[101,102] Pulmonary function abnormalities have also been reported in healthy adult volunteers exposed to aerosolized ribavirin.[103,104]

There is no OSHA standard specific to hazardous drugs, though OSHA has developed practice guidelines for personnel handling cytotoxic medications.[105] The guidelines recommend a written hazardous drug safety and health plan to address operating procedures; use of vertical flow biologic safety cabinets (Class II, type B or Class III) for preparation of drug solutions; and use of personal protective equipment including gloves, gowns, eye and face protection. They also specify practices around handling, administration and disposal of drugs, and outline guidelines pertaining to patient care and management of linen and other reusable items. Waste disposal, spill cleanup procedures, medical surveillance, hazard communication, training, and record keeping are also addressed.

Glutaraldehyde

Glutaraldehyde (1,5-pentenedial) is an effective microbiocide used for cold sterilization of endoscopes and bronchoscopes. It is also used for histologic tissue fixation and in the development of radiographs. Glutaraldehyde's antimicrobial activity stems from its ability to react with amino groups and cross-link proteins on cell surfaces. Glutaraldehyde is generally used as a 2% aqueous solution. Because it works more efficiently in an alkaline environment, sodium bicarbonate is added to achieve a pH of 7.5–8.0.

Technical personnel assigned to the cleaning and disinfection of endoscopes and bronchoscopes are commonly exposed, but nurses and physicians working within endoscopy or bronchoscopy suites may also have significant contact if fumes are not adequately ventilated or scopes are not adequately rinsed. Radiology and histology technicians have potential air or skin contact. Other hospital personnel may be exposed during glutaraldehyde spills. Use of inadequately rinsed endoscopes has caused adverse effects including tongue swelling and intestinal bleeding in patients undergoing procedures.[106]

Glutaraldehyde is a skin, eye, and respiratory tract irritant. Skin contact causes irritation, pruritis, and erythema. Eye contact may result in conjunctival swelling and erythema, and contact with high concentrations may result in corneal injury. Upper respiratory tract exposure may cause nasal irritation, throat irritation, and cough. Epistaxis has been reported rarely.[107,108]

Healthcare workers are also at risk for developing glutaraldehyde allergic conditions. Allergic contact dermatitis has been frequently reported and does not always abate following cessation of exposure.[109] An association between glutaraldehyde exposure and occupational asthma is well established.[110-112] Cases may occur at exposure levels below currently applicable guidelines. While the pathophysiology of glutaraldehyde-induced asthma is uncertain, IgE antibodies specifically directed at glutaraldehyde-modified albumin have been detected in some glutaraldehyde-exposed individuals with occupational asthma.[113] Although glutaraldehyde has mutagenic properties, human studies do not implicate it as a carcinogen, teratogen, or cause of spontaneous abortion.

There is no OSHA standard applicable to glutaraldehyde. A detailed set of recommendations for the safe handling of glutaraldehyde in healthcare facilities has been developed by the Association for the Advancement of Medical Instrumentation in conjunction with the American National Standards Institute. The recommendations address engineering and work practice controls, training of staff, and personal protective equipment. Local exhaust ventilation, routed either to a filtering system or an outside duct, is generally necessary to maintain air levels below recommended limits. Eye protection, impervious gowns, and nitrile or butyl rubber gloves are recommended to prevent skin or mucous membrane contact. Due to the potential hazard of eye contact, eyewash stations should be readily accessible to any personnel with potential for glutaraldehyde contact. Monitoring of workplace levels should take place after initiating use of glutaraldehyde; whenever a major change in protocol, work practices, or ventilation occurs; and on some regular basis based on volume of use and work practices.[107]

Formaldehyde

Formaldehyde is usually found as an aqueous solution ('formalin') containing 30–50% formaldehyde and 5–15% methanol (see Chapter 41). Exposure occurs among workers in anatomy, pathology, and histology laboratories, where formalin is used as a tissue fixative. Individuals who use formaldehyde to sterilize dialysis equipment and other medical devices may also be exposed. Elevated breathing zone exposures have been commonly reported. One study of an anatomy laboratory reported time-weighted average exposures up to 2.94 ppm (nearly four times the current OSHA permissible exposure limit), and a second reported peak exposures approaching 5 ppm.[114,115] Dissection tables which contain local exhaust ventilation systems are capable of reducing formaldehyde in gross anatomy laboratories to as low as 0.03–0.09 ppm.[116,117]

Inhaled formaldehyde is primarily absorbed by the upper respiratory tract. Exposures <10 ppm may cause intense irritation of mucous membranes, with few pulmonary effects in normal subjects. High exposure levels may cause tracheobronchitis, chemical pneumonitis and pulmonary edema. Among asthmatics, bronchospasm and airway inflammation may occur at levels as low as 0.3 ppm. Allergic reactions to formaldehyde are common, and skin contact or inhalation can result in urticaria, allergic contact dermatitis, or occupational asthma.[118]

There is limited evidence of formaldehyde's carcinogenicity in humans, but sufficient evidence in experimental animals.[119,120] The human cancer risks have been evaluated in numerous epidemiologic studies and several meta-analyses.[121-123] Differing abnormalities were found in two broadly defined groups: professionals (e.g., embalmers, anatomists, and pathologists) and industrial workers (e.g., workers making formaldehyde resins, plywood, particleboard, and apparel). Formaldehyde-exposed professionals had excess leukemia relative risks of 1.1–3.1; brain cancer relative risks of 1.2–3.3; and colon cancer relative risks of 1.1–2.3. None of these cancers was found in excess in the industrial workers, who suffered small, but significant excesses of lung cancer.[118]

The OSHA permissible exposure limit (PEL) for formaldehyde is 0.75 ppm as an 8-hour time-weighted average. OSHA requires that a baseline medical examination be offered to workers prior to first assignment to an area where formaldehyde levels are expected to be >0.5 ppm. An annual symptom questionnaire and periodic medical examination are required by OSHA to be offered to workers exposed to formaldehyde levels >0.5 ppm as an 8-hour time-weighted average, and to those exposed to formaldehyde levels >2 ppm on a 15-minute time-weighted average.

Ethylene oxide

Ethylene oxide exists at room temperature and standard pressure as a colorless gas. Because it is used as a cold sterilizing agent for medical supplies, exposures are of concern to those involved in surgical sterilizing, as well as to those who manufacture or package medical supplies and medical devices sterilized with ethylene oxide. Contact has been described in healthcare workers exposed to ethylene oxide off-gassing from recently sterilized medical devices. Nurses and hospital central supply workers may experience episodic exposures to high levels of ethylene oxide if closed sterilization equipment malfunctions or if an accidental release occurs.[124-126] Levels greater than 200 ppm have been described during such accidents.

The most important exposure route for ethylene oxide is inhalation, but contact with high concentrations of its vapor and splash exposures to liquid ethylene oxide can cause burns of the skin and eyes, and also initiate allergic reactions.

Bronchitis, asthma, and pulmonary edema have been associated with high level occupational exposures, and acute high level exposure can cause reactive airway dysfunction syndrome (RADS).[118,127] However, there are few reports of severe inhalation exposure in humans. Ethylene oxide-related occupational asthma has been reported in a chronically exposed worker with IgE against ethylene oxide–albumin complexes.[128] Sensitization can occur after skin and inhalation exposure, resulting in contact dermatitis, urticaria, periorbital edema, and allergic rhinitis.

CNS effects reported after acute or subacute inhalation exposure to ethylene oxide include drowsiness, incoordination, headache, nausea and vomiting, seizures, aseptic meningitis and coma. An association has been reported between chronic workplace exposures and progressive cognitive impairment, although these reports have been challenged.[118,129-132] Peripheral nervous system effects following high-dose exposure include delayed-onset toxic axonopathy and Wallerian degeneration. Sensorimotor disturbances of the lower limbs have been documented after subacute or chronic exposure to high and low concentrations.[133,134]

Ethylene oxide exposure can cause a variety of genotoxic effects after acute or chronic exposure. Chromosomal aberrations, including breaks, gaps, sister chromatid exchanges (SCE), unscheduled DNA repair supernumerary chromosomes, and suppression of DNA repair capacity, have been described in exposed workers.[135,136] Exposure of nurses to ethylene oxide has been associated with increased risks of spontaneous abortion.[137]

Ethylene oxide has been judged 'carcinogenic to humans' by IARC and 'known to be a human carcinogen' by the National Toxicology Program.[120,138] Epidemiologic studies of exposed workers have yielded inconsistent results. Most often cited is an increased incidence of hematopoietic cancers including leukemias of various types. Such cancers have been reported in some studies, but not in others.[139-142]

The OSHA PEL for ethylene oxide is 1 ppm as an 8-hour time-weighted average and 5 ppm as a 15-minute Excursion Limit. OSHA requires that a baseline medical examination be offered to workers prior to first assignment to an area where ethylene oxide levels are expected to be >0.5 ppm as an 8-hour time-weighted average. Annual medical surveillance, including a detailed work and medical history, physical examination, complete blood count and pregnancy or fertility testing if requested, must be offered to workers exposed to levels >0.5 ppm as an 8-hour time-weighted average for 30 or more days per year.

Elemental mercury

Healthcare workers may sustain exposures to elemental mercury in several settings (see Chapter 39.9). Dentists and dental technicians may contact mercury as a component of dental amalgam. In hospitals and other clinical settings, mercury may spill from broken thermometers or manometers. Mercury has also been used to fill balloons which serve as propulsive weights for bouginage dilators, Cantor tubes, and Miller–Abbott tubes.

The most important exposure route for elemental mercury is inhalation; about 80% of an inhaled dose is retained. The amount absorbed across the skin is estimated to be about 1% of that absorbed from the lungs. Only about 0.01% of an ingested dose is absorbed from the GI tract.[118]

Dental amalgams have contained as much as 50% elemental mercury.[143] When amalgam is mixed at the patient's side immediately before use, mercury vaporizes into room air and may also adhere to hands and clothing or spill onto surfaces. Potentially harmful exposures in dental offices have been documented in the past, and elevated mercury levels in urine and tissues have confirmed exposure among dental workers.[144] A study of British government dental clinics in the late 1970s found urine levels >30 µg/L in 8.2% of dentists and 27.4% of dental assistants.[143] Levels >100 µg/L were found in 6.5% of assistants. A US study from the 1960s found that 30% of dentists had urine mercury levels >50 µg/L.[145] Current exposure levels are better controlled due to improvements in ventilation and use of prepackaged alloys.

The principal effects of elemental mercury exposure involve the nervous system, but generally do not occur at urine mercury levels less than 100 µg/g creatinine. Neurologic effects include motor disorders; intellectual dysfunction; psychologic abnormalities; and peripheral sensorimotor neuropathy.[146] Subclinical changes have been demonstrated with urine levels of 35–50 µg/g creatinine, but such effects are usually reversed following removal from exposure.[147-149] Under conditions of heavy exposure, renal glomerular effects, due to mercury-induced immunologic mechanisms, may occur.[150] Tubular defects may lead to low-molecular-weight proteinuria.[151,152]

The OSHA PEL for elemental mercury is a ceiling limit of 0.1 mg/m³. Adequate spill management procedures in settings where mercury is used is an important method to minimize exposures to healthcare workers. In dental offices, proper training of personnel in preparation of amalgams and disposal of waste, use of precapsulated alloys, provision of adequate room ventilation, and avoidance of skin contact contribute to decreased workplace exposures.

PHYSICAL HAZARDS
Musculoskeletal injury

Healthcare workers have a high incidence of acute musculoskeletal injuries, especially in nursing care facilities (see Chapters 23 and 32). Higher injury rates in nursing care facilities are likely due to greater numbers of non-ambulatory patients compared to hospitals. Acute back disorders, in particular injuries of the low back, occur with high frequency during patient transfers, and are more likely when large non-ambulatory patients are moved by healthcare workers of smaller stature. Risk factors predisposing to injury include heavy patient weight, long horizontal distance between the lumbosacral spine and hands of the healthcare worker, and high frequency of lifting. A number of personal risk factors for back disorders have also been identified. They include increasing age, female gender, obesity, tobacco use, prior back injury, hypertension, systemic arthritis, job dissatisfaction, psychosocial stressors, and poor physical fitness.[153]

Ergonomic interventions in medical centers should consider both task-related and personal risk factors for injury. Proper ergonomics may reduce the incidence of acute injury as well as the incidence of disorders due to continuous repeated trauma. Tasks involving patient transfers, keyboarding, and material handling are reasonable targets of intervention. Increased use of lifting assistance devices has been demonstrated to reduce injury rates substantially.[154] Such devices may include portable total-lift hoists, ceiling mounted hoists, walking belts, shower chairs, shower gurneys, and devices to reposition patients in bed.

Hospitals rank as the third highest industry sector for non-fatal disorders associated with repeated trauma.[155] Clerical and administrative personnel are commonly affected, though risk factors for repetitive trauma disorders remain a subject of debate. Improving the ergonomics of a computer workstation generally increases comfort and decreases symptoms in those complaining of hand, wrist, and other musculoskeletal symptoms. A comprehensively designed ergonomics program has been shown to be effective in reducing upper extremity work related musculoskeletal disorders in a university medical center setting.[156]

OSHA has proposed an ergonomic standard, which was published for comment, promulgated, and later rescinded.[157]

Noise

Excessive noise exposure may be found in a number of settings involving healthcare workers including central sterile supply areas, operating rooms, food service areas, laundry, engineering, facilities maintenance, and print shops. For a discussion of the effects of noise and hearing loss, see Chapters 20.2 and 35.

OSHA has set 90 dB as the time-weighted average for an 8-hour work day and a maximum allowable exposure level of 115 dB for a short-term exposure. Noise levels in operating rooms have been measured at 118 dB when powered bone-cutting tools are in use,[158] and occupational hearing loss has been documented in operating room personnel.[159]

Noise has deleterious effects on health and performance unrelated to hearing loss, including elevation of heart rate and blood pressure.[160] It may also increase psychologic stress and impair concentration. Chronic over-exposure to noise should be avoided by the use of engineering controls and personal protective equipment when necessary. All areas within a medical center that may approach the OSHA limits for noise should be monitored for noise. Where noise levels exceed the OSHA threshold, a hearing conservation program should be initiated.[161]

Heat

Excessive heat exposure may occur in several areas in a medical center. Kitchen facilities, the boiler room, and laundry area are most common. Heat overexposure can cause a variety of health effects including dermatitis, syncope, heat cramps, heat exhaustion, and heat stroke (see Chapter 34). Engineering controls such as physically insulating sources of heat and enhancing ventilation provide the best strategy in medical centers to avoid heat stress. Providing water and allowing frequent breaks to those whose jobs require working in heat-exposed areas are other helpful controls in some circumstances.[162]

Lasers

Lasers (light amplification by stimulated emission of radiation) are used in hospital operating rooms, as well as in a number of outpatient settings (see Chapter 33.2). Laser types used include argon, carbon dioxide, dye, excimer, and Nd:Yag. Most lasers used in surgical procedures are considered class 4, which means that eye or skin exposure by direct beam is extremely dangerous, and that eye exposure by specular or diffuse reflection is also hazardous.

Lasers may cause harm via direct transmission of energy to eye or skin tissues, or through generation of potentially infectious or mutagenic aerosols. Damage is principally thermal, leading to vaporization of cells following rapid heating. Damage to the cornea, lens, or retina may lead in some cases to permanent visual field loss or blindness. Wavelengths less than 315 nm and greater than 1400 nm are absorbed primarily by the cornea and may cause a corneal burn. Those from 315 nm to 400 nm are absorbed by the lens and may induce cataracts with chronic exposure. Wavelengths from 400 nm to 1400 nm are transmitted to the retina where they may cause irreparable tissue burns.[163] Skin damage is a function of laser wavelength and depth of penetration. Wavelengths less than 400 nm cause primarily photochemical injury, while those between 400 nm and 1400 nm are more likely to result in thermal burns.

Lasers can also generate a smoke plume containing potentially infectious organisms or toxic byproducts of combustion when used on human tissue. Cellular residues and viruses, including human papilloma virus, have been detected in such aerosols. Studies have also demonstrated that pyrolysis products from laser-induced tissue vaporization may have mutagenic activity, as demonstrated by sister chromatid exchange and micronuclei assays.[164,165]

Operating suites where lasers are used are designed to prevent scatter of laser light. Such suites must also be kept well lit in order to minimize pupillary diameter. Eye protection designed to protect from the wavelengths of light produced by a specific laser type is imperative, as is skin protection. Local exhaust ventilation effectively reduces plume exposure.

The American National Standards Institute has published recommendations for safe practice around lasers, and for the medical evaluation and monitoring of personnel who routinely use Class 3b and Class 4 lasers. The recommendations call for evaluation of visual acuity and macular vision prior to job assignment, following a laser accident, and at the close of employment. Fundoscopic examination or further testing as determined by the examiner should be carried out if an abnormality is detected on the screening exam.[166]

Radiation

Healthcare workers represent the largest group of individuals occupationally exposed to radiation, most at levels well below the permissible yearly exposure limit of 50 millisievert (5 rem) (see Chapter 33.1). The average dose among healthcare workers has been reported to be 0.7 mSv/yr, with 53% of the occupationally exposed workforce receiving less than a measurable exposure, and 88% receiving less than 1 mSv/yr (100 mrem/yr). Less than 0.5% of the total workforce received greater than 20 mSv/yr, and less than 0.05% exceeded 50 mSv/yr.[167] Exposure of healthcare workers to radiation is regulated by OSHA, performance of radiation machinery is regulated by the Center for Radiologic devices of the FDA, and use of certain radioactive isotopes is regulated by the United States Nuclear Regulatory Commission. Radiation exposure may occur to individuals involved with diagnostic imaging procedures, radiation oncology treatments, or administration of radioactive isotopes.

In diagnostic imaging, fluoroscopic procedures such as cardiac catheterization, vascular procedures, and certain interventional radiologic procedures have the potential for highest individual exposures. Where staff are required to stand adjacent to a patient receiving x-rays, bodily protection with aprons containing 0.5 mm of lead is required. Substantial radiation doses may also occur to the hands of technicians who repeatedly stabilize body parts, such as the cervical spine of a trauma patient, and 0.5 mm lead-containing gloves should be used under such circumstances.[168] For imaging procedures which do not require staff to stand adjacent to the patient during x-ray use, most exposure to healthcare workers occurs through scatter of x-rays from the patient. A shielded barrier containing 0.5 mm lead or more provides adequate protection for staff.

Sources of exposure during radiation oncology treatment include external beams from linear accelerators, gamma knives or cobalt-60 therapy machines, and loading of radioactive sources for brachytherapy. External beam machines are housed within thick concrete walls to reduce outside scatter, and gamma knife procedures are performed in similar settings.[163] Staff who come into direct contact with radioactive sources, such as in the implantation of radioactive seeds for brachytherapy, should utilize bodily protection, such as lead-containing aprons, neck protectors, and gloves. To the extent possible, implantation of seeds should be accomplished quickly to minimize exposure to staff. Certain patients in whom seeds have been implanted may need to be hospitalized in radiation-shielded rooms to minimize exposure to others.

Patients who have undergone nuclear imaging procedures generally present minimal risk to those around them due to the low levels of radiation used in such imaging. Staff who administer radioactive isotopes must see that shielding is utilized for vials and syringes, and should don protection while handling isotopes. Certain patients who receive therapeutic doses of isotopes, such as iodine 125 or iodine 131, may require hospitalization immediately following treatment to minimize exposure to family or others.

Violence

Healthcare and social service workers have a high incidence of assault injuries.[169] Studies describe high incidences of verbal threat and other aggressive behaviors toward healthcare workers that may not result in physical injury. Healthcare workers may face threats from patients, patient family members, visitors or coworkers. The long-term consequences of threats or altercations that do not result in physical harm have not been well studied. Severe physical and emotional consequences of violence on the job have been documented.[170,171]

Several factors may contribute to the incidence of violence in the medical center workplace. They include de-institutionalization of the mentally disabled, inadequate staffing, weapons carriage into medical centers, presence of money and drugs, and ease of hospital entry.[172] Several medical center areas may be robbery targets due to perceived availability of money and drugs (i.e. pharmacy, emergency departments). Trauma centers and tertiary care facilities treating high acuity and critically ill patients often host frustrated family members and visitors, predisposing to confrontations with healthcare workers. Victims of intended homicide who are treated in medical centers may remain at risk from a perpetrator, placing staff at risk as well. Lack of training in recognizing and managing escalating hostility and aggressive behavior may also contribute to risk of violence.[173]

Shift work

Healthcare workers participate in shift work in a variety of ways (see Chapter 38). They may work on rotating shifts, moving between day, afternoon, and night shift, or they may work one shift continuously. The effects of shift work are to disrupt normal circadian physiologic rhythms leading to an altered sleep–wake cycle, in addition to social disruptions with family and friends.[174] Acute effects begin with disturbed sleep and lead to daytime sleepiness and decreased mental focus and performance. Individual variability among healthcare workers to adjust to shift work is important. Studies have shown an increased use of sick leave and, in general, decreased health status among shift workers when compared with day workers.[175] Shift workers who do not successfully adjust to shift work may develop a syndrome of chronic fatigue, sleep disturbance, depression, mood disturbance, and personality changes. There is also an increase in the incidence of cardiovascular diseases among shift workers.[176] Epilepsy can be exacerbated by sleep deprivation. Several studies have shown increased rates of gastrointestinal disorders including peptic ulcer disease. Those with underlying severe medical problems such as insulin-dependent diabetes or asthma may have significant problems with rotating shift work due to interference with medication dosing schedules.

Despite the need for shift work, there are strategies to reduce its ill effects. The natural sleep–wake cycle is approximately 25 hours. Therefore, work schedules that rotate clockwise, i.e. day to evening to night to day, are preferred over day to night to evening to day. In addition, it is preferable to have a slowly rotating schedule rather than weekly changes in rotating shift work.[177,178] Both the direction of shift change and the speed of rotation remain subjects of controversy.

ALLERGIES IN THE MEDICAL CENTER ENVIRONMENT
Allergies of animal workers

The use of a variety of laboratory animals in medical research is common, particularly in large academic medical centers. Employees who work with animals have an increased risk of developing hypersensitivities to allergens found in hair, dander, urine, serum, and saliva (see Chapter 37.1). Risk factors for allergies include a history of atopy, as well as exposure to laboratory or domestic animals.[179] Employee exposure via inhalation or direct skin contact to offending allergens sensitizes employees through an IgE antibody-mediated immediate hypersensitivity reaction. Symptoms typical of early allergy are rhinoconjunctivitis (80% prevalence), rashes and urticaria (40% prevalence).[180] More serious reactions, such as bronchospasm or anaphylaxis, occur less commonly.[181]

Preplacement screenings for employees who will work with animals should include history of allergy to domestic pets or laboratory animals, family history of allergy or asthma, as well as a personal history of asthma or other atopic conditions. In the event that the screening process identifies potential risk factors, specific testing (IgE) to allergens relevant for the work scenario should be considered. Employees who are identified on preplacement as having bronchospasm or asthma related to exposure to laboratory animals may be qualified to receive reasonable accommodation under the Americans with Disabilities Act.[182] Continued exposure to laboratory animal allergens may exacerbate their symptoms of bronchospasm and asthma and increase risk of anaphylaxis or life-threatening bronchospasm.

A number of individual animal factors are important in the development of allergy. Rats and mice are the most common animals causing allergy in laboratory workers, though this may result from increased use of such animals in medical research. The source of the protein and the nature of the employee's exposure to it must be considered. Hair and dander are ubiquitous in an animal facility, but it is believed that urine and, in some cases, saliva may be more allergenic.[183]

Efforts at exposure reduction have included use of hairless animals for experimentation, use of laminar flow cage racks, and establishment of ventilation systems equipped with HEPA filters. Dust-free bedding and biologic safety cabinets for manipulation of materials contaminated with animal secretions may also be useful.

The highest employee exposures are associated with tasks of direct animal handling, cage cleaning, and feeding.[179] Generally, researchers themselves have a lower risk of sensitization due to their intermittent animal exposure. Laboratory animal allergens may spread outside an animal facility when proper engineering and administrative controls are not in place, exposing employees who would not normally have direct animal contact. Administrative controls that may be useful to reduce exposure are the appropriate use of washing and showering facilities, and use of employer-provided clothes that are left at work and laundered by an appropriate facility.

Personal protective equipment may be effective in primary prevention of laboratory animal allergy. The use of gloves, gowns, respirators, and goggles as well as shoe coverings and hair coverings will reduce the allergen transport out of the animal facility and will reduce the total allergen accessible to the respiratory tract and mucus membranes of the employee. Rarely are respirators useful to decrease or eliminate symptoms once an animal worker has been sensitized.

Medical surveillance using a symptom questionnaire should be performed on a regular basis for employees at greatest risk of exposure,[184] namely those whose work involves direct handling of animal materials, cage cleaning, and feeding. In the event that symptoms of early laboratory animal allergy are detected, exposures should be reduced or eliminated, and personal protective equipment should be tried. If such efforts are not effective, medical removal of the employee from animal exposure may be necessary to avoid the risk of worsening symptoms.

Latex allergy

Large numbers of healthcare workers have become sensitized to natural rubber latex due to substantially increased glove use over the past 15 years. While prevalence estimates vary greatly due both to different methods of population selection, and various methods of testing,[185-188] it is generally believed that 5–10% of healthcare workers are sensitized to natural rubber latex. Risk factors for latex allergy include heavy glove use, frequent donning and doffing of gloves, history of atopy, food allergies, and history of surgical procedures early in life. The highest prevalence rates of latex allergy occur among spina bifida patients, due primarily to frequent early life contact between latex antigens and mucous membranes during surgical procedures.[189-191]

Latex is an elastic and durable material, which accounts for its continued widespread use in barrier protection for healthcare workers. As a naturally occurring material extracted from the commercial rubber tree, its sap is a complex mixture of protein, lipid, and phospholipid. Polyisoprene lends latex its strength and elasticity. The raw sap is often processed with ammonia or sodium sulfate and vulcanized with sulfur. Accelerants such as thiurams, carbamates, and mercapto compounds are used to decrease production time. Latex contains more than 200 proteins, at least 60 of which have been shown to cause type I hypersensitivity.

Three general patterns of clinical disease may result from latex glove exposure. Irritant contact dermatitis is most common, due to prolonged abrasion of gloves, sweating, and the alkaline pH of most powdered gloves. Allergic contact dermatitis, which may be resemble an irritant reaction clinically, is due to a delayed type IV hypersensitivity reaction to additives such as thiurams, carbamates, and mercaptobenzothiazole.[192] Chronic allergic contact dermatitis may be debilitating, and may also predispose to type I hypersensitivity reactions by allowing enhanced contact between latex protein antigens and the dermis. Type I immediate hypersensitivity reactions to soluble latex proteins may range clinically from localized urticaria to systemic urticarial reactions, conjunctorhinitis, angioedema, bronchospasm, or anaphylaxis. Life-threatening anaphylactic reactions have occurred in healthcare workers, and are more common in the spina bifida population. Anaphylaxis to latex proteins has occurred during dental and medical examinations and surgery as well as during the donning of latex gloves and in the presence of others donning gloves.[193] It is difficult to predict to which specific latex proteins allergic healthcare workers will become sensitized. Specific reactions to proteins hevB1 and hevB3 are common among spina bifida patients, but less so among healthcare workers.[194]

Route of exposure may play an important role in latex sensitization. Cornstarch powder is added to gloves to enhance the ease of removal from the mold and donning of the gloves. The powder has been shown to adhere to protein and contribute to its wide environmental distribution. In addition, it allows for respiratory exposure to bystanders who may not themselves have skin contact with latex protein. Cornstarch powder has been shown to be an irritant to the skin and may enhance the likelihood of latex protein entry into skin.[195] Levels of air-borne latex allergens are substantially reduced with discontinuation of powdered latex glove use.[196]

Preplacement evaluations, done for all healthcare workers, should include a latex allergy questionnaire.[197] Most latex-allergic healthcare workers can be accommodated in the medical workplace depending on area of specialty and level of reaction. Type 1 latex allergic personnel with histories of anaphylactic reactions, bronchospasm or hives caused by air-borne exposure should have no direct contact with latex and should work in environments free of air-borne latex proteins. Those with symptoms occurring only on direct contact of latex with the skin should use latex-free gloves, and should be monitored carefully for any symptoms resulting from other latex exposures in the workplace.

Identification of latex allergy early in its natural history provides an opportunity to halt progression of symptoms through reduction of exposure. Several non-latex gloves have been shown to provide comparable protection to that provided by latex gloves.[198]

References

1. Bell DM. Occupational risk of human immunodeficiency virus infection in healthcare workers: an overview. Am J Med 1997; 102(Suppl5B):9–14.
2. Centers for Disease Control and Prevention. Evaluation of blunt suture needles in preventing percutaneous injuries among healthcare workers during gynecologic surgical procedures – New York City, March 1993–June 1994. MMWR 1997; 46:25–9.
3. Quebbeman EJ, Telford GL, Hubbard S et al. Risk of blood contamination and injury to operating room personnel. Ann Surg 1991; 214:614–20.
4. Lynch P, White MC. Perioperative blood contact and exposures: a comparison of incident reports and focused studies. Am J Infect Control 1993; 21:357–63.
5. Centers for Disease Control and Prevention. Evaluation of safety devices for preventing percutaneous injuries among healthcare workers during phlebotomy procedures. Minneapolis-St. Paul, New York City, and San Francisco, 1993–1995. MMWR 1997; 46:21–9.
6. Mendelson MH, Short LJ, Schechter CB et al. Study of a needleless intermittent intravenous-access system for peripheral infusions: analysis of staff, patient, and institutional outcomes. Infect Control Hosp Epidemiol 1998; 19:401–6.
7. Gartner K. Impact of a needleless intravenous system in a university hospital. Am J Infect Control 1992; 20:75–9.
8. L'Ecuyer P, Schwab E, Iademarco E, et al. Randomized prospective study of the impact of three needleless intravenous systems on needlestick injury rates. Infect Control Hosp Epidemiol 1996; 17:803–8.
9. Hartley JE, Ahmed S, Milkins R et al. Randomized trial of blunt-tipped versus cutting needles to reduce glove puncture during mass closure of the abdomen. Br J Surg 1996; 83:1156–7.
10. Mingoli A, Sapienza P, Sgarzini G et al. Influence of blunt needles on surgical glove perforation and safety for the surgeon. Am J Surg 1996; 172:512–7.
11. Haiduven D, DeMaio T, Stevens D. A five-year study of needle stick injuries: significant reduction associated with commu-nication, education, and convenient placement of sharps containers. Infect Cont Hospl Epidemiol 1992; 13:265–71.
12. Linnemann C, Cannon C, DeRonde M, Lanphear B. Effect of educational programs, rigid sharps containers, and universal precautions on reported needlestick injuries in healthcare workers. Infect Cont Hospl Epidemiol 1991; 109:387–8.
13. Whitby M, Stead P, Nagman J. Needlestick injury: impact of a recapping device and an associated education program. Infect Cont Hospl Epidemiol 1991; 12:220–5.
14. White M, Lynch P. Blood contacts in the operating room after hospital-specific data analysis and action. Am J Infect Control 1997; 25:209–14.
15. Gerberding J. Procedure-specific infection control for preventing intraoperative blood exposures. Am J Infect Control 1993; 21:364–367.
16. Short L, Bell D. Risk of occupational infection with blood-borne pathogens in operating and delivery room settings. Am J Infect Control 1993; 21:343–50.
17. Federal Register. January 18, 2001; 66:5317–25.
18. Cardo DM, Culver DH, Ciesielski CA et al. A case control study of HIV seroconversion in healthcare workers after percutaneous exposure. N Engl J Med 1997; 337:1485–90.
19. Centers for Disease Control and Prevention. Updated US Public Health Service guidelines for the management of occupational exposures to HBV, HCV, and HIV and recommendations for postexposure prophylaxis. MMWR 2001; 50(RR11):1–42.
20. Centers for Disease Control and Prevention. Case-control study of HIV seroconversion in healthcare workers after percutaneous exposure to HIV-infected blood – France, United Kingdom, and United States, January 1988–August 1994. MMWR 1995; 44:929–33.
21. Conner EM, Sperling RS, Gelber R et al. Reduction of maternal–infant transmission of human immunodeficiency virus type 1 with zidovudine treatment. N Engl J Med 1994; 331:1173–80.
22. Balsley J. Efficacy of zidovudine in preventing HIV transmission from mother to infant. Am J Med 1997; 102(5B):45–6.
23. Sperling RS, Shapiro DE, Coombs RW et al. Maternal viral load, zidovudine treatment, and the risk of transmission of human immunodeficiency virus type 1 from mother to infant. N Engl J Med 1996; 335:1621–9.
24. Martin LN, Murphey-Corb M, Soike KF, Davison-Fairburn B, Baskin GB. Effects of initiation of 3'-azido,3'-deoxythymidine (Zidovudine) treatment at different times after infection of rhesus monkeys with simian immunodeficiency virus. J Infect Dis 1993; 168:625–35.
25. Van Rompay KKA, Otsyula MG, Marthas ML, Miller C, McChesney MB, Pedersen NC. Immediate zidovudine treatment protects simian immunodeficiency virus-infected newborn macaques against rapid onset of AIDS. Antimicrob Agents Chemother 1995; 39:125–31.
26. Tsai C-C, Emau P, Follis KE et al. Effectiveness of postinoculation (r)-9-(2-phosphonylmethoxypropyl) adenine treatment for prevention of persistent simian immunodeficiency virus SIV infection depends critically on timing of initiation and duration of treatment. J Virol 1998; 72:4265–73.
27. Ippolito G, Puro V. Zidovudine toxicity in uninfected healthcare workers. Am J Med 1997; 102(suppl 5b):58–62.
28. Russi M, Buitrago M, Goulet J, et al. Antiretroviral prophylaxis of healthcare workers at two urban medical centers. JOEM 2000; 42:1092–100.
29. Centers for Disease Control and Prevention. Serious adverse events attributed to nevirapine regimens for postexposure prophylaxis after HIV exposures – worldwide, 1997–2000. MMWR 2001; 49(51–52):1153–6.

30. Russi M, Hajdun M, Barry M. A program to provide antiretroviral prophylaxis to healthcare personnel working overseas. JAMA 2000; 283:1292–3.

31. West DJ. The risk of hepatitis B infection among health professionals in the United States: a review. Am J Med Sci 1984; 287:26–33

32. Beltrami EM, Williams IT, Shapiro CN, Chamberland ME. Risk and management of blood-borne infections in healthcare workers. Clin Microbiol Rev 2000; 13:385–407.

33. Hoofnagle JH. The clinical spectrum and course of chronic hepatitis B. In: Program of the workshop on management of hepatitis B. Bethesda MD, 2000;12–14.

34. Grady GF, Lee VA, Prince AM, et al. Hepatitis B immune globulin for accidental exposures among medical personnel: final report of a multicenter controlled trial. J Infect Dis 1978; 138:625–38.

35. Mahoney FJ, Steward K, Hu H, Coleman P, Alter M. Progress toward elimination of hepatitis B virus transmission among healthcare workers in the United States. Arch Intern Med 1997; 157:2601–5.

36. Alter MJ, Druszon-Moran D, Nainan DV, et al. The prevalence of hepatitis C virus infection in the United States, 1988 through 1994. N Engl J Med 1999; 341:556–62.

37. Centers for Disease Control and Prevention. Recommendations for follow-up of healthcare workers after occupational exposure to hepatitis C virus. MMWR 1998; 47:603–6.

38. Mitsui TK, Iwano K, Masuko C, et al. Hepatitis C virus infection in medical personnel after needlestick accident. Hepatology 1992; 16:1109–14.

39. Vogel W, Graziadei I, Umlauft F, et al. High-dose interferon-alpha2b treatment prevents chronicity in acute hepatitis C: a pilot study. Dig Dis Sci 1996; 41(Suppl. 12):81S–85S.

40. Camma C, Almasio P, Craxi A. Interferon as treatment for acute hepatitis C: a meta-analysis. Dig Dis Sci 1996; 41:1248–55.

41. Noguchi S, Sata M, Suzuki H, et al. Early therapy with interferon for acute hepatitis C acquired through a needlestick. Clin Infect Dis 1997; 24:992–4.

42. Jaeckel E, Cornberg M, Wedemeyer A, et al. Treatment of acute hepatitis C with interferon alfa-2b. N Engl J Med 2001; 345:1452–7.

43. Centers for Disease Control. Possible transmission of human immunodeficiency virus to a patient during an invasive dental procedure. MMWR 1990; 39:489–93.

44. Centers for Disease Control. Update: transmission of HIV infection during an invasive dental procedure – Florida. MMWR 1991; 40:21–33.

45. Centers for Disease Control and Prevention. Update: investigations of persons treated by HIV-infected healthcare workers – United States. MMWR 1993; 42:329–31, 337.

46. Ciesielski C, Marianos D, Ou C-Y et al. Transmission of human immunodeficiency virus in a dental practice. Ann Intern Med 1992; 116:798–805.

47. Ou CY, Ciesielski CA, Myers G et al. Molecular epidemiology of HIV transmission in a dental practice. Science 1992; 256:1165–71.

48. National Public Health Network of France. Roseau National de Sante Publique. HIV transmission from an orthopedic surgeon to a patient. Press Release 1997.

49. Lot F, Seguier J-C, Fegueux S et al. Probable transmission of HIV from an orthopedic surgeon to a patient in France. Ann Int Med 1999; 130:1–6.

50. Henderson DK. SHEA Position Paper: Management of healthcare workers infected with hepatitis B virus, hepatitis C virus, human immunodeficiency virus, or other blood-borne pathogens. Infect Control Hosp Epidemiol 1997; 18:349–62.

51. Harpaz R, Von Seidlein L, Averhoff FM. Transmission of hepatitis B virus to multiple patients from a surgeon without evidence of inadequate infection control. N Engl J Med 1996; 334:549–54.

52. Ross RS, Viazov S, Gross T, et al. Transmission of hepatitis C virus from a patient to an anesthesiology assistant to five patients. N Engl J Med 2000; 343:1851–4.

53. Esteban JI, Gomez J, Martell M. Transmission of hepatitis C virus by a cardiac surgeon. N Engl J Med 1996; 334:555–60.

54. Bell DM, Shapiro CN, Gooch BF. Preventing HIV transmission to patients during invasive procedures. J Public Health Dent 1993; 53:170–3.

55. Centers for Disease Control and Prevention. Recommendations for preventing transmission of human immunodeficiency virus and hepatitis B virus to patients during exposure-prone invasive procedures. MMWR 1991; 40:1–8.

56. Burris S. Human immunodeficiency virus-infected healthcare workers. Arch Fam Med 1996; 5:102–6.

57. AIDS/TB Committee of the Society for Healthcare Epidemiology of America. Management of healthcare workers infected with hepatitis B virus, hepatitis C virus, human immunodeficiency virus, or other blood-borne pathogens. Infect Control Hosp Epidemiol 1997; 18:349–63.

58. American College of Physicians and Infectious Diseases Society of America, Clinical Practice Subcommittee. Human immunodeficiency virus (HIV) infection. Ann Int Med 1994; 120:314–6.

59. Russi M. HIV and AIDS in the workplace. ACOEM position statement. J Occup Environ Med 2002; 44:495–502.

60. American College of Surgeons. Statement on the surgeon and hepatitis B infection. Bull Am Coll Surg 1995; 80:33–35.

61. American College of Surgeons. Statement on the surgeon and HIV infection. Bull Am Coll Surg 1991; 76:28–31.

62. American Hospital Association, Ad-Hoc Committee on AIDS Policy. Recommendations for healthcare practices and public policy. AIDS/HIV Infection 1992;11–14.

63. MacKay AP, Fingerhut LA, Duran CR. Health, United States, 2000. US Department of Health and Human Services, DHHS Pub. No. 00-1232. Hyattsville: National Center for Health Statistics, 2000

64. Centers for Disease Control and Prevention. Reported tuberculosis in the United States, 2000. Atlanta: CDC, 2000. Available at http://www.cdc.gov/nchstp/tb/

65. Centers for Disease Control and Prevention. Guidelines for preventing the transmission of mycobacterium tuberculosis in healthcare facilities, 1994. MMWR 1994; 43:RR-13.

66. Noskin GA, Peterson LR. Engineering infection control through facility design. Emerging Inf Dis 2001; 7(2).

67. Centers for Disease Control, National Institutes of Health. Biosafety in microbiological laboratories, 3rd edn. Atlanta: CDC and NIH, 1993.

68. DHHS (CDC). TB respiratory protection program in healthcare facilities: administrator's guide. DHHS Publication NIOSH No. 99-143. Atlanta: DHHS, 1999.

69. Asimos A, Kaufman J, Lee C et al. Tuberculosis exposure risk in emergency medicine residents. Acad Emerg Med 1999; 6:1044.

70. Ball R, Van Wey M. Tuberculosis skin test conversion among healthcare workers at a military medical center. Mil Med 1997; 162:338.

71. Occupational Health and Safety Administration. Proposed standard for occupational exposure to tuberculosis. Fed Reg 1997; 62:541–59.

72. Livornese LL, Dias S, Samuel C et al. Hospital-acquired infection with vancomycin-resistant Enterococcus faecium transmitted by electronic thermometers. Ann Intern Med 1992; 117:112–6.

73. Centers for Disease Control and Prevention. Immunization of healthcare workers: recommendations of the Advisory Committee on Immunization Practices (ACIP) and the Hospital Infection Control Practices Advisory Committee (HICPAC). MMWR 1997; 46(RR-18):1–44.

74. Guideline for infection control in healthcare personnel, 1998. Am J Infect Control 1998; 26:289–354.

75. Dames BL, McGlothlin JD. Controlling exposures to nitrous oxide during anesthetic administration. Publication no.

94–100. Cincinnati: National Institute for Occupational Safety and Health, 1994.

76. Westphal K, Byhahn C, Strouhal U, et al. Exposure of recovery room personnel to inhalation anesthetics. Anaesthesiol Reanim 1998; 23:157–60.

77. Hoerauf KH, Wallner T, Akca O, Taslimi R, Sessler DI. Exposure to sevoflurane and nitrous oxide during four different methods of anesthetic induction. Anesth Analg 1999; 88:925–9.

78. Boivin J-F. Risk of spontaneous abortion in women occupationally exposed to anaesthetic gases: a meta-analysis. Occup Environ Med 1997; 54:541–8.

79. Rowland AS, Baird DD, Weinberg CR et al. Reduced fertility among women employed as dental assistants exposed to high levels of nitrous oxide. N Engl J Med 1992; 327:993–7.

80. Ad Hoc Committee on the Effect of Trace Anesthetics on the Health of Operating Room Personnel, American Society of Anesthesiologists. Occupational disease among operating room personnel. Anesthesiology 1974; 41:321–40.

81. Cohen EN, Gift HC, Brown BW et al. Occupational disease in dentistry and chronic exposure to trace anesthetic gases. JADA 1980; 101: 21–31.

82. Guirguis S, Pelmear P, Roy M, Wong L. Health effects associated with exposure to anesthetic gases in Ontario hospital personnel. Br J Ind Med 1990; 47:490–4.

83. Cohen EN, Gift HC, Brown BW, et al. Occupational disease in dentistry and chronic exposure to trace anesthetic gases. J Am Dental Assoc 1980; 101:21–31.

84. Doll R, Peto R. Mortality among doctors in different occupations. Br Med J 1977; I:1433–6.

85. Hoerauf D, Lierz M, Wiesner G et al. Genetic damage in operating room personnel exposed to isoflurane and nitrous oxide. Occup Environ Med 1999; 56: 433–7.

86. Hoerauf KH, Wiesner G, Schroegendorfer KF et al. Waste anaesthetic gases induce sister chromatid exchanges in lymphocytes of operating room personnel. Br J Anaesthesia 1999; 82:764–6.

87. Husum B, Wulf HC, Mathiassen F, Niebuhr E. Sister chromatid exchanges in lymphocytes of dentists and chairside assistants: no indication of a mutagenic effect of exposure to waste nitrous oxide. Community Dent Oral Epidemiol 1986; 14:148–51.

88. McMartin HL, Rose VE, Smith DL et al. NIOSH criteria for a recommended standard. occupational exposure to waste anesthetic gases and vaports. Publication No. 77-140. Washington DC: DHWE (NIOSH), 1977.

89. Connor TH, Anderson RW, Sessink PJ, Broadfield L, Power LA. Surface contamination with antineoplastic agents in six cancer treatment centers in Canada and the United States. Am J Health Syst Pharm 1999; 56:1427–32.

90. Selevan SG, Lindbohm M-L, Hornung RW, Hemminki K. A study of occupational exposure to antineoplastic drugs and fetal loss in nurses. N Engl J Med 1985; 313:1173–8.

91. Stuecker I, Caillard J-F, Collin R et al. Risk of spontaneous abortion among nurses handling antineoplastic drugs. Scand J Work Environ Health 1990; 16:102–7.

92. Valanis B, Vollmer WM, Steele P. Occupational exposure to antineoplastic agents: self-reported miscarriages and stillbirths among nurses and pharmacists. J Occup Environ Med 1999; 41:632–8.

93. Hemminki K, Kyyroenen P, Lindbohm M-L. Spontaneous abortions and malformations in the offspring of nurses exposed to anaesthetic gases, cytostatic drugs, and other potential hazards in hospitals, based on registered information of outcome. J Epidemiol Commun Health 1985; 39:141–7.

94. Skov T, Maarup B, Olsen J, Rorth M, Winthereik H, Lynge E. Leukaemia and reproductive outcome among nurses handling antineoplastic drugs. Br J Ind Med 1992; 49:855–61.

95. Valanis B, Vollmer W, Labuhn K, Glass A. Occupational exposure to antineoplastic agents and self-reported infertility among nurses and pharmacists. J Occup Environ Med 1997; 39:574–80.

96. Saurel-Cubizolles MJ, Job-Spira N, Estryn-Behar M. Ectopic pregnancy and occupational exposure to antineoplastic drugs. Lancet 1993; 341:1169–71.

97. McDonald AD, McDonald JC, Armstrong B et al. Congenital defects and work in pregnancy. Br J Ind Med 1988; 45:581–8.

98. International Agency for Research on Cancer. IARC monographs on the evaluation of the carcinogenic risk of chemicals to humans: some antineoplastic and immunosuppressive agents. Vol. 26. Lyon, France: IARC, 1981.

99. International Agency for Research on Cancer. IARC monographs on the evaluation of the carcinogenic risk of chemicals to humans: overall evaluations of carcinogenicity: an updating of IARC monographs volumes 1 to 42. Vols 1–42(Suppl 7). Lyon, France: IARC, 1987.

100. International Agency for Research on Cancer. IARC monographs on the evaluation of the carcinogenic risk of chemicals to humans: pharmaceutical drugs. Vol. 50. Lyon, France: IARC, 1990.

101. Balmes JR, Estacio PL, Quinlan P et al. Respiratory effects of occupational exposure to aerosolized pentamidine. J Occup Environ Med 1995; 37:145–50.

102. Gude JK. Selective delivery of pentamidine to the lung by aerosol. Am Rev Resp Dis 1989; 139:1060.

103. California Department of Health Services Occupational Health Surveillance and Evaluation Program. Healthcare worker exposure to ribavirin aerosol: field investigation Fl-86-009. Berkeley: California Department of Health Services, 1986

104. Connor JD, Hintz M, Van Dyke R. Ribavirin pharmacokinetics in children and adults during therapeutic trials. In: Smith RA, Knight V, Smith JAD, eds. Clinical applications of ribavirin. Orlando: Academic Press, 1984.

105. US Department of Labor, Occupational Safety and Health Administration. OSHA Instruction CPL 2-2.20B CH-4, Directorate of Technical Support, April 14, 1995.

106. Lynch DA, Parnell P, Porter C, Axon AT. Patient and staff exposure to glutaraldehyde from KeyMed Auto-Disinfector endoscope washing machine. Endoscopy 1994; 26:359–61.

107. ANSI/AAMI. Safe use and handling of glutaraldehyde-based products in healthcare facilities. ANSI/AAMI 1996; ST58.

108. Wiggins P, McCurdy SA, Zeidenberg W. Epistaxis due to glutaraldehyde exposure. J Occup Med 1989; 31:854–56.

109. Nethercott JR, Holness DL, Page E. Occupational contact dermatitis due to glutaraldehyde in healthcare workers. Contact Derm 1988; 18:193–6.

110. Chan-Yeung M, McMurren T, Catonio-Begley F, Lam S. Occupational asthma in a technologist exposed to glutaraldehyde. J Allergy Clin Immunol 1993; 91:974–8.

111. DiStefano F, Siriruttanapruk S, McCoach J, Burge PS. Glutaraldehyde: an occupational hazard in the hospital setting. Allergy 1999; 54:1105–9.

112. Gannon PJ, Bright P, Campbell M, et al. Occupational asthma due to glutaraldehyde and formaldehyde in endoscopy and x-ray departments. Thorax 1995; 50:156–9.

113. Curran AD, Burge PS, Wiley K. Clinical and immunologic evaluation of workers exposed to glutaraldehyde. Allergy 1996; 51:826–32.

114. Akbar-Khanzadeh F, Vaquerano MU, Akbar-Khanzadeh M et al. Formaldehyde exposure, acute pulmonary response, and exposure control options in a gross anatomy laboratory. Am J Ind Med 1994; 26:61–75.

115. Uba G, Pachorek D, Bernstein J, et al. Prospective study of respiratory effects of formaldehyde among healthy and asthmatic medical students. Am J Ind Med 1989; 15:91–101.

116. Coleman R. Reducing the levels of formaldehyde exposure in gross anatomy laboratories. Anat Rec 1995; 243:531–3.

117. Martin WD, Nemitz JW, Hendley A, et al. Three years of experience with a dissection table ventilation sysstem. Clin Anat 1995; 8:297–302.

118. Russi M, Borak J. Chemical hazards of healthcare workers. In: Orford RR, ed. Clinics in occupational and environmental medicine. Occupational health in the healthcare industry. Philadelphia: WB Saunders, 2001.

119. International Agency for Research on Cancer. Wood dust and formaldehyde. Lyon, France: IARC, 1996; 62.

120. National Toxicology Program. Ninth report on carcinogens: 2000 summary. Research Triangle Park, NC: US Department of Health and Human Services, 2000.

121. Collins JJ, Acquavella JF, Esmen NA. An updated meta-analysis of formaldehyde exposure and upper respiratory tract cancers. J Occup Environ Med 1997; 39:639–51.

122. Blair A, Saracci R, Stewart PA, et al. Epidemiologic evidence on the relationship between formaldehyde exposure and cancer. Scand J Work Environ Health 1990; 16:381–93.

123. Partanen T. Formaldehyde exposure and respiratory cancer – a meta-analysis of the epidemiologic evidence. Scand J Work Environ Health 1993; 19:8–15.

124. Sobaszek A, Hache JC, Frimat P, et al. Working conditions and health effects of ethylene oxide exposure at hospital sterilization sites. J Occup Environ Med 1999; 41:492–9.

125. Wesolowski W, Sitarek K. Occupational exposure to ethylene oxide of hospital staff. Int J Occup Med Environ Health 1999; 12:59–65.

126. Zey JN, Mortimer VD, Elliott LJ. Ethylene oxide exposures to hospital sterilization workers from poor ventilation design. Appl Occup Environ Hyg 1994; 9:633–41.

127. Deschamps D, Rosenberg N, Soler P, et al. Persistent asthma after accidental exposure to ethylene oxide. Br J Ind Med 1992; 49:523–5.

128. Dechamp C, Dubost R, Forissier MF, et al Airway hyperreactivity to ethylene oxide with positive RAST (radio allergo sorbent test). Clin Exp Allergy 1990; 20:74.

129. Crystal HA, Schaumburg HH, Grober E, et al. Cognitive impairment and sensory loss associated with chronic low-level ethylene oxide exposure. Neurology 1988; 38:567–9.

130. Estrin WJ, Bowler RM, Lash A, et al. Neurotoxicological evaluation of hospital sterilizer workers exposed to ethylene oxide. Clin Toxicol 1990; 28:1–20.

131. Klees JE, Lash A, Bowler RM, et al. Neuropsychologic 'impairment' in a cohort of hospital workers chronically exposed to ethylene oxide. Clin Toxicol 1990; 28:21–8.

132. Dretchen KL, Balter NJ, Schwartz SL, et al. Cognitive dysfunction in a patient with long-term occupational exposure to ethylene oxide. J Occup Med 1992; 34:1106–13.

133. Finelli PF, Morgan TF, Yaar I, et al. Ethylene oxide-induced polyneuropathy. Arch Neurol 1983; 40:419–21.

134. Gross JA, Haas ML, Swift TR. Ethylene oxide neurotoxicity: report of four cases and review of the literature. Neurology 1979; 29:978–83.

135. Fuchs J, Wullenweber U, Hengstler JG, et al. Genotoxic risk for humans due to work place exposure to ethylene oxide: remarkable individual differences in susceptibility. Arch Toxicol 1994; 68:343–8.

136. Major J, Jakab MG, Tompa A. Genotoxicological investigation of hospital nurses occupationally exposed to ethylene-oxide: I. Chromosome aberrations, sister-chromatid exchanges, cell cycle kinetics, and UV-induced DNA synthesis in peripheral blood lymphocytes. Environ Molec Mutagen 1996; 27:84–92.

137. Hemminki K, Mutanen P, Saloniemi I, et al. Spontaneous abortions in hospital staff engaged in sterilizing instruments with chemical agents. Br Med J 1982; 20:1461–3.

138. International Agency for Research on Cancer. Some industrial chemicals. Ethylene oxide. Lyon, France: IARC, 1994; 60:73–159.

139. Hogstedt C, Malmqvist N, Wadman B. Leukemia in workers exposed to ethylene oxide. JAMA 1979; 241:1132–66.

140. Teta MJ, Benson LO, Vitale JN. Mortality study of ethylene oxide workers in chemical manufacturing: a 10-year update. Br J Ind Med 1993; 50:704–9.

141. Bisanti L, Maggini M, Raschetti R et al. Cancer mortality in ethylene oxide workers. Br J Ind Med 1993; 50:317–24.

142. Steenland K, Stayner L, Greife A et al. Mortality among workers exposed to ethylene oxide. N Engl J Med 1991; 324:1402–7.

143. Kelman G.R. Urinary mercury excretion in dental personnel. Br J Ind Med 1978; 35:262–5.

144. Buchwald H. Exposure to dental workers to mercury. Am Ind Hyg Assoc J 1972; 33:492–502.

145. Joselow MM, Goldwater LJ, Alvarez, A et al. Absorption and excretion of mercury in man. XV. Occupational exposure among dentists. Arch Environ Health 1968; 17:39–43.

146. Kishi R, Doi R, Fukuchi Y et al. Residual neurobehavioural effects associated with chronic exposure to mercury vapour. Occup Environ Med 1994; 51:35–41.

147. Chang Y-C, Yeh C-Y, Wang J-D. Subclinical neurotoxicity of mercury vapor revealed by a multimodality evoked potential study of chloralkali workers. Am J Ind Med 1995; 27:271–9.

148. Langworth S, Almqvist O, Soderman E et al. Effects of occupational exposure to mercury vapour on the central nervous system. Br J Ind Med 1992; 49:545–55.

149. Liang Y-X, Sun R-K, Sun Y et al. Psychological effects of low exposure to mercury vapor: application of a computer-administered neurobehavioral evaluation system. Environ Res 1993; 60:320–7.

150. Tubbs RR, Gephardt GN, McMahon JT et al. Membraneous glomerulonephritis associated with industrial mercury exposure. Am J Clin Path 1982; 77:409–13.

151. Cardenas A, Roels H, Bernard AM et al. Markers of early renal changes induced by industrial pollutants. I. Application to workers exposed to mercury vapour. Br J Ind Med 1993; 50:17–27.

152. Langworth S, Elinder CG, Sundquist KG et al. Renal and immunological effects of occupational exposure to inorganic mercury. Br J Ind Med 1992; 49:394–401.

153. Bernacki EJ, Schaefer JA. Human factors and ergonomics programming in the healthcare industry. In: Orford RR, ed. Clinics in occupational and environmental medicine. Occupational health in the healthcare industry. Philadelphia: WB Saunders, 2001;261–77.

154. Garg A. Long-term effectiveness of 'zero-lift program' in seven nursing homes and one hospital. DHHS, CDC, NIOSH, Technical Report. Contract No. 1160/CCU512089-02, Cincinnati: US Department of Health and Human Services, Public Health Service, Centers for Disease Control, National Institute for Occupational Safety and Health, 1999.

155. US Department of Labor, Bureau of Labor Statistics. Safety and Health Statistics 2000. Available at http://stats.bls.gov/news.release

156. Bernacki EJ, Guidera JA, Shaefer JA et al. An ergonomics program designed to reduce the incidence of upper extremity work related musculoskeletal disorders. J Occup Envir Med 1999; 41:1032–41.

157. Office of the Federal Register, National Archives and Records Administration. 29 CFR 1910.900, OSHA Ergonomics Program Standard (as amended). November 14, 2000; Vol 65, No. 220. Washington DC: OSHA.

158. Ray CD, Levinson R. Noise pollution in the operating room: a hazard to surgeons, personnel, and patients. J Spinal Disord 1992; 5:485–8.

159. Willett KM. Noise-induced hearing loss in orthopedic staff. J Bone Joint Surg 1991; 73B:113–5.

160. Belli S, Sani L, Scarfiiccia G, Borrentino R. Arterial hypertension and noise: a cross-sectional study. Am J Ind Med 1984; 6:59–65.

161. OSHA. Occupational Exposure to Noise. 29 CFR 1910.95. Washington DC: OSHA.

162. NIOSH. Criteria for recommended standard: occupational exposure to hot environments. Cinncinati: US Department of Health and Human Services, Public Health Service, Centers for Disease Control, National Institute for Occupational Safety and Health, 1986.

163. Vetter RJ, Classic KL. Ionizing radiation and laser safety. In: Orford RR, ed. Clinics in occupational and environmental

medicine. Occupational health in the healthcare industry. Philadelphia: WB Saunders, 2001;409–22.

164. Stocker B, Meier T, Fliedner TM, Plappert U. Laser pyrolysis products: sampling procedures, cytotoxic and genotoxic effects. Mutat Res 1998; 412:145–54.

165. Plappert UG, Stocker B, Helbig R, Fliedner TM, Seidel HJ. Laser pyrolysis products – genotoxic, clastogenic and mutagenic effects of the particulate aerosol fractions. Mutat Res 1999; 441:29–41.

166. American National Standards Institute. American National Standard for the Safe Use of Lasers in Healthcare Facilities. ANSI Z136.3. New York: ANSI, 1996.

167. Hendee WR, Edwards FM. Trends in radiation protection of medical workers. Health Physics 1990; 58:251–7.

168. Singer CM, Baraff LJ, Benedict SH, Weiss EL, Singer BD. Exposure of emergency medicine personnel to ionizing radiation during cervical spine radiography. Ann Emerg Med 1989; 18:822–5.

169. Department of Labor, Bureau of Labor Statistics. Survey of occupational injuries and illnesses, 1995. Summary 97-7. Washington DC: US Government Printing Office, 1997.

170. Caldwell ME. Incidence of PTSD among staff victims of patient violence. Hosp Commun Psychiatry 1992; 43:838–9.

171. Hales T. Occupational injuries due to violence. J Occup Med 1988; 30:483–7.

172. OSHA. Guidelines for preventing workplace violence for healthcare and social service workers. OSHA 3148.Washington DC: US Department of Labor, Occupational Safety and Health Administration, 1998.

173. Simonowitz JA. Healthcare workers and workplace violence. Occup Med 1996; 11:277–91.

174. Colligan MJ, Rosa RR. Shift work effects on social and family life. Occup Med 1990; 5:315–22.

175. Naitoh P, Kelly TL, Englund C. Health effects of sleep deprivation. Occup Med 1990; 5:209–38.

176. Knuttson A, Akerstedt T, Jonsson BG. Prevalence of risk factors for coronary artery disease among day and shift workers. Scand J Work Environ Health 1988; 14:317–21.

177. Knauth P. Speed and direction of shift rotation. J Sleep Res 1995; 4(suppl. 2):41–6.

178. Kecklund G, Akerstedt T. Effects of timing of shifts on sleepiness and sleep duration. J Sleep Res 1995; 4(suppl. 2):47–50.

179. Hollander A, Heederick D, Doeks G. Respiratory allergy to rats: exposure–response relationship in laboratory animal workers. Am J Respir Crit Care Med 1997; 155:562–7.

180. Hunskaar S, Fosse RT. Allergy to laboratory mice and rats: a review of the pathophysiology, epidemiology, and clinical aspects. Lab Anim 1990; 24:358–74.

181. Platts-Mills TA, Longbottom J, Edwards J, Crockcroft A, Wilkins S. Occupational asthma and rhinitis related to laboratory rats: serum IgG and IgE antibodies to the rat urinary allergen. J Allergy Clin Immunol 1987; 79:505–15.

182. Americans with Disabilities Act, 1990, 42 USC. 12101 et seq

183. Price JA, Longbottom J. Allergy to mice. Further characterization of two major mouse allergens (Ag1 and Ag3) and immunohistochemical investigations of their sources. Clin Exp Allergy 1990; 20:71–7.

184. Phipatanakul W, Wood RA. Allergens of animal and biologic systems. In: Fleming DO, Hunt D, eds. Biologic safety, principles and practice, 3rd edn. Washington DC: ASM Press, 2000.

185. Yassin M, Lierl M, Fischer T et al. Latex allergy in hospital employees. Ann Allergy 1994; 72:245–9.

186. Kaczmarek R, Silverman B, Gross T et al. Prevalence of latex-specific IgE antibodies in hospital jpersonnel. Ann Allergy Asthma Immunol 1996; 76:51–6.

187. Lagier F, Vervloet D, Lhermet I et al. Prevalence of latex allergy in operating room nurses. J Allergy Clin Immunol 1992; 90:319–22.

188. Toraason M, Sussman G, Biagini R, Meade J, Beezhold D, Germolec D. Latex allergy in the workplace. Toxicol Sci 2000; 58:5–14

189. Brehler R, Kuetting B. Natural rubber latex allergy. A problem of interdisciplinary concern in medicine. Arch Int Med 2001;161.

190. Hochleitner BW, Menardi G, Haussler B, Ulmer H, Kofler H, Reider N. Spina bifida as an independent risk factor for sensitization to latex. J Urol 2001; 166:2370–3.

191. Degenhardt P, Golla S, Wahn F, Niggemann B. Latex allergy in pediatric surgery is dependent on repeated operations in the first year of life. J Pediatr Surg 2001; 36:1535–9.

192. Conde-Salazar L, del-Rio E, Guimaraens D. Type IV allergy to rubber additives: a 10-year study of 686 cases. J Am Acad Derm 1993; 29:176–80.

193. National Institute for Occupational Safety and Health. NIOSH alert: preventing allergic reactions to latex in the workplace. Publication No. DHHS (NIOSH) 97–135. Cincinnati: NIOSH, 1997.

194. Wagner B, Buck D, Hafner C et al. Hev b7 is a Hevea brasiliensis protein associated with latex allergy in children with spina bifida. J Allergy Clin Immunol 2001; 108:621–7.

195. Brehler R, Voss W, Mueller S. Glove powder effects skin roughness, one parameter of skin irritation. Contact Derm 39:227–30.

196. Allmers H, Brehler R, Chen Z, Raulf-Heimsoth M, Fels H, Baur X. Reduction of latex aeroallergens and latex-specific IgE antibodies in sensitized workers after removal of powdered natural rubber latex gloves in a hospital. J Allergy Clin Immunol 1998; 102:841–6.

197. Sussman G, Gold M. Guidelines for the management of latex allergies and safe latex use in healthcare facilities. Ottawa: CHA Press, 1996

198. Hamann CP, Nelson JR. Permeability of latex and thermoplastic elastomer gloves to the bacteriophage phi X174. Am J Infect Control 1993; 21:289–96.

Chapter 18
Work Sectors of Emerging Importance

18.1 Emerging Technologies
Michael L Fischman, Daniel A Goldstein, Mark R Cullen

INTRODUCTION

While traditional manufacturing and agricultural work have engaged increasingly smaller percentages of workers in developed countries, newer production sectors, characterized by the utilization of rapidly evolving technologies, have gained increasing importance in the US and world economy. The most prominent of these are microelectronics, biotechnology, aerospace, and communications technologies. Compared to more traditional sectors, these activities involve different workforce demographics, novel environments, potential exposures to incompletely studied physical, chemical, and biologic hazards under rapid and changing workplace conditions. These characteristics require the development of new paradigms for occupational health practice and workplace hazard control. The purpose of this chapter is to outline some of the workplace health issues in these sectors, focusing on microelectronics and biotechnology, and to propose directions future practice might profitably evolve.

Workforce

Unlike conventional manufacturing, which may entail sharp distinctions between the work experience of minimally skilled hourly workers, skilled technicians, and supervisors, the new high technology workplace usually requires a substantially higher proportion of workers with advanced skills and integration. Engineers and scientists often work closely with skilled technicians. Many will perform multiple, complex tasks which are frequently changing. Moreover, for reasons including economic volatility, advancement opportunities, and competitive hiring practices, workers in these industries tend to change employers, job duties, and locations frequently, creating complex work histories. For obvious reasons, the workforce in most of the sector is relatively younger, more diverse in ethnicity and gender, and there are few unions or trade organizations relative to traditional sectors.

Work environment

The work environment can be even more radically different. Most new technologies involve manipulation of materials and products that are intrinsically costly, such as a silicon wafer or a genetically modified sow, so production systems are organized around product quality assurance. One consequence, evident in both the electronics and biotechnology industries, is the shift of production from factory environments to 'clean' rooms – specialized, limited-access work areas where workers wear protective clothing and equipment that limits the possibility of contaminating the product physically, chemically, or biologically. Lighting, ventilation and other ambient conditions are set to protect the product, creating environments with unusual characteristics.

For example, any particle inadvertently introduced into the air in semiconductor wafer fabrication rooms (fabs) is rapidly removed by filtration. Likewise, reverse isolation techniques are used to breed genetically engineered animals for biomedical uses. In each setting, the increasingly critical need to separate product (the wafers) from people to avoid particulate contamination – through automation, robotics, and separately exhausted enclosures – has led to reductions in the potential exposure to production chemicals. However, workers frequently wear uncomfortable personal protective equipment, have more limited opportunities for breaks, and have little flexibility to make environmental or task accommodations (such as opening windows) that can enhance and humanize the work experience in more traditional settings. Protection of the product may also impose constraints on the extent to which mechanical aspects of work can be modified, e.g., enhancing ergonomic risks, as occurs in the healthcare sector (see Chapter 17), although use of automation and robotics can reduce some ergonomic hazards.

Work hazards

Perhaps none of this would warrant unique consideration were it not for the nature of the hazards which have been introduced. For example, semiconductor wafer fabrication requires the use of a large number of chemicals, including inert, corrosive, and toxic gases, volatile organic compounds, polymers, and metals and metallic compounds. Many of these chemicals have not been well characterized toxicologically. Not only are there frequent introductions of new chemical agents in microelectronics and biohazards in biotechnology – often poorly tested or of unknown nature – but the exposure conditions can be unpredictable, sporadic, and generally hard to document.

In semiconductor manufacture, exposures are well controlled under usual conditions – samples typically contain very low or undetectable amounts of measured contaminants.[1] However, accidental leaks and spills occur infrequently which, as in other industries, are difficult to characterize and quantify. In biotechnology, as in other laboratory type settings, accidental exposures are the major concern, often controllable primarily by rigorous training and work practice measures, contrary to the traditional hierarchy of industrial hygiene controls. The potential for infectious, allergenic, or toxic reactions to inadequately characterized intermediate materials or end products is daunting, impeding design of meaningful surveillance programs or the diagnostic evaluation of worker complaints or illnesses. In addition, as in healthcare, there is the formidable task of preventing biologic contamination of the product, such as immunocompromised animals bred for biomedical or research purposes.

Finally, rapid advances in technology can result in frequently changing the materials and work processes. For example, in some parts of the semiconductor industry fabrication rooms are reconfigured every several years. Genetic manipulation of organisms may result in the introduction of numerous new strains and variants, rendering the usual notions of a 'complete' exposure history almost meaningless, let alone the feasibility of epidemiologic evaluation of the exposed workforce.

MICROELECTRONICS INDUSTRY
Work processes

Manufacture of computer chips on silicon wafers involves exotic multi-step processes, which change frequently. The following is a brief overview; more complete discussion can be found in the suggested readings.[2-4]

The first step is making the wafer – a large round platter of almost pure silicon or, less commonly, gallium arsenide. Wafer manufacturing occurs in a few separate dedicated manufacturing facilities, which are not part of the semiconductor wafer fabrication environment. To achieve this, quartz is reduced to silicon under very high temperature, ground to a powder then gassified in hydrogen and chlorine to trichlorosilane, which is reduced to pure silicon. A small crystal 'seed' is then dipped into the liquid silicon at the ends of a rod, allowing the crystal to grow while intentionally introducing very small quantities of impurities ('doping') such as boron, arsenic or phosphorus. These huge crystals are then machined (including grinding, slicing, and lapping), etched (in acid) and polished to form the wafer on which hundreds of chips (die) will then be fabricated.

The majority of the potentially toxic chemicals are introduced during fabrication. First a layer of silicon dioxide is applied, which is then protected by coating with a layer of photoresist. Photoresists contain light-reactive chemicals, polymers, and carrier solvents. As in conventional photography, the wafer is exposed to a light source, intense ultraviolet (UV) light. The light passes through a mask, containing the pattern for the circuitry, causing polymerization or solubilization of the exposed photoresist, dependent upon the type of photoresist (negative or positive). The resulting surface is developed, requiring use of chemicals, primarily strong bases. For the typical positive resist, exposed areas of solubilized photoresist are removed by the developer. The resulting unprotected silicon dioxide

surface can then be etched off by application of etchants – acids (wet etch) or excited gases (plasma etch).

Doping involves the introduction of desired chemical impurities into that portion of the surface of the wafer, which is now unprotected. This process may be accomplished by diffusion at high temperatures of dopant gases through the surface of the silicon or by ion implantation, in which the dopant ions are beamed, under vacuum and high electric fields, onto the wafer from heated filaments. In thin film, thin layers of materials, including silicon, silicon dioxide, and silicon nitride, are placed onto the surface of the wafer, in furnaces or chemical vapor deposition tools, to provide a layer that protects the underlying surface or serves as an insulator. Typically one wafer will go through repeated sequences of these steps to create multiple layers of complex circuitry.

When the circuits are complete, the wafer is metallized – the introduction of metallic circuit connectors, typically by vapor deposition. The fab and associated processes can thus be divided into four major functional areas, photolithography, etch, thin film (which includes ion implantation and metallization), and diffusion. Final processing includes inspection and chip separation, assembly into packaging, and testing, with the last three activities conducted outside the wafer fabrication facility, typically at a separate location.

Chemical/physical hazards

As noted, there is an extensive array of chemicals used in the manufacturing process, mostly, but not exclusively, in enclosed areas. Although a detailed review of the chemicals is beyond the scope of this chapter, some of the major chemical and physical hazards are shown in Tables 18.1.1 and 18.1.2.

Hazard	Reference
Organic solvents, including glycol ethers	Chapter 40
Inorganic acids	Chapter 47
Organic and inorganic silanes	Fischman, 2001[4]
Arsenicals	Chapter 39.2
Boron, gallium tungsten and other exotic metals and organometallic compounds	Chapter 39.9 and Fischman, 2001[4]
Hazardous gases including arsine phosphine, nitrous trifluorine and diboranes	Chapter 47 and Fischman, 2001[4]
Resins	Chapter 11
Diazonapthoquinones and other photoactive chemicals	Fischman, 2001[4]

Table 18.1.1 Chemical hazards in the microelectronics Industry

Hazard	Reference
Ionizing and non-ionizing radiation	Chapters 33.1 and 33.2
Ultraviolet light	Chapter 33.2
Noise	Chapter 34
Heat	Chapter 35
Low humidity	Chapter 50
Ergonomic stressors	Chapter 32

Table 18.1.2 Physical hazards in the microelectronics industry

Health risks and concerns

Despite the plethora of potential risk factors and the exotic nature of the chemicals and work, most health problems reported by physicians in the industry or practicing in areas where the industry is concentrated have been fairly commonplace. Skin irritation, possibly exacerbated by low humidity and protective clothing, is common. Eye irritation is also frequently encountered.[4,5] Respiratory complaints may be more common than in other industries,[5,6] although the majority are self-limited and poorly characterized irritative symptoms. Asthmatics and others with pre-existing airway disorders may find the environment problematic, perhaps due to the dry air in the fab or low-level irritation, although some allergic asthmatics report improvement in symptoms in an environment free of pollens and other particulates. Not surprisingly, syndromes resembling non-specific building-related illness and multiple chemical sensitivity have also arisen (see Chapter 49).

In addition to these medical reports, musculoskeletal problems have been encountered,[7] as might be expected from the complex and constantly changing organization of the clean rooms, although, compared with other industries, the work is not generally heavy or repetitive. Complaints related to heat and protective clothing occur, although significant heat-related illness does not. Complaints of difficulty hearing also occur in the fab environment, which is noisy but rarely exceeds noise action levels. Noise–related hearing loss does not appear to occur, with the possible exception of workers in mechanical support areas outside the fab.[4]

The greatest concerns in the industry have centered around reproductive health and cancer. Spontaneous abortion excess was first reported in a Massachusetts company in the mid 1980s.[8] This prompted two large studies on an industry-wide basis, which confirmed excesses of about 1.4-fold in the fab overall and ranging up to 70% in certain job categories.[9,10] Although the specific cause for the early fetal losses could not be ascertained with certainty, the clustering around jobs with exposure to photoresist solvents implicated ethylene glycol ethers because of their known reproductive/developmental toxicity in animals. In response, the industry has substituted less toxic glycol ethers, such as propylene glycol monomethyl ether acetate, or other alternative solvents, such as ethyl lactate, for these compounds. In addition, the industry has enhanced some engineering and other controls and generally created procedures that facilitate accommodations or transfers for concerned pregnant employees. Only a portion of the observed excess of spontaneous abortion in one of the studies could be explained on the basis of potential exposure to glycol ethers; excesses in other areas, such as etch, remain unexplained, raising the question of other contributing factors, e.g., unrecognized developmental toxicity of another agent or other factors, such as ergonomic factors or stress.

The issue of cancer risk remains unresolved. In addition to compounds which have been poorly studied, there are potential exposures, albeit well controlled, in the fabrication process to numerous known or suspect carcinogens, such as arsenic and sulfuric acid. The levels of exposure, however, are typically far below those observed in epidemiologic studies of other worker groups exposed to these materials. Only one small study of cancer has been undertaken among workers in this environment; it failed to show any consistent risk, although the power to detect an effect was very low.[11] Given the concerns, it is likely that further attempts to quantify cancer risks will be undertaken in the future.

Surveillance and control of occupational health and safety in the industry

Current practice in the industry is widely variable; a few companies have responded to public and worker concerns by instituting extensive medical monitoring, in some cases with data analysis for groups by job or work area. At present there is little data to support specific surveillance activities beyond those currently required in the US under OSHA, namely the reporting of occupational illnesses and injuries. Unfortunately, even the more intensive approach, providing questionnaire and medical information on a regular basis, will be of limited value in addressing the major unanswered questions about worker risks. For one thing, the outcomes of interest are not known with any certainty, and include a wide range of possible health effects; there is no single specific condition to perform surveillance around. Traditional health surveillance is intrinsically cross-sectional in nature, and therefore unlikely to provide a barometer to track more chronic effects of exposure should these occur. Moreover, the absence of linkage between symptoms or other health information and exposure reduces the ability to compare rates among groups with divergent exposures of interest. High employee turnover, combined with rapid changes in production processes and exposure patterns, further compound the difficulties associated with a traditional medical surveillance approach.

An alternative approach, perhaps in combination with ongoing symptom and health status surveillance, would be an aggressive 'sentinel event' approach. In this model, proactive scrutiny of all reported workplace events, combined with routine scrutiny of health insurance data to evaluate patterns of chronic diseases such as cancers among workers and retirees, may provide a more sensitive way to detect unsuspected adverse health consequences of the work. Although each observation would require confirmation by application of more formal epidemiologic methods, such an approach offers a coherent alternative when traditional surveillance strategies have limited efficacy given the nature of the exposures and the industry.

Any surveillance approach would require institution of three important prerequisites. First, it would be crucial that company personnel records are coded in such a way as to distinguish to the fullest extent possible the actual nature of an employee's job, rather than generic job titles which might be administratively simpler but inadequate for surveillance purposes. Second, records must be retained electronically, with appropriate documentation, for a minimum of three, and preferably four or five decades. This is crucial to evaluate the risks of chronic health effects. Finally, it would be desirable for health insurance records to be maintained by appropriate health data management companies, so that rates of illness and disease can be evaluated without complex and costly epidemiologic reconstructions as has been the case up until now.

BIOTECHNOLOGY

The advent of biotechnology allows us to move genetic material within and between species. In theory, this allows us to produce any desired gene product in the species of our choice, including the alteration of the human genome for therapeutic purposes. In practice, the applications of biotechnology have focused on certain key areas that show agronomic, economic, and/or therapeutic promise. This technology has created new potential hazards and newly exposed worker populations within the biotechnology industry.

Two key areas of concern will be addressed here: the handling of plants genetically modified for food and feed purposes, and the production of biopharmaceuticals. In the former circumstance, the inserted genes and their products are characterized and selected to be appropriate for human or animal consumption. Human health risks in this area appear to be of lesser concern and do not appear to differ qualitatively from the risks inherent in the conduct of conventional agriculture. Issues of ecologic harm, such as environmental changes in neighboring plants or organisms sharing the same ecosystem, continue to be hotly debated, given the vast and diverse settings in which these food crops may be introduced. In the pharmaceutical area, however, proteins with known or anticipated human pharmacologic activity are being produced in a wide variety of species, resulting in a higher potential for adverse effects upon worker health.

Food and feed crops

Genes may be inserted into food and feed crops for a variety of reasons – to confer selective resistance to herbicides; to confer resistance to pests; to confer agronomic traits such as drought or salt tolerance; to alter storage, processing, or cooking characteristics; or to improve the nutritional characteristics of a food or animal feed. In order to function, an inserted gene must be accompanied by gene regulatory sequences that allow expression of the gene within the plant. At present, many gene inserts also contain a marker for antibiotic resistance which is necessary to select for plant cells which have successfully acquired the desired gene insert, but such sequences are either not utilized in newer products or are removed from these products during development. The inserted gene is generally intended to produce a functional protein, although in some cases (antisense DNA mediated resistance to viral pathogens), no protein expression occurs. The protein products used in food and feed crops fall into several categories.[12] They may express pesticidal activity as in the case of the Bt (*Bacillus thuringiensis*) toxin, or confer resistance to herbicides by incorporating a resistant variant of a normally occurring enzymatic activity or by allowing a plant to degrade a particular herbicide. The inserted gene may result in new plant structural proteins, or may confer new or enhanced enzymatic activity upon the plant so that new nutrients or enhanced levels of nutrients are produced. Inserted genetic material may also act by down-regulating or up-regulating existing genes, and may potentially have unintended effects upon other genes within the plant cell either by direct insertion into those genes or by indirect regulatory (so-called pleotropic) effects.[13]

Potential novel occupational exposures resulting from the production of genetically modified feed and food crops include: (1) exposure to the novel protein; (2) exposure to the products of enzymatic activity conferred by the inserted protein, which may be either anticipated or unanticipated; (3) exposure to endogenous or novel plant toxins resulting from pleotropic effects; (4) effects mediated by antibiotic marker genes; and (5) effects of the inserted gene sequence itself.

Fortunately, food and feed products undergo safety evaluation prior to marketing,[12] greatly reducing some of these hypothetical risks. Although gene insertion is random, genetic events in crop plants are characterized to assure that normally expressed genes are not disrupted. Inserted novel genes and proteins are isolated and sequenced to assure that the intended material has been inserted without alteration. The novel proteins themselves are subjected to acute animal toxicology testing. Modified crops are characterized biochemically to assure appropriate nutrient properties and composition, feeding studies are performed in animal species, and levels of known toxins endogenous to the particular plant species quantified. To address food allergenicity concerns, inserted proteins are examined for structural similarity to known food allergens and to assure that they are readily digestible and heat labile; testing which is believed to reduce the likelihood of gastrointestinal allergy.[14] DNA itself is not likely to be directly harmful; thus far no transfer of plant DNA to human, animals, or bacterial species has been demonstrated.[15]

Currently available genetically modified crops are produced, processed, and sold in a manner identical to, and usually admixed with, conventional crop varieties. Thus, the worker population exposed to these materials and the modes of exposure are no different from those of the traditional food/feed workforce. An exception would be workers involved in the development of new and not yet fully characterized crops, whose exposure potential may be more like that in the biopharmaceutical industry discussed below.

Thus, the introduction of biotechnology crops, given the pre-market safety assessment of these products, does not appear to introduce significant novel risk to the food and feed production workforce. Toxic or other adverse effects from the gene insert, protein products, and products of enzymatic activity are not, in general, anticipated from a material suitable for food consumption. Any novel protein, even one which is not a gastrointestinal sensitizer, may be a potential human respiratory or skin allergen. Foods in general, particularly in the grinding or milling environment, are recognized occupational allergens, as are fungal and other contaminants of commodity crops.

Overall, the general nature of the hazards for workers employed in the food and feed production industries does not appear to be qualitatively altered by the introduction of marketed biotechnology crops, and it appears unlikely that quantitative risks are increased to any meaningful extent once one looks beyond the product development laboratory. The area of biopharmaceuticals presents a very different picture.

Biopharmaceuticals

Historically, development and production of pharmaceutical agents and biomedical devices involved well-delineated, traditional work activities readily identifiable by today's occupational physician. Compounds of interest were synthesized in chemistry laboratories, purified, and tested for their chemical properties. Using animal facilities, the products of these laboratories were then tested for therapeutic and adverse effects first in smaller, then in larger animals. If the results were satisfactory, production would begin, typically on a small scale at first, to provide enough material for further trials and testing. Finally, successful drugs went into large-scale production in chemical production facilities, unique only in that they are equipped as necessary to meet the standards of pharmaceutical production. Health hazards for each of these sets of activities – the chemistry lab, the vivarium, and the factory – could be addressed using relatively traditional industrial hygiene techniques, complicated perhaps by the novelty of some of the compounds tested, the need to utilize hazardous microorganisms to test antimicrobial agents; and the potential for zoonotic infections in animal facilities.

With the development of recombinant DNA technology and the explosion in knowledge of the genome, the traditional pathway to drug development is changing. Although chemistry laboratories have not disappeared, the 'source' of an increasing fraction of new pharmaceuticals is not organic synthesis but biologic synthesis, i.e., a protein product of a selected gene or a metabolic product resulting from gene insertion. In this new paradigm, the initial steps in drug development involve identification of a relevant DNA sequence which codes for a desired protein (or occasionally DNA or RNA) product. This sequence may be an existing gene from a plant or animal species, a modified gene, or even a fully synthetic DNA sequence. This DNA sequence, along with appropriate regulatory sequences (promoters, etc) is then inserted into the genome of an organism which will become, in effect, the 'factory' producing the desired agent.

Until recently, biosynthesis most often occurred in bacterial, mold, or yeast cultures or in immortalized lines of human or animal cells. The hazards of such classical 'fermentation-like' systems, regardless of scale, are reasonably well understood. However, in the coming decade, the organisms engineered to yield the voluminous quantities of proteins needed for commercial purposes will primarily be agricultural crops such as corn or tobacco. To accomplish plant-mediated synthesis, a gene of interest is inserted into plant cells under laboratory conditions using bacterial or viral vectors or mechanical (micro-projectile) means. Cells bearing the desired gene are identified, and the desired cells are grown into adult plants, from which further clones or stock can be obtained. Plants are then grown and selected to cull out offspring lacking desired expression of the trait of interest, typically at a seed production facility. Once the seed stock is established, 'production' occurs on a farm; the therapeutic agent is then isolated and purified from the harvested product.

Biotechnology is not limited to plants. Increasingly medical 'devices' may be grown in animals, such as the genetically modified swine expressing human rather than porcine cell surface markers, which may become the major source of organs for transplantation. As with drugs, breeding of these unique clones occurs in something resembling a laboratory, but once bred, the livestock are raised and harvested in a setting more like a farm. However, these highly specialized animals require more than just food and water; they require isolation from any organisms which could harm them and, especially, from any organisms which might persist in tissues, with or without harm to the pig, and subsequently harm an immunocompromised patient. Thus, the farm setting is modified to provide isolation from pathogenic organisms.

Undoubtedly, there will be many variations on these themes as the full potential of new genetic technologies becomes clear. The sea-change, however, has already occurred: the practice of occupational health and safety for the population of genetic technology workers will require coping with a new and rapidly changing set of hazards, with work occurring in surprising new settings, and with worker populations (e.g., farm workers) dealing with many hazards – both novel and traditional. At present there is virtually no road map for the practice of occupational medicine in this domain.

Hazards

Hazards in the biotechnology industry are best thought of in categories, since strategies for control are relatively unique to each class. The major groupings are: chemical, physical, and infectious and non-infectious biohazards. Since the first two groups are comprised of standard occupational health concerns, the focus of the discussion that follows will be on the infectious and non-infectious biologic risks. However, traditional health hazards (such as noise) can be easily overlooked when occurring in novel settings, and the need for continued vigilance for these traditional hazards cannot be overemphasized.

Infectious risks

Biomedical and pharmaceutical laboratories have a long tradition of utilizing infectious agents. The control of the associated hazards, using containment levels appropriate for the specific organism involved and for any genetic modifications present, has worked reasonably well over time. Existing documents[16,17] provide clear criteria for application of the different biosafety levels, and clear prescriptions as to the appropriate precautions. To date, there is no evidence that laboratory recombination per se has incrementally altered the risks from any organisms handled in the lab, although concerns about the potential of new strains, especially those with markers for antibiotic resistance, may pose new concerns about waste and environmental disposition.

Animal use in the laboratory is not new, although it has received proportionally less attention in occupational health than in the veterinary medicine literature. Traditional zoonotic infections such as Q-fever, while not novel, continue to be an issue. The risks of agents as Herpes B from primates and prion diseases from the handling of human or animal CNS tissue represent some of the most daunting new threats, requiring that any lab handling potentially infectious material have appropriate consultation and control mechanisms in place.

In addition, new possibilities are raised by the emerging genetic technologies. Foremost is the use of vectors for transfection of animal cells. Although usually harvested from wild-types with limited pathogenicity to human hosts, viral agents selected for this work are themselves modified in the process, but are typically not well studied, since their role in the research is circumscribed and generally short-lived. Whether, for example, a non-human adenovirus carrying one or more modified genes could pose a risk to workers remains unexplored, and is unlikely to be explored until an 'incident' occurs. Although viral and bacterial vectors are also utilized for plant transfection, these agents do not appear to have any propensity to infect humans or animals.

Of greater concern may be the viral vectors utilized for human gene therapy since, by design, these agents will infect the human host. These agents may be derived from a wide variety of viral strains including the retroviruses, adenoviruses, adenovirus-associated viruses, vaccinia, and the herpesviruses.[18] In general, these agents are replication deficient and thus cause only transient viremia. While most agents result in the transient, epichromosomal presence of the novel genes, some agents (primarily retroviruses) can permanently incorporate novel DNA into the human genome.[18] In general, large inocula are needed to have a significant effect, since the agents do not replicate. However, large accidental inoculations or inadvertent infection with replication-competent strains could cause serious occupational illness. Also the possibility remains that a replication-incompetent strain could acquire the ability to replicate via unintended genetic events or as a result of co-infection with another viral strain.[18]

Likewise, laboratories will likely utilize genetically modified, rather than traditional laboratory animals. Until now this has been largely limited to transgenic rodents whose potential to spread infection to humans appears limited. However, with the advent of larger genetically modified species, such as pigs, new possibilities arise, such as human transmission of new agents or more efficient transmission of old ones. Many if not most of the major viral infections of humans are suspected to have had animal origins, and many viruses are quite remarkable in the range of hosts they may infect. The 2003 outbreak of severe acute respiratory syndrome (SARS), traced to

food workers handling wild civet carcasses, is a compelling example. The emergence of prion variants in new host animals, as occurred in the 1980s with bovine spongiform encephalopathy (mad cow disease), indicates that particular caution is necessary regarding the handling of any CNS tissues or contaminated material.

Unfortunately, the range of possibilities is virtually infinite; possibilities specific to a given lab or technology will necessarily require detailed attention to the particular exposures, with broad appreciation for the 'possible'. The emergence of new human pathogens in animal species has been occurring as a natural phenomenon with great regularity, especially in the case of influenza viruses. It is not presently clear how the risks of this phenomenon in biotechnology systems compare with the risks inherent in the natural environment.

Non-infectious biohazards

A larger concern is the non-infectious occupational risk associated with genetically modified organisms and their products. Generally, these can be grouped into three classes. First are the potential toxicities of the protein products themselves. As discussed above, genetically modified plant products developed for human and animal consumption are of relatively limited concern in this regard, beyond the risk of newly introduced allergens and some alterations in plant composition.

We can be less confident about the risks of pharmaceutical protein products. Technology now allows constructs of various cytokines, cytokine inhibitors, agonists, and antagonists of numerous 'receptors' or other proteins in the body, including highly specific agents such as monoclonal antibodies. Although these proteins generally constitute a small portion of total protein production, many of these agents manifest remarkably high levels of biologic activity following parenteral administration, with effective doses in the microgram range. These proteins are unlikely to be well absorbed via the upper or lower respiratory tract, intact skin or gastrointestinal routes. However, some proteins and/or possibly peptide fragments may be absorbed, especially under dusty conditions. While some dust exposure may occur in the harvest or handling of whole crops, greater potential for dust exposure exists when crops such as corn or tobacco leaf are ground or milled to allow extraction of the desired material. Given the high biologic activity of these materials, systemic effects may be possible despite very low bioavailability.

It is possible that genetically modified agents may directly affect mucous membranes of the upper and lower respiratory tract and even the gastrointestinal tract. For example, a monoclonal antibody directed against inflammatory mediators, or cell surface markers, might precipitate lung injury by modulating pulmonary immune function of the airway epithelium. Although this risk is, at present, entirely theoretical, vigilance is required as we proceed into the future.

The majority of therapeutic proteins have undergone development in non-plant systems prior to initiating plant-mediated production, and many of these agents have undergone preclinical and early clinical testing either in animals and/or appropriate patient groups (often patients with rare or fatal conditions). However, the general safety of these materials for working adults typically has not been established. In particular, since protein agents must generally be administered parenterally for therapeutic purposes, these agents have rarely been studied via traditional routes of occupational exposure. Assessment of occupational risks is further complicated by the often high degree of biologic specificity of the proteins, which may have activity in only a limited number of species or be active only in humans. Thus, depending upon the degree of species specificity, traditional animal testing may fail to reveal hazards relevant to the workplace. The development of numerous such protein agents annually increases the likelihood of difficulties arising in exposed workers, but the ultimate magnitude of these difficulties remains undefined.

Another concern, and the one which has received the most attention in relationship to genetically modified foods, is the potential for exposed workers to develop allergic responses to new protein antigens. While proteins inserted into crops intended for food or feed use are selected to minimize the risk of gastrointestinal sensitization, the potential for pharmaceutical proteins to incite allergic pulmonary responses may be more substantial. Although there are algorithms and approaches for predicting gastrointestinal (i.e. food) allergenicity,[14] the predictive value of these algorithms for respiratory allergenicity is unknown, especially for workers who may be repeatedly exposed. Given that new proteins can potentially be allergenic, allergic responses such as dermatitis, urticaria, asthma, rhinitis, and anaphylaxis are potential adverse effects. It will generally not be feasible to screen workforces for sensitivity to these new products, since the antigens will likely be novel to humans and markers for sensitivity not developed until allergic responses occur and are fully evaluated.

The introduction of new or enhanced enzymatic activities and synthetic pathways may also introduce novel metabolic products, either intentionally or otherwise. Similarly, one may see so-called pleotropic effects in which the insertion of a foreign gene alters cell metabolism in unexpected ways as a result of changes in protein or cell function.[13] For example, a plant which previously expressed low levels of a toxin may express larger quantities of the toxin, or a previously unexpressed pathway may become active. Again, while food and feed products undergo substantial testing which may uncover such phenomena, such comprehensive testing is not necessarily undertaken for plants intended for biopharmaceutical production.

At this time, there is no simple way to look singly or collectively at these metabolic effects; singly, because it is unknown in advance what single product to study, and collectively because laboratory animals are limited in their food consumption. Even if a crop is tested, the animals may not consume enough of the whole plant product to assess the toxicity of a low-concentration material. Although there are presently no recognized cases of occupational illness resulting from pleotropic effects induced by modern genetic technologies, pleotropic effects of traditional breeding have, on at least one occasion, precipitated an outbreak of occupational illness in the form of photodermatitis resulting from unanticipated increases in psoralin levels in celery.[12] Hopefully, rapidly evolving technology in the area of gene expression profiling and metabolite analysis[13] will allow a more comprehensive approach to this area of hazard assessment in the near future.

Health studies in the biotechnology sector

For the reasons proposed above, current knowledge about occupational health for non-traditional hazards, particularly in the biopharmaceuticals area, remains extremely limited. There are a handful of reassuring reports that the recombinant DNA technologies in microbes of the last generation has not conferred important new infectious risks, as noted, but relevance to the new enterprises is unclear. Moreover, it appears inevitable that the production of new gene products will rise dramatically given the recent sequencing of the human genome and other advances in biotechnology. This assures that many workers will be working with unknown materials for the foreseeable future, many in novel workplace circumstances.

Occupational health surveillance – approaches

For workers in the traditional food and feed industries, including farming, the introduction of evaluated biotechnology crops will probably produce at most modest change in qualitative and quantitative health risk. This is in contrast to the evolving situation in the area of biotechnology research and biopharmaceuticals. Regarding these latter two areas, the potential for adverse outcomes, albeit remote in any single situation, is likely high in the aggregate, and the safety of the technology – given already high levels of public scrutiny – as well as the workers hangs in the balance.

The fact that there are neither well-defined surveillance approaches nor specific regulations should encourage higher, not lower, levels of professional input. Moreover, unlike some traditional aspects of occupational health in which intimate knowledge of modern medicine and biology is generally not critical, consultants in this industry will need to have substantial scientific expertise as they evaluate product by product, and class by class, the potential for human exposure and risk created by new developments. In these novel environments, care providers must be careful not to overlook obvious traditional risks like animal allergy, zoonoses, noise, and ergonomic issues. Beyond this, a number of suggestions from the authors may prove useful to the care provider in approaching the biotechnology work environment. The ultimate need for, and efficacy of, these approaches remain to be determined.
1. For farm workers and other food/feed industry workers handling approved genetically modified plants, no unique surveillance beyond usual measures appears to be mandated as this time. One plausible risk is allergy

to inserted proteins, a risk already common to foodstuffs and contaminants such as molds. If immunologic studies of exposed workers are performed, consideration should be given both to novel and to the far greater number of non-novel antigenic proteins present.

2. In evaluating and managing the infectious/transmissible risks of recombinant vectors and modified organisms in the laboratory setting – including microbes, plants, and animals – current guidelines from the National Institutes of Health[16] and the American Society for Microbiology[17] appear adequate. However, it is important to recognize that these criteria are based upon planned (or readily anticipated) and controlled events. Unanticipated genetic events may occur, particularly in animal species, with resulting novel pathogens, although the likelihood and extent of such events is unclear. Practitioners must therefore remain alert to the possibility of unique infectious presentations within the biotechnology workforce.

3. In evaluating the risks of biopharmaceutical products, the occupational physician should consider several characteristics which may not be evident on casual consideration of available toxicology data. These factors include the following.

   - Is the molecule biologically active as produced in the organism, or is further processing necessary to result in an active moiety?
   - Does the molecule produce biologic effects independently or is some other exogenous factor required for toxicity (i.e., an antibody designed to carry a radio-isotope to tumor cells would not likely present a hazard until radio-labeled)?
   - Does the target of the molecule occur in the general population, or is it only manifest in specific diseases?
   - Does the receptor for the protein exist on externally exposed surfaces such as the mucous membranes of the gastrointestinal or respiratory tract, or exist in the mucous coating of these surfaces?
   - What is known, if anything, about absorption of the particular molecule or about the activity and absorption of fragments derived from it?
   - Is the molecule known to have acute toxicologic effects (i.e., cholera toxin) or is it structurally or functionally analogous to a known toxin based upon bioinformatic (e.g., protein sequence homology) analysis?
   - What degree of species specificity does the molecule exhibit, and how will this affect the ability of animal testing systems to reveal useful information in regard to human hazards?
   - Given such specificity, can a sufficiently predictive animal model be developed (such as an animal transgenic for the human receptor, or a homologous molecule having a different species specificity to allow testing)?
   - Does a human disease model exist which may shed light on the possible effects of the product? For exam-ple, acquired immunodeficiency could model potential effects of a protein which eliminates T-cell function or interferes with interleukin-2 activity.
   - Is the protein a known human allergen and/or does it exhibit homology to known allergens?
   - Is the protein of human origin or has it been 'humanized' in sequence to reduce antigenicity?

4. In the absence of adequate predictive data, care should be exercised in the handling of biopharmaceutical proteins outside of the well-controlled laboratory environment. This is particularly true for dry operations such as grinding or milling. While it is highly likely that, in most situations, no unusual effect will arise, exposure should be carefully controlled using industrial hygiene and personal protective equipment as necessary. The occupational physician should be vigilant for anticipated and even unanticipated clinical effects, especially those which might be mediated by direct action of the product upon the lining of the respiratory and/or gastrointestinal tracts.

5. In assessing allergic responses in the workplace, one should consider both the novel and existing antigen potential of the biotechnology product.

Several additional administrative and technical practices may be helpful in addressing the occupational health needs of the biotechnology community.

First, we would propose that every development facility, including seed farms and other agricultural facilities where biotechnology products (other than approved food/feed products) are handled, have available internal and/or external medical resources whose responsibilities are separate from product development and production. Such groups would have regular meetings with investigators developing new products, and would have both the resources and authority to provide caution where unforeseen risks are contemplated. These resources should include consultants knowledgeable in the necessary areas of molecular biology, virology, infectious disease, etc, depending upon the nature of the hazards involved.

Secondly, we would recommend that each development facility constitute a biosafety committee to review the worker-related safety aspects of biotechnology projects before inception. While this function is mandated for facilities receiving Federal dollars in the USA, privately funded research groups would be advised to follow this model and to provide the committee sufficient resources and authority to assure effectiveness. Inclusion of occupational medicine on the IBC seems well advised. We believe that community member participation is an important aspect of biosafety committee function, and encourages community involvement with the need for business confidentiality and the freedom to disclose public hazards appropriately balanced.

Finally, institutional review boards (IRBs) can contribute to the oversight of biotechnology projects when those projects involve human subject research. Recent liability concerns, may, unfortunately, limit the access of private industry to independent IRBs in university settings.

Hopefully, a more systematic approach to occupational medicine in biotechnology will result, including productive and cost-effective approaches to surveillance, control and, if necessary, regulation.

References

1. Hallock MF, Hammond SK, Hines CJ et al. Patterns of chemical use and exposure control in the semiconductor health study. Am J Ind Med 1995; 28:681-97.
2. Harrison M. Semiconductor manufacturing hazards. In: Sullivan J, Krieger G, eds. Clinical environmental health and hazardous materials toxicology. Baltimore: Williams and Wilkins, 1992.
3. Van Zant P. Microchip fabrication: a practical guide to semiconductor processing, 3rd edn. New York: McGraw Hill, 1997.
4. Fischman M. Semiconductor manufacturing hazards. In: Sullivan J, Krieger G, eds. Clinical environmental health and hazardous materials toxicology, 2nd edn. Baltimore: Williams and Wilkins, 2001.
5. McCurdy SA, Pocekay D, Hammond SK et al. A cross-sectional survey of respiratory and general health outcomes among semiconductor industry workers. Am J Ind Med 1995; 28:847–60.
6. LaDou J, Rohm T. The international electronic industry. Int J Occup Environ Health 1998; 4:1–18.
7. Pocekay D, McCurdy SA, Samuels SJ et al. A cross-sectional study of musculoskeletal symptoms and risk factors in semiconductor workers. Am J Ind Med 1995; 28:861–72.
8. Pastides H, Calabrese EJ, Hosmer DW, Harris DR. Spontaneous abortion and general illness among semiconductor manufacturers. J Occup Med 1988; 30:543–51.
9. Schenker MB, Gold EB, Beaumont JJ et al. Association of spontaneous abortion and other reproductive effects with work in the semiconductor industry. Am J Ind Med 1995; 28:639–60.
10. Gray R. Final report. Retrospective and prospective studies of reproductive health among IBM employees in semiconductor manufacturing. Baltimore: Johns Hopkins University of Hygiene and Public Health, 1993.
11. Sorohan T, Pope DJ, McKiernan MJ. Cancer incidence and cancer mortality in a cohort of semiconductor workers: an update. Br J Ind Med 1992; 49:215–6.
12. Hammond BG, Fuchs RL. Safety evaluation for new varieties of food crops developed through biotechnology. In: Thomas JA, ed. Biotechnology and safety assessment, 2nd edn. New York: Taylor and Francis, 1998.
13. Kuiper HA, Kleter GA, Noteborn HP, Kok EJ. Assessment of the food safety issues related to genetically modified foods. Plant J 2001; 27:503–28.
14. Metcalf D, Astwood J, Townsend R, Sampson H, Taylor S, Fuchs R. 1996. Assessment of the allergenic potential of foods derived from genetically engineered crop plants. Crit Rev Food Sci Nutr 1996; 36(suppl):S165–S186.
15. AMA. Genetically modified crops and foods. Council on Scientific Affairs. Chicago: American Medical Association, 2001. http://www.ama-assn.org/ama/pub/article/2036-4030.html
16. NIH. NIH Guidelines for Research Involving Recombinant DNA Molecules. Washington DC: Government Printing Office, 2000. Updates available at http//:www.nih.gov/od/oba
17. Richmond JY, McKinney RW, eds. Biosafety in microbiological and biomedical laboratories, 4th edn. Washington DC: Government Printing Office, 1999.
18. Evans ME, Lesnaw JA. Infection control in gene therapy. Infect Control Hosp Epidemiol 1999; 20(8):568–76.

INTRODUCTION

The events of September 2001 dramatically highlighted the occupational hazards facing police and firefighters. Of the rescue workers fatally injured in the World Trade Center attacks in New York, 335 were firefighters and 61 were police officers or detectives.[1] The evolving homeland security roles of the public safety sector encompass domestic consequence management of a broad spectrum of threats of terrorist or trans-national attack. Clinicians evaluating police officers and firefighters either for preventive services, including fitness for duty determinations, or for acute or chronic medical complaints potentially related to work must take into account the unique aspects and expanding scope of firefighting and police duties. Even in the absence of major disasters, both professions experience high rates of work-related illness, injury and mortality. While many hazards of law enforcement and fire service work are by necessity sporadic and unpredictable, a more thorough understanding of the risks facing these public safety workers could lead to improvement in current preventive efforts.

This chapter will outline hazardous exposures faced by police and firefighters and summarize studies of health outcomes related to exposures and recommendations for preventive interventions. Many of the specific hazards are discussed in greater detail in other chapters of this book.

FIREFIGHTERS

There are approximately 1.1 million firefighters in the US, organized into more than 26,000 local fire departments.[2] Interior structural firefighting is a complex operation that can be divided into several stages. These include (1) alarm, during which personal protective equipment including self-contained breathing apparatus (SCBA) is donned prior to and during transportation to the incident scene; (2) entry, when the burning structure is breached and rescue operations begin; (3) suppression, involving venting and extinguishment of the fire; (4) overhaul, when the firefighters remove furnishings, open walls, and pull ceilings to ensure that the fire is completely extinguished, and (5) termination, during which equipment is recovered, and hundreds of feet of 1.5 to 6 inch diameter hoselines are drained and re-packed onto the engines. While fighting structure fires remains a core function of fire departments, the number of responses to medical emergencies and hazardous materials incidents has more than doubled in the past 20 years.[3] Other dangerous aspects of the firefighter's job include responding to emergencies using warning lights and sirens through traffic, operating in poorly controlled environments such as motor vehicle accident or crime scenes, and operating in a wide array of technical rescue situations, including working in confined spaces, high elevations, extremes of temperature, and urban environments.

Approximately three-fourths of firefighters are volunteers and the remainder are career personnel. The occupational hazards facing each group may differ in frequency and depend on the operational scope of the local department. Career fire departments generally respond to a greater number of calls, and typically protect larger populations and occupancies than volunteer departments.

As Figure 18.2.1 shows, there has been a 38.9% decrease in the number of US structure fires over the last 20 years.[4] This has been associated with a moderate decrease in total line-of-duty firefighter fatalities, though the occupational injury and mortality rates per fire appear to be stable or rising, with rates of 25 injuries per 1000 fires and 6.5 fatalities per 100,000 fires.[5-7]

Firefighting accounts for only 9% of fire service emergency call volume nationally, yet roughly 50% of line-of-duty deaths and 60-80% of injuries occur on the fire-ground[7] as shown in Figure 18.2.2. While the high rate of fatalities on the fireground might suggest that such deaths could be due to physical trauma or direct exposure to heat and smoke, in fact roughly half of firefighter deaths on the fireground are caused by heart attacks[6] or motor vehicle crashes (see below).

Specific hazards of firefighting

Table 18.2.1 summarizes the occupational hazards facing individuals in this profession and the possible health outcomes resulting from these exposures.

Physical hazards

Fighting structure fires involves many physically demanding and potentially hazardous tasks, including climbing ladders, crawling through confined spaces, lifting heavy tools and building materials, and maneuvering on elevated surfaces where there is a risk of falls. These activities must be performed while wearing heavy fire retardant clothing, a helmet, self-contained breathing apparatus (SCBA) respirator, and other protective gear that may weigh in excess of 50 pounds. There is consequently a need for physical fitness and a constant potential for traumatic injury or death. A study of National Fire Incident Reporting System data found that risk factors for acute injury while fighting fires included a greater than 5 alarm fire, structures greater than three stories, and at least one civilian being injured.[8] While there is a risk from physical assault violence by patients and others during provision of emergency medicine services (EMS), this risk has been found to be low.[9]

Heat is a critical exposure hazard when fighting fires. Interior structural firefighting can transiently involve exposures to temperatures exceeding 700°F, and the protective clothing worn by firefighters is designed to afford thermal protection from such environments in a time/dose-related manner[10] (see Chapter 34). Unfortunately, the heavy thermal and flame protective equipment adds significant weight and ergonomic disadvantage. It severely impairs the

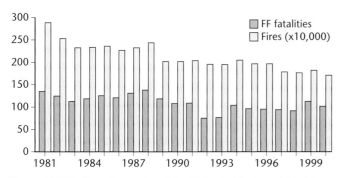

Figure 18.2.1: Twenty-year trends in US fire incidents and total line-of-duty firefighter (FF) fatalities, 1981–2000, based on data published by the US Fire Administration and National Fire Protection Association.[4]

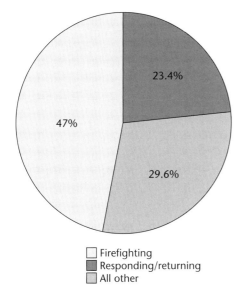

Figure 18.2.2: Ten-year pattern of firefighter activity at the time of death based on 1991–2000 fatality data.[5,6] Nearly three-fourths of line-of-duty deaths occur on the fireground or in motor vehicle crashes during emergency responses. The remaining fatalities are associated with training, EMS or rescue calls, and non-emergency fire service functions.

Hazard	Potential health outcome
Physical hazards	
Falls	Back and other musculoskeletal
Falling building material	injuries, other traumatic injuries
Ergonomic stressors	
Violence	
Heat and flame	Heat illness, cardiovascular demand, burns
Noise	Hearing loss
Chemical hazards	
Smoke inhalation	Inhalation injury, systemic exposure
Carbon monoxide	Hypoxia, myocardial ischemia, mental status impairment
Diesel fumes	Lung function, cancer
Hazardous materials	Systemic absorption and specific toxic effects
Psychologic hazards	
Traumatic events, shiftwork, other job stress	Post-traumatic stress disorder, suicide, sleep disturbances Possible link to hypertension, other cardiovascular disease
Biologic hazards	Tuberculosis, hepatitis, HIV, other respiratory and blood-borne infections
Other	
Motor vehicle accidents	
Traumatic injuries	

Table 18.2.1: Occupational hazards for firefighters

body's normal mechanisms for heat dissipation, and the inability to release heat generated by muscular activity during firefighting (despite profuse sweating) puts firefighters at increased risk for clinically significant heat stress. Even without thermal stress from a fire, the clothing has been shown to significantly increase core body temperature during physical activity.[11]

Typical noise exposures are of relatively short duration and high intensity, which may be different from the steady-state noise in many industrial environments. Amplified electronic or mechanical sirens are designed to be louder than background traffic noise, and are capable of sound pressure levels of 120 dB or more. The exposures to personnel riding in an ambulance or fire apparatus can exceed 100 dB. Since such exposures are short duration, the OSHA permissible exposure levels of 85 dBA may not be exceeded over an 8-hour time weighted average.[12–14] The high rate of hearing loss in firefighters, however,

suggests that such short exposures may be intense enough to cause lasting damage. Pump operators, who stand next to the diesel engines that are maintained in high idle throughout incidents to power the apparatus' water delivery capability, may experience the highest overall noise exposure during a shift. A number of engineering controls have been used to reduce siren noise exposures, so that the noise exposure may vary by the type and locations of sirens used by a particular department. In addition, active noise cancellation hearing protective devices employing radio communication can reduce noise exposures due to predictable sources such as sirens, but to date are not widely in use.

Chemical exposures

Smoke from burning materials exposes firefighters to a wide range of potentially toxic gases, fumes, vapors and particulates. The most common and significant is carbon monoxide.[15] The use of synthetic polymers and materials in building construction and interior furnishings since the 1930s has added to the complexity of the gases released during structural fires[16] (see Chapter 19.5). The exact mixture of chemicals depends on the material that is burning as well as the temperature of the fire. Materials that contain nitrogen, sulfur, and halogens can release hydrogen cyanide, nitrogen oxides, sulfur dioxide, ammonia, and halogen acids. Silk, polyvinyl chloride, plastics, wool, and insulation can release hydrogen chloride, hydrogen fluoride, isocyanates, and acrolein.[17] Other potential components of smoke include aldehydes, benzene, benzpyrenes and other polyaromatic hydrocarbons, phosgene, and particulates.[3] Until recently, training fires were often conducted using reclaimed oils from gas stations or industries and such oil fires may have contained PCBs, metals, and other contaminants. Additionally, stored chemicals like pesticides, manufacturing compounds or intermediates, and hydrocarbon fuels all produce toxic products of combustion in fires involving commercial, public and residential occupancies.

Since the 1970s, inhalation exposure has presumably decreased significantly due to the widespread use of SCBA for respiratory protection during firefighting and Hazardous Material (HAZMAT), emergency operations.[18] Recent studies suggest, however, that despite the use of protective equipment, there is ongoing evidence of exposure to polyaromatic hydrocarbons and other products of combustion during firefighting.[19,20] One reason may be the common practice of removing SCBA during overhaul operations, when the dense smoke and heat have cleared,[21,22] despite knowledge that the density of visible or carbonaceous smoke is not correlated with toxic gas concentrations in combustion environments.[17] Furthermore, recent testing of commercially available SCBAs for exclusion of weaponized chemicals by NIOSH has demonstrated that certain organic agents rapidly permeate some face pieces. HAZMAT responders use special protective equipment to provide an impermeable vapor–liquid barrier that completely encapsulates the wearer, including the SCBA. The implications for firefighters using SCBA alone for respiratory protection in fire environments with high concentrations of organic or non-polar gases require further investigation.

Most fire departments respond to HAZMAT incidents in their local jurisdictions, yet this function, when performed with proper protective equipment as described above, probably adds little to lifetime occupational chemical exposures in firefighters.[23,24] A recent study found that even though elevated levels of PCBs and polychlorinated dibenzofurans were found on the protective suits of firefighters, there was no evidence of significant exposure.[25]

Diesel fumes are a potentially significant hazard. Inadequate attention was paid to ventilation of fire stations when diesel engines replaced horses early in the last century. Traditionally, living and sleeping accommodations for on-duty firefighters have been located above apparatus floors with open stairwells and pole passages providing direct conduits for exhaust fumes and gases generated by the trucks. High ambient diesel emissions levels in fire station living quarters have been documented[26] leading to efforts to design fire stations with better separation of living quarters from apparatus bays. Many departments have also installed emissions management systems in their apparatus garages to actively vent each vehicle's exhaust. Despite availability of such solutions, many personnel are still headquartered in old construction fire stations where diesel fumes and other environmental threats persist.

Psychologic hazards
Firefighters routinely face both personal danger as well as exposure to potentially upsetting traumatic events in others. It has been proposed that these activities would predispose firefighters to post-traumatic stress disorders and other psychologic problems.[27] The need for functioning at high levels of physical exertion, even in the absence of physic danger, has been associated with psychologic strain.[28]

Biologic hazards
In their role as emergency medical responders, firefighters are at risk of exposure to blood-borne pathogens, tuberculosis, and other infectious disease agents.[29,30] Other potential biologic hazards include mold and bacterial growth from building materials.

Motor vehicle crashes
An important cause of line-of-duty fire service fatalities is motor vehicle accidents. As with many other hazards, the risk of motor vehicle accidents differs between career and volunteer departments. Career fire departments respond to a greater number of calls, and have significant losses due to apparatus accidents. Volunteer firefighters often respond to incident scenes in privately owned vehicles, and may be at increased risk for accidents due to excessive speed and crossing of intersections without sirens or warning lights. An additional cause of apparatus accidents in the volunteer fire service involves tanker trucks. Water for firefighting must be shuttled to incident scenes in rural areas without fire hydrants by water tankers. The high center of gravity and tendency of water loads to shift have contributed to incidents of tanker vehicle rollovers and volunteer fatalities.[31]

Studies of health outcomes in firefighters

A number of studies have examined patterns of morbidity and mortality in firefighters. The results of such studies must be viewed in light of at least two important epidemiologic aspects of firefighter health. First, career firefighters generally have to demonstrate above average physical stamina and strength at the time of entry into the profession. Individuals who remain actively employed as firefighters are also likely to be healthy enough to continue performing the physically demanding job duties. There is consequently a significant 'healthy worker effect' in cohorts of firefighters, and rates of illness would be expected to be lower than the general population due to this selection bias. Secondly, exposures to chemicals and particulates during firefighting operations should have decreased in recent decades due to the increased use of respiratory protection. Changes in patterns of diseases resulting from such exposures may only emerge slowly, over decades, due to the protracted latency of many of these conditions.

Musculoskeletal disorders
Acute musculoskeletal disorders are the most common type of line-of-duty injuries for firefighters, followed by lacerations and bruises. Together, these categories accounted for 77% of all reported US firefighter injuries in 2000.[7]

Muscular sprains, strains and chronic, recurring pain are also the leading causes of lost time and disability in the career fire service.[7,32] Back injuries are the most prevalent permanently disabling problem in most departments, accounting for over half of line-of-duty disability retirements of career firefighters.[33] The incidence may be higher in departments that provide emergency medical services.

Cardiovascular disease

As mentioned above, myocardial infarction and cardiac sudden death account for about half of line-of-duty deaths in firefighters. Workers' compensation statutes in many localities include a presumption that if heart disease or hypertension develops in a firefighter, a work-related association due to occupational stress is present. Cohort mortality studies have failed to consistently demonstrate that the rate of death from cardiovascular disease is greater than the general population,[34,35] although an apparent absence of the healthy worker effect has been noted in firefighter cardiovascular mortality rates.

Clearly, firefighting involves periods of extreme physical exertion, with high aerobic demands and static loads. The physiologic workload of fireground tasks may exceed 15–18 METs,[36] and typically involves asymmetric upper body work. Carbon monoxide exposures lead to tissue hypoxia and worsened cardiovascular demand. These factors alone or in combination could potentially unmask occult coronary artery disease not detected by standard cardiac stress testing. The sporadic nature of these occupational demands, however, is not sufficient to maintain either strength or aerobic fitness, and until recently little attention has been paid to the need for vigorous, ongoing, job-specific fitness programs. A study of body mass index in firefighters found that 87% were overweight, and the obesity was correlated with increased cholesterol and blood pressure.[37]

While the ranks of career firefighters thin rapidly over age 50, largely due to job-related disability retirements,[32,33] volunteer firefighters may remain active into their eighth decade, serving as fire police or otherwise assisting at emergency scenes. The data show that many of the fatal, line-of-duty heart attacks occur in these older, predominantly male volunteers. Most firefighters who die of heart attacks in the line of duty have a previous medical history of coronary artery disease.[5]

Cancer

A number of cohort studies have examined malignancy-related mortality in firefighters.[34,35,38–46] Increased standardized mortality ratios for malignant melanoma, multiple myeloma, leukemia, and cancers of the bladder, kidney, brain, and colon have been reported, although results have not been consistent among studies with respect to these cancers. Furthermore, many of these studies did not show an increasing risk with duration of employment.[3] The inconsistency of these studies must be viewed in light of the variability of individual and local exposure histories and the healthy worker effect discussed earlier. About one-third of the states in the US have presumptive occupational cancer statutes in place for firefighters.

Respiratory disorders

Despite the use of respiratory protection, firefighters continue to be at risk for respiratory effects of exposure to irritant chemicals and particulates. Severe smoke inhalation can lead to burns of the respiratory tract, pulmonary edema, and ARDS (see Chapter 19.5). Less severe exposures can cause significant irritant effects, including reactive airway dysfunction syndrome (RADS) and asthma. After the World Trade Center attacks, an increase of cough ('World Trade Center cough') and bronchial hyper-responsiveness was noted in firefighters exposed to high concentrations of particulates.[47]

In addition to airway irritation and asthma, other acute respiratory effects may result from exposure to particulates and smoke. A recent case report described acute eosinophilic pneumonia in a firefighter involved in the World Trade Center disaster.[48] An increased rate of sarcoidosis has been reported among firefighters compared to emergency medical service controls,[49] but this association remains unclear.

While respiratory hazards are also encountered in responding to hazardous materials incidents, a study of hazardous material firefighters found no excess of respiratory disease compared to other firefighters.[50]

Thermal injuries

The two main clinical results of heat and/or exposure in the fire service are burns and heat stress. For the past 10 years, burns have accounted for approximately 6% of firefighter line-of-duty injuries and fatalities.[6,32,33] First degree and small, second degree burns are probably vastly under-reported in the fire service, and are common during structural and wild land firefighting.

In recent years there have been several firefighter deaths due to heat stroke during training and emergency operations. The incidence of heat-related illness or symptomatic heat stress, like small burns, is undoubtedly underestimated by fire service statistics. Prevention of heat stress is discussed further below.

Psychologic disorders

High rates of post-traumatic symptoms have been noted in firefighter populations.[51,52] Following the 2001 World Trade Center attack, the rate of psychologic stress-related incidents among firefighter rescue workers increased 17-fold.[1] A study of firefighters with post-traumatic stress disorder complaints revealed an association of such symptoms with alcohol-related problems.[53] The efficacy of post-incident interventions aimed at reducing their psychologic impact on emergency services personnel is unproven.

Hearing loss

Despite the fact that firefighter noise exposures do not exceed OSHA limits when adjusted for intermittency, several studies have found that rates of hearing loss for firefighters are in excess of what would be expected from aging alone. Due to often asymmetric exposures such as sirens on vehicles, such hearing loss may exhibit a predominantly unilateral pattern more often than in other working populations.[54,55]

Occupational infections

Despite their risk of exposure to blood-borne pathogens, studies of public safety workers have not detected an elevated risk of hepatitis C above the background population.[56-58] Similarly, occupational transmission of HIV or tuberculosis to firefighters appears to occur infrequently.

Occupational medicine services for firefighters

Most fire departments require physician involvement in two very dissimilar roles. These are emergency medical services (EMS) medical direction and provision of occupational medical services. Some departments also include physician officer(s), referred to as fire surgeon(s) or chief medical officer(s). These individuals may serve in EMS, occupational medical, or other advisory capacity, but are distinguished by their status as sworn members of the department and their assigned responsibilities in emergency operations. In some small, rural departments, it may be necessary for a single community physician to provide both EMS medical direction and occupational medical services, although the qualifications are different, and there may be intrinsic conflicts between the roles.[59] Some fire service consensus standards require the occupational medical provider to serve on the department's safety committee.[60] This requires a level of operational involvement that has not been typical of contract medical providers, but is consistent with plant-based industrial occupational medical models.

A key aspect of providing occupational medicine services to firefighters is an awareness of existing guidelines for medical evaluations of fire service candidates and members. The International Association of Fire Fighters (IAFF)/International Association of Fire Chiefs (IAFC) Joint Labor-Management Fitness and Wellness Initiative[61] prescribes a comprehensive, annual program of medical and fitness evaluations for fire service personnel. Piloted by the fire departments in ten large, metropolitan areas in the US and Canada, this program's objectives include not only decreasing the morbidity and mortality of a career in firefighting, but also collection and analysis of the aggregate data to better define and track them. The second set of medical evaluation specifications for firefighters is published by the National Fire Protection Association (NFPA) in NFPA 1582, Standard on Medical Requirements for Fire Fighters and Information for Fire Department Physicians.[62] These standards are regularly updated, and serve as the basis for many individual health and safety programs for firefighters.

NFPA 1582 includes a model list of essential job tasks of interior structural firefighters that can be used by medical professionals to understand the demands of the job provided it has been validated by the administration of the contracting fire department. Efforts to merge the similar but distinct sets of requirements published by the IAFF/IAFC and the NFPA into a single, coherent standard are in progress.

Preplacement evaluations

In order to be eligible for hire, a prospective firefighter must generally pass a series of rigorous physical performance tests, requiring significant muscular strength and overall physical fitness. A preplacement evaluation by a clinician occurs after a candidate is accepted or hired by the department, but before beginning training or participating in emergency responses. The two main purposes for this initial evaluation are detection of any medical conditions that could interfere with the individual's ability to safely perform all of the essential job functions, and establishment of baseline values for a number of clinical parameters that should be followed throughout a firefighter's career.

Clinicians performing such preplacement examinations should attempt to get a detailed description of the duties required of firefighters or other members of fire departments, and customize the medical evaluation process to match the job. The most rigorous medical certification processes generally involve those whose essential job tasks include interior structural firefighting in urban environments, driving fire apparatus, and certain technical rescue specialists such as divers, flyers and others. In evaluating fitness for duty in such positions, the clinician must take into account the impact of any medical limitations on both the firefighter, as well as coworkers and the public.

Firefighters in departments that employ only defensive (exterior) fire suppression tactics, members of fire police squads, and command staff in many departments may not need to meet the same medical requirements as interior structural firefighters. Likewise, firefighters in small suburban jurisdictions may not need to be able to climb six or more flights of stairs carrying high-rise hose packs if there are no occupied structures more than three stories high.

A comprehensive discussion of the medical conditions that could compromise a firefighter's fitness for duty is beyond the scope of this chapter. Most of the potentially disqualifying conditions are readily recognized by medical providers, as they interfere with an individual's normal functioning, and it is clear that they could not routinely meet the physiologic demands of firefighting. The most common, problematic medical conditions confronted by fire department physicians include monocular vision, hearing deficits, diabetes mellitus, seizure disorders, and, of course, coronary artery disease. NFPA 1582 sets disqualification criteria for each of these conditions. The following brief discussion serves only to introduce some of the key issues related to these conditions.

New monocular vision results in impaired depth perception and narrows visual fields. These are significant concerns on the fireground, as awareness of surrounding hazards, and ability to negotiate ladders, crawl along floor joists and work on roofs are all essential job tasks. With training following loss of vision in one eye, firefighters can compensate for their impaired depth perception, but the loss of peripheral vision should disqualify them from driving fire department apparatus during emergency responses.

Unaided hearing in noisy conditions is a medical prerequisite for safe functioning on the fireground. There are a number of sounds at various volumes and frequencies that a firefighter must perceive on the fireground. It is essential that personnel be able to hear and communicate effectively over portable radios. They must also hear and localize calls or cries in fire rescue situations. Firefighters engaged in an interior fire attack are typically notified of the need for immediate evacuation due to untenable conditions or impending structure collapse by the sounding of apparatus air horns. All of these critical sounds must be detected and understood by firefighters in an environment of high background noise. Furthermore, this must be accomplished without the use of hearing aids, as there are currently none available that are certified to work when soaked in water, and this is a common condition during fireground operations.

Both epilepsy and insulin-requiring diabetes mellitus with a history of incapacitating hypoglycemia are associated with unpredictable episodes of impaired sensorium and functioning. Many individuals with these conditions, however, are fully capable of doing the physical work required of firefighters, although considerable clinical judgment is required to clear them for full duties. The emergency response and fireground environments may increase the risk and certainly compound the consequences of sudden incapacitation due to seizure or hypoglycemia. Shift work and night responses result in personnel fatigue while busy shifts or protracted incidents requiring personal protective equipment can result in transient dehydration and irregular food intake. Photic stimulation from flashing strobe lights together with the noise and emotional content of the fireground could serve as triggers for seizure activity. The early symptoms of hypoglycemia are indistinguishable from those experienced by many firefighters maximally exerting themselves under situational-induced catecholamine excess, and may be more likely ignored.

Coronary insufficiency or other cardiac condition that can compromise a firefighter's capacity to perform work requires comprehensive evaluation and definitive intervention. Once a diagnosis of cardiac disease has been established and treated, a candidate or firefighter can only be considered medically qualified for duty if there is no evidence of significant ongoing ischemic disease. The individual must be able to exercise to a high workload on cardiac stress testing without symptoms or electrocardiograph changes, and the left ventricular ejection fraction (LVEF) must be normal. This last requirement is a main reason for aggressive evaluation of personnel with cardiac risk factors and/or suggestive symptoms. Interventions such as revascularization, medication and modification of cardiac risk factors performed prior to actual myocardial infarction result in preservation of LVEF and may represent the difference between permanent medical disqualification and job retention for firefighters with cardiac disease.

Periodic examinations

Periodic, frequently annual, evaluations of firefighters are performed to detect early changes that could individually or in aggregate indicate interim exposures during emergency operations or failures in workplace occupational safety measures. These evaluations also screen for development of medical conditions that could compromise a firefighter's fitness for duty. OSHA requires a regular respiratory history and examination program for personnel using respirators, including SCBA, and this is conducted as part of the periodic medical evaluation in most departments. NFPA and IAFF/IAFC have developed guidelines for fire service-specific periodic examinations.

Return to duty examinations

Many fire departments also require firefighters to undergo medical evaluation prior to returning to duty following acute exposure to hazardous chemicals or certain infectious agents, after protracted absence for significant illness or injury, and prior to retirement, especially where service-connected disability may be involved. Medical and work capacity evaluation must consider the specific requirements of the individual's job. For example, following a cardiac or other systemic illness it may be advisable to refer a firefighter for exercise stress testing to ensure physiologic capacity to perform at high workloads. Prescriptive, job-specific work hardening with a physical therapist may be appropriate in some cases. It may also be necessary to recommend restricted duty for some firefighters during rehabilitation from injury or illness.

Other preventive services for firefighters

Occupational medical programs for fire departments should be more than just periodic, medical fitness-for-duty evaluations. Such programs should also help co-ordinate fitness and wellness initiatives for personnel, and should co-ordinate with fire department administrators to integrate traditional injury prevention strategies into departmental safety protocols. A physician should serve on the department's safety committee, which is mandated by NFPA 1500, Standard on Fire Department Occupational Safety.[60] In this capacity, the physician would participate in investigations of incidents that resulted in line-of-duty illness or injury to personnel, and should provide guidance for local programs requiring the use of hearing protection and vehicle restraints while riding in fire apparatus and hoods, gloves and SCBA during fire suppression.

Despite the rigorous physical fitness standards for initial hire into the fire service, many departments do not require that firefighters continue to maintain optimal physical conditioning. Inclusion of physical fitness initiatives in fire service occupational medical programs has been effective in reducing this toll in some studies.[63] Aerobic fitness is the best predictor of tolerance to heat,[64] adding even more incentive to fire departments to include physical fitness in their occupational medical programs. It is also vital that organized rehab sectors and procedures be established at fire incident scenes in order to rest and rehydrate crews, while sheltering them from environmental extremes, on a rotating basis. This will decrease the morbidity associated with uncompensable heat stress, especially in unacclimated personnel. Fire department occupational medical physicians may be contractually responsible for co-ordinating with EMS physician medical directors to develop rehab sector medical protocols.[62]

Fire department medical programs should include early access to specialty burn centers for definitive care of firefighters who sustain significant burn injuries, hyperbaric chambers for treatment of severe carbon monoxide intoxication, and other contingencies as dictated by local hazards.

Fire service occupational medical providers should maintain and compare records longitudinally in order to remain vigilant for clusters of medical conditions that may be related to a point source exposure, like a large pesticide fire, or ongoing exposure to environmental threats like asbestos, infectious organisms or noise. As in any industrial setting, such occurrences should be investigated, documented, reported as required or appropriate, and proactively mitigated where possible.

POLICE OFFICERS

As of 2000, there were 710,000 full-time sworn personnel in US state and local law enforcement agencies.[65] Police officers experience high rates of injuries and work-related fatalities. As an occupational group, however, they have not been as extensively studied as firefighters. Compared to firefighters, there is a lack of published guidelines regarding optimal occupational medicine services for police officers.

Occupational hazards of police work

Police officers, during the course of their career, encounter a variety of physical, chemical, and psychologic hazards. Many of these are similar to those faced by firefighters, and are listed in Table 18.2.2. Current understanding of the importance of these hazards and their impact on morbidity and mortality in this occupational group is limited due to a lack of carefully designed studies.

Hazard	Potential health outcome
Physical hazards	
Workplace violence	Injuries
Ergonomic stress	Back injuries
Traffic radar	? neoplasia
Chemical hazards	
Vehicle exhaust, other air pollutants	Respiratory disease
Psychologic hazards	
Traumatic events, shift work	Post-traumatic stress disorder, suicide, sleep disturbances ?Cardiovascular disease, motor vehicle accidents, sleep disturbances
Biologic hazards	
Blood-borne pathogens	Hepatitis, HIV
Respiratory pathogens	Tuberculosis, other

Table 18.2.2 Occupational hazards for police officers

Physical hazards

Police officers may experience direct physical violence such as gunshot or blunt trauma, resulting in injuries and death. In addition, pursuit of suspects may involve climbing, running and jumping, which further exposes them to risk of falls and acute musculoskeletal injuries.

Radar used for traffic surveillance is capable of emitting small amounts of microwave radiation. Actual measurements of microwave levels at the level of the testicles have indicated that exposure levels are minimal,[66] but efforts should be made to avoid excessive exposures.

Chemical exposures

Several studies have studied the effect of prolonged exposure to traffic fumes and other air pollutants for police officers engaged in traffic work. Elevated exposures to lead, polyaromatic hydrocarbons, and benzene have been reported.[67–69]

Psychologic stress

Psychologic stressors include the need for heightened awareness of potentially life-threatening dangers for prolonged periods of time, as well as the reaction to incidents of violence and other psychologically disturbing events. Such 'critical incidents' are considered to be a major risk factor for impaired psychologic functioning, including sleep disturbances and decreased functioning.[70] They are also potentially risk factors for cardiovascular conditions and motor vehicle accidents.

Infectious risks

Infectious disease risks encountered by policemen are similar to those reported for other emergency first responders, and include tuberculosis, hepatitis, and HIV exposures.[29,30,71,72]

Studies of health outcomes in police

Similar to firefighters, it is likely that studies of police cohorts are affected by both selection bias and the healthy worker effect. It has been noted that police workers differ anthropometrically from the general population, being taller and heavier than other occupational groups.[73] The level of physical conditioning required for entry into police work could select for individuals with lower overall risk for chronic disease, making it more difficult to detect occupation-specific increases in disease rates.

Cardiovascular disease

The psychologic stress experienced by police officers may lead to an increased risk of cardiovascular disease. As with firefighters, many workers' compensation statutes include presumptive compensation for heart disease or hypertensive conditions developing during the course of a police officer's career. While it seems biologically plausible that the psychologic stress of police work could lead to sympathetically mediated elevations in blood pressure and development of cardiovascular complications, there has been insufficient study of this association, and the existing studies provide conflicting results. A study of Iowa police officers found that the reported rate of cardiovascular disease was increased compared to the general population,[74] while a study of vital statistics found an increased risk of ischemic heart disease associated with the police profession.[75] A study of police officers in Rome did not demonstrate an elevated risk of cardiovascular mortality.[76]

Musculoskeletal disorders

Other occupational hazards linked to police work include back injuries and other musculoskeletal injuries due to ergonomic hazards. However, it is not clear that the overall risk and incidence of such injuries are greater than the general population. A 40-year follow-up study of a police cohort did not find an excess of death due to all accidents compared to the general population.[77]

Cancer

A recent report of a cancer cluster in police discussed the possibility of cancer effects due to police radar. Concern has been raised about risk of testicular and brain tumors due to microwave radiation from radar devices.[78] There is a lack of definite scientific evidence to support such an association (see Chapter 33)

Psychologic disorders

A study of 551 police officers found that while critical incidents predisposed to nightmares, the general work environment was associated with increased sleep disturbances compared to a reference population.[70] In a study of police work and aging, maladaptive behaviors such as gambling and drinking were associated with perceived work stresses.[79] A study of police officers who had experienced traumatic events found that 7% met criteria of post-traumatic stress disorder based on a structured interview, while 34% had post-traumatic stress symptoms.[80] Psychologic stress may also lead to an increase in the risk of suicide for police officers. A study which compared police workers to municipal workers found a relative risk of 2.65 for suicide over homicide and accidents combined;[81] however, a recent review of studies of suicide and police officers did not find strong evidence of an increased risk.[82]

Occupational medicine services for police

Clinicians providing occupational medicine services for police officers face many similar issues to their work with firefighters. There is a need for both initial preplacement screening to identify medical conditions that could interfere with the demands of the job, periodic medical surveillance for work-related conditions, and preventive programs to reduce morbidity due to medical and psychologic problems. For example, concern that acute exposure to traumatic events could lead to the development of post-traumatic stress disorder has led to the development of mental health interventions such as critical incident debriefing[83] although the effectiveness of such interventions is uncertain.[84] Ongoing programs to maintain physical fitness and reduce risk factors for cardiovascular disease have also been initiated. However, many police departments have not instituted such preventive services, and there is a dearth of published guidelines for police health and safety relative to those promulgated for firefighters.

SUMMARY

Occupational medical programs for fire and police department include initial and periodic medical evaluations to identify conditions that could interfere with a firefighter or police worker's ability to safely perform their duties. Occupational medical providers should also be actively involved in safety programs, including serving on health and safety committees and collaborating with administrators on policies and procedures relating to prevention of line-of-duty injuries and fatalities. Assistance in development of rehabilitation sector protocols, hearing conservation programs, physical fitness programs and investigating incidents involving injuries or deaths of firefighters and police, as well as clusters of suspected occupational disease, are examples of occupational medical support for these individuals. Ongoing research to better define the most important risks and adverse health outcomes for these professions will help focus future efforts toward enhanced prevention.

References

1. Anonymous. Injuries and illnesses among New York City Fire Department rescue workers after responding to the World Trade Center attacks. MMWR 2002; 51:1–5.
2. Karter MJJ. U.S. Fire Department profile through 2000. Quincy: National Fire Protection Agency, 2001.
3. Haas NS, Gochfeld M, Robson MG, Wartenburg D. Latent health effects in firefighters. Int J Occup Environ Health 2003; 9:95–103.
4. Ahrens M. The U.S. fire problem overview report: leading causes and other patterns and trends. Quincy: National Fire Protection Agency, 2001.
5. Fahy R, Leblanc PR. US firefighters fatalities. Natl Fire Protect Agency J 2001; 95:67–74.
6. FEMA. USFA firefighter fatalities in the United States in 2000. Emmitsburg: Federal Emergency Management Agency, 2001.
7. Karter MJJ, Badger SG. US firefighter injuries in 2000. Natl Fire Protect Agency J 2001; 95:50–54.
8. Fabio A, Ta M, et al. Incident-level risk factors for firefighter injuries at structural fires. J Occup Environ Med 2002; 44:1059–63.
9. Mechem CCD, Shofer FS, Jaslow D. Injuries from assaults on paramedics and firefighters in an urban emergency medical services system. Prehosp Emerg Care 2002; 6:396–401.
10. Lawson J. Firefighter's protective clothing and thermal environments of structural fire fighting. NISTIR 5804. Gaithersburg: National Institute of Standards and Technology, 1996.
11. Smith D, Petruzzello S, et al. Physiologic, psychophysical, and psychological responses of firefighters to firefighting training drill. Aviation Space Environ Med 1996; 67:1063–8.
12. NIOSH. Evaluation of noise and hearing loss in firefighters. HETA: 86-138-2017. Atlanta: NIOSH, 1990.

13. NIOSH. Evaluating risk of noise induced hearing loss for fire fighters in a metropolitan area, HETA: 88-0290-2460. Atlanta: NIOSH, 1994.

14. NIOSH. Evaluating risk of noise induced hearing loss for fire fighters, HETA: 89-0026-2495. Atlanta: NIOSH, 1995.

15. Alarie Y. Toxicity of fire smoke. Crit Rev Toxicol 2002; 32:259–89.

16. Hartzell G. Smoke toxicity in the 1990s. Adv Toxicol 1992; 3:1–22.

17. Brandt-Rauf PW, Fallon LF Jr, et al. Health hazards of fire fighters: exposure assessment. Br J Ind Med 1988; 45:606–12.

18. Brandt-Rauf PW, Cosman B, et al. Health hazards of firefighters: acute pulmonary effects after toxic exposures. Br J Ind Med 1989; 46:209–11.

19. Liou SH, Jacobson-Kram D, et al. Biologic monitoring of fire fighters: sister chromatid exchange and polycyclic aromatic hydrocarbon-DNA adducts in peripheral blood cells. Cancer Res 1989; 49:4929–35.

20. Caux C, O'Brien C, et al. Determination of firefighter exposure to polycyclic aromatic hydrocarbons and benzene during fire fighting using measurement of biologic indicators. Appl Occup Environ Hyg 2002; 17: 379–86.

21. Jankovic J, Jones W, et al. Environmental study of firefighters. Ann Occup Hyg 1991; 35:581–602.

22. Bolstad-Johnson DM, Crutchfield CD. Characterization of firefighter exposures during fire overhaul. Phoenix: Phoenix Fire Department, 2001.

23. Kales SN, Polyhronopoulos GN, et al. Medical surveillance of hazardous materials response fire fighters: a two-year prospective study. J Occup Environ Med 1997; 39:238–47.

24. Kales SN, Goldman RH. Mercury exposure: current concepts, controversies, and a clinic's experience. J Occup Environ Med 2002; 44:143–54.

25. Kelly KJ, Connelly E, et al. Assessment of health effects in New York City firefighters after exposure to polychlorinated biphenyls (PCBs) and polychlorinated dibenzofurans (PCDFs): the Staten Island Transformer Fire Health Surveillance Project. Arch Environ Health 2002; 57:282–93.

26. Froines JR, Hinds WC, et al. Exposure of firefighters to diesel emissions in fire stations. Am Ind Hyg Assoc J 1987; 48:202–7.

27. Regehr C, Hill J, et al. Individual predictors of traumatic reactions in firefighters. J Nerv Ment Dis 2000; 188:333–9.

28. Smith D, Manning T, et al. Effect of strenuous live-fire drills on cardiovascular and psychological responses of recruit firefighters. Ergonomics 2001; 44:244–54.

29. Lorentz J, Hill L, et al. Occupational needlestick injuries in a metropolitan police force. Am J Prev Med 2000; 18:146–50.

30. Kortepeter MG, Krauss MR. Tuberculosis infection after humanitarian assistance, Guantanamo Bay, 1995. Military Med 2001; 166:116–20.

31. Washburn AE, Fahy RF. 1996 Firefighter fatalities. Natl Fire Protect Agency J 1997; 91:46–60.

32. International Association of Fire Fighters. 1994 Death and injury survey. Washington: International Association of Fire Fighters, 1994.

33. International Association of Fire Fighters. Death and injury survey. Washington: International Association of Fire Fighters, 1995.

34. Guidotti T. Mortality of urban firefighters in Alberta 1927–1987. Am J Ind Med 1993; 23:921–40.

35. Tornling G, Gustavsson P, et al. Mortality and cancer incidence in Stockholm fire fighters. Am J Ind Med 1994; 25:219–28.

36. Manning JE, Griggs TR. Heart rates in fire fighters using light and heavy breathing equipment: similar near-maximal exertion in response to multiple work load conditions. J Occup Med 1983; 25:215–8.

37. Kales SN, Polyhronopoulos GN, et al. Correlates of body mass index in hazardous materials firefighters. J Occup Environ Med 1999; 41:589–95.

38. Heyer N, Weiss NS, et al. Cohort mortality study of Seattle fire fighters: 1945–1983. Am J Ind Med 1990; 17:493–504.

39. Howe GR, Burch JD. Fire fighters and risk of cancer: an assessment and overview of the epidemiologic evidence. Am J Epidemiol 1990; 132:1039–50.

40. Beaumont JJ, Chu GS, et al. An epidemiologic study of cancer and other causes of mortality in San Francisco firefighters. Am J Ind Med 1991; 19:357–72.

41. Demers PA, Vaughan TL, et al. A case-control study of multiple myeloma and occupation. Am J Ind Med 1993; 23:629–39.

42. Giles G, Staples M, et al. Cancer incidence in Melbourne Metropolitan Fire Brigade members, 1980–1989. Health Reports 1993; 5:33–8.

43. Aronson KJ, Tomlinson GA, et al. Mortality among fire fighters in metropolitan Toronto. Am J Ind Med 1994; 26:89–101.

44. Demers PA, Checkoway H, et al. Cancer incidence among firefighters in Seattle and Tacoma, Washington (United States). Cancer Causes Control 1994; 5:129–35.

45. Golden AL, Markowitz SB, et al. The risk of cancer in firefighters. Occup Med 1995; 10:803–20.

46. Baris D, Garrity TJ, et al. Cohort mortality study of Philadelphia firefighters. Am J Ind Med 2001; 39:463–76.

47. Prezant DJ, Weiden M, et al. Cough and bronchial responsiveness in firefighters at the World Trade Center site [comment]. N Engl J Med 2002; 347:806–15.

48. Rom WN, Weiden M, et al. Acute eosinophilic pneumonia in a New York City firefighter exposed to World Trade Center dust. Am J Respir Crit Care Med 2002; 166:797–800.

49. Prezant DJ, Dhala A, et al. The incidence, prevalence, and severity of sarcoidosis in New York City firefighters. Chest 1999; 116:1183–93.

50. Kales SN, Mendoza PJ, et al. Spirometric surveillance in hazardous materials firefighters: does hazardous materials duty affect lung function? J Occup Environ Med 2001; 43:1114–20.

51. Wagner D, Heinrichs M, et al. Prevalence of symptoms of posttraumatic stress disorder in German professional firefighters. Am J Psychiatry 1998; 155:1727–32.

52. Corneil W, Beaton R, et al. Exposure to traumatic incidents and prevalence of posttraumatic stress symptomatology in urban firefighters in two countries. J Occup Health Psychol 1999; 4:131–41.

53. McFarlane AC. Epidemiological evidence about the relationship between PTSD and alcohol abuse: the nature of the association. Addict Behav 1998; 23:813–25.

54. Tubbs RL. Noise and hearing loss in firefighting. Occup Med 1995; 10:843–56.

55. Kales SN, Freyman RL, et al. Firefighters' hearing: a comparison with population databases from the International Standards Organization. J Occup Environ Med 2001; 43:650 6.

56. Upfal MJ, Naylor P, et al. Hepatitis C screening and prevalence among urban public safety workers. J Occup Environ Med 2001; 43:402–11.

57. Averhoff FM, Moyer LA, et al. Occupational exposures and risk of hepatitis B virus infection among public safety workers. J Occup Environ Med 2002; 44:591–6.

58. Rischitelli G, McCauley L, et al. Hepatitis C in urban and rural public safety workers. J Occup Environ Med 2002; 44:568–73.

59. Bogucki MS. Medical support for fire service. Proceedings of the Symposium with Recommendations to the US Fire Administration. Prehosp Emerg Care 1997; 1:107–13.

60. NFPA. NFPA 1500 Standard on fire department occupational safety and health program. Quincy: National Fire Protection Agency, 2002.

61. IAFF/IAFC. Fire Service joint labor management wellness-fitness initiative. Fairfax, International Association of Fire Chiefs, 2000.

62. NFPA. NFPA 1582 Standard on medical requirements for fire fighters and information for fire department physicians. Quincy: National Fire Protection Agency, 2000.

63. Cady LD Jr, Thomas PC, et al. Program for increasing health and physical fitness of fire fighters. J Occup Med 1985; 27:110–4.

64. Kenney WL, Lewis DA, et al. A simple exercise test for the prediction of relative heat tolerance. Am Ind Hyg Assoc J 1986; 47:203–6.
65. Adams DB, Reynolds LE. Bureau of Justice Statistics 2002. At a glance. Washington DC, Department of Justice, Office of Justice Programs, Bureau of Justice Statistics, NCJ194449, 2002.
66. Fink JM, Wagner JP, et al. Microwave emissions from police radar. Am Ind Hyg Assoc J 1999; 60:770–6.
67. Crebelli R, Tomei F, et al. Exposure to benzene in urban workers: environmental and biologic monitoring of traffic police in Rome. Occup Environ Med 2001; 58:165–71.
68. Galati R, Zijno A, et al. Detection of antibodies to the benzo(a)pyrene diol epoxide-DNA adducts in sera from individuals exposed to low doses of polycyclic aromatic hydrocarbons. J Exp Clin Cancer Res 2001; 20:359–64.
69. Mortada WI, Sobh MA, et al. Study of lead exposure from automobile exhaust as a risk for nephrotoxicity among traffic policemen. Am J Nephrol 2001; 21:274–9.
70. Neylan TC, Metzler TJ, et al. Critical incident exposure and sleep quality in police officers. Psychosom Med 2002; 64:345–52.
71. Abel S, Cesaire R, et al. Occupational transmission of human immunodeficiency virus and hepatitis C virus after a punch. Clin Infect Dis 2000; 31:1494–5.
72. Rischitelli G, Harris J, et al. The risk of acquiring hepatitis B or C among public safety workers: a systematic review. Am J Prev Med 2001; 20:299–306.
73. Hsiao H, Long D, et al. Anthropometric differences among occupational groups. Ergonomics 2002; 45:136–52.
74. Franke WD, Collins SA, et al. Cardiovascular disease morbidity in an Iowa law enforcement cohort, compared with the general Iowa population. J Occup Environ Med 1998; 40:441–4.
75. Tuchsen F, Andersen O, et al. Occupation and ischemic heart disease in the European Community: a comparative study of occupations at potential high risk. Am J Ind Med 1996; 30:407–14.
76. Franke WD, Anderson DF. Relationship between physical activity and risk factors for cardiovascular disease among law enforcement officers. J Occup Med 1994; 36:1127–32.
77. Violanti JM, Vena JE, et al. Mortality of a police cohort: 1950–1990. Am J Ind Med 1998; 33:366–73.
78. van Netten C, Brands RH, et al. Cancer cluster among police detachment personnel. Environ Internat 2003; 28:567–72.
79. Gershon RR, Lin S, et al. Work stress in aging police officers. J Occup Environ Med 2002; 44:160–7.
80. Carlier IV, Lamberts RD, et al. Risk factors for posttraumatic stress symptomatology in police officers: a prospective analysis. J Nerv Mental Dis 1997; 185:498–506.
81. Violanti JM, Vena JE, et al. Suicides, homicides, and accidental death: a comparative risk assessment of police officers and municipal workers. Am J Ind Med 1996; 30:99–104.
82. Hem E, Berg AM, et al. Suicide in police – a critical review. Suicide & Life-Threatening Behav 2001; 31:224–33.
83. Mitchell AM, Sakraida TJ, et al. Critical incident stress debriefing: implications for best practice. Disaster Management Response 2003; 1:46–51.
84. Carlier IV, Voerman AE, et al. The influence of occupational debriefing on post-traumatic stress symptomatology in traumatized police officers. Br J Med Psychol 2000; 73:87–98.

Section 3

Occupational Diseases and Injuries

Chapter 19
Diseases of the Lung and Pleura

19.1 Approach to the Patient/Diagnostic Methods

Nargues A Weir, Mridu Gulati, Carrie A Redlich

INTRODUCTION

This chapter provides an overview of the different modalities available to assess patients with potential occupational or environmental respiratory illnesses. Regardless of the suspect etiology, a respiratory disease or symptoms should be characterized using the essential instruments of a pulmonary evaluation, including special features of the history and physical examination. Crucial to the assessment is also the understanding and implementation of radiography and lung function assessment. The chapters following will provide detailed discussions of specific pulmonary diseases of occupational or environmental etiology. This chapter will introduce the reader to the fundamental tools used to evaluate such respiratory diseases. Several recent publications provide a more detailed discussion of radiographic, physiologic, and pathologic methods used to evaluate occupational and environmental lung disorders.[1-5]

HISTORY

As with any occupational or environmental disease, the history is critical in evaluating a patient with a respiratory disorder. The causal occupational or environmental agent may be obvious from the initial assessment, but it is not uncommon to have a non-specific respiratory complaint without an evident etiology. The clinical history is important in better characterizing the disorder and its progression. A thorough occupational history should chronicle previous jobs, job titles, descriptions of job activities, years of employment, and potential toxins at each job, with a more detailed focus on the jobs most likely pertinent to the pulmonary problem. The duration and severity of the respiratory complaints, along with the presence of associated symptoms, should be determined.

As with other occupational and environmental diseases the temporal relationship between exposures of concern and symptoms or disease is critical. For most pneumoconioses the onset of respiratory illness occurs many years after the onset of exposure. Change in symptoms during vacations or weekends should be documented. Details of personal protective gear should be noted, with attention to proper fitting and appropriate use of equipment such as respiratory protective devices, as well as a description of the general ventilation and overall hygiene in the workplace. It is helpful to ask patients whether they believe their respiratory disorder is related to their job or environment. Presence of similar symptoms among coworkers should also be pursued.

In addition to the work history, an environmental history including the home environment and hobbies should be explored for potential exposures that may cause or exacerbate the respiratory disorder. The presence of pets, travel history, tobacco use, and military history should also be determined.

Obtaining a thorough history is not always possible. The latency of many respiratory diseases due to occupational exposures can be quite long, making it difficult to document important past clinical or exposure information. Medical records can be of assistance in such cases. These records may establish onset and duration of symptoms or potentially clarify the work history, as well as providing objective data such as previous radiographs and physiologic tests. This information may clarify temporal associations and providing a comparison for any current abnormalities found during the evaluation of a respiratory disorder. All of these clues may play an important role in establishing cause.

PHYSICAL EXAMINATION

As with other occupational or environmental diseases the physical findings in the patient with respiratory disease of occupational or environmental etiology rarely differ from the examination performed in non-exposure settings. The physical examination typically is most useful in detecting non-occupational disorders that may be causative of or contributing to the patient's respiratory condition, such as cardiac disease, connective tissue disorders or sinusitis. In addition to the lung and chest exam, particular attention should be given to the heart, skin, mucosal surfaces, and extremities. The physical exam can also help assess for severity of disease, i.e., breathlessness, cyanosis or clubbing.

Chest radiographs

Conventional chest radiography

Radiography is critical in the evaluation of the patient with respiratory complaints. Conventional chest radiography is the initial step in the radiographic assessment and can evaluate the lung parenchyma, pleura, hilum, and mediastinum. Patients with airway disease, such as asthma, rhinitis or bronchitis, as well as patients with early interstitial lung disease may have normal radiographs. Parenchymal opacities are a common feature of the pneumoconioses and other environmentally induced lung disorders, as well as non-occupational disorders.

Due to the variability in radiographic parenchymal and pleural changes, the International Labor Organization (ILO) classification was adopted to provide a standardized uniform system of reading chest radiographs and has enabled increased inter- and intra-observer reliability in epidemiologic investigations and in the clinical evaluation of patients. In the United States accreditation for the ILO classification is administered by NIOSH. The most current guidelines were adopted in 2000.[1] The ILO classification relies mainly on the posteroanterior radiograph at full inspiration on a 14 × 17 inch film and requires that readers have available to them the standard set of radiographs for comparison. Additional views may be obtained to aid the clinical assessment; however, these films are not incorporated into the classification. Film quality is also evaluated and graded as part of the system: grade 1 corresponds with excellent technique and quality, and grade 4 signifies an unreadable film.

Parenchymal opacities are categorized by size, shape, profusion, and extent of involvement. Size of the opacity is detailed as small, measuring up to 1 cm in diameter, or large, measuring greater than 1 cm. Small opacities are further subclassified according to their shape. Rounded opacities are represented by *p*, *q*, and *r* if they are up to 1.5 mm, 1.5–3 mm, and 3–10 mm in diameter respectively. Small irregular opacities are represented by *s*, *t*, and *u* to correspond with reticular or linear opacities of up to 1.5 mm, 1.5–3 mm, and 3–10 mm respectively. Not infrequently, there is more than one type of opacity seen on a radiograph. The system allows for two letters (e.g., *s/p*) describing the primary or prominent opacities, as well as the secondary opacities observed.

The classification arbitrarily divides each lung into three zones. The system allows designation of which zones are affected by the opacities, and the scoring system averages those zones most heavily involved. A profusion score indicates the concentration or aggregation of the opacities and is determined by comparison with a standard set of radiographs. The four main categories depicting profusion (0, 1, 2, 3) range from normal (category 0) to most affected (category 3), from which a 12-point scale is derived, ranging from 0/c (less than the profusion of a standard 0/0 radiograph) to 3/+ (more than the profusion on the standard 3/3 radiograph) (Figs 19.1.1 to 19.1.3). The following grid is used to score radiographs:

0/–	0/0	0/1
1/0	1/1	1/2
2/1	2/2	2/3
3/2	3/3	3/+

Large opacities (> 10 mm) are designated as category A, B or C depending on size. Large opacities usually are seen only in the setting of silica and coal dust exposure (Fig. 19.1.4).

Pleural abnormalities are also scored by the ILO classification. This is particularly important in the assessment of asbestos exposure. These abnormalities are characterized according to thickness, location (focal or diffuse), extent, presence or absence of calcification, and presence or absence of an effusion. Also, involvement of the chest wall, diaphragm or costophrenic angle is noted. The extent of

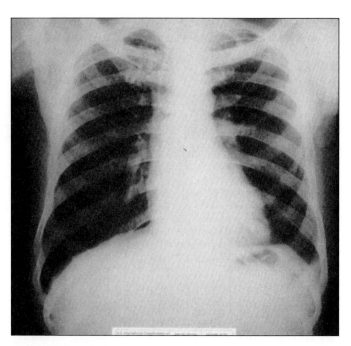

Figure 19.1.1: Category 1/1 film demonstrating small rounded opacities predominantly in upper lung fields. (Courtesy of ILO U/C International Classification of Radiographs of Pneumoconiosis.)

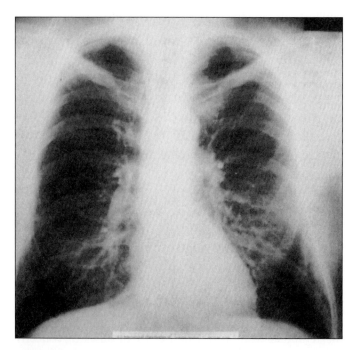

Figure 19.1.2: Category 1/1 film of small irregular opacities predominantly in lower lung fields. (Courtesy of ILO U/C International Classification of Radiographs of Pneumoconiosis.)

involvement and degree of pleural calcification are scored, with grade 3 being the most severe changes.

Computed tomography

While the plain chest radiograph remains an essential part of a diagnostic evaluation of occupational lung disease, computed tomography (CT) can provide clinicians with additional key information in selected patients. The CT

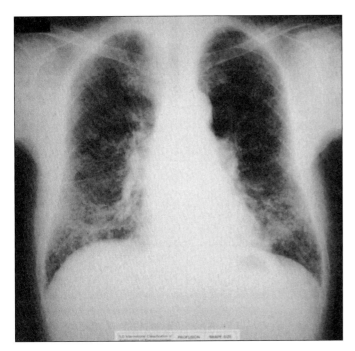

Figure 19.1.3: Category 3/3 film of small irregular opacities throughout both lung fields. (Courtesy of ILO U/C International Classification of Radiographs of Pneumoconiosis.)

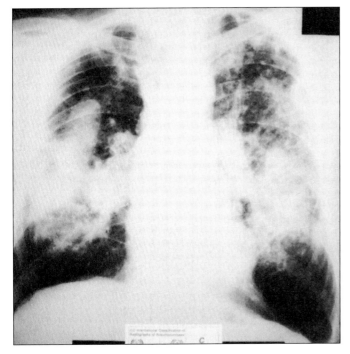

Figure 19.1.4: Chest x-ray study demonstrating progressive massive fibrosis (category C large opacities) and egg shell calcification of lymph nodes. (Courtesy of ILO U/C International Classification of Radiographs of Pneumoconiosis.)

scan findings of pneumoconioses such as asbestosis or silicosis typically follow the same patterns as seen on plain chest radiographs. However, the higher resolution of CT can provide a more sensitive and specific radiologic assessment of various abnormalities, including diffuse interstitial lung disease, lung masses, mediastinal and hilar lesions, and

pleural abnormalities. Certain findings on CT may provide diagnostic clues, but less commonly confirm a specific occupational etiology not suspected by plain chest radiograph. CT can also identify diseases that can coexist, such as emphysema and interstitial fibrosis.

Conventional CT is performed on the supine patient during an inspiratory breath-hold. Cross-sectional images are taken at 10 mm intervals and are collimated from the apex to the base. Two-dimensional imaging enables radiologists to more accurately and confidently identify the presence of abnormalities. High resolution computed tomography (HRCT) further modifies conventional CT by utilizing thin collimation (1–2 mm thickness). These slices are reconstructed at high spatial frequency, reducing the artifact seen with conventional CT. This method provides for sharper resolution and superior characterization of parenchymal abnormalities and is preferred over conventional CT in assessing diffuse lung disease. In addition, prone and end-expiratory HRCT images may further clarify early findings of interstitial lung disease and air trapping found in airways disease.

Radiologists use specific terminology to describe pulmonary abnormalities involving the alveoli, airways, and interstitium. For example, ground glass refers to a hazy opacity that does not obscure associated pulmonary vessels and is typically seen with an acute alveolitis, such as hypersensitivity pneumonitis (Fig. 19.1.5). Alveolar consolidation typically is more localized and obscures the underlying vascular structures. CT can define the extent of consolidation but is less useful in distinguishing the underlying cause. Honeycombing refers to extensive cystic radiolucencies and fibrosis, and typically is seen in advanced stages of interstitial lung diseases such as idiopathic pulmonary fibrosis or asbestosis (Fig. 19.1.6). CT findings of a specific disease can vary greatly, depending in part on the stage and severity of the disease. For example, a variety of HRCT patterns are associated with hypersensitivity pneumonitis including

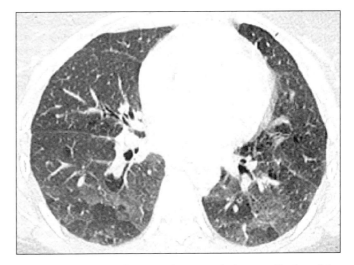

Figure 19.1.5: HRCT demonstrating ground glass opacification of the lungs in a patient with acute hypersensitivity pneumonitis. (From King TE. Classification and clinical manifestations of hypersensitivity pneumonitis (extrinsic allergic alveolitis). In: UpToDate, Rose BD (ed), Wellesley, MA, 2004. © 2004 UpToDate, Inc. For more information visit www.uptodate.com)

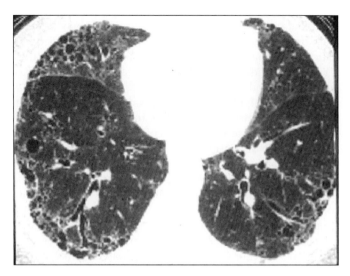

Figure 19.1.6: HRCT demonstrating interstitial pulmonary fibrosis with marked honeycombing and traction bronchiectasis in both lobes. The more peripheral regions of the lower lobes are typically involved. (From Stark P. High resolution computed tomography of the lungs. In: UpToDate, Rose BD (ed), Wellesley, MA, 2004. © 2004 UpToDate, Inc. For more information visit www.uptodate.com

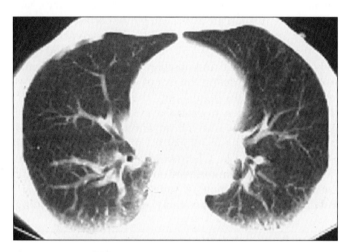

Figure 19.1.7: HRCT scan in a patient with asbestosis showing bibasilar opacities and thickened intralobular lines. There is a small pleural plaque in the right anterior hemithorax, which supports the diagnosis of asbestosis. (From Stark P. High resolution computed tomography of the lungs. In: UpToDate, Rose BD (ed), Wellesley, MA, 2004. © 2004 UpToDate, Inc. For more information visit www.uptodate.com

diffuse ground glass, multiple small nodules, honeycombing, and emphysema (discussed further in Chapter 19.6).

CT scans are especially useful in identifying early radiologic abnormalities in workers with normal chest radiographs. Thickened intralobular lines, subpleural curvilinear lines, and basilar abnormalities can identify early fibrosis in asbestos workers with normal chest radiographs[6] (Fig. 19.1.7). In a study of former coal miners with normal chest radiographs, more than half of the coal miners had nodules on HRCT.[1] The sensitivity of HRCT is substantially better than plain chest radiographs in hypersensitivity pneumonitis.[7,8] CT is also more sensitive than chest radiography in detecting emphysema,[9] and can identify mixed obstructive and interstitial processes.

Conventional CT may have a role in lung cancer screening. The National Cancer Institute sponsored trial of CT for lung cancer screening will provide further information regarding the utility of this screening modality in smokers with occupational exposures.[10]

Investigators have yet to establish a standard similar to the ILO classification system for HRCT. However, inter- and intra-observer agreement is superior[6] to conventional chest radiography. Several scoring systems have been proposed.[11,12] How well HRCT reflects lung function likely varies, but studies suggest that HRCT correlates with lung function in both obstructive and restrictive diseases.[12–14]

Although an important diagnostic modality, CT and HRCT have not replaced the normal chest radiograph. Despite limitations, chest radiography is widely available, relatively inexpensive, and remains the cornerstone of surveillance and screening programs, as well as being the initial imaging modality in evaluating clinical patients.

Positron emission tomography

While not an integral diagnostic modality in the assessment of occupational pulmonary disease, positron emission tomography (PET) may have an increasingly important role in the evaluation of malignancies related to work exposure. Chest radiography and CT are useful in the primary detection of nodules, but PET scan may better differentiate malignant from benign lesions. Subjects are injected with fluoro-deoxy-glucose (FDG), which is taken up by metabolically active lesions such as tumors. While PET can be more accurate in identifying cancer than CT, it has limitations.[15,16] PET's accuracy decreases significantly with smaller lesions (less than 10 mm) and with less metabolically active tumors. Inflammatory process can result in increased FDG uptake, raising the concern of false-positive results. Therefore, while the role of PET in the evaluation of suspicious lesions continues to evolve, its current application only complements the use of CT scans.[15]

Summary

In conclusion, radiography of the chest is a key part of the evaluation of occupational and environmental lung diseases. Familiarity with the different modalities, their strengths and shortcomings will help the provider make the appropriate test selection. Caution must be exercised, however, in the interpretation of these radiographs, and the radiography information should be synthesized with the clinical, occupational, physiologic, and other data obtained.

Physiologic assessment

Spirometry

The measurement of lung function is an important tool in the evaluation and management of patients with potential occupational and environmental lung diseases, impairment and disability assessments, as well as in the screening and surveillance of exposed workers. This important topic is discussed in greater detail in several recent publications.[2–5,17,18] The use of pulmonary function testing to assess pulmonary impairment is discussed in Chapter 8. Spirometry, a measure of dynamic lung volumes based on the forced vital capacity maneuver, is most commonly performed. The forced vital capacity (FVC), the forced expiratory volume in one second (FEV_1), and the FEV_1/FVC ratio are the measures most commonly evaluated from the FVC maneuver. Peak expiratory flow rate (PEFR), maximal mid-expiratory flow (MMEF or FEF_{25-75}) are also typically recorded. Spirometry can be performed in most outpatient settings as long as attention is paid to technique, instrument calibration, qualified technicians, equipment maintenance, and proper recording of collected data. Similar standards for the performance, standardization, and interpretation of spirometry are published by the American Thoracic Society and the European Respiratory Society.[19-22]

Interpretation of the test depends on the quality of the test, normative values, and criteria for determining abnormality. Reference values are typically derived from large population-based data sets, which traditionally included non-smoking, healthy Caucasians. Spirometry values are corrected for age, height, gender, and race. At extremes of height and age, these population values are less representative of the normal variation present. Individuals of Asian or African origin on average have lower FEV_1 and FVC than European and North American whites after adjusting for other factors, but normative data for various ethnic groups are limited. The third National Health and Nutrition Examination Survey (NHANES III) provided population data for more than 7000 healthy, non-smoking African-Americans, Mexican-Americans, and Caucasians as a more accurate estimation of normal spirometric values.[23] The American Thoracic Society (ATS) and American College of Occupational and Environmental Medicine (ACOEM) recommend using these reference values if possible. Population data for Asian-Americans and other ethnic groups are more limited. Underlying lung disease as well as suboptimal test performance can result in unacceptable spirograms and greater intra-subject test variability.[24]

Spirometry measurements are used to distinguish obstructive from restrictive or mixed disorders. The ratio of FEV_1/FVC is the best indicator of the presence of airflow obstruction. Because the FVC may be reduced with severe obstruction (due to trapping of gas), the severity of the obstruction cannot be reliably determined from this ratio. FEV_1 and FVC measurements that are > 80% of predicted values and FEV_1/FVC ratio > 70–75% are typically considered normal. However, the use of a lower limit of normal based on 5th percentile rather than a fixed cutoff is recommended by the ATS.[22] The severity of the obstruction is assessed by the degree of reduction in FEV_1. The pattern of reduced FEV_1 and FVC with a normal FEV_1/FVC ratio is suggestive of restrictive impairment. Reduction in MMEF or FEF_{25-75} is sensitive for mild airflow obstruction, but not very specific nor reproducible, and therefore the ATS does not recommend diagnosing obstruction solely on the basis of a reduced mid-flow rate.[22]

The flow–volume spirograms obtained during spirometry are also very helpful in determining the presence and severity of disease. Obstructive disorders result in concavity of the expiratory loop, with prolonged expiratory time seen in more advanced disease. Restrictive disorders result in a typical narrow, compressed spirogram. Information regarding the presence of upper airway obstructions such as vocal cord dysfunction can also be obtained from flow–volume loops. The interpretation of the respiratory spirograms is complementary to the evaluation of spirometry measurements.

In the setting of obstructive disease, reversibility of airflow obstruction can be assessed by performing postbronchodilator spirometry. A 12% increase in FEV_1 and a 200 ml increase in either FEV_1 or FVC are considered as a clinically significant bronchodilator response.[25] Bronchodilator response indicates airway hyper-responsiveness or asthma.

Lung volumes

Lung volume measurements are useful in assessing diseases with altered lung volumes, such as interstitial diseases or neuromuscular disease. Spirometry provides a reliable estimate of the vital capacity, but is unable to measure the volume remaining in the lungs at the end of expiration. Lung volumes can be measured using gas-dilution techniques or body plethysmography. The former is more commonly used and involves the helium or nitrogen washout methods to calculate the patient's functional residual capacity (FRC), which is used to determine the total lung capacity (TLC). Body plethysmography involves a chamber in which the patient sits; lung volumes are measured as a function of the pressure the patient generates against a closed mouthpiece, and provides a more accurate measure of lung volumes in severe obstructive disease, especially in bullous emphysema. However, availability is limited due to the space necessary for the equipment and the expense. TLC is used to both diagnose and assess the severity of restrictive disorders. Lung volumes can also document air trapping and hyperinflation.

Gas transfer

The gas exchange capacity of the lung can be measured using several techniques. Oxygen's ability to cross the alveolar–capillary membrane and be carried by blood is dependent on several factors, including surface area available in the lung, the thickness of the alveolar–capillary membrane, blood flow to the lung, and the hemoglobin concentration of the blood. The diffusion capacity of carbon monoxide (DLCO), a gas with much higher affinity for binding to hemoglobin, is most commonly measured since CO transfer is limited by diffusion only. The DLCO is usually determined by single-breath techniques. The DLCO is adjusted for hemoglobin concentration and alveolar volume. In its 1995 spirometry update the ATS reiterated that reference values for DLCO are problematic.[26] The lack of uniformity is due to large differences between population data available for comparison. Therefore, the ATS recommends using reference equations that are appropriate for the population being studied.[26] Finally, DLCO measurements will vary according to which calculation is utilized by the laboratory. Consistency in use of one method will lead to reproducible results.

A reduced DLCO can be an early manifestation of interstitial lung disease, such as asbestosis, silicosis or hypersensitivity pneumonitis. This reduction may precede other evidence of restrictive disease, making it more sensitive than lung volume or chest radiography in early disease.[13] Decreased DLCO also occurs with severe obstructive disease, pulmonary vascular disease, smoking, and anemia, among other causes. Increased DLCO is seen with asthma exacerbations, pulmonary hemorrhage, polycythemia, and altitude, in addition to other etiologies.

Gas transfer can also be assessed by measuring oxygenation by non-invasive oximetry or by arterial blood gas sampling. The former involves a near-infrared light that measures oxyhemoglobin and can reliably report arterial oxygen saturation within 3–5% of actual saturation. Its accuracy decreases below 70% saturation, and it cannot distinguish between oxyhemoglobin and other reduced hemoglobins. In the outpatient setting, it is a simple method of estimating gas transfer in the resting or ambulating patient. Arterial blood gas sampling is helpful in accurately measuring the partial pressure and saturation of oxygen, but involves arterial puncture. It also allows for calculation of the alveolar–arterial oxygen gradient and carbon dioxide.

Peak flow measurement

Peak expiratory flow rates (PEFRs) can be helpful in evaluating patients with possible work-related asthma and can be measured easily using portable inexpensive PEF meters (discussed further in Chapter 19.2). Serial PEFR measurements can be used to document increased diurnal variation (typically greater than 20%) and changes in PEFR in relationship to exposures. Optimum length and frequency of measurements at and away from work is unclear and has to take into account practical considerations. Careful patient education and compliance are essential. Three measurements should be recorded for each occasion, and concomitant medication use, symptoms, and exposures noted in the log. The patient has to still be in the workplace of concern, and clear improvement away from exposure is more likely earlier in the course of the disease. At least four daily measurements for a minimum of 2–3 weeks are likely necessary to be useful, including several consecutive days away from work, which can be problematic.

Problems with the use of PEFRs can include compliance, reproducibility, proper technique in performing the maneuver, and falsification of records.[25,27] Electronic devices can address many of these issues but are not widely available and are more costly. In addition, there are no uniformly accepted criteria for the interpretation of PEFRs, although qualitative interpretation has been shown to be comparable to quantitative analyses.[28] Computer programs are being developed to assist with interpretation.[25] Despite these limitations, careful records showing a clear pattern of work-related changes in PEFRs strongly support a diagnosis of work-related asthma, and have been found to have better sensitivity and specificity than spirometry.[29] Given that specific inhalation challenge is rarely available or feasible, PEFRs are usually the best hope of documenting work-related changes in lung function.

Cardiopulmonary exercise testing

Cardiopulmonary exercise testing (CPET) has a potentially informative role in the functional assessment of selected patients with suspected occupational respiratory disorders when specific questions persist after more standard cardiac and pulmonary evaluation. CPET can help evaluate unexplained dyspnea and exercise intolerance, and distinguish cardiac from respiratory causes of dyspnea. CPET can also provide objective data quantifying the degree of impairment. The indications for, methodology, and interpretation of CPET were thoroughly reviewed in a recent American Thoracic Society/American College of Chest Physicians statement on CPET.[30]

During CPET, a subject is asked to exercise on a cycle or treadmill at increasing work loads while electrocardiogram, heart rate, blood pressure, O_2 uptake from the air, and CO_2 output from the body and oxygenation (arterial blood gas measurements or oximetry) are monitored. Evaluation of the physiologic data derived from CPET can usually clarify whether the patient's exercise is limited by cardiac or pulmonary abnormalities or deconditioning. For example, Agostoni evaluated dyspnea in asbestos workers with a high prevalence of asbestosis (over 50%) and reported that almost 40% of the workers had a cardiac rather than respiratory exercise limitation.[31] The ATS and ACCP have endorsed a set of guidelines using pulmonary function testing as well as cardiopulmonary testing to classify the level of functional impairment based on VO_{2max}.[30] For most patients with occupational lung disorders respiratory impairment can be assessed with routine pulmonary function testing. CPET may be indicated when such testing does not appear to explain the patient's symptoms or adequately assess the degree of impairment. CPET is labor intensive and costly and should be used only when there is a clear indication.

Bronchoprovocation testing

Bronchoprovocation testing can provide useful information in the evaluation of patients with asthma or asthma-like symptoms (discussed further in Chapter 19.2). Methacholine or histamine challenge testing to assess non-specific bronchial hyper-responsiveness importantly can clarify the diagnosis of asthma in patients with normal spirometry. Serial changes in bronchial hyper-responsiveness in relationship to work can be used to support a diagnosis of occupational asthma. Specific inhalation testing is considered the gold standard for the diagnosis of immune mediated occupational asthma, but is rarely performed in most countries due to technical, financial, and practical considerations (discussed in Chapter 19.2).

Immunology testing

Immunology tests that demonstrate specific IgE antibodies or positive skin reaction to high molecular weight sensitizing agents can be helpful in confirming exposure and demonstrating immunologic sensitization to a specific agent, but are frequently not available, and by themselves do not confirm a diagnosis of occupational asthma (discussed further in Chapter 19.2). Such testing is typically less helpful with small molecular weight sensitizing agents, and has no role in the evaluation of RADS or irritant-aggravated asthma. Specific IgG antibodies in the evaluation of suspected hypersensitivity pneumonitis or asthma are typically found in asymptomatic exposed workers as well as those with disease, and more likely reflect exposure in most settings (see Chapters 19.3 and 19.6). However, they can be helpful in confirming sufficient exposure to the agent to generate a humoral immune response.

Bronchoscopy and surgical lung biopsy

Bronchoscopy and surgical lung biopsy can aid in the investigation of occupational and environmental interstitial disorders under certain circumstances. Several recent publications review the mineralogic analysis of lung tissue and bronchoalveolar lavage (BAL) specimens in greater detail.[3,4,32] Transbronchial biopsies yield small tissue samples that are most helpful in diagnosing granulomatous interstitial diseases, such as chronic beryllium disease or hypersensitivity pneumonitis. Such biopsies provide only limited amounts of lung tissue architecture for pathologic examination or mineralogic analysis. BAL cell analysis can aid in the evaluation of selected disorders such as hypersensitivity pneumonitis or chronic beryllium disease, for which the beryllium lymphocyte proliferation test is diagnostic (see Chapters 19.6 and 19.7).

Transbronchial biopsy and bronchoalveolar lavage are often insufficient to make a pathologic diagnosis of occupational lung disease. Lung biopsy is typically not needed when there is a clear exposure history and the clinical and radiographic presentation is characteristic of the pneumoconiosis caused by that exposure. However, lung biopsy can be helpful when the history is unclear, the individual is unaware of exposure or the presentation is atypical. In obtaining a lung biopsy, thoracoscopic or open procedures can be performed, with the former being less invasive. Lung biopsy provides superior size specimens for histologic and mineralogic analysis. The information obtained should be used in conjunction with the exposure history and other information known concerning the patient. Physicians should communicate in advance with pathologists to ensure that specialized analytic techniques are applied. At times pathologic examination may suggest an unanticipated diagnosis. For example, the presence of poorly formed non-necrotizing granulomas and lymphocytic interstitial infiltrates characteristic of hypersensitivity pneumonitis in a patient presumed to have usual interstitial pneumonitis may uncover unsuspected exposure to an agent associated with hypersensitivity pneumonitis.[33]

Light microscopy will demonstrate the pathologic changes, such as fibrosis or honeycombing, and can detect large, colored particles such as asbestos bodies or coal. Iron staining can better detect asbestos bodies. Light polarization techniques will detect birefringent silica particles, talc, and mica. X-ray diffraction and atomic absorption spectroscopy can detect minerals and elements such as different forms of silica, beryllium, titanium, and aluminum. Electron microscopy may help identify inhaled particulates and chemically similar fibers such as talc and anthophyllite asbestos, and can also provide important quantitative data.[32]

These techniques have limitations. The presence of a specific substance confirms exposure to that substance but does not prove causation. The concentration found in the lung may not reflect actual exposure, depending on issues such as clearance, durability, and solubility of the substance. Quantitative advanced techniques are not routinely available and standardization of techniques or 'normative' values are frequently limited. Regardless of these limitations, histopathologic examination and mineralogic assessment of lung biopsies may be invaluable in the diagnostic workup of suspected occupational lung disease.

References

1. Akira M. High-resolution CT in the evaluation of occupational and environmental disease. Radiol Clin North Am 2002; 40:43–59.
2. Chupp GL, ed. Pulmonary function testing. Philadelphia: WB Saunders, 2001.
3. Harber P, Schenker MB, Balmes JR, eds. Occupational and environmental respiratory disease. St. Louis: Mosby-Year Book, 1996.
4. Hendrick DJ, Burge PS, Beckett WS, Churg A, eds. Occupational disorders of the lung: recognition, management and prevention. London: WB Saunders, 2002.
5. Townsend MC. ACOEM position statement. Spirometry in the occupational setting. American College of Occupational and Environmental Medicine. J Occup Environ Med 2000; 42:228–45.
6. Begin R, Ostiguy G, Filion R, Colman N, Bertrand P. Computed tomography in the early detection of asbestosis. Br J Ind Med 1993; 50:689–98.
7. Akira M, Kita N, Higashihara T, Sakatani M, Kozuka T. Summer-type hypersensitivity pneumonitis: comparison of high-resolution CT and plain radiographic findings. Am J Roentgenol 1992; 158:1223–8.
8. Buschman DL, Gamsu G, Waldron JA Jr, Klein JS, King TE Jr. Chronic hypersensitivity pneumonitis: use of CT in diagnosis. Am J Roentgenol 1992; 159:957–60.
9. Klein JS, Gamsu G, Webb WR, Golden JA, Muller NL. High-resolution CT diagnosis of emphysema in symptomatic patients with normal chest radiographs and isolated low diffusing capacity. Radiology 1992; 182:817–21.
10. Garg K, Lynch DA. Imaging of thoracic occupational and environmental malignancies. J Thorac Imaging 2002; 17:198–210.
11. Gamsu G, Salmon CJ, Warnock ML, Blanc PD. CT quantification of interstitial fibrosis in patients with asbestosis: a comparison of two methods. Am J Roentgenol 1995; 164:63–8.
12. Jarad NA, Wilkinson P, Pearson MC, Rudd RM. A new high resolution computed tomography scoring system for pulmonary fibrosis, pleural disease, and emphysema in patients with asbestos related disease. Br J Ind Med 1992; 49:73–84.
13. Eterovic D, Dujic Z, Tocilj J, Capkun V. High resolution pulmonary computed tomography scans quantified by analysis of density distribution: application to asbestosis. Br J Ind Med 1993; 50:514–9.
14. Bergin CJ, Muller NL, Vedal S, Chan-Yeung M. CT in silicosis: correlation with plain films and pulmonary function tests. Am J Roentgenol 1986; 146:477–83.

15. Patz EF Jr, Lowe VJ, Hoffman JM, et al. Focal pulmonary abnormalities: evaluation with F-18 fluorodeoxyglucose PET scanning. Radiology 1993; 188:487–90.

16. Pieterman RM, van Putten JW, Meuzelaar JJ, et al. Preoperative staging of non-small-cell lung cancer with positron-emission tomography. N Engl J Med 2000; 343:254–61.

17. Sood A, Redlich CA. Pulmonary function tests at work. Clin Chest Med 2001; 22:783–93.

18. Evans SE, Scanlon PD. Current practice in pulmonary function testing. Mayo Clin Proc 2003; 78:758–63.

19. Quanjer PH, Tammeling GJ, Cotes JE, Pedersen OF, Peslin R, Yernault JC. Lung volumes and forced ventilatory flows. Report Working Party Standardization of Lung Function Tests, European Community for Steel and Coal. Official Statement of the European Respiratory Society. Eur Respir J 1993; 16(Suppl):5–40.

20. American Medical Association. Guides to the evaluation of permanent impairment, 5th edn. Chicago: American Medical Association, 2000.

21. American Thoracic Society. Standardization of spirometry, 1994 update. Am J Respir Crit Care Med 1995; 152:1107–36.

22. American Thoracic Society. Lung function testing: selection of reference values and interpretative strategies. Am Rev Respir Dis 1991; 144:1202–18.

23. Hankinson JL, Odencrantz JR, Fedan KB. Spirometric reference values from a sample of the general US population. Am J Respir Crit Care Med 1999; 159:179–87.

24. Humerfelt S, Eide GE, Kvale G, Gulsvik A. Predictors of spirometric test failure: a comparison of the 1983 and 1993 acceptability criteria from the European Community for Coal and Steel. Occup Environ Med 1995; 52:547–53.

25. Hankinson JL. Beyond the peak flow meter: newer technologies for determining and documenting changes in lung function in the workplace. Occup Med 2000; 15:411–20.

26. American Thoracic Society. Single-breath carbon monoxide diffusing capacity (transfer factor). Recommendations for a standard technique – 1995 update. Am J Respir Crit Care Med 1995; 152:2185–98.

27. Burge PS. Use of serial measurements of peak flow in the diagnosis of occupational asthma. Occup Med 1993; 8:279–94.

28. Cote J, Kennedy S, Chan-Yeung M. Quantitative versus qualitative analysis of peak expiratory flow in occupational asthma. Thorax 1993; 48:48–51.

29. Leroyer C, Perfetti L, Trudeau C, L'Archeveque J, Chan-Yeung M, Malo JL. Comparison of serial monitoring of peak expiratory flow and FEV1 in the diagnosis of occupational asthma. Am J Respir Crit Care Med 1998; 158:827–32.

30. ATS/ACCP. Statement on cardiopulmonary exercise testing. Am J Respir Crit Care Med 2003; 167:211–77.

31. Agostoni P, Smith DD, Schoene RB, Robertson HT, Butler J. Evaluation of breathlessness in asbestos workers. Results of exercise testing. Am Rev Respir Dis 1987; 135:812–6.

32. Churg A, Green FHY, eds. Pathology of occupational lung disease. New York: Igaku-Shoin, 1998.

33. Zacharisen MC. Idiopathic interstitial pneumonia: are we missing hypersensitivity pneumonitis? Ann Allergy Asthma Immunol 2002; 88:4–6.

19.2 Occupational Asthma

Susan M Tarlo, Moira Chan-Yeung

INTRODUCTION

Occupational asthma (OA) is defined as a disease characterized by variable airflow obstruction and/or airway hyper-responsiveness due to causes and conditions attributable to a particular working environment and not to stimuli encountered outside the workplace.[1] Agents can give rise to OA through immunologic and non-immunologic mechanisms. Pre-existing asthma aggravated by work exposure is usually considered as distinct from OA. However, the resulting disability to the worker can sometimes be as severe in asthma aggravated at work as for those with OA. Both OA as defined above and pre-existing asthma aggravated by work exposure can be grouped together as work-related asthma but it is important for the physician to make as accurate a diagnosis as possible since the management implications in respect to further work options often differ with the different forms of work-related asthma.

This section focuses on OA caused by sensitization to a substance and OA caused by exposure to high-level irritants encountered in the workplace. Work-related aggravation of asthma will also be discussed although there have been few studies to document the prevalence or optimal management of this condition. Asthma-like syndromes such as byssinosis are addressed separately in Chapter 19.3.

CAUSES

Sensitizer-induced OA (immunologically mediated)

Over 300 agents in the workplace have been implicated in causing asthma.[2] Table 19.2.1 summarizes some of the commonly recognized agents and workplaces associated with immune-mediated OA. These agents can cause asthma by immunoglobulin IgE-dependent or IgE-independent mechanisms. Although many of these have been confirmed by specific challenge tests, others have been less well investigated. Such a list serves a useful function in alerting physicians and other health professionals that their patients may be suffering from OA if they were exposed to one of the agents. Because new substances are introduced into industries, the absence of previous reports of association should not rule out the possibility of sensitizer-induced OA if diagnostic evidence is strong.

Irritant-induced OA (non-immunologically mediated)

The best example of occupational asthma caused by non-immunological mechanisms (i.e. irritant-induced asthma) is reactive airways dysfunction syndrome (RADS),[3] arising from exposure to a single, high level of exposure to irritant gases, fumes, and smoke. Any chemicals, irritant gases, fumes, and smoke, if present at very high concentrations, can give rise to RADS. There remains controversy as to whether moderate exposures to similar irritants can also induce new onset of asthma. Some examples of irritants which have been reported to cause RADS are given in Table 19.2.2.

Aggravation of asthma

Workplace aggravation of asthma can also be caused by irritants such as those listed in Table 19.2.3, but at exposure levels which can be far less than that usually associated with RADS. The reason is that the presence of airway hyper-responsiveness is a feature of established asthma (occupational and non-occupational) so that relatively low levels of irritants (both in workplace settings and outside the workplace) can provoke bronchoconstriction. This is illustrated in the laboratory setting by the increased responsiveness of asthmatics to inhaled histamine, methacholine, cold or dry air. In the workplace, this response may be provoked by second-hand smoke, dusts, fumes, and sprays, as well as by cold air, dry air and exercise – even in exposures low enough that they would not provoke symptoms in non-asthmatic workers.

PATHOPHYSIOLOGY

The pathophysiology of OA has been reviewed in depth by Fabbri and colleagues.[4]

Sensitizer-induced OA

Both environmental and genetic factors interact in the development and progression of asthma. Sensitizer-induced asthma results from a complex pathogenic cascade involving a number of different inflammatory cells and mediators. Exposure to inhaled allergens (which can include proteins and chemicals) results in sensitization to the allergen, chronic airway inflammation, and hyper-reactivity. Th2-like CD4 T cells (secrete IL-4, IL-5, and IL-13) play a key role in recognizing antigens and co-ordinating the complex acute and chronic asthmatic responses, including IgE production by B lymphocytes, airway inflammation and airway remodeling. Numerous mediators, including cytokines, growth factors, chemokines, leukotrienes, and reactive oxygen species are produced by a variety of lung cells, including epithelial cells, monocytes, mast cells, and lymphocytes. These mediators likely amplify recruitment of inflammatory cells such as eosinophils, basophils, neutrophils, and lymphocytes, as well as promoting airway remodeling. Active participation of the airway epithelium and oxidative stress in this process is an emerging concept.

High molecular weight compounds (>5 kDa) include flour, laboratory animal proteins, and detergent enzymes. They are usually proteins or polysaccharides, and induce

Agent	Common sources of exposure
High molecular weight agents	
Animal-derived material	Animal, poultry and insect
Dander	work, veterinary medicine,
Excreta	fishing and fish processing,
Secretions	laboratory work
Serum	
Plant-derived material	
Flour	Bakery
Grain	Grain elevator and terminal and feed mill
Castor bean	Oil manufacture
Coffee bean	Food processing
Wood dust	Sawmill, carpentry, furniture work
Vegetable gum	Printing
Psyllium	Healthcare
Latex	Latex
Enzymes	
α-amylase	Bakery
Papain	Food processing
Alcalase	Pharmaceutical industry
Bacillus subtilis derived enzyme	Detergent enzyme industry
Low molecular weight agents	
Spray paints	
Toluene diisocyanate	Manufacture of plastic, foam
Dimethylphenyl diisocyanate	Insulation
Hexamethylene diisocyanate	Automobile spray paint
Wood dust	
Western red cedar	Sawmill worker, carpenter, furniture maker
Acid anhydride	Users of plastics, epoxy resins
Biocides	
Formaldehyde	Healthcare workers
Glutaraldehyde	
Chloramine T	
Colophony – fluxes	Electronic workers
Irritant agents	
Chlorine	Pulp and paper mills
Acetic acid	Hospital setting
Isocyanates	Spray paint

For further information please refer to reference 2.

Table 19.2.1 Selected agents that cause immunologically mediated occupational asthma

Agents (with high-level exposures)	Exposure example
Volatile diisocyanates, e.g., TDI	Spills in polyurethane foam manufacture
Chlorine spills (puffs)	Paper mills
Acid spills, e.g., acetic acid	Hospital workers, metal platers
Hypochlorite fumes	Accidental mixing of bleach and ammonia while cleaning
Chemical fires	Industrial settings, firefighters
Calcium oxide	World Trade Center collapse with exposed aid workers and building occupants
Nitrogen oxides	Silo gas
Welding fumes	Welders
Tear gas	Police officers
Spray paint	Paint sprayers
Metam sodium	Pesticide use

Table 19.2.2 Selected causes of irritant-induced OA

Agent	Exposure example
Cigarette smoke	Bars or restaurant workers
Fumes from cleaning agents	Domestic cleaners
Dusts	Cleaners, factory workers, construction workers
Paint	Painters, secondary exposure during workplace renovations
Cold air	Outdoor workers in cold winter climates; grocery workers near refrigerators/freezers
Exercise	Manual workers
Any irritants from Table 19.2.2, even at relatively low levels of exposure	As in Table 19.2.2

Table 19.2.3 Common triggers to work-related aggravation of asthma

specific IgE antibodies that mediate the asthmatic response. These agents often affect atopic subjects and IgE specific antibodies can be detected in most affected asthmatics.

Low molecular weight agents such as platinum, anhydrides, and isocyanates likely act as haptens, combining with amino groups on proteins to form an antigen. The asthmagenic potency of a compound may be determined to a certain extent by its chemical structure. Some low molecular weight agents such as platinum induce specific IgE antibodies, similar to large molecular weight agents. Other low molecular weight compounds such as diisocyanates and plicatic acid (the agent responsible for Western red cedar asthma) may utilize IgE-independent mechanisms. In both diisocyanate and Western red cedar asthma, specific IgE antibodies have been found in only a small proportion of patients proven to have the disease, and non-atopic subjects are affected. Specific IgE antibodies to diisocyanate-HSA antigens are found in variable fractions of workers (5–50%) with proven occupational asthma induced by diisocyanates, depending in part on the type of diisocyanate, exposure setting, and technical aspects of the IgE assays.[5] In Western red cedar asthma, the significance of specific IgE antibodies is not clear since anti-IgE antibodies failed to inhibit the release of histamine by plicatic acid from granulocytes of patients with the disease.[6]

Antigen-specific T lymphocytes likely play a role in mediating the inflammatory response in the airways. Supporting evidence comes from studies of asthma induced by nickel, cobalt, diisocyanates, and Western red cedar demonstrating proliferation of peripheral blood lymphocytes from sensitized subjects upon stimulation with appropriate antigens.[4] CD 8 T cell clones derived from bronchial mucosa of two isocyanate asthmatics produced mixed Th1 (IL-2 and IFN-γ secreting) and Th2 cytokines.[7] Similarly in patients with Western red cedar asthma, peripheral blood lymphocytes released IL-5 and IFN-γ after stimulation with plicatic acid.[8]

There is no clear difference in the pathology of airways in patients with sensitizer-induced (immune-mediated) occupational asthma and non-occupational atopic asthma. Irrespective of the sensitizing agent, the final pathologic features in the airways are similar. There is subepithelial fibrosis, hypertrophy of airway smooth muscle, edema of the airway wall, accumulation of inflammatory cells and obstruction of the airway lumen by exudate and/or mucus. In both isocyanate-induced asthma and in Western red cedar asthma, T lymphocytes are found in the mucosa and submucosa.[4] Some studies have suggested that IgE-mediated OA is mostly associated with eosinophilic inflammation whereas OA due to low molecular weight sensitizers such as diisocyanates can be manifest in some patients predominantly as a neutrophilic inflammation. Cessation of exposure to the sensitizing agent is associated with a decrease in the number of inflammatory cells in the airway mucosa. In diisocyanate-induced asthma, some reversal of the subepithelial fibrosis has been found.[7]

Irritant-induced asthma

Classic RADS is caused by a single exposure to a high dose of irritant gases, fumes, or smoke in a previously healthy subject. The mechanism of irritant-induced asthma is not known. It has been postulated that RADS is a 'big bang' phenomenon. Exposure to high level of irritants leads to acute sloughing of the epithelium potentially exposing nerve endings, leading to neurogenic inflammation. In addition, there is airway edema and non-specific release of mediators from various cells including mast cells and macrophages, resulting in recruitment of cells into the airway, leading to airway inflammation.[3]

More controversial is the concept of 'low-dose RADS', suggested by Kipen[9] and by Brooks.[10] Kipen described workers who developed asthma during their working life, which coincided with exposures at varying times to agents including second-hand smoke, perfumes, and freshly cleaned carpets.[9] A larger group of asthmatics with similar exposure histories was described by Brooks[10] who reported an increased prevalence of underlying atopy and smoking history. He suggested that the relatively moderate to low irritant exposure may have 'unmasked' a tendency to asthma. It has been well described that smokers and individuals with allergic rhinitis are more likely than others to have airway hyper-responsiveness and therefore could have symptoms of asthma provoked by irritant exposures more easily than workers with normal airway hyper-responsiveness. Whether this is considered to be aggravation of subclinical asthma or new-onset asthma, or even with some reported cases coincidental onset of asthma, can be debated. Recent studies of firefighters following the collapse of the World Trade Center have documented the development and persistence of hyperactivity and RADS in these workers which was associated with the intensity of exposure to dust and smoke. Similarly it is not clear whether moderate or low irritant exposures can truly induce persistent increases in airway responsiveness (or long-term aggravation of asthma) rather than merely inducing a short-term exacerbation of asthma symptoms as has been previously believed.

The pathology of RADS is similar to that of typical asthma although the number of cases of RADS with reported histology is small. In some reports subepithelial fibrosis is more evident in RADS. The airway epithelium is extensively damaged and the submucosa infiltrated by mononuclear cells.[11]

Work-related aggravation of asthma

The pathogenesis of work-related aggravation of asthma does not differ from that of non-work-related aggravation of asthma. Airway hyper-responsiveness is a key feature of asthma such that relatively low levels of respiratory irritants will induce bronchoconstriction. In addition, some inhaled irritants such as ozone and cigarette smoke, and respiratory viral infections can induce an inflammatory response and transiently increase airway responsiveness which may produce a more symptomatic response in people with asthma due to their underlying airway hyper-responsiveness. While individuals with asthma can usually control their exposure in the home to irritants such as second-hand smoke, fumes from cleaning agents, strong perfumes, and dusts relatively easily, they often have less personal control of such exposures in the workplace and may develop worse asthma symptoms at work.

EPIDEMIOLOGY

Occupational asthma has become the most common occupational lung disease in developed countries.[12] Estimates of the incidence of OA have been made using registers based on mandated or voluntary physician reporting, medicolegal statistics, and various national or disability registries. There are considerable between-country differences in the estimated incidence of OA, ranging from 22 per million per year in the United Kingdom to 187 per million per year in Finland.[12] The differences are likely to be in part due to methods used to derive these estimates and in part to differences in local industries and employment opportunities.

In the United States, the 1978 Social Security Disability Survey showed that 7.7% of the participants identified asthma as a personal medical condition and 1.2% attributed it to workplace exposure.[13] Recent studies in the United States have shown that about 8% of adult patients with new-onset asthma, from community pulmonary physicians' practices, had a history of exposure to sensitizers and another 5% had exposure to irritants.[14] This finding was subsequently confirmed in asthma patients from physicians in primary care.[15]

Asthma affects 5–10% of the population worldwide and in developed countries. There has been an increase in prevalence during the past two decades in many industrialized countries.[16] There is a great deal of interest in determining whether the increase in prevalence of asthma can be partly accounted for by occupational exposure. Community-based studies on population attributable risk of occupational exposure for asthma carried out as part of the European Community Respiratory Health Survey have shown that there is considerable variation, from 5% in Spain to 41% in New Zealand, depending on local industries, options for employment, and population susceptibility.[17-20]

- Onset of asthma symptoms, usually within 24 hours following exposure to a high level of a respiratory irritant agent.
- Persistence of symptoms for at least 12 weeks.
- Objective evidence of asthma: airway hyper-responsiveness on histamine or methacholine challenge, or airflow limitation with significant bronchodilator responsiveness (at least 12% increase in FEV$_1$).
- No previously documented evidence of asthma or other chronic lung disease.

* Based on references 3, 34

Table 19.2.4 Criteria for diagnosis of irritant-induced asthma*

There is considerable variation in the prevalence of *sensitizer-induced OA* due to various industries from 2% in latex-exposed workers to 50% among detergent enzyme workers.[21] While between-workforce differences may due to methodology such as the definition of OA and the intensity of exposure, the asthmogenic potential of the agents is likely to be important.

There are fewer studies on the prevalence of *RADS or irritant-induced asthma*, and very little data on the preva-lence of aggravation of asthma at work. The definition of irritant-induced asthma has been modified from Brook's strict criteria for RADS in many reports (Table 19.2.4). Some variations include non-massive exposures on one or more occasions and some include asthma onset up to several days after the exposure incident(s). The prevalence clearly will be modified by such changes in definition. In an occupational lung disease clinic population 8% of patients with OA fulfilled criteria for RADS (3% of all consecutive referrals) while 17% of OA patients fulfilled expanded criteria for irritant-induced OA (6% of all referrals).[22] Similar findings, suggesting that irritant-induced OA accounts for a minority of all OA, were reported from compensation data in Ontario, Canada: 5% of all accepted work-related asthma claims were for irritant-induced OA (3% fulfilled RADS criteria).[23]

Among 623 inhalation accidents reported to the British Surveillance of Work-related and Occupational Respiratory Disease (SWORD) project, 9% had asthma-like symptoms which persisted for at least a month, of which 72% of those with further information were considered by their physician to have new-onset asthma (i.e. about 6%).[24] A report by Cone et al.[25] gives further information, both about the incidence of respiratory symptoms after an accidental exposure, and the natural history of irritant-induced asthma. They reported the effects of a pesticide spill (metam sodium) following derailment of a tank car, in which the plume traveled 40 miles over 3 days, exposing about 3000 people. About 7% of those exposed were referred for symptoms and 1.6% reported respiratory symptoms for at least 3 months. However, only 1% (30 subjects) fulfilled the historical criteria used in this study for irritant-induced asthma, even with expanded criteria for the time of onset of symptoms; their symptoms began between 4 hours and 7 days after the spill and they had no preceding respiratory history.

Although prevalence data for work-aggravated asthma are very limited and the condition frequently is not recognized by some compensation systems, it is likely quite common. This is supported by a recent study which found

that 50% of all accepted work-related asthma claims from the same compensation database in Ontario, Canada, were for work-related aggravation of asthma, i.e., the same number accepted as for OA[23] condition.

EXPOSURE FACTORS
Sensitizer-induced OA

Exposure is the single most important determinant of the incidence of OA. During the past decade, improved industrial hygiene techniques for measuring several low molecular weight compounds including diisocyanates, formaldehyde, and amines have become available. More importantly, immunochemical techniques have been developed for quantitating some aeroallergens.

Several studies have shown that there is a dose–response relationship between the level of exposure to occupational agents and the prevalence of sensitization and/or non-allergic bronchial hyper-responsiveness and/or asthma. These include exposure to high molecular weight allergens such as α-amylase, laboratory animal allergen, and low molecular weight compounds such as Western red cedar, acid anhydride, and colophony.[26-30]

The ability to measure exposure has led to the establishment of permissible exposure limits for some sensitizing agents. For OA, the minimum concentration or dose of the allergen that causes sensitization and the minimum concentration that causes symptoms after sensitization are likely different, and generally not well defined. There is a latency period during which time individuals become sensitized to the specific agent, usually more than a month and less than 2 years, but variable latency periods have been reported, and are likely related to the dose and timing of exposure, as well as host factors. Once an individual is sensitized to an agent, a minute dose can trigger an attack of asthma; the concentration necessary for sensitization is most likely greater. Although human data are limited, sensitization to certain agents such as isocyanates may occur through skin in addition to inhalational exposure, as has been shown in certain animal models.

Concomitant environmental exposures such as low levels of irritants and cigarette smoke may enhance sensitization to some occupational agents. As examples, it has been found that cigarette smoking is a significant risk factor for the development of sensitization and OA from exposure to complex platinum salts and to acid anhydrides as described below.[30,31] Diesel exhaust has been shown to have an adjuvant function in development of IgE-mediated sensitization to aeroallergens, and animal studies have also suggested an enhancing effect from ozone exposure. Further studies are required in this area as recently reviewed.[32]

Irritant exposures and RADS

Exposure conditions are central to the diagnosis of irritant-induced asthma and RADS. The more extreme an acute irritant exposure has been, and the shorter the period following this exposure that asthma symptoms have developed and been documented, the more credible is the diagnosis of irritant-induced asthma. Thus, the initial reports of RADS with new-onset asthma starting within 24 hours of a massive irritant exposure were very unlikely to be due to coincidental onset of asthma. Conversely, onset of asthma in a worker who has been exposed to presumed low to moderate concentrations of solvents or other potential respiratory irritants for several years could well be coincidental to the workplace exposures. Between these two extremes of exposure and symptom onset, the diagnosis of irritant-induced asthma is controversial.[32]

Exposure and work-aggravated asthma

In contrast to the exposure conditions for irritant-induced asthma, even low concentrations of respiratory irritants can aggravate pre-existing asthma. Second-hand cigarette smoke, cleaning agents, paints, and other fumes, as well as dust, can worsen symptoms and induce bronchoconstriction in individuals with asthma. Those who have mild asthma, well controlled with appropriate medications, may have no significant response to low concentrations of respiratory irritants while those with severe asthma (with severe underlying airway responsiveness) are more likely to have an exacerbation of asthma with lower exposure concentrations of irritants, or with exercise or cold air. Viral upper respiratory infections can increase airway responsiveness for up to 6 weeks and asthmatics who have or have recently had a cold may thus be worsened by irritant exposures at work which may not affect them at other times.

Similarly, a relevant allergen exposure can also increase airway responsiveness for several weeks. For example, a worker with asthma who is allergic to cats, after visiting a home with a cat on a weekend, might subsequently, for several weeks, notice that workplace irritants such as fumes from cleaning agents, which were previously tolerated, now worsen symptoms. If airway responsiveness improves, and/or asthma is well treated with medications and allergen avoidance measures, such patients may then be able to work with the same low-level irritant exposures without difficulty, unlike the patient with OA induced by a sensitizer which is still present in their work environment.

HOST DETERMINANTS

Not all subjects develop OA given the same degree of exposure. The following host susceptibility factors may be important in *sensitizer-induced OA*.

1. *Atopy.* Atopy (defined as positive skin test to one or more common allergens) has been shown to be associated with sensitization to some high molecular weight agents such as detergent enzymes[33,34] but not in others such as clams and snow crabs.[35,36]
2. *Smoking.* The effect of smoking appears to be dependent on the type of occupational agent. An interaction between smoking and atopy has been found in laboratory animal handlers[34] and in workers exposed to tetrachlorophthalic anhydride[30] atopic smokers had the

highest and non-atopic non-smokers had the lowest prevalence of sensitization. Among platinum workers, smoking, not atopy, is the most important risk factor for sensitization.[31] When agents cause OA by predominantly IgE-independent mechanisms, such as isocyanate-induced asthma and Western red cedar asthma, neither atopy nor smoking are important risk factors.[4]

3. *Non-allergic bronchial hyper-responsiveness.* The role of non-allergic bronchial hyper-responsiveness as a pre-existing risk factor for occupational asthma requires further study. In most instances, non-allergic bronchial hyper-responsiveness is the result rather than a predisposing host factor.[37]
4. *Genetic markers.* An association between certain HLA class II genes as well as other genes such as glutathione-s-transferases and diisocyanate, trimellitic anhydride, platinum or Western red cedar-induced asthma have been reported.[38,39] However, the results of such studies are preliminary and they cannot be used for screening of susceptible subjects. Moreover, asthma is likely to be a polygenic disease with multiple genes contributing to the disease rather than one.
5. *Upper airway symptoms* such as rhinitis and conjunctivitis often precede the lower airway symptoms. It has been suggested that they may be used as an early marker of OA.[40]

Little is known about the host determinants of *irritant-induced asthma*. RADS probably affects both atopic and non-atopic, smoking and non-smoking workers alike. Initial reports of RADS included more smokers than non-smokers. Recent studies have shown an increase in small particle deposition among smokers compared with non-smokers, and among those with baseline airflow limitation,[41] suggesting the possibility that such individuals might be more susceptible to airway effects of irritant small particulate inhalations. However, a history of smoking or the finding of atopy, while not excluding the diagnosis of irritant-induced asthma, may make the diagnosis somewhat less certain in that there may be more likelihood of previous underlying airway disease which may confound the diagnosis, even if not formally documented in medical records. This is particularly problematic in considering a diagnosis of new-onset irritant-induced asthma after moderate or low level irritant exposures.

Very little has been documented about the host determinants of *work-related aggravation* of asthma. However, as noted above, the response to non-occupational irritant exposures is known to relate to airway hyper-responsiveness (and asthma severity and control) and it is likely that the same factors are important in work-related aggravation of asthma.

CLINICAL FEATURES AND DIAGNOSIS
Sensitizer-induced OA

Occupational asthma is first suspected in clinical practice from the history. Any patient with a history suggestive of asthma (one or more symptoms of episodic cough, wheeze, retrosternal chest tightness, and dyspnea), which began during working life, should raise the diagnostic suspicion of OA. Suspicion increases if these symptoms are worse at work, and improve during weekends or holidays away from work.

Knowledge of the typical clinical features of sensitizer-induced asthmas is essential in obtaining and evaluating the occupational history. Sensitizer-induced asthma affects only a portion of exposed workers and develops after a variable latent period of exposure. Thus symptoms typically develop from several months to years after the onset of exposure. The typical asthma symptoms can occur within a few minutes of exposure, several hours after exposure, or in a biphasic or atypical more prolonged pattern. Allergic rhinitis type symptoms may predate asthmatic symptoms and symptoms commonly worsen over the week and improve away from work. Delayed symptoms after work in the evening suggest sensitizer-induced rather than irritant-induced asthma. The latency period and delayed evening symptoms can make the association with work less obvious to the patient and healthcare provider.

As asthma progresses, it is not uncommon for patients with sensitizer asthma to also respond to non-specific triggers that commonly affect typical atopic asthmatics such as cold air, irritants, and exercise. Improvement away from work may also become less dramatic. Thus careful documentation of the onset, timing, and progression of asthmatic symptoms in relationship to occupational and environmental exposures is essential for diagnosis. Particularly helpful is clarifying these patterns when the symptoms first started, when the association between work exposures and asthmatic symptoms may be more clear-cut.

The history of OA is a sensitive diagnostic tool for asthma related to a sensitizer, but has low specificity and requires additional investigative measures. Malo and colleagues[42] found the sensitivity and specificity of the clinical history to be 96% and 25% as compared with diagnoses based on objective investigations. The differential diagnosis includes asthma starting or worsening coincidental to the workplace, unrelated asthma aggravated by non-specific irritant exposures at work, and non-asthmatic causes of asthma-like symptoms (such as rhinitis with post-nasal drip, hypersensitivity pneumonitis, acute or chronic bronchitis, gastro-esophageal reflux, or cardiac asthma). Therefore the initial step in the investigation should be the objective confirmation of asthma by pre- and post-bronchodilator spirometry or methacholine or histamine challenge testing. These tests are best performed within 24 hours of the suspected work exposure, since if they are performed after a longer period, negative tests for asthma may be caused by an improvement away from exposure to a workplace sensitizer.

Although, in many cases the patient may not be aware of the exact chemical exposures at work, material safety data sheets can be requested from the workplace and may be of help in clarifying the presence of a workplace sensitizer. In this regard, the sheets should be requested not only for substances directly used by the patient but also for all agents to which there may be air-borne exposure, even intermittently. These sheets can be very helpful in assessing possible exposure agents, but they may be incomplete in respect to respiratory sensitizers since there is only the requirement to list known hazardous components of a compound, and only if these are present in amounts greater than 1%. Since new sensitizers are described each year, and once sensitized, respiratory responses to a sensitizer can occur at minute levels, a relevant exposure may not be detected unless the product manufacturer is specifically requested to provide full information.

Several studies have assessed the value of new and older investigations for occupational asthma, as reviewed in a consensus statement from the American College of Chest Physicians,[43] guidelines from the Canadian Thoracic Society,[44] and a recent review.[45] An objective assessment of asthma and its work relationships is generally accepted as necessary where possible for appropriate medical management but also for appropriate compensation decisions to be reached, although in practice this can sometimes be difficult to obtain. Non-occupational asthma is common and frequently has its onset in adult life. Each investigative measure used for OA can have false-positive and false-negative responses (Table 19.2.5), and therefore, it is advisable to combine as many investigations as are feasible in an individual patient.

Spirometry and non-specific challenge testing

An objective diagnosis of asthma is reached by pulmonary function tests (PFTs), pre- and post-bronchodilator, and/or a histamine or methacholine challenge test, using standard protocol.[46] If normal, these do not exclude OA if performed when the patient is off work and free of symptoms. However, whether they are normal or abnormal, they can serve as a baseline for comparison with subsequent spirometry and methacholine or histamine challenge responses after the patient returns to work, preferably performed towards the end of a typical work week and within 24 hours of the occurrence of symptoms. Results at this time which do not show evidence of asthma virtually exclude a diagnosis of OA, although a few such cases have been reported with diisocyanate-induced asthma.[47]

Serial monitoring of bronchial hyper-responsiveness

Alternatively, if the patient is working when first assessed, and if a methacholine or histamine challenge at that time confirms the presence of airway hyper-responsiveness, then repeat testing after a holiday period of 10–14 days before the patient returns to work is useful to objectively assess changes in reactivity while away from work. A significant improvement would support a diagnosis of occupational asthma unless explained by confounding factors. Depending on the individual pulmonary function laboratory, a minimum three-fold improvement in PC_{20} while off work is significant. However, lack of significant improvement in PC_{20} on holiday does not exclude OA since some sensitized asthmatics (perhaps those with longer duration of OA) can require a longer period away from exposure before

Assessment	False positive	False negative
History	Aggravation of coincidental asthma, rhinitis or other non-asthma diagnosis.	Uncommon. Lack of full weekends off work.
MSDS	Exposure does not prove sensitization.	Sheets may not list all sensitizers. Not all relevant sheets may be obtained by the worker.
PFTs pre- and post-bronchodilator, Methacholine or histamine challenge	Response indicates asthma, but not necessarily OA. Recent upper respiratory infection, significant COPD. True response indicates asthma, not necessarily OA.	Masking of variability by medications. Performed when asymptomatic or off work. Performed when asymptomatic or off work. Failure to stop asthma medications before the test.
Paired methacholine or histamine challenges	Intercurrent upper respiratory infection, or exposure to a non-occupational allergen trigger during period of work.	Insufficient time off work to see improvement. Intercurrent upper respiratory infection, or exposure to a non-occupational allergen trigger while off work. Masking of changes by asthma medications.
Peak expiratory flow readings	Work-related aggravation of asthma. Poor effort at the end of a work day: fabrication of results.	Only occasional exposure or no exposure to the sensitizer during the recording weeks at work.
Skin tests and in-vitro immunologic tests	Presence of immunologic sensitization without OA. Non-specific skin irritant effects of extract. Dermographism.	Inadequate or wrong allergenic extract. Masking of skin test response by antihistamines.
Workplace challenge	Coincidental aggravating exposures on the test day. Placebo effects.	Lack of exposure to the relevant sensitizer on the test day. Masking by medications.
Laboratory-specific challenges	Irritant exposure conditions. Placebo effect if not blinded. Unstable asthma or coincidental worsening on active exposure day.	Incorrect exposure agent, or inadequate concentration, duration of exposure, or absence of correct conditions such as heating, mixing with other chemicals. Masking by medications. Reduction of airway reactivity after a prolonged period off work. Failure to measure methacholine/histamine responses pre- and post-exposure.
Induced sputum and exhaled NO	Mainly research uses.	Mainly research uses.

Table 19.2.5 Some potential causes of false-positive and false-negative assessments in OA

significant improvement occurs. In the occurrence of a positive history, peak flow responses suggestive of an occupational component and a trend to improvement in histamine or methacholine PC_{20}, a longer period off work with repeat tests may help.

Serial monitoring of PEF

Serial peak expiratory flow (PEF) readings continue to be useful as a component of occupational asthma investigation.[48] Serial peak expiratory flow readings require careful patient instruction in the correct use of the peak expiratory flow meter. Suggested use is often three times on each occasion at least four times a day on working days and days off work, while also recording symptoms and medication use. However, optimum frequency to enhance compliance and accuracy of diagnosis remains unproven. Medications, other than as needed bronchodilators, are kept at a stable regular dosage during this time if possible, sufficient to control but not completely suppress symptoms. Compliance has been shown to be poor with such peak expiratory flow recording, especially when patients were asked to record values six times per day.[49] Nevertheless, if the patient does keep a record that has enough information over several weeks at work and over a holiday period, and if the record shows a clear pattern to support or refute asthma with a work relationship, then the sensitivity and specificity have been shown to be high compared with other tests for OA.

Electronic peak flow meters or portable spirometers give more objective information as to patient compliance but their current costs limit their practical usage. In a comparison with serial FEV_1 recordings using a portable ventilometer, Leroyer et al.[50] found better sensitivity and specificity of peak expiratory flow recordings. Using the best value at each time period, the sensitivity and specificity for occupational asthma were 73% and 100% for peak flow recordings, adding further validation to the use of this simple test as a component of investigations for OA.

There are no uniformly accepted criteria for the interpretation of peak expiratory flow recordings. Attempts have been made to develop objective criteria, but qualitative interpretation of plotted graphs by an experienced physician relates favorably to quantitative analyses.[51] If peak flow or portable spirometric recordings in work week periods show no significant changes of asthma, there may have been masking of such changes by regular asthma medications and the recordings should be repeated with use of less medication.

When interpreting changes in peak expiratory flow and methacholine or histamine responses during working weeks vs. weeks off work, consideration should be given to confounding factors. These include intercurrent respiratory viral infections within the preceding 6 weeks, or non-occupational relevant allergen exposures (as assessed from the history at the time of these tests, and from environmental allergy assessment, including skin prick testing to common aeroallergens).

Work-related changes in asthma severity, as assessed by serial peak expiratory flow monitoring and methacholine

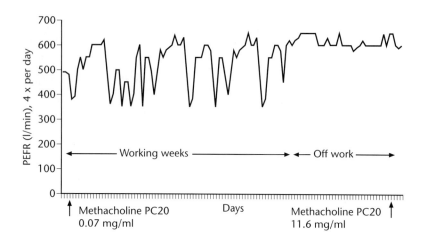

Figure 19.2.1: Serial PEF monitoring in a 42-year-old polyurethane foam worker (exposed to toluene diisocyanate) at work and off work showing improvement in PEF and methacholine PC20 while off work, supporting a diagnosis of sensitizer-induced OA.

or histamine challenges in combination, generally provide a clear objective method to confirm or refute the diagnosis of occupational asthma (e.g., Fig. 19.2.1). If peak flow monitoring can be adequately performed and interpreted, but not methacholine or histamine challenges, or vice versa, and the resulting changes are clearly positive or negative, although not ideal, this is usually sufficient to confirm or refute the diagnosis also. However, unfortunately in practice such data can be difficult to obtain. If the patient has left the implicated work exposure and cannot or will not return on a trial basis for such tests, or the work exposures in question have changed, then the diagnosis is more difficult to make.

Immunologic tests

Immunologic tests to demonstrate IgE antibodies in high molecular weight workplace sensitizers can be useful, when feasible, to confirm immunological sensitization, but are often limited by the lack of commercially available or standardized reagents. Hamilton and colleagues[52] have shown that a commercial skin prick test preparation of natural rubber latex at two different dilutions had a sensitivity and specificity between 95% and 100% relative to a history of latex allergy symptoms (combined with glove provocation tests when there was discordance between the history and skin test results). A positive skin test response supports a diagnosis of OA if associated with appropriate pulmonary function changes but as a sole investigation is not diagnostic. Similar conclusions could be drawn from a study by Bernstein and colleagues[53] in pharmaceutical workers sensitized to lactase: skin test-positive workers were nine times more likely to have upper or lower respiratory symptoms than skin test-negative workers but over 60% of skin test-positive workers had no respiratory symptoms.

Several methods are available to measure specific IgE antibodies in serum, with variable predictive value, depending on the workplace allergen and method used to measure specific IgE. Unfortunately there are relatively few well-characterized workplace allergen extracts for which reliable in-vitro allergen assays can be performed. Even for allergens such as those in natural rubber latex, which have been extensively studied and characterized, the role of in-vitro assay of IgE antibodies remains controversial since there can be significant cross-reactivity with non-occupational allergens.

An example of a useful assay in a university laboratory setting with careful controls is the assessment of specific antibodies to the occupational sensitizer trimellitic anhydride. The predictive value of in-vitro measures of serum IgE antibodies was assessed by Grammer and colleagues[54] using ELISA methods. Nine of 16 exposed workers with specific IgE antibodies either had asthma or developed it within 5 years of follow-up versus one of 165 without these antibodies. Similar predictive value for specific IgG antibodies was found for immunologic respiratory disease in that study although most studies of other sensitizers (e.g., of diisocyanates) have shown that IgG antibodies are more reflective of exposure than of occupational asthma. Therefore, when performed in the university research laboratory, the tests can be highly predictive but results cannot necessarily be extended to performance of these tests in other laboratories.

Other in-vitro tests to assess specific sensitization to occupational chemicals currently remain research tools but may become clinically useful in the future, e.g. assessment of mononuclear cell activation or chemokine production by diisocyanates[55,56] or by adducts of diisocyanates with epithelial cell proteins.[57]

Specific challenge tests

Occupational specific laboratory challenge tests are performed in very few centers, and generally are not available in many countries including the United States.[58] Nguyen et al.[59] have shown that a positive challenge response to high molecular weight occupational allergens in an individual sensitized patient relates to the total dose delivered rather than the concentration or duration of exposure alone. Therefore, a serial progressive increase in exposure duration can be used in such testing rather than progressive increases in concentration, potentially increasing the safety of the test. Although still considered to be a gold standard for diagnosis of OA, there are potential false-positive and false-negative responses.[60] A false-negative response may occur if the wrong agent is used or if the exposure conditions are not comparable to those in the workplace. For example, some patients can be sensitized to toluene diisocyanate (TDI), but not diphenylmethane diisocyanate (MDI), some to a prepolymer but not a monomer of a diisocyanate, and some to a specific isomer, e.g., 2,4-TDI but not 2,6-TDI. MDI is poorly volatile and therefore needs to be heated to generate respiratory exposure during a challenge test. After a long period away from exposure, sensitivity may be lost or there may be a need for multiple days of re-exposure to diisocyanates before measurable changes in peak flow, spirometry or methacholine/histamine responsiveness occur.

Laboratory-specific challenges can be useful in the following circumstances: when the diagnosis of OA remains in doubt despite other investigations; if other investigations could not be performed; or in the setting where a patient clearly has OA but it is necessary for their management to confirm what is their causative agent. These tests require specialized facilities which are only available in a few centers,[58] are time consuming and very costly, and false positives and false negatives can occur. Occupational hygienist support is necessary to generate, maintain and monitor appropriate exposure levels of the suspected sensitizer. During challenges, levels of exposure must be continuously monitored, since excessive levels could induce a severe asthmatic reaction, or can be irritating or potentially newly sensitize the patient.

New techniques
Two new techniques have been evaluated in the diagnosis and impairment assessment of OA: exhaled nitric oxide and induced sputum analysis. In patients with Western red cedar asthma, Obata et al.[61] found an increase in induced sputum eosinophils at 6 and 24 hours following a positive plicatic acid challenge but increases in exhaled nitric oxide at 6 and 24 hours after challenge did not correlate with a positive challenge. Similarly, in follow-up of patients with OA from Western red cedar, there was a significant association between respiratory impairment class and sputum eosinophils counts, but no correlation with exhaled nitric oxide.[62] Lemiere and coworkers[63] also reported a significant increase in induced sputum eosinophils and eosinophil cationic protein (ECP) in patients with OA

from various causes, during periods of work exposure as compared with periods off work, suggesting that in centers where this test can be performed, it can add to other tests in the investigation of OA.

Conclusion
The extent of objective testing and the choice of investigations will vary according to the degree of proof of diagnosis which is required and the facilities available. Depending on the assessment facilities and compensation system requirements, workplace exposure studies or laboratory chamber studies may be selected. It is recognized that objective proof or disproof of OA is not always feasible and less definitive evidence may be accepted by some compensation systems. However, the incorrect acceptance of a compensation claim may still lead to poor socioeconomic results for the patient by restricting their future employment options. A diagnosis which is confirmed as fully as possible by objective testing is recommended both for correct compensation decisions and for optimal medical management and occupational advice to the patient.

Irritant-induced OA

In contrast to the history of OA related to a sensitizer, the history may be of the acute onset of asthma symptoms within 24 hours of a high exposure to a respiratory irritant, raising the possibility of irritant-induced asthma/RADS.[3,22] This diagnosis should be suspected particularly if symptoms were severe enough to lead to an acute visit to a physician or hospital emergency department, persist for at least 3 months, and occur with no previous history of respiratory disease. Unfortunately, this remains a circumstantial diagnosis (Table 19.2.2). It relies largely on the history of exposure, and associated onset of symptoms, objective findings to support a diagnosis of asthma, and the lack of evidence of previous chronic respiratory disease. No prospective physiologic or histologic investigations can further prove the association with the workplace. Industrial hygiene data documenting the high exposure are rarely available as such events are frequently accidental or sporadic.

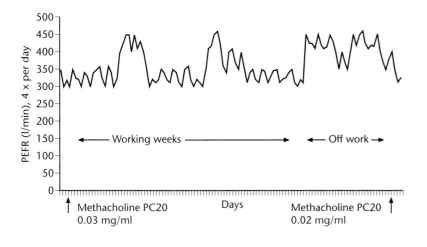

Figure 19.2.2: Serial PEF monitoring in a 50-year-old dry cleaner with asthma since childhood (exposed to solvents at work), at work and off work showing improvement in PEF but no change in methacholine PC20 while off work, supporting a diagnosis of work-related irritant aggravation of underlying asthma.

Work-related aggravation of asthma

The diagnosis of work-related aggravation of asthma is made on the following basis.

1. A history of asthma symptoms which worsen at work and improve to some extent after the work shift or on weekends or holidays off work, and a history of exposure at work to potential respiratory irritants such as fumes, sprays, or dusts.

2. Objective evidence of asthma based on a significant bronchodilator response or positive histamine or methacholine challenge test.

3. Objective demonstration of worsening of asthma at work by documented work-related changes in symptoms, medication requirements, and preferably peak expiratory flow recordings *without* other manifestations of sensitizer-induced OA as discussed above (i.e., not associated with changes in methacholine responsiveness at work versus off work, no findings of an immunologic response to an occupational sensitizer). Although the serial peak flow records may appear similar to those of patients with sensitizer-induced OA, it would be expected that an irritant aggravation of asthma would cause a reduction in peak flow results within minutes of exposure whereas some sensitizers (especially low molecular weight sensitizers) produce isolated late asthmatic responses starting several hours after exposure. In addition, the recovery from bronchoconstriction due to an irritant aggravation of asthma may occur sooner than the recovery from a sensitizer response. However, there may be significant overlap between the timing of these two types of response (e.g., Fig. 19.2.2).

The initial onset of asthma symptoms may have occurred prior to starting the current employment or during the current employment. If asthma began during a work period, careful assessment as to initial irritant-induced asthma or sensitizer-induced OA is appropriate since a diagnosis of current work-related aggravation of asthma does not exclude a previous work-related *cause* of asthma.

MANAGEMENT

A firm diagnosis as far as possible is essential for appropriate management of work-related asthma.

Sensitizer-induced OA

Workers with OA induced by a respiratory sensitizer who have had an objective diagnosis of OA should be removed from further exposure to that agent, in addition to receiving the same types of medical treatment as are given to non-occupational asthmatics. Removal from exposure to the sensitizer is sometimes achieved by a change in the work process. As an example, for a healthcare worker with OA from natural rubber latex, personal avoidance of contact with natural rubber latex gloves and other products, and use of only powder-free, low allergen latex gloves

by coworkers. Encapsulation of enzymes in the detergent industry, or removal of usage of epoxy glue can eliminate exposure to these sensitizers. If the sensitizer is only occasionally used in the workplace, then it may be feasible for the worker to wear protective equipment such as a helmet respirator with separate air supply, as has been shown to protect some workers sensitized to latex or farm allergens. Complete removal from exposure unfortunately is not always achieved due to variable workers' compensation systems and socioeconomic factors. As noted in the discussion of outcomes below, under select circumstances, very low exposures rather than complete removal may be adequate in some patients. Such workers require close monitoring to assess for worsening asthma.

The role of protective respiratory devices in farmers with OA has been considered for patients unable to leave areas of exposure to the workplace sensitizer. Muller-Wening and Neuhauss[64] show that use of three types of Racal respirators (including an 'Airstream helmet'), each with a P2 filter, worn during challenge tests with their workplace dusts reduced symptoms and responses but did not prevent them in most patients. In a workplace study of farmers with OA, Taivainen et al.[65] evaluated similar respirators, comparing symptoms and peak flows with the results from a period without the respirator. They found a significant improvement in symptoms and peak flow responses with the respirator use, but in only 8 of 33 patients did symptoms clear. These findings suggest that for farmers with OA who face severe financial consequences of avoiding allergen exposure, the use of a powered dust respirator helmet may limit the ongoing exacerbation of their asthma.

These studies recognize the real difficulties that may occur in providing complete avoidance of exposure to a sensitizer. Nevertheless, where feasible this remains the best option for sensitized patients. Laoprasert and colleagues[66] similarly assessed the use of HEPA-filtered helmets in preventing airway responses to natural rubber latex. Although the use of the respirator significantly reduced symptoms and FEV_1 changes during specific challenge tests, equivalent benefit was obtained by the use of powder-free low-allergen latex gloves. Substitution with these gloves would therefore appear to be a simpler solution to this problem. For patients with other causes of sensitizer OA, to remove the worker completely from exposure often requires a move to a different building at work, or a change in occupation.

Irritant-induced OA

Workers with OA induced by an irritant exposure at work should be managed in the same way as those with aggravation of underlying asthma (see below), except that appropriate precautions need to be in place to ensure that the patient is not at risk of further high-level irritant exposures. In some patients with irritant-induced OA who return to work, exposure to even relatively low levels of the same, or other, workplace irritants may induce asthma-like symptoms. This may be either on the basis of aggravation of asthma, as described above, or on the basis of vocal cord dysfunction/hyperventilation through a presumed subconscious response (see Chapter 49).

Work-aggravated asthma

Workers who have asthma which is not caused by their work may have their asthma aggravated by exposure to respiratory irritants at work, such as smoke, dusts, fumes, sprays, cold air, extremes of humidity, or marked exercise requirements. The degree of symptomatic exacerbation will depend not only on the severity of the airway non-specific triggering factor, but also on the severity of underlying asthma, and the adequacy of medical treatment and control of asthma. Therefore, the approach for these patients is to optimize the medical management of their asthma. This includes limiting exposure to relevant environmental allergens and non-occupational irritants such as tobacco smoke, and optimizing asthma medications, education, and compliance. In addition, reduced exposure to non-specific exacerbating triggers in the workplace should be attempted. Depending on the exacerbating triggers, recommendations may include a move to a different work area; changes in ventilation or process; the use of an appropriate respirator for short-term exposures to respiratory irritants; or work modification to avoid extreme cold or exercise. If asthma is severe, then a change in occupation to a relatively sedentary job in a clean environment may be needed to enable the patient to continue work.

COMPENSATION AND CONSIDERATION OF THE WORKPLACE

Many workers with asthma related to their workplace will be eligible for workers' compensation. Some workers' compensation systems are beginning to recognize and provide some degree of compensation for work-related aggravation of asthma as well as new-onset OA. The treating physician has a responsibility to submit the appropriate documentation for this and to ensure that as clear and objective a diagnosis has been achieved. An appropriate compensation decision is greatly facilitated if the patient has been thoroughly investigated with objective tests to confirm the diagnosis of asthma and demonstrate the work relationship. Early advice by the physician to leave the workplace before reaching an objective diagnosis will make further investigations more difficult to obtain, may unfairly deny the patient appropriate compensation for OA, and can have severe adverse socioeconomic consequences.

Healthcare providers should consider the public health implications when diagnosing a patient with work-related asthma. Once a diagnosis of OA due to a sensitizer has been reached, the treating physician should consider this as a 'sentinel event', suggesting that there may be others with OA or at risk for OA in the same workplace. Therefore there should be appropriate notification of public health officers and/or the company physician with the patient's consent. This may lead to further case-finding and preven-

tive measures. Similarly, if a diagnosis of RADS is reached, the healthcare provider should assess if other workers were similarly affected and ensure that the risk of future high irritant exposures is low.

IMPAIRMENT/DISABILITY EVALUATION

Evaluation of impairment for compensation purposes also requires objective criteria. Since asthma is characterized by variable airflow limitation, simple spirometry is usually not sufficient to reflect impairment. The American Thoracic Society guidelines for evaluating impairment in patients with asthma[67] have recommended that other factors also be considered: minimal medications required to control asthma, degree of airway hyper-responsiveness to histamine or methacholine when this can be safely assessed, and/or pre- and post-bronchodilator spirometric results (see Chapter 8). In addition, other factors to consider include: environmental control of non-occupational relevant allergens such as cats or dust mites, and triggers such as tobacco smoke at home, compliance with prescribed medications and correct usage of delivery devices for inhaled medications.

In addition to the assessment of medical impairment by objective assessment of asthma severity, for patients who have *sensitizer-induced OA* the degree of functional disability is affected by the need to completely avoid further exposure to the sensitizer. Thus a spray painter with OA from diisocyanate exposure in paints who has stopped working may have mild or no ongoing asthma but may still be disabled by the inability to return to his established trade. This needs to be considered in the physician's report to assist in the compensation system assessment of disability (which is a non-medical assessment, in contrast to the impairment assessment), and also needs to be considered in addition to the ongoing asthma severity if the physician is asked to provide advice as to future work restrictions.

OUTCOME
Sensitizer-induced OA

A number of studies have demonstrated that the majority of patients with OA fail to recover after removal from exposure, with worse outcomes associated with longer duration of symptoms and exposure, delayed diagnosis, and greater severity. Such studies support early recognition and removal from exposure. Recent studies provide additional insight into the outcome of OA. Perfetti et al.[68] have shown that among patients with OA from various causes, the outcome is significantly better in the group removed from relevant work exposure for over 5 years compared with those removed for 5 years or less. Their findings of continued improvement in outcome of asthma beyond 5 years of removal from exposure to the sensitizer suggest that permanent disability ratings of patients with OA should be periodically re-evaluated during this time period.

Although there are a few anecdotal reports of death from occupational asthma, there has been limited mortality data for these patients. In a preliminary report by Liss and colleagues,[69] three deaths from asthma were identified among workers previously compensated for OA. This led to a comparison of mortality between over 1000 patients compensated for work-related asthma (OA or work-related aggravation of asthma), compared with non-work related asthmatics from a secondary/tertiary referral clinic, and workers compensated for work-related injuries. Mortality from respiratory disease among compensated asthmatics was slightly greater than expected in the general population (SMR 1.3). Although reported mortality from respiratory causes except asthma was greater among the secondary/tertiary asthma clinic patients than among the work-related asthmatics, these findings indicate the potential serious consequences of work-related asthma.

Among the same population, Liss et al.[70] have also reported on the morbidity of patients with OA as assessed by hospital admissions for respiratory disease. Those with OA had a significantly high rate of hospitalization for asthma compared with other compensated workers, but as might be expected, the rate was less (about 50%) compared with asthmatic patients from a secondary/tertiary referral practice. In support of the findings from Perfetti et al.[68] suggesting an improvement in asthma severity over time, admissions for the OA group were mainly in the first 5 years after onset of asthma.

Merget and colleagues[71] report some unexpected findings in the follow-up of workers with confirmed OA induced by complex platinum salts. Most workers had transferred to work outside the plant production building but 11% continued to be exposed in the same area and 19% had been transferred to other areas within the production building. The follow-up was at a median period of 54 months after transfer of work site. Not surprisingly, those who remained in the same exposure area all continued to be symptomatic while 50% of those who left the production building had clearing of symptoms. Surprisingly, however, 50% of those transferred to other areas within the production building also had clearing of their asthma symptoms despite the likelihood that they still had exposure to low levels of platinum salts. This is contrary to previous studies, which have led to the conclusion that complete removal of exposure to the sensitizer is necessary in those with OA. Despite symptoms clearing and negative skin tests in many subjects, bronchial hyper-responsiveness to methacholine persisted in 91% of all subjects, perhaps on the basis of airway remodeling. The duration of exposure time with symptoms, among those who were transferred out of the production building, was 14 months for those moving to other buildings and 18 months for those who left the plant. This suggests that, at least for platinum-salt induced OA, the window of opportunity for reversing airway hyper-responsiveness by removing the worker from exposure after the onset of OA is very short, perhaps within a year of asthma onset. As the authors of this study discuss from their earlier work, this might be achieved by a medical surveillance program.

Despite the clearly improved medical outcome by removal from exposure to the workplace sensitizer, the socio-economic outcome of such removal is often worse (despite acceptance of a workers' compensation claim), especially if the patient is required to leave their company to avoid further sensitizer exposure. Changes in the exposure conditions within the same workplace are preferable if these can be achieved, as for example in healthcare workers with occupational asthma from natural rubber latex, where changes in glove use by the worker and coworkers to minimize air-borne allergen exposure may allow continued work[72] with better socioeconomic outcome.[73] However, for most occupational sensitizers there is no known safe exposure level for those with related OA and early removal remains the current medical advice after a confirmed diagnosis. If the patient is relocated within the same building where even very low exposures to the sensitizer may occur, they should be very carefully monitored (with serial peak expiratory flow recordings and methacholine challenges) to assess the effects on their asthma and should be removed from even very low exposure areas if asthma worsens in relation to those areas.

Irritant-induced OA

There is much less information available as to the outcome of irritant-induced OA as compared with information on sensitizer-induced OA. From the initial reports by Brooks on patients with RADS,[3] some individuals had persistence of asthma for several years while other had clearing within a few months (in his initial criteria, a minimum 3 month duration of asthma was required for diagnosis of RADS). Information from poison control centers and accidental spills suggests that short-term symptoms are more common than long-term asthma but prognostic factors have not been clearly identified to date. It is not known whether the duration of irritant-induced asthma relates to the degree of irritant exposure, and/or factors such as gender, smoking history and atopy.

Work-related aggravation of asthma

Similarly there is little published documentation as to the outcome of work-related aggravation of asthma. Clinical experience suggests that often there is a temporary aggravation of asthma at work if there have been unusually high exposures to irritants such as when the workplace is being repainted, or is under construction. Such exposures are not known to cause long-term worsening of asthma and clinically usually resolve within a few weeks after cessation of such exposures, so that the patient can return to their usual work. Workers' compensation data from a system where work-related aggravation of asthma was compensatable showed that the duration of work-attributed symptoms and time off work after a workplace accidental exposure was in the range of a few days to weeks for most patients with work-related aggravation of asthma as compared with several months for those with irritant-induced asthma.[74]

Some asthmatics have a long-term worsening of asthma which they may relate to a mild or moderate irritant exposure at work. Asthma severity is variable, often for no identified reason and currently it is not known whether mild or moderate workplace exposures can truly cause long-term or permanent asthma worsening or whether this represents the natural history of asthma in that patient for other/unknown reasons. Such questions might be resolved in the future by prospective studies of workplaces with and without irritant exposures.

PREVENTION
Sensitizer-induced OA

Primary prevention

Control of exposure in the form of substitution, improvement of ventilation, and change of process and enclosure have been used in occupational asthma. The most successful example is the virtual disappearance of detergent enzyme-induced asthma after the introduction of various forms of control.[75] Other studies also support a reduction in workplace aeroallergen exposure levels to prevent OA. For example, Houba et al.[76] in the baking industry showed a relationship between exposure levels and allergic symptoms. Reeb-Whitaker et al.[77] showed that in animal facilities aeroallergen levels could be significantly reduced by: (1) housing mice in cages with a filter-sheet top or a fitted filter-bonnet top, (2) using a negative pressure in the cage and (3) handling animals under a ventilated table.

Restriction of employment has been used with success in some instances in the primary prevention of OA, such as in the platinum refinery workers,[71] but knowledge of host susceptibility factors is limited. Atopy is a risk factor in asthma due to large molecular weight occupational allergens, but the positive predictive value is low. Moreover, over 30% of young adults are atopic subjects, thus screening for atopy is not recommended. Ensuring the workplace is free from tobacco smoke may be helpful in reducing sensitization to some allergens.

Secondary prevention
Medical surveillance programs for the early detection of OA have been suggested for occupational settings at high risk. However, there has been little published as to the effectiveness of these. In Ontario, a program of medical surveillance for diisocyanate-induced asthma was initiated in 1979 under government regulations. It has been reported that diisocyanate-induced OA is diagnosed earlier in Ontario than other causes of OA and these patients have a better outcome.[78] Nevertheless there has been no direct assessment of the program or its components.

A study by Kraw et al.[79] retrospectively assessed the outcome of 39 workers in one large foam-producing plant who were identified on the basis of the surveillance program and referred for specialist assessment. Only one was eventually found to have OA, although two who had a history of OA were quickly removed from exposure prior to assessment, and had resolution of their symptoms with no airway hyper-responsiveness. The questionnaire component in this study appeared to be the most useful screening measure. Spirometry did not add to the benefit of the questionnaire. However, further studies to assess the role of medical surveillance components are needed to more fully assess the value of such programs.

Irritant-induced OA

Some prevention of exposure to high concentrations of respiratory irritants in the workplace may be achieved by good occupational hygiene practices in the workplace and the inclusion of worker education as to the appropriate actions to take in the event of accidents, such as containment measures, appropriate respiratory protection and evacuation. However, because of the accidental nature of such exposures it may not be possible to prevent all cases of irritant-induced asthma.

Work-related aggravation of asthma

Unlike the preventive measures for irritant-induced asthma, which are indicated for all potentially exposed workers, the prevention of work-related aggravation of asthma is largely directed at the individual who has asthma, since they may not tolerate work environments which would be considered safe for non-asthmatics. The measures taken relate to the individual's asthma severity and control as well as to the work exposures.

Optimum non-occupational environmental control measures, asthma education, and pharmacologic control of underlying asthma are clearly beneficial to the patient to reduce the likelihood and severity of asthma exacerbations.

Patients with asthma would be expected to benefit from pre-employment counseling by their physician as to which types of occupation may aggravate their asthma symptoms, depending on the severity and control of asthma. Work in a relatively clean environment with limited expected exposure to dusts, smoke, fumes, and sprays, with moderate workplace temperatures and exertional requirements which are not known to trigger asthma in such a patient would be ideal. Conversely, shoveling snow in the winter months or work in an industrial setting with glues, solvents or irritant cleaning agents, for example, would be expected to exacerbate symptoms in most asthmatics. It is of interest that individuals with childhood onset of asthma may self-select to appropriate occupations. For example, a recent study[80] comparing medical x-ray technologists and physiotherapists found a significantly lower history of childhood asthma among the medical x-ray technologists (who had exposure to potential respiratory irritants in x-ray film processing and development).

There may be greater difficulty for adult-onset asthmatics who have already chosen their career path. They may have the option of primary prevention of work-related aggravation of asthma by moving to work in a relatively clean environment with moderate temperatures and exercise requirements as discussed above. If not, then secondary measures such as an adjustment in asthma control medications such as inhaled steroids and long-acting bronchodilators during work weeks in addition to short-acting bronchodilators as needed may prevent work-related exacerbations of asthma. Such patients should also be educated as to the likelihood of increased effects of workplace irritants at times of concurrent upper respiratory infections (at which time it may be appropriate for them to be off work or in modified duties until asthma control again improves), or at times after non-occupational allergen exposures.

SUMMARY AND CONCLUSIONS

Each year the number of causes of OA continues to increase, with new agents, or new occupational uses of previously recognized sensitizers. Prevalence rates of some of the causes have been studied in detail but rates for individual causes will vary with geographic region, depending on the local occupations, industrial practices, and industrial hygiene measures which will affect levels of exposure to respiratory sensitizers and irritants. As the prevalence of asthma in the general population has increased, more workers have asthma, thus increasing the population at risk for workplace aggravation of their asthma.

Work-related asthma should be considered in any adult with new onset or worsening asthma. Once the diagnosis of asthma is confirmed, investigations to clarify the presence and type of work-related asthma should be pursued. As objective a diagnosis as possible should be reached, as the management and prevention of sensitizer-induced, irritant-induced, and work-aggravated occupational asthma differ. Unfortunately there is no simple, readily available diagnostic test for occupational asthma. A careful occupational history is critical. Supportive or confirmatory investigations vary depending on the type of work-related asthma and, whenever possible, should be performed before the patient is removed from work. Improved preventive, surveillance, and diagnostic strategies are greatly needed. Ongoing research to better define the pathogenic mechanisms and host and exposure risk factors should lead to such strategies.

References

1. Bernstein IL, Chan-Yeung M, Malo JL, Bernstein DI. Definition and classification of asthma. In: Bernstein IL, Chan-Yeung M, Malo JL, Bernstein DI, eds. Asthma in the workplace. New York: Marcel Dekker Inc., 1999;1–4.
2. Chan-Yeung M, Malo JL. Tables of major inducers of occupational asthma. In: Bernstein IL, Chan-Yeung M, Malo JL, Bernstein DI, eds. Asthma in the workplace. New York: Marcel Dekker Inc., 1999;683–720.
3. Brooks S, Bernstein I. Reactive airways dysfunction syndrome. In: Bernstein IL, Chan-Yeung M, Malo JL, Bernstein DI, eds. Asthma in the workplace. New York: Marcel Dekker Inc., 1999;533–50.
4. Fabbri LM, Ciaccia A, Maestrelli P, Saetta M, Mapp CE. Pathophysiology of occupational asthma. In: Bernstein IL, Chan-Yeung M, Malo JL, Bernstein DI, eds. Asthma in the workplace. New York: Marcel Dekker Inc., 1999;81–110.
5. Cartier A, Grammer L, Malo J, et al. Specific serum antibodies against isocyanates: association with occupational asthma. J Allergy Clin Immunol 1989; 84:507–14.
6. Frew A, Chan H, Dryden P, Salari S, Lam S, Chan-Yeung M. Immunologic studies of the mechanisms of occupational asthma caused by Western red cedar. J Allergy Clin Immunol 1993; 92:466–78.
7. Mapp CE, Saetta M, Maestrelli P, Ciacia A, Fabbri LM. Low molecular weight pollutants and asthma: pathogenetic mechanisms and genetic factors. Eur Respir J 1994; 7:1559–63.
8. Frew AJ, Chan H, Chang JH, et al. T lymphocyte response to plicatic acid-albumin conjugate in occupational asthma due to Western red cedar. J Allergy Clin Immunol 1998; 108:841–7.
9. Kipen HW, Blume R, Hutt D. Asthma experience in an occupational and environmental medicine clinic: low dose reactive airways dysfunction syndrome. J Occup Med 1994; 36:1133–7.
10. Brooks SM, Hammad Y, Richards I, Giovinco-Barbas J, Jenkins K. The spectrum of irritant-induced asthma; sudden and not-so-sudden onset and the role of allergy. Chest 1998; 113:42–9.
11. Lemiere C, Malo J-C, Boulet L-P, Boutet M. Reactive airways dysfunction syndrome induced by exposure to a mixture containing isocyanate: functional and histopathologic behaviour. Allergy 1996; 51:262–5.
12. Meredith S, Nordman H. Occupational asthma: measures of frequency from four countries. Thorax 1996; 51:435–40.
13. Blanc P. Occupational asthma in a national disability survey. Chest 1987; 92:613–7.
14. Blanc PD, Cisternas M, Smith S, Yelin E. Occupational asthma in a community-based survey of adult asthma. Chest 1996; 109:56S–57S.
15. Blanc PD, Eisner MD, Israel L, Yelin E.H. The association between occupation and asthma in general medical practice. Chest 1999; 115:1259–64.
16. Burney PG J. Epidemiology trends. In: Barnes PJ, Grunstein MM, Leff AR, Woolcock A, eds. Asthma. Philadelphia: Lippincott-Raven, 1997;35–47.
17. Kogevinas M, Anto JM, Sunyer J, Tobias A, Kromhout H, Burney P, and the ECRHS Study Group. Occupational asthma in Europe and other industrialized areas; a population-based study. Lancet 1999; 353:1750–4.
18. Kogevinas M, Anto JM, Soriano JB, Tobias A, Burney P and the Spanish Group of the European Asthma Study. The risk of asthma attributable to occupational exposure. Am J Respir Crit Care Med 1996; 154:137–43.
19. Fishwick D, Pearce N, D'Souza W, et al. Occupational asthma in New Zealanders: a population based study. Occup Environ Med 1997; 54:301–6.
20. Johnson A, Dimich-Ward H, Manfreda J, et al. Occupational asthma in adults in six Canadian communities. Am J Respir Crit Med 2000; 162:2058–62.
21. Becklake M, Malo JL, Chan-Yeung M. Epidemiologic approaches in occupational asthma. In: Bernstein IL, Chan-Yeung M, Malo JL, Bernstein DI, eds. Asthma in the workplace. New York: Marcel Dekker Inc., 1999;27–66.
22. Tarlo SM, Broder I. Irritant-induced asthma. Chest 1989; 96:297–300.
23. Tarlo SM, Liss G, Corey P, Broder I. Classification and outcome of occupational asthma claims in Ontario. Chest 1995; 107:634–41.
24. Ross DJ, McDonald JC. Asthma following inhalation accidents reported to the Sword project. Ann Occ Hyg 1996; 40:645–50.
25. Cone JE, Wugofski L, Balmes JR, et al. Persistent respiratory health effects after a metam sodium pesticide spill. Chest 1994; 106:500–8.
26. Houba R, Heederik DJ, Doekes G, van Run PE M. Exposure sensitization relationship for alpha-amylase allergens in the baking industry. Am J Respir Crit Care Med 1996; 154:130–6.
27. Heederik D, Venables KM, Malberg P, et al. Exposure–response relationships for work-related sensitization in workers exposed to rat urinary allergens: results from a pooled study. J Allergy Clin Immunol 1999; 103:678–84.
28. Vedal S, Chan-Yeung M, Enarson D, et al. Symptoms and pulmonary function in western red cedar workers related to

duration of employment and dust exposure. Arch Environ Health 1986; 41:179–83.

29. Burge PS, Edge G, Hawkins R, White V, Taylor AN. Occupational asthma in a factory making flux-cored solder containing colophony. Thorax 1981; 36:828–34.

30. Venables KM, Newman-Taylor AJ. Exposure–response relationships in asthma caused by tetrachlorophthalic anhydride. J Allergy Clin Immunol 1990; 85:55–8.

31. Venables KM, Dally MB, Nunn AJ, et al. Smoking and occupational allergy in workers in a platinum refinery. Br Med J 1989; 299:939–42.

32. Tarlo SM. Workplace respiratory irritants and asthma. In: Banks D, ed. Occupational medicine: state of the art review. Philadelphia: Hanley and Belfus, 2000;471–83.

33. Mitchell C, Gandevia B. Respiratory symptoms and skin reactivity in workers exposed to proteolytic enzymes in the detergent industry. Am Rev Respir Dis 1971; 104:1–12.

34. Cullinan PLD, Nieuwenhuijsen MJ, Gordon S, et al. Work-related symptoms, sensitization, and estimated exposure in workers not previously exposed to laboratory rats. Occup Environ Med 1994; 51:589–92.

35. Desjardins A, Malo J-L, L'Archeveque J, Cartier A, McCants M, Lehrer SB. Occupational IgE-mediated sensitization and asthma caused by clam and shrimp. J Allergy Clin Immunol 1995; 96:608–17.

36. Cartier A, Malo J, Ghezzo H, McCants M, Lehrer S. IgE sensitization in snow crab-processing workers. J Allergy Clin Immunol 1986; 78:344–8.

37. Johnson AJ, Chan-Yeung M. Nonspecific bronchial hyper-responsiveness. In: Bernstein IL, Chan-Yeung M, Malo JL, Bernstein DI, eds. Asthma in the workplace. New York: Marcel Dekker Inc., 1999;173–92.

38. Newman-Taylor AJ. Genetics and occupational asthma. In: Bernstein IL, Chan-Yeung M, Malo JL, Bernstein DI, eds. Asthma in the workplace. New York: Marcel Dekker Inc., 1999;67–80.

39. Horne C, Quintana PJE, Keown P, Dimich-Ward H, Chan-Yeung M. Distribution of DRB1 and DQB1 HLA class II alleles in patients with western red cedar asthma. Eur Respir J 2000; 15:911–4.

40. Christiani D, Malo JL. Upper airways involvement. In: Bernstein IL, Chan-Yeung M, Malo JL, Bernstein DI, eds. Asthma in the workplace. New York: Marcel Dekker Inc., 1999;331–40.

41. Kim CS, Kang TC. Comparative measurement of lung deposition of inhaled fine particles in normal subjects and patients with obstructive airway disease. Am J Respir Crit Care Med 1997; 155:899–905.

42. Malo JL, Ghezzo H, L'Archeveque J, Lagier F, Perrin B, Cartier A. Is the clinical history a satisfactory means of diagnosing occupational asthma? Am Rev Respir Dis 1991; 143:528–32.

43. Chan-Yeung M. Assessment of asthma in the workplace. ACCP Consensus Statement. American College of Chest Physicians. Chest 1995; 108:1084–117.

44. Tarlo SM, L-P Boulet, Cartier A, et al. Canadian Thoracic Society Guidelines for occupational asthma. Can Respir J 1998; 5:289–300.

45. Tarlo SM. Recent advances in occupational asthma. Curr Opin Pulm Med 2000; 6:145–50.

46. American Thoracic Society. Guidelines for methacholine and exercise challenge testing–1999. Am J Respir Crit Care Med 2000; 161:309–29.

47. Banks DE, Barkman HW Jr, Butcher BT, et al. Absence of hyper-responsiveness to methacholine in a worker with methylene diphenyl diisocyanate (MDI) induced asthma. Chest 1986; 89: 389–93.

48. Cote J, Kennedy S, Chan-Yeung M. Sensitivity and specificity of PC 20 and peak expiratory flow rates in cedar asthma. J Allergy Clin Immunol l990; 85:592–8.

49. Moscato G, Godnic-Cvar J, Maestrelli P, Malo JL, Burge PS, Coifman R. Statement on self-monitoring of peak expiratory flow in the investigation of occupational asthma. Subcommittee on Occupational Asthma of the European Academy of Allergy and Clinical Immunology. J Allergy Clin Immunol 1995; 96:295–301.

50. Leroyer C, Perfetti L, Trudeau C, L'Archeveque J, Chan-Yeung M, Malo J-L. Comparison of serial monitoring of peak expiratory flow and FEV$_1$ in the diagnosis of occupational asthma. Am J Respir Crit Care Med 1998; 158:827–32.

51. Cote J, Kennedy S, Chan-Yeung M. Quantitative versus qualitative analysis of peak expiratory flow in occupational asthma. Thorax 1993; 48:48–51.

52. Hamilton RG, Adkinson NF Jr, and the Multi-Center Latex Skin Testing Study Task Force. Diagnosis of natural rubber latex allergy: multicenter latex skin testing efficacy study. J Allergy Clin Immunol 1998; 102:482–90.

53. Bernstein JA, Bernstein DI, Stauder T, Lummus Z, Bernstein IL. A cross-sectional survey of sensitization to Aspergillus oryzae-derived lactase in pharmaceutical workers. J Allergy Clin Immunol 1999; 103:1153–7.

54. Grammer L, Shaughnessy M, Kenamore B. Utility of antibody in identifying individuals who have or will develop anhydride-induced respiratory disease. Chest 1998; 114:1199–202.

55. Lummus ZL, Alam R, Bernstein DI. Diisocyanate antigen-enhanced production of monocyte chemoattractant protein-1, IL8 and tumour necrosis factor-L by peripheral mononuclear cells of workers with occupational asthma. J Allergy Clin Immunol 1998; 102:265–74.

56. Bernstein DI, Cartier A, Cote J, et al. Diisocyanate antigen-stimulated monocyte chemoattractant protein-1 synthesis has greater test efficiency than specific antibodies for identification of diisocyanate asthma. Am J Resp Crit Care Med 2002; 166:445–50.

57. Wisnewski AV, Lemus R, Karol M, Redlich CA. Isocyanate-conjugated human lung epithelial cell proteins: a link between exposure and asthma. J Allergy Clin Immunol 1999; 104:341–7.

58. Ortega HG, Weissman DN, Carter DL, Banks D. Use of specific inhalation challenge in the evaluation of workers at risk for occupational asthma. Chest 2002; 121:132–8.

59. Nguyen B, Weytjens K, Cloutier Y, Ghezzo H, Malo J-L. Determinants of the bronchial response to high molecular weight occupational agents in a dry aerosol form. Eur Respir J 1998; 12:885–888.

60. Banks DE, Tarlo SM, Masri F, et al. Bronchoprovocation tests in the diagnosis of isocyanate-induced asthma. Chest 1996; 109:1370–9.

61. Obata H, Dittrick M, Chan H, Chan-Yeung M. Sputum eosinophils and exhaled nitric oxide during late asthmatic reaction in patients with western red cedar asthma. Eur Respir J 1999; 13:489–95.

62. Chan-Yeung M, Obata H, Dittrick M, Chan H, Abboud R. Airway inflammation, exhaled nitric oxide, and severity of asthma in patients with western red cedar asthma. Am J Respir Crit Care Med 1999; 159:1434–8.

63. Lemiere C, Pizzichini MMM, Balkissoon R, et al. Diagnosing occupational asthma: use of induced sputum. Eur Respir J 1999; 13:482–8.

64. Muller-Wening D, Neuhauss M. Protective effect of respiratory devices in farmers with occupational asthma. Eur Respir J 1998; 12:569–72.

65. Taivainen AI, Tukiainen HO, Terho EO, Husman KR. Powered dust respirator helmets in the prevention of asthma among farmers. Scand J Work Environ Health 1998; 24:503–7.

66. Laopressert N, Swanson MC, Jones RT, Schroeder DR, Yunginger JW. Inhalation challenge testing of latex-sensitive healthcare workers and the effectiveness of laminar-flow HEPA-filtered helmets in reducing rhinoconjunctivitis and asthmatic reactions. J Allergy Clin Immunol 1998; 102:998–1004.

67. American Thoracic Society. Guidelines for the assessment of impairment/disability in patients with asthma. Am Rev Resp Dis 1993; 147:1056–61.

68. Perfetti L, Cartier A, Ghezzo H, Gautrin D, Malo J-L. Follow-up of occupational asthma after removal from or diminution of exposure to the responsible agent. Chest 1998; 114:398–403.

69. Liss G, Tarlo SM, Banks D, Yeung K-S, Schweigert M. Preliminary report of mortality among workers compensated for work-related asthma. Am J Ind Med 1999; 35:465–71.

70. Liss G, Tarlo SM, MacFarlane Y, Yeung K-S. Hospitalization among workers compensated for occupational asthma. Am J Respir Crit Care Med 2000; 162:112–8.

71. Merget R, Schulte A, Gebler A, et al. Outcome of occupational asthma due to platinum salts after transferal to low-exposure areas. Int Arch Occup Environ Health 1999; 72:33–9.

72. Tarlo SM, Easty A, Eubanks K, et al. Outcomes of a natural rubber latex control program in an Ontario teaching hospital. J Allergy Clin Immunol 2001; 108:628–33

73. Vandenplas O, Jamart J, Delwiche JP, Evrard G, Larbanois A. Occupational asthma caused by natural rubber latex: outcome according to cessation or reduction of exposure. J Allergy Clin Immunol 2002; 109:125–30.

74. Chatkin J, Tarlo SM, Broder I, Liss G, Banks D. Outcome of irritant-induced asthma in a workers compensation population. Chest 1999; 116:1780–85.

75. Venables K. Prevention of occupational asthma. Eur Respir J 1994; 7:768–78.

76. Houba R, Heederik D, Doekes G. Wheat sensitization and work-related symptoms in the baking industry are preventable. An epidemiologic study. Am J Respir Crit Care Med 1998; 158:1499–503.

77. Reeb-Whitaker CK, Harrison DJ, Jones RB, Kacergis JB, Myers DD, Paigen B. Control strategies for aeroallergens in an animal facility. J Allergy Clin Immunol 1999; 103:139–46.

78. Tarlo SM, Banks DE, Liss G, Broder I. Outcome determinants for isocyanate induced occupational asthma among compensation claimants. Occup Environ Med 1997; 54:756–61.

79. Kraw M, Tarlo SM. Isocyanate medical surveillance: respiratory referrals from a foam manufacturing plant over a five-year period. Am J Ind Med 1999; 35:87–91.

80. Liss GM, Tarlo SM, Doherty J, et al. Physician diagnosed asthma, respiratory symptoms and associations with workplace tasks among radiographers in Ontario, Canada. Occup Environ Med 2003; 60:254–61.

19.3 Byssinosis and Other Textile Dust-Related Lung Diseases

E Neil Schachter

For nearly 300 years, work in the textile industry has been recognized as an occupational hazard. In the early 18th century, Ramazzini described a peculiar form of asthma among those who card flax and hemp. The 'foul and poisonous dust' that he observed 'makes the workmen cough incessantly and by degrees brings on asthmatic troubles'.[1] That such symptoms did occur in the early textile industry has been illustrated by Bouhuys in his physiologic studies at Philipsburg Manor (a restoration project of life in the early Dutch colonies in North Tarrytown, New York).[2] In a primitive workshop where raw flax fiber was processed, this study documented objective lung function changes characteristic of those seen in modern textile workers.

The term byssinosis derives from a Greek (βνσσοζ) and a Latin (byssus) root first applied to the description of illnesses of textile workers by the Belgian public health physician Achille Adrien Proust in the late 19th century.[3] Although numerous authors throughout the 19th and early 20th centuries in both Britain and Europe[4-11] described the respiratory manifestations of work-related illness in textile mills with increasing frequency, the disease remained essentially unrecognized in the United States until the 1960s when studies under the direction of Richard Schilling indicated that despite pronouncements to the contrary by both industry and government, characteristic byssinosis did occur in the US.[12-16]

From this modest beginning, through the efforts of epidemiologic and clinical investigations, the United States not only recognizes the important prevalence of this illness among its textile workers, but has, as a result of these findings, developed some of the most stringent environmental standards in the world. Additionally, these cotton dust standards are coupled with medical surveillance within the industry. This approach begun in the 1970s promises to reduce the prevalence of byssinosis in the United States, although residual disease in older and retired workers may persist. Moreover, shifts in the textile industry to other centers throughout the world and particularly to developing countries have recently confirmed that with inadequate control, byssinosis will continue to be a important occupational illness of international concern (Table 19.3.1).

Niven et al.[140] report that: 'similar prevalence rates of byssinosis as experienced in the UK in the 1950s and 1960s are now being experienced in the developing countries where production is increasing. Prevalence rates of byssinosis of 30% in Indonesia, 37% in Sudan, 40% in Ethiopia and up to 50% in India have been reported, although the same criteria for diagnosing byssinosis have not been used in all these studies. It thus appears that while the disease is disappearing from the UK as a result of both lower dust exposures and because of industrial recession, it is becoming epidemic in parts of the world where cheap labor can be exploited'.

THE TEXTILE INDUSTRY

Natural fibers are common in the vegetable world, particularly among plants structured with cellulose (e.g., cotton, wood, straw); however, only a limited number of these natural fibers can be used for textile products based on their physical properties (e.g., length, strength, pliability, elasticity). The use of these vegetable fibers for the manufacture of textiles dates back to the third millennium BC. Cotton was processed in India, flax in Egypt, and silk in China. The manufacture of these textiles, however, remained relatively limited, and the processes for converting them to yarn and fabric were primitive until the Industrial Revolution, at which time the cleaning and spinning of textiles became automated and developed on a large scale. Despite a tremendous growth in the use of man-made fibers, natural fibers remain a major source of textiles.

Recent trends in the industry show that while worldwide consumption of cotton continues to grow in recent years, production in the US has stabilized or declined, as have exports of this commodity (Table 19.3.2). This trend is reflected by a drop in the current workforce, which is projected to continue, albeit at a slower rate, well into the next decade (Table 19.3.3).

Vegetable fibers are categorized according to the origin of the fiber within the plant (Table 19.3.4). The difficulty in physically separating cellulose fibers from other vegetable components explains in part why only a limited number of plants can be used for textile manufacture. Steps in the processing of the three major vegetable fiber groups are outlined in Table 19.3.5. The early phases of the process (e.g., opening, picking, carding) tend to be dustier and dirtier because during this phase, non-cellulose plant material is separated from the fibers to obtain a pure product. In this stage of processing, brittle components of the processed plant may be ground by the mechanical separator and disseminated in a fine dust that includes particles of respirable dimension. Inhalation of this material is associated with the clinical syndromes seen in textile workers. The description presented by Kay[8] in 1831 is particularly vivid: 'In the production of yarn, cotton is subjected to various processes, during the different stages of which, considerable quantities of dust and small filaments escape, are driven into the air by the circular motions of the machinery. I have ascertained by inquiries which I prosecuted extensively amongst the population engaged in cotton spinning, that those employed in the early processes, and particularly in the card rooms, are more subject to those affections of the lungs which are vulgarly classed under the symptomatic denomination of coughs, than the workmen engaged in the latter operations'.

PATHOGENESIS AND ETIOLOGIC AGENTS

Despite studies of workers, as well as in-vivo and in-vitro models, etiologic agent(s) and pathogenesis of byssinosis remain unclear. Identification of a specific agent could lead

Location	References
Europe	
Great Britain	85, 111, 113
France	148
Italy	136
Holland	149
Yugoslavia	150
Scandinavia	151
Spain	29
Africa	
Egypt	27
Sudan	152
Uganda/Kenya	83
Far East	
Indonesia	153
China	154
India	26, 96
North America	
United States	86, 87, 102
Canada	155
Mexico	156

Table 19.3.1 Worldwide recognition of byssinosis among textile workers

	1994	1996	1999
US cotton production	9.7	18.9	17.0
US cotton exports	9.4	6.9	6.7
Worldwide cotton consumption	84.3	89.8	91.5

Source: Cotton and Wool Yearbook Summary 1994–2000 in http://USDA.mannlib.cornell.edu/.

Table 19.3.2 Cotton industry: US and worldwide (millions of bales)

Industry segment	1988	1998	2008 (projected)
Weaving, finishing, yarn and thread mills	400	320	251
Knitting mills	215	159	128
Carpets and rugs	61	64	74
Miscellaneous goods	53	55	49
Textile mill products (total)	728	598	501

Source: US Department of Labor in ftp://ftp.bls.gov/pub/special. requests/ep/ind.employment/indout4.txt

Table 19.3.3 Number of workers employed in the US textile industry ('000).

to technology that would eliminate such a toxin (either during the growing of cotton or the processing of textiles) before it is spread by dust in the workplace. The most common hypotheses about the pathogenesis of byssinosis include: (1) the release of mediators, (2) immunologic mechanisms, and (3) airway reactions to specific cotton dust components.

Release of mediators

The release of pharmacologic mediators either preformed (e.g., histamine, serotonin) or synthesized de novo (e.g., leukotrienes) has been proposed to explain the mechanism of the acute (across-shift) changes seen with exposure to cotton dust.[16-24] The subacute changes have been associated with hyper-reactivity and sustained airway obstruction.

Source of fiber	Examples
Fibers originate from seeds or the inner walls of the fruit.	Cotton, kapok (kapok tree)
Each fiber is a single cell.	Coir (coconuts)
Fibers originate from the inner bast tissue of the plant stems. Each fiber consists of the overlapping cells.	Flax, hemp, jute
Fibers are part of the fibrovascular system of leaves.	Abaca, heneguen, sisal

Table 19.3.4 Classification of vegetable fibers by source

Cotton	Jute	Sisal
Ginning	Retting	Decoration
Grading	Grading	Grading
Baling	Baling	Baling
Marketing	Marketing	Marketing
Opening	Opening	Breaking
Picking	Spreading	Spinning
Carding	Carding	Weaving
Combing	Drawing	
Framing	Roving	
Roving	Spinning	
Spinning	Weaving	
Weaving		

Table 19.3.5 Schematic outline of some of the key steps in the processing of three major textile groups

In-vitro studies using both animal[16,17,19,22,24] and human tissue[20-23] demonstrate that exposure to cotton dust or extracts of cotton bracts (CBE) leads to the release of histamine and other mediators.[19] Although cotton dust may itself contain histamine and other mediators, the quantity of these agents has generally been considered too small to explain the physiologic phenomenon. Recent work in vivo with subjects not previously exposed to cotton dust demonstrates that CBE injected into the skin elicits a cellular reaction characteristic of non-immunoglobulin-related mediator release,[25] with the early appearance of mast cells, which degranulate, followed by prominent chemotactic effects. Similar findings of inflammation have been reported in the airways with the generation of mediators following CBE exposure.[22]

Elevated levels of histamine have been reported in the blood of both cotton and flax workers.[26] Levels usually are significantly higher on the first day of re-exposure after an absence from work, and in some studies, the amount of histamine appears to be related to the level of dust exposure.[27] Individuals continuously exposed to cotton dust were reported to have lower blood levels of histamine than those with interrupted exposure.[28] The histamine metabolite 1-methylimidazole-4-acetic acid has been found to be elevated in 24-hour urine samples of normal individuals challenged with cotton dust. This finding suggests that endogenously formed histamine is released following exposure to cotton dust.[29,30]

A host of other mediators have been associated with airway irritation due to cotton dust exposure. It has been suggested that a 5-hydroxytryptamine receptor agonist is released by cotton dust, an observation that may be related to the finding that circulating platelets decrease over the work shift in textile workers.[24] When they are incubated with gram-negative bacteria isolated from cotton, neutrophils induce platelets to release serotonin, probably as a result of the generation of platelet-activating factor (PAF).[31]

Products of arachidonic acid metabolism, prostaglandins, leukotrienes, and thromboxane have all been demonstrated following cotton dust and bract stimulation of cells and tissue in vitro.[32,33]

No single mediator can explain cotton dust-induced bronchial obstruction. Histamine, although ubiquitous in these reactions, in general is associated with only a short-lived airway response, and pretreatment with antihistamines has not consistently blocked byssinotic reactions.[34] In contrast, the mast cell stabilizer cromolyn blunts the response to CBE. Leukotrienes and PAFs may account for some of the delayed features of the response as well as the associated chemotactic phenomena. None of these mediators, however, explain the characteristic tachyphylaxis that occurs over the work week early in the course of the disease (see below).

Immunologic mechanisms

Immunologic mechanisms have been proposed to explain clinical findings in byssinosis. These include: (1) immediate hypersensitivity (immunoglobulin E [IgE] mediated), (2) immune complex formation, and (3) complement activation. In favor of an immune reaction is the relatively long period of time (usually years) required before workers begin to note symptoms, which could indicate sensitization. Clinical investigations, however, show that naive subjects develop airway obstruction when challenged with CBE,[35] as well as immediate and delayed skin reactions.[25] These lung function changes in naive subjects are, in general, not associated with symptoms, and the delayed onset of symptoms in workers may reflect slow progressive damage.

Studies of textile workers have suggested that IgE-mediated reactions might be involved in byssinosis,[36,37] and found that exposure to dust in textile mills can raise IgE levels.[38] The presence of specific allergy to fungal antigens in cotton dust has been reported. However, other studies[39] have found negative RAST and skin test results for cotton dust extracts in byssinotic workers. Non-specific allergy, produced by other antigens or airway hyper-reactivity, may play a role in predisposing workers to byssinosis.[40,41]

The early suggestions of an immune complex disease have not been borne out by subsequent investigations.[42,43] Extracts of cotton dust have been shown to activate the complement cascade in vitro.[44] However, in-vivo measurements of complement during the work shift do not show signs of activation.[39]

Specific cotton dust components

There are at least 50 biologically active components of cotton dust that could contribute to pathologic reactions. Two of these components have been extensively studied.

Endotoxin

Vegetable fibers are host to a variety of micro-organisms. Unopened cotton boles are sterile;[45] however, sterility quickly disappears after the bole opens, and bacterial contamination of baled cotton is widely recognized.[46] Of the bacterial flora that live on the plants processed by the textile industry, interest has focused on Gram-negative organisms. Measurements of airborne contamination in cotton mills suggest that concentrations of 10^2 to 10^5 organisms/m^3 were present, with higher concentrations being found in cardrooms.[47,48] Bacterial endotoxin is a biologically active organic constituent of the wall of Gram-negative bacteria and is now commonly measured in cotton dust as well as in the air of the mills.[49,50] It has been hypothesized that these endotoxins promote inflammatory reactions in humans that account for many of the features of byssinosis.[51]

Endotoxin that is composed primarily of bacterial lipopolysaccharides (LPS) induces a variety of in-vitro and in-vivo reactions when studied in various animal and human models. Alveolar macrophages are activated by LPS and respond by secreting lysosomal enzymes and neutrophil chemotactic factors and by increasing phagocytosis.[52,53] Platelets also are recruited in this response.[54,55] Additionally, histamine release[50] and fever have been associated with exposure to LPS.

In a model cardroom, Castellan and coworkers[56] demonstrated a strong correlation between lung function decrements (over a 6-hour exposure) with levels of endotoxin (6–779 ng/m^3), but not airborne dust concentrations (0.12–0.55 mg/m^3). A similar study[57] demonstrated that washing cotton resulted in reduced declines in FEV_1, which correlated with endotoxin concentrations. A group of investigators have proposed a standard for airborne endotoxin.[58] While these guidelines may prove useful (they are as yet untested) their potential is already limited by the fact that between laboratories comparisons of standardized endotoxin preparations yield very different measurements.[59]

In contrast, not all studies indicate that endotoxin is associated with bronchospasm.[60] Some of the exposure levels in these negative studies, however, were lower than may be necessary to produce bronchoconstriction.[17,50,51,61,62]

Recently a series of clinical studies such as those of Nightingale et al.[63] and Michel et al.[64] indicate that in asthmatic, atopic, and even healthy individuals, the inhalation of endotoxin is associated with neutrophil inflammation and the release of interleukins (e.g., IL8 and TNFα)and other mediators. In some but not all individuals, Kline et al.[65] have demonstrated dose-related drops in lung function following challenge with inhaled lipopolysaccharide. Despite the plausible hypothesis that, as in asthma, chronic inflammation (in this case associated with endotoxin exposure) is the causative agent of chronic lung disease in the textile industry, epidemiologic studies of textile workers, such as that reported by Christiani et al,[66] have not confirmed this. In their 11-year prospective study of cotton and silk workers in Shanghai, cumulative dust levels, but not endotoxin, were associated with a consistent 11-year loss in FEV_1 (after adjustments for confounders). The authors conclude that cotton dust is more strongly associated with chronic airflow limitation than with endotoxin.

Taken together, these studies suggest that although the presence and quantity of endotoxin in cotton dust may be a good index of acute bronchoconstrictor responses, endotoxin alone is not the principal bronchoconstricting agent. The role of endotoxin in the development of chronic byssinosis disease remains to be determined.

Tannins

This group of biochemical substances is widely distributed among plants, particularly in their roots, leaves, and fruits. Tannins have been documented in mill dust and aqueous extracts of bracts. Soluble tannin was found to constitute 4.2% of unsieved mill dust and 5.1% of respirable mill dust in one setting.[67] Studies suggest that the biologic activity of these tannins may explain some of the physiologic observations seen with byssinotic reactions.[24,68-75] Tannins have been shown to recruit neutrophils into the airways of different laboratory animals.[68,69] In vitro, tannins cause aggregation of platelets with the release of a number of mediators, including serotonin and thromboxane A_2.[23] These inflammatory responses tend to mimic the time course of the acute response to CBE extracts. In addition to stimulating inflammatory cells, tannins may have a toxic effect on respiratory epithelial and endothelial cells.[73,74]

Several additional interesting activities of tannins on airway cells have been described by Cloutier et al.[76,77] In vitro, tannin inhibits chloride secretion of airway epithelium in part by inhibiting protein kinase c (PKC). Such inhibition could result in mucus retention and decreased mucociliary transport. Additionally this group has shown that cotton bract tannin can blunt isoproterenol-stimulated cyclic AMP (cAMP) accumulation by desensitizing tracheal epithelial cells to beta agonists. Ultimately this also could affect chloride secretion and mucous content in the airways, a phenomenon demonstrated by Marom et al.[22]

Tannins, by contrast, do not produce direct airway smooth muscle contraction in animal models, as do extracts of cotton dust.[24,74] Laboratory studies using guinea pigs to observe neutrophil recruitment and cotton textile workers to measure lung function changes across a shift failed to demonstrate a clinical effect of tannins.[75] Hence, although the biologic activity of tannins remains impressive in vitro, there is little evidence to support the theory that these agents contribute to clinical findings.

Other agents

Examination of the biochemical constituents of cotton dust has shown that this byproduct contains more than 50 biologically active substances, including tannins, terpenoids, primary amines, endotoxins, glucans (a major biochemical component of fungi), and lacinelenes, many with known toxic properties.[19,67,78] Attempts to better define the nature of these active agents have met with varying degrees of success. An in-vivo assay with healthy human subjects was established by Buck[79,80] to determine the bronchoconstrictor potential of various fractions of the crude bract preparation. The majority of the extract activity was confined to low molecular weight substances (<1000 daltons). Removal of lacinelene and endotoxin activities in this analysis failed to significantly reduce the bronchoconstrictor activity of the extract. The active agent in this system was highly soluble in water (as the cotton washing trials suggest) and less so in organic solvents. This purified fraction contains glucose and possibly other hexoses as well as amino nitrogen, but the final identification of the active agent or agents remains elusive.

CLINICAL FEATURES OF TEXTILE WORKER'S DISEASE

Byssinosis is a disease of textile workers characterized by distinctive work-related respiratory complaints (often called Monday symptoms) as well as changes in pulmonary function. When they are processed to make textiles, many[81-83] but not all vegetable fibers may cause byssinosis (Table 19.3.6). The distinguishing feature of the clinical history in the patient with byssinosis is its relationship to the work week. The worker, typically after having worked a number of years in the industry, describes chest tightness beginning on Monday (or the first work day of the work week) afternoons. The tightness subsides that evening, and the worker is well for the remainder of the week, only to re-experience the symptoms on the following Monday. Monday dyspnea may continue unchanged for years or may progress with symptoms developing on subsequent workdays until tightness is present throughout the work week and ultimately while the person is away from work on weekends and vacation.

When the symptoms become chronic, dyspnea is described as effort dependent. At this stage, a non-productive cough may be present. Monday symptoms are accompanied by across-shift decreases in lung function. These decreases may be present on other work days even in the absence of symptoms, but the physiologic changes are not so marked (Fig. 19.3.1). Baseline (Monday pre-shift) lung function deteriorates as the disease progresses. The characteristic respiratory and physiologic changes seen in byssinosis workers have been standardized by Schilling[79,80] into a series of grades (Table 19.3.7), which currently form the basis of most clinical and epidemiologic investigations. Symptoms other than chest tightness are frequent among textile workers, particularly cough and bronchitis. These symptoms probably represent variants of the airway irritation brought on by dust inhalation.

Byssinosis	Non-specific airway irritation
Cotton	Jute
Flax	Sunn: Indian hemp
Soft hemp	Henequen
Sisal	Mauritius hemp
	Manila hemp
	St. Helena hemp

Table 19.3.6 Vegetable dusts causing byssinosis

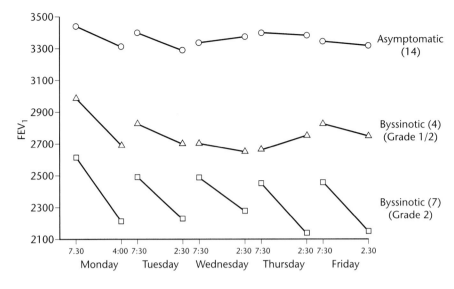

Figure 19.3.1: Forced expiratory volume in one second (FEV_1) during 5-day exposure of 25 carders classified according to symptoms of byssinosis. With permission from Merchant JA, Halprin GM, Hudson AR et al. Evaluation before and after exposure – the pattern of physiological response among cotton textile workers. Ann NY Acad Sci 1974; 221:38–43. © 1974 New York Academy of Sciences, USA.

Grade	Symptoms
Grade 0:	Normal – no symptoms of chest tightness or cough.
Grade 1/2:	Occasional chest tightness or cough or both on first day of working week.
Grade 1:	Chest tightness on every first day of the working week.
Grade 2:	Chest tightness on every first day and other days of the working week.
Grade 3:	Grade 2 symptoms, accompanied by evidence of permanent incapacity from ventilatory capacity.

Table 19.3.7 Grades of byssinosis

Many of the quoted epidemiologic studies note the high prevalence of bronchial irritability in workers with byssinosis. This finding tends to occur in older workers who frequently have a history of heavy smoking. Nevertheless, analysis of symptoms in non-smoking workers as well as pathologic findings suggest that chronic dust exposure is an independent risk factor for chronic bronchitis and, therefore, these symptoms are consistent with the diagnosis.

The prevalence of symptoms and lung function abnormalities is dose dependent and job dependent. For example, in a landmark study by Merchant et al.[86,87] involving North Carolina cotton textile workers, non-smoking workers in the yarn and cotton preparation areas had a byssinosis prevalence (all grades) of approximately 5% when they were exposed to median dust levels of 0.1 mg/m³; this rate rose to nearly 15% when the dust levels were 0.5 mg/m³. Among smokers, the prevalences were approximately 15% and 35% for similar exposure levels.

In different textile industries (e.g., hemp, cotton, flax) reported prevalences of byssinosis have varied greatly, as they have within a single industry. In a study by Valic and Zuskin[88] byssinosis prevalences were highest among hemp and flax workers (44% and 43%) and lower in cotton workers (20%). No specific byssinotic symptoms were elicited among the sisal or jute workers, although these workers experienced high prevalences of other non-specific respiratory symptoms. The absence of precise exposure data (e.g., dust and endotoxin levels) makes interpretation difficult.[88]

In addition to classic byssinosis, textile workers are subject to several other symptom complexes; in general, these problems are associated with fever and are not related to the initial day of the work week.

Mill fever (cotton fever, hemp fever) is associated with fever, cough, chills, and rhinitis that occurs with the workers' first contact with the mill or with return after a prolonged absence. Chest tightness does not appear to be associated with this syndrome. The occurrence of these findings is variable, from as low as 5%[85] of the workers to a majority of those employed.[89-91] Characteristically, symptoms subside after a few days despite continued exposure in the mill.

Weaver's cough[92] is primarily an asthmatic condition characteristically associated with fever; it occurs in both new and senior workers. The symptoms (unlike mill fever) can persist for months.

The third syndrome associated with textile processing is *mattress makers' fever*.[93] In its original description, it was characterized as an acute outbreak of fever and constitutional symptoms, including retrosternal discomfort in workers using low-grade cotton.

In general, the febrile syndromes are believed to be clinical entities distinct from byssinosis. For example, in studies of 528 cotton workers by Schilling,[88] 38 gave a history of mill fever. The prevalence among workers with classic byssinosis was 10% (14:134) compared with 6% (24:394) among workers without byssinosis (not significantly different).

As defined by historical criteria, chronic bronchitis is very prevalent among textile workers,[94,95] particularly among non-smoking textile workers.[89,96,97] This finding is not surprising because the most characteristic histologic feature of this disease is mucous gland hyperplasia.[98-100] The syndrome of chronic bronchitis should be distinguished carefully from the symptoms of classic byssinosis, although byssinotic and bronchitic complaints frequently overlap and are probably different pathophysiologic manifestations of airway inflammation in textile workers.

Pathologic studies of textile workers are limited, but reports have shown a consistent pattern of disease involving the larger airways but no evidence suggestive of destruction of lung parenchyma (e.g., emphysema).[99]

CLINICAL COURSE
Acute versus chronic disease

Implicit in the Schilling grading system (Table 19.3.7) is a progression from acute Monday symptoms to chronic and essentially irreversible respiratory disease in workers with byssinosis. That such a progression occurs has been suggested in cross-sectional data beginning with the early studies of Lancashire cotton workers, which found a shift toward higher byssinosis grades with increasing exposure (Table 19.3.8). Similar findings have since been reported by others.[101-102] Moreover, this progression may begin relatively soon after employment (e.g., within the first few years).[103]

Cross-sectional data[104,105] also have shown that other chronic respiratory symptoms such as wheezing or chronic bronchitis are much more prevalent in older cotton textile workers than in a similar control population. Table 19.3.9 shows the prevalence of chronic bronchitis in a population of cotton workers and in two control groups. In all cases, the cotton textile workers have more chronic bronchitis than do the controls, even when adjusting for sex and smoking status. Grade 3 byssinosis indicates that in addition to symptoms, textile workers demonstrate changes in respiratory function.

The progression from early byssinosis (grade 1) to late byssinosis (grade 3) is suggested by the association of lung function loss with the higher grades of byssinosis in cross-sectional studies of textile workers.[102,106] Several studies have given support to the concept that across-shift changes in lung function (which correlate with chest tightness) are related to chronic irreversible changes.[107]

Underlying the association between acute and chronic disease in textile workers is a dose–response relationship seen for acute symptoms. This relationship was first docu-mented by Roach and Schilling[108] who found a strong linear association between biologic response and total dust concentrations in the workplace. Based on their findings, they recommended 1 mg/m^3 gross dust as a reasonably safe level of exposure. This concentration, later adopted by the American Congress of Government Industrial Hygienists, was the value used as the threshold limit value (TLV) for cotton dust. The fine dust fraction (<7 μm) has been shown to account for practically all of the prevalence of byssinosis.[101,109,110] Merchant et al.[87] confirmed the association between byssinosis prevalence (as well as decrements in expiratory flows) and concentrations of lint-free dust in a study of cotton and other textile workers.

The validation of progressive changes in respiratory function suggested by cross-sectional studies has come from a number of longitudinal investigations that complement and extend the results of the earlier studies. These studies have highlighted the accelerated loss of lung function in cotton textile workers as well as the high incidence of new symptoms.[94,96,105,115,116]

Many authors have raised the potential confounding issue of cigarette smoking. Because many textile workers are cigarette smokers, it has been claimed that the chronic lung disease associated with exposure to textile dust can be attributed, in large part, to cigarette smoking. However, Beck et al.[117] demonstrated that the effects of cotton dust and smoking on lung function were additive, that is, the amount of lung function loss due to one factor (smoking or cotton dust exposure) was not changed by the presence or absence of the other factor. In a related study, Schachter et al.[118] demonstrated that using a parameter that described the shape of the maximum expiratory flow volume curve, angle beta, distinct patterns of lung function abnormalities could be shown for a smoking effect and for a cotton effect. Similar conclusions were also reached by Merchant.[86]

More recent studies have confirmed an association between acute, across-shift changes in lung function and chronic loss of lung function in textile workers. Glindmeyer et al.[119] found a significant association between acute and chronic effects of cotton dust extracts on lung function. While some shortcomings of this study have been pointed out by Becklake,[120] these observations are consistent with previous findings.

Years of exposure	Byssinosis grades 0	1	2	Total byssinotic (1 + 2)
0–9	14 (67%)	4 (19%)	3 (14%)	7 (33%)
10–19	22 (47%)	18 (39%)	7 (15%)	25 (53%)
10–29	22 (35%)	22 (35%)	19 (30%)	41 (65%)
30+	17 (29%)	23 (39%)	19 (32%)	42 (71%)

Table 19.3.8 Prevalence of byssinosis by length of work history

Sex	Smoking status	Columbia, SC, textile workers (1973)	Controls*	US HANES 1971–1975†
Male	Non-smoker	7.7	2.1	1.0§
	Smoker	36.6	21.1‡	13.6§
Female	Non-smoker	12.3	3.1	1.1§
	Smoker	21.4	7.6	7.1§

* Non-textile workers in Lebanon and Ansonia, Connecticut, and Winnsboro, South Carolina.
† Based on the Health and Nutrition Examination Survey of the National Center for Health Statistics to be representative of the US non-institutionalized population.
‡ Compared with cotton textile workers $P < 0.1$.
§ Compared with cotton textile workers $P < 0.05$.

Table 19.3.9 Prevalence of chronic bronchitis by sex and smoking status in three populations of whites aged 45–74 years

Mortality

Studies of cotton dust exposure on mortality rates have not consistently demonstrated an effect. Review of experience in the late 19th and early 20th centuries in England[121] suggested a high rate of cardiovascular mortality in older textile workers. In contrast, review of the experience in New England and Georgia mills failed to demonstrate high rates of mortality.[122,123] In contrast, a study of Dubrow and Gute[124] of male textile workers in Rhode Island using the proportionate mortality ratio (PMR), showed a significant PMR for non-malignant respiratory disease. These PMRs followed the trend of jobs with high dust exposure. An interesting finding of this and other studies[123,125] is the low mortality rates from lung cancer among these workers, which has been used to argue that smoking is not a major cause of mortality in these groups. Observations from a cohort in South Carolina[126] suggest that chronic lung disease is a major cause (or predisposing factor) for mortality in this population.

DIAGNOSIS

Unfortunately, there is no simple test to diagnose byssinosis. This diagnosis is made on the basis of worker symptoms and a consistent occupational exposure history. Although they are not always specific, lung function data may be helpful in establishing the diagnosis and in characterizing the degree of impairment.

History

Characteristic work-related symptoms found in the early stages of the disease (byssinosis grades 1/2, 1, and 2; Table 19.3.7) have served as a basis for establishing the clinical diagnosis. Chest tightness and breathlessness are associated with the first and possibly subsequent workdays following an absence from the workplace. These symptoms are characterized by substernal discomfort, which may be aggravated by exertion. The symptoms become progressively more prominent over the course of a work day, first being noted several hours after beginning work. The symptoms persist after leaving the mill but characteristically disappear by the evening. These grade 1 symptoms may persist for years or may advance rapidly to grade 2 symptoms.[85]

Confounding the clinical diagnosis of byssinosis is the frequent co-existence of cough and chronic bronchitis. These symptoms may result from dust exposure in combination with other risk factors, such as cigarette smoking, and the progression to grade 3 disease.

The importance of occupational history in the diagnosis of byssinosis needs to be emphasized. The early phases of the processing of cotton in the mill are those most likely to be associated with symptoms. Workers employed in maintaining and cleaning machinery (such as carding machines) may be at a particular risk. Also of interest when assessing exposure is the age of the equipment (many modern machines have built-in pollution control devices) and the layout of the mill; if the mill is small with different processing areas contiguous in one open space, dust levels and content may be similar in different processing areas.

A misconception that occasionally arises, even among otherwise sophisticated medical personnel, is that individuals may develop byssinosis from the end-product (cloth products). There is no evidence that these contain any of the toxicants of cotton dust, and hence neither fabricators of finished products (e.g., seamstresses) nor the general public are at risk.

Probably the most difficult differential diagnosis is in the older worker with irreversible lung disease. These workers with a variety of respiratory symptoms may describe 'Monday dyspnea,' which presumably occurred decades earlier. A history of cigarette smoking may confuse the issue because symptomatic findings may be identical in chronic smokers and workers with long exposures in the industry. Analysis of data from epidemiologic studies suggests that chronic exposures to cotton dust and cigarette smoke yield approximately equal physiologic impairment when measured by FEV_1.[111] A presumptive diagnosis should be made if the clinical, physiologic, and exposure data are consistent with byssinosis. This is particularly important in older workers with impairment of lung function in whom fixed symptoms are described and 'Monday dyspnea' may not be elicited.

Lung function

Monitoring of across-shift lung function changes and annual lung function testing are part of the mandated medical surveillance of workers in the United States.

In many workers with byssinotic symptoms lung function deteriorates over the Monday work shift. Characteristically, a 5% decrement or a loss of 0.2 liter of FEV_1 across a shift have been considered significant. More recently, the widespread availability of spirometric devices relating flow to volume has popularized the use of flow rates. Changes in flow rates at low lung volumes, such as the forced expiratory flow at 50% of the vital capacity (FEF_{50} or $Vmax_{50}$), show proportionally greater changes from baseline over a shift and have been used by some investigators[120] to characterize lung function changes. Despite the usefulness of spirometry in characterizing 'Monday dyspnea', there is not always a correlation between lung function and symptoms so that the absence of across-shift changes in FEV_1 does not exclude the diagnosis.

In addition to across-shift changes in spirometry, accelerated loss of lung function also is associated with work in the textile industry.[94] One proposed classification of respiratory impairment is shown in Table 19.3.10.[127] Other lung function measurements such as arterial blood gases[128] and nitrogen washout have been used to characterize byssinotic responses, but are not practical for diagnosis. Static lung recoil pressures[129] do not change with exposure. The diffusing capacity is usually unaffected in patients with byssinosis, consistent with the pathologic observations that chronic airway changes rather than emphysema are associated with byssinosis.[98-100,130] Overall, the physiologic picture suggests airways obstruction and, in particular, obstruction of smaller airways.[131] In some workers, however, a restrictive or mixed pattern also may be seen.[132]

Functional category	Across-shift change in FEV_1	Reduction in baseline FEV_1*
F0	None (less than 5%)	None (>80%)
F1/2	Slight (6–20%)	None
F1	Definite (>20%)	None
F2		Slight/moderate (60–75%)
F3		Moderate/severe (<60%)

* As a % of predicted

Table 19.3.10 Classification of respiratory impairment by functional grades in byssinosis

Physical examination

Physical findings in workers with byssinosis are non-specific. In workers with advanced disease, the stigmata of chronic obstructive airway disease (e.g., hyperinflation, cor pulmonale) may be elicited.

Laboratory evaluation

In general, routine laboratory examinations are not useful in the diagnosis of byssinosis. With advanced disease, the findings of respiratory insufficiency and cor pulmonale may be noted. The chest x-ray study usually is normal but may show changes caused by hyperinflation.

Challenge testing

A number of studies suggest that individuals with underlying hyper-responsiveness may be at greater risk for byssinosis. Among exposed individuals, atopic patients have been found to have greater declines in FEV_1 than non-atopic patients.[40] In studies of non-exposed individuals, responsiveness to a water-soluble extract of CBE produced lung function changes and symptoms similar to those of grade 1 byssinosis.[80] Similarly, non-exposed subjects who respond to CBE have been found to have a lower threshold to methacholine and a greater response to metaproterenol than those who do not respond to CBE.[41]

Immunologic testing

Extracts of various cotton byproducts have been shown to produce an immediate as well as a delayed reaction to skin testing[133] but have not proven to be useful diagnostically. Immediate sensitivity to skin testing has not been associated with airway reactivity. This finding is not surprising because the typical airway response to CBE is not immediate but subacute.[35,41] The delayed response on skin testing characterized by Schachter and colleagues,[25] may correlate with the airway inflammation and bronchoconstriction reported following airway challenge with CBE.[135] Skin testing and RAST testing for cotton dust have not been shown to be helpful in establishing the diagnosis of byssinosis.[39] Finally, workers with byssinosis do not have elevated levels of IgE.[136]

Other diagnostic tests

Routine blood and urine tests, chest x-ray studies, and ECGs are not helpful in diagnosing byssinosis. However, they may be useful in characterizing the complications of chronic lung disease, such as respiratory infection, respiratory failure, or cor pulmonale.

Blood histamine levels have been reported to correlate with the days of the week and the level of dust exposure,[26, 27] but have not been used routinely to diagnose this disease.

Pathologic studies of textile workers are limited, but reports have shown a consistent pattern of disease involving the airways without evidence suggestive of destruction of lung parenchyma (e.g., emphysema). Histologic evalua-tion is not indicated in the routine work-up of patients with suspected byssinosis.

Relatively little is known about the cellular constituents and inflammatory products associated with the airway disease of textile workers.[137] In a study of BAL in naive subjects prior to challenge with CBE, Merrill and coworkers[138] noted that the proportion of lymphocytes present in BAL correlated with the physiologic response. Subsequent studies by this group have demonstrated the inflammatory nature of the response to CBE[128] and the release of mediators. Experience is much too limited at present to advocate the use of this technique for either diagnosis or management.

Specific antigen inhalation tests have been used to characterize occupational lung diseases. Schachter and coworkers challenged seven senior textile workers with CBE[139] who all had severe impairment of respiratory function (mean FEV_1 52% of predicted) and carried a presumptive diagnosis of byssinosis. Four of seven workers responded to the extract (20% or greater decrease in maximal expiratory flow, measured on the partial flow volume curve [MEF] 40% [P]). These findings suggest that with chronic established disease, challenge with CBE may not be a sensitive method of diagnosis, because at this stage of the disease, reactivity to CBE may have waned in some workers.

TREATMENT AND PREVENTION

Byssinosis displays many of the physiologic features of asthma and chronic bronchitis. Therefore, it is not surprising that the administration of bronchodilating agents such as beta-adrenergic drugs can prevent bronchoconstrictor responses to textile dust exposure.

Antihistamines have been shown to modify byssinotic symptoms and airway obstruction.[18,34] This latter effect is not surprising given the histamine-releasing action of many textile dusts.[16,17] Disodium cromoglycate[34] has been shown to be a potent agent in preventing acute and delayed responses to organic dusts. Induced airway obstruction through extracts of CBE as well as bronchoconstriction in workers has been significantly reduced by pretreatment with disodium cromoglycate.[34,140] Finally, the administration of aerosolized steroids (e.g., beclomethasone) has proved beneficial.[140]

A comprehensive approach to medical management for the worker with byssinosis has not been formulated. Based on clinical studies, it would appear that beta-agonists (e.g., albuterol) are among the most effective agents for the management of acute respiratory symptoms. If the sensitive worker knows he or she will be exposed to a particularly dusty environment, pretreatment is indicated. The role of long-acting β-agonists such as salmeterol is unknown but is likely to be useful given the effectiveness in asthmatic individuals with persistent symptoms. Because most studies suggest that chronic airway disease in byssinosis is the result of a chronic inflammatory state, the use of aerosolized steroids for workers with symptoms who continue in a dusty environment may have short-term as well as long-term benefits. Other agents such as disodium cromoglycate and antihistamines also may play a role. To date, there are no controlled clinical trials indicating that long-term pharmacologic management alters the course of the disease.

Prevention of byssinosis is clearly preferable to medical management of the chronic condition. At present, recommended prevention strategies include: (1) dust abatement, (2) medical surveillance with transfer policies for affected workers, (3) treatment of raw cotton to eliminate toxic factors. Currently, preventive efforts are primarily directed at implementing the first two strategies. Pre-employment screening of workers to identify workers with airway hyper-reactivity or a pre-existing allergic condition has been considered but this has not been generally adopted. Finally, although a number of organic and biologic constituents of cotton dust have been implicated in byssinosis, this knowledge has not yet translated itself into an effective strategy for rendering the workplace less dangerous.

In view of the additive effect of cigarette smoking, smoking cessation should be promoted and a smoke-free workplace should be the norm, as recommended by NIOSH.[141]

Criteria for removal of the affected individual from the workplace, with or without transfer to less dusty areas, are not explicitly defined. Workers with a diagnosis of byssinosis, disabling symptoms, progressive lung function loss, or established obstructive airway disease should be considered for transfer or removal from high-risk areas.

COMPENSATION

Byssinosis was not commonly recognized as an occupational disease in the United States until the 1960s. In contrast, in Great Britain as early as 1927 governmental committees were set up to investigate the effects of dust in the cotton industry,[142] and as a result of one such effort, the Byssinosis (Workmen's Compensation) Scheme became effective in 1941. Under this policy, to be considered disabled, workers had to be male, employed on or after the date of adoption of the Scheme, and working in specified areas. It also was required that these workers be employed in the industry for at least 20 years and be totally and permanently disabled. Over the succeeding years, the terms for compensation were liberalized to include women, cover degrees of disability less than total, reduce the length of exposure necessary for claims, abolish the specific job requirements, and extend the regulations to include flax workers. By 1979, a total of 5045 textile workers had been accepted for compensation at a time when the average annual size of the eligible workforce was 14,700 (this number increased by 7500 in 1974 because of further changes in standards for eligibility).

SURVEILLANCE AND DUST CONTROL

In June 1978, the United States Occupational Safety and Health Administration (OSHA) issued a new cotton dust standard, based on a NIOSH criteria document. This standard proposed reductions in dust levels in the workplace to be implemented over a 4-year period. During this transition period, workers in high dust areas would wear respirators or masks. For those workers unable to wear respirators, the standard mandated transfer without loss of pay or seniority. In 1981, the United States Supreme Court upheld the more rigorous dust standards advocated by the Textile Worker's Union (ACTWU). At present, the principal provision requires that no more than 200 µg/m^3 respirable particles (measured over an 8-hour period as a time weighted average) be present in yarn manufacturing and cotton washing operations, and carding and spinning areas. For the textile mill waste house operations and lower grade washed cotton in the yarn manufacturing area, the level is 500 µg/m^3, and for slashing and weaving, 750 µg/m^3. The level is 1000 µg/m^3 for waste recycling and garnetting. Data are not readily available to confirm the common view that compliance is generally good.

The adequacy of the current standard has been challenged by the study of Glindmeyer et al.[147] indicating that exposure to dust concentrations below those specified by the current OSHA standard (i.e., <150 µg/m^3 in slashing and weaving areas) might be harmful, particularly in the case of workers who were smokers. They suggested that smokers be restricted from working in yarn manufacturing areas and that the feasibility of lowering allowable respirable dust levels for all yarn manufacturing be studied.

The OSHA standard mandates medical surveillance and specifies standards for the type of apparatus used, the measurement techniques, the interpretation of the tests, and the qualification of the personnel administering the tests. Current standards require that lung function tests be administered annually. If a worker's baseline is less than 80% of predicted or if the FEV$_1$ decreases by more than 5–10% over a work shift, retesting should be performed semiannually. If lung function is less than 60% of predicted, workers are referred to physicians for a complete examination. The consultant reports to the employer who then voluntarily initiates any necessary change in the employee's work status. Wage retention and transfer, however, are only guaranteed as specified by the employee's contract.[138] The standard does not address pre-existing airways disease. Recent studies suggest that prescreening workers with measurements of airway reactivity may be useful in identifying workers susceptible to byssinosis. Other studies suggest that airway hyper-reactivity may result from dust exposure.

The outcome of dust abatement on respiratory health in this country as a result of regulatory requirements is largely unknown. The one major study reported in the last decade which addresses this issue[147] indicates that overall byssinosis symptoms were less than 5% among the more than 2000 textile workers studied. There was nonetheless a significantly higher loss of lung function among textile workers due to dust exposure that was dose dependent. Despite clear-cut gains in worker safety in the United States, the problem of adequate and available medical, financial, and rehabilitative help for workers disabled by years of service in the textile industry remains to be resolved. Although the prevalence of byssinosis in developed countries has fallen, prevalence rates in the developing world remain high.

References

1. Ramazzini B. Diseases of workers. Translated from the Latin text De Morbis Artificum of 1713 by Wright WC. New York: Hafner Publishing Co., 1964.
2. Bouhuys A, Mitchell CA, Schilling RSF, Zuskin E. A physiologic study of byssinosis in colonial America. Trans New York Acad Sci 1973; 35:537–46.
3. Massoud A. The origin of the term 'byssinosis'. Br J Ind Med 1964; 21:162.
4. Collis EL. Report of the Inspector of Factory Workshops. London: His Majesty's Stationery Office, 1909.
5. Corn JK. Byssinosis. An historical perspective. Am J Ind Med 1981; 2:331–51.
6. Greenhow EH. Third Report of the Medical Officer of the Privy Council. Sir John Simon, Appendix 6. London: Her Majesty's Stationery Office, 1860;152.
7. Hill AB. Sickness among operatives in Lancashire cotton spinning mills. Industrial Health Research Board Report No. 59. London: His Majesty's Stationery Office, 1930.
8. Kay JP. Observations and experiments concerning molecular irritation of the lungs as one source of tubercular consumption; and on spinner's phthisis. North Engl Med Surg J 1831; 1:348–63.
9. Leach J. Surat cotton, as it bodily affects operatives in cotton mills. Lancet 1863; 2:648–9.
10. Patissier P. Traite des maladies des artisans. Paris: JB Baillière, 1822.
11. Proust AA. Traite d'hygiene publique et privee. Paris: Masson, 1877;171–4.
12. Schilling RSF. Worldwide problems of byssinosis. Chest 1981; 79:3S–5S.
13. McKerrow CB, Schilling RSF. A pilot enquiry into byssinosis in two cotton mills in the United States. JAMA 1961; 177:850–3.
14. Britten RH, Bloomfield JJ, Goddard JC. Health of workers in textile plant. US Public Health Service, Bulletin No. 207, 1933.
15. US Dept of Labor, Labor Standards Division. Special Bulletin No. 18, 1945.
16. Ainsworth SK, Neuman RE, Harley RA. Histamine release from platelets for assay of byssinosis substances in cotton mill dust and related materials. Br J Ind Med 1979; 36:35–42.
17. Antweiler H. Histamine liberation by cotton dust extracts: evidence against its causation by bacterial endotoxin. Br J Ind Med 1961; 18:130–2.
18. Bouhuys A, Ortega J. Improvement of 'irreversible' airway obstruction by thiazinamium (Multergan). Pneumologie 1976; 153:185–95.
19. Davenport A, Paton WDM. The pharmacologic activity of extracts of cotton dust. Br J Ind Med 1962; 19:19–32.
20. Evans E, Nicholls PJ. Studies of the mechanism of histamine release from lung tissue in vitro by cotton dust extracts. Agents Actions 1974; 4:304–10.
21. Hitchcock M, Piscitelli DM, Bouhuys A. Histamine release from human lung by a component of cotton bracts. Arch Environ Health 1973; 26:177–82.
22. Marom Z, Schachter EN, Goswami S, et al. The effect of cotton bract extract on respiratory glycoconjugate secretion from human airways in vitro. J Allergy Clin Immunol 1989; 84:710–7.
23. Rohrbach MS, Rolstad RA, Tracy PB, Russell JA. Platelet 5-hydroxytryptamine release and aggregation promoted by cotton bracts tannin. J Lab Clin Med 1984; 103:152–60.
24. Russell JA, Gilberstadt ML, Rohrbach MS. Constrictor effect of cotton bract extract on isolated canine airways. Am Rev Respir Dis 1982; 125:727–33.
25. Schachter EN, Buck MG, Merrill WW, et al. Skin testing with an aqueous extract of cotton bract. J Allergy Clin Immunol 1985; 76:481–7.
26. Parikh JR, Venkatakrishna-Bhatt H, Panchal GM. Blood histamine levels in cotton-dust exposed workers in a textile mill of Ahmedabad. Am J Ind Med 1987; 12:439–43.
27. Noweir MH, Abdel-Kader HM, Omran F. Role of histamine in the aetiology of byssinosis. Blood histamine concentrations in workers exposed to cotton and flax dust. Br J Ind Med 1984; 41:203–8.
28. Nicholls PJ, Evans E, Valic F, Zuskin E. Histamine-releasing activity and bronchoconstricting effects of sisal. Br J Ind Med 1973; 30:142–5.
29. Bouhuys A. Byssinosis in hemp workers. Arch Environ Health 1967; 14:533–43.
30. Edwards JH, McCarthy P, McDermott P, Nicholls PJ, Skidmore JW. The acute physiologic, pharmacological and immunological effects of inhaled cotton dust in normal subjects. J Physiol (London) 1970; 208:63–4.
31. Holt PG, Holt BJ, Beijer L, Rylander R. Platelet serotonin release by human polymorphonuclear leucocytes stimulated by cotton dust bacteria. Clin Exp Immunol 1983; 51:185–90.
32. Mundie TG, Ainsworth SK. Etiopathogenic mechanisms of bronchoconstriction in byssinosis. Am Rev Respir Dis 1986; 133:1181–5.
33. Cooper AD Jr, Merrill WW, Rankin JA, et al. Bronchoalveolar cell activation after inhalation of a bronchoconstricting agent. J Appl Physiol 1988; 64:1615–23.
34. Schachter EN, Brown S, Zuskin E, et al. The effect of mediator modifying drugs in cotton bract induced bronchospasm. Chest 1981; 79(Suppl):73s–77s.
35. Buck MG. A purified extract from cotton bracts induces airway constriction in humans. Chest 1981; 79(Suppl):43S–48S.
36. Oehling A, Gonzalez de La Reguera I, Viner Rueda JJ. A contribution to the allergic etiopathogeneity of byssinosis. Respiration 1972; 29:155–60.
37. Mundie TG, Pilia PA, Ainsworth SK. Serum immunoglobulin and complement concentrations in cotton mill workers. Arch Environ Health 1986; 40:326–9.
38. Salvaggio JE, O'Neil CE, Butcher BT. Immunologic responses to inhaled cotton dust. Environ Health Perspect 1986; 66:17–23.
39. Mundie TG, Osguthorpe JD, Martin C, Ainsworth SK. An investigation of atopy in byssinosis. Immunol Allergy Pract 1985; 7:367–72.
40. Jones RN, Butcher BT, Hammad YY, et al. Interaction of atopy and exposure to cotton dust in the bronchoconstrictor response. Br J Ind Med 1980; 37:141–6.
41. Schachter EN, Zuskin E, Buck MG, et al. Airway reactivity and cotton bract-induced bronchial obstruction. Chest 1985; 87:51–5.
42. Massoud A, Taylor G. Byssinosis: antibody to cotton antigens in normal subjects and in cotton and room workers. Lancet 1964; ii:607–10.
43. Edwards JH, Jones BM. Pseudoimmune precipitation by the isolated byssinosis antigen. J Immunol 1973; 110:498–501.
44. Mundie TG, Boackle RJ, Ainsworth SK. In vitro alternative and classical activation of complement by extracts of cotton mill dust: a possible mechanism in the pathogenesis of byssinosis. Environ Res 1983; 32:47–56.
45. Rylander R, Lundholm M. Bacterial contamination of cotton and cotton dust and effects on the lung. Br J Ind Med 1978; 35:204–7.
46. Rylander R, Imbus HR, Suh MW. Bacterial contamination of cotton as an indicator of respiratory effects among card room workers. Br J Ind Med 1979; 36:299–304
47. Cinkotai FF, Whitaker CJ. Airborne bacteria and the prevalence of byssinotic symptoms in 21 cotton spinning mills in Lancashire. Ann Occup Hyg 1978; 21:239–50.

48. Cinkotai FF, Lockwood MG, Rylander R. Airborne micro-organisms and the prevalence of byssinotic symptoms in cotton mills. Am Ind Hyg Assoc J 1977; 38:554–9.

49. Fischer JJ. The microbial composition of cotton dusts, raw cotton lint samples and the air of carding areas in mills. In: Wakelyn PJ, ed. Proceedings of the Third Special Session on Cotton Dust Research, Beltwide Cotton Research Conference, Phoenix, AZ, 1979;8–10.

50. Pernis B, Vigliani EC, Cavagnac, Finulli M. The role of bacterial endotoxins in occupational diseases caused by inhaling vegetable dusts. Br J Ind Med 1961; 18:120–129.

51. Rylander R. Bacterial toxins and etiology of byssinosis. Chest 1981; 79(Suppl):34s–38s.

52. Hudson A, Kilburn K, Halprin G, McKenzie W. Granulocyte recruitment to airways exposed to endotoxin aerosol. Am Rev Respir Dis 1977; 115:89–95.

53. Snella MC, Rylander R. Lung cell reactions after inhalation of bacterial lipopolysaccharides. Eur J Respir Dis 1982; 63:550–557.

54. Hinton DE, Lantz RC, Birch K, Burrell R. Quantitative morphologic studies of the lung following inhalation of bacterial endotoxin. In: Wakelyn PJ, Jacobs RR, eds. Proceedings of the Seventh Cotton Dust Research Conference, San Antonio, TX. National Cotton Council, 1983;39–44.

55. Rylander R, Beijer L. Inhalation of endotoxin stimulates alveolar macrophage production of platelet-activating factor. Am Rev Respir Dis 1987; 135:83–6.

56. Castellan RM, Olenchock SA, Kinsley KB, Hankinson JL. Inhaled endotoxin and decreased spirometric values. An exposure-response relation for cotton dust. N Engl J Med 1987; 317:605–10.

57. Petsonk EL, Olenchock SA, Castellan RM, et al. Human ventilatory response to washed and unwashed cottons from different growing areas. Br J Ind Med 1986; 43:182–7.

58. Rylander R. The endotoxin criteria document. The risk evaluation. Proceedings of the 21st Cotton and Organic Dusts Research Conference. New Orleans, 1997;153–6.

59. Chun DT. A quick summary of the highlights of parts 1 and 2 of the first round-robin endotoxin assay study and a brief preview of the next round. Proceedings of the 23rd Cotton and Other Organic Dusts Research Conference. Orlando, 1999;132–8.

60. Buck MG, Wall JH, Schachter EN. Airway constrictor response to cotton bract extracts in the absence of endotoxin. Br J Ind Med 1986; 43:220–6.

61. Jamison JP, Lowry RC. Bronchial challenge of normal subjects with the endotoxin of Enterobacter agglomerans isolated from cotton dust. Br J Ind Med 1986; 43:327–31.

62. Cavagna G, Foa V, Vigliani EC. Effects in man and rabbits of inhalation of cotton dusts or extracts and purified endotoxins. Br J Ind Med 1969; 26:314–321.

63. Nightingale JA, Rogers DF, Hart LA, Kharitonov SA, Chung KF, Barnes PJ. Effect of inhaled endotoxin on induced sputum in normal, atopic and atopic asthmatic subjects. Thorax 1998; 53:563–71.

64. Michel O, Nagy AM, Schroeven M, et al. Dose–response relationship to inhaled endotoxin in normal subjects. Am J Respir Crit Care Med 1997; 156:1157–64.

65. Kline JN, Cowden JD, Hunninghake GW, et al. Variable airway responsiveness to inhaled lipopolysaccharide. Am J Respir Crit Care Med 1999; 160:297–303.

66. Christiani DC, Ye TT, Zang S, et al. Cotton dust endotoxin exposure and longterm decline in lung function. Am J Respir Crit Care Med 1999; 35:321–31.

67. Bell AA, Stiponovic RD. Biologically active compounds in cotton: an overview. In: Wakelin PJ, Jacobs RR, eds. Proceedings of the 7th Cotton Dust Research Conference. Memphis: National Cotton Council, 1983;77–80

68. Kilburn KH, Lynn WS, Tres LL, McKenzie WN. Leukocyte recruitment through airway walls by condensed vegetable tannins and quecetin. Lab Invest 1973; 28:55–9.

69. Lauque DE, Hempel SL, Schroeder MA, et al. Evaluation of the contribution of tannin to the acute pulmonary inflammatory response against inhaled cotton mill dust. Am J Pathol 1988; 133:163–72

70. Rohrbach MS, Kreofsky T, Rolstad RA, Russell JA. Tannin-mediated secretion of a neutrophil chemotactic factor from alveolar macrophages. Am Rev Respir Dis 1989; 139:39–45.

71. Rohrbach MS, Rolstad RA, Russell JA. Tannin is the major agent present in cotton mill dust responsible for human platelet 5-hydroxytryptamine secretion and thromboxane formation. Lung 1986; 164:187–97.

72. Ayars GH, Altman LC, O'Neil CE, et al. Cotton dust mediated lung epithelial injury. J Clin Invest 1986; 78:1579–88.

73. Johnson CM, Hanson MN, Rohrbach MS. Toxicity to endothelial cells mediated by cotton bract tannin. Am J Pathol 1986; 122:399–409.

74. Antweiler H, Pallade S. Polyphenolic action on guinea pig smooth muscle and mast cells in the rat. Ann NY Acad Sci 1974; 221:132–6.

75. Rylander R. Plant constituents of cotton dust and lung effects after inhalation. Eur Respir J 1988; 1:812–7.

76. Cloutier MM, Guernsey L. Tannin inhibition of protein kinase C in airway epithelium. Lung 1995; 173:307–19.

77. Wakelyn PJ, Greenblatt GA, Brown DF, Tripp VW. Chemical properties of cotton dust. Am Ind Hyg Assoc J 1976; 37:22–31.

78. Cloutier MM, Schramm CM, Guernsey L. Tannin inhibits cAMP-a-adrenergic receptor pathway in bovine tracheal epithelium. Am J Physiol 1998; 274:L252–7.

79. Buck MG. Cotton bract and acute airway constriction in humans. ACS Symposium Series 1982; 189:187–202.

80. Buck MG, Bouhuys A. A purified extract from cotton bracts induces airway constriction in humans. Chest 1981; 79(Suppl):43s–49s.

81. Bouhuys A, Barbero A, Lindell SE, et al. Byssinosis in hemp workers. Arch Environ Health 1967; 14:533–44.

82. Bouhuys A, Duyn JV, Lennep HJV. Byssinosis in flax workers. Arch Environ Health 1961; 3:499–509.

83. Gilson JC, Stott H, Hopwood BEC, et al. Byssinosis: the acute effect on ventilatory capacity of dusts in cotton ginneries, cotton, sisal and jute mills. Br J Ind Med 1962; 18:9–18.

84. Bouhuys A. Breathing. New York: Grune & Stratton, 1974; 416–40.

85. Schilling RSF. Byssinosis in cotton and other textile workers. Lancet 1956; i:261–7, 319–24.

86. Merchant JA, Lumsden JC, Kilburn KH, et al. An industrial study of the biologic effects of cotton dust and cigarette smoke exposure. J Occup Med 1973; 15:212–21.

87. Merchant JA, Lumsden JC, Kilburn KH, et al. Dose–response studies in cotton textile workers. J Occup Med 1973; 15:222–30.

88. Valic F, Zuskin E. Effects of different vegetable dust exposures. Br J Ind Med 1972; 29:293–7.

89. Uragoda CG. An investigation into the health of kapok workers. Br J Ind Med 1977; 34:181–5.

90. Doig AT. Other lung diseases due to dust. Postgrad Med J 1949; 25:639–49.

91. Harris TR, Merchant JA, Kilburn KH, Hamilton JD. Byssinosis and respiratory diseases in cotton mill workers. J Occup Med 1972; 14:199–206.

92. Vigliani EC, Parmeggiani L, Sassi C. Studio de un epidemia di bronchite asmatica fra gli operai di una tessitura di cotone. Med Lav 1954; 45:349–78.

93. Neal PA, Schneiter R, Caminita BH. Report on acute illness among rural mattress makers using low grade, stained cotton. J Am Med Assoc 1942; 119:1074–82.

94. Beck GJ, Schachter EN, Maunder LR, Schilling RSF. A prospective study of chronic lung disease in cotton textile workers. Ann Intern Med 1982; 97:645–51.

95. Merchant JA, Kilburn KH, O'Fallon WM, et al. Byssinosis and chronic bronchitis among cotton textile workers. Ann Intern Med 1972; 76:423–33.

96. Kamat SR, Kamat GR, Salpekar VY, Lobo E. Distinguishing byssinosis from chronic obstructive pulmonary disease: results of a prospective five-year study of cotton mill workers in India. Am Rev Respir Dis 1981; 124:31–40.

97. Beck GJ, Schachter EN, Maunder LR. The relationship of respiratory symptoms and lung function loss in cotton textile workers. Am Rev Respir Dis 1984; 130:6–11.

98. Edwards C, Macartney J, Rooke G, Ward F. The pathology of the lung in byssinotics. Thorax 1975; 30:612–23.

99. Moran TJ. Emphysema and other chronic lung disease in textile workers: an 18-year autopsy study. Arch Environ Health 1983; 38:267–76.

100. Rooke GB. The pathology of byssinosis. Chest 1981; 79(Suppl):67s–71s.

101. Molyneux MKB, Tombleson JBL. An epidemiological study of respiratory symptoms in Lancashire mills, 1963–1966. Br J Ind Med 1970; 27:225–34.

102. Schrag PE, Gullett AD. Byssinosis in cotton textile mills. Am Rev Respir Dis 1970; 101:497–503.

103. Bouhuys A, Beck GJ, Schoenberg J. Epidemiology of environmental lung disease. Yale J Biol Med 1979; 52:191–210

104. Mustafa KY, Bos W, Lakha AS. Byssinosis in Tanzanian textile workers. Lung 1979; 157:39–44.

105. Bouhuys A, Schoenberg JB, Beck GJ, Schilling RSF. Epidemiology of chronic lung disease in a cotton mill community. Lung 1977; 154:167–86.

106. Zuskin E, Wolfson RL, Harpel G, et al. Byssinosis in carding and spinning workers. Arch Environ Health 1969; 19:666–73.

107. Imbus HR, Suh MW. Byssinosis: a study of 10,133 textile workers. Arch Environ Health 1973; 26:183–91.

108. Roach SA, Schilling RSF. A clinical and environmental study of byssinosis in the Lancashire cotton industry. Br J Ind Med 1960; 17:1–9.

109. McKerrow CB, Roach SA, Gilson JC, Schilling RSF. The size of cotton dust particles causing byssinosis: an environmental and physiologic study. Br J Ind Med 1962; 19:1–8.

110. Wood CH, Roach SA. Dust in cardrooms: a continuing problem in the cotton spinning industry. Br J Ind Med 1964; 21:180–6.

111. Fox AJ, Tombleson JBL, Watt A, Wilkie AG. A survey of respiratory disease in cotton operatives. Part I. Symptoms and ventilation test results. Br J Ind Med 1973; 30:42–7.

112. Fox AJ, Tombleson JBL, Watt A, Wilkie AG. A survey of respiratory disease in cotton operatives. Part II. Br J Ind Med 1973; 30:48–53.

113. Berry G, McKerrow CB, Molyneux MKB, et al. A study of the acute and chronic changes in ventilatory capacity of workers in Lancashire cotton mills. Br J Ind Med 1973; 30:25–36.

114. Merchant JA, Lumsden JC, Kilburn KH, et al. Intervention studies of cotton steaming to reduce biologic effects of cotton dust. Br J Ind Med 1974; 31:261–74.

115. Beck GJ, Doyle CA, Schachter EN. Smoking and lung function. Am Rev Respir Dis 1981; 123:149–55.

116. Beck GJ, Doyle CA, Schachter EN. A longitudinal study of respiratory health in a rural community. Am Rev Respir Dis 1982; 125:375–81.

117. Beck GJ, Maunder LR, Schachter EN. Cotton dust and smoking effects on lung function in cotton textile workers. Am J Epidemiol 1984; 119:33–43.

118. Schachter EN, Kapp MC, Beck GJ, et al. Smoking and cotton dust effects in cotton textile workers. Chest 1989; 95:997–1003.

119. Glindmeyer HW, Lefante JJ, Jones RN, Rando RJ, Weill H. Cotton dust and across shift changes in FEV1. Am J Respir Crit Care Med 1994; 149:584–90.

120. Becklake MR. Relationship of acute obstructive airway change to chronic (fixed) obstruction. Thorax 1995; 50 (Suppl 1): S16–D21.

121. Schilling RSF, Goodman N. Cardiovascular disease in cotton workers. Br J Ind Med 1951; 8:77–87.

122. Aldrich M. Mortality from byssinosis among New England cotton mill workers, 1905–1912. J Occup Med 1982; 24:977–80.

123. Henderson V, Enterline PE. An unusual mortality experience in cotton textile workers. J Occup Med 1973; 15:717–9.

124. Dubrow R, Gute DM. Cause-specific mortality among male textile workers in Rhode Island. Am J Ind Med 1988; 13:439–54.

125. Merchant JA, Ortmeyer C. Mortality of employees of two cotton mills in North Carolina. Chest 1981; 79(Suppl): 6s–11s.

126. Beck GJ, Schachter EN, Maunder LR, Bouhuys A. The relation of lung function to subsequent mortality in cotton textile workers. Chest 1981; 79(suppl):26s–30s.

127. Bouhuys A, Gilson JC, Schilling RSF. Byssinosis in the textile industry. Arch Environ Health 1970; 21:475–8.

128. Lopez-Merino V, Lombart RL, Marco RF, et al. Arterial blood gas tensions and lung function during acute responses to hemp dust. Am Rev Respir Dis 1973; 107:809–15.

129. Bouhuys A, van de Woestijne KP. Respiratory mechanics and dust exposure in byssinosis. J Clin Invest 1970; 49:106–18.

130. Zuskin E, Valic F, Butkovic D, Bouhuys A. Lung function in textile workers. Br J Ind Med 1975; 32:283–8.

131. Bouhuys A, Hunt VR, Kim BM, Zapletal A. Maximum expiratory flow rates in induced bronchoconstriction in man. J Clin Invest 1969; 48:1159–68.

132. Schachter EN, Maunder LR, Beck GJ. The pattern of lung function abnormalities in cotton textile workers. Am Rev Respir Dis 1984; 129:523–7.

133. Prausnitz C. Investigations on respiratory dust disease in operatives in the cotton industry. Medical Research Council, Special Report Series 212. London: His Majesty's Stationery Office, 1936;1–73.

134. Cayton HR, Furness G, Maitland HB. Studies in cotton dust in relation to byssinosis. Br J Ind Med 1952; 9:186–96.

135. Cooper JAD Jr, Merrill WW, Buck MG, Schachter EN. The relationship between bronchoalveolar neutrophil recruitment and bronchoconstriction induced by soluble extract of cotton bracts. Am Rev Respir Dis 1986; 134:975–82.

136. Petronio L, Bovenzi M. Byssinosis and serum IgE concentrations in textile workers in an Italian cotton mill. Br J Ind Med 1983; 40:39–44.

137. Reynolds HY. Bronchoalveolar lavage. Am Rev Respir Dis 1989; 135:250–63.

138. Merrill WW, Buck M, Cooper JAD, Schachter EN. Relationship of the ventilatory response to cotton bract extract and the cells and proteins of the lung. Chest 1987; 91:44–8.

139. Schachter EN, Buck MG. Newer approaches to the study of byssinosis. Proceedings of the 9th Cotton Dust Research Conference, New Orleans, 1985;108–10.

140. Niven RM CL, Pickering CAC. Byssinosis: a review. Thorax 1996; 51:632–37.

141. National Institute for Occupational Safety and Health. Current Intelligence Bulletin. Environmental tobacco smoke in the workplace. Lung cancer and other health effects. US Department of Health and Human Services Centers for Disease Control, Publication No. 91-108. Cincinatti: DHHS (NIOSH), 1991.

142. Rooke GB. Compensation for byssinosis in Great Britain. Chest 1981; 79(Suppl):124s–127s.

143. Bouhuys A, Beck GJ, Schoenberg JB. Priorities in prevention of chronic lung diseases. Lung 1979; 156:129–48.

144. Brown TC. Evaluating work relatedness of diseases. Chest 1981; 79:127s–129s.

145. Wegman DH, Levenstein C, Greaves IA. Byssinosis: a role for public health in the face of scientific uncertainty. Am J Public Health 1983; 73:188–92.

146. Bronstein JM. The effect of public controversy on occupational health problems: byssinosis. Am J Public Health 1984; 74:1133–7.

147. Glindmeyer HW, Lefante JJ, Jones RN, Rando RJ, Kader HMA, Weill H. Exposure-related declines in lung function of cotton textile workers. Am Rev Respir Dis 1991; 144:675–83.

148. Cinkotai FF, Emo P, Gibbs ACC, et al. Low prevalence of byssinotic symptoms in 12 flax scatching in Normandy, France. Br J Ind Med 1988; 45:325–8.

149. Bouhuys A, Lindell SE, Lundin G. Experimental studies on byssinosis. Br Med J 1960; 1:324–6.

150. Zuskin E, Ivankovic D, Schachter EN, Witek TJ. A ten year follow-up study of cotton textile workers. Am Rev Respir Dis 1991; 143:301–5.

151. Haglind P, Lundholm M, Rylander R. Prevalence of byssinosis in Swedish cotton mills. Br J Ind Med 1981; 38:138–43.

152. Khogali M. Byssinosis: a follow-up study of cotton ginnery workers in the Sudan. Br J Ind Med 1976; 33:166–74.

153. Lam TH, Ong SG, Baratawidjaja KG. A study of byssinosis in Hong Kong and Jakarta. Am J Ind Med 1987; 12:767–72.

154. Pei-Lian L, Christiani DC, Ting-ting Y, et al. The study of byssinosis in China. Am J Ind Med 1987; 12:743–54.

155. Holness DL, Taraschuk IG, Pelmear PL. Effect of dust exposure in Ontario cotton textile mills. J Occup Med 1983; 25:26–9.

156. Mayaudon EM. Estudio epidemiologico de personos ocupacionalmente expuestas al polvo de algodon. Salud Publica Mex 1972; 14:547–53.

19.4 **Chronic Obstructive Pulmonary Disease and Chronic Bronchitis**

Susan M Kennedy

Patients with chronic obstructive pulmonary disease (COPD) and chronic bronchitis are commonly encountered in clinical practice. COPD ranked as the fourth leading cause of death in 2000 and the prevalence of COPD morbidity is estimated at 4% in the United States.[1] In a report released in April 2001, the Global Obstructive Lung Disease Initiative of the US National Heart, Lung, and Blood Institute and the World Health Organization identified the major risk factors for COPD as 'tobacco smoke, occupational dust and chemicals, and indoor/outdoor air pollution'.[2]

Chronic bronchitis is defined clinically as the presence of cough with phlegm at least 3 months of the year, for at least 2 years. COPD is defined as 'airflow limitation that is not fully reversible, . . . progressive and associated with an abnormal inflammatory response of the lungs to noxious particles or gases'. COPD and chronic bronchitis are the functional and symptomatic consequences of chronic or repeated exposure to inhalation of pro-inflammatory agents from the combination of all sources of polluted air to which the patient has been exposed. These include voluntary sources (i.e., tobacco smoke) and sources present in the work and home environment.

Defining *occupational* COPD and *occupational* chronic bronchitis requires a consideration of this multifactorial etiology. Patients are often exposed to more than one source of polluted air, and the relative contribution of each may be impossible to disentangle. Thus, occupational COPD or chronic bronchitis is best defined as 'COPD or chronic bronchitis in a patient with a history of chronic exposure to pro-inflammatory agents in workplace air'. This definition is useful for clinical management and public health prevention as it points to the potential for eliminating or modifying occupational risk factors for the disease. Additional challenges with defining occupational COPD for legal or compensation purposes will be discussed below.

EPIDEMIOLOGY
Prevalence and population burden

The population prevalence of COPD and chronic bronchitis from all sources increases with age and varies with the distribution of risk factors in the population and with the definitions used. In the third US National Health and Nutrition Examination Survey (NHANES III), a large survey of a representative sample of the US population, the prevalence of low lung function among adults of all ages was 6.8% overall, with about equal prevalence among men and women.[3] The prevalence of COPD is increasing both in North America and worldwide, with the rate increasing fastest among women.[4] The direct and indirect costs to society are large, because the disease is prevalent, chronic, and contributes to considerable loss of work and productivity.

COPD was ranked as the 12th leading cause of disability-adjusted life years lost worldwide in 1990 (including all childhood and adult diseases and accidents).

The general population prevalence of *occupational* COPD and chronic bronchitis is difficult to estimate due to the lack of occupational exposure information in most population-based studies. After reviewing all available published evidence from general population epidemiologic studies, an ad hoc committee of the American Thoracic Society recently estimated the contribution of occupational exposure to the overall population burden of COPD to be at least 15%.[5] A recent study of 517 lifetime non-smokers referred to a hospital pulmonary function laboratory estimated the population attributable risk among non-smokers from occupational exposure to be 23.6% for bronchitis and 29.6% for obstructive lung disease.[6]

Specific occupational risk factors

Workplace-based studies can provide more precise estimates of the prevalence of occupational COPD and chronic bronchitis than population-based studies, due to more precise estimates of exposure. Occupations in which employees are more likely to develop occupational COPD and occupational chronic bronchitis are those associated with chronic or repeated exposure to organic particulate matter, bioaerosols, combustion products, mineral and/or metal particulate matter or fume, irritant gases and vapours, and combinations of these exposures. These exposures can be found in a wide variety of workplaces, including farming and food processing, wood and textile sector jobs, service occupations, and transportation, as well as the mining and metal processing jobs typically associated with occupational lung disease in the past.

Figure 19.4.1 shows prevalence rates for airflow obstruction (defined as FEV_1/FVC % below the age-adjusted lower 95% confidence limit) among non-smokers, aged 50 and over, from workplace-based cross-sectional studies, compared to a blue-collar 'control' population[7] and to 'expected rates',[8] from Canadian studies conducted by the UBC Occupational Lung Diseases Research Unit.[9–11] The sections that follow summarize some of the evidence showing work-relatedness of COPD in selected occupational groups.

Mineral particulate and fibers
Chronic or repeated exposure to mineral particulate matter is common in mining, tunnelling, mineral processing, excavating, and building and road construction. It can also be encountered in numerous other occupational settings such as cement work, stone carving, and even farming.[12] Patients with a history of chronic asbestos exposure are encountered in an even greater array of occupations

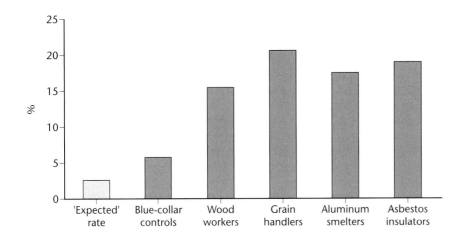

Figure 19.4.1: Prevalence rates for airflow obstruction (defined as FEV_1/FVC % below the age-adjusted lower 95% confidence limit) among non-smokers, aged 50 and over, exposed to mineral or organic dusts, or fumes, compared to a blue-collar 'control' population[7] and to 'expected rates';[8] from studies conducted by the UBC Occupational Lung Diseases Research Unit.[10,11,72]

including construction and maintenance work in all sectors.

Prevalence rates for COPD among miners range from 6 to 20% *among non-smokers*, and up to 60% among smokers[13–16] and the prevalence increases as exposure duration or intensity increases. Among non-smoking British coal miners, airflow obstruction was found in 10.5% of those exposed to low dust levels and 20.6% of those exposed to medium and high dust levels. Similarly, among non-smoking US underground coal miners the corresponding rates were 7.4% in the lower dust exposure category and 14.3% in the high dust exposure category.[17,18]

Among miners exposed to higher silica content dust, even higher COPD rates are seen. Among South African gold miners, the estimated effect of dust exposure on airflow obstruction was approximately 10 times greater than that seen among coal miners.[19] Increased mortality from bronchitis, emphysema, and asthma was associated with silica exposure among Norwegian smelter workers.[20]

COPD has also been clearly demonstrated in association with asbestos exposure.[21–24] From the evidence to date, airflow obstruction appears more pronounced among workers installing or handling asbestos products than among miners; however only few studies have looked specifically for airflow obstruction in these populations. Among miners and millers of wollastonite (another fibrous dust) significant dose–response relationships for cumulative dust and airflow obstruction were seen in both non-smokers and smokers.[25]

COPD is also linked to particulate exposure (with and without crystalline silica) in other industries, such as quarrying and carbon black manufacturing.[26,27]

Metal fumes, irritant gases, combustion products

Exposure to metal fumes, irritant gases, and combustion products appears to augment the effect of exposure to dust alone on COPD. This has been seen in mining and smelter workers,[28,29] workers in rubber manufacturing,[30] welders,[31–33] in tunnel workers,[34] and fire fighters.[35,36] There is some evidence that the risk of airflow obstruction in welders and smelter workers may be higher among atopic workers, raising the possibility that at least some of the excess airflow obstruction seen in these groups may be related to asthma.

Organic dusts – wood, textiles, grain, food processing

Although organic dust exposure is frequently associated with asthma and hypersensitivity pneumonitis, there is increasing evidence that chronic bronchitis and COPD are associated with exposure to both 'allergenic' and 'non-allergenic' organic dusts. For example, a recent study of non-asthmatic cedar sawmill workers found that the annual decline in FVC was significantly related to cumulative dust exposure, even when the average dust exposure was well below the accepted limit.[37] Studies of sawmill and furniture workers exposed to wood dusts from species not currently known to cause asthma also show exposure-related airflow obstruction.[38–40] Generally, in these studies, the excess airflow obstruction linked to dust exposure is similar among non-smokers and smokers.

There is also considerable evidence confirming a link between grain dust and COPD in both smokers and non-smokers, with consistent dose–response relationships found.[41–43] Among retired grain workers, moderate to severe airflow obstruction was found in 40% of non-smokers and 50% of smokers. Increased risk for chronic bronchitis was seen among food processing workers and highly elevated risk for chronic bronchitis and airflow obstruction was seen among bakers in a New Zealand population-based study.[44]

Textile workers exposed to cotton dust are also at risk for chronic bronchitis in addition to their increased risk for byssinosis (see Chapter 19.3). A large study of British cotton textile workers found about double the rate of chronic bronchitis among exposed workers, after taking into account the effects of smoking and age. The risk increased with longer exposure duration.[45]

Similar results have been seen in population-based studies. A large European population-based study of young adults found significantly increased chronic bronchitis (but not airflow obstruction) among workers exposed to organic dusts in textiles, agriculture, and wood and paper industries.[46] The fact that no association was seen between occupational exposures and lung function may have been due to the relatively young age of the subjects studied. In Spain, exposure to 'biologic dust' was associated with both chronic cough and airflow obstruction in a similar study.[47]

Agriculture

Agricultural exposures, including dusts from cereal grains, animal feed, and soils; gases and fumes, such as manure gases and fumes from disinfectants; and components from micro-organisms, such as endotoxin and fungal components, have all been suggested as potential initiators of the inflammatory process in the airways which may ultimately lead to chronic airway disease.

Mixed exposure to grains, other animal feeds, and animal by-products are found in animal confinement buildings and there is clear evidence of excess chronic bronchitis among farmers and workers in poultry and swine confinement buildings, with prevalence rates remarkably consistent across studies at about 25–35%.[19,48–52] Evidence for non-asthmatic chronic airflow obstruction in this industry is mixed. Some studies have reported reductions in airflow associated with duration of exposure[53,54] and accelerated decline in airflow over time among animal confinement farmers.[55]

Two population-based studies of retired workers have also shown increased respiratory morbidity from COPD and chronic bronchitis among agricultural workers. In the Dutch study of residents of Zutphen, among 824 men aged 65–84, increased chronic bronchitis was seen in association with agricultural work.[56] Among a random sample of French residents over age 65 ($n = 3777$), the occupational groups with the highest prevalence rates for dyspnea grade 3 or greater were farmworkers (37% with dyspnea) and farm managers (32%), compared to 31% among unskilled blue-collar workers, 25% among skilled blue-collar workers, and 15% among teachers.[57]

Environmental tobacco smoke in the workplace

There is growing evidence that exposure to tobacco smoke in the workplace contributes significantly to chronic bronchitis and COPD among non-smokers. A Scottish study of lifetime non-smokers revealed airflow obstruction (significantly reduced FEV_1 and FVC) among both men and women exposed to environmental tobacco smoke (ETS) at work compared to those not exposed at work;[58] similar results were found in a population-based study in China.[59] Occupational ETS exposure is particularly high among hospitality industry employees (e.g., waiters, bar tenders, casino workers) and hair levels of nicotine among non-smoking workers in these industries have been shown to be similar to those of active smokers.[60,61]

COMPARING THE EFFECT OF CIGARETTE SMOKING AND OCCUPATIONAL EXPOSURES

A growing body of research confirms that occupational exposure plays a clinically important role in the development of COPD in exposed workers. Among aluminum smelter workers, the impact of a 30-year working career with particulate exposure at the permitted level was about the same as smoking 75 grams/week (or about 1/2 pack of cigarettes per day).[62] Among tunnel workers exposed to dust and diesel exhaust, the decline in FEV_1 associated with each year of tunnel work was twice that associated with each pack year of cigarette smoking. Among fire fighters, the cumulative impact of 'being a fire fighter' on longitudinal decline in FEV_1 was about half as strong as the impact of cigarette smoking.[63]

Cigarette smoking and dust exposure appear to exert their effect on airways in a roughly additive fashion regardless of the dust type. There is a suggestion that the effect is more than additive in patients with marked airflow obstruction, and in the presence of high crystalline silica.[64]

NATURAL HISTORY, PATHOGENESIS

Most research indicates that the natural history of COPD is similar regardless of the source of the polluted air. Some evidence suggests that a rapid decline in airflow rates due to occupational exposures early in life may be linked to more pronounced airflow obstruction later. This has been seen in British, US, and Italian[65] coal miners, and among workers exposed to asbestos[66] and grain.

The specific mechanisms responsible for chronic airflow obstruction due to organic dust exposures are unclear. Autopsy carried out on three grain workers who died as a result of their illness showed that the lungs were not only emphysematous, but also had diffuse granulomata with fibrosis,[67] suggesting that grain dust may induce changes in both the airways and the parenchyma. Several of the studies cited above found that exposure to both grain and wood dust induced changes in FVC equal to the reductions in FEV_1, suggesting the possibility of alveolar duct or parenchymal involvement. Furthermore, some of the wood dust studies have implicated exposure to visible mold as well as dust in dose–response analyses. Immunologic mechanisms for airflow obstruction should be ruled out where possible in individual cases. However, in the absence of evidence of hypersensitivity, there is no clear way to determine the mechanism for chronic airflow limitation in workers exposed to organic dusts in the clinic or in epidemiologic studies.

ASSESSMENT OF EXPOSURE

Exposures in previous jobs as well as those in the current job are relevant for assessing the occupational contribution to COPD and chronic bronchitis. Therefore, the best clinical tool for assessing exposure is a detailed occupational history, augmented by specific enquiry about exposures to dusts, gases, and fumes. In fact, research has shown that a positive response to the simple question 'have you been exposed to dusts, gases, or fumes at work?' is linked to a more rapid decline in FEV_1 and increased prevalence of chronic bronchitis and airflow obstruction, in population studies.[68,69] Table 19.4.1 summarizes the results of population-based studies in which the exposure was assessed using a simple question about potential exposure to dusts, gases, or fumes in the usual or current job.

Country, year	Population	Measure of exposure	Risk estimate or effect
United States, 1987[73]	Sample of residents from 6 cities, $n = 8515$	Job with exposure to dust and gas or fume	Airflow obstruction: OR*: dust: 1.7 OR: dust/fumes: 1.6
France, 1988[74]	Residents from 7 cities (excluding 'manual workers'), $n = 12,182$	Exposed to dust, gases, chemical fumes in any job	Significant reduction in FEV_1/FVC ratio in exposed group
Poland, 1988[75]	Random sample of residents of Cracow, 13 yrs follow-up	History of exposure to dusts, variable temperature, chemicals	More rapid decline in FEV_1 in group with exposure to variable temperature, dusts, and irritating gases
Norway, 1991[76]	Random sample of residents from one county	Job with airborne exposure†	Chronic symptoms plus airflow obstruction: OR: high exposure: 3.6
China, 1992[77]	Residents of Beijing (not using coal heat), $n = 1094$	Exposure to dust, and gas/fume	Significant reduction in FEV_1/FVC ratio in exposed group
New Zealand, 1997[44]	Sample of residents from 3 areas, $n = 1132$	Everyone working with vapors, dusts, gases, fumes	Chronic bronchitis and airflow obstruction OR: exposed: 3.1

* OR: odds ratio; †based on job history.

Table 19.4.1 Summary of results of community-based studies using a simple occupational history and 'exposure to dust, gases, fumes' as the measure of exposure

If possible, the occupational history should be reviewed by a professional with knowledge of the typical occupational exposures in the region. However, this is seldom possible in clinical practice and evidence has shown that the patient is usually a reliable source for information about his or her exposures, both their duration and intensity. For each main job, the patient should be asked what year the job began and ended (to estimate duration of exposure); whether or not there was noticeable dust, fume, or gas exposure; and if so, how often it was present (to estimate intensity of exposure).

Although it is not possible provide a clear answer to the question, 'How much exposure is necessary before one should suspect an occupational contribution to COPD?', most research indicates that the relevant exposure duration is measured in years (or even decades), not months or days. Many patients will have held more than one job, and exposure duration should be summed over all jobs with relevant exposures. Time spent in irregular work environments should also be considered (e.g., in the armed forces, in the informal sector, in prison, during extended periods of casual or temporary employment), as hazardous exposures are common in these situations.

Exposures among women should be explored equally as for men, as chronic bronchitis prevalence has been shown to be similar in both sexes and many of the studies cited above have found increased rates associated with occupational exposures in women and men alike. Dust and fume exposures are seldom present every day, all day, so patients should be asked whether exposure occurred most days, only a few times a month, or only seldom (i.e., a few days a year). Exposures occurring at least a few times a month should be considered relevant.

Clinicians should not assume that if workplace exposures were within 'safe' limits or 'below regulatory standards' they were not high enough to produce disease. Many of the studies discussed above found significant airflow obstruction among workers exposed at or below regulated allowable limits. It is useful to consider the example of grain dust, which in many countries (including Canada and much of the United States) is still regulated with reference to the 'nuisance dust' standard, despite overwhelming evidence that this standard is unacceptable. The American Conference of Governmental Industrial Hygienists has adopted the term 'particulate not otherwise classified' rather than nuisance dust, to indicate 'that all materials are potentially toxic, to avoid the implication that these materials are harmless' and to emphasize that 'although these materials may not cause fibrosis and systemic effects, they are not biologically inert'.[70]

MANAGEMENT AND COMPENSATION

The evaluation of a patient with COPD (whether a smoker or non-smoker) should include consideration of occupational exposures that may have contributed to the disease. Continued occupational exposure may contribute to a worsening of the disease (in the patient, or in others in that workplace), if no preventive action is taken. For the patient still exposed to particulate or irritant gases or fumes, a recommendation should be made to reduce or eliminate the potential for the exposure. For the patient no longer exposed (or no longer working), the disease should be labelled as 'potentially occupational' in order that public health officials can assess the role of the occupational exposure and use this information to direct future prevention activities in the workplace.

Whether or not a patient with occupational COPD is entitled to compensation or disability benefits will depend on the specific requirements of the compensation or insurance carrier. These requirements vary across jurisdictions. *Disability* evaluation should be carried out without reference to etiologic agent, as the level of disability or impairment is unaffected by the cause. The decision to attach the label 'possibly occupational' to the diagnosis should be based on the occupational history. Although requirements vary among jurisdictions, it is the attending physician's role to raise the possibility of occupational etiology, not to make the final determination in law. General guidance can be found in the following statement from the Workers' Compensation Board (British Columbia, Canada) policy manual:[71]

'Since workers' compensation ... operates on an enquiry basis rather than on an adversarial basis, there is no onus on the worker to prove his or her case. All that is needed is for the worker to describe his or her experience of the disease and the reasons why they suspect the disease has an occupational basis. Then it is the responsibility of the Board to research the available scientific literature and carry out any other investigations into the origin of the worker's condition which may be necessary.'

That said, unfortunately, physicians do find themselves called upon by legal tribunals, to quantify the relative contribution of occupational exposure to COPD. This can be extremely difficult, if not impossible, in the absence of detailed exposure information and the expertise to interpret it. A useful benchmark may be the research among smelter workers, discussed earlier in this section, that found the effect of working for 30 years at today's 'accepted' exposure concentration had an impact on airflow of about the same magnitude as 30 years of cigarette smoking.[72]

PREVENTION

Some evidence suggests that a rapid decline in FEV_1 (but still in the 'normal' range) in young exposed workers may be associated with a worse prognosis. Therefore, although these workers are unlikely to seek treatment, if such a patient is encountered (e.g., as a result of routine screening or for other reasons) the index of concern should rise. The evidence is not strong enough to suggest that such a worker should be removed from exposure, but the patient should be made aware of his or her excess decline in lung function and the potential role of occupational exposure should be explored.

Global prevention of occupational COPD will require increased recognition of the disease (by physicians, by regulators, and by employers), and willingness by regulators and employers to act to reduce exposure to particulates and irritant gases and fumes in the work environment. Primary care and pulmonary physicians can play a major role in prevention by increasing the recognition of the disease, by reporting it, even if just as 'suspect' or 'possible' occupational COPD, to the local agency responsible for occupational disease prevention.

References

1. Hurd S. The impact of COPD on lung health worldwide: epidemiology and incidence. Chest 2000; 117:1S–4S.
2. Pauwels RA, Buist S, Calverley P, et al. Global strategy for the diagnosis, management, and prevention of chronic obstructive pulmonary disease: NHLBI/WHO Global Initiative for Chronic Obstructive Lung Disease (GOLD) Workshop Summary. Am J Respir Crit Care Med 2001; 163:1256–76.
3. Mannino DM, Gagnon RC, Petty TL, et al. Obstructive lung disease and low lung function in adults in the United States: data from the National Health and Nutrition Examination Survey, 1988–1994. Arch Intern Med 2000; 160:1683–9.
4. Soriano JB, Maier WC, Egger P, et al. Recent trends in physician diagnosed COPD in women and men in the UK. Thorax 2000; 55:789–94.
5. Balmes J, Becklake M, Blanc P, et al. American Thoracic Society Statement on Occupational Contribution to the Burden of Airway Disease. Am J Respir Crit Care Med 2003; 167:787–97.
6. Mak GK, Gould MK, Kuschner WG. Occupational inhalant exposure and respiratory disorders among never-smokers referred to a hospital pulmonary function laboratory. Am J Med Sci 2001; 322:121–6.
7. Kennedy SM, Chan-Yeung M, Marion S, et al. Maintenance of stellite and tungsten carbide saw tips: respiratory health and exposure–response evaluations. Occup Environ Med 1995; 52:185–91.
8. Crapo RO, Morris AH, Gardner RM. Reference spirometric values using techniques and equipment that meet ATS recommendations. Am Rev Respir Dis 1981; 123:659–64.
9. Kennedy SM, Dimich-Ward H, Desjardins A, et al. Respiratory health among retired grain elevator workers. Am J Respir Crit Care Med 1994; 150:59–65.
10. Kennedy SM, Vedal S, Muller N, et al. Lung function and chest radiograph abnormalities among construction insulators. Am J Ind Med 1991; 20:673–84.
11. Schenker M. Exposures and health effects from inorganic agricultural dusts. Environ Health Perspect 2000; 108(Suppl 4):661–4.
12. Fairman RP, O'Brien RJ, Swecker S, et al. Respiratory status of surface coal miners in the United States. Arch Environ Health 1977; 32:211–5.
13. Kibelstis JA, Morgan EJ, Reger R, et al. Prevalence of bronchitis and airway obstruction in American bituminous coal miners. Am Rev Respir Dis 1973; 108:886–93.
14. Marine WM, Gurr D, Jacobsen M. Clinically important respiratory effects of dust exposure and smoking in British coal miners. Am Rev Respir Dis 1988; 137:106–12.
15. Oxman AD, Muir DC, Shannon HS, et al. Occupational dust exposure and chronic obstructive pulmonary disease. A systematic overview of the evidence [see comments]. Am Rev Respir Dis 1993; 148:38–48.
16. Seixas NS, Robins TG, Attfield MD, et al. Exposure–response relationships for coal mine dust and obstructive lung disease following enactment of the Federal Coal Mine Health and Safety Act of 1969. Am J Ind Med 1992; 21:715–34.
17. Seixas NS, Robins TG, Attfield MD, et al. Longitudinal and cross sectional analyses of exposure to coal mine dust and pulmonary function in new miners. Br J Ind Med 1993; 50:929–37.
18. Hnizdo E. Combined effect of silica dust and tobacco smoking on mortality from chronic obstructive lung disease in gold miners. Br J Ind Med 1990; 47:656–64.
19. Kimbell-Dunn MR, Fishwick RD, Bradshaw L, et al. Work-related respiratory symptoms in New Zealand farmers. Am J Ind Med 2001; 39:292–300.
20. Hobbesland A, Kjuus H, Thelle DS. Mortality from nonmalignant respiratory diseases among male workers in Norwegian ferroalloy plants. Scand J Work Environ Health 1997; 23:342–50.
21. Kilburn KH, Warshaw RH, Einstein K, et al. Airway disease in non-smoking asbestos workers. Arch Environ Health 1985; 40:293–5.
22. Begin R, Boileau R, Peloquin S. Asbestos exposure, cigarette smoking, and airflow limitation in long-term Canadian chrysotile miners and millers. Am J Ind Med 1987; 11:55–66.
23. Kilburn KH, Warshaw RH. Abnormal pulmonary function associated with diaphragmatic pleural plaques due to exposure to asbestos. Br J Ind Med 1990; 47:611–4.

24. Demers RY, Neale AV, Robins T, et al. Asbestos-related disease in boilermakers. Am J Ind Med 1990; 17:327–39.
25. Hanke W, Sepulveda MJ, Watson A, et al. Respiratory morbidity in wollastonite workers. Br J Ind Med 1984; 41:474–9.
26. Gardiner K, Thethowan NW, Harrington JM, et al. Respiratory health effects of carbon black: a survey of European carbon black workers. Br J Ind Med 1993; 50:1082–96.
27. Malmberg P, Hendenstöm H, Sundblad BM. Changes in lung function in granite crushers exposed to moderately high silica concentrations: a 12-year follow-up. Br J Ind Med 1993; 50:725–31.
28. Kennedy SM, Wright JL, Mullen JB, et al. Pulmonary function and peripheral airway disease in patients with mineral dust or fume exposure. Am Rev Respir Dis 1985; 132:1294–9.
29. Manfreda J, Cheang M, Warren CP. Chronic respiratory disorders related to farming and exposure to grain dust in a rural adult community. Am J Ind Med 1989; 15:7–19.
30. Fine LJ, Peters JM. Respiratory morbidity in rubber workers: III. Respiratory morbidity in processing workers. Arch Environ Health 1976; 31:136–40.
31. Chinn DJ, Stevenson IC, Cotes JE. Longitudinal respiratory survey of shipyard welders: effects of trade and atopic status. Br J Ind Med 1990; 47:83–90.
32. Hjortsberg U, Orbaek P, Arborelius M. Small airways dysfunction among non-smoking shipyard arc welders. Br J Ind Med 1992; 49:441–4.
33. Bradshaw LM, Fishwick D, Slater T, et al. Chronic bronchitis, work related respiratory symptoms, and pulmonary function in welders in New Zealand. Occup Environ Med 1998; 55:150–4.
34. Ulvestad B, Bakke B, Melbostad E, et al. Increased risk of obstructive pulmonary disease in tunnel workers. Thorax 2000; 55:277–82.
35. Musk AW, Peters JM, Bernstein L, et al. Pulmonary function in firefighters: a six-year follow-up in the Boston fire department. Am J Ind Med 1982; 3:3–9.
36. Horsfield K, Guyatt AR, Cooper FM, et al. Lung function in West Sussex firemen: a four year study. Br J Ind Med 1988; 45:116–21.
37. Noertjojo HK, Dimich-Ward H, Peelen S, et al. Western red cedar dust exposure and lung function: a dose-response relationship [see comments]. Am J Respir Crit Care Med 1996; 154:968–73.
38. Chan-Yeung M, Wong R, MacLean L, et al. Respiratory survey of workers in a pulp and paper mill in Powell River, British Columbia. Am Rev Respir Dis 1980; 122:249–57.
39. Goldsmith DF, Shy CM. Respiratory health effects from occupational exposure to wood dusts. Scand J Work Environ Health 1988; 14:1–15.
40. Hessel PA, Herbert FA, Melenka LS, et al. Lung health in sawmill workers exposed to pine and spruce. Chest 1995; 108:642–6.
41. Enarson DA, Vedal S, Chan-Yeung M. Rapid decline in FEV$_1$ in grain handlers. Relation to level of dust exposure. Am Rev Respir Dis 1985; 132:814–7.
42. Huy T, De Schipper K, Chan-Yeung M, et al. Grain dust and lung function. Dose–response relationships. Am Rev Respir Dis 1991; 144:1314–21.
43. Peelen SJ, Heederik D, Dimich-Ward HD, et al. Comparison of dust related respiratory effects in Dutch and Canadian grain handling industries: a pooled analysis. Occup Environ Med 1996; 53:559–66.
44. Fishwick D, Bradshaw LM, D'Souza W, et al. Chronic bronchitis, shortness of breath, and airway obstruction by occupation in New Zealand. Am J Respir Crit Care Med 1997; 156:1440–46.
45. Niven RM, Fletcher AM, Pickering CA, et al. Chronic bronchitis in textile workers. Thorax 1997; 52:22–7.
46. Zock JP, Sunyer J, Kogevinas M, et al. Occupation, chronic bronchitis, and lung function in young adults. An international study. Am J Respir Crit Care Med 2001; 163:1572–7.
47. Sunyer J, Kogevinas M, Kromhout H et al. Pulmonary ventilatory defects and occupational exposures in a population-based study in Spain. Am J Respir Crit Care Med 1998; 157:512–7.
48. Iversen M, Dahl R, Korsgaard, J et al. Respiratory symptoms in Danish farmers: an epidemiological study of risk factors. Thorax 1988; 43:872–7.
49. Leistikow B, Pettit W, Donham K. et al. Respiratory risks in poultry farmers. In: Dosman JA, Dockcroft DW, eds. Principles of health and safety in agriculture. Boca Raton: CRC Press Inc., 1989;62–5.
50. Morris PD, Lenhart SW, Service WS. Respiratory symptoms and pulmonary function in chicken catchers in poultry confinement units. Am J Ind Med 1991; 19:195–204.
51. Zejda JE, Hurst TS, Rhodes CS, et al. Respiratory health of swine producers. Focus on young workers. Chest 1993; 103:702–9.
52. Choudat D, Goehen M, Korobaeff M, et al. Respiratory symptoms and bronchial reactivity among pig and dairy farmers. Scand J Work Environ Health 1994; 20:48–54.
53. Zejda JE, Pahwa P, Dosman JA. Decline in spirometric variables in grain workers from start of employment: differential effect of duration of follow up. Br J Ind Med 1992; 49:576–80.
54. Schwartz DA, Donham KJ, Olenchock SA, et al. Determinants of longitudinal changes in spirometric function among swine confinement operators and farmers. Am J Respir Crit Care Med 1995; 151:47–53.
55. Iversen M, Dahl R. Working in swine-confinement buildings causes an accelerated decline in FEV1: a 7-yr follow-up of Danish farmers. Eur Respir J 2000; 16:404–8.
56. Heederik D, Pouwels H, Kromhout H, et al. Chronic non-specific lung disease and occupational exposures estimated by means of a job exposure matrix: the Zutphen Study. Int J Epidemiol 18:382–9.
57. Nejjari C, Tessier JF, Dartigues JF, et al. The relationship between dyspnoea and main lifetime occupation in the elderly. Int J Epidemiol 1993; 22:848–54.
58. Chen R, Tunstall-Pedoe H, Tavendale R. Environmental tobacco smoke and lung function in employees who never smoked: the Scottish MONICA study. Occup Environ Med 2001; 58:563–8.
59. Xu X, Li B. Exposure–response relationship between passive smoking and adult pulmonary function. Am J Respir Crit Care Med 1995; 151:41–6.
60. Al Delaimy W, Fraser T, Woodward A. Nicotine in hair of bar and restaurant workers. NZ Med J 2001; 114:80–3.
61. Dimich-Ward H, Gee H, Brauer M, et al. Analysis of nicotine and cotinine in the hair of hospitality workers exposed to environmental tobacco smoke. J Occup Environ Med 1997; 39:946–8.
62. Soyseth V, Boe J, Kongerud J. Relation between decline in FEV$_1$ and exposure to dust and tobacco smoke in aluminium potroom workers. Occup Environ Med 1997; 54:27–31.
63. Sparrow D, Bosse R, Rosner B, et al. The effect of occupational exposure on pulmonary function. Am Rev Respir Dis 1982; 125:319–22.
64. Holman CD, Psaila-Savona P, Roberts M et al. Determinants of chronic bronchitis and lung dysfunction in Western Australian gold miners. Br J Ind Med 1987; 44:810–8.
65. Carta P, Aru G, Barbieri MT, et al. Dust exposure, respiratory symptoms, and longitudinal decline of lung function in young coal miners. Occup Environ Med 1996; 53:312–9.
66. Copes R, Thomas D, Becklake MR. Temporal patterns of exposure and non-malignant pulmonary abnormality in Quebec chrysotile workers. Arch Environ Health 1985; 40:80–87.
67. Cohen VL, Osgood J. Disability due to inhalation of grain dust. J Allergy 1953; 24:193–211.
68. Kauffmann F, Drouet D, Lellouch J, et al. Occupational exposure and 12-year spirometric changes among Paris area workers. Br J Ind Med 1982; 39:221–32.

69. Le Moual N, Bakke P, Orlowski E, et al. Performance of population specific job exposure matrices (JEMs): European collaborative analyses on occupational risk factors for chronic obstructive pulmonary disease with job exposure matrices (ECOJEM). Occup Environ Med 2000; 157:126–32.

70. American Conference of Governmental Industrial Hygienists. TLVs and BEIs: threshold limit values for chemical substances and physical agents. Biologic exposure indices. Cincinnati: ACGIH, 2000.

71. Rehabilitation Services and Claims Manual. British Columbia, Canada: Workers' Compensation Board, 2001.

72. Chan-Yeung M, Enarson DA, MacLean L, et al. Longitudinal study of workers in an aluminum smelter. Arch Environ Health 1989; 44:134–9.

73. Korn RJ, Dockery DW, Speizer FE, et al. Occupational exposures and chronic respiratory symptoms. A population-based study. Am Rev Respir Dis 1987; 136:298–304.

74. Krzyzanowski M, Kauffmann F. The relation of respiratory symptoms and ventilatory function to moderate occupational exposure in a general population. Results from the French PAARC study of 16,000 adults. Int J Epidemiol 1988; 17:397–406.

75. Krzyzanowski M, Jedrychowski W, Wysocki M. Occupational exposures and changes in pulmonary function over 13 years among residents of Cracow. Br J Ind Med 1988; 45:747–54.

76. Bakke PS, Baste V, Hanoa R, et al. Prevalence of obstructive lung disease in a general population: relation to occupational title and exposure to some air-borne agents. Thorax 1991; 46:863–70.

77. Xu X, Christiani DC, Dockery DW, et al. Exposure–response relationships between occupational exposures and chronic respiratory illness: a community-based study. Am Rev Respir Dis 1992; 146:413–8.

19.5 **Acute Inhalational Injury**

David A Schwartz

INTRODUCTION

The events in Bhopal, India, dramatically illustrate the potential consequences of acute exposure to toxic inhalants. In the workplace, toxic inhalants have been reported to cause a variety of clinical problems ranging from mild irritation of the upper airways to non-cardiogenic pulmonary edema (ARDS) and death. Exposure to toxic inhalants presents problems in clinical management for the following reasons:

1. exposures occur at infrequent, unpredictable intervals
2. exposures may involve large numbers of individuals
3. the exact toxic agent may not be known to the patient or physician
4. there are a broad range of acute clinical manifestations with a varying time of onset
5. the chronic effects of acute exposures have not been clearly characterized.

Despite these problems, knowledge of the basic principles underlying these acute parenchymal responses will allow the clinician to respond appropriately. Although many agents, such as asphyxiants (e.g., carbon monoxide and hydrogen cyanide), metal fumes (e.g., cadmium), and immunologically active inhalants (e.g., red cedar dust, animal dander, and grain dust), are potent mediators of acute lung injury, this chapter will focus attention on the agents which are capable of causing a toxic pneumonitis as well as inhaled toxins associated with systemic illnesses.

This discussion will focus on the perspective of a clinician who is faced with a patient with respiratory problems or concerns following exposure to a noxious agent. Importantly, many of the exposures that can result in acute toxic airway and parenchymal injury may also result in subacute and chronic abnormalities that can dramatically alter lung function. Although the long-term effects of acute inhalational injury are poorly understood, we will present this information since delayed effects from acute high-dose exposures regularly occur in the clinical setting. Specific agents are discussed further in Chapters 39 (metals) and 47 (toxic gases).

PROPERTIES OF IRRITANTS

Inhaled toxins exist in many forms and may be categorized by taking into account their physical properties. General categories include gases, vapors, fumes, aerosols, and smoke. Tables 19.5.1 and 19.5.2 summarize the physical properties of these inhalants. Table 19.5.3 lists selected agents that can cause acute inhalational injury to the lung. The initial pathologic responses to a harmful inhaled agent depend on a number of factors, including the concentration of the substance in the ambient air, the pH of the inhaled substance, the presence and size of particles, the relative water solubility of the inhaled agent, the duration of exposure, and whether the exposure occurs in an enclosed space versus an area with adequate ventilation and free circulation of fresh air. In addition, an undetermined number of host factors, including age, smoking status, the presence of pre-existing pulmonary or extrapulmonary disease, and the use of respirators or other protective breathing apparatus all impact upon an individual's response to the inhalation of a toxic substance.[1,2]

Inhaled gases with potential irritant effects manifest their actions at different anatomic locations in the respiratory system.[1,2] In general, substances that are highly water soluble, such as ammonia, sulfur dioxide, and hydrogen chloride, can cause immediate irritant injury to the upper airway. The acute effects of highly water-soluble irritants on the upper airway, exposed skin, and other mucous membranes often produce such unpleasant symptoms that exposed persons quickly leave the area of exposure, and avoid continued inhalation of the harmful toxins. In contrast, inhaled toxins that have low water solubility, such as phosgene, ozone, and oxides of nitrogen, often have little or no acute effect on the upper airway, and instead produce irritant effects at the level of the terminal bronchiole and alveolus. Because agents of low water solubility do not produce immediately noticeable upper airway irritation (except in episodes of massive acute exposure), exposed persons may inadvertently remain in the area of exposure, and thus increase their duration of exposure to harmful inhalants. Agents that exhibit intermediate water solubility, such as chlorine, can have pathologic effects throughout the respiratory system. However, extreme exposure to any one of these irritants may result in upper and lower respiratory tract involvement. Furthermore, absorption of any one of these irritants on particulate matter may also alter the area of involvement.

In addition to solubility, the size of inhaled particle is important in the pathogenesis of the toxic inhalation injury.[1] Aerosols, dusts, fumes, and smoke can produce upper airway injury as well as parenchymal damage. The location and extent of injury depend on the size of the inhaled particles as well as the intensity of the exposure. Particles that are 5.0 μm or less in diameter have the ability to penetrate into the lower respiratory tract, and often produce significant injury at the level of the terminal bronchioles and alveoli. Zinc chloride (hexite) particles, for example, have an average diameter of 0.1 μm and it is estimated that up to 20% of the inhaled zinc reaches the bronchiolar level, with the remainder deposited in more proximal airways.[3] The particles themselves may have direct toxic effects, or they may serve as vehicles for adsorbed gaseous agents that are carried more distally into the lungs and do harm when they interact with terminal bronchioles and alveolar cells.

Irritants directly injure cells through non-immunologically mediated mechanisms of injury and inflammation. Cell injury involves the deposition or formation of an acid (chlorine, hydrogen, chloride, oxides of nitrogen, phosgene, and sulfur dioxide), alkali (ammonia), or reactive oxygen species (ozone, oxides of nitrogen and possibly

Gas	a formless state of matter in which molecules move freely about and completely occupy the space of enclosure.
Aerosol	a relatively stable suspension of liquid droplets or solid particles in a gaseous medium.
Vapor	the gaseous form of a substance that normally exists as a liquid or solid and that generally can be changed back to a liquid or solid by either increasing ambient pressure or decreasing the temperature.
Fume	an aerosol of solid particles generally less than 0.1 μm in size that arises from a chemical reaction or condensation of vapors, usually after volatilization from molten materials.
Smoke	the volatilized gaseous and particulate products of combustion; the particles are generally less than 0.5 μm in size and do not settle readily.

Table 19.5.1 Definitions of types of inhaled substances[1]

Irritant gas	Water solubility	Mechanism of injury
Ammonia	high	alkali burns
Chlorine	intermediate	acid burns, reactive oxygen species
Hydrogen chloride	high	acid burns
Oxides of nitrogen	low	acid burns, reactive oxygen species
Ozone	low	reactive oxygen species
Phosgene	low	acid burns
Sulfur dioxide	high	acid burns

Table 19.5.2 Physical properties and mechanisms of lung injury of gaseous respiratory irritants[2]

Chemical	Properties and pulmonary sequelae
Gases	
Acetaldehyde	Strong oxidizer, upper airway irritant, delayed ARDS
Acrolein	Oxidizer, upper airway irritant, delayed ARDS
Ammonia	Alkali, water soluble, upper airway irritant
Boranes	Water insoluble, upper airway irritant
Bromine	Oxidizer, pneumonitis, ARDS
Chlorine	Intermediate solubility, upper and lower airway irritant
Hydrogen chloride	Water soluble, upper airway irritant
Hydrogen fluoride	Irritating odor, upper airway irritant, ARDS
Isocyanates	Reactive chemical, irritant, airway reactivity
Lithium hydride	Odorless, strong oxidizer, upper airway irritant
Oxide of nitrogen (NO, NO₂, N₂O₄)	Water insoluble, pneumonitis, ARDS, bronchiolitis obliterans
Ozone	Water insoluble, pneumonitis, ? ARDS
Phosgene	Water insoluble, pneumonitis, ARDS
Sulfur dioxide	Water soluble, pneumonitis, ARDS, bronchiolitis obliterans
Metals	
Antimony	Oxidizer, upper airway irritant
Cadmium	Odorless, pneumonitis, ARDS
Cobalt	Oxidizer, irritant, dyspnea
Manganese	Oxidizer, metal fume fever
Mercury	Odorless, pneumonitis, ARDS
Nickel	Musty odor, asthma, pneumonitis
Zinc	White aerosol, upper airway irritant, metal fume fever

Table 19.5.3 Selected agents known to cause acute pulmonary injury

chlorine).[2,4] The primary injury is localized in airway epithelial tissues, but extensive damage may also occur in subepithelial and alveolar regions. Acid injury results in coagulation of the underlying tissue, while acute injury due to alkali results in liquefaction of the mucosa and deep penetrating lesions in the airways. Reactive oxygen species include oxygen-derived metabolites (such as hydrogen peroxide and hydrochlorous acid), and oxygen-derived free radicals (such as superoxide anions and hydroxyl radicals). These reactive oxygen species may injure tissues and cells through lipid peroxidation that can directly injure cells as well as lead to elaboration of inflammatory mediators that can perpetuate the initial damage.[4] Regardless of the initial mechanism of irritant injury, inflammatory mechanisms that involve networks of pro-inflammatory cytokines may be subsequently initiated. The resultant inflammation may be important with regard to perpetuation of the acute injury as well as long-term sequelae. In addition, disruption and eventual repair of the airway epithelia may decrease the host's ability to defend against future inhaled infectious or irritant substances.

PATHOGENESIS AND CLINICAL PRESENTATION OF TOXIC INHALATIONAL INJURY

Inhaled toxic agents can cause a spectrum of airway and parenchymal pulmonary diseases that can be classified as acute disorders that occur within the first 1–2 days of exposure and chronic problems that develop weeks to months after the exposure (Table 19.5.4). This classification is clinically useful because it recognizes that the timing of the exposure in relationship to the onset of pulmonary disease is critical in assessing causality.

Upper airway

Acute injury

The potential for an inhaled substance to acutely injure the upper airway depends largely on that substance's irritant qualities. Water solubility and particle size, as well as duration and intensity of exposure, all influence the host response to a specific exposure. Upper airway injury due to the inhalation of toxic agents involves a number of pathophysiologic mechanisms. Irritants produce injury through

Acute (within 1–2 days of exposure)
Laryngeal edema
Airflow obstruction – asthma and bronchitis
Pneumonitis, pulmonary edema
ARDS
Persistent sequelae (weeks to months after the exposure)
COPD
Reactive airways dysfunction syndrome (RADS)
Bronchitis
Bronchiolitis obliterans
Bronchiolitis obliterans organizing pneumonia (BOOP)

Table 19.5.4 Classification of chemical injury to the lung

direct contact with the skin and mucous membranes. Tissue and cellular damage can result from the injurious effects of acid, alkali, or reactive oxygen species. Acidic substances or those that react to form acids coagulate the underlying tissue. In contrast, alkalotic substances cause liquefaction of the surface mucosa and lead to further penetrating injury of deeper structures.[2]

Reactive oxygen species are involved with a variety of cellular and tissue disruptions through lipid peroxidation.[4] The cellular injuries that result from the actions of acids, alkali, and reactive oxygen species may include loss of epithelial cell layer integrity, influx of inflammatory cells and mediators, and leakage of interstitial fluid. The initial insult to the airway epithelium decreases its ability to function as a protective barrier between the environment and the subepithelial layers. Disruption of the epithelium by inhaled toxins exposes underlying inflammatory cells, nerves, muscles, and blood vessels. The resulting inflammation, edema, and stimulation of neuronal afferent receptors may all contribute to the clinical manifestations.

Individuals exposed to irritants that injure the upper airway often have associated injury to exposed mucous membranes and skin. Clinical presentations include burns of exposed skin and corneas, rhinitis, conjunctivitis, tracheobronchitis, and oral mucositis. Persons exposed to upper airway irritants may experience burning sensations of the eyes, nasal passages and throat; profuse lacrimation and copious sputum production may also occur. Coughing and sneezing may be prominent symptoms. Upper airway injury from irritant inhalants is generally acute and self-limited. Life-threatening upper airway obstruction due to mucosal edema, large amounts of secretions and sloughed epithelial cells, or laryngospasm can occur in cases of massive acute exposure. Hoarseness or stridor may warn of impending airway compromise, and patients presenting with either of these physical findings must be carefully observed and may require emergent management of acute upper airway obstruction.

Treatment is not specific for most inhaled substances, but instead addresses removal of the patient from the exposure. Basic principles of airway management are paramount because the most likely acute life-threatening manifestation of this injury is upper airway obstruction due to a combination of tissue edema, thick secretions, and laryngospasm. Frequent suctioning of secretions is often required. Provision of adequate supplemental oxygen is necessary if there is evidence of hypoxemia. Inhaled racemic epinephrine may be useful for patients with potential for upper airway obstruction, but should not substitute for or delay emergent airway management by endotracheal intubation or tracheotomy if necessary. Corticosteroids have not been conclusively shown to influence outcome, but are suggested in cases with extensive upper airway edema. Toxic substances that remain present on the skin or mucosal surfaces should be removed via irrigation with large amounts of water. Basic principles of burn management should be applied to skin and mucosal surface burns. Ophthalmologic consultation is recommended for management of injuries to the cornea or other eye structures.

Conducting airways

Acute injury

Inhaled irritants that penetrate to the conducting airways are capable of inducing immediate as well as long-lasting injury through a variety of mechanisms. The airway epithelium provides a barrier that protects inflammatory cells and submucosal structures (nerves, vessels, and muscle) from direct exposure to environmental agents. Disruption of the integrity of this protective barrier can be caused by a variety of environmental agents and, importantly, may result in edema, inflammation, direct smooth muscle contraction, and stimulation of neuronal afferent receptors. Moreover, this primary lesion in the airway epithelium can facilitate stimulation by subsequent agents that come in contact with the denudated epithelial surface.

The tight junction interface between epithelial cells appears to be the primary site of injury following exposure to a variety of gases and aerosols. For instance, cigarette smoke has been shown to damage the airway epithelium by primarily disrupting the tight junctions between epithelial cells, resulting in increased permeability to other unrelated irritants, such as horseradish peroxidase.[5] Similarly, hamsters exposed to nitrogen dioxide gradually develop severe disruption of tight junctions between bronchial epithelial cells.[6] Ozone[7] has also been shown to increase airway epithelial permeability. Thus, damage to the airway epithelium, particularly at tight junctions, renders the respiratory mucosa permeable to other inhaled substances, which are then able to penetrate the subepithelial mucosal region. These agents may directly interact with effector cells in subepithelial mucosa. Thus, they may have direct smooth muscle bronchoconstrictive effects, and they may also stimulate parasympathetic sensory afferent nerve endings, resulting in extensive bronchoconstriction.[8]

Inhalation of irritant gases and aerosols may cause airway hyper-responsiveness by initiating a localized inflammatory response. Inhalation studies with allergens and specific environmental irritants have demonstrated that neutrophils and eosinophils are recruited within a few hours to the airway and alveolar surface, and this response has been shown to persist for at least 48 hours following this type of challenge.[9] Moreover, the number of mast cells, eosinophils, and airway epithelial cells obtained by bronchoalveolar lavage following an aerosol challenge has been found to correlate strongly with the degree of airway hyper-reactivity in mild atopic asthmatics.[10] Inflammatory cells such as neutrophils appear to be critical elements in the development of airway hyper-reactivity following exposure to ozone.[11]

Damage to the airway epithelium and inflammation of the subepithelial mucosa may contribute to the development of airway disease in persons exposed to irritant gases and aerosols. Inhaled agents, either allergens or irritants, may primarily cause mucosal inflammation that subsequently results in increased epithelial permeability. The altered epithelial permeability exposes subepithelial irritant receptors, which are subsequently at risk of being stimulated by a variety of agents including cold air, changes in humidity and temperature (exercise), and cigarette smoke. Damage to the airway epithelium by cigarette smoke is associated with increased epithelial permeability and an inflammatory reaction characterized by mucosal edema and infiltration of neutrophils.[12] In addition, direct damage to the airway epithelium may result in decreased production of epithelial-derived bronchodilating substances and neutral endopeptidases that would normally serve to reduce the effects of bronchoconstricting agents.[12]

The inflammatory response in the epithelial and subepithelial regions can result in chronic remodeling of the underlying airway architecture. Striking inflammatory changes, such as extensive collagen deposition beneath the epithelial basement membrane, eosinophil infiltration, and mast cell degranulation, are seen in transbronchial biopsy specimens obtained from asthmatic persons following aerosol challenges.[13] Chronic bronchitis, an inflammatory state characterized by neutrophil infiltration, is strongly associated with airway hyper-responsiveness and has been demonstrated in animals following exposure to irritant gases.[2] Release of mediators, such as histamine, leukotrienes, prostaglandins, neutrophil chemotactic factors, platelet activating factor, tachykinins, cytokines, and growth factors, from a variety of structural and inflammatory cells in the airway and subepithelial region may significantly contribute to the chronic inflammatory response that has been well documented in asthma and in other forms of chronic airway disease.

Changes in the structure of the airways may significantly enhance the development of airway reactivity and contribute to the development of respiratory symptoms. Baseline airway caliber appears to be an important determinant of airway hyper-responsiveness.[14] The airway caliber can be influenced by a variety of factors including the tone of the airway smooth muscle and the overall thickness of the subepithelial region. The thickness of the subepithelial region is influenced by edema and inflammation. Interestingly, inflammation and edema of the submucosal region not only may decrease airway caliber but also may alter airway smooth muscle mechanics, resulting in maximal contraction following stimulation of the airway smooth muscle. Similarly, chronic changes in the architecture of the basement membrane may also alter smooth muscle length-tension relations.

Lower airway injury resulting from irritant toxin inhalation can be manifested as transient or long-lasting intrathoracic airflow obstruction. The precise mechanism of the obstruction is not clear, but likely involves one or more inflammatory mechanisms. Exposed individuals who are cigarette smokers or who have pre-existing airway obstruction may be at increased risk for the persistence of toxin-induced airflow obstruction. Significant clinical manifestations of lower airway injury may not be initially recognizable, but may develop and worsen over the first 24–48 hours after exposure. Hospitalization for observation is indicated for initially asymptomatic exposed subjects who present with any objective evidence of respiratory compromise, such as decreased airflow, abnor-

malities of gas exchange, or an abnormal chest radiograph, or whose exposure history is suggestive of a relatively intense exposure. In addition, individuals who report respiratory symptoms including dyspnea or chest tightness should be hospitalized, followed closely with objective measures of respiratory function, and treated symptomatically, even in the absence of objective abnormalities.

Spirometry may initially be normal, but in some cases progressive airflow obstruction develops, and thus a case can be argued for obtaining baseline airflow indices and following the exposed individuals with spirometry over the first 24–48 hours after exposure. For individuals without significant decrements in airflow but with symptomatic chest tightness or wheezing, inhaled steroids are essential and bronchodilators may be useful. In cases that demonstrate airflow obstruction (FEV_1 of 80% or less than predicted, or 10% or less than the patient's initial baseline), a short course of systemic corticosteroids may be beneficial in addition to the use of inhaled steroids and bronchodilators. However, there is no definitive evidence that treatment with parenteral corticosteroids substantially improves the airflow obstruction or prevents the onset of bronchiolitis obliterans.

Chronic injury

Obstructive airway disease. Previously healthy individuals who experience acute toxin inhalation may go on to develop clinical and pathologic features of chronic obstructive pulmonary disease (COPD). Inhaled irritants most often implicated in the development of chronic bronchitis, emphysema, or reversible airflow obstruction include chlorine[15] and sulfur dioxide.[16] However, definitive evidence that demonstrates a causal relationship between a toxin exposure and resultant chronic respiratory disease is frequently difficult to elicit. This is often because of the frequent concomitant presence of potentially confounding factors, most prominently cigarette smoking, that independently increase any individual's risk for the development of COPD.

Nevertheless, there is some growing evidence that acute exposure to a number of inhaled irritants may produce conditions in the conducting airways that lead to a complex interaction of inflammation, smooth muscle activity, and neuronal inputs that are involved in the creation and perpetuation of varying degrees of fixed and reversible airflow obstruction. The initial irritant insult to epithelial cells appears to be central to subsequent abnormal function and continuing injury processes that involve the epithelium as well subepithelial structures. Repair of the acute injury may also contribute to resultant chronic airflow obstruction via scarring and other mechanical factors. Disruption of normal protective structures and mechanisms may also predispose exposed individuals to chronic pulmonary infections. In addition, damage to and destruction of functional alveoli may also involve ongoing inflammatory and repair processes that have been initiated by the acute irritant exposure.

The development of irritant-induced COPD appears to be dependent on the intensity of the exposure. In addition, underlying host factors, including cigarette smoking and pre-existing pulmonary disease, may increase an individual's likelihood of developing or worsening COPD. It is extremely difficult to accurately assess the potential contribution of acute irritant inhalation to chronic lung disease in individuals who smoke cigarettes. Baseline measures of pulmonary function can help determine the presence of pre-existing disease, but unfortunately this information is often unavailable, especially in cases of accidental acute exposure. Evaluation of possible irritant-induced COPD includes a thorough history, physical examination, radiographic evaluation, and objective measures of pulmonary function, including spirometry, measurement of lung volumes, determination of diffusing capacity, and assessment of gas exchange. Frequent measurement of spirometry may help determine progression or regression of airflow abnormalities. Treatment is as for COPD due to causes other than acute irritant exposure and includes bronchodilators, corticosteroids, smoking cessation, and supplemental oxygen if necessary. Occupational COPD and chronic bronchitis are discussed further in Chapter 19.4.

Reactive airways dysfunction syndrome (see also Chapter 19.2). The persistence of airway reactivity following acute exposure to respiratory irritants has been termed reactive airways dysfunction syndrome (RADS).[17] A variety of inhaled irritants have been associated with this syndrome, including sulfuric acid, chlorine, ammonia, household cleaners, and smoke. Most often, the initial inhalation injury is due to a single, acute, high-intensity exposure. Symptoms of airflow obstruction, including cough, dyspnea, and wheezing, are reported immediately or several hours after the end of the exposure, and may persist for months to years. Previous exposure or sensitization to the toxic agent does not appear to be necessary. By definition, individuals who develop RADS have no history of respiratory illness. Pulmonary function tests may be normal, or they may demonstrate airflow obstruction. Individuals with RADS have persistent, positive responses to methacholine challenge testing, even in the presence of normal pulmonary function tests. Non-specific bronchial reactivity may persist for months to years following the initial inhalation injury.

Bronchial biopsies of patients with RADS demonstrate an inflammatory response characterized by epithelial desquamation and mucus cell hyperplasia. The exact mechanisms of the pathophysiology of RADS are unclear, but implicated mechanisms include altered neural tone and vagal reflexes, modified beta-adrenergic sympathetic tone, and influences of a number of pro-inflammatory mediators. The direct irritant injury may expose and damage subepithelial irritant receptors. Subsequently, repair mechanisms which are not fully understood may result in alteration of the irritant receptor threshold and lead to airways hyper-reactivity. Changes in epithelial permeability may also contribute to the resultant hyper-reactivity. None of these proposed mechanisms is completely understood at this time.

Treatment of RADS includes the use of corticosteroids to help minimize inflammatory mechanisms, and bronchodilators to reverse bronchospasm. There is limited, mostly anecdotal, evidence for the efficacy of corticosteroids. Bronchodilators may only partially reverse airflow obstruction, especially in later, chronic stages of the syndrome.[18] Despite treatment with corticosteroids and bronchodilators, many exposed individuals may be left with persistent asthma-like symptoms, airflow obstruction, and non-specific bronchial hyper-reactivity.

Pulmonary parenchyma

Acute injury

Toxic inhaled agents that have relatively low water solubilities, such as phosgene, ozone, and nitrogen oxides, produce most of their irritant damage distal to the upper airway. Because of the relatively low solubilities of these substances, inhalation does not typically result in upper airway irritation and its associated symptoms. As a result, subjects may endure continued exposure to the toxic gases and thus increase the total time and resultant dose of exposure. In addition, massive acute inhalation of gases and aerosols that have intermediate (chlorine) or high water solubilities (ammonia, sulfur dioxide) can overwhelm the absorptive capacity of the upper airway and injure more distal structures. Damage may be particularly severe when particulates form part of the inhaled substance. The reasons for this are not fully understood, although it is possible that particle deposition in the alveoli might provide a nidus for ongoing inflammation and subsequent severe injury. Respirable particles with diameters in the 0.3–0.5 μm range can bypass the upper airways and deposit in the more distal airways and alveoli.[1]

The clinical consequences of these injuries include diffuse bronchiolar inflammation and obstruction as well as alveolar filling (pulmonary edema). Atelectasis may result from destruction or disruption of the surfactant layer. Individuals who have sustained an initial toxic insult to the lower airways and lung parenchyma may be more susceptible to subsequent pulmonary infections because of damage to inflammatory cells, including alveolar macrophages, that provide host defense against infectious agents.

The lower respiratory tract and alveoli are susceptible to injury from many inhaled toxins. In general, the extent and severity of acute lung injury due to a toxic inhalant appear to be dose related. The clinical and histopathologic features of toxin-associated pulmonary edema and ARDS are not unique to any particular inhalant. Instead, many different inhaled toxins can damage the pulmonary parenchyma via what appear to be common pathways that are identical or at least qualitatively similar to those that cause acute lung injury secondary to causes other than toxin inhalation. However, unlike some focal processes that progress to ARDS, the initial inhalation of toxins is more likely to produce a diffuse, relatively homogeneous acute lung injury.

Regions of the lower respiratory system that are susceptible to toxin injury include the airway epithelium, subepithelial mucosa, alveolar lining cells, and vascular endothelium. Alveolar type I epithelial cells seem particularly susceptible to acute injury from inhaled substances. Some of the mechanisms involved in the general epithelial injury described in the previous section also apply to injury to the epithelia of the lower airway and alveoli. Damage can result in focal and confluent areas of edema with protein-rich fluid in the alveolar spaces, hyaline membrane formation, and denudation of the alveolar epithelium. Mucous membranes of the bronchial and bronchiolar walls may be destroyed or denuded.

Pulmonary parenchymal injury that results from inhalation of irritant substances runs the spectrum of acute lung injury and includes pneumonitis, pulmonary edema, and the acute respiratory distress syndrome (ARDS). Pneumonitis is the most frequent parenchymal manifestation of inhalation injury. Clinical features include dyspnea, productive or dry cough, hypoxemia, mild restriction of ventilation, decreased alveolar gas diffusion, and diffuse bilateral infiltrates on the chest radiograph. Generally, pneumonitis caused by toxic inhalation is a self-limited process, with clinical improvement mirrored by rapid clearing of infiltrates seen on the chest x-ray. Treatment is supportive, usually includes supplemental oxygen, and may require mechanical ventilation. The use of corticosteroids has not been shown to be of significant benefit in the treatment of pneumonitis secondary to the inhalation of irritant gases such as chlorine, ozone, and phosgene, but may be indicated in cases of known inhalation of some metal fumes such as mercury, cadmium and zinc – all of which have been reported to progress to severe and sometimes fatal acute lung injury. As it is for toxic pneumonitis, the treatment of toxin-induced pulmonary edema and ARDS remains largely supportive, and may include hemodynamic monitoring and mechanical ventilation.

Chronic injury

Bronchiolitis obliterans. Bronchiolitis obliterans, an inflammatory reaction with obliteration of the small airways, can occur as a late consequence of the inhalation of several toxins. Exposures to ammonia, mercury, oxides of nitrogen, and sulfur dioxide have been associated with bronchiolitis obliterans.[19–22] High-intensity inhalation exposures can be followed by acute pulmonary edema and ARDS. Survivors of the acute lung injury may experience a relatively asymptomatic period that is followed by the development of irreversible airflow obstruction that often presents one to three weeks after the initial injury. Early inspiratory crackles are a characteristic physical exam finding. The appearance of the chest radiograph is variable, and may be associated with the degree of clinical severity. Mild cases can have normal chest x-rays, while more severely affected individuals may demonstrate hyperinflation. Infiltrates are generally absent. Pulmonary function tests typically demonstrate airflow obstruction that may

in some cases also be associated with restrictive defects. The histologic picture is characterized by the presence of granulation tissue plugs within the lumina of small airways and occasionally alveolar ducts, as well as by the destruction of small airways with obliterative fibrous scarring.

The pathophysiology of bronchiolitis obliterans due to toxin inhalation is not well understood. The predominance of neutrophils in the bronchoalveolar lavage fluid of some patients with bronchiolitis obliterans clearly identifies an active inflammatory process, but the exact mechanisms involved are not currently well defined. The process may not respond to treatment with corticosteroids; however, a 6-month trial of corticosteroids should be given. Bronchodilators may be efficacious in some symptomatic individuals, although clear-cut evidence of this potential benefit is not available.

Bronchiolitis obliterans organizing pneumonia (BOOP). Bronchiolitis obliterans organizing pneumonia (BOOP), a proliferative bronchiolitis with inflammation of the distal lung parenchyma, is an uncommon delayed consequence of the inhalation of toxic substances such as ammonia, mercury, and sulfur dioxide.[23,24] The clinical presentation is characterized by a persistent, non-productive cough, fever, sore throat, and malaise. The lung exam typically reveals late inspiratory crackles but no wheezes; many patients have no abnormalities on physical exam. The characteristic chest x-ray findings include bilateral, patchy, 'ground glass' densities which start as focal lesions but may coalesce with time. In contrast to patients with bronchiolitis obliterans, those with BOOP present with restrictive ventilatory physiology and decreased diffusing capacity.

The histology of BOOP includes the presence of granulation tissue in the small airways and alveolar ducts, as in bronchiolitis obliterans. In addition, however, the granulation tissue extends into the alveoli and may result in interstitial scarring. This distinction between the histologic features of BOOP and those of 'pure' bronchiolitis obliterans (without organizing pneumonia) may reflect different host responses to similar inhaled toxins.[24] Examination of the granulation tissue plugs from patients with BOOP demonstrates temporal uniformity in a patchy distribution with the preservation of background architecture. Bronchoalveolar lavage fluid demonstrates a neutrophilic alveolitis; lymphocytes may also be prominent. These findings suggest that the pathological process results from an initial insult (e.g., an inhaled toxin) with subsequent inflammatory and reparative processes.

Treatment of BOOP with corticosteroids often results in dramatic clinical improvement. Pulmonary function abnormalities can improve considerably, and in some cases may rapidly normalize. The radiographic abnormalities also rapidly clear. A small number of patients may not respond to corticosteroid therapy and may develop progressive fibrosis. Duration of therapy is generally at least 6 months but should be guided by the rate and extent of the clinical response.

CLINICAL COURSE AND EVALUATION

The development of a toxic pneumonitis indicates that the epithelia in the terminal bronchioles and alveoli have been acutely damaged and are no longer able to prevent fluid, inflammatory mediators, and cells from accumulating in the airways and alveoli. Importantly, the spectrum of disease is dependent on the extent and location of injury to the airway and alveolar epithelia. While brief exposures to soluble agents may result in only mild tracheal–bronchial irritation, more extensive exposure to insoluble aerosols and gases can cause diffuse alveolar injury and may present as acute respiratory distress syndrome (ARDS). Thus, the clinician should be aware of this spectrum in evaluating patients following exposure to potentially hazardous inhaled agents.

Among those surviving the acute symptomatic exposure, persistent airway hyper-reactivity and bronchiolitis obliterans have been reported in a few individuals. The term reactive airway dysfunction syndrome (RADS) has been applied to the persistence of airway reactivity following acute exposure to respiratory irritants. Although somewhat speculative, persistent airway hyper-reactivity is believed to result from continued epithelial cell inflammation, which causes either an increase in epithelial cell permeability or a decrease in the conduction threshold for subepithelial vagal afferent receptors.

BOOP is characterized by persistent respiratory symptoms and recurrent patchy infiltrates which wax and wane for several months prior to diagnosis. Although this represents an unusual manifestation of an inhalational injury, it should be included in the differential diagnosis given the proper clinical setting. The chest x-ray demonstrates areas of focal hyperinflation and, additionally, often has multiple patchy densities which appear as ground glass infiltrates. Physiologically most patients present with restrictive lung function and diminished diffusing capacity; however, occasionally airflow obstruction may also be present in this disease process. Lung biopsies, which are needed to definitively diagnose this condition, demonstrate extensive granulation tissue in the airways, alveolar ducts, and alveoli. Of note, organizing fibrosis is clearly identified in the peribronchial region and is typically of uniform age, suggesting a time-limited environmental or infectious insult. Corticosteroids appear to be effective in reversing the underlying inflammatory process in approximately 65% of the cases.

History

The medical history should take precedence and, given the potentially fatal outcome, initial attention should focus on the extent and pace of the parenchymal injury. Dyspnea is the most common symptom following inhalation of detrimental gases or aerosols. It is essential to grade the degree of dyspnea (at rest, with minimal exertion, or with extensive exertion) to both establish a new baseline and also determine the extent of the parenchymal injury. Clearly, the rate of change in dyspnea and specific signs of pulmonary disease are key features used to guide the clinical management. Other symptoms that have been observed in these patients include chest tightness and burning, a cough that may or may not be productive of sputum, and wheezing. Patients with dyspnea at rest and a cough with or without pink, frothy sputum should be assumed to have extensive parenchymal injury and are at high risk of developing (or having) ARDS. Other acute symptomatology may include asthma and bronchial inflammation or bronchitis.

Importantly, weeks to months after the exposure, individuals may first develop symptoms of asthma, bronchitis, or even bronchiolitis obliterans. These subacute symptoms will primarily develop from the delayed onset of airflow obstruction. Symptoms of airflow obstruction include wheezing, dyspnea with exertion, and cough with or without sputum production. However, unlike the acute symptomatology, these symptoms commonly develop 4–6 weeks following the exposure and may worsen over time.

The environmental or occupational history is critical since the clinical presentation can be confused with other more common forms of asthma, bronchitis, pneumonia, or ARDS. However, in many cases where symptoms develop acutely following exposure, the exposure history will be clearly evident. If questioned properly, patients can usually recall the specific exposure or event that was associated with the onset of symptoms. In most cases, there is a clear temporal relationship between exposure and symptom onset. However, with less soluble agents, such as nitrogen dioxide and phosgene, the onset of symptoms may occur hours to days after the exposure. In addition, the delayed or subacute symptomatology (asthma, bronchitis, and bronchiolitis obliterans) may take weeks to months to develop. Thus, clinicians need to aggressively pursue an occupational/environmental history in cases of non-bacterial pneumonia, adult onset asthma or bronchitis, and all cases of broncholitis obliterans and focus on relatively high exposures to the agents listed in Table 19.5.3.

Physical examination

Acutely following the exposure, the clinician needs to assess the pace and extent of the parenchymal injury. Given the potential life-threatening consequences of these exposures, the initial examination needs to be directed toward essential measures of cardiopulmonary function, such as gas exchange, pulmonary edema, and hemodynamic stability. In addition, if significant injury has occurred to the airway, signs of upper airway edema and stenosis along with generalized airflow obstruction may be present. Elevated temperatures are usually not part of the clinical picture; however, this may be present when diffuse parenchymal injury has occurred.

Weeks to months after the exposure, patients may present with signs of asthma, bronchitis, or even bronchiolitis obliterans. Thus, wheezing and rhonchi with patchy areas of rales are not infrequently observed. Since the onset of subacute airway and parenchymal disease can be quite insidious, the clinical evaluation should maintain a relatively low threshold for pursuing these delayed complications.

Substance	Acute clinical manifestations				Chronic clinical manifestations		
	Onset	Upper airway irritation	Pneumonitis, ARDS	Bronchiolitis obliterans, BOOP	Obstructive lung disease	RADS
Irritant gases							
Ammonia	minutes	severe	+	+	+	+
Chlorine	minutes to hours	moderate	+	–	+	+
Hydrogen chloride	minutes	severe	+	–	–	–
Oxides of nitrogen	hours	mild	+	+	+	+
Ozone	minutes to hours	mild	+	–	–	–
Phosgene	hours	mild	+	–	+	–
Sulfur dioxide	minutes	severe	+	+	+	+
Metals							
Cadmium	hours	mild	+	–	+	–
Mercury	hours	mild	+	+	–	–
Zinc chloride	minutes	mild	+	–	–	–
Zinc oxide	hours	mild	+	–	–	–

+ = exposure reported to be associated with clinical entity
– = exposure as yet not reported to be associated with clinical entity

Table 19.5.5 Pulmonary manifestations of toxin inhalation

Laboratory evaluation

Immediately following exposure, the clinician needs to be concerned with gas exchange and the extent of the parenchymal injury. Arterial blood gases (ABG) can adequately assess gas exchange and the chest radiograph will be helpful in determining the overall extent of the pulmonary injury. Since certain chemicals, particularly the less soluble ones, may have between 12 and 24 hours of delay between exposure and the full development of the lung injury, it is not unreasonable to observe patients for at least 12 hours following the exposure. Symptomatic patients should be hospitalized for a minimum of 24 hours, regardless of the initial chest radiogram and ABG. In the first 24–48 hours following exposure, pulmonary function tests are not needed and the results may be misleading. However, several days to weeks following the exposure, pulmonary function tests can be used to identify problems with airflow obstruction, restrictive lung function, or abnormal gas exchange. While airflow obstruction would be indicative of asthma or bronchitis, restrictive lung function with or without abnormal gas exchange (i.e., low diffusing capacity) would be most consistent with bronchiolitis obliterans.

Several weeks after the exposure, all patients should have a complete set of pulmonary function tests (spirometry, lung volumes, and diffusing capacity) to either document a return to baseline function or identify subclinical changes in lung function that may be related to the exposure. Occasionally methacholine challenge may be indicated to assess airway lability (RADs, for example). Rarely, an open lung biopsy is needed to establish the diagnosis of bronchiolitis obliterans in patients with patchy involvement of the lung parenchyma several months following the exposure.

Treatment

The treatments in the acute phases of these exposures are largely supportive. Specific attention needs to be directed toward bronchodilator therapy, adequate oxygenation, and the treatment of the non-cardiogenic pulmonary edema. Supplemental oxygen, intubation in severe cases, and ventilatory support with the use of positive expiratory pressure are the mainstays of treatment. If the patient has severe nasopharyngeal or pharyngeal edema, a tracheotomy may be needed. If bronchospasm is present, bronchodilators should be used and parenteral corticosteroids should be considered. In the absence of bronchospasm, the role of corticosteroids in the acute phase of pulmonary edema has not been definitively established and may place the patient at further risk for the complications of ARDS. Prophylactic antibiotics have not been proven to be helpful and should be reserved for those patients with evidence of overt infection. Beyond the acute phase, inhaled corticosteroids should be considered to diminish the local inflammation in the airway. Bronchodilators should only be used in patients with clinically significant airflow obstruction. Corticosteroids are clearly indicated in the treatment of bronchiolitis obliterans but have not been evaluated in effectively preventing the onset of this or any other late complication.

Prevention

Most toxic inhalational injuries occur as a result of accidental overexposures. Preventive measures can be taken to reduce the risks of such overexposures, such as better industrial hygiene and engineering controls, regular maintenance of equipment, and proper worker training. In addition, a comprehensive plan to handle accidents and emergencies is necessary, including appropriate evacuation plans and availability of necessary emergency provisions such as air supplying respirators, showers, and oxygen. Workers should be educated regarding potential risks, warning symptoms and the accident action plan, and regular practice drills be instituted.

EFFECTS OF SPECIFIC INHALED TOXINS ON THE RESPIRATORY SYSTEM

The following sections address the pulmonary effects of selective specific inhaled toxins. Table 19.5.5 summarizes the acute and long-term manifestations. Specific agents are discussed further in Chapters 39 (metals) and 47 (toxic gases).

Ammonia

Ammonia is a highly water-soluble substance that is extensively used in the manufacturing, chemical, and agricultural industries. Its uses are many, and include the manufacture of explosives, cyanides, synthetic fibers, and plastics. It also has applications in petroleum refining, as a cleaning agent and refrigeration system coolant. Its high nitrogen content makes ammonia a commonly used soil fertilizer; it can be applied in its liquid form, or as ammonia dissolved in water. Most inhalation exposures are the result of accidental releases, including tank leaks and transportation mishaps.[22,25,26]

Exposure to ammonia gas or vapors causes immediate irritation of the mucosal surfaces of the eyes, skin, nasopharynx, oropharynx, larynx, and trachea. Ammonia reacts with water that is present on mucosal surfaces to form ammonium hydroxide, which in turn forms hydroxyl ions. This exothermic reaction contributes to thermal burns that form part of the initial injury. In addition, chemical injury results from alkali burns that are deeply penetrating and result in tissue liquefaction. Cutaneous burns, which may be disfiguring, are deepest in areas with the highest moisture content. Burn injuries to the eyes may result in permanent visual impairment and include damage to the corneal endothelium, corneal stroma, iris, and lens; these burns are often more severe than those caused by other alkalis because of ammonia's ability to deeply penetrate tissues. Initial injury to the mucosa of the oropharynx may result in edema, hemorrhage, and sloughing of tissue and can result in fatal upper airway obstruction.

The severity of ammonia-induced injury depends on the concentration and duration of exposure. Lower airway and pulmonary parenchymal injury can occur acutely with high intensity exposures. It is characterized by pulmonary edema, hemorrhage, and atelectasis. A biphasic pattern of pulmonary response to ammonia inhalation has been reported, characterized by initial, acute pneumonitis that may clear over the next 2–3 days, followed in some individuals by the gradual development of airway obstruction and respiratory failure.[25] Bronchopneumonia due to superinfection with bacterial organisms is common. Bronchiectasis and focal bronchiolitis obliterans have been associated with this late phase.

Initial treatment of individuals exposed to ammonia gas or vapors includes immediate irrigation of all exposed surfaces, especially eyes, with copious amounts of water. The airway must be secured. Treatment of pulmonary involvement is supportive, and includes supplemental oxygen and mechanical ventilation if indicated. The use of corticosteroids is controversial, and prophylactic antibiotics have not been shown to clearly improve outcome.

Chlorine, chloramine, and hydrochloric acid

Chlorine (Cl_2) is a highly reactive gas that is widely found in industrial, environmental, and home settings. Its uses include as a bleaching agent in the textile and paper industries, and as part of water purification processes at swimming pools and sewage systems. Currently, episodes of toxic inhalation exposure are most often the result of accidental releases and spills.[27,28] Common settings for chlorine exposure are secondary to transportation accidents, accidental industrial releases or spills, and accidental spills or releases at swimming pools and sewage treatment facilities.[27,28]

Chlorine reacts with water to form hydrochloric acid (HCl) and hypochlorous acid (HOCl). These products, as well as elemental chlorine itself, exert various irritative effects on the respiratory system. Chlorine has intermediate water solubility, and its inhalation can therefore result in irritation of the upper and lower respiratory tracts. Its mechanism of cellular injury appears to involve the generation of oxygen free radicals. Hydrochloric acid and hypochlorous acid, on the other hand, are highly water soluble, and thus exert significant irritative effects on the mucous membranes of the upper respiratory tract and ocular conjunctivae. Lower respiratory irritation is less common with these acids, although it has been reported following acute, high-intensity exposures. Hydrochloric acid is an irritant and acts to coagulate underlying tissues.

The clinical manifestations of the inhalation of chlorine and its derivatives are similar to those of other inhaled gases that have similar solubility profiles. Because chlorine has intermediate water solubility, its irritant effects are manifested throughout the respiratory system, and include immediate rhinitis, conjunctivitis, and skin irritation, as well as cough, dyspnea, and chest tightness.

In addition to the toxic effects of chlorine and its derivatives discussed above, a significant number of toxic inhalation exposures involve the products that result from the mixing of chlorine compounds and other substances. Many of these exposures occur in the household setting and involve various cleaning agents.[29] Chloramine gas is formed when chlorine or hypochlorous acid are mixed with ammonia. Chloramine gas, in turn, decomposes to ammonia and hypochlorous acid or hydrochloric acid when it comes into contact with water. Ammonia, hypochlorous acid, and hydrochloric acid are all highly water soluble, and therefore have primarily upper respiratory tract irritative effects. Household bleach (which contains hypochlorous acid, or hypochlorite) reacts to form chlorine gas when it is mixed with phosphoric acid or hydrochloric acid. The resultant chlorine gas subsequently produces irritative symptoms throughout the respiratory tract.

Chlorine gas was one of several chemical warfare agents used in the First World War. Several follow-up studies of exposed military personnel report long-lasting pulmonary impairments, including chronic bronchitis and airflow obstruction, in some individuals. Others, however, apparently fully recovered from similar degrees of chlorine gas exposure. Total dose of exposure is probably the most significant determinant of long-term adverse respiratory effects following acute chlorine inhalation.[15]

Sulfur dioxide

Sulfur dioxide is a heavy, colorless gas that is widely used in many industrial processes, including mining, ore smelting, and the bleaching of wool and wood pulp.

Sulfur dioxide is highly water soluble and hydrolyzes to sulfuric acid upon contact with water on mucous membranes. While the acid injury to cellular components is not fully understood, it appears to involve direct damage via irritant mechanisms. In addition, subacute inflammation may contribute to long-term respiratory sequelae. Individuals who experience acute, high-intensity exposure report the immediate onset of symptoms that include burning of the eyes, nose, and throat, rhinorrhea, tearing of the eyes, dyspnea, chest tightness, and cough. Extremely high-intensity acute exposures can lead to death within minutes from respiratory failure due to a combination of alveolar hemorrhage and edema, possible reflex vagal stimulation, and the asphyxiating effect of high concentrations of sulfur dioxide.[16]

Significant extrapulmonary injuries include corneal injuries that can range in severity from superficial burns that resolve completely in days to weeks to permanent opacification; these injuries appear to be dose dependent. Less intense acute exposures can produce a broad range of upper and lower respiratory tract injury that also appear to occur in a dose-dependent manner. Acute pneumonitis can progress to ARDS. Survivors of the acute lung injury may experience a relatively asymptomatic period that is followed several weeks later by the onset of irreversible airflow obstruction due to bronchiolitis obliterans.[30] Other individuals may demonstrate immediate, persistent airflow obstruction and non-specific bronchial hyper-reactivity that is consistent with RADS.[17]

Treatment of inhalation injury due to sulfur dioxide and sulfuric acid is supportive and includes supplemental oxygen, maintenance of a patent airway, and mechanical ventilation if necessary. Corticosteroids have not been shown to alter the course of ARDS due to this toxic inhalation, and rarely provide significant benefit for patients who have developed bronchiolitis obliterans. However, a trial course of corticosteroids is not unreasonable. Bronchodilators may be helpful for those patients with symptomatic airflow obstruction.

Nitrogen oxides

Nitrogen oxides are major components of air pollution. In addition, accidental releases of nitrogen oxide gases can occur in occupational settings and result in high intensity exposures. Oxides of nitrogen are present in a number of industrial settings, including mining, acetylene welding, and explosives manufacturing. These gases can also be present in closed or poorly ventilated areas in which engines are operated. Perhaps the best recognized occupational exposure to nitrogen oxides occurs in agricultural workers ('silo filler's disease') who are exposed to silo gas that is formed via the decomposition of organic matter.[31]

Clinical manifestations of toxicity include signs and symptoms of a chemical pneumonitis, the severity of which is dose dependent and is influenced both by the time and concentration of the exposure. Severe cases progress to ARDS and sometimes lethal acute lung injury, while less severe cases can completely resolve or result in varying degrees of chronic airway obstruction and RADS. Bronchiolitis obliterans can be a late sequela and may develop following a relatively asymptomatic period after the resolution of ARDS.

The mechanism of injury due to the inhalation of nitrogen dioxide involves the production of nitric acid from the hydrolysis of nitrogen dioxide and water; this acid production occurs at the levels of the terminal bronchioles and alveolar membranes. Nitric acid can subsequently dissociate to nitrates and nitrites that can cause tissue injury through direct local cytotoxicity and inflammation, as well as via the formation of free oxygen radicals that can be involved with the peroxidation of lung lipids, with resultant disruption of cellular membranes. This constellation of toxin damage may explain the clinically recognized pulmonary edema and lower airway obstruction that often result from nitrogen oxide inhalation.

The treatment of the acute lung injury is supportive and includes supplemental oxygen and mechanical ventilation. In addition, awareness of the potential for the development of obstructive lung disease, including bronchiolitis obliterans, several weeks after initial apparent recovery is important. Individuals who survive the acute lung injury are at risk for these later complications and should be followed closely with serial assessment of pulmonary mechanics and gas exchange. Asymptomatic hypoxemia or decrements in airflow should be closely monitored since those individuals may also go on to develop bronchiolitis obliterans. Corticosteroids may be helpful in preventing or decreasing the severity of progressive airflow obstruction, and should be considered in asymptomatic individuals who demonstrate spirometric or gas exchange abnormalities.

Prevention of exposure includes the provision of adequate ventilation and appropriate respiratory protective equipment in all environments in which nitrogen oxides may be encountered.[31] Agricultural workers should be aware that the hazard from oxides of nitrogen in silos is greatest during the first week to 10 days after green ensilage has begun fermenting. Engineering controls can reduce the accumulation of harmful nitrogen oxides. Poorly ventilated silos should not be entered unless adequate respiratory protection is available.

Phosgene

Phosgene, another gaseous toxin that has relatively low water solubility, is perhaps most notorious for its role as a war gas. Its use in the First World War reportedly led to as many as 80% of all the gas deaths during that conflict. In modern times, phosgene is used to catalyze a number of industrial reactions including the production of polyurethane resin, toluene diisocyanate, pesticides, pharmaceutical products, and dyes. In addition, it is produced via heat decomposition of various solvents, paint removers, dry cleaning fluids, and methylene chloride.[32]

As for other inhaled toxins that have low water solubilities, phosgene produces its most recognized clinical effects through injury to the lower airway and lung parenchyma. A clinical picture of pneumonitis that can progress to the adult respiratory distress syndrome (ARDS) results. Phosgene is hydrolyzed to hydrochloric acid, and injury may occur via direct cytotoxicity or enzymatic poisoning. Phosgene is a colorless gas that at a concentration of one ppm has the odor of newly mown hay or grass. At higher concentrations it has a more pungent odor and can be mildly irritating to the upper airway. Concentrations of 5–10 ppm inhaled for as few as 5–10 seconds can cause immediate cough, lacrimation, and mucosal irritation. A latent period of 30 minutes to 8 hours can precede the onset of symptoms of lower airway and parenchymal irritation. The duration of the latent period is inversely proportional to the severity of exposure and is also thought to be inversely proportional to the subsequent severity of disease.

Clinical manifestations of the lower airway and parenchymal effects include dyspnea, chest tightness, and increasing respiratory distress. Physical exam may reveal cyanosis and rales. Chest radiograph can show diffuse bilateral infiltrates consistent with pulmonary edema. Treatment is supportive, and may include mechanical ventilation and supplemental oxygenation. Individuals that survive the acute injury can be left with chronic bronchitis or emphysema, although others may experience no long-lasting adverse clinical sequelae.[32]

Ozone

Ozone is recognized as a major constituent of environmental smog, and is also present as a naturally occurring gas in the upper atmosphere, where it has a protective effect against ultraviolet radiation from the sun. It is a colorless, odorless gas that has relatively low water solubility. Chronic and acute adverse health effects from the concentrations of ozone (0.05–0.8 ppm) that are commonly found in ambient air have been well described and include many respiratory symptoms as well as evidence of upper and lower airway irritation, inflammation, and airflow obstruction.[7] In the occupational setting, ozone has been implicated as a toxic inhalant in airplane cabins during high altitude flight, in industries where it is used as an oxidizing agent, and in arc welding where it can occur in association with oxides of nitrogen.[33]

Cadmium

Cadmium (Cd) is a highly corrosion-resistant metal that has many industrial applications. It is used in solder and brazing rods as well as in the manufacture of batteries, alkaline accumulators, and steel alloys. It is commonly used to electroplate or galvanize metal surfaces. In addition, cadmium-containing pigments are used widely including in paints, plastics, printing inks, leather, glass, and enamels.[34]

Most toxic exposures have been reported following exposure to cadmium vapors in enclosed spaces or poorly ventilated areas. Heating of cadmium-containing materials can release vapors and cadmium oxide fumes. The typical clinical presentation is similar to that for metal fume fever (see below), and includes an initial asymptomatic period that lasts several hours and is followed by fevers, chills, and myalgias. Unlike uncomplicated metal fume fever, after Cd exposure, these constitutional symptoms are often accompanied by or shortly followed by respiratory distress, including cough, chest tightness, and dyspnea. The chest x-ray reveals bilateral infiltrates consistent with pneumonitis. Initial pulmonary function tests can show a restrictive ventilatory defect and decreased diffusion. Fatal cases have been remarkable for initial pneumonitis that progresses to ARDS and eventual death from respiratory failure.[35] Individuals who survive the acute lung injury may be left with persistent ventilatory restriction.

The mechanisms involved with the acute lung injury due to cadmium inhalation are not well defined. Postmortem examinations of individuals who died after accidental acute inhalation exposure have revealed tracheobronchitis, consolidated lungs, denuded bronchial epithelium, intra-alveolar hemorrhage, and the presence of macrophages in the alveolar spaces.[35]

Treatment of acute lung injury due to the inhalation of cadmium fumes is supportive and common to treatment for other forms of acute lung injury and ARDS. Corticosteroids may help improve outcome, but their efficacy is not well established. Elevated blood and urine cadmium levels may help establish cadmium as the likely etiologic agent in cases in which the nature of the exposure is not clear. Blood levels may reflect acute exposure, while urine levels better reflect the total body burden. Monitoring of blood or urine levels during treatment has not been shown to influence the clinical outcome.[34]

Mercury

Acute mercury vapor inhalation occurs in occupational settings, including metal reclamation processing, fur and felt hat making, and dentistry. In addition, high exposures have occurred in the home during amateur attempts to extract precious metals from amalgams that also contain mercury.[36,37] Common to episodes of toxic mercury inhalation are settings that involve vapor generation in closed spaces or poorly ventilated areas.

Mercury vapor has little or no immediate upper airway or mucosal surface irritant effects, and as a result exposed individuals may inadvertently remain in an area where the harmful vapors are present. Typical clinical presentations include symptoms of cough, dyspnea, and respiratory distress that develop 12–24 hours post-exposure. These initial symptoms are sometimes accompanied by fever, nausea, vomiting, diarrhea, and a metallic taste in the mouth, similar to what is often experienced by individuals with metal fume fever. Symptoms of mercury vapor inhalation do not, however, spontaneously resolve in a pattern similar to that for metal fume fever. Instead, the pneumonitis may progress to ARDS. Death due to progressive respiratory failure may ensue; pneumothorax has been reported to be a preterminal event in several cases.

The severity of the injury appears to depend on the intensity of exposure and, possibly, the size and age of the exposed individual. Children and small household pets seem especially vulnerable to life-threatening acute lung injury after the inhalation of mercury, but death due to respiratory failure has also been reported in exposed adults.[37] Adults who survive the acute lung injury usually experience resolution of their symptoms from 2 to 7 days following onset, although longer courses of resolution have been reported for those who have sustained more severe injury.

The acute effects of inhaled mercury are usually confined to the respiratory system, although renal involvement with acute tubular necrosis has been reported.[20] The acute gastrointestinal and renal injuries that are seen after mercury ingestion are not typical of acute inhalation exposure. Chronic, low-intensity inhalation exposure may be associated with central nervous system and systemic symptoms and injury similar to that observed after ingestion.

Treatment of mercury inhalation is supportive and common to treatment for acute lung injury and ARDS. Corticosteroids have no proven benefit. Chelating agents, such as dimercaprol and d-penicillamine, frequently used to increase the rate of mercury excretion after ingestion, have not been shown to affect the outcome of the acute lung injury.[37]

Smoke bombs (zinc chloride)

Zinc chloride ($ZnCl_2$, or hexite) is a major ingredient of smoke bombs.[3,38] Oxides and chlorides of zinc and chloride are formed by the ignition of hexachlorethane, zinc oxide, and calcium chloride and are produced by some of the smoke-generating devices used by the military, in firefighter training, and for the generation of special effects in the entertainment industry. Toxic inhalations have occurred in settings where individuals have breathed in smoke in confined spaces (Fig. 19.5.1), in most instances without functional protective breathing apparatus. The smoke effect tends to contribute to the duration of exposure by obscuring vision, sometimes resulting in directional disorientation and the inability to quickly escape the area of exposure.

Zinc chloride is a hygroscopic, caustic salt that forms hydrochloric acid and zinc oxychloride upon contact with water on mucous membranes and other surfaces. The severity of injury appears to be related to the intensity of the exposure, and depends both on the duration of exposure and the concentration of zinc chloride in the smoke. Irritation and burning of the eyes, skin, and mucous membranes result. Zinc chloride is present in particulate form and the average size has been reported as 0.1 μm. This size makes it possible for relatively large amounts of the inhaled hexite to penetrate into the lower respiratory tract, and as much as 20% of the total may reach beyond the level of the respiratory bronchioles, while the remainder settles throughout the tracheobronchial tree. Deposition of particles in the lungs and subsequent forma-

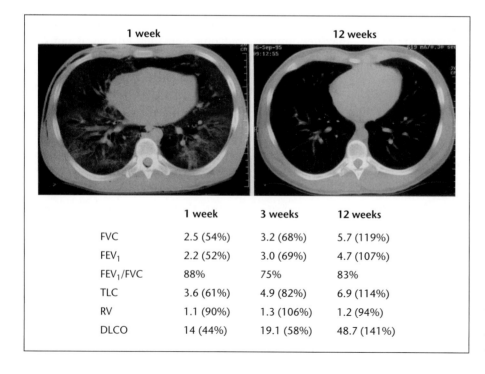

	1 week	3 weeks	12 weeks
FVC	2.5 (54%)	3.2 (68%)	5.7 (119%)
FEV$_1$	2.2 (52%)	3.0 (69%)	4.7 (107%)
FEV$_1$/FVC	88%	75%	83%
TLC	3.6 (61%)	4.9 (82%)	6.9 (114%)
RV	1.1 (90%)	1.3 (106%)	1.2 (94%)
DLCO	14 (44%)	19.1 (58%)	48.7 (141%)

Figure 19.5.1: Chest CT scan and pulmonary function tests obtained from an individual following an inhalation injury after a smoke bomb was ignited in an underground cave. The CT scans were obtained 1 week and 12 weeks after the accident and demonstrated the extensive interstitial lung disease that resolves radiographically. The pulmonary function tests obtained 1, 3, and 12 weeks after the exposure demonstrated marked restrictive lung function and abnormal gas exchange that also resolves within 3 months of exposure.

tion of hydrochloric acid may primarily be responsible for the diffuse lung injury.[38]

Signs and symptoms of tracheobronchitis and pneumonitis are common following inhalation of smoke that contains zinc chloride. Initial chest radiographs can be normal, but can also show diffuse bilateral infiltrates that are consistent with pneumonitis. Hypoxemia may not be present initially, but can develop over a course of several days after the exposure. Progression to ARDS following an initial period of clinical stabilization or partial resolution has been reported. Pneumothorax is a frequent complication of the acute lung injury due to subpleural emphysema.

The treatment of zinc chloride inhalation includes oxygen supplementation and mechanical ventilatory support if indicated. Corticosteroids have been used but it is unclear whether they alter the clinical course. N-acetylcysteine may minimize oxidant-induced lung injury, but it is not clear whether this influences the clinical outcome.[3] Exposed individuals who survive may have persistent ventilatory and diffusion defects.

Mace and tear gas

Chloroacetophenone (CN, or 'mace') and orthochlorobenzamalonitrile (CS) are crowd control agents commonly used by the military and law enforcement agencies. These inhaled agents, often referred to as 'tear gas', have immediate, profound, irritant effects on exposed mucous membranes and lacrimal glands and are used to incapacitate individuals. Exposure to either of these agents produces acute rhinorrhea, oral mucositis, conjunctivitis, and lacrimation. The severity of the effect is apparently dose related. Initial physical examination performed within hours of the inhalation exposure demonstrates findings consistent with irritant injury to mucous membranes and lacrimal glands, but no evidence of lower airway or parenchymal damage.

Several case reports describe varying degrees of pneumonitis and pulmonary edema, typically developing hours to several days after the inhalation exposure. The cases reported involved individuals who were exposed to tear gas for prolonged periods of time in poorly ventilated structures.[39,40] Controlled animal studies have also demonstrated delayed-onset pulmonary parenchymal injury and respiratory failure, with postmortem findings of pulmonary edema as well as hemorrhagic and atelectatic lungs following exposure to high concentrations of tear gas.[41]

Treatment of inhalation injury due to tear gas is supportive and includes management of the immediate mucous membrane irritant effects, with particular attention to maintenance of a patent upper airway with frequent suctioning if necessary. Infants and small children may be at particular risk for acute airway obstruction due to copious oral and nasal secretions. Corticosteroids have not been shown to be efficacious in this situation. Awareness of the potential for delayed evidence of acute lung injury is essential.

SYSTEMIC ILLNESS FROM INHALED TOXINS

A number of inhaled substances can cause extrapulmonary illness and injury. Metal fumes, fumes composed of heat-degraded fluorocarbons, and organic dusts have been implicated as causative agents in self-limited systemic syndromes (metal fume fever, polymer fume fever, and the organic dust toxic syndrome) that are notable for influenza-like illness with complete resolution within hours to days of exposure.[42–44] While some exposed individuals experience only constitutional symptoms, there appears to be a continuum of illness that extends to include significant pulmonary parenchymal injury in some exposed subjects. The mechanism or mechanisms of these syndromes are currently unknown, although recent human exposure–response studies have implicated cytokine-mediated inflammation as central to the pathogenesis of metal fume fever[45] and the organic dust toxic syndrome.

Metal fume fever

Metal fume fever is a self-limited syndrome characterized by the delayed onset of fever, chills, myalgias, and generalized malaise following exposure to fumes that contain metal oxides. The syndrome has acquired a number of names over time, including brazier's disease, spelter shakes, brass chills, zinc chills, welder's ague, copper fever, and foundry fever. Metalworkers with the syndrome sometimes describe their symptoms as being 'galvanized'. Welders are the workers most often reported to experience metal fume fever, although a variety of other metalworking occupations, including soldering, brazing, cutting, metallizing, forging, melting, and casting have been associated with exposures to metal fumes that are responsible for the syndrome.

A common scenario is that of exposure to metal oxide fumes generated by welding in a closed space or poorly ventilated area. Zinc oxide is often implicated as the toxic agent responsible for metal fume fever; however, fumes composed of oxides of copper, cadmium, mercury, aluminum, antimony, selenium, iron, magnesium, nickel, silver, and tin have also been implicated.[42]

Constitutional symptoms are often preceded or accompanied by complaints of dry throat and a sweet or metallic taste in the mouth. The characteristic fever, chills, and myalgias, which are sometimes accompanied by headache and nausea, usually develop 4–8 hours after exposure to metal fumes, and spontaneously resolve over the next 24–48 hours. Laboratory findings are remarkable for transient leukocytosis. Tachyphylaxis appears to occur in some individuals who are repeatedly exposed to metal oxide fumes, usually in occupational settings. These workers often report recurrent 'Monday fever' after returning to the workplace following weekend or vacation absences. Metal fume fever has been mistaken for influenza, atypical or community-acquired pneumonia, and a malaria-like illness because of overlapping presenting symptoms.

Some, but not all, individuals also complain of chest tightness, cough (usually non-productive), and varying degrees of dyspnea. The chest x-ray is typically normal, but in individuals with respiratory symptoms, a radiographic picture consistent with pneumonitis has been reported. Pulmonary function tests are usually normal, although in those with symptomatic and radiographic evidence of pneumonitis, obstructive and restrictive defects, as well as abnormalities of diffusion, have been reported. Human studies that have examined the systemic and pulmonary responses to exposure to zinc oxide fumes generated by welding in an environmental chamber suggest that cytokine-mediated inflammatory mechanisms are involved.[45] There appears to be a continuum of clinical severity that ranges from exposed persons who experience the classic, self-resolving, constitutional symptoms of metal fume fever, to those who also develop transient pulmonary impairment, to a group that experiences more severe, sometimes even life-threatening pulmonary injury.

The predisposition to developing these more serious manifestations of metal fume exposure appears to be related to the duration and concentration of the inhalation exposure, and also is most frequently reported after episodes involving fumes from zinc, mercury, and cadmium. The treatment of metal fume fever is supportive, and includes antipyretics and analgesics. Prevention involves provision of adequate ventilation, fume removal devices and respiratory protection for workers in environments where metal oxide fumes are generated.

Polymer fume fever

Polymer fume fever is a syndrome with many clinical similarities to metal fume fever. It results from the inhalation of pyrolysis products of fluoropolymers, the most often reported of which is polytetrafluoroethylene (PTFE, or Teflon).[43] In addition to their popularly recognized use as non-stick coatings on cooking equipment, fluorocarbon polymers are widely used in industrial settings as mold-release sprays, lubricants, and fabric or leather treatments. Heating of fluoropolymers to high temperatures results in the production of fumes composed of a vapor phase that can contain or ultimately produce carbonyl fluoride, perfluorinated alkanes, hydrofluoric acid, and carbon dioxide. Respirable particles may also contribute to the toxic elements in the heat-generated fumes.[43] The fumes produced may lead to the systemic and pulmonary toxicities through mechanisms that are not currently well understood.

The clinical presentation of polymer fume fever includes initial, sometimes immediate symptoms of upper airway irritation: dry throat, rhinitis, chest tightness, and conjunctivitis. Typically, constitutional symptoms consisting of fever, chills, and myalgias occur 4–8 hours after exposure and spontaneously resolve over the next 24 hours. Laboratory features include a transient leukocytosis. There is no consistent pattern of pulmonary function studies. However, individuals with pre-existing obstructive lung disease may experience worsening obstruction after recurrent exposures to polymer fumes.[46] Cough and dyspnea that are associated with wheezing and sometimes radiographic evidence of parenchymal consolidation can occur. Pneumonitis accompanies constitutional symptoms more often than is reported in cases of metal fume fever but is usually self-limited. The reasons for this difference are unknown, but may relate to the release of hydrofluoric acid. Unlike the decline in the severity of metal fume fever symptoms that is observed with frequent, repeated exposures to metal fumes, tolerance does not appear to develop in individuals repeatedly exposed to pyrolized fluoropolymers, implying possible qualitative differences in the mechanisms of injury and host response in these two syndromes.[46]

Exposure to pyrolized fluoropolymers occurs in home and industrial settings, often in poorly ventilated areas. Humans as well as animals may suffer the effects of this form of toxic inhalation; several case reports of polymer fume fever in humans also mention the sudden deaths of pet birds that were similarly exposed. Many workers who experience symptoms consistent with polymer fume fever are cigarette smokers, some of whom have reported the abrupt onset of symptoms immediately after smoking tobacco products. Several reports have suggested that these workers may have directly contaminated their smoking products with inert fluoropolymers that are subsequently pyrolized and inhaled in concentrated form along with the tobacco smoke. Alternatively, cigarette smoking may independently predispose individuals to the development of polymer fume fever and associated acute lung injury.

Treatment of polymer fume fever is supportive and similar to that for metal fume fever. Prevention includes provision of adequate ventilation. In addition, workers should adhere to strict hand-washing habits after handling products containing fluoropolymers, should not eat, drink, or smoke in the work environment, and should not carry smoking materials into the work setting.

Organic dust toxic syndrome

Organic dust toxic syndrome (ODTS), also referred to as silo unloader's syndrome, atypical farmer's lung, or pulmonary mycotoxicosis, is a self-limited illness characterized by fever, chills, myalgias, dry cough, headache, and dyspnea that occur 4–8 hours after exposure to large amounts of organic dusts.[44] These symptoms, although uncomfortable and sometimes transiently debilitating, usually spontaneously resolve over the next 36–48 hours with no long-term adverse sequelae. The etiologic agent or agents have not been fully characterized, but likely include substances that are present in moldy organic material, including fungal spores, actinomyces, bacteria, endotoxin, and other components of grain dusts. These air-borne substances are often encountered after uncapping silos that contain hay or corn silage, during the removal of layers of spoiled animal feed, or when working in swine confinement facilities. Agricultural workers are understandably at the highest risk for the development of ODTS, but others who are exposed to environments where large amounts of grains, hay, straw, or wood chips are present can also present with this syndrome. Although prior sensitization does not appear to be a characteristic feature in individuals who develop ODTS, those who have a history of atopy may manifest more severe symptoms compared to non-atopics.[47]

The physical exam in patients with ODTS is usually normal but can show the presence of bibasilar crackles and scattered wheezes. Laboratory studies reveal a neutrophil-predominant leukocytosis. Mild hypoxemia and infiltrates on chest x-ray have been reported. Bronchoalveolar lavage performed early in the course of the illness may reveal a predominance of neutrophils; with time, lymphocytes may dominate the BAL cellular population.[44] Open lung biopsy in ODTS reveals multifocal areas of acute inflammation with neutrophils and macrophages in terminal bronchioles, alveoli, and interstitial areas, but no evidence of granulomas. Human exposure–response studies have reproduced the characteristic symptoms and laboratory abnormalities, and have also demonstrated transient airflow obstruction.[48,49]

The initial symptoms of ODTS are sometimes confused with those of hypersensitivity pneumonitis. However, unlike hypersensitivity pneumonitis, ODTS is transient, can occur in previously unexposed individuals, and requires a relatively intense exposure. Bronchoalveolar lavage consistent with an acute neutrophilic alveolitis is different from the BAL lymphocytic predominance that has been reported in hypersensitivity pneumonitis. In contrast to what is often found in cases of hypersensitivity pneumonitis, serum allergic precipitins are usually negative in individuals with ODTS.[44]

The course of ODTS is benign, with spontaneous resolution of symptoms as well as laboratory and radiographic abnormalities within days of the exposure. Treatment is symptomatic. Steroids are not recommended. Long-term sequelae of repeated high-intensity exposures that lead to recurrent episodes of ODTS may be associated with chronic bronchitis and decrements in airflow, but these have not been clearly established. Prevention involves education of agricultural workers and other potentially exposed subjects regarding specific practices related to the handling of moldy hay, grains, and other organic materials. In addition, individuals who engage in activities known to produce large quantities of potentially harmful air-borne organic substances, such as weighing of swine and the intense handling of moldy grain, hay, straw, or wood chips, should be advised to wear respiratory protection.

Smoke inhalation

Inhalational injury due to smoke inhalation is the primary cause of morbidity and mortality in fire-exposed persons. The thermal and chemical content of the inhaled smoke accounts for the type and degree of respiratory injury. Direct thermal burns are usually limited to the supraglottic region because the nasopharnyx, larynx, and trachea are effective in cooling the hot, dry air. However, inhalation of steam and respiratory aspiration of hot liquids, which have a greater heat capacity, can cause direct pulmonary injury.

Toxic inhalant	Thermodecomposition source
Acrolein	Cellulosics and polyolefins
Ammonia	Inorganic combustion, melamine, nylon, silk and wool
Carbon monoxide	Incomplete combustion of hydrocarbons
Halogenated acids	Fire-retardant materials containing bromine and fluorinated resins and films
Hydrogen chloride	Chlorinated acrylics, polyvinyl chloride, and fire retardant-treated materials
Hydrogen cyanide	Acrylonitrile, nylon, polyurethane paper, silk and wool
Isocyanates	Urethane and isocyanate polymers
Nitrogen dioxide	Cellulose nitrites, and fabrics
Phosgene	Chlorinated acrylics, polyvinyl chloride, and fire retardant-treated materials
Sulfur dioxide	Combustion of compounds containing sulfur

Table 19.5.6 Toxic inhalants commonly encountered in fires

Of greater concern in fire victims is the large number of toxic gases and chemicals that can be generated in the fire environment. The particulates present in smoke are generally cleared by the respiratory tract. The toxic gases and chemicals resulting from the combustion of the numerous different materials and products that can be present in the fire environment are the major inhalational toxins. These gases and chemicals will vary from fire to fire as the materials that are burning differ in each fire. Major toxic inhalants commonly encountered in fires are listed in Table 19.5.6. The chemicals released in a fire fall into two broad categories – irritants and chemical asphyxiants. Irritants include acrolein, ammonia, chloride, hydrogen chloride, phosgene, and sulfur dioxide. The major chemical asphyxiants are carbon monoxide, produced by incomplete combustion of carbon-containing materials without adequate ventilation, and cyanide. Cyanide, produced by the combustion of materials such as polyurethanes, acrylics, and nylon, binds to mitochondrial cytochrome oxidase, resulting in anaerobic metabolism and lactic acidosis.

Smoke inhalation can result in a spectrum of clinical manifestations, depending on the toxic gases and chemicals present, and extent of exposure. The major acute effects are upper airway obstruction, bronchitis, and bronchospasm. Pulmonary edema and ARDS are less common. Recent studies of New York City fire fighters have shown persistent cough and bronchial hyper-responsiveness related to acute irritant exposures following the World Trade Center collapse.

Evaluation of those exposed to excessive smoke should proceed in a systematic fashion. Information about the fire environment, including potential combustion products, should be obtained. Risk factors predictive of clinically significant smoke inhalation include steam exposure, exposure in a closed space, exposure to plastic fumes, singed facial hair, oropharyngeal burns, altered consciousness, respiratory symptoms, an unexplained lactic acidosis, and a carboxyhemoglobin level higher than 20%. Initially, all smoke-exposed individuals should be treated with high concentrations of oxygen, and the carboxyhemoglobin level and serum pH should be measured.

Carbon monoxide poisoning can be assayed directly from the carboxyhemoglobin level, whereas an unexplained acidosis should raise the suspicion of cyanide intoxication. Upper airway burns are a marker of significant thermal injury and, under some circumstances, are an indication for early endotracheal intubation. In the event of clinically significant smoke inhalation, the patient should be hospitalized for at least 24 hours and observed for the potential delayed complications of chemical fume exposure. Symptomatic individuals should be hospitalized and treated supportively. Early treatment with steroids or prophylactic antibiotics has not been shown to be beneficial and generally is not recommended.

SUMMARY

Acute inhalation exposure to a number of substances produces a spectrum of pulmonary and systemic injuries. Physicians and other healthcare professionals may encounter individuals who have experienced acute inhalation exposure to unknown types or doses of toxic substances. Treatment is generally supportive and is not specific to any individual exposure. This chapter has described typical presentations of injury resulting from a number of inhaled toxins. Awareness of the patterns of presentation and potential consequences of irritant induced inhalation injury can help guide initial and subsequent management. Since the clinical course of these accidental inhalations are often unpredictable, it is prudent to carefully monitor, follow, and have a low threshold for hospitalization when managing these patients. Materials safety data sheets (MSDS) can furnish concise information about specific substances or products. Additional information is also available through computerized library search tools and online information services.

References

1. Kizer K. Toxic inhalations. Emerg Clin North Am 1984; 2:649.
2. Schwartz DA. Acute inhalational injury. In: Rosenstock L, ed. Occupational medicine: state of the art reviews, vol. 2. Philadelphia: Hanley and Belfus Inc., 1987;297.
3. Hjortso E, Qvist J, Bud M, et al. ARDS after accidental inhalation of zinc chloride smoke. Intens Care Med 1988; 14:17.
4. Barnes PJ. Reactive oxygen species and airway inflammation. Free Radical Biol Med 1990; 9:235.
5. Boucher R, Johnson J, Inoue S, Hulbert W, Hogg J. The effect of cigarette smoke on the permeability of guinea pig airways. Lab Invest 1980; 43:94.
6. Case B, Gordon R, Kleinerman J. Acute bronchiolar injury following nitrogen dioxide exposure: a freeze fracture study. Environ Res 1982; 29:399.
7. Menzel D. Ozone: an overview of its toxicity in man and animals. Toxicol Environ Health 1984; 13:183.
8. Holgate ST, Beasley R, Twentyman OP. The pathogenesis and significance of bronchial hyper-responsiveness in airways disease. Clin Science 1987; 73:561.
9. Metzger W, Richerson H, Worden K, Monick M, Hunninghake G. Bronchoalveolar lavage of allergic asthmatic patients following allergen bronchoprovocation. Chest 1986; 89:477.
10. Wardlaw AJ, Dunnette S, Gleich GJ, Collins JV, Kay AB. Eosinophils and mast cells in bronchoalveolar lavage in subjects with mild asthma: relationship to bronchial hyper-reactivity. Am Rev Respir Dis 1988; 137:62.
11. Fabbri LM, Aizawa H, Alpert SE, et al. Airway hyper-responsiveness and changes in cell counts in bronchoalveolar lavage after ozone exposure in dogs. Am Rev Respir Dis 1984; 129:288.
12. Hay DWP, Muccitelli RM, Wilson KA. Agonist specificity in the effects of epithelium removal on contradictions of the guinea pig trachea produced by leukotrienes, 5-hydroxytryptamine, and U-44069. Pharmacologist 1986; 28:141.
13. Beasley R, Roche WR, Roberts JA, Holgate ST. Cellular events in the bronchi in mild asthma and after bronchial provocation. Am Rev Respir Dis 1989; 139:806.
14. O'Connor G, Sparrow D, Taylor D, Segal M, Weiss S, Eleuteri D. Analysis of dose–response curves to methacholine: an approach suitable for population studies. Am Rev Respir Dis 1987; 136:1412.
15. Moore B, Sherman M. Chronic reactive airway disease following acute chlorine gas exposure in an aymptomatic atopic patient. Chest 1991; 100:855.
16. Charan N, Myers C, Lakshminarayan S, Spencer T. Pulmonary injuries associated with acute sulfur dioxide inhalation. Am Rev Respir Dis 1979; 119:555.
17. Brooks SM, Weiss MA, Bernstein IL. Reactive airways dysfunction syndrome (RADS). Persistent asthma syndrome after high level irritant exposures. Chest 1985; 88:376.
18. Gautrin D, Boulet L-P, Boutet M, et al. Is reactive airways dysfunction syndrome a variant of occupational asthma? J Allergy Clin Immunol 1994; 93:12.
19. Galea M. Case report. Fatal sulfur dioxide inhalation. Can Med Assoc J 1964; 91:345.
20. Kanluen S, Gottlieb C. A clinical pathologic study of four adult cases of acute mercury inhalation toxicity. Arch Pathol Lab Med 1991; 115:56.
21. McAdams A, Krop S. Injury and death from red fuming nitric acid. JAMA 1955; 158:1022.
22. Price S, Hughes J, Morrison S, Potgieter P. Fatal ammonia inhalation: a case report with autopsy findings. S Afr Med J 1993; 64:952.
23. Epler G. Bronchiolitis obliterans organizing pneumonia: definition and clinical features. Chest 1992; 102:2S.
24. Epler G, Colby T, McLoud T, Carrington C, Gaensler E. Bronchiolitis obliterans organizing pneumonia. N Engl J Med 1985; 312:152.
25. Arwood R, Hammond J, Ward G. Ammonia inhalation. J Trauma 1985; 25:444.
26. Montague T, Macneil A. Mass ammonia inhalation. Chest 1980; 77:496.
27. Das R, Blanc PD. Chlorine gas exposure and the lung: a review. Toxicol Ind Health 1993; 9:439.
28. Sabonya R. Fatal anhydrous ammonia inhalation. Hum Pathol 1977; 8:293.
29. Reisz G, Gammon R. Toxic pneumonitis from mixing household cleaners. Chest 1986; 89:49.
30. Woodford D, Coutu R, Gaensler E. Obstructive lung disease from acute sulfur dioxide exposure. Respiration 1979; 38:238.
31. NIOSH. Criteria for a recommended standard: occupational exposure to oxides of nitrogen (nitrogen dioxide and nitric oxide). Cincinnati: National Institute for Occupational Safety and Health, 1976.
32. Bradley B, Unger K. Phosgene inhalation: a case report. Texas Med 1982; 78:51.
33. Tashkin D, Coulson A, Simmons M, Spivey G. Respiratory symptoms of flight attendants during high-altitude flight: possible relation to cabin ozone exposure. Int Arch Occup Environ Health 1983; 52:117.
34. Barnhart S, Rosenstock L. Cadmium chemical pneumonitis. Chest 1984; 86:789.
35. Patwardham J, Finckh E. Fatal cadmium-fume pneumonitis. Med J Aust 1976; 1:962.
36. Moutinho M, Tompkins A, Rowland T, Banson B, Jackson A. Acute mercury vapor poisoning. Am J Dis Child 1981; 135:42.

37. Rowens B, Guerrero-Betancourt D, Gottlieb C, Boyes R, Eichenhorn M. Respiratory failure and death following acute inhalation of mercury vapor . A clinical and histologic perspective. Chest 1991; 99:185.

38. Homma S, Jones R, Qvist J, Zapol W, Reid L. Pulmonary vascular lesions in the adult respiratory distress syndrome caused by inhalation of zinc chloride smoke: a morphometric study. Hum Pathol 1992; 23:45.

39. Park S, Giammona S. Toxic effects of tear gas on infant following prolonged exposure. Am J Dis Child 1972; 123:245.

40. Stein A, Kirwan W. Chloroacetophenon-e (tear gas) poisoning: a clinicopathologic report. J Forensic Sci 1964; 9:374.

41. Cucinell S, Swentzel K, Biskup R, et al. Biochemical interactions and metabolic fate of riot control agents. Fed Proc 1971; 30:86.

42. Gordon T, Fine J. Metal fume fever. In: Rosenstock L, ed. Occupational medicine: state of the art reviews, vol. 8. Philadelphia: Hanley and Belfus Inc., 1993;505.

43. Shusterman D. Polymer fume fever and other fluorocarbon pyrolysis-related syndromes. Occup Med 1993; 8:519.

44. Von Essen S, Robbins RA, Thompson AB, Rennard SI. Organic dust toxic syndrome: an acute febrile reaction to organic dust exposure distinct from hypersensitivity pneumonitis. Clin Toxicol 1990; 28:389.

45. Blanc P, Boushey H, Wong H, Wintermeyer S, Bernstein M. Cytokines in metal fume fever. Am Rev Respir Dis 1993; 147:134.

46. Kales S, Christiani D. Progression of chronic obstructive pulmonary disease after multiple episodes of an occupational inhalation fever. J Occup Med 1994; 36:75.

47. Jacobs RR, Boehlecke B, Van Hage-Hamsten M, Rylander R. Bronchial reactivity, atopy, and airway response to cotton dust. Am Rev Respir Dis 1993; 148:19.

48. Clapp WD, Becker S, Quay J, et al. Grain dust-induced airflow obstruction and inflammation of the lower respiratory tract. Am J Respir Crit Care Med 1994; 150:611.

49. Larsson KA, Eklund AG, Hansson L-O, Isaksson B-M, Malmberg PO. Swine dust causes intense airways inflammation in healthy subjects. Am J Respir Crit Care Med 1994; 150:973.

19.6 Hypersensitivity Pneumonitis

Craig Glazer, Cecile S Rose

INTRODUCTION

Hypersensitivity pneumonitis (HP), also known as extrinsic allergic alveolitis, refers to a constellation of granulomatous, interstitial, bronchiolar and alveolar-filling lung diseases caused by repeated exposure and subsequent sensitization to a variety of organic and chemical antigens. Diagnosis relies on a constellation of findings including antigen exposure, characteristic signs and symptoms, pulmonary function abnormalities, radiologic abnormalities, and frequently, characteristic histologic findings.[1]

ETIOLOGY

The extensive list of agents known to cause hypersensitivity pneumonitis can be organized into three main categories: microbial agents, animal proteins, and low molecular weight chemicals (Table 19.6.1). Regardless of the antigen, typically only a minority of exposed and/or sensitized individuals will develop hypersensitivity pneumonitis.[2]

Microbial agents

As a group, various bacteria and fungi represent the most common causative agents.[1] Among bacteria, multiple species of thermophilic actinomyces are the most frequently reported. Thermophilic actinomyces contaminate decaying vegetable matter and are causally associated with farmer's lung (the prototypical example of HP), bagassosis, and composting (including mushroom worker's lung).[3–6] They may also contaminate ventilation systems and humidifiers, and cause disease through these exposure routes as well.[7] Other bacteria, including Bacillus, Klebsiella, and Epicoccum, have been causally associated with HP.[1] More recently, nontuberculous mycobacteria contaminating hot tubs and metal working fluids have been implicated as a likely cause of hypersensitivity pneumonitis.[8–11]

Multiple fungi have been shown to cause hypersensitivity pneumonitis including various species of Aspergillus, Mucor, Penicillium, Basidiospores, and Trichosporon. Summer-type hypersensitivity pneumonitis, the most common form of

Antigen	Exposure	Syndrome
Bacteria		
Thermophilic bacteria		
Micropolyspora faeni	Moldy hay	Farmer's lung
Thermoactinomycetes vulgaris	Moldy sugarcane	Bagassosis
T. sacchari	Mushroom compost	Mushroom worker's lung
T. candidus	Heated water reservoirs	Humidifier lung
		Air conditioner lung
Non-thermophilic bacteria		
Bacillus subtilis, B. cereus	Water	Humidifier lung
	Detergent	Washing powder lung
Fungi		
Aspergillus sp.	Moldy hay	Farmer's lung
	Water	Ventilation pneumonitis
Aspergillus _clavatus_	Barley	Malt worker's lung
Penicillium casei, P. roqueforti	Cheese	Cheese washer's lung
Alternaria sp.	Wood pulp	Wood pulp worker's lung
Cryptostroma corticale	Wood bark	Maple bark stripper's lung
Graphium, Aureobasidium pullulans	Wood dust	Sequoiosis
Merulius lacrymans	Rotten wood	Dry rot lung
Penicillium frequentans	Cork dust	Suberosis
Aureobasidium pullulans	Water	Humidifier lung
Cladosporium sp.	Hot tub mist	Hot tub HP
Trichosporon cutaneum	Damp wood and mats	Japanese summer-type HP
Amebae		
Naegleria gruberi		
Acanthamoeba polyphagia	Contaminated water	Humidifier lung
Acanthamoeba castellani		
Animal proteins		
Avian proteins	Bird droppings, feathers	Bird breeder's lung
Urine, serum, pelts	Rats, gerbils	Animal handler's lung
Wheat weevil (_Sitophilus granarius_)	Infested flour	Wheat weevil lung
Chemicals		
Toluene diisocyanate (TDI)	Paints, resins, polyurethane foams	Isocyanate HP
Diphenylmethane diisocyanate (MDI)	Paints, resins, polyurethane foams	Isocyanate HP
Hexamethylene diisocyanate (HDI)	Paints, resins, polyurethane foams	Isocyanate HP
Trimellitic anhydride	Plastics, resins, paints	TMA HP
Copper sulfate	Bordeaux mixture	Vineyard sprayer's lung
Sodium diazobenzene sulfate	Chromatography reagent	Pauli's reagent alveolitis
Pyrethrum	Pesticide	Pyrethrum HP

Table 19.6.1 Selected agents reported to cause hypersensitivity pneumonitis (HP)

HP in Japan, is caused by *Trichosporon asahii* (formerly *T. cutaneum*).[12] Rhizopus, Pullaria, Penicillium, Aspergillus, and Alternaria have all been implicated as causative agents in woodworker's HP.[13,14] In addition, both Aspergillus and Penicillium have been implicated in cases of farmer's lung disease.[15,16] Amebae such as *Acanthamoeba polyphagia* have been implicated in humidifier lung.[17]

Animal proteins

Avian antigens are the most common animal proteins associated with hypersensitivity pneumonitis. Interestingly, exposure to live birds is not required, as cases have been reported related to use of a feather duvet and with exposure to feather decorations.[18,19] Other implicated animal proteins include wheat weevil, rat, and gerbil proteins, and dust from mollusk shells.[5]

Low molecular weight chemicals

Isocyanates, reactive chemicals widely used in the production of polyurethane foams, elastomers, adhesives, and paints, are the most common cause of occupational asthma in developed countries.[20] In addition, these low molecular weight chemicals are known to cause hypersensitivity pneumonitis.[21] Acid anhydrides, another group of reactive chemicals widely used in industry, also cause an HP-like syndrome frequently accompanied by anemia.[22] In both circumstances the chemicals are thought to combine with endogenous proteins to form complete antigens.[5] Other rare chemical causes of HP include the pesticide pyrethrum, Pauli's reagent (sodium diazobenzene sulfate), and copper sulfate.[1]

EPIDEMIOLOGY

With the challenges of accurate diagnosis and disease reporting, reliable estimates of incidence and prevalence of hypersensitivity pneumonitis remain elusive and it is likely that hypersensitivity pneumonitis is more common than reported. Most studies have focused on farmer's lung, and estimates of incidence and prevalence vary significantly by region. In one study, the prevalence of farmer's lung in Scotland ranged from 23 to 86 per 1000 depending on the region investigated.[23] In Wyoming, the prevalence among dairy and cattle ranchers was found to be 3%, while in Wisconsin dairy farmers, prevalence rates as high as 12% have been reported.[24,25] The annual incidence of farmer's lung in Finland is 44 per 100,000.[26]

The prevalence of HP among bird hobbyists ranges from 0.5% to 21% depending on the study.[27] Among isocyanate workers, the prevalence of HP is approximately 1%.[21]

Importantly, attack rates in HP outbreaks may be significantly higher. Ganier et al reported an attack rate of 52% among office workers exposed to a contaminated humidification system.[7] Similarly, Rose et al described attack rates of 27% and 65% in sequential HP outbreaks among lifeguards at an indoor swimming pool.[28] Thus, hypersensitivity pneumonitis may be quite common in some high-risk settings.

PATHOGENESIS
Immunology

HP is characterized by the presence of activated T lymphocytes in bronchoalveolar lavage (BAL) and an interstitial mononuclear cell infiltrate on lung biopsy. The pathogenesis involves repeated antigen exposure leading to immunologic sensitization and subsequent immune-mediated lung inflammation. The mechanisms underlying this series of events appear primarily to involve cell-mediated immunity. Passive transfer of cultured lymphocytes from sensitized animals, including guinea pigs,[29] rats,[30] rabbits,[31] and inbred mice[32] to unexposed, non-sensitized animals results in disease similar to human HP when the naïve animals subsequently are challenged with inhaled or infused pulmonary antigens. More recent animal experiments have shown the specific cells responsible to be activated T-helper memory cells with Th1 differentiation.[33,34] Type 1 (Th1) cells are defined according to the primary cytokines secreted, interferon γ and IL-2,[35] and are the primary cells involved in cell-mediated immunity.

Data on the cytokines required for the manifestations of hypersensitivity pneumonitis confirm the importance of the cell-mediated immunity. Gudmundsson et al, using interferon γ knockout mice, proved that interferon γ is required for the development of HP in animals.[36] Overexpression of IL-12, a potent inducer of interferon γ production, modulates the expression of HP in various mouse strains.[37] Lymphocytes from BAL of patients with HP have been shown to overproduce interferon γ and to express high affinity IL-12 receptor, confirming the importance of these cytokines in human disease.[38]

Viral infection leads to activation of the cell-mediated immune system and may alter host susceptibility to HP. This is suggested by the clinical observation of a viral prodrome often preceding HP. Viral infections have been shown to enhance HP in animal models leading to both a more intense alveolitis and an increased granulomatous inflammatory response on pathologic specimens.[39] In addition, viral proteins have been found in the lower airways of patients with HP.[40]

The sequence of cellular and humoral events occurring in HP has been characterized using BAL. In a sensitized host, the initial response to antigen exposure is an influx of neutrophils.[41] This is followed by a T lymphocyte-predominant alveolitis, often with 60–70% lymphocytes.[42] Other cells found in increased numbers include natural killer cells and mast cells.[43,44] Alveolar macrophages play a pivotal role throughout this process. They act as antigen presenting cells and secrete a variety of cytokines which function to both enhance the inflammatory response and recruit lymphocytes into the lung.[45,46] In addition, activated macrophages release mediators of fibrosis including fibronectin and other matrix proteoglycans.[47]

Host factors

Although many people are exposed to environmental antigens associated with HP, typically only a small percentage develop disease. This suggests that host susceptibility or resistance factors may influence individual responses to inhaled antigens. Smoking is one such factor as multiple studies have shown that HP occurs more frequently in non-smokers.[48,49] However, smokers who do develop disease appear to have a worse prognosis than non-smokers. In one study, smokers with farmer's lung disease had lower vital capacities, more frequent clinical recurrences, and a poorer 10-year survival than non-smokers with farmer's lung disease.[50]

Other factors associated with differences in host susceptibility remain unclear. Despite multiple investigations, no association with HLA haplotypes and risk for HP has been discovered.[51,52] However, more recent work suggests polymorphisms in the tumor necrosis factor-α (TNF-α) gene may be associated with disease. A polymorphism at position 308 is associated with higher constitutive and inducible levels of TNF-α and was found more frequently in patients with pigeon breeder's disease than controls.[53] In addition, patients with the disease and the 308 polymorphism were younger, had increased mean lymphocyte percentage in BAL, and a reported shorter antigen exposure duration than those patients without the polymorphism.[53]

Exposure factors

Seasonal and geographic variations seen in most of the commonly recognized forms of HP indicate the importance of various exposure factors. Environmental risk factors such as antigen concentration, duration of exposure before symptom onset, frequency and intermittency of exposure, particle size, antigen solubility and potency, use of respiratory protection, and variability in work practices may influence disease prevalence, latency, and severity. Farmer's lung disease is most common in regions with heavy rainfall where feed is likely to become damp, and in harsh winter conditions where this damp hay is used to feed cattle in indoor barns with minimal ventilation. Pigeon breeder's lung is most common during the summer sporting season when exposures are at their highest.[54]

Indirect and apparently trivial antigen exposures may be important with some antigens. Bird breeder's lung has occurred in spouses of pigeon hobbyists exposed to dusty laundry and in individuals whose only known exposure was to down comforters or feather decorations.[18,19,55]

CLINICAL FEATURES
Signs and symptoms

Historically, the clinical presentation of hypersensitivity pneumonitis has been divided into acute, subacute, and chronic forms. However, significant overlap exists between these categories. In acute HP, systemic symptoms of fever, chills, and myalgias occur, along with respiratory symptoms of cough and dyspnea. These symptoms typically occur 4–12 hours after heavy exposure to the inciting antigen. Physical findings include fever and rales, and laboratory evaluation frequently reveals a peripheral leukocytosis. Recurrent acute symptom episodes should prompt consideration of HP and a careful historical search for relevant exposures.

The subacute and chronic forms typically present with an insidious onset of respiratory symptoms often with non-specific systemic symptoms such as malaise, fatigue, or weight loss. Usually, the temporal relationship between symptoms and exposure is difficult to elicit. A high degree of clinical suspicion is required to confirm the diagnosis and initiate appropriate management. In a case series from Japan, the most frequent symptoms in chronic HP were cough and dyspnea.[12] Fever (low-grade) occurred in only half of the patients. Physical examination may be normal or reveal basilar crackles. Wheezing may occur and thus should not be used to exclude the diagnosis. Cyanosis and right-sided heart failure are found in end-stage disease. Depending on the clinical presentation, the differential diagnosis of HP can be extensive and includes inhalation fevers, other granulomatous disorders such as sarcoidosis, immunologic diseases such as asthma, infections, and fibrotic lung diseases such as idiopathic pulmonary fibrosis.

Precipitating antibodies

The finding of specific IgG precipitating antibodies in the serum of a patient with suspected HP is a helpful diagnostic clue but is neither sensitive nor specific and is no longer considered a hallmark of HP. Serum precipitins are found in 3–30% of asymptomatic farmers, and in up to 50% of asymptomatic pigeon breeders.[56,57] Precipitins are thus a marker of exposure sufficient to generate a humoral immune response. However, they have no role in disease pathogenesis.

In addition, false-negative results can be common. In one study, 30–40% of patients with proven farmer's lung disease had no detectable precipitins to commonly tested antigens including *Saccharopolyspora rectivirgula*, *Aspergillus* species, and *Thermoactinomyces vulgaris*.[58] False-negative results may occur because of poorly standardized antigens, improper quality controls, insensitive techniques, the wrong choice of antigen, or underconcentrated sera.[59] They may also occur because serum precipitins may disappear over variable periods of time after cessation of exposure.[3]

Other laboratory studies

Mild elevations in erythrocyte sedimentation rate, C-reactive protein, and immunoglobulins of IgG, IgM, or IgA isotypes are occasionally evident, reflecting acute or chronic inflammation. Serum angiotensin-converting enzyme concentrations may be increased in patients with recurrent acute symptoms.[60] Antinuclear antibodies and other autoantibodies rarely are detected. Skin tests for both immediate and delayed-type hypersensitivity reactions are unhelpful in diagnosis. Recently, researchers have begun to investigate the utility of in-vitro lymphocyte proliferation tests to suspected antigens, with some success.[12,61] However, standardization of both methods and results interpretation awaits further investigation.

Physiology

There is no single characteristic pattern of pulmonary function abnormalities in hypersensitivity pneumonitis. The original descriptions emphasized restriction as the primary abnormality. Although this remains true in acute disease, more recent studies stress the importance of airways obstruction in subacute and chronic HP. Lalancette et al found obstructive abnormalities in 42% of farmers after six years of follow-up.[62] Others have confirmed the high prevalence of airways obstruction, even after accounting for the effects of smoking.[63,64] Methacholine challenge showing increased non-specific bronchial hyper-reactivity has been demonstrated in both acute and chronic disease.[65,66] Thus, patients with HP may exhibit obstructive, restrictive, or mixed patterns on pulmonary function testing. In early disease, normal values on spirometry and lung volumes are not uncommon.[67] Measures of gas exchange, particularly during exertion, are the most sensitive physiologic indicators of early HP abnormalities.[21,67]

RADIOGRAPHIC FEATURES
Standard chest radiographs

The radiographic findings of acute HP include diffuse ground glass opacification and a fine nodular or reticulonodular pattern, often with lower lung field predominance. Consolidation is rarely seen.[68] The reticulonodular pattern becomes more prominent in the subacute phase.[69] In chronic HP, fibrosis with upper lobe retraction, reticular opacity, volume loss, and honeycombing may be seen.[12,70] However, due to increasing awareness of disease preva-

lence and improved diagnostic techniques (especially fiberoptic bronchoscopy), the sensitivity of the chest radiograph has declined.[71] In fact, the sensitivity in recent population-based studies is only about 10%.[72,73] The sensitivity of high-resolution computed tomography (HRCT) is significantly better than plain radiographs.[74–76]

Computed tomography

A variety of HRCT patterns have been described in hypersensitivity pneumonitis, including ground glass, centrilobular nodules, fibrosis, and emphysema, discussed in more detail below.[77,78] Most of these patterns have been correlated with histologic findings and some with pulmonary function abnormalities.[77] In addition, up to 50% of patients have mediastinal lymphadenopathy.[79] However, the adenopathy typically is not diffuse and the enlarged nodes are almost always smaller than 20 mm (short axis diameter).[79]

Ground glass

Ground glass is defined as the presence of hazy increased opacity of the lung without obscuring underlying bronchial and vascular margins.[80] Ground glass is most common in acute hypersensitivity pneumonitis but may also be seen in subacute and chronic HP, especially if there is ongoing exposure (Fig. 19.6.1).[81] The ground-glass opacification may be patchy or diffuse and some authors report a middle lung zone predominance.[82] Ground-glass opacification may resolve with removal from exposure.[76]

Histologically, ground-glass opacification is thought to represent either active alveolitis or fine fibrosis.[76,83] This is

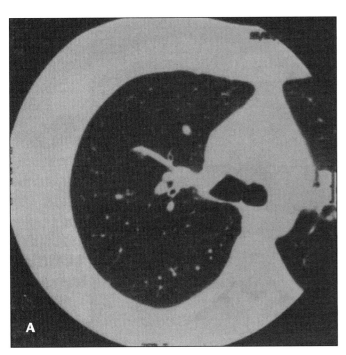
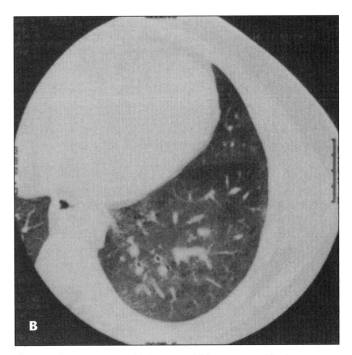

Figure 19.6.1: High-resolution (1.5 mm this section) CT images through the lungs of two patients with hypersensitivity pneumonitis show diffuse nodular densities in one (a) and generalized increase in attenuation of lung parenchyma with ground-glass opacification in the other (b).

consistent with the observed association with restriction and impaired gas exchange on pulmonary function testing.[84] Ground-glass opacification is frequently found in association with other radiographic abnormalities.

Centrilobular nodules

The nodules seen in hypersensitivity pneumonitis are round, poorly defined, and less than 5 mm in diameter (Fig. 19.6.1).[68] They are typically centrilobular[76] and profuse throughout the lung, but a middle to lower lung zone predominance has been variably reported.[82] A patchy or unilateral distribution is more consistent with infection than hypersensitivity pneumonitis.[85] In several series, centrilobular nodules are the most frequent HRCT finding in HP.[68,74,75,82] They are often found in association with ground-glass opacification, and the combination is highly suggestive of HP (Fig. 19.6.1).[77] As with ground glass, the nodules may regress with removal from exposure.[75,76]

Centrilobular nodules are the radiographic equivalent of the cellular bronchiolitis frequently seen on histology. Unlike ground-glass findings, centrilobular nodules have not been correlated with pulmonary function abnormalities.[76,84]

Airspace consolidation

Airspace consolidation differs from ground-glass opacity in that the underlying bronchial and vascular margins are obscured. Consolidation has only been reported in acute hypersensitivity pneumonitis,[68,75] but is uncommon.[76,85] When present, consolidation is the first abnormality to resolve with treatment.[75]

Fibrosis

The irregular linear opacities, traction bronchiectasis, and honeycombing that may be seen in hypersensitivity pneumonitis all signify fibrosis.[77] These changes are most often found in the chronic stage of HP,[75] and occasionally in subacute HP. They would be distinctly unusual in acute disease.[68] Fibrotic changes may spare the apices and the costophrenic angles.[82] In the transverse plane, the fibrotic changes are randomly distributed but a subpleural predominance has been described in some patients.[82] Honeycombing has been found in up to 50% of chronic bird fancier's lung[76] but may be less common in chronic HP of other etiologies.[12] In farmer's lung, radiologic emphysema may be more common than fibrosis.[78,81] Unfortunately, the presence and location of fibrotic changes remain non-specific, and HRCT cannot reliably distinguish chronic HP from idiopathic pulmonary fibrosis.[86]

Emphysema

Radiographic evidence of emphysema in patients with chronic HP was first noted by Barbee et al in 1968.[3] This finding was largely ignored until the early 1990s when Remy-Jardin et al noted emphysematous changes on HRCT in 50% of chronic bird fancier's HP.[76] In addition,

Lalancette et al reported that emphysema occurred more commonly than fibrosis in chronic farmer's lung.[62] A more recent study by Cormier et al confirmed that emphysema is more prevalent than fibrosis in chronic farmer's lung, even after accounting for the effects of tobacco abuse.[81] Another study showed an increased prevalence of emphysema in farmer's lung patients compared to control farmers matched for age, sex, and smoking status.[78] In that study, 13 of the 20 farmer's lung patients with emphysema were never smokers.

These findings indicate that hypersensitivity pneumonitis should be considered in the differential diagnosis of radiologic emphysema. While mechanisms for the development of emphysema in HP remain unclear, the bronchiolar inflammation and obstruction seen on pathologic examination are probably related.[2]

Mosaic pattern

High-resolution CT scans with a mosaic pattern display a patchwork of regions of differing attenuation.[80] In HP, this pattern is due to either patchy areas of ground glass or air-trapping. Air-trapping is best seen as a failure of an area to increase in attenuation on an expiratory scan.[87] A mosaic pattern is common in hypersensitivity pneumonitis. Nineteen of 22 patients in a series by Hansell et al displayed this finding.[84] Likewise, 15 out of 20 patients in Small et al's series had this pattern.[87] Thus, a mosaic pattern and air-trapping provide supportive evidence for the diagnosis of HP, especially when they occur in association with previously described abnormalities.[77]

Air-trapping does not have a proven histologic correlate but is probably associated with bronchiolitis.[84,87] HRCT evidence of air-trapping does correlate with evidence of obstruction on pulmonary function testing.[84,88]

Specific inhalation challenge

The use of specific inhalation challenge in the diagnosis of HP is limited by the lack of standardized antigens and methods. Inhalation of an aerosolized antigen suspected to be causative is most helpful when acute symptoms and clinical abnormalities are part of the disease presentation and occur within hours after exposure.[89] In experienced laboratories, provocative testing may be useful in discriminating chronic HP induced by avian antigens from other interstitial lung diseases.[90] In some patients with acute symptoms, exposure to the suspect environment with postexposure monitoring of symptoms, temperature, leukocyte count, spirometry, diffusing capacity, and chest radiograph may be preferable to laboratory challenge. Interpretation of results is often difficult, and routine inhalation challenge is not recommended in most patients with suspected HP.[91]

Histopathology

The classic histopathology of hypersensitivity pneumonitis features the triad of cellular bronchiolitis, lympho-

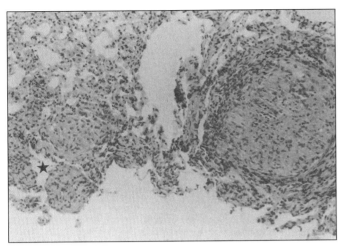

Figure 19.6.2: Photomicrograph (40 ×) of a hematoxylin and eosin-stained transbronchial lung biopsy from a patient with hypersensitivity pneumonitis shows interstitial pneumonitis containing ill-defined epithelioid macrophage aggregates involving a respiratory bronchiole at left (star in lumen) and a non-necrotizing interstitial granuloma at right.

Inhalation fevers	Humidifier fever
	Organic dust toxic syndrome
	Pontiac fever (non-pneumonic legionellosis)
Granulomatous disorders	Sarcoidosis
	Beryllium disease
	Drug-induced pneumonitis
	Granuloma-vasculitis syndromes
	Lymphatoid granulomatosis
	Eosinophilic granuloma
Immunologic diseases	Asthma
	Collagen-vascular diseases
	Allergic bronchopulmonary aspergillosis
	Eosinophilic pneumonias
Infections	Viral and mycoplasma pneumonias
	Psittacosis
	Fungal infections
	Mycobacterial infections
Fibrosing lung diseases	Idiopathic pulmonary fibrosis
	Bronchiolitis obliterans from other causes
	Inorganic dust pneumoconioses

Table 19.6.2 Differential diagnosis of hypersensitivity pneumonitis

plasmocytic interstitial infiltrate, and poorly formed non-necrotizing granulomas (Fig. 19.6.2).[92] Unfortunately, the complete triad is not always present and pathologic features may vary with disease stage. A fibrotic pattern very similar to usual interstitial pneumonitis (UIP) is frequently seen in chronic HP.[92] In addition, granulomas are only seen in 60–70% of acute cases and in less than 50% of chronic HP.[12,93] Giant cells, either alone or in clusters, airspace foam cells, and bronchiolitis obliterans with organizing pneumonia (BOOP) may also be seen.[92] Recently, Katzenstein et al added non-specific interstitial pneumonitis (NSIP) to the histologic spectrum of hypersensitivity pneumonitis.[94] In the original series describing NSIP, 18% of patients had exposures consistent with HP. Katzenstein et al concluded that a thorough search for exposures should be conducted upon diagnosis of NSIP.[94] The varied pathologic findings of HP have prompted multiple authors to conclude that histologic features are not pathognomonic, and additional clinical and radiologic data are needed to confirm the diagnosis.[1,5,91,92]

DIAGNOSTIC APPROACH

The diagnosis of HP remains challenging due to its varied presentation, wide spectrum of occupational and environmental exposure settings, and lack of a simple 'gold standard' and can include a large differential diagnosis (Table 19.6.2). The diagnosis should be considered in patients with both recurrent, more acute respiratory symptoms, as well as patients with insidious non-specific symptoms such as fatigue and weight loss. The differential diagnosis of HP includes a number of diseases. The following diagnostic studies are recommended on all patients with suspected HP: (1) *detailed* clinical history; (2) physical examination; (3) chest high-resolution computed tomography (unless the standard chest radiograph is clearly abnormal); (4) complete PFTs, including lung volumes, pre- and post-bron-

chodilator spirometry, and DLCO; and (5) fiberoptic bronchoscopy, usually with BAL and transbronchial biopsies.

The cornerstone of diagnosis and exposure prevention is a detailed history of symptoms plus occupational and environmental exposures. A clinical history suggesting a temporal relationship between symptoms and certain activities is often the first clue to the diagnosis of HP, although such a pattern may not occur in subacute or chronic forms of disease. The work history should include a chronology of current and previous occupations, with a description of specific work processes and exposures. Other important items in the work history include a list of specific chemicals, dusts, and other aerosol exposures, presence of persistent respiratory or constitutional symptoms in exposed coworkers, and whether respiratory protection was used. Review of Material Safety Data Sheets (MSDS) and any available industrial hygiene evaluations may supplement the work history.

The environmental history should explore exposure to pets and other domestic animals (especially birds); hobbies such as gardening and lawn care, which may involve sensitizing chemical exposures like pyrethrins; recreational activities, for example, use of hot tubs and indoor swimming pools from which microbial bioaerosols can be generated; use of humidifiers, cool mist vaporizers, and humidified air conditioners, which can be sources of microbial bioaerosols; moisture indicators such as leaking, flooding, or previous water damage to carpets and furnishings; and visible mold or mildew contamination in occupied spaces.

In patients whose detailed history is suggestive for HP but whose resting physiology is normal, exercise physiology can be helpful in detecting early abnormalities of gas exchange. Exercise testing can also help define impairment and guide treatment decisions, including the need for supplemental oxygen. Methacholine challenge does not distinguish asthma from HP and is generally not necessary. Serum precipitins are helpful when positive in supporting the diagnosis of bird breeder's lung, and in other circumstances in which the putative antigen has been identified.[95] However, negative precipitins should not be used to exclude the diagnosis, and positive precipitins can occur in exposed unaffected individuals.

DIAGNOSTIC CRITERIA

Although there are multiple published diagnostic criteria, none have been validated. Cormier proposes that all of the following features are required for diagnosis: appropriate exposure, dyspnea on exertion, inspiratory crackles, and lymphocytic alveolitis,[96] but that lymphocytic alveolitis is not required provided at least two of the following criteria are present: recurrent febrile episodes, infiltrates on chest radiograph, decreased DLCO, precipitating antibodies to causative antigens, granulomas on lung biopsy, or improvement away from the exposure.

A few points about these criteria deserve further emphasis. Unlike earlier criteria, precipitating antibodies are not essential for diagnosis due to limited sensitivity and specificity. Lymphocyte subset ratios are also not included as diagnostic criteria. Initial studies suggested a lymphocytic alveolitis with reduced CD4:CD8 ratio was diagnostic of hypersensitivity pneumonitis. Although lymphocytic alveolitis is common, more recent studies show that the CD4:CD8 ratio varies with phase of disease,[97] inciting antigen,[98] and time since last exposure,[99] limiting its utility as a diagnostic test.

Acute and subacute HP suspected from a careful history can usually be confirmed based on the radiographic features, physiology, and findings on bronchoscopy noted above. The diagnosis of chronic HP can be more challenging, and open lung biopsy may be indicated when the diagnosis remains uncertain.

NATURAL HISTORY AND PROGNOSIS

The clinical course of HP is variable but permanent sequelae may include persistent bronchial hyper-responsiveness, emphysema, or progressive interstitial fibrosis. An accelerated decline in lung function with continued antigen exposure has been demonstrated for most forms of HP, underscoring the importance of cessation of exposure. However, the clinical course of HP is variable even with antigen avoidance. Acute HP generally resolves without sequelae.[100] However, progressive impairment may occur with recurrent attacks or with a single severe attack.[3,101]

The subacute or chronic forms of HP present with insidious symptoms and more subtle clinical abnormalities, and are frequently recognized later in the disease course. The causative antigen cannot always be identified. As a result, these patients often have a poorer prognosis than those with acute disease. Symptomatic pigeon breeders monitored for 18 years showed a fourfold average rate of decline in pulmonary function in comparison with the expected rate.[102] Four children and five adults with chronic avian HP were monitored for up to 10 years after standard treatment

consisting of removal from exposure and corticosteroids. Four had persistent symptoms, three had persistent functional abnormalities, and one died after unsuccessful lung transplant.[103] In subacute and chronic HP, some patients may experience disease progression despite exposure avoidance while others do not, even with ongoing exposure.[99,104]

Long-term mortality rates for patients with chronic HP range from 1% to 10%.[105,106] Prognostic factors include age, duration of exposure after onset of symptoms, and time of exposure prior to diagnosis.[63,107] The specific antigen may also be important as some studies have shown prognosis is worse in avian HP than farmer's lung, with 5-year mortality rates approaching that of idiopathic pulmonary fibrosis (IPF).[108] Other potential prognostic factors include the ability to identify and thus avoid the relevant antigen and the presence of honeycombing.[108,109] BAL findings do not appear to predict prognosis.[110,111]

TREATMENT

The cornerstone of therapy for HP remains removal from exposure. Elimination of the antigen is the preferred approach and has the added benefit of preventing disease in other exposed individuals. For example, maple bark disease and bagassosis are now rare in the United States because changes in the handling of material resulted in diminished opportunity for microbial growth. Removal of damaged and colonized areas, disinfection, and elimination of conditions leading to seasonal mold contamination are effective in preventing recurrence of summer-type HP in Japan.[112] There are also numerous reports of patients with HP from other etiologies improving with removal from exposure alone.

In cases of home humidifier and hot tub-related HP, removal of the contaminated source is usually straightforward; however, on-site investigation of the work and home environments by an experienced industrial hygienist may be helpful in cases in which the exposure history is uncertain, particularly when disease is progressive. For fungal contaminants, both area and personal spore sampling and indirect immunofluorescence testing for spore-specific IgG have been used to assess indoor air quality and individual mold sensitization.[113] However, quantitative bioaerosol sampling for indoor microbial antigens is time consuming, expensive, and not readily available to most clinicians, and requires an experienced industrial hygienist and analytical laboratory. Even when properly performed, results are often difficult to interpret and the sensitivity is such that negative results should not be used to disprove disease or exposure.[114]

Unfortunately, antigen abatement may not always be feasible,[115] and removing the patient from the implicated environment may be necessary. In these cases, the social consequences and economic disruption to the affected individual may preclude strict abstinence from exposure. A long-term follow-up study of farmers found 70% had returned to farming by 15 years from diagnosis.[105] Respirators have been used when removal from exposure was impossible. Kusaka et al found that negative pressure respirators prevented recurrent episodes of acute HP in 20 of 21 farmers.[116] Nuutinen et al described the use of powered air-purifying respirators to protect farmers during indoor cattle feeding.[117] Although respirators may provide protection during inhalation challenge tests or in circumstances with limited exposure periods, verification of their efficacy in preventing new onset or recurrent HP awaits further investigation.[118,119] Moreover, respirators are difficult to wear for extended periods, require adequate fit testing and maintenance, and non-compliance with their use remains a significant problem.[120]

Oral corticosteroids are frequently used to supplement antigen avoidance in severe or progressive disease. In cases in which pulmonary function abnormalities are minor and spontaneous recovery is likely with removal from exposure, steroids are probably unnecessary. When used, doses typically begin at 40–60 mg/day of oral prednisone and continue at this level until significant symptomatic and objective functional improvement is seen. Pulmonary function should be monitored within the first 4 weeks after initiation of treatment.[65] If there is objective improvement, a gradual taper to minimum sustaining doses should follow; otherwise, steroids should be tapered and discontinued.

Corticosteroids may shorten the duration of acute illness but they have not been shown to affect long-term prognosis.[65,121] In patients suffering from acute HP, 2 months of corticosteroids therapy was compared to placebo; despite a more rapid resolution of functional and radiographic abnormalities in the steroid-treated group, long-term follow-up revealed no differences.[121]

Additional therapy includes supplemental oxygen in hypoxemic patients and other supportive measures. Inhaled steroids and β-agonists may be helpful in patients with airflow limitation.[122] In refractory cases, cytotoxic agents including cyclophosphamide and azathioprine have been used. As in IPF, regular monitoring for side effects and adverse reactions from these immunosuppressive agents is essential. The authors typically maintain cytotoxic therapy, if tolerated, for at least six months to assess functional improvement and efficacy in preventing disease progression. Prophylaxis for pneumocystis pneumonia, appropriate viral and pneumonia vaccination and prompt treatment of intercurrent infection are recommended.[1]

PREVENTION

Recognition of an index case of hypersensitivity pneumonitis may have considerable public health importance, since others exposed to the same environment are at risk for disease. Each case represents a sentinel health event, indicating the need for further investigation of the implicated environment where others may be at risk and where opportunities for prevention may be identified. Interventions may include control of moisture problems by preventing leaks and eliminating aerosol humidifiers or hot tubs. Dilution of contaminants can be affected by increasing the amount of outdoor air in a building, and high-efficiency filters can be added to the ventilation system.[114]

Altering work practices to reduce the prevalence of farmer's lung include efficient drying of hay and cereals before storage, use of mechanical feeding systems, and better ventilation of farm buildings.[123]

PEDIATRIC HYPERSENSITIVITY PNEUMONITIS

There have been several case reports and case series of HP occurring in children. The illness has been reported in all pediatric age groups from infant to adolescent.[124–127] Household birds are the most frequently reported antigenic exposure.[125,126,128,129] However, agricultural exposures, contaminated humidifiers, and mold damaged homes are also reported etiologies in children.[130–133] The clinical appearance of HP in children is similar to that of adults. Most reports describe repetitive episodes of acute disease that is often misdiagnosed as community acquired pneumonia, and clinical manifestations can be severe.[134] Children may also present with persistent unexplained respiratory symptoms.[129] Reported pulmonary function abnormalities include restriction, obstruction, and abnormal gas exchange.[125,131] Chest radiographs usually feature ground glass and reticulonodular infiltrates; HRCT findings are similar to those reported in adults.[135] Most reported childhood cases have improved with removal from exposure, but long-term functional abnormalities and lung fibrosis have been reported.[125,130] Fiberoptic bronchoscopy is usually not performed in children.

SUMMARY

Increasing recognition of the ubiquity of environmental antigen exposures and improved diagnostic tools, particularly HRCT and fiberoptic bronchoscopy, have led to increasing recognition of cases and outbreaks of HP in a wide variety of occupational and non-occupational settings. HP remains a diagnostic challenge because of the wide and varied spectrum of clinical findings and the lack of a simple 'gold standard' for diagnosis. The diagnosis depends on the combination of a strong clinical index of suspicion with a careful exposure history, and a constellation of radiographic, physiologic, and histopathologic findings. HP is both treatable and preventable but unrecognized disease may lead to permanent sequelae including asthma, emphysema, and interstitial fibrosis.[12] Confirmation of the diagnosis often generates broader public health implications regarding the potential risks from ongoing antigen exposure to others sharing the environment. Diagnosis of HP should prompt a search for additional cases in the shared environment as well as initiation of measures to eliminate further exposure.

References

1. Rose C. Hypersensitivity pneumonitis. In: Murray JF Nadel JA, eds. Textbook of respiratory medicine, 3rd edn. Philadelphia: WB Saunders; 2000;1867–84.
2. Lynch DA. Occupational and environmental lung disease. In: Lynch DA, Lee JS, eds. Imaging of diffuse lung disease. Hamilton: Decker Inc., 2000.

3. Barbee RA, Callies Q, Dickie HA, et al. The long-term prognosis in farmer's lung. Am Rev Respir Dis 1968; 97:223–31.

4. Buechner HPA, Thompson J, et al. Bagassosis: review with further historical data, studies of pulmonary function, and results of adrenal steroid therapy. Am J Med 1958; 25:234–7.

5. Grammer LC. Occupational allergic alveolitis. Ann Allergy Asthma Immunol 1999; 83:602–6.

6. Brown JE, Masood D, Couser JI, et al. Hypersensitivity pneumonitis from residential composting: residential composter's lung. Ann Allergy Asthma Immunol 1995; 74:45–7.

7. Ganier M, Lieberman P, Fink J, et al. Humidifier lung. An outbreak in office workers. Chest 1980; 77:183–7.

8. Khoor A, Leslie KO, Tazelaar HD, et al. Diffuse pulmonary disease caused by nontuberculous mycobacteria in immunocompetent people (hot tub lung). Am J Clin Pathol 2001; 115:755–62.

9. Case records of the Massachusetts General Hospital. Weekly clinicopathological exercises. Case 27-2000. A 61-year-old with rapidly progressive dyspnea. N Engl J Med 2000; 343:642–9.

10. Embil J, Warren P, Yakrus M, et al. Pulmonary illness associated with exposure to Mycobacterium-avium complex in hot tub water. Hypersensitivity pneumonitis or infection? Chest 1997; 111:813–6.

11. Shelton BG, Flanders WD, Morris GK. Mycobacterium sp. as a possible cause of hypersensitivity pneumonitis in machine workers. Emerg Infect Dis 1999; 5:270–3.

12. Yoshizawa Y, Ohtani Y, Hayakawa H, et al. Chronic hypersensitivity pneumonitis in Japan: a nationwide epidemiologic survey. J Allergy Clin Immunol 1999; 103:315–20.

13. Schlueter DP, Fink JN, Hensley GT. Wood-pulp workers' disease: a hypersensitivity pneumonitis caused by Alternaria. Ann Intern Med 1972; 77:907–14.

14. Dykewicz MS, Laufer P, Patterson R, et al. Woodman's disease: hypersensitivity pneumonitis from cutting live trees. J Allergy Clin Immunol 1988; 81:455–60.

15. Nakagawa-Yoshida K, Ando M, Etches RI, et al. Fatal cases of farmer's lung in a Canadian family. Probable new antigens, Penicillium brevicompactum and P. olivicolor. Chest 1997; 111:245–8.

16. Kaukonen K, Pelliniemi LJ, Savolainen J, et al. Identification of the reactive subunits of Aspergillus umbrosus involved in the antigenic response in farmer's lung. Clin Exp Allergy 1996; 26:689–96.

17. Edwards JH, Griffiths AJ, Mullins J. Protozoa as sources of antigen in 'humidifier fever'. Nature 1976; 264:438–9.

18. Haitjema T, van Velzen-Blad H, van den Bosch JM. Extrinsic allergic alveolitis caused by goose feathers in a duvet. Thorax 1992; 47:990–1.

19. Meyer FJ, Bauer PC, Costabel U. Feather wreath lung: chasing a dead bird. Eur Respir J 1996; 9:1323–4.

20. Mapp CE BB, Fabbri LM. Polyisocyanates and their prepolymers. In: Bernstein L, Chan-Yeung M, Malo JL, et al, eds. Asthma in the workplace, 2nd edn. New York: Marcel Dekker Inc., 1999;457–78.

21. Baur X. Hypersensitivity pneumonitis (extrinsic allergic alveolitis) induced by isocyanates. J Allergy Clin Immunol 1995; 95:1004–10.

22. Patterson R, Zeiss CR, Pruzansky JJ. Immunology and immunopathology of trimellitic anhydride pulmonary reactions. J Allergy Clin Immunol 1982; 70:19–23.

23. Grant IW, Blyth W, Wardrop VE, et al. Prevalence of farmer's lung in Scotland: a pilot survey. Br Med J 1972; 1:530–4.

24. Madsen D, Klock LE, Wenzel FJ, et al. The prevalence of farmer's lung in an agricultural population. Am Rev Respir Dis 1976; 113:171–4.

25. Marx JJ, Guernsey J, Emanuel DA, et al. Cohort studies of immunologic lung disease among Wisconsin dairy farmers. Am J Ind Med 1990; 18:263–8.

26. Terho I, Heinonen OP, Lammi S. Incidence of clinically confirmed farmer's lung disease in Finland. Am J Ind Med 1986; 10:330.

27. Christensen LT, Schmidt CD, Robbins L. Pigeon breeders' disease – a prevalence study and review. Clin Allergy 1975; 5:417–30.

28. Rose CS, Martyny JW, Newman LS, et al. 'Lifeguard lung': endemic granulomatous pneumonitis in an indoor swimming pool. Am J Public Health 1998; 88:1795–800.

29. Schuyler M, Cook C, Listrom M, et al. Blast cells transfer experimental hypersensitivity pneumonitis in guinea pigs. Am Rev Respir Dis 1988; 137:1449–55.

30. Richerson HB, Coon JD, Lubaroff D. Adoptive transfer of experimental hypersensitivity pneumonitis in the LEW rat. Am J Respir Crit Care Med 1995; 151:1205–10.

31. Bice DE, Salvaggio J, Hoffman E. Passive transfer of experimental hypersensitivity pneumonitis with lymphoid cells in the rabbit. J Allergy Clin Immunol 1976; 58:250–62.

32. Schuyler M, Gott K, Cherne A, et al. Th1 CD4+ cells adoptively transfer experimental hypersensitivity pneumonitis. Cell Immunol 1997; 177:169–75.

33. Schuyler M, Gott K, Edwards B. Experimental hypersensitivity pneumonitis: cellular requirements. Clin Exp Immunol 1996; 105:169–75.

34. Schuyler M, Gott K, Edwards B. Th1 cells that adoptively transfer experimental hypersensitivity pneumonitis are activated memory cells. Lung 1999; 177:377–89.

35. Mosmann TR, Cherwinski H, Bond MW, et al. Two types of murine helper T cell clone. I. Definition according to profiles of lymphokine activities and secreted proteins. J Immunol 1986; 136:2348–57.

36. Gudmundsson G, Hunninghake GW. Interferon-gamma is necessary for the expression of hypersensitivity pneumonitis. J Clin Invest 1997; 99:2386–90.

37. Gudmundsson G, Monick MM, Hunninghake GW. IL-12 modulates expression of hypersensitivity pneumonitis. J Immunol 1998; 161:991–9.

38. Yamasaki H, Ando M, Brazer W, et al. Polarized type 1 cytokine profile in bronchoalveolar lavage T cells of patients with hypersensitivity pneumonitis. J Immunol 1999; 163:3516–23.

39. Gudmundsson G, Monick MM, Hunninghake GW. Viral infection modulates expression of hypersensitivity pneumonitis. J Immunol 1999; 162:7397–401.

40. Dakhama A, Hegele RG, Laflamme G, et al. Common respiratory viruses in lower airways of patients with acute hypersensitivity pneumonitis. Am J Respir Crit Care Med 1999; 159:1316–22.

41. Fournier E, Tonnel AB, Gosset P, et al. Early neutrophil alveolitis after antigen inhalation in hypersensitivity pneumonitis. Chest 1985; 88:563–6.

42. Mornex JF, Cordier G, Pages J, et al. Activated lung lymphocytes in hypersensitivity pneumonitis. J Allergy Clin Immunol 1984; 74:719–27.

43. Denis M, Bedard M, Laviolette M, et al. A study of monokine release and natural killer activity in the bronchoalveolar lavage of subjects with farmer's lung. Am Rev Respir Dis 1993; 147:934–9.

44. Sutinen S, Reijula K, Huhti E, et al. Extrinsic allergic bronchiolo-alveolitis: serology and biopsy findings. Eur J Respir Dis 1983; 64:271–82.

45. Stankus RP, Cashner FM, Salvaggio JE. Bronchopulmonary macrophage activation in the pathogenesis of hypersensitivity pneumonitis. J Immunol 1978; 120:685–8.

46. Suga M, Yamasaki H, Nakagawa K, et al. Mechanisms accounting for granulomatous responses in hypersensitivity pneumonitis. Sarcoidosis Vasc Diffuse Lung Dis 1997; 14:131–8.

47. Teschler H, Thompson AB, Pohl WR, et al. Bronchoalveolar lavage procollagen-III-peptide in recent onset hypersensitivity pneumonitis: correlation with extracellular matrix components. Eur Respir J 1993; 6:709–14.

48. Warren CP. Extrinsic allergic alveolitis: a disease commoner in non-smokers. Thorax 1977; 32:567–9.

49. Baldwin CI, Todd A, Bourke S, et al. Pigeon fanciers' lung: effects of smoking on serum and salivary antibody responses to pigeon antigens. Clin Exp Immunol 1998; 113:166–72.

50. Ohtsuka Y, Munakata M, Tanimura K, et al. Smoking promotes insidious and chronic farmer's lung disease, and deteriorates the clinical outcome. Intern Med 1995; 34:966–71.

51. Flaherty DK, Braun SR, Marx JJ, et al. Serologically detectable HLA-A, B, and C loci antigens in farmer's lung disease. Am Rev Respir Dis 1980; 122:437–43.

52. Muers MF, Faux JA, Ting A, et al. HLA-A, C and HLA-DR antigens in extrinsic allergic alveolitis (budgerigar fancier's lung disease). Clin Allergy 1982; 12:47–53.

53. Camarena A, Juarez A, Mejia M, et al. Major histocompatibility complex and tumor necrosis factor-alpha polymorphisms in pigeon breeder's disease. Am J Respir Crit Care Med 2001; 163:1528–33.

54. McSharry C, Lynch PP, Banham SW, et al. Seasonal variation of antibody levels among pigeon fanciers. Clin Allergy 1983; 13:293–9.

55. Riley DJ, Saldana M. Pigeon breeder's lung. Subacute course and the importance of indirect exposure. Am Rev Respir Dis 1973; 107:456–60.

56. Roberts RC, Wenzel FJ, Emanuel DA. Precipitating antibodies in a midwest dairy farming population toward the antigens associated with farmer's lung disease. J Allergy Clin Immunol 1976; 57:518–24.

57. McSharry C, Banham SW, Lynch PP, et al. Antibody measurement in extrinsic allergic alveolitis. Eur J Respir Dis 1984; 65:259–65.

58. Cormier Y, Belanger J, LeBlanc P, et al. Bronchoalveolar lavage in farmers' lung disease: diagnostic and physiologic significance. Br J Ind Med 1986; 43:401–5.

59. Krasnick J, Meuwissen HJ, Nakao MA, et al. Hypersensitivity pneumonitis: problems in diagnosis. J Allergy Clin Immunol 1996; 97:1027–30.

60. Huls G, Lindemann H, Velcovsky HG. Angiotensin converting enzyme (ACE) in the follow-up control of children and adolescents with allergic alveolitis. Monatsschr Kinderheilkd 1989; 137:158–61.

61. Tanaka H, Sugawara H, Saikai T, et al. Mushroom worker's lung caused by spores of Hypsizigus marmoreus (Bunashimeji): elevated serum surfactant protein D levels. Chest 2000; 118:1506–9.

62. Lalancette M, Carrier G, Laviolette M, et al. Farmer's lung. Long-term outcome and lack of predictive value of bronchoalveolar lavage fibrosing factors. Am Rev Respir Dis 1993; 148:216–21.

63. Allen DH, Williams GV, Woolcock AJ. Bird breeder's hypersensitivity pneumonitis: progress studies of lung function after cessation of exposure to the provoking antigen. Am Rev Respir Dis 1976; 114:555–66.

64. Bourke SJ, Carter R, Anderson K, et al. Obstructive airways disease in non-smoking subjects with pigeon fanciers' lung. Clin Exp Allergy 1989; 19:629–32.

65. Monkare S. Influence of corticosteroid treatment on the course of farmer's lung. Eur J Respir Dis 1983; 64:283–93.

66. Freedman PM, Ault B. Bronchial hyperreactivity to methacholine in farmers' lung disease. J Allergy Clin Immunol 1981; 67:59–63.

67. Schwaiblmair M, Beinert T, Vogelmeier C, et al. Cardiopulmonary exercise testing following hay exposure challenge in farmer's lung. Eur Respir J 1997; 10:2360–5.

68. Silver SF, Muller NL, Miller RR, et al. Hypersensitivity pneumonitis: evaluation with CT. Radiology 1989; 173:441–5.

69. Matar LD, McAdams HP, Sporn TA. Hypersensitivity pneumonitis. Am J Roentgenol 2000; 174:1061–6.

70. Hargreave F, Hinson KF, Reid L, et al. The radiological appearances of allergic alveolitis due to bird sensitivity (Bird fancier's lung). Clin Radiol 1972; 23:1–10.

71. Hodgson MJ, Parkinson DK, Karpf M. Chest X-rays in hypersensitivity pneumonitis: a metaanalysis of secular trend. Am J Ind Med 1989; 16:45–53.

72. Lynch DA, Rose CS, Way D, et al. Hypersensitivity pneumonitis: sensitivity of high-resolution CT in a population-based study. Am J Roentgenol 1992; 159:469–72.

73. Fink JN, Schlueter DP, Sosman AJ, et al. Clinical survey of pigeon breeders. Chest 1972; 62:277–81.

74. Buschman DL, Gamsu G, Waldron JA Jr, et al. Chronic hypersensitivity pneumonitis: use of CT in diagnosis. Am J Roentgenol 1992; 159:957–60.

75. Akira M, Kita N, Higashihara T, et al. Summer-type hypersensitivity pneumonitis: comparison of high-resolution CT and plain radiographic findings. Am J Roentgenol 1992; 158:1223–8.

76. Remy-Jardin M, Remy J, Wallaert B, et al. Subacute and chronic bird breeder hypersensitivity pneumonitis: sequential evaluation with CT and correlation with lung function tests and bronchoalveolar lavage. Radiology 1993; 189:111–8.

77. Patel RA, Sellami D, Gotway MB, et al. Hypersensitivity pneumonitis: patterns on high-resolution CT. J Comput Assist Tomogr 2000; 24:965–70.

78. Erkinjuntti-Pekkanen R, Rytkonen H, Kokkarinen JI, et al. Long-term risk of emphysema in patients with farmer's lung and matched control farmers. Am J Respir Crit Care Med 1998; 158:662–5.

79. Niimi H, Kang EY, Kwong JS, et al. CT of chronic infiltrative lung disease: prevalence of mediastinal lymphadenopathy. J Comput Assist Tomogr 1996; 20:305–8.

80. Austin JH, Muller NL, Friedman PJ, et al. Glossary of terms for CT of the lungs: recommendations of the Nomenclature Committee of the Fleischner Society. Radiology 1996; 200:327–31.

81. Cormier Y, Brown M, Worthy S, et al. High-resolution computed tomographic characteristics in acute farmer's lung and in its follow-up. Eur Respir J 2000; 16:56–60.

82. Adler BD, Padley SP, Muller NL, et al. Chronic hypersensitivity pneumonitis: high-resolution CT and radiographic features in 16 patients. Radiology 1992; 185:91–5.

83. Leung AN, Miller RR, Muller NL. Parenchymal opacification in chronic infiltrative lung diseases: CT-pathologic correlation. Radiology 1993; 188:209–14.

84. Hansell DM, Wells AU, Padley SP, et al. Hypersensitivity pneumonitis: correlation of individual CT patterns with functional abnormalities. Radiology 1996; 199:123–8.

85. Tomiyama N, Muller NL, Johkoh T, et al. Acute parenchymal lung disease in immunocompetent patients: diagnostic accuracy of high-resolution CT. Am J Roentgenol 2000; 174:1745–50.

86. Lynch DA, Newell JD, Logan PM, et al. Can CT distinguish hypersensitivity pneumonitis from idiopathic pulmonary fibrosis? Am J Roentgenol 1995; 165:807–11.

87. Small JH, Flower CD, Traill ZC, et al. Air-trapping in extrinsic allergic alveolitis on computed tomography. Clin Radiol 1996; 51:684–8.

88. Lucidarme O, Coche E, Cluzel P, et al. Expiratory CT scans for chronic airway disease: correlation with pulmonary function test results. Am J Roentgenol 1998; 170:301–7.

89. Hendrick DJ, Marshall R, Faux JA, et al. Positive 'alveolar' responses to antigen inhalation provocation tests: their validity and recognition. Thorax 1980; 35:415–27.

90. Ramirez-Venegas A, Sansores RH, Perez-Padilla R, et al. Utility of a provocation test for diagnosis of chronic pigeon breeder's disease. Am J Respir Crit Care Med 1998; 158:862–9.

91. Richerson HB, Bernstein IL, Fink JN, et al. Guidelines for the clinical evaluation of hypersensitivity pneumonitis. Report of the Subcommittee on Hypersensitivity Pneumonitis. J Allergy Clin Immunol 1989; 84:839–44.

92. Colby TV, Coleman A. The histologic diagnosis of extrinsic allergic alveolitis and its differential diagnosis. Prog Surg Pathol 1989; 10:11–26.

93. Ando M, Arima K, Yoneda R, et al. Japanese summer-type hypersensitivity pneumonitis. Geographic distribution, home environment, and clinical characteristics of 621 cases. Am Rev Respir Dis 1991; 144:765–9.

94. Katzenstein AL, Fiorelli RF. Nonspecific interstitial pneumonia/fibrosis. Histologic features and clinical significance. Am J Surg Pathol 1994; 18:136–47.

95. Burrell R, Rylander R. A critical review of the role of precipitins in hypersensitivity pneumonitis. Eur J Respir Dis 1981; 62:332–43.

96. Cormier Y. Hypersensitivity pneumonitis. In: Rom W, ed. Environmental & occupational medicine, 3rd edn. Philadelphia: Lippincott-Raven, 1998;457–66.

97. Murayama J, Yoshizawa Y, Ohtsuka M, et al. Lung fibrosis in hypersensitivity pneumonitis. Association with CD4+ but not CD8+ cell dominant alveolitis and insidious onset. Chest 1993; 104:38–43.

98. Ando M, Konishi K, Yoneda R, et al. Difference in the phenotypes of bronchoalveolar lavage lymphocytes in patients with summer-type hypersensitivity pneumonitis, farmer's lung, ventilation pneumonitis, and bird fancier's lung: report of a nationwide epidemiologic study in Japan. J Allergy Clin Immunol 1991; 87:1002–9.

99. Yoshizawa Y, Miyake S, Sumi Y, et al. A follow-up study of pulmonary function tests, bronchoalveolar lavage cells, and humoral and cellular immunity in bird fancier's lung. J Allergy Clin Immunol 1995; 96:122–9.

100. Cormier Y, Belanger J. Long-term physiologic outcome after acute farmer's lung. Chest 1985; 87:796–800.

101. Chasse M, Blanchette G, Malo J, et al. Farmer's lung presenting as respiratory failure and homogeneous consolidation. Chest 1986; 90:783–4.

102. Schmidt CD, Jensen RL, Christensen LT, et al. Longitudinal pulmonary function changes in pigeon breeders. Chest 1988; 93:359–63.

103. Grammer LC, Roberts M, Lerner C, et al. Clinical and serologic follow-up of four children and five adults with bird-fancier's lung. J Allergy Clin Immunol 1990; 85:655–60.

104. Bourke SJ, Banham SW, Carter R, et al. Longitudinal course of extrinsic allergic alveolitis in pigeon breeders. Thorax 1989; 44:415–8.

105. Braun SR, doPico GA, Tsiatis A, et al. Farmer's lung disease: long-term clinical and physiologic outcome. Am Rev Respir Dis 1979; 119:185–91.

106. Kokkarinen J, Tukiainen H, Terho EO. Mortality due to farmer's lung in Finland. Chest 1994; 106:509–12.

107. de Gracia J, Morell F, Bofill JM, et al. Time of exposure as a prognostic factor in avian hypersensitivity pneumonitis. Respir Med 1989; 83:139–43.

108. Perez-Padilla R, Salas J, Chapela R, et al. Mortality in Mexican patients with chronic pigeon breeder's lung compared with those with usual interstitial pneumonia. Am Rev Respir Dis 1993; 148:49–53.

109. Coleman A, Colby TV. Histologic diagnosis of extrinsic allergic alveolitis. Am J Surg Pathol 1988; 12:514–8.

110. Cormier Y, Belanger J, Laviolette M. Prognostic significance of bronchoalveolar lymphocytosis in farmer's lung. Am Rev Respir Dis 1987; 135:692–5.

111. Cormier Y, Belanger J, Laviolette M. Persistent bronchoalveolar lymphocytosis in asymptomatic farmers. Am Rev Respir Dis 1986; 133:843–7.

112. Yoshida K, Ando M, Sakata T, et al. Prevention of summer-type hypersensitivity pneumonitis: effect of elimination of Trichosporon cutaneum from the patients' homes. Arch Environ Health 1989; 44:317–22.

113. Zwick H, Popp W, Braun O, et al. Personal spore sampling and indirect immunofluorescent test for exploration of hypersensitivity pneumonitis due to mould spores. Allergy 1991; 46:277–83.

114. American Conference of Governmental Industrial Hygienists. Developing an investigation strategy. In: Macher J, ed. Bioaerosols assessment and control. Cincinnati: American Conference of Governmental Industrial Hygienists, 1999.

115. Craig TJ, Hershey J, Engler RJ, et al. Bird antigen persistence in the home environment after removal of the bird. Ann Allergy 1992; 69:510–2.

116. Kusaka H, Ogasawara H, Munakata M, et al. Two-year follow up on the protective value of dust masks against farmer's lung disease. Intern Med 1993; 32:106–11.

117. Nuutinen J, Terho EO, Husman K, et al. Protective value of powered dust respirator helmet for farmers with farmer's lung. Eur J Respir Dis 1987; 152(Suppl):212–20.

118. Hendrick DJ, Marshall R, Faux JA, et al. Protective value of dust respirators in extrinsic allergic alveolitis: clinical assessment using inhalation provocation tests. Thorax 1981; 36:917–21.

119. Anderson K, Walker A, Boyd G. The long-term effect of a positive pressure respirator on the specific antibody response in pigeon breeders. Clin Exp Allergy 1989; 19:45–9.

120. Salazar MK, Connon C, Takaro TK, et al. An evaluation of factors affecting hazardous waste workers' use of respiratory protective equipment. Am Ind Hyg Assoc J 2001; 62:236–45.

121. Kokkarinen JI, Tukiainen HO, Terho EO. Effect of corticosteroid treatment on the recovery of pulmonary function in farmer's lung. Am Rev Respir Dis 1992; 145:3–5.

122. Carlsen KH, Leegaard J, Lund OD, et al. Allergic alveolitis in a 12-year-old boy: treatment with budesonide nebulizing solution. Pediatr Pulmonol 1992; 12:257–9.

123. Zejda JE, McDuffie HH, Dosman JA. Epidemiology of health and safety risks in agriculture and related industries. Practical applications for rural physicians. West J Med 1993; 158:56–63.

124. Eisenberg JD, Montanero A, Lee RG. Hypersensitivity pneumonitis in an infant. Pediatr Pulmonol 1992; 12:186–90.

125. Chiron C, Gaultier C, Boule M, et al. Lung function in children with hypersensitivity pneumonitis. Eur J Respir Dis 1984; 65:79–91.

126. Wolf SJ, Stillerman A, Weinberger M, et al. Chronic interstitial pneumonitis in a 3-year-old child with hypersensitivity to dove antigens. Pediatrics 1987; 79:1027–9.

127. El-Hefny A, Ekladious EM, El-Sharkawy S, et al. Extrinsic allergic bronchiolo-alveolitis in children. Clin Allergy 1980; 10:651–8.

128. Balasubramaniam SK, O'Connell EJ, Yunginger JW, et al. Hypersensitivity pneumonitis due to dove antigens in an adolescent. Clin Pediatr (Phila) 1987; 26:174–6.

129. Yee WF, Castile RG, Cooper A, et al. Diagnosing bird fancier's disease in children. Pediatrics 1990; 85:848–52.

130. O'Connell EJ, Zora JA, Gillespie DN, et al. Childhood hypersensitivity pneumonitis (farmer's lung): four cases in siblings with long-term follow-up. J Pediatr 1989; 114:995–7.

131. Miller MM, Patterson R, Fink JN, et al. Chronic hypersensitivity lung disease with recurrent episodes of hypersensitivity pneumonitis due to a contaminated central humidifer. Clin Allergy 1976; 6:451–62.

132. Johnson CL, Bernstein IL, Gallagher JS, et al. Familial hypersensitivity pneumonitis induced by Bacillus subtilis. Am Rev Respir Dis 1980; 122:339–48.

133. Hogan MB, Patterson R, Pore RS, et al. Basement shower hypersensitivity pneumonitis secondary to Epicoccum nigrum. Chest 1996; 110:854–6.

134. Krasnick J, Patterson R, Stillwell PC, et al. Potentially fatal hypersensitivity pneumonitis in a child. Clin Pediatr (Phila) 1995; 34:388–91.

135. Lynch DA, Hay T, Newell JD Jr, et al. Pediatric diffuse lung disease: diagnosis and classification using high-resolution CT. Am J Roentgenol 1999; 173:713–8.

19.7 Chronic Beryllium Disease and Cobalt-Related Interstitial Lung Disease (Hard-Metal Disease and Diamond Polisher's Lung Disease)

John R Balmes

Both beryllium and cobalt are relatively light metals that appear to have the potential to cause pulmonary toxicity through host immune responses because only a small percentage of exposed workers develop disease and relatively low level exposures can cause disease. Genetic susceptibility to interstitial lung disease from environmental exposure to these metals may involve either immunologically mediated sensitization (beryllium and possibly cobalt) or response to oxidant injury (possibly cobalt). Although much more is understood of host responses to inhaled beryllium than to inhaled cobalt, the interstitial lung diseases that result from chronic occupational exposure to these metals are important models of idiopathic sarcoidosis and giant cell interstitial pneumonitis, respectively.

BERYLLIUM DISEASE

Two different types of pulmonary disease can result from the inhalation of beryllium fumes or dust, or both. Short-term, high-intensity exposure ($\geq 25\ \mu g/m^3$) can cause acute lung injury that is clinically and pathologically indistinguishable from toxic pneumonitis caused by the inhalation of other chemically irritating materials (see Chapter 19.5).[1] Exposure to lower concentrations of beryllium in workplace air over months to years can lead to the development of a chronic granulomatous disease that is similar to sarcoidosis.

Acute toxic pneumonitis due to beryllium is now rare, at least in developed countries, because the primary production industry is aware of the metal's toxic potential and has taken steps to prevent massive exposures. However, many thousands of workers in the United States and elsewhere remain at risk for the development of chronic beryllium disease (CBD) because of relatively low-intensity exposures in industries involved in the fabrication and machining of beryllium-containing alloys. Because acute beryllium pneumonitis can be considered with other forms of toxic pneumonitis, this section is restricted to a discussion of CBD.

Epidemiology

It has been estimated that up to 800,000 persons in the United States have current or past occupational exposure to beryllium.[2] The reported prevalence of CBD in exposed workers ranges from 2% to 16%. For perspective, the reported prevalence of sarcoidosis is much lower in the general population.[3] That beryllium exposure can lead to granulomatous lung disease was established through investigation of an epidemic of sarcoidosis in the fluorescent lamp industry in Massachusetts during the 1940s.[4] Removal of beryllium from fluorescent lamp manufacture eventually ensued. Reports of cases of CBD among non-occupationally exposed residents of a neighborhood around a beryllium plant soon followed. The setting of an occupational exposure standard of 2 $\mu g/m^3$ by the US Atomic Energy Commission in 1952 led to a reduction of cases due to beryllium production, but continued use of the metal in the aerospace, electronics, nuclear energy/weapons industries, metal recycling, and other high-tech industries has continued to generate new cases of CBD in the subsequent decades.[5]

Several conclusions can be drawn from the epidemiological database on CBD. It is clear that host susceptibility is an important factor because most exposed workers never develop clinically manifest lung disease. The form of beryllium to which workers are exposed also is important because exposure to beryllium oxide or fine fumes from heated metal is associated with higher rates of disease than exposure during cold processing.[6] In addition to host susceptibility and the form of occupational exposure, there appears to be some relationship between dose of beryllium exposure and incidence of lung disease. Machinists of beryllium-containing materials in both the ceramics and nuclear weapons industries appear to have especially high rates of CBD.[7,8] Recent data suggest that genetic and exposure-related factors contribute independently to risk of CBD.[9]

Pathogenesis

The pathological hallmark of CBD is the formation of noncaseating granulomas, which are identical to those seen in sarcoidosis. These granulomas are typically confined to the lungs but also may be found in other organs such as the skin, liver, spleen, lymph nodes, heart, kidneys, and salivary glands. In addition to granulomas in the lungs, there usually is a coexistent diffuse mononuclear cell alveolitis.

The salient feature of CBD is its association with delayed hypersensitivity to beryllium salts. This delayed hypersensitivity can be demonstrated by the in-vitro response of cultured T lymphocytes from either bronchoalveolar lavage (BAL) fluid or peripheral blood and by skin patch testing. The concept that CBD represents a disorder of cell-mediated immunity is not a new one, but it is only in recent years that it has been fully appreciated. In addition to the presence of delayed hypersensitivity to beryllium, support for this concept comes from the following evidence:

1. a usual history of exposure to beryllium for months to years before the disease develops,
2. data from multiple animal models indicating that beryllium exposure can lead to a beryllium-specific cell-mediated immune response,[10]
3. proliferation and accumulation of beryllium-specific CD4$^+$ (helper) T lymphocytes in the lungs of patients with the disease,[11]

4. dependence of beryllium-induced proliferation of lung helper T cells on the presence of major histocompatibility complex (MHC) class II antigens,[12]

5. susceptibility to CBD is associated with particular human leukocyte antigen (HLA)-DP alleles (especially substitution of a glutamic acid in position 69 of the beta chain),[13] and

6. the finding of a limited subset of T-cell receptors in the lungs of patients with the disease.[14]

On the basis of this evidence, it is clear that CBD represents a cell-mediated hypersensitivity reaction to beryllium.

A plausible pathogenic sequence for chronic beryllium disease starts with phagocytosis of beryllium particles by alveolar macrophages, with beryllium acting as a hapten bound to some carrier protein (possibly even HLA-DP itself), followed by presentation of this new beryllium-induced antigen to T lymphocytes, which, in turn, leads to local clonal proliferation of sensitized CD4+ T cells. In response to subsequent inhalation of beryllium and further recognition of antigen, these helper T cells with memory for beryllium become activated and release various cytokines and chemokines consistent with a T-helper 1-type cytokine response (IFN-γ, TNF-α and IL-2). These mediators drive macrophage and other immune effector cell recruitment, giant cell and epithelioid cell formation, and ultimately, the creation of granulomas and surrounding fibrosis. Because the older term 'berylliosis' suggests a similarity to the mineral dust-induced pneumoconioses that are not characterized by an antigen-specific, cell-mediated immune response, the use of CBD is preferred.

Diagnosis

Patients with CBD typically present many years after initial exposure with respiratory symptoms of dyspnea and non-productive cough. Systemic complaints of weight loss, fatigue, and arthralgias also are frequent. The most common physical finding is inspiratory crackles at the bases, although skin lesions, hepatosplenomegaly, lymphadenopathy, and clubbing occasionally can be found.

The typical chest radiographic findings of chronic beryllium disease are diffuse interstitial infiltrates and mild bilateral hilar adenopathy, but can vary from normal to diffuse fibrotic changes. Hilar adenopathy is seen less impressively and frequently than in sarcoidosis (approximately 40% of cases) and rarely occurs in the absence of parenchymal changes (Fig. 19.7.1). The chest radiograph is an insensitive test for CBD. High-resolution computed tomography (HRCT) is more sensitive.[15]

Pulmonary function testing may demonstrate a restrictive pattern, an obstructive pattern, or a mixed restrictive-obstructive pattern. Occasionally, there may be an isolated impairment in diffusing capacity, especially in cases detected early. Mild hypoxemia is common. Pulmonary exercise testing is the most sensitive indicator of physiologic impairment in CBD, and an increased alveolar–arterial oxygen difference with exercise appears to have the greatest predictive value for the presence of the disease.[10]

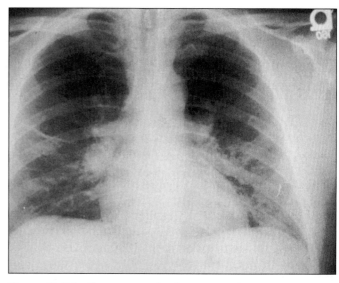

Figure 19.7.1: Chest x-ray study of a 40-year-old metal refiner exposed to beryllium fumes for 6 years.

The primary diagnostic challenge is to distinguish CBD from sarcoidosis, because virtually every clinical manifestation of sarcoidosis, with the exception of uveitis and erythema nodosum, has been reported with CBD.[16] A history of exposure is the most obvious clue, although patients may not be aware of exposure due to the fact that beryllium often is present in low percentage in alloys with copper or aluminum. There also may be a long latent period (from a few months to over 30 years) between beryllium exposure and clinical manifestations of disease, which can add to the difficulty of recognition of past exposure.

The histopathology of CBD is essentially identical to that of sarcoidosis so that transbronchial lung biopsy specimens showing non-caseating granulomas support either diagnosis (Fig. 19.7.2). Similarly, increases in the percentage of T lymphocytes and the ratio of helper to suppressor T cells on differential cell counting of BAL fluid are characteristic of both diseases. The results of other tests which may be used to help confirm a diagnosis of sarcoidosis, such as serum angiotensin-converting enzyme level and gallium scanning also do not distinguish chronic beryllium disease from its idiopathic counterpart.

Diagnostic criteria were developed for the US Beryllium Case Registry in 1952 to establish that a given patient had CBD.[16] These criteria consist of the following: (1) evidence of significant beryllium exposure; (2) presence of beryllium in lung tissue, lymph nodes, or urine; (3) a clinical picture consistent with beryllium disease; (4) radiologic evidence of a pulmonary interstitial inflammatory process; (5) pulmonary function abnormalities (restrictive or obstructive ventilatory defects, or impaired diffusion); and (6) histopathologic evidence of non-caseating granulomas in lung or lymph node tissue. These criteria have been replaced by a diagnostic approach informed by a greater understanding of the beryllium-specific cell-mediated immune response.

The current diagnostic approach to CBD involves demonstration of a beryllium-specific immune response

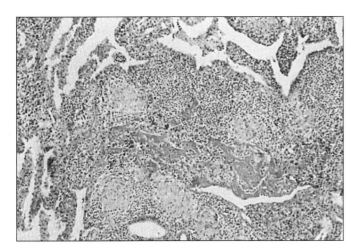

Figure 19.7.2: Open lung biopsy from patient in Figure 19.7.1, showing intense lymphocytic alveolitis and non-caseating granulomas.(H & E stain, low power.)

and histopathologic evidence consistent with CBD (non-caseating granulomas or mononuclear cell alveolitis).[17] The oldest test for beryllium hypersensitivity, the skin patch test, cannot be recommended because the test itself can induce beryllium sensitization in previously unsensitized individuals. Several groups of investigators have shown that the in-vitro proliferation of peripheral blood or BAL lymphocytes in response to beryllium salts is a specific test for beryllium hypersensitivity.[18,19] The test is called the beryllium lymphocyte proliferation test (BeLPT) and is available in a limited number of medical centers. The basic principle underlying the test is that T lymphocytes that have memory for beryllium antigen will proliferate when exposed to beryllium salts in cell culture. This beryllium-specific cellular immune response is quantitated based on cell uptake of radio-labeled DNA precursors.

The BeLPT using peripheral blood lymphocytes is both sensitive for beryllium sensitization and reasonably specific for CBD. The BeLPT using mononuclear cells obtained by bronchoalveolar lavage may be more sensitive. Virtually all patients with CBD have a positive BeLPT test using peripheral blood or bronchoalveolar lavage sample, and patients with other granulomatous diseases do not. Beryllium-exposed persons can have a positive BeLPT but no evidence of pulmonary disease on lung biopsy and are said to be 'beryllium sensitized'. Longitudinal follow-up of exposed populations has shown that such persons remain at risk for progression to CBD in the future.[20]

Fiberoptic bronchoscopy with multiple transbronchial biopsies is usually the best way to obtain adequate lung tissue to look for non-caseating granulomas and mononuclear cell infiltrates. The diagnosis of CBD can be confirmed in approximately 90% of patients with CBD by transbronchial biopsy, if a sufficient number of samples are taken,[10] similar to the yield in sarcoidosis. In patients for whom bronchoscopy is considered overly risky, the diagnosis of CBD can be made by chest imaging findings consistent with sarcoidosis/CBD in the setting of a positive BeLPT and a history of beryllium exposure.

Prognosis

The natural history of beryllium sensitization and chronic beryllium disease is under active investigation. In the past, when workers tended to be exposed to beryllium under poorly controlled conditions, it appeared that most persons who developed the disease progressed to pulmonary fibrosis. Spontaneous remission was believed to occur much less frequently than in idiopathic sarcoidosis, and the response to corticosteroids was characteristically poor. The mortality rate was noted to be as high as 35%.[21]

More recently, with generally lower levels of workplace exposure and the ability to detect beryllium-sensitized workers who have not developed clinical disease, evidence has emerged that challenges the traditional view of the natural history of CBD. First, some workers with the disease have improved after removal from further exposure.[22] Second, the clinical spectrum of CBD may be wider than previously recognized because in a report of a case series, in which the diagnosis was based on the results of BAL lymphocyte transformation testing and transbronchial biopsy, patients with disease were identified who were remarkably free of clinical manifestations.[23] Third, in most of the animal models of beryllium hypersensitivity reported to date, the inflammatory response resolves after cessation of exposure. These lines of evidence have prompted some investigators to call for the elimination of the usual modifier 'chronic' from the name given to the disease, as the disease may not become chronic in all workers, especially those detected early and with less beryllium exposure.

Although beryllium sensitization and CBD involve genetically mediated immune responses, there are exposure-related risks that suggest that improved industrial hygiene may decrease the likelihood of disease. The current OSHA standard of 2 µg/m³ (8-hour TWA) does not prevent CBD.[24] Continued vigilance to reduce beryllium contamination of workplace air to the lowest possible level, combined with careful medical surveillance using the BeLPT for early detection of sensitization, is required to prevent CBD.

Management

The cornerstone of treatment of CBD is prompt removal of the affected person from further exposure. As noted earlier, this intervention alone may lead to remission. In all other aspects, treatment should be modeled after that used for idiopathic sarcoidosis. Systemic steroid therapy clearly has a role in symptomatic patients with documented pulmonary physiologic abnormalities and in those rare patients with extrapulmonary disease involving vital organs. If steroid therapy is initiated, objective parameters of responses, such as chest radiographs, HRCT scans, and pulmonary function test results, should be serially monitored in order to adjust appropriately the dose and duration of treatment. Because beryllium is considered a probable lung carcinogen (see Chapters 30.2 and 39.3) and because of the potential for superimposed chronic obstructive pulmonary disease, cessation of smoking should be strongly encouraged.

Surveillance

As noted above, the blood BeLPT has high sensitivity and specificity for beryllium sensitization. Screening of beryllium-exposed workers with the blood BeLPT is recommended (see also Chapter 39.3). The test is a bioassay with some inherent variability, and a positive test is usually repeated to confirm sensitization. Because of the relatively low sensitivity of chest radiographic and pulmonary physiologic abnormalities for CBD, it is currently recomended that all sensitized individuals who have no contraindication undergo bronchoscopy for BAL and transbronchial biopsy.[10]

The results of population-based studies of beryllium-exposed workers that have employed blood BeLPT in conjunction with fiberoptic bronchoscopic diagnostic techniques suggest that such testing may prevent impairment due to CBD by identifying workers with subclinical disease. However, there is some evidence that progression to CBD may eventually occur in most sensitized workers. It has been recommended that beryllium-sensitized workers be re-evaluated (and considered for repeat bronchoscopy) every 1–3 years.[10] However, further longitudinal study of the natural history of beryllium sensitization without evidence of disease is necessary before this approach can be definitively supported. The genes which may modify risk of beryllium sensitization and CBD are under investigation. However, there currently is no clinical role for genetic testing for markers of CBD susceptibility.

COBALT-RELATED INTERSTITIAL LUNG DISEASE (HARD-METAL DISEASE AND DIAMOND POLISHERS' LUNG DISEASE)

One of the most intriguing causes of occupational lung disease is hard metal, a cemented alloy of tungsten carbide with cobalt (although other metals such as titanium, tantalum, chromium, molybdenum, or nickel may be added). Workers exposed to cemented tungsten carbide dust are at risk for the development of an interstitial lung disease, so-called hard metal disease. The use of this term tends to obscure the probable etiologic role of cobalt in the disease process. Workers in the diamond industry who were exposed to cobalt-containing dust from polishing disks have also developed interstitial lung disease identical to hard-metal disease, thereby confirming the likely role of cobalt.

A more prevalent occupational respiratory disorder than interstitial lung disease among hard metal workers is occupational asthma. Cobalt, which appears to induce specific sensitization of the airways, also is the etiologic agent of occupational asthma associated with exposure to hard metal dust. Because occupational asthma due to cobalt is similar to other types of occupational asthma (see Chapter 19.2), this section focuses on interstitial lung disease due to cobalt dust.

Epidemiology

Production of hard metal occurs worldwide. Exposure to hard metal is not confined to primary production workers; grinding of finished hard metal in the tool manufacturing industry is an important source of exposure. Thousands of workers in the United States have current or past exposure to tungsten carbide.[25] Despite the relatively large number of exposed workers, interstitial lung disease due to hard metal dust remains relatively rare. Only four (0.6%) of 700 employees at a Japanese production plant were found to have radiographic evidence of interstitial lung disease during a survey conducted from 1981 to 1990.[26] The prevalence of radiographic abnormalities suggestive of interstitial lung disease was somewhat higher (2.6%) in a cross-sectional study of 1039 hard metal production workers from 22 plants in the United States.[27] In fact, in one United States plant with extremely high cobalt dust concentrations, nine (6%) of 150 employees with heavy exposure had interstitial infiltrates.[28]

Workers are also exposed to cobalt dust alone, such as in the diamond polishing industry in Belgium which involves exposure to cobalt in the absence of tungsten carbide. Cobalt-induced lung disease has been reported in less than 1% of a workforce of approximately 5000 diamond polishers in Belgium.[29] A cross-sectional survey of 195 polishers working in 10 plants, however, did show a dose-response relationship for level of cobalt exposure and decrements in lung function.[30] Interstitial lung disease also has been recognized among dental technicians exposed to cobalt-chromium-molybendum alloys.[31]

Pathogenesis

The most characteristic histologic features of cobalt-induced interstitial lung disease are those of giant cell interstitial pneumonitis, with interstitial mononuclear cell infiltration and the accumulation of large, vacuolated mononuclear cells, as well as multinucleated giant cells in the alveoli.[32] In fact, a retrospective review of Liebow's original collection of 31 giant cell interstitial pneumonitis cases revealed that 27 had worked in the hard-metal industry.[33] Therefore, the finding of giant cell interstitial pneumonitis on lung biopsy strongly suggests exposure to hard metal or other cobalt-containing compounds. Electron microscopy has revealed that the giant cells can be either macrophages or type II alveolar epithelial cells. BAL fluid from patients with hard-metal disease may show a relative increase of other cells (lymphocytes, neutrophils, or eosinophils), but it is the presence of multinucleated giant cells that is the characteristic finding.

The relative proportions of desquamative alveolitis and interstitial fibrosis can vary from case to case, and if lung tissue is obtained late in the course of this disease or at autopsy, only the non-specific changes of end-stage fibrosis may be found.[32,34] In some cases of hard-metal disease, features of bronchiolitis obliterans also are observed. Most reported analyses of biopsied or autopsied lung tissue from hard-metal workers have demonstrated tungsten-containing particles but not cobalt accumulation. This lack of retained cobalt has been attributed to its solubility in body fluids and presumed rapid clearance from the lungs.

Animal toxicological studies conducted during the 1940s demonstrated that the intratracheal administration of either metallic tungsten or tungsten carbide dust produced little histologic change.[35] Similar studies demonstrated that the administration of a 10:1 mixture of tungsten carbide and cobalt induced acute pneumonitis and bronchiolitis.[35] Cobalt alone, whether administered by intratracheal injection or by inhalation, causes, in high concentrations, acute pulmonary edema or, in low concentrations, a granulomatous pneumonitis with progression to fibrosis.[36] More recent studies in rats have confirmed that the pulmonary toxicity of intratracheally administered cobalt is enhanced in the presence of metallic carbides such as tungsten carbide.[37]

The results of in-vitro studies have shown that cobalt and metallic carbides can interact to produce reactive oxygen species capable of causing oxidant injury.[38] The enhanced pulmonary toxicity of tungsten carbide-cobalt mixtures may be due to the ability of tungsten carbide to act as a conductor of electrons from cobalt to oxygen. It has even been suggested that genetically determined differences in antioxidant defense mechanisms may underlie the variable host susceptibility.[39]

To date none of the animal models have been shown to develop giant cell interstitial pneumonitis, the pathological hallmark of hard metal disease. Because cobalt is well documented to cause contact dermatitis via a type IV delayed hypersensitivity mechanism, a cell-mediated immune response has been suspected. Positive cobalt patch tests have been reported in hard-metal workers, and blast transformation of peripheral blood lymphocytes from sensitized individuals has been demonstrated with in-vitro culture in the presence of cobalt salts.[40] Moreover, susceptibility to develop cobalt-related interstitial lung disease among a group of exposed workers was associated with the same genetic polymorphism in the HLA-DP B1 alleles (Glu 69) associated with risk of CBD.[41]

Giant cell interstitial pneumonitis, however, is histologically distinct from granulomatous lung diseases involving cell-mediated immune responses such as hypersensitivity pneumonitis and CBD. Nonetheless, hard-metal disease must involve more than an acute chemical pneumonitis or a chronic dust accumulation mechanism because relatively low-level exposures can cause the disease and only a small number of exposed workers ever develop it. The possibility of an autoimmune process is suggested by the report of the recurrence of giant cell interstitial pneumonitis after lung transplantation in a patient with hard-metal disease.[42]

Any lingering debate over the primary etiologic role of cobalt in the interstitial lung disease seen among hard-metal workers would seem to be put to rest by reports from the Belgian diamond polishing industry. Both interstitial lung disease and occupational asthma have been described in workers using high-speed grinding tools with a polishing surface of microdiamonds cemented in very fine cobalt. No tungsten carbide is present in the dust generated by the diamond polishing process. The histologic findings on lung biopsy of diamond polishers with interstitial lung disease are identical to those of hard metal disease, including the virtually pathognomonic multinucleated giant cells.

Diagnosis

Workers who develop respiratory illness associated with occupational exposure to hard metal or other cobalt-containing dust present in several different ways.[10,25] A typical occupational asthma syndrome, characterized by decrements in expiratory flow rates during or after the work shift, is the most frequent occupational pulmonary disorder seen among hard metal workers. Positive specific inhalation challenges to either aerosolized cobalt powder or tungsten carbide powder containing cobalt have been reported. Interstitial lung disease, or classic hard-metal disease, may be associated with either rapidly progressive dyspnea or a slow, insidious course. Non-productive cough is common.

Constitutional symptoms such as fever and anorexia have been described and when these occur in association with interstitial infiltrates on chest radiographs, the diagnosis of an atypical pneumonia is suggested. However, when such acute or subacute episodes of pneumonitis recur in a worker exposed to grinding dust, the presence of hard-metal disease should be suspected. Some cobalt-exposed workers present with features of both asthma and interstitial lung disease.

On physical examination, crackles may be heard during acute episodes of interstitial pneumonitis or during late-stage fibrosis. Chest radiographs may be normal early in the course of the disease but typically show a diffuse reticulonodular pattern (Fig. 19.7.3). Pulmonary function tests usually show a restrictive ventilatory impairment with reduced diffusing capacity and increased elastic recoil. These abnormalities may be present even if the chest radiograph appears normal. If cobalt-induced asthma also is present, a mixed obstructive-restrictive picture may be noted. If the disease is allowed to progress, severe hypoxemia may develop, which, in turn, can lead to pulmonary hypertension and cor pulmonale.

As with other relatively rare occupational disorders, the key to the diagnosis is a high index of suspicion. Because the clinical features of cobalt-related interstitial lung disease are not particularly distinctive, the diagnosis usually is based on the history of exposure plus supportive laboratory data (Figs 19.7.3 and 19.7.4). BAL and lung biopsy are helpful if the characteristic multinucleated giant cells are revealed. However, if these procedures are

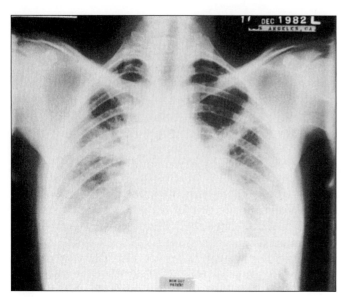

Figure 19.7.3: Chest x-ray of a 33-year-old grinder exposed to tungsten carbide dust for about 2 years.

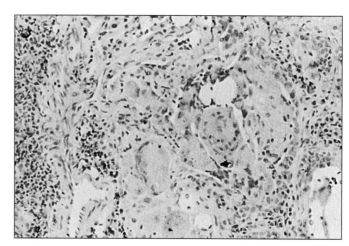

Figure 19.7.4: The transbronchial biopsy specimen of the patient in Figure 19.7.3, showing characteristic features of giant cell interstitial pneumonitis. Intense mononuclear cell infiltrate and fibrosis surround the numerous giant multinucleated cells. (H & E stain, high power.)

performed at a late stage in the disease process, non-specific findings are more likely to be demonstrated.

Although transbronchial biopsy specimens obtained via fiberoptic bronchoscopy may be adequate to show giant cell interstitial pneumonitis (Fig. 19.7.4), open lung biopsy has a greater yield.[10] Scanning electron microscopy with energy dispersive x-ray analysis typically demonstrates the presence of tungsten if the exposure has been to hard-metal dust, but cobalt usually is not found.

Prognosis

Once the diagnosis of hard-metal disease is made, the patient should be removed from further exposure. The natural history may vary from complete recovery to continued progression. Disabling pulmonary impairment can result from hard metal disease. Severe relapses on return to work with renewed exposure to cobalt-containing dust have been described in patients who initially recovered with removal from exposure. It seems likely that early diagnosis and removal from exposure leads to an improved prognosis, although there are limited data available to support such a statement.

Management

The primary treatment of cobalt-related interstitial lung disease is removal of the affected person from further exposure. Although some workers improve with cessation of cobalt exposure, others continue to worsen. The risk factors for continued progression are unclear. Corticosteroid therapy has been used successfully to treat persistent or severe disease in addition to removal from exposure, but there have been no controlled clinical trials of the efficacy of this treatment. There are also anecdotal reports of therapeutic success with cytotoxic agents such as cyclophosphamide in patients who do not respond to corticosteroids.[25]

Surveillance

Lower dust levels in modern hard-metal production facilities may have reduced the risk of classic hard-metal disease compared with past conditions in the industry,[43] but surveys in various settings have documented cases of both interstitial lung disease and occupational asthma when measured cobalt dust concentrations were below the current US OSHA threshold limit value time-weighted average of 50 $\mu g/m^3$.[27,28,30,44,45] These cross-sectional surveys have also shown that although cases of hard-metal disease with severe impairment are rare, increased interstitial markings on chest radiographs and lung function abnormalities occur in exposed workers who are asymptomatic. Medical surveillance using chest radiographs, review of respiratory symptoms and pulmonary function testing is recommended and may prove useful in preventing cases of severe interstitial fibrosis by leading to the removal of workers with early-stage disease or excessive cobalt exposure.

References

1. Kriebel D, Brain JD, Sprince NL, Kazemi H. The pulmonary toxicity of beryllium. Am Rev Respir Dis 1988; 137:464–74.
2. Jameson CW. Introduction to the conference on beryllium-related diseases. Environ Health Perspect 1996; 104:935–6.
3. American Thoracic Society. Statement on sarcoidosis. Am J Respir Crit Care Med 1999; 160:736–55.
4. Hardy HL, Tabershaw IR. Delayed chemical pneumonitis in workers exposed to beryllium compounds. J Ind Hyg Toxicol 1946; 28:197–211.
5. Eisenbud M. Origins of the standard for control of beryllium disease (1947–1949). Environ Res 1982; 27:79–88.
6. Cullen MR, Kominsky JR, Rossman MD, et al. Chronic beryllium disease in a precious metal refinery: clinical, epidemiologic and immunologic evidence for continuing risk from exposure to low level beryllium fume. Am Rev Respir Dis 1987; 135:201–8.
7. Kreiss K, Mroz MM, Zhen B, Martyny J, Newman LS. Epidemiology of beryllium sensitization and disease in nuclear workers. Am Rev Respir Dis 1993; 148:985–91.

8. Kreiss K, Wasserman S, Mroz MM, Newman LS. Beryllium disease screening in the ceramics industry: blood test performance and exposure-disease relations. J Occup Med 1993; 35:267–74.

9. Richeldi L, Kreiss K, Mroz MM, et al. Interaction of genetic and exposure factors in the prevalence of berylliosis. Am J Ind Med 1997; 32:337–40.

10. Newman LS, Maier LA, Nemery B. Interstitial lung disorders due to beryllium and cobalt. In: Schwarz M, King TE Jr, eds. Interstitial lung disease, 3rd edn. Hamilton, Ontario: Decker, 2003; 435–57.

11. Rossman MD, Kern JA, Elias JA, et al. Proliferative response of bronchoalveolar lymphocytes to beryllium: a test for chronic beryllium disease. Ann Intern Med 1988; 108:687–93.

12. Saltini C, Winestock K, Kirby M, et al. Maintenance of alveolitis in patients with chronic beryllium disease by beryllium-specific helper T cells. N Engl J Med 1989; 320:1103–9.

13. Richeldi L, Sorrentino R, Saltini C. HLA-DPb1 glutamate 69: a genetic marker of beryllium disease. Science 1993; 262:242-4.

14. Fontenot AP, Newman LS, Kotzin BL. Chronic beryllium disease: T cell recognition of a metal presented by HLA-DP. Clin Immunol 2001; 100:4–14.

15. Newman LS, Buschman DL, Newell JD Jr, et al. Beryllium disease: assessment with CT. Radiology 1994; 190:835–40.

16. Sprince NL, Kazemi H, Hardy HL. Current (1975) problem of differentiating between beryllium disease and sarcoidosis. Ann NY Acad Sci 1976; 278:654–64.

17. Newman LS, Kreiss K, King TE Jr, et al. Pathologic and immunologic alterations in early stages of beryllium disease: re-examination of disease definition and natural history. Am Rev Respir Dis 1989; 139:1479-86.

18. Mroz MM, Kreiss K, Lezotte DC, et al. Re-examination of the blood lymphocyte transformation test in the diagnosis of chronic beryllium disease. J Allergy Clin Immunol 1991; 88:54–60.

19. Stokes RF, Rossman MD. Blood cell proliferation response to beryllium: analysis by receiver-operating characteristics. J Occup Med 33:23–28, 1991.

20. Newman LS, Lloyd J, Daniloff E. The natural history of beryllium sensitization and chronic beryllium disease. Environ Health Perspect 1996; 104(Suppl 5):937–43.

21. Hardy HL, Rabe EW, Lorch S. United States Beryllium Case registry (1952–1966): review of its methods and utility. J Occup Med 1967; 9:271–6.

22. Sprince NL, Kanarek DJ, Weber AL, et al. Reversible respiratory disease in beryllium workers. Am Rev Respir Dis 1978; 117:1011–7.

23. Kreiss K, Newman LS, Mroz MM, Campbell PA. Screening blood test identifies subclinical beryllium disease. J Occup Med 1989; 31:603–8.

24. Kreiss K, Mroz MM, Newman LS, Martyny J, Zhen B. Machining risk of beryllium disease and sensitization with median exposures below 2 µg/m^3. Am J Ind Med 1996; 30:16–25.

25. Balmes JR. Respiratory effects of hard-metal dust exposure. Occup Med 1987; 2:327–44.

26. Kusaka Y, Fujimora N, Morimoto K. Hard metal disease: epidemiology and pathogenesis. In: Kobayashi S, Bellanti JA, eds. Advances in asthmology. Amsterdam: Elsevier Science, 1990; 271–6.

27. Sprince NL, Oliver LC, Eisen EA, et al. Cobalt exposure and lung disease in tungsten carbide production: a cross-sectional study of current workers. Am Rev Respir Dis 1988; 138:1220–6.

28. Sprince, N, Chamberlin R, Hales C, Weber A, Kazemi H. Respiratory disease in tungsten carbide production workers. Chest 1984; 86:549–57.

29. Demedts M, Gheysens B, Nayelo J, et al. Cobalt lung in diamond polishers. Am Rev Respir Dis 130:130–135, 1984.

30. Nemery B, Casier P, Roosels D, Lahaye D, Demedts M. Survey of cobalt exposure and respiratory health in diamond polishers. Am Rev Respir Dis 1992; 145:610–6.

31. Selden A, Sahle W, Johansson L, Sorenson S, Person B. Three cases of dental technician's pneumoconiosis related to cobalt-chromium-molybdenum dust. Chest 1996; 109:837–42.

32. Davison AG, Haslam PL, Corrin B, et al. Interstitial lung disease and asthma in hard-metal workers: bronchoalveolar lavage, ultrastructural, and analytical findings and results of bronchial provocation tests. Thorax 1983; 38:119–28.

33. Abraham JL, Burnett BR, Hunt A. Development and use of a pneumoconiosis database of human pulmonary inorganic particulate burden in over 400 lungs. Scanning Microsc 1991; 5:95–108.

34. Ohori NP, Sciurba FC, Owens GR, et al. Giant cell interstitial pneumonitis and hard metal pneumoconiosis. Am J Surg Pathol 1989; 13:581–7.

35. Harding HE. Notes on the toxicology of cobalt metal. Br J Ind Med 1950; 7:76–8.

36. Kerfoot EJ, Frederick WG, Domeier E. Cobalt metal inhalation studies on miniature swine. Am Ind Hyg Assoc J 1975; 36:17–25.

37. Lasfargues G, Lison D, Lardot C, Delos M, Lauwerys R. Comparative study in the rat of the long term pulmonary responses to pure cobalt metal and hard metal powder. Environ Res 1996; 69:108–21.

38. Lison D, Lauwerys R. In vitro cytotoxic effects of cobalt-containing dusts on mouse peritoneal and rat alveolar macrophages. Environ Res 1990; 52:187–98.

39. Lison D, Lauwerys R, Demedts M, Nemery B. Experimental research into the pathogenesis of cobalt/hard metal lung disease. Eur Respir J 1996; 9:1024–8.

40. Fischer T, Rystedt I. Cobalt allergy in hard metal workers. Contact Derm 1983; 9:115–21.

41. Potolicchio I, Mosconi G, Forni A, et al. Susceptibility to hard metal lung disease is strongly associated with the presence of glutamate 69 in HLA-DP beta chain. Eur J Immunol 1997; 27:2741–3.

42. Frost AE, Keller CA, Brown RW, et al. Giant cell interstitial pneumonitis: disease recurrence in the transplanted lung. Am Rev Respir Dis 1993; 148:1401–4.

43. Auchincloss JH, Abraham JL, Gilbert R, et al. Health hazard of poorly regulated exposure during manufacture of cemented tungsten carbides and cobalt. Br J Ind Med 1992; 49:832–6.

44. Meyer-Bisch C, Pham QT, Mur J-M, et al. Respiratory hazards in hard metal workers: a cross-sectional study. Br J Ind Med 1989; 46:302–9.

45. Kennedy SM, Chan-Yeung M, Marion S, et al. Maintenance of stellite and tungsten carbide saw tips: respiratory health and exposure–response relationships. Occup Environ Med 1995; 52:185–91.

19.8 Asbestosis and Asbestos-Related Pleural Disease

Carl A Brodkin, Linda Rosenstock

Asbestos is a term applied to a heterogeneous group of naturally occurring asbestiform minerals, characterized as hydrated silicates, with variable magnesium content. Asbestiform minerals have a fibrous structure, and tend to separate into distinct fibers, with length at least three times greater than width. Fibers are classified structurally, with serpentine fibers (i.e., chrysotile asbestos) representing curved structures, and amphibolic fibers (e.g., amosite, crocidolite, anthophyllite, actinolite, and tremolite asbestos) representing straight structures arranged linearly.[1,2] Fibers may also be classified by length, with fibers of greater than five microns in length identifiable by phase contrast microscopy (used in regulatory standards).

These six fibrous silicates are commonly referred to as asbestos, including the three most common commercial forms: chrysotile, or white asbestos; amosite, or brown asbestos; and crocidolite, or blue asbestos. Chrysotile is the most commonly used asbestos in North America, and accounted for more than 98% of asbestos consumption in the United States in the early 1990s.[3] Although some differences in biologic potency have been observed among various fiber types, from the point of view of the clinician, it should be recognized that the three main commercial types have been associated with all of the major malignant and non-malignant asbestos-related conditions.

Asbestos fibers are easily respirable, with inhalation representing the major route of exposure. The range of health effects from asbestos exposure is protean, including both pulmonary and non-pulmonary malignant and non-malignant conditions. This section focuses on two major non-malignant pulmonary sequelae: asbestosis and asbestos-induced pleural disease. Although these two types of outcomes, pleural and parenchymal, have distinct pathologic and physiologic manifestations, both represent dose-dependent outcomes of the same asbestos exposure. Pleural and parenchymal disease may occur either in isolation or together in the same individual.

ASBESTOS EXPOSURE SETTINGS

Worldwide use of asbestos increased steadily from the late 19th century, peaking in the early 1970s, with millions of tons of asbestos used in the United States since 1900.[4] Asbestos has been used in a wide variety of industrial products, including insulation, textiles, cement, friction products (such as brake linings), and many construction materials. Although consumption of asbestos in the United States and other developed countries has declined significantly over the past three decades, global production and use continue, with active mining in Russia, Canada, China, Kazakstan, and Brazil,[5] and export to developing countries, including South East Asia, Africa, South America, and Eastern Europe. Both the quantity and conditions of asbestos use in developing countries have led to substantial public health concerns internationally.[5] Many of the properties that make asbestos such an attractive industrial product, including durability, tensile strength, flexibility (allowing use in woven textiles), thermal resistance, and low electrical conductivity, are responsible for its hazardous properties and potency, as well as its environmental persistence.

Asbestos is ubiquitous in the environment of industrialized countries, and has become increasingly so in the developing world, where asbestos use has increased annually at a rate of approximately 7%. Historically, workers in industries involved in the production and use of asbestos products were at greatest risk for exposure, including asbestos mining and milling, friction products, asbestos cement, textile, shipyard, and construction industries. Specific trades considered at high risk for asbestos exposure include insulators, sheet-metal workers, plumbers and pipefitters, steamfitters, boilermakers, plasterboard workers, and numerous shipyard trades such as electricians and shipscalers.[6,7]

In addition to manufacturing settings, end-users or handlers of asbestos-containing materials and products are often at risk for exposure, and may be unaware of associated hazards. For instance, studies investigating the incidence of mesothelioma – a malignant outcome specific to asbestos exposure – have identified additional occupations, such as railway and power station workers, wharf laborers, brake mechanics,[8] transport drivers, welders, and metal workers[9] as being at risk for significant asbestos exposure. Similarly, needs assessment surveys of Department of Energy sites have identified former workers as an historic cohort having significant risk for asbestos exposure.[10] Mortality studies are also useful in identifying groups of workers at increased risk for asbestos-related diseases. For example, among 12,873 union construction plasterers and cement masons, a proportionate mortality ratio (PMR) of 1677 ($P < 0.01$) was observed for asbestosis.[11]

Asbestos frequently exists in older buildings, and may be present in machinery, pipes, or appliances. The Occupational Safety and Health Administration estimates that 1.3 million workers in construction and general industry encounter significant occupational exposure, most prominently during manipulation of asbestos during renovation or demolition.[12] In addition to occupational settings, many domestic products continue to contain asbestos, including brake pads and linings, vermiculite (which can be contaminated with tremolite asbestos), roofing products, gaskets, heat and acoustic insulation, fireproofing, and flooring material.[13]

EPIDEMIOLOGY

Following increased use of asbestos in the late 1800s, evidence began accumulating in the early 1900s of adverse respiratory effects related to exposure. Pulmonary fibrosis in asbestos-exposed workers was described at necropsy by 1906, radiographic changes by 1918, and a histopathologic description of pulmonary asbestosis provided by the

1920s.[14] Despite early clinical characterization of asbestos-related diseases, detailed information about populations at risk has been sporadic and largely confined to studies of occupational cohorts. Some variability in disease prevalence among different populations of workers with comparable cumulative asbestos exposure has been observed; factors to explain this are likely to include differences in fiber size, type, and distribution as well as individual host susceptibility factors. Nicholson and colleagues quantified the number of United States workers occupationally exposed to asbestos from 1940 to 1979, identifying about 19 million workers likely to have had significant occupational exposure. These exposures are estimated to result in several hundred thousand deaths, primarily due to lung cancer, as well as asbestosis, mesothelioma, and other cancers.[15]

The best evidence regarding the risk for the major non-malignant outcomes of asbestos remains those studies based on specific groups of exposed workers. There is reasonable evidence that, for asbestosis, there is a strong linear dose–response relationship between exposure and the proportion of the population affected. While it is likely that there is some exposure threshold, none has been demonstrated convincingly, such that individuals with low exposures or higher exposures of short duration (e.g., for a period of days to weeks) are not at risk. This pattern is probably different from the relation between exposure and asbestos-related malignancies, in which even low-level or brief exposures may confer at least some increased risk. Among South Carolina asbestos textile workers, Stayner and colleagues identified no evidence of a threshold for development of either asbestosis or lung cancer in relation to cumulative asbestos exposure.[16]

While a dose–response relationship is also observed for asbestos-related pleural disease, a clear threshold is even less apparent; pleural as well as parenchymal radiographic changes have been observed with exposure durations ranging from as little as one[17] to 12.7 months.[18] As with asbestosis, the prevalence of pleural disease increases with cumulative asbestos exposure, and is consistently observed in settings of high cumulative asbestos exposures.[19]

Asbestos-exposed workers with the highest level of exposures, such as asbestos insulators, accordingly bear the greatest burden of asbestos-related effects. Among workers certified by medical panels as having asbestosis, life expectancy has been found to be significantly shortened due to asbestos-related mortality, with 38% dying from lung cancer, 8% from mesothelioma, and 20% from asbestosis.[20]

Among populations of asbestos-exposed workers, prevalence rates for asbestosis and asbestos-related pleural thickening vary with intensity and duration of exposure, as well as time since initial exposure (disease latency). In a study of 2907 asbestos insulators, most with latencies of more than 30 years from first exposure, 12% had isolated radiographic fibrotic changes, 24% had isolated radiographic pleural changes, and 49% had both pleural and parenchymal changes.[21] Prevalence rates for both pleural and parenchymal outcomes are accordingly lower among those with lower exposures, as measured by both intensity and duration, and shorter latent periods.

Because latency plays such a major role in the radiographic appearance of non-malignant asbestos-related disease, which often occurs two decades or more following initial exposure, the mean age of populations studied is of major significance when considering whether populations have comparable outcomes. General population surveys may thus underestimate disease prevalence in high risk groups. In a review of chest radiographs from the first US National Health and Nutrition Examination Survey (NHANES) in the mid-1970s, 2.3% of men and 0.2% of women had occupationally related pleural thickening, extrapolated to a US population estimate of 1.3 million individuals, with a total of 8 million exposed to asbestos.[22]

Non-occupational environmental asbestos exposures occur, and are most concerning for malignant sequelae. Anderson and colleagues observed that both pleural and parenchymal changes were significantly more prevalent in exposed household contacts of asbestos workers than controls ($P < 0.001$), with 35% demonstrating pleural changes and 17% parenchymal changes, respectively.[23] Population surveys have identified higher rates of pleural abnormalities in locations where asbestos occurs naturally, ranging from 2% to 17% of individuals. An unfortunate sequela of such environmental contamination has occurred in Libby, Montana, where years of extensive environmental asbestos contamination resulted from vermiculite mining, processing, and commercial use. A cross-sectional investigation of 6668 adults from this community observed radiographic pleural thickening in 17.8% of individuals, with parenchymal changes in less than 1%.[24] In individuals with significant vermiculite exposure pathways identified, up to 34.6% had pleural abnormalities.

While air-borne asbestos is detectable at low concentrations in the ambient air of urban settings (e.g., 2×10^{-6} f/ml by phase contrast microscopy [PCM]), and to a lesser extent in rural areas (2×10^{-7} f/ml PCM),[25] this is unlikely to result in substantial risk for non-malignant asbestos disease in the absence of additional indirect exposures. These levels are orders of magnitude less than the current occupational exposure standard of 0.1 f/ml (PCM) for air-borne asbestos, that is predicted to result in an excess lifetime risk of 2/1000 for asbestosis and 5/1000 for lung cancer.

PATHOGENESIS AND PATHOLOGY

Asbestos fibers are inhaled deep into the respiratory tract, exerting their main influence at the level of the respiratory bronchioles and alveoli. Fibers migrate to the pulmonary interstitium via uptake by alveolar epithelial cells, with accumulation of macrophages leading to an inflammatory response, namely alveolitis and peribronchiolitis.[26] Despite activation of macrophages, many asbestos fibers are

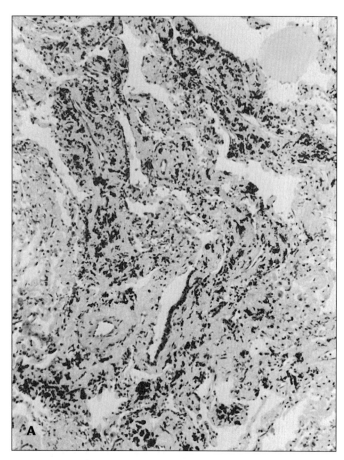
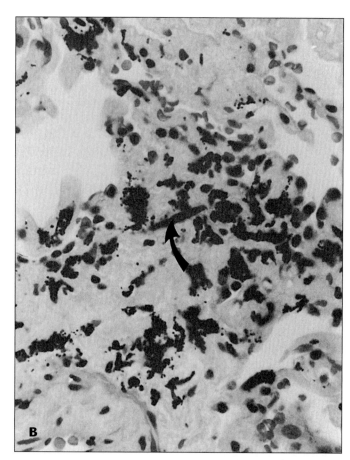

Figure 19.8.1: (a,b) Example of grade 1 asbestosis. This region of lung tissue shows peribronchiolar fibrosis in association with ferruginous bodies consistent with asbestos bodies *(arrow)*. ((a) × 125; (b) × 500.) (Courtesy of Sam Hammar, MD.)

retained in the pulmonary interstitium, or migrate to the pleura via lymphatic channels, causing a chronic inflammatory response.

Asbestos fibers cause direct cytotoxicity from generation of reactive oxygen intermediates,[27] with injury to intracellular macromolecules and associated lipid peroxidation. In addition, activated macrophages produce cytokines, interleukins, tumor necrosis factor, fibronectin, and other mediators, enhancing tissue inflammation and injury.[28] These inflammatory mediators stimulate granulocytic and fibroblastic responses, leading to tissue fibrosis.[29] This chronic inflammatory and fibrotic tissue response to asbestos represents the primary pathophysiologic mechanism for progressive lung injury.

Pathologic descriptions and diagnostic criteria for parenchymal and pleural asbestos-related diseases have been provided by the College of American Pathologists and NIOSH.[30] The macroscopic appearance of asbestosis (used here to refer only to parenchymal asbestos-induced fibrosis) is that of small, firm and brownish lungs, occasionally laced with gray fibrous streaks. Pulmonary fibrosis is linear and involves predominantly the lower (basilar) lung fields; honeycombing may be present. Histologically, the parenchymal interstitial fibrosis is similar to that observed in other diffuse interstitial lung diseases, except that asbestos bodies and elevated asbestos fiber content are typically present. The histologic diagnosis of asbestosis

is based on the minimal findings of fibrosis of the walls of the respiratory bronchioles, which may be the sole manifestation of early disease, in association with asbestos bodies (Fig. 19.8.1). The distribution of parenchymal fibrosis in early or mild disease is in subpleural regions, progressing centrally with more advanced disease.

Pleural plaques are discretely elevated gray-white areas of fibrous tissue, involving the parietal pleura in the region of the mid-thoracic chest wall and domes of the diaphragm. Plaques may be smooth or nodular, and round or irregularly shaped. Parietal plaques tend to calcify with time; histologically, there is no difference between non-calcified and calcified plaques, other than the presence of calcium. These sequelae have been collectively referred to as hyaline plaques. Diffuse pleural thickening results from thickening and fibrosis of the visceral pleura, often with fusion to the parietal pleura. Diffuse pleural thickening is also a common sequela of benign asbestos-induced pleural effusions. Diffuse pleural thickening and extensive pulmonary fibrosis are the classic features of advanced asbestosis.

In addition to the pathologic findings associated with pleural and parenchymal fibrosis, evidence of exposure itself can be found in sputum, lung tissue, and by bronchoalveolar lavage (BAL). The asbestos body or 'ferruginous body' represents an asbestos fiber coated with ferroprotein by macrophages (see figure 19.8.1B). Microscopically, asbestos bodies are brownish club-shaped and symmetrically nodular structures, that stain for iron due to high ferritin content. Because asbestos bodies are larger than fibers, they can be identified with light microscopy of lung and BAL specimens. Analysis of BAL in individuals with asbestosis may also identify a macrophage-predominant alveolitis, with some neutrophilia. While apparent asbestos bodies can arise in response to an array of foreign fibers, the large majority have asbestos cores, correlating with fiber lengths of greater than 10 microns. Asbestos bodies are a better reflection of amphibole than chrysotile asbestos lung burden, and represent only a small proportion of the total asbestos fiber load.

In contrast to asbestos bodies, quantification of asbestos fibers is generally performed by electron microscopy, and is not as widely available. Those with parenchymal asbestosis typically have the highest concentration of asbestos fibers in lung (number of fibers per weight of lung tissue); those with pleural plaques have higher numbers of fibers than those without, and those with occupational exposure have higher concentrations than those without, regardless of radiographic or functional manifestations of exposure. There is substantial variability among labs for quantitation of both asbestos bodies and tissue fiber concentration; interpretation generally requires specific knowledge of laboratory reference ranges.

CLINICAL EVALUATION OF THE PATIENT
Exposure history

Fundamental to the consideration of any of the asbestos-related outcomes and their probability is the occupational and environmental history of asbestos exposure. Three aspects of the history are essential: onset, duration, and intensity of exposure.

Exposure onset and latency

Exposure onset is of importance because of the characteristic latent period between first exposure and disease manifestation (termed 'latency'). For both interstitial fibrosis and pleural plaques, latencies are typically greater than 20 years.[31] Shorter latency periods do occur, and correlate with more intense and higher cumulative exposures. Shorter latent periods should heighten suspicion of other diagnostic entities. Diffuse pleural thickening, if it follows a benign asbestos effusion, is the one non-malignant outcome that may occur relatively early following exposure (e.g., several years), although mean latencies are still close to 20 years.

Exposure duration

The duration of exposure is also an important factor in determining whether or not abnormalities are attributable to asbestos exposure. Cumulative asbestos exposure durations are frequently greater than 6 months in individuals with asbestosis. If exposure has been intense, this duration may be shorter but evaluation should include

consideration for other causes of interstitial fibrosis. Similar exposure durations are observed in individuals with asbestos-related pleural thickening, although shorter exposure periods may be observed.

Exposure intensity

The intensity of asbestos exposure is best determined by information about the job or trade, the industry in which it was performed, and the circumstances of asbestos use or exposure and protection from it. While epidemiologic studies may characterize cumulative exposures quantitatively (e.g., fiber-year/ml of asbestos exposure), such measurements are rarely available for individual workers. Three general settings of exposure should be considered, namely direct, bystander, and indirect exposure. Direct exposure occurs with application, removal, or manipulation of asbestos or asbestos-containing materials. Bystander exposure occurs when a worker is exposed through proximity to coworkers generating asbestos dust through their direct activities. Indirect exposure occurs when asbestos is carried away from the worksite (e.g., dusty work clothing and shoes), exposing family members and other household contacts.

Asbestos insulation procedures, involving mixing and application of asbestos, provide a useful example of the range of exposure intensities encountered in industrial settings. Until the mid-1970s in the United States, it was common for asbestos insulators to work without respiratory protection, often in dusty, poorly ventilated environments, with resulting high intensity direct exposures. In a prospective study of 17,800 US and Canadian asbestos insulation workers, extremely high mortality rates for asbestosis were observed (e.g., 413–1187 deaths/10^5/year for those with more than 30 years from employment onset);[32] with 11% of deaths attributable to asbestosis in a sub-group of these workers.[33] Sheet-metal workers, who frequently worked in proximity to these insulators, also experienced high bystander exposures. In a US national survey of 9605 sheet-metal workers, 31% were identified as having asbestos-related radiographic changes.[34] Similarly, other trades, including electricians, carpenters, plumbers, and pipefitters, worked side by side with insulators, and although lower on average than the insulators, exposures were often of moderate to high intensity, through a combination of direct and bystander routes. The significant effect of indirect exposure related to asbestos insulation work is reviewed above, with highly prevalent radiographic changes among family members of these insulators.

An occupational history occasionally reveals unexpectedly high intensity asbestos exposures in unusual jobs, such as mixing asbestos powder into paints or glazing material. In taking the history, it is important to inquire about how asbestos was encountered, including work setting (indoor vs outdoors, enclosed vs open space), presence of engineering controls or personal protective equipment (e.g., exhaust hoses and use of fit-tested HEPA respirators), and observed levels of dust. While respirable asbestos fibers are not visible, the observed level of dust in the environment may serve as a qualitative index of exposure. For instance, diminished visibility (e.g., 'snow-storm' effects) in enclosed areas during application or removal of asbestos is indicative of very high intensity exposure (e.g., ship construction settings). Intact asbestos impregnated in material is not generally of concern, unless friable or otherwise disrupted to generate air-borne fibers. A partial list of occupations with common asbestos exposure is provided in Chapter 46.

Clinical history

The insidious onset of dyspnea, typically progressing over a number of years in association with diminished exertional tolerance, is the most common respiratory symptom in individuals with asbestosis. A non-productive cough may be present, and can progress to a productive cough later in the course of the disease, even in non-smokers. Wheezing and dyspnea are associated with significantly diminished ventilatory capacity in asbestos-exposed workers, with an 11–17% reduction observed in a cross-sectional study of 816 asbestos-exposed workers ($P <$ 0.001),[35] and a lesser 2–8% reduction observed for cough, phlegm and chronic bronchitis ($P < 0.001$). Development and progression of respiratory symptoms are associated with accelerated loss of lung function. In a longitudinal study of 446 asbestos-exposed workers, an excess decline in FEV_1 of 28 ml/year for development of dyspnea, and 67 ml/year for development of wheezing ($P < 0.01$), was observed relative to asymptomatic individuals.[36] Dyspnea was associated with an almost two-fold increased mortality from asbestosis in a 10-year follow-up of 2609 insulators from the North American insulator cohort (RR 1.9; 95% CI 1.10–3.28). Respiratory symptoms should be assessed in the context of pulmonary function testing and other objective parameters discussed below.

The individual with isolated pleural plaques usually is asymptomatic unless other sequelae, non-radiographically apparent, are present, or plaques are extensive. Patients with plaques may report episodic pleuritic or non-pleuritic chest pain, that has no other explainable cause. In cohort studies, presence of pleural thickening has been associated with increased dyspnea, for any given grade of radiographic fibrosis. Although individuals with diffuse pleural thickening often do not have symptoms, they more frequently report the presence of dyspnea, chest discomfort, or difficulty with full inspiration. These symptoms may be prominent in settings of bilateral diffuse thickening and fibrothorax. Among 64 individuals with bilateral diffuse pleural thickening, 56% reported chest pain, with 63% reporting moderate and 11% severe breathlessness.[37] Development of prominent or severe chest pain may indicate a pleuritis (e.g., asbestos-related pleural effusion), but should be evaluated further to rule out other causes, including malignancy (e.g., mesothelioma or lung cancer).

Asbestos exposure, independent of other pathologic endpoints, may also cause upper respiratory tract irritation,[38] and has been implicated as a cause of industrial bronchitis (e.g. asbestos insulators; see Chapter 19.4).

Physical examination

The major physical finding in asbestosis is basilar rales,[39] that may be pan-inspiratory or apparent only on end-inspiration. Rales are dose dependent, and can occur in the absence of radiographic changes. Finger clubbing or cyanosis may be present in advanced cases. When seen in patients with evidence of only mild interstitial fibrosis, clubbing should raise suspicion for possible malignancy. Physical findings are useful clinically; rales, clubbing, or cyanosis were associated with an almost two-fold increased mortality from asbestosis in the North American insulator cohort. The clinician should recognize that while useful when present, physical findings are not a sensitive indicator of asbestosis, particularly in early or mild disease, and may be minimal or absent even in patients with significant radiographic and functional abnormalities.

Radiographic features

While high-resolution CT (HRCT) scan of the chest has represented a major advance over the past 15 years, and is particularly valuable in equivocal cases, the plain chest roentgenograph remains the standard for radiographic evaluation of non-malignant asbestos-related disease.

Plain chest radiograph

On posteroanterior (PA) chest x-ray, pleural plaques have a variable appearance depending on their location in the chest, commonly having the density of pulmonary nodules at the lateral chest walls, and less density more medial to the chest wall. Non-calcified pleural plaques are difficult to detect in the medial two-thirds of the lungs, because they are then perpendicular to the x-ray beam and too thin for definition; calcified plaques, however, are sufficiently radiopaque to be detectable in all portions of the chest (Fig. 19.8.2). Plaques occur most commonly on the middle part of the diaphragm, on the posterolateral chest wall between the 7th and 10th ribs, and on the lateral chest wall between the 6th and 9th ribs. Plaques are often bilateral and symmetric in distribution, but asymmetric or unilateral pleural plaques are sufficiently common that they are indicative of past asbestos exposure, in the absence of other apparent causes, such as rib fractures.

The criterion of costophrenic angle blunting is required in the current 2003 ILO classification for reporting of diffuse pleural thickening.[40] In addition to costophrenic angle blunting, diffuse pleural thickening is characterized radiographically by a thickness of the pleura greater than 1 mm medial to the chest wall, often involving more than one-third the extent of the thoracic wall. Distinguishing discrete from diffuse pleural thickening is not always easy. Table 19.8.1 describes some characteristics helpful in making this determination.[41] Apical pleural thickening up to 10 mm (to the level of the 4th rib) can be a variant of normal; more pronounced apical thickening in asbestos-exposed individuals, with a mean of 21 mm, has been reported as an unusual complication in individuals with diffuse parenchymal fibrotic changes involving the upper

	Pleural thickening		Extrapleural shadows
	Discrete (plaques)	Diffuse	
Composition	Parietal pleura	Parietal and visceral pleura (affects only visceral pleura if interlobar fissures)	Muscles (serratus anterior, external oblique), intercostal extrapleural fat, companion shadows
Location*	Lateral and posterior chest wall at level of lower ribs (5–10) sparing costophrenic sulcus; can involve mediastinum, pericardium, middle third of diaphragm	Usually bilateral, along lateral chest wall; may involve costophrenic sulcus	Companion shadows; most prominent in association with upper ribs Muscle shadows: apparent pleural shadows are in continuity with well-developed muscle shadows along lateral chest wall
Appearance on posteroanterior chest x-ray study	May be calcified Uneven, sometimes with bizarre shape, well-defined medial border when seen in profile (tangential to x-ray beam), faint when seen en face (perpendicular to x-ray beam). May show abrupt change in density from dense, lateral to faint, medial shadow	Rarely calcified Ill-defined and irregular medial margin parallel to lateral chest wall; may show graded increase in density from medial to lateral border and widens inferiorly	Not calcified Pleural line along lateral chest wall often widens superiorly and tapers inferiorly. Muscles have rhythmic, symmetrical appearance of triangular, V, or quadrilateral shape, with one sharply defined border, often fading into adjacent soft tissue
Appearance on right and left anterior oblique chest x-ray	Shadow remains adjacent to lung field with similar appearance to posteroanterior film except for rotation in orientation (and hence density) to x-ray beam	Shadow remains adjacent to lung field within thoracic cage; identify if greater than 10 mm width	Shadows demonstrated to continue with those of adjacent soft tissue and may rotate outside of lung fields. Fat: rhythmic wavy appearance most prominent adjacent to rib rather than in intercostal space

* Apical pleural thickening alone (to level of 4th rib) is a variant of normal and should not be ascribed to asbestos unless associated with thickening below this level.
Adapted from Rosenstock L, Hudson LD. The pleural manifestations of asbestos exposure. Occup Med 1987; 2(2):383–407.

Table 19.8.1 Distinguishing pleural thickening from extrapleural shadows

lobes, and significant restrictive impairment[42] (Fig. 19.8.3). Interlobar tissue thickening may be the sole manifestation of asbestos exposure, but may also occur in association with other pleural abnormalities or interstitial fibrosis.

Parenchymal changes on posteroanterior chest radiographs are typically lower lobe (basilar) in location, and are described as a profusion of small irregular opacities. These opacities are present peripherally, beyond the normal bronchovascular markings of the lower lung fields. With more advanced disease, the middle and even upper lung fields may become involved. The small irregular opacities typical of asbestos-induced interstitial fibrosis are designated radiographically as 's' and 't' by the ILO classification (see also Introduction to Chapter 19). In advanced disease, opacities may have a honeycomb appearance (Fig. 19.8.4). When opacities are sufficiently dense and appropriately located, they may obscure the definition of adjacent structures, causing the appearance of an irregular diaphragm or heart border, the latter known as the shaggy heart sign. There has been no convincing evidence that asbestos itself can cause progressive massive fibrosis or large opacities. Although a few such cases have been reported in asbestos-exposed workers, it is likely that these manifestations are best explained by concomitant exposure to silica.

Even among heavily exposed cohorts with a high prevalence of interstitial changes, the large majority, often up to 90%, of abnormal chest radiographs fall in the mild grades of profusion by ILO criteria (1/0 and 1/1). Standard chest radiographs may have limited sensitivity in early or mild

parenchymal disease. For example, 25 of 138 (18%) asbestos insulation workers with histologic fibrosis on tissue specimens (obtained in the course of lung cancer resection) had no parenchymal changes apparent on chest radiograph.[43] Similarly, among 169 asbestos-exposed workers with normal chest radiographs, 57 (33%) had abnormal findings on HRCT consistent with asbestosis.[44]

Of interest to the clinician, most series have identified a non-concordance in individuals between the development of parenchymal versus pleural manifestations of asbestos exposure. Among those occupationally exposed who have radiographic evidence of interstitial fibrosis, about half will have concomitant pleural thickening; conversely, those with pleural thickening usually have a smaller proportion (less than 30%) of concomitant interstitial findings.

High-resolution computed tomography

High-resolution CT (HRCT) of the chest has become increasingly used in the radiographic assessment of asbestos-related pleural and parenchymal disease. While conventional CT has been shown to be a more sensitive indicator than standard chest radiographs in detecting asbestosis, rounded atelectasis, and pleural plaques, high-resolution techniques offer improved sensitivity for detection of asbestosis.[45–47] High-resolution CT studies should use algorithms with 2 cm or finer intervals. Because asbestosis is most prominent in basilar, posterior, and subpleural regions, it is important that prone views be

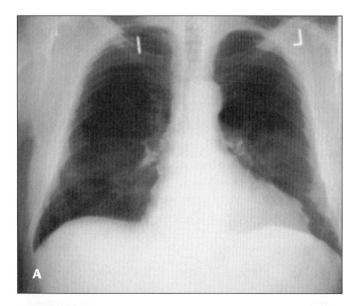

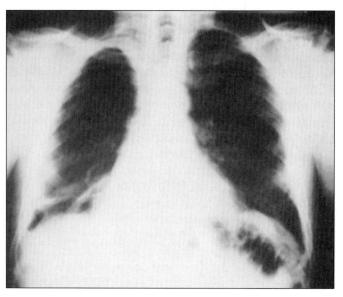

Figure 19.8.3: PA chest radiograph of 44-year-old asbestos insulator with diffuse bilateral pleural thickening and interstitial fibrosis (ILO 1/2).

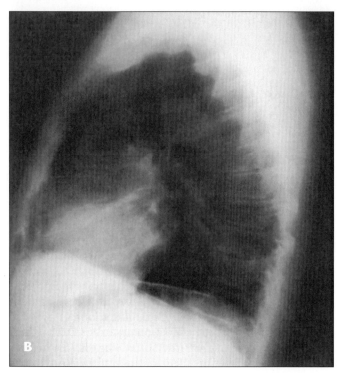

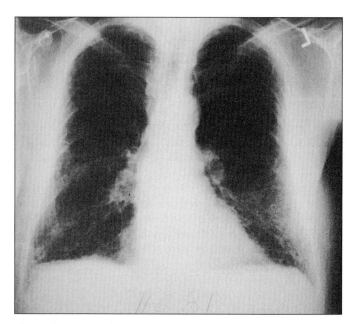

Figure 19.8.2: (a) PA chest radiograph of 70-year-old retired insulator with calcified diaphragmatic pleural plaques and normal parenchyma (ILO 0/1). (b) Lateral radiograph that better demonstrates calcified diaphragmatic plaques.

Figure 19.8.4: PA chest radiograph of 64-year-old painter with minimal diffuse bilateral pleural thickening and extensive fibrosis with honeycombing (ILO 3/3).

obtained to differentiate these fibrotic changes from dependent atelectasis in posterior fields. Characteristic features of asbestosis on HRCT include fibrotic intralobular interstitial thickening and interlobular septal thickening, subpleural lines and opacities, parenchymal bands, ground-glass opacities, and, in more severe disease, variable honeycombing.[48,49] A classification system for CT and HRCT findings in asbestos-related disease and other pneumoconioses, analogous to the ILO system, has been proposed.[50] Parenchymal fibrotic changes on HRCT have

correlated with other clinical parameters of asbestosis, including diminished vital capacity and diffusing capacity. Similarly, the extent of pleural thickening determined quantitatively by HRCT correlates strongly with diminished total lung capacity ($P = 0.002$).[51]

Pulmonary function

Pulmonary function tests are the most important tool for the functional assessment of non-malignant asbestos-related effects.

The pattern of pulmonary function abnormalities in individuals with asbestos-induced parenchymal disease (asbestosis) is classically described as a restrictive one. Typical findings include decreased ventilatory capacity on spirometry (diminished FVC and FEV_1, with well maintained FEV_1/FVC ratio); abnormal static lung volumes, with decreased total lung capacity (TLC) and residual volume, and abnormalities in gas exchange, characterized by reduced diffusing capacity (DLCO). A widened alveolar–arterial oxygen gradient, with or without hypoxemia, may be observed. The earliest and most sensitive finding in asbestosis is frequently a diminished diffusing capacity, which may occur in isolation or in combination with other findings.

While isolated restrictive impairment is the most common functional manifestation of asbestosis, a mixed restrictive and obstructive impairment is also common (with greater relative reductions in FEV_1 than FVC, resulting in a diminished FEV_1/FVC ratio). In addition to parenchymal effects, asbestos can cause airflow obstruction,[52–56] with pathophysiologic changes in the small airways. A consistent correlation between pathologic changes of fibrosis in respiratory bronchiolar walls and diminished FEV_1 and FEF_{25-75} has been observed.[57] The finding of diminished mid-expiratory flow rates (e.g., FEF_{25-75}) appears to be the most sensitive parameter for assessing early obstructive changes among asbestos-exposed workers,[58–60] reflecting small airways effects. Among 225 non-smoking female asbestos workers, with and without concomitant asbestosis, an increased RV/TLC ratio, suggestive of air trapping, and reduced airflow at mid to low lung volumes were observed, consistent with small airways obstruction. Asbestos-related airflow obstruction interacts with the effects of smoking, resulting in more pronounced obstructive changes.

Total lung capacity is generally an insensitive measure of functional impairment.[61] This is likely a result of the competing forces on TLC in mixed restrictive and obstructive impairment, with a reduction in TLC related to restrictive disease, and an increase in TLC related to concurrent obstructive air trapping. It is unlikely that isolated severe obstructive disease is attributable solely to asbestos exposure.

Pleural plaques have traditionally been viewed as markers of asbestos exposure; the isolated effects of asbestos-induced pleural disease on lung function have been more difficult to assess, due to the confounding effect of non-radiographically apparent interstitial disease. Evidence of an independent effect of pleural thickening on lung function was observed by Miller and associates among six asbestos-exposed workers with diffuse pleural thickening and minimal parenchymal disease on radiographic and pathologic examination.[62] A pattern characteristic of pleural-induced restriction was observed, with diminished vital capacity and DLCO, but increased DLCO/TLC ratio consistent with normal lung parenchyma that has become encased.

Several large cohort studies have subsequently provided additional evidence that pleural thickening is independently associated with functional respiratory impairment, most consistently affecting FVC.[63–65] In rare cases, isolated pleural disease may be sufficient to cause respiratory failure, with CO_2 retention and cor pulmonale. In those studies assessing the relative contribution to functional impairment of plaques versus diffuse pleural thickening, diffuse – particularly bilateral – pleural thickening was found to confer a greater adverse effect.[66]

Other laboratory tests

A number of other laboratory tests have been employed in assessing the pulmonary effects of asbestos exposure. Bronchoalveolar lavage (BAL) may demonstrate asbestos (ferruginous) bodies.[67,68] Neutrophilia, indicative of alveolitis, has correlated with objective findings of rales and diminished oxygenation, as well as accelerated loss of FEV_1 and DLCO.[69] While bronchoalveolar lavage findings in asbestos-exposed workers have demonstrated an altered immune response,[70] correlation between these findings and cumulative asbestos exposure has been variable, and BAL is appropriately reserved for excluding other etiologies.

The presence of pleural plaques indicates significant exposure to asbestos, and is associated with a more than 10-fold increased risk for development of mesothelioma compared to the general population.[71] In cases of prominent unilateral, progressive, or asymmetric pleural thickening, single positron emission computed tomography (e.g., SPECT with thallium-201 scintigraphy) may be useful in assessing metabolically active tumor such as mesothelioma.[72] Inflammatory changes associated with diffuse pleural thickening (e.g., pachypleuritis or 'crow's feet') may be characterized by gallium scanning. These scans do not have a role, however, in the routine evaluation of asbestos-exposed individuals.

Exercise testing has not proven useful as part of the routine evaluation of individuals with suspected or known asbestos-related non-malignant conditions, and is not required for diagnosis. Little correlation has been observed between the degree of respiratory impairment measured by static pulmonary function tests compared with maximal oxygen uptake (VO_{2max}) and other parameters of exercise testing.[73] Exercise testing is appropriately reserved for individuals who have dyspnea out of proportion to radiographic and static lung function findings.

CLASSIFICATION OF NON-MALIGNANT ASBESTOS-RELATED DISEASE

Pleura
    Pleural thickening
    Plaques (discrete pleural thickening)
    Diffuse pleural thickening
    Benign exudative pleuritis
    Rounded atelectasis
Parenchyma
    Asbestosis

Pleura

Pleural thickening

Pleural inflammation results from the migration of inhaled asbestos fibers to the pleura. Pleural thickening may be discrete (pleural plaques) or diffuse; both reflect significant prior exposure to asbestos and duration since initial exposure, with latency from exposure (often more than 20 years) being the most important determinant. These two abnormalities share many features in common, but are worth considering separately because they represent distinct pathophysiologic responses, with differential effects on pulmonary function and related symptoms. These distinct effects are coded separately in the current ILO classification of pneumoconiosis, and have been coded separately since 1980. Pleural thickening, when observed radiographically without other obvious cause, should always prompt a thorough occupational and environmental history to identify past asbestos exposure.

Plaques

Plaques represent areas of discrete or circumscribed thickening of the parietal pleura, and are the most common biologic effect of asbestos exposure. In contrast to the general population, plaques are highly prevalent in historically heavily exposed populations; for instance, plaques were identified in 82% of asbestos insulators with a latency of more than 40 years from exposure onset. Histologically, plaques are characterized by uniform hyaline connective tissue, classically described in a 'basket-weave' pattern, covered by normal mesothelial cells, without adhesions. Associated inflammatory cells may be present peripherally. Plaques are most frequently bilateral in location, a finding pathognomonic for asbestos exposure, but they may be unilateral. Calcification occurs over time, and is a function of duration from first exposure (latency).

Plaques are effectively identified on chest radiograph as discrete raised surfaces, with well-defined margins against the chest wall, frequently in the mid-thoracic or diaphragm region. Plaques may also appear 'en face' with serpiginous borders. It is useful to the clinician that the differential diagnosis of discrete pleural thickening is limited (Table 19.8.2). Subpleural fat pads are also located against the mid-thoracic wall, but typically have less distinct edges.[74] Plaques can be confirmed by conventional CT or HRCT when chest radiographic features are unclear. Features used to distinguish calcified asbestos plaques from those of other causes include the findings that non-asbestos plaques are more often unilateral, and more extensive than those due to asbestos; such plaques often involve the visceral pleural, so that a thickness of pleura is apparent between the calcification and the ribs.

The natural history of pleural plaques is one of slow progression. Since plaques do not form adhesions with the visceral pleura, they tend to have a minor impact on respiratory function. Studies of asbestos-exposed populations have variably observed small reductions in ventilatory capacity associated with plaques. Among 1211 sheet-metal

Discrete	Diffuse
Asbestos-related*	Asbestos-related
Mesothelioma	Loculated effusions
Lymphoma	Infectious processes* (e.g., tuberculosis,
Myeloma	paragonimiasis, bilateral empyema)
Metastatic cancer	Collagen vascular disease (e.g.,
Post-traumatic*	scleroderma, SLE, rheumatoid arthritis)
Post-infectious,	Sarcoidosis
e.g., tuberculosis*	Uremia
Mica and talc*	Drug reactions
Scleroderma*	Chronic beryllium disease
Chronic mineral oil	Silicosis
aspiration*	Mica and talc
* May calcify.	

Table 19.8.2 Differential diagnosis of pleural thickening

workers, circumscribed plaques were associated with a 140 ml reduction in FVC. A 6.5% average reduction in FVC associated with circumscribed plaques was similarly observed among 2611 asbestos insulators. However, in a clinic-based study of 1150 shipyard and construction workers, no reduction in FVC was observed in association with circumscribed plaques.[75] Interestingly, evidence of excessive and altered dead space ventilation was reported in 23 asbestos-exposed workers with dyspnea, pleural thickening and normal pulmonary function tests, suggestive of diminished chest wall or lung compliance.[76]

Plaques raise clinical concern as a marker of significant asbestos exposure, and have been associated with parenchymal changes of peribronchiolar fibrosis ($P < 0.001$) and alveolar fibrosis ($P < 0.05$) in autopsy series.[77] In addition to asbestosis, plaques are also associated with increased risk for the malignant outcomes of asbestos exposure, including mesothelioma and lung cancer. In a review of epidemiologic studies assessing relative risk of lung cancer in asbestos-exposed cohorts, Hillerdal and colleagues reported a 1.3–3.7-fold increase in risk for lung cancer in workers with radiographic evidence of plaques without fibrosis.[78]

Diffuse pleural thickening

In contrast to plaques, diffuse pleural thickening involves the visceral pleura, and may have more portentous clinical implications. In diffuse pleural thickening, adhesions frequently form with the parietal pleura, with radiographically indistinct borders, blunting of the costophrenic angle (Figure 19.8.5). Fibrous extensions into lung parenchyma, termed pachypleuritis (or 'crow's feet') may also occur. As noted above, diffuse pleural thickening is defined radiographically by involvement of the costophrenic angle. Rarely, isolated apical pleural thickening may occur, associated with fibrosis of the upper lobe, which must at times be distinguished from tuberculosis, mesothelioma, or other etiologies. Diffuse pleural thickening may occur in isolation, or in combination with pleural plaques. As with pleural plaques, diffuse thickening is associated with cumulative asbestos exposure and latency, but may also be seen following episodes of benign asbestos pleuritis.[79]

In contrast to the mild effect of plaques on lung function, diffuse pleural thickening may result in more significant restrictive respiratory impairment, with a 270 ml reduction in FVC observed among sheet-metal workers, an almost 20% predicted reduction in FVC among asbestos insulators, and a 13% decrement in FVC, on average, among shipyard and construction workers. Overall, restrictive ventilatory impairment is much more common than in circumscribed pleural disease, and may not correlate with extent of radiographic findings. In extreme cases, marked pleuritis and fibrothorax may occur, resulting in severe restrictive impairment and need for surgical decortication.

As discussed above, diffuse pleural disease may be associated with chest discomfort and associated respiratory symptoms. While this is typically mild or moderate, and frequently responds to non-steroidal anti-inflammatory therapy, in some patients chronic, severe, and disabling pleuritic pain can occur, prompting surgical pleurectomy in rare instances.[80] Once present, diffuse pleural thickening is likely to become more extensive with time.

The differential diagnosis of diffuse pleural thickening is broader than for plaques but it is often possible on the basis of radiographic findings and clinical history to exclude other likely causes (Table 19.8.2). Both mica and talc have been reported to be able to induce diffuse as well as discrete pleural lesions similar to those caused by asbestos, which may be explained by contamination of these products with asbestiform minerals.

For the clinician, identifying pleural thickening should serve as an added basis for increased vigilance in an asbestos-exposed individual at risk for other sequelae. In addition, the identification of otherwise clinically unimportant thickening may play a role in prompting greater attention by the physician and patient to the importance of prevention and specifically to smoking cessation. In addition to lung cancer risk, cigarette smoking diminishes mucociliary clearance of particulates such as asbestos, increasing the biologically available dose of fibers for a given level of exposure. An association between heavy cigarette smoking and mildly increased radiographic parenchymal changes in asbestos-exposed individuals has been observed;[81,82] interestingly, there is no evidence that cigarette smoke enhances risk for asbestos-related pleural thickening.[83]

Benign exudative pleuritis

The inflammatory effect of asbestos on the pleura may be manifest by an acute or sub-acute pleural effusion.[84,85] Effusions often last several months, with a mean duration of 4.3 months in one series of 22 patients, but may be persistent or recurrent in some cases.[86] The most common symptoms are pain, experienced by approximately one-third of individuals, and dyspnea reported by 6%; almost half are without any symptoms. Effusions are usually small, but may on occasion be up to several liters in volume. This asbestos-related outcome may be the sole manifestation of exposure.

Benign exudative pleuritis, also known as benign exudative pleurisy (BEP) or asbestos effusion, is defined as follows:

(1) history of asbestos exposure, (2) confirmation of effusion by radiographic studies or thoracocentesis, (3) absence of other diseases to better account for the effusion, and (4) no occurrence of associated malignancy within 3 years of diagnosis. Doseresponse relationships for asbestos pleural effusion have not been well characterized, and specific prevalence and incidence rates are unknown. The diagnosis is complicated by the fact that these effusions are usually transient, although they often leave the residua of diffuse pleural thickening, with obliteration of the costophrenic sulcus.

The clinical approach should include differential diagnostic considerations for exudative pleural effusion, including malignant, infectious (e.g., tuberculosis), and other inflammatory conditions (e.g., connective tissue disorders). Given the increased risk of pulmonary malignancy and mesothelioma in asbestos-exposed workers, excluding a malignant pleural effusion is essential. This frequently requires CT imaging of the chest, and direct examination of the pleura (e.g., thoracoscopy with biopsy of suspicious areas). While development of mesothelioma has been reported in individuals with chronic or recurrent asbestos-related pleural effusions, there is no evidence that this represents a direct progression of disease. Nevertheless, mesothelioma should be a concern in such individuals, because it can present with minimal evidence of a solid lesion and an exudative effusion that is indistinguishable from a benign one. Fluid characteristics are variable; commonly, the fluid is a sterile exudate that may be serosanguinous. In addition to neutrophils, lymphocytes and mesothelial cells, one of the more specific findings is an increased number of eosinophils (identified in pleural fluid and peripheral blood counts), that may be useful in establishing the diagnosis when present. The sensitivity for this finding is limited, however, with eosinophilic effusion reported in only 26% of cases in one series.

The reported mean latency for benign exudative pleuritis varies among series, ranging from 14 to 45 years. Importantly, BEP can be seen within the first 10 years of exposure and, given the longer minimum latencies for other non-malignant processes, it is not surprising that in one series, it was the most common asbestos-related abnormality within the first 20 years of asbestos exposure.[87] Pulmonary function may be abnormal, either as a consequence of mechanical restriction from the effusion or related to underlying pleural or parenchymal disease.

Rounded atelectasis

Rounded atelectasis, or pseudotumor, is thought to arise when pleural thickening of the visceral or parietal pleura, or both, compresses underlying parenchyma to form a radiographically appearing nodule or mass. In a series of 74 patients with rounded atelectasis, 64 (86%) had been exposed to asbestos.[88] Multiple or bilateral areas of involvement have been described.[89] This undoubtedly is the least common of the manifestations of exposure, although the exact prevalence is unknown. The radiographic appearance of these nodules is characteristically irregular, with a visible

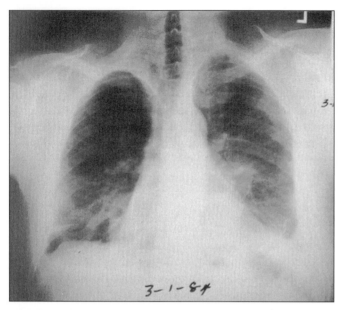

Figure 19.8.5: Posteroanterior chest x-ray of a 48-year-old insulator with a restrictive pulmonary impairment and exertional dyspnea, showing diffuse pleural thickening and bibasilar fibrosis (ILO 1/2).

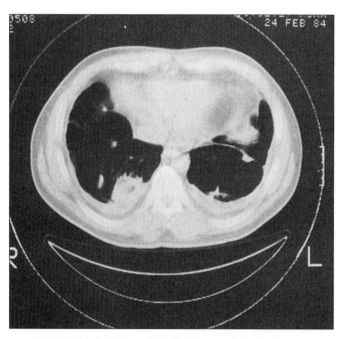

Figure 19.8.6: Chest CT of patient in Figure 19.8.5, showing right-sided posterior mass found at resection to be rounded atelectasis.

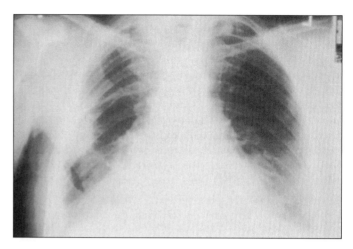

Figure 19.8.7: Posteroanterior chest x-ray of a 68-year-old brick mason with a restrictive pulmonary impairment and exertional dyspnea, and previous open thoracotomy, demonstrating the right pleural-based mass as pleural fibrosis; bilateral diffuse pleural thickening and bibasilar fibrosis are present.

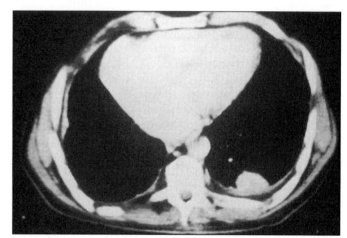

Figure 19.8.8: Chest CT of patient in Figure 19.8.7, showing left-sided posterior mass found at resection to be a well-differentiated adenocarcinoma.

Parenchyma

Asbestosis

Inhaled asbestos fibers cause an inflammatory response in the lung, characterized initially by alveolitis as well as peribronchiolitis, leading ultimately to persistent fibrotic parenchymal changes. Although some investigators have used the term asbestosis to encompass non-malignant asbestos-related pleural abnormalities, it is employed here to refer solely to the interstitial fibrosis and accompanying peribronchiolar fibrosis found in the parenchyma of affected individuals. Fibrosis may or may not be accompanied by pleural thickening and other pleural abnormalities. Among 4060 asbestos-exposed men enrolled in a randomized prospective chemoprevention trial (CARET Asbestos-Exposed Cohort), 18% had parenchymal opacities alone (ILO profusion score > 1/0), while 21% had both parenchymal opacities and pleural thickening.

band connecting the mass-like density to a region of pleural thickening. A more specific finding is the 'comet tail' or 'broom' sign, caused by pleura, bronchi, and blood vessels swirling from the hilum toward the rounded mass. CT scan (or occasionally bronchography) can provide adequate anatomic definition of the pleural base of the lesion and its distinctive features. Nonetheless, in the asbestos-exposed individual with pleural thickening and suspect rounded atelectasis, the risk for carcinoma remains high (Figs 19.8.6–19.8.8).

As noted above, all asbestos fiber types, including a wide spectrum of fiber lengths, cause asbestosis; there is thus no classification system based on fiber type or length. Further, it is often difficult to distinguish fiber types retrospectively, either historically, since many asbestos-containing materials represented a mixture of fiber types, or pathologically, due to variable biopersistence of specific fiber types in lung tissue. For example, chrysotile fiber bundles tend to fragment into narrower fibers in tissue, with leaching of magnesium, leading to greater degradation over time relative to amphibolic fibers but cumulative fibrogenic potential dose for dose is comparable.

The radiographic features of asbestosis, described in an earlier section, are similar to a number of other diffuse interstitial lung diseases, such as idiopathic pulmonary fibrosis. Concomitant pleural change, if present, increases the likelihood that the radiographic fibrosis is asbestosis; however, the absence of pleural change is not uncommon, and by no means excludes the diagnosis. It is useful for the clinician to consider the differential diagnosis of lower lobe (basilar) radiographic parenchymal fibrotic patterns, with associated volume loss or concomitant pleural thickening, listed in Table 19.8.3.

Asbestosis is classically described as a restrictive lung process, with impaired gas exchange manifest by diminished diffusing capacity. As discussed above (see Pulmonary Function), obstructive airway impairment also occurs, correlating with prominent and diffuse small airways changes.[90] Mixed obstructive and restrictive impairment is common, with bronchiolar effects of diminished mid-expiratory flow rates (e.g., FEF_{25-75}). Obstructive changes have been well documented in cohort studies after controlling for smoking, as well as in studies of non-smoking asbestos-exposed workers demonstrating airway dysfunction. The contribution of cigarette smoking, whether additive or synergistic, and the relative importance of parenchymal fibrosis versus dust load and concurrent occupational irritant exposures (e.g., welding fumes) are important factors contributing to risk for airflow obstruction.

The natural history of asbestosis is variable, and not always explained by exposure parameters, such as intensity, duration, and effect of exposure cessation. There is good evidence that a significant proportion of those with asbestosis will worsen clinically with time, even after exposure ceases; most, however, do not! Asbestosis is characterized by an accelerated loss of pulmonary function, that is likely mediated by an alveolitis, with asbestos-activated macrophages inducing inflammatory and subsequent fibrotic responses. Respiratory symptoms, particularly development or progression of dyspnea, correlate strongly with this accelerated ventilatory loss.

Asbestosis is associated with increased risk for lung cancer, mesothelioma, and other cancers. In a large prospective cohort study utilizing the Finnish Registry of Occupational Diseases, men with asbestosis ($n = 1376$) experienced a greater than sixfold increased risk for lung cancer (SIR 6.7; 95% CI 5.6–7.9), a 32-fold increased risk for mesothelioma (SIR 32: 95% CI 14–60), and a fourfold increased risk for laryngeal cancer (SIR 4.2; 95% CI 1.4–9.8).[91] Notably, among a subgroup of this cohort with identified progression of asbestosis radiographically, substantially increased lung cancer risk was observed (SIR 37; 95% CI 18–66).[92]

DIAGNOSIS AND TREATMENT

Many non-malignant asbestos-related pulmonary changes do not occur in isolation. The following discussion provides a general overview and summary of the approach to individual patients with asbestos exposure, at risk for a number of adverse outcomes. Criteria for the diagnosis of non-malignant asbestos-related diseases have been published,[93] and are currently being updated by the American Thoracic Society.

Diagnosis

The diagnosis of asbestosis, as with pleural thickening, rests on a history of sufficient exposure of appropriate latency and clinical, radiographic, and pulmonary function findings. The exposure history is a necessary but insufficient criterion. Suspicion for asbestos-related lung disease should be raised when moderate or greater exposure of more than six months duration, with latency of greater than 20 years from onset of exposure, has occurred. Rarely, high level exposures may be associated with shorter exposure durations and latencies.

Clinical, radiographic, and pulmonary function features are variably present. The patient with the classic presentation has basilar rales on physical examination, ILO profusion abnormalities of 1/0 or greater on chest radiograph (the minimal grade diagnostic of interstitial fibrosis), and restrictive or mixed restrictive-obstructive impairment on pulmonary function testing. A patient with asbestosis, however, may have the examination and pulmonary function findings just described, with an x-ray study not demonstrating significant parenchymal markings (e.g., ILO score 0/1). This is not surprising, given the non-concordance between histologically documented fibrosis and radiographic findings of parenchymal changes; such patients should be further evaluated with HRCT.

Asbestosis*‡
Idiopathic pulmonary fibrosis‡
Collagen vascular diseases‡
   Progressive systemic sclerosis
   Polymyositis
   Rheumatoid arthritis*
   Systemic lupus erythematosus*‡
Acute hypersensitivity pneumonitis**
Eosinophilic pneumonia
Lymphangitic carcinomatosis*

* Concomitant pleural involvement possible
† Variable mid-zone involvement with pneumonitis
‡ Diminished lung volumes often present
** Low lung volumes possible if persistent (chronic hypersensitivity reaction)

Table 19.8.3 Differential diagnosis of lower lobe (basilar) radiographic parenchymal fibrotic pattern

Although HRCT examination is more sensitive and specific than chest radiographs in detecting asbestos-related parenchymal disease, it is not required for diagnosis in most cases. Appropriate indications for HRCT in the diagnosis of non-malignant asbestos-related disease include equivocal chest radiographic findings, presence of significant respiratory symptoms and/or pulmonary function changes with an unremarkable chest radiograph, and the presence of extensive pleural abnormalities obscuring parenchymal markings.

The importance of diagnosing benign exudative pleuritis and rounded atelectasis rests largely on the need to exclude other diagnoses, particularly asbestos-related malignancies. The finding of isolated pleural thickening in an asbestos-exposed individual usually can be attributed to asbestos exposure when other causes are excluded, which is almost always possible by assessing clinical and radiographic findings.

Finally, invasive tissue sampling is virtually never required for the diagnosis of asbestosis or asbestos-related pleural disease. Pathologic assessment for parenchymal fibrosis, asbestos bodies, and fiber content may be useful, however, should tissue specimens become available from other therapeutic procedures (e.g., lung tissue obtained during thoracoscopic or open procedures for diagnosis and/or treatment of malignancy).

Treatment and management

As with a number of chronic interstitial lung diseases, asbestosis has an unfavorable clinical response to corticosteroids and other immunosupressive agents (e.g., cyclophosphamide and azathioprine). While it is possible that a subset of individuals with progressive alveolitis might benefit, no randomized clinical trials have established the efficacy of such therapy. The use of steroids is not routinely recommended, but may be considered on a case-by-case basis, with close monitoring of objective parameters (e.g., DLCO) to guide continuation of therapy.

Therapy for patients with asbestosis is supportive. Those with active respiratory symptoms and evidence of airflow obstruction may benefit from bronchodilators alone, or in combination with ipratropium or inhaled steroid therapy. In severe cases, oxygen saturation should be monitored periodically to assess need for supplemental oxygen. Bacterial infections should be promptly treated. Unlike silicosis, there is no evidence that asbestosis is associated with increased rates of tuberculosis or other atypical infections. Influenza and pneumococcal vaccines should be provided routinely.

Clinical management should focus on prevention, with smoking cessation being the primary emphasis, given the profound synergism between asbestos and smoking and lung cancer risk. Interestingly, evidence exists for a protective role of β-carotene on loss of ventilatory function in asbestos-exposed workers, with a 90 ml improvement in ventilatory capacity (FEV_1) associated with a 155 ng/ml increase in serum β-carotene concentration.[94] While this can be achieved with 15 mg/day β-carotene vitamin supplementation, routine supplementation cannot be recommended, due to the fact that participants in the trial taking 20–30 mg/day β-carotene experienced increased lung cancer and cardiovascular mortality. Given these findings, an adequate dietary intake of fruits and vegetables rich in β-carotene is prudent.

There is no evidence that removal of an affected individual from further exposure will alter the natural history of asbestos-related pleural or parenchymal fibrosis. Nonetheless, given the dearth of effective secondary interventions, it is prudent to eliminate or otherwise minimize all future asbestos exposures. Because of the economic ramifications, these decisions should be assessed on a case-by-case basis. Factors to be considered in whether or not even minimal exposure should continue include the extent of disease, and the intensity of exposure likely in the job. In developed countries, few jobs with exposures of fibrogenic potential still exist.

Although there is no clear evidence of the benefit of ongoing medical surveillance once a diagnosis of pleural or parenchymal abnormalities is made, the increased risk of lung cancer in this population, coupled with the benefits of early detection (e.g., surgical therapy for early stage cancer), has provided a cogent rationale for periodic examinations. Much recent interest has focused on the use of CT scan (e.g., spiral CT) to detect early asbestos-related cancers.[95] While the sensitivity of CT is excellent, high false-positive rates have limited the utility of CT lung cancer screening in asbestos-exposed workers. For example, a Finnish surveillance program reported 106 of 111 (95%) false positives among the nodular densities detected.[96] The benefits of early detection must therefore be weighed against the risks and costs of evaluating false positives (including invasive procedures). Routine CT screening is not recommended until prospective studies assessing impact on mortality are available.

Recommendations for periodic surveillance examinations for exposed workers without evidence of asbestos-related disease have ranged from every 2 to 5 years, and should be based on a consideration of latency from initial exposure. A Canadian task force on occupational respiratory diseases has made the following recommendations, which continue to provide useful guidelines, and which are required for some workers under regulatory standards (e.g., OSHA Regulations 29 CFR) (see Chapter 59): (1) occupationally exposed asbestos workers with normal chest radiographs and spirometry should receive an x-ray examination and spirometry every other year and (2) those with ILO category 1 profusion changes or greater, or suspicious symptoms or physical findings (e.g., increasing dyspnea or rales), should receive annual chest radiographs and spirometry, with full pulmonary function tests on alternate years. Medical monitoring for those with isolated pleural thickening should probably be no less than that recommended for those with normal radiographs, namely, biannual spirometry and x-ray studies, with more frequent testing in the presence of increasing symptoms or extensive pleural involvement.

Finally, the identification of these asbestos outcomes has the potential for affording affected individuals the benefit of compensation. Specific compensation systems vary within the United States and internationally,[97] depending on state or federal jurisdictions (see Chapter 57 Legal and Regulatory Issues in the Workplace). In general, workers' compensation covers the costs of medical care, including medical monitoring and treatment of complications, vocational rehabilitation, if needed, and the costs associated with attendant impairment and disability.

References

1. De Vuyst P, Karjalainen A, Dumortier P, et al. Guidelines for mineral fibre analyses in biologica samples: report of the ERS Working Group. Eur Respir J 1998; 11:1416–26.

2. United States Geologic Service (USGS) Minerals Information: Asbestos 2003. http://minerals.usgs.gov/minerals/pubs/commodity/asbestos/

3. Stayner LT, Dankovic DA, Lemen RA. Occupational exposure to chrysotile asbestos and cancer risk: a review of the amphibole hypothesis. Am J Public Health 1996; 86:179–86.

4. Committee on Nonoccupational Health Risks of Asbestiform Fibers. Asbestiform Fibers: Nonoccupational Health Risks. Board on Toxicology and Environmental Health Hazards, National Research Council. Washington DC: National Academy Press, 1984.

5. Collegium Ramazzini. Call for an international ban on asbestos. J Occup Environ Med 1999; 41:830–1.

6. Barnhart S, Keogh J, Cullen MR, et al. The CARET asbestos-exposed cohort: baseline characteristics and comparison to other asbestos-exposed cohorts. Am J Ind Med 1997; 32:573–81.

7. Omenn GS, Goodman GE, Thornquist MD, et al. Effects of a combination of beta-carotene and vitamin A on lung cancer and cardiovascular disease. N Engl J Med 1996; 334:1150–5.

8. Leigh J, Davidson P, Hendrie L, Berry D. Malignant mesothelioma in Australia, 1945–2000. Am J Ind Med 2002; 41:188–201.

9. Ferguson DA, Berry G, Jelihovsky T, et al. The Australian mesothelioma surveillance program 1979–85. Med J Aust 1987; 147:166–71.

10. Breysse PN, Weaver V, Cadorette M, et al. Development of a medical examination program for former workers at a Department of Energy national laboratory. Am J Ind Med 2002; 42:443–54.

11. Stern F, Lehman E, Ruder A. Mortality among unionized construction plasterers and cement masons. Am J Ind Med 2001; 39:373–88.

12. Safety and Health Topics: Asbestos. US Dept. of Labor Occupational Safety & Health Administration. August 28, 2003. http://www.osha.gov/SLTC/asbestos/

13. Asbestosis. American Lung Association, 2003 http://www.cheshire-med.com/programs/pulrehab/asbestosis.html

14. Selikoff IH, Lee DHK. Asbestos and disease. New York: Academic Press, 1978.

15. Nicholson WJ, Perkel G, Selikoff IJ. Occupational exposure to asbestosis: Population at risk and projected mortality, 1980–2030. Am J Ind Med 1982; 3:259–311.

16. Stayner L, Smith R, Bailer J, et al. Exposure–response analysis of risk of respiratory disease associated with occupational exposure to chrysotile asbestos. Occup Environ Med 1997; 54:646–52.

17. Ehrlich R, Lilis R, Chan E, Nicholson WJ, Selikoff IJ. Long term radiological effects of short term exposure to amosite asbestos among factory workers. Br J Ind Med 1992; 49:268–75.

18. Shepherd JR, Hillerdal G, McLarty J. Progression of pleural and parenchymal disease on chest radiographs of workers exposed to amosite asbestos. Occup Environ Med 1997; 54:410–5.

19. Jakobsson K, Strombert U, Albin M, Welinder H, Hagmar L. Radiological changes in asbestos cement workers. Occup Environ Med 1995; 52:20–27.

20. Berry G. Mortality of workers certified by pneumoconiosis medical panels as having asbestosis. Br J Ind Med 1981; 38:130–7.

21. Lilis R, Miller A, Bodbold J, Chan E, Selikoff IJ. Radiographic abnormalities in asbestos insulators: effects of duration from onset of exposure and smoking. Relationships of dyspnea with parenchymal and pleural fibrosis. Am J Ind Med 1991; 20:1–15.

22. Rogan WJ, Gladen BC, Ragan NB, Anderson HA. US prevalence of occupational pleural thickening: a look at x-rays from the first National Health and Nutrition Examination Survey. Am J Epidemiol 1987; 126:893–900.

23. Anderson HA, Lilis R, Daum SM, Selikoff IJ. Asbestosis among household contacts of asbestos factory workers. Ann NY Acad Sci 1979; 330:386–99.

24. Peipins LA, Lewin M, Campolucci S, et al. Radiographic abnormalities and exposure to asbestos-contaminated vermiculite in the community of Libby, Montana, USA. Environ Health Perspect 2003; 111:1753–9.

25. Agency for Toxic Substances and Disease Registry (ATSDR). Toxicological Profile for Asbestos (Update). Washington DC: DHHS, 1999.

26. Rom WN, Travis WD, Brody AR. Cellular and molecular basis of the asbestos-related diseases [State of the Art]. Am Rev Respir Dis 1991; 143:408–22.

27. Kienast K, Kaes C, Drumm K, et al. Asbestos-exposed blood monocytes-deoxyribonucleic acid strand lesions in co-cultured bronchial epithelial cells. Scand J Work Environ Health 2000; 26:71–7.

28. Quinlan TR, Berube KA, Marsh JP, et al. Patterns of inflammation, cell proliferation, and related gene expression in lung after inhalation of chrysotile asbestos. Am J Pathol 1995; 147:728–39.

29. Jaurand MC, Gaudrichet A, Atassi K, et al. Relationship between the number of asbestos fibres and the cellular and enzymatic content of bronchoalveolar fluid in asbestos exposed subjects. Bull Eur Physiopath Resp 1980; 16:595–606.

30. Report of the Pneumoconiosis Committee of the College of American Pathologists and the National Institute for Occupational Safety and Health. The pathology of asbestos-associated diseases of the lungs and pleural cavities: Diagnostic criteria and proposed grading schema. Arch Pathol Lab Med 1982; 106:544–96.

31. Selikoff IJ, Hammond EC, Seidman H. Mortality experience of insulation workers in the United States and Canada, 1943–1976. Ann NY Acad Sci 1979; 330:91–116.

32. Selikoff IJ, Seidman H. Asbestos-associated deaths among insulation workers in the United States and Canada, 1967–1987. Ann NY Acad Sci 1991; 643:1–14.

33. Markowitz SB, Marabia A, Lilis R, Miller A, Nicholson WJ, Levin S. Clinical predictors of mortality from asbestosis in the North American Insulator Cohort, 1981–1991. Am J Respir Crit Care Med 1997; 156:101–8.

34. Welch LS, Michaels D, Zoloth SR. The national sheet metal worker asbestos disease screening program: radiologic findings. Am J Ind Med 1994; 25:635–48.

35. Brodkin CA, Barnhart S, Anderson G, Checkoway H, Omenn GS, Rosenstock L. Correlation between respiratory symptoms and pulmonary function in asbestos-exposed workers. Am Rev Respir Dis 1993; 144:32–37.

36. Brodkin CA, Barnhart SB, Anderson G, et al. Longitudinal pattern of reported symptoms and accelerated ventilatory loss in asbestos exposed workers. Chest 1996; 109:120–6.

37. Yates DH, Browne K, Stidolph PN, Nevill E. Asbestos-related bilateral diffuse pleural thickening; natural history of radiographic and lung function abnormalities. Am J Respir Crit Care Med 1996; 153:301–6.

38. Kambic V, Radsel Z, Gale N. Alterations in the laryngeal mucosa after exposure to asbestos. Br J Ind Med 1989; 46:717–23.

39. Murphy RLH, Gaensler EA, Holford SK, Del Bono EA, Epler G. Crackles in the early detection of asbestosis. Am Rev Respir Dis 1984; 129:375–9.

40. International Labour Office. International Classification of Radiographs of Pneumoconioses. Geneva: International Labour Organization, 2003.

41. Rosenstock L, Hudson LD. The pleural manifestations of asbestos exposure. Occup Med 1987; 2:383–407.

42. Hillerdal G. Pleural and parenchymal fibrosis mainly affecting the upper lobes in persons exposed to asbestos. Resp Med 1990; 84:129–34.

43. Kipen HM, Lilis R, Suzuki Y, Valciukas JA, Selikoff IJ. Pulmonary fibrosis in asbestos insulation workers with lung cancer: a radiological and histopathological evaluation. Br J Ind Med 1987; 44:96–100.

44. Staples CA, Gamsu G, Ray CS, et al. High resolution computed tomography and lung function in asbestos-exposed workers with normal chest radiographs. Am Rev Respir Dis 1989; 139:1502–8.

45. Aberle DR, Gamsu G, Ray CS. High-resolution CT of benign asbestos-related diseases: clinical and radiographic correlation. Am J Roentgenol 1988; 151:883–91.

46. Genevois PA, De Vuyst P, Dedeire S, Cosaert J, Vande Weyer R, Sturyven J. Conventional and high-reolution CT in asymptomatic asbestos-exposed workers. Acta Radiol 1994; 35:226–9.

47. Neri S, Borashi P, Antonelli A, Falaschi F, Baschieri L. Pulmonary function, smoking habits, and high resolution computed tomography (HRCT) early abnormality of lung and pleural fibrosis in shipyard workers exposed to asbestos. Am J Ind Med 1996; 30:588–95.

48. Asbestosis and asbestos-related disease. In: Webb WR, Muller NL, Naidich DP, eds. High-resolution CT of the lung, 3rd edn. Philadelphia: Lippincott Williams & Wilkins, 2001;236–57.

49. Genevois PA, de Maertelaer V, Madani A, Winant C, Sergent G, De Vuyst P. Asbestosis, pleural plaques and diffuse pleural thickening: three distinct benign responses to asbestos exposure. Eur Respir J 1998; 11:1021–7.

50. Kraus T, Raithel HJ, Lehnert G. Computer-assisted classification system for chest X-ray and computed tomography findings in occupational lung disease. Int Arch Occup Environ Health 1997; 69:482–6.

51. Schwartz DA, Galvin JR, Yagla SJ, Speakman SB, Merchant JA, Hunninghake GW. Restrictive lung function and asbestos-induced pleural fibrosis. A quantitative approach. J Clin Invest 1993; 91:2685–92.

52. Jodoin G, Gibbs GW, Macklem PT, McDonald JC, Becklake MR. Early effects of asbestos exposure on lung function. Am Rev Respir Dis 1971; 104:525–35.

53. Kilburn KH, Warshaw RH, Einstein K, Bernstein J. Airway disease in non-smoking asbestos workers. Arch Environ Health 1985; 40:293–5.

54. Wang XR, Yano E, Wang M, Wang Z, Christiani DC. Pulmonary function in long-term asbestos workers in China. J Occup Environ Med 2001; 43:623–9.

55. Kennedy SM, Vedal S, Muller N, Kassam A, Chan-Yeung M. Lung function and chest radiograph abnormalities among construction insulators. Am J Ind Med 1991; 20:673–84.

56. Mohsenifar Z, Jasper AJ, Mahrer T, Koerner SK. Asbestos and airflow limitation. J Occup Med 1985; 28:817–20.

57. Churg A, Wright JL, Wiggs B, Pare PD, Lazar N. Small airways disease and mineral dust exposure. Am Rev Respir Dis 1985; 131:139–43.

58. Rodriquez-Roisin R, Merchant JE, Cochrane GM, Hickey BP, Turner-Warwick M, Clark TJ. Maximal expiratory flow volume curves in workers exposed to asbestos. Respiration 1980; 39:58–65.

59. Ohlson G, Rydman T, Sundell L, Bodin L, Hogstedt C. Decreased lung function in long-term asbestos cement workers: a cross-sectional study. Am J Ind Med 1984; 5:359–66.

60. Wang XR, Yano E, Nonaka K, Wang M, Wang Z. Pulmonary function of nonsmoking female asbestos workers without radiographic signs of asbestosis. Arch Environ Health 1998; 53:292–8.

61. Barnhart S, Hudson LD, Mason SE, et al. Total lung capacity. An insensitive measure of impairment in patients with asbestosis and chronic obstructive pulmonary disease? Chest 1988; 93:299.

62. Miller A, Teirstein AS, Selikoff IJ. Ventilatory failure due to asbestos pleurisy. Am J Med 1983; 75:911–9.

63. Schwartz DA, Fuortes LJ, Galvin JR, et al. Asbestos-induced pleural fibrosis and impaired lung function. Am Rev Respir Dis 1990; 141:321–6.

64. Jarvolm B, Sanden A. Pleural plaques and respiratory function. Am J Ind Med 1986; 10:419–26.

65. Miller A, Lilis R, Godbold J, Chan E, Selikoff IJ. Relationship of pulmonary function to radiographic interstitial fibrosis in 2611 long-term asbestos insulators Am Rev Respir Dis 1992; 145:263–70.

66. Hillerdal G, Malmberg P, Hemmingsson A. Asbestos-related lesions of the pleura: Parietal plaques compared to diffuse thickening studied with chest roentgenography, computed tomography, lung function, and gas exchange. Am J Ind Med 1990; 18:627–39.

67. Johnson NF, Haslam PL, Dewar Λ, Newman-Taylor AJ, Turner-Warwick M. Indentification of inorganic dust particles in bronchalveolar lavage macrophages by energy dispersive x-ray microoanalysis. Arch Environ Health 1986; 41:133–44.

68. Xaubet A, Rodriguez-Roisin R, Bombi JA, Marin A, Roca J, Agusti-Vidal A. Correlation of bronchalveolar lavage and clinical and functional findings in asbestosis. Am Rev Respir Dis 1986; 133:848–54.

69. Rom WN. Accelerated loss of lung function and alveolitis in a longitudinal study of non-smoking individuals with occupational exposure to asbestos. Am J Ind Med 1992; 21:835–44.

70. Sprince NC, Oliver LC, McCloud TC, Eisen EA, Christiani DC, Ginns LC. Asbestos exposure and asbestos-related pleural and parenchymal disease. Am Rev Respir Dis 1991; 143:822–8.

71. Hillerdal G. Pleural plaques and the risk for bronchial carcinoma and mesothelioma. Chest 1994; 105:144–50.

72. Watanabe N, Shimizu M, Kameda K, Kanazawa T, Seto H. Thallium-201 scintigraphy in malignant mesothelioma. Br J Radiol 1999; 72:308–10.

73. Cotes JE, Zejda J, King B. Lung function impairment as a guide to exercise limitation in work-related lung disorders. Am Rev Respir Dis 1988; 137:1089–93.

74. Sargent EN, Boswell WD, Ralls PW, Markovitz A. Subpleural fat pads in patients exposed to asbestos: distinction from non-calcified pleural plaques. Radiology 1984; 152:273–7.

75. Kee ST, Gamsu G, Blanc P. Causes of pulmonary impairment in asbestos-exposed individuals with diffuse pleural thickening. Am J Respir Crit Care Med 1996; 154:789–93.

76. Miller A, Bhuptani A, Sloane MF, Brown LK, Teirstein AS. Cardiorespiratory responses to incremental exercise in patients with asbestos-related pleural thickening and normal or slightly abnormal lung function. Chest 1993; 103:1045–50.

77. Sison RF, Hruban RH, Moore GW, Kuhlman JE, Wheeler PS, Hutchins GM. Pulmonary disease associated with pleural 'asbestos' plaques. Chest 1989; 95:831–5.

78. Hillerdal G, Henderson D. Asbestos, asbestosis, pleural plaques and lung cancer. Scand J Work Environ Health 1997; 23:93–103.

79. Lilis R, Lerman Y, Selikoff IJ. Symptomatic benign pleural effusions among asbestos insulation workers; residual radiographic abnormalities. Br J Ind Med 1988; 45:443–9.

80. Fielding DI, McKeon JL, Oliver WA, Matar K, Brown IG. Pleurectomy for persistent pain in benign asbestos-related disease. Thorax 1995; 50:181–3.

81. Barnhart S, Thornquist M, Omenn GS, Goodman G, Feigl P, Rosenstock L. The degree of roentgenographic parenchymal opacities attributable to smoking among asbetos-exposed subjects. Am Rev Respir Dis 1990; 141:1102–6.

82. Zitting AJ, Karjalainen A, Impivaara O, et al. Radiographic small lung opacities and pleural abnormalities in relation to smoking, urbainization status and occupational asbestos exposure in Finland. J Occup Environ Med 1996; 38:602–9.

83. Rosenstock L, Barnhart S, Heyer NJ, et al. The relation among pulmonary function, chest roentgenographic abnormalities, and smoking status in an asbestos-exposed cohort. Am Rev Respir Dis 1988; 138:272–7.

84. Robinson BWS, Musk AW. Benign asbestos pleural effusion: diagnosis and course. Thorax 1981; 36:896–900.

85. Hillerdal G, Ozesmi M. Benign asbestos pleural effusion: 73 exudates in 60 patients. Eur J Respir Dis 1987; 71:113–121.

86. Gaensler EA, Kaplan AI. Asbestos pleural effusion. Ann Intern Med 1971; 74:178–91.

87. Epler GR, McCloud TG, Gaensler EA. Prevalence and incidence of benign asbestos pleural effusion in a working population. JAMA 1982; 247:617–22.

88. Hillerdal G. Rounded atelectasis. Clinical experience with 74 patients. Chest 1989; 95:836–41.

89. Gamsu G, Aberle DR, Lynch D. Computed tomography in the diagnosis of asbestos-related thoracic disease. J Thoracic Imag 1989; 4:61–7.

90. Wright JL, Churg A. Severe diffuse small airways abnormalities in long term chrysotile asbestos miners. Br J Ind Med 1985; 42:556–9.

91. Karjalainen A, Pukkala E, Kauppinen T, Partanen T. Incidence of cancer among Finnish patients with asbestos-related pulmonary or pleural fibrosis. Cancer Causes Control 1999; 10:51–7.

92. Oksa P, Klockars M, Karjalainen A, et al. Progression of asbestosis predicts lung cancer. Chest 1998; 113:1517–21.

93. American Thoracic Society. The diagnosis of non-malignant disease related to asbestos. Am Rev Respir Dis 1986; 134:363–8.

94. Chuwers P, Barnhart S, Blanc P, et al. The protective effect of B-carotene and retinol on ventilatory function in an asbestos-exposed cohort. Am J Respir Crit Care Med 1997; 155:1066–71.

95. International expert meeting on new advances in the radiology and screening of asbestos-related diseases. Scand J Work Environ Health 2000; 26:449–54.

96. Tiitola M, Kivisaari L, Huuskonen MS, et al. Computerized tomography screening for lung cancer in asbestos-exposed workers. Lung Cancer 2002; 35:17–22.

97. Guidotti TL. Apportionment in asbestos-related disease for purposes of compensation. Ind Health 2002; 40:295–311.

19.9 Silicosis
Daniel E Banks

The most common health effect of occupational exposure to crystalline silica is silicosis, which remains the most common pneumoconiosis worldwide. This chapter will focus on the different clinical presentations and pathogenesis of silicosis, associated illnesses, their diagnosis and management. Silica exposure is discussed further in Chapter 46 and the health effects of coal mine dust which contains silica are addressed in Chapter 19.

Silicosis was first reported by the ancient Greeks and has been recognized throughout history.[1] The prevalence of this illness peaked in the last half of the 19th century and the early part of the 20th century, when mechanized industry was developing and the relationship between dust exposure and disease was less well understood. Yet, even today in developed countries, sporadic outbreaks of silicosis occur when workers are consistently exposed to silica particles of respirable size ($0.5–5.0$ µm in diameter)[2] at levels exceeding those recognized to be safe. The National Institute for Occupational Safety and Health reported that between 1968 and 1990 there were 13,744 deaths in the US where the death certificate mentioned silicosis. In more recent years the number attributable to silicosis appears to be lessening.[3]

Silicon dioxide, or silica, is the earth's most abundant mineral. Silica is considered to be either free (i.e., unbound to other minerals) or combined. Minerals with high amounts of free silica include quartz (including granite), flint, chert, opal, chalcedony, and diatomite. Combined forms of silica are called silicates and include, among others, asbestos, talc, and kaolin. This chapter will focus on the adverse pulmonary aspects of free silica exposure.[4]

Silica can exist in the crystalline or amorphous (non-crystalline) form. In the crystalline form, silica exists in different polymorphs (crystalline structures) as quartz, cristobalite, tridymite, coesite, and shistovite (Fig. 19.9.1). These are different in their structure, fibrogenicity, and biologic activity.[5] Of these, quartz is ubiquitous in the environment and occurs as sand as well as a constituent in many rocks. Cristobalite and tridymite occur naturally in lava and can be formed by the heating of quartz or amorphous silica. All but shistovite are arranged as a tetrahedral crystal.

Amorphous silica is non-crystalline and relatively less fibrogenic. It does not cause lung fibrosis. It occurs as diatomite (skeletons of prehistoric marine organisms) or as vitreous silica (glass), the result of carefully melting and then quickly cooling free crystalline silica. Heating diatomite (a process known as calcining), with or without alkali, forms cristobalite and adds the respiratory toxicity of free crystalline silica. Concerns regarding the impact of other minerals associated with the surface of the quartz particle on fibrogenicity have been considered, but have been inadequately researched.[6]

Many opportunities for occupational exposure to crystalline free silica of respirable size exist in the workplace. Some commonly encountered occupations in which the risk of silicosis exists are listed in Table 19.9.1. The Occupational

Safety and Health Administration permissible exposure limit (PEL) is 100 µg/m³ for an 8-hour work exposure.[7] There remains debate regarding whether this is a sufficiently protective standard.[8,9] In small, unregulated industries, as well as in numerous high-risk occupations, such as silica flour mill operations, sandblasting, drilling, and grinding, exposures have been documented to be excessive.[10]

The primary pulmonary illness attributable to silica exposure, silicosis, is caused by the inhalation of respirable size silica particles, and can be categorized by recognizable findings on the chest radiograph. The most typical presentations, simple silicosis and progressive massive fibrosis, appear different radiologically but are grouped under the category of classic silicosis because they are a part of the typical radiographic spectrum of this illness. Radiographically, simple silicosis appears as small (less than 10 mm in diameter) rounded opacities, typically predominant in the upper lung zones. Progressive massive fibrosis (also described as conglomerate silicosis) is the result of the coalescence of these small nodular opacities and appears as larger opacities (more than 20 mm in diameter), again typically distributed in the upper lung zones.

The other radiographic presentation of silicosis occurs only rarely and is referred to as silicoproteinosis, or acute silicosis. This condition appears as a basilar alveolar filling pattern following an overwhelming exposure to free crystalline silica over a short time span.

Bronchitis, a well-recognized effect of chronic dust inhalation, can occur with silica dust inhalation (see Chapter 19.4). Airway obstruction and lung function decline is most common with progressive fibrosis. In addition, silica exposure can be associated with autoimmune diseases (scleroderma, lupus erythematosus, rheumatoid arthritis (see Chapter 23.5)), nephropathy (see Chapter 25), tuberculosis (see Chapter 22), and lung cancer (see Chapter 30.1).[11]

CLASSIC SILICOSIS

Classic silicosis encompasses a continuum of severity ranging from simple silicosis (presenting as nodular pulmonary fibrosis with or without symptoms) to progressive massive fibrosis (severely disabling restrictive lung disease). These features usually develop slowly and frequently require a working lifetime to develop. However, in a small percentage of workers, the radiographic features of simple silicosis lead to progressive massive fibrosis in less than 10 years. Workers with these findings are described as having accelerated silicosis. Development of these radiographic features so soon after beginning exposure to silica means that progression of disease and severe respiratory impairment is very likely to occur.

The diagnosis of silicosis

There are three requirements for the diagnosis of silicosis. The first is a history of silica exposure sufficient to cause

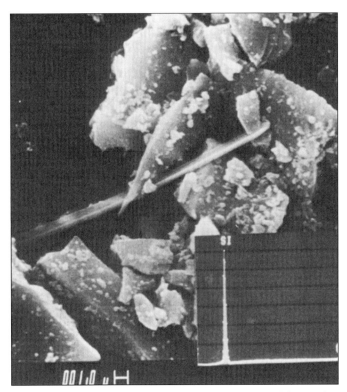

Figure 19.9.1: Scanning electron micrograph of a respirable sample of crystalline silica showing the diverse shape, size, and structure of these particles. Inset: An x-ray energy spectrometric analysis of a silica particle showing a distinct peak for silica (Si).

Occupation	Exposure
Mining	Silica contaminates the mined material
Milling	Dry, finely ground silica (silica flour) for abrasives and filler
Quarrying and stone work	Slate, granite, and sandstone exposures
Foundry work	Silica as a mold: fettling and chipping to make a better molded product
Sandblasting	Ship building, oil rig maintenance, preparing steel for painting
Pottery making	Crushing flint and fettling are major sources of exposure
Glass making	Sand used to polish and as an abrasive
Boiler work	Cleaning boilers may result in exposure to refractory brick and clouds of quartz dust

Table 19.9.1 Major industries with silica exposure

this illness. The second is the presence of chest radiograph features consistent with silicosis. The third is the absence of other illnesses that mimic silicosis. When all criteria are fulfilled, the diagnosis of silicosis can be made with confidence and additional clinical investigations are unnecessary. Uncommonly, particularly when other chest illnesses such as rheumatoid nodules, tumor, infection, other pneumoconiosis, or sarcoidosis cannot be clinically ruled out, and/or the exposure history is inconclusive, additional studies such as HRCT scan and lung biopsy are necessary to clarify the diagnosis.

When tissue for diagnostic analysis is required, an open lung biopsy is preferred, as more adequate tissue is obtained, and risk of pneumothorax from transbronchial biopsy is avoided. Because the silicotic lung is stiff in the upper zones and emphysematous in the lower zones, the incidence and morbidity associated with the development of pneumothoraces may be increased with a transbronchoscopic lung biopsy. However, transbronchial biopsy, in association with elemental analysis of bronchoalveolar lavage fluid for silica, has been used in the diagnosis of silicosis.[12]

Determining whether or not silica exposure in the workplace is sufficient to cause silicosis can be difficult and requires clinical judgment tempered by knowledge of the pitfalls in making the diagnosis. Silicosis generally requires prolonged exposure to respirable crystalline free silica at levels exceeding government standards. However, substantial individual differences in susceptibility exist. The most important factors in assessing exposure include the length of employment, exposure measurements (if available), and whether or not the worker was provided with effective respiratory protection. As a rule, the worker's silica exposure occurs as a part of a process that makes the silica particle respirable size. Without exposure to respirable size silica particles silicosis does not occur. The adequacy of respiratory protection devices is highly variable.

The diagnosis of silicosis should not be dismissed even if the worker provides a history of the use of a personal respirator. For example, a worker employed as a sandblaster for 15 years who had used respiratory protection might have a chest radiograph showing a background of small rounded opacities with superimposed bilateral upper zone masses (consistent with progressive massive fibrosis). In this case, the clinical picture would be very consistent with silicosis and the respiratory protection most likely was not adequate. Although respiratory protection has been thought of as an effective measure of preventing dust exposure, not infrequently workers who wear respiratory protection are not sufficiently protected.[13]

Data regarding the silica dust levels in the workplace, if available, can provide important information, but for many reasons may not accurately reflect a worker's exposure to silica over many years. Cases of acute silicosis in surface coal mine drillers have been reported where the measured dust levels were within normal limits. In this example, the measurements were not representative of the overwhelming dust exposures. Therefore, although dust measurements can be helpful, understanding the conditions under which the samples were collected and having confidence that these measurements represent the usual workplace environment are essential.

Individual differences in susceptibility to the effects of silica exposure remain poorly understood, with some workers developing much more severe disease than others employed in the same environment. Dufresne attempted to understand the silica dust burden and particle sizes in those with differing degrees of silicosis. The amount of quartz exposure retained and the length that the particles remained in the lung is important, but there was considerable variability and the investigators were unable to linearly correlate duration of dust in the lung and lung burden.[14] Recent studies suggest that the risk and severity of silicosis may be related in part to tumor necrosis factor-alpha (TNF-α) and interleukin-1 (IL-1) polymorphisms.[15,16]

Pathogenesis and histologic features of classic silicosis

Most forms of silicosis develop slowly. Usually 10 to 30 years are required from the beginning of exposure to the onset of clinical manifestations. Although host factors such as genetics, smoking, and underlying diseases may play a part in the development of silicosis, the most important factors include silica dust concentration in the air, duration of dust exposure, the crystalline structure of the silica particles, the percent of free silica, and the particle size.

Particles less than 5.0 μm in diameter are deposited in the alveoli, most often in the upper lung zones. Particles less than 1.0 μm in diameter are believed to be the most fibrogenic and most able to penetrate into the interstitium.[17] When lung cells in culture were exposed to equal masses of quartz, the smallest size fraction generated the most potent inflammatory response.[18] Depending on particle size, up to 80% of the silica dust is cleared quickly, with the small fraction of retained particles initiating the fibrogenic process.

The slow progression of simple silicosis in humans has made the study of the pathogenesis of this illness difficult. However, the use of animal models and in-vitro studies has made it possible to investigate the effects of exposure to silica particles. Studies of the factors in the BAL fluid collected from silica exposed workers have also provided insight into the pathogenesis of this illness.[19] The pathogenesis of silicosis has recently been reviewed.[20] Briefly, inhaled silica particles interact with alveolar macrophages and other lung cells in a complex cascade of events resulting in lung inflammation, fibrosis, and tissue remodeling forming silicotic nodules.[21,22] Key to the biologic response to silica appears to be its crystalline structure, highly reactive surface groups that generate free radicals and reactive oxygen species (ROS),[23,24] and persistence in lung tissue.

A complex cascade of events has been described.[21] Silica particles are directly cytotoxic and can react with cell membranes causing cell injury, oxidant damage, and release of inflammatory mediators. Silica particles can also react with scavenger receptors sites on alveolar macrophages, with the generation of ROS and inflammatory cytokines.

The primary cellular event in the pathogenesis of silicosis is the interaction between the silica particle and the alveolar macrophage. Retained silica particles are phagocytized by resident macrophages or penetrate the interstitium. Alveolar macrophages become activated, and an intense inflammatory response results with the production of ROS, activation of nuclear transcription factors NK-κB, and AP-1,[25,26] and release of a variety of inflammatory cytokines and mediators that recruit and activate inflammatory cells, including neutrophils and lymphocytes, promoting fibroblast proliferation and fibrotic responses. Key mediators include IL-1, TNF-α, transforming growth

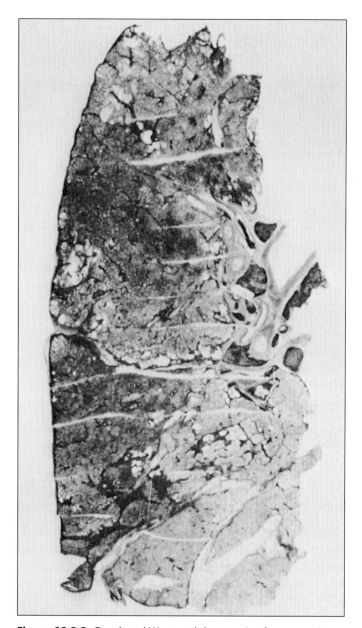

Figure 19.9.2: Gough and Wentworth lung section from a granite worker showing simple silicosis. Sparse silicotic nodules are present in the lung parenchyma. Hilar lymph nodes are more prominent and show silicotic lesions. Note the scattered changes of centrilobular and paraseptal emphysema.

factor-β, fibronectin, and chemokines, as well as cytokines which may downregulate inflammation such as IL-10.[27-35]

The net result of this ongoing inflammatory process is the silicotic nodule, the histologic hallmark of silicosis. This nodule usually forms near the small bronchioles. In some workers with relatively low silica exposure, inhaled silica is efficiently cleared from the lung and deposited in the lymph nodes. In this instance, presentation of calcified regional hilar lymph nodes on the chest radiograph may be noted without an extensive background of small rounded opacities (Fig. 19.9.2). In most cases, however, the lung cannot effectively clear the dust, and nodules begin to form by the arrangement of a collection of dust-laden

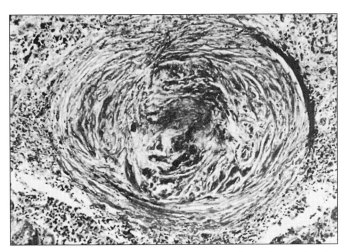

Figure 19.9.3: Photomicrograph (230×) of a well-developed silicotic nodule, with central hyalinization and concentrically arranged collagen fibers providing the onion-skin appearance. Peripherally, a rim of dust containing macrophages is seen.

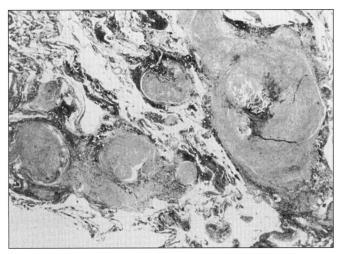

Figure 19.9.4: Photomicrograph (40×) of numerous silicotic nodules in close proximity that are beginning to coalesce, an early stage of the development of progressive massive fibrosis. The largest of these nodules shows central necrosis.

macrophages that is loosely surrounded by a reticulum of fibrous tissue. Eventually, a more defined central zone develops containing a mixture of hyalinized connective tissue and silica dust. This area becomes surrounded by relatively dust-free concentrically arranged fibrous tissue yielding an onion skin-like pattern (Fig. 19.9.3). Active inflammation and ongoing fibrosis occur at the periphery, a region composed of dust-laden macrophages, a halo of silica particles, and randomly arranged collagen fibers. As the nodules enlarge and coalesce, they form large conglomerate lesions typically found in the upper lobes (Fig. 19.9.4). These may encroach on the airways and pulmonary vasculature, and lead to a significant degree of pulmonary impairment. At some point, the central zone of this coalesced mass, now recognized as progressive massive fibrosis, may enlarge to a size exceeding its blood supply, resulting in central necrosis. Nodules may begin de novo or continue to enlarge even after exposure has ceased. Discontinuing silica exposure once silicosis is diagnosed is important but does not guarantee that the disease will not progress.

Polarized light microscopic examination reveals silica particles if they are present. Silica particles in tissue also may be demonstrated using the technique of scanning electron microscopy, and identified with mass spectrometry (Fig. 19.9.1).

Simple silicosis

Workers with simple silicosis usually do not have chest symptoms. Some, however, report a chronic productive cough, a feature likely similar to industrial bronchitis from dust exposure. Physical examination of the chest usually is unremarkable; audible coarse sounds are the result of coexisting bronchitis.

Roentgenographically, simple silicosis typically appears as an upper zone distribution of rounded opacities less than 1 cm in diameter (Fig. 19.9.5). These opacities are

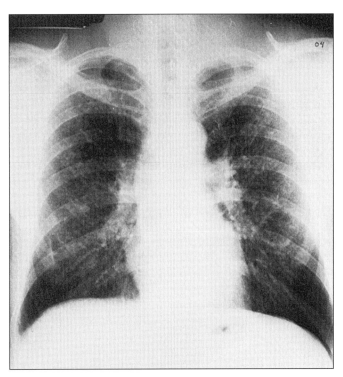

Figure 19.9.5: This PA chest radiograph is taken from a 24-year-old worker employed for 5 years as a bagger in the production of silica flour. Small rounded opacities (ILO 2/2) are diffusely present in both mid- and upper zones, consistent with simple silicosis. The development of this extent of simple silicosis in such a short time is consistent with accelerated silicosis that may rapidly progress toward respiratory impairment, progressive massive fibrosis, and premature death.

indistinguishable from those seen in simple coal workers' pneumoconiosis (see Chapter 19.10). Hilar lymph nodes are often enlarged with a distinctive peripheral calcification, described as eggshell calcification.

High-resolution CT scans have been to shown to have a good correlation with the nodular findings of silicosis on the chest radiograph, and a better description of the extent of emphysema compared to the chest radiograph.[36] Correlation between lung function tests and the chest radiograph and CT scan is variable. In simple silicosis it is primarily the degree of emphysema (in the presence of a history of cigarette smoking) rather than the extent of silicosis that determines pulmonary function.[37] Yet, the high-resolution CT scan has not been shown to clearly be more sensitive than the chest radiograph in the early detection of silicosis.[38] Gallium scanning has not been found to be sensitive or specific for silicosis.[39]

Pulmonary function studies in simple silicosis do not usually demonstrate functional impairment. There may be a trend for values to progress toward airways obstruction with a decrease in FEV_1 out of proportion to the decrease in FVC, a mild diminution in TLC and ventilatory capacities, and decreases in the helium equilibration time and compliance as the extent of profusion of small rounded opacities increases. This is most clearly exhibited in those with progressive massive fibrosis. As the disease progresses, reduction in compliance usually precedes the reductions in vital capacity or forced expiratory flow rate.

Among working South African middle-aged white gold miners, men with simple silicosis had lower FEV_1 values compared to those exposed without radiographic evidence of disease. The frequency of bronchitis was similar in the two groups. Those with silicosis missed work more often due to chest infections than their similarly exposed counterparts. Miners with silicosis appear to have the same or slightly more airway obstruction than men without silicosis who have had similar total exposure to dust.[40] Others have shown that silica dust exposure, independent of silicosis, is associated with chronic obstructive airways disease.[41] Pathologic studies demonstrating emphysematous changes support these findings.

Progressive massive fibrosis

Progressive massive fibrosis is the result of the conglomeration of small rounded opacities. It has been traditionally recognized that progressive massive fibrosis develops on a background of advanced simple silicosis. However, among coal workers who develop progressive massive fibrosis, not all have an advanced degree of simple coal workers' pneumoconiosis (see Chapter 19.10). Whether or not this also is the case in patients with silicosis is not clear.[42]

The respiratory symptoms present in a worker with progressive massive fibrosis can be variable. They range from only a chronic productive cough to exertional dyspnea and, in some persons, ultimately to respiratory failure. With time, however, the coalescence of silicotic nodules takes a toll on the underlying pulmonary parenchyma in all, with the usual result being progressive respiratory impairment.

Physical examination demonstrates decreased breath sounds on auscultation and, if the illness is extensive, signs of cor pulmonale and impending respiratory failure.

Crackles usually are not audible, and clubbing, if present, is attributable to another cause.

The chest roentgenogram reveals confluent nodules greater than 1 cm in diameter on a background of small rounded opacities characteristic of simple silicosis. The confluence of these nodules begins peripherally and migrates centrally. As with simple silicosis, progressive massive fibrosis develops most prominently in the upper lobes (Fig. 19.9.6). As these fibrous masses in the upper lobe progressively enlarge, the hila are retracted upward and the lower zones become hyperinflated and appear emphysematous (Fig. 19.9.7).

Pulmonary function studies initially demonstrate a decrease in compliance, followed by decreases in lung volumes and diffusing capacity. If bronchial distortion and lower zone hyperinflation are present, the forced expiratory time is likely to be prolonged and airflow obstruction is measurable.

Deterioration in lung function commonly occurs despite discontinuing silica exposure, and apparently unrelated to commonly measured immune markers.[43] The likelihood of

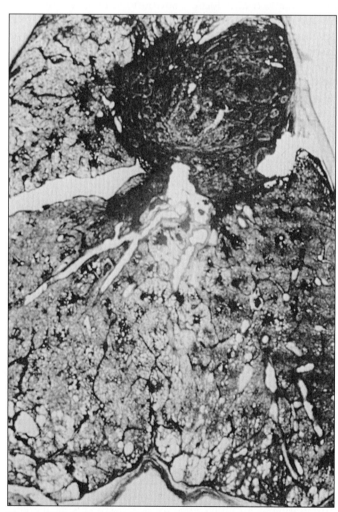

Figure 19.9.6: Gough and Wentworth whole lung section from a miner employed for many years as a motorman. This shows a large, dark upper zone mass consistent with progressive massive fibrosis and calcified lymph nodes. Scattered mid-zone nodules as well as basilar emphysema are present.

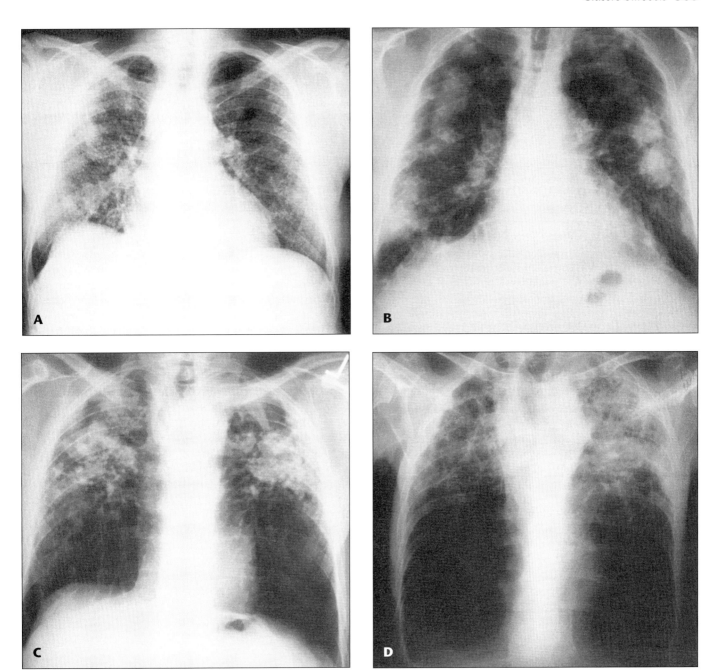

Figure 19.9.7: This series of chest radiographs reflects the different presentations of progressive massive fibrosis. (a) Chest radiograph from a 56-year-old man taken 7 years after ceasing employment at a silica flour mill where he had been employed for 6 years as a bagger. He complained of symptoms of dyspnea and chronic bronchitis. He had an 8-year smoking history. Spirometry showed borderline restriction. The chest radiograph showed profuse small rounded opacities and progressive massive fibrotic lesions in the right upper and mid-zones. (b) Chest radiograph from a surface mine driller who had smoked heavily for many years. Asymmetric bilateral upper zone progressive massive fibrotic lesions are present. The larger and denser left-sided mass lesion raises concern of a pulmonary malignancy. (c) Chest radiograph from a long-time underground coal miner who worked as a driller showing the 'angel wing' changes that occur with progressive massive fibrosis. The wings are the bilateral peripheral massive fibrotic lesions, and the body of the angel is the cardiac silhouette. (d) Chest radiograph from a worker employed for many years in a glass factory with silicosis who then experienced a relatively aggressive downhill course. Investigation revealed infection with *M. tuberculosis*. Although he responded to multiple drug therapy, he still had severe progressive massive fibrosis, extensive emphysema, and impaired function.

progression directly correlates with the duration and concentration of silica exposure, the amount of silicosis determined on the chest radiograph at the time of diagnosis, as well as the presence or absence of mycobacterium infection. In addition, black workers have been reported to progress more rapidly than their white counterparts.

Progression appears to slow as time from diagnosis increases.[44-46] Among non-smokers, it is usually those with progressive massive fibrosis who develop clinically important airflow obstruction and emphysema.

A recent report from Hong Kong reflects data from 648 workers with silicosis employed in numerous industries, but primarily caisson workers, hard rock drillers employed in bridge and building foundation construction, and stone splitters.[47] Workers with silicosis averaged 24 years of exposure. Most had simple silicosis with no significant lung function impairment but complained of respiratory symptoms. Nearly half of the silicotics had radiographic evidence of current or past tuberculosis. Approximately 70% had minimal (category 1) profusion of small rounded opacities, another 5% had more profuse radiographic findings, while 25% had progressive massive fibrosis.

Accelerated silicosis

Accelerated silicosis is characterized by the same features as classic silicosis except that the time from initial exposure to silica to the development of radiographic changes and ensuing respiratory impairment is much shorter. The chest radiograph may demonstrate rounded opacities as early as 4 years after initial silica exposure. This relatively early onset of silicosis occurs as a result of exposure to grossly excessive levels of dust. Accelerated silicosis is associated with frequent and relatively rapid progression to progressive massive fibrosis with severe respiratory impairment.

Seaton reported on an outbreak of silicosis among eight stonemasons working with sandstone on a cathedral. Although a number had accelerated silicosis, one with similar exposure had adenopathy alone.[48] The authors concluded that workers with accelerated disease had had chronic but relatively low-grade exposure to silica dust many years prior to the current substantial exposure. This previous exposure may have obstructed the lymphatics and caused an inability to clear the silica from the alveolar space.[49] There are correlates in animal models. In different rat species, the importance of lymphatic clearance of dust has been documented in the response to silica.[50] Substantial, but not well understood variation in the pulmonary pathologic response to aerosolized silica exposure has been shown in different strains of inbred rats.[51] It also appears that underlying epithelial injury accentuates the translocation of silica from the alveolus into the interstitium and lymphatic system.[52]

Acute silicosis

This most aggressive form of silicosis follows a short duration of exposure to overwhelmingly high concentrations of respirable free silica. The worker has a relatively rapid onset of chest symptoms and progressive respiratory impairment that invariably leads to death due to respiratory failure. Although patients with this form of silicosis may have some features of classic silicosis, there are distinct clinical, radiographic, and histologic differences.

In 1900 an illness referred to as 'chalicosis pulmonum', that developed after employment in a Nevada quartzite mill for only 3 months, was reported.[53] Deaths of a large number of these workers occurred within a year after the onset of symptoms. In 1929, Middleton described a febrile illness associated with progressive respiratory failure after exposures to overwhelming amounts of free crystalline silica among packers of abrasive soap powder in a London plant.[54] The first reported series of this aggressive manifestation of silicosis in the United States also involved exposure to abrasive soap powder. In 1932, Chapman described the death of three silica abrasive packers only 8–29 months after initial exposure.[55] Since these early reports, acute silicosis has been described in quartz tunnel drillers, sandblasters, silica flour workers, and surface coal mine drillers.

In each of these occupations, workers were exposed to high concentrations of fine, freshly fractured silica. As noted above, freshly fractured silica may well be more fibrogenic than 'stale' particles because of the ROS present on the freshly cut particles as described above.[56]

In 1969, Buechner reported four sandblasters with acute silicosis and coined the term 'silicoproteinosis' to describe these histologic findings.[57] At autopsy, these sandblasters had periodic acid-Schiff (PAS) positive-staining proteinaceous material filling the alveolar spaces, silica particles in the lung, and histologic changes of alveolar proteinosis (Fig. 19.9.8). However, a review of the literature prior to Buechner's description suggests that many of the earlier patients had similar histologic features.[58]

Workers with acute silicosis have been reported to present with an irritative, sometimes productive cough, weight loss, fatigue, and, occasionally, pleuritic pain.[59] The onset of symptoms usually is 1–3 years after the initial exposure; however, symptoms occurring less than a year after beginning sandblasting have been reported. Unlike the usually unremarkable chest examination of classic silicosis, crackles usually are present and likely reflect alveolar and airway fluid. Patients can rapidly develop cyanosis, symptoms of cor pulmonale, and respiratory failure. Survival after the onset of symptoms is typically less than 2 years. Infectious processes, particularly macrophage-mediated infections such as mycobacterial and fungal infections, frequently complicate the clinical course.

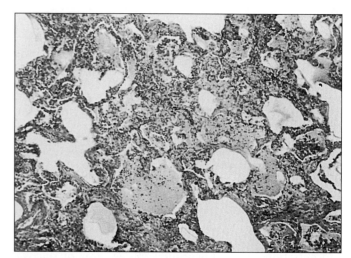

Figure 19.9.8: Photomicrograph (100×) of a lung section of a surface mine driller showing acute silicoproteinosis. Aveolar spaces are filled with a finely granular, PAS positive-staining exudate with eosinophils. Alveolar walls show thickening, with an infiltration of mononuclear cells and lymphocytes.

More recently, six cases of acute silicosis were described following varying times of excessive, overwhelming exposures to silica. Patients presented with cough and disabling dyspnea. Clubbing, not a typical feature in classic silicosis, was present in three and coarse chest sounds were audible in two. Lung function studies showed apparent restriction with severe decrease in diffusing capacity. BAL revealed lymphocytosis and neutrophilia. Four died of silicosis.[60]

The chest radiograph typically reveals diffuse alveolar infiltration and obliteration usually associated with air bronchograms.[61-63] The picture is one of a ground-glass appearance, and small rounded opacities are usually not seen. The chest radiographic progression is rapid. With time, these areas of alveolar filling progress to large masses consistent with progressive massive fibrosis. Cavity formation may occur and be difficult to distinguish from superimposed mycobacterial or fungal infection.

The alveoli are filled with lipid and proteinaceous exudative material, which under light microscopy is relatively acellular, with a granular, PAS-positive staining appearance. Silicotic nodules, if present, are smaller and more irregular than those seen in classic silicosis. Diffuse interstitial fibrosis is seen. Alveolar and vascular obliteration also occurs. Electron microscopy studies have demonstrated diffuse hyperplasia of type II pneumocytes, with hyperproduction of lipoproteins.[64] Within the alveolar spaces there are desquamated type II pneumocytes, macrophages, silica particles, and phospholipids.

Acute silicosis usually can be diagnosed on the basis of a history of overwhelming silica exposure, the above-described clinical features, and a chest radiograph consistent with this illness. However, the illness is relatively rare and often physicians find it difficult to believe that such extensive dust disease can occur in such a relatively short time. Rarely lung tissue may be needed for an accurate diagnosis, and an open lung biopsy is recommended. Frequently, workers with acute silicosis also have mycobacterial infection. Despite appropriate therapy, these workers continue to deteriorate. The differential diagnosis includes alveolar proteinosis, desquamative interstitial pneumonitis, and lipoid pneumonia, but these conditions can usually be excluded on the basis of the worker's history.

ASSOCIATED ILLNESSES
Silica exposure and mycobacterial infections

The association between silicosis and tuberculosis has been recognized since the mid 16th century and has been the subject of extensive epidemiologic studies. The reported prevalence of tuberculosis has varied from 75% in an autopsy study of silicotic South African gold miners in 1916[65] to 0.9% in 1975,[66] and to 3.9% in 1991,[67] and continues to increase in the face of silicosis and epidemic HIV infection. The incidence of tuberculosis is likely to be greater in workers with accelerated or acute silicosis.

Silica particles increase the susceptibility to mycobacterial infection by altering cell-mediated immunity[68] and macrophage function, diminishing the ability of the cellular milieu in the lung to defend itself against this infection.[69,70]

Several concepts are important to the understanding of the risk of mycobacterial infection, especially tuberculosis, in those with silica exposure. First, silica exposure, by itself and in the absence of silicosis, is a risk factor for tuberculosis.[71] Since only 34% of those with silicosis were recognized radiographically in one autopsy study, it is clear that recognizing silica exposure is important in determining risk.[72] Second, the frequency of mycobacterial infection appears to increase as the extent of radiographic change attributable to silicosis advances, and can develop after the worker ceases exposure.[73] Third, in the absence of radiographic evidence of silicosis, as silica exposure increases the risk for tuberculosis also increases.[74] Fourth, in a case-control study, those with silica exposure and tuberculosis died, on average, 4 years earlier than those with tuberculosis lacking silica exposure history.[75]

The diagnosis of tuberculosis in workers with silicosis sometimes can be difficult. Because tuberculous infections can be walled off in the lung by silica-induced fibrosis, a false-negative acid-fast-staining sputum smear may occasionally be present. Constitutional symptoms, such as fatigue, fever, dyspnea, and weight loss, can be seen in workers with worsening silicosis independent of a mycobacterial infection. Finally, the radiographic changes of tuberculosis may mimic advanced silicosis. The most important feature that enhances the clinician's suspicion for tuberculosis is radiographic progression over a short time period. This indicates superimposed mycobacterial infection until proven otherwise. A new infiltrate, coalescence of nodules in the upper lung fields, or cavitation of a pre-existing lesion mandates an aggressive search for mycobacterial organisms.

Recent studies have shown that the combination of silicosis and tuberculosis is more difficult to treat than tuberculosis alone, but multiple drug regimens achieve acceptable results. A 1989 study of South African gold miners compared multiple drug regimens.[76] A four-drug regimen for 4.5 months produced a relapse rate of only 3.8%. Other studies in which standard multi-drug anti-tuberculosis therapy was provided for 9–24 months have reported relapse rates of 0–5.1%. The epidemic of HIV infection in the South African gold mining population, in association with underlying silica dust exposure and silicosis, has led to epidemic mycobacterial transmission.[77-79]

Those with silicosis should undergo regular PPD skin testing. The frequency of this testing is not clear; however, in countries with a high endemic rate of tuberculosis, yearly testing is appropriate. If tuberculosis is less frequent, less frequent testing would be appropriate. If the results of the PPD test become positive without clinical evidence of active tuberculosis, at least 1 year of isoniazid therapy is indicated. Many advocate longer, even lifelong, antituberculosis prophylactic therapy in this setting because of the possibility of extensive irreversible damage to the silicotic lung by this organism.

Silicosis and carcinoma of the lung

Since the initial report by Goldsmith in 1982[80] linking silica and lung cancer, a number of articles and reports supporting or disputing this relationship[81-83] have been published. In 1997, the International Agency for Research on Cancer (IARC) reviewed the evidence and concluded that there is sufficient evidence to judge silica a carcinogen for humans.[84] The risk of lung cancer is highest in workers with silicosis who also smoke. The risk in those exposed to silica but without silicosis is less clear. See Chapter 30.2 for further discussion.

Connective tissue disease (see Chapter 23.5)

Silicosis is associated with an increased prevalence of autoimmune serology, elevated gamma globulin levels, and an increased frequency of connective tissue disease.[85-87] Although relatively infrequent, in one report of granite workers, approximately 1.5 per 100 workers with silica exposure developed morbidity due to arthritis, a prevalence greater than the general population.[88] Of the connective tissue diseases, scleroderma has probably been most commonly recognized in the past, with experimental data showing that silica dust is able to activate microvascular endothelial cells, mononuclear cells, and dermal fibroblasts in vitro in a fashion in common with pathophysiologic events known from idiopathic scleroderma.[89] This is recognized as a compensable occupational illness in several countries.[90] Steenland reported on a number of studies demonstrating increased rates of arthritis, scleroderma, rheumatoid arthritis, musculoskeletal disease, and renal insufficiency in silica exposed populations compared to non-silica exposed populations.[91] Of these, the least well associated with autoimmunity was renal disease.

More recently a review of 583 cases with death certificates identifying silicosis with scleroderma, lupus erythematosus, or rheumatoid arthritis showed that the risk was increased 2.5–15-fold greater than the general population, with rheumatoid arthritis occurring most frequently.[92] Importantly, these connective tissue diseases occurred in men, far different than the population of patients with connective tissue disease occurring in the absence of silicosis.[92]

In 1953, Caplan noted that the course of coal workers' pneumoconiosis in workers with dust exposure could be influenced by coexisting rheumatoid arthritis. In this group of workers, upper zone peripheral nodules appeared more frequently in the lungs of workers with rheumatoid arthritis. This presentation of rheumatoid nodules in workers with silica exposure has been termed Caplan's syndrome.[93]

Yet the role of the immune system is not well understood in silicosis. Antinuclear antibodies and elevated immunoglobulin levels have not correlated with the baseline profusion category of the chest radiograph, the rate of chest radiographic progression, or the rate of lung function decline in sandblasters with silicosis.[94]

Renal and extrapulmonary involvement (see Chapter 25)

Although the kidney may be the primary target organ for extrapulmonary involvement in silicosis, the data that relate renal changes to silica exposure are found mainly in a series of case reports and case series. Renal disease has been attributed both to a toxic effect or silica or an immunologically mediated process. The renal glomerular changes have not been consistent among the different workers with silica exposures, and there is no single clinical or laboratory finding of silica-induced nephropathy. We are unaware of reports showing increased levels of silica in the kidney or silicotic nodules in the kidneys of those with silicosis. It may be that the changes found in the kidney in these workers are immunologically mediated and are host- rather than silica-dose dependent.

One worker with acute silicosis developed acute glomerulonephritis and renal failure in the absence of underlying renal impairment.[95] The authors postulated a silica-induced defect in lipid metabolism in the renal cells. Six of 15 cases of silicosis in an autopsy study showed focal segmental glomerulosclerosis as well as pathology that included necrotizing and proliferative glomerulonephritis, mesangial hyperplasia, focal segmental obliteration of loops, and focal proliferative changes in Bowman's capsule.

A mortality study of silica-exposed workers found that mortality attributable to chronic nephritis was twice as high in silica-exposed workers compared with workers who had not been exposed to silica.[96] More recently, Rosenman showed that chronic kidney disease should be considered to be a complication of silicosis; however, it is not clear if this is a nephrotoxic or autoimmune effect.[97]

Silicotic lesions have also been described in the liver, spleen, bone marrow, and remote lymph nodes. These lesions are presumably the result of lymphatic or hematogenous spread and have not been recognized to affect the function of these organs.

PREVENTION, MANAGEMENT, AND TREATMENT

Prevention of silicosis remains the goal among exposed workers. Product substitution of silica with less toxic particles in abrasive blasting, control of air-borne dust concentration through engineering interventions, and appropriate use of respiratory protective devices are available and are effective in preventing the development of silicosis. Yet, new cases continue to develop.[98]

Since the initiation of dust control, the prevalence of silicosis has decreased dramatically.[99] In some mines and quarries, compliance with dust concentration has been achieved by instituting wetting techniques and improving ventilation. In other industries such as sandblasting, silica milling, and rock drilling, workers remain potentially exposed above the acceptable limit of respirable free silica. The use of silica sand for blasting has been banned in England. In the United States, particles less toxic than silica are available for blasting. Since 1974, the National Institute for Occupational Safety and Health (NIOSH) has recommended the substitution of non-silica-containing particles in abrasive blasting.[100,101] Yet, the use of silica for blasting continues and epidemics of acute silicosis recur among sandblasters.[102]

Medical screening of silica-exposed workers is generally recommended, using questionnaires, chest x-rays, and spirometry. Primary and secondary prevention are further discussed in Chapter 46.

Once silicosis develops, the primary risks to the worker are progression of disease with progressive decline of lung function and development of mycobacterial infection. Both conditions can hasten the development of respiratory impairment in these workers. Cowie assessed the rate of decline in silicotic compared to non-silicotic South African gold miners over a 5-year period. The rate of FEV_1 and FVC decline increased with profusion of opacities, increasing from a yearly rate of decline in FEV_1 of 37 mL and FVC of 15 mL in silica-exposed without silicosis, to a yearly rate of decline in FEV_1 of 128 mL and FVC of 116 mL in those with the most extensive disease.[103] In another study, the clinical and chest radiographic data from 64 silicotics was retrospectively assessed over 15 years.[104] Sixteen developed progressive massive fibrosis. The mean yearly FEV_1 decline was 71 mL in progressors compared to 43 mL per year in those who did not develop progressive massive fibrosis.

Once a diagnosis of silicosis is made the worker should be removed from further silica exposure. Clinical suspicion of the development of mycobacterial infection must be high, particularly when there has been a decline in lung function or rapid worsening of the chest radiograph. Standard tuberculosis treatment regimens are effective.[105] Regional differences in drug resistance should be considered. Regular chest radiographs and performance of PPD skin tests are recommended. Mycobacterial infections should also be suspected and their diagnosis aggressively pursued when acute chest illnesses occur. There is concern among some investigators that PPD conversion may require more than one year of INH prophylaxis.[106]

A number of treatment modalities specific for silicosis have been attempted in patients with the classic and acute forms of this disease.[107,108] Interpretation of the usefulness of these approaches has been hampered by the fact that these are single case reports or small clinical or animal trials. No single therapy has been proved effective.

Corticosteroid therapy has been tried in patients with acute and chronic forms of silicosis.[109,110] This approach may be helpful when silicosis is associated with autoimmune disease or in acute silicosis, and it may effectively improve lung function for a defined period of time. Isoniazid prophylaxis is appropriate when corticosteroid therapy is prescribed. Inhalation of aluminum powder has been shown not to be efficacious in inhibiting silicosis progression.[108]

Treatment of pneumoconiosis with whole lung lavage was described in 1982 by Mason et al.[111] Although dust was removed from the lung, improvement in pulmonary function was not demonstrated. Therapeutic whole lung lavage has been used for workers who developed acute silicosis and silicoproteinosis following massive silica inhalation, but improvement in lung function has not been clearly demonstrated.[112]

Tetrandrine, a plant alkaloid with antioxidant and anti-inflammatory properties, is an ancient Chinese remedy for rheumatic diseases.[113-115] It has been shown to arrest the progression of silicosis in small clinical trials.[116] Additional studies are needed to evaluate this agent for use in the treatment of silicosis.

As with other end-stage pulmonary diseases, lung transplantation has been performed on workers with extensive silicosis.[117] However, organ availability is limited and the treatment is usually offered to younger patients.

SUMMARY

Silicosis is a preventable interstitial occupational lung disease that has the potential to shorten a worker's life. Contraction of this illness results in an increased risk of mycobacterial infection, as well as the risk for progression despite ceasing exposure. Although further research on the mechanism of lung injury in silicosis and the potential modulation of this illness by different therapies will contribute to our therapeutic armamentarium for this disease, there are sufficient available data to protect workers. The extent to which current and future workers will be protected depends on the education of employers and employees, strict enforcement of industrial hygiene practices, and vigilance for circumstances where unacceptable exposures to respirable silica occur.

References

1. Agricola G. De re metallica, book I (1556). Translated by Hoover HC, Hoover L, vol. 12. San Francisco: Mining and Science Press, 1912.
2. Davies CN. Inhalation risk and particle size in dust and mist. Br J Ind Med 1949; 6:245–53.
3. NIOSH. Work-related lung disease surveillance report. NIOSH publication 94-120. Cincinnatti: National Institute for Occupational Safety and Health, 1994.
4. Ziskind M. Jones RN, Weill H. Silicosis. Am Rev Respir Dis 1976; 113:643–65.
5. Mandel G, Mandel N. The structure of crystalline SiO_2. In: Castranova V, Vallyathan V, Wallace WE, eds. Silica and silica-induced lung diseases. Boca Raton: CRC Press, 1996;63–78.
6. Donaldson K, Stone V, Duffin R, et al. The quartz hazard: effects of surface and matrix on inflammogenic activity. Environ Pathol Toxicol Oncol 2001; 20(Suppl 1):109–18.
7. Office of Federal Register. Code of federal regulations: Occupational safety and health standards. Subpart Z: Air contaminants – permissible exposure limits. Table 1-A. (29 CFR 1910.1000). Washington DC: Office of the Federal Register, National Archives and Records Administration, 1989.
8. Graham WG, Vacek PM, Morgan WK, et al. Radiographic abnormalities in long-tenure Vermont granite workers and

the permissible exposure limit for crystalline silica. J Occup Environ Med 2001; 43:412–7.

9. Kreiss K, Zhen B. Risk of silicosis in a Colorado mining community. Am J Ind Med 1996; 30:529–39.

10. Banks DE, Morring K, Boehlecke BA, et al. Silicosis in silica flour workers. Am Rev Respir Dis 1981; 124:445–50.

11. Craighead JE, Kleinerman J, Abraham JL, et al. Diseases associated with exposure to silica and nonfibrous silicate minerals. Arch Pathol Lab Med 1988; 112:673–720.

12. Nugent KM, Dodson RF, Idell S, et al. The utility of bronchoalveolar lavage and transbronchial lung biopsy combined with energy-dispersive x-ray analysis in the diagnosis of silicosis. Am Rev Respir Dis 1989; 140:1438–41.

13. Glindmeyer HW, Hammad Y. Contributing factors to sandblaster's silicosis: inadequate respiratory protection equipment and standards. J Occup Med 1988; 30:917–21.

14. Dufresne A, Loosereewanich P, Begin R, et al. Tentative explanatory variable of lung dust concentration in gold miners exposed to crystalline silica. J Exp Environ Epidemiol 1998; 8:375–98.

15. Yucesoy B, Vallyathan V, Landsittel DP, et al. Polymorphisms of the IL-1 gene complex in coal miners with silicosis. Am J Ind Med 2002; 39:286–91.

16. Yucesoy B, Vallayathan V, Landsittel DP, et al. Association of tumor necrosis factor-alpha and interleukin-1 gene polymorphisms with silicosis. Toxicol Appl Pharmacol 2001; 172:75–82.

17. Donaldson K, Stone V, Clouter A, et al. Ultrafine particles. Occup Environ Med 2001; 58:211–6.

18. Hetland RB, Schwarze PE, Johansen BV, et al. Silica-induced cytokine release from A549 cells: importance of surface area versus size. Hum Exp Toxicol 2001; 20:46–55.

19. Lugano EM, Dauber JH, Daniele RP. Acute experimental silicosis. Am J Pathol 1982; 109:27–36.

20. Mossman BT, Churg A. Mechanisms in the pathogenesis of asbestosis and silicosis. Am J Respir Crit Care Med 1998; 157:1666–80.

21. Lapp NL, Castranova V. How silicosis and coal workers' pneumoconiosis develop – a cellular assessment. In: Banks DE, ed. Occupational medicine: state of the art reviews, vol. 8. Philadelphia: Hanley and Belfus Inc., 1993;35–56.

22. Vallyathan V, Castranova V. Silicosis and coal workers' pneumoconiosis. Environ Health Persp 2000; 108(suppl 4):675–84.

23. Blackford JA, Jones W, Dey RD, et al. Comparison of inducible nitric oxide synthase expression and lung inflammation following intratracheal instillation of silica, coal, carbonyl iron or titanium dioxide in rats. J Toxicol Environ Health 1997; 51:203–18.

24. Wallaert B, Lassalle P, Fortin F, et al. Superoxide anion generated by alveolar inflammatory cells in simple pneumoconiosis and in progressive massive fibrosis of non-smoking coal workers. Am Rev Respir Dis 1990; 141:129–33.

25. Shi X, Dong Z, Huang C, et al. The role of hydroxyl radical as a messenger in the activation of nuclear transcription factor NF-KB. Mol Cell Biochem 1999; 194:63–70.

26. Driscoll KE, Hessenblein DC, Carter JM, et al. Macrophage inflammatory proteins 1 and 2 expression by rat alveolar macrophages, fibroblasts, and epithelial cells in rat lung after mineral dust exposure. Am J Respir Cell Mol Biol 1993; 8:311–81.

27. Rojansakul Y, Ye J, Chen F, et al. Dependence of NF-kappaB activation and free radical generation on silica-induced TNF-alpha production in macrophages. Mol Cell Biochem 1999; 200:119–25.

28. Takemura T, Rom WN. Ferrans VJ, Crystal RG. Morphological characterization of alveolar macrophages from subjects with occupational exposure to inorganic particles. Am Rev Respir Dis 1989; 140:1674–85.

29. Bowden DH, Adamson IYR. The role of cell injury in the continuing inflammatory response in the generation of silicotic pulmonary fibrosis. J Pathol 1984; 144:149–61.

30. Driscoll KE, Howard BW, Carter JM, et al. Mitochondrial-derived oxidants and quartz activation of chemokine gene expression. Adv Exp Med Biol 2001;500:489–96.

31. Bitterman PB, Wewers MD, Rennard SI, et al. Modulation of alveolar macrophage driven fibroblast proliferation by alternative macrophage mediators. J Clin Invest 1986; 77:700–8.

32. Jarirgar J, Begin R, Dufresne A, et al. Transforming growth factor-beta (TGF-beta) in silicosis. Am J Respir Crit Care Med 1996; 154:1076–81.

33. Arcangeli G, Cupelli V, Giuliano G. Effects of silica on human lung fibroblast in culture. Sci Total Environ 2001; 270:135–9.

34. Martin TR, Altman LC, Albert RK, Henderson WR. Leukotriene B production by the human alveolar macrophage: a potential mechanism for amplifying inflammation in the lung. Am Rev Respir Dis 1984; 129:106–11.

35. Driscoll KE, Carter JM, Howard BW, et al. Interleukin-10 regulates quartz-induced pulmonary inflammation in rats. Am J Physiol 1998; 275:L887–94.

36. Bergin CJ, Muller NL, Vedal S, Chan-Yeung M. CT in silicosis: plain films and pulmonary function tests. Am J Roentgenol 1986; 146:477–83.

37. Kinsella M, Muller N, Vedal S, et al. Emphysema in silicosis. A comparison of smokers with nonsmokers using pulmonary function and computed tomography. Am Rev Respir Dis 1990; 141:1497–500.

38. Takini D, Paggiaro PL, Falaschi F, et al. Chest radiography and high resolution computed tomography in the evaluation of workers exposed to silica dust: relation to functional findings. Occup Environ Med 1995; 52:262–7.

39. Bisson G, Lamoureux G, Begin R. Quantitative gallium 67 lung scan to assess the inflammatory activity in the pneumoconioses. Semin Nucl Med 1987; 17:72–80.

40. Irwig LM, Rocks P. Lung function and respiratory symptoms in silicotic and nonsilicotic gold miners. Am Rev Respir Dis 1978;117:429–35.

41. Wang M-L, Banks DE. Airways obstruction and occupational inorganic dust exposure. In: Occupational lung disease: an international perspective. London: Lippincott-Raven, 1998;69–82.

42. Hodous TK, Attfield MD. Progressive massive fibrosis developing on a background of minimal simple coal workers' pneumoconiosis. Proceedings of the VIIth International Pneumoconiosis Conference, Pittsburgh, DHS (NIOSH) publication number 90-108, Part 1; 123–6. Cincinatti: NIOSH.

43. Jones RN, Turner-Warwick M, Ziskind M, et al. High prevalence of antinuclear antibodies in sandblaster's silicosis. Am Rev Respir Dis 1976; 113:393–5.

44. Saiyed HN, Chatterjee BB. Rapid progression of silicosis in slate pencil workers: II. A follow-up study. Am J Ind Med 1985; 8:135–42.

45. Ng TP, Chan SL, Lam KP. Radiological progression and lung function in silicosis: a ten year follow up study. Br Med J (Clin Res Ed) 1987; 295:164–8.

46. Lee HS, Phoon WH, Ng TP. Radiological progression and its predictive risk factors in silicosis. Occup Environ Med 2001; 58:467–71.

47. Law YCS, Leung MCM, Leung CC, et al. Characteristics of workers attending the pneumoconiosis clinic for silicosis assessment in Hong Kong: retrospective study. Hong Kong Med J 2001; 7:343–9.

48. Seaton A, Legge JS, Henderson J, et al. Accelerated silicosis in Scottish stonemasons. Lancet 1991; 337:341–4.

49. Seaton A, Cherrie JW. Quartz exposures and severe silicosis: a role for hilar nodes. Occup Environ Med 1998; 55:383–6.

50. Eden K, Seebach HV. Atypical dust-induced pneumoconiosis in SPF rats. Virchows Arch (Pathol Anat) 1976; 372:1–9.

51. Davis GS, Leslie KO, Hemenway DR. Silicosis in mice: effects of dose, time, and genetic strain. J Exp Path Tox Oncol 1998; 17:81–97.

52. Adamson IY, Prieditis H. Silica deposition in the lung during epithelial injury potentiates fibrosis and increases particle translocation to lymph node. Exp Lung Res 1998; 24:293–306.
53. Betts WW. Chalicosis pulmonum or chronic interstitial pneumonia induced by stone dust. JAMA 1900; 34:70–74.
54. Middleton EL. The present position of silicosis in industry in Britain. Br Med J 1929; 2:485–9.
55. Chapman EM. Acute silicosis. JAMA 1932; 98:1439–41.
56. Vallyathan V, Shi X, Dalal NS, et al. Generation of free radicals from freshly fractured silica dust: potential role in acute silica induced lung injury. Am Rev Respir Dis 1988; 138: 1213–19.
57. Buechner HA, Ansari A. Acute silico-proteinosis. Dis Chest 1969; 55:274–84.
58. Gardner LU. Pathology of so-called silicosis. Am J Public Health 1933; 23:1240–9.
59. Suratt PM, Winn WC, Brody AR, et al. Acute silicosis in tombstone sandblasters. Am Rev Respir Dis 1977; 115:521–9.
60. Duchange L, Brichet A, Lamblin C, et al. Acute silicosis. Clinical, radiologic, functional, and cytologic characteristics of the broncho-alveolar fluids. Observations of 6 cases. Rev Mal Respir 1998; 15:527–34.
61. Sampson HL. The roentgenogram in so-called 'acute' silicosis. Am J Public Health 1933; 23:1237–9.
62. Banks DE, Bauer MA, Castellan RM, et al. Silicosis in surface coal mine drillers. Thorax 1983; 38:275–8.
63. Dee P, Suratt P, Winn W. The radiographic findings in acute silicosis. Radiology 1978; 126:359–63.
64. Hoffman EO, Lamberty J, Pizzolato P, Coover J. The ultrastructure of acute silicosis. Arch Pathol 1973; 96:104–7.
65. Watkins-Pitchford W, Moir J. Report no. 8. Johannesburg: South African Institute for Medical Research, 1916.
66. Murray J, Kielkowski D, Reid P. Occupational disease trends in black South African gold miners. An autopsy-based study. Am J Respir Crit Care Med 1996; 153:706–10.
67. Churchyard GJ, Kleinschmidt I, Corbett EL, et al. Factors associated with an increased case-fatality rate in HIV-infected and non-infected South African gold miners with pulmonary tuberculosis. Int J Tuberc Lung Dis 2000; 4:705–12.
68. Iyer R, Holian A. Immunological aspects of silicosis. In: Castranova V, Vallyathan V, Wallace E, eds. Silica and silica-induced lung diseases. Boca Raton: CRC Press, 1996;253–67.
69. Allison AC, D'Arcy Hart P. Potentiation of silica of the growth of Mycobacterium tuberculosis in macrophage culture. Br J Exp Pathol 1968; 49:465.
70. Gross P, Westrick ML, McNerney JM. Experimental tuberculosis. Am Rev Respir Dis 1961; 83:510.
71. Sherson D, Lander F. Morbidity of pulmonary tuberculosis among silicotic and nonsilicotic foundry workers in Denmark. J Occup Med 1990; 32:110–13.
72. Hnizdo E, Murray J, Sluis-Cremer, et al. Correlation between radiological and pathological diagnosis of silicosis: an autopsy population based study. Am J Ind Med 1993; 24:427–45.
73. Cowie RL. The epidemiology of tuberculosis in gold miners with silicosis. Am J Respir Crit Care Med 1994; 150:1460–2.
74. Hnizdo E, Murray J. Risk of pulmonary tuberculosis relative to silicosis and exposure to silica dust in South African gold miners. Occup Environ Med 1998; 55:496–502.
75. Chen GX, Burnett CA, Cameron LL, et al. Tuberculosis mortality and silica exposure: a case-control study based on national mortality database for the years 1983–1992. Int J Occup Environ Health 1197; 3:163–70.
76. Cowie RL, Langton ME, Becklake MR. Pulmonary tuberculosis in South African gold miners. Am Rev Respir Dis 1989; 139:1086–9.
77. Corbett EL, Churchyard GJ, Clayton TC, et al. HIV infection and silicosis: the impact of two potent risk factors on the incidence of mycobacterial disease in South African miners. AIDS 2000; 1:2759–68.
78. Churchyard GJ, Kleinschmidt I, Corbett EL, et al. Factors associated with an increased case-fatality rate in HIV-infected and non-infected South African gold miners with pulmonary tuberculosis. Int J Lung Dis 2000; 8:705–712.
79. Cowie RL. Short course chemoprophylaxis with rifampicin, isoniazid, and pyrazinamide for tuberculosis evaluated in gold miners with chronic silicosis: a double blind placebo controlled trial. Tuber Lung Dis 1996; 77:239–43.
80. Goldsmith DF, Guidotti TL, Johnston DR. Does occupational exposure to silica cause cancer? Am J Ind Med 1982; 3:423–40.
81. IARC. IARC Monograph on the evaluation of the carcinogenic risk of chemicals to humans. Volume 42: Silica and some silicates. Lyon: International Agency for Research on Cancer, 1987.
82. IARC. IARC Monograph on the evaluation of the carcinogenic risk of chemicals to humans. Volume 68: Silica, some silicates, coal dust, and para-aramid fibrils. Lyon: International Agency for Research on Cancer, 1997.
83. Weill H, McDonald JC. Exposure to crystalline silica and risk of lung cancer: the epidemiological evidence. Thorax 1995; 51:97–102.
84. Hessel PA, Gamble JF, Gee JB, et al. Silica, silicosis, and lung cancer: a response to a recent working group report. J Occup Environ Med 2000; 42:704–20.
85. Lippman M, Eckert HL, Hahon N, Morgan WKC. Circulating antinuclear and rheumatoid factors in coal miners. A prevalence study in Pennsylvania and West Virginia. Ann Intern Med 1973; 79:807–11.
86. Rodnan GP, Bendek TG, Medsger TA, et al. The association of progressive systemic sclerosis with coal miners' pneumoconiosis and other forms of silicosis. Ann Intern Med 1967; 66:323–329.
87. Haustein UF, Zeigler V, Hermann K, et al. Silica-induced scleroderma. J Am Acad Dermatol 1990; 22:444–8.
88. Klockards M, Kosela R, Jarvinen E, et al. Silica exposure and rheumatoid arthritis: A follow up study of granite workers, 1940–1981. Br Med J 1987; 294:997–1000.
89. Haustein UF, Anderegg U. Silica induced scleroderma – clinical and experimental aspects. J Rheumatol 1998; 10:1917-26.
90. Industrial Disease Standards Panel. Interim report to the Workers' Compensation Board (of Ontario) on Scleroderma. Toronto, Ontario: IDSP, 1992.
91. Stratta P, Canavese C, Messuerotti A, et al. Silica and renal diseases: no longer a problem in the 21st century ? J Nephrol 2001; 14:228–47.
92. Roseman KD, Moore-Fuller M, Reilly MJ. Connective tissue disease and silicosis. Am J Ind Med 1999; 35:375–81.
93. Caplan A. Certain unusual radiologic appearances in the chest of coal miners suffering from rheumatoid arthritis. Thorax 1953; 8:29–30.
94. Hughes JM, Jones RN, Gilson JC, et al. Determinants of progression in sandblasters' silicosis. Ann Occup Hyg 1982; 26:701–12.
95. Banks DE, Milutinovic J, Desnick RJ, Grabowski GA, Lapp NL, Boehlecke BA. Silicon nephropathy mimicking Fabry's disease. Am J Nephrol 1983; 3:279–84.
96. Collis EY. Mortality experience of an occupational group exposed to silica dust, compared with that of the general population and an occupational group exposed to dust not containing silica. J Indust Hyg 1933;395–417.
97. Rosenman KD, Moore-Fuller M, Reilly MJ. Kidney disease and silicosis. Nephron 2000; 85:14–9.
98. Glindmeyer HW, Hammad YY. Contributing factors to sandblasters' silicosis: inadequate respiratory protection equipment and standards. J Occup Med 1988; 30:917–21.
99. Hughes JM, Glazier JB, Maloney JE, West JB. Effect of extra-alveolar vessels on distribution of blood flow in the dog lung. J Appl Physiol 1968; 25:701–12.
100. Mackay GR, Stettler LE, Kommineni C, Donaldson HM. Fibrogenic potential of slags used as substitutes for sand in abrasive blasting operations. Am Ind Hyg Assoc J 1980; 41:836–42.

101. Stettler LE, Proctor JE, Platek SF, Carolan RJ, Smith RJ, Donaldson HM. Fibrogenicity and carcinogenic potential of smelter slags used as abrasive blasting substitutes. J Toxicol Environ Health 1988; 25:35–56.

102. Fleming DM, Mckinney B. Silicosis: clusters in sandblasters in Texas and occupational surveillence for silicosis. MMWR 1990; 39:433–7.

103. Cowie RL. The influence of silicosis on deteriorating lung function in gold miners. Chest 1998; 113:340–3.

104. Avashia SW, Parker JE. Clinical features associated with the development of progressive massive fibrosis. Chest 1996; 110.

105. Lin TP, Suo J, Lee CN, Lee JJ, Yang SP. Short-course chemotherapy of pulmonary tuberculosis in pneumoconiotic patients. Am Rev Respir Dis 1987; 136:808–10.

106. Morgan EJ. Silicosis and tuberculosis. Chest 1979; 75:202–3.

107. Banks DE, Cheng YH, Weber SL, Ma JK. Strategies for the treatment of pneumoconiosis. Occup Med 1993; 8:205–32.

108. Kennedy M. Aluminium powder inhalations in the treatment of silicosis of pottery workers and pneumoconiosis of coal miners. Br J Ind Med 1956; 13:85–101.

109. Goodman GB, Kaplan PD, Stachura I, Castranova V, Pailes WH, Lapp NL. Acute silicosis responding to corticosteroid therapy. Chest 1992; 101:366–70.

110. Sharma SK, Pande JN, Verma K. Effect of prednisolone treatment in chronic silicosis. Am Rev Respir Dis 1991; 143:814–21.

111. Mason GR, Abraham JL, Hoffman L, Cole S, Lippmann M, Wasserman K. Treatment of mixed-dust pneumoconiosis with whole lung lavage. Am Rev Respir Dis 1982; 126:1102–7.

112. Wilt JL, Banks DE, Weissman DN, et al. Reduction of lung dust burden in pneumoconiosis by whole-lung lavage. J Occup Environ Med 1996; 38:619–24.

113. Seow WK, Ferrante A, Li SY, Thong YH. Suppression of human monocyte interleukin 1 production by the plant alkaloid tetrandrine. Clin Exp Immunol 1989; 75:47–51.

114. Seow WK, Ferrante A, Li SY, Thong YH. Antiphagocytic and antioxidant properties of plant alkaloid tetrandrine. Int Arch Allergy Appl Immunol 1988; 85:404–9.

115. Ye J, Ding M, Zhang X, Rojanasakul Y, Shi X. On the role of hydroxyl radical and the effect of tetrandrine on nuclear factor – kappaB activation by phorbol 12-myristate 13-acetate. Ann Clin Lab Sci 2000; 30:65–71.

116. Chao DM, Berger MW. Enhancement of the in vivo action of tetrandine against silicosis by targeted drug delivery. Appl Occup Environ Hyg 1996; 11:1008–18.

117. Vermeire P, Tasson J, Lamont H, Barbier F, Versieck J, Derom F. Respiratory function after lung homotransplantation with a ten-month survival in man. Am Rev Respir Dis 1972; 106:515–27.

19.10 **Respiratory Diseases of Coal Miners**

Edward L Petsonk, Michael D Attfield

HISTORY
Coal production

The growth in coal mining was virtually coincident with the Industrial Revolution. Although shallow mining of coal seam outcrops is reported to have occurred since the 9th century, the 18th century brought increased demand for coal as well as the technology to pursue the mining of seams well below the earth's surface. By the early 1800s coal mining had become an important industry both in the United States and abroad. Employment in coal mining peaked about 100 years later in 1923, when over 800,000 coal miners were working in US mines. From that point, although production and consumption of coal continued to increase, mechanization progressively reduced the size of the work force. In 1999, average employment in coal mining work in the US was 108,244, down from 132,535 six years earlier. Between 1993 and 2002, annual US production remained stable at about 1 billion short tons of bituminous and 1.5 million tons of anthracite coal. Currently, about two-thirds of coal production is at surface mines, while about 57% of miners are employed at underground mining operations.[1]

The principal US coal deposits are shown in Figure 19.10.1. Coal production has recently been fairly evenly divided between Eastern and Western coalfields, but the proportion of production has been increasing in Western states and now exceeds that of the Appalachian coalfields.

Health effects

In Europe, recognition of the adverse health consequences of coal mining followed the marked increase in the number of miners. Wedel, in 1672, wrote of 'miners asthma', but was probably referring to hard rock miners. According to Kerr, the term was first applied to coal miners in 1822. Laennec described the black pigment in the lungs of coal miners as 'melanosis' in 1806, and by 1819 clearly differentiated the condition from malignant melanoma. Several years later, the term 'miners' black lung' was used to describe the disease in Scotland. In 1919, silicosis became a 'certifiable disease' in the UK, and British miners with pneumoconiosis became eligible for certain benefits. Based on studies among South Wales coal workers, a high prevalence of pneumoconiosis became evident in the 1930s, and the condition 'coal workers' pneumoconiosis' (CWP) was differentiated from silicosis in the early 1940s.

Unfortunately, this awareness of CWP failed to cross the Atlantic. A mine explosion in Farmington, West Virginia, on November 20, 1968, was widely reported on television, and graphically illustrated to the nation the plight of coal miners in the US. This tragedy added momentum to the movement to improve coal mine health and safety conditions. 'Black lung associations' were organized in the coalfields. A 3-week long strike in the West Virginia coal mines,

one of the largest and longest strikes ever called on the single issue of occupational health, ended when the state legislature passed a bill in 1969 making CWP a compensable disease. By the end of 1969 the Federal Coal Mine Health and Safety Act had been passed into law. Dust control and safe practices in coalmines were mandated and backed up by inspectors with the threat of fines or closures, and the right of the miners' representatives to participate in inspections.

MINING JOBS

An understanding of mining techniques is useful in the evaluation of respiratory diseases of miners, since different activities involve exposures to different degrees of risk. Activities at coalmines are generally classified into face, non-face, and surface work. By virtue of multiple activities, some workers spend portions of their workday in two or more of these mine locations.

Face workers

Miners working at the edge of the unmined coal seam, or coalface, are engaged in the actual removal of coal from the working 'section' of the mine. Face miners are generally exposed to the highest concentrations of respirable airborne dusts, particularly carbon, but may also be exposed to silica dust when the cutting bits strike silica-bearing rock immediately adjacent to or within the coal seams. There are three primary methods of mining coal underground that have been employed in the US. They are discussed below.

Continuous mining

Room and pillar mining with 'continuous mining' machines is one of the commonly used coal mining techniques in the US today. Continuous miner operators and their helpers direct the rotating bits on the machine into the coal seam to rip out the coal. The loosened coal is pushed to the back of the machine, where a loading machine operator and helpers use a large scoop to load the coal into a rubber-tired buggy (shuttle car), or directly onto a conveyor line.

Pillars of unmined coal are left at the sides of the advancing tunnel to help support the roof. As the continuous mining machine advances, roof bolters and their helpers install steel plates to strengthen the unsupported roof of the tunnel. Holes are drilled into the hard rock above the coal seam and long steel bolts inserted, along with glues, to anchor these plates. Silica exposure is common in roof bolting, and there may also be exposure to resins and plasticizers in glues. Timber men install wooden posts to further stabilize the roof of the tunnel. Brattice men install curtains or tubing to direct the flow of ventilation at the working face. Shuttle car ('buggy') operators transport newly mined coal in rubber-tired vehicles (Fig. 19.10.2). Scoop car oper-

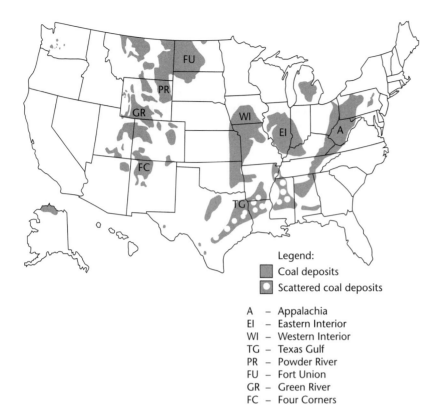

Figure 19.10.1: Map of United States coal deposits.

Legend:
■ Coal deposits
▣ Scattered coal deposits

A – Appalachia
EI – Eastern Interior
WI – Western Interior
TG – Texas Gulf
PR – Powder River
FU – Fort Union
GR – Green River
FC – Four Corners

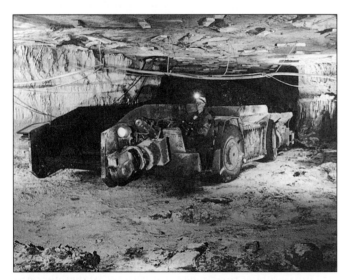

Figure 19.10.2: Coal miner operating rubber-tired shuttle car.

ators run battery-operated vehicles throughout the mine, transporting coal or mining supplies. Mobile bridge operators operate portable conveyor lines to move coal away from the face. Section maintenance workers repair and maintain the underground heavy equipment at the face in all mining methods.

Longwall mining
'Longwall mining' is currently the most cost-efficient and highly productive method of underground coal mining. Production using this technique is increasing as an alternative to room and pillar mining. The longwall machine spans several hundred to a thousand feet or more along the active coalface. A rotating drum (shear) or a plow moves back and forth along the face, breaking coal loose from the seam and allowing it to fall onto a conveyor line. A series of hydraulic 'jacks' support the roof along the face, and are advanced as the coal is removed. Behind the longwall device, the unsupported roof is simply allowed to fall. This minimizes the loss of the coal in pillars and the need for roof support activities, as in room and pillar mining. To develop the mining section in advance of the longwall machine, one or two continuous miner crews are generally operated. However, to run the longwall section itself, a smaller crew of longwall operators, mechanics, headgate operators, and jack setters is required.

Respirable dust exposures in longwall mining have been difficult to control. In recent years, nearly 40% of reported dust measurements on longwall sections have been over the 2 mg/m^3 respirable dust standard, compared with 10–15% on continuous mining sections.

Conventional mining
Little coal is mined in the US today using the 'conventional mining' technique, although many current miners have used this method in prior jobs. In this system, cutting machine operators and helpers make a deep cut in the coal face at the bottom of the seam. 'Shot firers' drill deep holes in the area of the cut and place explosive charges to blast the coal free. 'Hand loaders' or loading machine operators shovel the coal into vehicles, which then transport it away from the face. In addition to dust, important exposure to nitrogen oxides from the explosives may occur using this technique.

Non-face workers

Several underground mining activities relate to reducing dust or methane gas hazards. Masons construct plastic, cloth, or block barriers to keep the flow of air directed across the working face. Rock dusters scatter hygroscopic powdered limestone along the cut faces of the mine tunnels, to moisten and trap loose dusts and reduce the danger of explosion. Although this job may involve considerable visible dust and irritation, the lung toxicity of the limestone is considered to be lower than the other mine dusts. Electricians, mechanics, and welders may work with equipment throughout the mine.

Workers on non-face transportation have several types of exposure. The coal is loaded at the working face (see above) and transported to the main haulageways, where it is dumped into train cars or a conveyor belt and taken out of the mine. Motormen operate the train locomotives. To improve traction on the steel rails, motormen drop sand or other abrasives on the rails. The materials are fragmented into respirable particles and resuspended by passing trains, creating a mixed dust or silica exposure hazard. Belt men patrol the conveyor belts, assuring the continued movement of coal, and shoveling up spilled coal. In some mines, diesel exhaust exposure may be present from diesel-powered vehicles.

Surface workers

With a few important exceptions, surface workers generally are exposed to lower levels of respirable dust. Surface maintenance workers frequently perform welding and cutting on equipment, and may be exposed to welding fumes as well as asbestos from shields and gloves. Tipple operators and preparation plant workers are frequently exposed to higher levels of dust during the cleaning, processing, and loading of the coal. Lampmen and others at the mine portal often have little dust exposure.

Equipment operatives at surface coal mines, particularly high-wall drillers and their helpers, and to a lesser extent bulldozer operators, frequently experience important silica exposures while drilling and removing overburden. Surface coal miners have dust exposures that are generally lower than those of underground miners, but a risk of both simple and complicated pneumoconiosis remains.[2]

In summary, modern mining techniques bear little resemblance to the pick-and-shovel techniques of the early 1900s. Highly mechanized equipment allows mining more coal with far fewer miners. Unfortunately, the high production intrinsic to these operations may lead to dust levels that are difficult to control, and strict attention is necessary to avoid unhealthful conditions.

TERMINOLOGY
Overview

When dealing with respiratory diseases of coal miners, it is important to be familiar with disease definitions. Differing terms and different definitions have been used for clinical, epidemiological, pathological, and legal or legislative purposes.

In the clinical arena, use of the term 'pneumoconiosis' tends to be restricted to the radiologic or pathologic appearances relating to the accumulation of lung dust deposits and the associated tissue reactions. This usage is often interpreted to exclude other lung abnormalities, such as those associated with bronchitis or emphysema, although, as noted below, focal emphysema is often considered an integral component of the pathologic lesion of coal workers' pneumoconiosis. Such distinctions between the different mining-related disease processes may facilitate the diagnosis, treatment, and study of disease, but has tended to lead to fragmented understanding and assessment of the totality of lung disease associated with exposure to coal mine dust.

Generic definitions of pneumoconiosis, which include all dust-related effects on the lung, are also widely used. Some of these definitions are employed more in the non-clinical sphere, particularly with regard to legal/legislative activities, and include dust-related effects that may not be radiographically apparent, such as dust-induced chronic airflow obstruction. The lay term 'black lung' is a generic term used by miners for lung disorders associated with their work.

Since the radiographic pattern of CWP may be quite distinctive, pneumoconiosis in coal miners often has been defined based upon a radiographic appearance. For example, in research publications, confirmation of CWP may require that several readers concur in the finding of a certain shape and profusion on a chest film (for example, 1/0 rounded opacities using the International Labor Office system of classification of radiographs for pneumoconiosis) (for more detail, see Chapter 19.1). Although this approach increases precision, it may reduce sensitivity for several reasons: (1) it is recognized that readings of 0/1 rounded opacities also correlate with mine dust exposures; (2) the profusion of *irregular* as well as rounded opacities seen on the chest radiograph increases with increasing mining exposures; (3) the routine chest radiograph may be normal in the presence of clinically important and pathologically identifiable interstitial lung disease; and finally (4) several dust-related diseases, including bronchitis and emphysema, may not be apparent radiographically.[3] In spite of this, in the United Kingdom, for example, airflow obstruction among coal miners is compensable only for miners who also have radiographic evidence of pneumoconiosis.

Post-mortem lung pathology has shown that nodular radiographic changes correlate quite well with pathology: ILO q-type opacities on chest films are associated with coal macules and micronodules, while r-type opacities are associated with macronodules. The profusion of p opacities, and to a lesser extent q-type opacities, has been found to reflect the dust content of the lung at autopsy. With regard to large opacities, about two-thirds of those seen on chest films are subsequently confirmed on pathology. However, routine chest x-rays are not entirely sensitive for detecting CWP lesions, which may be found pathologically or on high-resolution computed tomography in miners with normal routine chest films. Among miners whose lungs revealed progressive massive fibrosis (PMF) on pathologic examination, 22% had prior chest x-rays showing no radiographic large opacities.[4,5]

In summary, for clinical purposes, coal miners with typical radiographic or pathological findings of pneumoconiosis are properly diagnosed as having coal workers' pneumoconiosis. For legal and compensation purposes, a broader definition of 'pneumoconiosis' is used, which includes dust-related effects that may not be radiographically apparent.

Specific medical terms relating to respiratory diseases in coal miners

Simple CWP. This lesion is defined clinically in miners showing multiple radiographic shadows up to 10 mm in diameter. These dust-related shadows are usually rounded, although irregular shadows may also be noted in combination with rounded opacities, or occasionally alone. The pathological correlates of the chest radiograph are discussed in the text.

Complicated CWP. This lesion is also defined clinically based on a chest radiograph showing a dust lesion or lesions over 10 mm in diameter. Complicated CWP is found most often on a background of smaller rounded opacities, with the risk increasing with increasing profusion. Progressive massive fibrosis (PMF) is a term often used interchangeably with complicated CWP, although not all of the larger rounded shadows seen in coal miners will progress with time.

Silicosis (see Chapter 19.9). This is the chronic interstitial lung disorder caused by the inhalation of respirable crystalline silica. Radiographically, silicosis is also characterized by small rounded opacities, which may coalesce to form shadows larger than 10 mm (complicated silicosis or PMF). Although silicosis is pathologically distinct from CWP, the two disorders often cannot be distinguished radiographically. The lungs of coal miners frequently show lesions consistent with both disorders.

Bronchitis (see Chapter 19.4). Sometimes referred to as industrial bronchitis, this dust-related disorder is characterized by excessive cough and sputum production. Sputum production is deemed excessive when it occurs on most days for at least three months a year for two or more years. The pathology of this disorder has been less well studied.

Focal emphysema. A form of airspace enlargement with tissue destruction, found in association with, and an integral part of the macular lesion of simple CWP.

LUNG PATHOLOGY
Pigmented lesions

The most characteristic and striking pathologic changes in the respiratory system of coal miners are associated with the accumulation of dark pigment, primarily located in lung macrophages. Localized dust macules are considered pathognomonic of CWP.[6] They are located at the level of the respiratory bronchioles, and are generally associated with deposition of reticulin, and with destruction of adja-

cent alveolar walls (focal emphysema), but with only minimal collagenous scarring (Fig. 19.10.3). With increasing dust deposition, the pigmented macule progressively enlarges, becoming solid and palpable. Adjoining macules may coalesce. At this stage, the lesions show clear collagen deposition, and are labeled nodular lesions. Destructive vascular lesions are commonly associated with nodules.

With further progression of the disorder, coalescence of nodules can result. The massive lesions of complicated CWP (progressive massive fibrosis) may also appear. These lesions are greater than 1–2 cm in diameter, and are usually seen in upper lobes or superior segments of lower lobes of lungs with extensive pigment deposition (Fig. 19.10.4). PMF lesions may be unilateral, bilateral, and multiple, and may show cavities containing black liquid. The lungs of miners with complicated CWP also usually show pathologic changes of bronchitis and extensive emphysema.

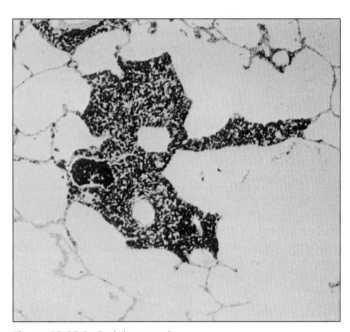

Figure 19.10.3: Coal dust macule.

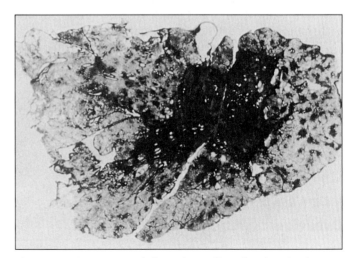

Figure 19.10.4: Gross pathology of complicated coal workers' pneumoconiosis

Cardiovascular changes consistent with cor pulmonale can also be seen. Right ventricular hypertrophy has been correlated with the thickening of pulmonary vessel walls seen in association with increasing severity of CWP, and emphysematous changes in miners' lungs.[7,8]

Factors facilitating progression to complicated CWP are not entirely understood. Excessive lung dust deposition is clearly the basis for the condition. The greatest risk factor for subsequent development of complicated CWP is the miner's radiographic category of simple CWP, with an additional effect of increasing age. The risk of progression to PMF in a miner with category 2 simple CWP is 3–4 times that of a miner with category 1. Exposures at a young age increase the duration of residence of the dust in the lung and also the risk of PMF.[9] In the past, mycobacterial infection was frequently associated with PMF, and was considered a precursor to its development. It is now accepted that PMF lesions often develop in the absence of infection. The role of excessive silica exposure is still debated, although PMF can clearly develop in workers with scant silica exposure. Miners, particularly those with simple or complicated CWP, have an increased frequency of autoantibodies and other serologic abnormalities. However, no clear role in disease pathogenesis of these findings has been defined.

Although it is rarely reported in the United States, dust-exposed miners with rheumatoid arthritis may develop a syndrome known as rheumatoid pneumoconiosis, or Caplan's syndrome (see Chapter 23.5). Features include multiple large (up to 5 cm) lung nodules developing rapidly, often over several months, with little or no background profusion of simple pneumoconiosis. The pulmonary lesions may cavitate, and occasionally will precede the onset of the joint disorder. Pathologically, the lesions are distinct from the typical lesion of PMF, and are similar to rheumatoid nodules.

Even in non-miners, the extent of pigment in the lungs generally increases with age. It is also greater in cigarette smokers than non-smokers. However, in the absence of occupational exposures, the deposition of pigment will very rarely be sufficient to form macular lesions.

Typical lesions of silicosis are described elsewhere (see Chapter 19.9). Overall, classical silicotic nodules have been reported at autopsy in the lung of 12.5% of coal miners. Higher prevalences are observed in certain jobs, such as motormen (25%), and in miners with complicated CWP (over 50%).[10]

Emphysema

The occurrence of emphysema in CWP has been recognized since the time of Osler, and is considered by some observers to be an integral component of the dust macule. Cigarette smoking may also result in emphysema of the centrilobular type, which differs from the emphysema due to coal dust only in the extent of lung involvement and the absence, in non-miners, of associated dust pigment. Generalized emphysema can be seen in the lungs of both smoking and non-smoking coal miners. After taking tobacco use into account, the extent of emphysema corre-lates with prior mine dust exposure, as well as the amount of dust retained in the lung. Opinions differ among pathologists as to whether the emphysema associated with the dust macule is different in any way from that related to tobacco use. However, the severity of airflow obstruction measured during life correlates significantly with the extent of pathologic emphysema in the coal miners' lungs at autopsy, suggesting an important functional effect.[11]

Bronchitis

The prevalence of chronic cough with sputum production is elevated in miners, increasing with mine dust exposure. It is generally accepted that coal mine dust deposition in the airways over prolonged periods of time leads to mucous gland enlargement and proliferation of goblet cells. However, few investigations have been performed regarding the histology of the airways and mucous glands in coal miners. The lungs of miners with complicated CWP frequently show the changes of chronic bronchitis. Some autopsy studies of miners have also shown a significant correlation between prior coal mine dust exposure and the proportion of mucous glands in the bronchial walls (the Reid Index). This is considered evidence that dust exposure contributes to the pathologic changes, as well as to the clinical symptoms, of chronic bronchitis. No significant relationship was found between airway mucous gland changes and the severity of pneumoconiosis.

In British coal miners there is a markedly different geographical distribution of mortality from pneumoconiosis versus chronic bronchitis and emphysema, suggesting that the exposures and mechanisms for these responses are different.[12]

Mycobacterial infection

Tuberculosis and non-tuberculous mycobacterial infections are seen in coal miners. The risk of these infections is generally considered to be increased with heavier dust exposures, particularly in miners with PMF. Some miners also have lesions of silicosis, which represent a greater risk factor than CWP alone for these infections. As in the general population, response to appropriate chemotherapy is usually good for tuberculous infections, and less satisfactory for most atypical mycobacterial disease. Tuberculosis is no longer considered an important factor in the development of complicated CWP in most countries, but is still associated with PMF onset and results in increased mortality among coal miners in some countries (e.g., China).[13]

Other conditions

Coal deposits also contain other variable components, including minerals such as crystalline silica and kaolin, as well as a polycyclic aromatic hydrocarbons (PAHs). In 1997, the International Agency for Research on Cancer determined that inhaled crystalline silica is a human carcinogen.[14] Thus, there has been an ongoing concern for a potential lung cancer risk among coal miners. In contrast to the finding

Pigmented lesions:
    Dust macule
    Coal nodule
    Progressive massive fibrosis (PMF)
    Silicotic nodule
Centrilobular emphysema
Bronchitis
Rheumatoid pneumoconiosis

Table 19.10.1 Pathologic classification of coal mine dust-induced changes

with crystalline silica, no consistent increase in lung cancer has been observed in relation to inhalation exposure to coal mine dust. However, several studies have reported an increased risk of gastric cancer among coal miners (see Chapter 30.5).[15]

Extracting coal requires the application of large amounts of mechanical energy to the coal, and injuries remain a constant threat to miners. In 2000, the US rates of fatal and non-fatal lost-time injuries in coal mining were 0.040 and 5.18 per 200,000 employee work-hours, respectively, or about three deaths and 356 non-fatal injuries per 10,000 miners annually. Discussion of injury risks is found in Chapter 31.

In summary, several pathological lesions have been identified in the lungs and airways of coal miners (Table 19.10.1). Some are rarely seen in the absence of extensive inhalation of coal mine dust, and therefore are accepted as generally related to occupational exposure. Some lesions have been correlated with the appearance of characteristic changes of CWP on the chest radiograph. Other lesions, while similar to those found in the general population, are seen with greater frequency in workers exposed to coal mine dusts. In the lungs of underground coal miners, macules, nodules, and massive lesions, as well as the emphysema associated with these lesions, and silicotic nodules, are accepted as almost uniformly related to mine dust exposures. In contrast, overall emphysema scores, carbon pigmentation, and possibly Reid indices are increased in miners' lungs in relation to their mine exposures, but can also be increased by other inhaled agents, depending on the relative exposures to mine dusts and other materials such as tobacco smoke.[11]

PATHOGENESIS

Observations from both human and animal studies have implicated overloading of lung clearance mechanisms in coal mine dust-related disorders. Excessive exposures trigger impairment of alveolar macrophage (AM)-mediated lung clearance, progressive accumulation of particle-laden macrophages, and subsequent inflammatory changes in the lung.[16] Once deposited, dust particles are thought to trigger release of mediators, including reactive oxygen species and related antioxidant protection mechanisms, as well as cytokines, growth factors, and related proteins. Tissue damage and remodeling in the respiratory tract results from modifications of the extracellular matrix. A number of animal and human studies have addressed these molecular mechanisms of lung injury from coal mine dust inhalation.

With dust exposure, increases in leukocyte recruitment as well as neutrophil adhesion have been observed, resulting in retention of inflammatory cells in the lung.[17]

Alveolar macrophages obtained from healthy subjects, exposed in vitro to coal dust particles, demonstrate release of tumor necrosis factor alpha (TNF-α) and interleukin-6 (IL-6). Alveolar macrophages from miners with CWP release higher levels of TNF-α and interleukin-1. Macrophages from dust-exposed workers with respiratory impairment also release increased amounts of oxidant species.[18] Bronchoalveolar lavage fluids from miners with CWP show an influx of mononuclear phagocytes, with an increased spontaneous production of oxidants, fibronectin, neutrophil chemotactic factor, and also of IL-6 and TNF-α. This spontaneous cytokine release is associated with an increased expression of cytokine messenger ribonucleic acid. Additional studies are needed to more fully characterize the cellular events and mediators responsible for the unique pattern of airway and parenchymal lung injury that is seen with coal mine dust inhalation.

RADIOLOGY
Radiographic changes in coal miners

Several patterns of abnormality on routine posteroanterior chest radiographs have been related to coal mine dust exposure. Most commonly, fairly discrete small nodular radiographic shadows are seen in the lung fields. These densities are usually rounded in shape, although they may be irregular, and are seen in greater numbers in the upper and middle, compared to the lower lung zones, with prominent lower zone involvement seen only occasionally. Typically the largest diameter of the small nodules categorized as simple CWP is 3 mm or less, but may be up to 10 mm. With increasing lung dust deposition, the number of opacities observed in a lung zone (profusion) increases. The normal vascular shadows of the lung become obscured.

Further progression may be indicated by a coalescence of the small opacities into a combined density, which may be quite homogenous. By convention, if a dust-related radiographic shadow is larger than 10 mm, it is categorized as complicated CWP or progressive massive fibrosis (PMF). Shadows of PMF are frequently bilateral, occurring in the upper and mid-lung zones. As they enlarge they may migrate toward the hilum, forming a sharp lateral margin delineated by a zone of emphysematous lung. Often the lesions are parallel to the chest wall, and are seen to have a greater diameter on the posteroanterior film than on the lateral view. If ischemic necrosis of the lesion occurs, a central cavitation or lucency may be noted.

Small irregularly shaped radiographic shadows are also observed in the lungs of miners. The finding of irregular densities, in contrast to small rounded densities, has more consistently been associated with a reduction in gas transfer and/or ventilatory lung function. The tissue pathology associated with these radiographic shadows is unclear. They have been correlated with increasing dust exposure, increasing age, and cigarette smoke, and are thought to have multiple causes, including both pathological emphysema and dust-induced fibrosis.

Under the ILO classification scheme, the small, rounded type of radiographic changes seen early in CWP are usually classified as 'p' or 'q' type opacities. The larger 'r' type opacities are more commonly associated with silicosis. As mentioned, irregular opacities (ILO type 's', 't', or 'u') may also be noted. A typical radiographic appearance of simple CWP is shown in Figure 19.10.5. The detail shows the opacities to be less than 3 mm in diameter ('q' type), and the profusion was interpreted as category 2.

Course and progression

Much of the information on the course and progression of radiographic changes in coal miners has been derived from long-term epidemiologic studies of coal miners in Britain. These were greatly facilitated by the concurrent collection of dust exposure data. In the main, these studies have shown that the overwhelming determinant of simple pneumoconiosis is the extent of exposure to coal mine dust per se. In addition, different coals are categorized by their 'rank', a characteristic which appears to have some influence on disease development. Rank is a factor which is related to the hardness and degree of metamorphosis of the coal due to heat and pressure.

High-rank coals, such as anthracite, have been associated with a greater risk of CWP and lung function deficits than lower rank and softer coals, such as bituminous coal or lignite. Silica may also play a role in the development of radiographic changes in underground coal miners, especially when experienced at high concentrations.[19] No other environmental factor has been shown to have a major effect. Tobacco use appears to have little effect on the development of the radiographic findings of CWP.

The main recognized risk factor for development of PMF is the category of simple CWP, particularly ILO categories 1/2 or greater.[20] Hence prevention of simple CWP must remain a priority. Recently it has been shown that there appears to be an exposure–response relationship between PMF and dust exposure in miners without radiographic evidence of simple CWP. Other factors pertinent to PMF development are coal rank, age of the miner, and residence time of dust in the lungs. Even though clear and consistent exposure–response trends have emerged from the many studies undertaken in the United Kingdom and elsewhere, much unexplained variability remains for both simple and complicated CWP. Large variations between mines in prevalence of diseases are seen that cannot be explained by recourse to available information on dust levels and composition.

The current federal dust standard in the US is 2 mg/m^3 (but may be further reduced when silica levels are high). This limit was derived from early British work which indicated that progression to category 2 or greater simple CWP would be prevented at this dust level. By this means, it was expected that further progression to PMF would be eliminated. As an additional health measure, an x-ray screening program was set up to identify miners with signs of CWP, and to offer them the right to work in a reduced dust envi-

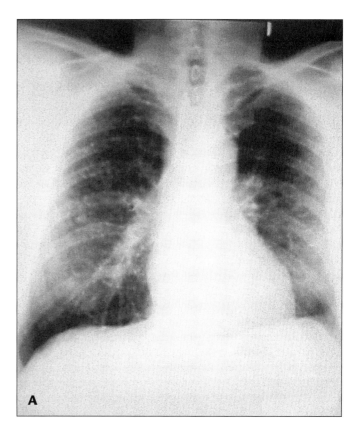

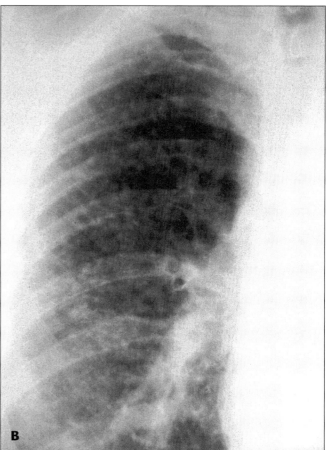

Figure 19.10.5: (a, b) Chest radiographic pattern of category 2 simple coal workers' pneumoconiosis with detail.

ronment, and have their work environment monitored more frequently. Dust-induced lung functional changes in the absence of radiographic changes were not considered during promulgation of the US standard.

Since the establishment of dust controls in the US, the prevalence of radiographically apparent CWP among underground miners has declined considerably.[21] Unfortunately, recent work from Britain and elsewhere suggests that the current US disease prevention strategy may be flawed. First, the more recent exposure–response models predict somewhat higher levels of disease than did the early work for the same dust exposure. In particular, 2 mg/m^3 is no longer associated with zero incidence of category 2 or greater (Fig. 19.10.6). Second, as noted earlier, it has been shown that PMF can develop when prior radiographs show no identifiable changes of simple CWP, and that this development is dose-related. Moreover, results from Britain have shown a substantial amount of PMF developing on a category 1 background. A survey of retired miners in Northern France also demonstrated the onset of simple or complicated CWP in 24% of miners who had normal radiographs at retirement. Finally, as discussed below, radiographic surveillance programs do not identify miners with dust-related reductions in ventilatory lung function that are not associated with radiographic changes of pneumoconiosis.

There is additional evidence that current US prevention strategies may not be entirely protective. Henneberger and colleagues found that, even after the establishment of a 2 mg/m^3 respirable dust standard, exposures among US coal miners were associated with an increased risk of respiratory symptoms.[22] As well, miners exposed for a working lifetime to the current US standard of 2 mg/m^3 respirable dust appear to have an elevated risk of dying from pneumoconiosis and COPD.[23]

In summary, there is no doubt that the current US health and environmental standard has led to a reduction in disease levels compared to those in the past, and there has been a significant decline in CWP mortality in the US, particularly among miners over age 45.[24] However, several recent reports have challenged the efficacy of the current US dust standard, and imply that it may be less protective than originally intended. A recent publication extensively reviewed current

knowledge of the health implications of coal mine dust exposures.[25] Based upon a critical review of the published scientific studies, the authors calculated the excess health risk (beyond that due to non-occupational factors including tobacco smoking) during work at the current US exposure limit for respirable coal mine dust (2 mg/m^3). Utilizing published exposure–response studies, it was estimated that for miners of low-rank bituminous coal working at the current exposure limit over a working life (45 years), 11–16.5% will develop pneumoconiosis, with 2–3% developing progressive massive fibrosis. Lower risks were projected for Western coal fields, and higher risks during the mining of Eastern higher rank and anthracite coals. In a similar calculation, clinically significant airflow obstruction (FEV$_1$ less than 65% of predicted normal) is projected to develop in 1–2% of miners working at the current dust exposure limit. Based upon these and other findings, a reduction in permissible exposures to 1 mg/m^3 was recommended. Additionally, since health risks would not be eliminated by the exposure reduction, medical monitoring was recommended using questionnaires and spirometry, in addition to chest radiographs.[25] However, at the time of writing, neither the exposure reduction nor monitoring recommendations have been implemented (see below)

Contemporary trends in CWP

Several radiographic surveys of selected mines, performed as part of the US National Coal Study, provide information regarding the prevalence of radiographic CWP in the US. The prevalence of the more advanced simple CWP (category 2 or greater) in miners with over 30 years tenure declined from about 11% in the first round of radiologic studies in 1971, to 8% in 1980, and to about 2% in 1988. The overall tenure-adjusted prevalence of CWP declined over the four surveys (Fig. 19.10.7). Some of the observed decline was found to be related to differences in the x-ray readers, as well as the use of a new version of the ILO chest

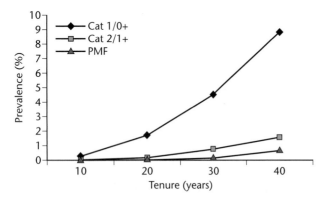

Figure 19.10.6: Predicted prevalence of radiographic coal workers' pneumoconiosis by mining tenure, assuming dust concentration of 2 mg/m^3, 83% carbon. Based upon British Field Research. (Adapted from Attfield[45] © 1992 American Public Health Association.)

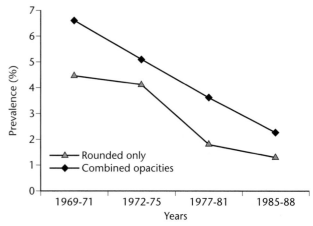

Figure 19.10.7: Trends in observed prevalence of radiographic category 1/0 or greater rounded only or combined opacities, adjusted to common job tenure. Based on the US National Study of Coal Workers' Pneumoconiosis. (Adapted from Attfield & Castellan[46] © 1992 American Public Health Association.)

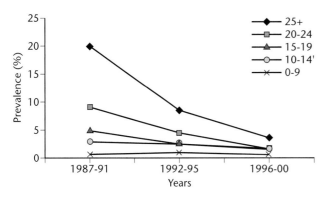

Figure 19.10.8: Recent trends in observed prevalence of radiographic category 1/0 or greater combined opacities by job tenure. Based on the US National Coal Workers' X-ray Surveillance Program. (Adapted from Wang ML, Petsonk EL: Pneumoconiosis prevalence among working US coal miners participating in federal chest x-ray surveillance programs: 1995 to 2000. Am J Epidemiol 153; 11:S127, by permission of Oxford University Press.)

radiograph classification system. When miners were grouped by mining tenure, and the proportion of miners with radiographic evidence of complicated CWP was analyzed, a clear decline was seen between the initial and final round of surveys. However, trends over the last decade were not as apparent.

In addition to the National Coal Study, an ongoing National Coal Workers' X-ray Surveillance Program is administered by NIOSH. Miners may participate in this program and receive chest radiographic examinations during the first 6 months and after 3 years of employment, and at approximately 3–5-year intervals thereafter. The classifications of radiographs taken under this program have been analyzed through 2000. The prevalence of category 1 or greater pneumoconiosis has generally declined for miners in each tenure category (Fig. 19.10.8). The proportion of participating miners showing complicated CWP also decreased since 1970 for all tenure groups. Thus, results of both the US National Coal Study and the US Coal Workers' X-ray Surveillance Program document a large reduction in the prevalence of radiographic changes of CWP in US coal miners since 1970.

Participation in the National Coal Study was over 90% in the first round, but was lower in later rounds. The US Coal Workers' X-ray Surveillance Program participation rates have been 50% or less. Although confidence in the analysis of trends is somewhat reduced by the participation rates, it does appear that the mandated programs of environmental and medical monitoring initiated under the Federal Coal Mine Health and Safety Act of 1969, in conjunction with transfer options and compensation of affected miners, have had an important effect in reducing the prevalence and incidence of CWP in US coal miners. Cases that continue to occur are more often noted in smaller mines and certain states.

Newer imaging techniques

In the past two decades, computerized radiographic techniques, gallium lung scanning, and magnetic resonance imaging have become widely available. Because traditional chest radiography is insensitive to early pathologic interstitial and emphysematous changes, interest has focused on these newer modalities in the non-occupational lung disorders. Limited evaluations of the usefulness of newer imaging techniques have been performed relative to the pneumoconioses. High-resolution computed chest tomography has been reported to be a more sensitive technique in identifying emphysema, as well as early pneumoconiosis among miners.[26] Coalescence of pneumoconiotic nodules and PMF lesions have been identified on CT scans when they were not apparent on routine radiographic evaluations.

Increased activity on gallium scanning of the lungs has been noted in several pneumoconioses, but this is nonspecific and may be less prominent in coal workers. Magnetic resonance imaging in the pneumoconioses has no currently demonstrated utility. Digital image processing has become widely used in the past few years for display, storage, and transmission of chest images. Computer-assisted pneumoconiosis interpretation of digitized images is being currently evaluated. However, at this time, additional studies are needed to define the role that digital processes should play in the evaluation of coal miners' lung diseases.

FUNCTIONAL CONSEQUENCES
Pathogenesis

The inhalation of sufficient coal mine dust affects the function as well as the structure of the lungs. Functional consequences can generally be divided into two categories: (1) effects related to the movement of gas into and out of the lungs (the 'bellows' function); and (2) effects related to the transfer of gases between the alveolar air and lung capillary blood.

Bellows function

Resistance to airflow into and out of the lungs of coal miners may be increased by bronchitic changes in the larger airways, by airway distortion, and by emphysematous destruction of elastic lung tissue at the level of the bronchioles and alveoli. These changes reduce the rate of maximal airflow, producing an obstructive ventilatory defect, demonstrated by reductions in the $FEV_1\%$ (FEV_1/FVC ratio) and the forced expiratory flow in the middle 50% of the vital capacity (FEF_{25-75}). In contrast, dilation of small air spaces can lead to overinflation and gas trapping, while fibrotic lesions, particularly of the massive type, reduce the volume of air contained in the lungs (total lung capacity).

Both of these latter changes can result in a reduction of the forced vital capacity (FVC) and forced expiratory volume in one second (FEV_1), producing a restrictive or mixed restrictive and obstructive pattern of abnormality on spirometry. It can be seen that, based on the predominant pathology, miners may show obstructive, restrictive, or often mixed patterns of dysfunction on spirometry related to their dust exposure. Recent studies have suggested that the loss of lung function due to dust exposure is not linear with time; rather, during the first months of exposure, there is an initial rapid loss of lung function, and subsequently a slower exposure-related decline.[27,28]

Gas exchange

Reduced ability to transfer gases in the lungs of miners can likewise result from multiple structural abnormalities. Dilation and distortion of small airways, as well as the fibrotic changes due to dusts, result in a heterogeneous delivery of inspired air into the alveoli. Destruction of capillaries and small vessels reduces the uniformity of lung perfusion. These effects combine to result in the mismatching of lung ventilation and perfusion and subsequent hypoxemia in the systemic arterial blood. The destructive loss of capillaries alone may also be sufficient to reduce the combined surface area of the alveolar-capillary membrane to an extent that gas transfer is impaired, particularly on exertion. In advanced disease, airflow obstruction may be so severe that alveolar ventilation is insufficient for metabolic demands. In this situation, hypoxia with hypercapnia results. An additional cause for hypoxia is reduced cardiac output, primarily seen in association with cor pulmonale and right ventricular dysfunction. Additionally, excessive ventilation on exertion has been associated with dyspnea in the presence of normal measures of lung mechanics.

INVESTIGATIONS OF COAL MINERS

The functional consequences of coal mine dust inhalation have been documented through both clinical and epidemiologic studies. Most studies of large groups of miners have used routine spirometry, evaluating the expiratory flows and forced vital capacity. Smaller groups have been studied utilizing other techniques. Series of miners have also been reported from clinics emphasizing disability/impairment evaluations. Although disability series are of interest, the representativeness of miners in these series is undetermined, exposure information is often scant or absent, and a control group is generally lacking. Their overall usefulness in the study of the effects of coal mine dusts on lung function is thus quite limited.

Epidemiologic studies

Most information regarding ventilatory effects of coal mining has been derived from large field studies of miners in the United States and the United Kingdom. Studies from other countries have been reported, and show generally very similar findings. Both cross-sectional and longitudinal evaluations of the US and British studies have been published. The lung function findings from both countries are quite consistent and are summarized below. The miners who were exposed to the dustiest environments show lower mean FEV_1 levels than those in less dusty mining jobs. More importantly, exposure–response rela-

tionships of FEV_1 with estimated dust exposure or with exposure surrogates such as tenure underground have been reported for miners in both countries. Other ventilatory function indices, such as FVC, FEV_1/FVC ratio, and flows at both higher and lower lung volumes have also been shown to be inversely related to estimated dust exposure.

Evidence of an effect on airflow at low lung volumes implies obstruction in small airways. In addition to the cumulative effects of dust, a large but non-progressive reduction in average lung function is seen in the group of miners who develop the symptom of a chronic productive cough. Groups of working miners from both the US and UK have been studied longitudinally over an approximately 11-year period. Results of these studies were quite similar, and showed that, as the miners' dust exposures increased, there was a resulting progressive decrement in lung function, as measured by the FEV_1, over the period of follow-up. Differences in the effects were seen between miners at different collieries. The effects on lung function associated with dust exposure were present after adjustment for smoking, and were typically observed to occur in all three smoking groups (never smokers, ex-smokers, and current smokers). The smoking and mine dust effects appeared to be independent and additive, but not synergistic. Thus, the average reduction in ventilatory function associated with exposure to mine dusts in smokers was similar to that in never-smoking miners. No disproportionate dust effects were noted in the smoking miners. In fact, the observed dust exposure effect, rather than being greater in current smokers, was often somewhat less.[29,30]

In miners who also smoke cigarettes, comparisons have been made between the excess reductions in lung function associated with mining exposures versus those associated with tobacco use. Since both effects are dose related, estimates of relative effect on lung function are conditional on the levels of exposure to tobacco smoke and to dust exposure chosen for the comparison. In the longitudinal study of US miners, for example, the average tobacco consumption in the smoking miners was 14 cigarettes per day. This was observed to result in an average excess loss of FEV_1 of 96 mL over 11 years in smoking miners compared to non-smoking miners. Eleven years of working at the coal face was associated with an average loss of FEV_1 of 84 mL in miners (non-smoking or smoking). For all miners, including those in less dusty work (average dust concentration 1.2 mg/m^3), the mean dust-related decline in FEV_1 over 11 years was 36 mL.

It has been suggested that although mean dust-related functional declines may be of similar magnitude to smoking effects, the tobacco and mining effects might be distributed differently. Under this hypothesis, tobacco effects among smokers are confined to large deficits in a small group of susceptibles, whereas mining effects are small but occur in most miners. Based on this hypothesis, equivalence in mean functional deficits attributed to dust and smoking could conceal very different functional consequences. However, several recent observations tend to contradict this hypothesis. Miners with non-specific airway hyper-responsiveness do show accelerated declines in lung function, but these miners do not appear to experience a disproportionate effect of dust exposure or smoking.[31] Miners with severe ventilatory deficits attributed to coal mine dust have also been identified, and studies of smoking and non-smoking miners have revealed similar increases in the proportions of severe impairments from dust- and smoking-related effects.[32,33]

Recent studies have demonstrated additional mine-related risk factors for lung function declines. Excess declines have been associated with exposures to explosive blasting and also to potentially contaminated water sprays used for dust suppression. Less steep rates of FEV_1 decline have been found among miners who use respiratory protective devices.[34] These findings suggest that additional health benefits can result from further improvements in the mine environment.

Miners' ventilatory lung function has also been compared to their chest radiographic changes of CWP, categorized using the ILO classification scheme. Higher categories of CWP, particularly complicated disease, are often associated with large reductions in FEV_1, and other functional consequences, as discussed below. Lower categories of simple CWP are not consistently associated with identifiable abnormalities on spirometry, after taking into account the functional losses associated with mine dust exposure, tobacco use, and the development of bronchitis. The relationship of the nodular lung disease of simple CWP and reduced lung function has repeatedly been investigated. Some studies observe a significant deficit in spirometry among miners who develop nodular simple CWP,[35] while others have not found an effect of nodular disease on lung function independent of the effects of emphysema.[36] Conversely, reduced lung function has repeatedly been observed among non-smoking miners without radiographic pneumoconiosis, and a negative x-ray does not exclude the possibility of occupationally related lung disease.[37,38]

Laboratory studies

Lung mechanics
Static lung compliance is often normal, but may be abnormally low or high in coal miners. High compliance, suggestive of emphysema, is the more common abnormality. Miners with PMF may have marked compensatory emphysema and high lung compliance; in others with PMF, the fibrotic process appears to predominate, and stiff lungs with low static compliance are seen. Miners with pinpoint ('p' type) opacities also appear to have dilation of peripheral airspaces.

Gas transfer
The transfer of gases in the lungs of coal miners has been evaluated using both the single-breath and the steady-state techniques to measure carbon monoxide diffusing capacity. Certain miners were found to have abnormalities on these tests. Reduced diffusing capacities are more commonly observed in miners with either pinpoint ('p' type) or irregular ('s' or 't' type) opacities of simple pneumoconiosis, and in those with complicated CWP, when compared to those with 'q' type opacities. Recent studies

among Chinese coal miners have found simple CWP to be a significant contributor to decrements in pulmonary function, including diffusing capacity.[39]

The findings related to gas exchange on exercise in coal miners are less well defined. Many authors have reported on highly selected groups of miners referred for disability evaluation. Estimated dust exposures were often not determined. Diminished gas transfer and/or excessive ventilation on exercise have been found in some groups, but not in others. Miners with PMF often have shown severe gas exchange abnormalities on exercise. Those with increasing airflow obstruction also generally have corresponding defects in gas exchange on exercise. When the functional correlates of radiographic pneumoconiosis have been carefully evaluated in miners without important airflow obstruction, it appears that simple pneumoconiosis, particularly categories 2 and 3, can lead to identifiable abnormalities of gas exchange on exercise. These changes have been attributed to the emphysema that often accompanies the radiographic changes.

In summary, low categories of pneumoconiosis, particularly the 'q' type opacities, in the absence of airflow obstruction, often appear to be associated with little or no gas exchange impairment. In contrast, miners with a finding of airflow obstruction, higher category of CWP, and either irregular or pinpoint opacities may show impairment of gas exchange, particularly on exertion.

Pulmonary hemodynamics
Increases in pulmonary artery pressure, at rest and on exercise, have been documented in some coal miners. Abnormalities are more commonly seen when the miners have measurable airflow obstruction. When the hemodynamics were compared to radiographic findings, abnormalities were most commonly seen in miners with complicated pneumoconiosis, silicosis, or pinpoint ('p' type) opacities of simple CWP. In the absence of airflow obstruction or one of these radiographic features, pulmonary hypertension appears uncommon in coal miners.

Summary

Miners may show several functional abnormalities in relation to the inhalation of coal mine dusts. Radiographic changes in PMF are often associated with multiple abnormalities. Certain patterns of simple pneumoconiosis (irregular and rounded pinpoint opacities) appear to be associated with gas exchange impairment. Studies of miners vary regarding the relationship between ventilatory function and radiographic category of simple CWP. In contrast, deficits in expiratory flow and volumes on spirometry appear to be related to the intensity and duration of dust exposures, independent of radiographic category of simple CWP. An additional reduction in ventilatory function is often seen in miners with symptoms of bronchitis. Spirometric abnormalities measured during miners' lives are correlated with pathologic changes in emphysema, which in turn have been correlated with measures of both dust exposure and lung dust retention.

The extent of pathologic emphysema is strongly related to coal dust content of the lungs, as well as to age and smoking. The dust effects in miners who smoke cigarettes appear to be additive to the effects of tobacco use; no disproportionate effect has been identifiable among coal miners who smoke. In smoking miners, FEV_1 reductions associated with a year of working at the mine face are of similar magnitude to the average annual smoking effect. When work at less dusty jobs is included, the average dust-associated reduction in ventilatory function over one year appears to be smaller than the average effect of a year of smoking. In addition, evidence indicates that dust exposure leads to severe lung function changes in some miners.

MORTALITY

A number of studies of coal miners from the US, the UK, and the Netherlands have investigated mortality rates among miners compared to the general population. These studies have identified increased deaths from pneumoconiosis, bronchitis, and emphysema, as well as accidents, but reduced mortality from a number of causes, including lung cancer and ischemic heart disease. The deficits observed in cause-specific mortality rates have been attributed to the strict prohibition of smoking in underground coal mines and to the healthy worker effect. As mentioned above, several studies have observed an elevated risk among coal miners for death due to gastrointestinal cancer (possibly related to incidentally ingested carcinogenic aromatic hydrocarbons in coal).

When mortality has been studied in relation to dust exposures, increasing mine dust exposure has been associated with risk of death from all causes, pneumoconiosis, bronchitis, and emphysema, after accounting for smoking and age. Mortality rates are also increased with the presence of radiographic pneumoconiosis, particularly PMF.[23,40] Miners who have deficits in FEV_1 or who experience accelerated losses of ventilatory lung function have an increased risk of death from cardiovascular and non-malignant respiratory diseases. A study from the Netherlands found that, in addition to a high standardized mortality rate for coal workers' pneumoconiosis, Dutch miners had significantly increased mortality from chronic airflow obstruction, and this was particularly evident among those without pneumoconiosis. Spirometric impairment was predictive of COPD mortality.[41]

A recent study reported mortality and questionnaire follow-up for 634 US coal miners whose lung function had been monitored over an average of 11 years. When evaluated after an additional 10–18 years, the group of miners with excessive FEV_1 losses reported a greater onset of respiratory symptoms and illness, and had experienced increased mortality from cardiovascular and non-malignant respiratory diseases, compared to their colleagues with more stable lung function.[42] Overall, the findings from the mortality studies among coal miners emphasize the importance of early detection of both radiographic abnormalities and lung function declines, as well as the initiation of effective interventions to prevent disease progression and death in affected miners.

DIAGNOSIS
Coal workers' pneumoconiosis

Pathologic changes of CWP may be found in the absence of radiographic evidence of pneumoconiosis. However, the radiographic picture of coal workers' pneumoconiosis is often sufficiently distinctive that, in the presence of an adequate exposure history, a diagnosis can be made with reasonable certainty. A lung biopsy is rarely needed. The question of what constitutes an 'adequate exposure history' is determined by the timing, duration, intensity, and other characteristics of the reported occupational exposures. Underground work prior to the institution of federal dust control regulations in 1970–73 likely represents a high risk of exposure. In this setting, pneumoconiosis developed in some miners with less than 5 years of exposure. Several jobs, as discussed above, offer recognized risks for silicosis. Face work, particularly in longwall mining, is still occurring with exposures commonly over the 2 mg/m^3 respirable dust standard. In the absence of these higher risk settings, a careful workup should be performed before diagnosing radiographic CWP in a miner with less than 5–10 years of coal mine exposure. Stability of the radiograph, or slow progression over a period of 2–5 years, is expected.

More rapid change should also prompt a search for alternative processes. Hilar or mediastinal adenopathy and pleural effusion are also not likely to be due to CWP alone. For example, the appearance in a coal miner with 10 or more years of underground mining experience of bilateral small rounded radiographic opacities in low profusion and principally in the middle and upper lung zones should be accepted as diagnostic of CWP. Some miners with this presentation have complaints of cough and sputum. Basilar lung crackles are usually scant or absent. Infectious processes, other interstitial lung disorders, and metastatic neoplasm should be carefully considered if fever, weight loss, clubbing, chest pain, hemoptysis, or progressive dyspnea or malaise are present. A broad list of differential diagnoses should be considered if the initial radiograph shows unilateral disease, predominant irregular opacities, or a high profusion of small rounded densities. Finally, prominent gas exchange abnormalities are also unusual early in the course of simple CWP.

Of great diagnostic concern is the development of a large radiographic opacity in a coal miner. The differential diagnosis must include malignancies and mycobacterial or fungal infections, as well as complicated CWP. PMF, which typically develops in the upper lung zones on a background of simple nodular densities, is often bilateral. Stability or slow progression over several years is consistent with complicated CWP. If doubt exists, then an appropriate workup should be completed before accepting the diagnosis of a dust-induced lesion. Caplan's syndrome (rheumatoid pneumoconiosis) may present as multiple larger nodules appearing without a definite background of simple CWP. The nodules may appear rapidly, i.e., over a period of weeks. A similar radiographic appearance may be seen with pulmonary metastases, but joint examination and serology will almost always reveal the confirming evidence of active rheumatoid disease.

MANAGEMENT
Medical screening and monitoring

Pre-placement medical testing is primarily intended to identify workers with existing medical conditions which would increase the health risk associated with coal mine employment. Periodic medical screening may utilize questionnaires, standard chest radiography, and spirometry. A program offering periodic chest radiographs to all underground coal miners in the US is currently mandated by federal regulations. This program serves to highlight potential areas of continuing medical and environmental problems. Due to the long latency of CWP, at times it can be difficult to relate contemporary environmental exposures to the cases identified. Miners with pneumoconiosis identified during screening qualify for administrative actions. They are entitled to increased frequency of personal environmental monitoring and offered the option to work in a reduced dust environment. This may require job transfer with maintenance of pay.

Periodic medical screening using spirometry is currently recommended, but not mandated. Pulmonary function testing is targeted toward identifying individuals with progressive airflow obstruction. To avoid the development of disabling lung impairment, workers with accelerated loss of lung function should be counseled regarding reducing current and future exposures to dust, if possible, as well as controlling other recognized risk factors (e.g., tobacco smoke).

General medical management

Medical management of a symptomatic coal miner with pneumoconiosis and/or airflow obstruction is similar in many ways to that of patients with non-occupational chronic lung diseases, but with emphasis on three principal areas: control of exposures, detection and treatment of complications, and compensation for disability. These are discussed below.

Exposure control

Control of symptoms in underground coal miners must address the mine environment, in addition to other potentially aggravating exposures, such as tobacco use. The miner should be encouraged to obtain and review the results of contemporary periodic air monitoring, to determine compliance of his or her work area with respirable dust and silica regulations.

A recommendation that the miner transfer to a surface job or a less dusty underground job is often the most viable option for reducing exposure to environmental dust.

Miners, particularly those not close to retirement, who have identifiable airflow obstruction, accelerated longitudinal decline in lung function, or radiographic changes of pneumoconiosis should be counseled regarding transfer to a less dusty environment. Miners who develop symptomatic bronchospasm in dusty environments can at times suppress the symptoms through the use of inhaled medications and oral bronchodilators. However, transfer is often necessary in order to control symptoms without resorting to more hazardous forms of therapy, such as systemic corticosteroid therapy. Transfer rights with retention of wage rates and benefits are available only for underground coal miners with radiographic abnormalities identified through radiographic surveillance, under current US mining regulations. Radiographs may be submitted to NIOSH for an official interpretation to determine eligibility.

In contrast to the situation in the US, dust control is less well established in coal mines in other countries. For example, in Poland, recommended dust levels may be exceeded in over 90% of measurements.[43]

Engineering controls are accepted as the primary method of exposure control, and recommendations for continuous use of respiratory protective equipment are rarely practical in underground coal mining. Occasionally, however, a miner with prominent cough or bronchospasm may be able to continue working underground while participating in a formal respiratory protection program. There is evidence that use of respirators can diminish the adverse respiratory health effects from exposure to current levels of coal mine dust.[34]

Attention should also be paid to non-occupational respiratory hazards. In smoking miners, recommending smoking cessation is an initial step in exposure management. Referral to volunteer organizations or other formal cessation programs, prescription of nicotine delivery systems when appropriate, and unambiguous advice from the healthcare provider are effective approaches.

Detection and treatment of complications

Dust-induced fibrosis, emphysema, and chronic airflow obstruction are irreversible changes. Interventions should be targeted toward detecting, treating, and preventing complications. Management of conditions etiologically unrelated to mine dust exposure may also be complicated by lung impairments related to dust effects.

Periodic monitoring of spirometry and chest radiographs is useful to determine the rate of progression of the disorder and to detect onset of complications. An initial electrocardiogram may be helpful for subsequent comparisons. In miners who present with symptoms and signs of illness, assessment of gas exchange at rest and exercise may be indicated. The subsequent performance of these evaluations must be tailored to the clinical course of the individual miner. Infectious exacerbations, including acute bronchitis and pneumonia, may occur in affected miners. Broad-spectrum antibiotics and physical therapies are helpful in reducing symptoms during episodes of purulent sputum production.

The treating clinician should take care to exclude both tuberculosis and non-tuberculous mycobacterial infections. Particularly in miners with silicosis, the risk of these infections is increased and the response to chemotherapy is less satisfactory (see Chapter 19.9). Tuberculin reactivity should be tested in all miners with CWP, since over 10% may have silicosis, which confers a 30-fold increased risk for development of active tuberculosis. In tuberculin-positive miners with radiographic pneumoconiosis, active disease must be carefully excluded. Once this has been accomplished, isoniazid preventative therapy is recommended for those with positive skin tests and no contraindications or risk factors for isoniazid-resistant infection. Nine months of daily treatment reduces the subsequent risk of developing active disease. Shorter regimens of chemoprevention including rifampin have also been effective but are not considered the first choice for miners with abnormal chest radiographs and a low risk of INH-resistant strains.

Inhaled and/or oral bronchodilator therapy should be attempted in most symptomatic miners. Prolonged courses of inhaled steroids have been shown to control symptoms and reduce non-specific bronchial hyper-responsiveness. Short, tapering courses of systemic corticosteroids may be helpful for acute exacerbations. However, it is rarely, if ever, justified to use long-term systemic steroids to allow a miner to remain working in a dusty environment.

Whole lung lavage, reported for two miners with silica exposure and pneumoconiosis, resulted in considerable removal of inorganic dust from the lungs.[44] However, there is currently no evidence that the course of disease is improved by this drastic measure.

Cor pulmonale with right heart failure due to CWP is treated the same as cor pulmonale due to other etiologies.

A coordinated rehabilitation program, with attention to nutrition, emotional stresses, pharmacologic and physical therapies, and judicious exercise may improve the clinical status of the disabled miner. As in patients with other irreversible disorders, discussions regarding the use of life-support and mechanical ventilation are appropriate in miners with severe but clinically stable lung disease.

Compensation/disability

Miners with lung impairments may be eligible for compensation under the Federal Black Lung Benefits Program, as well as through state pneumoconiosis and workers' compensation plans. In advising individual miners, the healthcare provider should be familiar with the specific requirements of the programs. Particular note should be taken of the statute of limitations, since the date of filing a claim relative to the establishment of a diagnosis of work-related disease may be critical in determining eligibility for benefits. Legal counsel often is necessary in establishing eligibility (see Chapter 57.1).

References

1. US Department of Labor, Mine Safety and Health Administration. Mine Industry Accident, Injuries, Employment, and Production Statistics. http://www.msha.gov/ACCINJ/accinj.htm [cited October 1, 2001]

2. Love RG, Miller BG, Groat SK, et al. Respiratory health effects of opencast coalmining: a cross sectional study of current workers. Occup Environ Med 1997; 54:416–23.

3. Attfield MD, Wagner GR. Chronic occupational respiratory disease. Occup Med 1996; 11:451–65.

4. Fernie JM, Ruckley VA. Coalworkers' pneumoconiosis: correlation between opacity profusion and number and type of dust lesions with special reference to opacity type. Br J Ind Med 1987; 44:273–7.

5. Vallyathan V, Brower PS, Green FH, et al. Radiographic and pathologic correlation of coal workers' pneumoconiosis. Am J Respir Crit Care Med 1996; 154:741–8.

6. Anonymous. Pathology standards for coal workers' pneumoconiosis. Report of the pneumoconiosis committee of the College of American Pathologists to the National Institute for Occupational Safety and Health. Arch Path Lab Med 1979; 103:375–432.

7. Ruckley VA, Gauld SJ, Chapman JS, et al. Emphysema and dust exposure in a group of coal workers. Am Rev Respir Dis 1984; 129:528–32.

8. Ruckley VA, Fernie JM, Chapman JS, et al. Comparison of radiographic appearances with associated pathology and lung dust content in a group of coal workers. Br J Ind Med 1984; 41:459–67.

9. Maclaren WM, Hurley JF, Collins HP, et al. Factors associated with the development of progressive massive fibrosis in British coal miners: a case-control study. Br J Ind Med 1989; 46:597–607.

10. Green FYH, Althouse R, Weber K. Prevalence of silicosis at death in underground coal miners. Am J Ind Med 1989; 16:605–15.

11. Leigh J, Driscoll TR, Cole BD, et al. Quantitative relation between emphysema and lung mineral content in coal workers. Occup Environ Med 1994; 51:400–7.

12. Coggon D, Inskip H, Winter P, et al. Contrasting geographical distribution of mortality from pneumoconiosis and chronic bronchitis and emphysema in British coal miners. Occup Environ Med 1995; 52:554–5.

13. Yi Q, Zhang Z. The survival analyses of 2738 patients with simple pneumoconiosis. Occup Environ Med 1996; 53:129–35.

14. IARC Working Group on the evaluation of carcinogenic risks to humans. Silica, some silicates, coal dust and para-aramid fibrils. Lyon, October 15–22, 1996. IARC Monographs on the Evaluation of Carcinogenic Risk to Humans. IARC: Lyon, 1997.

15. Swaen GM, Meijer JM, Slangen JJ. Risk of gastric cancer in pneumoconiotic coal miners and the effect of respiratory impairment. Occup Environ Med 1995; 52:606–10.

16. Oberdorster G. Lung particle overload: implications for occupational exposures to particles. Regul Tox Pharm 1995; 21:123–35.

17. Schins RP, Borm PJ. Mechanisms and mediators in coal dust induced toxicity: a review. Ann Occup Hyg 1999; 43:7–33.

18. Rom WN. Relationship of inflammatory cell cytokines to disease severity in individuals with occupational inorganic dust exposure. Am J Ind Med 1991; 19:15–27.

19. Miller BG, Hagen S, Love RG, et al. Risks of silicosis in coal workers exposed to unusual concentrations of respirable quartz. Occup Environ Med 1998; 55:52–8.

20. Gautrin D, Auburtin G, Alluin F, et al. Recognition and progression of coal workers' pneumoconiosis in the collieries of northern France. Exp Lung Res 1994; 20:395–410.

21. Goodwin S, Attfield M. Temporal trends in coal workers' pneumoconiosis prevalence. Validating the National Coal Study results. J Occup Environ Med 1998; 40:1065–71.

22. Henneberger PK, Attfield MD. Respiratory symptoms and spirometry in experienced coal miners: effects of both distant and recent coal mine dust exposures. Am J Ind Med 1997; 32:268–74.

23. Kuempel ED, Stayner LT, Attfield MD, et al. Exposure–response analysis of mortality among coal miners in the United States. Am J Ind Med 1995; 28:167–84.

24. Bang KM, Althouse RB, Kim JH, et al. Recent trends of age-specific pneumoconiosis mortality rates in the United States, 1985–1996: coal workers' pneumoconiosis, asbestosis, and silicosis. Int J Occup Environ Hlth 1999; 5:251–5.

25. National Institute for Occupational Safety and Health. Criteria for a recommended standard: occupational exposure to respirable coal mine dust. 1-9-95. DHHS (NIOSH) Publication No. 95-106. Cincinnati: US Department of Health and Human Services, Public Health Service, Centers for Disease Control.

26. Lamers RJ, Schins RP, Wouters EF, et al. High-resolution computed tomography of the lungs in coal miners with a normal chest radiograph. Exp Lung Res 1994; 20:411–9.

27. Seixas NS, Robins TG, Attfield MD, et al. Longitudinal and cross sectional analyses of exposure to coal mine dust and pulmonary function in new miners. Br J Ind Med 1993; 50:929–37.

28. Henneberger PK, Attfield MD. Coal mine dust exposure and spirometry in experienced miners. Am J Respir Crit Care Med 1996; 153:1560–6.

29. Love RG, Miller BG. Longitudinal study of lung function in coal miners. Thorax 1982; 37:193–7.

30. Attfield MD. Longitudinal decline in FEV1 in United States coal miners. Thorax 1985; 40:132–7.

31. Hodgins P, Henneberger PK, Wang ML, et al. Bronchial responsiveness and five-year FEV1 decline: a study in miners and non-miners. Am J Respir Crit Care Med 1998; 157:1390–6.

32. Marine WM, Gurr D, Jacobsen M. Clinically important respiratory effects of dust exposure and smoking in British coal miners. Am Rev Respir Dis 1988; 137:106–12.

33. Hurley JF, Soutar CA. Can exposure to coal mine dust cause a severe impairment of lung function? Br J Ind Med 1986; 43:150–7.

34. Wang ML, Petsonk EL, Beeckman LA, et al. Clinically important FEV1 declines among coal miners: an exploration of previously unrecognized determinants. Occup Environ Med 1999; 56:837–44.

35. Bourgkard E, Bernadac P, Chau N, et al. Can the evolution to pneumoconiosis be suspected in coal miners? A longitudinal study. Am J Respir Crit Care Med 1998; 158:504–9.

36. Gevenois PA, Sergent G, De Maertelaer V, et al. Micronodules and emphysema in coal mine dust or silica exposure: relation with lung function. Eur Respir J 1998; 12:1020–4.

37. Nemery B, Veriter C, Brasseur L, et al. Impairment of ventilatory function and pulmonary gas exchange in non-smoking coal miners. Lancet 1987; 2:1427–30.

38. Wang X, Yu IT, Wong TW, et al. Respiratory symptoms and pulmonary function in coal miners: looking into the effects of simple pneumoconiosis. Am J Ind Med 1999; 35:124–31.

39. Wang X, Yano E, Nonaka K, et al. Respiratory impairments due to dust exposure: a comparative study among workers exposed to silica, asbestos, and coal mine dust. Am J Ind Med 1997; 31:495–502.

40. Miller BG, Jacobsen M. Dust exposure, pneumoconiosis, and mortality of coal miners. Br J Ind Med 1985; 42:723–33.

41. Meijers JM, Swaen GM, Slangen JJ. Mortality of Dutch coal miners in relation to pneumoconiosis, chronic obstructive pulmonary disease, and lung function. Occup Environ Med 1997; 54:708–13.

42. Beeckman LA, Wang ML, Petsonk EL, et al. Accelerated declines in FEV1 and subsequent increased respiratory symptoms, illnesses, and mortality in US coal miners. Am J Respir Crit Care Med 2001; 163:633–9.

43. Marek K, Lebecki K. Occurrence and prevention of coal miners' pneumoconiosis in Poland. Am J Ind Med 1999; 36:610–7.

44. Wilt JL, Banks DE, Weissman DN, et al. Reduction of lung dust burden in pneumoconiosis by whole-lung lavage. J Occup Environ Med 1996; 38:619–24.

45. Attfield MD. British data on coal miners' pneumoconiosis and relevance to US conditions. Am J Pub Hlth 1992; 82:978–83.

46. Attfield MD, Castellan RM. Epidemiological data on US coal miners' pneumoconiosis, 1960 to 1988. Am J Pub Hlth 1992; 82:964–70.

47. Pon MRL, Roper RA, Petsonk EL, et al. Pneumoconiosis prevalence among working US coal miners participating in federal chest x-ray surveillance programs: 1996 to 2002. MMWR 2003; 52:336–400.

19.11 Other Pneumoconioses

James R Donovan Jr, James E Lockey

This chapter discusses less commonly seen chronic lung diseases caused by metals and minerals. The clinical evaluation of such patients is discussed briefly here and also in Chapter 19.1. Specific elements that can cause pneumoconioses are described. The fibrogenic potential of mineral dust is dependent on various physical and chemical properties of the dust, the dose retained in the lung, and specific physiologic and immunologic characteristics of the individual.[1] Silicon dioxide (SiO_2) as free silica is the most common naturally occurring fibrogenic dust. Silicates are silicon dioxide combined with various cations. The crystalline structure of silicates can vary from a platy occurrence or habit, such as mica, to a very fibrous habit, such as crocidolite or amosite asbestos.

Specific silicate ore sources such as talc can exist in a very pure deposit, or can contain minor concentrations of free silica or intergrowths of other minerals such as the amphibole tremolite. Proper mineralogic analysis of samples of an ore body taken from different locations and ongoing analysis of environmental samples from the workplace are crucial in the recognition, evaluation, and control of potential pulmonary health risks. Material Safety Data Sheets may not provide enough information to adequately characterize the physical and chemical properties of a specific silicate or potential contaminant minerals or metals.

Frequent natural contaminants of silicate ore bodies are the amphiboles tremolite, actinolite, and anthophyllite. These are considered non-commercial amphibole asbestos, in contrast to the commercial amphiboles amosite and crocidolite and the serpentine chrysotile asbestos. Other amphibole minerals such as winchite and richterite, that are not currently regulated by the Occupational Health and Safety Administration, can also be found as natural contaminants.[2] The non-commercial amphiboles exist in an asbestiform or highly fibrous habit or in a non-asbestiform or relatively non-fibrous habit. The term asbestiform refers to a fiber configuration, which is long and thin with high length-to-width ($>3:1$) or aspect ratios. When mechanical force is applied these amphiboles cleave along their specific crystalline planes and form short, squat cleavage fragments, mostly of a non-asbestiform variety, or long thin fibers, mostly of an asbestiform variety. Characterization of the mineralogy of the non-commercial amphiboles has been an area of ongoing confusion. The health implications of the non-commercial non-asbestiform amphiboles have not been adequately defined.

CLINICAL EVALUATION

The diagnosis of the pneumoconioses discussed in this chapter can be particularly challenging as exposures usually span many years and are rarely to a single agent, and the clinical features are usually non-specific. The radiographic and pulmonary function evaluation of patients for occupationally induced lung disease is covered in

Chapter 19.1. A standard posteroanterior chest radiograph should be interpreted for parenchymal and pleural changes by a physician trained and experienced in using the ILO International Classification of Radiography of the Pneumoconioses, the B-reader.

CT and high-resolution CT of the chest are more sensitive than the standard chest radiograph for detecting pleural changes, and for differentiating pleural adipose tissue from discrete and diffuse pleural thickening.[3] The sensitivity and specificity of high-resolution CT (HRCT) in the evaluation of diffuse interstitial fibrotic changes are excellent with a high degree of clinical application. Use of the high-resolution CT in the prone and supine positions will differentiate peripheral interstitial fibrotic changes from normal hydrostatic fluid changes that disappear with change in body position. HRCT has demonstrated predominant, sometimes characteristic findings for each type of pneumoconiosis, and represents a major advance in the accurate characterization of these parenchymal disorders.

Pulmonary function test results can be normal, or they may be of a restrictive, obstructive, or mixed obstructive-restrictive pattern, particularly in patients with progressive massive fibrosis. Progressive decrements of FVC over several spirometric measurements can be a sensitive indicator of an early and potentially progressive interstitial fibrotic process.

Although bronchoalveolar lavage (BAL) is not routinely indicated, it is a relatively non-invasive procedure and has been used in the evaluation of patients at risk for inorganic dust-induced lung disease with unusual presentations.[4,5] Evaluation of lavage fluid with energy dispersive spectrometry can provide information on the composition of inhaled dust. Cells obtained by BAL can be examined for the presence of dust particles. Such studies may confirm exposure, but it is unclear whether they correlate with exposure, tissue burden or disease. The BAL cell count and differential, and lymphocyte cell subset analysis into helper (CD4+) and suppressor (CD8+) T cells can suggest certain diagnoses, such as hypersensitivity pneumonitis, but are not diagnostic of any particular disease or pneumoconiosis.

Histologic examination of lung parenchyma generally provides the most definitive pathologic diagnosis, but frequently cannot determine etiology. Tissue obtained by open lung biopsy is less prone to sampling error than that obtained by transbronchial biopsy and is sufficient for qualitative and quantitative mineral dust analysis. Light microscopy with special staining techniques can detect parenchymal changes that develop in response to retained particles. Light microscopy is adequate for detecting ferruginous bodies. Phase-contrast light microscopy can detect uncoated fibers 0.2 mm or greater in diameter. Scanning electron microscopy can detect similar size particulates, and with energy dispersion x-ray analysis can identify elemental composition. Transmission electron microscopy can detect the smallest particulates, and with selected area electron diffraction it can characterize crystalline structure. Mineralogic analysis should always be interpreted in conjunction with the other information regarding the patient.

As with other more common pneumoconiosis, the diagnosis of diseases in this chapter depends on a careful occupational history documenting sufficient exposure to cause the disease, consistent clinical evaluation, including radiographic features and physiology, and the exclusion of any more likely non-occupational disorders. Mineralogic analysis, although not routinely available, is particularly helpful when the exposure history is inconclusive or the clinical presentation atypical.

SPECIFIC ELEMENTS THAT CAUSE PNEUMOCONIOSES
Aluminum (see Chapter 39.1)

Aluminum is derived from alumina (Al_2O_3), which is produced from the naturally occurring hydrous aluminum oxide ore, bauxite. Bauxite ore can contain various impurities, including quartz and cristobalite as well as clay minerals. The decomposition of alumina into metallic aluminum occurs in electrolytic cells known as pots located within potrooms. Aluminum metal powder is produced in a flake and granulated form. A lubricant oil such as stearin is added to the flake aluminum powder to permit easy separation of the aluminum particles. Uncertainties about aluminum-related pneumoconiosis are derived from the complexity of the exposure and the low prevalence of disease in spite of the extensive use of the metal.

A group of potroom workers involved in manufacturing alumina abrasives from bauxite developed diffuse progressive radiographic and pathologic fibrotic changes predominantly involving the upper lung fields. This rare condition, referred to as Shaver's disease, has been postulated by some investigators to be related to the silica present in the production process.[6]

Exposure to aluminum powder used in the manufacturing of explosives in Great Britain and Germany during the First World War has been associated with changes similar to the findings in Shaver's disease. These findings were most likely related to exposure to high levels of aluminum metal dust that was stamped and ground into a fine powder. Aluminum metal powder is considered more fibrogenic than aluminum oxides and silicates, but exposure is rare. A case study of an aluminum potroom worker with diffuse interstitial fibrosis and restrictive changes on pulmonary function tests demonstrated a markedly elevated aluminum particle burden as well as short aluminum fibers.[7]

Symptoms of reversible chest tightness, shortness of breath and wheezing have been reported by aluminum potroom workers, and have been termed potroom asthma. (see Chapter 39.2) Diagnostic criteria and good environmental measurements have not been standardized in many of the studies of this syndrome. Estimated annual incidence of potroom asthma varies from 0.06% to 4.0%. Exclusion of workers with a history of asthma or atopy in some of the studies may have caused these estimates to be artificially lowered. The role of smoking has not been determined. Causative factors that have been implicated include particulate and gaseous fluoride, total respirable dust, sulfur dioxide, and aluminum fluoride compounds.

Pneumoconiosis from exposure to aluminum metal or oxide of aluminum is rare. It would appear that high exposures with corresponding high lung burdens are required to induce pulmonary damage. A longitudinal study of nearly 1000 aluminum smelter workers demonstrated no accelerated decline in lung function.[8] The rarity of this particular pneumoconiosis is most likely a reflection of decreased exposure through improved working conditions and environmental control measures. Limited case reports have described a granulomatous alveolitis in workers exposed to aluminum, with increased CD4+ T lymphocytes, similar to sarcoid and chronic beryllium disease, and suggesting an immune-mediated response to aluminum.[9]

Antimony (see Chapter 39.10)

Antimony is mined and smelted in various areas of Central and South America, South Africa, the United States, China, and Russia. During the mining and milling process, there is potential for exposure to free silica. Within antimony smelting plants, the predominant exposure is to antimony trioxide and antimony pentoxide. Small amounts of free silica and arsenic oxide have also been identified in airborne dust samples of smelting plants.

Alloyed with lead or other metals, antimony is used in battery plates, solder, and pewter. Non-metallic uses include manufacturing flame-resistant fabrics, and pigments for ceramics, paints, and rubber compounds.

Exposure to antimony oxides during the smelting process can induce simple pneumoconiosis, particularly in those workers with 10 or more years of exposure. Small, round opacities with a diameter usually less than 1.0 mm are densely distributed in the middle and lower lung fields. Complicated pneumoconiosis has not been described, nor has progression after removal from exposure. Some airway obstruction with hyperinflation was identified in one study but without adjustment for tobacco use. No isolated restrictive abnormalities were noted, and the rest-and-exercise blood gas determination and diffusing studies were essentially normal.

Exposure to antimony ore during the mining and milling process can cause changes consistent with silicosis or mixed-dust pneumoconiosis (defined in a later section). Radiographic changes most commonly involve the upper and middle lung fields, and the round opacities usually are greater than 1.0 mm in diameter.

Exposure to antimony oxide has been associated with vesicular skin eruptions with residual hyperpigmentation as well as nasal septal perforation. Antimony trichloride and pentachloride are highly toxic and can cause acute pulmonary edema.

Barium

Barite, which is the natural form of barium sulfate ($BaSO_4$), is mined in the United States, Canada, Mexico, and Europe, and the source of the ore can often be contaminated with free silica and/or other minerals. The great majority of barite is processed into refined barium sulfate, which is used in oil and gas drilling. Approximately 10% of barite is converted into barium-containing compounds such as lithopone, which is used in the glass, paint, and rubber industries.

The inhalation of barite dust by miners or excessive exposure to barium-containing compounds can induce the pneumoconiosis baritosis (Fig. 19.11.1). The chest radiograph is striking due to the high radiodensity of barium, with small, round dense opacities that can involve all lung fields. Radiographic changes have been observed to diminish with cessation of exposure. Baritosis is not associated with any increased pulmonary morbidity or mortality and should be considered a benign pneumoconiosis. Fibrosis and accompanying respiratory symptoms apparently do not occur unless there is concomitant exposure to free silica. Barium sulfate contrast material used for radiographic procedures can be seen on chest x-ray if aspirated or instilled in the lung, but is considered inert.

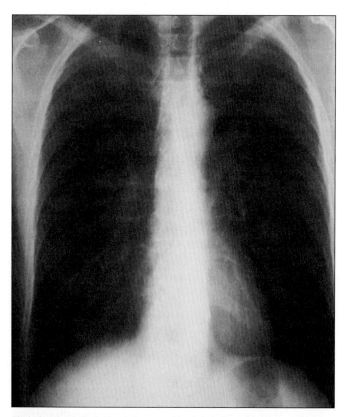

Figure 19.11.1: Baritosis is caused by inhalation of barium sulfate or barite ore. Patients are asymptomatic and the radiographic changes may improve after removal of the individuals from exposure. (Courtesy of Jerome F. Wiot, MD, University of Cincinnati.)

Graphite

Natural graphite exists as amorphous and crystalline carbon that is mined in North and South America, Europe, Asia, and Africa. Natural graphite contains various amounts of free silica as well as other impurities, including iron oxide, clay, mica, and other minerals. Synthetic graphite is produced by heating coal or coke higher than 2200°C (3992°F). Synthetic graphite is crystalline and contains only trace amounts of free silica. Historically, the mining and curing of natural graphite and the production of synthetic graphite was a dusty process in comparison to most current work practices.

Graphite is very resistant to thermal shock and is used in foundry facings and crucibles, in steel and cast iron manufacturing, as neutron moderators in atomic reactors, and in carbon electrodes.

Both simple and complicated pneumoconioses have been attributed to graphite dust exposure. The preponderance of cases are a mixed-dust pneumoconiosis, partially attributed to the free silica contaminant of the graphite dust. The role of silicon dioxide in graphite pneumoconiosis remains controversial, but both simple and complicated pneumoconioses have been reported in workers with only trace amounts of silica exposure or none at all. The clinical findings and pathogenesis of graphite pneumoconiosis are similar to coal worker's pneumoconiosis.[10]

Iron

Welders and other workers exposed to dust or fumes of metallic iron and iron oxide can develop a benign pneumoconiosis termed siderosis. Small, dense opacities distributed throughout the lung field can be demonstrated on chest radiograph, similar to simple silicosis. No symptoms or pulmonary function impairments are associated with pure siderosis. The pathologic findings in siderosis are perivascular and peribronchiolar aggregations of iron oxide dust particles, both in macrophages and in extracellular tissue.

A significant percentage of workers exposed to iron oxide encounter other occupational exposures that may represent a significant pulmonary hazard. Foundry workers, for example, are potentially exposed to various types of metal alloys as well as free silica, vermiculite, asbestos, and welding and oxyacetylene metal cutting fumes, as well as isocyanates. The resultant chest radiographic changes and pulmonary function abnormalities under these circumstances may be reflective of a mixed-dust pneumoconiosis rather than pure siderosis.

Kaolin

Kaolin, also called china clay, is a hydrated aluminum silicate that is found in the southeastern United States (primarily Georgia), and in Great Britain (Cornwall), Germany, Czechoslovakia, Egypt, and Japan. The principal industrial uses are in the manufacture of refractory ceramic bricks and fibers; as filler in plastics, rubber, paints, adhesives, and pharmaceuticals; and as an absorbent. Kaolin ore may contain appreciable quantities of free silica (quartz), micas, and feldspars, as well as various cations. Remarkably, Georgia kaolin contains very little free silica.

Simple and complicated pneumoconioses have been described in kaolin mine and mill workers, and can also be found in user industries. A 63-year-old male employed for 43 years in the polishing room of a clothes textile mill, who died of respiratory failure, was found on lung biopsy to have extensive fibrosis and substantial quantities of kaolin. Chest radiographs of kaolin workers have demonstrated predominantly irregular but also small, round opacities involving all lung fields at various levels of profusion. Large opacities have also been seen. Pleural thickening has been noted in mild kaolinosis. The overall prevalence of pneumoconiosis in current kaolin mine and mill workers has ranged from 7.2% to 13%.

Results of pulmonary function tests in kaolin workers with simple pneumoconiosis have tended to be normal or demonstrate a mild restrictive pattern. Workers with complicated pneumoconiosis may have normal pulmonary function or demonstrate an obstructive, restrictive, or mixed obstructive-restrictive pattern.

Pathologic examination of pulmonary tissue from (Cornish/china) (kaolin) clay and stone workers demonstrated both interstitial and nodular fibrosis. The interstitial fibrosis ranged from localized fibrosis around the respiratory bronchioles to diffuse fibrosis with obliteration of alveoli and honeycombing, and the severity of the conditions correlated with kaolin dust content of the lung. The nodular fibrosis varied in size (3 mm to 10 mm in diameter) and number (two to seven nodules per section), and correlated with quartz dust content of the lung. Complicated pneumoconiosis was seen in both groups. Histologic findings in five kaolin workers from Georgia with complicated pneumoconiosis demonstrated extensive kaolin deposition that was associated with peribronchiolar macules and nodules. Silica was not identified in the lung tissue from Georgia kaolin workers.

Synthetic vitreous fibers (see Chapter 46)

Man-made vitreous fibers (MMVF) are a generic group of synthetic amorphous glassy silicates fiberized from molten raw material.[12] Mineral wool includes slag and rockwool, and it is produced primarily from iron ore furnace slag and naturally occurring rock. Glass fiber includes glass wool, continuous glass filament, and special purpose glass fiber, and is produced from molten glass consisting of borosilicate and low alkaline silicate glasses with various amounts of stabilizers (aluminum, titanium, and zinc) and modifiers (sodium, calcium, barium, potassium, lithium, and magnesium). Refractory ceramic fiber is produced from kaolin clay or aluminum and silica.

Mineral wool is manufactured by a rotary or wheel centrifuge process. Glass wool is manufactured by a rotary and blowing process, continuous glass filament by drawing or extruding molten glass through set diameter holes, and special purpose glass fiber by a flame attenuation process. Refractory ceramic fiber is produced by a steam-blowing or wheel centrifuge process. A phenolic binder with oil as a lubricant and dust suppressor is commonly added in the manufacturing process of mineral and glass wool. During the curing process, the binder is normally fully polymerized and is chemically inert in the final product.

The average diameters of MMVF are dependent on the production process and end-use of the product. The average diameter for mineral wool is 3.5 to 7 µm; glass wool, 1 to 15 µm; special purpose glass fiber, less than 3 µm; and refractory ceramic fiber, 1 to 5 µm. Large variations in fiber diameter can occur for these classes of MMVF. Even though the average diameter may be set at 5 µm, a significant number of fibers have diameters within the respirable range of less than 3.5 µm diameter and less than 250 µm in length due to the nature of the production process. Continuous glass filaments average 3–25 µm in diameter and are manufactured by a method that maintains a more precise fiber diameter.

MMVF greater than 5 µm in diameter can cause mechanical skin irritation and itching, and irritation of the eyes and mucosal surfaces, especially in newly exposed individuals. Workers with atopic dermatitis or dermographism may not be able to tolerate MMVF exposure because of a lower itch threshold. A high concentration of fiber can cause upper and lower respiratory tract irritation that is transient in nature and resolves with removal of the affected individual from exposure.

There are two major ongoing mortality studies of United States and European mineral wool and glass fiber manufacturing workers. Within the United States the most recent study of the mineral wool and glass fiber cohort reported a small but statistically significant excess risk for lung cancer. This pattern, however, was not found to be associated with measures of exposure, such as duration of employment, fiber exposure estimates, or time since first employment.[13,14] An excess in lung cancer seen in one glass fiber manufacturing plant may have been due to differences in local versus the national prevalence of cigarette smoking.[15] The most recent analysis of the US workers from five rock and slag wool plants demonstrated an increased lung cancer mortality based on national but not local expected rates. The excess risk was concentrated in short-term workers and not related to measures of respirable fiber exposure. Interestingly there was an increased mortality from nephritis and nephrosis compared to both national and local rates, which needs to be further studied.[16]

The mortality study of European mineral and glass wool workers also demonstrated a significantly increased risk for lung cancer mortality compared against national mortality rates. For glass wool workers, however, there was no association with duration of employment or time since initial employment and with removal of short-term workers, no excess lung cancer was noted. In regard to the rock and slag wool cohort the investigators felt a possible relationship with exposures during the early phase of mineral wool production was not as clear as in previous studies but fiber exposure may have contributed non-specifically to the mortality results.[17-19] Within the European cohort there was no increased mortality from bronchitis, emphysema, or asthma.[20]

Clinical studies of workers involved with mineral wool and glass fiber manufacturing generally have not demonstrated any significant increase in chest radiograph or pulmonary function abnormalities. A morbidity study by Weill and Hughes in the United States in 1983 reported a possible relationship between exposure duration and ILO profusion categories 1/0 and 1/1. A follow-up survey in 1993 by Hughes et al. reported an overall prevalence of small opacities of 1.6%, which was similar to a non-fiber exposed comparison group. There was an association with indices of exposure at profusion level 1/0 but not 1/1. The authors concluded that there were no adverse clinical, functional, or radiographic effects of fiberglass and mineral wool manufacturing in the study population. Similar results have been found in other studies of mineral and glass wool manufacturing workers with the exception of a potential interaction between fiber exposure and heavy cigarette smoking and airway obstruction.[21]

End-user studies of mineral and glass wool exposure are limited. Workers using rotary spun fiberglass in appliance insulation for 15 years or longer were reported to demonstrate a 3.5% prevalence of irregular opacities at profusion level 1/1 to 2/1. Asbestos contamination within the plant site may have been a contributing factor.[22] Lower FEV_1 values in MMVF-exposed insulation workers, adjusted for self-assessed former asbestos exposure, have also been reported. The health risk to end-users from exposure to mineral and glass wool is certainly less than that associated with asbestos exposure. Further studies of end-users with no previous occupational exposure to asbestos are needed.

Refractory ceramic fiber (RCF) is primarily used in industrial environments requiring high temperature insulation, such as in oven and kiln wall linings and the aerospace industry. Extended use of RCF above 1000°C (1832°F) causes partial conversion to cristobalite, a type of crystalline silica. Animal inhalation studies at a maximum tolerated dose of 30 mg/m^3 of RCF have demonstrated the induction of mesothelioma, lung cancer, and interstitial and pleural fibrosis. Subsequent multiple-dose studies at 3, 9, and 16 mg/m^3 demonstrated minimal fibrosis at the two higher concentrations and one mesothelioma at the 9 mg/m^3 exposure.[23,25]

Within the US an initial cross-sectional evaluation of pulmonary function in workers involved with RCF manufacturing demonstrated a reduction in FVC in current (165 ml) and past (156 ml) male smokers and a reduction in FEV_1 (135 ml) in current male smokers and employment in production job tasks for 10 years. For females there was a reduction in FVC among non-smokers of 350mL per 10 years employment in production job tasks that was not seen in never-smoker males.[24] The results of European studies were similar indicating a probable interactive effect between smoking and RCF exposure and small decrements in FVC and FEV_1.[26] A longitudinal evaluation of pulmonary function obtained between 1987 and 1994 for those male workers with five or more tests demonstrated

no further decline in FVC or FEV_1 values that most likely was related to the lowering of workplace exposures.[27]

A recent chest radiograph analysis of US RCF manufacturing workers demonstrated an association between latency, duration of employment in a production job, and cumulative RCF exposure and pleural plaques. Of those workers with over 20 years in a production job task, 8% demonstrated pleural changes. The overall prevalence of pleural changes was 2.7%. There was a trend towards early interstitial changes but not at a statistically significant level.[28] A previous case-control study confirmed that potential previous asbestos exposure did not account for the changes. The European study indicated a relationship between time since first RCF exposure and pleural changes as well as a relationship with age and previous asbestos exposure.

The International Agency for Research on Cancer (IARC) classified biopersistent MMVF such as RCF and certain special-purpose glass wools as group 2B or possible human carcinogens. The more common insulating glass wool, rock and slag wool, and continuous glass filaments are group 3 or not classifiable as carcinogenic to humans.[29]

Ongoing animal and human studies will continue to refine knowledge concerning possible health risks associated with exposure to various types of MMVF. Maintaining exposure at 1 respirable fiber/cm^3 or less as a time-weighted average especially for biopersistent MMVF should help maintain a margin of safety for exposed workers. This is especially important for secondary and end-users when exposure levels may not be adequately controlled and where the data are inadequate to evaluate the potential health risk.

Mica

Micas are a group of complex aluminum silicates containing either alkaline metals or iron and magnesium. The muscovite form is a potassium aluminum silicate that is transparent and resistant to heat and electricity. It is used in stove windows and in the manufacture of paints, wallpaper, and lubricants. Other forms of mica are used as fillers in cements, asphalts, and pharmaceutical products; as a component of drilling muds in the oil industry; and within the electrical industry. Mica is mined in India, Canada, Brazil, Russia, and the United States. Human exposure is through mining and milling and through the application of micas in production processes.

Mixed-dust pneumoconiosis and silicosis in mica miners have been reported but appear related to contamination with free silica. The evidence that mica without silica can cause a pneumoconiosis with interstitial fibrosis is based largely on case reports and limited surveys of mica workers. Such reports have described pneumoconiosis secondary to grinding muscovite, which is believed to be nearly silica free. Objective findings have included: crackles involving the lung bases on chest auscultation, restrictive changes on pulmonary function tests, and small opacities on chest radiographs involving the lower lung fields. Pathologic changes noted are ill-defined fibrotic nodules as well as more widespread interstitial fibrosis. Mineralogic analyses of the lung tissues have demonstrated the muscovite form of mica free of other minerals.[30]

Mixed-dust pneumoconiosis

Mixed-dust pneumoconiosis is the terminology applied to lung disease caused by simultaneous exposure to crystalline silica and other dusts, such as iron oxides, coal, oil shale, and graphite. Anthracosilicosis and silicosiderosis are examples of specific mixed-dust pneumoconiosis. Occupations in iron, steel, and non-ferrous foundries and in arc welding and oxyacetylene metal cutting in an environment where there is free silica exposure have been associated with mixed-dust pneumoconiosis. The degree of fibrosis is related to the amount of free silica involved.

Classic whorled silicotic nodules are less common than in pure silicosis, perhaps secondary to a modifying effect on the free silica from an accompanying non-fibrogenic dust. Irregular peribronchiolar and perivascular collagen fibrosis is seen with increased content of iron, carbon, or other mineral dusts. The chest radiographic changes are isolated round or round and irregular opacities involving the upper lung or whole lung fields. Progressive disease can occur, but is less common than with silicosis. The occurrence of tuberculosis in mixed-dust pneumoconiosis is higher than that in the general population.

Oil shale

Oil shale is a sedimentary rock that contains oil. After being mined and crushed, the ore is heated to 350°C to 500°C (662°F to 932°F), releasing oil vapor, which is then condensed into liquid in a process called retorting. The oil shale industry existed in Scotland from 1850 until 1962. In the western United States, vast deposits of oil shale exist as a yet unused energy source. Oil shale contains minerals similar to low-rank coal, and can contain free silica, ash, kaolinite and mica.

A survey of Scottish oil shale workers demonstrated a prevalence of simple pneumoconiosis (ILO profusion category 2/1 or greater) ranging from 1.6% to 5.8% in miners and 0.6% to 3.6% in retort workers, and a few cases of complicated pneumoconiosis. Pulmonary function abnormalities of a mixed obstructive-restrictive pattern were identified in oil shale workers with simple pneumoconiosis. The decrements in lung function persisted after allowance for age and smoking status.[31]

In the early years of the industry, skin and scrotal cancer were described in workers producing paraffin products and in cotton mill workers using lubricating oils produced from oil shale. A mortality study by Seaton et al.[32] of oil shale workers first employed prior to 1953 demonstrated an excess of deaths from skin cancer.

Polyvinyl chloride (see Chapter 41)

Under normal temperature and pressure, vinyl chloride monomer is a gas and is used as a chemical intermediate in the polymerization of polyvinyl chloride (PVC) resin. A cross-sectional study by Soutar et al. of over 800 men in a PVC manufacturing facility demonstrated a relationship between PVC dust exposure and dyspnea, decrements in FEV_1 and FVC, and chest radiographic abnormalities. The changes in FEV_1 and FVC were small but consistent with a mixed obstructive-restrictive pattern. Chest radiographic changes were consistent with small, rounded opacities of ILO profusion category 1/1 or less.[33] Case reports with available pathology have demonstrated desquamative interstitial pneumonitis and interstitial fibrosis associated with a restrictive pattern on pulmonary function tests. Phagocytized PVC material in pulmonary macrophages has been seen in lung biopsy material. In a few instances, elevated urine and blood levels of phthalic acid derivatives were demonstrated.

Talc (see Chapter 46)

Talc is a hydrated magnesium silicate that exists in several crystalline forms, ranging from talc plates to the more uncommon talc fibers. Talc deposits can be mineralogically complex and, depending on the ore source, can range from pure talc to talc ore with intergrowths of the non-commercial amphibole asbestos minerals, tremolite, actinolite, and anthophyllite, as well as silica. The non-commercial amphiboles are primarily of the non-asbestiform variety that fracture into short prismatic and acicular cleavage fragments along their crystalline plane with the application of mechanical force. Longer fibers approaching a more asbestiform variety, however, have also been identified as well as occasional chrysotile asbestos.

When talc is discussed in the industrial setting, it can refer to a variety of minerals that have physical properties similar to talc, such as chlorites, pyrophyllite, and dolomite. The mineralogic variability of talc deposits as well as the use of the term talc to denote physical properties of various minerals rather than the specific hydrated magnesium silicate has caused persistent problems in interpreting the health effects from occupational exposures. A variety of minerals in addition to talc, including mica, kaolin, asbestos, and silica, have been identified on mineralogic analysis of lung biopsies from talc-exposed workers.

Within the United States, talc is predominantly produced from mines in New York, Vermont, North Carolina, Texas, Montana, and California. Talcs containing admixtures of previously listed minerals are used in industrial applications including the manufacturing of ceramics, paper, plastics, rubber, wall covering materials, asphalt, and electrical insulation. The pure talc deposits, such as those found in Montana, Vermont, and inland California, are used in consumer products such as cosmetics, deodorants, food processing, and as fillers in pharmaceuticals.

Three forms of pneumoconiosis have been associated with inhalational talc exposure: talcoasbestosis, talcosilicosis, and pure talcosis. A fourth form is associated with intravenous administration of medication intended for oral use in which pure talc is used as a filler. Talcoasbestosis has been associated with talc from the Gouverneur Talc District of upper New York State.[34] Miners exposed to talc mined near or in New York State have demonstrated radiographic and pathologic changes commonly associated with exposure to commercial asbestos. This includes irregular opacities involving the lower lung fields, and pleural and diaphragmatic plaques with calcification. Characterization of the mineralogy of the ore and the dust generated from the mining and milling processes has been a subject of ongoing debate.

Owing to the potential for mixed-dust exposure that includes the previously mentioned non-commercial amphibole asbestos, platy talc, homogeneous talc fibers, heterogeneous fibers composed of various elemental constituents, and in some circumstances, silica, the pathologic findings can be complex. Changes consistent with diffuse interstitial fibrosis with asbestos bodies, silicotic nodules, and granuloma formation with giant cells containing birefringent particles have been identified. Early mortality studies reported high mortality rates due to pneumoconiosis and lung cancer. Subsequent studies that were able to control for confounders such as smoking and previous occupational exposures have not substantiated an association with lung cancer.

Talcosilicosis is caused by the inhalation of talc associated with free silica. The free silica content of air during talc mining operations in Italy has been measured as high as 18%. Radiologic changes in cases from Italian and California coastal talc mining operations demonstrated diffuse round and irregular opacities, and peripheral conglomerate masses. The pathologic changes were consistent with silica exposure, with both silica and talc particles identified in the lung tissue. An increase in mortality from non-malignant respiratory disease in Italian miners was secondary to silicosis and silicotuberculosis.

Talcosis is caused by the inhalation of talc that is essentially free from other mineral contamination. Talcosis has been identified from occupational as well as non-occupational exposure, such as habitual use of excessive amounts of cosmetic talcum powder. An unusual case of pulmonary talcosis involved a respiratory technologist who admitted to regularly inhaling large amounts of hospital baby powder. This produced an asthma-like condition that was refractory to steroids and methotrexate, documented with lung biopsy.

Another example involved a 62-year-old woman who had been initially diagnosed with sarcoidosis until a biopsy revealed the presence of numerous birefringent particles in centrilobular lung zones, which were further characterized as impure talc, free of asbestos or silica. Her occupational history showed only that she had worked from age 14 to 18 in a factory making rubber hoses, with exposure to talc. This suggested that even a relatively short, but intense exposure to talc more than 40 years previously could be a cause of progressive lung fibrosis. Radiographic changes include round and irregular opacities that can be diffuse or limited to the upper (Fig. 19.11.2) or lower lung fields. Pathologic changes include focal fibrosis adjacent to small

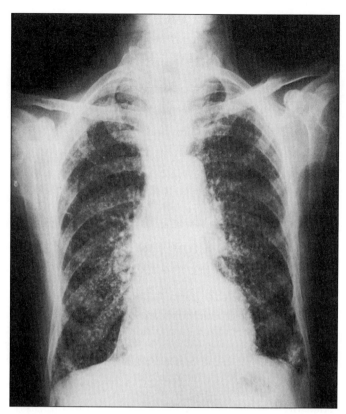

Figure 19.11.2: Talcosis is caused by inhalation of pure talc. This patient was employed in the Montana talc mines for 20 years and was asymptomatic, with normal pulmonary function tests. There are round opacities (ILO category 1/1) involving the upper lung fields.

airways and vessels to more diffuse fibrosis in workers with prolonged exposure to high concentrations of talc. Foreign body granulomas and multinucleated giant cells have also been identified. Chest radiographs can be normal in workers with focal pathologic changes. Pulmonary function tests in cases of talcosis range from normal to a restrictive or mixed restrictive and obstructive pattern. IARC reported that there was inadequate evidence for cancer in humans resulting from talc that does not contain asbestiform fibers.

Accidental aspiration of talc by infants or habitual use of excessive amounts of cosmetic talc can induce significant pulmonary disease, including bronchiolitis and extensive fibrosis with granuloma formation. When injected intravenously by individuals abusing oral medication in which talc is used as a filler, a foreign body granulomatous reaction can occur ultimately resulting in secondary cor pulmonale.

The spectrum of talc-related pneumoconiosis is associated with the heterogenicity and physical characteristics of the mineral, the intensity and duration of exposure, and individual differences in the pathologic reaction to the mineral. In general, it appears that higher concentrations of pure talc are required to induce pathologic changes in the lung in comparison to talc contaminated with asbestos and silica.

Tin

Tin occurs naturally in various tin-bearing minerals that are mined on several continents. Tin miners are exposed to silica, lead, arsenic, as well as other metals and are at risk for the development of nodular silicosis. Major industrial uses for tin include as a component of protective coatings, solder, jewelry, pewter, bronze, and various metal alloys.

Workers exposed to tin dust or fumes can develop radiographic changes consistent with dense small diffuse opacities. This condition, referred to as stannosis, is associated histologically with lung macules and macrophages laden with tin oxide particles (Fig. 19.11.3). Stannosis is considered a benign pneumoconiosis with no significant pulmonary symptoms or pulmonary function impairment associated with the radiographic findings.

Vermiculite

Vermiculite is a micaceous hydrated mineral with an aluminum-iron-magnesium silicate composition. With the application of heat, vermiculite expands up to 20 times its original size. Expanded vermiculite is used in insulating and fire-resistant materials, aggregates and filler in cements, plastic and flooring materials, agricultural products such as potting soil, and as carriers for fertilizers and other chemicals. The ore is shipped in an unexpanded form and is expanded at local facilities.

Vermiculite ore is frequently contaminated with various asbestiform minerals, mostly fibrous tremolite-actinolite, depending on the source of ore. The pulmonary health effects of vermiculite exposure appear related to the degree of contamination by these asbestiform fibrous amphiboles.

Vermiculite ore from a mine and mill near Libby, Montana (which closed in 1990), was contaminated with 5%–10% non-commercial fibrous asbestos, actinolite, and some tremolite. Other asbestiform minerals contaminating the Montana ore include winchite and richterite.[35] A morbidity and mortality study by Amandas et al. of the Montana vermiculite miners and millers demonstrated an increased risk of lung cancer, as well as pleural and parenchymal abnormalities on chest radiography, typical of those induced by asbestos,[36] as well as four persons with mesotheliomas.

A recent screening evaluation was completed of over 6000 current and former residents of the Libby, Montana, area, including former workers of the vermiculite mine or mill, as well as residents who lived in the area for 6 months or longer prior to 1991. Eighteen percent of participants had pleural abnormalities on chest radiographs, which increased to almost 40% in those individuals 65 years or older. The radiographic changes were noted not only in former mine and mill workers but also in residents with bystander exposure only.[34]

Vermiculite ore from the Enoree region, South Carolina, is believed to have low concentrations of the non-commercial asbestos tremolite and actinolite, mostly of the non-asbestiform variety. The mean concentration of fibers from bulk dust samples was 0.27 fiber per milligram of dust, with 37.9% fibers identified as tremolite-actinolite and 15.9% identified as talc anthophyllite. Air-borne fibers were thinner and shorter than the bulk dust samples, and air-borne concentrations were reportedly below 0.32 fiber/cc by transmission electron microscopy. A radiographic survey of 86 current and former employees demonstrated small opacities of ILO profusion category 1/0 or more in 4.7% and pleural thickening in 8.1%. However, a similar prevalence of radiographic findings was seen in a non-exposed group of employees.

Vermiculite from South Africa contains the non-commercial fibrous amphibole asbestos anthophyllite, as well as potentially small amounts of tremolite. A cross-sectional study of radiologic findings and lung function in 172 vermiculite workers demonstrated small opacities of profusion 1/0 or greater in 1.2%, pleural changes in 3.5%, and pleural calcifications in 1.7%. The changes were reportedly similar or lower than a comparison group not exposed to vermiculite.

Adverse health effects of vermiculite exposure may result when the vermiculite is contaminated with asbestiform minerals, primarily fibrous tremolite-actinolite. Routine monitoring of the source of the ore for amphibole contamination, and analysis of air-borne dust particulates can help limit tremolite-actinolite fiber exposure and the health risks known to be associated with asbestos exposure.

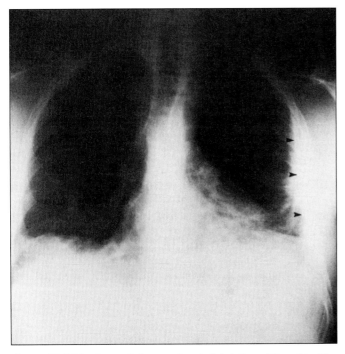

Figure 19.11.3: Stannosis is secondary to inhalation of tin oxide. The chest radiograph demonstrates multiple, round high-density shadows evenly distributed throughout both lung fields. (Courtesy of Jerome F. Wiot, MD, University of Cincinnati.)

Zeolite

Naturally occurring zeolites are a family of hydrated aluminum silicates that exist in approximately 40 non-fibrous and fibrous zeolite species. The main natural deposits in the western United States occur along the margins of the Great Basins (Utah, Nevada). Non-fibrous synthetic zeolite with no identifiable health risk is produced for its selective absorption and ion-exchange characteristics.

The fibrous zeolite species erionite morphologically resembles commercial amphibole asbestos fibers. Epidemiologic studies of several villages in the central Anatolia area of Turkey known as Cappadocia have identified an increased incidence of mesothelioma, lung cancer, and pleural and parenchymal changes commonly associated with commercial asbestos exposure.[37] The equal occurrence of mesothelioma in males and females at an unusually young age supports an environmental etiology. Mineralogic analysis of environmental samples and lung tissue demonstrated fibrous zeolite (erionite) as well as tremolite and chrysotile. Animal studies have confirmed that fibrous erionite is fibrogenic and carcinogenic.

Within the United States, a heavy equipment operator from Nevada with a pulmonary histologic pattern similar to asbestosis was found to have fibrous and non-fibrous aluminum silicate particles within the lung parenchyma. Using scanning electron microscopy with energy dispersion x-ray analysis, the particulates were found to be identical to a sample of fibrous erionite obtained from northern Nevada.

The health data associated with fibrous zeolite (erionite) exposure indicate that other naturally occurring fibrous minerals may, in fact, cause health abnormalities that are now associated with asbestos exposure. The occurrence of natural deposits of zeolite in certain areas of the western United States warrants caution during earth-moving construction projects, and other dispersive activities in areas with these types of geologic formations.

References

1. Potolicchio I, et al. Susceptibility to hard metal lung disease is strongly associated with the presence of glutamate G9 in HLA-DP beta chain. Eur J Immunol 1997; 27:2741–3.
2. Leake BE, et al. Nomenclature of amphiboles: Report of the subcommittee on amphiboles of the International Mineralogical Association, commission on new minerals and mineral names. Am Mineral 1997; 82:1019–37.
3. Akira M. High resolution CT in the evaluation of occupational and environmental disease. Radiol Clin North Am 2002; 40:43–59.
4. Rizzato G, et al. The differential diagnosis of hard metal lung disease. Sci Total Environment 1994; 150:77–83.
5. Costabel U, Bross KJ, Huck E, et al. Preliminary observations: lung and blood lymphocyte subsets in asbestosis and in mixed dust pneumoconiosis. Chest 1987; 91:110–2.
6. Shaver CG, Riddell AR. Lung changes associated with the manufacture of alumina abrasives. J Ind Hyg Toxicol 1947; 29:145–57.
7. Gilks B, Churg A. Aluminum-induced pulmonary fibrosis: do fibers play a role? Am Rev Respir Dis 1987; 136:176–9.
8. Chan-Yeung M, Enarson DA, MacLean L, Irving D. Longitudinal study of workers in an aluminum smelter. Arch Environ Health 1989; 44:134–9.
9. De Vuyst P, Dumortier P, Rickaert F, Van de Weyer R, Lenclud C, Yernault JC. Occupational lung fibrosis in an aluminium polisher. Eur J Respir Dis 1986; 68:131–40.
10. Hanoa R. Graphite pneumoconiosis: a review of etiologic and epidemiologic aspects. Scand J Work Environ Health 1983; 9:303–14.
11. Chaudhry BA, et al. Pleural thickening in mild kaolinosis. Southern Med J 1997; 90:1106–9.
12. Nomenclature Committee of TIMA, Inc. Nomenclature of man-made vitreous fibers. Stamford, Connecticut: TIMA, 1991.
13. Enterline PE, Marsh GM, Esmen NA. Respiratory disease among workers exposed to man-made mineral fibers. Am Rev Respir Dis 1983; 128:1–7.
14. Enterline PE, Marsh GM, Henderson VL, Callahan C. Mortality update of a cohort of US man-made mineral fiber workers. Am Occup Hyg 1987; 31:625–56.
15. Chiazze L, Watkins DK, Fryar C. A case-control study of malignant and non-malignant respiratory disease among employees of a fiberglass manufacturing facility. Br J Ind Med 1992; 49:326–31.
16. Marsh G, Stone R, Youk A, et al. Mortality among United States rock wool and slag wool workers: 1989 update. J Occup Health Safety Aust NZ 1996; 12:297–312.
17. Simonato L, Fletcher AC, Cherrie J, et al. The man-made mineral fiber European historical cohort study. Scand J Work Environ Health 1986; 12:34–47.
18. Boffetta P, Saracci R, Andersen A, et al. Cancer mortality among man-made vitreous fiber production workers. Epidemiology 1997; 8:259–68.
19. Boffetta P, Anderson A, Hansen J, et al. Cancer incidence among European man-made vitreous fiber production workers. Scan J Work Environ Health 1999; 25:222–6.
20. Sali D, Boffetta P, Anderson A, et al. Non-neoplastic mortality of European workers who produce man-made vitreous fibers. Occup Environ Med 1999; 56:612–7.
21. Weill H, Hughes JM, Hammond YY, et al. Respiratory health in workers exposed to man-made vitreous fibers. Am Rev Respir Dis 1983;128:104–112.
22. Hughes JM, Jones RN, Glindmeyer HW, Hammond YY, Weill H. Follow-up study of workers exposed to man-made mineral fibers. Br J Ind Med 1993;50:658–67.
23. Hansen EF, Rasmussen FV, Hardt F, Kamstrup O. Lung function and respiratory health of long-term fiber-exposed stonewool factory workers. Am J Respir Crit Care Med 1999; 160:466–72.
24. Bunn WB, Bender JR, Hesterberg TW, Chase GR, Konzen JL. Recent studies of man-made vitreous fibers. J Occup Med 1993; 35:101–13.
25. Mast RW, McConnell EE, Hesterberg TW, et al. Multiple-dose chronic inhalation toxicity study of size-separated kaolin refractory ceramic fiber in male Fischer rats. Inhal Toxicol 1995; 7:469–502.
26. Cowie HA, Wild P, Beck J, et al. An epidemiological study of the respiratory health of workers in the European refractory ceramic fibre industry. Occup Environ Med 2001; 58:800–10.
27. Lockey JE, Levin LS, Lemasters GK, et al. Longitudinal estimates of pulmonary function in refractory ceramic fiber manufacturing workers. Am J Respir Crit Care Med 1998; 157:1226–33.
28. Lockey JE, LeMasters GK, Levin L, et al. A longitudinal study of chest radiographic changes of workers in the refractory ceramic fiber industry. Chest 2002; 121: 2044–51.
29. IARC Monographs. Man-made Vitreous Fibres, Vol 81. Lyon, France: IARC, 2002.
30. Skulberg KR, Gylseth B, Skaug V, Hanoa R. Mica pneumoconiosis CA literature review. Scand J Work Environ Health 1985; 11:65–74.
31. Louw SJ, Cowie HA, Seaton A. Epidemiologic studies of Scottish oil shale workers: II. Lung function in shale workers' pneumoconiosis. Am J Ind Med 1986; 9:423–32.
32. Seaton A, Louw SJ, Cowie HA. Epidemiologic studies of Scottish oil shale workers: I. Prevalence of skin disease and pneumoconiosis. Am J Ind Med 1986; 9:409–21.

33. Soutar CA, Copland LH, Thornley PE, et al. Epidemiological study of respiratory disease in workers exposed to polyvinylchloride dust. Thorax 1980;35:644–52.

34. Abraham JL. Non-commercial amphibole asbestos fibers and cleavage fragments in lung tissues of New York State talc miners with asbestosis and talcosis. Am Rev Respir Dis 1990; 141:A244.

35. Medical Testing of Individuals Potentially Exposed to Asbestiform Minerals Associated with Vermiculite in Libby, Montana. A Report to the Community. Agency for Toxic Substances and Disease Registry. Atlanta, GA: US Department of Health and Human Services, 2001.

36. Amandus HE, Althouse R, Morgan WKC, et al. The morbidity and mortality of vermiculite miners and millers exposed to tremolite-actinolite: Part III. Radiographic findings. Am J Ind Med 1987; 11:27–37.

37. Baris YI, Saracci R, Simonato L, et al. Malignant mesothelioma and radiological chest abnormalities in two villages in central Turkey. Lancet 1981; i:984–7.

Chapter 20
Disorders of the Eye, Ear, Nose and Throat

20.1 Ophthalmologic Disorders

Lea Hyvärinen, Susan H Forster

INTRODUCTION

Ophthalmologic disorders can occur in a variety of different work environments. Visual and ergonomic issues impact on a large number of office workers. Ergonomic problems and injuries caused by poor ergonomics are not reported as effectively as cases related to trauma and toxic exposures. The reported incidence of occupational injuries that lead to temporary or permanent visual disability approaches 70,000 workers in the United States each year.[1] Many of these injuries are preventable.

Diagnosis is often challenging as signs or symptoms may be subtle and not clearly attributable to a given cause. Work-related disorders of the eyes and visual pathways often mimic other diseases. Underlying eye and visual pathway disorders may increase susceptibility to workplace exposures. Health professionals need to be informed of the working conditions or the hazards that exist in the workplace. Allergic reactions are common in industrial, agricultural, and office settings but are also attributable to exposure in non-work environments, which often present a confounding factor. An affected group of workers from the same industry may seek medical help from a variety of different sources, which makes identification of clusters of work-related disorders difficult. Thus, there remains an important role for specialists who are knowledgeable about the work environment and potential work-related risks. In addition to accurate diagnosis of individual cases, clinical investigations of groups of workers are important to document a causal relationship between ocular or visual changes and work.

Finding an occupational link to illness sometimes requires ingenuity. For example, recent investigation by Schuman et al.[2] showed an increase in the incidence of visual field defects in wind instrument players presumably secondary to the transient elevation of intraocular pressure while playing high resistance wind instruments.

Assessment of visual function is an important part of pre-employment medical screening and monitoring of the workforce. Assessment techniques used today do not cover important visual functions, like motion perception in traffic-related occupations or contrast sensitivity in monitoring exposure to toxic substances.[3]

CLINICAL EVALUATION

An evaluation of a worker with a possible eye disorder or vision problem consists of a careful history and an examination. In addition to assessment of individuals and clusters of workers with presumed work-related exposures, evaluation prior to employment is important to determine the worker's capacity to perform in that work and to consider its possible ill effects to each given worker's health. In the evaluation not only are measurements made but also the worker's vision is assessed in terms of the requirements of each particular occupation.

In most occupations visual tasks are related to four main functional areas: (1) orientation and mobility; (2) tasks resembling activities of daily life, i.e., finding objects at work and using tools and instruments; (3) communication; and (4) sustained near-vision tasks like reading and writing. In cases of evaluation of visually impaired workers their special ergonomic needs require consultation with local and nationwide services.[4]

History

An occupational case history should include pertinent symptoms and their onset and duration. Certain symptoms should always lead to questioning about possible exposures, and exposure to a known toxic substance should lead to questions about specific symptoms. An exposure may result in acute or chronic symptoms with a latency period between exposure and onset of symptoms from seconds to years. Visual symptoms are often vague and can sound like psychogenic complaints. When a worker complains of blurred vision or a change in the quality of vision, the physician should consider the possibility of a neurologic disorder or a reaction caused by an environmental exposure or pharmaceutical agent.[3] Color vision and contrast sensitivity are often first affected. The treating physician should have access to information on all chemicals that the worker may be or has been exposed to and their known effects on the eyes and vision.

Physical examination

Patients may complain of ocular pain, irritation, itching, or periocular swelling. Severe pain and photophobia (light-induced pain) in a red eye suggest intraocular involvement and warrant immediate ophthalmologic evaluation. Discharge from the eye is caused by conjunctival irritation or conjunctivitis. Itching is typical of allergic reactions. Blurred vision, difficulties in seeing, ergonomic and spectacle problems are other common complaints.

The physical examination should include the following: (1) testing of visual acuity and color vision, (2) visual field testing, (3) testing of ocular motility, (4) external examination, (5) fundus examination, (6) laboratory and electrophysiologic tests. Many tests are beyond the scope of the occupational physician and require referral to a neurologist or an ophthalmologist with special interest in occupational health.

Visual acuity

Measurement of visual acuity is nearly always included in an examination of the eyes and vision. Although it does not define the pathology or state of health of an eye or of visual pathways,[5] it provides some basic information about visual functioning. Testing should be done at the distance marked on the test. If the patient generally wears distance glasses, testing should be done using the glasses unless documentation of uncorrected vision is specifically required. Visual acuity is tested first binocularly, and then for each eye separately. The Landolt C optotype and number charts are universally accepted, but the EDTRS and the old Snellen chart are also acceptable in the United States. Luminance at the chart needs to be 80 candelas per square meter or higher. Lightboxes make it possible to have standard luminance wherever the test is used.

Visual acuity is recorded for binocular vision and each eye separately. If glasses are used this is noted. Visual acuity values can be recorded in one of two ways, i.e., (1) as the last line read correctly (for example, if a person reads the 20/30 line and two letters on the 20/25 line, the result is given as 20/30, ignoring the partially correct line); or (2) more precisely, the last line read correctly plus the number of letters read correctly on the following line (in the previous example, as 20/30 +2). Visual acuity measurements with a near card complete testing at distance. Near vision is particularly relevant in assessment of vision ergonomics of office workers, although an office worker with asthenopic symptoms (eye strain) needs referral to an eye care professional for thorough evaluation of the refractive correction and demands of the working conditions.

Visual acuity is measured at low contrast for quick detection of early changes in the optics of the eye, changes in the function of the retina or subtle pathway damages. In most occupations measurement at 2.5% contrast is sufficient, but in occupations that require visual functions at very low contrast levels, such as quality control or handling large white surfaces, regular measurements at 1% contrast are warranted. The occupational low contrast tests are used in lightboxes.

In visual acuity testing the threshold of recognition is measured. However, it is not possible to function at acuity threshold. A reserve capacity two to three times greater than the threshold is needed to work comfortably. This can be easily measured at the workplace by asking the employee to move backward and measure the distance from which he or she can read the text with which he or she works. For example, many computer screen texts can be read with distance glasses at a distance of 2–4 m. Thus there is a 3–6 times reserve capacity in visual acuity.

Color vision

Color vision appears to be particularly sensitive to toxic exposures, including a number of different solvents, mercury,

and certain pharmaceuticals. There are two types of color vision tests: screening tests and quantitative tests. Screening tests such as Ishihara pseudoisochromatic plates and Waggoner H-R-R plates are designed to detect even minor inherited deviations of color perception. The Ishihara plates detect only red–green confusion while the Waggoner H-R-R plates detect blue–yellow defects also. These tests are not quantitative. The severity of color vision deficiency of a healthy worker is assessed using the Farnsworth Panel D-15 test, the Good-Lite 16 Hue test or the Lanthony desaturated test that utilize arranging color pigments so they are adjacent to colors of similar hue. The Farnsworth-Munsell 100 Hue test is used in diagnostic work when lesions in the retina or in the pathways are suspected. Each eye is tested separately. This test is more cumbersome and time consuming to administer and more costly to run, but is helpful in assessing changes due to neurotoxic substances.

All color vision tests must be used under daylight type illumination, either at a window facing north or using a blue incandescent bulb. A wrong color temperature of light may lead to incorrect test results. During the last 10 years color vision changes have continued to be reported due to exposure to styrene, toluene, perchlorethylene, carbon disulfide, metallic mercury, and mercury vapor.

Visual field testing

Visual field tests can be divided into two types: those that test peripheral field and those that examine central field. Though only roughly quantitative, confrontation fields are the most frequently used visual field test in occupational medicine. They are easy to administer and do not require the use of any specialized equipment. Each eye is tested separately with the patient facing the examiner. After occluding one eye the patient is asked to look at the examiner's opposing eye. The examiner then brings his hands or a test object slowly into view from the periphery, from an area of non-seeing to an area of seeing, and asks the patient to report when the test object is seen. This should be done in all four quadrants of peripheral vision. Binocular testing, that is with neither eye occluded, is helpful in the assessment of a worker's functional vision.

Automated visual fields and Goldmann visual fields provide quantitative techniques to evaluate visual fields; islands of loss of vision (scotomas) within the visual field can be documented. Field defects in the lower part of the visual field increase risk of accident, especially if work areas are poorly lit and tools or other materials obstruct walkways.

In cases of homonymous hemianopia it is important to know that a test result from Goldmann or automated perimetry can be misleading. In lesions of the posterior part of the visual pathway, motion perception may be present in the 'blind' hemifield and thus the worker is not visually impaired.[6] This is important to know when assessing vision for a driver's license.

The Amsler grid test, used in some places, is a simple, rough way of evaluating function in the optic pathways and macula. Subtle changes are not detected with this test. Distortion or missing individual letters and irregularities in straight lines are subjective symptoms of minute changes in central visual field. Consultation by an ophthalmologist is necessary, even if visual acuity is unchanged.

Ocular motility and pupils

Disturbances in eye movements are followed especially in workers exposed to neurotoxins. Early signs are difficult to note because the change may be only in saccade accuracy and in reduction of saccade maximum velocity. They can be measured using quantitative eye-tracking equipment. Paresis of an extraocular muscle causes diplopia that increases when the head is turned in the direction of the paretic muscle. Convergence insufficiency and the presence of nystagmus should be noted, as well as pupillary reactions to light and convergence.

External and fundus examination

The physical examination in occupational healthcare should start with observation of the outer eye using a penlight. If the lid margins are erythematous, it is worth compressing the meibomian glands to see whether they produce clear oil, a thick whitish or yellowish mixture, or, sometimes, pus. The cornea's clarity and its epithelial surface can best be seen through a magnifying device. Fluorescent staining of the cornea is helpful and should be used frequently. The examination should also assess the depth of the anterior chamber after trauma, pupillary reactions to light, convergence and the red reflex. Also, obvious pathologic changes in the nerve head or macula should be noted.

Electrophysiologic and other laboratory testing

Laboratory testing is uncommon at the initial stage of an evaluation of potentially work-related ocular and visual symptoms. Infections of the lid margins may require bacterial culture in resistant cases. When exposure to a chemical is suspected, measurement of the chemical and its metabolites in body fluids (when available) may be performed. If exposure to neurotoxins presents a risk, photographic documentation of the retina or optic nerve head is indicated, even if color vision, visual acuity, and contrast sensitivity with best optical correction are normal.

CLASSIFICATION OF OPHTHALMOLOGIC DISORDERS
Disorders of the cornea and conjunctiva

Allergic conjunctivitis

Allergic conjunctivitis occurs in nearly all occupations and is caused by a long list of workplace and other environmental allergens. The clinical picture is often complicated by postinfection allergic reactions. When allergic conjunctivitis occurs in conjunction with systemic allergic manifestations, it becomes a part of a more extensive clinical evaluation related to the other affected organs, and is discussed in Chapters 19.2 (Asthma), 20.3 (Upper airway disorders), and 29 (Dermatologic disorders).

The role of work-related factors is the first question to be considered. If there are no known workplace antigens or irritants but symptoms worsen at work, dry eyes from low humidity in the workplace or decreased blinking during near work activities may be contributing to the symptoms.

Clinical features Symptoms of allergic conjunctivitis are not specific, i.e., mucous discharge, dryness, itching, burning, foreign body sensation, and tearing. Thin threads of mucus in the lower fornix are almost pathognomonic of an allergic reaction. Symptoms are caused by the changes in the quality of the tear layer overlying the cornea and conjunctiva. Mucus that normally protects the cornea as an even layer becomes thick and uneven. Small areas of the cornea remain unprotected and dry quickly. Nerve endings located in the superficial layers of the cornea are stretched and cause a foreign body sensation. It is important to explain the symptoms to the patient because the pain can be intense and the irregular tear film can blur vision transiently.

Diagnosis In making a diagnosis, it is important to make sure that there is no infection complicating the picture. Chronic blepharitis is common and must be treated before diagnostic testing for allergic conjunctivitis is possible. Treatment includes warm compresses and ointments, which contain hydrocortisone, gently rubbed on the lid margin in the evening. If thick cheesy discharge can be expressed from the meibomian glands the use of systemic tetracycline is considered.

Although blepharitis is not a work-related disease, nor does it necessarily disturb work, it should be treated because the chronic inflammation slowly closes the ducts of the meibomian glands. When this happens, the protective oil layer disappears, and the person is left with irritated eyes because of an abnormal tear layer. This in turn may lower the patient's resistance to mucous membrane irritants.

The case history is key in determining the likely etiology of allergic conjunctivitis. The type and duration of symptoms during working days and weekends should be recorded. Environmental factors should be noted, including ventilation, sources of irritating and allergic exposures, such as carpeting, cleaning agents, smoking, various chemicals used in the workplace (including those used by adjacent workers). Suspicion about workplace factors, as opposed to non-occupational environmental irritants or allergens, should heighten if the patient reports resolution of symptoms after a temporary change in the workplace, or during a vacation or sick leave. Through careful investigation, it may be possible to narrow the number of suspected allergens or irritants to a few. If the employee is entitled to compensation because of work-related disease, the diagnosis needs to be confirmed using exposure in well-controlled laboratory conditions.

Treatment Often a single specific allergen or irritant cannot be identified and empirical treatment is a reasonable approach to the problem. Reduction or prevention of exposure to the allergen or irritant is preferred, but often this is not possible, or only to a certain extent. Uncertainty defining a single specific agent should not prevent appropriate reasonable interventions to reduce exposure to allergens. Allergic conjunctivitis is frequently treated symptomatically: cool compresses may provide relief in acute reactions, artificial tears are also helpful. In any treatment, avoidance of any preservatives in the medications used, especially benzalconium chloride, is important. Topical mast-cell stabilizers and antihistamines are effective. Systemic antihistamines may be helpful, particularly when systemic allergic symptoms coexist. Because of the possibility of increased intraocular pressure, potentiation of herpetic or fungal keratitis, and of cataract formation, topical steroids should be prescribed only by an ophthalmologist.

Dry eye syndrome

Dry eye syndrome is common. Though not caused by the work, the symptoms are often worsened by low humidity at the workplace. Symptoms are similar to those of allergic conjunctivitis and generally worsen as the day goes on and with near vision tasks. Treatment with artificial tears is helpful. Use of a humidifier may be helpful in low humidity environments such as can occur with air-conditioning or forced hot air heating. Punctal plugs may be indicated if symptoms persist.

Other disorders of the conjunctiva and cornea

Irritation of the cornea resulting from chemicals, high or low temperature, dust, and other irritant exposures should be distinguished from an allergic reaction. Exposure to irritating agents may worsen an underlying allergic condition. Chemical irritation may lead to accumulation of fluid under the corneal epithelium, as is the case after exposure to triethylamine. Resultant minute subepithelial corneal vesicles, which can be seen only on microscopic examination, can cause blurred, hazy vision.[7] Exposure to tertiary amines may cause corneal opacities.[8]

Ultraviolet (UV) light-induced keratoconjunctivitis is still a common problem, despite awareness of the condition and exposure risks. The symptoms first appear within hours after UV exposure and vary from a slight irritation to severe sloughing of the epithelium with intense pain and tearing. UV light is absorbed in the cornea and the lens, with only minimal amounts reaching the retina in normal eyes. Regular plastic lens materials absorb UV light. Those working in areas with potential UV exposure should use protective lenses with side shields. Glass lenses vary in their transmission of UV light and should have UV coating when needed.

UV burns of the cornea should be treated with sterile ointment, tight bandaging and pain medication. In addition to acute corneal damage, subacute damage may also occur from lower levels of exposure to UV light. Symptoms include dryness or foreign-body sensation in the late night and early morning hours. Chronic exposure may lead to thickening of the conjunctiva and changes in the corneal surface. Since it is often difficult to find an eye drop that protects the irritated cornea well enough to make the patient symptom free, prevention measures are important.

Disorders of the lens

Some epidemiologic studies of workers with UV-B light exposure support the correlation between a high level of exposure to UV-B light and cortical and posterior subcapsular cataracts. Since most eyeglass materials effectively absorb UV light, workers who wear regular glasses are less exposed to environmental UV radiation outside their working hours than are those who do not use spectacles or sunglasses. Eyeglass use should thus be carefully evaluated in studies on work-related lens changes to correctly assess the role of exposure to UV radiation at work. Because there are so many contributing factors involved, the role of work-related radiation in cataracts is usually hard to prove.

Exposure to organic nitrate explosives has been reported to be associated with cataract formation.[9] In the 1980s increased prevalence of cataracts was noted in glass and metal workers, felt to be related to short-wave infrared radiation.[10]

Disorders of the retina and optic pathways

Chemicals with potential for affecting retinal function are commonly used, but in most developed countries exposure is well below the levels that are toxic to the retina. Light-induced retinal damage can occur from phototoxicity or thermal injury.[11] The former is typically caused by short-wavelength light, the latter by visible and infrared light. Short-wavelength blue light also causes degradation in the image quality. This can be prevented by absorbing the blue light using special filter lenses. Blue light seems to have particularly unfavorable effects on the elderly retina.

Exposure to lasers can cause serious, permanent loss of central vision. The damage is usually caused by the energy absorption within the melanin granules of the retinal pigment epithelium. Laser burns are classified into four categories: Grade 1, retinal edema; Grade 2, retinal coagulation necrosis; Grade 3, necrosis with hemorrhage; and Grade 4, hemorrhage bursts into the vitreous. Small laser burns have clinical importance only when they occur in the center of the macula. It is advisable to take photographs of the maculae of workers at risk and to record any lesions in the retinas of workers prior to working in areas where there is risk of exposure, to avoid confusion with future laser light-induced scars. Extended exposure to very low-level laser energy may cause subtle damage to the retina; this has been reported in ophthalmologic surgeons who perform laser coagulations regularly over a period of several years. The damage is measurable only with extremely sensitive techniques and does not lead to functional losses.[12]

A number of solvents have been reported to cause altered color vision, most commonly in the blue–yellow axis, even at relatively low levels of exposure. Impaired color vision has been reported following chronic exposure to styrene, toluene, perchloroethylene, n-hexane, carbon disulfide and solvent mixtures.[13–17] Carbon disulfide has also been reported to cause changes in the retinal capillary bed resembling diabetic retinopathy.[18,19] In one follow-up study, such changes persisted four years after exposure had ceased.[18]

Eye strain and visual ergonomics

Many occupations have become more and more office based, using computers instead of manual labor. Therefore visual ergonomics have become important, especially in planning the working conditions of presbyopic employees. Their spectacles need to be fitted so that the reading addition in the lens is placed at a height that corresponds to the direction used in reading the computer screen and other materials. Presbyopic technicians, librarians, nurses, etc. – all employees who have need to read while looking upwards – need specially fitted glasses in order to see properly.

Symptoms of eyestrain include sore eyes, headaches, and fatigue, often associated with intensive close work, including reading and use of video display terminals.[20–23] Environmental and ergonomic factors are important contributors. Poor contrast or small text may force workers to function too close to their visual threshold.

If the direction of gaze is too high, blinking decreases, and dry spots appear now and then on the cornea, causing discomfort. Computer tasks may require long periods of intensive attentional search, leading to fatigue. Employees working under pressure may feel tense and fail to relax neck, facial, and eye muscles for micropauses (2 to 5 seconds).

Poor placement of a video display terminal may cause glare from a window or artificial lighting (Fig. 20.1.1a). Elevated placement of a video display terminal may require the worker to look up, causing neck muscle tension. All visual target areas should be placed so that the head posture is comfortable and nodding is avoided (Fig. 20.1.1b). This usually means that surfaces to be read are placed lower in the visual field. When visual targets are placed lower, not only is the head posture better, but also eye irritation becomes less common as the lid aperture becomes smaller, blinking more frequent, and thus the tear layer on the cornea more stable. Existing office furniture seldom makes good visual ergonomics possible.

Visual comfort requires pleasant luminance levels. Illumination should be adjustable at each workstation. Glare sources should be avoided, as glare degrades visual function. Workers with eyestrain should also have their eyes checked for a change in refractive error or the need for reading glasses. Eyestrain increases with increased duration of time working at a video display terminal, and the near point of accommodation increases and convergence decreases in parallel with these symptoms.[20]

Shared workstations need to be adjustable so that workers of different heights may be positioned comfortably for the task. Nowadays, most workstations require looking at several distances. Regular bifocal glasses with small reading additions may cause an uncomfortable neck posture if the screen is placed too high. From the large selection of progressive lenses, only lenses with a large area for near work and a broad enough progression area should be fitted for office work.

An intelligent choice of lenses is possible only when the structure of work is described clearly enough to the ophthalmologist or optometrist. This means that the workers need to have charts to mark their different working distances. When the new glasses are used at work, fine-tuning of distances and heights of visual target areas is often needed before head posture and movements are comfortable – glasses need to fit the work and the work must be arranged to fit the glasses. When both adjustments are done, even demanding office work is comfortable while the worker uses regular progressive lenses.

Accidents

The CDC indicates that eye injuries are a leading cause of work-related diseases and injuries in the United States.[24] Between 5% and 19% of all industrial accidents involve eye injuries.[25] NIOSH estimates that approximately 900,000 occupational eye injuries occurred in the United States in 1983, 84% of which were considered minor. The incidence of occupational injuries that lead to temporary or permanent visual disability approaches 70,000 workers each year,[1] and many of these are preventable. Appropriate eye protection is commonly not worn. According to the National Eye Trauma System Registry, only 1.5% were wearing safety glasses.[26] In a West Virginia study, a rate of 567 compensable ocular injuries per 100,000 workers was reported, most injuries occurring in the areas of agriculture, construction, and manufacturing, with a large predilection for males.[27] Time lost from work varies with the severity and type of injury.

Superficial foreign bodies

Superficial foreign bodies are the most commonly occurring work-related eye injuries.[28] A foreign body may cause

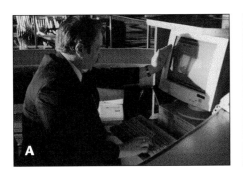

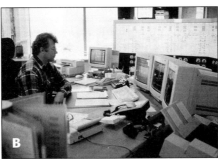

Figure 20.1.1 Work at VDU with poor (a) and good (b) visual ergonomics. (a) Large window behind the worker makes the text on the screen nearly impossible to read. (b) Workstation for office work is designed to fit presbyopic as well as younger workers. The computer screens are placed low and at a distance that makes shifting of gaze from one screen to another easy. Regular progressive, multifocal lenses can be fitted to function well in this kind of workstation.

a corneal or conjunctival abrasion or become embedded in the cornea or conjunctiva. Fluorescein stains the damaged epithelium and helps to locate the foreign body. After it is removed, antibiotic ointment is applied. Corneal abrasions usually heal within 48 hours but it is wise to use ointment nightly for a week.

Complications of corneal abrasions include infection and recurrent erosions. Infection should be suspected if a discharge develops and immediate referral to an ophthalmologist is required. Recurrent erosion is a common complication and occurs when the basement membrane that underlies the superficial epithelium of the cornea is disrupted. This prevents firm adherence of the corneal epithelium to the basement membrane and the corneal epithelium then breaks down after minor trauma, such as rubbing of the eye. Therefore it is wise to cover the eye with a patch for the first few nights.

Penetrating ocular foreign bodies

If a penetrating injury is suspected, the eye should be covered with a sterile patch when the patient is sent to the emergency clinic. No medications are used. Though only representing a small proportion of work-related eye injuries, penetrating eye injuries represent a substantial portion of work-related permanent severe vision loss.[28] The incidence of occupational injuries leading to temporary or permanent visual disability approaches 70,000 workers each year.

Safety should be an integral part of vocational training. According to the National Eye Trauma System Registry, 2939 penetrating eye injuries were reported between 1985 and 1991. Of these, 21% occurred at the workplace, fewer than 10% of the injured were wearing eyeglasses or goggles, and only 1.5% were wearing safety glasses.[26] Comprehensive workplace strategies to prevent eye injuries are essential, including workplace modifications, use of appropriate personal protective equipment, worker education, and appropriate trained personnel. Prevention of traumatic injuries is discussed further in Chapter 31 (Traumatic Injuries).

Chemical injuries

Though less frequent than mechanical eye injuries, chemical injuries may occur in laboratory, agricultural, or industrial settings and represent a significant threat to vision. Numerous chemicals can cause serious ocular injury, especially strong acids and bases. Immediate irrigation is essential to minimize permanent vision loss. Therefore bottles with irrigation fluid must be near all workstations where dangerous chemicals are used and the workers must be trained to find and open the bottle even when they cannot open their eyes. Irrigation is continued until the worker is brought to the health station or the ambulance arrives. The full extent of the injury may not be apparent at the time of the initial assessment. Irrigation is continued while transporting the patient to an emergency room for further treatment.

Alkali burns tend to be more caustic and thus more damaging than acid injuries. However, both have the potential to cause severe vision loss. Prevention of accidents is important. Protective eyewear should always be worn when handling corrosive or caustic fluids and gases, preferably behind a protecting window or screen.

Electromagnetic radiation

Visible, ultraviolet, infrared, microwave, and laser energy have all been implicated in work-related eye injuries. Visible and ultraviolet wavelengths have been associated with pterygium and macular degeneration. Infrared exposure in glass and metal workers has been associated with cataract formation.

Microwaves may be associated with cataract formation. In workplaces where microwave exposure is possible and where maximum exposure is kept below the World Health Organization exposure limit of 10 $mW/cm^2/0.1$ hour, no cataractous changes have been found. The various lasers used today in industry pose different risks of morbidity to the eye depending on wavelength and type of laser. Workers should have an eye examination and photographic documentation of any eye pathology prior to working in places where there is risk of exposure to laser. Protective shields or goggles need to be used.

Prevention

Prevention is the most important consideration in occupational eye disorders and damage to the visual pathways. According to the Bureau of Labor statistics, 60% of workers who suffer eye injuries did not wear eye protection at the time of the injury; 40% of those who wore protection wore the wrong kind of protection. Appropriate eye protection is probably the most important single intervention to decrease the incidence of eye injury in workplaces. Eye disorders related to exposure to allergens and irritating substances, chemicals and radiation are preventable.

Recommendations to prevent eye injuries and disorders at work include: (1) making an assessment of operations and exposures that pose a risk; (2) checking for visual problems in routine health exams; (3) reducing exposures by requiring the use of appropriate protective eyewear, and worksite and engineering modifications; (4) planning for eye emergencies; (5) reviewing written procedures and strategies for preventing and dealing with eye injuries. These efforts should minimize the number of eye injuries and disorders that occur in the worksite. Similarly, all neurotoxic chemicals in the environment should be known and carefully avoided in the workplace.

The other important area in prevention of work-related vision and ergonomic problems is better planning of workstations and improvement in the fitting and quality of glasses of presbyopic office workers. With good planning of working posture and glasses, neck and lower back problems in office workers are fully preventable. At the same time, working capacity improves.

SUMMARY

There are many etiologies for occupational eye disorders including injuries, exposures, inappropriate spectacle correction for the task, and ergonomic factors. Sensitivity to these factors may help avoid occupational eye disorders and damage to visual pathways. An important factor in decreasing the incidence of occupationally related eye pathology is the use of eye protection in the workplace. The ophthalmologic effects of potentially neurotoxic chemicals are a more difficult problem. Each year thousands of new chemicals are introduced with unknown effects on the eyes or visual pathways. These potentially harmful chemicals warrant further investigation.

References

1. Accident Facts. Chicago: National Society to Prevent Blindness/National Safety Council, 1989.
2. Schuman JS, Massicotte EC, Connolly S, Hertzmark E, Mukherji B, Kunen MZ. Increased intraocular pressure and visual field defects in high resistance wind instrument players. Ophthalmology 2000; 107:127–33.
3. Jarvinen P, Hyvarinen L. Contrast sensitivity measurement in evaluations of visual symptoms caused by exposure to triethylamine. Occup Environ Med 1997; 54:483–6.
4. Lighthouse International, Information and Recourses Center, (800) 829 0500.
5. Lamble D, Summala H, Hyvarinen L. Driving performance of drivers with impaired visual acuity. Accident Analysis Prev 2002; 34:711–6.
6. Hyvärinen L, Raninen AN, Näsänen RE. Vision rehabilitation in homonymous hemianopia. Neuro-Ophthalmology 2002; 27:97–102.
7. Jarvinen P, Engstrom K, Riihimaki V, Ruusuvaara P, Setala K. Effects of experimental exposure to triethylamine on vision and the eye. Occup Environ Med 1999; 56:1–5.
8. Page EH, Cook CK, Hater MA, Mueller CA, Grote AA, Mortimer VD. Visual and ocular changes associated with exposure to two tertiary amines. Occup Environ Med 2003; 60:69–75.
9. Lewis-Younger CR, Mamalis N, Egger MJ, Wallace DO, Lu C. Lens opacifications detected by slitlamp biomicroscopy are associated with exposure to organic nitrate explosives. Arch Ophthalmol 2000; 118:1653–9.
10. Lydahl E. Infrared radiation and cataract. Acta Ophthalmol Suppl 1984; 166:1–63.
11. Magnavita N. Photoretinitis: an underestimated occupational injury? Occup Med (Lond) 2002; 52:223–5.
12. Frennesson C, Bergen J. Retinal function in Swedish ophthalmologists using argon lasers as reflected in colour contrast sensitivity. Normal thresholds in the great majority of the cases. Acta Ophthalmol Scand 1998; 76:610–2.
13. Iregren A, Andersson M, Nylen P. Color vision and occupational chemical exposures: I. An overview of tests and effects. Neurotoxicology 2002; 23:719–33.
14. Gobba F. Color vision: a sensitive indicator of exposure to neurotoxins. Neurotoxicology 2000; 21:857–62.
15. Gong YY, Kishi R, Katakura Y, et al. Relation between colour vision loss and occupational styrene exposure level. Occup Environ Med 2002; 59:824–9.
16. Issever H, Malat G, Sabuncu HH, Yuksel N. Impairment of colour vision in patients with n-hexane exposure-dependent toxic polyneuropathy. Occup Med (Lond) 2002; 52:183–6.
17. Wang C, Tan X, Bi Y, et al. Cross-sectional study of the ophthalmological effects of carbon disulfide in Chinese viscose workers. Int J Hyg Environ Health 2002; 205:367–72.
18. De Rouck A, De Laey JJ, Van Hoorne M, Pahtak A, Devuyst A. Chronic carbon disulphide poisoning: a 4 year follow-up study of the ophthalmological signs. Int Ophthalmol 1986; 9:17–27.
19. Eskin TA, Merigan WH, Wood RW. Carbon disulfide effects on the visual system. II. Retinogeniculate degeneration. Invest Ophthalmol Vis Sci 1988; 29:519–27.
20. Bergman T. Eye care: health effects of video display terminals. Occup Health Safety 1980; 49:6–8, 53–5.
21. Travers PH, Stanton BA. Office workers and video display terminals: physical, psychological and ergonomic factors. AAOHN J 2002; 50:489–93.
22. Nakazawa T, Okubo Y, Suwazono Y, et al. Association between duration of daily VDT use and subjective symptoms. Am J Ind Med 2002; 42:421–6.
23. Thomson WD. Eye problems and visual display terminals – the facts and the fallacies. Ophthalmic Physiol Opt 1998; 18:111–9.
24. Morbidity Mortality Weekly Report 1984; 33:16–7.
25. Belfort R Jr, Bonomo PP, Neustein I. Industrial eye injuries – analysis of 500 cases. Ind Med Surg 1972; 41:30–2.
26. Dannenberg AL, Parver LM, Brechner RJ, Khoo L. Penetration eye injuries in the workplace. The National Eye Trauma System Registry. Arch Ophthalmol 1992; 110:843–8.
27. Islam SS, Doyle EJ, Velilla A, Martin CJ, Ducatman AM. Epidemiology of compensable work-related ocular injuries and illnesses: incidence and risk factors. J Occup Environ Med 2000; 42:575–81.
28. Saari KM, Parvi V. Occupational eye injuries in Finland. Acta Ophthalmol Suppl 1984; 161:17–28.

20.2 Occupational Hearing Loss

Peter M Rabinowitz, Thomas S Rees

'Artillerymen, blacksmiths, and the blasters in mines often become deaf, and this seems to be dependent upon defective energy of the acoustic nerve, from having been so frequently over excited.'[1]

INTRODUCTION

Noise-induced hearing loss (NIHL) is the second most common form of acquired hearing loss, after age-related loss (presbycusis),[2] and has long been recognized as a problem in occupations associated with prominent noise. Noise is the most pervasive hazardous agent in the workplace. In 1981, there were an estimated 9 million US workers exposed to hazardous occupational noise levels.[3] Despite job loss in noisy industries and the widespread institution of hearing conservation programs, NIHL is currently one of the most common occupational diseases and the second most frequently self-reported occupational injury. NIHL is listed as one of the eight most critical occupational diseases and injuries requiring research and development activities within the framework of the National Occupational Research Agenda (NORA).

Even when away from the workplace, people have exposure to hazardous noise levels from recreational, social, and community sources[4] (see Chapter 35). Although NIHL is permanent, irreversible, and prevalent,[5] it is preventable.[6] In addition to the major problem of NIHL, the ear is susceptible to other environmental factors, both physical and chemical, that are of potential clinical significance. The most important of these are summarized in Table 20.2.1. While a wide range of factors can affect hearing, this chapter will focus on the effects of excessive noise on the auditory system.

Mechanisms of hearing

The ear is a complex organ, capable of transforming airborne sound waves into mechanical energy, transferring this mechanical energy into electrochemical signals and then to neural impulses, which are processed as auditory information. The external ear collects sound waves and funnels them through the 2.5–3 cm long external ear canal to the tympanic membrane. The tympanic membrane, approximately 9 mm in diameter, transforms the air-borne sound waves into mechanical vibrations, which are transmitted through the ossicular chain of the middle ear (malleus, incus, and stapes).

The mechanical transmission of energy through the ossicular chain is mediated by the tensor tympani and stapedius muscles, which act as a damper for excessive sound energy. The stapes, the smallest bone in the body, rests in the oval window of the cochlea (inner ear). The transduction of mechanical energy to electrochemical neural potentials takes place in the cochlea. Physical displacement of the oval window sends a fluid wave through the cochlea. There are approximately 16,000 sensory hair cells in the cochlea, asso-ciated with approximately 31,000 sensory nerve fibers. The hair cells are stimulated by the fluid wave within the cochlea and nerve impulses are then transmitted via the 8th cranial nerve to the auditory centers of the brain.

CLINICAL EVALUATION OF HEARING LOSS
Otologic evaluation

It is the healthcare provider's responsibility to determine whether or not the worker has incurred an occupationally related hearing loss. This opinion can only be formulated after obtaining a detailed work and health history, complete otologic examination, audiologic examination, and, if indicated, specialized testing.

The history should include age, family history, ototoxic drug use, presence of tinnitus, vestibular symptoms, noise exposure (occupational and non-occupational), neurologic symptoms, aural fullness, ear pain, ear discharge, as well as hearing loss onset, progression, fluctuation, and symmetry. Past and present occupational and non-occupational noise exposure must be documented. The type of noise exposure and duration should be determined. The use of hearing protection devices should also be documented. The patient should be questioned regarding non-occupational noise exposure including use of firearms, power tools, chain saws, snowmobiles, motorcycles, small aircraft noise, and other sources. Other possible causes of sensorineural hearing loss including ototoxic drugs, central nervous system infections, radiation to the head and neck, head injury, and family history should be explored.

The healthcare provider should ideally seek information about the work environment, such as noise levels, characteristics of the noise, and audiograms taken prior to employment, periodically during employment, and at the time of termination of employment. Unfortunately, such information is often not available, thus requiring the examiner to depend on the patient's self-report of the noise exposure. It is estimated that workers in an 85 dB environment will have to speak loudly, while those in 85–90 dB will have to shout to communicate at arm's length. As the surrounding noise reaches 95 dB, communication only occurs with shouting, even if the workers stand next to each other. Certain environments are known to be inherently very noisy, such as saw mill or chain saw work, metal chipping in foundries, and various construction jobs. Questionnaires can be quite helpful in documenting details of the otologic history and ensuring that important questions are not omitted.

The physical examination should include a head and neck examination, with special attention to the external ear and tympanic membrane. The mobility of the tympanic membrane is assessed with pneumo-otoscopy. Evaluation of the cranial nerves and cerebellar function should be included in patients with suspected neurologic

Disorder	Causes
Noise-induced hearing loss	Chronic noise exposure
Noise-induced tinnitus	
Acoustic trauma	Sudden intense noise or excessive pressure
Ototoxicity due to chemicals including medications	Organic solvents, heavy metals, carbon monoxide, NSAIDS, ASA, cisplatin, aminoglycosides, furosemide
Damage to auditory cortex	Neurotoxins
Ear disorders due to diving	Noise, barotrauma, air embolism
Radiation-induced damage	Radiation to head and neck
Trauma to external and middle ear	Slag burns, foreign objects

Table 20.2.1 Hearing disorders caused by environmental agents

	Hertz (Hz)						
	500	1000	2000	3000	4000	6000	8000
Right ear (dB)	25	35	35	45	50	60	45
Left ear (dB)	25	35	40	50	60	70	50

1. Unilateral impairment:
(Average dB at 500, 1000, 2000, 3000 Hz) – 25 dB (low fence) × 1.5% = Percentage of unilateral impairment
Right ear = (25 + 35 + 35 + 45 ÷ 4) – 25 × 1.5% = 15%
Left ear = (25 + 35 + 40 + 50 ÷ 4) – 25 × 1.5% = 18.8%
2. Bilateral impairment:
(Percentage of unilateral impairment in better ear x 5) + (Percentage of unilateral impairment in poorer ear) ÷ 6 = Percentage of bilateral impairment
(15 × 5) + (18.8%) ÷ 6 = 15.6%

Table 20.2.2 Sample audiogram and calculation of impairment (AAO-79 method)

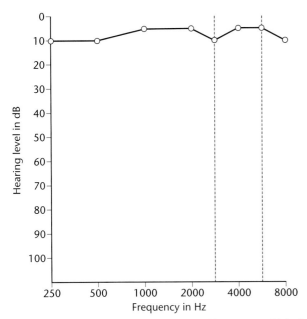

Figure 20.2.1: An audiogram showing normal hearing sensitivity in the right ear.

disease. Laboratory and radiologic studies are useful in the evaluation of some otologic conditions.

Audiologic evaluation

Basic evaluation

The clinical assessment of hearing loss includes the completion of an audiogram (Fig. 20.2.1). The frequency scale along the abscissa is measured in hertz (Hz) for the octave frequencies of 250 Hz through 8000 Hz. The most critical frequencies for speech reception and understanding are 500, 1000, 2000, and 3000 Hz; these frequencies are used in the AMA computation of binaural hearing impairment (Table 20.2.2), as will be discussed later.

The intensity scale on the ordinate of the audiogram is measured in decibels (dB), ranging from a very faint hearing level (HL) of –10 dB up to a very loud level of 110 dB HL. Sensitivity thresholds are obtained for each frequency,

and for each ear separately using earphones. This air conduction (AC) testing measures the responsiveness of the entire auditory system, from the ear canal through the middle ear to the cochlea and associated neural pathways to the brain; any loss by air conduction testing may be due to a disorder anywhere in the entire auditory system.

The use of pure tone bone conduction (BC) audiometry defines the general anatomic location of the hearing disorder, since sound transmission by bone conduction bypasses the outer and middle ear. An oscillator is placed behind the ear to be tested and sensitivity thresholds are obtained for the frequencies 250 Hz through 4000 Hz.

Many factors can affect the quality of audiometric data. Audiometric equipment requires annual electroacoustic calibration and routine biologic checks. The testing environment necessitates a very quiet room without excessive ambient noise levels per ANSI S31-1999. The competence and experience of the test examiner are of paramount importance. While certified audiometric technicians can adequately perform routine hearing tests, certified clinical audiologists should be used for difficult cases as well as all compensation claims.

In addition to pure tone threshold measurements, the basic audiologic evaluation includes the measurement of threshold sensitivity for speech and the assessment of word recognition abilities. The speech reception threshold (SRT) test serves primarily as a reliability check on the pure tone threshold levels. Familiar two-syllable words are presented to each ear separately through earphones and the intensity level at which 50% of the words are correctly repeated is defined as the SRT. The SRT should agree within ±10 dB with the pure tone average (PTA) threshold levels at 500, 1000, and 2000 Hz. When the SRT and PTA do not agree, an exaggerated hearing loss should be considered. The SRT is most often obtained at a softer dB level than the PTA in persons who exaggerate their hearing loss. Careful re-instruction and the use of modified test procedures are warranted in such cases, in an effort to obtain a valid test.

A hearing impairment may be reflected not only in a sensitivity loss but also in impairment in the ability to

Pure tone average (dB HL)	Classification	Effects on speech understanding
0–25	Normal	No significant difficulty
25–40	Mild	Difficulty with soft speech
40–55	Moderate	Difficulty with normal speech
55–70	Moderately severe	Difficulty with loud speech
70–90	Severe	Can only understand shouted or amplified speech
90–110	Profound	Usually cannot understand even amplified speech

Table 20.2.3 An example of a classification system for degree of hearing loss

understand speech, even when speech is sufficiently loud. The assessment of word recognition (speech discrimination) analyzes the patient's ability to understand speech when presented at comfortably loud levels; it is not a threshold or sensitivity test. Standardized lists of 25–50 single-syllable words (i.e., darn, art, chief, etc.) are presented to each ear separately at comfortably loud intensity levels. These words are repeated back by the patient and the percentage of correct responses is the word recognition score. Scores may range from 0% to 100%; scores of 90–100% are considered normal.

Special evaluation

Additional audiologic tests are sometimes needed in hearing assessment; these tests are used to rule out exaggerated hearing loss or to define the site of the hearing loss in the auditory system. If concern exists for an embellished response, additional tests may be utilized to identify true organic hearing levels. The use of tympanometry provides information regarding the mobility of the middle ear system. This is an objective test procedure, which measures the middle ear pressure, the ear canal volume and the mobility of the tympanic membrane/middle ear system. Since NIHL is due to sensorineural pathology, abnormal tympanometric results may suggest middle ear (conductive) involvement contributing to the patient's hearing loss.

Electrophysiologic measurements, such as brainstem auditory evoked potentials (BAEPs; also known as auditory brainstem response, ABR), can help in determining the general degree of a hearing loss without requiring a subjective response from an individual. Electrocochleography measures the electrophysiologic activity originating within the cochlea and can supplement information provided by BAEP/ABR audiometry, but is less commonly used in clinical practice.

Transient and distortion product otoacoustic emissions (OAEs) is another objective measure of hearing function that is gaining wider acceptance. The outer hair cells of a healthy ear emit faint sounds (echoes) when moderate-level clicks or tones are presented to the ear. Robust OAEs are usually obtained in ears with thresholds less than or equal to 30 dB HL. Voluntary thresholds in excess of 30 dB HL with normal OAEs suggest exaggerated hearing loss. While OAEs do not quantify the exact amount of hearing loss, they do provide the clinician with a means of validating the voluntary audiometric results.

The evaluation of asymmetric sensorineural hearing loss, or clinical suspicion of 8th nerve or central auditory involvement, requires special audiologic procedures to define the site of auditory impairment. The evaluation of the integrity of the stapedius (acoustic) reflex by impedance measurement is a helpful test in differentiating between cochlear and 8th nerve involvement. BAEPs are also used to differentiate cochlear involvement from 8th nerve involvement.

Audiometric test interpretation

Degree of hearing loss

The results obtained from the air conduction evaluation provide quantitative information as to the amount of hearing loss. Classification systems have been devised in an effort to relate the amount of air conduction hearing loss to the expected degree of handicap imposed by a hearing loss. Such systems typically use the PTA to estimate various hearing loss categories and the expected effects of the loss upon speech understanding. An example of such a classification system is shown in Table 20.2.3.

Further discussion of the interpretation of the degree of hearing loss will be presented in the section dealing with hearing loss impairment assessment.

Location of auditory impairment

The general anatomic area of the hearing loss can be determined by comparing the air conduction and bone conduction thresholds. A conductive hearing loss is present when air conduction results demonstrate a hearing loss but bone conduction results are within the normal range (Fig. 20.2.2). The etiology of the conductive loss cannot be determined by the audiogram alone, as any obstruction in the sound-conducting mechanism of the ear, from the external canal (e.g., cerumen impaction, foreign body) through the middle ear (e.g., middle ear effusion, otosclerosis), may be the cause of the conductive hearing loss.

When a hearing loss is detected by air conduction and similarly by bone conduction, a sensorineural hearing loss is present. The hearing disorder could be located in the cochlea, the associated neural pathways, or in both sensory and neural auditory system (Fig. 20.2.3). NIHL presents as a sensorineural hearing loss. A loss in hearing sensitivity for bone conduction with a greater loss by air conduction represents a mixed hearing loss (Fig. 20.2.4). Correction of the conductive component by medical or surgical treatment should result in a sensorineural hearing loss alone, as reflected by the bone conduction thresholds.

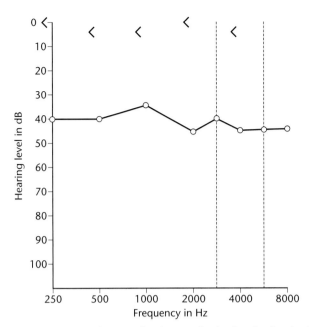

Figure 20.2.2: An audiogram showing conductive hearing loss in the right ear. (o = air conduction; < = bone conduction)

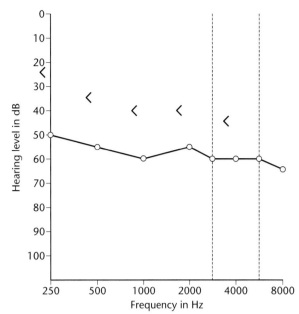

Figure 20.2.4: An audiogram showing mixed hearing loss in the right ear. (o = air conduction; < = bone conduction)

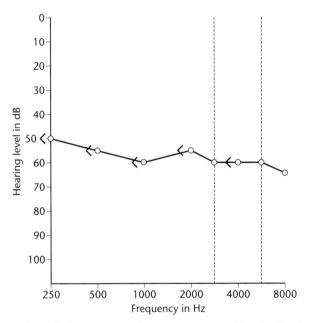

Figure 20.2.3: An audiogram showing sensorineural hearing loss in the right ear. (o = air conduction; < = bone conduction)

Noise-induced hearing loss (NIHL)

Clinical effects

In general, NIHL is related to significant sensory cell loss within the cochlea. The mechanism by which the sensory cells are lost is probably a combination of physical and metabolic stress. In the case of temporary threshold shifts, metabolic exhaustion of the sensory hair cells is likely. A growing body of literature suggests that reactive oxygen species produced in response to noise overexposure play a

role in this process.[7] Nerve fiber degeneration also appears to take place secondary to the loss of the inner hair cells of the cochlea.

Early NIHL in the 3000–4000 Hz region of the audiogram correlates with hair cell degeneration in the region of the organ of Corti, located near the base of the cochlea. Sensory and neural elements are progressively destroyed in the basal and more apical regions following continued noise exposure, with resultant hearing deterioration in the adjacent low and high frequency ranges.

Sounds of sufficient intensity and duration will damage the ear and result in temporary or permanent hearing impairment. The hearing loss may range from mild to severe and may also be accompanied by tinnitus. Tinnitus can be experienced in many forms, such as ringing, hissing, buzzing or clicking, etc. It can be disabling, dramatically affecting and diminishing the quality of life. It is estimated that as many as 36 million Americans have tinnitus, with 7 million experiencing severe tinnitus.[8] The effects of noise on hearing can be divided into several categories.

1. *Acoustic trauma* is the sudden loss of hearing caused by an intense single incident noise blast or explosion. Most cases of acoustic trauma are caused by impulses from explosions, such as bombs, blasts, and gunfire. There have been reports recently of airbag-induced otologic injuries, characterized by a variety of otologic pathologies, including sensorineural hearing loss, conductive hearing loss, mixed hearing loss, tinnitus, and disequilibrium.[9] Due to the very high sound intensity, the auditory system may be damaged both in the middle ear and the cochlea, since the acoustic insult may exceed the physiologic protective capabilities of the auditory system. In addition to tympanic membrane rupture, the middle ear ossicles may become dislocated, causing a conductive hearing loss. A

sensorineural hearing loss can often occur due to direct mechanical injury to the sensory cells of the cochlea, or fistulas between the inner and middle ear. Acoustic trauma can produce hearing losses that are more severe than seen with NIHL, especially in the low and middle frequencies. In addition to immediate hearing loss, affected individuals may also complain of vertigo, tinnitus, and pain. The injury may be unilateral or bilateral, depending upon the direction of the blast. Sensorineural hearing loss from acoustic trauma may exhibit some recovery from initial levels; patients need to be followed for 4 to 6 months to determine if the hearing loss is permanent. The precipitating episode is usually very dramatic, with onset of hearing loss apparent to the patient.

2. *Temporary threshold shift* (TTS) is a temporary hearing decrease following noise exposure. Following loud noise exposure, the individual reports a high frequency tinnitus, a feeling of aural fullness, and a sensation of muffled hearing. These symptoms gradually resolve after removal from the noise, and hearing recovers to baseline within hours. With repeated exposure to the offending noise, hearing recovery may be slower and may not be complete. If the hearing recovery is incomplete, a permanent threshold shift has occurred. The industrial worker who is exposed to loud noise and has TTS after each workday and on weekends is a typical example. The hearing usually recovers initially; however, repeated noise exposures result in diminished hearing recovery and permanent NIHL.

3. *Permanent threshold shift* (PTS) is a persistent and irreversible hearing decrease following repeated exposures to loud noise. It is the result of an accumulation of noise exposures repeated on a regular basis over a number of years. It is usually bilaterally symmetric and often accompanied by high frequency ringing tinnitus. While persons who experience acoustic trauma can define the exact time of onset of the hearing loss, those with PTS cannot report a time of onset, since the hearing loss is insidious and gradually worsens over years. PTS usually occurs without the affected individual being aware of it until the hearing loss progresses to involve the critical frequencies for speech understanding. Since PTS is permanent, it is referred to as a NIHL.

Clinical presentation of NIHL

Noise over-exposure typically causes a high frequency hearing loss. The earliest effects tend to occur in the regions around 4000 Hz, with recovery at higher frequencies. This creates a characteristic 'notching' of the audiogram.[10] The exact location of the 'notch' depends on multiple factors including the frequency of the damaging noise, the shape of the ear canal, and cochlear sensitivity.[11] This 'notching' is in contrast to age-related hearing loss (presbycusis), which also produces high frequency hearing loss but in a down-sloping pattern without recovery at 8000 Hz. Therefore, in early noise-induced hearing loss, the average hearing thresholds at 500, 1000, and 2000 Hz are better than the average at 3000, 4000, and 6000, and the hearing level at 8000 Hz is usually better than the deepest part of the 'notch'.

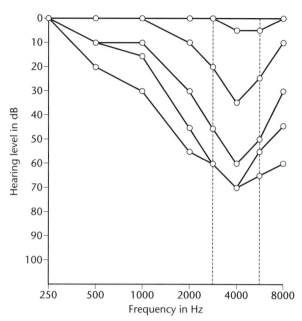

Figure 20.2.5: An audiogram showing the progression of noise-induced hearing loss, from a mild high-frequency impairment to a severe hearing impairment.

Early NIHL, producing a mild sensorineural loss in the 4000–6000 Hz region, has little effect upon the individual's ability to understand speech. However, if the hearing impairment extends to the important speech frequencies at and below 3000Hz, the individual will begin to experience increasingly greater difficulties in speech understanding. Continued progression of NIHL due to cumulative effects of loud noise exposure results in a more severe hearing loss in the 3000–6000 Hz area, and may extend into the middle and lower audiometric frequencies (Fig. 20.2.5). This may reduce the prominence of the 'notch' and, in conjunction with the progressive effect of aging, make it difficult to distinguish between age-related and noise-induced loss without access to previous audiograms.

NIHL initially affects the perception of the high frequency consonant sounds (such as s, f, th, sh). Speech may seem to be garbled and indistinct. The presence of competing background noises and voices, such as in restaurants and groups, further reduces speech understanding. Persons with NIHL typically complain of being able 'to hear but not understand speech'. Such difficulties in speech understanding increase with the spread of the hearing impairment into the frequencies of 500 through 3000 Hz. While initially many persons with noise-induced hearing loss may not seek help for their condition,[12] the difficulties in speech understanding can lead to fatigue, anxiety, stress, and reduced quality of life. The eventual result of progressive hearing loss is social withdrawal and isolation.[13] Other associated conditions may be depression and increased risk of accidents.[14]

Progression of hearing loss after removal from noise

Recent reports from audiometric examination of individuals in the Framingham Study suggest that individuals with notched audiograms, presumably due to noise exposure, may continue to have progression of these notches later in life.[15] However, there is no firm evidence that previously noise-exposed ears are either more sensitive to future noise exposure or that hearing loss due to noise progresses once the exposure to noise is discontinued. It is clear that NIHL can interact with presbycusis, exacerbating age-related effects.

Asymmetric hearing loss

When an individual has incurred greater noise exposure in one ear than in the other ear, the audiogram may show an asymmetry in hearing threshold levels for the two ears. When evaluating asymmetric sensorineural hearing loss, it is necessary to determine whether or not the working environment was such that the working conditions exposed one ear to more noise than the other ear. For example, truck or tractor drivers may suffer greater hearing loss in the ear closest to the engine exhaust, and a worker whose ear is facing a particularly offending noise source during work may also experience greater hearing loss in the ear closest to the noise source. Most indoor factory environments, however, are highly reverberant so that one ear rarely receives significantly more noise than the other.

The examiner must also be aware that there are various non-occupational noise sources that typically result in hearing asymmetry. The most common cause of asymmetric NIHL relates to the firearm user who typically demonstrates a greater hearing loss in the ear contralateral to the trigger finger. That is, right-handed hunters most often demonstrate a greater high frequency NIHL in the left ear. Of particular concern in the evaluation of asymmetric hearing loss are those conditions that reflect non-NIHL otologic pathology. Etiologies such as Meniere's disease, sudden idiopathic sensorineural hearing loss, and acoustic neuromas most often present unilaterally and require otologic evaluation. Such is also the case with allied otologic asymmetric complaints such as unilateral tinnitus, unilateral aural fullness, and vestibular symptoms.

Tinnitus

The problem of assessing injury and damages without the assistance of objective standards is particularly challenging where claims of tinnitus are included. Some compensation agencies allow a percent rating for the presence of tinnitus, in addition to the amount of hearing impairment. The lack of reliability of measurement of tinnitus and the prevalence of tinnitus in the population compounds the problem. Glorig has described a guideline used by the Veterans Administration that may be useful to experts in forming opinions as to the clinical significance of tinnitus complaints.[16] These include criteria that the treatment history must include one or more attempts to alleviate the perceived disturbance by medication, prosthetic management, or psychiatric intervention, and that the complaint of tinnitus must be supported by statements from family or significant others.

Comparing a patient's tinnitus to audiometric tones or noises (tinnitus matching) may be helpful in assessing a complaint of tinnitus. Noise-induced tinnitus is usually at or above 3000 Hz, or at least no more than an octave below the noise-affected frequencies. Its loudness is typically only 3–5 dB and very rarely more than 15 dB above audiometric threshold, and usually varies by no more than 2 dB on repeat audiometric measurements within a single session. Tinnitus loudness is not a reliable indicator of annoyance or disability, and tinnitus matching tests have potential value only in documenting the existence of tinnitus, not its severity.

Susceptibility to NIHL

The development of NIHL is dependent upon a number of factors, including the intensity of the noise, the length of time a person is exposed to the noise, and individual susceptibility. The more intense the noise, the more likely it will produce hearing loss. In addition, the longer a person is exposed to a particular noise, the greater the probability of injury to the auditory system. A long-standing observation in the field of NIHL has been that some individuals' ears are more easily damaged by noise than others. There are some persons with 'tough' ears whose hearing seems to withstand prolonged loud noise levels and others with relatively 'tender' ears that develop hearing loss greater than the norm. There is a broad range of individual differences in sensitivity to any given noise exposure and individual varying susceptibility to NIHL.

It is commonly assumed that variability in susceptibility is a manifestation of biologic factors that are unique to each individual. Some have proposed that imperfections in the physical characteristics of the cochlea and variability in cochlear structure contribute to the susceptibility. Recent research has examined the role of antioxidant status in mediating susceptibility.[17] A number of potentially important variables have been examined, including age, gender, cardiovascular disease, race, previous inner ear damage, efficiency of the acoustic reflex, smoking, and pigmentation. At present, the data are inconclusive in specifying variables related to susceptibility.

A relationship between TTS and PTS has been sought for many years, since it has been hoped that the amount of TTS could be used to predict the risk of PTS. Unfortunately, the relationship between TTS and PTS is by no means clear, since no straightforward relationship between TTS and PTS has been delineated. This issue of individual susceptibility is a strong reason for annual audiometric monitoring of all employees in loud noise environments. Those persons who experience hearing deterioration require greater noise protection and possible change of work location to a less hazardous noise environment.

Audiometric surveillance for NIHL

The OSHA hearing conservation amendment mandates audiometric surveillance of workers who are exposed to noise levels equal to or exceeding 85 dBA on an 8-hour time-weighted average (TWA).[18] The standard requires testing when beginning work in a noisy area, and yearly testing thereafter. While this routine audiometric testing can be performed by an audiometric technician who has completed the necessary education and training requirements, any individual who needs to be referred for additional testing should be evaluated by an audiologist. In the US, audiometric technicians are certified by the Council of Accreditation in Occupational Hearing Conservation (CAOHC); and audiologists are certified by the American Speech-Language-Hearing Association (ASHA).

Surveillance audiograms should be performed in a sound-controlled acoustic environment. The OSHA standard provides guidelines for acceptable ambient noise levels inside a testing booth; slightly more stringent criteria are listed in the ANSI standard S3.1 1977. For the baseline audiogram, the individual should not have been exposed to loud noise for at least 16 hours prior to testing, to avoid temporary threshold shifts. Subsequent surveillance tests, however, do not require the noise-free interval. OSHA regulations require testing at the frequencies of 500, 1000, 2000, 3000, 4000 and 6000 Hz, but it is advisable to test at 8000 Hz as well to look for a 'recovery pattern' at that frequency. The results of the periodic audiogram should be compared to the baseline. If the employee's test shows a 'shift' from baseline in excess of 10 dB for the average hearing level at 2000, 3000, and 4000 Hz in either ear (a '10 dB shift' or 'standard threshold shift'), a retest may be performed within 30 days. If the shift persists, the employee must be informed in writing within 21 days, fitted with hearing protectors if not already using them, refitted and counseled if already using protectors, and referred for a clinical audiologic evaluation and/or otologic evaluation if appropriate. While OSHA requires use of the 10dB shift criteria, other shift criteria have been proposed. These include NIOSH '10 dB twice', or a shift from baseline of 15 dB at any frequency on two subsequent tests.[19]

Although OSHA has not recommended specific otologic referral criteria, the American Academy of Otolaryngology – Head and Neck Surgery (AAO/HNS) has previously proposed criteria for referral of individuals to an otolaryngologist.[20]

1. Baseline audiogram
   a. Average hearing levels at 500, 1000, 2000, and 3000 Hz greater than 25 dB in either ear.
   b. Difference in average hearing level between the better and poorer ears of more than 15 dB at 500, 1000, and 2000 Hz, or more than 30 dB at 3000, 4000, and 6000 Hz.
2. Periodic audiograms
   a. Change for the worse in average hearing level in either ear compared to the baseline audiogram of more than 15 dB at 500, 1000, and 2000 Hz, or more than 20 dB at 3000, 4000, and 6000 Hz.

Other criteria that may indicate a need for physician referral include ear pain, drainage, dizziness, severe persistent tinnitus, fluctuating or rapidly progressive hearing loss, or a presence of accumulated cerumen or other foreign material within the ear canal. If the employee presents with other more non-specific complaints, including aural fullness or discomfort, or if audiometric findings are inconsistent, an otolaryngology referral may also be prudent.

Age correction of the periodic audiogram may be performed under the OSHA standard to allow for the contribution of aging to the change in hearing level. The standard provides an appendix of age correction values. The process of applying population-derived norms to an individual audiogram is a method of indirect standardization, and allows for comparison of hearing loss rates between different worker populations. Age correction, however, has been criticized as decreasing the sensitivity of medical surveillance,[19] and some hearing conservation programs such as that of the US Air Force do not use an age correction.

Treatment

While conductive hearing losses are often amenable to medical or surgical treatments, hearing loss due to the effects of prolonged loud noise exposure causes a permanent and irreversible sensorineural hearing impairment, for which no specific treatment is currently available. As is the case with most types of sensorineural hearing impairments, the most common and effective remediation is hearing aid amplification. Hearing aids are simply miniature personal amplifiers, and are chosen on the basis of responses shaped to provide the necessary amplification for the frequencies affected by the hearing loss. Persons with high frequency hearing losses are fitted with hearing aids incorporating only high frequency amplification. Most hearing aids are custom made to fit within the ear and are individually programmed for the particular hearing loss.

Persons requiring hearing aids should be referred to certified dispensing audiologists, as they are the professionals who possess the necessary expertise to fit and counsel the hearing-impaired person. If a hearing loss is related to a compensation claim, hearing aid rehabilitation should be included in any settlement. Since hearing aids have a limited life expectancy (4–6 years), compensation for future hearing aids should also be considered in compensation settlements. In addition, devices such as amplified telephones, infrared TV transmitters, and other personal assistive listening devices should be considered for the hearing-impaired individual.

Accommodation of the hearing-impaired worker

If an employee is determined to have a significant hearing loss at the time of employment or subsequently, the occupational medicine clinician faces several issues regarding accommodation of a hearing-impaired employee. Considerations include risks to the individual due to inability to hear auditory warning signals, interference of hearing protection with high frequency hearing acuity, and risk of further loss due to noise or ototoxic exposures. The hearing-impaired worker who requires hearing aids presents a difficult challenge also. While hearing aids are needed by the individual to hear and understand others, the use of amplification in noise environments may cause additional hearing damage. The clinician must also consider whether the individual is sufficiently impaired to pose a risk to others if operating machinery or performing other safety sensitive jobs. The Department of Transportation has published guidelines for acceptable hearing levels for operators of commercial vehicles. In addition to ensuring that an individual receives adequate evaluation and treatment of the hearing loss, reasonable accommodation for hearing-impaired individuals can include special warning devices relying more on visual signals, flat attenuation hearing protectors, and avoidance of safety sensitive tasks requiring auditory acuity.

Prevention

A hearing conservation program has historically consisted of at least seven identifiable elements: monitoring hearing hazards; engineering and administrative controls; audiometric evaluation; personal hearing protective devices; education and motivation; record keeping; and program evaluation. When engineering and administrative controls fail to reduce noise to an acceptable level, personal hearing protective devices (HPDs) are vital to prevent NIHL. Personal hearing protection can be an effective means of noise reduction if appropriately worn. There are a number of different types of HPDs that may be considered depending on the individual's occupation. The attenuation characteristics of the HPD must be appropriate for the characteristics of the noise environment.

HPDs are generally of two types – earplugs and earmuffs. There are many different varieties of earplugs, from custom molded to disposable types. Flanged pre-molded earplugs provide satisfactory attenuation if properly fitted. Ear discomfort may encourage a more compliant 'one size fits all' plug. An expandable foam plug is available which can be compressed and inserted; it expands in the ear canal resulting in an effective seal. These expandable earplugs are usually quite comfortable to wear and they also can provide high noise attenuation values. Custom-fitted earplugs will yield excellent sound protection if properly fitted. Retention of the plug may be a problem and a poor fit will result in discomfort. Custom plugs require cleaning and maintenance and, in fact, offer few advantages over the less expensive foam plugs. All earplugs need to fit snugly into the ear canal so that there is no sound leakage around the plug; training in correct insertion is important.

Circumaural hearing protectors or muffs fit over the outer ears to reduce acoustic levels outside the ear canal. The device must be designed to provide for a compliant fit and effective seal around the ear. The cup material should be rigid and of large volume so as to provide the best low frequency attenuation levels. Since earmuffs do not require insertion into the ear canal, they are perhaps more hygienic and less likely to cause external ear canal infections. They are also easier to remove and replace in conditions of intermittent noise exposure. The singular disadvantage to these devices is that they are cumbersome and bulky. In conditions of extremely high noise, it may be necessary to wear both earplugs and earmuffs together.

The amount of actual or real ear attenuation of HPDs depends on a number of factors including the design, material, and fit of the device. Protection is greatest in the high frequencies for most devices. In conditions of high noise exposures or when significant communication demands exist, it may be helpful to determine the frequency characteristics of the environmental noise, along with the intensity, in order to select a HPD with the exact appropriate attenuation characteristics.

Workers' compensation and assessment of impairment

Assessment of impairment

Following the history, otologic examination, and audiologic evaluation, it must be determined if the individual's hearing status has been adversely affected, on a 'more probable than not' basis, by occupational loud noise exposure.[21] If the audiometric configuration shows greater thresholds in the 3000–6000 Hz range with some recovery at 8000 Hz (i.e., 'notching'), the presumption of NIHL is strengthened significantly. Older persons, however, may not show this characteristic high frequency notch, due to the effects of aging (presbycusis) causing deterioration of the high frequency thresholds.[22] While there is no universally accepted method to separate the effects of noise exposure from the effects of presbycusis upon auditory function, an approach using clinical data and epidemiologic models has been proposed.[23] Many compensation agencies therefore consider the two etiologies together, with the loss being appraised as if it were entirely caused or exacerbated by a confirmed history of noise exposure. While it is extremely helpful to have access to a baseline audiogram prior to the initiation of employment, as well as annual audiograms, to characterize the history of the hearing loss, such records are often not available.

The presence of conductive hearing loss, unilateral hearing loss, visible otologic abnormalities (i.e., chronic otitis media, eardrum perforations), and unusual audiometric configurations would suggest non-industrial etiologies. Of course, if an industrial accident such as an aural slag burn occurred, a conductive hearing loss could be present. Such cases are usually rather straightforward, due to the clear-cut history and physical findings. A greater challenge is to determine the contribution of non-occupational noise exposures to the development of NIHL in compensation cases, since such exposures may be difficult to quantify. The task of the examining medical provider is to form a judgment 'to a reasonable degree of medical probability' or more likely than not, whether a given noise exposure significantly contributed to the overall hearing loss.

Workers' compensation statutes

Although US workers' compensation programs were initially established in the early 1900s, it was not until the late 1940s that industrial claims for NIHL were first filed. In 1953 New York became the first state to draft proposals for provisions dealing specifically with NIHL. Today, most states treat NIHL as an occupational disease with scheduled awards based upon the degree of hearing loss, although some states still require the claimant to show 'incapacity to work', 'disablement' or some other reason for economic disability. States also vary widely on such critical compensation issues as hearing impairment formulas, waiting periods for filing, presbycusis corrections, filing time limits, and whether willful failure to use hearing protection voids an employee's right to file for compensation.

Workers' compensation laws exist in all 50 states and for most federal workers. Unfortunately, these laws are not uniform, particularly with respect to hearing loss claims, and employ a bewildering array of schemes to determine whether compensation is appropriate and, if so, how much is due.[24] To make matters worse, some states apparently administer their systems in ways that are not entirely consistent with their 'governing' legislation. Before becoming involved with a workers' compensation case, the professional should obtain a copy of the appropriate state statute, and seek advice from another professional experienced with the system, as statutes are frequently amended.

Many methods have been used over the years to calculate impairment ratings for hearing loss. The majority of compensation formulas use the pure tone audiogram to determine eligibility for compensation awards, although the frequencies used to arrive at the amount of compensation may be different. Since NIHL typically first affects the frequencies in the 3000–6000 Hz range, a critical factor is whether or not frequencies above 2000 Hz are included in the averaging process. Compensation formulas include a specification of the frequencies that will be averaged, a low and a high fence (the decibel criterion threshold level at which impairment is assumed to begin, and the level at which it is assumed to be complete), and a method of averaging the better and poorer ears.

The most widely accepted formula at the present time is that proposed in 1979 by the American Academy of Otolaryngology ('AAO-79' method), and subsequently accepted by the American Medical Association.[25] This formula averages the frequencies of 500, 1000, 2000, and 3000 Hz. Prior to this, only the frequencies of 500, 1000, and 2000 Hz were used in the 1959 AMA formula. The low fence, or beginning of impairment, is 25 dB HL. The better ear is weighted to be five times more important than the poorer ear.

While the AAO-79 method is perhaps the most widely accepted compensation formula, some states have no recommended formula, but leave impairment ratings to the discretion of the examining physician. The Veterans Administration (VA) incorporates speech discrimination (understanding) scores into a compensation schedule. Many states include a provision that excludes a claim when the occupational noise exposure is below a specified level, such as 90 dBA TWA. The statutes of limitations for filing claims vary from jurisdiction to jurisdiction, and are as short as 30 days to as long as 5 years. Over 40 states and provinces permit some type of deduction in impairment award for presbycusis (hearing loss attributed to aging). In other jurisdictions, the use of the AAO-79 low fence of 25 dB HL is considered to account for the effects of aging on hearing. Although tinnitus typically accompanies NIHL, only about one-half of US states permit additional impairment for tinnitus. Some states deny compensation or penalize workers for failure to use protective devices. A few states reduce the compensation award if the claimant

shows improvement with the use of hearing aids. Due to these many differences in hearing impairment calculation and awards, individuals with the exact same audiograms can receive entirely different hearing loss ratings and compensation, dependent upon the jurisdiction and governmental agency responsible for NIHL claims.

Non-noise-induced hearing loss

Head trauma

Hearing loss, tinnitus, facial nerve injury, and/or dizziness can be caused by blunt or penetrating trauma to the head. Motor vehicle accidents, industrial accidents, falls, and recreational injuries can result in fractures of the temporal bone. The large majority (80%) of temporal bone fractures are classified as longitudinal and are typically caused by a direct blow to the lateral skull, usually the parietal region. Longitudinal fractures pass through the ear canal and the middle ear but bypass the inner ear structures. These fractures typically produce conductive losses by lacerating the ear canal, rupturing the tympanic membrane, causing blood accumulation behind the tympanic membrane (hemotympanum), and/or dislocating the ossicular chain. Even though the inner ear structures are not directly involved in longitudinal fractures, a high frequency sensorineural hearing loss with tinnitus may sometimes occur, with an audiometric configuration resembling NIHL. These losses are believed to be caused by 'labyrinthine concussion' and may or may not improve over subsequent months.

Transverse fractures of the temporal bone are seen in association with intense blows to either the occiput or a direct frontal blow. The fracture usually passes through the vestibule of the inner ear resulting in complete and permanent loss of cochlear and vestibular function. The hearing loss is a severe/profound sensorineural impairment; 10–20% of longitudinal and 40–50% of transverse temporal bone fractures are associated with facial nerve injury.

A history of head injury with loss of consciousness is strongly correlated with a risk for hearing loss.[26] Injuries too mild to cause loss of consciousness will rarely cause permanent hearing loss.

Penetrating trauma to the temporal bone can range from a simple Q-tip injury to a life-threatening emergency due to a gunshot wound to the temporal bone. Penetrating temporal bone trauma is generally more destructive than blunt trauma, as vascular and other intracranial injuries are more commonly effected in penetrating injuries. Hearing loss is related to the site of damage to the auditory system, from external canal injury up to the central auditory system. Facial nerve trauma is present approximately half of the time and tends to be severe, as the nerve may be transected and large segments of the nerve may be missing or damaged.

Most patients experience some degree of balance disturbance after temporal bone trauma. Causes of post-traumatic vertigo include postconcussive syndrome, concussive injury to the labyrinth, cupulolithiasis, massive and disruptive injury to the labyrinth, and traumatic perilymphatic fistula.

Inner ear disorders of diving

A professional diver's hearing is at risk for multiple reasons, and studies of divers have suggested increased rates of hearing loss.[27] Noise-induced hearing loss is possible due to high intensity noise generated by compressed air entering the diver's helmet or decompression chambers. Divers may also be exposed to high noise levels from nearby ship engines or power tools. Additionally, sensorineural hearing loss may be due to barotrauma and decompression sickness.[28] Decompression sickness of the inner ear must be considered as a potential cause for sensorineural hearing loss following a dive if the diver has been close to or exceeded the safe depth and time limits of the United States Navy Dive Tables (see Chapter 36). Vertigo is a frequent concomitant symptom.

Sensorineural hearing loss following diving may also be caused by labyrinthine membrane rupture. This is usually caused by pressure disequilibrium between the inner and middle ear and may be the result of a strong Valsalva maneuver used by the diver to clear an unobstructed ear during the dive. A sudden pop may be experienced followed by hearing loss and vertigo. The membrane rupture may occur anywhere within the labyrinthine membranes or at the oval or round window membrane. The evaluation of vertigo or hearing loss following a dive should include an audiogram as soon as possible.

Decompression sickness is best treated by immediate recompression in a chamber. In some cases, hyperbaric oxygen may be helpful even though the diving profile does not suggest decompression sickness. As a temporizing measure, oxygen should be administered and a benzodiazepine will provide vestibular sedation. If decompression sickness is unlikely, sensorineural hearing loss following a dive is considered secondary to labyrinthine membrane rupture. There are no pathognomonic findings, and the fistula may only be identified at the time of surgical exploration of the middle ear. The hearing loss of many patients with suspected fistulas may improve on simple bed rest. If the hearing loss persists or is progressive, or if vertigo is present, surgical exploration of the middle ear for closure of the labyrinthine fistula at either the oval or round window, is generally required.

Prevention of labyrinthine injuries related to diving includes strict adherence to the profiles established by the United States Navy Dive Tables. Pressure disturbances in the middle ear cannot always be avoided, but are more common in cases of poor eustachian tube function. A documented sensorineural hearing loss after diving is a contraindication to further diving.

Radiation-induced hearing loss

Radiation exposures during treatment of head and neck cancers have been associated with sensorineural hearing loss. This appears to be a direct result of radiation injury to the cochlea, and should be considered in the differential of sensorineural hearing loss.[29,30]

Other non-noise-induced trauma

The external and potentially the middle ear may be traumatized by debris and other contaminants generated in the industrial setting. Specifically, slag burns of the external canal, tympanic membrane, and even the middle ear have historically been a frequent source of permanent tympanic membrane perforations and conductive hearing loss. The frequency with which this type of injury occurs has declined as a result of the increased use of noise protection devices. The history is diagnostic. The welder will report a foreign body sensation in the ear followed by intense pain and burning sometimes accompanied by a sizzling. If the slag comes in contact with the tympanic membrane, perforations of almost any size may result in any quadrant. Large perforations are not uncommon, and at times portions of the slag will contaminate the middle ear. The amount of conductive hearing loss that results will depend on the size and location of the perforation. Infection following contamination of the middle ear may ensue and will be manifested by drainage.

Initial treatment generally includes an antibiotic to discourage infection; drops may be used if there is no tympanic membrane perforation. Unfortunately, and in contrast to burns caused by caustic agents, thermal burns of the tympanic membrane are very slow to heal and are likely to become chronic. This being the case, surgical closure is generally required, and foreign material may be removed from within the middle ear cleft at the time of tympanic membrane repair.

Prevention of slag burns may be accomplished by using appropriate protective hoods. As mentioned above, the consistent use of noise protection devices in conjunction with welding hoods has reduced the incidence of this form of industrial injury.

Hearing loss due to chemicals

In addition to well-known ototoxic drugs such as aminoglycosides and cisplatin, clinical and experimental studies indicate a potential harmful effect of chemicals, especially organic solvents, on the auditory system. The mechanism of such damage is considered to be through direct neurotoxic mechanisms. Known neurotoxins, such as the organic solvents toluene and styrene, have been shown to cause hearing loss in both animal models and human studies. Metals with neurotoxic properties such as lead, methyl mercury, and arsenic have also been reported as ototoxicants. Such toxins may affect hearing by direct cochlear damage or by retrocochlear action on the auditory nerve and auditory cortex. Carbon monoxide may predispose to hearing loss through an asphyxiant mechanism.[31]

Recent studies have suggested that certain ototoxic chemicals may damage hearing or potentiate the effect of noise on hearing. Solvents and metals are most likely to exacerbate noise-induced hearing loss, as they have well-established neurotoxic effects.[32] While a direct causal relationship between sensorineural hearing loss and exposure to these substances has yet to be definitively established in humans, animal studies indicate that there may be a synergistic effect between noise and chemical exposure.[33]

References

1. Williams J. Treatise on the ear; including its anatomy, physiology, and pathology. London: Churchill, 1860.
2. Brookhouser PE. Prevention of noise-induced hearing loss. Prev Med 1994; 23:665–9.
3. EPA. Noise in America: the extent of the noise problem. Washington DC: US Environmental Protection Agency,1981.
4. Clark WW, Bohne BA. Effects of noise on hearing. JAMA 1999; 281:1658–9.
5. Niskar AS, Kieszak SM, Holmes AE, et al. Estimated prevalence of noise-induced hearing threshold shifts among children 6 to 19 years of age: the Third National Health and Nutrition Examination Survey, 1988–1994, United States. Pediatrics 2001; 108:40–3.
6. Berger E, Royster LH, Royster JD, Driscoll DP, eds. The noise manual, 5th edn. Fairfax: American Industrial Hygiene Association, 2000.
7. Kaygusuz I, Ozturk A, Ustundag B, et al. Role of free oxygen radicals in noise-related hearing impairment. Hear Res 2001; 162: 43–7.
8. Shulman A. Epidemiology of tinnitus. In: Shulman A, Tonndorf J, Feldman H, et al, eds. Tinnitus, diagnosis/treatment. Philadelphia: Lea & Febiger, 1991;237–47.
9. Morris MS, Borja LP. Air bag deployment and hearing loss. Arch Otolaryngol 1998; 124:507.
10. McBride DI, Williams S. Audiometric notch as a sign of noise induced hearing loss. Occup Environ Med 2001; 58:46–51.
11. Suter A. Hearing conservation manual, 4th edn. Milwaukee: Council for Accreditation in Occupational Hearing Conservation, 2002;78.
12. Hetu R, Riverin L, Getty L, et al. The reluctance to acknowledge hearing difficulties among hearing-impaired workers. Br J Audiol 1990: 24:265–76.
13. Hetu R, Getty L, Quoc HT. Impact of occupational hearing loss on the lives of workers. Occup Med 1995; 10:495–512.
14. Zwerling C, Whitten PS, Davis CS, et al. Occupational injuries among older workers with visual, auditory, and other impairments. A validation study. J Occup Med 1998; 40:720–3.
15. Gates GA, Schmid P, Kujawa S, et al. Longitudinal threshold changes in older men with audiometric notches. Hear Res 2000; 141: 220–8.
16. Glorig A. Tinnitus: suggested guidelines for determining impairment, handicap and disability. In: Annual meeting of the American Academy of Otolaryngology-Head and Neck Surgery. Alexandria: American Academy of Otolaryngology-Head and Neck Surgery, 1987.
17. Henderson D, McFadden S L, Liu CC, et al. The role of antioxidants in protection from impulse noise. Ann NY Acad Sci 1999; 884:368–80.
18. OSHA. 1910.95 CFR Occupational noise exposure: hearing conservation amendment (final rule). Fed Reg 1983; 48:9738–85.
19. NIOSH. Criteria for a recommended standard: occupational noise exposure revised criteria. Cincinnati: DHHS, 1998.
20. Simpson TH, Stewart M, Blakley BW. Audiometric referral criteria for industrial hearing conservation programs. Arch Otolaryngol 1995; 121:407–11.
21. Dobie RA. Compensation for hearing loss. Audiology 1996; 35:1–7.
22. Consensus conference. Noise and hearing loss. JAMA 1990; 263:3185–90.
23. Dobie RA. Medical-legal evaluation of hearing loss, 2nd edn. San Diego: Singular, 2001;398.
24. American Speech-Language-Hearing Association. A survey of states' workers' compensation practices for occupational hearing loss. Ad Hoc Committee on Worker's Compensation. ASHA J 1992; 8(Suppl):2–8.
25. Anonymous. Guide for the evaluation of hearing handicap. JAMA 1979; 241:2055–9.
26. Neuberger M, Korpert K, Raber A, et al. Hearing loss from industrial noise, head injury and ear disease. A multivariate analysis on audiometric examinations of 110,647 workers. Audiology 1992; 31: 45–57.
27. Molvaer OI, Albrektsen G. Hearing deterioration in professional divers: an epidemiologic study. Undersea Biomed Res 1990; 17:231–46.
28. Talmi YP, Finkelstein Y, Zohar Y. Barotrauma-induced hearing loss. Scand Audiol 1991; 20:1–9.
29. Mencher GT, Novotny G, Mencher L, Gulliver M. Ototoxicity and irradiation: additional etiologies of hearing loss in adults. J Am Acad Audiol 1995; 6:351–7.
30. Chen WC, Liao CT, Tsai HC, et al. Radiation-induced hearing impairment in patients treated for malignant parotid tumor. Ann Otol Rhinol Laryngol 1999; 108:1159–64.
31. Fechter LD, Chen GD, Rao D, et al. Predicting exposure conditions that facilitate the potentiation of noise-induced hearing loss by carbon monoxide. Toxicol Sci 2000; 58:315–23.
32. Morata TC. Assessing occupational hearing loss: beyond noise exposures. Scand Audiol 1998; 48(Suppl):111–6.
33. Morata TC. Chemical exposure as a risk factor for hearing loss. J Occup Med 2003; 45: 676–82.

20.3 **Upper Airway Disorders**

Rebecca Bascom, Maadhava Ellaurie

Upper airway disorders are among the most common chronic conditions challenging clinicians, with diverse etiologies including allergic and non-allergic mechanisms. The range of dysfunction[1] includes impaired mucociliary clearance, nasal passage obstruction, upper airway collapse during sleep, and paradoxical vocal fold motion during the respiratory cycle. Upper airway disorders lead the differential diagnosis for patients presenting with typical symptoms of headache, nasal congestion, rhinorrhea, postnasal drip, sneezing, nasal burning, and dysphonia. Upper airway disorders may also explain cough, dyspnea, chest tightness, stridor, snoring, non-restful sleep, sleep disruption, and daytime hypersomnolence.

Allergic upper airway disorders are apparently increasing in frequency, in parallel with the worldwide increase in atopic asthma. The prevalence of rhinitis in 55,000 Swedish conscripts rose from 4.4% in 1971 to 8.4% in 1981. The attributable fraction of rhinitis caused by occupational factors is about 5% to 15%, admittedly a rough estimate. High-risk persons are those with allergy and/or hyperactivity and allergic diseases in the family. High-risk occupations are in industries involving exposure to highly active allergens, such as animal products, chemicals, latex, and flour.

The most common occupational or environmental upper respiratory condition is mucous membrane irritation. Surveys of adults in the past decade indicate 12-month cumulative prevalence rates ranging from 28% to 62%.[2,3] Mucosal irritation occurs in domestic, industrial, and office settings; controlled human challenges show that the upper respiratory inflammatory responses differ among irritants, and collectively these are distinct from the inflammatory responses to allergens or infectious agents. Despite the clinical impression of a high prevalence of irritant rhinitis, few studies have addressed possible long-term effects by comparing the effects of medical removal versus continued symptomatic exposure. Determinants of susceptibility to chronic effects, such as squamous metaplasia, are also poorly understood, but animal studies have developed a robust chronic exposure data-set enabling new dosimetric models.

An important function of the upper airway is communication.[4,5] Work-related hoarseness may significantly impair communication, especially by telephone or in a high-noise environment. Hoarseness, therefore, ranges from a nuisance to a distinct disability. 'Professional voice users' include singers, but also teachers, telephone operators, telemarketers, customer relations staff, and sales personnel.

The upper respiratory tract enables olfaction; vapors entrained in the nasal passages move turbulently to the superior part of the nasal cavity and bind to diverse receptors in the olfactory epithelium. Direct toxicity to olfactory epithelium clearly occurs for some, but not all, inhaled agents.[6] Acquired olfactory impairment may be due to traumatic damage to the olfactory nerve, direct toxicity to olfactory epithelium, alterations in the surface fluid overlying the epithelium, and nasal pathology that obstructs airflow to the olfactory epithelium.[7]

Effective functioning of the upper respiratory tract directly influences job performance and worker morale. Studies have shown that the domains of physical limitation, physical functioning, pain, social functioning, emotional limitation, mental health, and general health perceptions are all significantly worse in rhinitis patients compared to controls. Upper respiratory tract symptoms often influence a worker's perception of risk. Office workers may notice work-associated mucosal irritation and mistakenly fear they are suffering from asbestos poisoning. The physician must develop an organized and effective approach to diagnosing, treating, and explaining these disorders.

PATHOPHYSIOLOGY

The upper airway serves several critical functions. It warms and humidifies inhaled air and filters large particles, including many common allergens. It is the primary adsorptive surface for water-soluble gases, such as sulfur dioxide, and removes substantial quantities of less soluble gases, such as ozone. Obstruction of the nasal passages may result in a change from nasal to oral respiration. Oral breathing bypasses the filtering functions of the nose, increasing the hazard to the lower airways and lungs. An interesting study by Lehmann in 1935 (cited by Proctor[8]) assessed the nasal filtering capacity in miners with and without advanced silicosis. Miners with the most effective nasal filters seemed to have least disease, except for those few miners who had highly effective filtration but were mouth breathers.

The epithelium of the upper airway ranges from the stratified squamous epithelium of the nasal alae, to the transitional epithelium of the antrum, to the pseudostratified columnar epithelium of the nasal passages. Additional transitional zones occur in the oropharynx and glottis. The four functional components of the nasal mucosa are venous sinusoids, postcapillary venules, glands, and the nervous system.[9,10] The venous sinusoids swell and constrict in response to sympathetic tone and other stimuli, and thus regulate nasal airflow and patency. Postcapillary venules are present in the superficial lamina propria, where plasma extravasation and diapedesis of leukocytes occur. Their endothelial cells respond to mediators by contracting, opening gaps in the basement membrane and expressing adhesion molecules and releasing nitric oxide (NO), endothelin, and other mediators that regulate vascular tone. The seromucous glands release antimicrobial factors such as lysozyme, lactoferrin, secretory immunoglobulin (Ig) A, hyaluronic acid, and neutral mucins. Mucous cells and goblet cells release acidic mucins coated with sialic acid and sulfate groups that enable them to adsorb particulate or irritant chemicals on the mucosal surface. Innervation of these structures is by sympathetic, parasympathetic, and type C nerves. Non-myelinated type C nociceptive nerves are present in the epithelium and mediate sensations of itch and burning pain by H1 and capsaicin receptors, respectively.[11] Parasympathetic nerves include cholinergic nerves that mediate glandular secretion,[12] and sympathetic fibers are responsible for vasodilation of the venous sinusoids. Sympathetic fibers contain either norepinephrine or norepinephrine and neuropeptide Y (NPY). Norepinephrine causes vasoconstriction and collapse of the sinusoids and an increase of nasal patency, while NPY reduces vascular permeability.

Cardinal nasal symptoms of congestion, pruritus, sneezing, and secretions occur through these mechanisms.[10] Congestion results primarily from venous sinusoidal pooling and secondarily from subepithelial vasodilation, increased vascular permeability, and glandular secretion. Pruritus, burning, and sneezing result from sensory nerve stimulation, though these responses can be dissociated.[13] Secretions are the result of glandular stimulation and increased vascular permeability. Some of the components of nasal secretions that have been studied are prostaglandin D2 (PGD2), tosyl-arginine methyl ester (TAME) esterase activity, kinins, albumin, immunoglobulins, lactoferrin, lysozyme, tryptase, and major basic protein. Asthma and rhinitis often coexist[14] and basement membrane thickening, eosinophilic inflammation, and epithelial shedding are present on biopsies obtained from both sites, though typically are worse in the lower airway.

Subclasses of T-helper (TH) lymphocytes have been identified among antigen-specific T cells by measuring the profile of cytokines that they produce. TH1 cells are characterized by production of interleukin (IL)-2, interferon (IFN)-gamma, and tumor necrosis factor (TNF)-beta, and evoke cell-mediated immunity and phagocyte-dependent inflammation. TH1 responses are highly protective against infections mounted by the majority of microbes, especially the intracellular parasites. TH1 cytokines activate phagocytes and promote B lymphocytes to produce opsonization and complement-fixing antibodies. TH2 cells represent a polarized form of the T-helper cell-mediated immune response that is characterized by the production of IL-4, IL-5, IL-6, IL-9, IL-10, and IL-13 but not of IFN-gamma and TNF-beta. TH2 cells evoke strong antibody responses (including the IgE class) and eosinophil accumulation, but inhibit several functions of the phagocytic cells. The TH2 cytokines induce the differentiation, activation, and the in-situ survival of the eosinophils (through IL-5), promote the production by B lymphocytes of high amounts of antibodies including IgE (through IL-4 or IL-13), as well as promoting the growth of mast cells and basophils (through IL-4, IL-5, and IL-10). It appears that both environmental and genetic factors act in concert to determine the TH1/TH2 profile.

The allergic reaction appears to be the result of a TH2-type T-cell response to one or more common environmental allergens. Circulating IgE binds to high-affinity Fc epsilon receptor 1 on mast cells and basophils. Re-exposure to allergen leads to cross-linking of these Fc receptors and degranulation of these cells. The preformed and newly formed mediators lead to an immediate hypersensitivity reaction and a late-phase response. Histamine plays the most important role in the immediate reaction, together with TAME esterase, PGD2, and kinins. Four to 6 hours following the immediate phase, a late-phase response occurs with an accumulation of eosinophils, basophils, and TH2 cells together with increased levels of histamine, TAME esterase, and kinins. Nasal levels of NO, too, are elevated in patients with allergic rhinitis and appear to correlate with inflammation.[15,16] Levels rise further during the pollen season and may be modulated by nasal steroids.

CLINICAL EVALUATION

The initial evaluation of a patient with upper respiratory symptoms consists of a careful history and physical examination (Table 20.3.1). A careful history is the single most important diagnostic tool for evaluating upper respiratory tract disease. Many centers base the initial empiric treatment of rhinitis solely on the history. This is probably reasonable for cases with mild symptoms or an evident etiology, provided that there is follow-up to verify the efficacy of treatment. Temporal patterns of irritation, congestion, rhinorrhea, or sneezing often suggest likely etiologies. As with asthma, the response to allergen exposure can occur within minutes of exposure (acute response), can occur hours later (isolated late response), can be a biphasic response, or an acute, sustained response. A symptom diary may be useful to clarify these patterns. The evaluation of asthma in the occupational setting emphasizes the importance of observation and measurement with 2-week intervals of exposure and removal from exposure (see Chapter 19.2). A similar 'longer-view' approach will clarify some complex cases of upper airway diseases.

The history should also pay particular attention to symptoms suggesting sinusitis (facial pain and pressure, fever, discolored mucus), or asthma or reactive airways (paroxysmal cough, episodic chest discomfort, exercise or nocturnal dyspnea, or wheezing). Upper chest or xyphosternal discomfort accompanying dyspnea may indicate laryngeal dysfunction instead of asthma. Hyperfunctional voice disorder can also cause dyspnea and upper chest discomfort, often with cough. Treatment of the upper airway disease can improve asthma and seems to reduce sinusitis risk. If the evaluation suggests concomitant lower respiratory tract disease, further workup should proceed, as described elsewhere in this text (see Chapter 19.1).

If the history is strongly suggestive of IgE allergies, a referral should be made directly for allergy skin testing. If an allergist is not available, radioallergosorbent tests (RAST) may be performed on sera to a panel of allergens appropriate for the region. Allergy reference laboratories exist that allow serum samples to be mailed in for analysis. A less desirable approach is to obtain a multiallergen RAST and then to refer patients for allergy skin testing if the screening multi-RAST has positive results. False-negative results limit the applicability of this approach; also, targeted environmental modification needs cannot be determined. If the physical examination indicates pharyngitis, cultures of the throat may be taken. Nasal cultures are not indicated routinely. A nasal swab test may help assess the nature of the cellular influx.

History

1. Symptoms (symptom diary)
   Nature: Congestion, rhinorrhea, sneezing, itching, hoarseness, coughing, headache, postnasal drip, burning, irritation, and dryness
   Timing: Seasonal, perennial, episodic, weekends, and vacations
   Severity: 0–5 (absent, mild, mild-moderate, moderate, moderate-severe, or severe). Number and length of attacks, boxes of tissue used.
   Precipitants: Specific environments, odors, or exposures
   Past symptom patterns: Childhood respiratory symptoms
2. Environmental
   Home: Age, structure, dampness, insulation type(s), heating and air-conditioning, carpets, renovations or remodeling, environmental tobacco smoke, roaches, rodents, dust, visible mold, history of leaks, or standing water. Have allergen reduction measures been taken (e.g., carpet removal or encasement of mattress and pillow)?
   Pets: Dogs, cats, or birds
3. Occupational
   Type of work and length at past and present jobs, materials used, and known exposures
   Industrial hygiene sampling results and material safety data sheet information
   Other employee problems
4. Hobbies
   Materials: Solvents, finishes, pesticides, herbicides, exotic plants, prints, glues, epoxies, paints, and lubricants
   Activites: Grinding, spraying, gluing, soldering, welding, or cleaning
5. Habits and medications
   Habits: Tobacco smoke, cocaine, or other drugs
   Medications: Prescription drugs or intranasal decongestants

Physical examination

1. Ears: Erythema, tympanic light reflex, mobility, and air–fluid levels
2. Nasal mucosa (pre- and posttopical decongestants):
   Color: Red, pale, or bluish.
   Exudate: Amount and nature.
   Abnormal features: Swelling, polyps, septal deviation, ulcers, or pigmentation
3. Pharynx: As with nasal mucosa plus tonsils and dentition
4. Sinuses: Localized tenderness, transillumination, and osteal or posterior pharyngeal purulence
5. Neck: Thyroid, lymphadenopathy, and muscle trigger points
   Vocal performance: Habitual pitch, pitch range, phonation times on /a/, /s/, and /z/
6. Lungs: Presence and quality of spontaneous cough, size and shape of rib cage, breathing pattern (inspiratory to expiratory ratio), accessory muscle use, percussion, wheezes, rales, ronchi, and e-to-a changes

Diagnostic measures

1. Nasal swab: Number of eosinophils, neutrophils, and basophils per high-power field
2. Serology/hematology: Total and allergen-specific IgE, and eosinophil count
3. Pulmonary functions: Spirometry, flow volume loops, diffusing capacity, and serial peak flows
4. Antigen skin testing
5. Environmental sampling results: Dusts, mists, fumes, and vapors

Diagnostic adjuncts

1. Computed tomography scans
2. Fiberoptic rhinoscopy and videostroboscopy
3. Rhinometry: Acoustic rhinometry, nasal rhinomanometry
4. Methacholine reactivity
5. Antigen challenge/symptom provocation
6. Special procedures: Nasal lavage, biopsy, and mucociliary transport

Table 20.3.1 Components of upper airway symptom evaluation

Further diagnostic studies that may be initiated at the initial visit include a request for information about the work environment, including material safety data sheets and air sampling information. House dust analysis may be ordered through specialized facilities to identify the presence of specific antigens. A literature search may be needed to identify laboratories capable of measuring antibodies to unusual antigens. A judgment must be made at the initial visit as to the severity of the health effects that are occurring. Any lower respiratory symptoms should prompt additional evaluation. Interim work placement recommendations should be made, and recommendations for work modification or respiratory protection should be given to the patient in writing at the time of the office visit.

A provisional diagnosis is often made at the initial visit. Medication may be prescribed as a therapeutic trial or for symptomatic relief. Allergen avoidance, nasal corticosteroids, and non-sedating antihistamines are prescribed for allergic rhinitis. Nasal cromolyn sodium (Nasalcrom) relieves symptoms in some patients. For irritant rhinitis, avoidance of irritant triggers is advisable but may be difficult. If nasal dryness or irritation is the dominant complaint, saline lavage (1/4 of a teaspoon of salt in one cup of warm water, snuffled, then expelled) or oral guaifenesin (Robitussin) may be tried. Pharmacotherapy is difficult for vasomotor rhinitis. Nasal ipratropium bromide (Atrovent) for runners and sneezers, and oral alpha-agonists demonstrate limited success. Antihistamines do not appear to help in this condition. Low-dose tricyclic antidepressants at bedtime have been suggested. If a bacterial infection is suspected, a course of antibiotics is prescribed.

Charcoal-impregnated paper masks intended for use against nuisance volatile organic compounds (VOCs) should be used only if exposures are clearly low level. The psychosocial impact of putting someone in a respirator should be considered. Local-air cleaners may provide symptomatic relief when office or home ventilation is inadequate and point sources (such as tobacco smoke) cannot be controlled. The performance characteristics of air cleaners are highly variable. A combination high-efficiency particulate air (HEPA) filter and charcoal (or other VOC-adsorbing substance) is most appropriate for most office environments. Anecdotal data suggest that portable air cleaners worn around the neck may provide symptomatic improvement for some sensitive patients.

We recommend a follow-up visit 2 to 4 weeks after the initial visit. At that time, the results of laboratory studies and the response to treatment are evaluated. Workplace data are assessed. Further recommendations after discussion with the patient may include additional treatment or testing, source reduction, respiratory protection, medical removal, or job modification.

History

The history seeks to establish the presence and nature of upper respiratory symptoms, to gauge their severity, and to seek evidence for the major causes of rhinitis. A patient who is distraught with concern about an occupational or environmental exposure is often reassured by a thorough medical history, including an occupational and environmental history, and rational plan for longitudinal evaluation and monitoring. The initial visit is also a time to help the patient distinguish between the actual events and symptoms that occurred, and the subsequent interpretations and conflicts that may affect his or her perception of the health problem.

Environmental history

The environmental history should include a description and sketch of the home. Adjacent structures should be noted. Note the age, type of structure, and building materials in the home. Determine the type and age of insulation, the type of heating and air-conditioning systems, whether wall-to-wall carpets are present, and, if present, their age and whether they are on a concrete slab (a situation leading to high concentrations of house-dust mites). If there is a forced-air system, focus on the type of humidification system and how it is maintained. Determine whether there is a wet basement or crawl space and the history of leaks. Ask whether there have been renovations to the home. Determine the presence of pets (cats, dogs, and birds), cockroaches, and rodents. Hobby-rooms and workrooms should be identified and the specific nature of the activity and materials. Responses to these questions may alert the physician to possible causes of symptoms. Animals, roaches, or rodents are important sources of allergens. Excess dampness as well as water (basement, forced-air system, or leaks) can be a source of bioaerosols and is a strong determinant of respiratory symptoms (even in the absence of identifying a specific pathogen or allergen). VOCs arise from hobbies, cleaning, or new furnishings. New carpets can be a source of irritants; old carpets, especially those on concrete, can be a reservoir for house-dust mites or molds. If an outside dog uses a rug, the rug can be damp and can develop high mold counts.

Occupational history

In addition to a routine screening occupational history (see Chapter 3), the physician should focus on the current or most recent job. Central functions of the job that require upper airway functioning typically include speaking (specify needed volume, intelligibility, and duration) and, less likely, olfaction. The ability to wear a respiratory mask may be compromised by sinus pressure or pain. Requirements for sustained alertness are important to assess the impact of diseases such as sleep apnea and to predict the impact on job performance of medications such as antihistamines.

Allergy and symptom history

A careful allergy history also should be obtained, because the temporal pattern of symptoms will identify likely seasonal allergic causes for further diagnostic evaluation. Seasonal exacerbations can be readily shown with a retrospective diary or patient history. In general, early spring rhinitis relates to local tree pollens, late spring rhinitis relates to grass pollen, and fall rhinitis relates to weed pollen. A local allergist can provide more specific information about regional allergens and typical patterns of pollen dispersal. Patients are less able to link perennial rhinitis symptoms with exposure to relevant antigens such as dust mites, cats, rodents, or cockroaches.

Patients should be specifically questioned about their childhood health, whether they had childhood respiratory troubles, and whether they were raised with household smokers, because adult respiratory problems are associated with childhood exposure to environmental tobacco smoke (ETS). Immunodeficiency diseases such as secretory IgA deficiency may present with childhood infections.

The examiner should question the patient about any exposures that trigger symptoms, including cold air, ETS, perfumes, cleaning materials, and other household products. In more complex cases, a daily symptom diary may provide additional clues to environmental precipitants and document particular patterns of reaction. The diary should encompass 2 weeks of usual activities and should include symptoms such as congestion, rhinorrhea, sneezing, and other sentinel symptoms. Rough quantification helps discern any patterns and can be recorded as the severity of congestion or headache on a five-point scale. Quantifying the number and length of sneezing attacks and the approximate number of tissues used during an episode of rhinorrhea may be helpful.

Physical examination

The face is inspected for periorbital or facial swelling. Sinuses are palpated by applying gentle pressures. The maxillary sinuses are palpated below the orbits, the frontal sinuses over the eyebrows, and the ethmoid sinuses over the bridge of the nose. Non-specific hyperesthesia or tenderness may be noted, but the finding of differential or localized tenderness raises the suspicion of sinusitis. Sinus transillumination is an insensitive procedure, particularly for maxillary sinus disease.

The ears are examined and tympanic membranes inspected for erythema or fluid by insufflation. The patient should blow against his or her pinched-closed nose while the physician looks for motion of the light reflex on the tympanic membrane. This maneuver provides additional information about middle ear fluid and eustachian tube function. In the absence of formal hearing tests, patients can be asked about the quality of the voices they hear (muffled voices suggest fluid in the middle ear). The physician can ask questions in a quiet voice when positioned behind the patient. Inability to hear in the simple scenario suggests a need for hearing tests and possible assistive devices (see Chapter 20.2).

Many physicians do not inspect the nasal passages. This can be done readily using the speculum from the ear examination. Landmarks to recognize include the nasal septum and turbinates. The mucosa is inspected for the presence, color, and thickness of secretions; mucosal ulcers; the color of the mucosa (pale, bluish, or red); bogginess; swollen turbinates; and polyps. A stream of purulent mucus descending over the inferior turbinate confirms sinusitis. Since the nasal speculum provides only a partial view, patient referral for an otolaryngology examination is indicated if the inspection of the nasal passage does not correlate with the history, if treatment failure suggests structural disease, or if strongly unilateral symptoms raise a suspicion of neoplasm.

Otolaryngologists typically inspect the mucosa using a headlamp, and increasingly with a fiberoptic rhinoscope. The mucosa should first be inspected without the application of decongestants. A topical vasoconstrictor can then be applied (e.g., oxymetazoline [Afrin]), with repeat inspection 2 to 15 minutes later. Decongestion should not be performed in the case of poorly controlled hypertension or in the rare case of allergy to the vasoconstrictor. The main reason for visualization after decongestion is that a swollen inferior turbinate can obstruct the view of posterior polyps or of purulent discharge, which is often seen inferior to the middle meatus in early sinusitis.

The oral mucosa is visualized with particular attention to the presence and nature of secretions in the posterior pharynx, one of the most sensitive signs of draining sinuses. The salivary pool is noted, and absence of saliva under the tongue suggests a sicca syndrome.

The quality of the voice and presence of spontaneous cough are noted. Screening for hyperfunctional voice disorder can be done at the initial visit as follows. Listen to phonation at the patient's habitual pitch on /a/ (the sound 'ahhh'); a normal voice produces a single sustained tone without pitch breaks, excess tremor, or dysphonia (hoarseness). Ask the patient to repeat the /a/ on his or her lowest pitch, and then on his or her highest pitch. The habitual pitch should be just above the bottom third of the pitch range, and the pitch range should exceed one, preferably 1.5, octaves. The patient should then be instructed to phonate on /a/ for as long as he or she can. Normal values exceed 15 seconds. Patients with hyperfunctional voice disorder may phonate only 3 seconds and dissolve in a paroxysm of coughing and discomfort. These same patients can typically speak in full sentences during conversation without inducing discomfort. The abnormality is only demonstrable during the sustained phonation on a single sound. Maximal phonation times on the phonemes /s/ and /z/ will complete the screening examination. An s/z ratio of 1.4/1 is typical. Patients with hyperfunctional voice disorder will often have an increased s/z ratio, meaning that they have adequate breathing capacity but demonstrate abnormalities of the phonatory apparatus.

The neck is palpated for adenopathy, and the thyroid is palpated for tenderness, nodules, or enlargement. Lung examination is included to identify concomitant lower tract findings.

Diagnostic procedures

Direct assessment of upper respiratory function remains limited because of the lack of commonly available meas-ures of physiologic response. Nonetheless, when directed by the history and physical examination, the tests identified may play a role in the diagnostic workup. Selectively applied, they may either clinch a particular diagnosis or can at least raise the level of confidence enough to allow a provisional diagnosis, with subsequent treatment and workplace recommendations.

Nasal swab

Samples of nasal mucosa can be obtained with a swab or a curette. The most comfortable procedure for the patient is to use a flexible, disposable plastic scoop (Rhinoprobe). The probe is inserted in the nose under direct vision and pulled gently for 0.5 cm along the middle turbinate. The contents of the probe are then spread on a slide. Alternatively, a Calge swab may be inserted approximately 3 cm and gently pulled along the septum of the nasal cavity below the inferior or medial turbinate. Once off the mucosa, the swab is rotated, and a second pull is made, for a total of five passes. This is somewhat less comfortable. One swab from each nostril is rolled onto two glass slides, air dried, and stained. Commonly available stains, such Wright–Giemsa stain or Diff Quik, will identify neutrophils and eosinophils on one slide; alcian blue will best pick up basophils on the other. The slide is examined, and the presence and proportions of inflammatory cells (particularly neutrophils and eosinophils) are noted. Eosinophils are characteristic of allergic diseases, and a high correlation has been found between nasal eosinophils and signs and symptoms of allergy. Eosinophilic rhinitis that occurs without an identifiable allergic cause is termed non-allergic rhinitis with eosinophilia syndrome. Increased metachromatic cells (basophils or mast cells) also have been observed with in-season allergic patients. Neutrophils are more commonly seen with infections or irritant exposures. They may also be present in association with eosinophils in allergic rhinitis. Population-based epidemiologic studies have not been performed with nasal swabs; therefore, the distribution of the findings of neutrophils in a normal population is unknown. Generally, the normal nasal mucosal cytologic findings consist of numerous epithelial cells with perhaps a few neutrophils and bacteria but no eosinophilic or basophilic cells. A qualitative and quantitative grading scheme has been used for both clinical medicine and pharmaceutical studies (Table 20.3.2).[17]

Pulmonary function

Spirometry with flow volume loops should be performed on all individuals who are being evaluated for work-related upper respiratory disease. Attention to the entire flow volume loop (slow inspiration followed by maximal exhalation followed by maximal inspiration) enables assessment of extrathoracic airflow obstruction. A ratio of the FEF50/FIF50 of greater than 1 suggests extrathoracic airflow obstruction. Early termination of the inspiratory flow loop or marked asymmetry suggests laryngeal dysfunction.

The expiratory portion of the test establishes a critical baseline value for the patient without lower respiratory

Grade	Cytologic findings		
	Inflammatory cells	Neutrophils/eosinophils	Basophils
0	None	0–1	0–0.3
1	Few scattered cells or clumps	1–5	0.4–1.0
2	Moderate	6–15	1.1–3.0
3	Many cells or large clumps	16–20	3.1–6.0
4	Large numbers	>20	>6

Table 20.3.2 Qualitative and quantitative grading scheme for cytologic findings in rhinitis. The values represent the mean of cells per 10 high-powered fields (×1000).

symptoms and begins the diagnostic evaluation for patients with concomitant chest symptoms. In workers exposed to protein allergens, spirometry and 2 weeks of peak flow tracings are usually sufficient to exclude significant illness (see Chapter 19.2). For symptomatic exposure to irritants or low-molecular-weight sensitizers, a complete set of pulmonary function studies, including spirometry, diffusing capacity, and serial peak flow measures, is advised, given the potential for hypersensitivity pneumonitis and interstitial inflammation.

Allergy testing

Serum IgE is not a good screening test for allergic disease; although allergic disease is distinctly uncommon in the presence of a low IgE level, it may occur in the presence of a normal serum IgE concentration. Age-specific reference values should be used to evaluate the total IgE. The presence of eosinophils on a nasal swab or a history of perennial rhinitis should prompt a referral for skin testing.

If the history suggests that nasal symptoms are related to exposure to low-molecular-weight compounds, obtaining serum IgE levels against such compounds should be considered only in unusual cases. Antibodies to toluene diisocyanate are often undetectable despite clinical sensitization; antibodies to hexamethylene diisocyanate and methylene bisphenyl diisocyanate appear to be more sensitive. It is not appropriate to obtain antibodies to evaluate symptoms resulting from a single exposure. Technical factors may significantly affect the laboratory results, and caution is advised in the selection of a reference laboratory.

If a patient previously had skin tests, these results should be obtained for review. Indicators of good-quality skin tests include the explicit measurement of the response to a negative control (saline) and a positive control (histamine). If saline causes a wheal and flare, then RAST rather than skin prick testing is the test of choice. If the histamine skin test is negative, then the medication history should be reviewed for unrecognized antihistamines, or failure to stop medications far enough in advance of the skin testing. Local allergists are usually familiar with the major allergy seasons in each community. There is usually a spring season related to trees and grasses, and a late summer or fall season occurring with ragweed. The primary perennial allergens are cats, house-dust mites,

and, in some cases, mold spores. In an urban setting, cockroach and rodent allergens may be important. If skin test results were previously negative but the symptoms are strong and increase in the middle of a known allergy season, repeat skin testing may be warranted at the time of the symptoms. Fungi may cause allergic disease despite negative skin tests because such tests assess only some of the many species that exist.

Skin tests are generally accepted for IgE-mediated protein allergens. There is no established value for skin tests against chemicals, such as formaldehyde, and cigarette smoke. An etiologic role for these latter agents remains best established by a combination of clinical evaluation, symptom diary, and environmental assessment. Provocation testing is not a practical clinical tool in most cases.

Fiberoptic rhinoscopy and videostroboscopy

Fiberoptic rhinoscopy is rarely part of the initial workup, although it is increasingly used by allergists and otolaryngologists.[18] For difficult cases and in consultation with experienced operators, however, it may usefully identify polyps, sinusitis (through purulence at the ostia), septal deviation, and posterior nasopharyngeal lesions, and provide excellent visualization of the vocal cords and glottis. The procedure is well tolerated by patients, and clinicians find it superior to laryngoscopy in cases of suspected unilateral vocal cord paralysis.

Fiberoptic rhinoscopy is key to diagnosing laryngeal dysfunction (also called vocal cord dysfunction or vocal fold dysfunction). The hallmark of this group of disorders is paradoxical vocal fold motion, asynchronously with the respiratory cycle. The normal pattern is vocal fold abduction during inspiration and a return to neutral position during exhalation; the abnormal pattern is adduction of the vocal folds during inspiration. A posterior chink, stippling of the epiglottis, and interarytenoid edema are often seen. With practice, the clinician can position the rhinoscope so the patient can breathe comfortably without gagging.

Videostroboscopy provides even clearer visualization of the larynx, but does not allow concomitant visualization of the nasal passages.

Radiography and computed tomography (CT)

The diagnosis of sinusitis, when accompanied by classic symptoms, presents little difficulty. The presence of fever, frontal headache or facial pain, and purulent nasal discharge, supported by opacity on transillumination, tenderness to palpation, nasal neutrophilia, and/or visible sinus drainage, dictates the presumptive diagnosis of sinusitis and a trial of antibiotics. More diffuse and puzzling symptoms, however, or upper airway symptoms recalcitrant to treatment may demand further workup. CT of the sinuses has replaced the sinus X-ray series since the latter may show maxillary or frontal sinusitis, but it typically misses ethmoid or sphenoid disease. Cost-effective imaging of the sinuses can be obtained by a limited, dry (non-contrast) CT, performed at the end of a course of antibiotics. This will demonstrate osteomeatal disease, masses, congenital abnormalities, and refractory inflammation.

Rhinometry

Rhinometry is not widely available and it is unclear whether it will ever have the wide clinical application and utility that exists with spirometry. Nasal airway dimensions and physiology can be repeated after decongestants, helping to separate fixed lesions (e.g., deviated septum) from vascular congestion.

Acoustic rhinometry can document surgical correction of septal deviations. Acoustic rhinometry measures the cross-sectional area of each nasal passage as a function of the distance from the nasal antrum.

Nasal resistance is calculated by measuring the pressure and flow at the nose during gentle panting efforts. For anterior rhinomanometry, one side of the nasal cavity is occluded to monitor nasopharyngeal pressure by a differential pressure transducer. Airflow through the other nares is measured with a pneumotachometer.[6] From the relationship between flow rate and pressure, one can derive nasal airway resistance. Commercially available anterior rhinomanometers measure airflow through one nares by means of a closely fitting face mask, while the other nares is sealed with a small tube to measure nasopharyngeal pressure. The technique is easy to perform, requires very little patient cooperation, and is convenient for nasal provocation. Posterior rhinomanometry is also available, but the procedure is difficult to perform for some patients. The test consists of placing a modified diving or anesthesia mask on the patient, having the patient close his or her mouth over a tube, and then having the patient perform panting maneuvers through the nose.

Nasal inspiratory peak flow meters have been used in some epidemiologic studies. These measures may provide confirmation of congestion and document the possible association with workplace exposures. They can also be used as an outcome measure during challenge studies.

Nasal reactivity by methacholine and histamine challenge

Nasal reactivity can be assessed using methacholine, histamine, or capsaicin challenge. A variety of techniques have been employed; however, this test has primarily been used in a research setting. An increase in secretions has also been demonstrated following capsaicin or methacholine challenge in subjects with vasomotor rhinitis when compared with unaffected subjects. In the experimental setting, cholinergic nasal reactivity increases following antigen challenge. A new method for methacholine challenge, utilizing impregnated paper discs, obviates the need for mist inhalation, making the procedure considerably safer, more comfortable, and more convenient. The clinical utility of the test is limited by the narrow separation of nasal reactivity between patient groups.

Challenge by specific suspected agents

Nasal challenge with antigen is used in some countries, such as Finland, to establish a diagnosis of occupational nasal allergy. The use of provocation with other agents (e.g., cold air, ozone, or ETS) may demonstrate hyper-responsiveness in some people, but its use has been limited to a few centers. It remains primarily a tool for research settings.

Nasal lavage

Nasal lavage has been used as a research tool to define the inflammatory response to specific agents. As the inflammatory patterns with different nasal conditions are defined, a screening instrument may be feasible akin to the 'dipstick' screening of urine samples.

Nasal biopsy or cytology

Nasal biopsy is rarely performed unless the physical examination suggests granulomatous disease, such as sarcoidosis or Wegener's granulomatosis, or malignancy. Improved techniques of nasal cytologic examination are being developed and may play a role in occupational medicine. These are being used initially to study pathogenesis and may later be used to indicate dose, host response, or susceptibility. Nasal mucosal cytologic testing by scraping has been used successfully in studies of formaldehyde-exposed workers to detect squamous metaplasia as a possible precursor of dysplastic transformation.

Mucociliary transport

The mucociliary apparatus clears both soluble and insoluble materials. The sugar test quantifies the mucociliary transport of soluble substances: a small quantity of sucrose is placed on the inferior turbinate, and the subjects are instructed not to sniff or blow and to indicate when they taste sweetness. Intervals greater than 30 minutes are considered abnormal. In the research setting, insoluble radiotracers and charcoal powders have been used to assess clearance, and may show reduced clearance despite the presence of a normal sugar test.

CLASSIFICATION OF DISORDERS

This section describes specific types of upper respiratory tract disease. The individual patient may have one or more conditions simultaneously, and the physician must tailor the therapy and work recommendations accordingly. The interested reader is referred to an excellent classic textbook on the nose,[8] a more recent clinical rhinitis text,[19] and a classic nasal toxicology text.[20] A review by Harkema discusses the comparative pathology of the nasal mucosa in laboratory animals exposed to inhaled irritants, highlighting problems of cross-species comparisons.[21]

Rhinosinusitis

Rhinosinusitis is an inflammation of the paranasal sinuses and the nose and occurs frequently in patients with perennial rhinitis. Acute rhinosinusitis commonly follows a viral upper respiratory infection (URI) and lasts for up to 3 weeks. Chronic rhinosinusitis is inflammation of the sinuses that lasts longer than 3 months. Common causes are infection, mechanical obstruction, allergy, and primary eosinophilic inflammation of the nasal and sinus mucosa. Other causes include fungal infections such as aspergillus or an immune response to a fungus. More than 50% of asthmatics have chronic rhinosinusitis. Local, systemic, and environmental factors all contribute to the development of rhinosinusitis. Local risk factors include URIs, allergic rhinitis, non-allergic rhinitis, deviated nasal septum, tumors, and nasal polyps. Environmental risk factors include cigarette smoke, swimming and diving, barotraumas, and overuse of topical decongestants. Systemic factors include IgG and IgA deficiency, cystic fibrosis, bronchiectasis, diabetes, Wegener's granulomatosis, immotile cilia syndrome, immunosuppressive therapy, HIV infection, and Kartagener's syndrome.

The signs and symptoms of rhinosinusitis are facial pain, pressure, or fullness, nasal obstruction, purulent nasal discharge and discolored postnasal drip, hyposmia, anosmia, cough, headache, halitosis, dental pain, fever, fatigue, and pressure, pain, and fullness in the ears. Plain sinus X-rays are not useful in the diagnosis of recurrent and chronic rhinosinusitis in adults. A coronal CT scan can identify involved sinuses, define pathologic changes, and is necessary when the diagnosis is in question, complications are suspected, and when surgical intervention is being considered. Nasal endoscopy can identify anatomic abnormalities, pinpoint the source of infection within the middle meatus, and is useful in obtaining nasal cultures from the osteomeatal complex. Allergy skin tests, mucociliary clearance measurements, and nasal airway measurements are other useful diagnostic tests.

Management of rhinosinusitis includes using appropriate medications to control infection and reduce inflammation, palliative measures, and surgery when aggressive medical management has failed. Palliative treatment consists of nasal lavage with warm salt water and inhalation of warm mist through the nose for 15 minutes three to four times a day. The choice of antibiotic therapy for rhinosinusitis depends on local sensitivity patterns, potential for resistance, suspected bacteria, and the patient's allergy history. Common bacterial pathogens in acute rhinosinusitis are *Streptococcus pneumoniae* and other streptococcal species, *Haemophilus influenzae*, and *Moraxella catarrhalis*. Treatment of acute rhinosinusitis is typically 10–14 days, but up to 3 weeks of treatment is sometimes necessary. Chronic infectious rhinosinusitis may need up to 6 weeks of antibiotic treatment, and anaerobes, staphylococcus, and gram-negative pathogens may be present in addition to pneumococcus. Antibiotics used for repeated episodes of acute or recurrent rhinosinusitis include amoxicillin/clavulanate, azithromycin, clarithromycin, levofloxacin, and loracarbef. Intranasal steroids are indicated to treat allergic and non-allergic rhinitis and nasal polyps, and are useful in the maintenance therapy for chronic rhinosinusitis. Oral and topical decongestants can alleviate symptoms and oral mucolytics may help to thin discharge and promote drainage. Surgery is considered when appropriate medical management of rhinosinusitis has failed. The goals of surgery are to reduce recurrences of

rhinosinusitis, remove obstruction to sinus drainage, and alleviate acute complications. Mucociliary clearance defects are often present in patients with persistent symptoms post sinus surgery, and bacterial testing may show clearance of infection.

Rhinitis

A simple classification of rhinitis lists four groups:
- infectious (purulent) rhinitis;
- seasonal allergic rhinitis (also called pollinosis or hay fever);
- perennial allergic rhinitis; and
- perennial non-allergic rhinitis (eosinophilic or non-eosinophilic).[22]

Absent from this scheme is episodic rhinitis related to specific stimuli, rhinopathies which typically show intra-subject consistency but inter-subject variation. Irritant rhinitis, cold air-induced rhinitis, and gustatory rhinitis are examples of episodic rhinitis. The clinical history points to the link between a stimulus and the rhinitic response.

Infectious rhinitis

Respiratory tract infections result in billions of dollars of direct medical costs and indirect costs (e.g., lost time). The effect of environmental exposures on infectivity and rates of infection is therefore of interest. Oxides of nitrogen (produced as the combustion products from gas stoves, welding, and smelting operations) have been associated with increased respiratory infections in some, but not all, studies. Samet and associates reviewed the epidemiologic studies and concluded that 'evidence implies that clinically relevant effects of NO_x from gas stoves are uncommon at the concentrations found in most US homes'.[23]

Energy conservation measures that reduce ventilation may increase infectious respiratory diseases that are spread through droplet nuclei. One study demonstrated consistently higher rates of febrile acute respiratory disease among army trainees occupying modern (energy-efficient design and construction) barracks compared with old barracks.[24] Immunization of military trainees against adenovirus has been associated with reduction in acute respiratory disease rates.

Allergic rhinitis

Epidemiology Allergic rhinitis is a common condition with prevalence estimates ranging between 5% and 25% of the population. Both seasonal and perennial antigens may cause allergic rhinitis, with dominant antigens varying by region. Recent research has focused on the home as an important source of exposure to antigens such as cats, mites, cockroaches, and rodents. The non-industrial work environment (e.g., schools or office buildings) can also be a clinically important source of these allergens. Even less is known about the entrapment of seasonal pollens into buildings. It is plausible that, as has been shown in relation to IgE-mediated asthma, upper respiratory tract exposure to irritants (e.g., ozone) will enhance the likelihood of allergic rhinitis. Tobacco smoke is a major indoor pollutant and is strongly associated with allergic sensitization. Increased serum IgE levels and an increased prevalence of positive skin tests to aeroallergens and occupational allergens have been shown in several studies. Smokers are sensitized more easily to occupational allergens than are non-smokers exposed to allergens to the same degree.

Allergic rhinitis also appears to increase the likelihood of developing viral respiratory infections. The allergen exposure maintains a persistent inflammation that upregulates the expression of intercellular adhesion molecule (ICAM)-1 and vascular cell adhesion molecule (VCAM)-1 in the inflamed epithelium. Since ICAM-1 is the ligand for almost 90% of the rhinoviruses, the upregulation may explain the increase in viral respiratory infections.

Work-related allergic rhinitis is well documented. Common symptoms are sneezing, rhinorrhea, and nasal congestion. The prevalence of occupational rhinitis is unknown, but limited data indicate that occupational allergic rhinitis is more common than occupational allergic asthma. Symptoms may be immediate (within an hour of exposure) or delayed (late-onset symptoms 8 to 24 hours after exposure). Prolonged removal from work and re-exposure under close observation may be necessary to establish the link with the workplace. An IgE mechanism is likely for most rhinitis caused by exposure to high-molecular-weight protein allergens. The mechanism of rhinitis associated with low-molecular-weight chemicals is less certain, because skin tests and IgE antibodies may be negative in the presence of clinical sensitization. When possible, skin testing should be performed to establish the presence of a specific IgE allergy.

In Finland, nasal provocation testing is performed routinely at the Institute of Occupational Health. Of 300 to 400 annual provocation tests for rhinitis, occupational causes are diagnosed in approximately 10%, with flour dust being the primary allergen. Nasal provocation is rarely performed for occupational diagnosis in the US at present.

The prevalence of occupational allergic rhinitis is estimated to be 10% to 40% among exposed workers. It may occur alone or in conjunction with occupational asthma. Symptoms of rhinitis are less pronounced with low-molecular-weight agents, but more often appear before occupational asthma in the case of high-molecular-weight agents. In a survey of 474 laboratory animal workers, 17% had nasal symptoms repeatedly within 12 hours of contact with animals, with chest symptoms occurring in 9% and eye symptoms in 10%. Over 80% of patients with rat or mouse allergy have IgE antibodies to Rat n 1 or Mus m 1, which are lipocalin rodent urinary protein allergens. A cross-sectional study of 218 dock workers occupationally exposed to green coffee beans reported a 9% prevalence of work-related oculorhinitis, a 4% prevalence of both oculorhinitis and asthma, and a 1% prevalence of asthma.[25] A cross-sectional study of workers exposed to phthalic anhydride showed symptoms of rhinitis in 40% of the heavily exposed workers and 20% of the low-exposure workers.[26] Specific IgG antibodies were significantly elevated in the former group. Guar gum causes rhinitis.[27]

Limited studies have focused on the pathogenesis of occupational rhinitis. Studies of rat-allergic workers showed that challenge in a rat vivarium was associated with nasal symptoms and increases in nasal lavage histamine and TAME esterase activity, indicating mast cell activation.[28] The allergenic agent is a protein in rat urine, and immediate skin test results were positive in sensitized individuals. The studies confirm that laboratory animal rhinitis is a classic IgE-mediated reaction. A dose–response relationship was demonstrated between the allergen concentration and the response. Cage cleaning resulted in the highest air-borne concentrations of allergen. Recently, it has been recognized that galactomannans, high polymer carbohydrates, may also trigger an IgE-mediated response.

Articles describing occupational asthma commonly allude to the presence of concomitant upper respiratory symptoms. The list of causative agents for occupational asthma (see Chapter 19.2) should be considered a list of potential agents for occupational allergic rhinitis.

Inhalation of latex from powdered gloves can cause rhinitis in latex-sensitive persons. These reactions have been described in workers in healthcare and rubber-glove manufacturing facilities. The majority of latex-allergic individuals are atopic, with seasonal allergic rhinitis and allergic asthma.

Diagnosis Diseases such as occupational allergic rhinitis are recognized by the clinical pattern and confirmed by specific skin tests. When sensitization to a workplace agent is suspected, the causative agent may be a well-established sensitizer (see Table 20.3.3). However, new sensitizers are still being reported; therefore, a clinical diagnosis of sensitization may necessitate an evaluation of a compound.

Protein allergens
Laboratory animals
Guar gum (galactomannans)
Psyllium
Coffee beans
Grain mites
Grain dust
Flour dust

Low-molecular-weight chemicals
Western red cedar (plicatic acid)
Trimellitic anhydride
Phthalic anhydride
Isocyanates

Other
Sodium isononanyl oxybenzene sulfonate
Carbonless copy paper
Permanent wave solution

The list of agents causing occupational asthma (see Chapter 19.2) should be consulted for other possible causative agents. Common environmental allergens that may be present in the occupational environment include cat (brought in on the clothes of workers with domestic cats), dust mite, roach, rodents, and pollens from grasses, trees, and weeds. A local allergist should be consulted about the regional allergens and their expected seasons.

Table 20.3.3 Upper respiratory sensitizers

Companies should be notified when their products trigger specific reactions in patients. Permissible exposure limits are essentially irrelevant in evaluating cases of allergic rhinitis or other sensitization because exposure well below allowable limits may cause significant disease.

Treatment and prevention For occupational asthma, allergen avoidance is recommended because the prognosis is related to the duration of symptomatic exposure. It is plausible that a similar relationship for prognosis exists for occupational rhinitis, but this has not been established. It is our impression that, at present, medical removal for occupational allergic rhinitis occurs only sporadically. Environmental control measures can include providing adequate ventilation, enclosing open operations, automating hand operations, supplying space suits, and providing glove boxes.

The first line of treatment for allergic disease is allergen avoidance. This standard recommendation needs to be placed in the context of the realities of the workplace. Antihistamines are most helpful for the treatment of allergic symptoms and may be tried for chronic rhinitis. They are ineffective for the treatment of chronic nasal congestion unless combined with a decongestant. The sedating side effects of antihistamines may create a workplace hazard. Jobs should be reviewed to determine whether motor coordination or alertness is important. Problems with sedation can be minimized by using desloratidine (Clarinex), fexofenadine (Allegra), azatadine (Trinalin), or antihistamines from the alkylamine or ethylenediamine classes, administering a long-acting antihistamine at bedtime, or combining a decongestant with an antihistamine.

Avoidance of antihistamines can often be achieved by the use of inhaled nasal corticosteroids. The topical steroids have been shown to be safe and highly effective. They block the inflammatory cell influx that occurs in the late-phase IgE response. Intranasal antihistamines such as azelastine hydrochloride (Astelin) are effective in treating the symptoms of allergic rhinitis. Intranasal cromolyn sodium (Nasalcrom), too, is safe and effective in the management of seasonal and perennial allergic rhinitis, and is considered first-line treatment for managing allergic rhinitis during pregnancy. A trial of cromolyn sodium is merited in cases of non-allergic rhinitis with eosinophilia because there are mixed opinions as to its efficacy in this condition.

Allergen immunotherapy is effective in the treatment of seasonal allergic rhinitis caused by pollens and in perennial allergic rhinitis caused by dust mites and molds. It can affect the natural course of the disease and is indicated in allergic individuals who are inadequately controlled on medications or who experience undesirable side effects from medications. Such therapy is given for a period of 3 to 5 years.

Irritant rhinitis
Epidemiology Irritant rhinitis is defined as rhinitis symptoms induced by dusts, chemicals, or fumes that are noxious to tissues. Irritation can occur to a wide range of aerosols, gases, and vapors, including inert dusts. The

mechanisms of activation of the sensory irritant receptor are reviewed in detail by Nielsen.[26] Irritation can describe only a symptom, but usually it also implies a non-specific inflammatory response. A respiratory irritant that mainly affects deeper structures, such as ozone, often causes large airway and nasal inflammation characterized by plasma exudation. Very soluble gases and dusts with a diameter greater than 10 μm tend to produce sinusitis and nasal irritation.

Mixtures of chemicals may induce symptoms and/or nasal neutrophilia, although individual components of the mixture would be expected to be inert. Sick-building syndrome is a term that applies to a constellation of symptoms occurring in non-industrial worksites, for which the cause is unknown (see Chapter 50). The symptoms encountered in the sick-building syndrome include irritation of the eye, nose, and throat; dry mucous membranes and skin; erythema; mental fatigue; headache; airway infections; cough, hoarseness of the voice, and wheezing; unspecific hyper-reactivity reactions; nausea; and dizziness. Studies point to a high prevalence of work-associated upper respiratory symptoms in some office buildings. The mechanism of these symptoms is often unknown, but nasal symptoms consistent with an irritant mechanism may be a prominent part of the symptom complex.

Exposure to a common mixture, ETS, provokes symptoms of irritation in many individuals. Eye irritation is more common than nose and throat irritation, although both have been demonstrated at low concentrations of smoke (e.g., 1 ppm of carbon monoxide [CO]). Many patients also report that they are allergic to tobacco smoke. Studies of this condition have confirmed ETS-induced rhinitis in some subjects but indicate that an allergic mechanism is not responsible. A history of one or more symptoms of rhinitis (rhinorrhea or congestion) with historic ETS exposure was reported by one-third of a group of healthy young adults.[29] Controlled challenge studies with a brief high level of smoke confirmed the occurrence of nasal congestion in the subjects with a history of ETS sensitivity but not in historically ETS-non-sensitive individuals. Nasal lavage studies following smoke exposure did not show elevations of histamine (indicating that mast cell activation was not occurring), or of albumin (indicating that an increase in vascular permeability was not occurring), or of TAME esterase activity (indicating that glandular secretion was not occurring). These data suggest that non-allergic vascular congestion is responsible for the increased nasal resistance. Controlled challenge to tobacco smoke at moderate doses of smoke (15 ppm CO for 1 hour) caused congestion in both study groups; HEPA filtration of the smoke decreased congestion only in ETS-non-sensitive individuals. The urinary cotinine/creatinine ratio did not correlate with the magnitude of the congestive response, suggesting that host factors, not altered dose, were responsible for the differential response. It is unknown whether differential acute responsiveness relates to a differential risk of chronic exposure.

Some individuals report the onset of chronic rhinitis following an acute high-level irritant exposure. One example was a 16-year-old youth who opened a container of large swimming-pool chlorine tablets that had been left in the sun. He had immediate nose and chest irritation with paroxysmal coughing. Since that time (2-year follow-up), he has had chronic non-allergic rhinitis without lower respiratory symptoms or methacholine hyper-reactivity. Greater than 95% of inhaled chlorine is absorbed in the upper airway. In animal studies, nasal lesions were observed following chlorine exposure.

Exposure limits for some irritants were established based on the relative potency of the chemical as determined by the animal model of Yves Alarie.[30,31] The concentration of a chemical causing a 50% inhibition in the respiratory rate (RD50) was established in a mouse inhalation challenge model. The threshold limit value was set as 10% of that value. The rank order of chemicals by RD50 in mice has been shown to be fairly similar to the rank order of chemicals by irritant symptoms in humans. It is interesting to note that differences exist in the RD50 of different inbred strains of mice to a single chemical. Differential sensitivity to irritants in humans has also been documented. It is also worth mentioning that the Alarie RD50 mouse bio-assay does not consider the ability of the chemical to induce inflammation or long-term tissue damage. Despite these limitations, the Alarie method has provided a practical approach to ranking irritants and suggesting exposure levels.

Changes in air quality related to air-borne pollutants may be a factor contributing to the severity of upper airway disorders (see Chapter 51). Chronic alterations of the normal structure of the nasal mucociliary apparatus may have adverse effects on the nasal defense mechanisms that protect the upper respiratory tract tissues from potentially harmful levels of inhaled irritant gases, dusts, and bacteria. The nature of the lesions in toxicity studies with volatile chemicals in rodents varied with the duration of exposure.[20] In short-term exposures, degeneration and regeneration of the affected olfactory mucosa were frequently seen. With long-term exposure, basal cell hyperplasia and respiratory metaplasia were observed. The human nasal mucosa is susceptible to ozone toxicity. Acute inflammation is induced in the nasal airways after exposure to this highly reactive irritating gas. Long-term ozone exposure causes mucous cell metaplasia and epithelial hyperplasia in the surface nasal epithelium of rats. These changes persist for weeks and months after the end of a chronic exposure. A study in a Mexico City population showed a strong correlation between histopathologic changes in the nose and nasal symptoms.[32] Residents complained of epistaxis, rhinorrhea, nasal crusting, dryness, and nasal obstruction. Nasal biopsies showed patchy shortening of cilia, basal cell hyperplasia, deciliated areas, and squamous metaplasia. Dysplastic lesions were predominantly located on antral squamous epithelium and in squamous metaplastic epithelium of the posterior inferior turbinates, and they exhibited p53 nuclear accumulation. Individuals with more than 10 hours of daily outdoor exposure for 5 years or more had the highest rate of dysplasia. Subjects with epistaxis were more likely to

have dysplasias and neovascularization. The results of this study suggest that nasal lesions in Mexico City residents are possibly related to toxic and carcinogenic pollutants such as ozone, aldehydes, and particulate matter.

Major sources of inhaled pollution in industrialized cities are diesel exhaust particles (DEPs) and their associated polyaromatic hydrocarbons (PAHs). DEPs make up 40% of the particles less than 10 μm (PM10) in a big city. In-vitro models of human airway epithelial cells have shown that DEPs undergo phagocytosis and induce a specific inflammatory response, with an increase in IL-8, granulocyte-macrophage colony-stimulating factor, and IL-1 beta. Experiments in guinea pigs have shown that DEPs significantly enhance histamine-induced vascular permeability and increase eosinophil infiltration into the nasal mucosa. Thus, DEPs may play an important role in promoting nasal hyperactivity by enhancing antigen absorption through the nasal mucosa and increasing eosinophil-induced inflammation. DEPs also upregulate histamine H1 receptor expression in human nasal epithelial cells and mucosal endothelial cells. DEPs have several effects on the human in-vivo allergic response. They enhance local mucosal IgE production, induce an inflammatory response of cells, chemokines, and cytokines, and thereby exacerbate allergic inflammation. PAHs enhance local mucosal IgE production without a measurable cellular inflammatory response. DEPs in combination with an allergen such as ragweed enhanced local antigen-specific IgE production.[33] Following the combined challenge, there was a deviation of cytokine production toward a TH2 profile with an increase in IL-4 and a decrease of IFN-gamma. Exposure to DEPs can enhance the clinical symptoms to an allergen by enhancing mast cell degranulation as well as modify the nature of the subsequent immune response. In humans with ragweed allergy, a combination of DEPs and ragweed allergen is capable of driving in-vivo isotype switching to IgE. DEPs also act as mucosal adjuvants in a de-novo IgE response in humans and increase allergic sensitization. Thus, DEPs not only play a role in exacerbating pre-existing allergic antibody responses and allergic inflammation but can also be a factor in driving primary sensitization to inhaled allergens in human subjects.

Diagnosis Work-related mucosal irritation is a diagnosis that must often be made on a clinical basis alone because there are few diagnostic tools and the symptoms are often non-specific. Clinical findings of irritant rhinitis include erythemal obstruction, rhinorrhea, and postnasal drainage. Nasal cytologic findings are unremarkable or show neutrophils.

The occupational physician should interpret the recommended or legal limits for a chemical in the context of an assessment of an individual's sensitivity. Exposure levels below the recommended exposure limits may present problems for some otherwise healthy people and may additionally aggravate patients with any pre-existing conditions.

Periodic medical screening of groups of workers for upper respiratory irritant symptoms is indicated when a known irritant is present or a new mixture or process is being used. The presence of symptoms can focus industrial hygiene attention on areas needing additional air sampling or ventilation. Physicians are often the ones who identify and recommend air sampling for a worst-case scenario. Industrial hygienists usually have an established sampling strategy for a specific area and try to define a representative exposure. Physicians should be aware that each of these approaches has merit.

Table 20.3.4 lists selected compounds that are nasal or respiratory irritants at varying levels of exposure. The compounds are grouped according to the permissible exposure limits as a rough guide to irritant potential. Carcinogens are so noted because this designation will lower the recommended exposure level independent of the irritant potential. Material safety data sheets should be consulted for information about other compounds. In the authors' experience, almost any substance may provoke symptoms in one individual or another. The symptoms, and the risk of continued exposure, must be weighed against existing information about the irritant potential of these agents. The occurrence of symptoms with low-level irritant exposures should provoke evaluation for mucosal inflammation of other causes (e.g., IgE-mediated disease). A professor of pulmonary medicine has remarked that, 'Each spring, when my hay fever acts up, I can't stand my wife's perfume'.

Treatment Meltzer and coworkers advise the practice of 'consistent avoidance of the irritant or nonspecific factors that may trigger symptoms in patients with chronic rhinitis'.[34] This recommendation needs to be placed in the context of the realities of the workplace and the options for alternative work.

The physician may believe it to be in the best interests of a patient to recommend adjustments in workplace ventilation or altered work practices, even when environmental assessment finds no evidence of increased concentrations of specific chemicals above threshold limit values. Medical removal may be indicated, particularly if the irritant symptoms are linked with other symptoms, such as severe headache, visual disturbances, or neurologic symptoms. An industrial worker who is significantly intolerant of the irritants or VOCs in his or her workplace may find the best long-term success by retraining for a non-industrial position.

Removal from irritant exposure may also be necessary when mucosal inflammation is severe. Adequate respiratory protection may be temporarily productive, but it should not substitute for engineering and process controls; one patient's problems with a particular process or material may herald a widespread future problem for other workers.

In the industrial setting, a fundamental preventive strategy is to follow the motto 'The solution to pollution is dilution'. However, if the point source is being handled by the worker, general ventilation may not reduce breathing-zone exposure. Irritating materials may be replaced by less toxic ones, or process enclosure can occur. Respiratory protection may be effective when these strategies are impractical.

The relative efficacy of strategies to avoid widespread mucosal irritation in office buildings continues to be debated. There is general agreement that ventilation should meet the new American Society of Heating, Refrigerating and Air Conditioning Engineers standards, and point sources should be minimized (see Chapter 50). Strategies to accommodate sensitive or allergic individuals in the office setting may include bans on workplace smoking, the use of low VOC-emitting products, or the provision of individual offices with high-capacity portable air cleaners.

Air cleaners should be recommended only after careful thought. Improperly chosen air cleaners result in unnecessary expenditure and divert resources from more effective treatments. Anecdotal evidence suggests that properly chosen air cleaners can produce significant symptomatic improvement for some individuals with rhinitis triggered by specific exposures, such as ETS, or in buildings where cleanup is delayed. They also may be effective against small point source VOCs. However, a wide range of so-called air cleaners are marketed, and many are ineffective because of low flow rates or inadequate removal of pollutants. The recommended commercial testing program for air cleaners determines their efficacy for removal of particulates only. This ignores the important contribution of irritating vapors to indoor air symptoms. Some commercial air cleaners actually generate ozone to purify the air and may seriously exacerbate symptoms. Portable air cleaners usually have limited utility in pollen allergy because their capacity for particle filtration is often overwhelmed by the influx of allergen from the outside.

Other standard recommendations for medical management of upper respiratory disease are outlined subsequently. Vigorous exercise is a decongestant, and 15 to 30 minutes of exercise once or twice daily has been recommended for the nasal congestion that occurs in chronic rhinitis. Elevation of the head of the bed 30 degrees may reduce the nasal congestion that occurs with recumbency.

Nasal saline is an effective treatment for irritated tissue. Two sprays of commercially available buffered saline spray may be used four times daily. A less expensive option is to have patients mix one-quarter teaspoon of table salt with one cup (8 oz) of warm tap water and to snuffle it into the nose. A bulb syringe is preferred by some patients. A third option is a longer, higher-volume saline lavage using one teaspoon of salt with 800 ml of water administered with the nasal adapter of the Water Pik. Some physicians recommend putting petroleum jelly proximal to the nasal antrum to reduce irritant symptoms; it is unclear how this affects nasal epithelial morphology and nasal airflow. It should not be used as a substitute for point source reduction.

Intranasal decongestants are not advised for chronic use because they may induce rhinitis medicamentosa, which is iatrogenic nasal vasodilation and obstruction caused by the overuse of topical sympathomimetics. Topical decongestants may be used for 3 days for an acute viral illness,

At Levels < 1 ppm	Terphenyls	Furfuryl alcohol	Chlorobromomethane
Antimony oxide	Thiram	Glycidol	Cyclohexane
Azinphos-methyl	Toluene 2,4-diisocyanate	Hydrogen sulfide	Cyclohexene
Barium compounds	Tributyl phosphate	Messityl oxide	1, 2-Dichloroethylene
Benzoyl peroxide	2,4,6-Trinitrotoluene	Methyl acrylate	Dichlorotetrafluoroethane
Bromine	Vanadium pentoxide	Methylamine	Ethyl acetate
Bromoform	Zinc chloride	5-Methyl-3-heptanone	Ethyl bromide (NIOSH D)
tert-Butyl chromate	Zirconium compounds	Morpholine	Ethyl ether (NIOSH D)
Calcium oxide		1,2,3-Trichloropropane	Fluorotrichloromethane
Camphor	**At Levels of 1 to 9 ppm**	Triethylamine (NIOSH D)	Isopropyl acetate (NIOSH D)
Chlorine	Acetic anhydride (NIOSH D)		Isopropyl alcohol
Chlorine dioxide	Acetylene tetrabromide	**At Levels of 50 to 99 ppm**	Isopropyl ether
Chlorine trifluoride	Allyl alcohol	n-Butyl alcohol	Methyl acetate
Chlorobenzylidene malonitrile	Allyl chloride	Chlorobenzene (NIOSH D)	Methyl acetylene
Copper dusts, mists, and fume	Allyl glycidyl ether	Cumene	Methylal
Cotton dust	Benzyl chloride	Cyclohexanol	Methylcyclohexane
Demeton	Boron oxide	Cyclopentadiene	n-Propyl acetate
Diazomethane	Boron trifluoride	Diacetone alcohol	n-Propyl alcohol
Dibutyl phthalate	n-Butylamine	o-Dichlorobenzene	Tetrahydrofuran
1,3 Dichloro-5,5-dimethylhydantoin	Chloroacetaldehyde	Ethyl butyl ketone	
Dichlorvos	Crotonaldehyde	n-Hexane	**Irritants which are also NIOSH Ca**
Dimethylphthalate	Dibutylphosphate	Hexone	Acetaldehyde
Dinitrobenzene	Ethanolamine	sec-Hexyl acetate	Acrolein
Diphenyl	Ethylene chlorohydrin	Isobutyl alcohol	Acrylonitrile
2-Ethoxyethylacetate	N-Ethylmorpholine	Isopropyl glycidyl ether	Arsenic
Ethyl mercaptan	Formic acid	Methylcyclohexanol	Benzene
Ferbam	Furfural (NIOSH D)	o-Methylcyclohexanone	beta-Chloroprene
Ferrovanadium dust	2-Hexanone	alpha-Methyl styrene	1,3,-Butadiene
Fluorine and fluorides	Hydrogen bromide	Mineral spirits	Cadmium
Hafnium	Hydrogen chloride	Octane	bis-Chloromethylether
Hydrogen selenide	Hydrogen fluoride	Petroleum distillates (Naphtha)	Chloromethyl methyl ether
Iodine	Hydrogen peroxide	Styrene	Chromic acid and chromates
Ketene	Isophorone		1,2 Dibromo-3-chloropropane
Lindane	Isopropylamine (NIOSH D)	**At Levels of 100 to 199 ppm**	p-Dichlorobenzene
Maleic anhydride	Magnesium oxide fume	N-Amyl acetate	3,3'-Dichlorobenzidine
Manganese compounds	(NIOSH D)	sec-Amyl acetate	Dichloroethylether
Methyl Cellosolve® acetate	Nitric acid	n-Butyl acetate	Diglycidyl ether
Methylene bisphenyl isocyanate	Nitrous oxide	Dibromodifluoromethane	Dimethyl sulfate
Methyl isocyanate	Perchlorylfluoride	Dipropylene glycol methyl ether	Di-sec octyl phthalate
Molybdenum (NIOSH D)	Phenol	Ethyl benzene	Dioxane
Organotins	Phenyl ether	Ethylformate	Ethyl acrylate
Oxalic acid	Phenylether-biphenyl mixture	Isoamyl acetate	Ethylene dibromide
Oxygen difluoride	Phenyl glycydyl ether	Isoamyl alcohol	Ethylene imine
Ozone	Phthalic anhydride	Isobutyl acetate	Ethylene oxide
Paraquat	Sulfur dioxide	Methyl (n-amyl) ketone	Formaldehyde
Parathion	Sulfur monochloride	Methyl formate	Hydrazine
Pentachlorophenol	Sulfuryl fluoride	Methyl methacrylate	Methyl hydrazine
Perchloromethyl mercaptan	Tetranitromethane	Naphtha (coal tar)	2-Nitropropane
Phosgene		N-Pentane	Propylene oxide
Phosphoric acid	**At Levels of 10 to 49 ppm**	2-Pentanone	Tetrachloroethylene
Phosphorus	Acetic acid	Turpentine	(perchloroethylene)
Phosphorus pentachloride	Ammonia	Vinyl toluene	1,1,2-Trichlorethane
Phosphorus pentasulfide	2-Butoxyethanol	Xylenes	Trichloroethylene
Phosphorus trichloride	Cyclohexanone		
Pindone	Diethylamine	**At Levels of 200 ppm or More**	**Other**
Platinum	2-Diethylaminoethanol	2-Butanone	Tobacco dust (tobacco factory)
Selenium	Diisobutylketone	sec-Butyl acetate	Carbonless copy paper
Sulfur pentafluoride	Dimethylamine	tert-Butyl acetate	Grain dust

Note: This list is primarily drawn from the NIOSH Pocket Guide to Chemical Hazards[40] and includes substances listed as causing 'irritation, laryngeal, mucous membrane, pharyngeal, or respiratory'. Compounds are grouped by the exposure limits (see text for explanation). NIOSH Ca means the substance should be considered a possible carcinogen (see Acheson[41] for additional discussion of upper airway carcinogens). NIOSH D indicates substances for which NIOSH has questioned whether the permissible exposure limits are adequate to protect workers from recognized health hazards (see Pocket Guide, Appendix D).

Table 20.3.4 Upper respiratory irritants

for air travel, or at the initiation of steroid or cromolyn sodium therapy. Combination oral antihistamines and oral decongestants may be useful in the treatment of allergic rhinitis, eosinophilic non-allergic rhinitis, and nasal hyper-reactivity characterized by increased secretions.

Vasomotor rhinitis
Vasomotor rhinitis is characterized by nasal symptoms of vasomotor and secretory instability occurring in the absence of any defined cause or disorder. Clear rhinorrhea is present, IgE is low, and nasal cytologic findings are unre-

markable. Some physicians use this term to describe rhinitis provoked by a range of low-level VOCs. In this case, avoidance may decrease symptoms. Oral alpha-agonist decongestants can be helpful, but they remain unsatisfactory in 50% to 70% of patients. Runners (i.e., patients with predominant rhinorrhea) benefit from nasal ipratropium bromide. Low-dose tricyclic antidepressants show a response rate on the constellation of symptoms from 60% to 80%. Nasal steroids and antihistamines are not significantly useful. Saline lavage and exercise are also recommended.

Atrophic rhinitis

Atrophic rhinitis is defined as nasal symptoms resulting from aging or as normal nasal mucosa is replaced by squamous epithelium. Studies by Broder and coworkers of people living in homes with formaldehyde insulation demonstrated an increase in squamous metaplasia among the subset of people intending to remediate their homes. These individuals had an excessive range of symptoms, although patch tests were negative and nasal resistance was similar to controls.[35] More information is needed on the histology of the nasal mucosa in other populations chronically exposed to irritants.

Nasal ulcers

The compounds most commonly associated with nasal ulcers and perforations are listed in Table 20.3.5. Ulcers, other sores, and leukoplakia indicate potentially serious exposures. The characteristically painless and non-necrotic, non-heaped-out punch lesions of chromium exposure may

| *Ulcers/perforated nasal septum* |
| Arsenic |
| Calcium oxide |
| Chromic acid and chromates |
| |
| *Epistaxis* |
| Warfarin |
| Pindone (tert-Butyl valone) |
| |
| *Rhinorrhea (with miosis, lacrimation, and salivation)* |
| Carbaryl |
| EPN (Ethyl p-nitrophenyl benzene thionophosphonate) |
| Malathion |
| Parathion |
| Phosdrin |
| Pyrethrum |
| TEDP (Tetraethyl dithiopyrophosphate) |
| TEPP (Ethyl pyrophosphate) |
| |
| *Blue-gray nasal septum* |
| Silver |
| |
| *Numb mucous membrane* |
| Rotenone |
| DDT (Dichlorodiphenyltrichloroethane) |
| |
| *Edema on nasal folds* |
| Nitramine |
| |
| *Stomatitis* |
| Mercury vapor |
| |
| Note: Data obtained from the NIOSH Pocket Guide to Chemical Hazards.[40] |

Table 20.3.5 Miscellaneous occupational upper respiratory effects

indicate the need for hematologic and air monitoring (see Chapter 39.5). Painful exudative lesions may indicate infection requiring antibiotics. All lesions not substantially resolved in 2 weeks and persistent leukoplakia merit referral to an otolaryngologist for evaluation and possible biopsy.

Periodic medical screening for workers exposed to substances affecting the upper respiratory tract may be indicated when the experience at a worksite indicates a risk. An example would be monthly inspection of the nasal septum in workers exposed to chromium dust. Topical anti-inflammatory treatment, respiratory protection, and medical removal are options when nasal ulcers are found. Formal group evaluation also becomes an important adjunct to individual assessment when screening workers routinely exposed to known irritants.

Laryngitis and related disorders

Laryngitis and cough

Laryngitis, or inflammation of the larynx, can be caused by the same list of conditions and exposures that cause rhinitis. A similar diagnostic approach is recommended, with two modifications. Symptoms of vocal abuse or gastric reflux should be sought in the history, and patients should be referred to an otolaryngologist for adequate visualization of the vocal cords. The primary differential diagnosis of persistent paroxysmal non-infectious cough includes cough-variant asthma, postnasal drip, and gastroesophageal reflux.

Voice disorders

Occupational voice disorders among speech and voice professionals are very common and these disorders often constitute a barrier to work performance. The primary risk factor in voice and speech professions is the need for prolonged use of the voice. Males have a 50% lower total number of vibrations than females. This may explain why female teachers report significantly more voice problems than males. Vocal nodules are also almost exclusively seen in females. Air quality, dryness, dust, and allergies can cause hoarseness. Exposure to ETS may contribute to some minor changes in vocal fold structure and physiology.[36] Videostroboscopic evaluation revealed mild edema and erythema in passive smokers. Smoking cigarettes leads to chronic irritation and an increase in vocal fold mass. Sidestream smoke carries more free nicotine and higher values of such substances as CO, benzene, NO, and ammonia. ETS has also been linked to the development of laryngeal carcinoma. Vocal cord paralysis has also been reported following lymph node involvement by silicosis.

Upper airway obstruction

Laryngeal edema is a potentially life-threatening complication of inhalation injury caused by thermal burns, irritant chemicals, and smoke inhalation The obstruction may develop up to 48 hours after the injury, and in-hospital observation is prudent. A case report described reversible obstructive sleep apnea caused by occupational exposure to guar gum dust, presumably related to pharyngeal edema.[37]

A case report by Sales and Kennedy details epiglottic obstruction related to diisocyanate exposure.[38] A 34-year-old non-atopic, non-smoker began making award plaques with 65% methylene diisocyanate (MDI). One week later, he was treated for fever, diaphoresis, chest pain, and nasal congestion. Subsequent evaluation showed persistent asthmatic symptoms and marked epiglottic dysfunction with aspiration demonstrated by barium contrast cineradiography. Total epiglottectomy resolved the upper airway symptoms without altering asthmatic symptoms. Histologic examination of the excised epiglottis showed marked chronic submucosal inflammatory changes with focal fibrosis, edema, and reactive changes.

Extrathoracic airflow obstruction and chronic laryngotracheitis have been described in some Persian Gulf War veterans.[39] Veterans complained of cough, shortness of breath on exertion, and sleep disturbances. Histologic examination of the upper airways showed chronic inflammation with mononuclear cells and thickening of the basement membrane; sampling data indicated exposure to PM10 (fine particulate) levels seven- to eightfold higher than the Environmental Protection Agency standards.

Biologic weapons such as anthrax can also affect the airways, and physicians should be aware of that potential.

References

1. Feron VJ, Arts JH, Kuper CF, et al. Health risks associated with inhaled nasal toxicants. Crit Rev Toxicol 2001; 31:313-47.
2. American Thoracic Society. What constitutes an adverse health effect of air pollution? Official statement of the American Thoracic Society. Am J Respir Crit Care Med 2000; 161(2 Pt 1):665-73.
3. Keles N, Ilicali OC, Deger K. Impact of air pollution on prevalence of rhinitis in Istanbul. Arch Environ Health 1999; 54:48-51.
4. Rantala L, Paavola L, Korkko P, et al. Working-day effects on the spectral characteristics of the teaching voice. Folia Phoniatr Logop 1998; 50:205-11.
5. Vilkman E, Voice problems at work: a challenge for occupational safety and health arrangement. Folia Phoniatr Logop 2000; 52:120-5.
6. Hardisty JF, RH Garman, JR Harkema, et al. Histopathology of nasal olfactory mucosa from selected inhalation toxicity studies conducted with volatile chemicals. Toxicol Pathol 1999; 27:618-27.
7. Doty RL, Mishra A. Olfaction and its alteration by nasal obstruction, rhinitis, and rhinosinusitis. Laryngoscope 2001; 111:409-23.
8. Proctor D, Andersen I. The nose: upper airway physiology and the atmospheric environment. New York: Elsevier Biomedical; 1982.
9. Baraniuk JN. Pathogenesis of allergic rhinitis. J Allergy Clin Immunol 1997; 99:S763-72.
10. Eccles R. Pathophysiology of nasal symptoms. Am J Rhinol 2000; 14:335-8.
11. Sanico AM, Atusta S, Proud D, et al. Dose-dependent effects of capsaicin nasal challenge: in vivo evidence of human airway neurogenic inflammation. J Allergy Clin Immunol 1997; 100:632-41.
12. Philip G, Jankowski R, Baroody FM, et al. Reflex activation of nasal secretion by unilateral inhalation of cold dry air. Am Rev Respir Dis 1993; 148:1616-22.
13. Bascom R, Kagey-Sobotka A, Proud D. Effect of intranasal capsaicin on symptoms and mediator release. J Pharmacol Exp Ther 1991; 259:1323-7.
14. Togias A. Mechanisms of nose–lung interaction. Allergy 1999;54 Suppl 57:94-105.
15. Kharitonov SA, Rajakulasingam K, O'Connor B, et al. Nasal nitric oxide is increased in patients with asthma and allergic rhinitis and may be modulated by nasal glucocorticoids. J Allergy Clin Immunol 1997; 99:58-64.
16. Henriksen AH, Sue-Chu M, Holmen TL, et al. Exhaled and nasal NO levels in allergic rhinitis: relation to sensitization, pollen season and bronchial hyperresponsiveness. Eur Respir J 1999; 13:301-6.
17. Meltzer EO, Orgel HA, Jalowayski AA. Cytology. In: Naclerio RM, ed. Allergic and non-allergic rhinitis. Clinical aspects. Copenhagen: Munksgaard; 1993:66-81.
18. Stammberger H. Rhinoscopy. In: Naclerio RM, ed. Allergic and non-allergic rhinitis. Clinical aspects. Copenhagen: Munksgard; 1993:51-7.
19. Mygind N, Naclerio RM, eds. Allergic and Non-allergic Rhinitis. Philadelphia: WB Saunders; 1993.
20. Barrow C. Toxicology of the nasal passages. In: Chemical Industry Institute of Toxicology Series. Washington, DC: Hemisphere Publishing Corporation; 1986:317.
21. Harkema JR. Comparative structure, function and toxicity of the nasal airways. Predicting human effects from animal studies. In: Gardner DE, ed. Toxicology of the lung, 3rd edition. New York: Taylor & Francis; 1999: 55-83.
22. Mygind N, Naclerio RM. Definition, classification, terminology. In: Naclerio RM, ed. Allergic and non-allergic rhinitis. Clinical aspects. Copenhagen: Munksgard; 1993:11-14.
23. Samet JM, Marbury MC, Spengler JD. Health effects and sources of indoor air pollution. Part I. Am Rev Respir Dis 1987; 136:1486-508.
24. Brundage J, Scott R, Lednar W, et al. Building associated risk of febrile acute respiratory disease in army trainees. JAMA 1988; 259:2108-12.
25. DeZotti R, Patussi V, Fiorito A, et al. Sensitization to green coffee bean (GCB) and castor bean (CB) allergens among dock workers. Int Arch Occup Environ Health 1988; 61:7-12.
26. Nielsen G. Mechanisms of activation of the sensory irritant receptor by air-borne chemicals. Crit Rev Toxicol 1988; 21:183-208.
27. Kanerva D, Tupasela O, Jolanki R, et al. Occupational allergic rhinitis from guar gum. Clin Allergy 1988;18: 245-52.
28. Eggleston PA, Ansari AA, Ziemann B, et al. Occupational challenge studies with laboratory workers allergic to rats. J Allergy Clin Immunol 1990;86: 63-72.
29. Bascom R, Kulle T, Kagey-Sobotka A, et al. Upper respiratory tract environmental tobacco smoke sensitivity. Am Rev Respir Dis 1991; 143:1304-11.
30. Alarie Y. Sensory irritation by air-borne chemicals. Crit Rev Toxicol 1973; 2:299.
31. Alarie Y, Luo JE. Sensory irritation by air-borne chemicals: a basis to establish acceptable levels of exposure. In: Barrow CS, ed. Toxicology of the nasal passages. Washington, DC: Hemisphere Publishing Company; 1986:91-100.
32. Calderon-Garciduenas L, Rodriguez-Alcaraz A, Villarreal-Calderon A, et al. Nasal epithelium as a sentinel for air-borne environmental pollution. Toxicol Sci 1998; 46:352-64.
33. Diaz-Sanchez D, Garcia MP, Wang M, et al. Nasal challenge with diesel exhaust particles can induce sensitization to a neoallergen in the human mucosa. J Allergy Clin Immunol 1999; 104:1183-8.
34. Meltzer EO, Schatz M, Zeiger RS. Allergic and nonallergic rhitis. In: Middleton E Jr, Reed CE, Ellis EF, et al, eds. Allergic principles and practice, 3rd edn. St Louis: CV Mosby; 1988:1253-89.

35. Broder I, Corey P, Cole P, et al. Comparison of the health of occupants and characteristics of houses among control homes and homes insulated with urea formaldehyde foam. II. Initial health and house variables and exposure-response relationships. Environ Res 1988; 45:156-78.

36. Lee L, Stemple JC, Geiger D, et al. Effects of environmental tobacco smoke production on objective measures of voice production. Laryngoscope 1999; 109:1531-4.

37. Leznoff A, Haight JS, Hoffstein V. Reversible sleep apnea caused by occupational exposure to guar gum dust. Am Rev Respir Dis 1986; 133:935-6.

38. Sales J, Kennedy K. Epiglottic dysfunction after isocyanate inhalation exposure. Arch Otolaryngol Head Neck Surg 1990; 116:725-7.

39. Das AK, Davanzo LD, Poiani GJ, et al. Variable extrathoracic airflow obstruction and chronic laryngotracheitis in Gulf War veterans. Chest 1999; 115:97-101.

40. US Department of Health and Human Services, Public Health Service, Centers for Disease Control, National Institute for Occupational Safety and Health. NIOSH Pocket Guide to Chemical Hazards. DHHS (NIOSH) Publication No. 90-117. Washington, DC; US Government Printing Office, July 1990.

41. Acheson ED. Epidemiology of nasal cancer. In: Barrow CS, ed. Toxicology of the nasal passages. Washington, DC: Hemisphere Publishing Company; 1986:135-41.

Chapter 21
Disorders of the Blood and Blood-Forming Organs

Ben Hur P Mobo Jr, Mark R Cullen

The vulnerability to exogenous poisons of the circulating blood cells and the stem cells from which they evolve has been well established for over a century. Heavy metals, solvents, ionizing radiation, pesticides, and a wide range of reactive organic chemicals have all been implicated in the cause of primary hematologic disturbances. Although not all of the major hematologic diseases have established environmental or occupational causes, many do.[1,2] The most important of these are summarized in Table 21.1, along with a list of agents known to cause them.

Although the mechanisms of injury for most of the diseases remain incompletely understood, the basis for prevalent and well-recognized effects on this target organ is apparent. First, although circulating cells and the bone marrow are not intimately connected to a portal of entry for toxins like lung or skin, all agents that enter the systemic circulation have at least brief contact with blood and marrow at concentrations reflecting systemic absorption, which are considerably higher than those that reach other targets such as the nervous system or other visceral organs. Second, because all cell lines except for some lymphocytes are extremely short lived and turn over rapidly, even mild effects on cell survival or production are likely to result in measurable abnormalities. Finally, because blood is so readily and frequently subject to evaluation, and because normal values are so tightly controlled under physiologic conditions, subclinical effects are more readily detected than for virtually any other organ system.

Many of the toxins that have an impact on hematologic function also have effects on other target organs, as is evident from Table 21.1. However, circulating blood cells or bone marrow often represent the first and/or most severely affected tissues, even in systemic poisonings. Appropriate evaluation of hematologic disturbances, however apparently mild or inconsequential, merits consideration of occupational or environmental causes. Moreover, identification of a cause, such as an abnormal hemoglobin or congenital enzymatic defect, should not discourage a thorough examination of environmental factors. As will be seen, individuals with such underlying host factors are potentially more susceptible to exogenous insult that may at once be life threatening and readily amenable to amelioration by environmental control or avoidance.

CLINICAL EVALUATION
History

Hematologic disorders may have protean clinical presentations, ranging from asymptomatic to the conspicuous and life-threatening consequences of markedly depressed levels or function of one or more cell lines. Although classic symptoms of anemia (fatigue, pallor, dyspnea), neutropenia (infection, fever, sore throat), and thrombocytopenia (ecchymoses, bleeding) may be evident in severe cases, other manifestations also must be considered, including skin discoloration (jaundice, acrocyanosis), change in urine color (hemoglobinuria), or abdominal pain associated with hemolysis or enlargement of the liver and spleen. Often, the history alone is inadequate to target hematologic dysfunction, which becomes apparent based on physical and laboratory findings.

The search for environmental etiologies depends on the nature of the disturbance identified or suspected. Clues should always be sought to effects on other organs such as the nervous system, gastrointestinal (GI) tract, and skin, that might turn suspicion toward heavy metals, solvents, or pesticides. Another important issue is the timing of possible exposures of interest. Acute or subacute disturbances of circulating cells, such as hemolysis, usually can be traced to very recent exposures if the environment is responsible. Recent changes in job or activity, the introduction of a new chemical into the environment, or the occurrence of an accidental overexposure or spill should be actively sought in the history and pursued if the sequence of events suggests a cause-and-effect relationship. Because the circulating cells have half-lives that are measurable in hours (for neutrophils), days (for platelets), and months (for red cells), historic or more chronic exposures are unlikely to be the cause unless some change in dose or form of exposure has occurred. However, with the exception of massive or accidental overexposures, the temporal association between exposure to agents with potent effects on circulating cells and consequent clinical manifestations is rarely so obvious – unlike the case with some occupational lung or skin disorders – that it will occur to the patient. For example, a worker newly hired in a lead-exposed job may not develop hemolysis until enough lead has accumulated to cause acute poisoning, typically after several weeks or months. Similarly, a glucose-6-phosphate dehydrogenase (G6PD)-deficient

Disorder	Representative causes
Methemoglobinemia	Aniline, nitrites
Hemolytic anemia	Arsine, lead, trinitrotoluene
Hypoproliferative anemia	Lead, trimellitic anhydride
Secondary polycythemia	Cobalt, carbon monoxide
Thrombocytopenia	Turpentine, chlordane, polyurethane
Aplastic anemia	Benzene, ionizing radiation
Myelodysplastic syndrome	Benzene, nitrogen mustard
Myelofibrosis	Ionizing radiation

Table 21.1 Hematologic disorders caused by environmental agents

person beginning employment in a pharmaceutical house may work for months before having contact with a potent oxidant that precipitates an acute hemolytic crisis. In general, therefore, the task of connecting the environment to the disturbance, however acute, requires thoughtful reconstruction by the treating physician.

At the other end of the disease spectrum, effects on the bone marrow itself, such as hypoproliferative, dysplastic, or neoplastic processes, are more consistent with a long-standing exposure to a culprit known or suspected to be causal, such as benzene or ionizing radiation. It also must be remembered that unlike the circulating cells, the response of bone marrow to injury at one point in time may result in later consequences that follow a prolonged period of apparently normal hematologic function. Thus, it is well described that individuals who have worked in the past with potent leukemogens such as benzene may appear well by all parameters for many years, only to develop subsequently a myeloproliferative process or leukemia.

For such chronic conditions, questions such as 'Have you *ever* been exposed to. . .?' are appropriate, and a thorough lifetime review is in order when evaluating those conditions that have well-established environmental causes. Whenever possible, additional historical clues to possible dose of exposure should be sought as well. For example, if someone had been exposed to benzene, it would be valuable to know whether or not he or she had experienced any of the typical acute solvent effects on the central nervous system (CNS). The early occurrence of GI or dermal effects likewise is a clue to an excessive dose of arsenicals in the appropriate settings. Most often, unfortunately, such historical exposures can only be indirectly inferred from the nature of the patient's contact, its duration, and the physician's knowledge of the particular industry or environmental setting.

Physical examination

The physical examination may offer valuable clues to both the presence of a hematologic disorder and its etiology. Pallor, jaundice, or signs of high-output congestive heart failure suggest the possibility of severe anemia. Disorders of platelets usually result in petechiae or ecchymoses when the absolute count drops below $20,000/mm^3$ or when platelets are functionally impaired. Splenic enlargement, with or without coincident hepatic enlargement, is a hallmark of many myeloproliferative disorders

and also is evident in certain chronic hemolytic anemias. Acrocyanosis is the major clue to the presence of methemoglobinemia that might elude detection if this sign is overlooked.

Because the agents that most predictably cause hematologic disturbances may affect other organs as well, a careful search for signs of these effects may be rewarding. Examples include the dermal effects of arsenicals (hyperkeratoses, pigmentary changes) and organochlorine pesticides (chloracne, porphyria cutanea tarda), or the neurologic effects of arsenic or lead (peripheral neuropathy). On the other hand, the sensitivity of most such signs in the setting of hematologic disorders is low, so the absence of such signs should not discourage careful history taking and the appropriate use of laboratory tests to identify causal agents or markers of their effects.

Laboratory evaluation

As noted earlier, hematologic function is highly amenable to laboratory investigation because of its constancy over time (i.e., the timing of samples is generally unimportant), and, because of the uniformity of most parameters in the healthy population, the ranges of normal generally are narrow. For these reasons, one rarely needs multiple specimens or access to a previous specimen from the same individual to interpret a complete blood count (CBC), differential count, or peripheral blood smear. On the other hand, rarely does this basic test battery provide strong evidence of an environmental basis for disease. Although such findings as basophilic stippling (due to lead) or Heinz bodies (due to oxidant stresses) may point toward a toxic etiology, these findings are non-specific.

Beyond the CBC, a wide range of tests are readily available that may allow precise definition of a disease process if not its cause. Evaluation of reticulocyte count, serum and urine hemoglobin, haptoglobin, and direct and indirect bilirubin generally allows classification of anemias into those that are hemolytic and those that result from inadequate marrow production. Various immunologic tests such as the direct Coombs' test may allow differentiation of peripheral destructive processes into immune versus non-immune bases; similar tests now exist for evaluating rapid platelet turnover. The effects of nutritional deficiencies and chronic disease states, such as chronic inflammatory processes or renal, endocrine, and liver disease, generally can be excluded by simple blood tests as well. Bone marrow aspiration discriminates major causes at that site, where the production and maturation of myeloid and megakaryocyte precursors to neutrophils and platelets occur. The addition of a biopsy and cytogenetic study may provide highly accurate pathophysiologic classification and prognostication. Unfortunately, environmental effects on blood are so similar to the effects caused by infection, systemic disease, and idiopathic disorders that none of these more sophisticated tests provides direct evidence of a toxic etiology. Rather, the role of such testing is to establish the basis of the lesion physiologically and to exclude non-environmental causes, if possible. The laboratory must be used in a different way if etiologic clues to an environmental factor on the history or the physical examination are to be confirmed. For many agents of interest, such as heavy metals or pesticides, the most valuable approach is direct assessment of the toxin or its metabolites in blood or other body fluids. Indirect evidence may be obtainable by examination of metabolic consequences associated with the agent, for example, the inhibition of various enzymes of porphyrin synthesis caused by lead or organochlorine compounds.

Although these approaches to confirmation of an etiologic agent are useful for culprits that are either long lived in the body (e.g., organochlorine pesticides, heavy metals) or produce their effects very shortly after exposure occurs (e.g., aromatic amines), the laboratory is less useful for pinpointing historical causes of chronic diseases, such as the myeloproliferative states caused by benzene or ionizing radiation. At the present time, there are no specific markers for these important etiologies and evaluation ultimately hinges on recognition of the appropriate disease state combined with knowledge of exposure parameters, including intensity, duration, and latency.

CLASSIFICATION

A classification of non-malignant hematologic disorders follows.

DISORDERS OF SINGLE CELL LINES

Red cells
Methemoglobinemia
Anemias
    Hemolytic anemias
        Intravascular hemolysis
        Extravascular hemolysis
    Hypoproliferative anemia

Polycythemia

Platelets
Thrombocytopenia
    Peripheral destruction
    Hypoproliferation
Other platelet disorders

Disorders of white blood cells
Neutrophils
Eosinophils
Lymphocytes

DISORDERS OF STEM CELLS AND MICROENVIRONMENT

Hypoplastic and aplastic anemia

Myelodysplastic syndromes

These disorders are discussed in detail throughout the rest of this chapter.

DISORDERS OF SINGLE CELL LINES

The most frequently encountered environmental effects on blood are those that affect circulating cells. Injury may occur at any stage in the lifespan, ranging from maturation within the bone marrow through premature senescence within the vasculature or in the reticuloendothelial system. Because all the major cell lines turn over rapidly, these disorders almost invariably reflect the recent effects of toxins or other injurious agents; often, the culprit is still detectable in body tissue, which may aid the examining physician considerably in the differential diagnosis.

Disorders of red blood cells

Methemoglobinemia

Oxidation of the iron in hemoglobin without oxygen binding results in an altered hemoglobin molecule that is almost black in color and functionally limited. A wide range of organic chemicals, mostly of the aromatic nitro and amino groups, are capable of causing the formation of methemoglobin in clinically significant quantities.[3] Although the condition has been best described in workers making dyestuffs and explosives, a wide range of chemicals have been implicated, including phenylpropanolamine.[4] More common causes of chemical-induced methemoglobinemia are listed in Table 21.2.

Pathogenesis The iron in hemoglobin is normally maintained in the reduced state, as ferrous or Fe^{+2} iron. Although iron in hemoglobin has the remarkable property

Agent	Setting of exposure
Aromatic nitro and amine compounds	
Aminophenol	Fur making
Aniline	Dyes, pharmaceuticals
Chloroaniline	Plastics
Dinitrobenzene	Dyes, explosives
Dinitrotoluene	Dyes, explosives
Naphthalamine	Dyes, explosives
Nitroaniline	Dyes
Nitrobenzene	Dyes, explosives
Nitrotoluene	Dyes, explosives
Phenylpropanolamine	Pharmaceuticals
Trinitrotoluene	Explosives
Toluidine	Dyes, chemicals
Aliphatic nitro compounds, nitrates, nitrites	
Ethylene glycol dinitrate	Explosives
Nitroglycerin	Explosives, pharmaceuticals
Nitropropane	Chemicals, coating
Organic and inorganic nitrites	Pharmaceuticals, chemicals
Miscellaneous	
Antimalarials	Pharmaceuticals
Chloramphenicol	Pharmaceuticals
Sulfa drugs	Pharmaceuticals
Naphthalene	Moth balls
Nitrofurantoin	Pharmaceuticals

Table 21.2 Environmental causes of methemoglobinemia and/or oxidant-induced hemolysis

of being able to combine directly with oxygen while maintaining this reduced form, other oxidants (see Table 21.2) may directly oxidize the iron to the ferric or Fe^{+3} state without binding of oxygen. Unopposed, this alteration leads to two important functional changes:

- a sharp leftward shift in the oxygen dissociation curve of neighboring normal hemoglobin molecules (limiting delivery of oxygen to tissues); and
- denaturation of hemoglobin altogether, leading to development of inclusions called Heinz bodies, which can destabilize the red cell membrane and lead to hemolysis (see the section on Hemolytic Anemias).

Obviously, if the proportion of hemoglobin in the Fe^{+3} state rises, the total oxygen-carrying capacity of blood also is directly decreased, because methemoglobin is unable to carry oxygen.

In the normal person, there are no fewer than four separate enzyme systems that may oppose the oxidation of hemoglobin to methemoglobin.[5] The most important system is rate-limited by the enzyme nicotinamide-adenine dinucleotide (NADH) methemoglobin reductase, or cytochrome $b5$ reductase. Under normal circumstances, this system scavenges almost all of the methemoglobin formed by physiologic oxidants or low-level chemical exposures. Rare individuals with congenital methemoglobinemia have deficiencies in this system and are somewhat blue in color.

When the NADH methemoglobin reductase system is overwhelmed, NADPH generated by the alternative glucose-metabolizing pathway (Embden–Meyerhof pathway or hexose monophosphate shunt) may reduce methemoglobin. However, to be quantitatively effective, an additional redox transfer factor is necessary. Methylene blue is the usual therapeutic choice (see later) to serve this role. The shunt must be intact to work, however, because once methylene blue is oxidized, it can serve as a further oxidant stress itself unless it is quickly reduced by NADPH. The rate-limiting enzyme in this pathway is G6PD, which is, unfortunately, congenitally deficient in a high proportion of black and Middle Eastern populations.

Two other pathways exist to reduce methemoglobin back to the ferrous form. One involves reduced glutathione, and the other involves ascorbic acid. These pathways are probably of limited physiologic importance and as yet have not been found to have any therapeutic applications.

Clinical manifestations and diagnosis The major effects of methemoglobin in increased concentrations are acrocyanosis and asphyxiation. The onset often is insidious because exposure may result transdermally or through gradual accumulation over several days. Fatigue, dyspnea, palpitations, headache, or abdominal distress may precede recognition of cyanosis.[6]

The hallmark for diagnosis is recognition of cyanosis, which begins in acral areas. Blood obtained from an artery or a vein is very dark and *does not turn red on exposure to the air,* a distinguishing feature of cyanosis due to hypoxemia. Arterial blood gases may reveal a normal PO_2 even when

the amount of methemoglobin starts to exceed 30% of total hemoglobin, the level at which major organ damage becomes likely in otherwise healthy individuals. Usual tests such as blood chemistries and an electrocardiogram generally do not help distinguish between hypoxemia and methemoglobinemia. The most important test is direct measurement of methemoglobin – a test that is fast, easy, and cheap, but it is not routine and must be ordered. Another important diagnostic test is a CBC and reticulocyte smear, which is used to search for evidence of hemolysis that often is caused by the same oxidants, as indicated by Heinz body formation (see the section on Hemolytic Anemias).

Having confirmed the diagnosis, there is generally little reason to identify the causal agent in body fluids, although the agent usually still is present. When there is no clear history of exposure or when multiple possible agents are present in the environment, samples of blood and urine and a gastric aspirate may be helpful. The gastric aspirate is particularly useful for the detection of covert or accidental ingestion, which is well described.

Management The principles of management are straightforward. First, 100% oxygen should be delivered while results of tests are pending. Next, the patient should undergo skin decontamination by thoroughly washing the entire body because dermal contact is an important route of exposure in the industrial setting. If there is suspicion of ingestion, gastric lavage, followed by the administration of charcoal and cathartics, is appropriate.

If the methemoglobin level exceeds 20% or the patient is markedly symptomatic, methylene blue should be administered in 1% intravenous solution, over about 10 to 15 minutes, to a dose of 1 to 2 mg/kg. The medication must be given with some caution, especially in patients who may be G6PD deficient, in whom it could cause the formation of more methemoglobin or precipitate further hemolysis.[7] The effect is rapid, peaking within 1 hour, at which point the dose may be repeated orally or intravenously. Patients should be monitored closely until the methemoglobin levels are well below 20% and to ensure that no rebound effect has occurred after stopping the methylene blue.

Finally, evidence of coincident hemolysis must be searched for and managed, as discussed later. The key is maintenance of adequate hemoglobin and good renal function. When methemoglobinemia and hemolysis coexist in major degrees, consideration should be given to exchange transfusion as a lifesaving means to establish adequate tissue oxygenation.

Prevention The key to prevention is the use of primary strategies – strict control of air levels and scrupulous measures to avoid skin contact because many of these agents, such as aniline, are rapidly absorbed through intact skin. As a backup strategy, it is appropriate to measure CBC, reticulocyte counts, and methemoglobin levels periodically and even more frequently in new workers whose sensitivity to the effect is not characterized and whose experience with these toxins may not be adequate. There is debate in the literature regarding the efficacy of excluding individuals from exposure altogether based on baseline or pre-placement levels of the enzyme G6PD. Many, if not most, with mild-to-moderate deficiencies, as are common in the black population, have worked around these chemicals without any adverse or disproportional effect, probably owing to the complexity of the heme reduction mechanism. On the other hand, it is probably reasonable to exclude from further exposure any G6PD-deficient individual who has developed a significant degree of methemoglobinemia under routine working circumstances (i.e., levels > 5% to 10%). In such cases, the worker has provided biologic evidence of sensitivity and further exposure presents an unacceptable level of risk.

Anemias

Hemolytic anemias   Hemolysis, or shortened red cell lifespan, is a common effect of a diverse range of environmental and occupational exposures. Following the usual clinical convention, we classify them here based on their clinical presentations.

Intravascular hemolysis   Premature destruction of red blood cells within the vasculature has been described in three important environmental or occupational exposure settings:

- as a consequence of overexposure to the gases *arsine* (AsH_3) and *stibine* (SbH_3) (Chapter 39.2);
- in association with other clinical consequences of *acute lead poisoning* (Chapter 39.7); and
- as a consequence of *repetitive trauma of the hands or feet against a hard surface,* so-called march hemoglobinuria.

Because the mechanisms and presentations differ markedly, these conditions are discussed separately. Intravascular hemolysis also has been reported in association with *angiosarcoma of the liver,* a rare tumor usually associated with an environmental cause such as vinyl chloride monomer, arsenicals, and thorium (see Chapter 30.6).

HEMOLYSIS DUE TO ARSINE AND STIBINE

Pathogenesis   These gaseous metal compounds (AsH_3, SbH_3) are highly reactive and bind to multiple sites in the red cell, including the membrane, oxyhemoglobin, and virtually all free sulfhydryl groups.[8] The integrity of the membrane is impaired by disruption of sodium–potassium pump channels, as well as by depletion of glutathione. The net effect is loss of osmotic balance of the cells, swelling, and intravascular lysis. Although some portion of these compounds is oxidized to the highly toxic metals arsenic and antimony, the role that these metals play in the acute hemolytic reactions is unclear but is probably of secondary importance.[9] In most cases, the acute hemolytic effects and their consequences, such as reduction in effective oxygen transport, sludging of red cell debris in the circulation, and the outpouring of free hemoglobin into plasma, dominate the clinical picture, which bears little resemblance to acute poisonings with these metals in other forms (see Chapter 39.2).

Clinical manifestations and diagnosis   Because these gases are not particularly irritating, there may be no evidence of an acute reaction for several hours after an accidental exposure. The onset of hemolysis is heralded by non-specific GI and neurologic symptoms such as headache, dizziness, nausea, and abdominal or flank pain. Shortly thereafter, the evidence of darkened urine and a jaundiced appearance to the skin marks the classic clinical presentation of acute intravascular hemolysis.[10] There is no clinical history or physical examination findings that distinguish the picture from acute hemolysis of other causes, such as transfusion reaction.

Initial laboratory evaluation is consistent with intravascular hemolysis: low hematocrit, low or absent haptoglobin, free hemoglobin in plasma and urine, and dramatic elevation of lactate dehydrogenase (LDH). The peripheral smear initially may show fragmentation of cells, as well as anisocytosis and poikilocytosis. There may not be striking reticulocytosis early in the course of the disease in view of the rapidity of onset of the reaction and possibly also the myelosuppressive effects of arsenic itself; leukocytosis is commonly seen, but platelet count may be low, suggesting disseminated intravascular coagulopathy or hemolytic-uremic syndrome. Diagnostic tests such as direct Coombs' or tests for fibrinolytic factors (e.g., fibrin split products) are negative.

The most striking and clinically important extra-hematologic signs and laboratory findings are related to renal function, which is generally affected early by hemoglobin in plasma. Evidence of early acute tubular necrosis may be seen by rising blood urea nitrogen (BUN) or serum creatinine and failure to conserve sodium appropriately; oliguria or even anuria is usually evident within a day. There are no pathognomonic findings for a toxic etiology unless a sample of urine is sent to the laboratory for measurement of levels of the base metals, which may be elevated if determined before renal failure is profound.

In addition to renal injury, other findings may include hepatomegaly with slightly elevated enzymes and diffuse CNS dysfunction, including alterations of mental status. Occasionally, evidence of acute myopathy is seen with muscle tenderness and elevations of creatine phosphokinase (CPK). Whether these additional findings are related to the toxicity of the base metals or to the acute hemolytic reaction itself is unclear.

In addition to the acute hemolytic syndrome described earlier, a more chronic variant of hemolysis has been described in an outbreak among workers with repeated low-level exposures to arsine. These individuals had anemia with reticulocytosis and basophilic stippling similar to that seen in subacute lead intoxication (see later). The occurrence of this syndrome has not been reported for over 50 years.

Course and management   The mainstay of treatment includes steps to ensure an adequate hematocrit and to preserve renal function. Oxygen and alkaline diuresis are appropriate immediately. If oliguric renal failure ensues, exchange transfusion is considered the treatment of choice because the hemolytic reaction itself may persist for up to 4 days after a single acute exposure. There is no role in acute management for chelating agents such as British Anti-Lewisite because it cannot bind arsine or stibine to any appreciable degree.

After these steps are taken, treatment depends on the clinical course. If renal failure is profound, hemodialysis is generally indicated for as long as necessary; chronic dialysis may be needed in severe cases in which renal function fails to recover. Late manifestations of arsine poisoning may include evidence of bone marrow depression, peripheral or central neuropathy, and GI manifestations typical of arsenic poisoning. In such cases, there may be a role for chelating agents (see Chapter 39.2) although the literature has not established their utility in this setting.

Prevention   Because the major risk of arsine and stibine gas is accidental overexposure, the thrust of prevention must be primary: real-time, continuous monitoring for leaks wherever the gases are used and intense education in industrial operations in which arsine or stibine may be generated by faulty work practices such as the addition of acids to tanks in which traces of the metals may be found. The routine use of surveillance, including CBCs and reticulocyte counts in workers who have regular opportunities for exposure, may be of some value in detecting early or chronic low-level failures of primary prevention, but it is a meager substitute.

HEMOLYSIS IN ACUTE LEAD POISONING   Individuals who rapidly accumulate lead over a period of days to months may develop the insidious syndrome called acute lead poisoning. This syndrome is classically characterized by abdominal pain or colic, intravascular hemolysis, and peripheral or central neurologic symptoms and signs.[11,12] Although it is called acute, the designation has been applied to distinguish the picture from the more indolent picture of chronic lead intoxication, which occurs in individuals with regular, longstanding exposures (see Chapter 39.7). In no sense is acute lead poisoning truly acute like the syndrome caused by arsine (above); it is virtually impossible to absorb enough lead fast enough to cause such an immediate reaction.

Pathogenesis   Lead causes many alterations in red cell function, most classically by interference with enzymes in the cascade of porphyrin and heme synthesis (see the section on Hypoproliferative Anemia). However, the effect of lead that leads to hemolysis is unrelated to porphyrins and is probably due to the inhibition of the enzyme pyrimidine 5′ nucleotidase, leading to destabilization of membrane function with the formation of basophilic inclusions within the cells (stippling) and premature destruction within the vasculature.[13] The role of other lead–red cell interactions in the pathogenesis of the hemolysis is unclear, as is the marked variability in host responses to lead, such as why some individuals can have prolonged intense exposures sufficient to cause chronic lead poisoning without ever manifesting the acute syndrome.

Clinical presentation and diagnosis   Rarely is hemolysis the major presenting sign of acute lead poisoning. Typically, patients seek attention for GI or neurologic complaints and the usually mild-to-moderate anemia is discovered as part of the workup. Basophilic stippling usually is seen, although it is non-specific for lead, and the reticulocyte count is elevated. Contrary to the information contained in the old literature on this subject, the average red cell size (mean corpuscular volume [MCV]) is normal or even elevated if reticulocytosis is pronounced; microcytosis should suggest either another diagnosis or the coexistence of a second problem such as iron deficiency or thalassemia trait.[11] In children, for example, both iron deficiency and thalassemia trait are common in the population at risk for acute lead poisoning. Haptoglobin may be low but rarely is nil, and free hemoglobin in plasma or urine is not seen. Tests for other causes of hemolysis, such as Coombs' and G6PD tests, are negative. The diagnosis of acute lead poisoning is made by measurement of the whole blood lead level, which is generally very high in this setting, usually over 70 μg/dl. The zinc or free erythrocyte protoporphyrin (ZPP or FEP) levels also are usually very high because of concomitant inhibition of heme synthetase, leading to an accumulation in the red cell of heme's precursor. Because only iron deficiency also is known to cause such elevations of red cell protoporphyrins (with the exception of the rare hereditary condition erythroporphyria), the combination of high protoporphyrin levels and hemolysis is almost pathognomonic for lead poisoning.

Because the rate of hemolysis is low even in severe cases compared with that induced by intense exposures to arsine, for example, renal injury due to free pigment is not a problem. However, acute accumulation of lead may itself affect renal function, with development of Fanconi's syndrome, which includes proximal tubular injury with renal tubular acidosis, aminoaciduria, phosphaturia, uricosuria, and glycosuria.

Management and course   The presence of significant hemolysis in acute lead poisoning is a compelling reason to initiate aggressive chelation therapy, which might otherwise be a judgment call. This therapy is described in Chapter 39.7. Usually, the hemolysis responds rapidly, with decrements in reticulocyte count and a rise in hematocrit occurring within days. There is no need to take additional steps such as transfusion or diuresis unless the level of hematocrit presents a threat to the patient's immediate health, such as in the presence of ischemic heart disease. As a caution, because blood lead levels generally rise again after completion of a course of chelation with CaEDTA or BAL, it can be expected that hemolysis also may return in a milder form and the patient must be watched carefully. Avoidance of any lead exposure in this setting is crucial to successful management.

Prevention Regular blood lead levels, ZPPs, and CBCs are an essential part of surveillance for anyone, either adult or child, who may have had significant lead exposure.

HEMOLYSIS DUE TO COPPER Copper has been implicated in rare cases of acute hemolysis in the setting of Wilson's disease, suicide attempts, and dialysates contaminated with copper from copper pipes.[14] In 1995, a case of acute hemolysis complicated by acute renal failure was reported in a Nigerian man living in the US.[15] The patient had ingested a green-colored 'spiritual drink' containing copper as part of a cleansing ritual practiced by some Nigerians. He underwent hemodialysis and subsequently stabilized with improvement in hematocrit, indirect bilirubin, and lactate dehydrogenase (LDH) levels.

The mechanism of copper-induced hemolysis is thought to be due to inhibitions of glycolysis, NADPH, and G6PD systems.[16] Treatment is generally supportive care.

TRAUMATIC HEMOLYSIS (MARCH HEMOGLOBIN-URIA, SPORTS ANEMIA) An appreciable fraction of individuals participating in activities that bring body surfaces repeatedly and forcefully against hard external objects will lyse red cells.[17] In a small fraction of the population, this lysing of red cells may be sufficient to lead to mild anemia, hemoglobinuria, or both. In addition, plasma volume expansion contributes to 'pseudoanemia'.[18] Either condition usually is transient. Rarely are there any clinical signs or symptoms other than the pigmentary change in urine.

The major importance of this disorder is its exclusion from more serious causes of hemolysis or intrinsic renal disease. Exclusion of intrinsic renal disease is effectively accomplished by demonstrating that red cells are absent in urine – the pigment arises from hemoglobin, which occasionally is mixed with small amounts of myoglobin from the same trauma. Exclusion of more serious forms of hemolysis, such as paroxysmal cold or nocturnal hemoglobinurias or that induced by toxins or drugs, relies on the fact that almost all abnormal laboratory tests – reduced haptoglobin, increased free hemoglobin, and mild elevations of muscle enzymes – return to normal within a day or two after an episode. Reticulocytosis is demonstrable only with frequent, repeated bouts. The peripheral blood smear may be normal or may show macrocytosis.[19] Physical examination may be normal as well. The history of long runs, military activities, karate, conga drumming, or other physical contact with hard surfaces is essential to the diagnosis.

Treatment consists largely of reassurance. Whenever possible, further episodes should be controlled by efforts to reduce the degree of trauma between the body surface and external objects to the greatest extent possible, often by using appropriate protective equipment.

Extravascular hemolysis Certain environmental exposures may lead to alterations of the red cell that decrease its survival because of enhanced splenic destruction. In almost every case, the cause is a combination of an external environmental factor and a host factor. The first important group includes those caused by potent *oxidants*. For these conditions, host deficiencies of enzymes such as G6PD are important co-factors in disease. The second group is *immune mediated*; presumably, affected subjects carry some predisposition for development of an immunologic response to an external agent that directly or indirectly disturbs red cell membrane integrity. Finally, certain exposures have been demonstrated to accelerate or *exacerbate the hemolytic process due to abnormal hemoglobin* structure. Individuals with hereditary variants may be at risk for environmental exposures that are unimportant to hosts with typical AA hemoglobin patterns.

OXIDANT HEMOLYSIS

Pathogenesis A large and somewhat eclectic group of chemical agents, including pharmaceuticals and reactive compounds used in plastics, explosives, and dyes, are potent chemical oxidants. Important environmental agents have been listed previously in Table 21.2. As noted in the earlier discussion on methemoglobinemia, these compounds may directly oxidize heme iron to form methemoglobin, or they may bind to the protein moiety of hemoglobin, generally at a sulfhydryl group. If this binding is not reversed by reduced glutathione, hemoglobin may precipitate, forming hyperpigmented vesicular structures in the red cells called Heinz bodies. Unfortunately, the presence of Heinz bodies, in turn, makes these cells less distensible as they traverse the sinusoids of the spleen, and premature destruction results.

The natural defenses of the red cell are complex. It remains unclear why one single oxidant compound may induce clinically significant methemoglobinemia in one individual, with minimal hemolysis, while causing the reverse in another person. Based on clinical reports, it seems likely that individuals with hereditary deficiencies of the enzyme G6PD are at increased risk for hemolysis, as are some individuals with congenital variants of this and other enzymes in the hexose monophosphate shunt.[20] In some individuals, both reactions may occur and some investigators believe that methemoglobin formation may be the precursor of the denatured hemoglobin, which leads to hemolysis.

Clinical manifestations and diagnosis Irrespective of underlying enzyme status, subjects who develop acute hemolytic crises after exposure to oxidants are clinically normal and well prior to the offending exposure. The onset of illness usually is abrupt and may occur hours to several days after initial contact with the offending agent. Because the host may be unusually susceptible, the exposure need not entail unusual circumstances such as a spill, ingestion, or the like; others similarly exposed may be fine. The onset usually is marked by fever, systemic complaints, and, often, pigmenturia; infection is likely to be the first diagnostic consideration.

Physical examination typically reveals pallor, tachycardia, fever, and, sometimes, mild jaundice. The spleen, liver, or both may be tender and somewhat enlarged. The primary clue to acute hemolytic crisis and its possible underlying cause comes from the laboratory. Low hematocrit with reticulocytosis is the rule. The smear may reveal Heinz bodies, but schistocytes, spherocytes, or nucleated red cells typically are not seen. The white count and platelets generally are unremarkable. Liver and muscle enzymes are normal. Urinalysis is most remarkable for occult blood without red cells. Tests for specific causes of extravascular hemolysis, such as Coombs' or hemoglobin electrophoresis, are normal.

There are several clues to the roles of oxidants and underlying enzyme abnormalities. Measurement of methemoglobin may yield evidence of a more generalized oxidant effect. Heinz bodies, if present, are strongly suggestive of this diagnostic consideration. Confirmation ultimately may require measurement of red cell levels of enzymes such as G6PD or others in the Embden–Meyerhof pathway. However, these measurements must be interpreted with caution because:

- the most deficient cells (generally older cells) are the first to be hemolyzed, hence the measured levels during or immediately after a crisis are falsely high;
- there is marked populational heterogeneity, making establishment of normal levels for an individual subject precarious; and
- the defect may be in any of several enzymes, at least in theory.

For these reasons, the most important diagnostic feature in the usual case of oxidant hemolysis is the history of new or very recent onset of exposure to a potential oxidizing agent. In the occupational setting, a careful history of recent work, including changes in job or activity, is most likely to be revealing. It is especially important to remember, however, that the intensity of the exposure of concern may be unremarkable in and of itself because the crisis may involve a susceptible host, not necessarily overexposure per se.

Management, course, and prevention Because oxidants are rapidly bound or metabolized and because the levels of protective enzymes are higher in newly made cells, hemolytic crises from oxidants are generally self-limited. Although in severe cases there may be need for exchange transfusion to support oxygen transport and to minimize the resultant acute renal failure from pigmenturia, these measures are rarely necessary. No steps other than supportive care and observation generally are required or beneficial.

Obviously, it is imprudent to return an individual to a potentially similar exposure situation after recovery from an episode of hemolytic crisis; if exposure cannot be reduced sharply, permanent transfer or job change is indicated. Less clear are the roles for:

- pre-placement screening of workers likely to be exposed to oxidants; and
- routine surveillance with examinations and blood testing for those who are exposed.

Unfortunately, there are insufficient data on which to make strong judgments.[21] Although pre-placement blood studies are likely to prevent exposure of most of those at the highest risk for hemolytic crisis, they do not exclude all and they undoubtedly exclude many who could work with perfect safety in the environment. There is no credible reason to exclude individuals based on any less specific characteristic than a documented low level of G6PD or related enzymes, such as all members of an ethnic or racial group known to have high carrier rates of enzyme variants, or all those with any other hematologic disturbance. Whether or not pre-placement studies are chosen, periodic CBCs with methemoglobin levels and reticulocyte counts are probably advisable because they may help detect excessive exposures or overly susceptible individuals.

In any event, it should never be forgotten, however relevant host factors may be, that the oxidant class of chemicals includes extremely potent and reactive agents, and many are capable of causing devastating effects in any host at sufficiently high levels of exposure. Primary control of exposure, therefore, remains the sine qua non of prevention of disease from these compounds.

IMMUNE-MEDIATED HEMOLYSIS Although there is a long list of drugs that can cause immune-mediated hemolysis (e.g., by serving as haptens on red cell membranes, by forming immune complexes that, in turn, bind red cells, or by inducing autoantibodies), environmental exposures that cause similar effects have not been clearly identified. Hemolysis is a prominent component of the hemorrhagic pneumonitis and anemia syndrome described in workers exposed to the plastic component *trimellitic anhydride,* or *TMA* (see Chapter 41). Workers with this syndrome typically have gamma G immunoglobulin (IgG) antibodies directed against TMA–red cell adducts but are not predictably Coombs' positive on direct testing.[22,23] Whether this is a variant of the innocent bystander mechanism of hemolytic anemia described with quinidine and other drugs remains to be elucidated. In any event, the hemolysis behaves much like quinidine-induced cases and responds to removal of the individual from exposure. The therapeutic role of steroids in this setting is unclear, but all patients should be evaluated for iron deficiency because they generally have had significant hemoptysis, the usual presenting and predominating complaint.

A case of Coombs-positive anemia related to exposure to the pesticide *dieldrin* was reported in 1978.[24] An IgG anti-dieldrin antibody was identified. The patient required splenectomy for cure.

The only other well-documented setting in which an environmental exposure may lead to immune-mediated hemolysis is in association with malignant mesothelioma due to asbestos exposure. Study of case reports suggests that tumor antigens cause the relevant immunologic reaction, not antigens associated with asbestos per se. Treatment with corticosteroids is supportive during management of the otherwise lethal tumor.

HEMOGLOBINOPATHIES AND ENVIRONMENTAL EXPOSURES
Sickle cell anemia and trait For reasons familiar to victims of SS disease, many aspects of the work and ambi-

ent environment represent potential threats for sickle cell crises. These include exertional stresses, with attendant dehydration and hemoconcentration; exposures to oxygen-deficient atmospheres, leading to hypoxemia; and exposure to chemicals that could impair oxygen transport, such as asphyxiants. Unfortunately, much has been written but little proved regarding substantive risks to the much larger population of individuals who carry the sickle cell trait (hemoglobin AS). Although historically excluded from exertional sports, aviation, diving, and other activities because of theoretic effects on renal and other target tissues, there are no credible data to support the view that sickle cell trait substantially alters an individual's responses to any environmental stress of relevance.[25] In fact, recent studies suggest that such individuals handle barometric changes, hypoxia, and exertion no less well than age- and sex-matched counterparts. Any occupational exclusion, including aviation, sports, or diving, that is not based on physiologic demonstrable abnormalities in such individuals is inappropriate.

Other hemoglobinopathies   There are no reliable data on special risks of carriers of thalassemia traits or other major hemoglobin variants. These factors should not be used for the purpose of job placement or risk determinations. Their only importance at present is in the differential diagnosis of environmental effects, a reason why baseline CBCs are of value in surveillance for any suspected agent that affects the peripheral blood.

Hypoproliferative anemias   Anemias caused by inadequate production of red cells are of two broad types. First are those due to alterations in the bone marrow stem cells, which ultimately differentiate into the red cell series, or in the microenvironment of the marrow, which supports the growth and normal differentiation of the bone marrow stem cells. These disorders include aplastic anemia, myelodysplastic syndromes (MDS, refractory anemias), myeloproliferative diseases, and diseases associated with infiltration of bone marrow by infection, granuloma, or tumor. Although anemia often dominates in clinical presentation, in general, such disorders affect multiple cell lines, which becomes apparent on examination of the peripheral smear or, if necessary, the marrow itself. For this reason, and because this group of diseases are of special importance in occupational and environmental medicine practice, the subject is considered in detail separately later in this chapter.

On the other hand, inadequate production of red cells also may occur because of more specific lesions that affect the development of red cells. These may include inadequate stimulation by the hormonal mediator erythropoietin, as in chronic renal insufficiency; inability to respond to stimulation, as in chronic inflammatory or malignant disease states; or inability to synthesize hemoglobin or one of its constituents because of nutritional deficiency or metabolic blockade, either acquired or congenital.

Outside the context of another disease of occupational or environmental origin, such as renal insufficiency due to solvents or lung cancer due to asbestos, the environmental causes of this group of disorders are relatively few. Iron deficiency with microcytic anemia may be an integral part of the pulmonary hemorrhage–anemia syndrome seen in some individuals exposed to TMA; however, as noted earlier, immune-mediated hemolysis is probably more important clinically when patients are first seen.[22,23]

A single case of megaloblastic anemia with normal levels of folate and B_{12} has been described following exposure to the pesticide *chlordane*.[26] The clinical picture was identical to that seen in pernicious anemia, and all manifestations reversed on removal of the individual from exposure. Complicating acceptance of a causal relationship, however, was the occurrence in this case of cholestatic hepatitis, likely due to the exposure. Because malabsorption was documented, the role of chlordane as a primary cause of megaloblastic change in the erythron must be questioned despite the measured nutrient levels.

Pernicious anemia also has been linked to longstanding *work in textile mills* by epidemiologic studies of mortality.[27] No obvious biologic basis for this link is known, so it is unclear whether it relates to the well-characterized immune-mediated gastric injury leading to vitamin B_{12} deficiency or whether there may be some environmental factor in this work setting that causes a similar clinical picture of megaloblastic anemia.

Macrocytosis without anemia has been described recently in *organic solvent*-exposed workers believed not to have been exposed to benzene or other myelotoxic compounds, but the significance of this observation remains obscure.[28]

The best-described cause of hypoproliferative anemia due to an environmental factor is the effect of *lead* on heme synthesis.

Anemia of chronic lead intoxication   The mechanism and presentation of hemolysis that occurs when individuals are heavily exposed to lead above their accustomed burden has been described earlier in this chapter. Accumulated body lead also has a subtle but measurable effect on the proliferation of red cells from the marrow irrespective of the rate of accumulation and unrelated to any of the acute manifestations of lead poisoning. Although clinically far less important than the hemolytic episodes or other organ system effects of lead, the inhibition of heme synthesis has been long understood and forms the basis for much of our knowledge of the mechanisms of lead poisoning at the cellular level, as well as the development of an important biomarker to assess lead burden, the whole blood ZPP or FEP level.[11]

PATHOGENESIS   The pathway by which glycine, succinyl coenzyme A (CoA), and iron are converted into heme for incorporation into hemoglobin is illustrated in Figure 21.1. Two enzymes in this pathway are markedly lead-sensitive in readily demonstrable fashion. d-Aminolevulinic acid (ALA) dehydratase, which synthesizes the first porphyrin ring, is exquisitely sensitive, with decreases in the bioactivity of the enzyme measurable once

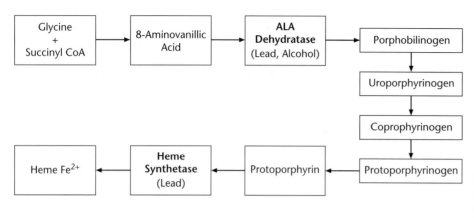

Figure 21.1: The heme synthesis pathway in red cell precursors. Lead inhibits the enzyme ALA dehydratase, as does alcohol. Lead also inhibits the rate-limiting enzyme heme synthetase.

whole blood level exceeds about 10 µg/dl; similar inhibition is conferred by low levels of alcohol, but there is no evidence of synergy between the two. This enzyme is not rate limiting, however, and even marked depression, as may be seen with low levels of lead, is rarely associated with any other measurable biochemical change. At somewhat higher body burdens, usually when the whole blood level approaches 35 or 40 µg/dl, there is inhibition of the more important enzyme ferrochelatase, or heme synthetase, which incorporates iron into the protoporphyrin ring to form heme. This blockade leads to the accumulation of protoporphyrin in the red cells, the basis for the ZPP or FEP blood screen. With progressive inhibition of heme synthetase, there is a gradual inhibition of the proliferative process, with small incremental decreases in hemoglobin production. The marrow, in turn, compensates with an increased stimulation of red cell production, causing compensatory erythroid hyperplasia, as would be seen in iron deficiency.

DIAGNOSIS AND CLINICAL MANIFESTATIONS The hematologic picture associated with elevated lead burden is unimpressive unless accompanied by acute hemolysis, as described previously. Although slightly lower than may be predicted, the hematocrit and hemoglobin are usually well within the normal range. The MCV and red cell morphology usually are normal, although a few basophilic stippled cells may be identified. The only relevant abnormal laboratory tests are the whole blood lead level and the protoporphyrins, ZPP or FEP, assuming that they have been ordered.

Because the hematologic disturbance associated with chronic lead poisoning tends to be very mild, the most important clinical issue is recognition of the underlying cause, which may be associated with far more important renal, neuropsychiatric, reproductive, or other manifestations of lead poisoning. For this reason, lead poisoning should remain in the differential diagnosis of normochromic, normocytic anemias in both children and adults who may have had significant exposures. Perhaps more important, because peripheral blood findings in lead poisoning are so frequently normal, a CBC and smear should never be used as a screening test for lead poisoning,

nor should a normal CBC ever be used to exclude the diagnosis, which may be suggested by other clinical features or by virtue of known exposure.

Polycythemia

As with the hypoproliferative anemias discussed earlier, polycythemia may be primary, a myeloproliferative disorder of stem cells, or secondary to other factors. Consideration of environmental causes of primary polycythemia or polycythemia vera is discussed in Chapter 30.3. Here, we shall consider two causes of secondary increases in blood hemoglobin:

- the metal *cobalt*; and
- chronic exposure to asphyxiants, especially carbon monoxide.

Although secondary polycythemia also may be seen with lung diseases due to environmental factors, this form is no different from that seen with chronic obstructive pulmonary disease.

Cobalt-induced polycythemia

It has long been recognized that cobalt is a potent stimulus for red cell production, even beyond its important role as a co-factor for vitamin B_{12}. Years ago, cobalt salts were used therapeutically in the treatment of sickle cell and other congenital anemias. The mechanism for erythrocytosis appears to be inhibition of oxidative metabolism, with induction of tissue hypoxia resulting in stimulation of erythropoietin.

From a clinical point of view, the only environmental demonstration of this effect of cobalt occurred in association with consumption of cobalt-contaminated beer in Canada several decades ago.[29] The major clinical manifestation was the development of a congestive cardiomyopathy, but many of those affected also had evidence of an increased red cell mass. Both problems ameliorated when cobalt was removed as a foaming agent from the beer. Similar effects on the blood and the heart have not been seen in the major occupational settings where cobalt is used and where the serious respiratory effects are seen, namely in hard metal manufacture and grinding and in diamond cutting (see Chapter 39.3). To date, no case of an exposed individual with significant polycythemia in these settings has been reported. Increased hemoglobin is not part of the clinical picture of cobalt-induced asthma or parenchymal lung disease.

Polycythemia secondary to asphyxiants

The occurrence of increased red cell mass in response to tissue hypoxia is appropriate, probably regulated in the kidney, where erythropoietin is produced. Not surprisingly, regular exposure to oxidative uncouplers such as cyanide or significant levels of carbon monoxide has, as a consequence, elevated erythropoietin levels and, therefore, elevated hemoglobin levels. Rarely is this manifestation serious in itself compared with the life-threatening risk of the exposure on cardiovascular function. For this reason, the main importance of the association is as an indirect sign that leads to suspicion of regular overexposure to a lethal compound rather than to its hematologic consequences, which are slight, rarely much exceeding that seen, for example, in very heavy smokers.

Disorders of platelets

Thrombocytopenia

Far less is known about environmental causes of thrombocytopenia than anemia, at least in part for reasons related to detection: the normal number of cells varies far more than the normal hematocrit, counts are less frequently obtained, and profound derangement of function or counts is necessary before clinical symptoms or signs of bleeding ensue. It may, of course, also be true that platelets are less susceptible to environmental alteration or damage, but this seems unlikely in view of the sensitivity of platelets to the effects of drugs, infectious agents, and other physiologic disturbances.

As with anemia, there are two broad possibilities for a decrease in platelet count: decreased production and increased destruction. Isolated decreases in platelet production have been described after intense exposure to a number of the complex *organochlorine pesticides*.[30] More diffuse damage to stem cells in marrow or the marrow microenvironment also may affect platelets along with other cell lines, the subject of a subsequent section. Decreased survival of platelets may be on an immune or a non-immune basis. Immune destruction has been described in association with *isocyanates* and *turpentine*. Non-immune destruction has been described in workers who have developed advanced hepatic dysfunction from *vinyl chloride monomer* exposure; the mechanism of vinyl chloride monomer exposure that dominates the clinical picture is presumably hypersplenism associated with portal hypertension (see Chapter 26.1).

Megakaryocyte hypoplasia due to organochlorine pesticides Sporadic reports have appeared over the years associating these suspect myelotoxic compounds with selective thrombocytopenia. Vacuolated megakaryocytes have been reported in two individuals with otherwise normal bone marrow, suggesting an effect specific to production of platelets. However, the natural history of these lesions is not clear, nor is the relationship to the more diffuse effects of these compounds on bone marrow function, which is more frequently described (see later).

Immune thrombocytopenic purpura due to organic chemicals Two cases of an idiopathic thrombocytopenic purpura (ITP)-like illness were reported in 1963 from a single polyurethane insulation process.[31] Each person had developed a sudden onset of asthma, presumably due to toluene diisocyanate (TDI) exposure, which was uncontrolled. One patient responded promptly to removal from exposure, whereas the other required prolonged medical treatment, including steroids and, ultimately, splenectomy. However, despite extensive subsequent experience with TDI asthma, no further cases of thrombocytopenia have been documented, suggesting that the cause was a factor unique to this work environment. In 1991, a case of recurrent polyurethane-induced thrombocytopenia was reported in a young girl who was re-exposed during home renovation.[32] In both instances, thrombocytopenia responded to cessation of exposure and systemic steroid.

Two cases of self-limited thrombocytopenia also have been described after intense exposure to turpentine; both cases occurred in children.[33] In each child, platelet counts rebounded promptly once the exposure was discontinued.

Other platelet disorders

Functional disturbances of platelets, as seen with various drugs and metabolic disturbances, have not been described in relation to specific environmental agents or exposures. Similarly, no agent is known to cause thrombocytosis or a hypercoagulable state except in the setting of a primary marrow disorder (see later) or an injury to another organ system, such as in lung cancer.

Disorders of white blood cells

Neutrophils

Although transient neutrophilia is common in a host of acute occupational and environmental illnesses, such as metal fume fever or alveolitis caused by irritant gases, it is neither specific nor important as a feature in differential diagnosis. Persistent neutrophilia or evidence of early forms in the periphery should suggest a chronic inflammatory disorder or a myeloproliferative disease; environmental agents are not known to cause such changes directly. Neutropenia may be seen in the setting of injury to the bone marrow due to ionizing radiation, arsenic, benzene, or other agents affecting stem cells or the marrow microenvironment. However, the isolated neutropenia seen in response to various drugs and infections has not been described in the occupational or environmental setting unrelated to more diffuse marrow effects, which can readily be demonstrated either on peripheral smear or, if necessary, by examination of the bone marrow itself.

Eosinophils

Mild eosinophilia may be seen in the range of environmental allergic disorders that are gamma E immunoglobulin (IgE) mediated, including rhinitis and conjunctivitis and asthma, especially when caused by large antigenic molecules such as proteins. Importantly, eosinophilia is not always present in asthma due to small molecules such as isocyanates or Western red cedar, but mild elevations, especially in atopic individuals, should not be used as strong evidence against these considerations either. Eosinophilia also may be seen in association with delayed-type hypersensitivity immune disorders, including contact dermatitis and hypersensitivity pneumonitis. In hypersensitivity pneumonitis, eosinophils may be seen variably in peripheral blood and bronchoalveolar lavage fluid.

An outbreak of eosinophilia associated with acute respiratory illness was reported in 1986 among rubber workers.[34] A careful hazard evaluation revealed that cases were largely limited to employees associated with the thermoinjection process, but a specific causal agent could not be isolated in the neoprene rubber plant. Both eosinophilia and respiratory symptoms responded to removal of individuals from exposure but recurred in some on re-exposure; long-term follow-up has not been published.

The most notable environmental disease associated with more striking eosinophilia (i.e., >1000 cells/mm^3) is the toxic oil syndrome (see Chapters 23.5 and 44). In this disease, the early manifestations include fever, pneumonitis, and eosinophilia, sometimes as high as 50% of the total white count. Eosinophilia also was very prominent in the closely related disorder eosinophilia–myalgia syndrome, caused by ingestion of contaminated L-tryptophan preparations. Neurologic, dermal, and musculoskeletal sequelae of the two disorders also are indistinguishable, suggesting a related or possibly common causal agent.

Exogenous agents have not been implicated in the hypereosinophilic syndrome, nor is persistent eosinophilia an important sign in any other toxicologic illnesses. Its presence should suggest parasitic, autoimmune, or malignant disease.

Lymphocytes

Benzene causes mild depressions of total lymphocyte counts, usually in a dose-related fashion. Depression of lymphocyte counts is an early peripheral finding and portends depression of the bone marrow, which is more serious. Occasionally, a paradoxical absolute lymphocytosis is seen in this setting. Beyond this, environmental agents, including other marrow toxins such as arsenicals, do not have significant effects on lymphocyte numbers. Even the several lymphoproliferative diseases that have been most strongly associated with environmental or occupational exposures, such as multiple myeloma or non-Hodgkin's lymphoma (see Chapter 30.3), generally are not associated with major changes in lymphocyte counts or changes in their appearance on peripheral smear.

On the other hand, changes in technology have led to considerable interest in the lymphocyte family as a target for toxic injury. Two groups of effects are worthy of mention. The first are immunologic. It is now clear that in several environmental diseases of importance, delayed-type hypersensitivity is of central pathogenic importance. Disorders include allergic contact dermatitis (Chapter 29.1), extrinsic allergic alveolitis of all causes (Chapter 19.6), and chronic beryllium disease (Chapter 19.7). For the respiratory diseases, the most specific test for diagnosis is based on identification of a subgroup of sensitized lymphocytes in peripheral blood or bronchoalveolar lavage, which reacts in vitro to stimulation by the causal agent. Further, in chronic beryllium disease, at least, this specific reactivity is associated with depression of function of lymphocytes globally, which is clinically recognizable by anergy.

At present, possible roles for lymphocytes in the pathogenesis of many other occupational and environmental diseases are being explored, including asthma, pneumoconioses, malignancies, and multiple chemical sensitivities. In the attempt to study these conditions, various populations and individuals are having a variety of sophisticated studies performed on lymphocytes from peripheral blood and other internal sites. Tests may include in-vitro responses to various antigens, subtyping by measurement of receptors on cell surfaces, and others. In general, these tests are research tools that at present have virtually no direct clinical application in medicine except when gross alterations are seen, as with various infections like the human immunodeficiency virus (HIV). For now, it is premature to attempt to interpret more subtle changes as either indicative of an effect of an environmental agent in an individual or predictive of risk for later health effects.

A second important area of focus on lymphocytes has been on the integrity of their genome. Because lymphocytes have very long lives in the body and are very accessible to study, evolving technologies have begun to look at aberrations of chromosomes in lymphocytes as a function of environmental exposures. This approach may be accomplished either by direct staining of the cells (banding) and performance of routine cytogenetic analysis or by co-culture with DNA base-pair analogs, which allows detection of more subtle sister chromatid exchanges. At present, the state of the art is such that several established human carcinogenic agents, including ionizing radiation, chemotherapeutic alkylating agents, cigarette smoke, and benzene, have been proved to increase the background rates of these chromosomal changes. Several other exposures also have been shown consistently to enhance the rate of such changes, such as ethylene oxide and some pesticides. What has not been demonstrated is any causal connection between increased rates of chromosomal alterations in these long-lived cells and any direct health effect, malignant or otherwise. Therefore, at the present time, these effects on lymphocytes, while interesting and possibly helpful in determining the range of biologic effects of an agent, cannot be equated with early effects themselves or even act as clear markers of early effects. Furthermore, the level of such alterations measured in a subject who may have been exposed to one or more agents of interest cannot be equated with a risk for any outcome of importance or interest at this time.

DISORDERS OF BONE MARROW STEM CELLS AND MICROENVIRONMENT

Disorders of the blood-forming organ in bone marrow are typically recognized when signs or symptoms develop that are referable to a deficiency of one or more cell lines or when a CBC demonstrates such deficiencies of multiple lines in an asymptomatic person. Examination of bone marrow may reveal that the marrow is impaired secondary to an external or systemic disease, such as infiltration with granulomas and tumor or blood-borne infection, or the marrow itself may be the problem. Secondary involvement of the marrow can be distinguished by examination of a bone marrow aspirate and a biopsy, combined with a culture for viral, mycobacterial, fungal, or bacterial organisms. The following section considers the primary disturbances of the marrow that may be produced by environmental toxicity. As will be apparent, these disorders range over a spectrum from those that are clearly benign (i.e., they are not associated with the presence of a malignant clone of cells) to those that are obviously neoplastic (i.e., myeloproliferative diseases and leukemias). Between these two extremes are a collection of conditions that share features of both. We consider here all of those conditions that are not frankly neoplastic. Hematopoietic malignancies are considered separately in Chapter 30.3.

Aplastic anemia (bone marrow hypoplasia)

Aplastic anemia is an imprecise but time-honored term that refers to the primary depression of the precursors of multiple cell lines, usually all of them. When the defect is limited to erythropoietic cells only, with normal cellularity in other lines, the term pure red cell aplasia is used; similar isolated defects of the other cell lines also have occasionally been described.[35] The hallmark of aplastic anemia is decreased cellularity of the bone marrow, in which the cellular material (if any can be found) generally is normal morphologically and the remainder of the marrow space is occupied by fat.[36]

Although aplastic anemia is rare (affecting about three persons per 100,000 per year), a substantial fraction of all cases appear to occur as a result of an identifiable event or exposure, including certain infections, drugs, and environmental agents. Established and suspect environmental agents are listed in Table 21.3. A small fraction of cases occur in young individuals with apparent chromosomal instability syndromes such as Fanconi's anemia.

Pathogenesis

Aplastic anemia may be induced by injury to the marrow in one of three ways. First, the primitive stem cells, which differentiate into all cell lines, may be directly destroyed or

Known causes
Trinitrotoluene
Dinitrotoluene
Benzene
Lindane (gamma-benzene hexachloride)
Ionizing radiation
Arsenic/arsenicals
Alkylating agents
Suspect causes
2,3,7,8 TCDD (Dioxin)
Chlordane
DDT
Ethylene glycol ethers
Paradichlorobenzene
Pentachlorophenol
Reported causes
Diclorvos
Organophosphate insecticides
Stoddard solvent
Methoxychlor
Chlorophenothane
Toxaphene

Table 21.3 Environmental causes of aplastic anemia

inhibited. Second, an immunologic reaction may be initiated, which secondarily leads to cell-mediated or antibody-mediated attack on these primitive stem cells. Third, the mesenchymal stromal cells, which appear necessary to support the growth and differentiation of stem cells, may be injured. Although many of the functions of these slowly replicating cells remain to be elucidated, it is known that they secrete many of the cytokines and other factors, such as interleukins, that are obligate growth factors for stem cells.

The sites and mechanisms of injury are not completely understood for any of the agents known or suspected to cause aplastic anemia, which are listed in Table 21.3. Using available in-vitro culture techniques to grow marrow stem cells in their own or autologous environments, it appears likely that direct injury to stem cells is a major dose-related consequence of ionizing radiation and radiomimetic chemotherapeutic drugs. By interaction of radical metabolites with stem cell chromosomes, benzene probably also disrupts the function of stem cells directly. The apparent reversibility of the effects of many of the toxins in animal experiments and human experience suggests a primary role for the rapid turnover of stem cells, which return to normal or apparently normal kinetics after removal of the toxin from the marrow. One could infer that failure of the condition to reverse in more severe cases or with higher experimental doses may be related to total or near-total eradication of the vital stem cell line.

Substantial experimental evidence is mounting, however, to support the view that stromal injury may be as important or even more important than injury to stem cells themselves. Stem cells from irradiated animals do not replicate normally in the environment of irradiated marrow despite their return to normal numbers and full growth and differentiation potential when transplanted into non-irradiated animals. Similar results also have been found with alkylating agents, distinguishing them from various antimetabolites, which depress stem cells only transiently. This factor is extremely important because it may explain the long delay in recovery from even sublethal marrow injuries. Further, damage to the microenvironment of the marrow may explain the emergence of late consequences of aplastic anemia that occur up to many years after apparently normal recovery.

However, aplastic anemia does not appear to occur unless there is injury to the stem cell, either directly or via immunologic attack. Further, damaged stromal cells themselves do not appear capable of causing this type of injury de novo, although they may participate in the occurrence or unmasking of malignant clones (see later). Thus, aplastic anemia itself is not a late consequence of environmental damage to the bone marrow, unlike the myelodysplastic and myeloproliferative syndromes, which do occur later. Excess cases of aplastic anemia have not been seen in populations that have been subjected to ionizing radiation after the initial period, nor do cases spontaneously occur long after exposure to chemotherapy, benzene, or other primary causes, such as drugs or viruses.

Presentation and diagnosis

The diagnosis of aplastic anemia is suggested by the finding of depressed counts of two or more cell lines on the peripheral smear of an individual, with or without clinical symptoms. Generally, the physical examination is normal except for the effects of low cell counts, such as fever, pallor, and petechiae. In particular, lymphadenopathy and splenomegaly usually are absent; their presence should raise alternative considerations. However, because a bone marrow examination is necessary in any event, the differential diagnosis usually revolves around the result of this examination.

Even when the typical findings of aplastic anemia are present on evaluation of the marrow – hypocellularity with normal or near-normal cell morphology and absence of infiltrating cells or fibrosis – there remain two important tasks in the differential diagnosis. First, the diagnosis of aplastic anemia must be confirmed. Second, a detailed search for the cause must be undertaken. Confirmation of the diagnosis of aplastic anemia requires exclusion of diseases that may closely mimic it, including certain infections (typical and atypical tuberculosis, HIV, cytomegalovirus [CMV] infection) and leukemia occurring without blasts, so-called aleukemic leukemia, now generally called myelodysplastic syndrome (MDS). Rarely, carcinomatosis may be missed on a single biopsy. Exclusion of these possibilities with obviously different indications for treatment generally requires careful culture of the marrow and other specimens, performance of stem cell cytogenetic tests, and examination of multiple specimens if suspicion lingers. Once the diagnosis is secure, the search may begin for a causal agent. In addition to the environmental agents listed in Table 21.3, two other categories are important – viral infection and drugs. The viruses include infectious mononucleosis and hepatitis, especially non-A, non-B (the role specifically for hepatitis C in aplastic anemia has not yet been confirmed). The drug list is lengthy and includes antibiotics, anti-inflammatory drugs, and a host of others. For each of these possibilities, it must be kept clearly in

mind that there generally is not a significant latency period between exposure to a causal agent for aplastic anemia and the resultant syndrome. For this reason, the search should be confined largely to events and environments to which the patient has been exposed over the previous 6 months.

Given the severity of the disorder, the public health implications if others have been exposed, and the danger of continued exposure during treatment if the cause is not found, a full evaluation of the individual's home and workplace environment is warranted in every case in which the cause is not obvious, such as the administration of a drug with high potential for this effect. When appropriate, clinical evaluation of coworkers or co-inhabitants may provide valuable clues. Unfortunately, although recent exposures are sought, there is rarely any diagnostic utility to blind testing of biologic specimens for toxic agents unless the history itself is suspicious. The unanticipated presence of inorganic arsenic in urine may be the single exception to this rule (see Chapter 39.2).

Clinical course and treatment

The natural history of aplastic anemia follows one of four pathways.

1. Some cases reverse spontaneously, usually after the discovery of a causal agent that can be removed, such as a drug.
2. Most cases persist and require long-term support or a trial of curative bone marrow transplantation.
3. Some cases evolve directly into a myeloproliferative syndrome or acute leukemia within months to years.
4. Among those who appear to recover, late consequences such as the development of a myelodysplastic or myeloproliferative syndrome may occur.

The treatment for all but very mild cases of aplastic anemia is independent of the specific cause; all patients should avoid exposure to myelotoxic agents. Among patients who recover spontaneously or after transplant, it is not clear whether continued surveillance of blood counts or even bone marrow examinations are of any value in preventing late complications.

Prevention

Because it seems very likely that subacute injury with marrow toxins carries a far better prognosis than more profound injury, workers with even a slight risk of exposure to myelotoxic substances should be under very careful hematologic surveillance. This surveillance should include a pre-placement evaluation of CBC, platelet count, differential counts, and reticulocyte counts. These tests should be repeated at least yearly and each individual should serve as his or her own control, which permits a search to be performed for subtle changes in cell size or count that may long precede frank abnormalities. Individuals with unanticipated variations during exposure should have a full diagnostic evaluation and assessment to determine whether excessive exposure is occurring before they are returned to the same environment.

At present, there is no rational basis for the exclusion of anyone from jobs involving possible risk of marrow toxin exposure except individuals who have had prior marrow injuries or reactions to the agent in question.

Myelodysplastic syndromes

In the early 1980s, the term MDS came into vogue to describe a group of apparently related disorders of the bone marrow with the following characteristics:

- anemia, usually with macrocytosis on peripheral smear;
- abnormal numbers (increased or decreased) of platelets and leukocytes with morphologic abnormalities, but not frank blasts;
- a hypercellular bone marrow with sideroblastic or megaloblastic morphology in the red cell line and often abnormalities of myelocytic cells and megakaryocytes;
- absence of metabolic disturbances or nutritional deficiencies, such as folate, B_{12}, and iron; and
- frequent abnormalities on marrow cytogenetic studies suggesting the presence of a malignant clone.[37]

Because many patients with MDS are asymptomatic, many are elderly, and the nomenclature and International Classification of Disease (ICD) coding of the disorder have been inconsistent, our knowledge of MDS has been largely derived from well-described case series. From these studies, we can infer that MDS is not rare and probably precedes leukemia in a substantial proportion of all cases. There has been enough careful follow-up of patients who have been exposed to ionizing radiation and chemotherapy to know that these agents strongly predispose individuals to the delayed occurrence of MDS, usually 3 to 10 years after treatment with apparently normal intervening marrow recovery.[38] Further, the occurrence of fairly unique patterns of cytogenetic abnormalities in such cases, as opposed to those that occur de novo, has facilitated the search for other environmental causes.[39,40] From this viewpoint, it appears that organic solvent exposure may be an important risk for MDS. This impression is strongly reinforced by a review of well-described cases of benzene-related disease, over half of which now appear to be most consistent with MDS as opposed to aplastic anemia.[41,42] It is likely, therefore, that agents that may cause aplastic anemia during exposure can cause MDS later, but full epidemiologic and experimental confirmation of these relationships is still needed.

Pathogenesis

The careful prospective observation of cancer patients treated with radiation and chemotherapy has generated knowledge of the sequence of events in MDS. The primary lesion appears to lie in the stromal cells, which support stem cell growth and differentiation. Later, a malignant clone or clones emerge. Whether the primary occurrence of a transformed cell line, independent of the damage to stromal cells, is necessary for the development of MDS is uncertain. Also, it remains possible that the primary lesion is, in fact, a malignant transformation with the secretion of paracrine factors that secondarily impede the function of the stroma, but serial marrow studies suggest that the stromal injury is the underlying lesion and not a reaction to abnormal stem cells.

Over time, the malignant clone or clones appear to grow, with progressive deterioration of marrow function and evolution of progressively more transformed cells. Leukemia develops in 10% to 20% of cases studied.

Clinical presentation and differential diagnosis

About half of the affected patients are discovered by routine CBC, whereas the rest present with signs and symptoms referable to a deficiency of a blood cell line, as with aplastic anemia. Some patients have enlargement of the spleen and liver. Bone marrow examination and cytogenetic studies, combined with routine exclusion of other causes of hematologic disease, are generally diagnostic, although classification may be difficult if malignant features are already apparent.

Attribution of cause requires proof of substantial exposure to a myelotoxic agent at some time prior to onset, generally with a latent interval of 3 to 10 years but longer periods are well recognized. Evidence that the prior exposure was sufficient to cause even transient bone marrow injury, as would be seen with chemotherapy or high-dose benzene exposure, provides very strong support for an etiologic relationship, but this evidence frequently is not available. Further, it must be remembered that between the time of putative injury and the later development of MDS, all peripheral blood studies and bone marrow examinations may be normal. In other words, the availability of a normal CBC between the time of an exposure of interest and the occurrence of MDS does not exclude a causal relationship.

It appears that the presence of abnormalities on chromosome 5 or 7 or both also suggests previous exposure to a marrow toxin as causal. Most of the cases of MDS that have occurred after exposure to radiation or chemotherapy have had such changes while few others do. Further, in some case series, those individuals who have been previously exposed to myelotoxic agents have a far higher prevalence of such cytogenetic abnormalities than those without. Although over-reliance on cytogenetics would be premature at present, the data are very useful, especially for focusing the search for a causal factor in cases in which chromosome 5 or 7 or both are affected when otherwise none might be apparent.

Clinical course and management

MDS either smolders for a long time or evolves into frank leukemia. There is no evidence that the disease is reversible, so spontaneous remission should raise questions about the diagnosis itself. Further, no form of therapy other than support appears to offer any change in the natural history of the disease. More disturbingly, when acute leukemias do emerge, they tend to be very poorly responsive to any modality of treatment. This appears especially true for those patients who have evidence of prior mutagenic exposure.

Prevention

At this point, only reduction in exposure to myelotoxic agents appears at all likely to reduce the occurrence rate of

MDS. There is no evidence that close follow-up of individuals who have had marrow injuries offers any long-term advantage other than reassurance and early detection of MDS so that supportive care can be initiated before a life-threatening complication occurs.

References

1. Rugo HS, Damon LE. Occupational hematology. In: LaDou J, ed. Occupational medicine. Stamford, Connecticut: Appleton and Lange; 1997.
2. Testa NG, Dexter TM. Long-term hematopoietic damage: concepts, approaches, and results relevant to the study of environmental toxins. Environ Health Perspect 1989; 82:51-6.
3. French CL, Yaun SS, Baldwin LA, Leonard DA, Zhao XQ, Calabrese EJ. Potency ranking of methemoglobin-forming agents. J Appl Toxicol 1995; 15:167-74.
4. Wax PM, Hoffman RS. Methemoglobinemia: an occupational hazard of phenylpropanolamine production. J Toxicol 1994; 32:299-303.
5. Beutler E. Methemoglobinemia and other causes of cyanosis. In: Beutler E, Lichtman M, Coller B, Kipps T, Seligsohn U, eds. Williams' hematology, 6th edn. New York: McGraw-Hill; 2001.
6. Wright RO, Lewander WJ, Woolf AD. Methemoglobinemia: etiology, pharmacology, and clinical management. Ann Emerg Med 1999; 34:646-56.
7. Harvey JW, Keitt AS. Studies of the efficacy and potential hazards of methylene blue therapy in aniline-induced methaemoglobinaemia. Br J Haematol 1983; 54:29-41.
8. Klimecki WT, Carter DE. Arsine toxicity: chemical and mechanistic implications. J Toxicol Environ Health 1995; 46:399-409.
9. Hatlelid KM, Carter DE. Reactive oxygen species do not cause arsine-induced hemoglobin damage. J Toxicol Environ Health 1997; 50:463-74.
10. Franzblau A, Lilis R. Acute arsenic intoxication from environmental arsenic exposure. Arch Environ Health 1989; 44:385-90.
11. Cullen MR, Robins JM, Eskenazi B. Adult inorganic lead intoxication: presentation of 31 new cases and a review of recent advances in the literature. Medicine (Baltimore) 1983; 62:221-47.
12. Schwartz J, Landrigan PJ, Baker EL Jr, Orenstein WA, von Lindern IH. Lead-induced anemia: dose-response relationships and evidence for a threshold. Am J Public Health 1990; 80:165-8.
13. Valentine WN, et al. Lead poisoning: association with hemolytic anemia, basophilic stippling, erythrocyte pyrimidine 5'-nucleotidase deficiency, and intraerythrocytic accumulation of pyrimidines. J Clin Invest 1976; 58:926-32.
14. Manzler AD, Schreiner AW. Copper-induced acute hemolytic anemia: a new complication of hemodialysis. Ann Intern Med 1970; 73:409-12.
15. Sontz E, Schwieger J. The "green water" syndrome: copper-induced hemolysis and subsequent acute renal failure as consequence of a religious ritual. Am J Med 1995; 98:311-15.
16. Fernandes A, Mira ML, Azevedo MS, Manso C. Mechanisms of hemolysis induced by copper. Free Radic Res Commun 1988; 4:291-8.
17. Erslev AJ. March hemoglobinuria, sports anemia, and space anemia. In: Beutler E, Lichtman M, Coller B, Kipps T, Seligsohn U, eds. Williams' hematology, 6th edn. New York: McGraw-Hill; 2001:627-8.
18. Oscai LB, Williams BT, Ghetig BA. Effect of exercise on blood volume. J Appl Physiol 1968; 24:622-4.
19. Dang CV. Runner's anemia. JAMA 2001; 286:714-16.
20. Djerassi L. Hemolytic crisis in G6PD-deficient individuals in the occupational setting. Int Arch Occup Environ Health 1998; 71(Suppl):S26-8.
21. Beutler E. Glucose-6-phosphate dehydrogenase deficiency [comment]. N Engl J Med 1991; 324:169-74.
22. Ahmad D, Morgan WK, Patterson R, Williams T, Zeiss CR. Pulmonary haemorrhage and haemolytic anaemia due to trimellitic anhydride. Lancet 1979; 2:328-30.
23. Patterson R, Addington W, Banner AS, et al. Antihapten antibodies in workers exposed to trimellitic anhydride fumes: a potential immunopathogenetic mechanism for the trimellitic anhydride pulmonary disease–anemia syndrome. Am Rev Respir Dis 1979; 120:1259-67.
24. Hamilton HE, Morgan DP, Simmons A. A pesticide (dieldrin)-induced immunohemolytic anemia. Environ Res 1978; 17:155-64.
25. McKenzie JM. Vocational options for those with sickle cell trait: questions about hypoxemia and the industrial environment. Am J Pediatr Hematol Oncol 1982; 4:172-8.
26. Lisiewicz J. Immunotoxic and hematotoxic effects of occupational exposures. Folia Med Cracov 1993; 34:29-47.
27. Roman E, Beral V, Sanjose S, Schilling R, Watson A. Pernicious anaemia in the textile industry. Br J Ind Med 1991; 48:348-52.
28. Larese F, Fiorito A, De Zotti R. The possible haematological effects of glycol monomethyl ether in a frame factory. Br J Ind Med 1992; 49:131-3.
29. Weber KT. A Quebec quencher. Cardiovasc Res 1998; 40:423-5.
30. Lundholm CE, Bartonek M. A study of the effects of p,p'-DDE and other related chlorinated hydrocarbons on inhibition of platelet aggregation. Arch Toxicol 1991; 65:570-4.
31. Jennings GH, Gower ND. Thrombocytopenic purpura in toluene di-isocyanate workers. Lancet 1963; I:406.
32. Michelson AD. Thrombocytopenia associated with environmental exposure to polyurethane. Am J Hematol 1991; 38:145-6.
33. Pedersen LM, Rasmussen JM. The haematological and biochemical pattern in occupational organic solvent poisoning and exposure. Int Arch Occup Environ Health 1982; 51:113-26.
34. Thomas RJ, Bascom R, Yang WN, et al. Peripheral eosinophilia and respiratory symptoms in rubber injection press operators: a case-control study. Am J Ind Med 1986; 9:551-9.
35. Baer MR, Dessypris EN. Deletion of the long arm of chromosome 5 (5q-) as a secondary event in the course of refractory anemia. Cancer Genet Cytogenet 1986; 22:169-76.
36. Young NS. Acquired aplastic anemia [published erratum appears in JAMA 2000; 283:57]. JAMA 1999; 282:271-8.
37. Heaney ML, Golde DW. Myelodysplasia. N Engl J Med 1999; 340:1649-60.
38. Nakanishi M, Tanaka K, Shintani T, Takahashi T, Kamada N. Chromosomal instability in acute myelocytic leukemia and myelodysplastic syndrome patients among atomic bomb survivors. J Radiat Res 1999; 40:159-67.
39. West RR, Stafford DA, White AD, Bowen DT, Padua RA. Cytogenetic abnormalities in the myelodysplastic syndromes and occupational or environmental exposure. Blood 2000; 95:2093-7.
40. Nisse C, Lorthois C, Dorp V, Eloy E, Haguenoer JM, Fenaux P. Exposure to occupational and environmental factors in myelodysplastic syndromes. Preliminary results of a case-control study. Leukemia 1995; 9:693-9.
41. Hayes RB, Songnian Y, Dosemeci M, Linet M. Benzene and lymphohematopoietic malignancies in humans [comment]. Am J Ind Med 2001; 40:117-26.
42. Cullen MR, Solomon LR, Pace PE, et al. Morphologic, biochemical, and cytogenetic studies of bone marrow and circulating blood cells in painters exposed to ethylene glycol ethers. Environ Res 1992; 59:250-64.

Chapter 22
Occupational Infectious Diseases

Adelisa L Panlilio, Julie Louise Gerberding

Infections acquired in the work setting represent an eclectic group that is seldom, if ever, considered together as a single category. Occupational infections involve several organ systems, respiratory, enteric, and skin infections being particularly common. Transmission involves not only casual person-to-person contact, but also a variety of other routes in special work environments. It is thus important to consider what unique features characterize the infectious diseases that can be considered occupational.

Perhaps one useful way of thinking about these diseases is that, as a group, they tend to be transmitted during work schedules or practices that are systematized. Therefore, they can be anticipated, and to the extent that unsafe infection-prone practices can be identified and modified, they can be systematically prevented. Another common feature is that many of the occupational infectious diseases can be regarded as behavioral. To the extent that unsafe practices have been defined, and practice policies modified to reduce infection risk, continued transmission often represents failure to follow accepted standards. Although certain occupational infections can be prevented by vaccines (e.g., hepatitis B), prevention often depends on simple behavioral changes, such as hand hygiene, use of gloves, and not working while ill. Finally, the anthrax cases during the fall of 2001 in the United States demonstrate the possibility of intentional (and criminal) exposure to infectious agents in the workplace, in this instance among those handling mail.[1] These intentional exposures, fortunately, are rare events, but should be considered in assessing sources of exposure for unexpected illnesses.

Prevention depends primarily on defining risky occupational practices or environments, clearly articulating policies for preventing communicable disease acquisition; removing structural barriers to compliance with policies (e.g., providing soap, hand cleansers, and gloves; allowing time away from work during periods of illness); and promoting healthy practices through behavioral change. Because infectious diseases may represent the most common cause of time lost from work, it is important for the clinician concerned with occupational medicine to understand the relationship of specific infections to specific work environments and practices, and to give at least as much attention to prevention as to diagnosis and treatment.

INFECTIOUS DISEASES TRANSMITTED IN THE WORKPLACE

Occupationally acquired infections have historically been associated with animal exposures and unsanitary work environments. Modernization of agrarian techniques and improvement in sanitation have markedly decreased the incidence of these infections in the developed world, though they remain problematic in developing countries. While nearly all infectious diseases could conceivably be transmitted in the workplace, the emphasis here is on those that can be transmitted by casual contact or by specific work-related exposures, with emphasis on diseases that are most common, most serious, or most readily prevented. Health-care settings pose a unique challenge because of the proximity of infectious patients, susceptible patients, and healthcare personnel. Infections transmitted from personnel may have devastating effects on certain groups of patients, particularly the immunosuppressed. Likewise, certain infections transmitted to personnel, such as multidrug-resistant tuberculosis, may have serious or even fatal, consequences. Table 22.1 summarizes the microbial etiology, sources, routes of infection, categories of workers at risk, and clinical manifestations of selected infectious diseases that have occupational predilections. A detailed discussion of waterborne microbial diseases is also provided in Chapter 54. Because the treatment of occupationally acquired infections does not differ from that of infections acquired non-occupationally,[2] the emphasis of this chapter is on the recognition and prevention of these infections.

Air-borne/droplet infections

The common cold

Epidemiology The common cold is the most frequent illness causing absenteeism from work. Rhinoviruses cause up to 30% of cases, coronaviruses approximately 10%, and other pathogens – including influenza virus, parainfluenza virus, respiratory syncytial virus, and adenoviruses – 15–20% of cases. In about 40% of cases, the cause cannot be determined. The large number of viral subtypes within each

Condition	Organism	Source	Route	Workers at risk	Clinical manifestations
Anthrax	Bacillus anthracis (gram-positive rod)	Herbivores (goats, sheep), hides, wool, bones	Inhalation	Veterinarians, wool sorters, weavers	Lung: Biphasic upper respiratory infection, pneumonia
		Contaminated soil	Cutaneous inoculation		Cutaneous: Papules (painless) Ulcer (large) Necrotic eschar
Blastomycosis	Blastocystis dermatitidis (yeast with broad-based buds)	Soil, dogs	Inhalation, cutaneous inoculation, bite	Outdoorsmen exposed to soil	Lung: Acute and chronic pneumonia Skin: verrucous lesions ulcers, subcutaneous nodules Bone: osteolytic with draining sinuses
Brucellosis	Brucella abortus, B. melitensis, B. suis, B. canis (gram-negative coccobacilli)	Contaminated milk products, swine, cattle, goats	Ingestion, cutaneous inoculation, inhalation	Abattoir workers, farmers, dairy workers, veterinarians	Lymphadenopathy, chronic hepatitis
Cat-scratch fever	Afipia spp. (bacilli on Warthin-Starry stain)	Cats, dogs	Bite, scratch	Animal handlers	Skin: Papules, pustules, regional inflammation, lymphadenopathy Ulcero-glandular syndrome
Coccidioido-mycosis	Coccidioides immitis	Soil, fruit, cotton, landfill	Inhalation	Visitors to endemic areas, healthcare personnel exposed to infective spores (e.g., inside moist casts), archeologists	Lung nodule or cavity, disseminated disease
Colorado tick fever	Orbivirus	Small rodents	Tick bite (D. andersoni)	Travelers to mountains in the United States	Biphasic fever, rash, pain, vomiting, leukopenia
Dengue	Aedes aegyptii flavivirus	Primates	Mosquito bite	Travelers to tropics, military personnel	Fever, severe muscle and bone pain, hemorrhagic signs (petechiae, purpura, gastrointestinal bleeding), lymphadenopathy, rash
Encephalitis La Crosse	Bunyaviridae, California serogroup	Chipmunks, squirrels	Mosquito bite	Animal handlers, campers	Encephalitis
Equine (eastern and western)	Alphaviridae	Wild swamp-associated birds, horses	Mosquito bite	Animal handlers, campers	Encephalitis
Erysipelothrix	Erysipelothrix rhusiopathiae	Animals, birds, fish, decaying matter	Direct inoculation	Fishermen, poultry workers, farmers, abattoir workers, housewives	Local inflammation with pruritus, suppuration not present, sepsis with endocarditis
Histoplasmosis	Histoplasma capsulatum	Soil in areas with avian and bat excrement	Inhalation	Soil movers, construction workers, spelunkers, pigeon and chicken handlers	Asymptomatic pneumonitis, acute pneumonitis, mediastinal lymphadenopathy, mediastinal collagenosis, histoplasmoma, disseminated disease

Table 22.1 Infectious diseases transmitted occupationally to selected workers

Condition	Organism	Source	Route	Workers at risk	Clinical manifestations
Leptospirosis	*Leptospira* spp. (motile spirochete)	Domestic and wild animals	Inoculation of infected urine, direct mucocutaneous inoculation	Abattoir workers, veterinarians, farmers	Icteric fever: hepatitis renal failure, uveitis, meningitis Anicteric fever
Lyme disease	*Borrelia burgdorferi*	Ixodes tick from deer, other mammals	Bite	Outdoorsmen	Early: erythema chronicum migrans Delayed: meningitis and encephalitis, myocarditis, arthritis
Melioidosis	*Pseudomonas pseudomallei*	Soil	Direct inoculation	Military troops, travelers in Southeast Asia	Acute: localized nodule Latent: asymptomatic (years) Acute pneumonitis, sepsis, chronic suppuration
Monkeypox	Monkeypox virus	Infected animals or humans	Direct inoculation, bite	Animal handlers, veterinarians	Rash, fever, chills, sore throat, lymphadenopathy
Nocardiosis	*Nocardia* spp.	Soil	Direct inoculation, inhalation	Outdoor workers	Mycetoma, pneumonia with cavity and empyema, brain abscesses, skin and visceral abscesses
Orf	Orf virus	Sheep	Direct inoculation	Sheep raisers	Local lesion (hyperplastic mass)
Pasteurella	*Pasteurella multocida*, *P. haemolytica*, *P. pneumotropica* (gram-negative coccobacilli)	Domestic and wild animals	Bite, cutaneous inoculation, inhalation	Children, animal handlers	Skin: focal soft tissue with serosanguineous discharge, rapidly progressive cellulitis Lung: pneumonia Sepsis
Plague	*Yersinia pestis* (gram-negative rod)	Mammals (deer, mice, rodents, squirrels, chipmunks), carnivores, pets	Flea bite, direct inoculation, inhalation	Animal handlers	Bubonic: regional lymphadenopathy Pneumonic: pneumonia, disseminated intravascular coagulation Septicemic: pneumonia DIC
Psittacosis	*Chlamydia psittaci*	Psittacine birds, fowl, ducks, sparrows, canaries, pigeons	Inhalation of bird feces, mouth-to-beak, direct inoculation of infected tissues	Bird handlers, turkey processors	Pneumonitis, fever, headache, myalgia, arthralgia, hepatosplenomegaly
Rabies	Rabies virus	Wild animals, dogs, cats, livestock, some rodents	Direct inoculation	Animal handlers, veterinarians, children	Prodrome: fever, URI symptoms, local paresthesias Acute neuro: altered mental status, seizure, hyperactivity, laryngospasm, fasciculations, coma
Rat-bite fever	*Streptobacillus moniliformis*, *Spirillum minus*	Rats, laboratory mice, turkeys	Direct inoculation, bites, ingestion	Animal handlers	Fever, rash, arthralgia, arthritis
Relapsing fever	*Borrelia hermsii* and *Borrelia recurrentis*	Lice from humans, ticks from rodents	Bites	Campers, travelers	Relapsing fever, rash, hemorrhagic complications
Severe acute respiratory syndrome (SARS)	SARS coronavirus	Humans, animals?	Droplet, direct contact with respiratory secretions, air-borne?	Healthcare personnel	Asymptomatic to severe respiratory illness with fever, headache, dry non-productive cough, malaise, dyspnea, progressing to pneumonia

Table 22.1 (Cont'd) Infectious diseases transmitted occupationally to selected workers

Condition	Organism	Source	Route	Workers at risk	Clinical manifestations
Sporotrichosis	Sporothrix shenckii	Soil, plants	Direct inoculation	Plant handlers, miners, lumber workers	Ulcer, lymphatic nodules
Spotted fever	Rickettsia spp.	Rodents, dogs	Tick bite, mite bite	Campers, travelers	Fever, headache, rash
Tetanus	Clostridium tetani (gram-positive rod)	Soil	Direct inoculation	Unimmunized travelers to endemic areas, laborers, drug addicts	Tetanus (local, cephalic, generalized)
Tularemia	Francisella tularensis (gram-negative coccobacilli)	Wild mammals (rabbits, muskrats), domestic animals, ticks, mosquitoes	Bites, direct inoculation, inhalation, rarely ingestion	Hunters, trappers, laborers, farmers	Depends on route of entry. Ulceroglandular, glandular, oculoglandular, oropharyngeal, pneumonic, typhoidal, and septic forms
Typhus	Rickettsia spp.	Humans, flying squirrels, rodents	Louse and flea or mite bites, direct inoculation, inhalation in laboratories	Outdoors workers, granary workers, laboratory technicians, soldiers	Fever, headache, rash, central nervous system
Whitlow	Herpes simplex virus type 1 (HSV-1)	Humans	Direct contact with infected secretions	Contact sports, healthcare personnel	Localized vesicles, regional lymphadenopathy (may recur)
Yellow fever	Flavivirus	Primates	Mosquito bite	Travelers to endemic areas	Biphasic fever, jaundice, hemorrhagic complications, vascular collapse
Yersiniosis	Yersinia enterocolitica, Y. pseudotuberculosis (gram-negative rod)	Rodents, lagomorphs, domestic animals, fowl	Direct inoculation ingestion via water/food	Animal handlers, campers	Gastrointestinal: enterocolitis mesenteric adenitis Skin: erythema nodosum Exudative pharyngitis Sepsis

Table 22.1 (Cont'd) Infectious diseases transmitted occupationally to selected workers

etiologic category, as well as the potential for recurrences, account for the high incidence of the common cold, even among healthy adults. Colds are more common in the fall, winter, and early spring, perhaps because of increased crowding among children during the colder seasons.

Workers are most apt to acquire colds from exposure to young children in the home. Secondary cases among coworkers may then develop. Adults experience two to four colds each year, although the incidence among adult women exceeds that of men by a small margin, and smokers have a substantially increased risk.

The modes of transmission of cold viruses are not entirely elucidated. For rhinoviruses, transmission among experimental subjects occurs most readily by direct hand-to-hand contact, with a case followed by autoinoculation of the mucous membranes of the eye or nose. Such finger-to-mucous membrane contact is ubiquitous and unavoidable. Other viruses are transmissible by aerosolized droplets. The importance of fomites (such as drinking glasses, telephone receivers, and shared office equipment) as vectors of transmission has not been determined.

Clinical manifestations Typical cold symptoms include nasal congestion, coryza, non-productive cough, sneezing, pharyngitis, and laryngeal irritation. Fever is often low grade, or may be absent. Viral upper respiratory infections usually resolve within 7–10 days, but longer durations are not uncommon.

Treatment, prevention, and control Treatment for uncomplicated infections is symptomatic. Decongestants are more useful in relieving symptoms than are antihistamines. Expectorants, saline gargles, and other non-prescription remedies are useful in some cases. Antibiotics should not be prescribed for the treatment of colds.

Colds are difficult to prevent. A policy of work restriction until symptoms improve may prevent the spread of colds but is likely to be impractical (Table 22.2). The cost–benefit analysis of such an approach could be useful, especially in childcare and healthcare settings. Hand washing after contact with nasal secretions may be helpful. Care should be taken to use tissues when coughing or sneezing and to dispose of soiled tissues after use.

Influenza

Epidemiology Influenza is a self-limited respiratory illness caused by types A and B influenza virus. Epidemics of influenza occur annually in the winter months. Adults remain susceptible to the illness despite prior episodes of infection because the antigenic structure of influenza viruses changes frequently, leading to new epidemics.

Influenza is spread from person to person, primarily by the coughing and sneezing of infected persons or sometimes by direct contact, either with infected persons or a contaminated surface. The disease is easily transmitted, and a single index case may transmit to a large number of susceptible persons in a short period of time. Adults and children typically are infectious from 1–2 days before through 5–6 days after the onset of symptoms.

Clinical syndromes An attack of influenza starts abruptly with fever, malaise, myalgia, and headache. Respiratory symptoms mimicking those of the common cold and lower respiratory symptoms including dry cough also are frequent. Fever resolves in uncomplicated cases in 48–72 hours, but other symptoms may persist for days to weeks. Influenza pneumonia, associated with hypoxemia, cough, and interstitial infiltrates, is not common in healthy adults. Elderly patients and those with underlying immunodeficiencies and chronic pulmonary diseases are at high risk for secondary bacterial pneumonias, often caused by *Streptococcus pneumoniae* and less often by *Haemophilus influenzae* and *Staphylococcus aureus*.

The diagnosis of influenza frequently is made on the basis of clinical symptoms and signs. However, influenza is very difficult to differentiate from respiratory illnesses caused by other pathogens on the basis of clinical symptoms alone. Other pathogens that can cause similar symptoms include, but are not limited to, *Mycoplasma pneumoniae*, adenovirus, respiratory syncytial virus (RSV), rhinovirus, parainfluenza viruses, and Legionella species. Many pathogens, including influenza, RSV, and parainfluenza, cause outbreaks in a seasonal pattern. Laboratory confirmatory tests can be performed to differentiate influenza from other illnesses. Appropriate patient samples to collect for laboratory testing can include a nasopharyngeal or throat swab from adults, or nasal wash or nasal aspirates, depending on which rapid test is used. Samples should be collected within the first 4 days of illness. Rapid influenza tests provide results within 24 hours; viral culture provides results in 3–10 days. Most of the rapid tests are more than 70% sensitive for detecting influenza and more than 90% specific. Because as many as 30% of samples that would be positive for influenza by viral culture may give a negative rapid test result, negative rapid tests should be followed by viral culture in a sample of the swabs collected. Viral culture can also identify other causes of influenza-like illness when influenza is not the cause.

Serum samples can be tested for influenza antibody to diagnose acute infections. Two samples should be collected per person: one sample within the first week of illness and a second sample 2–4 weeks later. If antibody levels increase from the first to the second sample, influenza infection likely occurred. Because of the length of time needed for a diagnosis of influenza by serologic testing, other diagnostic testing should be used for rapid detection of possible outbreaks. During community outbreaks, specific virologic or serologic diagnosis is not necessary once the type(s) of influenza virus causing the outbreak have been identified.

Treatment, prevention, and control Persons at high risk for serious morbidity (persons aged 65 and older, persons with chronic underlying diseases) should receive influenza vaccine annually. Immunization also is recommended for healthcare personnel and others at risk for transmitting influenza to high-risk patients (Table 22.3). While annual immunization of healthcare personnel is recommended, the National Health Interview Survey indicated vaccination rates of only 34% and 37% in the 1997 and 2000 surveys, respectively.[3] Vaccination of healthcare personnel

Disease/problem	Work restriction	Duration
Conjunctivitis	Restrict from patient contact	Until discharge ceases
Cytomegalovirus infections	No restriction	
Diarrheal diseases		
Acute stage (diarrhea with other symptoms)	Restrict from patient contact, contact with the patient's environment, or food handling	Until symptoms resolve
Convalescent stage, Salmonella spp.	Restrict from care of high-risk patients	Until symptoms resolve; consult with local and state health authorities regarding need for negative stool cultures
Hepatitis A	Restrict from patient contact, contact with patient's environment, and food handling	Until 7 days after onset of jaundice
Herpes simplex		
Hands (herpetic whitlow)	Restrict from patient contact and contact with the patient's environment	Until lesions heal
Measles		
Active	Exclude from duty	Until 7 days after the rash appears
Postexposure (susceptible personnel)	Exclude from duty	From the 5th day after the 1st exposure through the 21st day after last exposure
Meningococcal infections	Exclude from duty	Until 24 hours after start of effective therapy
Mumps		
Active	Exclude from duty	Until 9 days after onset of parotitis
Postexposure (susceptible personnel)	Exclude from duty	From 12th day after 1st exposure through 26th day after last exposure or until 9 days after onset of parotitis
Pertussis		
Active	Exclude from duty	From beginning of catarrhal stage through 3rd week after onset of paroxysms or until 5 days after start of effective antimicrobial therapy
Postexposure (asymptomatic personnel)	No restriction, prophylaxis recommended	
Postexposure (symptomatic personnel)	Exclude from duty	Until 5 days after start of effective antimicrobial therapy
Rubella		
Active	Exclude from duty	Until 5 days after rash appears
Postexposure (susceptible personnel)	Exclude from duty	From 7th day after 1st exposure through 21st day after last exposure
Staphylococcus aureus infection		
Active, draining skin lesions	Restrict from contact with patients and patient's environment or food handling	Until lesions have resolved
Tuberculosis		
Active disease	Exclude from duty	Until proved non-infectious
TST converter	No restriction	
Varicella		
Active	Exclude from duty	Until all lesions dry and crust
Postexposure (susceptible personnel)	Exclude from duty	From 10th day after 1st exposure through 21st day (28th day if VZIG given) after last exposure
Viral respiratory infections, acute febrile	Consider excluding from the care of high-risk patients or contact with their environment during community outbreak of RSV and influenza	Until acute symptoms resolve
Zoster		
Localized, in healthy person	Cover lesions; restrict from care of high-risk patients	Until all lesions dry and crust
Generalized or localized in immunosuppressed person	Restrict from patient contact	Until all lesions dry and crust
Postexposure (susceptible personnel)	Restrict from patient contact	From 10th day after 1st exposure through 21st day (28th day if VZIG given) after last exposure or, if varicella occurs, until all lesions dry and crust

Modified from Bolyard et al. 1998[19]

Table 22.2 Summary of suggested work restrictions for healthcare personnel exposed to or infected with infectious diseases of importance in healthcare settings, in the absence of state and local regulations

Immunogen	Indications	Schedule	Major precautions and contraindications	Special considerations
Anthrax vaccine adsorbed (AVA)	US military personnel; selected laboratory personnel	Primary vaccination, three SQ doses at 0, 2, and 4 weeks, followed by doses at 6, 12, and 18 months. Annual boosters recommended by manufacturer	Severe allergic (anaphylactic) reaction following a previous dose of AVA or a vaccine component	No studies of vaccine use during pregnancy Vaccine not recommended during pregnancy Vaccinate during pregnancy only if the potential benefits of vaccination outweigh the potential risks to the fetus
Haemophilus influenzae type b vaccine		Dose not established		
Hepatitis A vaccine	Consider for adults at high risk (HIV infection, asplenia) Persons who work with HAV-infected primates or with HAV in a laboratory setting; persons at increased risk for HAV infection, or who are at increased risk of complications of HAV infection; travelers to countries where hepatitis A is endemic; not routinely indicated for US healthcare personnel	Two doses of vaccine IM, either (HAVRIX) 6–12 mos apart or (VAQTA) 6 mos apart	History of anaphylactic reaction to alum or preservative 2-phenoxy ethanol Vaccine safety during pregnancy not evaluated. Risk to fetus is likely low and should be weighed against the risk of hepatitis A in women at high risk	
Hepatitis B recombinant vaccine	Adults at increased risk of occupational, social, environmental, or family exposure	IM injections at 0, 1, and 6 months; indications for boosting are not established	No apparent adverse effects to fetus; not contraindicated in pregnancy. History of anaphylactic reactions to common baker's yeast	Test persons with ongoing risk of exposure 1–2 months after completing the primary series to assess serologic response
Influenza vaccine	Adults with cardiopulmonary disease, chronic care facility residence, medical care provider, older than 65 years	Annual immunization	History of anaphylactic hypersensitivity after eating eggs	No evidence of maternal or fetal risk when given during pregnancy; recommended after 1st trimester
Measles vaccine	All born after 1956 unless: 1. MD diagnosed measles 2. live vaccine on or after first birthday 3. laboratory evidence of immunity	1 SQ dose; second dose at least 1 month later, at entry to college, on employment in healthcare setting, or before travel	Pregnancy; immunocompromised state (including HIV-infected persons with severe immunosuppression); history of anaphylactic reactions after eating gelatin or receipt of neomycin; recent receipt of immune globulin	MMR is vaccine of choice if recipients likely to be susceptible to rubella and/or mumps Persons vaccinated between 1963 and 1967 with killed measles vaccine alone or a vaccine of unknown type should be revaccinated with two doses of live measles vaccine May be useful in some outbreak situations
Meningococcal vaccine (tetravalent A, C, W135, Y)	Travelers to areas where disease is epidemic, consider for laboratorians working with aerosolizable solutions with *N. meningitidis*	One dose; need for boosting not established	Vaccine safety in pregnant women not evaluated; vaccine should not be given during pregnancy unless risk of infection high	
Mumps live vaccine	All susceptible adults; if person was born before 1957, assume immunity	One SQ dose	Pregnancy; immunocompromised state; history of anaphylactic reaction after gelatin ingestion or receipt of neomycin	MMR is vaccine of choice if recipients likely to be susceptible to rubella and/or measles
Pneumococcal vaccine (23 valent)	Adults with underlying disease or immunodeficiency predisposing to pneumococcal infection; adults older than 65 years	One dose IM or SQ; repeat after 6 years for high-risk patients	Serious allergic reaction to a dose of pneumococcal vaccine or a vaccine component is a contraindication to further doses of vaccine	The safety of vaccine in pregnancy not studied. Women at high risk of pneumococcal disease and who are candidates for pneumococcal vaccine should be vaccinated before pregnancy, if possible
Polio vaccine inactivated (IPV) live oral (OPV)H	Not routinely recommended for unimmunized adults over 18 years unless traveling to endemic area or in healthcare occupation	IPV preferred (2 doses 4–8 weeks apart, and then 3rd dose 6–12 months later); use OPV if exposure is possible within next 4 weeks (single oral dose). Booster doses may be IPV or OPV	History of anaphylactic reaction after receipt of streptomycin or neomycin. Safety of vaccine during pregnancy not evaluated; do not give during pregnancy	Use only IPV for immunosuppressed persons or personnel who care for immunosuppressed patients. Use OPV if immediate protection against polio needed

Table 22.3 Recommended adult immunizations against selected infections

Immunogen	Indications	Schedule	Major precautions and contraindications	Special considerations
Rabies human diploid cell vaccine (HDCV), rabies vaccine adsorbed (RVA), purified chick embryo cell (PCEC) vaccine	Personnel who work with rabies virus or infected animals in diagnostic or research activities	Primary, HDCV, RVA, PCEC IM, 1 ml (deltoid), one each on days 0, 7, and 21 or 28, or HDCV, ID 1 ml, one each on days 0, 7, and 21, or 28. Booster HDCV or RVA, IM, 0.1 ml (deltoid) day 0 only, or HDCV ID 0.1 ml day 0 only	Corticosteroids, other immuno-suppressive agents, antimalarials, and immunosuppressive illnesses can interfere with the development of active immunity after vaccination	The frequency of booster doses should be based on frequency of exposure. Vaccine may be given during pregnancy if risk of exposure warrants vaccination
Rubella vaccine (live)	All adults lacking prior live vaccine or laboratory evidence of immunity	One SQ dose	Pregnancy; immunocompromised state; history of anaphylactic reaction after receipt of neomycin	Women pregnant when vaccinated or who become pregnant within 3 mos of vaccination should be counseled on the theoretic risks to the fetus; the risk of rubella vaccine-associated malformations is negligible. MMR is vaccine of choice if recipients likely to be susceptible to mumps and/or measles
Tetanus and diphtheria toxoid (Td)	All adults, prophylaxis for wound management	Two IM doses 4 weeks apart, third dose 6–12 months later, booster every 10 years	First trimester of pregnancy; history of neurologic reaction or immediate hypersensitivity reaction; persons with severe local (Arthus-type) reaction after previous dose of Td vaccine should not be given further routine or emergency doses of Td for 10 years	
Typhoid vaccine, SQ, oral	Personnel in laboratories who frequently work with *Salmonella typhi*. Travelers to areas where exposure risk is present	Two 0.5 ml doses SQ > 4 weeks apart; booster every 3 years; or four oral doses on alternate days; repeat every 5 years	History of severe local or systemic reaction to a previous dose of typhoid vaccine; Ty21a should not be given to immunocompromised persons	Vaccination should not substitute for proper procedures when handling specimens and cultures in the laboratory
Vaccinia (smallpox)	Laboratory workers who directly handle cultures or animals contaminated or infected with non-highly attenuated vaccinia virus, recombinant vaccinia viruses derived from non-highly attenuated vaccinia strains, or other orthopoxviruses that infect humans (e.g., monkeypox, cowpox, vaccinia, and variola), workers investigating or caring for animal or human monkeypox cases	One dose administered with a bifurcated needle; boosters every 10 years	Vaccinia vaccine should not be administered for routine non-emergency indications if these conditions are present among either recipients or their household contacts: eczema, pregnancy, immunosuppression, anaphylactic reactions to neomycin, polymyxin, streptomycin, and chlortetracycline	Recently vaccinated healthcare personnel should avoid contact with unvaccinated patients, particularly those with immunodeficiencies, until the scab has separated from the skin at the vaccination site
Varicella	Healthcare personnel without reliable history of varicella or laboratory evidence of immunity	Two 0.5 ml doses SQ, 4–8 weeks apart if ≥ 13 years of age	Pregnancy, immunocompromised state, history of anaphylactic reaction after receipt of neomycin or gelatin; salicylate use should be avoided for 6 weeks after vaccination	Serologic testing before vaccination may be cost-effective because up to 93% of persons with history of varicella are immune

Adapted from Bolyard et al. 1998[19] and CDCP 1997.[54]

Table 22.3 (Cont'd) Recommended adult immunizations against selected infections

had been associated with reduced work absenteeism and fewer deaths among nursing home patients.[3,4] Most employers do not provide influenza prevention programs for workers outside the healthcare field.[3]

Amantadine and rimantadine can reduce the duration of uncomplicated influenza A illness when administered within 2 days of onset of illness in otherwise healthy adults. Zanamavir and oseltamivir can reduce the duration of uncomplicated influenza A and B illness by approximately 1 day compared with placebo. None of these antiviral agents has been shown to be effective in preventing serious influenza-related complications. To reduce the emergence of antiviral drug-resistant viruses, the duration of therapy should typically be no longer than 5 days.

Both amantadine and rimantadine are indicated as prophylaxis for influenza A, but not for influenza B infection. Oseltamivir has been approved as prophylaxis for influenza A and B. Zanamivir has not been approved for prophylaxis, but has been shown to be as effective as oseltamivir in preventing febrile, laboratory-confirmed influenza illness. They are approximately 70–90% effective in preventing illness from influenza A. Chemoprophylaxis can be a component of influenza outbreak control programs.[3]

Measles

Epidemiology The incidence of measles (rubeola) has steadily declined in the United States during the last decade and is no longer considered endemic. Measles is a major cause of morbidity and mortality worldwide. The majority of cases in the United States in recent years have been imported or secondary cases epidemiologically linked to imported cases.[5]

Infected persons are highly contagious by the air-borne route during the viral prodrome, and when cough and coryza are prominent, until about 2 days after the rash appears. Infection confers lifelong immunity. Although most adults born prior to 1957 experienced childhood infection and are no longer susceptible, up to 10% may lack natural immunity. In recent epidemics, cases occurred among unimmunized children, as well as children and young adults who had received a single vaccination with live virus, and among older adults.[5]

Clinical syndromes Measles progresses in several phases. Initial virus replication occurs in the respiratory tract and leads to a primary viremic phase, which usually is asymptomatic. Release of virus from infected reticuloendothelial cells produces secondary viremia and infection of the entire respiratory system, accompanied by symptoms of coryza, cough, and in some, bronchiolitis or pneumonia. Koplik's spots, a bluish-gray enanthem most prominent on the buccal mucosa, precede development of the rash. In a typical case of measles, the rash begins on the face, then progresses to the trunk and distal extremities, and disappears in the same sequence after 5–6 days.

Treatment, prevention, and control Live-attenuated vaccine for prevention of measles became available in the early 1960s. All healthy children should receive the vaccine at age 15 months. Because 10% do not respond to a single dose of vaccine, a second dose is now recommended to improve vaccine efficacy.[7]

All healthy adults born after 1957 who have not received two doses of live virus vaccine or have not experienced measles also are advised to receive vaccine (Table 22.3). Persons who received killed vaccine have a risk of developing atypical measles, and require re-immunization with live virus vaccine. Live virus vaccine is contraindicated in infants, pregnant women, and immunosuppressed persons. Passive immunization with γ globulin is available for unimmunized persons exposed to infected individuals, but is not routinely recommended for adults. Measles rarely can exacerbate tuberculosis and cause a temporary inhibition of delayed hypersensitivity. Vaccine administration should be delayed for 1 month after tuberculin testing, and until treatment is under way in persons with active tuberculosis.

Mumps

Epidemiology Mumps is a viral illness transmitted by the oral or respiratory route during contact with contaminated fomites or aerosolized droplet secretions. Mumps is less contagious than measles or rubella but produces significant morbidity, especially among adults. The incubation period ranges from 2 to 3 weeks. Virus is detectable for 6 days prior to and 9 days after the appearance of symptoms. Most adults are immune to mumps, but 10–20% of unimmunized adults have no serologic evidence of prior infection and are considered susceptible. Mumps incidence is now very low in all areas of the United States. The substantial reduction in mumps incidence during the past few years likely reflects the change in the recommendations for use of measles mumps rubella (MMR*) vaccine.[6]

Clinical syndromes Parotitis typically is bilateral, but unilateral disease and involvement of other salivary glands occurs in some persons. Localized parotid tenderness and swelling, fever, and painful swallowing suggest the diagnosis. Aseptic meningitis is common but benign. Encephalitis is a rare but serious manifestation. About 25% of affected postpubescent men develop orchitis, epididymitis, or both, which is bilateral in 15% of cases and may be the sole manifestation of mumps infection. About 50% of cases of mumps orchitis result in testicular atrophy, but neither sterility nor impotence are common sequelae. Oophoritis occurs in about 5% of women with mumps.

Treatment, prevention, and control Two doses of MMR vaccine separated by at least 1 month (i.e., a minimum of 28 days), and administered on or after the first birthday, are recommended for all children and for certain high-risk groups of adolescents and adults.[6] Adult men and healthcare personnel with no history of mumps or mumps immunization should be screened for immunity and

---

* The use of trade names and commercial sources is for identification only and does not imply endorsement by the Public Health Service or the US Department of Health and Human Services.

vaccinated if they are susceptible. Immunization is contraindicated in persons with immunosuppression and in pregnant women (Table 22.3). Passive immunization with mumps immune globulin decreases the incidence of orchitis and is recommended for mumps in adult men with a single testis. Individuals with active mumps should be excluded from work until 9 days after the onset of parotitis to avoid transmission to others in the workplace (Table 22.2).

Parvovirus (fifth disease)

Epidemiology Fifth disease, also called erythema infectiosum or 'slapped cheek disease', is an infection caused by parvovirus B19. It is a common rash illness that is usually acquired in childhood, but can be an occupational risk for school and childcare personnel. It has been transmitted to personnel in healthcare settings.

Clinical syndromes Symptoms begin with mild fever and symptoms of fatigue. After a few days, the cheeks take on a flushed 'slapped' appearance. There may also be a lacy rash on the trunk, arms, and legs. Not all infected persons develop a rash. The child is usually not very ill, and the rash resolves in 7–10 days. Most persons who get fifth disease are not very ill and recover without any serious consequences. An adult who is not immune can be infected with parvovirus B19 and either have no symptoms or develop the typical rash of fifth disease, joint pain or swelling, or both. Usually, joints on both sides of the body are affected. The joints most frequently affected are the hands, wrists, and knees. The joint pain and swelling usually resolve in a week or two, but they may last several months. About 50% of adults, however, have been previously infected with parvovirus B19, have developed immunity to the virus, and cannot get fifth disease. Fifth disease is believed to be spread through direct contact, fomites, or large droplets. The period of infectivity is before the onset of the rash. Once the rash appears, a person is no longer contagious. The incubation period is 4–14 days but may be as long as 20 days.

Treatment, prevention, and control Symptomatic treatment for fever, pain, or itching is usually all that is needed for fifth disease. Adults with joint pain and swelling may need to rest, restrict their activities, and take anti-inflammatory medications to relieve symptoms. Transmission can be prevented by careful attention to hygiene, especially hand washing. No special precautions are necessary. Excluding persons with fifth disease from work, childcare centers, or schools is not likely to prevent the spread of the virus, since people are contagious before they develop the rash.

Pertussis

Epidemiology Pertussis, or whooping cough, is an acute infectious disease caused by the bacterium *Bordetella pertussis*. Pertussis continues to be an important cause of mortality in the United States. A dramatic decline in the incidence followed the widespread use of whole-cell pertussis vaccines in the mid-1940s. However, since the early 1980s, the reported pertussis incidence has increased cyclically with peaks occurring every 3–4 years.[7,8] Contributing to this increase in incidence is the waning of immunity over time following vaccination, particularly in older age groups. Transmission most commonly occurs by contact with respiratory secretions or large aerosol droplets from the respiratory tracts of infected persons and less frequently by contact with freshly contaminated articles of an infected person. Analysis of national surveillance data for pertussis during 1997–2000 indicates that pertussis incidence continues to increase in infants too young to receive three doses of pertussis-containing vaccine and in adolescents and adults.[7]

Clinical syndromes The incubation period of pertussis is commonly 7–10 days. Pertussis begins insidiously with non-specific upper respiratory symptoms including coryza, sneezing, low-grade fever, and a mild, occasional cough, similar to the common cold. The cough gradually becomes more severe, and after 1–2 weeks, the second, or paroxysmal stage, begins. Characteristically, the patient has paroxysms of numerous, rapid coughs generally with a characteristic high-pitched whoop, commonly followed by vomiting and exhaustion. The patient usually appears normal between attacks. Older persons (i.e., adolescents and adults), and those partially protected by the vaccine may become infected with *B. pertussis*, but usually have milder atypical disease. Pertussis in these persons may present as a more persistent cough of greater than 7 days duration, and may be indistinguishable from other upper respiratory infections. Inspiratory whoop is uncommon. *B. pertussis* is estimated to account for up to 7% of cough illnesses per year in older persons. Even though the disease may be milder in older persons, these infected persons may transmit the disease to other susceptible persons, including unimmunized or underimmunized infants.

Treatment, prevention, and control The medical management of pertussis cases is primarily supportive, although antibiotics are of some value, with erythromycin being the drug of choice. This therapy eradicates the organism from secretions, thereby decreasing communicability and, if initiated early, may modify the course of the illness. There is no pertussis-containing vaccine (including DTaP) currently licensed for persons 7 years of age or older, and vaccination with DTaP currently is not recommended after the 7th birthday. Vaccine reactions are thought to be more frequent in older age groups, and pertussis-associated morbidity and mortality decrease with increasing age. Studies are currently under way to determine if a booster dose of acellular pertussis vaccine administered to older children or adults may reduce the risk of infection with *B. pertussis*. This may in turn reduce the risk of transmission of *B. pertussis* to infants and young children who may be incompletely vaccinated. Studies among older children, adolescents, and adults examining pertussis disease burden and transmission of disease to infants might guide future policy decisions on the use of acellular pertussis vaccines among persons more than seven years of age. Currently, vaccination of children more than 7 years of age, adolescents, and adults is not recommended either routinely or as an outbreak control measure. In the future, licensure of pertussis vaccines for adolescents or adults may lead to new recommendations for the use of vaccines in outbreaks.[9]

Pneumonias

Epidemiology   Most epidemics of bacterial pneumonia in the workforce are due to community-acquired infections. However, legionellosis is one type of pneumonia which can be transmitted in the workplace. *Legionella pneumophila* is an important cause of both epidemic and endemic adult pneumonia, and it can be associated with outbreaks in the workplace. This organism colonizes aquatic ecosystems and potable water, and it is transmitted to humans by the air-borne route. Contaminated air conditioners, humidifiers, and shower heads have been implicated in outbreaks among workers and hospital patients. Outbreaks of legionellosis have occurred after persons have breathed mists that come from a water source (e.g., air conditioning cooling towers, whirlpool spas, showers) contaminated with Legionella bacteria. Persons may be exposed to these mists in homes, workplaces, hospitals, or public places. Legionellosis is not passed from person to person.

A careful occupational history should be obtained from all adults who present with pneumonia, because occupational exposures cause many otherwise rare pneumonias. Public health authorities should be notified if an occupational source is suspected so that an epidemiologic investigation to identify transmission routes and other susceptible individuals may commence.

Clinical pneumonia syndromes   Community-acquired bacterial pneumonia usually is exhibited acutely, with fever, chills, productive cough, and often, pleurisy. Chest examination demonstrates signs of consolidation that may be confirmed radiologically. Sputum examination may aid implementation of empiric therapy by suggesting the etiologic pathogen. Blood cultures should be obtained when invasive disease is suspected, and lumbar puncture to evaluate meningeal fluid is indicated when symptoms or signs of meningitis are present.

Patients with legionnaire's disease usually have fever, chills, and a cough, which may be dry or productive. Some patients also have muscle aches, headache, tiredness, loss of appetite, and, occasionally, diarrhea. Chest x-rays often show pneumonia but are not pathognomonic. It is difficult to distinguish legionnaire's disease from other types of pneumonia by symptoms alone; other tests are required for diagnosis. The definitive test is culture isolation of the organism in sputum, bronchoalveolar fluid, or pleural fluid.

Other useful diagnostic tests detect the bacteria in sputum by specialized stains, identify Legionella antigens in urine samples, or compare antibody levels to Legionella in two blood samples obtained 3–6 weeks apart. The time between the patient's exposure to the bacterium and the onset of illness for legionnaire's disease is 2–10 days.

Treatment, prevention, and control   Empiric ambulatory therapy of acute community-acquired bacterial pneumonia, not requiring hospitalization, should include coverage for pneumococcus and *H. influenzae*, if the patient has a history of chronic obstructive lung disease. Amoxicillin, trimethoprim-sulfamethoxazole and cefixime are reasonable choices, unless atypical pneumonia caused by *M. pneumoniae* or *C. pneumoniae* is suspected, in which case erythromycin is preferred. Erythromycin is the antibiotic currently recommended for treating persons with legionnaire's disease. In severe cases, a second drug, rifampin, may be added.

Preventing bacterial pneumonia is a difficult challenge. Workers at risk for pneumococcal and Haemophilus infections should be immunized, although the efficacy of this approach among patients at highest risk is debated (Table 22.3). Influenza immunization could eliminate a major risk factor for both primary and secondary bacterial pneumonias. Occupational exposures to potential pathogens should be minimized with proper ventilation. Prevention of legionellosis is achieved by maintaining an environment that is not conducive to survival or multiplication of Legionella. The necessary preventive measures may involve water treatment or modification of air conditioning and ventilation systems.[10] These preventive steps, which may be costly, should be directed at healthcare facilities, and occupational settings where cases have been identified.[11]

Rubella

Epidemiology   Rubella (German measles) virus is transmitted person to person by mucosal exposure to infected droplets of respiratory secretions. Since 1969, children in the United States have been routinely immunized against rubella at age 15 months, so that the majority of recognized cases today occur in adults and unimmunized children. Since 1992, reported indigenous rubella has continued to occur at a low but relatively constant endemic level with an annual average of less than 200 rubella cases.[7] Recent data indicate that the rate of rubella susceptibility and risk for rubella infection are highest among young adults. No large epidemics have occurred since the vaccine was licensed for use in 1969. However, outbreaks continue to occur among groups of susceptible persons who congregate in locations that increase their exposure, and among persons with religious and philosophic beliefs against vaccination. Several recent outbreaks have occurred in workplaces where most employees are foreign born, particularly from Latin America.[6] Reinfection can occur following natural or acquired immunity, but it is usually asymptomatic and only rarely accompanied by viremia.

Rubella virus is shed from the respiratory tract of infected persons beginning 10 days before the development of rash and for several days after the rash appears. The onset of the rash coincides with the period of maximal contagiousness, and infected persons are not considered infectious for more than 7 days after the rash appears. Infected infants shed virus for several months despite the presence of antibody.

Clinical syndromes   Adult rubella is often asymptomatic. Symptoms occur 12–23 days after exposure. Following a prodrome of fever and malaise, adults exhibit a maculopapular rash that begins on the face and extends downward, persists for 3–5 days, and often is accompanied by regional lymphadenopathy of the head and neck, which persists for days to weeks. One-third of adult women may develop arthritis in the fingers, knees, and wrists during the exanthematous phase of illness. Children develop hemorrhagic complications more often than adults. In contrast, encephalitis, albeit rare, is more common in adults and is fatal in 20–50% of cases.

Maternal rubella infection acquired in the first 20 weeks of gestation frequently results in congenital rubella. The earlier in pregnancy rubella occurs, the more severe the fetal consequences. Infection in the first trimester results in deafness, congenital heart disease, cataracts or glaucoma, endocrine abnormalities, and mental retardation in up to 60% of newborns. Spontaneous abortion also occurs commonly.

Treatment, prevention, and control   Immunization of children and susceptible adults with live attenuated rubella virus effectively prevents rubella and accounts for the dramatic decline in the incidence of this disease in the United States. However, many adult women of childbearing age remain susceptible to rubella and require immunization prior to conception to prevent congenital rubella. The hemagglutination-inhibition serologic assay detects natural or acquired immunity. The Advisory Committee on Immunization Practices (ACIP) recommends screening of healthcare personnel who have not been vaccinated, and immunization of susceptible individuals.[7] Complications of rubella vaccine occur among adults and include low-grade fever, symmetric polyarthralgias, distal paresthesias, lymphadenopathy, and rash. Vaccine is contraindicated in immunosuppressed persons and pregnant women. Pregnancy should be avoided for 3 months after vaccination (Table 22.3).

Susceptible household contacts of infected adults and children pose a transmission risk in the workplace during the period of virus shedding, beginning about 10 days before the development of rash (about 1 week after exposure) until 7 days after rash appears. Therefore, susceptible individuals should not report to work during this time interval (Table 22.2).

Tuberculosis

Epidemiology   Tuberculosis (TB) is caused by *Mycobacterium tuberculosis* and, rarely today, by *M. bovis*. The incidence of tuberculosis (TB) in the United States declined steadily until the mid-1980s, but then sharply increased, especially in urban areas. The resurgence of TB in the United States in the late 1980s and early 1990s was associated with the emergence of multidrug-resistant TB (MDR-TB) and the HIV/AIDS epidemic. With this resurgence of TB in the United States came several high-profile nosocomial outbreaks associated with lapses in infection control practices and delays in diagnosis and treatment of persons with infectious TB, as well as

the appearance and transmission of MDR-TB strains. Since 1992, the declines in the overall number of reported TB cases, including the level of MDR-TB, appear to reflect successful efforts to strengthen TB control following the resurgence of TB and the emergence of MDR-TB.[12]

Activities emphasizing the first priority of TB control (i.e., promptly identifying persons with TB, initiating appropriate therapy, and ensuring completion of therapy) have been the most important factors in achieving this improvement. Such activities reduced community transmission of *M. tuberculosis*, particularly in areas with a high incidence of AIDS. Improvements in implementation of infection control measures in healthcare settings, concurrent with mobilization of the nation's TB control programs, succeeded in reversing the upsurge in reported cases of TB, and case rates have declined to their lowest levels to date. The threat of MDR-TB is decreasing, and the transmission of TB in healthcare facilities continues to abate due to implementation of infection controls and reductions in community rates of TB.

Nevertheless, some healthcare personnel are at risk for acquiring TB. Pulmonary TB is most commonly transmitted in healthcare settings by inhalation of aerosolized droplet nuclei derived from the respiratory secretions of patients with active respiratory TB. Close contact usually is required. Most other categories of workers generally are not at risk without close and sustained workplace contact with a person who has active untreated disease. Ingestion of unpasteurized milk from cows infected with *M. bovis* is no longer an important source of TB in most industrialized countries.

Clinical syndromes   Primary infection usually is asymptomatic in adults. Teenagers and young adults are at higher risk for rapid progression to active disease, usually characterized by apical cavitary disease, than are older adults. Primary infection in the elderly usually is exhibited as lower lobe consolidation with hilar adenopathy. Primary tuberculosis in persons with advanced HIV infection is commonly symptomatic and progressive.

Once infection occurs, the organism may disseminate from the lungs to other sites, including the gastrointestinal and genitourinary tracts, and bone. Normally, the infection is contained by the host's immune response at this stage. The risk for reactivation is highest in the first year after exposure and declines thereafter. However, aging and stressors such as immunosuppression, intercurrent illness, and chronic malnutrition may increase the risk for reactivation or dissemination of the disease later in life. Clinically, reactivation tuberculosis usually is exhibited as upper lobe pulmonary cavitary disease, but virtually any organ system may be involved.

Treatment, prevention, and control   Tuberculin skin testing allows determination of prior exposure to TB in immunologically healthy adults, by assessing delayed hypersensitivity to tuberculin antigens using purified protein derivative. The tuberculin skin test (TST) is the only proven method for identifying infection with *M. tuberculosis* in persons who do not have TB disease. Although the available TST antigens are neither 100% sensitive nor specific for detection of infection with *M. tuberculosis*, no better diagnostic methods have yet been devised.

The preferred skin test for diagnosing *M. tuberculosis* infection is the Mantoux test. It is administered by injecting 0.1 ml of 5 tuberculin units (TU) PPD intradermally into the dorsal or volar surface of the forearm. Tests should be read 48–72 h after test administration, and the transverse diameter of induration should be recorded in millimeters. There are three cut-off levels recommended for interpretation of the TST results.[14] In HIV-infected persons, any reaction resulting in an induration larger than 5 mm is read as positive. Among others, the presence of 15 mm or more of induration always indicates a positive test, 5–10 mm indicates a positive result in persons at risk for TB, and less than 5 mm is negative.

A positive TST means an individual has been exposed to TB in the past and is at risk for reactivation. A baseline chest radiogram should be performed on all persons with newly diagnosed TST positivity. If the x-ray study suggests active disease, sputum samples should be obtained, stained for acid-fast bacilli, and cultured for mycobacteria. Treatment should be implemented immediately if the index of suspicion is high. Public health officials should be notified to institute case management and evaluation of contacts in the home and work environment. If the x-ray study is negative, treatment with isoniazid to suppress or eradicate latent organisms may be recommended, especially in persons younger than age 35 and for those who have recently converted to positive TSTs.[13]

Although BCG vaccine is the most widely administered of all vaccines in the world, and has the highest coverage of any vaccine in the WHO Expanded Programme on Immunization, it appears to have had little epidemiologic impact on TB. Despite its shortcomings, and because of its beneficial effect in children and against leprosy, BCG vaccine likely will remain a component of childhood vaccination strategies in developing countries. However, because of questions about the vaccine's efficacy, and because it induces dermal hypersensitivity to purified protein derivative (PPD) tuberculin in most recipients, BCG has never been recommended for programmatic use in the United States.[14]

Healthcare providers should follow appropriate infection control procedures, including use of isolation rooms and respiratory protection, when caring for patients with active tuberculosis.[15,16]

Varicella/zoster

Epidemiology   Varicella virus, the causative agent of chickenpox and zoster, is a highly contagious herpes virus spread by the respiratory route from person to person. The incubation period is about 14 days, and the period of infectivity begins a few days prior to the onset of the rash to about 6 days after the first crop of vesicles appears. Immunosuppression usually prolongs the period of infectivity, especially if varicella zoster immune globulin (VZIG) has been administered. Zoster represents reactivation of

varicella virus that is latent in sensory nerve ganglia, and it is not a manifestation of primary infection except in newborns infected in utero. The incidence of zoster increases with age and immunosuppression. Susceptible persons in direct contact with zoster lesions risk developing primary varicella.

In the prevaccine era, varicella was endemic in the United States, and virtually all persons acquired varicella by adulthood. As a result, the number of cases occurring annually was estimated to approximate the birth cohort, or approximately 4 million per year. This incidence has likely decreased since licensure of the vaccine in 1995. Varicella is not a nationally notifiable disease, and surveillance data are limited.[17]

Clinical syndromes   Varicella in otherwise healthy children usually is a benign, self-limited disease characterized by low-grade fever and vesicular rash, often preceded by a viral prodrome. Varicella vesicles of primary infection appear first on the scalp and trunk and disseminate in crops showing various stages of development over the next 3–4 days. Healing results in crusting accompanied by intense pruritus. Manifestations of varicella are more severe in adults than in children. About 15% of adults with varicella show radiographic evidence of pulmonary involvement, but this is rarely clinically significant. However, cough, tachypnea, and impaired gas exchange can occur and persist for months after infection. Varicella during pregnancy can produce congenital varicella. In its most severe form, this infection can result in mental retardation, blindness, growth retardation, deafness, chorioretinitis, and a peculiar dermatomal lesion of the upper or lower extremity associated with limb atrophy.

Zoster, the most common manifestation of varicella infection among adults, characteristically produces unilateral vesicular eruptions preceded by pain in one to three dermatomes. Disseminated zoster, which is more likely in immunosuppressed patients, probably poses the same risk of infection transmission as primary varicella infection. The major complication of zoster is postherpetic neuralgia, which is especially common in the elderly and may be extremely debilitating. Zoster frequently produces cerebrospinal fluid pleocytosis and occasionally encephalitis. Immunologically healthy persons may experience recurrences of zoster, usually in the same dermatome as the initial outbreak. Zoster is a marker of deteriorating cell-mediated immunity among HIV-infected patients, and it may disseminate.

Treatment, prevention, and control   Passive immunization with VZIG is recommended for immunosuppressed susceptible persons, children with leukemia and other malignancies, and neonates exposed in utero within 5 days before delivery.[18]

Several antiviral drugs are active against varicella zoster virus, including acyclovir, valacyclovir, famciclovir, and foscarnet.[18] Famciclovir and valacyclovir are approved for use only in adults. Clinical studies indicate that these drugs may be beneficial if given within 24 hours of onset of rash, resulting in a reduction in the number of days new lesions appeared, in the duration of fever, and in the severity of cutaneous and systemic signs and symptoms. Antiviral drugs have not been shown to decrease transmission of varicella, reduce the duration of absence from school, or reduce complications. Oral acyclovir can be considered in otherwise healthy adolescents and adults or secondary cases in the household, because of the increased risk of severe illness in these groups. Antiviral therapy may also be considered for persons with chronic cutaneous or pulmonary disorders, persons receiving long-term salicylate therapy, and for children receiving short, intermittent or aerosolized courses of corticosteroids. Antiviral drugs are not recommended for routine postexposure prophylaxis. Systemic steroids in older adults (more than 60 years old) may reduce the incidence and severity of postherpetic neuropathy if started early (within 5 days of skin manifestations).

Varicella has been difficult to prevent because of the high degree of contagion in households, schools, and healthcare settings. Live attenuated virus vaccines have demonstrated efficacy in preventing primary infection, and one was licensed for use in the United States in 1995. Routine immunization is now recommended for children less than 18 months of age.[17] Varicella vaccination should be given to susceptible adolescents and adults who are at high risk of exposure to varicella. This group includes persons who live or work in environments in which there is a high likelihood of transmission of varicella, such as teachers of young children, residents and staff in institutional settings, and military personnel. Varicella vaccination is also recommended for susceptible adolescents and adults who will have close contact with persons at high risk for serious complications of acquired varicella, including healthcare personnel and susceptible family contacts of immunocompromised individuals. The ACIP recommends that all healthcare personnel be immune to varicella, either from a reliable history of prior varicella infection or vaccination, to reduce the risk of infection and its complications, and to decrease the possibility of transmission of varicella zoster virus to patients (Table 22.3).

Susceptible adults exposed to children with varicella or with disseminated zoster pose a risk of transmitting varicella to non-immune coworkers, and they should not work until the incubation period is over or, if they become ill, until all lesions are crusted (Table 22.2). Dermatomal zoster is not spread efficiently by the air-borne route and otherwise healthy adults afflicted with this illness may be allowed to work if they can avoid touching the lesions and contaminating the work environment. The role of vaccine in the postexposure management of susceptible employees needs to be elucidated. Data from the United States and Japan in a variety of settings indicate that varicella vaccine is effective in preventing illness or modifying the severity of illness if used within 3 days, and possibly up to 5 days, of exposure. ACIP recommends vaccine be used in susceptible persons following exposure to varicella.[17] Personnel should be excluded from work who have onset of varicella until all lesions have dried and crusted (Table 22.2).

Following exposure to varicella, personnel who are not known to be immune to varicella (by history or serology) should be excluded from duty beginning on the 10th day after the first exposure until the 21st day after the last exposure (28th day if VZIG was given).

Enteric infections

Acute gastrointestinal infection

Epidemiology Acute gastrointestinal infection follows upper respiratory illness as the next leading category of infectious diseases causing absenteeism among adult workers. A wide array of pathogens, including viruses, bacteria, and protozoa, can result in acute infections of the stomach, small bowel, or colon. A comprehensive discussion of enteric pathogens is provided in Chapter 54 (Waterborne Microbial Diseases). Most of the etiologic agents are acquired by the fecal–oral route; produce mild, self-limited diseases; and resolve without specific therapy. Agents of dysentery (e.g., Shigella spp.) often are highly transmissible through low-inoculum exposures. Occupational transmission of food-borne or water-borne illnesses occurs; person-to-person transmission has propagated outbreaks of many of these illnesses in healthcare settings, daycare and nursery schools, and institutions where sanitation is poor. Instances of such transmission have generally involved food handlers, who are often poorly trained and short-term employees, serving as sources of transmission to others. Occupations requiring travel to countries with poor sanitation present a major risk for gastrointestinal infections. Poultry workers are frequently exposed to salmonella infections.

Avoidance of oral contact with sources of fecal contamination is the most important strategy for preventing transmission of pathogens associated with intestinal infections. Maintaining good personal hygiene, including careful hand hygiene after using restrooms and before food preparation; proper cooking and storage of foods; and avoidance of contaminated foods and water when traveling are essential prevention strategies. Food handlers with diarrheal illnesses should not work until symptoms have resolved, and cure of bacterial infections should be documented by obtaining negative stool cultures more than 48 hours after antimicrobial therapy is completed (Table 22.2). The only vaccines for any of the etiologic agents for acute enteric infections are for typhoid and hepatitis A, which are recommended for personnel in laboratories who frequently work with *Salmonella typhi* or hepatitis A virus (Table 22.3).

Blood-borne infections

Cytomegalovirus

Epidemiology Cytomegalovirus (CMV) is a ubiquitous herpes virus transmitted by direct inoculation with infected body fluids (including blood, blood products, respiratory secretions, saliva, and urine) and through sexual contact with infected partners. At least 40% of healthy adults have serologic evidence of prior CMV infection. Infection can be acquired perinatally, in utero during maternal primary infection, during birth by passage through infected vaginal secretions, or through ingestion of infected breast milk. CMV is known to be highly transmissible in daycare centers and nursery schools. Sexually active adults and recipients of blood products are also at high risk for infection.

Infants and young children excrete CMV in their urine, saliva, and respiratory secretions for several months after infection. Virus is much less readily detected in healthy adults, but intermittent shedding has been documented. Like all herpes viruses, CMV remains latent in the host after initial infection. Previously infected persons may be reinfected with new strains of CMV.

Occupational transmission of CMV has been documented in childcare settings, where person-to-person spread through exposure to infected secretions and urine is believed to provide an efficient mode of transmission. Up to 50% of seronegative workers in preschool daycare centers have acquired CMV infection in some studies, indicating a potentially serious risk to women of child-bearing age, because of the adverse effects of primary maternal CMV infection on the fetus. At one time, employment in healthcare settings also was believed to pose a high risk for CMV acquisition. However, epidemiologic investigations suggest that most infections in healthcare personnel are acquired sexually, or from exposure to young children in the home, and not from work-related contact.

Clinical syndromes Initial infection with CMV usually is asymptomatic in healthy persons. A self-limited mononucleosis-like illness occurs in a minority, which may be complicated by hepatitis, pneumonitis, hematologic abnormalities, and myocarditis.

Immunosuppressed children and adults with primary CMV infection, reactivation, or reinfection may develop severe sequelae. Organ transplant recipients, HIV-infected patients, and persons with malignancies have a risk of developing CMV viremia, pneumonia, hepatitis, pancreatitis, enteritis, and retinitis.

Primary CMV infection at any stage of pregnancy carries a greater risk to the fetus than does recurrent CMV infection during pregnancy. Symptoms of congenital CMV infection may be present at birth, and are due to the consequences of active virus replication and resultant end-organ damage. Congenital cytomegalic inclusion disease, the most severe form of this entity, includes central nervous system disease, respiratory distress, hepatitis, hepatosplenomegaly, rash, and multi-system failure. Infection acquired from exposure to cervical CMV during birth usually is asymptomatic and detected by the onset of virus shedding 4–8 weeks postpartum.

Treatment, prevention, and control Antiviral therapy with ganciclovir or foscarnet for CMV infection is reserved for immunosuppressed persons at high risk for severe complications. The safety and effectiveness of these agents in preventing congenital CMV have not been established.

Avoidance of mucosal contact with infected body fluids is the best strategy for preventing CMV transmission. Hand washing after contact with secretions and fomites is essential, especially in nurseries and daycare settings.

The presence of persons at risk for CMV shedding in the workplace does not pose a hazard to other employees unless direct contact with infected secretions is anticipated. Isolation of infected neonates or children is not essential if hand washing is performed after contact with secretions, blood, and urine. Pregnant healthcare providers compliant with hand washing protocols can generally safely care for patients with CMV infection.[19-21] No work restriction is necessary for individuals with CMV infection (Table 22.2).

Hepatitis B

Epidemiology Hepatitis B virus (HBV) is transmitted by direct exposure to blood and other infected body fluids. Children born to infected mothers are at high risk for HBV infection. Persons parenterally exposed to blood, including multi-transfused patients, hemophiliacs, dialysis patients, and injection drug users, also are at significant risk. Sexual contact with infected partners is another efficient mode of HBV spread. In most industrialized countries, adult infections usually are acquired sexually or by injection drug use.

HBV is a relatively hardy virus capable of surviving on environmental surfaces and fomites. Transmission in households is well documented and may, in part, be attributable to mucosal contact with fomites contaminated with secretions or blood from infected persons.

Healthcare personnel and others at risk for occupational blood exposure through percutaneous, mucosal, or dermal routes can acquire HBV infection. The risk associated with accidental needle-stick inoculation of infected blood to susceptible healthcare personnel varies between 5% to 35%, depending on the hepatitis B e antigen (HBeAg) status, and hence the viral titer of the source. In up to 50% of occupational infections, a discrete exposure cannot be identified.

Hepatitis B has an incubation period of 40–180 days. The period of infectivity precedes the development of jaundice by 2–7 weeks and correlates with the presence of hepatitis B surface antigen (HBsAg) in the serum; 5–10% of persons with acute (but often clinically silent) infection develop chronic antigenemia. In the United States, up to 1% of adults are carriers of HBV, and provide a reservoir for maintenance of the disease in the population.

Clinical syndromes HBV infection results in clinically apparent hepatitis in about one-third of acutely infected adults. Clinical hepatitis may be preceded by a prodrome of fever, malaise, urticarial or maculopapular rash, and arthralgias for several days. Fever usually resolves before the onset of jaundice. Jaundice, dark urine, and scleral icterus usually are present by the time patients seek medical attention. Right upper quadrant tenderness, mild hepatic enlargement, and occasionally, splenomegaly are signs that should suggest the diagnosis. The most striking laboratory abnormality is the finding of extreme elevations in the aminotransferase enzymes. Alanine aminotransferase (ALT) and aspartate aminotransferase (AST) may be elevated to more than 10 times the normal levels, whereas the bilirubin and alkaline phosphatase levels are increased to a much lesser extent.

Fulminant liver involvement occurs in about 1% of adults and may be complicated by more serious abnormalities, including hypoglycemia, coagulopathy, and hypoalbuminemia. Hepatic encephalopathy, hepatorenal syndrome, and bleeding diatheses are life-threatening complications seen in these patients. About 10% of adults with clinically apparent acute HBV infection proceed to chronic HBs-antigenemia, and are at risk for chronic hepatitis, postnecrotic cirrhosis, and primary hepatocellular carcinoma.

Patients with asymptomatic primary HBV infection are at higher risk for chronic infection than those with symptomatic infection. While chronic persistent hepatitis, a benign illness of little clinical consequence except for the potential for HBV transmission to susceptible individuals, may occur, the major health concern is chronic active hepatitis, which eventually may produce cirrhosis, liver failure, and hepatoma.

Hepatitis B is differentiated from other causes of hepatitis by serologic assays.[23] A positive hepatitis B surface antigen (HBsAg) test identifies patients with current infection and correlates with infectivity during acute and chronic infection. Titers of HBsAg in the chronic phase of illness may wax and wane and occasionally fall below the limits of laboratory detection, so sequential testing should be performed if chronic HBV is suspected. The presence of HBeAg correlates with active virus replication and is a marker of high infectivity and high titer of HBV in the liver and blood. Antibody to hepatitis B surface antigen (HBsAb) appears when HBsAg is cleared and is positive in individuals with immunity after recent or prior infection or immunization. Persons with HBsAb are not susceptible to acute infection or chronic hepatitis B, except in the very rare case in which reinfection occurs with a strain of hepatitis B against which the normal antibody response does not provide cross-protection. Hepatitis B core antibody (HBcAb) appears before HBsAb and just after HBsAg is cleared from the serum, and this is a useful test for diagnosing acute hepatitis B in the window period before HBsAb appears. High titers of HBcAb persist in chronically infected persons and obviously do not predict immunity from further liver disease.

Treatment, prevention, and control　There currently is no treatment for acute hepatitis B. Alpha interferon and lamivudine have been licensed for the treatment of persons with chronic hepatitis B. These drugs are effective in up to 40% of cases.

HBV infection is largely preventable. Inoculation with recombinant vaccines containing HBsAg components is safe and highly immunogenic, and appears to confer protection from infection for at least 12 years (Table 22.2). Postvaccination testing should be done 1–2 months after completion of the three-dose series to document an appropriate response (i.e., > 10 mIU/ml).[23] More than 90% of

persons immunized with three properly timed doses (e.g., 0, 1, and 6 months) of vaccine administered intramuscularly in the deltoid region develop protective HBsAb levels. Factors associated with a lack of response include improper vaccination (improperly stored vaccine, gluteal inoculation, subcutaneous injection), obesity, older age, and smoking. Persons who do not respond to the primary vaccine series should receive a second three-dose series or be evaluated for HBsAg positivity.

Since 1982, substantial progress has been made toward eliminating HBV transmission in children and reducing the risk for HBV infection in adults.[24] Recommendations of ACIP have evolved from universal childhood vaccination, to prevention of perinatal HBV transmission, vaccination of adolescents and adults in high-risk groups, and catch-up vaccinations for susceptible children in high-risk populations.[25,26] The ACIP vaccination strategies for children and adolescents have been implemented successfully in the United States, and routine immunization of all children is now recommended. The Occupational Safety and Health Administration's (OSHA's) Blood-borne Pathogen Standard mandates provision of vaccine at no cost to all healthcare employees and others at occupational risk for blood exposure.[27] Substantial declines in the incidence of acute hepatitis B have occurred among highly vaccinated populations, such as young children and healthcare personnel. Vaccine should also be provided to susceptible individuals before sexual maturity, particularly to teenagers in those settings (e.g., inner cities, concentration of poverty) where HBV is highly prevalent, and to all adults at risk for sexual or occupational exposure.

Preimmunization screening for evidence of prior or persistent infection usually is not cost effective. However, postimmunization testing for antibody response is recommended 1-2 months after the 3rd dose to detect nonresponders among persons at high risk for exposure. Titers of HBsAb fall over time and may be undetectable after 5–10 years. The duration of vaccine protection is under investigation. Most data suggest that protection persists even when HBsAb titers fall below the level of detection, and routine screening and boosting are not recommended.

The need for prophylaxis for persons sustaining accidental percutaneous or mucosal exposures to blood should be based on several factors, including the HBsAg status of the source, and the hepatitis B vaccination and vaccine-response status of the exposed person. Such exposures usually involve persons for whom hepatitis B vaccination is recommended. Any blood or body fluid exposure to an unvaccinated person should lead to initiation of the hepatitis B vaccine series. A summary of prophylaxis recommendations for percutaneous or mucosal exposure to blood according to the HBsAg status of the exposure source and the vaccination and vaccine-response status of the exposed person is shown in Table 22.4.[23]

When hepatitis B immune globulin (HBIG) is indicated, it should be administered as soon as possible after exposure (preferably within 24 hours). The effectiveness of HBIG when administered more than 7 days after exposure is unknown. When hepatitis B vaccine is indicated, it

Vaccination and antibody response status of exposed healthcare personnel*	Treatment		
	Source HBsAg† positive	Source HBsAg† negative	Source unknown or not available for testing
Unvaccinated	HBIG§ × 1 and initiate hepatitis B vaccine series	Initiate hepatitis B vaccine series	Initiate hepatitis B vaccine series
Previously vaccinated			
Known responder¶	No treatment	No treatment	No treatment
Known non-responder**	HBIG × 1 and initiate revaccination or HBIG × 2††	No treatment	If known high risk source, treat as if source were HBsAg positive
Antibody response unknown	Test exposed person for anti-HBs:§§	No treatment	Test exposed person for anti-HBs:
	1. If adequate,¶ no treatment is necessary		1. If adequate, no treatment is necessary
	2. If inadequate** HBIG × 1 and vaccine booster		2. If inadequate, administer vaccine booster and recheck titer in 1–2 months

* Persons who have previously been infected with HBV are immune to reinfection and do not require postexposure prophylaxis.
† Hepatitis B surface antigen.
§ Hepatitis B immune globulin; dose is 0.06 ml/kg intramuscularly.
¶ A responder is a person with adequate levels of serum antibody to HBsAg (i.e., anti-HBs ≥10 mIU/ml).
** A non-responder is a person with inadequate response to vaccination (i.e., serum anti-HBs <10 mIU/ml).
†† The option of giving one dose of HBIG and reinitiating the vaccine series is preferred for non-responders who have not completed a second vaccine series but failed to respond, two doses of HBIG are preferred.
§§ Antibody to HBsAg.

Table 22.4 Recommended postexposure prophylaxis for exposure to hepatitis B virus

should also be administered as soon as possible (preferably within 24 hours) and can be administered simultaneously with HBIG at a separate site (vaccine should always be administered in the deltoid muscle).

For exposed persons who are in the process of being vaccinated but have not completed the vaccination series, vaccination should be completed as scheduled, and HBIG should be added as indicated (Table 22.4). Persons exposed to HBsAg-positive blood or body fluids who are known not to have responded to a primary vaccine series should receive a single dose of HBIG and reinitiate the hepatitis B vaccine series with the first dose of the hepatitis B vaccine as soon as possible after exposure. Alternatively, they can receive two doses of HBIG, one dose as soon as possible after exposure, and the second dose 1 month later. The option of administering one dose of HBIG and reinitiating the vaccine series is preferred for non-responders who did not complete a second three-dose vaccine series. For persons who previously completed a second vaccine series but failed to respond, two doses of HBIG are preferred.[23]

Hepatitis C

Epidemiology Hepatitis C virus (HCV) infection is the most common chronic blood-borne infection in the United States. It is estimated that 1.8% of Americans have been infected with HCV. HCV-associated end-stage liver disease is the most frequent indication for liver transplantation among US adults.[28]

The incubation period for acute HCV infection ranges from 2 to 24 weeks (averaging 6–7 weeks). HCV transmission occurs primarily through exposure to infected blood, such as through injection drug use, blood transfusion, solid organ transplantation from infected donors, unsafe medical practices, occupational exposure to infected blood, and birth to an infected mother (i.e., vertical transmission). HCV may also be acquired through sexual contact, but the importance of this mode of transmission in the United States is not well characterized. HCV is not transmitted efficiently through occupational exposures to blood. Healthcare personnel who are parenterally exposed to infected blood through needlestick injuries may acquire HCV infection, but the magnitude of risk (approximately 2 in 100 HCV needlesticks) is less than that associated with HBV exposure. One epidemiologic study indicated that transmission occurred only from hollow-bore needles compared with other sharps. Transmission rarely occurs from mucous membrane exposures to blood, and no transmission in HCV has been documented from skin exposures to blood. Data are limited on survival of HCV in the environment.

In contrast to HBV, the epidemiologic data for HCV suggest that environmental contamination with blood containing HCV is not a significant risk for transmission in the healthcare setting, with the possible exception of the hemodialysis setting where HCV transmission related to environmental contamination and poor infection control practices have been implicated. The risk for transmission from exposure to fluids or tissues other than HCV-infected blood also has not been quantified but is expected to be low. HCV is not known to be transmissible through the airborne route, through casual contact in the workplace, or by fomites.

Clinical syndromes Hepatitis C virus infection produces a spectrum of clinical illness similar to HBV and is indistinguishable from other forms of viral hepatitis based on clinical symptoms alone. Serologic tests are necessary to establish a specific diagnosis of hepatitis C. Most adults acutely infected with HCV are asymptomatic. After acute infection, 15–25% of persons appear to resolve their infection without sequelae as defined by sustained absence of HCV RNA in serum and normalization of ALT levels.[28] Chronic HCV infection develops in most persons (75–85%), with persistent or fluctuating ALT elevations indicating active liver disease developing in 60–70% of chronically infected persons. No clinical or epidemiologic features among patients with acute infection have been found to be predictive of either persistent infection or chronic liver disease. Moreover, various ALT patterns have been observed in these patients during follow-up, and patients might have prolonged periods (greater than or equal to 12 months) of normal ALT activity even though they have histologically confirmed chronic hepatitis. Thus, a single ALT determination cannot be used to exclude ongoing hepatic injury, and long-term follow-up of patients with HCV infection is required to determine their clinical status and prognosis.

The course of chronic liver disease is usually insidious, and progresses slowly without symptoms or physical signs in the majority of patients during the first two or more decades after infection. Chronic hepatitis C frequently is not recognized until asymptomatic persons are identified as HCV positive during blood donor screening, or elevated ALT levels are detected during routine physical examinations. Most studies have reported that cirrhosis develops in 10–20% of persons with chronic hepatitis C over a period of 20–30 years, and HCC in 1–5%, with striking geographic variations in rates of this disease. However, when cirrhosis is established, the rate of development of HCC might be as high as 1–4% per year. Longer follow-up studies are needed to assess lifetime consequences of chronic hepatitis C, particularly among those who acquired infection at young ages.

Although factors predicting severity of liver disease have not been well defined, recent data indicate that increased alcohol intake, being aged greater than 40 years at infection, and being male are associated with more severe liver disease. In particular, among persons with alcoholic liver disease and HCV infection, liver disease progresses more rapidly; among those with cirrhosis, a higher risk for development of HCC exists. In addition, persons who have chronic liver disease are at increased risk for fulminant hepatitis A.

Screening enzyme immunoassay (EIA) and supplemental confirmatory immunoblot tests are licensed and commercially available to detect antibodies to HCV (anti-HCV). Anti-HCV may be detected within 5–6 weeks after the onset of infection but a single anti-HCV test cannot distinguish between acute, chronic, or past infection. HCV RNA can be detected within 1–2 weeks of exposure to the virus and several weeks before elevations of ALT and detection of anti-HCV. Testing for anti-HCV by EIA is recommended 4–6 months after an exposure to detect infection; testing for HCV RNA may be performed 4–6 weeks after exposure if earlier detection of infection is desired.[23]

Treatment, prevention, and control HCV-positive patients should be evaluated for the presence and severity of chronic liver disease. Initial evaluation for presence of disease should include multiple measurements of ALT at regular intervals, because ALT activity fluctuates in persons with chronic hepatitis C. Patients with chronic hepatitis C should be evaluated for severity of their liver disease and for possible treatment. Alpha interferon (with or without ribavirin) treatment of HCV appears to prevent HCV replication, decrease hepatic inflammation, and improve symptoms among chronically infected persons. Persons with chronic HCV have undergone successful liver transplantation, although recurrences have been documented in this setting.

Antiviral therapy is recommended for patients with chronic hepatitis C who are at greatest risk for progression to cirrhosis. These persons include anti-HCV-positive patients with persistently elevated ALT levels, detectable HCV RNA, and a liver biopsy that indicates either portal or bridging fibrosis or at least moderate degrees of inflammation and necrosis. Therapy for hepatitis C is a rapidly changing area of clinical practice and consultation with a knowledge specialist (e.g., hepatologist) is recommended.[29]

No clinical trials have been conducted to assess postexposure use of antiviral agents (e.g., interferon with or without ribavirin) to prevent HCV infection, and antivirals are not FDA approved for this indication. Available data suggest that an established infection might need to be present before interferon can be an effective treatment.[23,29]

Because there is currently no postexposure prophylaxis (PEP) for HCV, the intent of recommendations for postexposure management is to achieve early identification of infection and, if present, referral for evaluation of treatment options. In addition, no guidelines exist for administration of therapy during the acute phase of HCV infection. However, limited data indicate that antiviral therapy might be beneficial when started early in the course of HCV infection. When HCV infection is identified early, the person should be referred for medical management to a specialist knowledgeable in this area.[23]

At present, avoidance of parenteral exposure to blood is the only available strategy for preventing HCV infection.

Human immunodeficiency virus

Epidemiology It is estimated that more than 60 million persons worldwide had been infected by HIV and that 40 million were living with HIV/AIDS by the end of the year 2000.[30] In the United States, almost 1 million persons are living with HIV.[30] Most individuals with HIV infection are active adults employed in the workforce. The primary means of acquiring infection among adults is either through behaviors such as unprotected homosexual or heterosexual intercourse with an infected partner, involving the exchange of body fluids, or injecting drug use involving shared needles and syringes. The virus also is perinatally transmitted to approximately 20–40% of children born to infected mothers, (e.g., vertical transmission). Breastfeeding is a bidirectional mode of transmission, to nursing infants of infected mothers and, rarely, to mothers of nursing infants when nipple maceration and biting occur. Since 1985, all donated blood in the United States has been screened for HIV infection. The risk of HIV infection due to transfusion of blood products screened by current methods is estimated to be 1 in 1,900,000 units transfused.[32] Screening does not completely eliminate the potential for a seronegative but infected unit from a recently infected donor to escape detection.

HIV is not transmitted by the air-borne route, by household or workplace contact with infected persons, by exposure to contaminated environmental surfaces, or by insect vectors. The virus is easily inactivated by most common disinfectants, including household bleach (diluted 1:100).

Commercial sex workers are at the greatest risk of acquiring HIV infection occupationally. The other group of workers at risk for acquiring HIV infection occupationally is healthcare personnel. Healthcare providers and other workers in contact with blood or other body fluids who sustain accidental percutaneous or mucosal inoculations with virus-infected material are at risk for infection. The magnitude of risk depends on the severity of exposure, but on the average, about 1 in 300 HIV needlesticks results in infection. The risk for infection following mucosal exposures is estimated to be lower at approximately 0.09%. In the absence of direct exposure, healthcare providers are not at occupational risk for HIV infection. In the United States, through December 2002, there have been 57 cases of occupationally acquired HIV infection reported with an additional 139 possible cases.[32]

Clinical syndromes The clinical course of HIV infection is variable and changing with the advent of antiretroviral therapy, as well as treatment and prophylaxis for infectious complications. Early after infection, within a few weeks to months, an acute febrile illness characterized by malaise, pharyngitis, lymphadenopathy, maculopapular rash, and headache may occur. The frequency of this mononucleosis-like illness has varied widely in reports of seroconverting individuals. At initial presentation of such patients, HIV antibody screening tests (enzyme immunoassay (EIA)) may be negative, but viral antigen (p24 antigen) and serologic reactivity to one or more viral components (Western blot test) allows the diagnosis to be established at this stage. HIV infection should be suspected in any person with a mononucleosis syndrome lacking a positive heterophil antibody response (monospot test).

Following initial infection, most persons have generalized asymptomatic lymphadenopathy and appear well. However, laboratory tests document a gradual decline in the number of circulating T-helper lymphocytes (CD4 cells), beginning soon after infection and continuing over the next several years. T-helper cells are essential components of the immune system and mediate aspects of both cellular and humoral immunity.

Symptoms, signs, and illness suggestive of mild to moderate immunodeficiency appear after about 5 years, when CD4 cells decrease by about 50%, to less than 500 cells/dl. Intermittent fever, oral thrush, bacterial pneumonia, enteric infections, and reactivated TB are typically diagnosed at this time. Signs suggestive of more rapid deterioration include oral hairy leukoplakia (a wart-like white growth in the oral cavity), shrinking lymphadenopathy, fever, weight loss, and elevated erythrocyte sedimentation rate. When CD4 cell counts fall below 200, serious opportunistic infections can be anticipated. Pneumocystis pneumonia (PCP) was the most common index diagnosis in the first 5 years of the epidemic, but the advent of effective PCP prophylaxis has altered the picture. Other opportunistic infections and malignancies, including Kaposi's sarcoma, lymphoma, disseminated TB, toxoplasmosis, and cryptococcal meningitis, now account for the majority of index HIV diagnoses.

With the exception of TB, the infectious complications of HIV infection generally are not transmissible to healthy individuals and pose no risk in the workplace. Indeed, the causative organisms are ubiquitous and most adults have already been exposed. Opportunistic infections in HIV-infected patients usually represent reactivation of dormant organisms when the immune system can no longer keep them inactive.

Treatment, prevention, and control Treatment should be offered to all patients with symptoms ascribed to HIV infection.[34] Recommendations for offering antiretroviral therapy in asymptomatic patients require analysis of many real and potential risks and benefits. Information regarding treatment of acute HIV infection from clinical trials is very limited. Ongoing clinical trials are addressing the question of the long-term clinical benefit of potent treatment regimens for primary infection. In general, treatment should be offered to individuals with fewer than 350 CD4 T cells/mm or plasma HIV RNA levels exceeding 55,000 copies/rnL (by RT-PCR or bDNA assay). Once the decision has been made to initiate antiretroviral therapy, the goals should be maximal and durable suppression of viral load, restoration and/or preservation of immunologic function, improvement of quality of life, and reduction of HIV-related morbidity and mortality.[33] HIV-infected individuals found to have latent TB infection should be treated with antituberculous therapy to prevent activation of disease.[13]

Persons at risk for direct contact with blood and other potentially infected materials should receive specific instruction in universal/standard precautions for infection control, as recommended by the Centers for Disease Control and Prevention[34,35] and mandated by the Occupational Safety and Health Administration.[27] For most environments outside healthcare settings, common sense and attention to personal hygiene are adequate to protect workers. Gloves should be worn to clean up visible sites of blood contamination. Environmental surfaces can then be decontaminated with disinfectant solutions or household bleach (diluted 1:100).[34,36]

Individuals sustaining accidental parenteral exposures to HIV should be counseled to undergo baseline and follow-up testing for 6 months after exposure (e.g., 6 weeks, 3 months, and 6 months) to diagnose occupational infection. Postexposure chemoprophylaxis with antiretroviral agents has been recommended by the US Public Health Service since 1996 after certain exposures to HIV-infected sources which pose a risk of infection transmission, such as needlesticks, mucous membrane, and non-intact skin exposures (Tables 22.5 and 22.6). Data from animal models of prophylaxis with these agents suggest that antiviral activity is diminished when treatment is delayed for more than 24 hours. For this reason, immediate reporting and access to chemoprophylaxis is recommended. Occupational exposure is a frightening experience. Consultation with clinicians knowledgeable about HIV transmission risks who can provide supportive counseling to the worker is essential during the follow-up interval. CDC recommends that occupationally exposed workers refrain from unsafe sexual practices, pregnancy, and blood and organ donation for 6 months after exposure to minimize the risk of transmission.

Occupational zoonoses

Zoonoses are infections that are maintained in nature by transmission between vertebrate animals, and they can be transmitted from other vertebrates to humans or from humans to other vertebrates. Zoonotic pathogens can be divided into two major groups: (1) those transmitted primarily among wild animals (e.g., *Yersinia pestis*, rabies), and (2) those transmitted primarily among domestic animals (e.g., *Sporothrix schenkii*, non-typhoid Salmonella spp.). Other infections not properly classified as zoonoses can result from working directly with animals (e.g., infected wounds resulting from animal bites) or with animal products (e.g., anthrax in carpet weavers). Many zoonotic infections present occupational risks, not only to those who work with live or dead vertebrate animals or animal products but also to workers exposed to certain environments contaminated by animals or animal products.

Thus, workers in veterinary medicine, animal husbandry, and animal research are at risk for acquiring a host of zoonotic infections specific to the type of live animal exposure, just as those involved in healthcare work with humans are at risk for infections acquired from humans. Examples of such zoonotic infections include Q fever in veterinarians, psittacosis (caused by *Chlamydia psittaci*) in duck farmers, orf (contagious ecthyma) in shepherds, lymphocytic choriomeningitis (e.g., leptospirosis) in laboratory workers who handle rodents, fatal herpes virus simiae infection in primate handlers, and more recently, monkeypox in veterinarians and pet store owners.[37,38]

Influenza A (H5Nl) (avian flu) infection was shown to have been transmitted from ducks and chickens to poultry workers in Hong Kong and has become an important source of epidemic infection in various international

Exposure type	HIV positive, Class 1*	HIV positive, Class 2*	Infection status of source		HIV negative
			Known source, unknown HIV status†	Unknown source§	
Less severe	Recommend basic 2-drug PEP	Recommend expanded 3-drug PEP	Generally, no PEP warranted; however, consider basic 2-drug PEP** for source with HIV risk factors††	Generally, no PEP warranted; however, consider basic 2-drug PEP** in settings where exposure to HIV-infected persons is likely	No PEP warranted
More severe§§	Recommend expanded 3-drug PEP	Recommend expanded 3-drug PEP	Generally, no PEP warranted; however, consider basic 2-drug PEP** for source with HIV risk factors††	Generally, no PEP warranted; however, consider basic 2-drug PEP** in settings where exposure to HIV-infected persons is likely	No PEP warranted

* HIV positive, Class 1 – asymptomatic HIV infection or known low viral load (e.g., <1500 RNA copies/ml). HIV positive, Class 2 – symptomatic HIV infection, AIDS, acute seroconversion, or known high viral load. If drug resistance is a concern, obtain expert consultation. Initiation of postexposure prophylaxis (PEP) should not be delayed pending expert consultation, and, because expert consultation alone cannot substitute for face-to-face counseling, resources should be available to provide immediate evaluation and follow-up care for all exposures.
† Source of unknown HIV status (e.g., deceased source person with no samples available for HIV testing).
§ Unknown source (e.g., a needle from a sharps disposal container).
¶ Less severe (e.g., solid needle and superficial injury).
** The designation 'consider PEP' indicates that PEP is optional and should be based on an individualized decision between the exposed person and the treating clinician.
†† If PEP is offered and taken, and the source is later determined to be HIV negative, PEP should be discontinued.
§§ More severe (e.g., large-bore hollow needle, deep puncture, visible blood on device, or needle used in patient's artery or vein).

Table 22.5 Recommended HIV postexposure prophylaxis (PEP) for percutaneous injuries

Exposure type	HIV positive, Class 1†	HIV positive, Class 2†	Infection status of source		HIV negative
			Known source, unknown HIV status§	Unknown source¶	
Small volume**	Consider basic 2-drug PEP††	Recommend basic 2-drug PEP	Generally, no PEP warranted; however, consider basic 2-drug PEP†† for source with HIV risk factors§§	Generally, no PEP warranted; however, consider basic 2-drug PEP†† in settings where exposure to HIV-infected persons is likely	No PEP warranted
Large volume¶¶	Recommend basic 2-drug PEP	Recommend expanded 3-drug PEP	Generally, no PEP warranted; however, consider basic 2-drug PEP†† for source with HIV risk factors§§	Generally, no PEP warranted; however, consider basic 2-drug PEP†† in settings where exposure to HIV-infected persons is likely	No PEP warranted

*For skin exposures, follow-up is indicated only if there is evidence of compromised skin integrity (e.g., dermatitis, abrasion, or open wound).
†HIV positive, Class 1 – asymptomatic HIV infection or known low viral load (e.g., <1500 RNA copies/ml). HIV positive, Class 2 – symptomatic HIV infection, AIDS, acute seroconversion, or known high viral load. If drug resistance is a concern, obtain expert consultation. Initiation of postexposure prophylaxis (PEP) should not be delayed pending expert consultation, and, because expert consultation alone cannot substitute for face-to-face counseling, resources should be available to provide immediate evaluation and follow-up care for all exposures.
§ Source of unknown HIV status (e.g., deceased source person with no samples available for HIV testing).
¶ Unknown source (e.g., splash from inappropriately disposed blood).
** Small volume (i.e., a few drops).
†† The designation 'consider PEP' indicates that PEP is optional and should be based on an individualized decision between the exposed person and the treating clinician.
§§ If PEP is offered and taken, and the source is later determined to be HIV negative, PEP should be discontinued.
¶¶ Large volume (i.e., major blood splash).

Table 22.6 Recommended HIV postexposure prophylaxis (PEP) for mucous membrane exposures and non-intact skin* exposures

settings;[39] lyssavirus (related to rabies virus) infections have been transmitted from bats to humans in Australia,[41] and a large outbreak of febrile encephalitic and respiratory illnesses among workers who had exposure to pigs was shown to be due to infection with a previously unrecognized paramyxovirus (formerly known as Hendra-like virus, now called Nipah virus).[41] Brucellosis is an example of a zoonotic infection in abattoir workers exposed to live or dead animals or animal products. Examples of zoonotic infections acquired by workers exposed to environments harboring or contaminated by contagious animals include leptospirosis in rice field workers, and Argentine hemorrhagic fever typically acquired by adult males harvesting corn in cornfields inhabited by rodents, which serve as the reservoir for Junin or Machupo virus.

It is beyond the scope of this chapter to review the large number of zoonoses (about 200 have been described) that could pose a risk to workers in unique jobs that involve contact with various animals or environments. For each type of occupation that involves regular animal contact, it is important to recognize the types of infectious disease risks involved, consider baseline studies and storage of serum for future serologic tests if risks are high, plan preventive measures when possible, and prepare for early diagnosis and treatment of such infections when illness occurs.[42] Some of the zoonoses, the occupational groups they affect, and their clinical presentations are included in Table 22.1.

Emerging occupational infectious issues

Infectious diseases continue to emerge, posing threats to the health of workers in numerous settings. A prime example of such a threat is severe acute respiratory syndrome or SARS, first identified in early 2003 and responsible for illness and death primarily among exposed healthcare personnel.[43] Emerging infectious issues which may prove to be challenges for occupational health include those posed by bioterrorism, biotechnology,[44] and emerging and re-emerging infections. These emerging infections emphasize the need for continued vigilance and for careful history taking about occupational exposures when evaluating individuals for illnesses that could possibly be occupationally acquired. Timeliness in identification and reporting of cases assists in the accurate estimation of the magnitude of the infectious disease problem and in the development of additional preventive and therapeutic measures.

PRIMARY PREVENTION: SCREENING, IMMUNIZATION, AND SURVEILLANCE
Initial employee screening and immunization

Screening of employees for infection with or susceptibility to infectious diseases is an important part of healthcare maintenance, especially when the occupational setting poses a significant risk of transmitting or acquiring infections. Screening also is warranted if specific interventions are available to prevent disease transmission among workers. Assessment of behaviors, such as smoking, that increase the risk of acquiring infections also is valuable so that employees can be provided educational and other interventions to modify risks.

Preventing infectious diseases in workers can decrease absenteeism and financial costs associated with disability, sick leave, and health insurance, even if the primary source of infection is non-occupational. Attending to these issues at the time of employment obviates the need for ongoing surveillance of many infections and simplifies outbreak investigations by documenting the pre-exposure immune status of contacts.

TST screening for active disease identifies those persons who would benefit from prophylaxis (Tables 22.5 and 22.6).[14] TB vaccination with bacillus of Calmette-Guerin (BCG) vaccine, a live attenuated strain of *M. bovis*, is provided for children and some workers in most European countries, but it is not recommended in the United States because of its unproven efficacy when used in adults and because it induces dermal hypersensitivity to purified protein derivative (PPD) tuberculin in most recipients, impeding the usefulness of TST as a screening tool.

Persons age 65 years and older, persons with chronic diseases or pulmonary disorders, and healthcare personnel should be offered pneumococcal vaccine and annual influenza vaccine (Table 22.3).[45]

Rubella immune status should be ascertained and men and women immunized in settings where women of child-bearing age are employed (Table 22.3). Even though rubella is not often transmitted in the workplace, outbreaks can occur among susceptible individuals and vaccination is an important public health intervention. Medical personnel should demonstrate proof of rubella immunity or vaccination prior to patient contact.

Measles vaccine should be provided to all workers born after 1957 with no documented history of measles who have not received two injections of live virus vaccine (Table 22.3). Screening for immunity to varicella and mumps is not routinely recommended, except for healthcare providers and adults with no history of infection with these agents who are exposed to young children.

All adults require tetanus immunization. Tetanus diphtheria toxoid (Td) boosters should be administered every 10 years to adults who have completed primary immunization (Table 22.3). Employees with no prior history of tetanus diphtheria immunization or with uncertain histories should receive a series of three primary vaccine injections.[45] Similarly, adults with no history of polio immunization should undergo primary immunization with inactivated polio vaccine, especially if they are employed in healthcare settings or when travel to endemic areas is anticipated.

Persons employed in occupations that pose a risk for parenteral contact with blood and other body fluids should be offered hepatitis B immunization (Table 22.3). Healthcare personnel, laboratory workers, animal handlers, first responders, and personal service workers such as barbers, tattooists, and cosmetologists are included in this category. Adults with multiple sexual partners also should be encouraged to undergo immunization. Serum banking to allow documentation of baseline serostatus is useful for laboratory and healthcare personnel at risk for other blood-borne infections such as HIV or more exotic infections.

Special immunizations

Laboratory workers and animal handlers may be at risk for unusual infectious diseases. Q fever, a rickettsial disease transmitted by the air-borne route, is a special risk encountered by handlers of sheep and similar animals. Serologic testing for Q fever titers prior to occupational exposure is important to document baseline status and to detect seroconversion at follow-up testing. Although smallpox vaccine is no longer recommended routinely, genetically engineered vaccines prepared from vaccinia may pose a risk to researchers and clinicians treating patients enrolled in vaccine trials. Laboratory workers who handle vaccinia or recombinant vaccinia preparations in culture or in animals should receive vaccinia vaccine. Healthcare personnel caring for patients immunized with vaccinia or other orthopoxviruses or tissues and specimens from patients with these infections also should be immunized. A program for smallpox vaccination for selected individuals who may be in the frontline for responding to a bioterrorist attack has recently been initiated in the United States.[46] Consultation should be obtained to determine the need for screening, immunization, and testing for other exotic infections.

Some animal handlers are at risk of acquiring rabies through bites or exposure to infected secretions and tissues. Immunization with human diploid cell vaccine (three 1-ml intradermal doses on day 0, 7, and 21 or 28) should be provided to workers at risk for rabies and for persons traveling for more than 1 month to areas where rabies is endemic (Table 22.3). Booster injections should be provided every 2 years for those with continuing exposure.

Routine surveillance and outbreak investigation

Surveillance of infectious diseases is conducted to detect increased occurrence of disease so that preventive interventions can be initiated. Surveillance can be passive (based on employee health consultations or reports from contractual providers or supervisors) or active (actual monitoring of disease occurrence).

Active surveillance for infectious diseases is not required in most occupational settings. In work environments where exposure to *M. tuberculosis* may occur – such as healthcare settings, residential care facilities, shelters, and correctional facilities – active TST surveillance among susceptible individuals is indicated. Periodic TSTs are especially important in the wake of several recent outbreaks associated with drug-resistant strains of *M. tuberculosis* in hospitals, adult care settings, and home healthcare settings.[16] Skin testing should be performed at least annually in these settings, and perhaps as often as every 6 months, for personnel at high

risk for exposure to active TB. Surveillance of teachers, travelers to endemic areas, and employees in other institutional settings where close contact with infected individuals is possible also may be warranted, depending on the local prevalence of TB.[14]

Surveillance for infections among laboratory workers and animal handlers exposed to specific pathogens should be individualized in accordance with standard guidelines for biosafety in microbiologic and biomedical laboratories.[47]

Maintaining standardized records of reportable infectious diseases is an important component of passive surveillance in the workplace. Centralized collection and assessment of these records at regular intervals may allow early detection of outbreaks of occupational infections amenable to specific control interventions. Geographic or temporal clusters of cases or clustering among persons with similar attributes or occupational tasks suggest a common source of exposure and infection and warrant investigation. Local public health officials and regulatory agencies should be consulted promptly when an outbreak is initially suspected. Reporting of occupationally acquired infections permits public health agencies to identify clusters of old and emerging illnesses and ultimately prevent them. These events should be reported as mandated by state and local regulations.[48,49]

Return-to-work criteria

Employees diagnosed with communicable infectious diseases should not return to work until the period of infectivity is past. Specific guidelines should be consistent with local public health regulations. Some workers, for example food handlers with certain diarrheal illnesses, cannot resume their duties until culture evidence of cure is obtained. Employees should be advised of the return-to-work policies at the time of employment and when illness is diagnosed. A table for length of work restriction for healthcare personnel can be used to guide return-to-work policies for the workplace (Table 22.2).[19]

PRIMARY PREVENTION: INFECTION CONTROL PRECAUTIONS
General infection control in the workplace

Common sense dictates attention to personal hygiene among all workers. Hand washing after using the bathroom and before handling food is essential. The mouth should be covered while sneezing or coughing, and soiled tissues and dressings should be disposed of in trash containers.

Employers have a responsibility to minimize crowding in the work setting. Facilities for hand washing should be available in bathrooms and food preparation areas. Proper ventilation also is important. Trash should be emptied at regular intervals, and work areas should be clean and free of pests. Smoking should be prohibited in common work areas.

Spills of blood, body fluids, and other potentially infectious substances should be removed with disposable paper towels or other suitable procedures. Contaminated areas should then be disinfected with commercial products or with a solution of household bleach (diluted 1:100).[34,36]

Infection control in healthcare settings

Infection control programs in healthcare settings are necessary to prevent transmission of healthcare-related infections to patients and healthcare personnel. The CDC has established a two-tiered system of infection control precautions.[16] The first tier consists of 'standard precautions' which are precautions recommended for delivery of care to all patients regardless of diagnosis or presumed infection status. They are designed to limit exposure to blood or other body substances and include elements such as hand hygiene and use of appropriate protective barriers, e.g., masks, eye protection, and gloves, as needed to prevent direct contact. The second tier of precautions recommended by CDC are 'transmission-based precautions', designed for the management of patients known or suspected to be infected with pathogens whose transmission can be limited by the adoption of additional measures beyond those which are part of standard precautions. They apply to pathogens transmitted by the air-borne or aerosol routes, droplets, and by direct and indirect contact.

Respiratory precautions are employed for patients with infections communicable by the air-borne route. Such patients are housed in private rooms with special ventilation and should wear surgical masks when leaving their rooms. Respiratory protection (i.e., N-95 respirators) also are advised for providers in close contact with patients on respiratory precautions. However, the re-emergence of epidemic and MDR-TB has led to a re-emphasis of other fundamentals for prevention of transmission of tuberculosis in healthcare and other settings. Early identification of TB allows early indication for therapy, and requires alertness in considering TB in high-risk patients with pulmonary symptoms, especially those with HIV infection. Special ventilation measures and respiratory protection are especially important for cough-inducing procedures, such as sputum induction and aerosolized pentamidine administration. Healthcare personnel who have the potential for being exposed to *M. tuberculosis* should be screened on employment and at least annually thereafter by PPD skin testing, comparing previous test results to current results to identify those who have converted to skin test positivity.[15]

Procedures for disposal of infectious wastes have been developed by the CDC.[36] Needles and other sharp objects should be sterilized prior to disposal. Liquid and laboratory wastes may be dumped into sewage systems. Materials heavily contaminated with bacteria or blood should be placed in special bags that are specifically labeled for infectious waste and should be disposed of according to community standards for such materials.[36]

Employers have a responsibility to educate employees about infection control. Barriers to prevent exposure, including masks, gowns, eye protection, and gloves, should be readily available to workers at risk. Hand washing facilities and hand hygiene supplies are essential. Where access to sinks or running water is not feasible, alcohol hand rubs or packaged towels containing disinfectants should be provided.

Impervious containers for the disposal of needles and other sharp objects are essential.[50] Such containers should be made available on ambulances and provided to home health aides and other visiting healthcare personnel. Personal service workers who use needles, razors, and other sharp objects also should have access to safe disposal units. Persons receiving care at home who require injections or other procedures that demand the use of needles also should be provided with impervious disposal containers and instructed in proper disposal methods to protect sanitation workers and others in contact with waste.

Infection control in laboratory settings

Despite improvements in engineering controls, work practices, and personal protective equipment, laboratory personnel are nevertheless at risk for occupationally acquired infections. Laboratory personnel may acquire infection by aerosolization of specimens, mouth pipetting, or percutaneous injury or mucocutaneous contact. Methods of infection control applicable to laboratory settings are described in the CDC document entitled 'Biosafety in Microbiological and Biomedical Laboratories'.[47]

Infection control in childcare settings and schools

By 1995, it was estimated that 14.5 million children were attending out-of-home daycare in a variety of settings including licensed child daycare centers, regulated daycare homes, and unregulated family daycare homes.[51]

Many serious infections occur as endemic or microepidemic problems in the daycare setting. These include *H. influenzae* type b, hepatitis A, cytomegalovirus, parvovirus B 19, and enteric infections (Shigella, Giardia, rotavirus, *Clostridium difficile*, Campylobacter, Cryptosporidium, calcivirus, Salmonella, enteric adenovirus, astrovirus, and several types of *E. coli* infections). In addition, the high rate of acute respiratory infections leads to early onset of otitis media, frequent antibiotic use, and emergence of multidrug-resistant enteric pathogens.

Thus, workers in close contact with children risk exposure to a wide variety of communicable pathogens contained in secretions, urine, and stool. All such personnel, as well as all children in schools and daycare centers, should be screened for immunity to common childhood infections and vaccinated if immunity is not present (Table 22.2).

Regulation of childcare facilities is essential to reduce risks to children and workers. National standards for infection control in childcare facilities were promulgated in 1990.[52] Hand washing facilities and policies are the most important component of disease prevention in school and daycare settings. Hands should be washed after contact with mucous membranes and potentially infected body fluids. Older children should be instructed in personal hygiene. Children with fever or diagnosed infections should be excluded from attending daycare or school until transmission risk is no longer present, and policies for such exclusion should be in place. Prompt reporting of disease outbreaks and prompt involvement of public health authorities are essential. Employees should be instructed in common-sense first aid procedures for handling wounds, bites, and other situations in which exposure to infected blood or tissues is possible. Barrier protection is rarely required in schools, but gloves should generally be available for emergencies requiring first aid.

Infection control for special occupational groups

Pregnant workers

Infection with a variety of agents during pregnancy has the potential to cause fetal damage, especially when primary infection occurs. While a number of these infections can be community acquired, the likelihood of exposure to certain of these pathogens can be greater in healthcare settings. Infections with as rubella, CMV, and parvovirus are among the infectious agents which may be of special concern to pregnant healthcare personnel. In general, adherence to standard precautions as well as pre-exposure immunizations when available and appropriate are the best way of preventing the devastating effects of such infections (Table 22.2).[19,21]

Immunodeficient workers

Immunodeficient workers are at increased risk of devastating infections, particularly with opportunistic agents. The greatest risk for such workers is likely in the healthcare setting where there can be ample opportunity for exposure to these agents. Many immunocompromising illnesses would be viewed by the US legal system as disabilities and therefore, individuals with those conditions would be covered under the provisions of the Americans with Disabilities Act of 1990 (see Chapter 57.1).[53] Such persons should be informed about their risks and furthermore, their employers should make reasonable accommodations to allow their employees to continue to perform their jobs, taking into consideration the provisions of applicable federal, state, and local regulations.

CONCLUSIONS

Occupational infectious diseases encompass a large variety of infections which can involve many organ systems. They include some common infections, such as influenza, that pose a special problem in the workplace because of close interpersonal contact and crowding, and that taken together account for a large proportion of time lost from work. Many of these infections are preventable by policies that promote hygiene and provide exclusion from work during periods of contagion. In addition, a variety of less common, but sometimes serious, infections are particularly associated with specific occupations. Recognition of the types of infection risk associated with specific occupations can, in most cases, lead to effective, often simple steps for primary prevention, as well as opportunities for early diagnosis and treatment.

References

1. Jernigan JA, Stephens DS, Ashford DA, et al. Bioterrorism-related inhalational anthrax: the first 10 cases reported in the United States. Emerg Infect Dis 2001; 7:933–44.
2. Mandell GL, Douglas RG, Bennett JE, eds. Principles and practice of infectious diseases, 5th edn. New York: Churchill Livingstone, 2000.
3. Centers for Disease Control and Prevention. Prevention and control of influenza: recommendations of the Advisory Committee on Immunization Practices (ACIP). MMWR 2002; 51(RR-3):1–31.
4. Potter J, Stott DJ, Roberts MA, et al. Influenza vaccination in long-term-care hospitals reduces the mortality of elderly patients. J Infect Dis 1997; 175:1–6.
5. Centers for Disease Control and Prevention. Measles – United States, 2000. MMWR 2002; 51:120–3.
6. Centers for Disease Control and Prevention. Measles, mumps, and rubella – vaccine use and strategies for elimination of measles, rubella, and congenital rubella syndrome and control of mumps: recommendations of the Advisory Committee on Immunization Practices (ACIP). MMWR 1998; 47(RR-8):1–57.
7. Centers for Disease Control and Prevention. Pertussis – United States, 1997–2000. MMWR 2002; 51:73–6.
8. Güris D, Strebel PM, Bardenheier B, et al. Changing epidemiology of pertussis in the United States: increasing reported incidence among adolescents and adults, 1990–1996. Clin Infect Dis 1999; 28:1230–7.
9. Centers for Disease Control and Prevention. Guidelines for the control of pertussis outbreaks. Atlanta, Georgia: CDC 2000. Available at http://www.cdc.gov/nip/publications/pertussis/guide.htm. Accessed July 2002.
10. American Society for Heating, Refrigerating, and Airconditioning Engineers. ASHRAE Guideline 12-2000: Minimizing the risk of legionellosis associated with building water systems. Atlanta, Georgia: American Society for Heating, Refrigerating, and Airconditioning Engineers, 2000;1–17.
11. Tablan OC, Anderson LJ, Arden NH, Breiman RF, Butler JC, McNeil MM. Guideline for prevention of nosocomial pneumonia. The Hospital Infection Control Practices Advisory Committee, Centers for Disease Control and Prevention. Infect Control Hosp Epidemiol 1994; 15:587–627.
12. Centers for Disease Control and Prevention. Progressing toward tuberculosis elimination in low-incidence areas of the United States: recommendations of the Advisory Council for the Elimination of Tuberculosis. MMWR 2002; 51(RR-5):1–16.
13. Centers for Disease Control and Prevention. Targeted tuberculin testing and treatment of latent tuberculosis infection. MMWR 2000; 49(RR-6):1–54.
14. Centers for Disease Control and Prevention. The role of BCG vaccine in the prevention and control of tuberculosis in the United States: a joint statement by the Advisory Council for the Elimination of Tuberculosis and the Advisory Committee on Immunization Practices. MMWR 1996; 45(RR-4):1–18.
15. Centers for Disease Control and Prevention. Guidelines for preventing the transmission of tuberculosis in health-care facilities, 1994. MMWR 1994; 43(RR-13):1–132.
16. Garner JS. Guideline for isolation precautions in hospitals. The Hospital Infection Control Practices Advisory Committee. Infect Control Hosp Epidemiol 1996; 17:53–80.

17. Centers for Disease Control and Prevention. Prevention of varicella: update recommendations of the Advisory Committee on Immunization Practices (ACIP). MMWR 1999; 48(RR6):1–12.

18. Atkinson W, Wolfe C, eds. Epidemiology and prevention of vaccine-preventable diseases. Atlanta, Georgia: US Department of Health and Human Services, CDC, 2002.

19. Bolyard EA, Tablan OC, Williams WW, et al. Guideline for infection control in healthcare personnel, 1998. Infect Control Hosp Epidemiol 1998; 19:407–63.

20. Centers for Disease Control and Prevention. Guideline for hand hygiene in health-care settings: recommendations of the Healthcare Infection Control Practices Advisory Committee and the HICPAC/SHEA/APIC/IDSA Hand Hygiene Task Force. MMWR 2002; 51(RR-16):1–45

21. Siegel JD. Infection control precautions for the pregnant healthcare worker. Bailliere's Clin Infect Dis 1999; 5:439–61.

22. Beltrami EM, Williams IT, Shapiro CN, Chamberland ME. Risk and management of bloodborne infections in healthcare workers. Clin Micro Rev 2000; 13:385–407.

23. Centers for Disease Control and Prevention. Updated US Public Health Service guidelines for the management of occupational exposures to HBV, HCV, and HIV and recommendations for postexposure prophylaxis. MMWR 2001; 50(RR-11):1–52.

24. Centers for Disease Control and Prevention. Achievements in public health: hepatitis B vaccination – United States, 1982–2002. MMWR 2002; 51:549–52, 563.

25. Centers For Disease Control. Hepatitis B virus: a comprehensive strategy for eliminating transmission in the United States through universal childhood vaccination: recommendation of the Immunization Practices Advisory Committee (ACIP). MMWR 1991; 40(RR13).

26. Centers For Disease Control. Protection against viral hepatitis: recommendations of the Immunization Practices Advisory Committee (ACIP). MMWR 1990; 39(RR-2):1–26.

27. Occupational Safety and Health Administration, Department of Labor. 29 CFR Part 1910.1030, Occupational exposure to bloodborne pathogens; final rule. Fed Reg 1991; 56:64004–182.

28. Centers for Disease Control and Prevention. Recommendations for prevention and control of hepatitis C Virus (HCV) infection and HCV-related chronic disease. MMWR 1998; 47(RR-19):1–39.

29. National Institutes of Health Consensus Development Conference Panel Statement. Management of Hepatitis C. Hepatology 2002; 36:S3–20.

30. DeCock KM, Janssen RS. An unequal epidemic in an unequal world. JAMA 2002; 288:236–8.

31. Schreiber GB, Busch MP, Kleinman SH, Korelitz JJ. The risk of transfusion-transmitted viral infections. N Engl J Med 1996; 334:1685–90.

32. Centers for Disease Control and Prevention. Surveillance of healthcare personnel with HIV/AIDS, as of December 2002. Fact sheet. Available at http://www.cdc.gov/ncidod/hip/BLOOD/hivpersonnel.htm. Accessed December 19, 2003.

33. Department of Health and Human Services, Panel on Clinical Practices for the Treatment of HIV Infection. Guidelines for the use of antiretroviral agents in HIV-infected adults and adolescents. US Department of Health and Human Services, March 23, 2004. Available at http://aidsinfo.nih.gov/guidelines/adult%5CAA_032404.pdf. Accessed March 25, 2004.

34. Centers For Disease Control. Recommendations for prevention of HIV transmission in healthcare settings. MMWR 1987; 36(Suppl 2S):15–18S.

35. Centers for Disease Control. Update: universal precautions for prevention of transmission of human immunodeficiency virus, hepatitis B virus, and other bloodborne pathogens in health-care settings. MMWR 1988; 37:377–82, 387–8.

36. Centers for Disease Control and Prevention. Guideline for environmental control in healthcare facilities. MMWR 2003; 52(RR-10):1–44.

37. Centers for Disease Control and Prevention. Monkeypox home page at http://www.cdc.gov/ncidod/monkeypox/index.htm. Accessed August 6, 2003.

38. Centers for Disease Control and Prevention. Multistate outbreak of monkeypox – Illinois, Indiana, and Wisconsin, 2003. MMWR 2003; 52:537–40.

39. Bridges CB, Lim W, Hu-Primmer J, et al. Risk of influenza A (H5N1) infection among poultry workers, Hong Kong, 1997–1998. J Infect Dis 2002; 185:1005–10.

40. Mackenzie JS. Emerging viral diseases: an Australian perspective. Emerg Infect Dis 1999; 5:1–8.

41. Centers for Disease Control and Prevention. Outbreak of Hendra-like virus – Malaysia and Singapore, 1998–1999. MMWR 1999; 48:265–9.

42. Weber DJ, Rutala WA. Risks and prevention of nosocomial transmission of rare zoonotic diseases. Clin Infect Dis 2001; 32:446–56.

43. Drazen J. SARS – looking back over the first 100 days. N Engl J Med 2003; 349:319–20.

44. Eckebrecht T. Occupational standards for the protection of employees in biotechnology. Int Arch Occup Environ Health 2000; 73(Suppl):S4–7.

45. Centers for Disease Control and Prevention. General recommendations on immunization: recommendations of the Advisory Committee on Immunization Practices (ACIP) and the American Academy of Family Physicians (AAFP). MMWR 2002; 51(RR–2).

46. Centers for Disease Control and Prevention. Recommendations for using smallpox vaccine in a pre-event vaccination program: supplemental recommendations of the Advisory Committee on Immunization Practices (ACIP) and the Healthcare Infection Control Practices Advisory Committee (HICPAC). MMWR 2003; 52(RR-7):1–16.

47. Centers for Disease Control and Prevention/National Institutes of Health. Biosafety in microbiological and biomedical laboratories, 4th edn. HHS Publication no. (CDC) 93-8395. Atlanta, Georgia: US Department of Health and Human Services. Public Health Service, 1999.

48. Centers for Disease Control. Case definitions for public health surveillance. MMWR 1990; 39(RR-13):1–43.

49. Centers for Disease Control. Mandatory reporting of infectious diseases by clinicians. Mandatory reporting of occupational diseases by clinicians. MMWR 1990; 39(RR-9):1–28.

50. NIOSH. Selecting, evaluating, and using sharps disposal containers. DHHS (NIOSH) Publication No. 97-111. Cincinnati, Ohio: US Department of Health and Human Services, Public Health Service, Centers for Disease Control and Prevention, National Institute for Occupational Safety and Health, 1998.

51. US Census Bureau. Child care arrangements for preschoolers by family characteristics: Fall 1995. Available at http://www.census.gov/population/socdemo/child/ppl-138/tab01a.txt. Accessed September 13, 2002.

52. Giebink GS. National standards for infection control in out-of-home child care. Semin Pediatr Infect Dis 1990; 1:184–94.

53. Americans with Disabilities Act of 1990, 104 Stat. 327, 42 U.S.C. sec. 12101 et seq

54. Centers for Disease Control and Prevention. Immunization of health-care workers: recommendations of the Advisory Committee on Immunization Practices (ACIP) and the Hospital Infections Control Practices Advisory Committee (HICPAC). MMWR 1997; 46(RR-18):1–42.

Chapter 23
Musculoskeletal Disorders

23.1 Overall Approach to Managing Musculoskeletal Disorders
David M Rempel, Bradley A Evanoff

The musculoskeletal disorders considered in this section are conditions with typically long natural histories such as tendonitis, rotator cuff syndrome, low back pain, osteoarthritis, and entrapment neuropathies. They are usually not acute injuries, preceded by a single high-force event, but rather are associated with weeks, months or years of exposure to rapid motions or repeated forceful tasks. In the past these disorders have been labeled with various terms, such as cumulative trauma disorders (CTD), repetitive strain injuries (RSI), and repetitive motion disorders (RMD). However, the term musculoskeletal disorders (MSDs) is preferred as it does not focus on causation in the name. These conditions may be due to rapid, repeated motions or forceful pinching, or a medical condition, such as pregnancy. Each must be evaluated for causation separately.

In the US, almost 1 million workers annually report taking time away from work for treatment and recovery from musculoskeletal pain or loss of function due to overexertion or repetitive motion of the back or upper extremities.[1] Estimated workers' compensation costs for these lost workdays range from $13 to $20 billion.

Medical management

Good medical management of MSDs includes: (1) early reporting of symptoms, (2) timely access to healthcare providers and appropriate medical treatment, (3) rapid evaluation and modification of job risk factors, (4) the provision for limited or modified work duties when necessary, and (5) close medical follow-up. Comprehensive programs that integrate ergonomic evaluations with medical treatment are effective in reducing the incidence and severity of work-related musculoskeletal disorders.

The goals of a medical management program should be to reduce or eliminate symptoms, prevent progression of the disorder, and reduce the duration and severity of functional impairment and related disability. In other words, to keep the patient functional at work and prevent disease progression. The long-term goals of treatment and prognosis should be discussed with the patient, and the workers' compensation carrier. Employers should be notified of any necessary time-loss or work restrictions. Modifications to the treatment plan or work expectation should be communicated.

Encourage early reporting of symptoms

Appropriate treatment and workplace interventions should be implemented promptly. A delay in treatment can contribute to the severity and duration of disability. If the patient presents early, when the symptom intensity is mild, it may be possible to manage the disorder without lost time or without limiting the employee's essential job duties.

Conservative treatment is most effective when begun in the early stages of these disorders. Patients who are treated after a prolonged symptomatic period are less likely to respond favorably than those treated earlier.[2-5] With some disorders, such as carpal tunnel syndrome, patients can often be treated conservatively in the early stages of disease, while surgery is usually necessary when patients present with advanced disease.[6]

Healthcare providers

The choice of healthcare providers for treating the injured workers is important. The healthcare provider should have training or experience in ergonomics and the role of work modifications in the treatment of work-related musculoskeletal disorders. Effective treatment requires an accurate diagnosis and identification of aggravating factors including home and work mechanical factors, psychosocial factors and other aggravating medical factors (e.g., diabetes mellitus, pregnancy, etc). Treatment and determination of work-relatedness also require knowledge of specific job duties.

The best way for a healthcare provider to obtain knowledge of job duties is through a worksite visit. Since this is impractical in many clinical settings, information about exposures and job duties can also be obtained through a written work description, a videotape of the job tasks, or even a picture of the employee working at the workstation. The physician should have access to a person at the workplace with knowledge of job activities and the ability to coordinate a job evaluation and facilitate modifications of the job. If modifications are not possible, then the person may facilitate appropriate job placement during the recovery period. Working knowledge of the industry and the specific workplace is also needed in order to make appropriate recommendations regarding temporary or permanent job modifications. Many employers will provide detailed information about job duties and physical exposures to the treating physician. It is difficult to provide optimal care for employees when this information is not available.

Ergonomic interventions

A number of studies have documented the importance of ergonomic changes in treating workers with work-related musculoskeletal disorders.[7-14] Comprehensive ergonomic programs that incorporate primary prevention of MSDs through ergonomic changes in jobs, early detection of MSDs through surveillance, and early treatment of MSDs with an emphasis on early return to modified work have been endorsed by many corporations, professional guidelines and the National Research Council.[1,15] The approach involves the application of ergonomic principles to job design for primary and secondary prevention.

The majority of injured or symptomatic employees require no lost time and are able to return to productive work quickly, as long as their work is modified to reduce physical exposures to the affected body part. Job modifications which reduce physical exposures can be inexpensive and simple. Examples of job modifications include training or retraining, modifications of the job to reduce awkward postures (e.g., tilted work surfaces, change in work surface height), changes in tool design or maintenance, and changes in work procedures (job rotation, work–break pattern, limit overtime).

Where it is difficult to reduce risk factors through engineering modifications, temporary job transfer or restrictions may be necessary. Examples of temporary restrictions include restriction of specific tasks, reduction in pace or quantity of work, or limitation of hours worked. If an employee is to be transferred to a different job, the new job should be assessed by the employer and the healthcare provider to be sure that the employee will not be exposed to aggravating factors. In most cases, keeping an injured or symptomatic employee at work in an appropriate, modified duty position is preferable to time loss.

Examples of successful programs

The medical literature has examples of successful programs which have decreased the length or severity of disability resulting from injuries, through integrating ergonomic interventions as part of medical treatment of injured workers. One such study evaluated workers from a variety of industries who had lost more than 4 weeks of work due to back injuries.[16] Workers were randomly assigned to receive an ergonomics intervention, an intensive clinical and rehabilitation intervention, neither, or both. The ergonomics intervention consisted of a worksite ergonomics evaluation that included labor and employer representatives in determining the need for job modification. After observation of a worker's tasks with a trained ergonomist, these parties determined the need for modifications to improve the worksite. Implementation of the modifications remained the employer's responsibility. The clinical and rehabilitation intervention consisted of patient education ('back school'), referral to a back pain specialist, and a multidisciplinary work rehabilitation intervention. Combination of the rehabilitation intervention along with the ergonomics intervention was the most successful in returning injured workers to work. The ergonomics intervention was the most effective element of the program, resulting in more than a two-fold increase in the rate of return to usual work. By facilitating return to usual work, the ergonomics

intervention reduced the rate of long-term disability. In this study, the intensive clinical and rehabilitation intervention did not significantly reduce the time of absence from regular work when applied separately from the ergonomics intervention.

Another example of an integrated program was reported for sheet metal workers at an aircraft manufacturer.[7] This program combined pre-placement evaluations of workers with ongoing surveillance for symptoms and signs of upper extremity musculoskeletal disorders. Job modification was implemented for those with signs of early disorders, through restriction of work hours and restriction of use of vibrating hand tools. This program reported decreased workers' compensation costs, decreased time loss, and decreased severity of injury.

Other authors have described comprehensive initiatives to manage the incidence and cost of occupational injuries, that included an ergonomics component directed specifically toward injured workers. One such program has been described among hospital employees at an academic health center.[17] This study demonstrated decreases in musculoskeletal injuries, lost time (change from 10.4 days to 6.6 days average time loss), and total case costs (18% cost reduction) following the implementation of a comprehensive intervention that included case management, treatment by physicians experienced with work injuries, and the use of ergonomic worksite evaluation and modification. A later report from this group described elements of the program aimed at the early diagnosis and treatment of work-related upper extremity disorders. The program included ergonomic assessment and abatement of the affected employees' work areas, and close coordination between the treating physicians and the ergonomists. The program resulted in pronounced decrease in the number of work-related upper extremity MSDs and a virtual elimination of cases which required surgery.[18]

These and other peer-reviewed studies indicate that a multifaceted program can reduce the cost and burden of MSDs in different working populations. Many corporations have ergonomics programs based on the efficacy of such programs in reducing injuries.[19] Successful approaches have most often used a combination of ergonomic principles for prevention, as well as improved recognition and management of MSDs.

Patient education

Patient education is critical to successful management of MSDs. Since many MSDs are chronic, a successful outcome would be one where the patient knows enough about the aggravating factors and methods of treatment so that he or she can participate in management independently with minimal disruption of essential work and home duties. It is critical that the patient hears a consistent message from all involved healthcare providers. Since much of the recovery is dependent on appropriate patient behavior (home exercise program, modifying home activities, modifying work pattern) contradictory messages will interfere with recovery. If the physician tells the patient to reduce forward bending, and this is not reinforced by the therapist, then there will likely be little effect on patient behavior.

Splints for the thumb, wrist or elbow may be useful to immobilize and protect a joint during the acute phase of injury. However, the use of the splint should be reduced relatively rapidly, within weeks, in order to avoid complications. Prolonged splint usage can lead to muscle atrophy, joint stiffness, or splint dependency. Exceptions are sprains (ligament), which may require splinting for longer periods. Some splints are worn to protect the underlying soft tissue (e.g., soft elbow splint for ulnar neuropathy).

Splints should be relatively loose and comfortable and not so snug that they restrict circulation or cause localized pressure. Generally, splints should not be worn during work. In order to accomplish the work task, the patient may 'fight' the splint and thereby aggravate the condition.

Therapy modalities

Physical therapy modalities include immobilization, traction, massage, passive range-of-motion, ultrasound, heat, cold, the percutaneous delivery of medications with electrical charge of ultrasound (ionto- and phonophoresis), work conditioning, and patient education. The most valuable of these may be patient education directed at modifying daily activities at home and work. Improper therapy can delay recovery.

Not all therapists have the same approach to treating patients. In some cases, this is based on maintaining outdated ideas that places the patient in a passive role, as the 'recipient' of hot packs, massage, and other ineffective treatments. Successful practices of occupational and physical therapy are based on an active approach that incorporates graded exercise and increasing the level of responsibility on the part of the patient to protect and rehabilitate the injured area.

Home exercise program

Some conditions (e.g., wrist tendinitis, epicondylitis, low back pain) may benefit from a progressive home exercise program, following the acute phase of injury. The general strategy is to transition rapidly from immobilization to stretching, then slowly advance the strengthening protocol. For example, after the acute phase of tendonitis, when the pain becomes intermittent and dull, passive tendon stretching should be initiated. This stretching should continue even after symptoms have resolved. When the pain has become infrequent and of low intensity, strengthening should begin. The weights initially used should be small and increased very gradually. For example, for epicondylitis, initially 1/4 kg weights can be used during wrist extension and flexion with 10 to 20 repetitions, twice daily. The motions should be performed slowly. The load may be increased gradually every 2–4 weeks. There may some discomfort after strengthening. If the discomfort lasts more than an hour then the load or repetition rate should be decreased.

Case management

Three of the most common barriers to improvement are: (1) a delay in implementing prescribed workplace modifications, (2) a delay in starting therapy, and (3) poor patient compliance. Much of this is due to poor communication between the involved parties: employee, human resources contact, claims examiner, employer, and healthcare providers. Case managers, who are usually nurses, can help coordinate communication to address these barriers.[20]

Appropriate administration of paperwork with the workers' compensation carrier can lead to more rapid approval for treatments. Case managers can assist with arranging specific referrals (e.g., occupational therapist, ergonomist, medical specialist) in unison with the treating physician. They can also help in scheduling appointments to minimize time loss. The case manager can expedite obtaining items, such as special tools or chairs recommended by an ergonomist, through direct communications with the claims examiner. In order to facilitate return to work, the case manager can clarify or negotiate modified duty with the employer and treating physician, and assist the employer in maintaining compliance with prescribed workplace modifications.

The case manager can also maintain regular contact with the patient to improve compliance with home treatments. Employees usually need help understanding the abilities and limitations of workers' compensation.

OSHA 300 Log

After the physician evaluation, the employer must make a determination of whether the case should be recorded as an injury or illness in the OSHA Log. As of January 1 2002, the rules for reporting an injury or illness on the OSHA Log have changed (www.osha-slc.gov/recordkeeping/index.html). The old OSHA 200 Log has been replaced by the OSHA 300 Log. An injury or illness is now considered work related if work 'caused or contributed to the condition or significantly aggravated a preexisting condition'. It is recorded on the Log if any of these occur:
• death,
• loss of consciousness,
• restricted work activities or job transfer,
• days away from work,
• medical treatment beyond first aid, or
• a significant work-related injury or illness is diagnosed by a physician or other licensed healthcare professional.

The distinction between a 'new' case and a 'recurring' case has also changed. A 'new' case is one in which there is no previously recorded injury or illness of the same type affecting the same body part, or if signs and symptoms reappear after complete recovery from a previous injury or illness. Other cases are 'recurring pre-existing conditions' and include signs and symptoms that are associated with chronic illnesses.

For some companies the addition of a recordable case on their Log has serious ramifications. These companies may be concerned that they will be targeted for an OSHA inspection if their recordable rate is high. Or they may link management bonuses to low recordable rate. A more progressive approach places emphasis on controlling lost time and less on the recordable rate. This approach encourages early reporting of symptoms in order to prevent disability, even if this increases OSHA recordables.

Psychosocial factors

Psychosocial factors at work such as high job demands, high job stress, lack of job satisfaction, deadline work, lack of support from coworkers or supervisor should also be addressed. If these factors interfere with recovery, it may be necessary to discuss them with the supervisor or someone from the company's human resources office to attempt to resolve the problem. Other psychosocial factors may also interfere with recovery or be of concern to the patient. These include job insecurity, concern about future employment, financial consequences of the disorder, lack of support from family members, and depression. These should be dealt with directly.

Success

A successful outcome is one in which the patient is able to perform the essential duties of the job and desired home activities with minimal symptoms and limitations. Given the chronic nature of these conditions, the patient may continue to have episodes of pain. However, he or she will understand how to minimize the impact of a pain flare. Generally, this point is achieved when the employee: (1) has an intimate knowledge of activities that aggravate the condition, (2) identifies ways of avoiding or reducing those activities, (3) has support from the supervisor and coworkers, (4) has knowledge of pacing and pain management techniques, and (5) participates in daily home exercises.

The symptoms may resolve rapidly or may take months or even years to reach an acceptable outcome. During this time the healthcare providers play an essential role in continuing patient education, providing encouragement, and setting reasonable expectations.

References

1. National Research Council and Institute of Medicine. Musculoskeletal disorders and the workplace. Washington DC: National Academy Press, 2001.
2. Gelberman RH, Aronson D, Weisman MH. Carpal-tunnel syndrome: results of a prospective trial of steriod injection and splinting. J Bone Joint Surg 1980; 62A:1181–4.
3. Dellon AL. Review of treatment results for ulnar nerve entrapment at the elbow. J Hand Surg 1989; 14A:688–700.
4. Stern PJ. Tendinitis, overuse syndromes, and tendon injuries. Hand Clin 1990; 6:467–76.
5. Rystrom CM, Eversmann MW. Cumulative trauma intervention in industry: a model program for the upper extremity. In: Kasdan ML, ed. Occupational hand and upper extremity injuries & diseases. Philadelphia: Hanley & Belfus, 1991;489–505.
6. Dammers JWHH, Veering MM, Vermeulen M. Injection with methylprednisolone proximal to the carpal tunnel: randomized double blind trial. Br Med J 1999; 319:884–6.
7. Melhorn JM. A prospective study for upper-extremity cumulative trauma disorders of workers in aircraft manufacturing. J Occup Environ Med 1996; 38:1264–71.
8. Higgs PE, Mackinnon SE. Repetitive motion injuries. Ann Rev Med 1995; 46:1–16.
9. Norris RN. Applied ergonomics: adaptive equipment and instrument modification for musicians. Md Med J 1993; 42:271–5.
10. Feuerstein M, Huang GO, Ortiz JM, et al. Integrated case management for work-related upper-extremity disorders: impact of patient satisfaction on health and work status. J Occup Environ Med 2003; 45:803–12.
11. Evanoff B, Wolf L, Aton E, et al. Reduction in injury rates in nursing personnel through introduction of mechanical lifts in the workplace. Am J Ind Med 2003; 44:451–7.
12. Travers PH. Implementing ergonomic strategies in the workplace – an occupational health nursing perspective. AAOHN J 1992; 40:129–37.
13. Evanoff BA, Bohr PC, Wolf LD. Effects of a participatory ergonomics team among hospital orderlies. Am J Ind Med 1999; 35:358–65.
14. Herbert R, Gerr F, Dropkin J. Clinical evaluation of work-related carpal tunnel syndrome. Am J Ind Med 2000; 37:62–74.
15. Glass LS, ed. Occupational medicine practice guidelines: a quick reference. Evaluation and management of common health problems and functional recovery in workers. OEM Press, 2004.
16. Loisel P, Abenhaim L, Durand P, et al. A population-based, randomized clinical trial on back pain management. Spine 1997; 22:2911–8.
17. McGrail MP Jr, Tsai SP, Bernacki EJ. A comprehensive initiative to manage the incidence and cost of occupational injury and illness. J Occup Environ Med 1995; 37:1263–8.
18. Bernacki EJ, Guidera JA, Schaefer JA, Lavin RA, Tsai SP. An ergonomics program designed to reduce the incidence of upper extremity work related musculoskeletal disorders. J Occup Environ Med 1999; 41:1032–41.
19. GAO. Worker Protection: Private Sector Ergonomics Programs Yield Positive Results. GAO/HEHS-97-163. Washington DC: General Accounting Office, 1997.
20. Shaw WS, Feuerstein M, Lincoln AE, Miller VI, Wood PM. Case management services for work-related upper extremity disorders: integrating workplace accommodation and problem solving. Am Acad Occup Health Nurs J 2001; 49: 378–89.

23.2 Neck and Shoulder Disorders
Mats Hagberg

Disorders of the shoulder and neck region are a common problem in the general population and among industrial workers. In the general population, as many as one in every third woman and one in every fourth man report pain in the neck and shoulder that is present on a near daily basis. Pain in the neck region in the past year was reported by 34% of British workers.[1] Reported neck and shoulder pain is often non-specific and may not correlate with a pathoanatomic process. Both physical and psychosocial factors have been reported as risk factors.[2]

Several reviews have addressed the association between occupational stressors and disorders of the neck and shoulder.[3-5] The most common specific disorder of the neck and shoulder region is shoulder tendinitis. The revalence of shoulder tendinitis in the general population is approximately 2%. Among US workers, the prevalence of shoulder tendinitis was 8% for those exposed to highly repetitive or forceful upper extremity and hand motions compared with 1% among non-exposed workers. Similarly in sport, the pattern of usage and cumulative trauma has been associated with disorders of the neck and shoulder. Thus there is a consistency between both occupational and non-occupational activities for work-related disorders in the neck and shoulder.[6] The importance of preventative measures to address ork-related neck and shoulder dis-orders has been recognized in Canada, the USA and in the European Union.[3,4,7]

CLINICAL EVALUATION

Accurate assessment of neck and shoulder symptoms is essential, because shoulder symptoms may be referred from processes of pulmonary, cardiac or abdominal origin. Neck symptoms may also be related to cranial disorders.[8] Neck and shoulder disorders may also cause symptoms to the upper extremity and hand, as frequently occurs with compression of cervical nerve roots. Patients seeking medical attention for persistent musculoskeletal illness should thus be examined comprehensively in these anatomic regions.

History

The type, onset, and localization of symptoms should be explored in great detail. Visual aids, such as the use of a diagram or manikins to let the patient mark the type and location of pain, have demonstrated reliability.[9] It is important to distinguish between nociceptive and neurogenic pain.[10] Nociceptive pain usually originates from peripheral pain receptors reacting to mechanical or chemical stimuli. Muscle pain can be regarded as a nociceptive pain. Neurogenic pain is caused by a dysfunction in the nervous system, commonly causing sensory disturbances, as occurs with entrapment of nerves. Whereas neurogenic pain may follow the sensory distribution of a nerve, noci-ceptive pain may be more diffuse and correlate poorly with a specific nerve distribution.

Radiating pain in a dermatomal distribution may indicate a cervical root process (radiculopathy). The character, quality, distribution, intensity, frequency and duration of symptoms should be described. Information should be elicited about the relationship between symptoms and posture, movements, and physical loading during occupational activity. The temporal relation between symptoms during recreational activities and rest should also be explored.

General medical history should also be addressed. Concerns for systemic disease include weight loss, severe pain or morning stiffness which may indicate an endocrine disorder, infection, or tumor. Family and past medical history addressing rheumatologic disorders should also be addressed.

Individual susceptibility factors, such as genetic factors or lack of fitness, should be elicited, as they may result in a lower than normal threshold for related musculoskeletal injury. Furthermore, local strain may trigger symptoms early in an individual with a preclinical systemic disease. Important individual factors that may increase the risk of contracting a work-related musculoskeletal disorder in the neck and shoulder include congenital malformations, age, smoking, inflammatory, and endocrine disorders.

Work and exposure history

Job title alone offers insufficient information to determine whether neck and shoulder disorders are work related, and whether the patient can return to his or her job. Specific work tasks should be delineated, including work posture, repetition, weight and nature of material handled, and work organization. A history of sudden high energy transfers or precipitating events or accidents resulting in clinical or subclinical injury should be elicited.[11]

While the work and exposure history will assist the clinician in determining work relatedness in most cases, direct evaluation of the workplace may be useful in some cases, particularly regarding job redesign and return-to-work programs for rehabilitation. Such evaluations can be performed by direct observation at the work site or representative video recordings.

Work postures and repetition
Special attention should be directed to the frequency and duration of extreme positions of the head and arms. The examiner should inquire about the duration and frequency of work done with hands at or above the shoulder level. Specific inquiry regarding maintaining the head in a flexed or twisted position should be addressed. Even a position with a slightly flexed neck may result in severe discomfort if sustained for a significant period of time. It is possible that discomfort during work hours will progress to more persistent or chronic pain for some workers over time (Fig. 23.2.1).

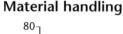

Neck flexion

Percent of operators
with reported pain

Neck flexion > 66 degrees

Neck flexion 56-65 degrees

Neck flexion < 55 degrees

0 10 20 30 40 50 60

Figure 23.2.1: The relation between forward flexion in the neck, and pain and stiffness in the neck.

Material handling

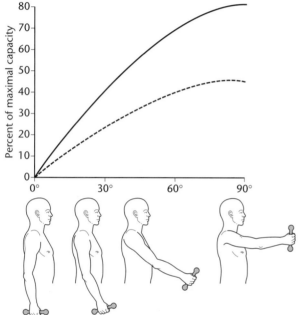

Figure 23.2.2: The strength utilization ratio for a woman (sold line) and a man (dotted line) when holding a 1 kg tool in the hand with a straight arm at different angles of shoulder flexion. The strength utilization ratio is the fraction of the maximal capacity that is needed to perform the contraction.

The degree of shoulder flexion during lifting, in addition to the actual weight lifted, determines the physical load on the shoulder. Figure 23.2.2 presents the utilization ratio of each lift in relation to the individual maximal capacity. For instance, lifting a 2-pound weight (1 kg) by hand with a straight arm at 90 degrees of forward flexion required 45% of maximal muscular capacity in an average man and 81% of capacity in a woman. Material handling performed near maximal capacity (80–100% of maximal) will increase the risk for strain injuries due to poorly controlled movements.

The strength utilization ratio in the shoulder for a given position can be calculated by simple biomechanical principles. The shoulder joint torque is obtained by adding the torque produced by the lifted object and the torque produced by the weight of the arm. The torque of the lifted object is calculated by multiplying the weight of the object in newtons (kilograms × 10) by the length of

the lever arm in meters. The torque produced by the weight of the arm is calculated the same way, by multiplying the weight of the arm in newtons by the lever arm (the weight of the arm is 5% of the body weight). The center of gravity for the weight of the arm is located approximately at half the distance of the arm (upper arm + forearm) from the shoulder joint (0.6 meters is a typical measure for the length of the arm for average-sized men and women). At 90 degree of forward flexion, the torque in the shoulder joint produced by the weight of the arm would be about 12 newton-meters in a 80 kg man (5% × 80 kg × 10 × 0.6 × 1/2 m) and 10 newton-meters in a 65 kg woman. The maximal capacity for shoulder joint torque is 27 newton-meters for women and 53 newton-meters for men. Hence the strength utilization ratio when holding the arm in 90 degrees of forward flexion without any load would be on average 37% for a woman (60 kg) and 23% for a man.

Work organization

A self-regulated work pace may result in a different exposure compared with that determined by preset machine-paced work. The patient should be asked about the frequency, distribution, and duration of pauses and breaks. Working in the same position for sustained periods of time, even when work posture is not extreme, may result in a static loading of muscles and an increased risk of muscle strain injuries. Psychosocial factors such as psychological job demands, decision latitude, social support, and job satisfaction are all variables with a strong influence on symptoms.[2] These variables may also influence shoulder muscle tension, directly affecting discomfort and pain. In computer-based work, the type of work (e.g., data entry, information retrieval, or programming) results in different pause patterns and exposures on the neck and shoulder. Continuous data entry work for more than 4 hours per day, without significant pauses, increases the risk of discomfort and muscle pain syndromes in the shoulder and neck region.

Physical examination

The physical examination of the shoulder and neck includes the following steps: (1) inspection for local swelling, erythema, and muscle atrophy; (2) testing the range of motion; (3) testing for muscle contraction pain and muscle strength; (4) palpation of muscle tendons and insertions; (5) specific provocative maneuvers.

Testing the range of motion

When the active range of motion is impaired, passive range of movement should also be tested. The passive range of motion is the range that the patient can achieve when assisted by the examiner. The following movements should be tested in the neck (cervical spine): forward flexion-extension, rotation and lateral flexion. In the shoulder, testing of forward flexion-extension, abduction, internal and outward rotation should be performed. Descriptions of range of motion limits are provided in the useful reference 'The Clinical Measurement of Joint Motion' published by the American Association of Orthopedic Surgeons.[12]

Determination of contraction pain and muscle strength in the neck

The examiner puts a firm grip on the head of the patient and then asks the patient to tilt his/her head to the side, to rotate, and to flex and to extend. The patient is instructed to report any feeling of discomfort during contraction. In the shoulder, forward flexion, abduction at 30 degrees, and outward and inward rotation in the neutral position are tested against the resistance of the examiner's hands. The best position for the examiner is to stand behind the standing or seated patient during these isometric maneuvers.

Palpation

Palpation of the bony structures, tendons, and muscles is performed while the patient is standing or sitting. By comparing right and left sides, abnormal tenderness is effectively identified. Palpation of the neck is most easily performed with the patient in the supine position with the shoulder at the top end of the examination table. With the patient relaxed, the head should be held by the examiner with one hand while the other hand examines the bony structures and muscles of the neck. If the patient experiences pain in the forearm and hand during compression maneuvers, a cervical hernia may be present, particularly if this pain is relieved by traction applied to the patient's head. In contrast, when traction of the cervical spine results in pain, this may indicate strain or damage to other musculoskeletal structures of the cervical spine, such as ligaments, articular capsules, or muscles.

Specific provocative maneuvers

The foramen compression test is performed with the patient in the sitting position. The examiner rotates the patient's head, while at the same time flexing it laterally to the same side. This maneuver results in narrowing of the intervertebral cervical foramina allowing detection of a nerve root compression and irritation (cervical radiculopathy). A positive test result occurs when the patient experiences pain or numbness in the forearm and hand of the side to which the head is rotated and flexed.

In the same position, the *Arm-Lasegue test* is performed by the examiner who tilts the patient's head to one side (lateral flexion) and, on the other side, depresses the shoulder girdle. In this test, the nerves of the cervical brachial plexus are stretched and abnormal irritation to these structures will result in pain or paresthesias in the forearm and hand on the side of the depressed shoulder.

Another test of compression of the nerve roots of the brachial plexus is the *Roos test,* which additionally allows assessment of thoracic outlet syndrome. The patient is again in a sitting position and elevates both the arms to 90 degrees abduction with external rotation ('hands up' position). The patient is instructed to open and clench the hands at a rate of once per second for 3 minutes. The normal experience during the test is a forearm tightness and neck and shoulder fatigue. Patients with abnormal irritation involving the lower trunk of the brachial plexus develop progressive tingling and pain of the ulnar side of the forearm and hand.

The *bursa test* for shoulder bursitis is performed by compressing the upper arm against the coracoacromial arch. The presence of shoulder pain during this maneuver may indicate subacromial bursitis, frequently associated with shoulder tendinitis. The *Yeargason maneuver* is an isometric test to assess bicipetal tendinitis. With the upper arm along the body, in 90 degrees flexion at the elbow joint, the examiner takes the hand of the patient and asks him or her to supinate the forearm. A positive result is elicited if this contraction evokes pain in the shoulder, as the biceps is the main supinator of the forearm.

Laboratory tests

Blood tests such as erythrocyte sedimentation rate and rheumatoid factor may be useful to assess inflammatory and rheumatologic disorders. Imaging tests such as radiographs, ultrasound, CT, and MRI to detect anatomic abnormalities should be performed as directed by the clinical findings reviewed above. Radiographic findings must be placed in the context of clinical findings. For instance, degenerative changes are common, and may not be related to the neck–shoulder symptoms.

CLASSIFICATION

A common nosology for disorders of the neck and shoulder does not currently exist. This has impeded agreement on the associations between these disorders and specific occupations or stresses. Criteria for various musculoskeletal disorders have been proposed as case definitions for surveillance and epidemiological studies.[13] The use of terms such as RSI (repetitive strain injuries) and CTD (cumulative trauma disorders), while useful for general characterizations, should be avoided as specific diagnoses.

In industrial settings, the ergonomic exposure may modify symptoms and signs of disorders and diseases.[14] For instance, in job tasks involving repetitive arm elevations, signs of both tendinitis and non-specific regional pain may be present, related to both repetitive strain on rotator cuff tendons and static strain on neck and shoulder muscles. If the presence of musculoskeletal symptoms and signs does not correlate with criteria for a specific disease diagnosis, an ICD label that focuses on the symptoms rather than the pathology is recommended.[15] An example of a non-specific neck–shoulder pain condition is the label 'cervicobrachial syndrome' M53.1 (ICD-10). For simplicity, we discuss disorders based on anatomy, beginning with syndromes with clearly defined anatomic relations. The major disorders include:

- rotator cuff disorders and biceps tendinitis
- cervical spondylosis and osteoarthritis of the shoulder and acromioclavicular joints
- cervical radiculopathy
- thoracic outlet syndrome
- cervicobrachial pain syndromes.

Rotator cuff disorders and biceps tendinitis

Tendinitis and tenosynovitis are inflammatory conditions of the tendon and the synovial membrane of tendon sheath. Common sites for inflammation of the shoulder are the tendons to the rotator cuff muscles (supraspinatus, infraspinatus, subscapularis, and teres minor muscles), and long head of the biceps brachii. At these locations the tendons perform large movements as they pass through relatively narrow spaces in the periarticular regions of the shoulder joint.

Inflammation of a tendon can be part of a general inflammatory disease such as rheumatoid arthritis, but is most frequently caused by local inflammation as a result of mechanical irritation and friction. For the latter, signs of inflammation may be subtle, and some advocate use of the term tendopathies or tendalgias rather than tendinitis.

Epidemiology and work relatedness

Posture and force are the main risk factors for shoulder tendinitis. For instance, automobile assemblers with acute shoulder pain and tendinitis have higher frequency and longer duration of elevation of the arms during work compared to controls. Among exposed US industrial workers, there was a 7.8% prevalence of shoulder cumulative trauma disorders, involving both should tendinitis and degenerative joint disease. Work tasks with high force and/or repetition on the wrist and hands were associated with a greater than five-fold risk of injury. Similarly, female students performing repetitive shoulder flexion developed shoulder tendinitis frequently. Among professional pitchers, approximately 10% had experienced shoulder tendinitis. In a survey of swimmers in Canadian swimming clubs, 15% reported having significant shoulder disability, primarily due to impingement syndromes related to the butterfly and freestyle strokes. Tendinitis of the biceps brachii was identified in 11% of elite tennis players.

Pathophysiology of shoulder tendinitis

The pathophysiologic process for shoulder tendinitis involves tendon degeneration. Degeneration of the tendon is caused by impairment of perfusion and nutrition, in addition to mechanical stress. Cellular injury within the tendon results in debris formation progressing to calcium deposition over time. The tendons to the supraspinatus, the biceps brachii (long head), and the upper parts of the infraspinatus muscle groups have a zone of avascularity. Signs of degeneration, including cell death, calcification, and microruptures are located predominantly in this region of avascularity. Impairment of circulation, and accelerated degeneration is caused by compression and static tension of these shoulder tendons. Compression of tendons occurs when the arm is elevated. During elevation of the arm, the rotator cuff tendons and the insertions on the greater tuberosity are forced under the coracoacromial arch, resulting in impingement. Compression of the rotator cuff tendons, particularly the supraspinatus tendon, results from the narrow space between the humeral head and the tight coracoacromial arch (Fig. 23.2.3). Chronic bursitis, as well as complete or partial tears of the rotator cuff tendons or biceps brachii, may result in a chronically disabling impingement syndrome.

In addition to impingement, circulation of the tendon may also be affected by muscle tension. Circulation in the tendon is inversely proportional to muscle tension, and ceases at higher tension levels. Studies have demonstrated that when the intramuscular pressure in the supraspinatus muscle exceeds 30 mmHg at 30 degrees of forward flexion or abduction in the shoulder joint (Fig. 23.2.4), an impairment of blood circulation occurs at this level. Because the major blood vessel supplying the supraspinatus tendon runs through the supraspinatus muscle, it is likely that circulation of the tendon is disturbed under these conditions. It is thus not surprising to find a high risk of shoulder tendon lesions in activities involving static contractions of the supraspinatus muscle, or repetitive shoulder forward flexions and abductions. Occupational groups with static tension of the supraspinatus muscle include welders and seamstresses. Groups that perform repetitive shoulder joint movements include assembly line workers in the automotive industry, painters, and athletes such as swimmers.

Degenerative changes in the tendon may trigger an inflammatory 'foreign body' response to the debris of dead cells, resulting in an active tendinitis. Additionally, infection (e.g., viral, urogenital) or systemic inflammation may precipitate an episode of tendinitis in the shoulder, likely representing an immune-mediated response.

Clinical effects and course

Degenerative changes beginning in the avascular zone of tendons progress to calcium deposition, associated with increased friction between the humeral head and the coracoacromial arch. Progressive calcification may result in tendon rupture with subacromial bursitis. Rotator cuff tendon rupture may be partial or complete. Tendinitis is classified into different stages.[16] Stage I is characterized by edema and hemorrhage, often seen acutely after excessive tendon stress during overhead use. Stage II is characterized by fibrotic and degenerative changes resulting from

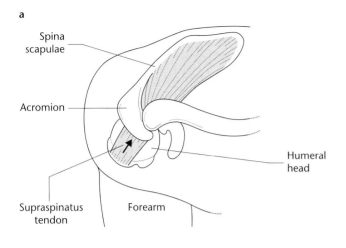

a

Spina
scapulae

Acromion

Humeral
head

Supraspinatus
tendon

Forearm

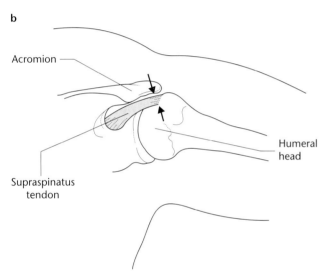

b

Acromion

Humeral
head

Supraspinatus
tendon

Figure 23.2.3: Impingement. (a) The distal part of the supraspinatus tendon will slide under the anterior part of the acromion (arrow). (b) During this process impingement occurs against the undersurface of the anterior aspect of the acromion. The pressure and mechanical friction are centered on the supraspinatus tendon.

repeated episodes of mechanical inflammation. More extensive calcification, often accompanied by bone spurs and tendon rupture, is associated with tendinitis.

Diagnosis

The diagnosis of rotator cuff and bicepetal tendinitis is based on typical distinct shoulder complaints, such as pain with isometric abduction, flexion, inward and outward rotation in the shoulder, and tenderness over the tendons at the humeral head. Limitation of the active range of shoulder motion is included in the diagnostic criteria. Evidence of calcium deposition at the shoulder joint radiographically may support the diagnosis of tendinitis. Tendinitis appearing in a worker with high local load on the shoulder can be considered work related, in the absence of systemic inflammatory conditions or infection (reactive tendinitis). High local load of the shoulder can occur in job tasks requiring repetitive shoulder flexions (or abductions), or work with the hands at or above shoulder level. Leisure time activities should be reviewed, as both sport and household work can precipitate tendinitis. While no established threshold limit levels exist for shoulder load, high local load on the shoulder is considered present when the hand is kept one hour per working day at or above shoulder level, or when repetitive flexions or abductions more than 60 degrees in the shoulder joint are performed frequently and regularly during the working day.

Management

Conservative measures including rest, ice application to tendons following exertion, and use of non-steroidal anti-inflammatory therapy should be initiated. Efficient treatment for more persistent shoulder tendinitis following these conservative measures is a single subacromial steroid injection mixed with local anesthetics. In chronic severe shoulder tendinitis, surgical removal of the lateral part of the acromion may ameliorate pain. A change in workplace design or work task may be necessary if the tendinitis is related to high local shoulder load. A history of prior shoulder tendinitis (stages I or II) results in increased risk

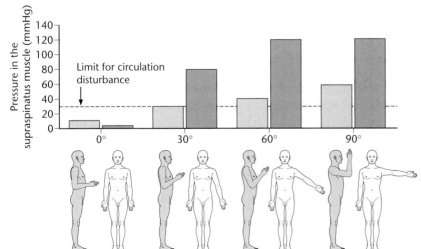

Figure 23.2.4: Intramuscular pressure in the supraspinatus muscle at different angles of abduction and forward flexion. Pressure exceeding 30 mmHg may impair blood circulation.

for relapse among workers continuing to perform repetitive or forceful movements.

Prognosis

The clinical course may progress from stage I to III, but recovery of the tendon can also occur within each stage. A stage III impingement may lead to progressive disability. In a study of assembly workers with chronic tendinitis (stage II and III) a 2-year follow-up revealed that only 8 out of 20 patients had experienced significant recovery.

Cervical spondylosis, shoulder joint and acromioclavicular joint osteoarthritis

Cervical spondylosis and shoulder joint osteoarthritis (OA) are degenerative changes of cartilage and bone in the joints and intervertebral discs.

Epidemiology and work relatedness

Cervical spondylosis is common in the general population. More than 80% of the population over the age of 50 years have radiographic signs of cervical spondylosis. Dentists and miners have been reported to have an increased risk of spondylosis (age-standardized odds ratio 2 to 5). Notably, referent groups (frequently representing office workers) have also had a high prevalence of cervical spondylosis (14–38%). Loading of the cervical spine by extreme position of the head may represent the pathogenic mechanism for spondylosis among dentists and miners. This is consistent with a finding of increased cervical spondylosis in a Jamaican rural population where loads were carried on the head.

OA in the shoulder joint usually occurs late in life, and is often bilateral. Shoulder joint osteoarthritis was found more commonly in dentists compared to farmers, however specific ergonomic exposures related to shoulder joint OA have not been well characterized. Occupations with high physical demand have been associated with degenerative changes in the shoulder joint (see Chapter 23.3). An increased risk for acromioclavicular OA has been reported among construction workers. Heavy lifting and handling of heavy tools with hand-arm vibration have been suggested as the exposure-related factors for development of acromioclavicular joint OA.[17]

Pathogenesis

The pathogenesis of primary OA is frequently not known. Primary (idiopathic) OA is the most common diagnosis, in the absence of predisposing factors such as previous fractures. If such predisposing factors exist, the OA is termed secondary. There are disputes regarding the pathogenic mechanism for work-related OA, with hypotheses including metabolic trauma, or microfractures due to sudden impact or repetitive impact loading.

Clinical presentation

The clinical presentation of OA is variable. While there may be a discrepancy between radiographic findings and patients' symptoms and signs, there is frequently strong correlation in advanced disease. Symptoms may include pain during movement, and when loading the joint during forceful or repetitive activities. In severe osteoarthritis the range of motion is diminished.

Diagnosis

The diagnosis of osteoarthritis relies mainly on imaging techniques. In the shoulder joint, arthroscopy may reveal early signs of osteoarthrosis.

Management

Symptoms of inflammation may be ameliorated by oral non-steroidal anti-inflammatory medications. Local steroid injections should generally be avoided, since the degenerative process is accelerated by steroids. Loading of the osteoarthritic joint should be minimized by work redesign.

Prognosis

Osteoarthrosis usually occurs late in life, but may result in substantial limitations on work activities in younger individuals. Symptomatic improvement is often seen with NSAIDs and reduction of joint load (e.g., work restrictions).

Cervical radiculopathy

Radiculopathy represents a compression of the nerve root caused by a herniated disc or narrowed intervertebral foramen.

Epidemiology and work relatedness

Cervical radiculopathy has a prevalence of 1–5%. In studies of data entry operators, dock workers, and assembly line packers, a risk ratio below one was observed. Cervical radiculopathy has not been well characterized in terms of physical or other work stresses, though it clearly represents a complication of traumatic cervical spinal injury.

Pathogenesis and clinical effects

The etiology of cervical herniation and narrowed intervertebral foramen remains obscure. Symptoms include severe pain, with distinct radiation of the pain to specific dermatomes. Tingling and numbness may be present. Wasting of muscles can occasionally be seen, as in a C7 syndrome where atrophy of the first dorsal interosseus muscle may occur. Loss of muscle strength may result in impairment.

Diagnosis

The diagnosis of cervical radiopathy may be established by clinical examination, where the findings are specific sensory loss in affected dermatomes, diminished motor reflexes, and a positive result on testing of compression of the cervical spine or the intervertebral foramina. Radiographic examination with CT scan, MRI or myelography may show the hernia or the impingement on a spinal nerve. Nerve conduction studies may demonstrate changes in nerve function.

Management

Surgical release of the herniation is rarely required, as traction therapy of the cervical spine is sufficient (e.g., with use of a soft cervical collar).

Prognosis

The prognosis is good in most cases. At least partial recovery with improved symptoms is often observed within several weeks or months following initiation of treatment.

Thoracic outlet syndrome

The diagnosis of thoracic outlet syndrome (TOS) has generated much controversy regarding definition and treatment. TOS has been associated with several syndromes of distinct etiology and clinical course.[18,19]

Pathogenesis

TOS is a neurovascular impingement syndrome occurring at different anatomical levels where the brachial plexus and the subclavian vessels may be entrapped as they pass en route from the cervical spine to the upper extremity. TOS can be divided into neurogenic and vascular etiologies. Neurogenic symptoms and signs result from compression of the brachial plexus at various levels, and is more prevalent than vascular compression. The level of compression is described as subtypes of TOS, including: (1) cervical rib or fibrous band syndrome, (2) scalenus syndrome, (3) costoclavicular syndrome, and (4) hyperabduction syndrome (or pectoralis minor syndrome).

Epidemiology and work relatedness

The prevalence rate of neurogenic TOS varies considerably among industrial workers, ranging from reported rates of 44% for female assembly line workers, to 0.3% for industrial workers in the USA. Differences in reported prevalences may reflect variable and poorly characterized diagnostic criteria for TOS. In a prospective study, a positive Roos test (abduction external rotation maneuver) for neurogenic TOS predicted a slowing of the nerve conduction velocities in the wrist region.[20]

Clinical presentation

Shoulder and neck pain of variable character, with or without radiation to the arm and hand, is the hallmark of TOS. Symptoms reflect the degree to which particular nerves are compressed. A common type of neurogenic TOS is caused by a cervical rib or a fibrous band that may impinge the lowest part of the brachial plexus, causing pain radiating down the ulnar side of the arm, forearm and hand. This pain may be exacerbated by strenuous use of the hand.

Diagnosis

The diagnosis of TOS is based on history and clinical examination. Roos test (or abduction external rotation – AER – maneuver) is typically positive. In epidemiologic studies, diagnostic criteria of neurogenic TOS have included positive outcomes of the Roos test in association with shoulder and arm pain. These diagnostic criteria are criticized by

some because they do not require more quantitative physiologic measures such as NCV/EMG abnormalities. Vascular forms of TOS are rare. Radiographic findings may include identification of a cervical rib.

Management

Surgery may be indicated in severe cases, with progressive neuropathy or vascular symptoms. Conservative management with strength training, work redesign, or work transfer is often sufficient to allow significant recovery.

Cervicobrachial pain syndromes

Cervicobrachial pain syndrome, characterized by nonlocalized pain in the neck and shoulder, is among the most common work-related conditions involving the neck and shoulder. Cervicobrachial pain syndrome is defined as pain in the shoulder and neck, with or without radiation to the arm and hand, where the anatomic basis for the pain cannot be identified. Symptoms and signs may resemble or overlap those associated with TOS and primary fibromyalgia. However, the condition does not conform totally to any specific diagnosis. The term cervicobrachial pain syndrome may include different entities such as myofascial pain syndrome, cervical spondylosis, tension neck syndrome, or enthesopathy (periarticular inflammation).

The following discussion focuses on regional muscle pain syndrome, since it probably represents the majority of cases of cervicobrachial pain syndrome. Regional muscle pain syndrome is often termed myofascial syndrome. Tension neck syndrome is a term widely used in epidemiologic studies of work-related pain, localized to the shoulder and neck region. The criteria for tension neck syndrome are usually pain in the shoulder or neck in addition to tenderness over the descending part of trapezius muscle (shoulder–neck area).

Epidemiology and work relatedness

Non-specific neck and shoulder pain syndrome is more common among females than males, with an almost sixfold increase in females observed in some studies of industrial workers. The occupational groups with repetitive arm work task and constrained work postures showed high rates of the syndrome, often exceeding 50% prevalence.

Pathogenesis

Prolonged static contraction of the trapezius muscle during work or in daily activity results in an overload of the type 1 muscle fibers, and may represent the pathogenetic mechanism for non-specific neck shoulder pain syndrome. The type 1 muscle fibers are used in low static contractions. In biopsies from patients with chronic trapezius muscle pain, findings of 'ragged red fibers' involving large type 1 fibers were observed. This may be one explanation of the rapid fatigue and pain in such patients. When the demand for energy in the muscle fiber is higher than available, muscle pain may occur. Postural pain syndrome associated with sagging shoulders is a type of cervicobrachial syndrome that may be caused by prolonged stretching of the trapezius muscle or the brachial plexus.

Common to the cervicobrachial pain syndrome is that discomfort may be triggered by a pain locus in muscles, tendons, joint capsules, or ligaments in the shoulder–neck area. Nociceptors (pain receptors) in these loci may be the origin of not only the neck–shoulder pain, but also diffuse referred pain to the arm and hand. The nociceptive pain may trigger a chronic pain syndrome that can effect the sympathic nervous system. A possible pathogenic mechanism for chronic pain is that an initial injury caused by strain (e.g., microrupture) does not recover fully, and is followed by subsequent injury events. Pain receptors induce a pathway of signals to the central nervous system, with progressively increasing susceptibility to stimuli. The neurologic response to normal activity is eventually perceived as a painful stimulus (e.g., chronic pain syndrome). Psychosocial factors at home and at work may represent contributing factors, by stress alone or by psychologically mediated muscle tension.

Clinical effects

The predominant clinical symptom is activity-related pain. Stiffness and severe pain at extreme postures are also common. A chronic pain syndrome should be recognized as soon as possible for proper treatment and rehabilitation, preferably in a multidisciplinary pain clinic, with emphasis on maximizing function.

Diagnosis

It is important to rule out specific lesions, which may include neurodiagnostic, imaging, or other laboratory studies. Rarely does a muscle biopsy yield important diagnostic information. Often there is a significant discrepancy between the patient's significant level of symptoms and minimal objective findings by the physician. Blood test and radiographic examination are typically normal. In many patients, the Roos test for TOS may be positive, although a true TOS with mechanical compression on the neurovascular bundle does not exist. In this case the test may indicate an increased sensitivity and irritability of the brachial plexus or adjacent muscular structures. More generalized muscle pain indicates primarily fibromyalgia. Specific criteria have been set by the American College of Rheumatology.

Management

A thorough examination is necessary to exclude other diagnoses related to the neck and shoulder (see sections above). Emphasis is placed on maintaining the patient's functional status. This may include ergonomic modifications, job redesign, and technique training to minimize strain during work by avoiding prolonged static contractions. Physical training reduces pain and increases performance, although an initial pain increase is often experienced when training is started.[21] Management of chronic pain may include physical therapy, acupuncture, use of local anesthetics, or biofeedback. Psychosocial factors at work and at home can be the obstacle to successful management.

Prognosis

The prognosis for cervicobrachial pain syndrome is variable. The general experience is that pain and discomfort may be decreased, but not eliminated, in the majority of cases. It is important to initiate rehabilitation early, with the goal of minimizing time loss and disability.

References

1. Palmer KT, Walker-Bone K, Griffin MJ, et al. Prevalence and occupational associations of neck pain in the British population. Scand J Work Environ Health 2001; 27:49–56.
2. Warren N, Dillon C, Morse T, Hall C, Warren A. Biomechanical, psychosocial, and organizational risk factors for WRMSD: population-based estimates from the Connecticut upper-extremity surveillance project (CUSP). J Occup Health Psychol 2000; 15:164–81.
3. Bernard BP, ed. Musculoskeletal disorders and workplace factors. Cincinnati: National Institute for Occupational Safety and Health, 1997.
4. Hagberg M, Silverstein B, Wells R, et al. Work related musculoskeletal disorders (WMSDs): a reference book for prevention. London: Taylor & Francis, 1995.
5. Keyserling WM. Workplace risk factors and occupational musculoskeletal disorders, Part 2: A review of biomechanical and psychophysical research on risk factors associated with upper extremity disorders. Am Ind Hygiene Assoc J 2000; 61:231–43.
6. Fulcher SM, Kiefhaber TR, Stern PJ. Upper-extremity tendinitis and overuse syndromes in the athlete. Clin Sports Med 1998; 17:433–48.
7. Buckle P. Risk factors for work-related neck and upper limb musculoskeletal disorders. European Agency for Safety and Health at Work, 1999;1-93. www.osha.eu.int
8. Piligian G, Herbert R, Hearns M, Dropkin J, Landsbergis P, Cherniack M. Evaluation and management of chronic work-related musculoskeletal disorders of the distal upper extremity. Am J Ind Med 2000; 37:75–93.
9. Ohnmeiss DD. Repeatability of pain drawings in a low back pain population. Spine 2000; 25:980–8.
10. Lundeberg T. Pain physiology and principles of treatment. Scand J Rehabil Med 1995; 32(Suppl):13–41
11. Hagberg M, Christiani D, Courtney TK, Halperin W, Leamon TB, Smith TJ. Conceptual and definitional issues in occupational injury epidemiology. Am J Ind Med 1997; 32:106–16.
12. Greene WB, Heckman JD, eds. The clinical measurement of joint motion. Rosemont: American Academy of Orthopedic Surgeons, 1994.
13. Harrington JM, Carter JT, Birrell L, Gompertz D. Surveillance case definitions for work-related upper limb pain syndromes. Occup Environ Med 1998; 55:264–71.
14. Hagberg M. Exposure considerations when evaluating musculoskeletal diagnoses. In: Mital A, Kreuger H, Kumar S, Menozzi M, Fernandez J, eds. Advances in occupational ergonomics and safety. Cincinnati: International Society for Occupational Ergonomics and Safety, 1996;411–5.
15. Norregaard J, Jacobsen S, Kristensen JH. A narrative review on classification of pain conditions of the upper extremities. Scand J Rehab Med 1999; 31:153–64.
16. Kainberger F, Mittermaier F, Seidl G, Parth E, Weinstabl R. Imaging of tendons – adaptation, degeneration, rupture. Eur J Radiol 1997; 25:209–22.
17. Hagberg M. Clinical assessment of musculoskeletal disorders in workers exposed to hand-arm vibration. Int Arch Occup Environ Health 2002; 75:97–105.
18. Parziale JR, Akelman E, Weiss AP, Green A. Thoracic outlet syndrome. Am J Orthop 2000; 29:353–60.

19. Wilboum AI. Thoracic outlet syndromes. Neurol Clin 1999; 17:477–97.

20. Toomingas A, Nilsson T, Hagberg M, Lundstrom R. Predictive aspects of the abduction external rotation test among male industrial and office workers. Am J Ind Med 1999; 35:32–42.

21. Hagberg M, Harms-Ringdahl K, Nisell R, Hjelm EW. Rehabilitation of neck-shoulder pain in women industrial workers: a randomized trial comparing isometric shoulder endurance training with isometric shoulder strength training. Arch Phys Med Rehabil 2000; 81:1051–8.

23.3 Upper Extremity Disorders
Martin Cherniack

Because the upper extremity frequently manipulates and contacts the work environment, it is not surprising that signs and symptoms affecting the hand and arm are frequent in clinical occupational medicine practice. Evaluation and treatment of acute traumatic events, such as crush injuries, burns, amputations, and lacerations, have been characterized in the hand surgery literature and are beyond the scope of this text. Unlike acute injuries, activity-related disorders of the musculoskeletal and neuromuscular systems, acquired in the course of adult working life, are often not attributable to a single traumatic event, but rather repetitive trauma. In the past decade, public controversies over issues such as work attribution in carpal tunnel syndrome and the government's role in enforcing ergonomic principles in the workplace have been challenged with evolving medical consensus on causation, etiology and treatment.

In the 1990s, the incidence of repetitive trauma disorders (RTDs) affecting the upper extremity reported by the US Department of Labor surpassed all other occupational disorders, in both frequency and cost.[1] While there is no single comprehensive data source that reliably records medically diagnosed musculoskeletal disease, analyses of National Health Interview Survey have suggested that chronic muculoskeletal diseases of the upper extremity effect approximately 10% of the population. A similar fraction of work-associated cases appears to be reported to either the Bureau of Labor Statistics or to State Workers Compensation authorities.[2,3] One difficulty encountered in characterizing this phenomenon is the abundance of terms that have been applied to symptoms associated with cumulative or repetitive work.[4,5] They include cumulative trauma disorders (CTDs), repetitive trauma disorders (RTDs), repetitive strain injuries (RSIs), overuse syndrome, and repetitive stress disorders (RSDs) (Table 23.3.1).[6,7]

Since clinicians are often faced with problems of attribution of work-related upper extremity disease and with providing recommendations for workplace modification, it is worthwhile to address the question of risk or exposure factors. For MSDs, microanatomic injury and repair is often subclinical and in its early stages may not be associated with objective findings.[8,9] Although the object of much active research, the relationship between subthreshold injury and the onset of recognized clinical disorders is imprecisely understood.[10-12] It is thus particularly important to identify workplace factors that may contribute to disease progression. In the past 5 years, extensive structured reviews of the peer review literature by the National Institute of Occupational Safety and Health,[13] the Institute of Medicine and the National Research Council,[14,15] and the Occupational Safety and Health Administration[16] have generated a consensus on known ergonomic risk factors for musculoskeletal disease. These are summarized in Table 23.3.2.

CLINICAL EVALUATION

Establishing an etiology for complaints affecting the upper extremity requires careful assessment of the pathophysio-logic basis of signs and symptoms.[17-19] Prior to attributing an upper extremity disorder to workplace factors, the clinician must address two basic clinical questions.

1. Is the process local, involving anatomically isolated structures or groups of structures; is it regional, involving an area of the arm and shoulder without anatomic focus; or is it systemic, involving multiple discrete or more distal organ systems?

2. What is the specific site of disturbance? For example, can pain be assigned to joints, entrapped nerves, tendon dysfunction or vascular insufficiency?

Behind this are important distinctions between inflammation and chronic degeneration, in tendons for example, or between nerve entrapment and intrinsic neuropathy. Since muscle, tendon, and nerve have considerable plasticity, the delineation between reversible symptomatic disorders and more persistent pathological changes is important.

History

Because symptoms affecting the upper extremity are relatively common and are frequently chronic, the medical history must concentrate on prior symptoms as well as the presenting complaint. A history that includes previous trauma, use of medications, and other medical conditions is essential.[20-23] Because joint pain, neuritic symptoms, myalgias, and cold-related symptoms may overlap with rheumatologic illnesses, particularly collagen vascular diseases, a review of constitutional, dermatologic, and other internal organ system disease or symptoms should be elicited. The importance of identifying previous trauma, particularly for proximal upper extremity disorders, cannot be overstated.

General medical history
Frequency and duration of symptoms are especially important. Because many upper extremity complaints are chronic, the eliciting event initiating a visit to the physician's office may be only indirectly related to the natural history of the condition. This poses particular problems for accurately defining the interval between the initial occurrence of symptoms and their clinical recognition. Temporal considerations also apply to the frequency of symptoms, whether they are episodic or continuous, and whether there is a seasonal or climatic component. Because distinctions between pain, numbness and dysesthesias, loss of sensation, and loss of function may be critical for both staging and diagnosis, specialized questions should be addressed, including daily performance skills, such as dressing, grasping slippery objects, and using fine implements. Shift work deserves special consideration, because unusual sleep patterns may be the result of a change in schedule or physical discomfort.

Work-related factors such as repetitive and forceful motion may interact with non-work-related factors to injure the upper extremity. The medical history should emphasize systemic disorders associated with neuropathy,

Repetitive strain injury
Repetitive motion injury
Diseases of acquired function
Cumulative musculoskeletal disorder
Computer-related health epidemic
Cumulative trauma disorder
Overuse syndrome
Occupational myalgia
Video display terminal (VDT) syndrome

Table 23.3.1 Common synonyms for disorders associated with repeated or cumulative mechanical stress

Basic biochemical risk factors
  Force
  Awkward postures
  Static postures
  Repetition
  Dynamic factors
  Compression
  Vibration
Modifying factors
  Intensity
  Duration
  Temporal profile
  Cold temperatures

Table 23.3.2 Ergonomic risk factors for musculoskeletal disease

articular, and periarticular disorders.[24,25] For instance, a mild diabetic neuropathy may have a more pronounced symptomatic expression in a heavily used upper limb. Alternatively, clinicians have often recognized that patients with musculoskeletal pain report local or referred phenomena such as paraesthesias or numbness in the hands. Common work-related musculoskeletal disorders such as epicondylitis without nerve entrapment have been associated with reduced subjective sensory perception.[26,27]

Predisposing conditions for tendinitis include rheumatoid arthritis, gout, pseudogout, Ehlers–Danlos syndrome, hypothyroidism, diabetes, Dupuytren's contractures, and infections, such as tuberculosis and atypical *Mycobacteria*. Rheumatoid arthritis and other collagen vascular disorders also have been associated with secondary Raynaud's phenomenon, mononeuritis, and synovial inflammatory conditions causing nerve compression. Hepatitis B and C are also relatively common in some industrial populations and are associated with muscle and joint complaints. Although these disorders account for less than 5% of presenting patients evaluated for work-related upper extremity disorders, their potential presence should be elicited, particularly because continuous occupational exposures may aggravate underlying disease.

A history of hand injuries, including those due to frostbite, crush, penetrating trauma, and fracture, is important, because callosities and nerve and vascular injury may be independently associated with physiologic impairment or increase susceptibility to workplace factors.[28,29] Personal habits, including tobacco and alcohol use, should be assessed. Tobacco use may significantly complicate and exacerbate vasospastic episodes[30,31] (e.g., Burger's disease) and alcohol use is an important source of metabolic neuropathies.

The occupational history

In selected settings, a single traumatic episode or recent change in work organization may obviate the need for comprehensive history taking, but in most instances, particularly in cases in which the onset is more insidious, a full occupational history is essential. Because job titles may not accurately describe job activity, particularly in the building trades, it is essential that tasks be described in detail, even acted out. This accounting should include identifying specific tools, fittings, and uses, and weekly or monthly hours of total use. Tool weight, time in overhead postures, and approximate force and strength requirements should be characterized. Handedness and hand position are particularly important, and symptoms that are unilateral may not always follow the predicted pattern.

Although symptoms in the dominant tool-wielding hand predominate among poultry workers,[32-34] a high incidence of carpal tunnel syndrome (CTS) in the non-dominant (carcass-supporting) hand has been described in butchers.[35] Similarly, although vibration-induced symptoms are usually bilateral, the plane of vector forces may be greater in the non-dominant supporting hand. The dramatic transition to the electronic office also requires greater detail than 'computer work' or 'data entry'.[36,37] Office-related musculoskeletal disorders usually involve reversible pathology, and worksite modification is frequently a key component of cure (see Chapter 15). Accordingly, the history should include an estimate of actual hours spent in keying or inputting, and descriptions of work surface height, position and type of input device, and adjustability of chairs and work surfaces.[38,39]

The following points should be included in the occupational history.
1. Symptoms in previous jobs.
2. Previous occupations and job responsibilities and tasks.
3. Home and ambient use of tools such as chain saws and other power tools.
4. The duration between employment and symptom onset.
5. The presence and description of symptoms in coworkers.
6. The relationship between symptom onset and temperature, and stage of the work shift.
7. The presence of symptoms on vacations and time off.
8. Previous diagnosis, treatment, and response.
9. Broader changes in work equipment, management organization, materials and products, and organization of teams and work assignments.
10. Individual factors such as the initiation of bonus or incentive programs; recent return to work following pregnancy, illness, or lay-off; and the quality of training.

While a history of hobbies and other non-work activities is important, such risk factors are as likely to exacerbate existing or work-related disease as to cause new disorders.[40,41] Most non-work activities are not performed with the duration or intensity, or under the time constraints characteristic of occupational exposures. In addition, certain industries, such as meatpacking, demonstrate disease clusters and rates of disease that are substantially above population background rates and rates found in other industries. Investigators in Washington State found that, compared to industry-wide carpal tunnel syndrome (CTS) incidence rates, oyster and crab packers demonstrated a relative risk (RR) of 14.8 (95% CI: 11.2–19.5) and the meat and poultry industries had a relative risk of 13.8 (95% CI: 11.6–16.4).[3] Thus, the likelihood of detecting the presence of disease rises with recognition of high risk within an industry.

Although the general elements of the occupational history cannot be overemphasized, there are some specific exposures, chemical and physical, that require special inquiry, because upper extremity tissue damage may actually be worse than can be determined from physical inspection alone. A distant history of cold injury may clarify contemporary dysesthesias and cold intolerance. Sensory abnormalities in workers exposed to extreme cold have persisted for years after pertinent exposures. Microwave radiation exposure, which may occur from unexpected sources, such as food preparation, drying or kilning of wood products, sealing of packaging, and rubber and polymer curing, may cause significant soft tissue injury, including surgical emergencies requiring decompression with trivial skin damage. Similar considerations apply to thermal and electrical burns, particularly in cases in which the injury is not circumscribed by an area of direct contact. The occupational history should attempt to differentiate between trivial first aid and extended medical evaluation and observation.

Physical examination

Despite notable advances in imaging, the physical examination of the upper extremity is the most important component of upper extremity assessment and definition of treatment course. While inherent limitations in reliability, sensitivity and specificity of clinical testing exist, there have been several consensus reviews on the utility of clinical tests and their administration.[19,42,125]

The examination should include inspection of the neck, shoulder girdle, upper arm, forearm, wrist, and hand. In the absence of obvious anatomic change, injury, or abnormal movement, a detailed examination should follow, focusing on patterns of weakness, swelling, numbness, and paresthesias. Provocative tests are highly important: they highlight the important distinction between pain syndromes and painless dysfunction. Because pain syndromes associated with repetition and chronicity are frequent, there should be special consideration to palpation of muscle bellies and musculotendinous junctions, as well as to joint capsules and ligaments. Pain during active isometric resistance of wrist and forearm flexion and extension, respectively, is indicative of tenosynovitis.

Bilateral examination is important, even when symptoms are unilateral. Delayed arterial refill in the hand (assessed by Allen's test) or pulse drop on neck and shoulder manipulation may suggest a vascular cause of unilateral dysesthesias, but contralateral delay in the absence of symptoms may suggest an alternate diagnosis. The pattern of elicited pain also may be useful in differentiating a diagnosis. Tendon ruptures, inflammatory tenosynovitis, and

arthritides should be sharply localized. More diffuse pain is characteristic of cervical disease, tumors, and dislocations. Retrograde pain suggests a distal nerve entrapment.

Anatomically well-defined nerve entrapment disorders are detected by tapping over the nerve (e.g., Tinel's sign for carpal tunnel syndrome), demonstration of motor weakness, and dermatomal patterns of abnormal sensation in involved nerves.[42,43] Stretching an entrapped nerve may exacerbate symptoms, as in the wrist flexion maneuver of Phalen's test. Physical examination may be less sensitive in milder cases. Provocative tests must, however, be put in a context. Reviews of the ability for Phalen's test to distinguish between subjects with and without carpal tunnel syndrome (CTS) have varied in the published literature, although they generally do not exceed 80%.

Usually, physical examination provides little insight into the cause of the injury. However, there are some characteristic physical findings that may directly suggest an association with a work-related source.

Hand, wrist, and forearm

A cool cyanotic hand may be the result of arterial damage from repeated percussion (e.g., ulnar hammer syndrome) or traumatically induced vasospasm, as is seen in vibration-induced Raynaud's phenomenon. In cases in which vascular insufficiency is severe, trophic changes at the fingertips may be visualized.

A claw hand implicates brachial plexus compression or proximal median nerve injury. Acute injury or chronic supportive wrist abduction from climbing may be important associations. Wrist drop, characterized by extensor weakness, is rarely seen in the context of a metabolic neuropathy but has classic associations with arsenic and lead. Trigger digits, caused by narrowed flexor sheaths or tendon thickening, produce an audible snapping and are associated with repetitive work and forceful grasping of hand tools, such as pliers. Dupuytren's contractures, although more often associated with liver disease and alcohol consumption, have been linked to percussive work. In these examples, it is important to differentiate between fixed anatomic conditions and conditions which are transient. Transient flexor contraction, usually in the early morning, is common following trauma or surgery, but it is mechanical rather than neurologic in nature. Hyperkeratoses of the palms usually reflect the existence of callosities; the association with arsenic toxicity is less common than in previous eras.

The forearm

Forearm pain in extensor and flexor compartments is common and usually related to muscle and tendon dysfunction, strain or shortening. Forearm pain has been attributed to median nerve compression – the so-called pronator syndrome – associated with muscle hypertrophy and overuse. Nerve entrapments in the forearm are much less common than at the wrist or elbow.[44,45]

The elbow

Extensive leaning on the elbows and forceful manipulation, such as in slaughterhouse work, has been associated with nerve compressions at the elbow. The evaluation of occupational elbow pain should merit a search for motor weakness in the hand. Chronic injury at the lateral epicondyle can be confirmed by eliciting tenderness over the common extensor origin, which frequently radiates toward the wrist on resisted extension. Although lateral epicondylitis has been associated with tennis playing (e.g., 'tennis elbow'), traumas other than racquet sports have been implicated. The presence of radiating pain emanating from the medial elbow suggests possible ulnar nerve compression, especially after forceful elbow extension.

Shoulder

Impingement syndromes, characterized by limited range of motion of the shoulder, are common where overhead work is a frequent activity. It is important to recognize that in almost all cases, impairment guidelines, such as the AMA Guide, suppose structural pathology, and are not suitable for establishing normal range of motion. Physical therapy guidelines are a more useful source of reference values for range of motion.

In summary, the physical examination remains a critical component of the evaluation of the upper extremity and should include the following components useful for diagnosis. An organized approach may be useful. Either proximal to distal (neck–shoulder to digit) or distal to proximal (digit to neck–shoulder) is practical, but it is usually more efficient to progress from anatomic region. The following sequence may prove helpful.
1. General inspection
2. Local inspection and physical examination (color, temperature, tissue integrity)
3. Derivation of pain – static or in movement
4. Measurement of range of motion
5. Provocative tests
6. Motor and sensory exam
7. Preliminary diagnoses

Laboratory evaluation

Laboratory evaluation is important in diagnosing upper extremity disorders. In general, in the past decade there have been few significant additions to laboratory medicine which bear directly on occupational disorders of the upper extremity. Principal modalities include radiographs, electrophysiologic tests, vascular tests, quantitative sensory tests such as vibrometry, and serologic, hematologic, and blood chemistry profiles. In general, the more mechanistic tests have application to local disorders, whereas serology and blood chemistries have relevance to systemic disorders. There are substantial areas of overlap and potential differentiation. Joint pain and motor disturbances from lead toxicity may be exhibited by anemia. Diabetes is a great masquerader and may be confused with or complicate occupationally induced neuropathy. Cold intolerance and peripheral nerve dysfunction due to vibration may be complicated by thyroid disorders. Vascular imaging plays an important role in detecting uncommon but important disorders such as distal arterial obstruction or vascular thoracic outlet compression.

Radiographic studies

X-ray studies of the hands and joints may be critical in the diagnosis of arthritides and traumatic synovitis. Calcification of ligaments can reflect overuse as well as fluorosis. Bone cysts appear more commonly in manual workers, although neither the pathology nor clinical significance is clear.[21] The presence of epicondylar bone spurs may clarify a suspicion of epicondylitis, but their absence does not exclude the diagnosis. Abnormal neck films are notoriously imprecise localizers of cervical spine radicular disease; however, normal films are a useful screen. There appears to be a relatively good assessment of patency of the carpal tunnel by CT, and the median nerve is well visualized by MRI. The diagnostic utility may be compromised by cost, institutional experience, and the greater physiologic relevance of electrodiagnostic studies.

MRI has an important place, particularly in more complex diagnosis. For example, the relative morbidity of angiographic studies of hand circulation discouraged vascular studies in the past. MR(A) currently provides excellent resolution and is the test of choice, unless an intervention such as thrombolytic therapy is considered. MRI of peripheral nerves is also an important potential diagnostic tool. Recurrent symptoms following carpal tunnel release present problems of management, because of the high morbidity associated with repeated surgery. Visualization of nerve flattening or scar formation provides an objective basis for re-instrumentation. MRI has an important role in hand pain. Carpal ischemia, ligamentous injuries and erosions of carpal bones, and early breakdown of repetitively stressed joints, such as the CMC joint of the thumb, will elude standard x-ray diagnosis. They are often highly responsive to conservative therapeutic intervention, when diagnosed at an early stage.

Electrophysiologic studies

The laboratory is essential for the diagnosis of entrapment neuropathies, peripheral and polyneuropathies due to diabetes, and metabolic and inflammatory diseases.[46-49] Certain electrodiagnostic patterns may be helpful in differentiating a distal exposure-related neuropathy,[50] such as that seen with vibration, and the EMG can be specific in conditions such as delayed organophosphorus-induced neurotoxicity. Two common uses in an industrial cohort are for diagnosis of CTS, in which sensory or motor median nerve conduction may be focally blocked at the wrist, and in cervical radiculitis, in which denervation on the EMG may present a diagnostic pattern. Cross-elbow studies are also commonly ordered in the assessment of ulnar nerve entrapment at the elbow, although these studies have a limited sensitivity, even when compression is identified at surgery. F waves and somatosensory-evoked responses have been used in the diagnosis of the thoracic outlet syndrome, although their interpretation has been questioned. The wide disparity in reported results would indicate that they are not an efficacious diagnostic tool.

In earlier studies of American hand surgeon practice, it appeared that CTS was diagnosed in the absence of nerve conduction studies about one-third of the time.[12,51]

However, in a recent study of the practices of physicians certified in physical medicine, rehabilitation and electrodiagnostic medicine, electrophysiologic testing substantially altered 42% of diagnostic decisions.[50] The recognition among many physicians that carpal tunnel release is performed too frequently, and the requirement by some insurance carriers that nerve conduction studies always precede release surgery, may exert impact on the standard of practice. While electronegative carpal tunnel syndrome has been frequently described in the clinical literature, population-based studies have conversely demonstrated that as many as 40% of workers with heavy use patterns may have delayed median nerve latencies in the absence of significant symptoms.[12,52] There is controversy over the sensitivity of electrophysiologic studies because there is no pathologic or other gold standard for CTS (see Chapter 19.2). One difficulty is the age specificity of the tests as well as the wide variation of reported normal values.

There is also the important recognition that conventional nerve conduction studies are summaries of function. The onset latency of the action potential relates only to the fastest conducting fibers, while its waveform reveals the functional status of the remaining, slower conducting fibers. Slowed conduction itself leads to few, if any, clinical symptoms, as long as all the impulses arrive at the target organ. It is also widely recognized that the relative degree of slowing does not correspond with clinical severity. Conduction block, however, is often accompanied by symptoms of major loss of strength. In summary, the EMG indicates the need for therapeutic intervention when there is evidence of cervical root irritation or when specific motor branches of the ulnar nerve demonstrate denervation. However, slowing at the carpal tunnel, the most frequently utilized finding, usually does not require a specific generic intervention. It should be remembered that paresthesias (ectopic peripheral nerve activity), functional deficits, positional or nocturnal brachalgias, and digital cramping require a differential diagnosis, and the nerve conduction study provides a physiologic measurement, not an anatomic image.

Quantitative sensory tests
Tests for vibrotactile threshold at single or multiple frequencies and tests of thermographic threshold have become available for use in the industrial setting and have been the subject of international standardization.[53,54] Their simplicity and portability define them as potentially powerful surveillance instruments, and in principle they can measure specific mechanoreceptor thresholds and different fiber types (heat and cold) in the digit.[50,55,56] Moreover, certain mechanoreceptor populations appear to be age specific, whereas others are not age sensitive.

Vibrometry alone may not differentiate between focal receptor injury, such as can be caused by cold and vibration, and more proximal compression neuropathy. There is convincing evidence that while these are preferred tests for small fiber nerve injury, they provide insensitive measures of nerve compression, which will be the more common concern in most work settings. The testing algorithm should be carefully reviewed before initiating screening

programs in working populations. Although not currently available, it would be highly attractive to have a portable, simply operated, and relatively inexpensive device that differentiates cervical myelopathy, median nerve mononeuropathy and small fiber dysfunction with a high level of sensitivity and reliability.

Blood testing
Elevated muscle enzymes (creatine kinase [CK], aldolase) have been reported in industrial workers with acute neck and shoulder disorders, but a more conventional use of muscle enzymes is in the identification of inflammatory myositis, particularly as it may coexist with degenerative upper extremity diseases. Rheumatoid arthritis, collagen vascular diseases, and gout all merit the appropriate serologic and chemistry studies (see Chapter 23.5). An elevation in the sedimentation rate is both common and non-specific, limiting its diagnostic value.

Raynaud's phenomenon, attributable to impact and vibration from power tools, will usually not require an extensive rheumatologic workup when workplace risk factors are identified, and when signs and symptoms are confined to the hands and have a gradual onset of expression. However, since isolated Raynaud's may precede a full presentation of an autoimmune disorder by several years, specialized laboratory tests (e.g., anti-centromere antibody, anti-topoisomerase I) are warranted at baseline, particularly when cases are sporadic. In the past decade, Lyme disease and hepatitis C have also been recognized in the differential diagnosis of generalized joint or muscle pain.

Classification

Because diagnostic criteria have varying levels of specificity, even for the most frequently diagnosed upper extremity diseases, there have been significant challenges for case definitions. For this reason it is useful to aggregate soft tissue disorders affecting the upper extremity into the categories outlined in Table 23.3.3 and discussed below.

DISORDERS OF DEFINED ANATOMY AND QUANTIFIABLE PATHOPHYSIOLOGY BY OBJECTIVE MEASUREMENT
Hand–arm vibration syndrome

Vibration exposure to the hands and arms associated with pneumatic hand tools and larger stationary tools, such as rock drills, has been associated with a characteristic pattern of neurologic, peripheral vascular, and musculoskeletal signs and symptoms.[57-59] Outcomes involving measurable neurologic and arterial dysfunction have added substantially to clinical assessment of pain and function. Tools implicated in the disorder include chain saws, rock drills, grinders, pneumatic hammers, and jackhammers. Changes in disease prevalence associated with the chainsaw, the hallmark vibratory tool, has been due to industrial modifi-

I Disorders of defined anatomy and quantifiable pathophysiology by objective measurements
Hand–arm vibration syndrome – vasospasm and small fiber neuropathy
Nerve entrapment and occlusion disorders which can be assessed by electrophysiologic tests
Median nerve
Carpal tunnel syndrome
Anterior interosseous nerve syndrome
Ulnar nerve
Cubital tunnel syndrome (entrapment at the elbow)
Ulnar nerve syndrome (canal of Guyon)
Radial nerve
Radial tunnel syndrome – posterior interosseous nerve (motor)
Radial tunnel syndrome – posterior interosseous nerve (sensory)
Wartenburg's syndrome
Occupationally induced distal polyneuropathy
Vaso-occlusive disorders and disorders of peripheral circulation
II Anatomically defined and semiquantified disorders based on clinical assessment
Tendinitis of the hand and wrist
Extensor and flexor tendinitis of the forearm
Trigger digits
Tendinitis of the elbow
Lateral epicondylitis
Medial epicondylitis
III Entrapment syndromes which suggest multilevel disease and symptoms without anatomic localization
Multiple site or multinerve compression syndromes
Neurogenic thoracic outlet syndrome
Diffuse myalgia

Table 23.3.3 Classification of disorders of the upper extremity

cation. While the emphasis on air-powered and electrical tools increases power and portability, these modifications may also result in increasing risk for disease.

The most commonly described symptom has been cold-induced vasospasm, detectable as finger blanching, which is often indistinguishable from Raynaud's phenomenon of primary and secondary origin. The most frequent clinical abnormality has been a quantifiable deficit in cutaneous sensory performance; another common occurrence has been pain and paresthesias suggestive of peripheral neuropathy or focal compression, which greatly complicates differentiation from the CTS. A pattern of declining hand strength and electromyographically defined early fatiguability is common. Because of the involvement of multiple organ systems, a more general acronym, HAVS (hand–arm vibration syndrome), has come into common usage.

The contribution of small fiber injury to deficits in touch and temperature sensation is consistent with the observation that the tissues of the digit and palm absorb well over 90% of transmitted energy from a conventional vibrating tool, contributing to small fiber nerve injury.

Pathogenesis

The principal clinical presentations of HAVS – vasospasm, quantitative cutaneous sensory deficits, and nerve conduction abnormalities, frequently at the wrist – involve different anatomic sites and, accordingly, different mechanisms of injury. Vibration is measured in terms of the frequency distribution of oscillations; the direction, velocity, and

acceleration of those oscillations; and the impulsivity, or force range (amplitude), expressed in each impact cycle. Each of these physical characteristics has a bearing on symptoms and tissue injuries that may occur, particularly in the palms and digits, but also more proximally in the shoulder and neck when frequencies are very low. For example, large impact tools, such as jackhammers, produce tissue waves that can affect the shoulder and neck. On the other hand, electric rotary tools can produce energies that are entirely absorbed in the hand and wrist. Although cold-related vascular symptoms frequently follow neurologic symptoms chronologically, the vascular and neurovascular symptoms appear to be independent, and pure vasospastic disease is common.

Quantitative sensory abnormalities, presumed to be due to injury to local fingertip receptors, represent the most common abnormality.[60,61] There is controversy over the prevalence of nerve conduction abnormalities in workers exposed to vibration, as about 20% of symptomatic cases may have median nerve slowing at the wrist, which is indistinguishable from CTS.[62-64] Because HAVS more frequently involves the palm and the distal ulnar nerve, there is usually a poor response to carpal tunnel release, particularly if there is a return to the former worksite. In each case, the common etiology is vibration, predominantly in the 30–500 Hz range, although there is debate about the identity and weighting of the most damaging frequencies. The role of very high frequencies (above the 1500 Hz 'upper limit' of conventional measurement) from high-speed tools, including medical and dental drills, saws, and ultrasonic devices, is uncertain. Several studies have indentified small fiber and vascular dysfunction but the mechanisms have not been defined.[65]

Clinical course

There is little evidence that tolerance plays a major role in vibratory disorders, and vascular attacks may affect the majority of dedicated workforce within a decade of exposure. Over time attacks generally increase in frequency and are elicited by milder temperatures. There are two predominant patterns – diffuse attacks and a cold-intolerant pattern. These patterns do not differ on quantitative tests, and the delineating factor may be the ability to seek cold protection. Unlike Raynaud's phenomenon resulting from other causes, trophism and gangrene are extremely rare. In cooler climates, the onset of summer markedly attenuates the vascular condition. It is also important to recognize that cold-related pain is a hallmark of chronic peripheral nerve injury. Symptoms that follow the dermatome of an established peripheral nerve injury should be confirmed by laboratory testing, or a history which indicates a well-circumscribed blanching pattern.

A traditional distinction has been made between HAVS and an 'acute vibration syndrome', where hand paresthesias induced by power tool use will remit symptomatically after several hours. However, more recent information has associated the severity of these paresthesias with the duration and intensity of exposure, suggesting that even apparent reversibility may disguise a cumulative disease process.

Because anti-vibration gloves do not effectively protect the hands, clinical management involves work attenuation or removal, if tool types remain unchanged. Since small fiber nerve injury appears to be largely irreversible, and Raynaud's is at best partially reversible, there is a compelling case for termination of exposure. On the other hand, industrial indemnification policies in the United States provide limited material support, even when disease is advanced. The decision to remove from work is therefore complicated and frequently involves a balance between risk for disease progression and implications of disability.

Diagnosis

Although history and clinical presentation are important, there should be particular emphasis on quantitative testing, to reinforce a decision on the individual's removal from exposure, assess intervention, and to stage subclinical disease. Digital vasospasm has been traditionally tested by cold water immersion, but temperature recovery testing appears to be without value. Cold challenge plethysmography, where available, offers greater precision with reliable quantitation. Workers with non-detectable finger systolic blood pressures or with reductions of more than 30–40% with moderate cold stimulation have vasospastic disease that will become aggravated by further exposure.[30,66] In contrast, vascular tests, such as brachial/digital blood pressure comparisons, doppler and pulse-volume plethsymo-graphy at ambient temperatures, and temperature recovery following cold challenge, have no significant role in the diagnosis of cold-induced vasospastic disease.

Nerve conduction studies, particularly segmental studies, can delineate isolated median nerve wrist abnormalities from more diffuse neuropathies and systemic polyneuro-pathies. Cutaneous neurologic abnormalities are well assessed by quantitative sensory tests, particularly vibrotactile thresholds that are abnormal in a majority of exposed workers.[60,67] Hand weakness is a common complaint, and is often influenced by diffuse slowing of myelinated nerves.[68] Because there is great age and population specificity to these tests, they should not be used for pre-employment or cross-sectional screening without a well-documented parameter for normalcy. Hand x-ray studies frequently are abnormal in manual workers, with degenerative joint disease, trauma, and bone cysts a common finding; these conditions rarely contribute to the diagnosis.[21,69]

Differential diagnosis

Principal competing diagnoses include Raynaud's phenomenon (both primary and secondary), peripheral obstructive arterial disease, associated systemic conditions such as diabetes and rheumatoid arthritis, and peripheral neuropathy.[70] Occlusive disease, such as the ulnar hammer syndrome, will often present as a Raynaud's pattern, but the distribution and onset usually make diagnosis clear. Routine vascular laboratory studies will generally establish the diagnosis. The differentiation from other entrapment neuropathies (e.g., CTS) and more proximal lesions is

particularly important.[71] There has been considerable attention in the vibration literature to differentiating entrapment neuropathies such as CTS from distal small fiber nerve injuries in the digits. In the past 15 years, most investigators have recognized that small fiber injury to fingertip nociceptors is distinctly more common than CTS in vibration-exposed workers, that electrodiagnostic studies are insensitive measures of this type of injury, and that quantitative sensory testing is essential if unnecessary carpal tunnel surgery is to be avoided. These tests, particularly measurement of vibrotactile thresholds, have consistently demonstrated deficits in perception in both symptomatic and asymptomatic patients exposed to vibration.

As noted, a suspicion for collagen vascular disease warrants laboratory studies. Screening laboratory studies should include a complete blood count, blood chemistry studies, ESR, rheumatoid factor, ANA, thyroid function tests, and in some settings, cold agglutinins, cryoglobulins, and assays for Lyme disease. There are good reasons to obtain specific antibodies for collagen vascular disease that may present as isolated Raynaud's phenomenon. Degenerative conditions, such as rheumatoid arthritis, usually preclude significant vibratory exposure from heavy tools.

Treatment and prognosis

For established disease with positive plethysmography, abnormal vibrotactility, functional interference with perception, and increasing pain, exposure removal is generally necessary for effective management. A decade ago, NIOSH recommended mandatory work removal at a specified symptom level. Because removal from exposure may mean loss of employment, alternative approaches may be necessary. These alternative approaches include calcium channel blockers, including sublingual administration to abort attacks in extreme conditions, and liberal use of hand warmers in cases in which vascular symptoms predominate. In general, however, medication is poorly tolerated at doses needed to eliminate Raynaud's attacks, and is therefore not a practical option. Anti-vibration gloves, particularly those with wrist supports, should be used regardless of the presence of symptoms as they block higher frequencies, but are ineffective against the most damaging frequencies. Until it can be demonstrated that higher frequencies are benign, the role of gloves is justified.

Smoking reduction reduces the frequency and intensity of vascular attacks. Continued smoking prolongs measurable vascular dysfunction when exposure is terminated. A restrictive program of administrative controls that reduces exposures to less than 2 hours per day, coupled with vigorous tool maintenance and replacement with less vibration-producing machines, may abort clinical and subclinical progression. Fortunately, if exposures are attenuated or eliminated, the prognosis for milder cases is relatively good, with almost 50% of patients improving to near their baseline in about 5 years following last exposure. Unfortunately, when neurologic disease is well established, improvement is more modest.

Carpal tunnel syndrome

Carpal tunnel syndrome (CTS) (Fig. 23.3.1) is identified by a characteristic pattern of pain, paresthesias, and weakness following the distribution of the median nerve distal to the transcarpal ligament in the wrist. Along with tenosynovitis, it is one of the two diagnoses most frequently ascribed to repetitive workplace injury.[72] Although the median nerve provides only limited motor innervation to the hand, in the earliest accounts by surgical pioneers, such as Paget and Hunt (1911), thenar atrophy and compressive neuritis were the predominant described pathologies.[73] Despite clinical series evolving over the past 40 years that include several thousands of patients, aggressive carpal tunnel release is a relatively new surgical procedure.[74] Allowing for the earlier misdiagnosis as TOS for conditions which would currently be called CTS, only 12 releases were described in the surgical literature prior to 1950. It is now an extremely frequent procedure, with the average American hand surgeon performing more than 100 per year, more than 90% on an outpatient basis.

There appears to be widespread confidence in the clinical presentation among specialists, independent of nerve conduction studies. Although in the 1960s Phelan, who

Seamstresses and sewing machine operators
Packinghouse workers
Fish processing workers
Poultry workers
Quarry workers
Electronics assemblers
Dental hygienists
Forestry workers
Furniture assemblers
Automobile and aircraft workers
Grocers and checkout clerks
Letter sorters and optical scanners
Butchers and boners
Clerical workers
Restaurant and hotel employees
Clerks

Table 23.3.4 Occupations associated with carpal tunnel syndrome

did much to advance surgical technique and recognition in the United States, denied a particular role for occupation,[75] there is substantial recent literature that associates CTS with work.[70,76-78] Because of the strong association of carpal tunnel syndrome with repetitive and forceful activities and awkward postures, there has been particular attention to the process by which joint deviation, loading and repetitive muscle contraction may raise pressure within the carpal tunnel. Table 23.3.4 lists occupations with increased risk of CTS.

In spite of the wide acceptance of the diagnosis and the availability of confirmatory electrodiagnostic testing, recent studies have provided evidence for potential confusion. Motor and sensory nerve conduction delays have been described in 25% of asymptomatic individuals in workforces with primary repetitive manual tasks.[79] In some workforces, when classic paresthesias are present, positive nerve conduction studies are recognized in less than 60% of cases. Intermittent nocturnal brachalgias, which are a hallmark of carpal tunnel syndrome, when routinely screened, may be recognized commonly in adults over 60 years of age. In short, both the basis for and consequences of diagnosis are ambiguous. Even when the pattern of nerve injury distinctly implicates a focal site of compression, the indication for surgical decompression may be unclear.

Pathogenesis

Because of its tight internal dimensions and prodigious content of nine flexor tendons enclosed in synovial sheaths, the carpal canal offers little tolerance for volume change. In principal, median nerve compression can result from space-occupying lesions, such as neuromas; expansion of soft tissues, as with synovitis or accessory muscles; bony protrusions,[80] such as calluses; or intrinsic susceptibility from primary nerve pathology, as in diabetic neuropathy. Many systemic diseases, including amyloidosis, hypothyroidism, acromegaly, and Paget's disease, have been associated with CTS. With the exception of rheumatoid arthritis, diabetes, and pregnancy, underlying conditions have been relatively infrequent in large case series. Such conditions are even rarer in occupational cohorts, usually involving less than 5% of cases.

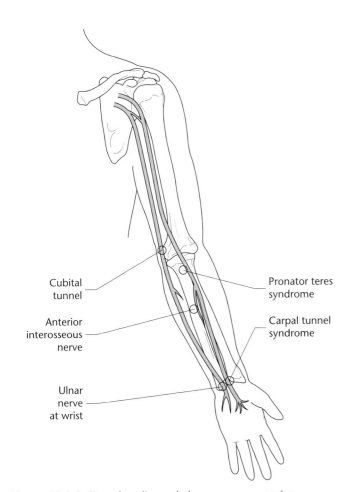

Cubital tunnel

Anterior interosseous nerve

Ulnar nerve at wrist

Pronator teres syndrome

Carpal tunnel syndrome

Figure 23.3.1: Sites of median and ulnar nerve compression. (Adapted from Harter BT. Indications for surgery in work-related compression neuropathies in the upper extremity. J Occup Med 1989; 4:484–95.)

Recent efforts at defining CTS in the workplace have focused on extrinsic cumulative trauma to soft tissues in the wrist. Force, repetition, and vibration have emerged most consistently as relevant job risks. No simple correlation exists between force and symptoms. Newer data have cast doubt on a single mechanism involving extrinsic compression caused by an inflamed synovium. For example, force exerted over the base of the palm during assembly tasks may cause mechanical damage to the median nerve in the palm, causing signs and symptoms of carpal tunnel syndrome. Internal responses may include inflammatory responses to tissue injury, neurochemical changes, and altered metabolism. Force and vibration may cause an intrinsic and reversible swelling of myelinated nerves, and in some cases, more distal injury to glabrous skin receptors or small nerve fibers with a carpal tunnel-like pattern.[77,81,82]

The narrow anatomic confines of the carpal canal lends credence to the presumption that extreme postures would be a risk factor. Studies of intracarpal pressure in these more exaggerated or non-neutral positions have been consistent, generally demonstrating large increases in pressure, when the wrist is forcefully stressed, particularly in hyperextension. Relatively low fingertip loads also raise carpal pressure. Pinching, grasping and wrist angulation are often accompanied by classic symptoms in diagnosed cases.

Clinical course

Because clinically identified CTS represents a spectrum of diseases ranging from vague paresthesias in a median nerve distribution to frank thenar atrophy, there is no universal clinical course. The literature on outcomes is limited, mostly characterizing results of surgical interventions. The condition is often progressive, unless there is medical intervention or, in the occupational setting, workplace alterations are made. However, intermittent symptoms, particularly if they occur during sleep or if they are positional, will often resolve with only modest intervention. Because long-standing paresthesias and muscle atrophy bring a worse prognostic outcome, an argument exists for early surgical intervention. While plausible, many cases will persist at a low level without aggravation for many years. Alternatively, the rapid relief that may accompany rest or a work change, and the frequent necessity for job change even after surgery, complicates the decision on intervention. Given the potentially benign course of uncomplicated nerve compression, and access to ergonomic interventions, conservative management can and should play a larger role. It is also important to recognize that accompanying symptoms, such as painful tendons and joints, limited range of motion and diminished wrist mechanics, and problems with dexterity, will usually not be addressed by surgery. If these are the main source of disability, the limits of carpal tunnel release require consideration.

Diagnosis

Because compressive neuropathy can result in local demyelination or more serious axonal degeneration, a differentiation between paresthesias (numbness and tingling) and loss of sensation is important. Clumsiness due to sensory and proprioceptive impairment suggests a more serious condition. A history of night-time and morning symptoms, sometimes occurring with driving, and relief by shaking or movement, is particularly useful in differentiating CTS from cervical myelopathy and more diffuse processes that involve small nerve fibers. The classic physical diagnostic tests, Phelan's maneuver and Tinel's sign, are positive in many asymptomatic individuals and correlate poorly with nerve conduction tests.

Electrodiagnostic studies are at the core of clinical decision making, although reports of surgical amelioration in patients with negative electrodiagnostic results is well established when other clinical evidence is documented. Muscle wasting can be difficult to determine clinically, so reports of thenar weakness should warrant full EMG studies. Because rheumatoid arthritis, thyroid disease, and diabetes mellitus have all been associated with CTS, and because they are relatively common disorders, screening tests are often warranted, even when a secondary etiology seems improbable. The coexistence of a work-related disorder and neuropathy from another disease process is important, as additive insults may significantly limit future function.

Differential diagnosis

The diagnosis of CTS poses three difficulties for the clinician: (1) differentiation from musculoskeletal pain syndromes and other anatomically non-specific soft tissue disorders, (2) differentiation from other entrapment neuropathies with a peripheral presentation, and (3) differentiation of purely localized nerve compression from systemic disorders.

Systemic causes of CTS include conditions producing edema (pregnancy, cirrhosis, and the nephrotic syndrome); infiltrative disorders such as amyloidosis, myxedema, and acromegaly; and soft tissue inflammatory states, such as rheumatoid arthritis. One of the most important causes is diabetic neuropathy, which may place the nerve at increased risk of injury, causing a more severe pattern of pain and sensory loss in the upper extremity than in the lower extremity. In most working cohorts, systemic diseases are uncommon. Differentiation of CTS from other causes of nerve entrapment and neuropathy is summarized in Table 23.3.5.

Treatment

In the absence of gross weakness or atrophy, conservative management, including hand splints at night, is the first line of treatment.[83] Job task modification is often critical in this phase. Corticosteroid injection into the carpal tunnel may have some short-term value while carrying a small risk of nerve injury. The role of physical and occupational therapy is equivocal. However, many cases of carpal tunnel syndrome are accompanied by significant wrist and flexor inflammation with associated compression. These associated structural abnormalities may benefit from physical therapy, including iontopheresis. Persistent pain, progres-

Disorder	Similarities	Differences
Vibration neuropathy	Finger paresthesias	Exposure history; sensorineural distribution beyond median nerve
	Reduced grip, Nerve conduction abnormalities	
Radiculopathies		
C6	Paresthesias of digits I and II	Neck, shoulder, chest wall pain; Use pain, night improvement, normal nerve conduction at wrist, abnormal EMG
C7	Paresthesias, Pain on dorsum of hand	Decreased elbow extension and finger extension and flexion, abnormal EMG
Neurogenic TOS	Paresthesias relieved by position or shaking	Association with arm elevation
Reflex sympathetic dystrophy	Pain and paresthesias, sensation of edema, reduced flexion	Rubor, cyanosis, trophic finger changes
Diabetic mononeuritis	Pain and weakness	Asymmetry, diffuse reduction in nerve conduction

Table 23.3.5 Differential diagnostic considerations for carpal tunnel syndrome

sive symptoms, and EMG abnormalities are indications for surgery, which is usually successful in relieving nighttime and positional paresthesias. A common postsurgical complaint of diminished hand strength must be weighed in the management of manual workers. A minority of occupationally induced cases are initially surgical candidates, and in almost all cases, a return to the previous conditions of employment will prove painful, if not impossible, after surgery.[84] Therefore, hand rehabilitation and worksite assessment are key components of clinical management.

Anterior interosseous syndrome (Fig. 23.3.1)

The anterior interosseous nerve arises distal to the lateral epicondyle as the last major branch of the median nerve. It contains no superficial sensory fibers but innervates the long flexor of the thumb, the deep flexors to the second and third digits, and the pronator quadratus. The classic clinical findings are forearm pain and diminished pinch.[85] The EMG is the definitive diagnostic test, and the differential diagnosis includes tendon rupture and repetitive injury. Occupational etiologies are prominent, particularly in jobs requiring repetitive flexion and pronation of the elbow. Workers at risk include butchers, carpenters, and leather cutters; heavy lifting also has been implicated. Except in acute rupture, rest and immobilization rather than surgery is the primary intervention, with work reassignment frequently necessary. Recovery may be slow, and rehabilitation needs are extensive. These conditions are relatively rare compared with the more common entrapment neuropathies.

Cubital tunnel syndrome (Fig. 23.3.1)

Ulnar nerve compression at the elbow may be caused by acute or chronic trauma and the condition has been associated with chronic upper body weight bearing by the elbow, and has been frequently diagnosed in computer use. It is the second most common entrapment neuropathy. Diagnosis may be challenging, as paresthesias in an ulnar distribution and positive percussion signs (Tinel's at the triceps sulcus, medial epicondyle, and cubital tunnel) are rather common. Because of the extensive motor inner-

vation to the hand from the ulnar nerve, functional limitations may be very significant and may be manifested by diminished hand strength. The ulnar nerve supplies the adductor pollicis brevis, a portion of the flexor pollicis brevis, the digital flexors in the ulnar hand, and the first dorsal interosseous muscle. In classic ulnar nerve compression, the loss of pinch function may be almost complete; however, a more generalized weakness is the usual pattern. Digital coordination may be limited. Because of diminished innervation of the hypothenar muscle group, opponens function may be significantly reduced. Nerve conduction studies applied above and below the elbow can localize the lesion and differentiate ulnar nerve compression at the wrist, which may have a similar presentation. Because splinted immobilization may require many weeks of observation and because surgery often has little success, the clinician has limited courses for action.

The principal diagnostic challenge is that nerve conduction studies are normal as much as 50% of the time, even when symptoms are classic.[86] Occupational therapy is often highly effective, particularly when there are mechanical limitations in the pronator–flexor complex. In many cases, the exposed ulnar nerve is irritated by pressure at the elbow and the simple modification of posture or provision of protection is sufficient. When motor lesions are expected, however, it is important that an EMG is performed to identify affected motor groups. Because of a problematic surgical success rate, ulnar nerve compression at the elbow requires careful management.

Ulnar tunnel syndrome (Fig. 23.3.1)

Ulnar nerve compression at the wrist (Guyon's canal) is associated with repetitive blunt trauma to the hypothenar region, and it may occur in carpentry, auto repair, and polishing, as well as from handle pressure from hand tools. Many cases are attributable to the workplace. However, compared to carpal tunnel syndrome and cubital tunnel syndrome, it is rather uncommon. Accordingly, the tendency to simultaneously release the canal of Guyon during carpal tunnel syndrome should be discouraged.

Depending on the branches affected, loss may be motor, sensory, or combined. Nerve conduction studies are diagnostic and assist in the differentiation from ulnar nerve entrapment at the elbow and from C8 to T1 radiculopathy. Pisiform fracture is one reason for surgical intervention, although the presenting complaint will be pain. However, in general, ulnar tunnel syndrome is relatively rare, and combined carpal tunnel and ulnar tunnel releases for hand paresthesias probably involve misdiagnosis of a more general peripheral neuritic pattern.

Radial tunnel syndrome

Posterior interosseous nerve motor branch compression in the radial forearm is a relatively uncommon condition. While pain below the radial head of the humerus may be present, the primary finding is incomplete paralysis of the wrist extensors. It is a surgical condition that is confirmed by electrodiagnostic studies. A more controversial and common disorder involving the sensory branch of the posterior interosseous nerve is so-called 'resistant tennis elbow'. The predominant symptom, pain distal to the lateral epicondyle, complicates differentiation from lateral epicondylitis. The syndrome is most common in manual workers performing repetitive tasks involving forceful twisting pronation, supination, elbow flexion and extension.

Pain in lateral epicondylitis is more often provoked by forceful grip and wrist extension, but differentiating nerve entrapment from tendinitis may prove difficult. There are significant implications for clinical management. Radial tunnel syndrome affecting the motor branch is often a surgical condition, whereas lateral epicondylitis is probably best treated with rest and physical therapy. While an anatomic band at the arcade of Frohse may affect the sensory branch and is a disorder subject to release, the more common presentation is a combination of pain distal to the lateral epicondyle accompanied by a positive provocative test (resisted middle finger extension and resisted supination). Radial sensory nerve conduction studies correlate poorly with symptoms. This presentation occurs commonly in the setting of apparent multiple entrapments and should be categorized as such when multiple compression signs are present.

Because of its superficial course through the wrist, the radial nerve is susceptible to entrapment and injury, causing dorsal and radial wrist pain. Although associated with iatrogenic interventions from tenosynovectomy and tight casting, Wartenburg's syndrome may evolve from wristbands and tight industrial gloves. The latter is an important consideration, given the recent introduction of splinted industrial gloves for carpal tunnel prevention support. Relief from external compression is generally curative.

Occupationally induced distal neuropathies

Toxic neuropathies are addressed in Chapter 28.2. The preeminence of hand symptoms in manual workers may make differentiation from entrapments difficult. The neuropathies caused by lead, arsenic, some organophosphorus pesticides, and n-hexane, although involving both upper and lower extremities, may be more obvious in the upper extremity because of interference with fine coordinative tasks. There may be the additional problem of local trauma to an injured nerve.

Vasoocclusive disorders and disorders of peripheral circulation

Arterial occlusive disease, expressed as either Raynaud's phenomenon or digital pain, has been described in a variety of hand-intensive tasks. Palmar and digital artery occlusion that is work induced is usually due to traumatic ulnar artery occlusion, the so-called *hypothenar syndrome* or *ulnar hammer syndrome*.[87,88] The general mechanism causing thrombotic emboli in the palm and fingers is blunt trauma, caused by using the hand as a percussive object or by aggressively twisting hard objects. The disorder has also been described, although uncommonly, with the use of hand-held pneumatic tools. The usual mechanism is ascribed to trauma and abrupt endothelial injury, with the ulnar artery being bludgeoned against the hook of the hamate. Contraction around the ulnar artery by an anatomic muscle sling or anomalous hypothenar muscle have also been described. Physiologically the lesion is the consequence of thrombi or small clots that lodge in smaller or more peripheral vessels. This can occur because of pressure, the abruption of blood flow, and stasis-related clot formation.

It is also hypothesized that shear forces injure the blood vessel lining or endothelium, with repair mechanisms within the vascular intima leading to clot formation. The use of large vibratory tools, such as jackhammers and posting drills, can produce a combined disorder of traumatically induced arterial vasospasm and occlusion. Diagnostic tests include clinical assessment of refill time, plethysmography, Doppler studies, MR(A) and arteriography. The acute presentation of Raynaud's, particularly in an ulnar distribution, is grounds for immediate intervention, with thrombolytic therapy.[89] Given the irreversibility of symptoms when clot is organized, even a moderate level of suspicion warrants immediate imaging.

ANATOMICALLY DEFINED AND SEMIQUANTIFIABLE DISORDERS BASED ON CLINICAL ASSESSMENT
Tendinitis of the hand and wrist (Fig. 23.3.2)

To assist in their gliding movement, tendons are surrounded by a layer of tenosynovium, which in the flexor and extensor hand compartments become synovial sheaths.[90] These sheaths are a frequent site of inflammation and tendinitis. Pathophysiologically, four main types of non-acute tendon disorders have been suggested.[9] Paratenonitis (tenosynovitis) is the inflammation of the paratenon with symptoms including pain, swelling, warmth and tenderness. Tendinosis

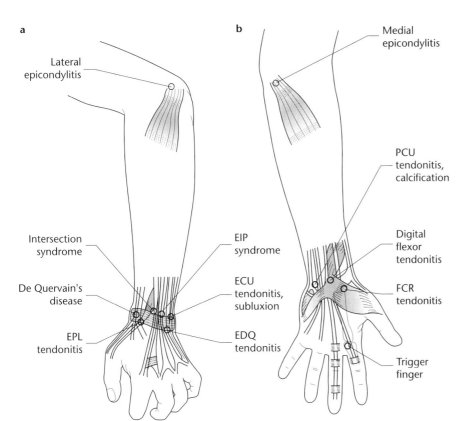

Figure 23.3.2: Dorsal (a) and volar (b) locations of tendinitis in the upper extremity. (Adapted from Thorson EP, Szabo RM. Tendinitis of the wrist and elbow. J Occup Med 1989;4:419–31.)

involves intratendinous degeneration with fiber disorientation, scattered vascular ingrowth, occasional necrosis and calcification. Tendon nodularity may be noted, but swelling of the tendon sheath is absent. Paratenonitis may be observed with tendinosis and corresponding signs of inflammation and nodularity.

Tendinitis (tendon strain or tear) may range from inflammation with acute hemorrhage and tear to inflammation with chronic degeneration. While this classification is not universally accepted, the basic distinctions between inflammation, degeneration and nodularity have treatment consequences. Local tissue pressure and pain also may accompany inflamed synovium at the elbow, wrist, and finger joints. Two anatomically specific and discrete disorders are tenosynovitis – inflammation of synovial linings, confined to the wrist and hand, and peritendinitis crepitans – inflammation of musculotendinous junctions that may extend into the muscle bellies themselves. The cardinal tenet of diagnosis is anatomic localization, through stretching and isometric resistance of the tendon. Treatment includes rest and non-steroidal anti-inflammatory therapy.

Although poorly localized pain syndromes are sometimes labeled as tendinitis or tenosynovitis, this practice is inappropriate and leads to incorrect management and prevention. A history of previous injury should be pursued, and radiographic evaluation is sometimes merited, because even minor anatomic anomalies may become a focus for inflammation due to repetition. Particular problems have been associated with sharp handle edges and excessive deviations from a neutral axis in either a radial–ulnar or flexor–extensor plane.

Extensor and flexor tendinitis of the forearm

The most important extensor tendinitis involves the long abductor of the thumb and its short extensor.[91-93] This inflammatory condition, called de Quervain's syndrome, is characterized by pain and swelling over the radial styloid process. The classic physical diagnostic maneuver, Finkelstein's test, involves elicitation of typical pain with the hand in ulnar deviation and the thumb adducted to the palm. A palpable nodule in the first dorsal compartment or early ganglion cyst formation may be diagnostic. Included in the differential diagnosis is arthritis of the first metacarpal phalangeal joint that may arise from repetitive tasks, such as are found in light assembly. Fractures, sprains, ligamentous tears, and avascular necrosis also may cause a similar pattern of pain over the dorsum of the hand. Immobilization, thumb splints, and NSAIDs may be curative in conjunction with job modification. Injection of the tendon sheath with steroids is effective and benign and an alternative first-line treatment in severe cases. Fibrosis may warrant surgery, but surgery should not be a first line of approach.

An intersection syndrome involving tendinitis of both the extensor carpi radialis longus and brevis may involve pain and crepitus over the distal extensor forearm.[94] This is a relatively common disorder, which has been associated with repetitive wrist movement, weight training, and rowing. This is a non-surgical condition, which responds to the familiar triad of rest, NSAIDs, and injection of corticosteroids, if necessary.

Tendinitis of the flexor carpi ulnaris is characterized by wrist pain with flexion and extension. It is associated with repetitive use and racquet sports. Pain and weakness should be reproduced by forced ulnar deviation. Conservative management usually is effective. A less common condition involves the flexor carpi radialis, which may impede wrist flexion, causing a trigger wrist. Tendinitis of the digital flexors may occur in the setting of CTS, with palmar pain exacerbated by digital flexion against resistance. Treatment is part of general carpal tunnel therapy discussed above. Wrist range of motion, defined by flexor and extensor tendons, is a good gauge of overall dynamic function.

A principle of hand therapy is that restoration of normal wrist dynamics is central to the treatment of nerve compression and soft tissue hand pain. Although 60 degrees of flexion and extension is often described as normal, a healthy wrist should be capable of 80 degrees of active motion. A subset of individuals will have wrist hyperlaxity with flexion well in excess of 90 degrees, MCP extension in excess of 45 degrees, and hyperextensibility of the IP of the thumb and DIPs of the four digits. 'Double jointedness' or hyperlaxity also poses risks of injury because of the tendency to eccentrically contract small muscle groups. Intrinsic muscle training with a hand therapist is critical, as conventional exercises that promote range of motion may exacerbate this problem.

Involvement of the musculotendinous junction of the extensor muscle mass in the forearm is common in workers performing intensive manual tasks. It is important that localization distinguishes pain in the muscle body from tendon pain and tendon insertion pain at the lateral epicondyle. Vague forearm functional pain can often be localized to these structures and may be accompanied by tendon tautness, provoked by direct palpation. These types of trigger points (tendon jump signs) may be mistaken for a multiple trigger point syndrome; but they respond well to manual therapy. Pain at the musculotendinous junction may mimic a nerve compression disorder (radial tunnel syndrome, ulnar nerve compression, pronator syndrome). Provocative testing of the muscle tendon groups against resistance is an important feature of diagnosis.

Experience indicates that tendinitis can resolve with surprising slowness. The reasons can be found in the pathophysiology of tendon repair. Exercise and movement are fundamental to the therapeutic process of an injured tendon; however, movement of a deformed, devascularized, or inflamed tendon will provoke further injury and breakdown. A knee injury may take up to 2 years to fully repair, and the same mechanisms prevail in the upper extremity.

Trigger digits

A snapping sound, usually of the first and third digit, is commonly related to nodular enlargement of the tendon or narrowing of the flexor tendon sheath.[95] Severe pain is uncommon, although clicking or snapping is often alarming. Because of the intrinsic strength in finger flexors, a locked flexed position may occur. Local steroid injection may abort an early presentation, but elimination usually

requires surgery, which is usually successful and minimally traumatic. There are several considerations for prevention when early nodularity occurs at a threshold where surgery is not yet required. Friction is generated at these locations as the tendon slides against adjacent surfaces, causing a shearing force. Higher levels of muscle tension are required to achieve a specific level of strength at the fingertip during non-neutral wrist postures, and tendons are subject to greater shear stress with non-neutral wrist postures. Similarly, compressive force in the A1 pulley has been demonstrated to dramatically rise from the neutral posture to full flexion. In short, although attention is usually paid to the digit itself, many of the same measures that may prevent carpal tunnel syndrome and flexor tendinitis are pertinent to the avoidance of trigger digits.

Lateral and medial epicondylitis

Lateral epicondylitis usually is attributed to tears and associated inflammation in the common extensors at elbow level. It is this anatomic location that is useful in the differentiation from radial tunnel syndrome, because pain is often reproducible with firm palpation over the lateral epicondyle and extensor muscle mass.[96] The condition has been associated with heavy lifting and occurs most frequently in the fourth and fifth decades of life. The characteristic symptoms are pain with lifting, gripping, and wrist extension. The popular epithet of tennis elbow notwithstanding, it is a common condition among industrial workers. In the case of epicondylitis, the insertional tears seen in young athletes playing racket sports have little in common with the non-inflammatory degeneration seen in older populations, whether or not work is implicated as a risk factor. Restrictions from lifting and gripping are common approaches to care, with immobilization and steroid injection being more aggressive, though frequently necessary treatments. Because the condition is usually non-inflammatory, NSAIDs are usually of limited value; however, limiting wrist flexion and stabilizing the forearm extensor insertion at the lateral elbow with a support strap may be helpful. Because grip and extension are so central to many jobs, lateral epicondylitis is a condition that can be irreconcilably chronic and produce major and undesirable changes in life and work.

Skilled occupational therapy has a distinctive place, particularly since limited mobility of forearm extensors is often a precipitating condition. Medial epicondylitis (golfer's elbow) is attributable to tears or chronic inflammation of the common flexors or pronator teres at the level of the elbow. The same considerations articulated for lateral epicondylitis apply to medial involvement of the elbow, except that extension limitations at the wrist may be more important. Medial epicondylitis is also important because of intermittent trapping or stretching of the ulnar nerve. This complex is particularly common in keyboard use, and its identification is important, since surgical release is almost never warranted. For both lateral and medial epicondylitis, equal attention should be paid to muscle and musculotendinous units as to elbow insertions. For this reason elbow injection accompanied by muscle stretching and strengthening is often an effective therapeutic strategy.

ENTRAPMENT SYNDROMES WHICH SUGGEST MULTILEVEL DISEASE AND SYMPTOMS WITHOUT ANATOMIC LOCALIZATION
Multiple site or multinerve compression syndromes

At times, workers may experience anatomic and tissue changes with multiple sites of nerve compression, that cause greater symptoms than would be experienced with a single site of compression. Many patients with diffuse upper extremity symptoms may also experience problems with nerve compression that appear to arise at multiple levels. The best-known manifestation is the so-called 'double crush' syndrome, which can be a consequence of degenerative cervical spine disease or acquired postural torsion at the brachial plexus.[97,98] In the classic 'double crush' syndrome, there is compression at the carpal tunnel as well. Other potential scenarios could include ulnar nerve entrapment at the brachial plexus and cubital tunnel, or at the cubital tunnel and Guyon's canal. The delineation of multiple compression abnormalities most often arises in the distribution of the ulnar nerve. Since Tinel's sign at the elbow is easily elicited, and ulnar nerve compression at the elbow often eludes electrodiagnostic verification, the presence of a multiple site disorder is easily missed.

Nerve compression at the neck, and especially postural nerve compression at the brachial plexus, may lead to peripheral nerve impairment distally, expressed as symptoms or through provocative palpation or extended movement, as with Adson's test. These observations can be significant in situations where work postures place muscles in shortened positions. For example, workers who perform tasks requiring prolonged or resisted pronation may develop pronator muscle shortening that compresses the median nerve in the forearm when the forearm is placed in supination. Alternatively, prolonged and static work postures that result in pectoralis minor or scalene muscle tightness can compress the brachial plexus. Alterations in axoplasmic flow and transport of nutrient substances has been proposed as the mechanism of this injury.[8,99] Metabolic abnormalities (e.g., diabetes, alcoholic neuropathy, collagen vascular disease) can contribute to nerve dysfunction and make it more susceptible to injury. Recognition is important, because even provocatively derived symptoms that appear anatomically specific are unlikely to be alleviated by surgery when there are signs of multiple compression. Postural therapy, particularly oriented to the cervical spine, scapula, and brachial plexus, is usually the first treatment option.

Neurogenic thoracic outlet syndrome

Thoracic outlet syndrome (TOS), presumed compression of the brachial plexus, subclavian artery, or both at the level of the shoulder, is often suspected and diagnosed. It is a diagnosis with a history of broad application to a wide variety of upper extremity symptoms and signs, and it is discussed in detail in Chapter 23.2. True vascular TOS that compresses the subclavian artery is rather rare,[100,101] and even the apparent loss of pulse with shoulder abduction may not be clinically significant. On the other hand there is a distinctive postural pattern of shoulder protraction, neck immobility with head forward projection, shortening and pain in the pectoralis minor muscles, and trigger points in the scalene muscles that has been associated with positional paresthesias.[102] This has been called *neurogenic thoracic outlet syndrome* and it is relatively common in industrial workers performing extended overhead work and in computer workers with weakened proximal musculature.[103,104]

The pattern of cold clammy hands, and dermal mottling in the hands, is an accompanying observation of TOS. The latter has been attributed to sympathetic ectopic activity rather than to true vascular compression. These presentations usually respond to stretching and upper back strengthening. It is important to recognize that the controversies over thoracic outlet syndrome are decidedly semantic and the distinction is between a rare and fixed neurovascular compression and a much more common acquired postural syndrome.[105] Some proponents argue that congenital and acquired fibrous bands or anomalous muscle slings, discovered at surgery, are fairly common and form a predisposition to symptom presentation.[106] In any event, postural issues are frequently important, and even in classic presentations, physical therapy is the first line of treatment.

Diffuse myalgias

Diffuse myalgias in general, and fibromyalgia in particular, remain controversial. What is less controversial is the patient presenting with multiple areas of soft tissue pain, that are aggravated by use, and lack localizing signs. This minority of patients that present with multiple signs represents a therapeutic dilemma. In some settings, the localization in muscle bellies associated with measurable levels of activity suggests an inflammatory state.

Increasing attention has been paid to metabolic and neuroregulatory factors to better understand the relationship between acute muscle fatigue and the development of chronic muscle disorders, as well as to characterize the pattern of pain symptoms that affect the neck, shoulders, forearms, wrists, and fingers in manually intensive tasks that occur well below the muscles' maximum voluntary contraction (MVC). Neurohumoral substances are chemicals that affect cell membranes and function, and excite afferent nerves. Muscle pain, inflammation, and ischemia, or sustained static contraction, lead to release of potassium chloride, lactate, arachidonic acid, bradykinins, serotinin, and histamine. In addition to producing pain, these agents can excite chemosensitive afferents – gamma muscle spindles – that respond to stretch. It is hypothesized that increased spindle excitation can cause the stiffness and pain of 'myalgia'.

Reduced blood flow that is characteristic of static contraction and increased transmural pressure is reversible, but there is additional evidence that the pattern of reduced flow, injury and diminished repair, and chronic fiber damage all contribute to muscle pain. Higher subjective levels of fatigue, as well as electrophysiologic evidence of fatigue, are more common in large muscle groups, such as the neck and shoulder muscles, when activities are static and repetitive rather than dynamic. While the links between physiology and clinical diagnosis are sometimes obscure, a therapeutic program which emphasizes pharmacologic control of nerve pain with increasing exercise tolerance offers a basis for improvement. It is also important to recognize that in a dynamic view of nerve and muscle dysfunction, the generation of pain from multiple symptoms is not surprising and necessitates a dynamic therapy.

Regional complex pain and vascular pain

Pain syndromes are beyond the scope of this chapter, but there are several relevant observations that pertain to the management of upper extremity disorders. Patients meeting clinical criteria for complex regional pain syndrome (CRPS) present rather uncommonly, representing less than 1% of all patients with upper extremity disorders. Conversely, the presentation of cool mottled hands may occur in as many as 20% of patients, and symptoms of neurogenic thoracic outlet syndrome signs may be present in more than half of patients. The critical distinction is between mild and relatively easily reversed proximal compressive disorders and major regional and vascular pain syndromes. Intransigent pain, the presence of edema, and severe mottling aggravated by exertion suggest a shift in the axis from mild autonomic dysfunction to vascular pain.[107] Recognition and early treatment, including physical therapy and ganglion blockade in more severe cases are important, because of the evidence that significant sympathetic dysfunction is a precursor of full-blown CRPS.

CUMULATIVE TRAUMA DISORDERS REPRESENTING PARTICULAR CLINICAL CHALLENGES
Cumulative trauma disorders in the office environment

A virtual epidemic reporting of computer-related upper extremity injuries in public sector workers in New South Wales and Victoria gave birth to the term RSI in the early 1980s.[108-111] Subsequently the electronic office has been associated with frequent upper extremity syndromes but limited lost work time. There are compelling arguments that biomechanical factors lie at the root of these computer-

related syndromes.[77,112-114] Physical risk factors include entry speed and duration, insufficient rest cycles, and non-neutral joint postures; intrinsic risk factors include anthropometry, age and gender; and work organizational factors have also been ascribed (see Chapter 15).

Etiology

Common triggering factors in office work usually include static loading of the neck, shoulder, and proximal upper extremity, coupled with dynamic, repetitive loading of the wrist and hand. Neck and shoulder complaints have been particularly common among video display terminal (VDT) operators, and have been attributed to prolonged isometric muscle contraction.[115-118] There is more ambiguity in identifying the pathologic mechanism associated with repetitive wrist and finger movement, pinching and grasping, wrist extension and flexion, and ulnar deviation because of the intrinsic complexity of hand movements, particularly in office work, and because of the difficulty in quantifying variables of exposure in hand pain syndromes. Stereotypy appears to be an important factor in wrist complaints, reflected in symptom prevalence among mail sorters and supermarket checkout workers,[76] although evidence for more anatomically defined disorders exists in these settings. The high proportion of proximal disorders, such as neurogenic TOS, in office workers, and relatively high level of ulnar nerve compression syndromes are somewhat surprising given the hand intensity of work. However, the relationship between individual posture and anthropometry and the work surface and seating suggest an etiology that requires a multilevel approach.

Investigations of the relationship between duration of employment and symptoms are contradictory and complicated.[119,120] Because arm and hand pain problems tend to emerge early in employment, programs emphasizing job training and adaptation are justified. Work organization has been interpreted as a source of psychosocially driven symptoms. There is a companion viewpoint that automation of the office, carried out rapidly and driven by technology and organizational needs, rather than the experience of the semiskilled workforce, is a contributory social factor.

Treatment

Although there are few treatment recommendations unique to office work, job uniformity in the office often obviates the types of transfer or reassignment that are practical in other work settings.[83] For VDT operators, the balance lies between individual job modification and the kind of generic adaptations that have occurred in Australia. These include providing comfortable workstation design, limiting the keystroke rate and duration, and providing regular, frequent rest breaks. There are some excellent materials available through the internet and OSHA for optimizing the office set-up. Moreover, because the physical inputs are limited – chairs, keyboards, monitors, trays, pads, headsets, and their placement – the electronic office may be an ideal environment for retraining and reacclimatizing individuals with upper extremity disorders, even when derived from the office. That is, while job content may be difficult to modify, there are many opportunities for manipulating hardware in the office.

Cumulative trauma disorder in the heavy industrial environment

Hand and wrist problems, loosely diagnosed as CTS, have been observed among garment workers and meatpackers, and in a variety of manufacturing settings. More than is the case with white collar work, industrial CTDs have a substantial overlap with some of the anatomically specific disorders, especially CTS. In general, work involving dynamic loading, force, and stereotypy is somewhat easier to detail in manufacturing, although with changes in work organization, the distinctions elude a simple exposure classification. A challenging set of findings, enhanced by aging of the workforce, involves industrial workers who present with combined disorders affecting muscle, nerve, tendon and joint.

Epidemiology

When jobs have been compared cross-sectionally, symptoms are more common among the most physically demanding job categories. When white and blue collar incidence rates have been compared within the same facility, there is a clear gradient indicating a greater incidence of symptoms among manual workers. However, associations between specific causative factors and symptoms have been difficult to substantiate in many analyses. Similarly, force and repetition, two putatively strong causal factors, have been implicated with variable weight (see Chapter 32). There is, however, considerably greater prevalence in largely female occupations, such as textiles manufacture, in which symptoms have been widely reported.

Etiology

Very different symptom rates within the same plant and reduction by ergonomic intervention support a causative role for specific processes. Stereotypy, coupled with forceful exertions and postures requiring static loading, has been identified as a prominent risk factor. The association between symptoms and a specific job has focused on biomechanics (centered on the worker) and ergonomics (centered on the task). Forceful exertion, repetition rate, and awkward postures, such as hyperflexion or ulnar deviation, are frequent biomechanical factors.

Ergonomic considerations have included workstation design, tool construction, and physical factors, such as temperature, lighting, and humidity. Particularly troublesome are hand tools that extend physical strength by requiring resistance against the base of the palm. Thus, screwdrivers, scrapers, buffers, and polishing tools have been implicated. In physically demanding and stereotyped jobs, such as in the meat processing industry, a particularly high incidence of symptoms is common early in employment, implicating overexertion, if not overuse, and the importance of training and experience. In many metal trades prolonged work at shoulder height is common.

Treatment and ergonomics

The approach to individual therapy is complicated by social considerations, usually the need for continued employment, limited modified duty, and insufficient impairment to merit sufficient income replacement.[121-124] Aggressive physical therapy is helpful, although with involvement of multiple anatomic sites, the prospects for full alleviation may be limited. Job analysis can range from simple time and motion and postural checklists, to more sophisticated slow motion videotape studies and translation of specific tasks into quantitative components. EMGs may be recorded for specific work processes. Because of the complexity and academic nature of these investigations, they generally have limited practical application, and the absence of a reference standard places great weight on the experience of the clinician. Nevertheless, some job modification may be useful, including the following.

1. Identification and attenuation or elimination of offending tasks or equipment.
2. Reduction of work rate, overtime hours, and pain-inducing activities.
3. Job rotation or reassignment, at least until symptoms abate.
4. Investigation of job retraining, while function is maintained.

In general, ergonomic assessment has a clearer focus in industrial or other physical work than in office work, particularly when symptoms occur primarily in specific departments or processes.

References

1. Bureau of Labor Statistics. Occupational injuries and illnesses in the United States by industry. Bulletin 2399. Washington DC: US Department of Labor, 1992.
2. Bureau of Labor Statistics. BLS Survey of occupational injuries and illnesses in 1977–1995. Washington DC: US Department of Labor, 1995.
3. Franklin GM, Haug J, Heyer N, Checkoway H, Peck N. Occupational carpal tunnel syndrome in Washington State, 1984–1988. Am J Public Health 1991; 81:741–6.
4. Chatterjee DS. Repetitive strain injury. J Soc Occup Med 1987; 37:100–15.
5. Cunningham LS, Kelsey JL. Epidemiology of musculoskeletal impairments and associated disability. Am J Public Health 1984; 74:574–9.
6. McDermott FT. Repetition strain injury: a review of current understanding. Med J Aus 1986; 144:196–200.
7. Maeda K, Horiguchi S, Hosokawa M. History of the studies on occupational cervicobrachial disorders in Japan and remaining problems. J Hum Erg 1982; 11:17–29.
8. Lieber RL, Friden J. Muscle damage is not a function of muscle force but active muscle strain. J Appl Physiol 1993; 74:520–6.
9. Leadbetter WBC. Cell-matrix response in tendon injury. Clin Sports Med 1992; 11:533–78.
10. Asbury AK. Numbness, tingling and sensory loss. In: Fauci AS, Braunwald E, Isselbacher KJ et al, eds. Harrison's principles of internal medicine. New York: McGraw Hill, 2000;1–7.
11. Johansson H, Sojka P. Pathosphysiological mechanisms involved in genesis and spread of muscle tension in occupational muscle pain and in chronic musculoskeletal pain syndromes: a hypothesis. Med Hypoth 1991; 35:196–203.

12. Werner R, Franzblau A, Albers J, Armstrong T. Median mononeuropathy among active workers: are there differences between symptomatic and asymptomatic workers? Am J Ind Med 1998; 33: 374–8.

13. National Institute for Occupational Safety and Health. Musculoskeletal disorders and workplace factors. DHHS (NIOSH) Publication 97-141. Cincinnati: US Department of Health and Human Services, Public Health Service, Centers for Disease Control, National Institute for Occupational Safety and Health, 1997.

14. National Academy of Sciences. Work-related musculoskeletal disorders: a review of the evidence. Washington DC: National Academy Press, 1998.

15. National Research Council and the Institute of Medicine. Musculoskeletal disorders and the workplace: low back and upper extremities. Washington DC: National Academy Press, 2001.

16. Ergonomics Program Standard. USDOL, 2000.

17. Kasdan ML, ed. Occupational hand injuries: state of the art reviews. Philadelphia: Hanley & Belfus, 1989.

18. Pascarelli EF, Hsu Y-P. Understanding work-related upper extremity disorders: clinical findings in 485 computer users, musicians, and others. J Occup Rehab 2001; 11:1–21.

19. Sluiter BJ, Rest KM, Frings-Dresen MH. Criteria document for evaluating the work-relatedness of upper-extremity musculoskeletal disorders. Scand J Work Environ Health 2001; 27(Suppl 1):1–102.

20. Anderson JAD. Arthrosis and its relation to work. Scand J Work Environ Health 1984; 10:429–33.

21. Gemne G, Saraste H. Bone and joint pathology in workers using hand-held vibrating tools. Scand J Work Environ Health 1987; 13:290–300.

22. Hernberg S. Work-related diseases: some problems in study design. Scand J Work Environ Health 1984; 10:367–72.

23. Kuorinka I, Koskinen P. Occupational rheumatic diseases and upper limb strain in manual jobs in a light mechanical industry. Scand J Work Environ Health 1979; 6(Suppl 3):39–47.

24. Farkkila M, Pyykko I, Jantii V, Aatola S, Starck J, Korhonen O. Forestry workers exposed to vibration: a neurological study. Br J Ind Med 1988; 45:188–92.

25. Feldman RG, Goldman R, Keyserling WM. Peripheral nerve entrapment syndromes and ergonomic factors. Am J Ind Med 1983; 4:661–81.

26. Lindblom U, Ochoa J. Somatosensory function and dysfunction. In: Asbury A, McKhann G, McDonald I, eds. Diseases of the nervous system. Clinical neurobiology. London: WB Saunders, 1992;213–28.

27. Leffler AS, Kosek E, Hansson P. The influence of pain intensity on somatosensory perception in patients suffering from subacute/chronic lateral epicondylalgia. Eur J Pain 2000; 4:57–71.

28. Collins ED, Novak CB, Mackinnon SE, Weisenborn SA. Long-term follow-up evaluation of cold sensitivity following nerve injury. J Hand Surg 1996; 21:1078–85.

29. Viikari-Juntura E. Neck and upper limb disorders among slaughterhouse workers. Scand J Work Environ Health 1983; 9:283–90.

30. Olsen N, Nielsen SI, Voss P. Cold response of digital arteries in chain saw operators. Br J Ind Med 1982; 39:82–8.

31. Pyykko I, Starck J. Pathophysiologic and hygienic aspects of hand–arm vibration. Scand J Work Environ Health 1986; 12:237–41.

32. Armstrong TJ, Foulke J, Joseph B, Goldstein S. Investigation of cumulative trauma disorders in a poultry processing plant. Am Ind Hyg Assoc J 1982; 43:103–16.

33. Marklin RW, Monroe JF. Quantitative biomechanical analysis of wrist motion in bone-trimming jobs in the meat packing industry. Ergonomics 1998: 41:227–37.

34. Masear VR, Hayes JM, Hyde AG. An industrial cause of carpal tunnel syndrome. J Hand Surg 1986; 11:222–7.

35. Falck B, Aarnio P. Left-sided carpal tunnel syndrome in butchers. Scand J Work Environ Health 1983; 9:291–7.

36. Amick BC, Damron J. A three-year longitudinal assessment of changes in office activities following the introduction of microcomputers into a multinational bank. App Ergonomics 1993; 24:397–404.

37. Berqvist U, Wolgast E, Nilsson V, Voss M. The influence of VDT work on musculoskeletal disorders. Ergonomics 1995; 38:754–62.

38. Armstrong TJ, Fine L, Goldstein S. Ergonomic considerations in hand and wrist tendinitis. J Hand Surg 1987; 12A:830–7.

39. Lundervold A. Electromyographic investigations during typewriting. Ergonomics 1985; 1:226–39.

40. Bongers PM, de Winter CR, Kompier MAJ, Hildebrandt VH. Psychosocial factors at work and musculoskeletal disease. Scand J Environ Health 193; 19:297–312.

41. Houtman ILD, Bongers PM, Smulders PGW, Kompier MAJ. Psychosocial stressors at work and musculoskeletal problems. Scand J Work Environ Health 1994; 20:139–45.

42. Kuhlman KA, Hennessey WJ. Sensitivity and specificity of carpal tunnel syndrome signs. Am J Phys Med Rehab 1997; 76:451–7.

43. Goldring DN, Rose DM, Selvarajan K. Clinical tests for carpal tunnel syndrome: an evaluation. Br J Rheumatol 1986; 26:388–90.

44. Dellon LA. Radial sensory nerve entrapment in the forearm. J Hand Surg 1986; 11:199–205.

45. Howard FM. Controversies in nerve entrapment syndromes in the forearm and wrist. Orthop Clin North Am 1986; 17:375–81.

46. Eisen A, Schomer D, Melmed C. The application of F-wave measurement in the differentiation of proximal and distal upper limb entrapment. Neurology 1977; 27:662.

47. Kimura J. Electrodiagnosis in diseases of nerve and muscle: principles and practice. Philadelphia: FA Davis, 1984.

48. Kimura J. Principles and pitfalls of nerve conduction studies. Electroencephalogr Clin Neurophysiol 1999; 50(Suppl):12–15.

49. Ma DM, Liveson JA. Nerve conduction handbook. Philadelphia: FA Davis, 1983.

50. Haig AJ, Tzeng HM, LeBreck DB. The value of electrodiagnostic consultation for patients with upper extremity nerve complaints: a prospective comparison with the history and physical examination. Arch Phys Med Rehab 1999; 80:1273–81.

51. Spindler HA, Dellon AL. Nerve conduction studies and sensibility testing in carpal tunnel syndrome. J Hand Surg 1982; 7:260–3.

52. Grundberg AB. Carpal tunnel decompression in spite of normal electromyography. J Hand Surg 1983; 8:348–9.

53. Bove FJ, Letz RE, Baker EL. Sensory thresholds among construction trade painters: a cross-sectional study using new methods for measuring temperature and vibration sensitivity. J Occup Med 1989; 31:320–5.

54. Johannson RS, Vallbo AB. Tactile sensory coding in the glabrous skin of the human hand. Trends Neurosci 1983; 6:27–32.

55. Cherniack M, Moalli D, Viscoli K. A comparison of traditional electrodiagnostic studies, electroneurometry and vibrometry in the diagnosis of carpal tunnel syndrome. J Hand Surg 1996; 21A:122–31.

56. Maeda S, Yonekawa Y, Kanada K, Takahashi Y. Vibrotactile TTS of fingertip vibratory sensation from hand-transmitted vibration having the same equal equivalent tool vibration levels according to the JIS B 4900 determination method. Ind Health 1996; 34:257–66.

57. Cherniack MG, Letz R, Gerr F, et al. Detailed clinical assessment of neurological function in symptomatic shipyard workers. Br J Ind Med 1990; 47:566–72.

58. NIOSH. Criteria for a recommended standard occupational exposure to hand–arm vibration. DHHS 89-106. Cincinnati: NIOSH, 1989.

59. Pelmear PL, Taylor W. Hand–arm vibration syndrome. J Family Pract 1994; 38.

60. Farkkila M, Pyykko I, Jantti V, et al. Forestry workers exposed to vibration: a neurological study. Br J Ind Med 1988; 45:188–92.

61. Brammer AJ, Piercy JE, Auger PL, Nohara S. Tactile perception in hands occupationally exposed to vibration. J Hand Surg 1987; 12:870–5.

62. Brammer AJ, Pyykko I. Vibration-induced neuropathy: detection by nerve conduction measurements. Scand J Work Environ Health 1987; 13:317–22.

63. Koskimies K, Farkkila M, Pyykko I, et al. Carpal tunnel syndrome in vibration disease. Br J Ind Med 1990; 47:411–6.

64. Wieslander G, Norbäck D, Göthe CJ, Juhlin L. Carpal tunnel syndrome (CTS) and exposure to vibration, repetitive wrist movements, and heavy manual work: a case-referent study. Br J Ind Med 1989; 46:43–7.

65. Cherniack M, Mohr S. Raynaud's phenomenon associated with the use of pneumatically powered surgical instruments. J Hand Surg 1994; 19A:1008–15.

66. Nielsen SL. Raynaud's phenomenon and finger systolic blood pressure during cooling. Scand J Clin Lab Invest 1980; 38:765–70.

67. Ekenvall L, Gemne G, Tegner R. Correspondence between neurologic symptoms and outcome of quantitative sensory testing in the hand–arm vibration syndrome. Br J Ind Med 1989; 46:570–4.

68. Farkkila M, Pyykko I, Korhonen O, Starck J. Vibration-induced decrease in the muscle force in lumber jacks. Eur J Appl Physiol 1980; 43:1–9.

69. James PB, Yatyes JR, Pearson JCG. An investigation of the prevalence of bone cysts in hands exposed to vibration. In: Taylor W, Pelmear PL, eds. Vibration white finger in industry. New York: Academic Press, 1975: 43–51.

70. Rosen I, Stromberg T, Lundborg G. Neurophysiological investigation of hands damaged by vibration: comparison with idiopathic carpal tunnel syndrome. Scand J Plast Reconstr Surg Hand Surg 1993; 27:209–16.

71. Juntunen J, Matikainen E, Seppalainen Am, Laine A. Peripheral neuropathy and vibration syndrome. Int Arch Environ Health 1983; 52:17–24.

72. Gainer JV, Nugent GR. Carpal tunnel syndrome: report of 430 operations. South Med J 1977; 3:325–8.

73. Hunt J. The thenar and hypothenar types of neural atrophy of the hand. Am J Med Sci 1911; 141:224–41.

74. Pfeiffer GB, Gelberman RH, Boyes JH, Rydevik B. The history of carpal tunnel syndrome. J Hand Surg 1988; 13:28–34.

75. Phelan G. The carpal tunnel syndrome. J Bone Joint Surg 1966; 48A:211–28.

76. Margolis W, Kraus JF. Prevalence of carpal tunnel syndrome in female supermarket checkers. J Occup Med 1987; 29:953–6.

77. Rempel D, Keir PJ Smutz WP, Hargens AR. Effects of static fingertip loading on carpal tunnel pressure. J Orthop Res 1997; 15:422–6.

78. Silverstein BA, Fine LJ, Armstrong TJ. Occupational factors and carpal tunnel syndrome. Am J Ind Med 1987; 11:343–58.

79. Louis DS, Hankin FM. Symptomatic relief following carpal tunnel decompression with normal electroneuromyographic studies. Orthopedics 1987; 10:434–6.

80. Dekel S, Papaioannou T, Rushworth G, et al. Idiopathic CTS caused by carpal stenosis. Br Med J 1980; 280:1297–303.

81. Faithfull DK, Moir DH, Ireland J. The micropathology of the typical carpal tunnel syndrome. J Hand Surg 1986; 11:131–2.

82. Lundborg G, Myers R, Powell H. Nerve compression injury and increased endoneurial pressure: a 'miniature compartment syndrome'. J Neurol Neurosurg Psychiatry 1983; 46:1119–24.

83. Rempel D, Jamojilovic R, Levinsohn DG, et al. The effects of wearing a flexible wrist splint on carpal tunnel syndrome pressure during repetitive hand activity. J Hand Surg 1994; 19A:106–10.

84. Kulick MI, Gordillo BS, Javidi T, et al. Long-term analysis of patients having surgical treatment for carpal tunnel syndrome. J Hand Surg 1986; 11A:59–66.

85. Rask MR. Anterior interosseous nerve entrapment (Kiloh–Nevin syndrome). Clin Orthop 1979; 142:176.

86. Miller RG. The cubital tunnel syndrome: diagnosis and precise localization. Ann Neurol 1979; 6:56.

87. Duncan WC. Hypothenar hammer syndrome: an uncommon cause of digital ischemia. J Am Acad Dermatol 1996; 34:880–3.

88. Kreitner K-F, Duber C, Muller L-P, Degreif, J. Hypothenar hammer syndrome caused by recreational sports activities and muscle anomaly in the wrist. Cardiovasc Intervent Radiol 1996; 19:356–9.

89. Wheatley MJ, Marx VM. The use of intra-arterial urokinase in the management of hand ischemia secondary to palmar and digital arterial occlusion. Ann Plast Surg 1996; 37:356–63.

90. Kurppa K, Waris P, Rokkanen P. Peritendinitis and tenosynovitis. Scand J Work Environ Health 1970; 5(Suppl 3):19–24.

91. Denman EE. Rupture of the extensor pollicis longus crush injury. Hand 1979; 11:295.

92. Luopajarvi T, Juorinka I, Virolainen M, et al. Prevalence of tenosynovitis and other injuries of the upper extremities in repetitive work. Scand J Work Environ Health 1979; 5:48–55.

93. Thompson AR, Plewes LW, Shaw GE. Peritendinitis crepitans and simple tenosynovitis: a clinical study of 544 cases in industry. Br J Ind Med 1951; 8:150–60.

94. Grundberg AB. Pathologic anatomy of the forearm: intersection syndrome. J Hand Surg 1985; 10A:299–302.

95. Bennett B. Dupuytren's contracture in manual workers. Br J Ind Med 1982; 39:98–100.

96. Coonrad RW. Tennis elbow: its course, natural history, conservative and surgical management. J Bone Joint Surg 1973; 55A:1177.

97. Hurst LC, Weissberg D, Carroll RE. The relationship of the double crush to carpal tunnel syndrome (an analysis of 1000 cases of carpal tunnel syndrome). J Hand Surg 1985; 10B:202–4.

98. Mackinnon SE. Double and multiple 'crush' syndromes. Hand Clin 1992; 8:369–90.

99. Leiber RL, Friden J. Skeletal muscle metabolism, fatigue and injury. In: Gordon SL, Blair SJ, Fine LJ, eds. Repetitive motion disorders of the upper extremity. Rosemont: American Academy of Orthopedic Surgeons, 1994.

100. Mackinnon SE, Novak CB. Evaluation of the patient with thoracic outlet syndrome. Semin Thorac Cardiovasc Surg 1996; 8:190–200.

101. Wilbourn AJ. Thoracic outlet syndrome is overdiagnosed. Muscle Nerve 1999; January:130–8.

102. Toomingas A, Hagberg M, Jorulf L, et al. Outcome of the abduction external rotation test among manual and office workers. Am J Ind Med 1991; 19:215–27.

103. Roos DB. Thoracic outlet syndrome is underdiagnosed. Muscle Nerve 1999; January:126–9.

104. Sallstrom J, Schmiddt H. Cervicobrachial disorders in certain occupations with special reference to compression in the thoracic outlet. Am J Ind Med 1984; 6:45–52.

105. Smith T, Trojaberg W. Diagnosis of thoracic outlet syndrome: value of sensory and motor conduction studies and quantitative electromyography. Arch Neurol 1987; 44:1161–63.

106. Roos DB. Congenital anomalies associated with thoracic outlet syndrome. Am J Surg 1976; 132:771–8.

107. Veldman PH, Reynen HM, Arntz IE, Goris RJ. Signs and symptoms of reflex sympathetic dystrophy: prospective study of 829 patients. Lancet 1993; 342:1012–6.

108. Awerbach M. RSI or 'kangaroo paw.' Med J Aust 1985; 142:237–8.

109. Green RA, Briggs CA. Anthropometric dimensions and overuse injury among Australian keyboard operators. J Occup Med 1989; 31:747–50.

110. Hadler NM. Clinical concepts in regional musculoskeletal illness. Orlando: Grune & Stratton, 1987.

111. Kiesler S, Finholt T. The mystery of RSI. Am Psychol 1988; 43:1004–15.

112. Armstrong TJ, Foulke JA, Bernard J, Gerson J, Rempel DM. Investigation of applied forces in alphanumeric keyboard work. Am Ind Hyg Assoc J 1994:55:30–5.

113. Feuerstein M, Armstrong T, Pickey P, Lincoln A. Computer keyboard force and upper extremity symptoms. J Occup Environ Med 1997; 39:1144–53.

114. Hunting W, Laubli T, Grandjean E. Postural and visual loads at VDT workplaces. Ergonomics 1981; 24:917–31.

115. Lindman R, Eriksson A, Thornell LE. Fiber type composition of the human female trapezius muscle: enzyme-histochemical characteristics. Am J Anat 1991; 190:385–92.

116. Tola S, Riihimaki H, Videman T, et al. Neck and shoulder symptoms among men in machine operating, dynamic physical work and sedentary work. Scand J Work Environ Health 1988; 14:299–305.

117. Hagberg M, Wegman DH. Prevalence rates and odds ratios of shoulder-neck diseases in different occupational groups. Br J Ind Med 1987; 44:602–10.

118. Larsson B, Jensen BR, Nemeth B, Sjogaard S. EMG-driven shoulder model in three dimensions. In: Book of Abstracts: 15th Congress of the International Society of Biomechanics. Jyvaskyla, Finland: University of Jyvaskyla, 1995; 532–3.

119. Middlestadt SE, Fishbein M. Health and occupational correlates of perceived occupational stress in symphony orchestra musicians. J Occup Med 1988; 30:687–92.

120. Ostberg O, Nilsson C. Emerging technology and stress. In: Cooper CL, Smith MJ, eds. Job stress and blue collar work. New York: John Wiley & Sons, 1985; 149–69.

121. Leino P, Hasan J, Karppi S-L. Occupational class, physical workload, and musculoskeletal morbidity in the engineering industry. Br J Ind Med 1988; 45:672–81.

122. Lutz G, Hanford T. Cumulative trauma disorder controls: the ergonomics program at Ethicon, Inc. J Hand Surg 1987; 12A:863–6.

123. Meagher SW. Tool design for prevention of hand and wrist injuries. J Hand Surg 1987; 12A:855.

124. Armstrong TJ. Ergonomics and cumulative trauma disorders. Hand Clin 1986; 2:553–64

125. Praemer A, Furner S, Rice DP. Musculoskeletal conditions in the United States. Rosemont: American Academy of Orthopedic Surgeons, 1999.

23.4 **Back and Lower Extremity Disorders**
Bradley A Evanoff

Low back pain is among the most common health complaints among working-aged populations around the globe, ranking second only to respiratory illnesses as a symptom-related reason for visits to a physician.[1] In the United States 70–80% of adults will experience a significant episode of low back pain at least once in their lives;[2] similar levels of lifetime prevalence are reported from other industrialized countries.[3] Data from the National Health Interview Survey (NHIS) indicate that there are over 22 million cases of back pain annually in the US that last 1 week or more, resulting in almost 150 million lost workdays.[4]

Although common, low back pain is usually a benign condition. Only a small fraction of back pain episodes involve nerve root impingement and even for those cases, the natural history favors recovery.[5] Only rarely does back pain herald a significant infection, malignancy, or systemic rheumatologic disorder.[6]

Nonetheless, low back pain is a major cause of disability, limitation of activity, and economic loss in western, industrialized countries. Disability due to low back pain is a complicated phenomenon influenced not only by the physical condition of an individual person, but by other personal factors and by societal factors including medical care, the work environment, and the workers' compensation system. Rapid rises in reported disability due to low back pain in the 1970s and 1980s led some authors to describe an 'epidemic' of low back pain. More recent data have shown a 34% decrease in the number of low back pain claims and an even sharper decline in compensation payments for low back pain in the US between 1987 and 1995.[7] Data from the Bureau of Labor Statistics (http://bls.gov.oshhome.htm) have shown a decline over the past decade in the number of reported cases of back or spinal injury associated with lost work days.

Despite apparent improvements over the past decade, low back pain accounts for a substantial burden of cost and disability. It has been estimated that approximately 1% of the US working-aged population is permanently disabled due to back pain, while at any given time up to 1% of workers are temporarily disabled due to back pain.[8] Back impairments remain the most common chronic conditions causing activity limitation in persons under age 45 in the United States. Back pain is the most common reason for filing a workers' compensation claim,[9] reportedly accounting for 16–25% of all workers' compensation claims and 23–33% of all workers' compensation claim costs.[4,7,9,10] Annual costs of low back pain in terms of workers' compensation claims have been estimated at over $9–11 billion, while the total economic impact of low back pain in the US, including lost earnings and other uncompensated losses, has been estimated at $75–100 billion.[2,11]

While there is widespread agreement about the severity and widespread nature of low back pain, there is much less agreement concerning the etiology, or even the definition, of low back pain. One of the difficulties in interpreting the literature on low back pain is the plethora of clinical definitions and the different ways in which patients can be identified, e.g., by symptoms, by medical treatment, or by disability. Most people with symptoms of low back pain do not come to medical attention; most episodes of low back pain which come to medical attention result in no change in work status; most alterations of work status due to low back pain do not lead to long-term disability. Very different pictures of low back pain may thus emerge from differing case definitions. Interpretation of the literature is further complicated given the multifactorial origin of low back pain. In a given patient, the onset, severity, reporting, and prognosis of low back pain may be influenced by a variety of work and non-work factors. The presence of personal risk factors in a patient does not rule out work-relatedness, just as work may not be the sole cause of an individual patient's symptoms.

Studies of the epidemiology of back pain have linked the frequency and severity of low back pain with a variety of personal, lifestyle, and occupational factors. A number of non-work factors have been associated with low back pain. These include age, gender, overall level of physical fitness, lumbar mobility, lumbar strength, tobacco use, non-work physical activities, past history of low back disorders, and congenital structural abnormalities such as spondylolisthesis.[3,6,12]

Recent comprehensive reviews of the scientific literature on work-relatedness of low back pain have been conducted by NIOSH and by the National Academy of Sciences.[3,13,14] These reviews have concluded that there is strong evidence that low back pain disorders are associated with work-related lifting and forceful movements, and with whole-body vibration. There is also evidence that work in awkward postures (bending and twisting) and heavy physical work are associated with increased risk for low back pain disorders. These reviews have also noted that psychosocial factors such as job satisfaction, personality traits, perception of intensified workload, and job control are associated with low back pain.

Identified workplace factors include frequent bending and twisting, heavy physical labor, and prolonged sedentary work. Jobs requiring frequent lifting of objects weighing 25 pounds or more seem to be associated with an increase in risk, as are sudden, unexpected maximal lifting efforts. The effect of lifting may be modified by individual fitness and strength capability, and by the rate, position, distance, and height of the lifting task. The exposure to vibration that accompanies motor vehicle operation (4–6 Hz) also has been shown to be a risk factor for low back pain. Truck drivers, manual material handlers, and nursing personnel are among the occupations with the highest rates of compensable back pain episodes.

CLINICAL EVALUATION

Low back pain may arise from any of a host of structures comprising the lumbosacral spine and its associated soft tissues or from abdominal, retroperitoneal, or pelvic structures. It may be the result of local or systemic processes. With current clinical tests and imaging procedures, however, the cause of most episodes of low back pain remains unclear, and perhaps 85% of patients cannot be given a precise pathoanatomic diagnosis.[15] Pain in these cases is typically assumed to be related to soft tissue injury or to degenerative changes, and non-specific terms such as sprain or strain are commonly used to describe the etiology of low back pain.

Given the idiopathic nature of most episodes of low back pain, the primary goals of the evaluation are to identify: (1) any systemic or visceral cause of pain, (2) any neurologic compromise requiring urgent surgery, (3) any other findings that influence the choice of therapy or prognosis, including workplace exposures which may incite or exacerbate symptoms. A limited diagnostic evaluation, combined with strong reassurance regarding prognosis and careful attention to the patient's concerns, best serves the needs of most patients. In cases of back pain which are work related, it is also important to define work exposures which may need modification in order to improve functional recovery or prevent recurrence.

HISTORY

Current consensus guidelines and expert opinion on the appropriate diagnostic evaluations of low back pain (LBP) recommend that the evaluation focus on three questions: (1) Is the pain caused by a systemic disease? (2) Is there neurologic compromise that may require surgical evaluation? (3) Is there social or psychological distress that may amplify or prolong the pain?[15] These guidelines, intended for general medical practice, give scant attention to issues of work-relatedness or fitness for work. Thus, like Ramazzini, the physician treating a patient with low back pain should 'venture to add one more question: What occupation does he follow? Though this question may be concerned with the exciting causes, yet I regard it as well timed or rather indispensable, and it should be particularly kept in mind when the patient to be treated belongs to the common people.'[16]

The most important immediate goal of the history is to determine if a patient has pain related to a serious local condition such as a fracture, a systemic disorder such as malignancy or infection, or a neurologic disorder requiring surgical evaluation, such as cauda equina syndrome. The history should focus on 'red flags' which indicate the possible presence of a disorder more serious than non-specific LBP. These red flags include a history of trauma, age >50 or <20, history of malignancy or immune compromise, pain which worsens when supine, recent onset bowel or bladder dysfunction, saddle anesthesia, and severe or progressive neurologic deficit of the lower extremities.[6,17,18]

Other history which may suggest a medically serious cause of low back pain includes age over 70 or a history of corticosteroid use (suggesting compression fracture), unexplained weight loss (suggestive of malignancy), IV drug use or recent urinary tract infection (which raise suspicion for spinal infection), pain of over 1 month duration, or failure to improve with conservative therapy. A history of prolonged early morning back pain and stiffness, especially in persons under age 40, may be a clue to inflammatory spinal arthritis. These conditions, exemplified by ankylosing spondylitis (AS), are often associated with insidious onset and symptomatic improvement with exercise.

The vast majority of cases seen in a primary care setting or in an occupational medicine clinic will present with non-specific low back pain or with symptoms of sciatica. Past history of low back disorders should be sought, as should information on the onset and time course of symptoms, and any functional limitations due to symptoms. Location of symptoms should be determined, specifically radiation of pain or paresthesias to the distal lower extremity. Other important historical points include the temporal pattern, relation to work or other daily activities, other precipitating factors, and evidence of functional disability related to the syndrome. These factors are particularly important in planning the individual's return to work. Inquiry about alcohol or drug abuse and depressive symptoms may identify factors that amplify or prolong pain and are amenable to specific intervention.

Often neglected in the history is a description of the patient's work activities, including descriptions of awkward working postures, lifting requirements, other forceful movements, whole body vibration, and need for bending and twisting of the back. Information on monotonous work, job control, and job satisfaction should also be sought. This information is essential for making determinations about work-relatedness, as well as for planning work restrictions and return to full work.

PHYSICAL EXAMINATION

As with the history, the most important immediate goal of the physical examination is to seek physical signs which may indicate a serious medical condition. Severe localized tenderness or percussion tenderness may indicate fracture, infection, or a tumor. Fever or tachycardia may indicate a systemic or local infection. Cauda equina syndrome is indicated by laxity of the anal sphincter, perineal or perianal sensory loss, major motor weakness or paraparesis, and hyperactive or hypoactive reflexes. Progressive neurologic deficit is indicated by new or progressive motor weakness, and increased sensory loss. Tenderness at the costovertebral angle may suggest renal colic or pyelonephritis, while a pulsatile abdominal mass indicates an abdominal aortic aneurysm. In older patients with a suggestive history, breast or prostate examination may be appropriate to look for evidence of malignancy.

Examination of the lumbosacral spine includes musculoskeletal and neurologic components, and should proceed according to an organized routine. Unfortunately, most of the items commonly assessed on physical examination have limited reproducibility between different examiners, as well as having limited prognostic significance.[19] However, in addition to excluding the serious disorders listed above, a careful baseline physical examination is necessary to allow clinical progression to be assessed. Beginning with the patient disrobed and standing, the alignment, curvature, and symmetry of the spine, pelvis, and lower extremities are evaluated. The range of motion of the lumbosacral spine is assessed in flexion and extension. Visual estimation of range of motion is adequate for general clinical purposes, though goniometers can also be used for more precise measurement. Measurement of minimum distance from fingertips to floor is useful to assess the effect of treatment on combined lumbar and hip mobility. A lateral bending maneuver is performed to each side to assess symmetry and any resultant effect on symptoms. Toe raises, heel walking, and standing on one leg (Trendelenburg's test) assist the evaluation of lower extremity muscle weakness.

A thorough neurologic examination is essential in patients with sciatica or lower extremity neurologic complaints. With the patient sitting, patellar and Achilles reflexes are tested. Strength of the quadriceps and psoas muscles is assessed. With the patient supine, the straight leg raising maneuver is performed. Radicular symptoms extending into the lower leg and foot, as opposed to increased back or thigh pain, suggest compression and inflammation of the L4, L5, or S1 spinal nerve root (sciatic nerve). Radicular symptoms should not be produced until the leg is raised to 30 or 35 degrees, at which point dural movement begins. No further tension is applied beyond 60 to 70 degrees. Confirmation of a positive finding is elicited if the leg is lowered to an asymptomatic angle and radicular symptoms are reproduced by passive dorsiflexion of the foot. Pain in the contralateral leg on straight leg raising (crossed straight leg raising sign) is highly specific for nerve root impingement.

Another widely used root tension sign consists of flexing the hip to 90 degrees, then slowly extending the knee until sciatic pain is elicited. Hip joint range of motion should be assessed. Circumferential measurements of the thigh and calf aid in the detection of muscle atrophy. A dermatomal sensory and motor examination of the lower extremities also is performed. Painful areas in the lower extremities are palpated to identify any locally inflamed structures requiring specific treatment.

Palpation is continued in the prone position and includes the spine, paravertebral musculature, and sciatic notches. Localized tenderness or reproduction of referred symptoms typically is noted. These findings help confirm the mechanical nature of the symptoms.

A number of other examination techniques for spinal motion, muscle spasm, sacroiliac joint function, and facet joint disease are recommended by various experts but are not in wide clinical use, and have limited documentation of their diagnostic utility. Non-organic physical signs, including observed pain behavior and a non-anatomic distribution of tenderness and neurologic findings, are widely used to identify magnified illness behavior. Although clinically useful in individual patients, these signs should not be taken to establish an artificial distinction between organic and psychogenic contributions to pain, because the two almost always coexist.

LABORATORY EVALUATION AND DIAGNOSTIC IMAGING

Diagnostic tests play a very limited role in the initial management of acute low back pain. In the absence of 'red flags' on history as discussed above, plain radiographs of the lumbosacral spine are unlikely to change diagnosis or therapy, and are widely overused. Radiographs are appropriate in cases of chronic or recurrent low back pain, but should be ordered acutely to rule out fracture or systemic disorder only if suggested by the history. For patients aged 20 to 50 with non-radicular back pain and no suggestive history of potentially serious underlying condition, it is most appropriate to wait 4 weeks before obtaining AP radiographs. If symptoms have not improved in 4 weeks, plain radiographs of the lumbar spine should be obtained, along with a complete blood count and erythrocyte sedimentation rate in order to help rule out occult neoplasm or osteomyelitis.[6,20,21] If osteomyelitis or neoplasm is suspected but not detected on the plain radiographs, these tests should be followed by a bone scan or by MRI of the spine.

Patients with radicular back pain may also derive little benefit from early diagnostic imaging, since many of these patients will have spontaneous resolution of their symptoms, and early surgical management is indicated only in cases of severe or progressive neurological deficits. Patients with persistent or progressive neurological deficits and an exam consistent with a nerve root impingement should be referred for MRI to evaluate the anatomic basis of the nerve root symptoms. Patients with more ambiguous nerve root involvement may benefit from electromyography in order to determine if nerve root impingement is present. Counseling and education of patients are important, as patients may request imaging which is inappropriate. The use of MRI is especially problematic because a substantial proportion of persons without back pain have disk abnormalities revealed by MRI. Among asymptomatic adults, studies have shown a prevalence of disk herniation of 22–40%, and a prevalence of bulging disk of 24–79%.[22-24] Anatomic abnormalities seen on MRI must be evaluated critically for their clinical importance in each patient.

Older adults with symptoms suggestive of spinal stenosis (pain or paresthesias in the legs relieved by spinal flexion, pseudoclaudication) should be evaluated for the presence of this disorder. The diagnosis can usually be made on the basis of CT or MRI; electromyography may be useful to determine the extent of neurologic impairment.[25]

THERAPY
Non-specific low back pain

Management

Evidence-based guidelines for the treatment of low back pain have been provided by several expert panels and should be referred to for the management of most cases.[6,21,26] For acute cases, the provider should offer a confident and positive approach, which is justified by the generally good prognosis of acute low back pain. Reassurance regarding prognosis should be provided, as many workers with low back pain are apprehensive about the potentially disabling nature of their injury. Early return-to-work activities, with work modifications as necessary, and re-establishment of normal or near-normal activities of daily living are important aspects of care. Efforts to alter lifestyle factors associated with low back pain (smoking, sedentary lifestyle, obesity) should be made, although these efforts are unlikely to be of short-term benefit.

Non-steroidal anti-inflammatory drugs (NSAIDs) are effective for relief of symptoms and provide adequate relief in most patients. Opioid analgesics may be considered in the small minority of patients who do not attain adequate symptom relief from NSAIDs; opioid drugs should be used with caution and for a clearly limited time. Muscle relaxants may also be of use in relief of symptoms, though clinical studies do not clearly identify which patients will benefit from these drugs. Sedation is a common side effect, though in patients who are having trouble sleeping due to back pain this can be used to therapeutic advantage through evening dosing. Physical therapy and spinal manipulation are also effective in providing temporary symptom relief in patients with acute or subacute low back pain.[27]

Many experts believe that use of manipulation or physical therapy should be delayed until 2–3 weeks following the onset of symptoms, because a substantial fraction of patients will improve spontaneously within this time. Back exercises do not seem to be useful in the acute phase, though there is evidence that exercise is helpful in chronic back pain and in the prevention of recurrence. Massage therapy has not received extensive study but shows promise in clinical trials.[28] A wide array of alternative therapies are advocated by practitioners but lack consistent evidence of effectiveness in clinical trials. These treatments include laser stimulation of trigger points, various injection therapies, acupuncture, reflexology, traction, and corsets.

In cases of chronic low back pain, current clinical judgment favors use of an active exercise program. Treatment of chronic cases emphasizes strengthening and range-of-motion exercises and aerobic conditioning in the context of formal assessment of baseline and progressive function (physical capacities evaluation). Maintaining patient adherence to an intensive exercise regimen may be difficult. Referral to a multidisciplinary pain center may be beneficial to some patients with low back pain. Such centers usually employ multiple, simultaneous treatments including supervised, graded exercise, cognitive or behavioral therapy, and patient education in concert with medical therapies. Antidepressants are useful in patients with depression (one-third of patients with chronic low back pain), though there is conflicting evidence about their use in patients without clinical depression.[15] Tricyclic antidepressants may be more effective than serotonin reuptake inhibitors in the treatment of chronic pain patients.

In workers who have been temporarily disabled from work due to low back pain, decisions about return to work cannot be made in isolation from knowledge about their work and their workplace. The modification of physical job demands to facilitate early return to work is felt by many experienced clinicians to be a critical element in the prevention of longer-term disability. Such a view is supported by a study of work-related back pain among workers from a variety of industries who had been away from work for more than 4 weeks due to their back injuries.[29] Workers were randomly assigned to receive an ergonomics intervention, an intensive clinical and rehabilitation intervention, neither, or both (see study description in Chapter 23.1). The ergonomics intervention was the most successful element of this program, resulting in more than a two-fold increase in the rate of return to usual work. By facilitating return to usual work, the ergonomics intervention appeared to reduce progression to long-term disability. In this study, the intensive clinical and rehabilitation intervention did not significantly reduce the time of absence from regular work when applied separately from the ergonomics intervention.

Herniated intervertebral disk

Management

In the absence of cauda equina syndrome or progressive neurologic deficit, conservative (non-surgical) management should be pursued for at least a month in the majority of cases. After 6 weeks of treatment, only about 10% of patients still have sufficient symptoms that surgical management is considered. Early treatment parallels the treatment of non-specific low back pain, with the caveat that the safety and effectiveness of spinal manipulation are not clear. Epidural corticosteroid injections offer temporary symptomatic relief in some patients, and their use may reduce rates of surgery in patients who otherwise would be candidates for surgical decompression.[30]

In patients who still have significant pain or neurologic deficits after 4 weeks, diskectomy should be considered in order to provide quicker symptom relief and return to function. Patients with herniated disks who undergo surgery do not return to work more quickly than those treated with non-surgical therapy, though surgery appears to lead to improved functional and symptomatic outcomes at 1 year.[31,32] Long-term outcomes are similar among patients treated surgically and non-surgically.[33,34] The result of surgical treatment of these patients is strongly related to the findings at surgery. The better defined the clinical syndrome is, the better the surgical outcome will be, with at least partial relief of sciatica in up to 90% of carefully selected patients. Approximately 70% of patients experience relief of back pain. Surgical outcomes also can be adversely affected by unrealistic patient expectations, depression, and substance abuse.

Determination of work-relatedness

The determination of work-relatedness of this common condition often is a substantially more complex matter. The onset of symptoms after an obvious physical stress or impact, such as a fall, blunt trauma, or sudden, unaccustomed lifting, is usually accepted as prima facie evidence of work-relatedness. This is probably appropriate in most cases. However, the unfounded assumptions that back pain must result from an injury and that work-related back pain implies an injury in the workplace underlie these determinations in many jurisdictions. As a result of this misconception, onset of back symptoms in association with an obvious physical insult in the workplace often is considered a necessary condition for acceptance of work-relatedness.

This approach misses an important distinction between the back injury with immediate onset of symptoms following (and presumably due to) a physical insult and the painful condition of the low back that may result from repetitive exposure to physical or other stressors in the workplace. Either scenario is consistent with a work-related back condition, and the circumstances surrounding the onset of back symptoms have relatively little to contribute to etiologic attribution in the latter case.

That said, the scientific basis for work attribution is limited due to the absence of useful means to measure in the workplace the actual load on the lumbar spine and to correlate measured load with risk of back pain in a given case. Careful assessment of job activities interpreted in light of available epidemiologic and biomechanical evidence can be used to arrive at the best estimate of the associated risk of back pain.

The job activities assessment should, to the greatest extent possible, quantify the worker's exposure to the variety of factors found to be associated with an increased risk of back pain. Quantitative assessment of these risk factors in the workplace remains difficult, and definitions of what constitutes high versus low risk on these parameters have yet to be clarified. The National Institute for Occupational Safety and Health has published guidelines for manual lifting in industry.[35,36] These guidelines are based on relative risk estimates derived from detailed biomechanical analyses of simplified lifting models. Further work is needed to make this approach more clinically applicable.

Potential interactions among these risk factors and possible effects of longstanding exposure to one or more of them also require further research. In addition to these physical factors, some studies of the psychosocial environment in the workplace have found markedly increased relative risks for back-related disability claims associated with such factors as job monotony and poor work satisfaction. Few studies have adequately measured both physical and psychosocial risk factors for low back pain. One such study in transport workers found that physical workloads and psychosocial factors were independent risk factors for the development of back pain.[37]

In sum, difficulties with exposure assessment and exposure–response estimation substantially complicate the determination of work-relatedness for low back pain. In the absence of an acute physical insult, the challenge to the clinician is to: (1) ascertain the frequency and intensity of exposure to one or more identified risk factors, (2) interpret the exposure in light of available biomechanical and epidemiologic evidence, and (3) estimate the likely effect of that exposure relative to the legal standard for occupational causation operative in a given jurisdiction.

Prevention of low back pain

The use of preplacement screening with low back radiographs should not be employed, as plain radiographs are not a useful predictor of future low back disorders.[38] There is some evidence that exercise programs which combine aerobic conditioning with specific strengthening of the back and legs can reduce the frequency of recurrence of low back pain.[39,40]

Lifting education programs have generally been ineffective at reducing the frequency of occurrence of low back pain.[39,41,42] Lumbar corsets or back belts do not seem to be effective in reducing the occurrence of low back pain.[42-44]

A growing body of evidence suggests that ergonomic interventions that reduce physical exposures can lead to reduced frequency or severity of low back pain disorders in high-risk jobs. Although few high-quality studies currently exist to assess the effectiveness of such interventions, a number of retrospective analyses and case studies have shown that engineering changes that alter the physical aspects of work can reduce the frequency of low back disorders.[14] Appropriate interventions must be specific to the biomechanical risk factors encountered in a particular work-place. In addition to engineering controls (incorporating ergonomic design), there is evidence to support the effectiveness of administrative controls (changing workplace culture), modification of individual risk factors (through exercise programs), and the use of programs utilizing a combined approach. Multidisciplinary, participatory approaches which involve employers and employees appear to be successful at reducing back pain and disability, and foster compliance and acceptance of changes.[45-47]

Guidance on the design of safer lifting jobs is provided by NIOSH (www.cdc.gov/niosh/lifitng1.html) and by other organizations.

References

1. Andersson GBJ. Epidemiologic features of chronic low-back pain. Lancet 1999; 354:581–5.
2. Frymoyer JW. Back pain and sciatica. N Engl J Med 1988; 318:291–300.
3. Bernard B, ed. Musculoskeletal disorders and workplace factors. NIOSH Publication no. 97-141. Cincinnati, OH: National Institute for Occupational Safety and Health, US Department of Health and Human Services, 1997.
4. Guo HR, Tanaka S, Halperin WE, Cameron LL. Back pain prevalence in US industry and estimates of lost workdays. Am J Pub Health 1999; 89:1029–35.
5. Atlas SJ, Deyo RA, Patrick DL, Convery K, Keller RB, Singer DE. The Quebec task force classification and the severity, treatment, and outcomes of sciatica and lumbar spinal stenosis. Spine 1996; 21:2885–92.
6. Bigos S, Bowyer O, Braen G, et al. Acute low back pain problems in adults. Clinical practice guidelines no. 14. AHCPR Publication no. 95-0642. Rockville, MD: Agency for HealthCare Policy and Research, Public Health Service, US Department of Health and Human Services, 1994.
7. Murphy PL, Volinn E. Is occupational low back pain on the rise? Spine 1999; 24:691–7.

8. Rosomoff HS, Rosomoff RS. Low back pain: evaluation and management in the primary care setting. Med Clin North Am 1999; 83:643–62.

9. Hashemi L, Webster BS, Clancy EA, Volinn E. Length of disability and cost of workers' compensation in low back claims. J Occup Environ Med 1997; 39:937–45.

10. Webster BS, Snook SH. The cost of 1989 workers' compensation low back pain claims. Spine 1994; 19:1111–6.

11. Webster BS, Snook S. The cost of compensable low back pain. J Occup Med 1990; 32:13–15.

12. Dempsey PG, Burdorf A, Webster BS. The influence of personal variables on work related low back disorders and implications for future research. J Occup Environ Med 1997; 39:748–59.

13. National Academy of Sciences. Work-related musculoskeletal disorders: report, workshop summary, and workshop papers. Washington, DC: National Academy Press, 1999.

14. National Academy of Sciences. Musculoskeletal disorders and workplace: low back and upper extremities. Washington, DC: National Academy Press, 2001.

15. Deyo RA, Weinstein JN. Low back pain. N Engl J Med 2001; 344:363–70.

16. Ramazzini B. Diseases of workers. Translated from the Latin text De Morbis Artificum of 1713 by Wilmer Cave Wright. New York Academy of Medicine/The History of Medicine Series. New York: Hafner Publishing, 1964.

17. Harris JS, ed. Occupational practice guidelines. Beverly, MA: OEM Press, 1997.

18. Johanning E. Evaluation and management of low back disorders. Am J Ind Med 2000; 37:94–111.

19. Deyo RA, Rainville J, Kent DL. What can the history and physical examination tell us about low back pain? JAMA 1992; 268:760–5.

20. Staiger TO, Paauw DS, Deyo RA, Jarvik JG. Imaging studies for acute low back pain. Postgrad Med J 1999; 105:161–72.

21. Harris JS, ed. ACOEM Committee on Practice Guidelines. Occupational medicine practice guidelines. Low back complaints. Beverly, MA: OEM Press, 1997.

22. Boden SD, Davis DO, Dina TS, Patronas NJ, Wiesel SW. Abnormal magnetic-resonance scans of the lumbar spine in asymptomatic subjects: a prospective investigation. J Bone Joint Surg Am 1990; 72:403–8.

23. Jensen MC, Brant-Zawadski MN, Obuchowski N, Modic MT, Malkasian D, Ross JS. Magnetic resonance imaging of the lumbar spine in people without back pain. N Engl J Med 1994; 331:69–73.

24. Weishaupt D, Zanetti M, Hodler J, Boos N. MR imaging of the lumbar spine: prevalence of intervertebral disk extrusion and sequestration, nerve root compression, end plate abnormalities, and osteoarthritis of the facet joints in asymptomatic volunteers. Radiology 1998; 209:661–6.

25. Katz JN, Dalgas M, Stucki G, et al. Degenerative lumbar spinal stenosis: diagnostic value of the history and physical examination. Arthritis Rheum 1995; 38:1236–41.

26. Waddell G, Feder G, McIntosh A, Lewis M, Hutchinson A. Low back pain evidence review. London: Royal College of General Practitioners, 1996. www.rcgp.org.uk/backpain/index.htm

27. Cherkin DC, Deyo RA, Battie M, Street J, Barlow W. A comparison of physical therapy, chiropractic manipulation, and provision of an educational booklet for the treatment of patients with low back pain. N Engl J Med 1998; 339:1021–9.

28. Ernst E. Massage therapy for low back pain: a systematic review. J Pain Symptom Manage 1999; 17:65–9.

29. Loisel P, Abenhaim L, Durand P, et al. A population-based, randomized clinical trial on back pain management. Spine 1997; 22:2911–8.

30. Riew KD, Yin Y, Gilula L, et al. The effect of nerve-root injections on the need for operative treatment of lumbar radicular pain. A prospective, randomized, controlled, double-blind study. J Bone Joint Surg Am 2000; 82A:1589–93.

31. Atlas SJ, Deyo RA, Keller RB, et al. The Maine Lumbar Spine Study. II. One-year outcomes of surgical and nonsurgical management of sciatica. Spine 1996; 21:1777–86.

32. Atlas SJ, Keller RB, Robson D, Deyo RA, Singer DE. Surgical and nonsurgical management of lumbar spinal stenosis: four-year outcomes from the Main Lumbar Spine Study. Spine 2000; 25:556–62.

33. Gibson JNA, Grant IC, Waddell G. The Cochrane review of surgery for lumbar disc prolapse and degenerative lumbar spondylosis. Spine 1999; 24:1820–32.

34. Weber H. Lumbar disk hernation: a controlled, prospective study with ten years of observation. Spine 1983; 8:131–40.

35. Waters TR, Putz-Anderson V, Garg A, Fine LJ. Revised NIOSH equation for the design and evaluation of manual tasks. Ergonomics 1993; 36:749–76.

36. Waters TR, Putz-Anderson V, Garg A. Application manual for the revised NIOSH lifting equation. PB94-176930. Cincinnati, OH: National Institute for Occupational Safety and Health, 1994.

37. Krause N, Ragland DR, Greiner BA, Syme SL, Fisher JM. Psychosocial job factors associated with back and neck pain in public transit operators. Scand J Work Environ Health 1997; 23:179–86.

38. Himmelstein JS, Anderson GB. Low back pain: risk evaluation and preplacement screening. Occup Med 1988; 3:255–69.

39. Lahad A, Malter AD, Berg AO, Deyo RA. The effectiveness of four interventions for the prevention of low back pain. JAMA 1994; 272:1286–91.

40. Frost H, Lamb SE, Klaber Moffett JA, Fairbank JC, Moser JS. A fitness programme for patients with chronic low back pain: 2-year follow-up of a randomized controlled trial. Pain 1998; 75:273–9.

41. Daltroy LH, Iversen MD, Larson MG, et al. A controlled trial of an educational program to prevent low back injuries. N Engl J Med 1997; 337: 322–8.

42. van Poppel MN, Koes BW, van der Ploeg T, Smid T, Bouter LM. Lumbar supports and education for the prevention of low back pain in industry: a randomized controlled trial. JAMA 1998; 279:1789–94.

43. NIOSH. Workplace use of back belts. Review and recommendations. DHHS 94-122. Cincinnati, OH: US Department of Health and Human Services, Public Health Service, Center for Disease Control and Prevention, National Institute for Occupational Safety and Health, 1994.

44. NIOSH. Back belts – do they prevent injury? Cincinnati, OH: US Department of Health and Human Services, Public Health Service, Center for Disease Control and Prevention, National Institute for Occupational Safety and Health, 1997. www.cdc.gov/niosh/backbelt.html

45. Johanning E, Landbergis P, Geissler H, Karazmann R. Cardiovascular risk and back disorder intervention study of mass transit operators. Int J Occup Environ Health 1996; 2:79–87.

46. Johanning E. Back disorder intervention strategies for mass transit operators with whole-body vibration – comparison of two transit system approaches and practices. J Sound Vibration 1998; 215:629–34.

47. Evanoff BA, Bohr PC, Wolf LD. Effects of a participatory ergonomics team among hospital orderlies. Am J Ind Med 1999; 35:358–65.

23.5 **Systemic Rheumatologic Disorders**
Paul S Darby, Carl A Brodkin

Work-related musculoskeletal disorders (MSDs) comprise a substantial portion of the cost of occupational illness. The National Institute for Occupational Safety and Health (NIOSH) in 1996 estimated the US cost to be $13 billion annually, while the AFL-CIO in 1997 estimated the annual cost at $20 billion.[1] As of 1999, MSDs accounted for one in every three injuries and/or illnesses that resulted in lost time.[2] In a recent US survey of persons more than 18 years of age, the leading reported cause of disability significant enough to interfere with daily life and/or work was arthritis and rheumatism (non-back or spine).[3]

The implications, then, of rheumatologic conditions on the practice of occupational medicine are substantial. In contrast to the previous chapters in this section, this chapter will not focus on ergonomic issues and localized injury associated with repetitive movements. Rather, the concern here will be systemic inflammatory diseases that traditionally fall under the realm of the subspecialty of rheumatology. Clinically apparent rheumatologic disease may, of course, be limited to a single body location. The usual characteristic, whether manifestations are localized or systemic, is chronic pain and progressive physical impairment of the musculoskeletal system. Disease may also involve numerous other body systems, including the hematopoietic, cardiopulmonary, vascular, central nervous, genitourinary, and dermatologic systems. As summarized in Table 23.5.1, some rheumatologic conditions are associated with workplace or environmental exposures. Other pre-existing conditions may be exacerbated by the workplace. This chapter covers the major rheumatologic diseases that may arise from workplace or environmental exposures.

EVALUATION OF THE WORKER WITH SUSPECTED MUSCULOSKELETAL OR RHEUMATIC DISEASE

The cornerstones of the evaluation of a patient with musculoskeletal or rheumatic complaints are a careful history and physical examination. The history should distinguish inflammatory and non-inflammatory conditions. Inflammatory conditions, such as rheumatoid arthritis (RA), are generally accompanied by significant (often greater than 1 hour) of morning stiffness, a sensation of gelling after inactivity, and, frequently, systemic symptoms such as fatigue and malaise. In contrast, patients with non-inflammatory, mechanical conditions, such as osteoarthritis (OA), generally have less than a half hour of morning stiffness and are more symptomatic with prolonged joint use toward the end of the day. The history also should elicit other symptoms that may provide a clue that a systemic illness is present. For example, RA and

systemic lupus erythematosus (SLE) can involve the skin, cardiac or pulmonary systems.

The goal of the physical examination is to identify organs involved, and to distinguish between intra-articular and periarticular conditions. Periarticular disorders, such as tendinitis and bursitis, are characterized by pain or focal tenderness with movement of the joint in the specific planes that stress the involved structure, with additional objective findings of stiffness, or localized pain during isometric loading of the tendon. Inflammatory synovitis, in contrast, is accompanied by pain on movement of the affected joint in all directions, with warmth and swelling. Testing for joint stability and noting deformities document the consequences of underlying joint pathology. Particular attention should be directed towards the hands, one of the most fruitful areas of examination in systemic inflammatory disease, especially given the occupational implications.

The laboratory evaluation, though often informative, must be based upon a careful history and physical examination. Nevertheless, certain laboratory tests are of definite value. An elevated erythrocyte sedimentation rate (ESR) may help distinguish between inflammatory and non-inflammatory conditions, although elevated sedimentation rates can be seen in association with age, infections, cancer, and other disorders. C-reactive protein (CRP) levels respond more rapidly than the ESR to changes in inflammatory activity, and thus CRP is probably a more sensitive early measure of inflammation.[4] A plethora of autoantibody tests are available for the assessment of rheumatic diseases. Rheumatoid factor, while a useful screening test for RA, has limited efficacy due to a very high false-positive rate. Interpretation of findings of low serologic titers represents a challenge. Antinuclear antibodies (ANA) are highly sensitive for SLE, but are also limited by low specificity. ANA subsets such as anti-smooth muscle antibody (Sm) and double-stranded DNA (dsDNA) are highly specific for SLE and are useful ancillary tests when ANA is positive. When the ANA is negative, and the diagnosis of SLE is strongly suspected, anti-Ro antibody and a CH50 should be ordered, as some patients will be anti-Ro positive or complement deficient.[4–6] Assays for complement components and immune complexes are expensive, and are seldom helpful in the initial evaluation of patients with suspected rheumatic disease. Despite the strong association between the HLA-B27 allele and the seronegative spondyloarthropathies such as ankylosing spondylitis, the high background prevalence of this genetic marker, particularly in Caucasians, limits its usefulness. X-ray studies may suggest destruction of cartilage or bone but are only occasionally useful in the initial management of atraumatic rheumatologic conditions. Aspiration of synovial fluid can be very informative: fluid containing more than 2000 white cells per cubic centimeter is considered inflammatory. Synovial fluid white blood cell counts of less than 2000 are typically seen in OA.

Rheumatic condition association	Exposure	Strength of association
Osteoarthritis	Repetitive trauma	Suspected
Rheumatoid arthritis	Silica	Reported
	Agricultural work	Reported
Systemic lupus erythematosus	Hydrazine	Reported
Systemic sclerosis	Silica	Suspected
Scleroderma-like disorders	Vinyl chloride monomer	Known
	Solvents	Suspected
	L-Tryptophan (contaminant)	Known
Fibromyalgia	Chemical or factory work	Reported
Gout	Lead	Known
Brucellosis	Sheep, dogs, cattle	Known
Lyme disease	Outdoor work	Known
Parvovirus infection	Day care	Suspected
Osteonecrosis	Diving	Known
	Tunnel work	Known
Osseous fluorosis	Fluoride	Known
Muscle disorders	Halogenated hydrocarbons	Known
	Firefighting	Reported

Table 23.5.1 Associations between rheumatic conditions and occupational or environmental exposures

OSTEOARTHRITIS

OA is the most common form of arthritis, and it is seen radiographically in at least one joint in more than 80% of individuals over 70 years of age. The lifetime prevalence of involvement of weight-bearing joints exceeds 40%. Although the precise pathogenesis of OA is unknown, several etiologic factors are well recognized. Age is the strongest risk factor,[7] although it is unclear whether the age-related changes are primarily biochemical or mechanical. Alterations in the cartilage matrix may occur with acute trauma, infection, calcium pyrophosphate dihydrate (CPPD) deposition disease, acromegaly, hemochromatosis, Wilson's disease, and gout. It also has been proposed that repetitive forceful loading of joints in occupational settings leads to cartilage injury and the development of OA.[8] While there remains some controversy over specific pathogenic theories, the epidemiologic studies reviewed below clearly document OA in joints exposed to repetitive stress trauma.

Occupational epidemiology

People with pre-existing OA often experience work disability, especially when faced with physically demanding jobs in which they have little control over the pace or the specific physical demands of work.[9] Felson and colleagues observed an association between occupations that require repetitive knee bending, such as mining and farming, and OA;[10-13] farming was also associated with hip OA. Several reports suggest that occupational repetitive trauma may cause OA in joints generally unaffected by idiopathic OA. For example, Hadler and colleagues investigated three groups of females employed for at least 20 years in textile manufacturing jobs requiring repetitive winding, burling, or spinning.[14] The burlers and spinners had more radiologic evidence of OA in the dominant second and third distal interphalangeal joints than had the winders, suggesting that repetitive use may cause distinct osteoarthritic syndromes in the hand.

Obesity has been demonstrated to predispose individuals to OA of the knee, suggesting that mechanical loading is associated with an excess of OA.[15] In a large Scandinavian study, radiographic evidence of OA of the knee was found in 3.9% of laboring dock-workers as compared with 1.4% of white-collar shipyard workers and 1.6% of community controls, a significant difference.[16] Similarly, among a well-studied group of 347 Swedish men, there was a strong association between radiographic evidence of OA of the hip and exposure to heavy labor, heavy lifting, and much tractor driving.[17] These studies are limited because radiographic studies were not obtained routinely on all workers. A recent study from Japan, where obesity is rare, nonetheless found an association between hip OA and heavy occupational lifting.[18] The association between hip OA and heavy work has been well demonstrated in case-control studies controlling for obesity and participation in sports, with a 2.4-fold increase in hip OA in workers performing heavy compared to light work.[19]

A number of uncontrolled observations also point to the role of repetitive trauma in the pathogenesis of OA in joints not usually affected in idiopathic OA. For example, eight foundry workers who sustained considerable repetitive forces at the elbow joint have been reported with clinical and radiographic evidence of OA of the elbow.[20] Classic clinical and radiographic changes of OA in the metacarpophalangeal joints of seven manual laborers who gripped with their hands repeatedly and intensively for prolonged periods also have been reported,[21] as has a case of severe OA of the metacarpophalangeal joints and elbow in a 62-year-old man who worked 27 years as a jackhammer operator.[22] In a study of 20 pianists averaging 33.9 years of age who had practiced piano at least 2 hours a day for at least 5 years, radiographic evidence of OA at the third, fourth, or fifth metacarpophalangeal joints was noted in eight (40%).[23] However, a report of 16 patients with OA of the elbow who were not exposed to repetitive elbow trauma underscores the need for controlled studies.[24] In a large series of patients undergoing shoulder arthroscopy, a significant association between type III and IV superior labrum anterior posterior (SLAP) lesions and a high-demand occupation was found.[25]

In summary, there is growing evidence over the past decades that repetitive loading of joints in occupational settings leads to OA in joints rarely affected by idiopathic OA. Repetitive trauma is associated with an increased risk of OA in the knee and hip.

Clinical features

OA is generally classified as idiopathic or secondary. Secondary OA results from metabolic, infectious, and inflammatory diseases; acute trauma; epiphyseal diseases; congenital hip dysplasia; and other conditions. Idiopathic

OA is age related, with a striking prevalence for particular joints, including the distal interphalangeal joints of the hand, and the knee, hip, lumbar spine, and feet. Some joints are less frequently involved in idiopathic OA, including the metacarpophalangeal joints of the hand, and the elbow, shoulder, and ankle. Involvement at these sites should raise concern of secondary OA, including an occupational association.

Symptoms of OA usually progress insidiously. Patients experience dull aching pain in the affected joint(s) that is generally exacerbated by prolonged use and improved by resting the joint. As noted above, morning stiffness usually lasts less than 30 minutes; stiffness that lasts longer suggests inflammatory arthritis. Physical examination reveals bony enlargement of the joint, limitation in range of motion variable, joint line tenderness, and, in advanced disease, crepitus and joint deformity. Radiographs reveal characteristic joint space narrowing, subchondral sclerosis, cysts adjacent to the joint, marginal osteophytes, and other degenerative changes.

Treatment

Symptomatic relief can usually be obtained by resting affected weight-bearing joints or splinting other joints, such as the first carpal metacarpal. Pharmacologically, non-steroidal anti-inflammatory drugs (NSAIDs) are the first-line treatment of choice, although gastric irritation, including gastrointestinal bleeding, is a concern, as well as renal insufficiency with chronic administration. Cyclo-oxgenase (COX)-2 inhibitors show promise for their decreased risk of gastrointestinal bleeding, though renal insufficiency remains a concern. A recent randomized double-blind trial, conducted in 29 clinical centers in the US, found that rofecoxib, 25 mg/day, provided advantages over acetaminophen, 4000 mg/day, celecoxib, 200 mg/day, and rofecoxib, 12.5 mg/day, for symptomatic knee OA.[26] Intra-articular injections of corticosteroids and/or hyaluronic acid can be useful in refractory cases.[27] Use of some herbal preparations in the treatment of OA has been reported in a recent review.[28] A Cochrane review found the evidence for the use of avocado–soybean unsaponifiables in the treatment of OA convincing, but found the evidence for other herbal interventions insufficient to either recommend or discourage their use.[29] Many patients take intensively advertised and unregulated supplements such as glucosamine and chondroitin sulfate. Advocates of these alternative modalities cite reports of progressive and gradual decline of joint pain and tenderness, improved mobility, sustained improvement after drug withdrawal, and a lack of significant toxicity associated with short-term use. Critics point out that in the great majority of the relevant clinical trials, sample izes were small, and follow-up was short term.[30] In advanced disease, many joints can be approached surgically, with arthroplasty or arthrodesis. Surgical modalities under investigation also include autologous chondrocyte transplantation.[31]

RHEUMATOID ARTHRITIS

RA is a chronic, systemic inflammatory disorder characterized by symmetric polyarthritis and, occasionally, extra-articular manifestations.

Epidemiology

The prevalence of RA is approximately 1%, with women affected two to three times more frequently than men; the peak incidence occurs between the fourth and sixth decades. An estimated 2.1 million US adults have RA,[32] with medical costs of approximately $8.7 billion annually.[33]

The literature on the association between specific occupations and RA is conflicting. Studies that do not use standard classification criteria for RA further limit interpretation. Major studies from the National Center for Health Statistics and others[34] have demonstrated no statistically significant correlation between occupation and the onset of RA. Other investigators have suggested that RA in males is associated with agricultural work.[35] A Swedish registry-based cohort study found an increased risk of RA in farmers, upholsterers, lacquerers, concrete workers, and hairdressers, as well as in several 'white-collar' trades.[36] Substantial handling of organic solvents was also associated with an increased relative risk for RA.

Exposure to silica and established silicosis have been associated with extrapulmonary conditions, including scleroderma and RA. Rheumatoid pneumoconiosis (Caplan's syndrome) is a syndrome of nodular fibrosis of the lung and RA in coal workers.[37] In an early population-based study of an entire community in South Wales, there was no increased prevalence of RA among miners and ex-miners.[38] A Finnish cohort of 1026 granite workers hired between 1940 and 1971 was followed until the end of 1981.[39] The incidence of awards for disability related to RA, the prevalence of RA, and the prevalence of individuals receiving medication for RA were significantly higher among granite workers than in the general male population of the same age. A retrospective analysis of all patient records was used to verify diagnoses according to standardized criteria and showed a predominance of severe seropositive erosive RA, especially when the onset of the disease occurred after 50 years of age or older. None of the patients had Caplan's syndrome, and only a few had evidence of silicosis at the onset of RA.

The pathophysiologic basis for the association between RA and occupational exposure to dust such as silica remains unclear. Exposure to silica may facilitate entry of infectious agents, or increase an individual's susceptibility to them. Pulmonary silicosis and RA share some immunochemical features, such as the serologic findings of rheumatoid factor and ANA, circulating immune complexes, and decreased resistance to infectious diseases.

Clinical features

Clinically, RA is characterized primarily by symmetric polyarthritis most commonly involving the metacarpophalangeal and proximal interphalangeal joints, wrists, neck, hips, knees, elbows, and metatarsophalangeal joints. With continued synovitis, cartilage and, ultimately, bony destruction may occur, resulting in deformity and disability.

Extra-articular manifestations may include subcutaneous nodules, pleuritis, pericarditis, interstitial lung disease, mononeuritis multiplex, compression neuropathies such as the carpal or tarsal tunnel syndromes, Sjögren's syndrome, and episcleritis. Laboratory features include anemia of chronic disease, elevated sedimentation rate, and, in about two-thirds of patients, positive rheumatoid factors, which are antibodies to the Fc portion of IgG. Radiographs reveal periarticular osteopenia and soft tissue swelling early in the disease, with characteristic joint space narrowing and bony erosions with progressive disease.

The diagnosis of RA is made clinically. The most important step in the diagnosis is to exclude other causes of inflammatory polyarthritis. The revised classification criteria for RA that were published in 1987 were found by a large academic rheumatology practice to have a diagnostic sensitivity of 95% and a specificity of 73%.[40]

Treatment is usually initiated with an NSAID. If these drugs fail to relieve the pain and inflammation, disease-modifying antirheumatic drugs (DMARDs) are generally offered, such as hydroxychloroquine, oral or intramuscular gold, sulfasalazine, and methotrexate. Promising advances in the treatment of RA using various biologic therapies have been made.[41] Clinical trials testing the transfer of anti-arthritic protein coding genes to the synovial lining of human joints are in progress.[42]

SYSTEMIC LUPUS ERYTHEMATOSUS

SLE is a chronic inflammatory disease of unknown etiology with protean manifestations. The prevalence of SLE varies greatly among populations. In the US, the prevalence in women is 1 in 700, and among black women, 1 in 250. There is a marked female predominance of approximately 9:1.

Occupational epidemiology

A variety of drugs can cause a lupus syndrome, autoantibodies, or both, which suggests that environmental and occupational etiologies may exist for this disorder. The two most thoroughly studied medications associated with SLE are procainamide and hydralazine, which contain aromatic amino and hydrazine groups, respectively. Slow or rapid acetylation of these drugs is genetically determined; and a person of the slow-acetylator phenotype is more likely to develop autoantibodies and a lupus-like syndrome from exposure to these drugs. Procainamide-induced SLE can remit when *N*-acetylprocainamide is substituted for procainamide, providing presumptive evidence of the etiologic role of the amino group.

At the present time, however, associations between environmental agents and SLE are speculative, based only on case reports. In the US, hydrazine use exceeds 30 million pounds a year. Hydrazine and its derivatives are used in the synthesis of such diverse products as plastics, anticorrosives, rubber products, herbicides, pesticides, photographic supplies, rocket fuel, preservatives, textiles, dyes, and pharmaceuticals. Hydrazine sulfate has additionally been investigated as an anticancer and anticachexia agent, with unconvincing results, and is marketed in the US as an unregulated dietary supplement.[43] Hydrazine itself occurs naturally in tobacco and tobacco smoke, and a number of aromatic hydrazines are present in mushrooms. A laboratory worker exposed to hydrazine sulfate developed fatigue, photosensitive rash, a positive ANA, arthralgias, photosensitivity, and periungual telangiectasias, which resolved with cessation of the exposure.[44] When evaluated, it was determined that she had a slow-acetylator phenotype, and many of her healthy family members also had antibodies to nuclear constituents. Tartrazine (FD&C yellow #5) is an azo dye present in thousands of foods and drugs which can be broken down to hydrazine compounds and has been implicated in one case of pruritus, photosensitivity, arthralgia, and myalgia.[45,46] Alfalfa sprouts, which contain a highly basic amine, canavanine,[47] have caused a lupus-like disease in monkeys.[48] A case report described a hairdresser with acute exacerbations of SLE which coincided with periods of intense work with aromatic coloring agents.[49] The disorder disappeared completely after a period of 4 years following a change of occupation.

A case-control study was completed in a small four-county area in Southeast Georgia to identify risk factors for SLE and other connective tissue diseases.[50] The investigators found that a family history of connective tissue diseases and the use of hair dyes were associated with connective tissue disorders.

After a cluster of three cases of SLE were noted in workers at one US Army ammunition plant, a cross-sectional study was performed to determine whether or not there was an excess of autoimmune disease.[51] Using serologic criteria only, however, no rheumatologic, hepatic, or renal abnormalities were noted in employees with 8-hour time-weighted exposures to cyclotrimethalintrinitamine (RDX) of up to 1.57 mg/m^3.

Clinical features

Arthritis occurs in over 90% of patients with SLE and is generally non-destructive. Skin lesions, including the typical erythematous malar rash, occur in about 50% of patients, as do pleuritis and pericarditis. Renal disease, central nervous system involvement, and hematologic abnormalities occur frequently, and may complicate management of these patients.

The etiology of SLE is unknown, but appears to involve both genetic and environmental factors. The disease is characterized by autoantibodies, including ANA, which likely have a role in pathogenesis. Pathologically, involvement in most organs relates to vasculitis or mononuclear cell infiltrates. Diagnosis is made on the basis of clinical features. The treatment of SLE is complex and has undergone major advances, which are reviewed elsewhere.[52]

SYSTEMIC SCLEROSIS

Systemic sclerosis, or scleroderma, is a systemic disorder characterized by fibrosis of the skin, blood vessels, and internal organs. The incidence is estimated at 4–12 cases per million annually, with peak onset in the fourth through sixth decades, and a female-to-male ratio of approximately three to one. A variety of occupational and environmental exposures have been associated with the development of scleroderma or related fibrosing conditions.[53]

Occupational epidemiology

Exposure to silica has been associated with increased risk of systemic sclerosis. A case-control study revealed that South African gold miners with systemic sclerosis had significantly greater exposure to silica dust than age-matched miner referent groups.[54] In a study conducted in Pittsburgh, 47% of patients admitted to the hospital with systemic sclerosis had heavy exposure to silica dust from local coal mines, whereas just 19% of hospitalized controls were similarly exposed.[55] Although case reports of scleroderma-like syndromes arising in the setting of silicone implantations (such as in cosmetic augmentation mammoplasty) have suggested an etiologic association,[56] a recently convened National Science Panel found no evidence to support an association between silicone breast implants and connective tissue diseases.[57] The pathogenesis of silica-associated scleroderma is unknown. Interestingly, the clinical findings in this syndrome are indistinguishable from idiopathic systemic sclerosis, except for a male predominance and earlier age of onset.

Clinical features

Systemic sclerosis is generally characterized as limited or diffuse, based on the extent of skin involvement. In limited cutaneous scleroderma, skin involvement is confined to the distal extremities and face. The CREST syndrome (*C*alcinosis, *R*aynaud's phenomenon, *E*sophageal dysmotility, *S*clerodactyly, and *T*elangiectasias) is common in this group. Visceral involvement generally does not occur until after a decade of skin disease in limited systemic sclerosis, and renal disease occurs in just 1% of individuals. Diffuse cutaneous systemic sclerosis is characterized by the rapid progression of skin thickening, including the proximal extremities and trunk. Raynaud's phenomenon, arthritis, tendon contractures, esophageal disease, and interstitial lung disease are common. Sclerodermal renal crisis, characterized by hypertension and azotemia, may occur in 15% of patients.

The diagnosis of systemic sclerosis generally is made on the basis of the history and physical examination. A useful physical finding is dilation of periungual vessels on capillary microscopy. Hand radiographs may reveal lesions of the distal tufts later in the course of disease.

Advances in organ-specific therapy, particularly calcium channel antagonists in Raynaud's phenomenon, proton pump inhibitors in esophageal reflux, intravenous iloprost and endothelin receptor antagonists in pulmonary hypertension, and angiotensin-converting enzyme (ACE) inhibitors in renal crisis, have decreased morbidity and mortality in patients with scleroderma.[58]

Scleroderma-like disorders

A scleroderma-like syndrome has been well documented in workers exposed to vinyl chloride.[59] Polyvinyl chloride is widely used in the plastics industry and is produced by polymerization of gaseous monomeric vinyl chloride. Between 1% and 3% of workers exposed to vinyl chloride monomer at concentrations of 300 to 500 ppm have been affected. The syndrome consists of Raynaud's phenomenon, thickening of the skin over the dorsum of the hand and distal forearm, acro-osteolysis, and other derangements of internal organs, including fibrosis of the lung and liver, splenomegaly, and thrombocytopenia. Angiosarcoma of the liver has been noted in isolated reports.[60] The diagnosis is made on the basis of an individual's medical history, occupational history, and physical examination. Capillary microscopy of the nail beds may reveal dilated or deformed capillary vessels, as seen in systemic sclerosis. Angiography reveals tortuosities and obstruction of digital arteries, reflecting the primary vascular pathophysiology of the hand lesions.

The bony lesion of vinyl chloride disease, acro-osteolysis, begins with small erosions, which progress to transverse defects in the distal phalanges (Fig. 23.5.1).[61] Bony resorption is also seen in approximately half of patients with idiopathic systemic sclerosis; however, in these patients, resorption is primarily in the distal tuft, whereas in vinyl chloride disease, the central shaft of the distal phalanx is involved. Other sites of bony resorption in vinyl chloride disease include the metatarsals, sacroiliac joints, distal clavicles, and mandible. Lesions may heal when the exposure to vinyl chloride is discontinued. The differential diagnosis of acquired acro-osteolysis in workers includes vinyl chloride toxicity, thermal injury, and trauma,[62] in addition to non-occupational etiologies, such as mixed connective tissue disease, sarcoidosis, and hyperparathyroidism.[63]

The etiology and pathogenesis of vinyl chloride disease are obscure. Some evidence suggests that metabolites of vinyl chloride may represent the toxic intermediates, and that genetic susceptibility and immunologic mechanisms may be involved.[64]

Management involves symptomatic treatment and, most importantly, elimination of exposure. Since recognition of this syndrome in the 1960s, regulatory levels of monomeric vinyl chloride have been reduced to 5 ppm or less in most settings, with a resulting decline in the incidence of this disorder. Although many patients have

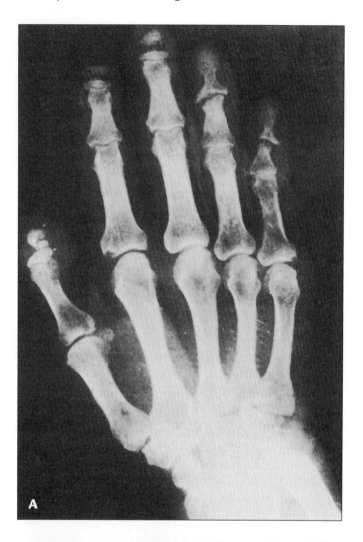

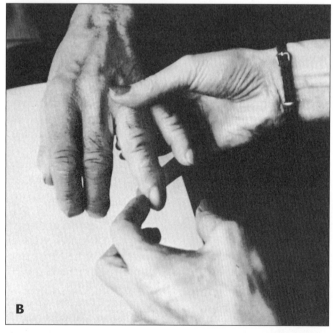

improved or recovered completely upon removal from the exposure, disabling symptoms may persist.

Scleroderma-like syndromes have also been reported with exposure to epoxy resins and organic solvents. Six patients engaged in the polymerization of epoxy resins developed sclerodermatous skin changes, muscle weakness, and fatigue.[65] Visceral involvement was not observed. The syndrome was characterized by rapid onset within months of exposure, as compared with many years of exposure in cases of vinyl chloride disease. Interestingly, the chlorinated alkene solvents trichloroethylene and perchloroethylene, which are structurally similar to vinyl chloride, have been associated with the development of scleroderma-like syndromes.[66,67] Scleroderma-like skin induration has been reported in therapy with bleomycin, and with the abuse of pentazocine and cocaine.[68]

Two epidemics in the 1980s identified other chemicals associated with scleroderma-like disorders. In 1981, toxic oil syndrome (TOS) affected thousands of previously healthy Spaniards, who developed a syndrome of acute and often fulminant pneumonitis followed by chronic sclerodermatous skin changes, myopathy, and sicca syndrome. Extensive investigation revealed that the offending agent was contained in rapeseed oil, denatured with aromatic amines, and sold as inexpensive cooking oil.[69] In 1989, the eosinophilia–myalgia syndrome (EMS), including eosinophilia, severe myalgia, sclerodermatous skin changes, fasciitis, and myopathy and neuropathy, was recognized in users of certain lots of L-tryptophan;[70] this syndrome appeared to be caused by one or more contaminants formed during the preparation of L-tryptophan by one company in Japan.[71] Removal of the contaminated preparation from circulation ended the epidemic.

The mechanisms by which contaminated oil and L-tryptophan led to clinical syndromes similar to scleroderma and eosinophilic fasciitis are not known, although a common aniline-derived or related indole ring-containing compound is suspected (Fig. 23.5.2). The initial manifestations of TOS included fever, headaches, cough, dyspnea, skin eruptions, intense myalgias, and eosinophilia. Edematous skin changes gave way to sclerodermatous lesions, neuropathy, and chronic neuromuscular disability. The presentation and evolution of EMS were strikingly

A. Aniline

B. Tryptophan

Figure 23.5.1: A: X-ray views of hands of long-term vinyl chloride worker showing loss of bone in distal phalanges. B: Finger shortening and pseudoclubbing associated with acro-osteolysis. (Courtesy of Ruth Lilis, MD.)

Figure 23.5.2: Chemical structures of (A) aniline, the parent compound of contaminants found in toxic oil syndrome, and (B) L-tryptophan, the parent compound associated with the eosinophilia–myalgia syndrome.

similar to those of TOS, as were the histopathologic features. In both epidemics, most patients had complete resolution of symptoms following exposure but some were left with chronic disability; a mortality rate of approximately 1% was observed for TOS and about 0.1% for EMS. No therapy, including corticosteroids, was of proven efficacy in these syndromes.

FIBROMYALGIA

Fibromyalgia syndrome (FMS) is a common disorder of unknown etiology, characterized by diffuse and chronic musculoskeletal pain, discrete tender points on physical examination, profound fatigue, and sleep disorder. Fibromyalgia is estimated to affect from 1% to 5% of the population of industrialized societies.[72–74] There is considerable overlap between FMS, chronic fatigue syndrome (CFS), and certain psychiatric disorders, which continues to engender controversy.[74–77]

Epidemiology

Trauma through 'overuse' or 'repetitive strain' has been reported to be associated with the development of FMS.[78,79] The prevalence of trauma as an initiating event in FMS has been reported to range from 11% to 24%; however, no formal studies have adequately examined this relationship.[74] Etiologic associations between occupational exposure and FMS therefore remain speculative.[80]

Clinical features

The clinical picture is dominated by pain, which is diffuse and primarily affects the axial skeleton, shoulder, and pelvic girdles, as well as soft tissues.[81] Patients with FMS may have a biologic predisposition to more sensitive pain perception than people without FMS.[82] Stiffness is also common, lasting up to 1 to 2 hours daily. Fatigue is one of the most debilitating symptoms of fibromyalgia, and it seems to be closely related to non-restorative sleep. It is estimated that 70% of patients have a sleep disorder.[83] Symptoms occurring in at least 25% of patients include paresthesias, arthralgias and subjective stiffness, headaches, irritable bowel syndrome, Raynaud's syndrome, sicca syndrome, palpitations, dizziness, and psychologic disturbances. The disease may be exacerbated by weather, temperature, exercise, stress, and acute trauma.

The clinical examination of the patient with fibromyalgia is remarkable only for tender points (Fig. 23.5.3). These are symmetrically distributed in characteristic locations, including the intertransverse or interspinous ligaments of C4 to C6, the upper border of the trapezius, the inner scapula, the origin of the supraspinatus, the upper outer quadrant of the buttocks, the lateral epicondyle, and the medial fat pad of the knee. Laboratory examinations are generally unremarkable except for sleep studies, which reveal an 8 to 10 cycle/sec interference pattern superimposed on the usual 1 to 2 cycle/sec wave pattern characteristic of stage IV non-rapid eye movement sleep.

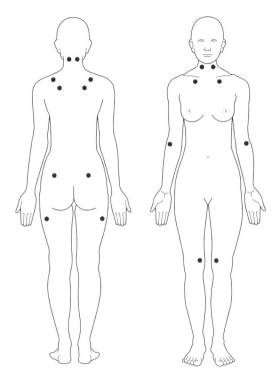

Figure 23.5.3: Location of typical tender points in patients with fibromyalgia.

The diagnosis of fibromyalgia is made on the basis of a characteristic history, with physical examination revealing tender points, and the absence of other notable physical or laboratory findings. A variety of other disorders, including systemic rheumatic diseases, must be excluded. The pathogenesis of fibromyalgia is largely unknown. Possible mechanisms, including post-traumatic neurologic changes, which have been demonstrated in animal models, as well as psychological etiologies, wherein minor trauma triggers FMS, have been posited.[74] The adjudicative difficulties inherent in the trauma–FMS–disability association have been summarized in a consensus report.[84] Classification criteria for fibromyalgia[85] are listed in Table 23.5.2.

The treatment of FMS should ideally entail a multidisciplinary program. Treatment should address physical fitness, work and other functional activities, mental health, and other commonly associated conditions such as irritable bowel syndrome, interstitial cystitis, migraine headaches, and temporomandibular joint dysfunction.[86] Tricyclic antidepressants such as amitriptyline have been used successfully to treat pain associated with FMS; NSAIDs and systemic corticosteroids have typically been ineffective. Promising medications include 5-HT$_3$ receptor antagonists such as odansetron[87] and the serotonin/dopamine receptor antagonist olanzapine.[88] The avoidance of dietary monosodium glutamate and aspartame has been beneficial in some patients.[89]

GOUT

Gout has been described since antiquity. The prevalence of gouty arthritis is 2–2.6 per 1000 persons and increases

1. History of widespread pain.
   Definition: Pain is considered widespread when all of the following are present: pain in the left and right side of the body, above and below the waist. In addition, axial skeletal pain must be present. Shoulder and buttock pain is considered as pain for each involved side. Low back pain is considered lower segment pain.
2. Pain in 11 of 18 tender point sites on digital palpation.
   Occiput: bilateral, at the suboccipital muscle insertions.
   Low cervical: bilateral, at the anterior aspects of the intertransverse spaces at C5–C7.
   Trapezius: bilateral, at the midpoint of the upper border.
   Supraspinatus: bilateral, at origins, above the scapula spine near the medial border.
   Second rib: bilateral, at the second costochondral junctions, just lateral to the junctions of upper surfaces.
   Lateral epicondyle: bilateral, 2 cm distal to the epicondyles.
   Gluteal: bilateral, in upper outer quadrants of buttocks in anterior fold of muscle.
   Greater trochanter: bilateral, posterior to the trochanteric prominence.
   Knee: bilateral, at the medial fat pad proximal to the joint line.

Digital palpation should be performed with an approximate force of 4 kg.

* For classification purposes, patients are said to have fibromyalgia if both criteria are satisfied. Widespread pain must have been present for at least 3 months. The presence of a second clinical disorder does not exclude the diagnosis of fibromyalgia.
From Wolfe F, Smythe HA, Yunus MB, et al.[85] © 1990 John Wiley & Sons, Inc. Reprinted with permission of Wiley-Liss, Inc., a subsidiary of John Wiley & Sons, Inc.

Table 23.5.2 The American College of Rheumatology 1990 criteria for the classification of fibromyalgia*

steadily with age and serum uric acid concentration. It is predominantly a condition of males, but also occurs in elderly women with renal dysfunction, diuretic use, or both. Gout is an important disorder in occupational medicine because of its association with lead intoxication.

Occupational epidemiology

The association between lead ingestion and gout has been recognized for over two centuries. Lead toxicity may result from inhalation of fumes from radiator recycling operations or ingestion of lead-containing materials such as paints, water from lead pipes, and historically, with the use of illicit alcohol (moonshine) distilled in lead-containing car radiator stills.[90] Patients with saturnine gout may exhibit other symptoms of lead toxicity for months or years before developing gouty arthritis.[91] Classic findings, as well as the diagnosis and treatment of lead intoxication, are discussed in Chapter 39.7.

The occurrence of gout in lead-intoxicated individuals also suggests that prior lead exposure at a subclinical dose may explain some of the renal disease commonly observed in patients with gout.[92] However, it has also been shown that patients with gout, renal impairment, and a history of lead exposure may have normal EDTA chelation tests, indicating that concurrent disease entities (e.g., hypertension, diabetes) may explain the renal insufficiency observed in gouty patients with moonshine exposure.[93] Chronic low-level environmental lead exposure may interfere with urate excretion in patients with renal insufficiency. This inhibition may be markedly improved by lead-chelating therapies.[94]

Clinical manifestations

Acute gouty arthritis is characterized by episodes of exquisitely painful monoarthritis with a predilection for lower extremity joints, particularly the first metatarsophalangeal joint (podagra). Untreated attacks last up to 2 weeks but usually resolve completely. Attacks become more frequent and prolonged over time, often involving multiple joints. Chronic tophaceous gout generally occurs after many years of untreated disease and is characterized by deposits of uric acid in the helix of the ear, extensor surfaces of the forearm, olecranon bursa, and other sites.

Gouty arthritis results from an inflammatory response to monosodium urate crystals deposited in joints and periarticular structures. Monosodium urate crystals may form when the serum urate concentration exceeds the solubility threshold of approximately 7 mg/dl. Hyperuricemia occasionally arises from overproduction due to enzymatic defects in purine metabolism. Over 80% of cases, however, are due to undersecretion of urate because of proximal tubular dysfunction, likely representing the pathophysiologic process in saturnine gout.

The clinical features of saturnine gout do not differ substantially from idiopathic gout. A greater predilection for knee involvement, as well as polyarticular disease, has been observed. Treatment of acute saturnine gout is the same as for idiopathic gout, including NSAIDs or colchicine in acute cases and urate-lowering agents on a chronic basis. Because renal dysfunction is often present in saturnine gout, doses of colchicine and allopurinol should be reduced. Uricosurics are less effective in the setting of renal dysfunction. Removal of the affected individual from exposure to lead is imperative, but the role of chelation is uncertain if signs of acute intoxication are absent.

ANKYLOSING SPONDYLITIS AND THE SPONDYLOARTHROPATHIES

As discussed in Chapter 23.4, millions of workers in the US are evaluated annually for low back complaints. Although most low back syndromes are mechanical in nature, inflammatory back disease occurs in 0.1% to 1% of the population and, therefore, must be considered in the differential diagnosis. The spondyloarthropathies are related disorders characterized by inflammation of the spine, sacroiliac joints, peripheral joints, and, variably, the eye, skin, and other organs. Specific spondyloarthropathies include ankylosing spondylitis (AS); Reiter's syndrome and other reactive arthritides; psoriatic arthritis; and enteropathic arthritis, including Crohn's disease and ulcerative colitis. These diseases have no known occupational associations, although Reiter's syndrome and other reactive arthritides have been reported in outbreaks of enteritis in settings such as military camps. Patients with AS who have physically demanding jobs are more likely to experience permanent or temporary work disability, or require accommodation than those with less physically demanding jobs.[95]

Spondylitis can usually be distinguished from mechanical back pain by history. Patients with AS have the insidious onset of back discomfort before age 40, generally in the late teens or twenties. Mechanical pain seldom starts in the teens and generally has an acute or subacute rather than insidious onset. Spondylitis also is associated with morning stiffness, usually lasting for more than 30 to 60 minutes, which is improved with exercise. Mechanical back pain usually causes just a few minutes of stiffness, which worsens with exercise. The physical examination is generally unrewarding in distinguishing early spondylitis from mechanical back pain. Although sacroiliitis and ligamentous calcification are characteristic radiographic findings in spondylitis, they generally do not appear in the initial years of disease.

Mechanical back pain has an excellent prognosis, with 90% of patients being symptom free 3 months following an episode. Spondylitis, particularly AS, has a less favorable natural history. Spontaneous remissions are uncommon, and progressive disability with deforming spine fusion may occur. For this reason, it is critical to diagnose spondylitis early, and institute a physical therapy program directed at maintaining lumbar and cervical extension, preventing fusion in a stooped posture. NSAID therapy is appropriate, especially to improve exercise tolerance and physical capacity. Recently, clinical responses have been reported with tumor necrosis factor (TNF)-alpha antagonists such as etanercept and infliximab.[96,97] The risk of activating an occult infection with these agents, however, demands that they be used with great care.

INFECTIOUS DISEASES

Rheumatic conditions caused by infectious diseases (see Chapter 22) may be acquired in occupational settings,[98] and include the following common conditions.

Septic bursitis

Bursae are synovia-lined cavities. The prepatellar and olecranon bursae are superficial and frequently traumatized. Resultant skin lesions provide a portal of entry for purulent organisms, particularly *Staphylococcus aureus*, which is involved in 80% of cases of septic bursitis. Workers exposed to repeated knee or elbow trauma, including carpenters, carpet layers, and other laborers, are at risk for septic bursitis.[99]

Symptoms include pain, swelling, and diminished range of motion. Associated cellulitis is common. Systemic symptoms and fever occur occasionally. Diagnostic aspiration should be performed and appropriate antibiotics initiated. Hospitalization and intravenous antibiotics are advisable in patients with systemic features or impaired host defenses. In many patients, outpatient oral antibiotic therapy (e.g., penicillinase-resistant penicillins) is adequate, because the olecranon and prepatellar bursae do not communicate with the joint space.

Brucellosis

Brucella are non-encapsulated gram-negative aerobic bacilli. There are four species: *B. melitensis* found in goats, sheep, and camels; *B. abortus* in cattle; *B. suis* in hogs; and *B. canis* in dogs. The organisms may cause infection by direct contact (through abraded skin or exposed conjunctivae), inhalation, or ingestion. Thus, workers in contact with dogs, sheep, or cattle, such as farmers, slaughterhouse workers, and veterinarians, are at risk. Brucellosis also may be acquired through ingestion of unpasteurized milk. There were 82 cases of brucellosis reported in the US for 1999. The usual incubation period is 10 to 21 days. The characteristic tissue reaction to *Brucella* is the formation of a non-caseating granuloma.

The most common clinical features are fever, fatigue, anorexia, and weight loss. Arthritis and spondylitis may occur, particularly in association with *B. melitensis* and *B. suis* infections. Arthritis is generally polyarticular and migratory, affecting the knees, sacroiliac joints, shoulders, hips, sternoclavicular joints, elbows, ankles, and manubriosternal joints. Arthritis develops in 10% to 20% of acute, self-limited cases of brucellosis and in 50% to 65% of patients with chronic infections.[100]

Lyme disease

Lyme disease was initially described in 1977 and has become a significant source of morbidity in endemic areas.[101] The initial cluster was located in Lyme and surrounding towns at the mouth of the Connecticut River. Currently, the disease is endemic in the northeastern, mid-Atlantic, and north-central regions of the US, as well as in portions of the West Coast states. From 1991 to 2000, the annual incidence has nearly doubled to an all-time high of nearly 18,000 cases, with a bimodal age distribution peaking at 5 to 9 and 50 to 59 years of age.[102]

Among workers studied in an endemic area of southeastern New York, most of whom were employed outdoors, 6% were seropositive, compared with 1.1% of 362 New York blood donors.[103] Outdoor leisure activity was a significant risk factor (odds ratio [95% confidence interval (CI)] = 2.5 [1.2, 5.2]); while outdoor employment was associated with increased risk (odds ratio [95% CI] = 2.0 [0.3, 12.0]), this was not statistically significant. In multivariate analyses of outdoor workers in New Jersey, adjusting for age, sex, and recreational activities, a history of tick bites on the job conferred a significant risk of seropositivity (odds ratio [95% CI] = 5.1 [1.1, 23.6]).[104] Another study found an incidence of Lyme disease of 3.8 per 100,000 persons in Monmouth County, New Jersey, from 1980 to 1982, and 0.5 per 100,000 persons in the rest of the state.[105] The incidence at the Naval Weapons Military Reserve was over 1000 per 100,000 persons. Outdoor workers had a fivefold higher risk than indoor workers of contracting disease. These data point to substantial occupational risk.[106]

The infectious agent in Lyme disease is the spirochete *Borrelia burgdorferi*. *Borrelia* are transmitted by *Ixodes* ticks. The ticks feed on white-footed mice in the larval and nymph stages, allowing for horizontal transmission from nymphal to larval generations and consequent perpetuation of *Borrelia* infection. Adult ticks feed on white-tailed deer and a variety of other wild animals and birds. The disease is transmitted to humans by nymphal and, occasionally, adult forms. When the nymph feeds, the organism migrates from the tick midgut to the salivary glands and is transmitted in saliva. The tick must remain attached to its host for as long as 24 hours for migration and transmission to occur.

Clinical features of Lyme disease generally are classified in three stages. Stage I, or localized Lyme disease, occurs within 3 to 30 days of infection and consists of erythema migrans, an enlarging erythematous circular lesion with a clearing center, often accompanied by mild constitutional symptoms and regional lymphadenopathy. Of note, 20% to 35% of patients with Lyme disease do not experience erythema migrans, and only a minority of patients actually remember a tick bite. Stage II, disseminated infection, occurs weeks to months after the initial infection. Although multiple organ systems may be involved, the most common manifestations are neurologic, which occur in 10% to 20% of cases and include meningoencephalitis, cranial neuritis, radiculoneuritis, and myelitis. Cardiac involvement, including abnormal conduction and other arrhythmias, occurs in up to 10% of patients. Stage III, chronic persistent infection, may occur months to years following the initial infection and generally involves arthritis, nervous system involvement, or both. The knee is the most commonly involved site, followed by the shoulder, ankle, and elbow.

The diagnosis of Lyme disease is based on clinical features and supporting serologic tests. The serologic diagnosis of Lyme disease is a two-stage process in which a positive or equivocal result by an enzyme-linked immunosorbent assay (ELISA) or immunofluorescent assay is then followed by Western blot; a rapid assay has also been reported.[107] Sensitive techniques such as the polymerase chain reaction are also available, though no single diagnostic modality is suitable for detection of *Borrelia burgdorferi* in every patient with erythema migrans.[108] Negative results from US laboratories should be interpreted cautiously when tick exposure occurred in Europe or other regions of the world. Better recognition of two emerging tick-borne zoonoses (babesiosis and human granulocytic ehrlichiosis) that can also be co-transmitted with Lyme disease is changing the approach to diagnosis and treatment of Lyme disease.[109]

The treatment of Lyme disease really begins with prevention of infestation through proper use of protective clothing and repellants, followed by careful body inspection and removal of any attached ticks with tweezers, grasping only the head. A tick bite should not be treated with antibiotics, but cleansed and observed. Erythema migrans should be treated with oral amoxicillin, doxycycline, or cefuroxime. The treatment algorithm for various stages of disease is complex and beyond the scope of this text. These and further detailed treatment guidelines have been published recently by the Infectious Diseases Society of America.[110]

OSTEONECROSIS

Osteonecrosis, ischemic necrosis of bone, and avascular necrosis are terms used interchangeably to denote a painful disorder associated with inadequate vascular supply to bone. Numerous conditions may impair circulation to bone, causing osteonecrosis. For example, dislocation or fracture of the hip may disrupt blood supply to the femoral head. Corticosteroids and alcohol use appear to cause hypertrophy of intramedullary fat cells with consequent impairment of intramedullary fat metabolism. Sickle cell disease may cause sludging in bony sinusoids with attendant ischemic necrosis. Exposure to deep-sea pressures and compressed air are important occupational exposures that may also predispose an individual to osteonecrosis. Approximately 20% of cases are idiopathic.

Occupational epidemiology

Osteonecrosis is a significant occupational hazard in workers exposed to compressed air, such as tunnel workers,[111] or elevated ambient pressures, such as deep-sea divers (see Chapter 36).[112] A report from the British Decompression Sickness Central Registry and Radiological Panel indicates that the prevalence of dysbaric osteonecrosis among commercial divers is 4.2%.[113] Gaseous nitrogen solubilizes and accumulates in vascular tissues, including bone, during exposure to elevated pressure. When workers return to normal ambient pressures, nitrogen becomes insoluble, forming gaseous bubbles. These nitrogen bubbles may occlude osseous capillary flow, increase intramedullary pressure, and exert a direct toxic effect on osteocytes.

Dysbaric osteonecrosis involves two distinct syndromes: juxta-articular lesions, which involve the humeral and femoral heads, and shaft lesions, which typically involve the distal femoral shaft.[114] Juxta-articular lesions are much more important because they can lead to joint destruction and significant disability. Shaft lesions, in contrast, are generally asymptomatic. The presence of shaft lesions, however, has been used to disqualify workers from further hyperbaric exposures.[115]

Several risk factors have been identified for the development of dysbaric osteonecrosis. The duration of an episode of diving is strongly associated with osteonecrosis. Radiologic osteonecrosis occurs in 0.7% of divers with less than 4 years of experience and in 10.7% of divers with 12 or more years of experience. The depth of diving also is a strong risk factor; osteonecrosis rarely occurs in divers at a maximum depth of less than 30 meters, compared with a 15.8% prevalence at a maximum depth greater than 200 meters. The rate of decompression also is a strong risk factor; gradual adjustment is much safer than abrupt exposure to normal atmospheric pressure. Age and obesity also appear to be independent risk factors (see Chapter 36).[116]

Clinical features

Divers and compressed air workers may experience decompression sickness on return to ambient pressures. The characteristic symptom is limb pain, which may be relieved by bending the extremity – thus, the colloquial term, 'the bends'. More severe symptoms of decompression sickness include pulmonary edema and neurologic symptoms. It is presumed that these acute symptoms of decompression also result from the formation of nitrogen bubbles in the microcirculation.

Physical examination is non-specific until actual joint destruction occurs, at which point, range of motion is limited. Radiographs are generally normal until late in the disease process, when areas of sclerosis appear. The collapse of subchondral bone is evidenced by a lucency or crescent sign (Fig. 23.5.4). Flattening of the articular surface appears subsequently, followed by secondary degenerative changes. Radionuclide bone scanning is much more sensitive than routine radiography, showing increased activity, which reflects the initial repair phase. Magnetic resonance imaging (MRI) is the most sensitive test for osteonecrosis (Fig. 23.5.5), showing changes due to necrosis of bone before sclerotic changes are evident.

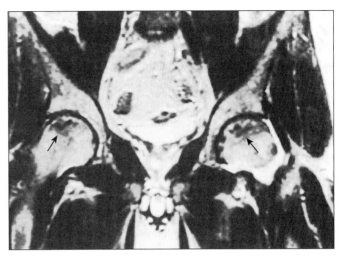

Figure 23.5.5: MRI of the hip, showing osteonecrosis in a patient with a normal plain radiograph. It demonstrates areas of lucency (*arrows*) in both femoral heads, corresponding to necrotic bone. The left hip has a moderate effusion, which appears as a bright signal in this T_2-weighted scan.

Management

Despite increased recognition of the problem over the last two decades, and continued attempts to improve decompression protocols, dysbaric osteonecrosis remains a significant hazard among compressed air workers. Multinational experience over many years indicates that all current air decompression schedules for caisson and compressed air tunnel workers are inadequate to prevent osteonecrosis.[117] Hyperbaric oxygen decompression seems to be the only viable method for safely decompressing tunnel workers. This technique has been successfully used in Germany, where only hyperbaric oxygen decompression of compressed air workers is permitted, as well as in France and Brazil. Once osteonecrosis has occurred, hyperbaric oxygen therapy has been demonstrated to limit bony destruction in animal studies.[118] Elimination of weight bearing on joints offers symptomatic relief and may retard progression of joint destruction. NSAIDs are of modest value. Aggressive surgical approaches, including arthroplasty, are effective but involve considerable rehabilitation. Many surgeons recommend core decompression for the treatment of osteonecrosis in the early stages of hip and knee involvement.[119] The rationale is that early ischemic changes result in elevated pressures within the affected bone, which further compromise the vascular supply. The procedure allows histologic confirmation of osteonecrosis, measurement of pressure within the affected bone, and therapeutic decompression. The efficacy and safety of the procedure are debatable.[120] Affected workers require long-term follow-up, as lesions can develop in previously normal areas and progression of previously identified lesions may occur, even in the absence of further exposure to hyperbaric pressures.[121]

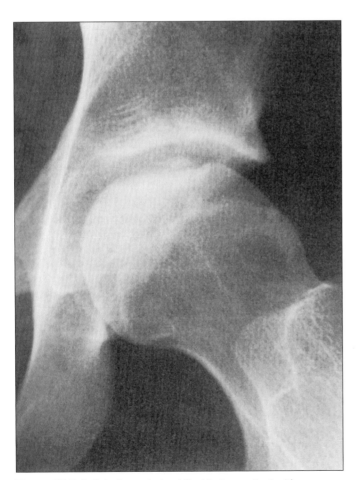

Figure 23.5.4: Plain X-ray study of the hip in a patient with osteonecrosis, revealing a crescent sign, indicating bone infarction without collapse of subchondral bone.

FLUOROSIS

Musculoskeletal manifestations from exposure to fluoride were initially described by Moller and Gudjonsson in 1932.[122] During the winter of 1931 to 1932, these authors investigated employees of a factory that processed cryolite, which contains sodium, fluoride, and aluminum, and which is frequently mixed with quartz. The investigators were struck by the abnormal appearance of the thoracic vertebrae, clavicles, and ribs on chest X-ray studies of these exposed workers. The bone appeared peculiarly dense and coarse. Moller and Gunjonsson performed skeletal surveys of 78 workers and found that among 30 (38%), there were distinct osseous changes. The workers also complained of acute nausea, vomiting, and anorexia with cryolite dust exposure, which predictably disappeared when the exposure was removed.

Seventy years later, the spectrum of fluorosis has been recognized in other industries and with other environmental exposures, but the clinical syndrome remains essentially as that described by Moller and Gudjonsson.[123] Significant fluoride exposure may occur in the mining and processing of cryolite, fluorspar, and apatite, which occur in sedimentary rock. Fluorides are used in the processing and manufacture of aluminum, nickel, copper, gold, and silver.[124,125] Fluoride also is used as a preservative and a bleaching agent, and is a component of certain pesticides.

Epidemiology

At the present time, the most common exposures include fluoridated drinking water and the manufacture of aluminum, fertilizer, and glass. It is estimated that around 350,000 workers in the US are exposed to fluoride. The number of individuals exposed to fluoride in drinking water is more difficult to estimate. However, excessive levels have been noted in parts of India, China, Africa, and South America.[126] Because fluoride intake is related to both the concentration and the amount of water consumed daily, environmental fluorosis occurs more commonly in hot climates, with increased water consumption. Fluorosis has been noted in 3000-year-old human mandibles from the Arabian Gulf region.[127] In China, the risk of fluorosis is elevated in areas where high-fluoride coal is burned indoors.[128,129]

Metabolism and pathogenesis

Fluoride may be inhaled or ingested. Ninety percent of fluoride taken by mouth is absorbed through the gastrointestinal tract. Systemic absorption of inhaled fluoride depends largely on the particle size. Of absorbed fluoride, 50% is excreted in the urine within 24 hours. Of the remainder, 99% is taken up by the bones. The half-life of fluoride in bone may reach 8 years. In bone, fluoride displaces hydroxy residues from apatite, forming fluorohydroxyapatite.

The mechanism of fluoride's toxic effect is not well understood. Recently, hyperparathyroidism was correlated with an increase in fluoride ingestion, and the severity of skeletal fluorosis was observed to parallel an increase in parathyroid hormone (PTH) concentration.[130] Fluoride has been observed to stimulate osteoblasts, resulting in new bone formation. With increasing concentrations of fluo-

Daily exposure	Sequelae
1 to 2 mg	None
2 to 4 mg	Tooth mottling
	No skeletal changes
8 mg	Skeletal changes rare
20 to 80 mg	Crippling skeletal disease

Table 23.5.3 Sequelae of increasing exposure to fluoride

ride, the new bone is woven rather than lamellar. At 1 to 2 mg/day, a typical dose achieved in water fluoridation programs, no adverse effects are seen. At 2 to 4 mg/day, the dental enamel becomes mottled, but no skeletal changes are observed. At approximately 8 mg/day, osteosclerosis has been observed in a small fraction of exposed individuals. Crippling fluorosis with advanced bony changes has been observed following exposure to 20 to 80 mg/day of fluoride for 10 to 20 years. Workers exposed to less than 8 mg/day of fluoride have had no skeletal changes following as much as 14 years of observation. The Occupational Safety and Health Administration (OSHA) has established a limit of 2.5 mg of fluoride per cubic meter of air averaged over an 8-hour shift (Table 23.5.3).

Clinical manifestations

Early diagnosis of fluorosis is made on the basis of history of exposure, with concomitant musculoskeletal and, often, gastrointestinal symptoms. Musculoskeletal symptoms include vague joint pains and restriction of movement. Pain in the heel, hand, and other sites may arise from bony exostoses at the sites of ligamentous or muscular attachments. Bone pain may become diffuse. Gastrointestinal symptoms include nausea, loss of appetite, and vomiting, which occur acutely on exposure to fluoride. Some adaptation to these effects has been noted over time. Short-term exposure also may cause irritation of the eyes and respiratory tract. Advanced cases may be accompanied by kyphosis, limitation of chest expansion, and severe contractures of joints, including the knee and hips. Spinal stenosis may result from impingement of the spinal cord and roots by exostoses in the spinal canal. Radiographic changes occur after significant exposure and are less useful in diagnosing early disease. Characteristic findings include sclerosis and coarsened trabeculae of the vertebrae, along with vertebral fusion (Fig. 23.5.6). Bony exostoses are noted at the attachments of muscles, ligaments, and tendons. Bony overgrowths also may be noted in joint capsules and interosseous membranes. The differential diagnosis of these radiographic findings include AS and other spondyloarthropathies, diffuse idiopathic skeletal hyperostosis, and vitamin A intoxication.

Prompt removal from exposure is mandatory for workers with fluorosis and was until recently the only available treatment. A double-blind, controlled trial was conducted to examine the effect of a combination of calcium, vitamin D3, and ascorbic acid supplementation in fluorosis-affected children.[131] A significant improvement in dental

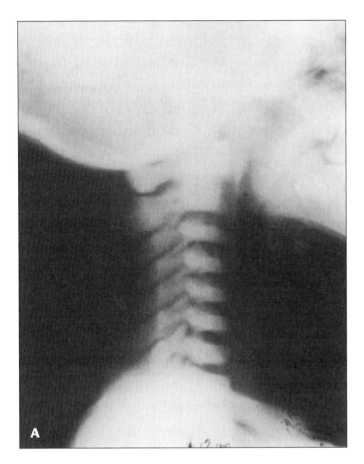

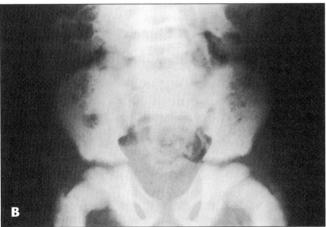

Figure 23.5.6: A: Cervical spine: 12-year-old child affected by endemic osteofluorosis. Note increased sclerosis of vertebral bodies and base of skull, with abnormal bone formation evidenced by decreased height of vertebral bodies. B: Pelvis: note unusual trabecular pattern and early sclerosis of pubic and ischial bones. The sacroiliac joints and Y cartilages are prominent, and the lumbar bones are of decreased height in this young child affected by endemic osteofluorosis. (A and B courtesy of David Christie, MD.)

MUSCLE DISORDERS

Muscle may be the target of inflammatory, infectious, metabolic, traumatic, and toxic insults, including environmental exposures. Most muscle disorders are associated with weakness, pain, or clinical evidence of muscle damage. Inflammatory muscle disease is termed polymyositis if there is no evidence of characteristic skin lesions over the hands and extensor surfaces, and dermatomyositis if such lesions are present. These disorders are generally idiopathic. However, cimetidine and D-penicillamine may induce a polymyositis syndrome, suggesting that environmental agents may do likewise, although specific evidence is currently lacking. A variety of drugs cause myopathy associated with myalgia and weakness, including chloroquine, colchicine, and the HMG-CoA reductase inhibitors, particularly when combined with lipid-lowering therapy.

Rhabdomyolysis refers to acute destruction of muscle cells, leading to weakness and marked elevation of creatine kinase. Rhabdomyolysis may occur in response to a variety of agents, including alcohol, drugs, prominent overexertion, thermal stress and infection. The urine is characteristically darkened by myoglobin. Treatment consists of removing the offending agent, hydrating, alkalinizing the urine, and providing supportive care.

Malignant hyperthermia is a group of inherited disorders that are characterized by rapid increases in core temperature from 39°C to 42°C in response to inhalation anesthetics such as halothane, methoxyflurane, cyclopropane, and diethyl ether; or muscle relaxants, most commonly succinylcholine. In the autosomal dominant variety, individuals are normal between attacks, but 50% of patients may have an elevation in creatinine phosphokinase and 90% experience muscle contractions following exposure to concentrations of caffeine, halothane, or hexamethonium that would not normally cause symptoms. A recessive form of the disease is associated with a number of congenital musculoskeletal abnormalities. It is believed that this disorder results from the release of calcium from muscle endoplasmic reticulum on exposure to the triggering agents. The endoplasmic reticulum is believed to be defective in storing the calcium ion. The result is a sudden increase in myoplasmic calcium, which activates myosin ATPase, which, in turn, converts adenosine triphosphate to adenosine diphosphate, phosphate, and heat. This disorder is exceedingly rare but may arise in occupational settings. Denborough and associates reported a case of a worker involved in the production of fire extinguishers who complained of malaise, stiffness, and weakness in his forearms and hands during the work week which improved on weekends.[132] His serum creatinine kinase was markedly elevated. The plant used bromochlorodifluoromethane, which has a structure similar to halothane. The worker had rhabdomyolysis due to recurrent exposures to this agent. Avoiding occupational exposure to halogenated hydrocarbons resulted in improvement in symptoms.

Metallic poison from lead, arsenic, and antimony produces two types of striated muscle lesions. One is muscular atrophy secondary to neuritis, and the other is a fibrous

and skeletal fluorosis was noted in these children. This study suggests that fluorosis may be somewhat reversible, at least in children. Further studies are needed in adults. Gradual improvement in symptoms has been noted in some exposed workers upon retirement.

pattern of degeneration. No proliferation of sarcolemmal nuclei or other reactive changes have been observed, even in the most chronic stages of lead poisoning, and the significance of these changes and their clinical importance are not clear.

References

1. US Department of Health and Human Services. Musculoskeletal Disorders and Workplace Factors. DHHS (NIOSH) Publication No. 91-141. Cincinnati: National Institute of Occupational Safety and Health; 1997:1-6.
2. US Department of Labor BoLS. Workplace Injuries and Illnesses in 1999. Vol. USDL 00357. Washington, DC: US Government Printing Office; 1999.
3. Anonymous. Prevalence of disabilities and associated health conditions among adults – United States, 1999. Morb Mortal Wkly Rep 2001; 50:120-5.
4. Shmerling R, Liang M. Evaluation of the patient: B. Laboratory assessment. In: Klippel J, ed. Primer on the rheumatic diseases, 11th edn. Atlanta: Arthritis Foundation; 1997.
5. Maddison P, Provost T, Reichlin M. Serologic findings in patients with "ANA-negative" systemic lupus erythematosus. Medicine (Baltimore) 1981; 60:87-94.
6. Atkinson JP. Complement deficiency. Predisposing factor to autoimmune syndromes. Am J Med 1988; 85:45-7.
7. van Saase JL, van Romunde LK, Cats A, Vandenbroucke JP, Valkenburg HA. Epidemiology of osteoarthritis: Zoetermeer survey. Comparison of radiological osteoarthritis in a Dutch population with that in 10 other populations. Ann Rheum Dis 1989; 48:271-80.
8. Panush RS. Occupational and recreational musculoskeletal disorders. In: Ruddy S, Harris ED, Sledge CB, eds. Kelley's textbook of rheumatology, 6th edn. Philadelphia: WB Saunders; 2001:429-38.
9. Felson DT. Do occupation-related physical factors contribute to arthritis? Baillière's Clin Rheumatol 1994; 8:63-77.
10. Felson DT, Zhang Y. An update on the epidemiology of knee and hip osteoarthritis with a view to prevention. Arthritis Rheum 1998; 41:1343-55.
11. Felson DT, Zhang Y, Hannan MT, et al. Risk factors for incident radiographic knee osteoarthritis in the elderly: the Framingham Study. Arthritis Rheum 1997; 40:728-33.
12. Felson DT, Hannan MT, Naimark A, et al. Occupational physical demands, knee bending, and knee osteoarthritis: results from the Framingham Study. J Rheumatol 1991; 18:1587-92.
13. Anderson JJ, Felson DT. Factors associated with osteoarthritis of the knee in the first national Health and Nutrition Examination Survey (HANES I). Evidence for an association with overweight, race, and physical demands of work. Am J Epidemiol 1988; 128:179-89.
14. Hadler NM, Gillings DB, Imbus HR, et al. Hand structure and function in an industrial setting. Arthritis Rheum 1978; 21:210-20.
15. Felson DT, Anderson JJ, Naimark A, Walker AM, Meenan RF. Obesity and knee osteoarthritis. The Framingham Study. Ann Intern Med 1988; 109:18-24.
16. Lindberg H, Montgomery F. Heavy labor and the occurrence of gonarthrosis. Clin Orthop 1987; (214):235-6.
17. Jacobsson B, Dalen N, Tjornstrand B. Coxarthrosis and labour. Int Orthop 1987; 11:311-13.
18. Yoshimura N, Sasaki S, Iwasaki K, et al. Occupational lifting is associated with hip osteoarthritis: a Japanese case-control study. J Rheumatol 2000; 27:434-40.
19. Roach KE, Pewrsky V, Miles T, Budiman-Mak E. Biomechanical aspects of occupation and osteoarthritis of the hip: a case-control study. J Rheumatol 1995; 21:2334-40.
20. Mintz G, Fraga A. Severe osteoarthritis of the elbow in foundry workers. Arch Environ Health 1973; 27:78-80.
21. Williams WV, Cope R, Gaunt WD, et al. Metacarpophalangeal arthropathy associated with manual labor (Missouri metacarpal syndrome). Clinical, radiographic, and pathologic characteristics of an unusual degeneration process. Arthritis Rheum 1987; 30:1362-71.
22. Fam AG, Kolin A. Unusual metacarpophalangeal osteoarthritis in a jackhammer operator. Arthritis Rheum 1986; 29:1284-8.
23. Bard CC, Sylvestre JJ, Dussault RG. Hand osteoarthropathy in pianists. J Can Assoc Radiol 1984; 35:154-8.
24. Doherty M, Preston B. Primary osteoarthritis of the elbow. Ann Rheum Dis 1989; 48:743-7.
25. Kim TK, Queale WS, Cosgarea AJ, McFarland EG. Clinical features of the different types of SLAP lesions: an analysis of 139 cases. Superior labrum anterior posterior. J Bone Joint Surg Am 2003; 85-A:66-71.
26. Geba GP, Weaver AL, Polis AB, Dixon ME, Schnitzer TJ. Efficacy of rofecoxib, celecoxib, and acetaminophen in osteoarthritis of the knee: a randomized trial. JAMA 2002; 287:64-71.
27. Ayral X. Injections in the treatment of osteoarthritis. Best Pract Res Clin Rheumatol 2001; 15:609-26.
28. Long L, Soeken K, Ernst E. Herbal medicines for the treatment of osteoarthritis: a systematic review. Rheumatology (Oxford) 2001; 40:779-93.
29. Little CV, Parsons T. Herbal therapy for treating osteoarthritis. Cochrane Database Syst Rev 2001; (1):CD002947.
30. Brief AA, Maurer SG, Di Cesare PE. Use of glucosamine and chondroitin sulfate in the management of osteoarthritis. J Am Acad Orthop Surg 2001; 9:71-8.
31. Anders S, Schaumburger J, Grifka J. [Surgical intra-articular interventions in arthrosis]. Orthopade 2001; 30:866-80 (in German).
32. Lawrence RC, Hochberg MC, Kelsey JL, et al. Estimates of the prevalence of selected arthritic and musculoskeletal diseases in the United States. J Rheumatol 1989; 16:427-41.
33. Yelin E. The costs of rheumatoid arthritis: absolute, incremental, and marginal estimates. J Rheumatol Suppl 1996; 44:47-51.
34. Wysocki Z, Janas Z, Cichon L, Sikorzewski M, Gregorowicz H. [Rheumatoid arthritis and morbidity among wet spinning factory women workers]. Med Pr 1977; 28:515-7 (in Polish).
35. Leistner K. Occupational aspects of rheumatoid arthritis. Baillière's Clin Rheumatol 1989; 3:211-18.
36. Lundberg I, Alfredsson L, Plato N, Sverdrup B, Klareskog L, Kleinau S. Occupation, occupational exposure to chemicals and rheumatological disease. A register based cohort study. Scand J Rheumatol 1994; 23:305-10.
37. Miall W, Caplan A, Cochrane A. An epidemiological study of rheumatoid arthritis associated with characteristic chest x-ray appearances in coal-workers. BMJ 1953; 11:1231-6.
38. Miall W. Rheumatoid arthritis in males. An epidemiological study of a Welsh mining community. Ann Rheum Dis 1955; 14:150-8.
39. Klockars M, Koskela RS, Jarvinen E, Kolari PJ, Rossi A. Silica exposure and rheumatoid arthritis: a follow up study of granite workers 1940-81. BMJ (Clin Res Ed) 1987; 294:997-1000.
40. Levin RW, Park J, Ostrov B, et al. Clinical assessment of the 1987 American College of Rheumatology criteria for rheumatoid arthritis. Scand J Rheumatol 1996; 25:277-81.
41. Skapenko A, Kalden JR, Schulze-Koops H. Treatment of rheumatoid arthritis in the third millennium. Scand J Rheumatol 2001; 30:249-54.
42. Evans CH, Ghivizzani SC, Palmer GD, Gouze JN, Robbins PD, Gouze E. Gene therapy for rheumatoid arthritis. Expert Opin Biol Ther 2001; 1:971-8.
43. Web document. National Cancer Institute Studies of Hydrazine Sulfate. Located at

http://cis.nci.nih.gov/fact/9_18.htm, updated 02/12/2001, last accessed on 11/28/2003.

44. Reidenberg MM, Durant PJ, Harris RA, De Boccardo G, Lahita R, Stenzel KH. Lupus erythematosus-like disease due to hydrazine. Am J Med 1983; 75:365-70

45. Lee M, Gentry AF, Schwartz R. Tartrazine-containing drugs. Drug Intell Clin Pharm 1981; 15:782-8.

46. Pereyo N. Tartrazine and drug-induced lupus. Schoch Lett 1980; 30:1.

47. Alcocer-Varela J, Iglesias A, Llorente L, Alarcon-Segovia D. Effects of L-canavanine on T cells may explain the induction of systemic lupus erythematosus by alfalfa. Arthritis Rheum 1985; 28:52-7.

48. Malinow MR, Bardana EJ Jr, Pirofsky B, Craig S, McLaughlin P. Systemic lupus erythematosus-like syndrome in monkeys fed alfalfa sprouts: role of a nonprotein amino acid. Science 1982; 216:415-7.

49. Camus JP, Prier A. [Occupational systemic lupus due to cosmetics (author's translation).] Ann Med Interne 1980; 131:279-80 (in French).

50. Arnett FC, Bias WB, McLean RH, et al. Connective tissue disease in southeast Georgia. A community based study of immunogenetic markers and autoantibodies. J Rheumatol 1990; 17:1029-35.

51. Hathaway JA, Buck CR. Absence of health hazards associated with RDX manufacture and use. J Occup Med 1977; 19:269-72.

52. Ruiz-Irastorza G, Khamashta MA, Castellino G, Hughes GR. Systemic lupus erythematosus. Lancet 2001; 357:1027-32.

53. Haustein UF, Ziegler V. Environmentally induced systemic sclerosis-like disorders. Int J Dermatol 1985; 24:147-51.

54. Sluis-Cremer GK, Hessel PA, Nizdo EH, Churchill AR, Zeiss EA. Silica, silicosis, and progressive systemic sclerosis. Br J Ind Med 1985; 42:838-43.

55. Rodnan GP, Benedek TG, Medsger TA Jr, Cammarata RJ. The association of progressive systemic sclerosis (scleroderma) with coal miners' pneumoconiosis and other forms of silicosis. Ann Intern Med 1967; 66:323-34.

56. Varga J, Schumacher HR, Jimenez SA. Systemic sclerosis after augmentation mammoplasty with silicone implants. Ann Intern Med 1989; 111:377-83.

57. Tugwell P, Wells G, Peterson J, et al. Do silicone breast implants cause rheumatologic disorders? A systematic review for a court-appointed national science panel. Arthritis Rheum 2001; 44:2477-84.

58. Steen VD. Treatment of systemic sclerosis. Am J Clin Dermatol 2001; 2:315-25.

59. Walker AE. Vinyl chloride disorder. Br J Dermatol 1981; 105(Suppl 21):19-21.

60. Binns CH. Vinyl chloride: a review. J Soc Occup Med 1979; 29:134-41.

61. Preston BJ, Jones KL, Grainger RG. Clinical aspects of vinyl chloride disease: acro-osteolysis. Proc R Soc Med 1976; 69:284-6.

62. Murphy OB, Bellamy R, Wheeler W, Brower TD. Post-traumatic osteolysis of the distal clavicle. Clin Orthop 1975; 109:108-14.

63. Destouet JM, Murphy WA. Acquired acroosteolysis and acronecrosis. Arthritis Rheum 1983; 26:1150-4.

64. Black CM, Welsh KI, Walker AE, et al. Genetic susceptibility to scleroderma-like syndrome induced by vinyl chloride. Lancet 1983; 1:53-5.

65. Yamakage A, Ishikawa H, Saito Y, Hattori A. Occupational scleroderma-like disorder occurring in men engaged in the polymerization of epoxy resins. Dermatologica 1980; 161:33-44.

66. Sparrow GP. A connective tissue disorder similar to vinyl chloride disease in a patient exposed to perchlorethylene. Clin Exp Dermatol 1977; 2:17-22.

67. Lockey JE, Kelly CR, Cannon GW, Colby TV, Aldrich V, Livingston GK. Progressive systemic sclerosis associated with exposure to trichloroethylene. J Occup Med 1987; 29:493-6.

68. Mainardi C, Trajkovic S. Fibrosing conditions associated with organic solvents and drugs. In: Kaufman L, Varga J, eds. Rheumatic diseases and the environment. London: Arnold; 1999:75-80.

69. Kilbourne EM, Rigau-Perez JG, Heath CW Jr, et al. Clinical epidemiology of toxic-oil syndrome. Manifestations of a new illness. N Engl J Med 1983; 309:1408-14.

70. Medsger TA Jr. Tryptophan-induced eosinophilia-myalgia syndrome. N Engl J Med 1990; 322:926-8.

71. Belongia EA, Hedberg CW, Gleich GJ, et al. An investigation of the cause of the eosinophilia-myalgia syndrome associated with tryptophan use. N Engl J Med 1990; 323:357-65.

72. Goldenberg D, Bennett R. Fibromyalgia. Rheum Dis Clin North Am 1989; 15: Preface.

73. Wolfe F, Ross K, Anderson J, Russell IJ, Hebert L. The prevalence and characteristics of fibromyalgia in the general population. Arthritis Rheum 1995; 38:19-28.

74. Wolfe F, Pollina D, Krupp L. Environmental factors in fibromyalgia and chronic fatigue syndrome. In: Kaufman L, Varga J, eds. Rheumatic diseases and the environment. London: Arnold; 1999:161-7.

75. Goldenberg DL. Fibromyalgia, chronic fatigue syndrome, and myofascial pain syndrome. Curr Opin Rheumatol 1997; 9:135-43.

76. Hudson JI, Goldenberg DL, Pope HG Jr, Keck PE Jr, Schlesinger L. Comorbidity of fibromyalgia with medical and psychiatric disorders. Am J Med 1992; 92:363-7.

77. Goldenberg DL, Simms RW, Geiger A, Komaroff AL. High frequency of fibromyalgia in patients with chronic fatigue seen in a primary care practice. Arthritis Rheum 1990; 33:381-7.

78. Wolfe F. The clinical syndrome of fibrositis. Am J Med 1986; 81:7-14.

79. Littlejohn GO. Fibrositis/fibromyalgia syndrome in the workplace. Rheum Dis Clin North Am 1989; 15:45-60.

80. Donnay A. Carbon monoxide as an unrecognized cause of neurasthenia: a history. In: Penney D, ed. Carbon monoxide toxicity. Boca Raton: CRC Press; 2000:231-60.

81. Goldenberg DL. Fibromyalgia syndrome. An emerging but controversial condition. JAMA 1987; 257:2782-7.

82. Clauw DJ. Elusive syndromes: treating the biologic basis of fibromyalgia and related syndromes. Cleve Clin J Med 2001; 68:830, 832-4.

83. Moldofsky H. Sleep and fibrositis syndrome. Rheum Dis Clin North Am 1989; 15:91-103.

84. Wolfe F. The fibromyalgia syndrome: a consensus report on fibromyalgia and disability. J Rheumatol 1996; 23:534-9.

85. Wolfe F, Smythe HA, Yunus MB, et al. The American College of Rheumatology 1990 criteria for the classification of fibromyalgia. Report of the Multicenter Criteria Committee. Arthritis Rheum 1990; 33:160-72.

86. Barkhuizen A. Pharmacologic treatment of fibromyalgia. Curr Pain Headache Rep 2001; 5:351-8.

87. Moulin DE. Systemic drug treatment for chronic musculoskeletal pain. Clin J Pain 2001; 17(4 Suppl): S86-93.

88. Kiser RS, Cohen HM, Freedenfeld RN, Jewell C, Fuchs PN. Olanzapine for the treatment of fibromyalgia symptoms. J Pain Symptom Manage 2001; 22:704-8.

89. Smith JD, Terpening CM, Schmidt SO, Gums JG. Relief of fibromyalgia symptoms following discontinuation of dietary excitotoxins. Ann Pharmacother 2001; 35:702-6.

90. Ball GV, Sorensen LB. Pathogenesis of hyperuricemia in saturinine gout. N Engl J Med 1969; 280:1199-202.

91. Halla JT, Ball GV. Saturnine gout: a review of 42 patients. Semin Arthritis Rheum 1982; 11:307-14.

92. Batuman V, Maesaka JK, Haddad B, Tepper E, Landy E, Wedeen RP. The role of lead in gout nephropathy. N Engl J Med 1981; 304:520-3.

93. Wright LF, Saylor RP, Cecere FA. Occult lead intoxication in patients with gout and kidney disease. J Rheumatol 1984; 11:517-20.

94. Lin JL, Yu CC, Lin-Tan DT, Ho HH. Lead chelation therapy and urate excretion in patients with chronic renal diseases and gout. Kidney Int 2001; 60:266-71.

95. Ward MM, Kuzis S. Risk factors for work disability in patients with ankylosing spondylitis. J Rheumatol 2001; 28:315-21.

96. Braun J, de Keyser F, Brandt J, Mielants H, Sieper J, Veys E. New treatment options in spondyloarthropathies: increasing evidence for significant efficacy of anti-tumor necrosis factor therapy. Curr Opin Rheumatol 2001; 13:245-9.

97. Barthel HR. Rapid remission of treatment-resistant ankylosing spondylitis with etanercept – a drug for refractory ankylosing spondylitis? Arthritis Rheum 2001; 45:404.

98. Madkour MM. Occupation-related infectious arthritis. Baillière's Clin Rheumatol 1989; 3:157-92.

99. Ho G Jr, Tice AD, Kaplan SR. Septic bursitis in the prepatellar and olecranon bursae: an analysis of 25 cases. Ann Intern Med 1978; 89:21-7.

100. Goldenberg D. Bacterial arthritis. In: Kelley W, Harris E, Ruddy S, Sledge C, eds. Textbook of rheumatology, 3rd edn. Philadelphia: WB Saunders; 1989.

101. Steere AC. Lyme disease. N Engl J Med 1989; 321:586-96.

102. [No authors listed].Lyme disease – United States, 2000. Morb Mortal Wkly Rep 2002; 51:29-31.

103. Smith PF, Benach JL, White DJ, Stroup DF, Morse DL. Occupational risk of Lyme disease in endemic areas of New York State. Ann N Y Acad Sci 1988; 539:289-301.

104. Schwartz BS, Goldstein MD. Lyme disease in outdoor workers: risk factors, preventive measures, and tick removal methods. Am J Epidemiol 1990; 131:877-85.

105. Bowen GS, Schulze TL, Hayne C, Parkin WE. A focus of Lyme disease in Monmouth County, New Jersey. Am J Epidemiol 1984; 120:387-94.

106. Schwartz BS, Goldstein MD. Lyme disease: a review for the occupational physician. J Occup Med 1989; 31:735-42.

107. Gomes-Solecki MJ, Wormser GP, Persing DH, et al. A first-tier rapid assay for the serodiagnosis of Borrelia burgdorferi infection. Arch Intern Med 2001; 161:2015-20.

108. Nowakowski J, Schwartz I, Liveris D, et al. Laboratory diagnostic techniques for patients with early Lyme disease associated with erythema migrans: a comparison of different techniques. Clin Infect Dis 2001; 33:2023-7.

109. Terkeltaub RA. Lyme disease 2000. Emerging zoonoses complicate patient work-up and treatment. Geriatrics 2000; 55:34-5, 39-40, 43-4 passim.

110. Wormser GP, Nadelman RB, Dattwyler RJ, et al. Practice guidelines for the treatment of Lyme disease. The Infectious Diseases Society of America. Clin Infect Dis 2000; 31(Suppl 1):1-14.

111. Kindwall EP, Nellen JR, Spiegelhoff DR. Aseptic necrosis in compressed air tunnel workers using current OSHA decompression schedules. J Occup Med 1982; 24:741-5.

112. Calder IM. Bone and joint diseases in workers exposed to hyperbaric conditions. Curr Top Pathol 1982; 71: 103-22.

113. Aseptic bone necrosis in commercial divers. A report from the Decompression Sickness Central Registry and Radiological Panel. Lancet 1981; 2:384-8.

114. Davidson JK. Dysbaric disorders: aseptic bone necrosis in tunnel workers and divers. Baillière's Clin Rheumatol 1989; 3:1-23.

115. Heard JL, Schneider CS. Radiographic findings in commercial divers. Clin Orthop 1978;(130):129-38.

116. Lam TH, Yau KP. Dysbaric osteonecrosis in a compressed air tunnelling project in Hong Kong. Occup Med (Lond) 1992; 42:23-9.

117. Kindwall EP. Compressed air tunneling and caisson work decompression procedures: development, problems, and solutions. Undersea Hyperb Med 1997; 24:337-45.

118. Levin D, Norman D, Zinman C, et al. Treatment of experimental avascular necrosis of the femoral head with hyperbaric oxygen in rats: histological evaluation of the femoral heads during the early phase of the reparative process. Exp Mol Pathol 1999; 67:99-108.

119. Hungerford DS. Role of core decompression as treatment method for ischemic femur head necrosis. Orthopade 1990; 19:219-23.

120. Colwell CW Jr. The controversy of core decompression of the femoral head for osteonecrosis. Arthritis Rheum 1989; 32:797-800.

121. Van Blarcom ST, Czarnecki DJ, Fueredi GA, Wenzel MS. Does dysbaric osteonecrosis progress in the absence of further hyperbaric exposure? A 10-year radiologic follow-up of 15 patients. Am J Roentgenol 1990; 155:95-7.

122. Moller P, Gudjonsson S. Massive fluorosis of bones and ligaments. Acta Radiol Scand 1932; 13:269.

123. Grandjean P. Occupational fluorosis through 50 years: clinical and epidemiological experiences. Am J Ind Med 1982; 3:227-36.

124. Dinman BD, Bovard WJ, Bonney TB, Cohen JM, Colwell MO. Prevention of bony fluorosis in aluminum smelter workers. Absorption and excretion of fluoride immediately after exposure – Pt. 1. J Occup Med 1976; 18:7-13.

125. Dinman BD, Elder MJ, Bonney TB, Bovard PG, Colwell MO. Prevention of bony fluorosis in aluminum smelter workers. A 15-year retrospective study of fluoride excretion and bony radiopacity among aluminum smelter workers – Pt. 4. J Occup Med 1976; 18:21-3.

126. Singh A, Malhotra KC, Singh BM, Mathur OC. Endemic fluorosis. Indian J Med Sci 1966; 20:569-74.

127. Nayeem F. The mandible – an analysis. Acta Anat 1992; 145:132-7.

128. Ando M, Tadano M, Yamamoto S, et al. Health effects of fluoride pollution caused by coal burning. Sci Total Environ 2001; 271:107-16.

129. Finkelman RB, Belkin HE, Zheng B. Health impacts of domestic coal use in China. Proc Natl Acad Sci USA 1999; 96:3427-31.

130. Gupta SK, Khan TI, Gupta RC, et al. Compensatory hyperparathyroidism following high fluoride ingestion – a clinico-biochemical correlation. Indian Pediatr 2001; 38:139-46.

131. Gupta SK, Gupta RC, Seth AK, Gupta A. Reversal of fluorosis in children. Acta Paediatr Jpn 1996; 38:513-9.

132. Denborough MA, Hopkinson KC, Banney DG. Firefighting and malignant hyperthermia. BMJ (Clin Res Ed) 1988; 296:1442-3.

Chapter 24
Cardiovascular Disorders

Lawrence J Fine, Linda Rosenstock

Despite the marked decline between 1985 and 1997 of about 30% in the age-adjusted death from coronary heart disease in white men and women, coronary artery disease (CAD) remains the leading cause of death in the United States.[1] Although identification and modification of cardiovascular risk factors is an ongoing area of intense investigation, the contribution of known major risk factors (advanced age, male gender, hypertension, low serum HDL-cholesterol and high serum LDL-cholesterol, smoking, physical inactivity, and type II diabetes mellitus) does not explain a significant fraction of the cases of coronary artery disease.[2] There is active research on a variety of other risk factors from socioeconomic status to genetic factors.[3] Research during the last 50 years has established that a limited number of chemical exposures directly cause or substantially contribute to coronary artery disease.

In the last two decades, there has been increased interest in the possibility that other aspects of work play a role in causing heart disease. The psychosocial or work organization characteristics of work are examples of non-chemical exposures that are the focus of research studies. In some of the research the significant relative risks are modest in magnitude, but because these psychosocial exposures are common, from a public health perspective, they may still be important. With common conditions like CAD, modest additional increases in risk may lead to a substantial number of potentially preventable cases. One of the complexities of investigating a common disease of multifactorial causation is that the suspected occupational risk factor can either directly or indirectly contribute by affecting one of the causal factors. Lead, for example, may cause systolic arterial hypertension even at low levels of exposure and, thus, indirectly contribute to CAD.

Several occupational exposures have been definitively linked to cardiovascular conditions, including CAD and dysrhythmias. A larger number of occupational exposures have been implicated in at least one investigation as causally related to a wide range of cardiovascular conditions such as hypertension, and it is possible that with further study additional occupational and environmental exposures may be similarly implicated. Cohort studies have found modest elevations in the rate of coronary artery disease in workers very highly exposed to 2,3,7,8-tetrachlorodibenzo-p-dioxin and very modest elevations for some groups of cardiovascular diseases in workers from mercury mining and refining facilities.[6,7] Several agents are definite cardiac toxins at high levels of exposure, such as carbon monoxide or fluorocarbons, but their effects at more typical levels of industrial use are less clear.

Suggestions about occupational risk for CAD also come from studies which either (1) examined a wide range of occupations in order to identify occupations associated with elevated rates of cardiovascular diseases, or (2) were primarily undertaken to study the relationship between cancer and occupation and observed significant increases in cardiovascular mortality. In European studies of the latter type the occupation with the most consistent elevated risk for CAD not explained by traditional risk factors is urban professional drivers such as truck drivers or bus drivers.[4] Occupational psychosocial stressors may explain this association.[5] Consideration of psychosocial stressors at work is increasingly being integrated with the large body of research on heart disease and the social determinants of health such as education, socioeconomic status, gender and ethnicity. Investigators in Denmark postulated that 16% of the premature cardiovascular mortality in men and 22% in women in Denmark might be related to occupational factors. The three most common suspected factors were monotonous high-paced work, shift work, and passive smoking.[8] A similar estimate was adopted by The European Heart Network in July 1998.[9]

CLINICAL EVALUATION
History

The medical history will usually direct the clinician to suspect correctly the presence of heart disease in the symptomatic patient. A careful history should include a search for symptoms suggesting myocardial ischemia, especially exertional chest pain (angina). Cardiac dysrhythmias are often asymptomatic but may be associated with palpitations and, if cardiac output is compromised, dyspnea, light-headedness, and syncope. Right, left, or biventricular dysfunction, regardless of cause, will often produce symptoms of fatigue and dyspnea. Non-coronary vascular disease secondary to atherosclerosis is suggested by symptoms consistent with end-organ ischemia, such as claudication or transient cerebral ischemia (TIA).

The occupational history should focus on eliciting possible exposures to known or suspected occupational cardiovascular toxins or risk factors. This aspect of the history should identify any changes in symptoms relative to variations in time at work or type of work. A foundry worker, for example, who is exposed to carbon monoxide and heat might complain of angina at the end of a workday at the time when his carboxyhemoglobin levels would be highest.

Any clues in the history that are reliable indicators about the level of exposure are important. In terms of chronic effects, a careful determination not only of the intensity but the duration of exposure is particularly important.

Examination

A routine, comprehensive cardiovascular examination should be performed, including a thorough evaluation of the peripheral vascular system with a description of the presence, strength, symmetry, and auscultatory findings of peripheral pulses. A search for end-organ effects should include a careful fundoscopic evaluation of retinal blood vessels. The physical examination should also include evaluation of other organ systems that may explain the patient's symptoms, such as the respiratory system, or that may in turn show evidence of the sequelae of cardiovascular dysfunction, such as hepatic enlargement in congestive cardiomyopathy. Rarely, findings in other organ systems may also implicate an occupational etiology; for example, the presence of polyneuropathy in a worker who has been heavily exposed to carbon disulfide and who has symptoms of coronary heart disease.

Laboratory evaluation

The laboratory evaluation, as is the case for cardiovascular disease of any cause, should be a directed one and based on symptoms and signs and suspected or known physiologic abnormalities. The resting electrocardiogram (ECG) may be helpful in evaluating ischemia, dysrhythmias, and hypertension. Continuous ambulatory rhythm monitoring may identify abnormalities not seen on the resting ECG and may allow for an assessment of the relationship among exposures, symptoms, and dysrhythmias. Chest radiography aids in the evaluation of heart chamber size and other anatomic abnormalities, such as valvular calcification or enlarged pulmonary arteries. Cardiac imaging techniques and catheterization play important roles in the assessment of cardiac function and the evaluation of coronary artery disease. In seeking evidence of current exposure, specific tests, such as carbon disulfide metabolites (2-thiothiazolidine-4-carboxylic acid), carboxyhemoglobin levels, or carbon monoxide in exhaled air, should be undertaken based on the exposure history and degree of suspicion about its relation to the identified abnormalities.

CLASSIFICATION

The following is a classification of occupational cardiovascular disorders. These disorders are discussed in detail throughout the rest of this chapter.
1. Coronary artery disease.
2. Dysrhythmias.
3. Hypertension.
4. Cardiomyopathy.
5. Peripheral vascular disease.
6. ECG abnormalities.
7. Cor pulmonale.

CORONARY ARTERY DISEASE

Cardiac ischemia, which results from an imbalance between the heart's demand for oxygen and the delivery of oxygen to the myocardium, most often is caused by CAD. Causes of cardiac ischemia may be either acute, which transiently result in increased demands for oxygen (such as during vigorous work in a hot humid climate), or chronic, which contribute directly or indirectly to the development of CAD. Among occupational exposures, only carbon disulfide (CS_2), carbon monoxide, methylene chloride, nitrate esters, and physical inactivity at work have been definitely linked to acute cardiac ischemia or CAD, with strong causal associations established for CS_2 and physical inactivity at work. There is substantial scientific evidence that non-occupational exposure to sidestream smoke from cigarettes is causally related to a moderate increase in the risk of dying from CAD among spouses of cigarette smokers, and there is some evidence that occupational exposures to sidestream smoke have been higher than home exposures.

Other occupational factors for which there is considerable evidence for a relationship are adult social class linked to occupation and possibly psychosocial stressors, such as monotonous high-paced work where the employees also have little control over the pace or methods of work. For a much larger group of exposures there is either less evidence, or they simply have been proposed as possible causes of cardiac ischemia, either by their acute effects or by contributing to the development of CAD. This group of occupational exposures includes arsenic, cobalt, inorganic mercury, high temperature, shift work, standing at work, and low-frequency noise. The occupational factors most strongly associated with cardiac ischemia are discussed separately.

CS_2

A solvent and chemical intermediate known to be neurotoxic for more than a century, CS_2 has been implicated as the cause of chronic cardiovascular disease since the 1940s. An increase in CAD mortality has often been observed in a number of CS_2-exposed populations from different countries; however, the findings of these studies are sometimes in conflict. Overall, the trend over time has been a declining risk for exposed workers because levels of exposure have declined from earlier levels. For example, a 10-year prospective Finnish study found a two- to five-fold greater relative risk of dying from CAD in workers exposed to CS_2 before 1970. This increased risk was noted by age 50 years in workers with 15 years of exposure.[10] A Japanese study found no evidence of increases in CAD, but a substantial increase in the frequency of retinal microaneurysms was observed.[11] This marked difference between the Japanese and Finnish studies led to an interesting collaborative research effort. Joint teams of Japanese and Finnish investigators studied workers from their respective countries. They confirmed that Japanese CS_2 workers have a high rate (25%) of retinal microaneurysms; their Finnish counterparts have a low rate (4%) of such hemorrhages. The reason for this disparate result may reflect the interaction between such factors as exposure, diet, and the difference in the prevalence of CAD or hypertension between the countries and other lifestyle variables.

Since the publication of the first mortality studies, several of the earlier cohorts have been updated, and other cohorts have been reported, including a large American cohort.[12,13] Together these studies confirmed the definite association between exposure to CS_2 in the production of rayon and excess mortality from CAD. The follow-up of the Finnish cohort documents the success of their intervention program, instituted after 1972, which included substantial reductions in the level of exposure to CS_2. This is an example of the effectiveness of primary and secondary prevention triggered by a research study and effective implementation of a control program.[14]

Several important questions remain inadequately answered. The precise shape of the relationship between exposure and effect and the mechanism of the action of CS_2 are unknown. There is a difference of opinion whether long-term exposure below the TLV-TWA (threshold limit value/time-weighted average) (31 mg/m^3) may cause increased mortality from CAD.[15-17] More precise elucidation of the exposure–response relationship for cardiovascular mortality will require studies with more detailed characterization of lifetime exposures at the lower (current levels) of exposure. Another important issue is whether CS_2 exposure contributes to atherosclerosis at locations other than the coronary arteries; the potential to do so is suggested by the elevated rate of retinal microaneurysms in the studies from Japan. The largest American mortality study, however, did not find an increase in the mortality rate from cerebrovascular disease, suggesting that, if there is a general atherosclerotic effect in US workers, it is not marked at the average duration and level of exposure studied.[8]

In addition to mortality from CAD, several studies have addressed the possible mechanisms, pathways, and cardiovascular morbidity from CS_2 including changes in blood lipids, heart rate, diastolic blood pressure, and carotid artery distensibility. While the results of the studies are not consistent, a few investigations identified absence of mortality effects below the TLV-TWA. Some findings indirectly support the validity of the older NIOSH recommendation, an exposure one-tenth of the TLV-TWA, of 1 mg/m^3.[18] One study found in a population with geometric mean exposures in the range of less than 2.2 to 13.0 mg/m^3 that CS_2 may have caused significant decrement in carotid artery wall distensibility and an increase in heart rate but no changes in level of blood pressure or blood lipids.[19] Another study in the United States found a significant and positive linear trend between low density lipoprotein cholesterol (LDL) and exposure after adjustment for confounders.[20] In this study the low exposed workers had median CS_2 exposures of 3.1 mg/m^3, moderate exposed had exposures of 13 mg/m^3, and high exposed had exposures of 24 mg/m^3.

A large Japanese study found no differences in blood lipids, blood pressure, or carotid artery wall stiffness, but did find the prevalence of microaneurysm of the retinal artery was significantly higher in workers exposed to CS_2.[21]

The median current exposure was 13 mg/m^3 for CS_2 and 1.5 mg/g Cr for 2-thiothiazolidine-4-carboxylic acid (TTCA) levels in the urine post-shift. Overall the research on CS_2 shows that exposures have been reduced over the last few decades, with a resulting reduction in the level of risk for mortality from work-related CAD in Europe and United States. Nevertheless at current levels of exposure, which in general seem to be below the TLV of 31 mg/m^3, there is some evidence of exposure-related abnormalities or dysfunction which may be harbingers of a possible remaining low level of risk for work-related cardiovascular disease in long-term exposed workers at current levels of exposure. There are also few animal studies of the adverse toxic effects of exposures above and below the TLV level.[22,23] These animal studies confirm that CS_2 interacts with a diet high in saturated fat to accelerate the arteriosclerotic process at levels of exposure similar to those found in epidemiological studies. Animal studies suggest that the interaction between non-work-related and work-related factors is substantial. Like lead, CS_2 appears to operate by several pathways or mechanisms by which damage or dysfunction occur.

Diagnosis and treatment

The diagnosis of CS_2-related CAD rests on the documentation of exposure by the work history and, when available, biologic monitoring of exposed workers through direct measurements of CS_2 in the blood or urine or by urine metabolites. The duration of exposure probably needs to be at least several years before adverse cardiovascular effects occur, and the adverse effects are dependent on the intensity of the exposure. Treatment does not differ from the usual treatment of CAD, although further exposure should be eliminated. TTCA measurements in the urine are an effective method of biomonitoring and have been used in the United States.[24,25] Whether elimination of further exposure halts progression is unclear. Prevention generally can best be accomplished by engineering means, with complete enclosure of any operation using CS_2 to minimize human exposure. The NIOSH recommends an exposure limit of 1 ppm or 3.1 mg/m^3; the exposure limit set by the Occupational Safety and Health Administration (OSHA) is 10 ppm or 31 mg/m^3. There are diverse views about whether the present exposure standard in the United States is sufficiently protective.[12,13]

Nitrate esters

Nitrate esters, of which nitroglycerin (NTG) is the most well known, have a long history of use both as pharmaceuticals and explosives. Exposures to NTG and ethylene glycol dinitrate (EGDN) in the explosives industry are the most extensively studied. In addition to their oxidant properties and potential to induce methemoglobinemia, nitrates have acute effects of variable onset and duration as arterial vasodilators. Among regularly exposed workers, these vasodilatory effects may result in headaches. Commonly, a tolerance develops so that the headaches occur only after re-exposure after several days away from work. Sufficiently high acute exposures can also cause systemic hypotension and confusion.

In older studies, the association between episodes of anginal pain, myocardial infarction, and cardiovascular death and acute occupational exposures to nitrate esters in the manufacture of explosives was convincing.[26,27] Nevertheless, these studies have provided conflicting evidence about whether, in addition to these acute effects, there are additional chronic sequelae. Hogstedt and colleagues studied two cohorts of Swedish workers exposed to NTG and EGDN.[28,29] Both cohorts had significantly increased death rates of about two-fold from CAD; the elevated rate continued even after exposure had ceased, suggesting a delayed chronic effect. Because these exposures were in the past, they most likely were higher than current exposures, although a precise determination of levels of exposure is difficult to obtain because EGDN and NTG can be absorbed through the skin.

However, an epidemiologic study in the United States involving exposure to NTG and dinitrotoluene found no evidence for a delayed chronic effect of NTG exposure on the risk for mortality from cardiovascular disease, but it did find a three-fold increased risk in younger men for acute cardiac deaths. However, after the start of a more comprehensive screening program for CAD in this workforce, no more excessive cardiac deaths were observed.[30] Most of these deaths occurred in men with current exposure. It is possible that a chronic effect on cardiovascular disease is restricted to exposures involving EGDN but not NTG. Earlier clinical reports had suggested that sudden death in exposed workers could occur in workers without pre-existing clinical CAD. The findings of the US cohort may not be consistent with this observation.

When, after 1970, exposed members of the cohort were screened every 6 months for hypertension, resting ECG abnormalities and treadmill ECG, the risk of death from CAD declined to normal. Although the association between exposure to NTG and EGDN or other nitrates in the explosives industry and death from adverse cardiac effects is convincing, prospective studies are needed of currently exposed workers who would likely have substantially lower exposures to determine whether excess cardiac deaths are still occurring, and whether there are chronic persistent effects from low-level exposures. Nevertheless, convincing case reports suggest some current exposures are hazardous.[31]

Pathogenesis

While the specific pathogenic mechanism of nitrate-induced cardiac ischemia is unknown, two types of acute cardiac effects have been described. The first is rebound vasospasm. This may occur up to several days following cessation of exposure. Coronary artery spasm induced in this fashion can result in myocardial ischemia and necrosis, dysrhythmias, and sudden death. The second acute effect of exposure to nitrates is the paradoxical occurrence of dysrhythmias after re-exposure to nitrates after a period away from work, typically on Monday or after vacations.

Diagnosis

The diagnosis of the nitrate-induced ischemic disease depends on the patient's history and, in particular, the timing of exposures in relation to symptoms. The cases in the scientific literature have been reported only from the explosives industry.

Prevention

Prevention of acute and postulated chronic effects of nitrates depends on the reduction of all exposures. Although some explosives producers have attempted to eliminate all at-risk workers from exposed areas by identifying all workers with evidence of CAD with medical screening, this may not identify all susceptible workers. It is not known whether workers with stable CAD are at elevated risk from exposure to nitrate esters. Neither is it clear how to mitigate routinely the effects of exposure–re-exposure transitions. It is possible that workers without CAD also may be at elevated risk. Non-lethal symptoms, like headache, should alert all to the potential for more serious sequelae.

Carbon monoxide

In contrast to CS_2 or nitrate esters, carbon monoxide exposure is more common. It exerts its primary adverse health effects through its avid binding to hemoglobin, with a resultant decrease in tissue oxygen delivery. Carbon monoxide also binds to the cytochrome oxidase system in the mitochondria of cardiac muscle and may, thereby, directly decrease myocardial contractility. The potential effects of single excessive exposures include myocardial ischemia or infarction, dysrhythmias, and sudden death. It is not until higher levels of carboxyhemoglobin are reached, usually above 25%, that manifestations of ischemia, dysrhythmias, and ECG abnormalities are likely to be observed in otherwise healthy workers. Most of these acute high exposures will occur from combustion sources, such as during firefighting.[32,33]

The consequences of repeated low-dose exposures are not completely understood. Two types of studies have been conducted, i.e., experimental studies in which patients with CAD are exposed to low levels of carbon monoxide and epidemiologic studies of cohorts of exposed workers. Workers exposed on a continuous basis to levels of carbon monoxide within current OSHA-allowable limits (50 ppm) may achieve carboxyhemoglobin levels of 5% or more, levels comparable to those achieved by moderate to heavy cigarette smokers. Levels of non-exposed non-smokers will generally be below 1%. The most common source of exposure is the exhaust from gasoline engines.[34] The current OSHA permissible exposure limit (PEL) for CO is 50 ppm as an 8-hour time-weighted average (TWA). The NIOSH recommended exposure limit (REL) for CO is 35 ppm as an 8-hour TWA and a ceiling limit (CL) of 200 ppm. The American Conference of Governmental Industrial Hygienists (ACGIH) has adopted a threshold limit value (TLV) for CO of 25 ppm as an 8-hour TWA.[30]

NIOSH recommended immediately dangerous to life and health concentration (IDLH) for CO is 1200 ppm. The IDLH is the concentration that could result in death or irreversible health effects, or prevent escape from the contaminated environment within 30 minutes.

The acute cardiac effects of carbon monoxide are likely to be principally dependent on the ability of coronary arteries to increase blood flow to the myocardium in response to the hypoxic stress of carbon monoxide. As a result, the effects of relatively low-level exposure to carbon monoxide may be substantially different in individuals with CAD than in those without CAD. Experiential studies in patients with CAD who are exposed to low levels of carbon monoxide during exercise have identified acute adverse effects at elevated carboxyhemoglobin levels of 2–6%; these adverse effects include limitations of exercise capacity as indicated by ST-segment depression, development of angina, or increase in the frequency of multiple ventricular premature depolarizations.[35-38]

Overall, mortality studies of workers exposed to carbon monoxide provide some evidence to support the hypothesis that the adverse effect of chronic carbon monoxide exposure is acute or subacute only and does not persist many years after exposure ceases. Cohort mortality studies of two groups of workers with intermittent exposure have been reported, i.e., iron foundry workers, and tunnel workers. The carbon monoxide exposures in iron foundries are highest in the furnace and pouring areas. Most mortality studies of foundry workers focus on non-malignant respiratory disease or cancer. Several, however, also examined cardiovascular mortality in the furnace and pouring operations, where the carbon monoxide levels are likely to be the highest. Four of these latter studies demonstrate increased risk for either CAD or total cardiovascular mortality for workers in the furnace, melting or pouring operations,[39-42] with one of the positive studies documenting carbon monoxide levels in the range of 85–110 mg/m^3 (75–96 ppm).[35]

In an earlier morbidity study of this cohort, there was suggestive evidence of an interaction between smoking and carbon monoxide exposure in causing angina.[43] In another of the positive foundry studies, the median levels were from 20 ppm to over 100 ppm.[36] One of the few additional studies with more detailed information on exposure is a study of New York tunnel workers who collect tolls and walk the tunnels. This study found a significant increase of 35% in the mortality rate from CAD in the tunnel workers.[44] The excess appeared to decline after 1970, when the carbon monoxide levels were reduced by improved ventilation. Prior to 1970, the levels averaged more than 50 ppm, with some peaks above 400 ppm. The study noted that the excess mortality was limited to the first few years after employment; as a result, the authors concluded that the risk declined after cessation of employment (i.e., a cessation of occupational exposures). In a more recent investigation of this cohort, the exposure levels for carbon monoxide were very low and therefore it is not surprising that there was also no carbon monoxide exposure disease relationship in active workers.[45]

If older study findings such as the Stern investigation of tunnel workers are correct, that the increased risk from carbon monoxide exposure is moderate, it is not surprising that the other mortality investigations of other occupations with intermittent exposures have not detected the increased risk. The Stern study was more likely to detect an effect because it used an internal comparison group (i.e., the bridge workers who were hired in a similar manner to the tunnel workers). This study also may have had less misclassification of exposure with a higher fraction of those who were considered exposed by the investigators actually being exposed. In summary, the Stern study and the two foundry studies provide evidence that exposures to carbon monoxide above 50 ppm are associated with an increased risk of death from CAD. The effect most likely involves acute or subacute mechanisms. However, the acute effects in experimental studies in patients with CAD at lower levels of exposure to carbon monoxide suggest caution in assuming that there are no effects at low levels for workers with CAD and ischemic-related arrhythmias or angina.

Pathogenesis

The two most likely mechanisms for the acute effects of carbon monoxide involve the indirect effect of reducing the oxygen-carrying capacity of hemoglobin by the formation of carboxyhemoglobin, as well as the direct effect on cellular metabolism.

Diagnosis and treatment

Recognition of carbon monoxide-induced cardiovascular toxicity relies on the exposure history and clinical setting. Acute exposures that produce carboxyhemoglobin levels above 25% may pose a cardiac hazard even for individuals with a normal cardiovascular system; lower levels pose primarily a cardiac hazard for individuals with significant CAD. This is presumably because workers with normal coronary arteries can increase the oxygenated blood supply to the heart to compensate for the reduced capacity related to the carboxyhemoglobin level. It is likely that exposure to low levels of carbon monoxide, such as 35 ppm, causes a reduced exercise tolerance and reduced threshold for angina. Many cigarette smokers have a carboxyhemoglobin level of 5%, which is the level that a non-smoker would reach if exposed to 35 ppm for 8 hours a day.

Acute cardiac events occurring under circumstances in which carbon monoxide exposure is suspected, such as smoke inhalation or work in an enclosed space with an operating fuel-burning engine or furnace, could be causally related: carboxyhemoglobin levels should be obtained, and oxygen therapy immediately begun. With very high level of exposure, treatment with hyperbaric oxygen may be indicated[46] (see Chapter 36).

Patients with new-onset angina or exacerbations of angina at work should be closely questioned regarding possible exposure. Checking a carboxyhemoglobin level after a typical work shift may be helpful. Treatment is the prevention or reduction of exposure.

Methylene chloride

A solvent in common use, methylene chloride (dichloromethane) has cardiotoxicity because of its metabolic conversion to carbon monoxide. The biologic half-life of carbon monoxide from this source is longer than that of the inhaled gas. Methylene chloride exposure should be considered in any individual with a clinical presentation consistent with carbon monoxide toxicity, such as anginal symptoms worsening at work, and should be recognized as additive to other occupational and environmental sources of exposure to carbon monoxide. Stewart and colleagues described an individual who had three myocardial infarctions, each following an exposure to methylene chloride in a confined space.[47]

Exposed workers in a triacetate fiber production process had average values of COHb ranging from 1.77% to 4% in the non-smoking group, and between 4.95% and 6.35% in a smoking group, with individually measured methylene chloride exposures averaging up to 99 ppm (8-hour TWA).[48] While there was no simple relationship between the workers who were smokers and their COHb levels, there was a linear relationship between exposure and COHb level in the non-smokers that were not influenced by exposures on the previous day.[49] NIOSH and OSHA have documented high exposures to methylene chloride in the furniture-stripping industry and other industries.[50,51] Several epidemiologic studies have not found an association between mortality from heart disease and methylene chloride in the chemical industry.[52-54] The clinical evaluation needs to focus on the intensity and duration of the exposure, as well as on the carboxyhemoglobin level of an acutely exposed employee.

Passive smoking

There is substantial epidemiologic evidence that exposure to environmental tobacco smoke (ETS) is an important public health factor in deaths from CAD.[55] Most studies have found that non-smokers living with smokers have about a 30% increased risk of death from CAD. While there is some difference of opinion about the strength of the epidemiological evidence for the risk of cardiovascular disease from occupational passive smoking exposure, a meta-analysis of eight studies yields a significant relative risk of 1.21.[56,57] While the median levels of workplace concentrations of nicotine in areas where smoking is allowed are lower than in homes where smoking occurs, the range of level of exposures is larger in workplaces (with some having very high levels of exposure).[58,59] According to the NHANES III study (1988–1991), a representative sample indicated that nearly 40% of US workers report being exposed to ETS in the workplace.

The 1999 data from NHANES suggest that for the entire US population there has been a 75% reduction in the average level of exposure to ETS based on serum cotinine levels. Some of this reduction may be the result of changes in workplace smoking policies. There are a variety of possible biologically plausible explanations for the effect of ETS,

ranging from effects on platelet aggregation to small increases in the level of blood carboxyhemoglobin.[60] In summary, environmental tobacco smoke is likely one of the most common workplace exposures to a potential occupational cardiac toxin. In 1999, Steenland estimated that approximately 1700 deaths from CAD per year may be related to occupational ETS exposure among non-smoking US workers 35–69 years of age.[52]

Arsenic

Arsenic exposure during the manufacture of pesticides and smelting of copper has been associated with an increased risk of developing lung cancer. In one of these mortality studies there was also an increase in the exposure-related risk of dying from cardiovascular disease, although additional follow-up of this Swedish cohort did not demonstrate an exposure-'heart' disease relationship, despite a strong relationship between arsenic and lung cancer.[61] Current levels of exposure are substantially lower than the levels to which these Swedish workers were exposed formerly. One of two recent re-analyses of United States copper smelters cohorts also found evidence of exposure-related excess mortality for cardiovascular but not cerebrovascular disease.[62,63] It seems possible that the high levels of exposure to arsenic during the smelting of copper in the past may have been associated with an increased rate of cardiovascular disease. This premise is supported by the observed acute toxic effect of arsenic compounds on the heart in patients treated with arsenic trioxide and cardiovascular diseases, and also seen in populations chronically exposed to drinking water with high levels of arsenic contamination.[64,65] It also has been proposed that arsenic at current exposure levels may increase the risk of cardiovascular disease by increasing blood glucose levels.[66]

Air particle pollution and cardiovascular disease

There is increasing evidence that links intermittent increases in the level of fine particulate air pollution to acute increases in the risk of mortality or morbidity from cardiovascular disease in the general population. One recent study concluded that elevated concentrations of fine particles may transiently elevate the risk of myocardial infarctions within a few hours to one day after exposure.[67] In a Swedish case referent investigation of myocardial infarction and occupational exposure to motor exhaust and other organic combustion products, a significant and dose-related risk for myocardial infarction was observed.[68] The relative risk was 2.1 among those who were highly exposed after adjustment for a variety of other risk factors such as tobacco smoking, obesity, and physical inactivity in leisure time. Since exposure to combustion products is common, this research study warrants follow-up, particularly since the levels of fine particle exposure are likely higher in some occupational groups than in the urban population.

Stress: physical, thermal and psychologic

Physical and thermal stresses have been implicated in aggravating myocardial ischemia, with or without concomitant clinical CAD. Among physical stress factors, although regular high levels of physical activity mostly likely reduce the risk of dying from CAD, unusually heavy exertional activities, particularly episodic ones, may increase the risk of acute ischemic events among those with underlying CAD.[69,70] The risk of sudden death in individuals free from clinical CAD, however, was very low at about one sudden death per 1.51 million episodes of exertion. Routine vigorous exercise reduced the risk further but did not eliminate it.[65] Epidemiologic studies support both the detrimental effect of the lack of physical activity at work (sedentary) and the protective effect of moderate to very high levels of physical activity at work or at leisure (such as brisk walking for 30 minutes each day of the week).[64,71,72] It is clear that benefits of physical activity clearly outweigh the small risks of transient increase in sudden death associated with vigorous physical activity.

Thermal stress

In the last decade there has been increased interest in the modest acute elevations in mortality rates for CAD in middle-aged and elderly populations associated with ambient temperatures below 18 degrees C.[73] The transient increased peak for CAD occurred 2 days after the temperature change and is postulated to be partially related to thrombosis, due to hemoconcentration in the cold, and from other consequences of cardiovascular reflexes that are acutely induced by cold.[69] These elevations interestingly are greater in regions with warm winters like Greece rather than in cold ones like Finland. In fact, in the coldest city in Siberia, Yakutsk, there was no winter increase in CAD mortality.[74]

The risk seems higher in populations who wear less protective clothing and are less active outdoors and with cooler homes. These population-based studies, which show a relationship between exposure to cold ambient temperatures and mortality from CAD, raise the issue of whether occupational exposures to cold temperatures less then –18 degrees C, particularly when sedentary or inadequately clothed, might increase the transient risk for middle-aged workers with some degree of clinically silent coronary atherosclerosis or clinically evident CAD. Two studies suggest that this may be a useful question to investigate for occupationally exposed workers. A study in Pennsylvania found significant transient increases in the death rate from CAD in men aged 35–49 for either low temperature less than 7 degrees C (RR 2.08) and further increases on cold days with snow fall of more than 3 cm (RR 3.54).[75] The latter observation could be a combined effect of the cold weather and unusual exertion.

In the CORDIS study, significant increases in the rate of asymptomatic ST-segment depressions during ambulatory electrocardiac monitoring were found among women workers working at ambient temperatures lower than 20 degrees C after adjusting for traditional CAD risk factors.[76] Cold temperatures may also aggravate angina, presumably by inducing an increase in peripheral vascular resistance at the same time that myocardial oxygen demand is increased. The cold effect is likely a transient risk factor for CAD mortality. The magnitude of effect in the European studies is very modest and only detectable with very large samples; however, the magnitude noted in the Pennsylvania study is larger.[71]

Rarely, acute myocardial infarction may occur after severe heat stroke in young individuals.[77] In periods of extreme hot weather, the mortality from cardiovascular disease increases; however, compared to cold weather the increases are more clearly linked to those with definite pre-existing risk factors such as old age, pre-existing heart disease, living alone, and being confined to bed.[78] Two of the three epidemiological studies of heat-exposed workers provide evidence that the longer the duration of exposure to hot working environments, the lower the CAD mortality, presumably because of worker selection or the benefits of physical conditioning.[79,80] One of the studies did observe an increase in the risk for CAD mortality with increasing duration of employment in a hot mining environment.[81] One new physical factor has been proposed: in one investigation, standing at work was related to the progression of carotid atherosclerosis, particularly in men with CAD or carotid stenosis.[82] In summary, with regard to the thermal association with CAD mortality, because the impact of colder temperatures on CAD mortality occurs over a broader range of temperatures, it may be a more important issue than occupational exposures to hot environments.

Psychosocial stress

The interplay between socioeconomic factors and work environment in the pathogenesis of CAD has been actively explored by a number of investigators. This body of research divides into two principal areas. The first investigates the role of factors such as income, education, and other socioeconomic determinants in the traditional risk factors for CAD and the mortality from CAD. The second examines the psychosocial occupational environment and the development of CAD. The association between CAD or heart disease mortality and socioeconomic measurements has been investigated. Since two-thirds of all heart disease deaths result from CAD, the socioeconomic pattern for total heart disease mortality is likely similar to CAD mortality.[83] In 1997 in the United States for working age men (25–64), persons with incomes under $10,000 had death rates from heart disease 2.5 times higher than persons with incomes over $25,000.[79]

Gradients of similar magnitude were observed for most of the other gender, race and ethnic groups in the United States. In the United Kingdom, Ireland, and Nordic countries manual workers compared to non-manual workers have higher mortality from CAD, while in France, Switzerland, and Southern Europe the manual workers had similar or lower rates than the non-manual workers.[84] In the United States compared to Northern Europe, differences were smaller for US manual workers aged 30–44 years old, but as large for older American manual workers (aged 45–64).[80] In both England and United States, while the prevalence of CAD risk factors is higher in lower socioeconomic (SES) groups, the SES gradient for risk factors may not be increasing or fully explain the SES gradient in CAD mortality.[85,86] In addition to the importance of these SES studies because of their public health significance, from a research perspective they suggest that SES factors must be addressed carefully in studies of the psychosocial characteristics of work and CAD.

There are two common hypotheses that have been proposed for psychosocial characteristics of work that may contribute substantially to an increased risk for CAD. The first, proposed by Robert Karasek in 1979 and later modified by Johnson and Hall, is that the incidence of CAD will be elevated in occupations characterized by low levels of social support (workplace isolation), by jobs with low control or decision latitude (little influence over work methods and opportunities to use skills or learn new skills), and by jobs with high levels of psychological demands (such as deadlines or high work pace).[87,88] This model is called the job strain or demand–control–support model (DCS) (see Chapter 38).[89] In many of these studies, the job characteristics are defined based on questionnaire responses from employees (Table 24.1). In this model, the highest risk jobs will be those with low social support, low control, and high demands (job strain).

The second model, proposed by Johannes Siegrist, has three key components. It is called the effort–reward–imbalance (ERI) model. The first component is the rewards of a job. Rewards are measured by level of financial rewards, esteem (similar to prestige and social support), and job security and promotion opportunities.[90] The second component is job efforts that are related to the level of physical and mental workload. The third component is the

individual's response (personal pattern of coping) to the balance between the effort and reward of his or her jobs. The psychological stress of a job that is related to the imbalance between high demands and low rewards is increased if an individual uses a coping strategy called 'overcommitment'. This strategy involves attitudes, behaviors, and emotions involving excessive effort and a strong need for approval and support from the work situation.[86] The most adverse or stressful situations thus involve jobs with high demands and low rewards for workers who exhibit the coping strategy of overcommitment. Siegrist believes this model may be particularly useful during difficult economic periods, when some workers may have few alternatives to jobs with low rewards, job security and other job benefits, including downward mobility. Each of these models focuses on identifying common work-related conditions (exposures) that may elicit chronically stressful reactions in workers.

Although the DCS model is sometimes measured subjectively based on workers' questionnaires, theoretically its focus is the objective conditions of work and does not address directly the issue of job security or pay. The ERI model differs in that it addresses the subjective reactions and coping strategy of the worker to the psychosocial working conditions, the level of job insecurity, and salary.

More epidemiological studies have been performed to evaluate the DCS than the ERI model. There are several European studies that have found that either jobs with high demands and low control or jobs with low control regardless of the level of demands are associated with higher rates of CAD morbidity.[91] The earliest European studies had the highest relative risks, and generally provide stronger support for low job control in association with CAD rather than the job strain hypothesis (low control/high demands).[87] However, findings of only one of the five studies conducted in the United States are clearly supportive of the hypothesis.[87,92] Most of the earlier European and United States studies involved only male working populations. Three of the largest and most recent European studies of men, which also adjusted for traditional CAD risk factors and socioeconomic status, reported significant relative risks for low job control or job strain in range of 1.3–2.5, depending on the health endpoint and subsample of the population examined.[93–95]

Two of these European studies also examined the job control or job strain aspect of the DCS model in women workers. They found significant relative risk for job control or job strain in the range of 1.5–1.7, with adjustment for some of the traditional CAD risk factors.[90–96] While over 20 investigations have examined the DCS model and some measure of CAD, many fewer studies have examined the ERI model.[83,87] The three prospective studies of this model also adjusted for traditional risk factors, and found significant relative risks between 2 and 4.5.[83,97] One of these studies compared the relative risks between the alternative job stress models in both women and men. This report also adjusted the relative risks by employment grade, a measure of socioeconomic status, and by traditional CAD risk factors. The significant resulting relative risks for new CAD when both

Job demands scale (0 = yes, 1= no)
  Is your job hectic?
  Is your job psychologically demanding?
Work control scale (0 = never, 1= sometimes, 2 = often)
  Influence over the planning of work?
  Influence over the setting of the workplace?
  Influence over how time is used in work?
  Planning of breaks?
  Planning of vacations?
  Flexible work hours?
  Freedom to receive a phone call during work hours?
  Freedom to receive a private visitor at work?
  Varied task content?
  Varied work procedures?
  Possibilities for ongoing education as a part of the job?
Work social support scale (0 = no, 1= yes)
  Could talk to coworkers during breaks?
  Could leave their job to talk with coworkers?
  Could interact with coworkers as part of their work?
  Met with coworkers outside of the workplace?
  Had met with a coworker during last 6 months?

Table 24.1 Questions used to measure job strain and work support

job stress measures were simultaneously included in the analysis were 2.15 for ERI model and 2.38 for low job control (self measured) and 1.56 for low job control (externally assessed by supervisors).[83] The authors suggested that future studies need to further understand the overlapping and unique features of each model. The implication of this study is that a model that focuses both on workers' reactions and the 'objective assessment' of the psychosocial characteristics of jobs, and considers additional factors such as job insecurity, may be a superior model.

Other researchers have also described the important relationship between 'occupational exposure' and subsequent onset of disease. Non-occupational factors affecting this relationship include earlier events in childhood or adult life (life course perspective), the interaction between genetic and environmental factors, the interaction between non-occupational and occupational exposures like social support at work or outside work, personal health habits and ties, and a wide variety of community and societal factors.[98,99] Because of the complex nature of the interaction with these factors and earlier mentioned socioeconomic and cultural factors, generalizations across groups that vary substantially in socioeconomic or cultural attributes may not hold for either the DCS or ERI model. While some occupational factors may be associated with the development of CAD, others likely will be associated with the promotion of health and possibly reduction of the risk for CAD. While childhood socioeconomic determinants may be related to the subsequent risk of developing CAD, adult exposures including occupational factors appear more important with CAD.[100,101]

In summary, several reviewers and investigators have concluded that the European studies provide support for the hypothesis that psychosocial aspects of work are related to the risk of developing CAD.[83,84,88,93] Although this is a potentially important hypothesis from a public health perspective, for this hypothesis to gain more support, particularly in the United States, several additional factors or questions will need to be addressed. Studies in the United States similar to the European studies would add more weight and acceptance of the evidence if they confirmed the findings of the European studies. A basic question is whether there is selection of individuals at high risk into high-strain jobs or selection of individuals at low risk into other jobs. This selection might be the result of a variety of factors, such as educational level. Individuals in these high-risk jobs, for example, might have different access to medical care, or different levels of non-work social support. Because socioeconomic status is associated with cigarette smoking, in some studies the investigators have examined these traditional CAD risk factors as potential confounders, and in general, have concluded that they are not the principal explanation for the differences in CAD mortality or morbidity between high- and low-strain occupations.[83,91,92]

Another major issue is that the exposure variable in these studies is usually the current job, not an individual's entire occupational experience. Another possible limitation of many of these studies is that the exposure classification is based on questionnaire data rather than direct observation of the workplace by the investigators. Finally, the application of these concepts to clinical decision making remains difficult because of the complex interaction between the individual, culture, and work.

Pathogenesis

The mechanism for the potential adverse cardiac effects of psychologic stress is an area of active investigation. Several mechanisms have been proposed.[102] First, specific working conditions, such as time pressure, could cause activation of the hypothalamic-pituitary-adrenal (HPA) axis leading to elevation of hormones such as catecholamines. Second, increased activity in the sympathetic nervous system together with alterations in the regulation of the HPA axis could result either in elevated blood pressure or more frequent dysrhythmias. Third, the work stresses could lead to adverse lifestyle behaviors, such as increased cigarette smoking or obesity. Fourth, work stress may change the rate of progression of precursors of CAD. For example, psychosocial stress in monkeys causes exacerbation of diet-related atherosclerosis, with activation of the sympathetic nervous system; stress also induces endothelial injury mediated by beta-1-adrenoceptor activation, even without an atherogenic diet.[103] The interaction between the acute and chronic effects of psychosocial stress, and the endocrine, endothelial, and nervous systems, is likely to be complex. Nevertheless, these animal studies suggest biologically plausible mechanisms by which chronic exposure to adverse psychosocial factors could be related to CAD.[104]

The diagnosis of stress-related ischemia should be limited to circumstances in which the stressors are clearly identifiable and for which there is strong scientific evidence. Acute events, especially myocardial infarction and sudden death, occurring in the setting of unaccustomed and severe thermal stress associated with heat stroke can be work related. In individuals without clinical CAD, one study estimated the occurrence of one sudden death per 1.51 million episodes of substantial physical exertion, and that routine vigorous exercise reduced the risk further but did not eliminate it.[65] Anginal patterns temporally related to certain work activities also suggest stress as a precipitant, but chemical factors like carbon monoxide must first be excluded.

Management and prevention

Patients with severe or unstable CAD should avoid episodic, severe unaccustomed work stresses. Cardiac rehabilitation programs and enhancing fitness may be valuable for such workers.

Shift work

Shift work is work occurring outside the normal daytime shift, particularly work between midnight and 6am. The evidence for a possible link between shift work and CAD was recently reviewed; however, findings were inconsistent.[105] One of the most recent prospective studies did not find evidence of a relationship between shift work and mortality from CAD after adjustment for socioeconomic status.[106] Despite the large number of workers who regularly perform shift work, a clearer picture of whether shift work is related indirectly or directly to the risk of CAD will require further investigation.

DYSRHYTHMIAS

Abnormal cardiac rhythms secondary to ischemia may result from the agents discussed previously. In addition, a number of chemicals have been associated with atrial and ventricular dysrhythmias by mechanisms largely unrelated to ischemia. Such events may occur even in individuals with anatomically normal coronary vessels; however, they are rarely fatal. The levels of exposure that preceded these deaths were not well documented but likely were high. The agents of concern are organic solvents, with both halogenated (particularly fluorocarbons) and non-halogenated chemicals. Evidence for the association between these chemicals and dysrhythmias comes from compelling case reports, clinical studies, and experimental animal investigations.[107–110] Many of the case reports have been of intentional overexposures, such as glue sniffing (toluene), but a few have also come from occupational settings, including chlorofluorocarbon.[111,112] With very high levels of exposure, the animal studies and case reports of human inhalant abuse suggest that a wide range of solvents are cardiac toxins.[113] In addition to the association of acute exposure to high levels of non-halogenated and halogenated solvents and acute dysrhythmias, there is more limited and inconsistent evidence for a chronic effect or an effect at lower levels of exposure.[113–115]

Several epidemiologic studies have been conducted of solvent-exposed workers, principally in rubber, chemical, and dry-cleaning industries. Each of these studies has limitations for evaluating the association between acute intense solvent exposure and CAD mortality. Most of these studies had limited information on the fluctuating level of acute exposures and were designed as cancer mortality studies, not as studies of heart disease. A review of the literature showed no consistent association between solvents with the exception of CS_2 and CAD.[105] One study of trichloroethylene found a modest significant increase in mortality for CAD (SMR of 108) but this association was not dose related and has not been consistently found in other studies.[116,117] In summary, there is considerable evidence that after high levels of exposure, some non-halogenated and halogenated industrial solvents cause serious dysrhythmias in some individuals. The results of the older studies of moderate levels of exposure to fluorocarbons are in conflict with those of newer studies, which include better measurements of exposure and the finding of no effect. In contrast to the acute effects of high-level exposure, most of the epidemiologic studies on cohorts of workers exposed to industrial solvents have not found evidence of an increased risk of death from heart disease.

Pathogenesis

The pathogenesis of solvent-related dysrhythmias is likely to involve the sensitization of the myocardium to endogenously secreted catecholamines. Direct effects of some of these substances on myocardial contractility may also play a role. In addition, it is possible that with high exposure hypoxia also plays a role because these agents, in general, are also respiratory depressants in animals. The greatest risk for dysrhythmias occurs in situations of overexposures. Other factors that may increase the risk for occurrence of these events include those associated with increased catecholamine production, including physical, psychologic, and thermal stress, or the use of sympatho-mimetic medication. It is plausible that, if these co-factors are present, the level of exposure that would trigger a dysrhythmia may be lower.

Diagnosis

An evaluation should be undertaken for any patient presenting with cardiac dysrhythmias without a known cardiac cause and a history of high levels of exposure to suspected toxic agents. The role of solvents should also be considered in patients with known or suspected rhythm disturbances who experience palpitations or syncope temporally related to exposure. Ambulatory rhythm monitoring may be used to document the presence of dysrhythmias and assess their relation to time at work. If dysrhythmias are present, re-assessment several days after cessation of exposure can provide additional evidence implicating the role of solvents. The role of other possible workplace factors that may be contributing to dysrhythmias should also be assessed.

Management

When workplace exposures are considered to be contributing to observed dysrhythmias, all efforts to reduce exposures should be made. Removal from all further exposure should be recommended when exposure reduction measures fail or the dysrhythmias cause substantial symptoms or hemodynamic effects.

Prevention

Patients with known serious ventricular rhythm disorders should be cautioned about substantial solvent exposure, either occupational or non-occupational (e.g., hobbies). Advising patients who have myocardial disease and are at risk for such disturbances must be done on a case-by-case basis.

HYPERTENSION

A number of occupational factors may play a role in the development of hypertension. These include workplace psychosocial stress, physical factors, such as noise, and chemical exposures, including lead and CS_2. The most extensively studied exposure is lead. Although blood pressure effects may occur at low levels of exposure, the specific effect of lead on blood pressure is still not clearly defined.[118] It is not clear if the lead-related effect is only on systolic or diastolic pressure or both, or whether it is an acute or chronic effect. The distinction between acute or chronic effect is complicated because up to 95% of total body lead burden accumulates in the skeleton with a constant influence on the levels of serum and plasma blood lead. The plasma lead, which constitutes less than 1% of whole blood lead level, may be the biologically relevant lead for effects on the vascular system.[114] Overall the evidence suggests a modest increase in either systolic or diastolic blood pressure.

The increase in blood pressure probably occurs at lower levels of environmental or occupational exposure, and the rate of increase may be non-linear with the principal effect occurring at low exposure levels.[119,120] The increases in blood pressure have been associated with blood lead levels between 7 and 35 μg/dL and bone lead levels of 10 to 50 μg/g.[121] These levels are common in occupationally exposed workers. The potential public health importance of the blood pressure and lead relationship is illustrated by the results of one prospective study of hypertension, a community study of the elderly which found a significant rate ratio of 1.7 for new hypertension cases in highly exposed versus low exposed subjects based on bone lead levels.[114] The high exposed group had a mean patellar lead level of 53 μg/g and no subject had a blood lead above 35 μg/dL. Based on animal studies, two mechanisms have been proposed.[114] One involves action on arterial smooth muscle, and the other on the renin-angiotensin axis. In contrast to lead, there is little evidence that current exposures to CS_2 are a significant factor in hypertension. At exposures below the TLV value for CS_2 there does not appear to be an acute or subacute effect on blood pressure, although there still may be an effect on carotid artery distensibility.[9,15]

The relation between chronic exposure to noise and hypertension remains an active area of research. In the last 10 years, studies have yielded inconsistent results for a relation between exposures above 90 dB and increased risk of hypertension or an elevation in either the systolic or diastolic blood pressure, generally after many years of exposure.[122–127] An interesting recent study of chronic noise exposure reported transient increases in systolic and diastolic pressures and heart rate in exposed workers less than age 50. This increase in blood pressure persisted for several hours after exposure; it is postulated that these changes over time might lead to more permanent changes in blood pressure.[128] Studies of chronic noise exposure and the risk for increased blood pressure are difficult because they require careful prospective assessment of blood pressure and cumulative assessment of noise exposures in a large number of subjects.

The same models of psychosocial stress and job strain that have been used in studies of CAD also have been applied to blood pressure and psychosocial working conditions. Interestingly, ambulatory blood pressure measurements generally are higher on work days compared to non-work days.[129] In a review of the studies examining the relationship between blood pressure and job strain model, the reviewers concluded that studies using measures of ambulatory blood pressure were more useful than studies of routine blood pressure measured in clinical settings.[87] These reviewers also concluded that there is substantial

evidence to support the association between psychosocial stress or job strain and significant elevation of blood pressure; however, since the strongest US studies have largely been done by one group, confirmatory studies by other investigators would reinforce their hypothesis.

One of the most interesting studies found a three-fold increased risk for job strain and hypertension during routine screening. In this case-control study, it was possible to consider several potential confounders, including 'type A' behavior, 24-hour sodium excretion, physical activity level of the job, educational level, and smoking. None of these variables explained the relationship between job strain and hypertension. Age, body mass index, and regular drinking of alcoholic beverages were additional risk factors assessed in this study. The possible relation between job strain and hypertension was supported by two additional findings from this group of researchers. One study found both ambulatory monitoring of diastolic pressure and left ventricular mass measured by echocardiography were related adversely to job strain.[130] A later longitudinal study found that interval changes in blood pressure were significantly related to job strain.[131] The possible mechanisms for the elevation of blood pressure by job strain include stimulation of the sympathetic nervous system, as well as the hypothalamic-pituitary-adrenal and renin-angiotensin systems.[122]

The ERI model has also begun to be applied to studies of blood pressure and psychosocial characteristics with some positive cross-sectional associations.[92] A recent study of the coping strategy used by workers who perceived that they had been treated unfairly found a complex relation between coping strategies, psychosocial working conditions, gender, age and hypertension.[132] Although the diagnostic importance of these factors in an individual patient with hypertension is unclear, if additional studies confirm these findings, then preventive action may be warranted. Current research also seems to be increasingly focused on the interaction among personality, psychologic coping strategy, psychosocial work stressors, gender, and blood pressure. The nature of these inter-relationships is not clear and may be quite complex. As a result, translating the results into effective prevention strategies will be challenging.[132,133]

CARDIOMYOPATHY

Only one environmental exposure (cobalt) has been linked directly to the development of cardiomyopathy. The association with cobalt, observed in heavy consumers of beer (for a period in the late 1960s, cobalt was added to beer to stabilize foam formation), may be confounded by other factors, such as alcohol and diet. However, only subclinical cardiac muscle dysfunction has been reported after cobalt exposure in industrial settings, and these changes could be related to hard metal lung disease.[134] A recent epidemiological study of men exposed to hard metal which consists of tungsten carbide and cobalt powders found no excess mortality from heart disease.[135] Antimony has also been anecdotally linked with the development of cardiomyopathy and ECG abnormalities. One of two epidemiologic studies of exposed workers provides equivocal evidence of risk of increased mortality from heart disease.[136,137] Similarly, there are several case reports of cardiomyopathy following intense exposure to solvents. Other occupational factors to be considered are those associated with the development of CAD, such as CS_2, which in turn can result in ischemic cardiomyopathy.

PERIPHERAL VASCULAR DISEASE

There is very limited evidence that occupational factors may be related to peripheral vascular disease. In countries where there are high levels of arsenic in the drinking water, there have been reports of an association between 'black foot disease' and environmental arsenic exposure but no reports of an elevated prevalence of peripheral vascular in occupationally exposed workers.[138] There is one study of peripheral vascular disease in young workers exposed to CS_2, which found evidence of damage to retinal vessels but little evidence for damage to peripheral vessels at current levels of exposure.[139]

ECG ABNORMALITIES

Abnormalities found on the resting ECG are neither sensitive nor specific for diagnosing many cardiovascular diseases. In most cases in which occupational exposures have been associated with ECG abnormalities, these findings simply reflect the underlying disease problem, such as that between CS_2 and CAD or that between some high-level solvent exposures and premature ventricular contractions.[140] Arsine, for example, in addition to its hemolytic effect, may have a detrimental effect on the myocardium after a high level of exposure. Temporary ECG abnormalities were noted in all survivors of an arsine poisoning episode in 1949. These changes resolved within 10 months, and they were characterized by large T waves in the V_2 through V_5 leads.[141] Overexposure to arsine, and perhaps arsenic, may cause the prolongation of the Q-T interval.[142] In each case, removal from exposure is indicated; the role of chelation is less clear.

COR PULMONALE AND OCCUPATIONS AND OTHER CARDIOVASCULAR DISEASES

The effects of respiratory insufficiency on pulmonary arterial pressures and subsequent right-sided ventricular failure are well recognized. As discussed in Chapter 19, a wide range of occupational exposures may cause severe respiratory dysfunction, which may be associated with this secondary effect on the heart.

References

1. McGovern PG, Jacobs DR, Shahar E, et al. Trends in acute coronary heart disease mortality, morbidity, and medical care from 1985 through 1997; the Minnesota Heart Survey. Circulation 2001; 104:19.
2. Fuster V, Gotto AMJ. Risk reduction. Circulation 2000; 102:IV-94.
3. Marmot M, Shipley M, Brunner E, Hemingway H. Relative contribution of early life and adult socioeconomic factors to adult morbidity in the Whitehall II study. J Epidemiol Commun Health 2001; 55:301–307.
4. Netterstrom B, Knud J. Impact of work-related and psychosocial factors on the development of ischemic heart disease among urban bus drivers in Denmark. Scand J Work Environ Health 1990; 14:231.
5. Tuchsen F. High risk occupations for cardiovascular disease. In: Schnall P, Belkic K, Landsbergis P, Baker D, eds. The workplace and cardiovascular disease. Occup Med 2000; 15:57–60.
6. Steenland K, Piacitelli L, Deddens J, Fingerhut M, Chang LI. Cancer, heart disease, and diabetes in workers exposed to 2,3,7,8-tetrachlorodibenzo-p-dioxin. J Natl Cancer Inst 1999; 91:779–86.
7. Boffetta P, Sallsten G, Garcia-Gomez M, et al. Mortality from cardiovascular diseases and exposure to inorganic mercury. Occup Environ Med 2001; 58:461–6.
8. Olsen O, Kristensen TS. Impact of work environment on cardiovascular disease in Denmark. J Epidemiol Commun Health 1991; 45:4–9.
9. Social Factors, Work, Stress and Cardiovascular Disease Prevention in the European Union – The European Heart Network – July 1998. Report prepared by the European Heart Network's Expert Group on Psychosocial and Occupation Factors. http://www.ehnheart.org/.
10. Tolonen M, Nurminen M, Hernberg S. Ten-year coronary mortality of workers exposed to carbon disulfide. Scand J Work Environ Health 1979; 5:109.
11. Sugimoto K, Goto S, Taniguchi H. Ocular fundus photography of workers exposed to carbon disulfide: a comparative epidemiological study between Japan and Finland. Int Arch Occup Environ Health 1977; 39:97.
12. MacMahon B, Monson R. Mortality in the US rayon industry. J Occup Med 1988; 30:698.
13. Kotseva K. Occupational exposure to low concentration of carbon disulfide as a risk factor for hypercholesterolaemia. Int Arch Occup Environ Health 2001; 74:38.
14. Nurminen M, Hernberg S. Effects of intervention on the cardiovascular mortality of workers exposed to carbon disulfide: a 15 year follow up. Br J Ind Med 1985; 42:32.
15. American Conference of Governmental Industrial Hygienists. Threshold limit values for chemical substances and physical agents. Cincinnati OH: ACGIH, 1998.
16. Swaen GM, Braun C, Slangen JJ. Mortality of Dutch workers exposed to carbon disulfide. Int Arch Occup Environ Health 1994; 66:103–10.
17. Price B, Bergman TS, Rodriguez M, Henrich RT, Moran EJ. A review of carbon disulfide exposure data and the association between carbon disulfide exposure and ischemic heart disease mortality. Reg Tox Phar 1997; 26:119–28.
18. NIOSH. Occupational exposure to carbon disulfide: criteria for a recommended standard. Washington DC: US Government Printing Office, 1977.
19. Kotseva K, Braeckman L, Duprex D, et al. Decreased carotid artery distensibility as a sign of early atherosclerosis in viscose rayon workers. Occup Med 2000; 51:223–9.
20. Egeland GM, Burkhart GA, Schnorr TM, Hornung RW, Fajen JM, Lee ST. Effects of exposure to carbon disulphide on low density lipoprotein cholesterol concentration and diastolic blood pressure. Br J Ind Med 1992; 49:287–93.
21. Omae K, Tabebayashi T, Nomiyama T, et al. Cross sectional observation of the effects of carbon disulphide on arteriosclerosis in rayon manufacturing workers. Occup Environ Med 1998; 55:468–72.
22. Antov G, Kazakova B, Spasovski M, et al. Effects of carbon disulphide on the cardiovascular system. J Hyg Epidemiol Microbiol Immunol 1985; 29:329–35.

23. Wronska-Nofer T, Laurman W, Nofer JR, et al. Carbon disulfide-induced modification and cytotoxicity of low-density lipoproteins. Toxicol Vitr 1996; 10:423–9.

24. Kivistö H. TTCA measurements in biomonitoring of low-level exposure to carbon disulphide. Int Arch Occup Environ Health 2000; 73:263.

25. Cox C, Que Hee SS, Tolos WP. Biologic monitoring of workers exposed to carbon disulfide. Am J Ind Med 1998; 33:48.

26. Lange RL, Reid MS, Tresch DD, et al. Non-atheromatous ischemic heart disease following withdrawal from chronic industrial nitroglycerin exposure. Circulation 1972; 46:666.

27. Morton WE. Occupational habituation to aliphatic nitrates and the withdrawal hazards of coronary disease and hypertension. J Occup Med 1977; 19:197–200.

28. Hogstedt C, Axelson O. Nitroglycerin-nitroglycol exposure and the mortality in cardiocerebrovascular diseases among dynamite workers. J Occup Med 1977; 19:675.

29. Hogstedt C, Andersson K. A cohort study of mortality among dynamite workers. J Occup Med 1979; 21:553.

30. Stayner L, Dannenberg A, Thun M, et al. Cardiovascular mortality among munitions workers exposed to nitroglycerin and dinitrotoluene. Scand J Work Environ Health 1992; 18:34–43.

31. RuDusky BM. Acute myocardial infarction secondary to coronary vasopasm during withdrawal from industrial nitroglycerin exposure. A case report. Angiology 2001; 52:143.

32. Barnard RJ, Weber JJ. Carbon monoxide: a hazard to fire fighters. Arch Environ Health 1979; 34:255.

33. NIOSH. Warehouse fire claims the life of a battalion Chief – Missouri. Report 99F-48. Cincinnati OH: NIOSH.

34. NIOSH, CDPHE, CPSC, OSHA, EPA. Preventing carbon monoxide poisoning from small gasoline-powered engines and tools. DHHS (NIOSH) Publication No. 96-118. Cincinnati OH: NIOSH, 1996.

35. Sheps DS, Herbst MSN, Hinderliter MD, et al. Production of arrhythmias by elevated carboxyhemoglobin in patients with coronary artery disease. Ann Intern Med 1990; 113:343.

36. Allred EN, Bleecker ER, Chaitman BR, et al. Effects of carbon monoxide on myocardial ischemia. Environ Health Perspect 1991; 91:89–132.

37. Leaf DA, Kleinman MT. Urban ectopy in the mountains: carbon monoxide exposure at altitude. Arch Environ Health 1996; 51:283–290.

38. Kleinman MT, Leaf DA, Kelly E, Caiozzo V, Osann K, O'Neill T. Urban angina in the mountains: effects of carbon monoxide an hypoxemia on subjects with chronic stable angina. Arch Environ Health 1998; 53:388–97.

39. Koskela RS, Mutanen P, Sorsa JUA, Klockars M. Factors predictive of ischemic heart disease mortality in foundry workers exposed to carbon monoxide. Am J Epidemiol 2000; 152:628–32.

40. Silverstein M, Maizlish N, Park R, Silverstein B, Brodsky L, Mirer F. Mortality among ferrous foundry workers. Am J Ind Med 1986; 10:27–43.

41. Andjelkovich DA, Mathew RM, Yu RC, Richardson RB, Levine RJ. Mortality of iron foundry workers II. Analysis by work area. J Occup Med 1992; 34:391–401.

42. Park RM. Mortality at an automobile engine foundry and machining complex. J Occup Environ Med 2001; 43:483–93.

43. Hernberg R, Karava R, Koskela RS, et al. Angina pectoris, ECG findings and blood pressure of foundry workers in relation to carbon monoxide exposure. Scand J Work Environ Health 1976; 2(Suppl 1):54.

44. Stern FB, Halperin WE, Hornung RW, et al. Heart disease mortality among bridge and tunnel officers exposed to carbon monoxide. Am J Epidemiol 1988; 128:1276.

45. Herbert R, Schechter C, Smith DA, et al. Occupational coronary heart disease among bridge and tunnel officers. Arch Environ Health 2000; 55:152–63.

46. Juurlink DN, Stanbrook MB, McGuigan MA. Hyperbaric oxygen for carbon monoxide poisoning (Cochrane Review). In: The Cochrane Library Issue 3. Oxford: Update Software, 2001.

47. Stewart RD, Fisher TN, Hosko MJ, et al. Experimental human exposure to methylene chloride. Arch Environ Health 1972; 25:342.

48. Soden KJ, Marras G, Amsel J. Carboxyhemoglobin levels in methylene chloride-exposed employees. J Occup Environ Med 1996; 38:367–71.

49. Amsel J, Soden KJ, Sielken RL, Valdez-Flora C. Observed versus predicted carboxyhemoglobin levels in cellulose triacetate workers exposed to methylene chloride. Am J Ind Med 2001; 40:180–91.

50. OSHA. Regional news release, US Department of Labor Office of Public Affairs. OSHA cites Alabama firm for over-exposing employees to methylene chloride. Region 4 News Release: USDOL: 01-16. Feb 12, 2001.

51. Estill CF, Kovein RJ, Jones JH, Morton A. Assisting furniture strippers in reducing the risk from methylene chloride stripping formulations. Report No 170-20a. Cincinnati OH: NIOSH, 1999.

52. Hearne FT, Pifer JW. Mortality of two overlapping cohorts of photographic film base manufacturing employees exposed to methylene chloride. J Occup Environ Med 1999; 41:1154–69.

53. Tomenson JA, Bonner SM, Heijne CG, Farrar DG, Cummings TF. Mortality of workers exposed to methylene chloride employed at a plant producing cellulose triacetate film base. Occup Environ Med 1997; 54:470–6.

54. Gibbs GW, Amsel J, Soden K. A cohort mortality study of cellulose triacetate-fiber workers exposed to methylene chloride. J Occup Environ Med 1996; 38:693–7.

55. Ducatman AM, McLellan RK. Epidemiological basis for an occupational and environmental policy on environmental tobacco smoke. Arlington Heights IL: American College of Occupational and Environmental Medicine, 2000.

56. Kawachi I, Coiditz GA. Workplace exposure to passive smoking and risk of cardiovascular disease: summary of epidemiological studies. Environ Health Perspect 199; 107(Suppl 6):847–51.

57. Steenland K. Risk assessment for heart disease and workplace ETS exposure among non-smokers. Environ Health Perspect 1999; 107(Suppl 6):859–63.

58. Hammond SK. Exposure of US workers to environmental tobacco smoke. Environ Health Perspect 1999; 107(Suppl 2):329–40.

59. Trout D, Decker J, Mueller C, Bernert JT, Pirkle J. Exposure of casino employees to environmental tobacco smoke. J Occup Environ Med 1998; 40:270–6.

60. Otsuka R, Watanabe H, Hirata K, et al. Acute effects of passive smoking on the coronary circulation in healthy young adults. JAMA 2001; 286:436–41.

61. Jarup L, Pershagen G, Wall S. Cumulative arsenic exposure and lung cancer in smelter workers: a dose–response study. Am J Ind Med 1989; 15:31.

62. Hertz-Picciotto I, Arrighi HM, Hu SW. Does arsenic exposure increase the risk for circulatory disease? Am J Epidemiol 2000; 151174–81.

63. Lubin JH, Fraumeni JF. Does arsenic exposure increase the risk for circulatory disease? Am J Epidemiol 2000; 152:290–2.

64. Ohnishi K, Yoshida H, Shigeno K, et al. Prolongation of the QT interval and ventricular tachycardia in patients treated with arsenic trioxide for acute promyelocytic leukemia. Ann Intern Med 2000; 133:881–5.

65. Rahman M, Tondel M, Ahmad SA, Chowdhury IA, Faruquee MH, Axelson O. Hypertension and arsenic exposure in Bangladesh. Hypertension 1999; 33:74–8.

66. Jensen GE, Hansen ML. Occupational arsenic exposure and glycosylated haemoglobin. Analyst 1998; 123:77–80.

67. Peters A, Dockery DW, Muller JE, Mittleman MA. Increased particulate air pollution and the triggering of myocardial infarction. Circulation 2001; 103:2810–15.

68. Gustavsson P, Plato N, Hallqvist J, et al. A population-based case-referent study of myocardial infarction and occupational exposure to motor exhaust, other combustion products, organic solvents, lead, and dynamite. Stockholm Heart Epidemiology Program (SHEEP) Study Group. Epidemiology 2001; 12:222–8.

69. Albert CM, Mittleman MA, Chae CU, Lee IM, Hennekens CH, Manson JE. Triggering of sudden death from cardiac causes by vigorous exertion. N Engl J Med 2000; 343:1355–61.

70. Sesso HD, Paffenbarger RS, I-Min L. Physical activity and coronary heart disease in men The Harvard Alumni Health Study. Circulation 2000; 102:975–80.

71. D'Avanzo B, Santoro L, La Vecchia C, et al. Physical activity and the risk of acute myocardial infarction. GISSI-ERFIM Investigators. Gruppo Italiano per lo Studio de Sopravvivenza nell'Infarto-Epidemiologia dei Fattori di Rischi dell'Infarto Miocardico. Ann Epidemiol 1993; 3:645–51.

72. Brand RJ, Paffenbarger RS, Sholtz RI, Kampert JB. Work activity and fatal heart attack studied by multiple logistic analysis. Am J Epidemiol 1979; 10:52–62.

73. The Eurowinter Group. Cold exposure and winter mortality from ischemic heart disease, cerebrovascular disease, respiratory disease, and all causes in warm and cold regions of Europe. Lancet 1997; 349:1341–6.

74. Donaldson GC, Ermakov SP, Komarov YM, McDonald CP, Keatinge WR. Cold related mortalities and protection from cold in Yakutsk, eastern Siberia. Br Med J 1998; 317:978–82.

75. Gorjanc ML, Flanders WD, VanDerslice J, Hersh J, Malilay J. Effects of temperature and snowfall on mortality in Pennsylvania. Am J Epidemiol 1999; 149:1152–60.

76. Green MS, Peled I, Harari G, Luz J, Akselrod S, Norymberg M, Melamed S. Association of silent ST-segment depression on one-hour ambulatory ECGs with exposure to industrial noise among blue-collar workers in Israel examined at different levels of ambient temperature – the CORDIS Study. Public Health Rev 1991; 19:277–93.

77. Garcia-Rubira JC, Aguilar J, Romero D. Acute myocardial infarction in a young man after heat exhaustion. Int J Cardiol 1995; 47:297–300.

78. Semenza JC, Rubin CH, Falter KH, et al. Heat-related deaths during the July 1995 Heat Wave in Chicago. N Engl J Med 1996; 335(2):84–90.

79. Redmond CK, Emes JJ, Mazumdar S, Magee PC, Kamon E. Mortality of steelworkers employed in hot jobs. J Environ Pathol Toxicol 1979; 2:75–96.

80. Moulin JJ, Wild P, Mantout B, Fournier-Betz M, Mur JM, Smagghe G. Mortality from lung cancer and cardiovascular diseases among stainless-steel producing workers. Cancer Causes Control 1993; 4:75–81.

81. Wild P, Moulin JJ, Ley FX, Schaffer P. Mortality from cardiovascular diseases among potash miners exposed to heat. Epidemiology 1995; 6:243–7.

82. Krause N, Lynch JW, Kaplan GA, et al. Standing at work and progression of carotid atherosclerosis. Scand J Work Environ Health 2000; 26:227.

83. Pamuk E, Makuc D, Heck K, Reuben C, Lochner K. Socioeconomic status and health chartbook: United States, 1998. Hyattsville, MD: National Center for Health Statistics, 1998.

84. Kunst AE, Groenhof F, Andersen O, et al. Occupational class and ischemic heart disease mortality in the United States and 11 European countries. Am J Public Health 1999; 89:47–53.

85. Bartley M, Fitzpatrick R, Firth D, Marmot M. Social distribution of cardiovascular disease risk factors: change among men in England 1984–1993. J Epidemiol Commun Health 2000; 54:806–6.

86. Iribarren C, Luepker RV, McGovern PG, Arnett DK, Blackburn H. Twelve-year trends in cardiovascular disease risk factors in the Minnesota Heart Survey – are socioeconomic differences widening? Arch Intern Med 1997; 157:873–81.

87. Bosma H, Peter R, Siegrist J, Marmot M. Two alternative job stress models and the risk of coronary heart disease. Am J Pub Health 1998; 88:68–74.

88. The European Heart Network. Social factors, work, stress and cardiovascular disease prevention in the European Union. July 1998. http://www.ehnheart.org/

89. Karasek R, Theorell T. The demand-control-support model and CVD. In: Schnall P, Belkic K, Landsbergis P, Baker D, eds. The workplace and cardiovascular disease. Occup Med 2000; 15:78–83.

90. Siegrist J, Peter R. The effort-reward-imbalance model In: Schnall P, Belkic K, Landsbergis P, Baker D, eds. The workplace and cardiovascular disease. Occup Med 2000; 15:83–7.

91. Belkic K, Landsbergis P, Schnall P, et al. Psychosocial factors: review of the empirical data among men. In: Schnall P, Belkic K, Landsbergis P, Baker D, eds. The workplace and cardiovascular disease. Occup Med 2000; 15:24–46.

92. Steenland K, Johnson J, Nowlin S. A follow-up study of job stain and heart disease among males in the NHANES population. Am J Ind Med 1997; 31:256–9.

93. Teorell T, Tsutsumi A, Hallquist J, et al. Decision latitude, job strain, and myocardial infarction: a study of working men in Stockholm. Am J Public Health 1998; 88:382–8.

94. Bosma H, Marmot MG, Hemingway H, Nicholson AC, Brunner E, Stansfeld SA. Low job control and risk of coronary heart disease in the Whitehall II (prospective cohort) study. Br Med J 1997; 314:558.

95. Sacker A, Bartley MJ, Firth D, Fitzpatrick RM, Marmot MG. The relationship between job strain and coronary heart disease: evidence from an English sample of the working male population. Psychol Med 2001; 31:279–90.

96. Reuterwall C, Hallqvist J, Ahlbom A, et al. Higher relative but lower absolute risks of myocardial infarction in women than in men: analysis of some major risk factors in the SHEEP study. J Int Med 1999; 246:161–74.

97. Peter R, Siegrist J. Psychosocial work environment and the risk of coronary heart disease. Int Arch Occup Environ Health 2000; 73(Suppl): S41–5.

98. Levi L. Stressors at the workplace: theoretical models – a historical overview In: Schnall P, Belkic K, Landsbergis P, Baker D, eds. The workplace and cardiovascular disease. Occup Med 2000; 15:69–73.

99. National Research Council. Singer BH, Ryff CD, eds. New horizons in health: an integrative approach. Committee on Future Directions for Behavioral and Social Sciences Research at the National Institutes of Health. Washington DC: National Academy Press, 2001.

100. Marmot M, Shipley M, Brunner E, Hemingway H. Relative contribution of early life and adult socioeconomic factors to adult morbidity in the Whitehall II study. J Epidemiol Commun Health 2001; 55:301–7.

101. Wamala SP, Lynch J, Kaplan GA. Women's exposure to early and late life socioeconomic disadvantage and coronary heart disease risk: the Stockholm Female Coronary Risk Study. Int J Epidemiol 2001; 30:275–84.

102. McEwen BS. Allostasis and allostatic load: implications for neurophyschopharmacology. Neuropsychopharmacology 2000; 22:108–24.

103. Skantze HB, Kaplan J, Petterson K, et al. Psychosocial stress causes endothelial injury in cynomonglus monkeys via beta-1-adrenoceptor activation. Atherosclerosis 1998; 136:153–61.

104. Rozanski A, Blumenthal JA, Kaplan J. Impact of psychological factors on the pathogenesis of cardiovascular disease and implications for therapy circulation 1999; 99:2192–217.

105. Steenland K. Shift work, long hours and CVD. In: Schnall P, Belkic K, Landsbergis P, Baker D, eds. The workplace and cardiovascular disease. Occup Med 2000; 15:7–17.

106. Boggild H, Suadicani P, Hein HO, Gyntelberg F. Shift work, social class, and ischaemic heart disease in middle aged and elderly men; a 22 year follow up in the Copenhagen Male Study. Occup Environ Med 1999; 56:640–5.

107. Antti-Poika M, Heikkila J, Saarinen L. Cardiac arrhythmias during occupational exposure to fluorinated hydrocarbons. Br J Ind Med 1990; 47:138.

108. Edling C, Ohlson C-G, Ljungkvist G, et al. Cardiac arrhythmia in refrigerator repairmen exposed to fluorocarbons. Br J Ind Med 1990; 47:207.

109. Wilcosky TC, Simonsen NR, Solvent exposure and cardiovascular disease Am J Ind Med 1991; 19:569–86.

110. Egeland GM, Bloom TF, Schnorr TM, et al. Fluorocarbon 113 exposure and cardiac dysrhythmias among aerospace workers. Am J Ind Med 1992; 22:851–7.

111. Kaufman JD, Silverstein MA, Moure-Eraso R. Atrial fibrillation and sudden death related to occupational solvent exposure. Am J Ind Med 1994; 25:731–5.

112. Bowen SE, Daniel J, Balster RL. Deaths associated with inhalant abuse in Virginia from 1987 to 1996. Drug Alcohol Depend 1999; 53:239–45.

113. Egeland GM, Bloom TF, Schnorr TM, Hornung RW, Suruda AJ, Wille KK. Fluorocarbon 113 exposure and cardiac dysrhythmias among aerospace workers. Am J Ind Med 1992; 22:851–7.

114. Speizer FE, Wegman DH, Ramirez A. Palpitation rates associated with fluorocarbon exposure in a hospital setting. N Engl J Med 1975; 292:624–6.

115. Edling C, Ohlson CG, Ljungkvist G, Oliv A, Soderholm B. Cardiac arrhythmia in refrigerator repairmen exposed to fluorocarbons. Br J Ind Med 1990; 47:207–12.

116. Blair A, Hartge P, Stewart PA, McAdams M, Lubin J. Mortality and cancer incidence of aircraft maintenance workers exposed to trichloroethylene and other organic solvents and chemicals: extended follow up. Occup Environ Med 1998; 55:161–71.

117. Wartenberg D, Reyner D, Scott CS. Trichloroethylene and cancer: epidemiological evidence. Environ Health Perspect 2000; 108(Suppl):161–76.

118. Cheng Y, Schwartz J, Sparrow D, Aro A, Weiss ST, Hu H. Bone lead and blood lead levels in relation to baseline blood pressure and the prospective development of hypertension. The Normative Aging Study. Am J Epidemiol 2001; 153:164–71.

119. Schwartz BS, Stewart WF, Todd AC, Simon D, Links JM. Different associations of blood lead, meso-2,3-dimercaptosuccinic acid (DMSA)-chelatable lead, and tibial lead levels with blood pressure in 543 former organolead manufacturing workers. Arch Environ Health 2000; 55:85–92.

120. Tepper A, Mueller C, Singal M, Sagar K. Blood pressure, left ventricular mass, and lead exposure in battery manufacturing workers. Am J Ind Med 2001; 40:63–72.

121. Hu H. Exposure to metals. Prim Care 2000; 27:983–96.

122. Talbott EO, Gibson LB, Burks A, Engberg R, McHugh KP. Evidence for a dose–response relationship between occupational noise and blood pressure. Arch Environ Health 1999; 54:71–8.

123. Tomei F, Fantini S, Tomao E, Baccolo TP, Rosati MV. Hypertension and chronic exposure noise. Arch Environ Health 2000; 55:319–25.

124. Fogari R, Zoppi A, Vanasia A, Marasi G, Villa G. Occupational noise exposure and blood pressure. J Hypertension 1994; 12:475–9.

125. Hessel PA, Sluis-Cremer GK. Occupational noise exposure and blood pressure: longitudinal and cross-sectional observations in a group of underground miners. Arch Environ Health 1994; 49:128–34.

126. Hirai A, Takata M, Mikawa M, et al. Prolonged exposure to industrial noise causes hearing loss but not high blood pressure: a study of 2124 factory laborers in Japan. J Hypertension 1991; 9:1069–73.

127. Yiming Z, Shuzeng Z, Selvin S, Spear RC. A dose–response relationship for noise-induced hypertension. Br J Ind Med 1991; 48:179.

128. Fogari R, Zoppi A, Corradi L, Marasi G, Vanasia A, Zanchetti A. Transient but not sustained blood pressure increments by occupational noise. An ambulatory blood pressure measurement study. J Hypertension 2001; 19:1021–7.

129. Pickering T. The effects of occupational stress on blood pressure in men and women. Acta Physiol Scand 1997; 161:125–8.

130. Schnall PL, Pieper C, Schwartz JE, et al. The relationship between 'job strain' workplace diastolic blood pressure and left ventricular mass index. JAMA 1990; 11:1929–35.

131. Schnall PL, Landsbergis PA, Schwartz J, et al. A longitudinal study of 'job strain,' workplace diastolic blood pressure, and ambulatory blood pressure: results from a 3-year follow-up. Psychosom Med 1998; 60:697–708.

132. Theorell T, Alfredsson, Westerholm P, Falck B. Coping with unfair treatment at work – what is the relationship between coping and hypertension in middle-aged men and women? An epidemiological study of working men and women in Stockholm (the Wolf Study). Psychother Psychosom 2000; 69:86–94.

133. Friedman R, Schwartz JE, Schnall PL, et al. Psychological variables in hypertension: relationship to causal or ambulatory blood pressure in men. Psychosom Med 2001; 63:19–31.

134. Horowitz SF, Fischbein A, Matza D, et al. Evaluation of right and left ventricular function in hard metal workers. Br J Ind Med 1988; 45: 742–6.

135. Wild P, Perdix A, Romazini S, Moulin JJ, Pellet F. Lung cancer mortality in a site producing hard metals. Occup Environ Med 2000; 57:568–73.

136. Jones RD. Survey of antimony workers mortality 1961–1992. Occup Environ Med 1994; 51:772–6.

137. Schnorr TM, Steenland K, Thun MJ, Rinsky RA. Mortality in a cohort of antimony smelter workers. Am J Ind Med 1995; 27:759–70.

138. Wu MM, Kuo TL, Hwang YH, Chen CJ. Dose–response relation between arsenic concentration in well water and mortality from cancers and vascular diseases. Am J Epidemiol 1989; 130:1123–32.

139. Maugeri U, Iovicic M, Cavalleri A, et al. The peripheral vascular system in young workers exposed to the risk of carbon disulfide. Med Lav 1966; 57:709–14.

140. Cunningham SR, Dalzell GWN, McGirr P, et al. Myocardial infarction and primary ventricular fibrillation after glue sniffing. Br Med J 1987; 294:739.

141. Josephson CJ, Pinto SS, Petronella SJ. Arsine: electrocardiographic changes produced in acute human poisoning. Arch Ind Hyg 1951; 4:43.

142. Glazenes FS. Electrocardiographic findings with arsenic poisoning. Calif Med 1968; 109:158.

Chapter 25
Renal and Bladder Disorders

Caroline S Rhoads, William E Daniell

Toxins that gain access to the circulation have the potential to cause significant damage to the urinary tract. The kidneys provide a major route for the excretion of these substances, and normal renal function (glomerular ultrafiltration of blood, proximal tubular secretion and reabsorption, and medullary tubular concentration) can produce intracellular, interstitial, and intratubular concentrations of chemicals that exceed those found in the blood and other tissues. Some chemicals, particularly low molecular weight compounds of neutral pH, may accumulate within the renal interstitium in a manner analogous to urea. Other chemicals, such as cadmium, may be concentrated intracellularly through sequestration and molecular binding. The kidneys are also a site for enzymatic detoxification of a wide variety of chemical classes, and the generation of reactive intermediate compounds with increased toxicity poses an additional risk. At the distal end of the urinary tract, concentrated and excreted chemicals may rest for hours in contact with bladder mucosa.

While the risk for urinary tract injury from exogenous chemicals is theoretically high, the actual incidence and prevalence of occupational renal disease are not known. About 20% of acute renal failure is attributable to the toxic effects of chemicals but most of these cases involve the adverse effects of pharmaceutical agents administered for clinical purposes. At the present time, the United States Renal Data System does not include nephrotoxicity as a distinct category in its listing of causes of end-stage renal disease. It is thus equally difficult to estimate the prevalence of chronic occupational renal disease. The infrequent recognition of nephrotoxicity, particularly that attributable to occupational or environmental chemicals, is unlikely to reflect the true rate of occurrence.

Clinical recognition of occupational renal disease is challenging. Clinicians may have a low index of suspicion for chemical causes of disease in general, and patients may lack symptoms and signs that would alert the clinician to the presence of early renal disease. Normal kidneys have a large functional reserve and the glomerular filtration rate (GFR) may be preserved during early renal damage. Once the GFR begins to decline, adult patients may remain asymptomatic despite having GFRs as low as 30 mL/minute. An individual can thus sustain substantial acute or chronic renal injury without associated symptoms or changes detectable by laboratory tests and can subsequently have progressive renal dysfunction long after exposure to an injurious factor ceases.

When chemical toxicity is suspected and renal damage detected, it may be difficult to prove chemical causation. The available assays for direct measurement of industrial chemicals in body fluids and tissues commonly have little utility in ascertaining the clinical relevance of historically remote, temporally variable, or mixed chemical exposures. In addition, early histopathologic changes of renal disorders attributable to workplace chemicals typically have no pathognomonic features, and the pathologic features of renal diseases in general become increasingly non-specific with disease progression.

Finally, there may be little incentive for a clinician to identify a specific chemical cause for a patient's renal disease as this usually has little therapeutic benefit beyond ensuring that the exposure has ceased. There are few workplace chemicals for which there are known to be effective antidotal treatments, and identification of historically remote exposures may allow no meaningful opportunity for exposure prevention or modification.

Epidemiologic investigation of occupational renal disorders and other disorders of the urinary tract has been subject to the same limitations faced at the clinical level, principally the lack of tests to detect dysfunction prior to advanced stages of disease. As a consequence, there have been relatively few studies in this area, with most having concentrated on a limited spectrum of occupational exposures, chiefly certain metals and organic solvents. However, the continuing development of new and increasingly sensitive assays for markers of nephrotoxicity, such as plasma and renal proteins in urine, offers increasing potential for epidemiologic identification of possible nephrotoxic effects of occupational chemical exposures, particularly those involving the renal tubules.

The personal and social costs of urinary tract disorders are high. In the United States the annual cost of providing healthcare for individuals with end-stage renal disease is estimated to exceed 13 billion dollars, and the costs in terms of reduced quality of life are incalculable. While it is likely that occupational urinary tract disorders do not account for a major proportion of these overall costs, the absence of incidence and prevalence data does not allow an assessment of their contributions to these disorders. The personal risk and social costs for workers exposed to chemicals with potential but yet uncharacterized toxicity for the urinary tract could still be substantial. Clinical and epidemiologic investigations are needed to define the extent of occupational urinary tract disorders.

CLINICAL EVALUATION
Clinical history and physical examination

The medical and exposure histories are critical to the evaluation of patients suspected of having occupational urinary tract disease. Virtually every component of the urinary tract has been found to be susceptible to injury following acute or chronic exposures to specific toxic chemicals, particularly if consideration is extended to pharmacologic agents. Therefore, in the evaluation of unexplained disorders at any level of the urinary tract, any recent or remote chemical exposures that fall outside the range of usual population experience should be given consideration as possible causative or contributory factors. It is critical that consideration not be restricted to lists of chemicals with known potential to injure the urinary tract. Currently identified urotoxins should be regarded as exemplifying pathophysiologic mechanisms that, at least theoretically, might also be inducible by other chemicals with yet unrecognized potential for urinary tract toxicity.

The key feature to be determined in the exposure history; beyond the qualitative assessment of exposure dose, is the temporal relationship between the exposure and the probable onset of the condition under evaluation. For acute conditions (such as acute renal failure) or for conditions with relatively abrupt onsets (such as rapidly progressive glomerulonephritis), exposures occurring within hours to days or possibly weeks are more likely to be of clinical significance than are exposures that occurred remotely in time. In contrast, for chronic conditions with relatively indolent onsets (such as chronic renal failure), recent exposures may have minimal relevance in comparison to historically remote or cumulative longer-term exposures. Substantial exposures that occurred and ended early in a working career should still be considered as potential causative or contributing factors in the development of chronic urinary tract disorders that occur in older persons. Finally, general statements such as these should be treated as guides and not as absolute rules because remote exposures may serve as predisposing factors for acute conditions, and recent short-term exposures may precipitate the clinical manifestation of an otherwise slowly progressive disorder.

Information regarding the frequency and usual intensity of exposure to suspected occupational toxins, and the degree of personal protection, allows some estimate of the relative dose in comparison with the range of occupational, domestic, and general environmental experience. Exposure patterns characterized by variability or intermittent high peaks across a workshift may potentially have greater biologic significance than would uniform exposure to the comparable cumulative amount. In addition, consideration should be given to the potential for skin exposure; for some agents, such as organic solvents, dermal absorption can potentially contribute more to the total dose received than the associated inhalation exposure.

The possibility of a chemical etiology should be considered for any patient with renal dysfunction, even in the presence of other presumptive pathogenic processes.

Clinical experience with drug-induced nephrotoxicity shows that numerous factors (e.g., age, genetic predisposition, hypertension, diabetes, gout, pre-existing chronic renal disease, and transient factors such as intravascular fluid depletion or co-administered drugs) can enhance a drug's intrinsic nephrotoxicity. Such factors are likely also to influence any acute or chronic renal effects of workplace chemicals, and conversely, exogenous chemicals might worsen pre-existing renal disease of non-toxic etiology.

The physical examination is unlikely to reveal information that is directly pertinent to the urinary tract, but associated findings involving other organ systems including skin and mucous membrane changes associated with metals (see heavy metals) and neurologic changes associated with organic solvents may be helpful in identifying an etiologic factor.

Laboratory testing

Laboratory tests are essential for characterizing the nature and severity of renal dysfunction. However, most clinical tests have limited utility in the consideration of occupational factors, either in etiologic evaluation of renal disease or in screening or surveillance for renal dysfunction. Measurements of serum electrolyte concentrations or osmolality generally contribute little to these occupational goals. While the serum creatinine level and to a lesser degree the blood urea nitrogen (BUN) level are the conventional clinical tools used to screen for and monitor reductions in GFR, these tests are insensitive to mild renal dysfunction. Dynamic tests of renal concentrating ability after fluid deprivation potentially provide a sensitive measure of distal tubular function; however, these tests have limited applicability outside of a clinical research setting.

In general, urinary sediment examination is an insensitive and non-specific indicator of suspected occupational urinary tract disease or injury, and has little applicability outside of situations involving known or suspected risk for urinary tract tumor (see Chapters 30.3 and 30.4). Imaging studies and tissue examination can provide anatomic and pathologic classification, and can lead to diagnoses that reduce the likelihood of occupational contribution, but these studies do not commonly yield information that is otherwise helpful in identifying an occupational etiology. Tissue findings are rarely pathognomonic for the effects of chemical toxins or other occupational factors. In addition, kidney biopsy is invasive and expensive. In contrast to the limited clinical utility of the tests noted above, measurements of plasma and renal proteins in the urine offer broad potential for occupational epidemiologic studies and surveillance programs to detect the subclinical renal effects of chemical exposures.

A variety of factors determine the applicability of laboratory tests to clinical, screening, or surveillance situations, and the limitations of a test must be considered accordingly when ordering a test or interpreting its result in relation to an individual or group. Tests that lack normal reference ranges based on appropriate comparison populations or have substantial degrees of interindividual variability will have little diagnostic value in the non-serial evaluation of an individual and should be interpreted cautiously. However, tests that have limited degrees of interindividual variability but low degrees of intraindividual variability, such as the serum creatinine level, can provide useful information regarding an individual even when small changes are found on serial measurements or in comparison to a previous value. The potential for chronologic variability (e.g., diurnal or seasonal effects and temporal variation in laboratory methods) should always be considered when screening groups or serially monitoring individuals. The influence of urine flow rate on a urine test result may be at least partially controlled by standardization relative to an indirect measure of urine concentration, such as urine creatinine, specific gravity or osmolarity. The practice of urine concentration adjustment, however, is based largely on convention and has undergone only limited scrutiny for most specific urine analytes; unadjusted urine analyte values should always be considered and reported concurrently.

Glomerular filtration rate

Invasive functional studies (such as intravenous injection of inulin or *p*-aminohippurate [PAH] to measure GFR or renal plasma flow, respectively) may allow definitive characterization of exposure-related reductions in renal excretory function. Such studies have been used to describe functional decrements in association with occupational carbon disulfide exposure and hypertension; however, the logistic difficulties of these procedures normally limit their use to clinical research settings. Creatinine clearance is potentially useful as an alternative measure, but the necessity for timed collection of blood and urine specimens limits its applicability in surveillance programs. Serum measurements of creatinine and BUN levels are the most commonly used alternatives to provide indirect estimates of GFR.

Serum creatinine level measurements, unfortunately, have little value in the detection of early stages of chronic renal injury because of the large functional reserve of the kidneys. Serum creatinine levels show an inverse, hyperbolic relationship with GFR, such that small increases in creatinine above normal can represent major functional loss. An individual's serum creatinine level may not convincingly exceed the upper normal reference range until up to one half of renal function is lost.

While there is little reassurance to be gained from a normal serum creatinine level, the detection of an elevated creatinine level (or even a small mean increment when evaluated among exposed workers and non-exposed controls) is strong evidence of renal dysfunction. Furthermore, because the degree of intraindividual variability in the serum creatinine level is normally much less than interindividual variability, small increases in an individual's creatinine level over time should be regarded as potentially significant.

Urine proteins

Urine contains proteins of plasma and renal origin. Normally, no more than 150 mg of protein are excreted each day. The glomerulus presents a charge and size selective barrier to the filtration of plasma proteins that excludes the majority from the ultrafiltrate. Both high molecular weight (HMW) proteins such as albumin (about 65,000 daltons) and low molecular weight (LMW) proteins such as β-2-microglobulin (<40,000 daltons) are able to cross the glomerulus to varying degrees. Reabsorption of the two predominant LMW proteins, β-2-microglobulin (β2M) and retinol binding protein (RBP), is nearly complete, with a fractional reabsorption of 99.97%. LMW proteins normally account for about 20% of the daily protein excretion. Reabsorption of albumin and other HMW proteins is less complete, with a fractional reabsorption of between 90 and 99%. HMW proteins normally account for about 40% of the daily protein excretion. Renally derived glycoproteins (including Tamm-Horsfall protein) which are secreted by the renal tubular epithelial cells during the course of tubular work constitute another 40% of the normal daily protein excretion. Against this background, changes in the level of excretion of HMW and LMW plasma proteins can serve as approximate markers of glomerular and tubular dysfunction, respectively.

In the absence of acute illness or unusually intense activity, protein excretion in excess of 150 mg per day is a reliable indicator of kidney damage. Excessive excretion of albumin and other HMW proteins such as transferrin is indicative of glomerular damage. In this setting there is increased filtration of HMW plasma proteins without any accompanying change in the normally total filtration of LMW plasma proteins. The relatively low affinity of HMW proteins for tubular reabsorption sites is aggravated by the filtrate overload, and the HMW protein excess appears to provide little competition for LMW protein reabsorption. Consequently, HMW protein excretion increases without substantial increase in the urinary LMW protein concentration.

In contrast, the proteinuria associated with proximal tubular damage and dysfunction (with preservation of glomerular function) is characterized by absolute increases in excretion of both LMW and HMW plasma proteins, but with markedly greater relative increase in LMW protein excretion. LMW proteins provide the better indicator of tubular proteinuria because, although HMW proteins still comprise the major proportion of total urine protein, the increases in concentrations of LMW proteins are more readily detectable in comparison to their low normal concentrations than are the increases in HMW proteins.

A wide variety of urine proteins have been investigated as markers for occupational renal disease (Table 25.1).[1] Urine proteins can potentially serve as markers of renal injury from low or short-term chemical exposures, but toxin-induced proteinuria is most likely to be persistent after long-term exposures and to be most representative of a cumulative exposure effect. At the earliest stages of renal damage, the specific proteins present may localize the site of damage to either the glomerulus or the tubule. When more advanced disease is present, however, multiple classes of proteins may be present, reflecting more widespread damage. Patterns of proteinuria may suggest a

Markers of effects at the glomerular level
High molecular weight plasmaproteins (>40,000 D) in urine: albumin, transferrin, IgG
Components of glomerular structure in urine or plasma: fibronectin, laminin, sialic acids, anti-glomerular basement membrane antibodies; prostanoids: thromboxane B_2, 6-keto-prostaglandin $F_{1\alpha}$
Markers of early effects at the proximal tubule
Low-molecular weight proteins in urine: β-2-microglobulin, retinol binding protein, α-1-microglobulin
Enzymes:
N-acetylglucosaminidase (NAG), total non-specific alkaline phosphatase (TNAP), human intestinal alkaline phosphatase (HIAP), gamma glutamyl transferase (GGT), alanine aminopeptidase (AAP)
Kidney antigens:
Brush border BB-50
Marker of the distal tubule
Kallikrein
Marker of the loop of Henle
Tamm-Horsfall glycoprotein
Markers of the collecting tubule and interstitium
Prostaglandin$_{2\alpha}$, prostaglandin E_2
Site-unrelated markers
Glycosaminoglycans

* Adapted from Mutti[1]

Table 25.1 Site selectivity of biomarkers of early renal effects*

specific toxin but are not pathognomonic; the causative agent is usually inferred from the exposure history and further documented by direct measurement in blood or urine. The sensitivity of urinary markers for detecting renal damage varies widely and it is possible that urine protein abnormalities may not be detected until a cumulative dose threshold or period of latency has occurred. In addition, both intersubject and intrasubject variations can be substantial, further complicating the interpretation of these tests.[2] Nonetheless, these markers allow for the detection of early renal damage and are useful for surveillance, monitoring, and risk reduction in the industrial setting, and there is some evidence that low level LMW proteinuria may be reversible when workers reduce their exposure to occupational toxins.[3]

High molecular weight plasma proteins

Albumin is the most abundant high molecular weight (HMW) plasma protein in urine, and it is the urine protein that is measured most commonly to assess proteinuria. It is stable in urine, even with prolonged frozen storage, and can be quantified readily across the full range of concentrations found in urine. Complicating its role as a marker of possible nephrotoxicity is the fact that albuminuria also can result from chemically unrelated, non-disease factors, such as heavy exercise, severe heat stress, and orthostatic postural influences. Mild degrees of albuminuria (less than 0.5 g/day) can arise with either glomerular or tubular damage, and the site of dysfunction can potentially be distinguished by the absence or presence, respectively, of low molecular weight proteinuria. Higher degrees of albuminuria are generally attributable to a predominantly glomerular defect, particularly when albuminuria reaches the nephrotic range

(urine total protein more than 3.5 g/day). Nephrotic syndrome has only rarely been described in association with occupational chemicals, most notably with mercury exposure (discussed later in this chapter).

Other HMW plasma proteins have been used or suggested for characterization of proteinuria. Transferrin has been reported to be more sensitive than albumin in the early detection of glomerular defects in diabetic and cadmium nephropathies. It is less stable than albumin, however, and urine samples can be stored reliably only for short periods before analysis.

Low molecular weight plasma proteins

The protein β2M (molecular weight, 12 kD) appears in the urine when tubular absorption of protein is impaired. It has been used extensively in epidemiologic investigations and ongoing surveillance of workers with selected chemical exposures, most notably cadmium. In workers chronically exposed to cadmium, an increase of urine β2M concentration to critical threshold levels can signal an irreversible cadmium effect on the kidney before any remarkable changes appear in other clinical test parameters (discussed later in this chapter). The widespread use of β2M reflects its historically early use as a renal marker, more than its suitability for occupational exposure surveillance, because β2M is unstable at acid pH or with prolonged storage. Even with neutralization of the urine at the time of sample collection, the degree of degradation in the bladder can be significant. Retinol binding protein RBP (21 kD) is a practical substitute for β2M, in view of its comparable renal handling, its relative stability, and the existence of reliable assays for its quantification. Increases in RBP excretion have been reported among workers with chronic exposure to cadmium and chromium. α-1-microglobulin (30 kD) has also been considered as a marker of tubular dysfunction, primarily because of its higher concentration in urine (and consequently greater technical ease of quantification). However, the available evidence indicates that it may be a less accurate marker of tubular function than β2M or RBP.

Proteins of renal origin

Enzymes. A number of enzymes found in renal (and non-renal) cells have been suggested as urine protein markers of renal injury. These enzymes are all HMW proteins, and it is assumed that, in the absence of evidence for glomerular dysfunction, their increased presence in urine reflects release from damaged tubular tissue. Examples include the lysosomal enzyme, *N*-acetylglucosaminidase (NAG), and the luminal brush border enzyme, human intestinal alkaline phosphatase (HIAP). These assays have been used increasingly in studies of occupational exposures, and both NAG and HIAP have been found to be sensitive markers of early renal damage.[4]

Increases in urine NAG and HIAP have been detected in workers chronically exposed to cadmium and mercury. Urine NAG may also be elevated in workers exposed to lead. The initial evidence suggested that urine NAG and other enzyme activities were less sensitive indicators of renal tubulotoxicity than the LMW proteins β2M and RBP, but more recent studies have variably described comparable or improved sensitivity. Furthermore, in contrast to β2M, the enzyme NAG is unstable only in alkaline conditions (pH greater than 8), which are not usually found in urine, and there exists an automated assay for urine NAG activity. Day to day differences in enzyme excretion may be significant and thus it is critical that serial specimens be collected under the same conditions. Age, sex, body mass index, blood pressure, and smoking and drinking habits all impact measurements between individuals.[2]

The onset and persistence of enzymuria will vary with the nephrotoxin, the exposure pattern, and the specific enzyme. There is generally limited understanding of the temporal relationships between these markers and the renal injury that may occur in occupational exposure situations, particularly in the absence of ongoing exposure. In general, acute renal injury will produce detectable increases in these markers within hours or days, with increases that last only several days or 1 week with limited injury. Enzymuria may even normalize during short-term nephrotoxin exposures, and it has been speculated that tissue stores of enzyme may become depleted or that tissue regeneration may lead to some degree of resistance. Enzymuria has been reported to become persistently abnormal after chronic or high-level acute exposures to nephrotoxic drugs.

Antigens. Renal tubular antigens have also proven to be sensitive indicators of tubular damage in workers exposed to heavy metals. For example, a monoclonal antibody for a proximal tubular brush border protein (BB-50) detected increased antigen excretion in the urine of chromium-exposed workers and patients with cancer who were receiving cisplatin. Drug-related increases have also been reported for other renal tubular antigens in urine; however, antigen assays are not yet standardized and their utility for the clinical evaluation of workers is yet to be established.

Circulating immune markers
Antiglomerular basement membrane (anti-GBM) antibodies occur in association with one class of immune-mediated glomerulonephritis. The etiology of this uncommon condition is unknown, although epidemiologic evidence indicates organic solvent exposures may increase the risk for this and other types of glomerulonephritis (discussed later in this chapter). Other than the use of anti-GBM antibody titers in case studies of solvent-associated glomerulonephritis, this assay has had limited application in occupational investigations. Another assay for circulating antibody directed against renal tissue (antilaminin antibody) was used to demonstrate an increased prevalence of antibody among hydrocarbon-exposed refinery workers and cadmium-exposed, but not lead-exposed, workers. The presence of antibody in these studies showed no correlation with renal dysfunction. The utility of circulating immune markers for occupational studies is generally not established.

DISORDERS OF THE KIDNEY AND URINARY TRACT
Acute renal disorders

A broad array of industrial toxins has been associated with acute renal failure, typically in the setting of severe short-term overexposure. It is likely that acute nephrotoxic exposures can produce any degree of excretory insufficiency, but the cases that ultimately come to clinical recognition usually involve acute renal failure, either of an oliguric or non-oliguric nature. Chemically induced acute renal failure may be produced either through direct toxic actions on renal tissue, or indirectly through systemic, prerenal mechanisms.

Postrenal or obstructive mechanisms have generally not been described in association with acutely toxic exposures. However, for example, the acute renal dysfunction associated with ethylene glycol poisoning is at least partially attributable to the obstructive effects produced by intratubular crystallization of calcium oxalate, a major metabolite of ethylene glycol. In addition, certain other chemicals, notably cadmium, place chronically exposed workers at increased risk for urolithiasis; affected workers face at least the theoretic possibility of obstructive renal dysfunction, particularly in the context of anatomic anomalies, such as a solitary kidney.

Only a small proportion of chemicals associated with acute renal failure have their primary or most severe toxic effects directly on the kidneys. Chemically induced acute renal failure commonly occurs in the context of multiple organ system dysfunction, and it can be difficult or impossible in an acute poisoning to ascertain whether renal dysfunction is a direct or indirect consequence of the toxin involved. Fortunately, the issue is more of general toxicologic interest than clinical concern. Clinical management of acute renal dysfunction in such settings is generally supportive. Selection of toxin-specific treatments (in the limited number of situations where antidotal or chelation regimens, or facilitated toxin removal through extracorporeal technologies are known to be efficacious) is generally dictated by the overall severity of systemic illness rather than the primacy or degree of renal dysfunction.

Pigment nephropathy
Chemical and physical factors with no inherent potential to cause renal cell injury through direct toxic action may indirectly cause acute renal insufficiency through pigmenturias generated by chemically induced rhabdomyolysis or hemolysis (Table 25.2). Myoglobin and, to a lesser degree, hemoglobin have toxic effects on the renal tubular epithelium.

Rhabdomyolysis. Most cases of toxin-induced rhabdomyolysis occur in the setting of intentional ingestion or abuse of a variety of drugs and chemicals and thus have limited pertinence to industrial exposures.[5] Many of the reported cases, however, involve chemicals that are used in industry and are capable of producing, or are known to have produced, some degree of systemic toxicity with skin

Systemic disorders/hemodynamic insufficiency
 Heat stress
 Circulatory depression
Hemolysis/hemoglobinuria-associated factors
 Heat stroke
 Arsenic trioxide
 Arsine
 Aniline
 Benzene
 Coal tar derivatives
 Copper sulfate
 Cresol
 Ethylene glycol dinitrate
 Hydroquinone
 Ispropyl alcohol
 Methyl chloride
 Methylparaminophenol sulfate
 Naphthalene
 Phenol
 Phenylhydrazine
 Phosphine
 Potassium/sodium bromate
 Potassium dichromate
 Propylene glycol
 Sodium chlorate
 Stibine
 Tribromoethanol
 Trinitrotoluene
Rhabdomyolysis/myoglobinuria-associated factors
 Vigorous physical exertion
 Repeated impact trauma
 Electrical or crush injury
 Systemic infection
 Arsenic trioxide
 Carbon monoxide
 Copper sulfate
 Dinitrophenols
 Ethanol
 Ethylene glycol
 Ispropyl alcohol
 Lindane
 Mercuric chloride
 Methanol
 p-Phenylenediamine
 Zinc phosphide
Methemoglobinemia (and secondary hemolysis)-associated factors
 Aniline (and analogues)
 Carbon monoxide
 Dinitrophenol
 Ethylene glycol dinitrate
 Sodium chlorate
 Trinitrophenol (picric acid)

Table 25.2 Reported indirect causes of acute renal failure

or inhalation exposure. Chemical ingestions that are severe enough to produce rhabdomyolysis are frequently accompanied by severe metabolic derangements, seizures, and prolonged immobilization, all of which may themselves produce muscle injury and exacerbate rhabdomyolysis. In a given case it is frequently difficult to determine whether the rhabdomyolysis is primarily due to a direct effect of the toxin or whether it is primarily due to systemic illness induced by the toxin.

Non-chemical factors have generally been identified more commonly than have chemical substances as occupational causes of rhabdomyolysis and acute renal failure. Rhabdomyolysis is a well-recognized possible consequence of electrical and crush injuries and has also been seen with lesser degrees of trauma, such as repeated impact trauma

experienced during the operation of jackhammers or other physical impact tools. Vigorous physical exertion, particularly in relatively hot environments, can also be a cause. The risk for exertional rhabdomyolysis has not shown any clear association with the degree of premorbid physical fitness, but it has been speculated that fitter individuals may be at greater risk because of their greater muscle mass and potentially greater willingness to attempt extreme exertion. In severe cases, heat stroke can produce rhabdomyolysis (or hemolysis), and these factors and the usually concomitant hemodynamic insufficiency can lead to renal failure. Systemic infections (e.g., viral syndromes) can also result in varying degrees of rhabdomyolosis, with associated renal failure. Finally, it should be noted that the venoms of certain snakes, spiders, and hymenoptera are capable of causing acute renal failure along with rhabdomyolysis and/or hemolysis, and in some instances, direct nephrotoxicity.[6]

Hemolysis. Although free myoglobin is inherently more nephrotoxic than free hemoglobin, hemolysis and resultant acute renal failure have been more clearly linked with occupational chemical exposures than has rhabdomyolysis. Arsine (AsH_3) is a dense, colorless, non-irritating gas with a faint garlicky odor that causes hemolysis during both acute and chronic exposure. It may be generated incidentally as a refining byproduct from arsenic-contaminated non-ferrous metals, including the common and usually benign practice of spraying water on metal dross. Arsine is also used routinely as a source material for arsenic dopant in semiconductor manufacturing, in which even with appropriate precautions, the potential remains for accidental release of large quantities of arsine during use or transport. Acute exposure to very high levels of arsine may cause massive acute hemolysis, acute tubular necrosis, and even death. Arsine exposures and their clinical manifestations may be abrupt or insidious. The severity and rapidity of the onset of arsine poisoning manifestations show some correlation with the concentration and duration of exposure.[7]

Milder cases may not be apparent until 24 hours after exposure, and the initial presentation may be non-specific, with headache, weakness, and abdominal complaints. With severe poisoning, however, the symptoms may appear within 2 hours, followed by hemoglobinuria within 4–6 hours, jaundice at 24–48 hours, and anuria or oliguria within 2–3 days. Acute renal failure is the most common cause of death in fatal arsine poisonings. The renal failure has been attributed to acute tubular necrosis induced indirectly by hemolysis and mediated through tubular accumulation of hemoglobin casts or through anemia, hemodynamic insufficiency, and consequent renal tubular ischemic injury. However, there are reports of severe tubular necrosis occurring out of proportion to the degree of hemolysis and hemoglobinuria, and even mild cases may show evidence of tubular dysfunction. Experimental evidence further indicates that arsine, or arsenic complexed with hemoglobin, has directly nephrotoxic properties.

Survivors of arsine-induced renal failure commonly have persistent abnormalities of renal function for months and up to 1 year afterward. Hypertension and chronic interstitial nephritis have been reported as long-term outcomes. Delayed recovery may reflect sequestration of hemoglobin-arsenic complex in renal lysosomes with subsequent slow release and prolonged nephrotoxicity. Consequently, although chelating agents such as dimercaprol (BAL) have generally not been effective in modifying the course of arsine-induced hemolysis and acute renal failure, it has been speculated that BAL or another appropriate chelating agent may have a longer-term benefit in reducing residual renal dysfunction. Exchange transfusion has also been reported to be beneficial in managing acute arsine hemolysis.[8]

Arsine is probably the most potent hemolytic substance found in industrial settings, but other industrial chemicals are also known or suspected to cause hemolysis. Two other gaseous hydrides of Group V elements (phosphine, PH_3, and stibine, AbH_3) have acute toxic properties that are similar to, although less severe than, those of arsine. Arsenic trioxide, or white arsenic, typically has minimal hematologic effects with acute or chronic poisoning, but has been reported in isolated cases of acute ingestion to cause hemolysis with associated renal dysfunction. Hemoglobinuric renal failure has also been reported with cresol skin burns in industrial accidents. Table 25.2 lists examples of other commercial and industrial chemicals that have been associated with hemoglobinuric renal failure, primarily in cases involving chemical ingestion.

Methemoglobinemia. Certain chemicals that either bind to or oxidize hemoglobin may produce hemolysis with acute overexposure, and they have at least the potential to cause secondary acute renal insufficiency. Although this is not a common phenomenon with carbon monoxide poisoning and carboxyhemoglobinemia, it has been reported in a limited number of cases. Methemoglobinemia also is typically not associated with hemolysis. However, some industrial chemicals that can generate methemoglobinemia with overexposure have been reported either experimentally, or in case reports of poisonings, to produce oxidative hemolysis, and poisonings, with certain of these chemicals also have been associated with renal failure. Chlorate salts produce prominent intravascular hemolysis and an extracellular methemoglobinemia, and acute hemoglobinuric renal failure has been reported to occur with poisoning by a sodium chlorate weed killer. Methemoglobinemia is a central feature of poisoning with aniline and its homologues, many of which are used extensively as synthetic precursors in the chemical industry. Hemolysis is not a common feature of poisoning with these aromatic nitro and amine compounds (See Chapter 42), but it has been described in association with acute renal failure following poisonings.

Dinitrophenol, which is used as an herbicide, and trinitrophenol (picric acid), which is used in the explosives industry, each produce methemoglobinemia with intoxication, and trinitrophenol can cause intravascular hemolysis. These agents are highly toxic and may cause multiple organ system failure, including renal failure; however, the relative contribution of the methemoglobinemia and hemolysis cannot be distinguished from broad systemic effects associated with poisonings. Ethylene glycol dinitrate, another explosives agent, also has been reported to cause methemoglobinemia and acute renal failure.

Genetic deficiencies. Individuals with certain genetic enzyme deficiencies, such as glucose-6-phosphate dehydrogenase (G6PD) deficiency, may experience acute hemolysis and secondary renal dysfunction with exposure to specific chemical substances that, for the general population, may not be toxic (e.g., fava bean ingestion) or are toxic at much higher levels of exposure. While this has been described infrequently in industrial settings, the potential for unrecognized predisposition to hematologic toxicity exists.

Phenylhydrazine is an oily, relatively non-volatile liquid used as a precursor in the manufacture of dyes and pharmaceuticals; it is also a reagent in chemical analysis. It can produce marked hemolysis, anemia, and decreased urinary output in experimentally poisoned rabbits and guinea pigs, and it produces a low-grade hemolytic anemia when used medically in humans for the treatment of polycythemia vera. There are no reports of fatalities or acute renal failure from industrial exposures. However, phenylhydrazine is absorbed readily across the skin, and the potential exists for such occupational toxicity. Another aromatic nitro compound, trinitrotoluene, has produced acute hemolytic episodes in explosives workers with G6PD deficiency and no prior history of hemolytic anemia, although no renal dysfunction was reported in the described cases.[9] The polyaromatic compound naphthalene can induce hemolysis after metabolism to naphthol and naphthoquinone intermediates, and subsequent metabolic detoxification can be slowed by deficiency of G6PD or glutathione. Ingestion of naphthalene has led to hemolytic anemia and renal dysfunction.

It is at least a realistic consideration that genetic deficiency traits or disorders, such as G6PD deficiency, might place affected individuals at increased risk for hemolytic (or rhabdomyolytic) effects of specific industrial chemical exposures. In general, however, this is a rare mechanism, and the human experience is based on isolated case reports. Despite the broad prevalence of certain genetic enzyme deficiencies, such as the 15% prevalence of G6PD deficiency among African-Americans, no identified genetic deficiencies have been linked to any predictable or significant risk for occupational renal toxicity. There is presently no need to restrict selected individuals from specific chemical exposures on the basis of isolated genetic enzyme deficiencies.

Acute interstitial nephritis

Certain pharmacologic agents may cause an acute hypersensitivity nephritis characterized by renal enlargement, diffuse interstitial infiltration by mononuclear cells, relative non-prominence of tubular or glomerular necrosis, and frequent coexistence of non-renal signs of hypersensitivity. The drug-induced form generally follows a second or later administration of the causative drug, and the degree of dysfunction shows little correlation with the recent or cumulative drug dose. This phenomenon has not been reported as a consequence of occupational chemical exposures, but it is theoretically feasible that the operative mechanism could occur in the context of occupational chemical exposure. Occupational exposures should a least be considered when evaluating individuals with no readily apparent cause for either acute interstitial nephritis or acute nephropathy in the setting of an allergic reaction.

Nephrotoxic acute renal injury and renal failure

The predominant pathogenic mechanism in most cases of acute renal failure induced by chemicals is tubular injury, and the most prevalent pathologic appearance is tubulointerstitial nephritis with associated inflammation or necrosis. While primary nephrotoxic action at the level of the glomerulus is less common, as the clinical course of tubulointerstitial injury progresses, there develops an increasing degree of histologic change or necrosis involving nontubular renal structures, including the glomerulus. With some noteworthy exceptions, such as lead and oxalate-producing toxins, the histologic appearance of nephrotoxic acute renal failure is relatively non-specific. The extent of histologic change and the clinical pattern do, however, show some correlation with the toxin dose. Most patients have some degree of oliguria beginning within hours to days of exposure. With higher doses, the poisoned individual is more likely to be anuric.

Milder cases may have little or no decrease in urinary output and may show only minimal or selective changes in renal excretory pattern, such as aminoaciduria. Many of these mild cases might easily escape detection. Most of the published clinical and experimental experience with nephrotoxic acute renal injury pertains to heavy metals and organic solvents, particularly the halogenated hydrocarbon solvents, but a wide variety of chemicals have been identified or suspected as having potential to produce acute nephrotoxicity (Table 25.3). Similar to the acute pigment nephropathies, however, it is sometimes difficult to characterize the relative nephrotoxicity of many of the individual chemicals for which there is only limited clinical evidence because of the frequent simultaneous toxic effects on other organs.

Metals and other elements

Arsenic. Acute arsenic intoxication, which may occur with ingestion or through inhalation of dusts or fumes, produces a potentially severe multisystem disorder. Trivalent arsenic (e.g., arsenic trioxide) and the generally less toxic pentavalent forms (e.g., arsenates) have limited inherent toxicity for the proximal renal tubules. Acute tubular and cortical necrosis have been observed with acute poisoning, and one case report describes the development of an acute exacerbation of chronic interstitial nephritis with ongoing arsenic ingestion, but in general, nephrotoxicity is not a central feature.[10] Treatment is dictated by the severity of the poisoning. The high potential for inhalation of arsine gas to cause acute renal injury is described above.

Tubulointerstitial nephropathy
Metals and elements
  Antimony*
  Arsenic
  Barium*
  Bismuth*
  Cadmium
  Chromium
  Copper*
  Iron*
  Lead
  Lithium*
  Mercury
  Platinum*
  Silver
  Thallium
  Uranium
  White phosphorus
Metal chelation therapy
  Ethylenediaminetetraacetic acid
  Penicillamine
Glomerular nephropathy
Metals
  Mercury
  Silica/silicon
Organic solvent mixtures
Halogenated hydrocarbons
  Carbon tetrachloride
  Chloroform
  Methylene chloride
  Tetrachloroethane
  1,1,1-Trichloroethane
  Tetrachloroethylene
  Trichloroethylene
  Ethylene dibromide
  Ethylene dichloride
  Allyl chloride[†]
  Chloroprene[†]
  Dibromochlorpropane[†]
  Dichloropropene[†]
  Hexachlorobutadiene[†]
  Vinylidene chloride[†]
Glycols and derivatives
  Ethylene glycol
  Propylene glycol
  Dialkyl glycols
    Diethylene glycol
    Dipropylene glycol
  Monoalkyl glycol ethers
    Methyl cellosolve[‡]
    Ethyl cellosolve[‡]
    Butyl cellosolve[‡]
  Dialkyl glycol ethers
  Dioxane
  Ethylene glycol diacetate
  Ethylene glycol dinitrate
Organic solvent mixtures
  Petroleum distillates
    Diesel oil
    Turpentine
    Gasoline
  Abusive solvent inhalation
Pesticides
  Bipyridyls
    Paraquat
    Diquat
    Morfamquat[†]
  Dinitrophenols and dinitro-o-cresols
  Organic mercurials

* Evidence from pharmacologic use.
† Evidence from experimental animal studies.
‡ Ethylene glycol monomethyl ether.

Table 25.3 Reported nephrotoxic causes of acute renal failure

Cadmium Acute cadmium toxicity, which may occur occupationally with inhalation of fumes produced by welding or burning cadmium-containing metals, primarily and most severely affects the lungs. However, absorbed cadmium rapidly and preferentially accumulates in the liver and kidneys, and renal injury also may occur with acute intoxication, potentially resulting in marked proteinuria or acute tubular or cortical necrosis with renal failure. Use of the chelating agent BAL is contraindicated for acute cadmium toxicity because of its tendency to increase renal cadmium concentrations after acute overexposure and because of the apparent greater nephrotoxicity of the cadmium-BAL complex than of cadmium alone. Other currently available chelating agents either have no ability to extract cadmium from intracellular sites (e.g., ethylenediaminetetra-acetic acid, EDTA) or have been principally studied in animal models of cadmium intoxication (dimercaptosuccinic acid, DMSA, and 2,3-dimercapto-1-propanesulfonic acid, DMPS).[11] Treatment should be supportive.

Chromium. Chromium, particularly in the form of potassium dichromate, is a potent proximal tubular toxin in animal models. In humans, acute renal failure has been produced by ingestion of hexavalent chromium compounds and also through skin burns caused by accidental contact with chromic acid, covering as little as 10% of body surface area.[12] Chromium is dialyzable, and dialysis is recomended for treatment of acute chromium poisoning. Both hemodialysis and continuous peritoneal dialysis have been reported to enhance chances of survival without residual renal dysfunction. Chelating agents have no demonstrated efficacy in chromium intoxication.

Lead. Severe lead poisoning in children is commonly accompanied by transient toxic nephropathy, particularly when blood lead levels exceed 60 μg/dL, and acute encephalopathy. The primary functional abnormality is a proximal tubule reabsorptive defect, which manifests clinically with a Fanconi-like syndrome (generalized aminoaciduria, phosphaturia, glycosuria, increased fractional excretion of urate resulting in hypouricemia, and various degrees of bicarbonate wasting [renal tubular acidosis]). The Fanconi syndrome induced by lead, in contrast to the primary and other secondary forms, also is associated with fructosuria and citraturia. The phosphaturia can be sufficient to cause rickets.

Pathologic evaluation of affected kidneys typically reveals non-specific cytomegaly, mitochondrial morphologic changes, and a relatively characteristic abnormality, acid-fast intranuclear inclusion bodies in the proximal tubule epithelial cells. The glomeruli are generally unaffected or show only minimal, non-specific changes. The inclusion bodies, which consist of a lead-protein complex, can also be demonstrated in urinary sediment and in other non-renal tissues. Both the tubular histologic changes and the reabsorptive defects have been produced experimentally in rats fed dietary lead. Similar intranuclear inclusions have also been described in the kidneys of occupationally lead-exposed workers with evidence of mild renal insufficiency, but they are generally not seen with more advanced stages of chronic lead nephropathy. While the inclusion bodies of acute lead nephropathy resolve during and after the course of chelation treatment and exposure cessation, recent evidence suggests that the proximal tubule resorptive defect can persist for years after the acute exposure.[13] The clinical significance of this persistent resorptive defect remains unclear as it has not been associated with reduced renal function.

Acute lead nephropathy may require specific therapy in the form of electrolyte or bicarbonate replacement to restore metabolic balance, but otherwise, therapy is generally dictated by the severity of manifestations in other organs, which typically present greater acute clinical significance than the nephropathy. Treatment for clinically significant lead intoxication with or without acute nephropathy should include a chelating agent, usually EDTA. When lead nephropathy is present, EDTA therapy should not be withheld because of concern about possible additional nephrotoxicity from EDTA. Although it has not been demonstrated consistently in clinical follow-up investigations, repeated episodes of acute lead intoxication in children may result in a chronic nephropathy and, ultimately, renal failure (discussed in Chronic Renal Disorders Section).

Mercury. The potential for mercury to produce acute nephrotoxicity depends on its chemical form and the nature of the exposure. Mercury poisoning in occupational settings most commonly involves inhalation of elemental mercury, which is highly volatile. Elemental mercury has its primary effects on the lungs and nervous system, and although it is preferentially accumulated in the kidneys, it rarely produces significant renal injury. A variety of organic mercury compounds are used widely as fungicides, and in general, they may be absorbed readily by any route of exposure. While their primary toxic effect is also on the central nervous system, they may also affect the kidneys. It is speculated that the nephrotoxic potential of organic mercury compounds correlates with their tendency to undergo metabolic transformation to inorganic mercury. The phenyl and methoxymethyl mercuric salts have been described in animal models as having nephrotoxic properties similar to those of mercuric chloride (described below). However, there have been only a small number of reports linking organomercurial agents to nephrotoxic injury in humans, with these reports pertaining to chronic rather than acute manifestations.

The soluble inorganic salts of mercury, which are absorbed best by ingestion and weakly with dermal exposure, rarely cause poisoning in occupational settings. Severe renal injury is a major manifestation of accidental or suicidal ingestions, although such poisonings with these agents are uncommon. The mercurous salt (Hg_2Cl_2) is minimally toxic and has even been used as a medicine in the past, but the mercuric salt ($HgCl_2$) is extremely nephrotoxic. If an individual survives the corrosive gastrointestinal injury from an acute ingestion, the major systemic toxic effect is acute proximal tubular necrosis. Severe poisonings progress to oliguric renal failure within several days and generally require dialysis to ensure survival. If a patient survives the initial clinical course, the recovery phase is characterized initially by polyuria and then by progressive resolution of renal impairment toward normal over a course lasting up to several months. Residual renal dysfunction is common, occurring in association with persistent interstitial nephritis, dystrophic calcification of the renal tubules, and end-stage renal disease.

The clinical course of acute poisoning in humans parallels that seen in experimental animal models of acute mercuric chloride nephrotoxicity. In animals, mercury avidly binds to sulfhydryl groups of proteins such as albumin and metallothionein. Within a few hours of exposure, inorganic mercury begins to accumulate in proximal tubular epithelial cells complexed with metallothionein. It is postulated that toxicity occurs when sulfhydryl binding sites on buffering proteins such as metallothionein and glutathione are saturated. At that point mercuric or mercurous ions may bind to more critical cell components and cause dysfunction or damage. When mercury exposure ceases, bound mercury is released slowly with reported half-lives ranging from 10 days to 4 months.[14]

A chelating agent should be administered as early as possible after acute mercury poisoning to bind competitively with free mercury and minimize protein binding and tissue accumulation. In the presence of anuric renal failure, BAL can accumulate to toxic levels and, even in the absence of renal failure, it has the potential to increase central nervous system levels of mercury. Thus, DMPS and DMSA, the water-soluble derivatives of BAL, are now more commonly used. Early hemodialysis, in combination with chelation therapy, has been reported to reduce dramatically the acute mortality of mercury poisoning and the risk of subsequent chronic renal failure.[15]

Silver. There have been reports of acute renal failure among photographic film developers, with the presumed cause being silver exposure. Injections of silver salts in animals have confirmed the ability of silver to induce tubular degeneration associated with renal interstitial silver deposits and relative glomerular sparing.[16]

Uranium. Uranium is a highly potent nephrotoxin, with relatively high specificity for the proximal tubules, and uranyl nitrate injections are used routinely to induce acute tubular necrosis in experimental animals. However, acute renal failure has only rarely been described in humans with overexposure to uranium. One incident involved three workers exposed to a uranium cloud, with each developing transient proteinuria, diminished urine output, and slight increases in BUN levels, but no long-term residual dysfunction. In a case of deliberate overdose, chelation therapy proved ineffective and chronic renal failure with an incomplete Fanconi syndrome resulted from the ingestion.[17] Exposure to low levels of uranium in drinking water was associated with increased urinary excretion of tubular proteins in another study, but no clinical renal disease was detected.[18]

Pharmaceutical agents. A number of metals and other elements are recognized as having the potential to cause nephrotoxic side effects when used as pharmaceutic agents. In general, there are limited parallels between the therapeutic administration (or intentional excessive ingestion) of such agents and occupational exposure to the same or related compounds. The former typically involves ingestion or injection of agents at higher doses and, often, as uniquely different chemical compounds relative to those found in industry. However, their adverse clinical effects should at least be recognized in considering occupational exposures to related compounds. Oral use of *bismuth* compounds, which were used formerly as antisyphilitic therapy, frequently caused acute renal failure or nephrotic syndrome. Renal failure was the most common cause of death with bismuth poisoning. However, metallic bismuth and bismuth oxide are poorly soluble in plasma and are rapidly excreted in the urine and have not been associated with occupational nephrotoxicity. Analogous to lead intoxication, bismuth induces the development of distinctive, refractile inclusion bodies in the epithelial cells of the proximal tubules and causes tubular degeneration. Dialysis has been reported to be beneficial in the treatment of acute poisoning.

Lithium carbonate, which is used widely for the treatment of manic-depressive and other psychiatric disorders, interferes with ion transport in both the proximal and distal tubules and is capable of causing nephrogenic diabetes insipidus and an incomplete distal renal tubular acidosis (impaired urinary acidification after an acid challenge). Diabetes insipidus may be produced or precipitated in chronically exposed individuals by acute lithium overdosage, which may not be completely reversible. However, other than the strong irritant properties and flammability of lithium hydride, industrial experience with lithium has been relatively benign.

Certain organometallic complexes and their salts commonly have adverse renal effects when used as pharmaceutic agents. These effects may have no relevance for industrial situations involving the same metals, particularly in view of the general lack of any recognized human or experimental nephrotoxicity associated with the metallic or inorganic forms of those metals. Three examples are presented here.

Organic *gold* salts, used for the treatment of rheumatoid arthritis, can cause hematuria and proteinuria to nephrotic proportions. The condition is generally at least partially reversible with cessation of therapy and is rarely fatal. Gold toxicity may involve the renal tubules or the glomeruli, depending on the specific compound involved and the dose and chronicity of exposure; gold toxicity has not been described with industrial exposures.

The primary limitation to the use of the cancer chemotherapeutic drug, *cisplatin*, is its potent and dose-related nephrotoxicity. The primary renal sites of involvement are the distal and collecting tubules. Although platinum binding to cytosolic components in dosed animals is usually maximal within 24 hours and urine abnormalities (casts, enzymuria, and proteinuria) may be detected soon after a nephrotoxic dose, azotemia develops slowly in association with polyuria and may take more than 1 week to reach peak levels. Industrial exposures to platinum compounds have been associated with irritant and sensitization effects on mucocutaneous barriers and the respiratory tract, but there have been no reports of acute or chronic renal effects.

Organic *antimony* compounds, which have been used to treat helminthic infections, commonly produce cardiac, hepatic, and to a lesser degree, renal adverse effects, and large doses have produced acute renal failure. Acute industrial inhalation exposures to inorganic antimony compounds have generally been associated with mucocutaneous, respiratory, and gastrointestinal irritant conditions, and rarely, sudden death, but there are no reports of significant renal effect. The hemolytic and secondary renal effects of exposure to stibine, the gaseous anhydride of antimony, were described previously.

Accidental or intentional ingestions. Certain metal compounds, such as inorganic mercury, are potentially nephrotoxic at large doses that are generally only achieved through accidental or intentional ingestion and that are relatively unlikely to occur in industrial settings. Acute thallium poisoning, which has occurred historically through ingestion of rat poisons or depilatory agents, usually affects multiple organ systems and may cause albuminuria, diminished renal concentrating ability, or renal failure. Transient albuminuria occurred in each of six workers poisoned while recovering thallium from flue dust at a sulfuric acid plant. Other examples include copper sulfate, iron (as the pharmaceutical preparation, ferrous sulfate), barium chloride, and elemental white phosphorus. Each of these has produced acute renal failure with massive oral ingestion; however, renal impairment is generally only one feature of severe multisystemic poisoning with these agents, and their inherent nephrotoxicity is relatively low, at the exposure levels expected in most industrial processes.

Metal chelation therapy. It should be recognized that some chelating agents used therapeutically for metal intoxications, EDTA and penicillamine (Cuprimine) for example, have intrinsic potential to cause nephrotoxic injury. In general, however, their use is not contraindicated in metal intoxications in which acute renal insufficiency is not prominent. The primary factors in deciding whether or not to initiate chelation therapy should remain the identity of the metal involved and the overall degree of systemic toxicity.

Halogenated hydrocarbons

Carbon tetrachloride. Carbon tetrachloride is historically the most nephrotoxic of the halogenated hydrocarbons. It was formerly used widely as a cleaner and degreaser but has largely been replaced, other than for use as an intermediate in the synthesis of fluorochlorocarbon compounds. Accidental inhalational poisonings were not uncommon in industrial and domestic settings during previous periods of higher use. Acute overexposure to carbon tetrachloride primarily affects the kidneys and liver, and is accompanied by transient depression of the central nervous system. Kidney damage is relatively more pronounced after inhalation exposure, and liver damage after oral ingestion. Toxicity is mediated by metabolism to a reactive intermediate, probably a free radical, and the kidneys and liver appear to be injured by different mechanisms.

While liver injury is usually maximal within 1–2 days after exposure, renal dysfunction is generally most severe 7–10 days after the exposure, at a time when the liver abnormalities may have nearly resolved. The proximal tubules and loop of Henle are most affected, although the distal tubules also may be involved. In survivors, a subsequent diuretic phase may last for several weeks, and renal function may not return to normal for up to 6 months. Some have suggested that the acute tubular necrosis results from volume depletion during the period of liver injury and that careful volume repletion early in the course may prevent or reverse kidney damage. Despite appropriate treatment with supportive measures and hemodialysis when necessary, carbon tetrachloride poisonings have been fatal in up to 30% of cases. Interestingly, it has been observed clinically and further documented experimentally that acute or chronic ethanol use and acute simultaneous exposure to other alcohols and ketones may worsen the acute toxicity of carbon tetrachloride.[19]

Chloroform. Chloroform is also capable of causing liver and renal injury with acute overexposure, but its toxicity for both organs is much less than that of carbon tetrachloride, and its central anesthetic properties are much greater. Despite extensive use of chloroform as an anesthetic in the past, reports of chloroform nephropathy are relatively uncommon in humans. As is the case with carbon tetrachloride, renal toxicity is more pronounced after inhalation and hepatotoxicity after ingestion.

Others. Although many chlorine and bromine derivatives of LMW aliphatic hydrocarbons are known to be nephrotoxic when administered by inhalation or other routes to experimental animals, clinically significant renal injury is less common and occurs generally in settings of high exposure. Acute inhalation overexposures to the chlorinated solvents in common contemporary use, including tetrachloroethylene, trichloroethylene, and 1,1,1-trichloroethane, typically produce transient abnormalities in BUN or creatinine levels. However, renal tubular and hepatic necrosis have been reported in association with occupational use of tetrachloroethylene in a degreasing tank, and abusive inhalation of trichloroethylene has produced hepatic injury and acute renal failure. Workers exposed to tetrachloroethylene in the dry cleaning industry have been found to have increased urinary excretion of tubular proteins and enzymes in a number of studies, but without significant functional impairment.[20] Ingestion of ethylene dichloride (EDC), which has been used as a solvent, a fumigant, and a chemical intermediate, has produced both liver and kidney injury in humans and animals, but the reports of EDC inhalational poisoning through occupational exposure generally have described liver toxicity without prominent renal involvement.

Ethylene dibromide (EDB), which has been used as a gasoline additive and also as a fumigant, is associated with both acute and chronic renal injury. In animal models, EDB was more toxic with acute inhalation or ingestion exposure than was carbon tetrachloride, and resulted in early hepatic injury and a prolonged course of nephrotoxicity. In humans, there is one case report of overexposure to EDB by inhalation in a confined space that resulted in marked liver necrosis and less severe, proximal renal tubular defects.[21] Other case reports involve suicidal ingestions which are commonly fatal due to liver and renal failure. Treatment is supportive.

Experimental nephrotoxicity. In experimental animal studies, the most acutely toxic halogenated hydrocarbon compound is hexachlorobutadiene (HCBD). Regardless of the route of administration, HCBD exposure results in prominent proximal tubular injury. HCBD has been used as a solvent, a fumigant, and an intermediate in rubber and lubricant production. It is a probable human carcinogen, and its use is now much less than in the past. HCBD is commonly an unwanted byproduct in syntheses of certain chlorinated compounds, and the potential remains for inadequately controlled exposures. HCBD-associated nephrotoxicity has not been documented in humans. In rodents, inhalation of dibromochloropropane (DBCP), a fumigant, primarily affects the testes and kidneys, with single experimental exposures being capable of producing permanent renal injury. DBCP has been established as a human sterilant in both manufacturing and field application settings, but human nephrotoxicity has not been described.

Other halogenated hydrocarbons showing highly potent nephrotoxicity in experimental animals include 1,3-dichloropropene, vinylidene chloride, and allyl chloride (3-chloro-1-propene). The latter is unusual for producing characteristic glomerular changes and interstitial tissue proliferation in addition to tubular injury. Chloroprene is relatively less nephrotoxic in experimental animals but has produced moderate to severe tubular degeneration with single administered doses.

Glycols

Ethylene glycol is classically cited as a severe acute nephrotoxin, and the kidney is in fact the major target organ following ethylene glycol ingestion. However, inhalation or dermal exposures to ethylene glycol are typically limited to mucocutaneous irritation and acute central nervous system intoxication. Consequently, despite common use as a chemical manufacturing substrate, a solvent, and an antifreeze agent, occupational exposures to ethylene glycol have only been associated with acute renal injury in situations of accidental or intentional ingestion. It is theoretically possible, however, that extreme exposure situations such as heating ethylene glycol within a confined space could produce vapor concentrations sufficient to produce systemic and specifically renal toxicity.

Acute ethylene glycol intoxication manifests clinically in three phases. Initial inebriation with central nervous system depression is followed by cardiovascular dysfunction within about 12 hours. Survivors of the acute phase may then go on to develop proteinuria and acute renal failure within 24–72 hours. Anuria may develop and be relatively prolonged. Although ethylene glycol shows some direct effect on the central nervous system, most of its systemic toxicity is attributable to its metabolites. With clinically significant ethylene glycol intoxication, metabolic disturbance including an osmolar gap and a severe anion gap metabolic acidosis results, with accumulation of lactate and consumption of bicarbonate, as well as production of glycine from glycolate and glyoxalate. The end-metabolite oxalate forms calcium oxalate crystals which may cause tissue injury within multiple organs. Renal injury appears to be primarily attributable to intratubular deposition of crystalline oxalate, which is associated with acute tubular necrosis, interstitial nephritis, and focal cortical hemorrhagic necrosis. Oxalate crystals may be demonstrable in urine microscopically or grossly as precipitates.[22]

Early treatment of ethylene glycol intoxication with either ethanol, a competitive inhibitor of the alcohol dehydrogenase enzyme, or 4-methylpyrazole (Fomepizole), a direct inhibitor of the enzyme, may avert the development of acidosis and the need for hemodialysis, though the efficacy of these therapies has not been definitively established. Most patients, however, develop acidosis and renal failure prior to presentation and, for these patients, hemodialysis and aggressive management of acidosis are also critical components of initial treatment. Large cumulative doses of sodium bicarbonate may be necessary to treat the acidosis, and calcium supplementation is often necessary to reverse hypocalcemia. Pyridoxine and thiamine stimulate the metabolism of glyoxalate and have been proposed as additional treatment agents; their use is relatively benign and, therefore, advisable. While dialysis dependence may be prolonged, renal failure frequently reverses.

The derivatives of ethylene glycol include diethylene glycol, dipropylene glycol, the monoalkyl and dialkyl glycol ethers (cellosolves), ethylene glycol diacetate, and dioxane (diethylene dioxide). These derivatives are used in industry, most commonly as solvents, and are known to have analogous and even more severe potential to cause renal injury than ethylene glycol. At least one of these compounds (dioxane) has been linked to deaths related to severe renal and hepatic injury following occupational exposures at relatively high levels for periods of 1 week to 2 months. More commonly, their toxicity is manifested following acute ingestion. The inherent nephrotoxicity of these derivatives may be compounded by the effects of concomitant intravascular hemolysis, particularly with the ether derivatives. It has not been established whether therapy with ethanol or 4-methylpyrazole is efficacious in the management of intoxications with these agents.

Petroleum distillates

Acute tubular necrosis has been produced by short-term exposures to a variety of petroleum distillate fractions. Several case reports have described strong temporal associations between acute oliguric renal failure and short-term exposure to diesel oil. In one case, biopsy-confirmed acute tubular necrosis developed abruptly and then progressively resolved following a several-week period of frequent hand washing with diesel oil. Other cases of acute renal failure with dermal exposure occurred after immersion in seawater contaminated with diesel oil and after hair washing with diesel oil. Isolated reports have described acute nephritic changes and acute renal failure with heavy skin exposure to turpentine and gasoline. One case report described oliguric acute renal failure after exposure to petroleum naphtha, which is widely used as a paint thinner. While renal function returned to normal within 2 weeks, the patient experienced a second episode of acute renal failure several months later after again exposing himself to the same product.[23]

Commercially available petroleum distillates may include more than 100 individual solvent compounds in various proportions, and it is impossible to implicate any specific compound as the nephrotoxic agent in cases involving such mixed exposures. In some instances, however, the reported exposure has involved specific petroleum-derived solvent compounds.

Abusive inhalation of glues and other solvent-based consumer substances results in levels of exposure that far exceed the occupational exposure limit. The abused substances commonly include toluene, as the single or predominant solvent compound, or petroleum distillates. While exposure to toluene at levels below the occupational limit has not been associated with renal toxicity, the more intense exposures associated with abuse can induce acute tubular injury with renal tubular acidosis and renal failure.[24,25] In some but not all reported cases, rhabdomyolysis preceded the renal failure and was undoubtedly a contributing factor.

Bipyridyl herbicides

Poisoning with paraquat, a non-selective herbicide, is most remarkable for the production of profound pulmonary toxicity, including non-cardiogenic pulmonary edema and progressive pulmonary fibrosis. If victims survive the acute systemic and pulmonary effects, proximal tubular dysfunction (including glycosuria, aminoaciduria, and phosphaturia), clinically significant levels of proteinuria, or acute renal failure may develop within 2 to 6 days.[26] Poisonings have been reported most often as a consequence of accidental or intentional ingestion but have also resulted after dermal exposures, generally involving sites with skin abrasions or other lesions, and after inhalation exposure. Early hemodialysis, hemoperfusion, or both, have been recommended to expedite removal of paraquat from the blood, enhance chances of survival, and minimize subsequent chronic pulmonary disease. Peritoneal dialysis appears to be ineffective. The renal effects of diquat poisoning are generally more pronounced than those of paraquat, and

the pulmonary toxicity is generally less;[27] the treatment is the same. Another bipyridyl herbicide, morfamquat, has been used less extensively, and there is no human experience relating to its toxicity to date; however, it is known to cause renal damage in experimental animals and should be regarded as a likely human nephrotoxin.

Biologic toxins

Exposures to biologic toxins can occur with greater prevalence in some occupations, although these generally do not represent singularly occupational hazards. Environmental factors associated with allergic reactions, including poison ivy, poison oak, hymenoptera (e.g., bees and wasps) stings, certain snake bites, and plant allergens, have produced the nephrotic syndrome, presumably involving an immunologic mechanism. Other environmental factors, including the venoms introduced by the bites or stings of certain arthropods, hymenoptera, and snakes, have direct toxic effects which may produce multisystem injury, in many cases including acute renal failure. Ingestion of certain mushrooms and plants also may produce such clinical pictures. Hemolysis or rhabdomyolysis may be involved. These biologic toxins will not be discussed in further detail.[6]

Acute toxic glomerulonephropathy

Glomerulonephropathies have developed relatively abruptly in the setting of chronic or subchronic exposures to mercury, silica, and mixtures of organic solvents. These are discussed in greater detail subsequently. It is noteworthy that a number of case reports have described the onset of rapidly progressive glomerulonephritis or specifically anti-GBM glomerulonephritis (both with pulmonary involvement [Goodpasture's syndrome] and without) within periods as short as days following short-term exposures to various organic solvent mixtures.[28] It has also been reported that individuals with glomerulonephritis may show exacerbations and improvements in renal function, respectively when increasing, resuming, or discontinuing occupational solvent exposures. This temporal association supports a causative or aggravating role for acute solvent exposures or in the clinical manifestations of some glomerulonephritides. The available evidence for an acute solvent-induced glomerulonephritis is limited to case reports at this time. In contrast, a much larger body of epidemiologic evidence indicates there is likely a causal association between chronic occupational solvent exposures and the development of glomerulonephritis (described in the next section).

Chronic renal disorders

Chronic tubulointerstitial nephropathy

Data from experimental exposure situations identify the proximal tubule as the primary target for many occupational nephrotoxins. In the absence of close surveillance, early renal damage from these agents generally escapes detection, however, and by the time a patient presents for evaluation the primary lesions have usually been obscured by other direct and indirect toxic effects. Histopathologic studies generally reveal only non-specific abnormalities of renal architecture, particularly diffuse interstitial fibrosis.

Cadmium. The kidney is the primary target organ for cadmium toxicity. Cadmium has an exceptionally long half-life in the body of greater than 10 years. After initial accumulation in the liver, chronic, low-level exposure results in up to 50% of the cadmium body burden being concentrated in the kidneys, primarily in the renal cortex bound to metallothionein. Urine cadmium levels serve little purpose in evaluating recent cadmium exposures, but can serve as an indicator of the cumulative body burden, long after cadmium exposures have ceased. Cross-sectional studies of occupationally and environmentally exposed populations, using either historic information or urine cadmium concentrations as measures of long-term exposure, have repeatedly documented cumulative exposure-related increases in serum creatinine concentration and in urinary excretion of tubular proteins.[29]

A majority of these studies have examined urine β2M levels, but urine measurements of many other tubular proteins and enzymes such as RBP and NAG have also been utilized to demonstrate the effect of cadmium on renal function. Epidemiologic studies indicate that the relationship between cadmium exposure and tubulotoxic effects follows a threshold pattern, with estimates of the necessary cumulative cadmium exposure ranging between 5 and 20 years at current permissible exposure levels. Findings from animal and in-vivo human investigations support the concept of a critical concentration for cadmium in the renal cortex, and suggest that renal tubular dysfunction is likely to occur when the renal cortical concentration of cadmium reaches 200 μg/g. Urinary cadmium concentrations generally exceed 10 μg/g creatinine at this point.[29]

The most common manifestations in both early and late stages of cadmium nephrotoxicity are deficiencies of proximal tubular reabsorption. The first sign is usually a tubular proteinuria, but glycosuria, phosphaturia, calciuria, and generalized aminoaciduria also may be evident. HMW proteinuria also may occur, although it rarely achieves clinically significant levels. Albuminuria may occur in the absence of significant tubular proteinuria, suggesting that cadmium may have adverse effects at both glomerular and tubular levels of the nephron. It should be noted that the absolute urine concentration of albumin, which is normally present in the urine in measurable levels, will invariably exceed those of smaller molecular weight proteins, even in the context of substantial tubular proteinuria. The relative increase of albumin or total protein in the urine compared with normal values, however, is usually orders of magnitude less than the relative increases in low molecular weight proteins, which may be increased 1000-fold in chronically exposed workers. Therefore, qualitative and quantitative measurements of urine total protein or albumin have little utility in the early or preclinical stages of cadmium nephropathy.

Urine measurements of LMW proteins have proved effective in monitoring cadmium-exposed workers and are routinely employed in industries using cadmium. Urine cadmium can serve as a marker of both cumulative exposure and the presence of renal disease; for an assessment of recent cadmium exposure, blood measurement may be more useful. The biologic standards adopted by the Occupational Safety and Health Administration (OSHA) in 1999 require more intensive monitoring and follow-up of workers who have screening urine cadmium levels > 3 μg/g creatinine, urine β2M > 300 μg/g creatinine, or blood cadmium > 5 μg/L whole blood. Medical removal of workers may be required when urine cadmium levels are > 7 μg/g creatinine, β2M > 750 μg/g creatinine, or blood cadmium > 10 μg/L whole blood. The complete OSHA standard and monitoring protocol should be consulted and utilized to guide individual patient care.[30,31]

Abnormal proteinuria is rarely observed when the urine cadmium concentration is below 5–10 μg/g creatinine, but urine cadmium levels at or above this threshold are associated with a higher risk for renal tubular dysfunction. The risk of renal involvement increases progressively with higher urine cadmium levels. It has been well established that the nephrotoxic effects of cadmium can be irreversible and can progress even after cessation of exposure. Periods of follow-up extending for 5 or more years after workers have been removed from exposure because of increased urine β2M levels have demonstrated significant average increases in urine proteins and serum creatinine, as well as progressive nephrocalcinosis. Nevertheless, exposure cessation may delay the development of clinically significant abnormalities in these parameters.

The natural history of cadmium toxicity is characterized by gradual progression of proteinuria with renal failure or osteomalacia described only in isolated cases among occupationally exposed workers. Environmental studies have generally demonstrated progressive but persistent subclinical tubular damage, manifested by increasing excretion of tubular proteins and enzymes. In contrast, urinary calculi are not uncommon among long-term cadmium-exposed workers; the prevalence is undetermined but was reported to be as high as 44% in one series. The dramatic Itai-Itai disease, which affected individuals who consumed food contaminated by cadmium in one region of Japan, is characterized by painful bone disease, osteomalacia, and pseudofractures attributed to disordered calcium, phosphate, and vitamin D metabolism caused or influenced by the cadmium-induced renal damage.

Renal pathologic findings in advanced cases have included frank kidney contraction, tubular atrophy and dilation, interstitial fibrosis, with relative sparing of glomeruli at the microscopic level. Varying degrees of proteinuria occur with some cases progressing to renal failure. The significance of minor signs of renal dysfunction attributable to cadmium may have greater significance in the context of other diseases. For example, one study of individuals residing in areas of Belgium with relatively high levels of environmental cadmium contamination found that those with diabetes were more susceptible to chronic cadmium nephrotoxicity. Other groups at potentially higher risk include women, the elderly, smokers, and those with iron deficiency.

Historic cohort mortality studies of cadmium-exposed working populations have yielded mixed results in studying end-stage renal disease as a cause of death. At least two studies of worker cohorts have reported greater than expected numbers of deaths from renal disease, with insufficient power to demonstrate statistical significance. Two larger mortality studies found no cadmium-associated risk after adjustment for potential confounding factors, but a nested case-control study conducted within the combined cohorts from those two studies found a two-fold increased risk of death from nephritis and nephrosis among workers with relatively high career exposure to cadmium. Several studies have demonstrated increased all-cause mortality in environmentally exposed subjects, with evidence of cadmium-induced kidney damage at baseline; however, the proportion of these deaths that is attributable to renal disease is not known.[29,32]

There is no established treatment for cadmium-induced tubular nephropathy beyond removal from further exposure. Reductions in urine protein excretion have been described when individuals with mild and presumably early dysfunction reduce or cease their exposure to cadmium. One retrospective study found that workers whose urine β2M levels were less than 1000 μg/g creatinine and whose urine cadmium levels never exceeded 20 μg/g creatinine when exposure was reduced or stopped, showed evidence of reversible toxicity.[3] The long-term significance of this initial improvement is questionable in light of multiple studies describing slow progression of dysfunction. It has also been reported that calcium and vitamin D replacement can slow the progression of associated osteomalacia, but such treatment is probably contraindicated other than in severe cases because of the risk for nephrocalcinosis. Chelating agents have no demonstrated effectiveness for the condition.[11]

Lead. Lead remains a widely used metal, and toxic exposures still occur commonly in both occupational and general environments. Chronic renal failure and the pathologic manifestations of end-stage renal disease were identified as late manifestations of chronic occupational lead exposure during the 19th and early 20th centuries, but with improved control of lead exposures in contemporary workplaces in the developed world, chronic lead nephropathy has become a relatively rare clinical diagnosis. The progression from acute and reversible lead nephropathy to the chronic and irreversible form has been demonstrated reproducibly in rodent models, and there are several lines of human evidence that indicate that lead exposure causes or contributes to chronic renal disease.[33]

The strongest evidence for the existence of a chronic lead nephropathy comes from clinical and pathologic investigations in Queensland, Australia. At the turn of the last century, chronic nephritis occurred there with excessive frequency among young adults, particularly those with histories of childhood lead poisoning. For at least 10

years before the recognized increase in renal disease, acute lead poisoning had been a problem among children in this region who played on and under wooden verandas that were routinely coated with lead-containing paints. The use of lead paint was prohibited there in 1922, and the occurrence of chronic renal disease progressively declined, approaching the rates seen in other provinces by the 1940s and 1950s. A retrospective follow-up study of children hospitalized for plumbism between 1915 and 1935 established the status of 352 (of 401) former patients in 1954 and found that 165 had died by age 40 years or younger, including 107 who had died with causes of death listed as nephritis variants.

A 1956 autopsy study, which included 67 Queensland natives who died between the ages of 20 and 50 years with chronic nephritis, found the lead content of skull and rib bones to be twice as high among cases of idiopathic renal disease than among cases with non-renal disease or renal disease of other established causes. A follow-up study of childhood lead poisoning victims from the 1920s and 1930s in Boston, however, did not reveal either any significant predilection for renal disease or premature death. It has been hypothesized that chronic renal disease was averted because these children received chelation therapy.[34] Other supportive clinical evidence comes from the historically observed cases of chronic renal failure among moonshine drinkers. In addition to having impaired renal function, drinkers of lead-contaminated alcohol had evidence of high total body lead by EDTA lead mobilization testing; renal biopsy specimens revealed intranuclear inclusion bodies in renal epithelial cells, a characteristic of acute lead nephropathy in children.

The other major body of evidence for a chronic lead-induced nephropathy comes from studies of occupationally exposed individuals. One study of 140 deaths among a subcohort of 241 Australian lead smelter workers, who had formerly been acutely lead poisoned, found a five-fold increased risk of death from chronic renal disease in comparison to other lead-exposed, but never acutely poisoned, workers from the same smelter. In addition, three large historic cohort studies of battery or smelter workers exposed to lead demonstrated twice the expected risk for mortality from chronic renal disease (and some hypertension-related diseases), with 20 years of exposure being associated with a four-fold increased risk for death from renal disease. With extended follow-up, however, this excess mortality from non-malignant renal disease became attenuated.[35,36] Many epidemiologic studies have documented an association between higher blood lead levels (greater than 60 μg/dL) and elevated serum creatinine in lead-exposed workers.[37] Low level environmental lead exposures have been associated with elevated blood lead levels and increases in serum creatinine as well, although the magnitude of the rise in creatinine is small and the clinical significance uncertain.[38]

In general, clinical tests have not been valuable in assessing asymptomatic lead-exposed workers. Cross-sectional studies have not found clinical parameters, such as BUN, to be higher than laboratory reference values, or to correlate with historic or laboratory measures of lead exposure. A number of studies have demonstrated increased excretion of tubular proteins such as NAG by patients with elevated blood lead levels, but the clinical significance of these findings remains unclear.

A comprehensive clinical evaluation of 140 lead-exposed workers (only five of whom were symptomatic) found 57 who had abnormally high lead excretion (>650 μg) with EDTA chelation challenge and no other disease. Of these 57 workers, 21 had reduced GFRs (less than 87 mL/min/1.73m^3 body surface area, by iodothalamate clearance) and comparable reductions in effective renal plasma flow (by PAH clearance), with no obvious alternative explanation for renal dysfunction.[39] Only three had elevations of serum creatinine or BUN. Six of 12 asymptomatic subjects with abnormal kidney function underwent renal biopsy, with light microscopic changes demonstrating focal tubular atrophy, interstitial disease, and generally normal glomeruli. Two subjects had some evidence of glomerular sclerosis. Fluorescence microscopy revealed various patterns of immunoglobulin deposition in tubular and glomerular basement membranes in the seven cases so studied. Among eight subjects who had reduced GFRs and who underwent thrice weekly EDTA chelation treatment for 6 to 50 months, four showed 20% or greater improvements in GFR (two worsened and two showed no change), with normalization of EDTA-mobilized lead excretion. The authors characterized the observed treatment response as evidence of probable lead causation and as effective reversal of preclinical lead-induced renal dysfunction. They did not, however, recommend EDTA therapy for established lead nephropathy. In another study, the same investigators also found that the degree of EDTA-mobilized lead excretion correlated highly with increases in serum creatinine among 44 men with gout (including 26 with histories of industrial lead or moonshine exposure), a condition that historically has been associated with lead exposure. The investigators speculated that, not only some proportion of non-specific or idiopathic chronic renal disease cases, but also some cases with an identifiable cause, such as gout or hypertension, may be primarily attributable to chronic lead toxicity.[40]

Once diagnosed, the treatment for chronic interstitial nephritis attributed to lead is non-specific, other than elimination of further lead exposure. There is no clear evidence that long-term EDTA chelation therapy improves the course of clinically established chronic lead nephropathy. The possibility exists that long-term EDTA administration in renally compromised patients may itself have an adverse renal effect. Wedeen and coworkers recommend that such treatment only be undertaken with careful follow-up and with a clearly defined endpoint, such as normalization of EDTA-challenge response or improvement in renal excretory function within an a priori designated time frame.[39]

Mercury. Acute poisoning with mercuric salts, described previously, can result in persistent renal impairment characterized primarily by tubular dysfunction. Workers chronically exposed to mercuric salts have been reported to have increased urinary excretion of certain lysosomal enzymes,

particularly NAG, suggesting the presence of proximal tubular dysfunction or injury. Tubular proteinuria also occurs with Minamata disease, a severe neurotoxic disorder that occurred in an outbreak caused by dietary ingestion of seafood contaminated by methyl mercury. However, despite the generally higher affinity of methyl mercury for renal than neurologic tissues, the proteinuria of Minamata disease was not associated with marked azotemia and renal impairment.

Beryllium. Chronic beryllium exposure is well established as a cause of granulomatous pneumoconiosis (berylliosis) or chronic beryllium disease (CBD) and has also been associated with extrapulmonary involvement; skin and, to lesser degrees, liver and lymph nodes are the most commonly described extrapulmonary sites of beryllium deposition and pathologic changes. There have been reports of pathologic changes in other organs, including the kidneys. Renal pathologic changes consistent with old or scarred granulomas (Schaumann bodies associated with local beryllium deposition) have been reported. Most of the reported cases with renal pathologic changes have described hyperemia and intrarenal calculi. Hypercalcemia and hypercalciuria have also been reported frequently with CBD, and nephrolithiasis has been present in as many as 10% to 30% of cases, with passage of calcium oxalate- (and beryllium-)containing urinary stones.[41]

Other elements. Cross-sectional epidemiologic studies of chrome platers and of workers with long-term exposures to uranium dust have found slight but statistically significant increases in urine tubular protein excretion. However, no links have been established between chronic exposures to either of these agents and development of clinically significant renal dysfunction. Germanium is sometimes used (in inorganic forms, such as germanium oxide) as a component of folk remedies or health elixirs. There have been at least 13 reported cases of nephropathy associated with regular ingestion of such mixtures over periods spanning 6 to 20 months. The pathologic findings on renal biopsy have uniformly appeared as chronic tubulointerstitial nephritis, typically with proximal or distal tubular degeneration and interstitial fibrosis, and without significant glomerular injury or evidence of immunologic mechanism. The systemic toxicity of germanium in experimental exposures is low, but the kidneys and liver are usually affected.[42]

Chronic glomerulonephropathy

Mercury. Chronic elemental mercury poisoning primarily affects the central nervous system but also may produce proteinuria. There is human and animal evidence that elemental and inorganic mercury are capable of inducing an immunologically mediated glomerular abnormality and proteinuria that occasionally may reach nephrotic proportions. Young children with exposure to mercury ointment may have acrodynia, an idiosyncratic and presumably allergic reaction whose central features are dermatologic, but which may be associated with proteinuria. There have also been a number of reports of transient proteinuria and overt nephrotic syndrome occurring idiosyncratically among workers with chronic or subacute exposure to metallic or inorganic mercury. The syndrome has occurred with various degrees of mercury exposure but, typically, without other manifestations of mercury toxicity. Most of the reported cases have resolved completely after cessation of exposure.

The most frequent pathologic pattern on renal biopsy has been a membranous-like glomerulonephropathy, with deposits of immune complex in the glomerular basement membrane, although normal and other immunofluorescent patterns have also been described. An analogous phenomenon can be induced experimentally in rodents by repeated subcutaneous or intramuscular injection of mercuric chloride or by injection or inhalation of a variety of organic mercury compounds, with glomerular deposition of antiglomerular antibodies. A progressive membranous nephropathy with glomerular deposition of immune complexes ensues, followed by resolution of both immunologic and histopathologic changes. Despite consistent reproducibility in selected genetically susceptible experimental animals, it appears that the mercury-induced proteinuric syndrome occurs rarely in humans. Recent cross-sectional studies of exposed workers have found no increase in urinary albumin, anti-GBM antibodies or other autoantibodies.[43,44]

Other metal exposures have been reported in association with proteinuria of probable glomerulotoxic origin. As discussed earlier, organic gold salts, used for the treatment of rheumatoid arthritis, can cause hematuria and proteinuria up to nephrotic proportions. A pharmacologic preparation of bismuth (bismuth tartrate), which previously also was used in the treatment of rheumatoid arthritis, reportedly caused nephrotic syndrome. Nickel carbonyl inhalation in experimental rats produced proteinuria.

Silica. There is mounting evidence that silica exposure increases the risk for renal disease. Animals exposed to silica under experimental conditions have developed a variety of nephrotoxic effects, including glomerulosclerosis. Three studies have documented subclinical renal dysfunction in silica-exposed workers as evidenced by increased urinary excretion of both glomerular (albumin and transferrin) and tubular (RBP and NAG) proteins. These abnormalities were found independent of silicosis, and with either short- or long-term exposure.

Numerous case reports have described biopsy proven proliferative glomerulonephritis in persons exposed to silica (either with silicosis or without any pulmonary disease), and two recent studies document an increased risk for end-stage renal disease (particularly due to glomerulonephritis) in silica-exposed workers.[45,46] In addition, two case-control studies of patients with either rapidly progressive glomerulonephritis and antineutrophil cytoplasmic antibodies (ANCA) consistent with Wegener's granulomatosis found an increased incidence of silica exposure in these patients compared with controls.[47,48] The mechanism

for this putative nephrotoxicity is not well understood and may involve both a direct nephrotoxic effect as well as an immune-mediated mechanism of injury.

Supporting the argument for a direct toxic effect is a case report of acute renal failure following acute overexposure to silica without associated immune deposits on renal biopsy. However, the lack of a clear dose–response relationship and the frequent finding of immune deposits on biopsy specimens argue in favor of an immune-mediated mechanism. In all likelihood, both mechanisms of injury may play a role. Silica-related nephrotoxicity may progress to chronic renal failure and even death, despite steroid treatment and hemodialysis. In one reported case, aggressive immunosuppressive therapy was judged to be helpful.

Organic solvents. Organic solvents have been implicated as either causative or contributing agents in the development of a variety of primary glomerular disorders. While this has not been replicated in studies, a number of investigations have described increased levels of selected urine proteins among groups of workers with chronic exposure to solvents. Cohort mortality studies have not revealed clearly increased risk for death from primary glomerular diseases.

The main evidence in support of there being a causal association between organic solvents and glomerulonephritis comes from an extensive series of case reports and case-control epidemiologic investigations.[49] The case reports have generally described instances of anti-GBM glomerulonephritis occurring in the context of either chronic, subchronic, or acutely excessive exposures to a variety of organic solvents in both occupational and domestic settings. The predominance of anti-GBM glomerulonephritis among reported cases has indicated an anti-GBM immunopathogenic mechanism, possibly initiated by interactions between inhaled solvent vapors and pulmonary alveolar basement membrane, which share common antigenic properties. However, the findings of case-control studies indicate that the increased risk for glomerulonephritis associated with solvent exposure is greater than can be explained by anti-GBM glomerulonephritis alone, indicating a broader association with many types of primary glomerulonephritis.

At least 15 case-control studies have examined the relationship between solvents and glomerulonephritis, and many have described significantly increased risks, ranging up to nine-fold increases, for solvent exposures that exceed the usual population experience.[50] The studies have included all types of primary glomerulonephritis, suggesting either that the estimated risk extends to all types or that an even greater risk may be attached to some subgroup of glomerulonephritis. Two studies that examined single categories of glomerular disease, proliferative in one study and membranous in the other, both found substantially increased risks associated with solvent exposure. The case-control studies have been criticized for methodologic limitations, such as the recall bias inherent to retrospective interview studies. However, the credibility of these studies is supported by the consistency and reproducibility of findings across numerous investigations (each having different types and degrees of methodologic limitation), the high magnitude and statistical significance of the risk estimates, and the evidence for a dose–response relationship in each study that examined subgroups defined by time or intensity of exposure.[28]

The chemical structural diversity of the associated solvent compounds, the widespread prevalence of solvent use, and the relative rarity of primary glomerulonephritis suggest that any pathogenic mechanism involving organic solvents is probably multifactorial or relatively idiosyncratic. Although the risk for glomerulonephritis may be greater with solvent exposure, solvent exposures appear to be involved in only a small proportion of glomerulonephritis cases. The weight of evidence favors any effect of solvents being non-specific and not limited to specific solvent compounds. Immune mechanisms are probably involved, and it is plausible that there is an immunogenetic predisposition. It may be that potentially glomerulotoxic immune factors arise independently of solvent exposure and that solvents interact with those factors or with renal tissue to precipitate or facilitate the development of glomerulonephritis. For example, when anti-GBM antibodies were injected into rabbits, the antibodies adhered to alveolar basement membrane after intratracheal instillation of gasoline, but not after saline instillation. Other than cessation of further exposures, there is no specific treatment for cases of glomerulonephritis associated with organic solvents. The clinical severity of primary glomerulonephritis has been observed to fluctuate adversely with variations in intensity of continued solvent exposure, and it is prudent to recommend avoidance of non-incidental solvent exposure for any individual with glomerulonephritis.

Vascular nephropathy

Chronic exposure to carbon disulfide may accelerate atherosclerosis, and epidemiologic studies of chronically exposed workers have demonstrated significantly increased risks for cardiovascular disease. In addition, an increased prevalence of hypertension has been reported among exposed workers. One study of artificial silk workers reported that half of those with 20 or more years exposure were hypertensive. Carbon disulfide-induced renovascular disease has been invoked to explain this observation. This hypothesis is supported by one clinical study that evaluated 26 carbon disulfide-exposed workers, 16 of whom were hypertensive or had a history of hypertension. The effective renal plasma flow (ERPF, as measured by PAH clearance) was significantly lower on average in the entire group in comparison to eight normotensive and non-exposed control subjects. When creatinine clearance was measured in the five subjects with the lowest ERPFs, four had normal creatinine clearances and relatively high filtration ratios (creatinine clearance/ PAH clearance). These findings support the presence of intrarenal vascular changes.

Renal papillary necrosis

Renal papillary necrosis is an uncommon condition that may occur in association with a variety of intrarenal, urologic, and systemic conditions. In clinical series, it has been associated most often with diabetes mellitus and, in others, with excessive analgesic use. It is particularly strongly associated with excessive use of phenacetin-containing analgesics, although most, if not all, analgesics and non-steroidal anti-inflammatory agents have the potential to cause this condition in humans and animals. Other medical agents also have been incriminated as possible causes, including phenothiazines, cyclophosphamide (Cytoxan), and radiocontrast agents, and it has been speculated that other drugs and chemicals may also contribute to or cause renal papillary necrosis. Although it has not been demonstrated to occur in humans with occupational exposures to many chemicals, it has been produced in experimental animal exposures using a variety of chemicals that either have been used in industry, are structurally related to industrial chemicals, or are recognized as industrial pollutants. These include methylaniline, tetrahydroquinoline, ethylenimine, bromoethanamine, diphenylamine, diphenylmethyl alcohol, phenylanthranilic acid, aminopyrene, dioxin, and PCBs (specifically, Aroclor 1242). In managing cases of renal papillary necrosis, therefore, it is reasonable at least to consider the possible role of antecedent occupational chemical exposures.

Renal cystic disease

Renal cystic disease (RCD) in humans is most often attributable to heritable conditions, particularly autosomal dominant polycystic kidney disease. It is clear, however, from clinical experience and animal experiments that heritable factors are not solely involved in the development of RCD and that cyst development can occur in the absence of heritable factors. For example, RCD occurs in up to 40% of patients undergoing chronic dialysis therapy, including patients with previously non-cystic kidneys. Chemical factors have been considered as possible causes of this acquired condition. Although certain experimental animal species have been identified as having inherited predispositions to renal cyst development, renal cyst formation can be induced reproducibly and in a dose-related manner by experimental exposures to a variety of drugs and chemicals, independent of identifiable predisposition.

Diphenylamine and diphenylthiazole are well characterized experimentally as cystogenic agents. Diphenylamine also produces renal cysts in the offspring of female rats exposed during pregnancy. Cyst formation has also been produced experimentally by lead acetate, diethylhexyl phthalate, dibutyl phthalate, 2,4,5-trichlorphenoxyacetic acid, alloxan, biphenyl, lithium (lithium chloride), and cisplatin, the latter two of which are pharmaceutic agents that have been related adversely to cyst formation in humans. RCD has not been recognized to occur in association with any occupational chemical exposure, but the possibility should be considered in patients with RCD and no family history or obvious alternative explanation.

Radiation nephritis

Renal involvement is generally not a direct feature of ionizing radiation exposure produced either by internal emitters, which gain entry to the body, or by acute whole-body external radiation (radiation sickness). Renal injury commonly occurs following excessive partial-body external radiation exposure to sites including the retroperitoneum; however, this is described only with therapeutic radiation and usually at cumulative doses exceeding 2300 rads (23 Gy) over a several-week period. Such exposure produces no clinically detectable acute changes other than local skin changes, but it may result in acute radiation nephritis up to 6–12 months later.

The acute nephritis usually manifests with hypertension, which in turn, may produce proteinuria, microhematuria and azotemia. It may occur in the setting of cardiac failure and a relatively refractory anemia. The initial renal pathologic injury includes degenerative changes of the tubular epithelial and glomerular endothelial cells and may progress (as the chronic condition) to include extensive atrophic changes and interstitial fibrosis. The mortality rate is generally high, and survivors often have persistent proteinuria or renal insufficiency. Chronic radiation nephritis may develop years after exposure, with or without acute radiation nephritis in the interim. It is characterized by clinical features similar to the acute condition, although the condition is generally slowly progressive and does not show spontaneous improvement. Malignant hypertension and its complications are common, particularly in the chronic syndrome.

Hypertension

Lead. Chronic lead exposure is associated with subclinical increases in blood pressure and may also increase the risk for developing hypertension. By the early 20th century, it was generally accepted that hypertension was a clinical manifestation of chronic lead poisoning. However, subsequent controlled epidemiologic studies of lead-exposed working populations have generally not demonstrated substantial increases in either hypertension or mortality from hypertensive diseases. Many authorities now question the existence, or at least the clinical significance, of any inherent hypertensive effect of lead beyond that secondarily attributable to lead-associated chronic renal insufficiency. There is, however, evidence indicating that lead exposure has some degree of hypertensive effect. Each of two large population-based studies in the United States and Great Britain found that higher blood lead levels were significant predictors of hypertension, and that the blood lead level showed a statistically significant, although small, positive association with both systolic and diastolic blood pressure.[51,52] Experimental animal studies have demonstrated that dietary lead can increase blood pressure and that lead, even at low levels, may produce changes in the balance of renin and angiotensin.

Blood lead appears to make a small proportional contribution to blood pressure in the general population, relative to other risk factors. However, in situations that differ from the general population experience, lead may be a more substantial contributor to blood pressure elevation. For example, a study in the west of Scotland, where plumb-

ing systems commonly contain lead parts, found significantly higher blood lead levels among 130 hypertensive subjects than among matched normotensive subjects. Blood lead levels also were higher among normotensive individuals with elevated serum urea levels. Another study that included 20 men with essential hypertension and normal renal function observed significantly higher blood lead levels among hypertensive subjects than the normotensive controls.[53] In each study, occult lead exposure was presumed to be a contributing factor to the development of hypertension. Duration of lead exposure may be more strongly associated with blood pressure than elevations in blood lead levels. Because of this, the EDTA lead mobilization test has been suggested as one potentially helpful test for evaluating selected patients with essential hypertension, but it is not broadly accepted as such. In the absence of other manifestations of lead intoxication, there is no indication for chelation treatment for hypertension associated with increased body burden of lead.

Cadmium. Cadmium has also been linked with hypertension. Some, but not all, animal experiments have demonstrated a cadmium hypertensive effect at levels of exposure below those producing evident renal damage. Studies of industrially and environmentally exposed individuals, however, have generally found no substantial increase in hypertension. In summary, the data regarding a possible cadmium hypertensive effect are equivocal, but this issue has not been addressed as closely for cadmium as for lead.[54]

Carbon disulfide. Chronic exposure to carbon disulfide is associated with an increased risk for hypertension and hypertensive diseases. The hypertensive effect is presumed to be the result of vascular nephropathy (discussed earlier).

Non-renal urinary tract disorders

Urolithiasis

The acute toxic nephropathy induced by ethylene glycol is mediated in part by the intratubular concentration and crystallization of calcium oxalate (described earlier). Although it is believed that tubular obstruction by these crystals is the major mechanism by which renal injury is produced, acute oxalate crystal formation is not associated with clinically significant obstruction distally in the urinary tract. There is no reported increase in risk for stone formation among individuals with chronic ethylene glycol exposure in the occupational setting.

Urinary calculi have been reported with high frequency in some studies of long-term cadmium-exposed workers, with prevalence reported as high as 44% in one series involving Swedish workers. This risk for stone formation has not been observed in all series of cadmium-exposed workers, however, and the wide differences in prevalence remain unexplained. Hypercalciuria is usually present with cadmium-associated urolithiasis, and it is believed to play a primary role in stone formation. Other possible contributory effects of cadmium include its interference with calcium-binding proteins and calcium deposition in bone.

There are a variety of other uncommon or speculative causes of urolithiasis. Chronic beryllium exposure is rarely associated with chronic tubulointerstitial nephritis (described earlier), and this may be accompanied by passage of small calcium oxalate stones, which may contain beryllium. Silica stones are common in domestic grazing animals, particularly in regions where the amount of silicon in forage is high. However, although silicon is a common component of calcium oxalate, uric acid, and phosphate stones in humans, silica-predominant stones occur rarely in humans and are only known to occur with chronic magnesium trisilicate antacid use. It should be noted that, although primary gout may lead to urate nephrolithiasis, there is no identified risk for stone formation with saturnine (lead-induced) gout, even though it may produce hyperuricemia and hyperuricosuria. There is also no evidence that manganese causes urolithiasis, but it may be noteworthy that manganese can interfere with the synthesis of glycosaminoglycans, which have been hypothesized to play inhibitory roles in calcium oxalate crystal growth and aggregation in urine. Bilateral renal calculi and aminoaciduria have been reported with excessive intake of Worcestershire sauce, representing a suspected environmental lithogen. No specific component of the sauce was identified as the possible cause.

Bladder disorders

Neurogenic bladder. A number of pharmacologic agents are capable of causing bladder dysfunction. In the late 1970s, neurogenic bladder associated with the polyurethane foam catalytic agent dimethylaminoproprionitrile (DMAPN) occurred in epidemic proportions at two separate polyurethane manufacturing plants following introduction of the agent, and additional symptomatic cases were later identified at five other plants.[55] Although DMAPN had already been used as a catalyst in an acrylamide waterproofing process for more than 10 years without any recognized problem, more than one-half of the exposed workers at the polyurethane plant had symptomatic bladder dysfunction, most often manifested as urinary retention. Of individuals referred for neurologic evaluation, seven of eight reported cases lacked either a detrusor reflex or normal sensation of bladder filling, and three had prolonged sacral latencies, with two of those three having evidence of partial denervation on external anal sphincter examination.

Electrophysiologic findings of distal extremity peripheral neuropathy were also present in most members of this selected subgroup. Broad surveys at the affected plants also revealed symptomatic evidence of sexual dysfunction (partial impotence and increased libido) and non-specific symptoms of irritability, insomnia, and headaches. The symptoms of urinary retention occurred as early as 1 week after the first exposure, and persisted without improvement in most cases until the DMAPN exposure ceased. About one-half of cases improved within 1–2 weeks after the agent was withdrawn, and of the 14% who were still symptomatic after 3 months, nearly all were still symptomatic 2 years later. Several individuals still had objective findings on cystometric and electrophysiologic examinations.

Experimental animal studies and isolated reports of human pathologic studies of biopsied sural nerves indicate that the primary site of DMAPN action is probably the neuronal axon. The predominance of genitourinary over extremity dysfunction is unusual for toxic neuropathies and is still not fully explained. Urinary difficulties have also been described in a few cases of neuropathy from acrylamide, another nitrile compound, but these manifestations of autonomic involvement have only appeared late in the course of peripheral neuropathy. Rodents can develop urine retention in less than 12 hours after oral doses of DMAPN, and then bladder function returns to normal within 2 to 3 days. A study of rats exposed separately to equimolar doses of DMAPN, cyanoacetic acid, and dimethylamine found urinary retention in 100%, 50%, and 25%, of animals respectively. The relevance of these additional findings is not established for human exposures.

Cystitis. Acute hemorrhagic cystitis and urinary irritative symptoms (e.g., dysuria and frequent urination) have occurred in humans with exposures to formamidine pesticides, toluidines (methyl aniline homologues), and chlorotoluidines. The conditions have generally cleared promptly after exposure cessation. As an illustration, two individuals had abdominal pain, dysuria, and gross hematuria during the evening after having cleaned a water tank earlier that day. Cystoscopic bladder biopsies demonstrated hemorrhagic cystitis. Hematuria resolved within 2 days and dysuria within about 1 week. Based on the presence of a metabolite of the chlorotoluidine pesticide chlordimeform (chlorphenamidine) in the serum and urine specimens, it was determined that the tank had been used previously to haul chlordimeform, resulting in this acute exposure. Lower urinary tract symptoms have also been reported among jewelers exposed to cadmium in brazing materials. Consideration should always be given to the possibility that hematuria of bladder origin, particularly in instances of suspected chronic chemical exposures, could represent an initial manifestation of malignant or premalignant disease.

References

1. Mutti A. Biologic monitoring in occupational and environmental toxicology. Toxicol Lett 1999; 108:77–89.
2. Stengel B, Watier L, Chouquet C, Cenee S, Philippon C, Hemon D. Influence of renal biomarker variability on the design and interpretation of occupational or environmental studies. Toxicol Lett 1999; 106:69–77.
3. Roels HA, Van Assche FJ, Oversteyns M, De Groof M, Lauwerys RR, Lison D. Reversibility of microproteinuria in cadmium workers with incipient tubular dysfunction after reduction of exposure. Am J Ind Med 1997; 31:645–52.
4. Taylor SA, Chivers ID, Price RG, et al. The assessment of biomarkers to detect nephrotoxicity using an integrated database. Environ Res 1997; 75:23–33.

5. Koffler A, Frieler RM, Massry SG. Acute renal failure due to non-traumatic rhabdomyolysis. Ann Intern Med 1976; 85:23–8.

6. Abuelo JG. Renal failure caused by chemicals, foods, plants, animal venoms, and misuse of drugs. Arch Intern Med 1990; 150:505–10.

7. Fowler BA, Weissberg JB. Arsine poisoning. N Engl J Med 1974; 291:1171–4.

8. Romeo L, Apostoli P, Kovacic M, Brugnone F. Acute arsine intoxication as a consequence of metal burnishing operations. Am J Ind Med 1997; 32:211–6.

9. Djerassi L. Hemolytic crisis in G6PD-deficient individuals in the occupational setting. Int Arch Occup Environ Health 1998; 71(Suppl):S26–28.

10. Prasad GV, Rossi NF. Arsenic intoxication associated with tubulointerstitial nephritis. Am J Kidney Dis 1995; 26:373–6.

11. Kelley C, Sargent DE, Uno JK. Cadmium therapeutic agents. Curr Pharm Des 1999; 5:229–40.

12. Wedeen RP, Qian L. Chromium-induced kidney disease. Environ Health Perspect 1991; 92:71–4.

13. Loghman-Adham M. Aminoaciduria and glycosuria following severe childhood lead poisoning. Pediatr Nephrol 1998; 12:218–21.

14. Zalups RK. Molecular interactions with mercury in the kidney. Pharm Rev 2000; 52:113–43.

15. Graeme KA, Pollack CV. Heavy metal toxicity, Part I: arsenic and mercury. J Emerg Med 1998; 16:45–56.

16. Rosa RM, Brown RS. Acute renal failure associated with heavy metals and organic solvents. In: Brenner BM, Lazarus MJ, eds. Acute renal failure, 2nd edn. Edinburgh: Churchill Livingstone, 1988;353–69.

17. Pavlakis N, Pollock CA, McLean G, Bartrop R. Deliberate overdose of uranium: toxicity and treatment. Nephron 1996; 72:313–7.

18. Zamora ML, Tracy BL, Zielinski JM, Meyerhof DP, Moss MA. Chronic ingestion of uranium in drinking water: a study of kidney bioeffects in humans. Toxicol Sci 1998; 43:68–77.

19. Manno M, Rezzadore M, Grossi M, Sbrana C. Potentiation of occupational carbon tetrachloride toxicity by ethanol abuse. Hum Exp Toxicol 1996; 15:294–300.

20. Verplanke A, Leummens M, Herber R. Occupational exposure to tetrachloroethene and its effects on the kidneys. J Occup Environ Med 1999; 41:11–16.

21. Letz GA, Pond SM, Osterloh JD, Wade RL, Becker CE. Two fatalities after acute occupational exposure to ethylene dibromide. JAMA 1984; 252:2428–31.

22. Jacobsen D, McMartin KE. Methanol and ethylene glycol poisonings: mechanisms of toxicity, clinical course, diagnosis and treatment. Med Toxicol 1986; 1:309–34.

23. Landry JF, Langlois S. Acute exposure to aliphatic hydrocarbons: an unusual cause of acute tubular necrosis. Arch Intern Med 1998; 158:1821–3.

24. Stengel B, Cenee S, Limasset JC, et al. Immunologic and renal markers among photogravure workers exposed to toluene. Scand J Work Environ Health 1998; 24:276–84.

25. Kamijima M, Nakazawa Y, Yamakawa M, et al. Metabolic acidosis and renal tubular injury due to pure toluene inhalation. Arch Environ Health 1994; 49:410–13.

26. Vaziri ND, Ness RL, Fairshter RD, Smith WR, Rosen SM. Nephrotoxicity of paraquat in man. Arch Intern Med 1979; 139:172–4.

27. Jones GM, Vale JA. Mechanisms of toxicity, clinical features, and management of diquat poisoning: a review. J Toxicol Clin Toxicol 2000; 38:123–8.

28. Daniell WE, Couser WG, Rosenstock L. Occupational solvent exposure and glomerulonephritis. JAMA 1988; 259:2280–3.

29. Jarup L, Berglund M, Elinder CG, Nordberg G, Vahter M. Health effects of cadmium exposure – a review of the literature and a risk estimate. Scand J Work Environ Health 1998; 24(Suppl 1):1–51.

30. http://www.osha-slc.gov/OshStd_data/1910_1027.html This site contains a complete description of the OSHA cadmium standard.

31. http://www.osha-slc.gov/dts/osta/oshasoft/gocad2.html This site provides resources to facilitate the implementation of OSHA's biologic monitoring protocol for cadmium.

32. Nishijo M, Nakagawa H, Morikawa M, et al. Relationship between urinary cadmium and mortality among inhabitants in a cadmium polluted area in Japan. Toxicol Lett 1999; 108:321–7.

33. Loghman-Adman M. Renal effects of environmental and occupational lead exposure. Environ Health Perspect 1997; 105:928–39.

34. Wedeen RP. Nephrotoxicity secondary to environmental agents and heavy metals. In: Schrier RW, Gottschalk CW, eds. Diseases of the kidney, 6th edn. Boston: Little, Brown & Co., 1996;1231–47.

35. Cocco P, Hua F, Boffetta P, et al. Mortality of Italian lead smelter workers. Scand J Work Environ Health 1997; 23:15–23.

36. Steenland K, Selevan S, Landrigan P. The mortality of lead smelter workers: an update. Am J Public Health 1992; 82:1641–4.

37. Chia KS, Jeyaratnam J, Lee J, et al. Lead-induced nephropathy: relationship between various biologic exposure indices and early markers of nephrotoxicity. Am J Ind Med 1995; 27:883–95.

38. Kim R, Rotnitzky A, Sparrow D, Weiss ST, Wager, Hu H. Longitudinal study of low-level lead exposure and impairment of renal function. JAMA 1996; 275:1177–81.

39. Wedeen RP, Malik DK, Batuman V. Detection and treatment of occupational lead nephropathy. Arch Intern Med 1979; 139:53–7.

40. Wedeen RP, D'Haese P, Van de Vyver FL, Verpooten GA, DeBroe ME. Lead nephropathy. Am J Kidney Dis 1986; 8:380–3.

41. Stoeckle SD, Hardy HL, Weber AL. Chronic beryllium disease: long-term follow-up of sixty cases and selective review of the literature. Am J Med 1969; 46:545–61.

42. Hess B, Raisin J, Zimmermann A, Horber F, Bajo S, Wyttenback A, Jaeger P. Tubulointerstitial nephropathy persisting 20 months after discontinuation of chronic intake of germanium lactate citrate. Am J Kidney Dis 1993; 21:548–52.

43. Barregard L. Enestrom S, Ljunghusen O, Wieslander J, Hultman P. A study of autoantibodies and circulating immune complexes in mercury-exposed chloralkali workers. Int Arch Occup Environ Health 1997; 70: 101–6.

44. Ellingsen DG, Barregard L, Gaarder PI, Hultberg B, Kjuus H. Assessment of renal dysfunction in workers previously exposed to mercury vapor at a chloralkali plant. Br J Ind Med 1993; 50:881–7.

45. Rapiti E, Sperati A, Miceli M, et al. End-stage renal disease among ceramic workers exposed to silica. Occup Environ Med 1999; 56: 559–61.

46. Calvert JM, Steenland K, Palu S. End-stage renal disease among silica-exposed gold miners. JAMA 1997; 277:1219-23.

47. Gregorini G, Ferioli A, Donato F, et al. Association between silica exposure and necrotizing crescentic glomerulonephritis with P-ANCA and anti-MPO antibodies: a hospital based case-control study. In: Wolfgang G, ed. Advances in experimental medicine and biology. New York: Plenum Press, 1993.

48. Nuyts GD, VanVlem E, DeVos A, et al. Wegener granulomatosis is associated to exposure to silicon compounds: a case-control study. Nephrol Dial Transplant 1995; 10:1162–5.

49. Hotz P. Occupational hydrocarbon exposure and chronic nephropathy. Toxicology 1994; 90: 163–283.

50. Ravnskov U. Hydrocarbons may worsen renal function in glomerulonephritis: a meta-analysis of the case-control studies. Am J Ind Med 2000; 37:599–606.

51. Schwartz J. The relationship between blood lead and blood pressure in the NHANES-II survey. Environ Health Perspec 1988; 78:15–22.

52. Pocock SJ, Shaper AG, Ashby D, Delves HT, Clayton BE. The relationship between blood lead, blood pressure, stroke, and heart attacks in middle-aged British men. Environ Health Perspec 1988; 78:139–55.

53. Granadillo VA, Tahan JE, Salgado O, et al. The influence of the blood levels of lead, aluminum and vanadium upon the arterial hypertension. Clin Chem Acta 1995; 233:47–59.

54. Staessen JA, Kuznetsova T, Roels HA, Emelianov D, Fagard R. Exposure to cadmium and conventional and ambulatory blood pressures in a prospective population study. Am J Hypertens 2000; 13:146-56.

55. Kreiss K, Wegman DH, Niles CA, Siroky MB, Krane RJ, Feldman RG. Neurological dysfunction of the bladder in workers exposed to dimethylaminoproprionitrile. JAMA 1980; 243:741–5.

Chapter 26
Gastrointestinal Disorders

26.1 Liver Diseases
Carl A Brodkin, Stan Lee, Carrie A Redlich

Occupational and environmental liver diseases include acute and chronic liver injury caused by workplace or environmental exposure(s). In the first half of the 20th century, a number of case reports and series documented liver injury following exposure to now well-recognized hepatotoxins such as carbon tetrachloride, trinitrotoluene, tetrachloroethane, and yellow phosphorus. The use of such agents has been reduced or eliminated in most workplace settings. However, liver injury associated with exposure to chemicals used in the workplace still occurs and may be underdiagnosed. Hepatotoxic exposures also can be encountered in the environment by contact with contaminated water, air, soil, or food, or with naturally occurring hepatotoxins such as aflatoxins.

Occupational and environmental liver injury can be challenging to recognize, diagnose, and manage for several reasons. The incidence, etiologic agents, natural history, diagnostic criteria and management strategies for occupational liver disease have not been fully characterized. Acute toxic liver injury frequently has a non-specific clinical presentation, whereas chronic liver injury usually remains asymptomatic until it reaches an advanced stage. It is unknown how often occupational liver disease goes unrecognized, is attributed to other etiologies, or is misclassified as idiopathic.

Once liver disease is recognized, it must be distinguished from non-occupational or non-environmental etiologies on the basis of clinical presentation, exposure history, laboratory findings, and pathologic findings when available. The existence of two common causes of liver disease, namely alcohol and hepatitis viruses, must be considered. Although exposure to alcohol and hepatitis viruses may be more frequent in certain occupations, the majority of liver disease caused by these two entities occurs outside the workplace. However, even the separation between occupational and non-occupational liver disease is not absolute. For example, a study of cirrhosis mortality and occupation in California from 1979 to 1981 found the highest cirrhosis mortality rates among "blue-collar" occupations (construction workers, carpenters, painters, machinists). Notably, these occupations often carry greater exposure to hepatotoxic chemicals that may directly contribute to cirrhosis or potentially interact with alcohol consumption, to increase risk.[1]

The diagnosis of occupational liver injury is facilitated by human and toxicologic data. The information available is based on the following sources: (1) isolated case reports of liver injury, usually following obvious overexposure; (2) epidemiologic studies demonstrating liver function test abnormalities or increased incidence of chronic liver disease in certain groups (frequently with multiple, poorly characterized exposures); and (3) animal toxicology studies documenting hepatotoxic responses to specific agents. Because of limited human data, the hepatotoxic potential of a given substance frequently is determined based on animal studies. Such studies often focus on effects of a single acute high exposure rather than on chronic low-level or simultaneous multiple exposures that reflect most occupational exposure conditions. Significant interspecies differences in susceptibility, possibly related to variable hepatic metabolism, also limit the applicability of animal findings to the prediction of human hepatotoxicity.

The diagnosis of occupational liver disease is complicated by several host and acquired factors, discussed later, that can potentiate hepatotoxic effects and may result in enhanced or unexpected toxicity. Thus, a high level of suspicion is required to recognize and diagnose liver disease of occupational or environmental origin; the diagnosis need not be dismissed because liver injury associated with a given substance has not been reported previously.

This chapter reviews acute and chronic non-malignant occupational and environmental liver injury, including clinical features, known and suspected causative agents, strategies for diagnosis, screening for preclinical disease, and management.

ROLE OF THE LIVER IN METABOLISM

The liver is the major site for the biotransformation of exogenous substances such as chemicals, drugs, and dietary factors, and it is a frequent site of toxicity. These exogenous substances, or xenobiotics, are generally lipophilic and not easily cleared from the body. They are metabolized primarily by the cytochrome P-450 mono-oxygenase enzyme system, a large family of related enzymes located in the smooth endoplasmic reticulum of the hepatocyte. There are additional hepatic enzyme systems that metabolize certain alcohols, nitrogen and sulfur compounds, oxides, and other xenobiotics (see Chapter 5). Hepatotoxicity may result from the xenobiotic directly, or from its metabolism to toxic intermediates – often electrophilic compounds or free radicals. Normally these intermediates are detoxified by conjugation or transferase reactions to less toxic, water-soluble compounds and excreted in the urine or bile.[2]

The toxicity of a given substance may be assessed by the activity of the specific hepatic enzyme system responsible for its bioactivation and detoxification, as well as by factors affecting the substance's absorption, storage, and excretion. Significant interindividual variation in these enzyme systems can occur. Such differences are determined by (1) host factors, including genetically inherited polymorphisms, age, and sex, and (2) acquired or exogenous factors, such as medication, ethanol or cigarette use, diet, and pre-existing liver disease. All of these factors may contribute to individual differences in susceptibility to exogenous chemicals and drugs.

Numerous drugs (including barbiturates, phenytoin, and steroids), foreign chemicals (including organic solvents, polycyclic aromatic hydrocarbons in cigarette smoke, halogenated pesticides, dioxins, and polychlorinated biphenyls [PCBs]), and dietary factors (such as ethanol or vegetable indoles) are potent inducers of the cytochrome *P*-450 enzymes. Metals, antibiotics, cimetidine, carbon monoxide, ethanol, and altered nutritional status can inhibit the cytochrome *P*-450 system. The ability of many of these exogenous agents to potentiate hepatotoxicity has been well documented in animal studies and human case reports. In animals, the administration of alcohols (e.g., ethanol, isopropanol), ketones (e.g., acetone), trichloroethylene (TCE), medications (e.g., phenobarbital), and PCBs have been shown to potentiate the hepatotoxicity of carbon tetrachloride and other chlorinated hydrocarbons. In humans, ethanol administration has been shown to increase the toxicity of TCE, carbon tetrachloride, and drugs such as acetaminophen. Recent human exposure studies have shown that ethanol can alter the metabolism of a number of chemicals including styrene, methyl ethyl ketone, and toluene. Similar interactions probably occur with many occupational, environmental, and dietary substances, and these interactions may be important determinants of hepatic toxicity.

These findings have an impact on the evaluation of occupational liver disease, because workers are frequently exposed to multiple chemicals, alcohol, medications, cigarettes, and varied diets. Interactions between these factors may potentiate hepatotoxic effects and must be considered in evaluating patients with possible occupational or environmental liver injury.

CLASSIFICATION OF OCCUPATIONAL HEPATOTOXINS AND MECHANISMS

Hepatotoxins can be classified as either intrinsic or idiosyncratic toxins. Most hepatotoxins are intrinsic toxins, that is, their hepatotoxicity is a predictable property of the substance itself, and most individuals will be affected if the dose is sufficient. Most intrinsic toxins (e.g., carbon tetrachloride) also are classified as direct toxins, namely, the substance or its metabolite directly injures the liver. Acute and subacute injury by such toxins usually produces varying degrees of dose-dependent hepatocellular injury with necrosis and steatosis.

The mechanism of hepatic injury related to alcohol and other organic solvents, representing a large class of intrin-

sic hepatotoxic agents, is illustrative. An etiologic model of alcohol-induced hepatocellular damage involving oxidative stress has been demonstrated in animal studies. In addition to ethanol,[3] the microsomal ethanol oxidizing system (MEOS) has a high capacity to oxidize numerous solvent substrates including halogenated compounds such as carbon tetrachloride[4] and non-chlorinated solvents including acetone,[5] butanol, pentanol, and benzene.[6] Potentiation of hepatotoxicity from solvent mixtures has been demonstrated with the induction of microsomal cytochrome P450IIE1 by alcohol consumption in the presence of bromobenzene.[7] This solvent inducible enzyme system can produce highly reactive intermediates, leading to peroxidation of lipid membranes[8] such as endoplasmic reticulum, and covalent binding to cellular macromolecules (DNA, RNA, and proteins). Support for a mechanism of direct biologic injury includes (1) the anatomic association between selective centrizonal injury and enhanced microsomal P450IIE1 activity in this region,[9] and (2) animal models demonstrating marked enhancement of ethanol-induced hepatic injury with carbon tetrachloride, with striking activation of P450IIE1.[10]

In contrast to intrinsic hepatotoxins, a few hepatotoxins (e.g., beryllium) are idiosyncratic in that they cause liver injury that is sporadic and generally not dose related, possibly by a hypersensitivity or other immunologic reaction. Typically, granulomas or eosinophilic infiltrates are found on liver biopsy.

Hepatotoxins can also be classified by the pathologic or clinical syndrome they cause, although exposure to a specific hepatotoxin can result in more than one type of liver injury. For example, acute exposure to the solvent carbon tetrachloride can result in acute necrosis, whereas chronic exposure results in steatosis, fibrosis, and cirrhosis in animals. In Table 26.1.1, occupational and environmental liver disorders are classified based on both their clinical

Type of injury	Selected agents
Acute/subacute	
Acute or subacute hepatic necrosis (± steatosis)	Halogenated aliphatics (CCL₄, tetrachloroethane, trichloroethylene, ethylchloroform) Nitro compounds (dimethylformamide, trinitrotoluene, 2-nitropropane) Aromatic hydrocarbons (toluene) Metals (arsenic, lead, phosphorus)
Acute viral hepatitis	Viral agents (hepatitis A, B, C) (see Chapter 22)
Acute cholestatic hepatitis	Methylene dianiline
Chronic	
Steatosis	See acute necrosis
Chronic hepatocellular disease (fibrosis/cirrhosis)	CCL₄ and other chlorinated organic solvents, arsenic, mixed solvents
Chronic hepatitis	Viral agents (hepatitis B, C)
Granulomatous hepatitis	Beryllium, copper
Hepatoportal sclerosis	Vinyl chloride monomer, arsenic, thorium

Table 26.1.1 Classification of non-malignant occupational liver disease

presentation and pathologic processes, with examples of proven or suspected etiologic agents.

Table 26.1.2 lists the major known or suspected occupational and environmental hepatotoxins associated with non-malignant liver injury. The toxicity of certain agents is predicted on the basis of their chemical structure. An agent that has documented hepatotoxicity in animal studies should be considered a possible human hepatotoxin.

Hepatotoxic substances may be encountered in a variety of occupations, including construction activities, electronic manufacturing, farming, painting, and textile and dye manufacturing. Epidemiologic studies of workers in such occupations have shown variable evidence of liver injury. Contributing to this variability is the lack of sensitivity and specificity of current screening tests for subclinical liver disease and imprecise exposure assessment.

Exposure to hepatotoxic substances also can occur in a number of home or environmental settings such as with cleaning agents, paints or paint removers, chemical contaminants, or natural toxins in the environment. Dramatic instances of liver disease associated with massive environmental contamination have been reported, such as cooking oil heavily contaminated with PCBs (Japan, 1968), wheat with hexachlorobenzene (Turkey, 1955 to 1957), and flour with 4,4'-diaminodiphenyl-methane (England, 1965). There is often little information available on the effects of low-level exposure to the numerous natural and man-made substances present in the environment and food chain.

GENERAL EVALUATION
Clinical history

As with most environmental illnesses, a careful medical, occupational, and exposure history is the key to suspecting and diagnosing work-related or environmental hepatotoxicity. The clinical presentation of acute and chronic toxic liver injury can range from no symptoms to acute nausea, abdominal pain, and jaundice. Occasionally, it presents insidiously as end-stage liver disease. Most hepatotoxins also affect other organs, including the central and peripheral nervous systems, kidney, and mucous membranes. Symptoms related to these organs may predominate, and information on these symptoms should be elicited from the patient and coworkers. Central nervous system symptoms (e.g., euphoria, headaches, and dizziness), mucosal irritation, and disulfiram-like reactions following alcohol ingestion suggest excessive solvent exposure. The temporal relationship between the exposure and onset of symptoms is essential to diagnosing acute hepatotoxicity but is less helpful in diagnosing chronic disorders. Symptoms usually develop within days to weeks following acute solvent exposure, depending on the extent of poisoning. Exposure to solvents, pesticides, and heavy metals should be specifically assessed.

Further information about potential hepatotoxic exposures can be obtained from material data safety sheets, the employer, Occupational Safety and Health Administration (OSHA), and industrial hygiene monitoring. A description of the workplace, including the use of protective equipment and ventilation systems, is helpful in assessing the mode (dermal, inhalation, or ingestion) and extent of exposure. The introduction of any new chemicals and the occurrence of unusual or accidental exposures also should be investigated. A prior history of liver and biliary disease, medication and alcohol use, obesity, diabetes, and risk factors for viral hepatitis (blood transfusions, sexual practices, and intravenous drug abuse) should be ascertained to rule out other contributing causes of hepatic injury. Alternative hepatotoxic exposures, such as hobby or other home chemical use, and additional jobs, should also be excluded.

Halogenated hydrocarbons
Carbon tetrachloride
Tetrachloroethane
Tetrachloroethylene
Trichloroethylene
1,1,1,-Trichloroethane
Chloroform
Vinyl chloride
Anesthetic gases
Hydrochlorofluorocarbons (HCFCs)
Halothane
Methoxyflurane
Alcohols
Ethyl alcohol
Aromatic hydrocarbons
Styrene
Toluene
Xylene
Plasticizers
Methylenedianiline
Nitro compounds
Trinitrotoluene
Dinitrobenzene
2-Nitropropane
N,N-Dimethylformamide
Pesticides
Organochlorine insecticides
　　Chlordecone
Fungicides
　　Hexachlorobenzene
Herbicides
Paraquat
Chlorphenoxy acids (2, 4, 5-T, Agent Orange)
Chlorinated aromatic compounds
Polychlorinated biphenyls
Chloronaphthalenes
2, 3, 7, 8-Tetrachlorodibenzo-p-dioxin (TCDD)
Dibenzofurans
Metallic compounds
Arsenic
Beryllium
Cadmium
Copper
Iron
Thallium
Lead
Phosphorus
Environmental agents
Aflatoxin
Amanita phalloides toxin

Table 26.1.2 Partial list of known or suspected human hepatotoxins associated with non-malignant liver disease

Physical examination

Although typical signs of hepatic injury or dysfunction may be present (right upper quadrant tenderness, hepatosplenomegaly, jaundice), the physical examination is not a sensitive indicator of liver disease. The examination should not be limited to the abdomen; evidence of toxicity to other organ systems, such as mucous membranes and nervous system, and extra-abdominal manifestations of liver disease should be evaluated.

Laboratory and radiographic assessment of hepatotoxicity

Tests for evaluating hepatotoxicity fall into four general categories: (1) serum markers of hepatobiliary disease, (2) biochemical tests of liver function, (3) imaging tests, and (4) liver biopsy.

Serum markers of hepatobiliary disease

Most useful in the evaluation of hepatotoxicity are markers of hepatocellular necrosis, which reflect the release of intracellular enzymes into serum following cytotoxic injury.[11] Enzyme release results from increased hepatocyte membrane permeability. The most important of these tests are aspartate aminotransferase (AST or SGOT), a mitochondrial and cytosolic enzyme, and alanine aminotransferase (ALT or SGPT), a cytosolic enzyme. AST also is present in muscle, heart, and kidney, whereas ALT is more specific for liver. Both markers have been validated in a wide variety of clinical and experimental settings. Severe elevation (> 8–10 times normal) may occur in acute toxic and viral injury. Mild elevation (< 2–3 times normal) is generally seen in chronic or resolving hepatocellular injury or less severe acute injury. ALT activity is reduced in alcohol-related liver disease;[12] levels of greater than 300 are uncommon in alcoholic liver injury. The pattern of transaminase elevation also can be helpful in distinguishing alcohol from other hepatotoxic injury. Since alcohol selectively inhibits ALT activity, a high AST/ALT ratio (greater than one) is often seen in this setting.[13] In contrast, other toxin- and viral-induced hepatic injury usually results in an AST/ALT ratio of less than one.[14] It is important to recognise that subclinical disease can occur despite normal aminotransferases, especially with chronic liver injury.

A second group of serum markers include enzymes whose synthesis is induced by cholestasis. The most important of these are alkaline phosphatase (AP) and γ-glutamyl transpeptidase (GGT). The specificity of AP for liver disease is reduced by the presence of other AP isoenzymes in bone, intestine, and placenta. AP is useful in assessing hepatotoxic exposures associated with cholestasis, such as methylenediamine. Although GGT is sensitive for hepatocellular injury, it lacks sufficient specificity to be useful diagnostically. This lack of specificity is due to its presence in several organs (kidney, seminal vesicles, pancreas, spleen, heart, brain, and common bile duct), its inducibility by alcohol and other medications, and its long half-life in serum (26 days).

Biochemical tests of liver function

Measurements to assess various functions of the liver include tests of hepatic clearance, tests of hepatic metabolism, and tests of synthetic function.

Tests of hepatic clearance Clearance tests dynamically assess three levels of hepatocyte function simultaneously: uptake, metabolism, and excretion. These tests assess the liver's ability to clear exogenously introduced or endogenously produced organic anions. Hepatic clearance was traditionally assessed by the sulfobromophthalein sodium test (BSP). BSP is eliminated by biliary excretion following conjugation with glutathione in the liver. The irritative effects of BSP during infusion have limited its clinical utility.

Indocyanine green (ICG) dye is excreted without conjugation by the liver, reducing biologic variability due to enzyme induction (e.g., from diet and medications). Increased retention of ICG thus reflects diminished hepatic clearance. The utility of ICG clearance in detecting occupational liver injury has been evaluated primarily in workers exposed to vinyl chloride monomer. ICG clearance is believed to be the most specific test in detecting early liver injury in this population. The utility of the ICG test in other exposure settings is unclear. The test also is limited by cost, availability, and cumbersome administration.

Cholic and chenodeoxycholic bile acids, which are included in the bile, are endogenously produced organic anions. Bile acids are cleared exclusively by the liver; thus, their serum concentrations reflect hepatic function, analogous to serum creatinine in the assessment of renal function. Measurement of fasting serum bile acids (SBA) avoids the administration of exogenous agents, and has been advocated as a sensitive screening test for hepatobiliary disease. Conjugated cholic acid (CCA) appears to provide high positive predictive value for hepatobiliary disease.[15] Serum bile acids more specifically reflect excretory function than serum bilirubin, and in occupational settings, several studies have revealed increased serum bile acid levels in workers exposed to mixed solvents as well as styrene.[16–19] Bilirubin levels may be elevated in cholestasis, severe acute hepatitis, and chronic liver injury; conjugated (direct) bilirubin and direct/total bilirubin may be useful in assessing early hepatic dysfunction on a population basis in solvent-exposed workers.[20,21]

Tests of hepatic metabolism The hepatic biotransformation system, composed predominantly of cytochrome P-450 (microsomal) enzymes, is the major site of metabolism for exogenous compounds such as drugs or chemicals. Measurement of an exogenous substance's clearance can be used to assess hepatic metabolic enzyme activity. Changes in metabolism may reflect (1) advanced hepatocellular injury, resulting in reduced enzyme activity, or (2) the induction or inhibition of certain hepatic metabolic enzymes by xenobiotic agents. The metabolism of radiolabeled antipyrine and aminopyrine, both of which can be measured non-invasively, most frequently has been used in research settings. Several studies have reported altered antipyrine metabolism in workers exposed to solvents and pesticides. However, the significance of such findings is unclear.

The liver and erythropoietic systems are organs of heme synthesis, via porphyrin intermediates. Accumulation of several porphyrin metabolites, which are measurable in urine, can occur with hepatic dysfunction. Coproporphyrinuria has been demonstrated in the setting of alcohol, lead, and hexachlorobenzene exposure. Although urinary porphyrin levels have not been validated clinically, they may provide a useful biologic marker of exposure in the future.

Tests of hepatic synthetic function

Hepatic function can be assessed grossly by serum measurement of proteins synthesized and secreted by the liver, such as serum albumin, ferritin, urea, and coagulation factors, measured indirectly by prothrombin time (PT). These tests are limited clinically by poor sensitivity. This poor sensitivity is due to the large functional reserve of the liver; generally more than 90% of hepatic parenchyma must be destroyed before measurable changes in protein synthesis occur.

Imaging tests

Imaging studies provide a clinically useful, non-invasive means of hepatic tissue characterization. Ultrasonography compares sonic penetration of hepatic and renal parenchyma: steatosis and fibrosis increase liver echogenicity relative to the kidney. In a prospective, controlled study of 85 patients with biopsy-proven hepatic disease, Saverymuttu observed a sensitivity of 94%, and specificity of 84% in detecting hepatic parenchymal changes.[22] A significant exposure–response relationship between sonographic parenchymal changes and hepatotoxic exposure to vinyl chloride monomer and perchloroethylene has also been observed in occupational settings.[23–25] Neither ultrasound nor CT distinguishes steatosis from fibrosis with precision. Ultrasound is preferred in the initial evaluation of biochemical abnormalities, to assess biliary as well as parenchymal disease. In patients with chronic hepatic injury, magnetic resonance imaging (MRI) may be useful in distinguishing inflammatory and necrotic changes (patchy enhancement) from fibrosis (linear enhancement) using a gadolinium-enhanced technique.[26]

Liver biopsy

Histopathologic examination offers the most precise assessment of hepatotoxic parenchymal changes, such as hepatocellular injury, inflammation, steatosis, and fibrosis. Thus, it is considered the definitive "gold standard" test for liver disease and can be helpful both diagnostically and prognostically in characterizing the type, extent, and activity of liver injury. In experienced hands, percutaneous liver biopsy is a safe procedure that can be performed on an outpatient basis. However, as with any invasive procedure, it does carry some risks (e.g., hemorrhage, infection). Indications for liver biopsy include persistently elevated aminotransferases of unclear etiology, unexplained hepatomegaly, and anatomic abnormalities. Histologic evidence of hepatocellular injury such as necrosis or regen-

eration and steatosis (microvesicular, macrovesicular, or both), although not unique for toxic liver injury, are suggestive of the condition. Centrizonal (perivenular or Zone 3) distribution of injury within the hepatic lobule is characteristic of solvent-induced injury, though this may be diffuse in more severe cases. Such findings may be subtle, especially if the biopsy is performed weeks to months after the exposure of concern, as frequently occurs, and they are not specific for a given substance. Ultrastructural examination may provide further, or confirmatory, findings suggestive of a toxic injury, such as small droplet fat formation and prominent vesicular endoplasmic reticulum. If environmental liver injury is suspected prior to biopsy, part of the tissue should be fixed in glutaraldehyde, because it enables the evaluation of both fat content and ultrastructure. The lack of certain findings on biopsy, such as Mallory's hyaline and ground glass hepatocytes, also can be helpful in ruling out alternative diagnoses such as alcohol- or viral-induced injury.

Overview of laboratory tests

In summary, of the numerous laboratory and imaging tests available, serum aminotransferases (ALT and AST) are most helpful in the evaluation of patients with hepatocellular injury and in screening exposed populations. However, such tests may not be sensitive enough to detect mild acute injury, and are much less useful in the detection of chronic liver injury. They also are not specific for chemical or occupational-induced injury. Although liver biopsy is useful in evaluating individual cases of suspected hepatotoxicity, it is an invasive procedure that carries cost and some risk for morbidity (and in rare instances, mortality), making it impractical as a screening test. See Table 26.1.3 for further comments regarding these diagnostic tests.

ACUTE OCCUPATIONAL AND ENVIRONMENTAL LIVER DISORDERS
Acute and subacute hepatocellular diseases

Acute and subacute hepatocellular injuries are the most commonly recognized occupational liver disorders. They include a spectrum of liver injury ranging from acute injury following a single massive hepatotoxic exposure, as occurs in accidental poisoning, to repeated hepatotoxic exposures over days to weeks. Although numerous suspected and known animal hepatotoxins, primarily organic solvents, are widely used throughout industry today, there is a limited amount of human data on the effects of such exposures. The incidence of acute and subacute occupational and environmental hepatotoxicity is unknown.

Pathogenesis

The typical pathologic findings are varying degrees of hepatocellular necrosis and steatosis. Neither of these

Test	Type of injury	Comments
Serum markers		
Aminotransferases (AST, ALT)	Acute/subacute hepatocellular injury.	Best available test for acute/subacute hepatocellular injury Not sensitive for fatty liver
Alkaline phosphatase	Cholestatic injury (i.e., methylenediamine)	High sensitivity for cholestatic injury; not very specific
γ-glutamyl transpeptidase (GGT)	Cholestatic and hepatocellular injury	Elevated with ethanol consumption, hepatobiliary disease, low specificity
Tests for function		
Tests of hepatic clearance		
Indocyanine green (ICG)	Early hepatobiliary injury	Useful for vinyl chloride toxicity Requires IV infusion and multiple blood samples
Bile acids (SBA) (cholic, chenodeoxycholic acid)	Early hepatobiliary and hepatocellular injury	Not readily available. Improved sensitivity compared to AST, ALT for hepatobiliary and hepatocellular disease in some settings (e.g., vinyl chloride)
Bilirubin	Cholestatic with hepatocellular injury	Elevated conjugated (direct) bilirubin, conjugated (total bilirubin ratio observed with styrene and other solvent exposure) Less specific than SBA or AST, ALT
Tests of hepatic metabolism		
Antipyrine clearance	Early hepatocellular injury	Not readily available, high test individual variability. May be marker of exposure rather than toxicity
Tests of synthetic function		
Albumin, PT	Late hepatocellular injury	Low sensitivity for early disease
Imaging tests		
Ultrasound	Biliary disease, fatty change, hepatocellular injury	High sensitivity and specificity for biliary disease. Efficacy not established for parenchymal disease
CT scan	Fatty change, hepatocellular injury	Efficacy not established for parenchymal disease
MRI scan	Chronic hepatocellular injury and fibrosis	Fibrosis observed by linear enhancement using gadolinium
Liver biopsy	Subacute/chronic hepatocellular injury	Gold standard for the diagnosis of parenchymal disease. Centrizonal (Zone 3) changes in solvent-induced injury

Table 26.1.3 Diagnostic tests for occupational liver disease

conditions is specific for occupational or environmental toxins. Necrosis can occur with either a zonal pattern (usually centrizonal) or more diffusely, depending on the toxic agent and degree of exposure. Some degree of inflammatory response, with a lymphocytic infiltrate, also may be seen. Agents causing acute hepatocellular injury also may result in more chronic hepatocellular disease following repeated exposure, and are discussed in the following section. Some established and suspected human hepatotoxic agents, grouped by classes of substance, are listed in Table 26.1.2.

Clinical features

The clinical effects of acute and subacute hepatic necrosis may vary greatly in severity from asymptomatic histologic or functional abnormalities to manifestations of severe hepatic necrosis, depending on the intrinsic toxicity of the hepatotoxic agent, the degree of exposure, and host susceptibility factors (either genetic or acquired). Fulminant hepatic injury, with abdominal pain, nausea, and jaundice, may occur following heavy acute. Historically, exposures have frequently involved chlorinated organic compounds (e.g., carbon tetrachloride).[27] Most recently reported cases have occurred following accidental overexposure, ingestion,

abuse (e.g., sniffing), extensive dermal contact, or respiratory exposure in a closed or poorly ventilated area. Agents have included dimethylformamide, 2-nitropropane, 1,1,1-trichloroethane, or trichloroethylene (TCE). Such acute hepatic injury usually is part of a multisystem disease, with prominent central nervous system and renal involvement. With less extensive exposure, asymptomatic elevations in liver aminotransferases may be noted. A clinical presentation between these extremes, with non-specific gastrointestinal symptoms, also occurs. Individual host factors, or additional exposures such as alcohol, medications, or other chemicals in the workplace may alter the severity of the toxic hepatic injury.

Physical findings depend on the severity and duration of the hepatocellular injury. They range from a normal examination, to right upper quadrant tenderness, hepatomegaly, jaundice, and signs of hepatic failure in extreme cases.

Diagnosis

In acute fulminant cases, the diagnosis of hepatitis and the specific etiology usually are not difficult to determine. Often, there is a history of an unusual overexposure occurring immediately prior to the onset of symptoms (1–3 days). Markedly elevated liver aminotransferase and bilirubin levels are noted, along with other findings of hepatic failure, such as coagulopathy, renal, and neurologic dysfunction. The specific hepatotoxin(s) usually can be determined from occupational and environmental history. Occasionally, blood or urine testing can be performed to identify a particular chemical or its metabolite. Less severe clinical presentations, such as that following subacute poisoning, can be more difficult to recognize and diagnose. Symptoms and physical findings may be unremarkable so liver function tests are not obtained. The clinician must therefore have a high level of suspicion for occupational liver disease. Elevated aminotransferase levels (ALT and/or AST) are the best available indicator of acute hepatic injury, but other causes for hepatic injury should be excluded before attributing the injury to a workplace exposure.

A thorough exposure history is essential to recognising an occupational etiology. A medical history, physical examination, and blood tests help exclude other causes of elevated levels of liver enzymes, including medications; hypervitaminosis (due to megavitamins); obesity; metabolic disorders, including diabetes hypertriglyceridemia, and hemochromatosis; pregnancy; viral hepatitis; and alcohol. Serologic tests for hepatitis A and B are useful in detecting acute viral hepatitis; in hepatitis C, the serologic test may take up to 6 months after infection to become positive. Polymerase chain reaction (PCR) tests for both hepatitis B DNA and hepatitis C RNA are extremely sensitive for viral hepatitis in both the acute and chronic setting (see Chapter 22). The possibility of unrecognized alcohol use or idiopathic liver injury are usually the most difficult differential diagnoses to definitively rule out. With alcohol-induced liver injury, AST levels greater than 300 are uncommon and the AST/ALT ratio usually is greater than one. An occupational or environmental etiology is strongly suggested if aminotransferase levels improve within 2–6 weeks following removal from the exposure(s), but it is not ruled out if the aminotransferase levels remain elevated (see later).

If liver aminotransferases remain elevated, a liver biopsy should be considered. Findings of hepatocellular injury and steatosis are consistent with a hepatotoxic etiology, whereas marked inflammation is more suggestive of a viral one.

Natural history and management

Acute occupational hepatitis is a severe, potentially fatal disease that usually occurs 1–3 days following a massive accidental hepatotoxic exposure. Multiorgan system failure, including central nervous system depression (i.e., coma) and renal failure, is frequently present, particularly in fulminant cases. Acute occupational hepatitis should be treated in a similar manner to any other type of severe hepatitis, with appropriate supportive measures. Referral to a liver transplant center may be required in fulminant cases. If the patient recovers from the acute episode, the prognosis is usually good. Aminotransferase elevations and symptoms generally improve within days, with resolution over weeks, but the time course is variable.

Subacute hepatocellular injury may develop weeks to months following the hepatotoxic exposure, depending on the nature and extent of the exposure. If the patient is diagnosed or strongly suspected of having undergone toxic exposure, he or she should be removed from the suspected exposure and observed. Exposure to other risk factors such as alcohol consumption should be minimized. The workplace and environment should be evaluated for hepatotoxins, and appropriate measures taken to reduce exposures. Elevated aminotransferase levels and symptoms generally improve 1–4 weeks following removal from exposure, but the time course is variable, depending on the specific hepatotoxin; persistent elevations that last for months have been documented in outbreaks. Whether chronic liver disease may result following subacute hepatotoxic injuries is unclear.

Acute cholestatic injury

Acute cholestatic liver injury is rare following occupational or environmental exposures but has been reported following exposure to methylene dianiline, an aromatic amine used as an epoxy resin hardener.[28] An epidemic of cholestatic jaundice occurred in Epping, England (so-called Epping jaundice) in 1965 after bread made from flour contaminated with methylene dianiline was ingested. Similar cases have been reported following occupational exposure during the manufacture or handling of methylene dianiline.

The clinical, laboratory, and pathologic findings are consistent with a mixed cholestatic-hepatocellular injury,[29] that is dose dependent rather than idiosyncratic. Symptoms may include abdominal pain, pruritus, fever, and jaundice. Laboratory studies show elevated bilirubin, alkaline phosphatase, and aminotransferase levels. A consistent pattern of injury with bile stasis, portal inflammation, and variable hepatic necrosis is found on liver biopsy. The diagnosis depends on an appropriate exposure history, clinical and laboratory presentation, and elimination of other causes of acute cholestatic injury, such as drugs or biliary obstruction. Resolution of liver injury following removal typically occurs from exposure has not been reported.

CHRONIC (NON-MALIGNANT) OCCUPATIONAL AND ENVIRONMENTAL LIVER DISORDERS
Fatty liver (steatosis) and steatohepatitis

Fatty change in the liver, termed steatosis, was first characterized in alcohol-related liver disease. Steatosis is defined morphologically as greater than 5% hepatocytes containing fat, or quantitatively as greater than 5 g lipid per 100 g hepatic tissue. Steatosis occurs in other disorders, including diabetes mellitus, hypertriglyceridemia, obesity[30] (with 90% prevalence in the morbidly obese); with various medications; and as a normal variant, with up to 20% prevalence in some series.[31] Some degree of steatosis usually is found accompanying acute hepatocellular necrosis. Marked steatosis is more commonly seen in chronic toxin-induced liver injury, frequently as the predominant finding. Steatosis may be accompanied by varying degrees of inflammation, termed steatohepatitis. There is good evidence that this can be multifactorial, thus industrial hepatotoxins may interact with underlying metabolic disorders and other causes of non-alcoholic steatohepatitis (NASH).[32]

Pathogenesis

Steatosis results from the pathologic alteration of hepatic fat metabolism. Dietary fat normally is transported to the liver via the portal vein as chylomicrons containing fatty acids. Hepatocytes convert free fatty acids to a transportable form, very low-density lipoprotein (VLDL), which is secreted into the circulation. Hepatotoxins can block fat metabolism at several steps, resulting in intrahepatic accumulation of free fatty acids and triglycerides, producing lipid droplet formation at the cellular level and diffuse or focal steatosis at the tissue level.

Clinical presentation

Fatty liver associated with occupational exposure was first described with yellow phosphorus poisoning in the 19th century, with pronounced steatosis and necrosis found at autopsy. Similar cases of acute massive necrosis and steatosis have been described with trinitrotoluene in munitions industries, arsenical pesticide use in vintners, and the use of certain chlorinated aliphatic solvents (such as carbon tetrachloride, methyl chloroform, and tetrachloroethane), usually following accidental massive exposures. More subtle microsteatosis was recently described following routine short-term exposure to dimethylformamide in a fabric-coating factory.

The prevalence of fatty changes related to chronic, low-level, chemical exposure is not known. Patients are usually asymptomatic. Screening tests (AST, ALT) may not detect steatosis in the absence of inflammation and necrosis. Investigation of steatosis is usually limited by strong reliance on histologic diagnosis, which is invasive and may not be available. Diagnosis is further complicated by the confounding etiologies of fatty liver, including alcohol consumption, obesity, diabetes, medications, and their interactions with suspected toxins.

Chronic exposure to chlorinated solvents such as carbon tetrachloride can cause varying degrees of steatosis and hepatocellular injury. Although the evidence is less consistent with non-chlorinated solvents, several studies have found steatosis in workers exposed to non-chlorinated solvents, including dimethylformamide, toluene, and mixed aliphatic and aromatic solvents. The relative degree and severity of steatosis and necrosis found on histopathologic examination is likely related to the chronicity and extent of the exposure, as well as the hepatotoxic characteristics of the particular exposure. Acute high-level exposures tend to be associated with greater amounts of necrosis, whereas steatosis tends to predominate with more chronic exposures.

Natural history

The natural history of chemically induced hepatic steatosis has not been well characterized. Histopathologic data from animal models indicate that fatty change occurs as part of a continuum of reversible, morphologic changes: cloudy swelling is followed by hydropic changes and, finally, steatosis. In humans, the reversibility of alcohol-related fatty change with abstinence has been well documented. Acute solvent-related steatosis is generally associated with necrosis and elevated aminotransferase levels. The elevated aminotransferase levels generally resolve within weeks to months of removal from exposure. Because of the need for histologic evidence, the natural history of the accompanying acute steatosis is less clear, but the condition most likely also resolves over time. Steatosis following acute exposures is thus likely to represent subclinical injury at a reversible stage.

At present, there are no human longitudinal studies addressing the sequelae of isolated steatosis with prolonged or ongoing occupational exposure. Necrosis, steatosis, and fibrosis can be induced in animals by the chronic administration of carbon tetrachloride. Evidence exists in both animal and human studies that steatosis can occur in the absence of elevated serum hepatic transaminase levels. Balazs demonstrated that rats exposed to low doses of carbon tetrachloride had no ALT elevation, despite marked fatty and hydropic changes histologically.[33] Similarly, longitudinal follow-up of individuals with alcohol-induced or metabolically induced (diabetes and obesity) hepatic injury have demonstrated significant progression of steatosis to fibrosis histologically, termed 'steatocirrhosis',[34] often in the absence of an inflammatory response and associated transaminase elevation.[35,36] In one study, seven workers exposed to dimethylformamide over a 3-month to 10-year period, with persistently elevated aminotransferase levels, underwent liver biopsy. Variable degrees of steatosis, which was greatest in those with longer periods of exposure, were found; there was no evidence of progression to fibrosis or cirrhosis at the time of biopsy.

Diagnosis

Laboratory tests may not be helpful in diagnosing fatty liver, because they frequently do not detect steatosis in the absence of inflammation. Non-invasive anatomic evaluation of the liver by ultrasonography and CT scan can suggest hepatic steatosis. The definitive diagnosis of steatosis depends on histopathologic examination of a liver biopsy specimen.

When significant steatosis is found, either incidentally or in the work-up of elevated serum aminotransferases, evaluation should attempt to differentiate occupational from other known causes of steatosis, as discussed earlier. The history should include a review of the following: medications associated with steatosis (such as phenytoin [Dilantin], tetracycline, isoniazid, nitrofurantoin, and phenylbutazone) and the presence of hyperlipidemia, diabetes mellitus, obesity or pregnancy, and substance abuse, such as glue sniffing. Laboratory evaluation should include measurements of fasting blood sugar and triglyceride levels.

Management

The presence of steatosis without other obvious etiologies, associated with exposure to hepatotoxic agents, is suggestive of occupational or environmental liver disease. Although the natural history of steatosis in such settings is unclear, further toxic exposure should be minimized, and removal of the person from the workplace should be considered. Resolution of any concomitant elevation of aminotransferase levels after removal from exposure supports an occupational etiology.

Chronic hepatocellular injury

Chronic hepatocellular injury can occur after prolonged exposure to agents that cause acute and subacute hepatic injury or steatosis. Human data are limited to a few case reports of liver injury following chronic exposure to various hepatotoxic agents (including dimethylformamide, carbon tetrachloride, and mixed solvents) and cross-sectional surveys reporting elevated liver enzyme levels in exposed cohorts such as painters, print or shoe repair workers[20] compared with controls. The clinical presentation may range from minimal to pronounced symptoms and aminotransferase elevations. Liver biopsy may show varying degrees of necrosis, regeneration, inflammation, and steatosis.

The diagnosis of chronic hepatocellular injury is made based on the guidelines given earlier for acute and subacute liver injury. However, the diagnosis frequently is more difficult to determine than that of acute or subacute injury. Exposure assessment frequently is complicated by multiple, poorly defined exposures over many years, and it must be differentiated from other etiologies. Resolution of enzyme elevations after removal of the person from exposure is helpful. However, the natural history is not well defined, and aminotransferase abnormalities appear to resolve more slowly than with acute hepatocellular injury. It is unclear whether progression to cirrhosis or increased risk for hepatoma occurs.

Granulomatous hepatitis

Exposure to pathogenic dusts that cause pulmonary granulomatous lesions also may result in hepatic granulomas. Hepatic granulomas also may result from drug-induced hepatic injury or may be a non-specific finding in almost any setting. Hepatic granulomas have been described in chronic beryllium disease, silicosis, vineyard sprayer's lung (presumed secondary to copper exposure), and following mica and cement exposure. The hepatic lesions usually are asymptomatic and functionally not important, but rarely can be accompanied by hepatomegaly, necrosis, or fibrosis. Diagnosis depends on the appropriate exposure history and finding granulomatous changes on liver biopsy. The inhaled foreign particles may be detected in the biopsy specimen. The natural history of such lesions is not well defined but is most likely benign. As with the underlying granulomatous disorder, the lesions may progress after exposure has ceased. It is unclear whether or not the administration of steroids is beneficial. Exposure to additional hepatotoxic agents should be minimized.

Hepatoportal sclerosis

Hepatoportal sclerosis is a rare form of non-cirrhotic periportal fibrosis, which can lead to portal hypertension. It has been described most commonly as a consequence of exposure to vinyl chloride monomer,[37,38] inorganic arsenicals, and thorium compounds. Inorganic arsenicals and thorium compounds are no longer in common use.

Vinyl chloride monomer, a chlorinated hydrocarbon, is used in the production of polyvinyl chloride (PVC), a widely manufactured plastic. Hepatoportal sclerosis has been documented in several studies of workers exposed to vinyl chloride, primarily in PVC polymerization manufacturing plants.[39] Liver histology has shown hyperplasia of hepatocytes and sinusoidal cells, with dilatation of sinusoids and progressive subcapsular, portal, perisinusoidal, and, occasionally, intralobular fibrosis, which is accompanied by portal hypertension and splenomegaly. Workers with hepatoportal sclerosis have a markedly increased risk of developing angiosarcoma of the liver, a rare liver cancer seen almost exclusively in the setting of vinyl chloride or arsenic exposure;[40] greater than threefold increases in liver cancer (SMR 333; 90% CI 202–521) have been observed in vinyl chloride polymerization plant workers.[41] Hepatoportal sclerosis usually is found in tumor-free areas of the liver in patients with angiosarcoma and may be a premalignant promoting factor (see Chapter 30.6).

Vinyl chloride-induced liver injury presents insidiously, with the diagnosis made frequently 15–20 years after the first exposure.[42] Portal hypertension with periportal fibrosis may develop eventually. The diagnosis is made on the basis of a consistent exposure history and characteristic findings on liver biopsy. Standard liver function tests usually are of limited value in detecting vinyl chloride-induced liver injury. Several studies have indicated that ICG clearance and serum bile acids provide improved sensitivity and specificity in screening exposed workers.[43]

There have been a few case reports suggesting that exposure to polymeric vinyl chloride also may be associated with hepatic angiosarcoma. Whether exposure to PVC also can cause non-malignant liver injury is unclear. There generally is little release of vinyl chloride monomer from solid PVC materials, although significant amounts may be released with combustion of PVC products and possibly in the processing or some applications of PVC materials.

Cirrhosis

Cirrhosis, or end-stage liver disease, is defined as a chronic, irreversible condition in which the normal lobular architecture is replaced by fibrous tissue and regenerating nodules derived from the remaining hepatocytes. Cirrhosis is most commonly due to alcohol or viral infection but also may be caused by chronic biliary disease, metabolic diseases such as hemochromatosis, and congestive heart failure. Cases of cirrhosis sometimes are idiopathic. Animal studies have shown that hepatotoxic exposures such as carbon tetrachloride, arsenic, and aflatoxins can result in cirrhosis. The role of occupational or environmental substances in the development of cirrhosis, either alone or interacting synergistically with other etiologic agents has not been well characterized in humans. Whatever the initial cause, the pathogenesis involves hepatocellular necrosis, with subsequent deposition of large amounts of connective tissue and nodular regeneration of hepatocytes.

There have been isolated, often not well-documented, case reports of cirrhosis associated with repeated exposure to several occupational agents, most of them no longer in use, including carbon tetrachloride, arsenicals, tetra-chloroethane, trinitrotoluene, and trichloroethylene (TCE).[44] Increased mortality due to cirrhosis has been noted in several cohorts of workers with known or suspected hepatotoxic exposures (primarily solvents), including pressmen, shipyard workers, marine inspectors, metal fabrication employees, anesthesiologists, vineyard workers exposed to arsenical pesticides, and PCB workers. Mortality studies have also suggested increased risk for chronic hepatic injury in occupational groups with long-term daily exposure to organic solvents. These studies have observed relative risks for cirrhosis ranging from 1.6 to 2.1 in automobile spray painters and newspaper printers.[45–48] However, in many of these studies, confounding factors, such as ethanol or viral hepatitis, were not accounted for.

In patients with idiopathic cirrhosis, the diagnosis of an occupational or environmental etiology should be considered if there has been a history of repeated exposure to known or suspected hepatotoxins. Further hepatotoxic exposures should be minimized.

MAJOR HUMAN HEPATOTOXINS

Several specific environmental agents that have been reported to cause liver injury in humans are discussed in this section.

Solvents

Carbon tetrachloride and other chlorinated solvents

Carbon tetrachloride is the classic example of an intrinsic occupational hepatotoxin. The hepatotoxicity of carbon tetrachloride was first recognized in the 1920s, when it was frequently used as a solvent, dry-cleaning agent, fire extinguisher, and anthelmintic. As with most hepatotoxic solvents, acute intoxication results in multisystem disease, with central nervous system depression and acute necrosis of the renal tubules and the liver. Symptoms and liver aminotransferase abnormalities usually occur 1–2 days following the acute exposure and resolve in 1–2 weeks, but the time course may vary depending on the dose and length of exposure. Histology reveals centrilobular necrosis and steatosis; cirrhosis following carbon tetrachloride exposure is well established in animal models, and there are a few case reports in humans. Carbon tetrachloride-related hepatotoxicity is potentiated by ethanol consumption.[49] Because of renal and hepatic toxicity, use of carbon tetrachloride has decreased greatly, but cases of hepatotox-

icity still are reported. Tetrachloroethane and chloroform also are no longer in general use because of their recognized hepatotoxicity.

1,1,1-Trichloroethane and TCE are widely used chlorinated solvents with documented animal hepatotoxicity. Although they are less hepatotoxic than carbon tetrachloride, exposure to both agents has been associated with case reports of hepatic necrosis and steatosis.[50–53] Perchloroethylene, a popular dry-cleaning solvent, is also hepatotoxic in animal studies and historical case reports.[54] Elevations in GGT, in the absence of other liver function test abnormalities have been observed in surveillance of exposed workers.[55] A cross-sectional field investigation of 29 dry-cleaning operators observed mild to moderate hepatic parenchymal changes in echogenicity, as determined by hepatic ultrasonography, in two-thirds of dry cleaners compared with only one-third of referents (OR 3.2, 95% CI 1.04–9.8),[25] with minimal associated changes in transaminase levels.

Dimethylformamide

Dimethylformamide is a widely used hepatotoxic solvent. Several recent reports have documented acute and chronic liver injury in workers exposed to dimethylformamide.[56] In addition to typical gastrointestinal symptoms, a disulfiram-type reaction (acquired alcohol intolerance) is frequently reported following acute exposure. Elevated serum aminotransferase levels, with an increased ALT/AST ratio, have been found. Liver biopsy following acute exposure (less than 2 months) has shown variable degrees of hepatic necrosis, regeneration, and microvesicular and macrovesicular steatosis, whereas marked steatosis without fibrosis has been found on biopsy following longer exposures[57] (Fig. 26.1.1). Elevated liver enzyme levels may persist weeks to months after removal of the person from further exposure. The long-term effects of dimethylformamide exposure are not known.

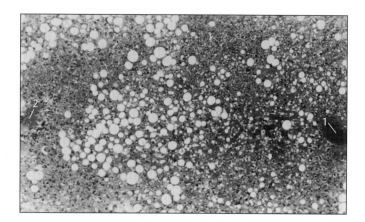

Figure 26.1.1: Liver histology from a patient who had been exposed to the solvent demethylformamide for several years. Liver architecture is normal, but there is moderate to severe steatosis, mainly in zones 2 and 3. 1, central vein; 2, a portal tract. (Carnoy's fixation, H & E, original magnification × 130.) (From Redlich CA, West AB, Fleming LE, et al. Clinical and pathological characteristics associated with occupational exposure to dimethylformamide. Gastroenterology 1990; 99:748–57, with permission from American Gastroenterological Association.)

Aromatic and other solvents

Toluene is one of the most frequently used solvents in industry, and it is a known animal hepatotoxin. Elevated serum transaminase and GGT levels have been found in print workers exposed to toluene[58,59] and after exposure to glues.[60] Liver biopsies reveal fatty liver with mild non-specific inflammation. The long-term hepatic effects of toluene exposure are not known.

Several investigations of workers exposed to relatively high levels of styrene (e.g., 50–300 ppm) observed elevations in serum hepatic transaminase[61] and GGT levels,[62–64] suggesting hepatic necrosis and cholestasis, respectively. Two independent cross-sectional studies of workers exposed to lower levels of styrene, including fiberglass reinforced plastics workers and boat and tank fabricators, observed increased direct bilirubin and AP levels compared to non-exposed referent groups, consistent with diminished hepatic clearance of conjugated bilirubin with associated cholestasis.[21] The absence of similar elevations in hepatic transaminase levels in these studies suggests that low-level styrene exposure results in mild metabolic dysfunction without significant hepatic parenchymal necrosis.

There are isolated case reports of acute hepatotoxic injury following acute exposure to several other solvents, including 2-nitropane,[65,66] methyl chloride, tetrahydrofuran, carbon tetrabromide, and xylene.[67]

Mixed solvents

Exposure to solvent mixtures is more common than isolated single exposures. Several epidemiologic studies have reported elevated liver enzyme levels in workers such as painters, print workers, and chemical workers exposed to various solvents including toluene, acetone, benzene, methyl ethyl ketone, and styrene. Typically, aminotransferase levels have been elevated compared with control groups, with AST/ALT ratio less than one. Dossing observed that 13 of 156 (8.3%) career painters with chronic encephalopathy due to 'white spirit' (mixed aliphatic and aromatic hydrocarbons) exposure had elevated serum transaminases.[68] Liver biopsy revealed that 11 of these 13 painters (85%) had moderate steatosis and focal hepatic necrosis. Evidence of hepatotoxicity has also been demonstrated in painters exposed chronically to solvents, with elevated alkaline phosphatase levels observed in a cross-sectional study of Swedish house painters.[69] Elevated GGT levels also have been reported in solvent-exposed groups such as paint manufacturers and sprayers,[70] as well as necrosis and steatosis on liver biopsies of selected subjects.[71] Severe liver injury with centrilobular and hemorrhagic necrosis has been observed in chemical plant workers exposed to mixtures of carbon disulfide, isopranolol, toluene, and acrylonitrile.[72] In some of these studies, other competing etiologies, such as alcohol, viral hepatitis, or obesity, were not well controlled.

Solvent mixtures may interact to enhance hepatotoxicity, as demonstrated by Charbonneau and colleagues in rodents exposed to CCl_4, acetone, and corn oil.[73,74] In human volunteers, altered oxidative hepatic metabolism during mixed solvent exposure has also been demonstrated with toluene,[75,76] as well as methyl ethyl ketone (MEK) and various alcohols,[77] and may explain the variable hepatotoxicity observed with mixed solvent exposures.[11]

Halothane and other anesthetic solvents

Halothane is a general anesthetic agent that can cause hepatitis in patients undergoing general anesthesia, and in occupationally exposed workers, such as anesthetists and operating room personnel.[78,79] Halothane-induced hepatitis is not dose dependent, and significant liver injury is rare, usually occurring following repeated exposures. Serum aminotransferase levels are elevated, and liver biopsy shows spotty to massive necrosis, frequently with steatosis and eosinophilic infiltration. Fever and eosinophilia usually are present. There are rare case reports of cirrhosis and chronic active hepatitis following halothane exposure. A few epidemiologic studies have reported an increased frequency of liver disease among operating room personnel.[80] Methoxyflurane, another widely used anesthetic, also has been reported to cause liver injury similar to halothane-induced hepatitis.

Organochlorine pesticides and related polychlorinated compounds

Several non-specific liver abnormalities have been associated with exposure to pesticides. A massive outbreak of acquired porphyria cutanea tarda and hepatomegaly occurred in Turkey following the ingestion of grain contaminated with the fungicide hexachlorobenzene. Chronic hepatic sequelae were not well documented. The organochlorine pesticide chlordecone has been reported to cause hepatomegaly, non-specific changes on liver biopsy, and marked proliferation of smooth endoplasmic reticulum on electron microscopy, consistent with induction of P-450 enzymes.[81] These changes resolved following removal of the affected individuals from exposure. The use of organochlorine pesticides has been limited because of potential carcinogenicity, including liver and biliary tract cancer among DDT-exposed workers.[82]

2,3,7,8-Tetrachlorodibenzo-*p*-dioxin (TCDD), or dioxin, is a contaminant of chlorophenoxy herbicides that can cause chloracne and liver injury.[83] Mildly elevated liver aminotransferase and GGT levels have been reported following TCDD exposure, with necrosis and steatosis on liver biopsy. Persistent liver injury has been reported by a European group who found elevated transaminases, GGT, and urinary porphyrins in Austrian chemical workers 25 years after their main exposure to dioxin.[84] Because of its storage in body fat, dioxin has an extremely long half-life of many years. Persistently elevated transaminase levels have also been documented among Vietnam veterans exposed to Agent Orange.[83,85]

PCBs and chlorinated naphthalenes have been used widely as insulating liquids in electrical systems. While no longer manufactured because of concerns about their biopersistence and carcinogenicity,[86] exposure continues to be documented in inhabitants living near electrochemical factories.[87] Heavy occupational exposure or accidental oral ingestion of these agents has been reported to cause hepatic necrosis and, in some cases, subsequent subacute hepatic necrosis and cirrhosis. Among workers manufacturing capacitors and transformers, elevations in LDH and GGT correlated with PCB levels.[88]

Halogenated pesticides such as DDT and hexachlorobenzene, chlorinated dioxins such as TCDD, and polychlorinated biphenyls (PCBs) are all potent inducers of various cytochrome *P*-450 mono-oxygenases, and they may potentiate the hepatotoxicity of other exposures by enhancing metabolism of toxic intermediates.

Metals

Arsenic

Accidental arsenic ingestion can result in acute hepatic injury with necrosis and steatosis. Chronic exposure to arsenic has been seen in vintners,[89] farmers, and miners, with variable hepatotoxcity. Arsenic in insecticide sprays has been associated with an increased incidence of cirrhosis and hepatoportal sclerosis. Such arsenical compounds are no longer in use. Besides its hepatic effects, arsenic also affects the gastrointestinal tract, central nervous system, and cardiovascular system. Hemorrhagic necrosis of the GI tract, nausea, vomiting, CNS depression, and vascular collapse are frequently seen.[90] Environmental arsenic poisoning from ground-water sources has been an important public health problem in endemic areas such as Bangladesh and West Bengal, where hepatic abnormalities are frequently seen as part of a multisystemic illness.[91]

Lead

Elevated aminotransferase levels have been reported with acute inorganic lead intoxication, usually with lead levels in the range of 80 μg/dl or greater. Levels promptly improve following chelation treatment and removal from further exposure. The presence of liver injury may explain some of the gastrointestinal toxicity found in acute poisoning cases.

Other environmental agents

Although they are primarily industrial hepatotoxins, many of the agents discussed earlier and listed in Table 26.1.1 also are potential environmental toxins. Hepatotoxic exposures could potentially occur through contact with contaminated water, air, soil, or food. Such environmental contamination is of particular concern with chemicals such as DDT or PCBs, which are very stable, resist biodegradation, and accumulate in the environment and food chain. Notably, the substitution of hydrochlorofluorocarbons (HCFC) for ozone-depleting chlorofluorocarbons has resulted in prominent hepatic injury among groups of exposed workers.[92] In addition, several naturally occurring toxins produce marked hepatotoxicity on ingestion.

Aflatoxins

The fungus *Aspergillus flavus* produces toxins, termed aflatoxins, that can contaminate food products, including nuts, corn, and wheat. The fungus is abundant in tropical and subtropical regions, and thrives under moist, warm conditions. Aflatoxin B1 is a potent inhibitor of RNA synthesis and the most hepatotoxic of these compounds.[90] Acute exposure has been reported to cause necrosis, steatosis, and inflammation. Chronic exposure is associated with an increased risk of hepatic carcinoma; the risk of malignancy is directly proportional to the amount of toxin ingested.[90]

Mushroom poisoning

Ingestion of *Amanita phalloides* (death cap) mushrooms can result in fatal poisoning, with massive hepatic necrosis. Fulminant hepatic failure is seen, with coma and renal failure common. These mushrooms contain several toxins, with α-amanitin being the most toxic. Amatoxin is thermostable, and can remain active for years. A fatal dose has been estimated to be in the range of 7 mg, or three mushrooms.[90]

Viral agents

Hepatitis A, B, or C can occur as an occupational disease in healthcare workers and others in contact with the excreta or blood from patients or carriers infected with these viruses. Hepatitis A causes an acute hepatitis, typically with no long-term sequelae. Hepatitis B and hepatitis C may cause both acute and chronic hepatitis. A full discussion of viral hepatitis is provided in Chapter 22.

MEDICAL SURVEILLANCE FOR OCCUPATIONAL LIVER DISEASE
Surveillance strategies

Strategies for controlling occupational liver disease follow the general principles of primary and secondary prevention. Primary preventive strategies attempt to identify and remove (or reduce) hepatotoxic exposures. Hepatotoxic substances are identified by review of the chemicals used and assessment of industrial hygiene to limit exposure. Hepatotoxic exposures can be minimized by substituting less toxic agents and by using engineering controls (e.g., improved ventilation) and personal protective equipment.

Secondary preventive strategies involve the screening of workers actively exposed to known or suspected hepatotoxins. This approach is appropriate when exposure is unpredictable or unavoidable (i.e., not amenable to primary prevention). Such strategies attempt to identify hepatic disease at an early, reversible stage.

Screening tests for occupational hepatotoxicity

Screening tests for occupational liver disease include the biochemical, clearance, and metabolic tests described earlier.[93] Despite high sensitivity and specificity in particular settings, all tests are potentially limited by low predictive value.[11,94] Because of a low prevalence of hepatic disease in the general population, only a small percentage of individuals who have positive test results actually have liver disease. For example, serum aminotransferase levels, which are more than 90% accurate in the diagnosis of acute viral hepatitis, have a predictive value of less than 10% in screening for chronic liver disease in the general population.

Determining the predictive value of screening tests is complicated by the lack of prevalence data for occupational liver disease. A notable exception is vinyl chloride monomer, with a 2–3% prevalence of chronic liver disease in exposed workers. The most accurate test for such disease is ICG clearance, with a predictive value of 20%. In most industries, however, the prevalence of hepatic disease is unknown and probably variable; the efficacy of a screening test in one setting cannot be assumed to be the same in another.

Screening of healthy workers is recommended only when there is exposure to known or strongly suspected hepatotoxic agents. Because no ideal screening test for occupational liver injury exists, serum aminotransferase tests (AST and ALT) remain the best practical choice at present. They are inexpensive, available, and clinically validated. Combination testing, namely requiring positive results on two different tests, may enhance predictive value, but this approach has not been validated and may result in high rates of false-negative results. Metabolic tests such as antipyrine clearance should be considered markers for specific exposures rather than for actual hepatic injury.

Clinical management of abnormal liver function tests

Management of abnormal liver function tests depends on the clinical presentation (the extent and type of liver injury) and exposure setting (the likelihood and extent of hepatotoxic exposure).[95] In acute and subacute settings, with well-documented exposure to a known or suspected hepatotoxin, an association between the liver injury and hepatotoxic exposure frequently can be determined, once other possible etiologies have been excluded. Prompt removal of the affected individual from exposure to any workplace or environmental hepatotoxin is indicated. Transaminase levels are generally elevated several fold and should be monitored closely, with the use of early hepatic ultrasound to rule out biliary obstruction. Supportive care, including hospitalization, may be required in severe cases.

On the other hand, in the setting of chronic low-level exposures, as often occurs in mass screening of healthy workers, the relationship between elevated hepatic transaminase levels and specific exposures may be much more difficult to determine. Because low predictive values, in the range of 5–20% for available tests, generate high rates of false-positive findings, emphasis should be placed on distinguishing true from false-positive results. Removal of the affected individual from work should be considered only after alternative etiologies, such as medications, non-occupational liver disorders, and excessive alcohol use

have been excluded.[96] For example, mild hyperbilirubinemia in an otherwise healthy worker likely represents Gilbert's syndrome and usually does not warrant further evaluation. There are no strict guidelines for the management of abnormal serum aminotransferase levels, which are often minimally elevated. In situations in which significant exposure is unlikely and transaminase levels are between one and two times normal, repeat testing in 4 weeks has been advocated, with further investigation reserved only for persistent elevations.

A general approach for evaluating possible occupational or environmental liver disease is summarized in the following list, although modifications are needed, depending on the particular clinical and exposure setting.

1. Assess both occupational and non-occupational causes of liver disease, including significant alcohol use, viral hepatitis (A, B, and C), biliary disease, medications, blood transfusions, and hepatotoxic exposures from work, hobbies, the home, and second jobs (see item 3). Potential hepatotoxic medications are numerous[97] (e.g., acetaminophen, isoniazid, erythromycin, estrogens, phenytoin, and megavitamins such as vitamin A) and should be discontinued, when possible. The abnormal liver tests should be repeated in 2–4 weeks. Metabolic etiologies including diabetes mellitus, hemochromatosis, hypertriglyceridemia and obesity should be considered.

2. Consider the AST/ALT ratio. Ratios less than one are suggestive of viral or toxic exposures rather than alcohol use.

3. Attempt to determine the presence of any known or suspected hepatotoxins in the workplace or environment. Sources of such information may be obtained from material data safety sheets, the worker, the employer, the manufacturer, and industrial hygiene sampling, if available.

4. If a significant hepatotoxic exposure is identified, the individual should be removed from further exposure and his or her AST and ALT should be rechecked in 2–4 weeks. Recovery suggests an occupational or environmental etiology, but persistent elevations do not rule it out. Such persons may return to work or the same environmental setting on a trial basis if appropriate controls or exposure modifications have been implemented. Close follow-up, with continued monitoring of AST and ALT levels, is necessary in these situations.

5. Persistent elevation of AST and ALT levels greater than twice normal for over 2 months warrants further investigation; referral to a hepatologist should be considered. Such individuals have an increased likelihood of chronic active hepatitis, steatohepatitis, and fibrotic changes.[98] Hepatic ultrasonography, liver biopsy, or both, may be indicated. Findings of steatosis and necrosis are particularly suggestive of an occupational etiology. A trial entailing removal of the affected individual from hepatotoxic exposures, even if they are only suspected, should be considered. Because various hepatotoxins may interact, alcohol use and potentially hepatotoxic medications should be minimized.

In the end, the diagnosis of occupational or environmental liver injury must integrate the clinical data discussed above with knowledge regarding the intrinsic hepatotoxicity and nature of the exposure(s). Limited knowledge regarding hepatotoxicity, particularly for new or poorly characterized chemicals, as well as a determination of the nature and extent of exposure, especially with more chronic presentations, frequently represent challenges to the clinician.

References

1. Harford TC, Brooks SD. Cirrhosis mortality and occupation. J Stud Alcohol 1992; 53:463–8.
2. Batt A-M, Ferrari L. Manifestations of chemically induced liver damage. Clin Chem 1995; 41:1882–7.
3. Reinke LA, McCay PB. Free radicals and alcohol liver injury. In: Watson RR, ed. Drug and alcohol abuse reviews, vol. 2: liver pathology and alcohol. Totawa: The Humana Press, 1991;133–68.
4. Johansson I, Ingelman-Sundberg M. Carbon tetrachloride-induced lipid peroxidation dependent on an ethanol-inducible from of rabbit liver microsomal cytochrome P-450. FEBS Lett 1985; 183:265–9.
5. Koop DR, Casazza JP. Identification of ethanol-inducible P-450 isozyme 3A as the acetone and acetol monooxygenase of rabbit microsomes. J Biol Chem 1985; 260:13607–12.
6. Koop DR, Orlandi CL, Schnier GG. Ethanol-inducible P450 isozyme 3a is a benzene hydroxylase. FASEB J 1988; 2:A1012(abstract).
7. Hetu C, Dumont A, Joly JG. Effect of chronic ethanol administration on bromobenzene liver toxicity in the rat. Toxicol Appl Pharmacol 1983; 67:166–77.
8. Ingelman-Sundberg M, Johansson I. Mechanisms of hydroxyl radical formation and ethanol oxidation by ethanol-inducible and other forms of rabbit liver microsomal cytochromes P-450. J Biol Chem 1984; 259:6447–58.
9. Tsutsumi M, Shimizu M, Lasker MJ, Lieber CS. Intralobular distribution of ethanol-inducible cytochrome P450IIE1 in liver. Hepatology 1988; 8:1237A.
10. Hasumara Y, Teschke R, Lieber CS. Increased carbon tetrachloride hepatotoxicity, and its mechanism, after chronic ethanol consumption. Gastroenterology 1974; 66:415–22.
11. Harrison R. Medical surveillance for workplace hepatotoxins. State Art Rev 1990; 5:515–30.
12. Matloff DS, Selinger MJ, Kaplan MM. Hepatic transaminase activity in alcoholic liver disease. Gastroenterology 1980; 78:1389–92.
13. Cohen JA, Kaplan MM. The SGOT/SGPT ratio – an indicator of alcoholic liver disease. Dig Dis Sci 1979; 24:835–8.
14. Fleming LE, Shalat SL, Redlich CA. Liver injury in workers exposed to dimethylformamide. Scand J Work Environ Health 1990; 16:289–92.
15. Ferraris R, Fiorentini M, Galatola G, et al. Diagnostic value of serum immunoreactive conjugated cholic or chenodeoxycholic acids in detecting hepatobiliary disease. Dig Dis Sci 1987; 32:817–23.
16. Edling C, Tagesson C. Raised serum bile acid concentrations after occupational exposure to styrene: a possible sign of hepatotoxicity. Br J Ind Med 1984; 41:257–9.
17. Franco G, Fonte R, Tempini G, Candura F. Serum bile acid concentrations as a liver function test in workers occupationally exposed to organic solvents. Int Arch Occup Environ Health 1986; 58:157–64.
18. Franco G, Santagostino G, Lorena M, Imbriani M. Conjugated serum bile acid concentrations in workers exposed to low doses of toluene and xylene. Br J Ind Med 1989; 46:141–2.
19. Franco G. New perspectives in biomonitoring liver function by means of serum bile acids; experimental and hypothetical biochemical basis. Br J Ind Med 1991; 48:557–61.
20. Tomei F, Giuntoli P, Biagi M, Baccolo TP, Tomao E, Rosati MV. Liver damage among shoe repairers. Am J Ind Med 1999; 36:541–7.
21. Brodkin CA, Moon JD, Camp J, Echeverria D, Redlich C, Checkoway H. Serum hepatic biochemical activity in two populations of styrene-exposed workers. Occup Environ Med 2001; 58:95–102.
22. Savertymuttu SH, Joseph AEA, Maxwell JD. Ultrasound scanning in the detection of hepatic fibrosis and steatosis. Br Med J 1986; 292:13.
23. Williams DMJ, Smith PM, Taylor KJW, Crossley IR, Duck BW. Monitoring liver disorders in vinyl chloride monomer workers using greyscale ultrasonography. Br J Ind Med 1976; 33:152–7.
24. Taylor KJW, Williams DMJ, Smith PM, Duck BW. Grey-scale ultrasonography for monitoring industrial exposure to hepatotoxic agents. Lancet 1975; i:1222–4.
25. Brodkin CA, Daniell W, Checkoway H, et al. Ultrasonic detection of occult hepatotoxicity in perchloroethylene-exposed workers. Occup Environ Med 1995; 52:679–85.
26. Semelka RC, Chung JJ, Hussain SM, et al. Chronic hepatitis: correlation of early patchy and late linear enhancement patterns on gaddinium-enhanced MR images with histopathology initial experience. J Mag Res Imag 2001; 13:385–91.
27. Brautbar N, Williams J. Industrial solvents and liver toxicity: risk assessment, risk factors, and mechanisms. Int J Hyg Environ Health 2002; 205:479–91.
28. Bastian PG. Occupational hepatitis caused by methylenedianiline. Med J Aust 1984; 141:533–5.
29. Kopelman H, Scheuer PJ, Williams R. The liver lesion of the Epping jaundice. Q J Med 1977; 35:553–67.
30. Wanless IR, Lentz JS. Fatty liver hepatitis (steatohepatitis) and obesity: an autopsy study with analysis of risk factors. Hepatology 1990; 12:1106–10.
31. Nomura H, Kashiwagi S, Hayashi J, et al. Prevalence of fatty liver in a general population of Okinawa, Japan. Jpn J Med 1988; 27:142–9.
32. Chitturis, Farrel GC. Etiopathogenesis of nonalcoholic steatohepatitis. Semin Liver Dis 2001; 21:27–41.
33. Balazs T, Murray TK, McLaughlan JM, Grice HC. Hepatic tests in toxicity studies on rats. Toxicol Appl Pharmacol 1961; 3:71–9.
34. Harinasuta U, Chomet B, Ishak KG, Zimmerman HJ. Steatonecrosis-mallory body type. Medicine 1967; 46:141–61.
35. Diehl AM, Goodman Z, Ishak KG. Alcohol-like liver disease in nonalcoholics: a clinical and histologic comparison with alcohol-induced liver injury. Gastroenterology 1988; 195:1056–62.
36. Powell EE, Cooksley WGE, Hanson R, Searle J, Halliday JW, Powell LW. The natural history of nonalcoholic steatohepatitis: a follow-up study of forty-two patients for up to 21 years. Hepatology 1990; 11:74–80.
37. Thomas LB, Popper H, Berk PD, et al. Vinyl chloride induced liver disease. N Engl J Med 1975; 292:17–22.
38. Tamburro CH, Mack L, Popper H. Early hepatic histologic alterations among chemical (vinyl monomer) workers. Hepatology 1984; 4:413–8.
39. Falk H, Creech JL, Heath CW, et al. Hepatic disease among workers at a vinyl chloride polymerization plant. JAMA 1974; 230:59–63.
40. Wagoner JK. Toxicity of vinyl chloride and poly (vinyl chloride): a critical review. Environ Health Persp 1983; 52:61–6.
41. Wu W, Steenland K, Brown D, et al. Cohort and case-control analyses of workers exposed to vinyl chloride: an update. J Occup Med 1989; 31:518–23.
42. ATSDR (Agency for Toxic Substances and Disease Registry) case studies in environmental medicine. Vinyl chloride toxicity. Clin Toxicol 1990; 28:267–86.
43. Liss GM, Greenburg RA, Tamburro CH. Use of serum bile acids in the identification of vinyl chloride hepatotoxicity. Am J Med 1985; 78:68–76.

44. Thiele DL, Eigenbrodt EH, Ware AJ. Cirrhosis after repeated trichloroethylene and 1,1,1-trichloroethane exposure. Gastroenterology 1982; 83:926–9.

45. Dossing M, Skinhoj P. Occupational liver injury: present state of knowledge and future perspective. Int Arch Occup Environ Health 1985; 56:1–21.

46. Lloyd JW, Decoufle P, Salvin LG. Unusual mortality experience of printing pressman. J Occup Med 1977; 19:543–50.

47. Paganini-Hill A, Glazer E, Henderson BE, Ross RK. Cause-specific mortality among newspaper web pressmen. J Occup Med 1980; 22:542–44.

48. Chiazze L, Ference LD, Wolf PH. Mortality among automobile assembly workers. J Occup Med 1980; 22:520–6.

49. Hasumura Y, Teschke R, Lieber CS. Increased carbon tetrachloride hepatotoxicity, and its mechanism, after chronic ethanol consumption. Gastroenterology 1974; 66:415.

50. McCunney RJ. Diverse manifestations of trichlorethylene. Br J Ind Med 1988; 45:122–6.

51. Nakayama H, Kobayashi M, Takahashi M, et al. Generalized eruption with severe liver dysfunction associated with occupational exposure to trichloroethylene. Contact Derm 1988; 19:48–51.

52. Hodgson MJ, Heyl AE, Van Thiel DH. Liver disease associated with exposure to 1,1,1-trichloroethane. Arch Int Med 1989; 149:1793–8.

53. Texter EC Jr, Grunow WA, Zimmerman HJ. Massive centrizonal necrosis of the liver due to inhalation of 1,1,1-trichloroethane. Gastroenterology 1979; 76:1260.

54. Meckler LC, Phelps DK. Liver disease secondary to tetrachloroethylene exposure. A case report. JAMA 1966; 197:662.

55. Gennari P, Massimo N, Motta R, et al. Gamma-glutamyltransferase isoenzyme pattern in workers exposed to tetracholorethylene. Am J Ind Med 1992; 21:661–71.

56. Redlich CA, Beckett WS, Sparer JS. Liver disease associated with occupational exposure to the solvent dimethylformamide. Ann Intern Med 1988; 108:680–6.

57. Redlich CA, West AB, Fleming LE, et al. Clinical and pathological characteristics associated with occupational exposure to dimethylformamide. Gastroenterology 1990; 99:748–57.

58. Guzelian P, Mills S, Fallon HJ. Liver structure and function in print workers exposed to toluene. J Occup Med 1988; 30:791–6.

59. Boewer C, Enderlein G, Wollgast U, Nawka S. Epidemiological study on the hepatotoxicity of occupational toluene exposure. Int Arch Environ Health 1988; 60:181–6.

60. Knight AT, Pawsey CG, Aroney RS, et al. Upholsterers' glue associated with myocarditis, hepatitis, acute renal failure and lymphoma. Med J Aust 1991; 154:360–2.

61. Axelson O, Gustavson J. Some hygienic and clinical obersvation on styrene exposure. Scand J Work Environ Health 1978; 4(Suppl 2):215–9.

62. Thiess AM, Friedheim M. Morbidity among persons employed in styrene production, polymerization and processing plants. Scand J Work Environ Health 1978; 4(Suppl 2):203–14.

63. Triebig G, Lehrl S, Weltle D, Schaller KH, Valentin H. Clinical and neurobehavioural study of the acute and chronic neurotoxicity of styrene. Br J Ind Med 1989; 46:799–804.

64. Lorimer WV, Lilis R, Fischbein A, et al. Health status of styrene-polystyrene polymerization workers. Scand J Work Environ Health 1978; 4(Suppl 2):220–6.

65. Harrison R, Letz G, Pasternak G, Blanc P. Fulminant hepatic failure after occupational exposure to 2-nitropropane. Ann Int Med 1987; 107:466–8.

66. Hine CH, Pasi A, Stephens BG. Fatalities following exposure to 2-nitropropane. J Occup Med 1978; 20:333–7.

67. Morely R, Eccleston DW, Douglas CP, et al. Xylene poisoning: a report on one fatal case and two cases of recovery after prolonged unconsciousness. Br Med J 1970; 3:442–3.

68. Dossing M, Arloen-Soberg P, Peterson LM, et al. Liver damage associated with occupational exposure to organic solvents in house painters. Eur J Clin Invest 1983; 13:151–7.

69. Lundberg I, Nise G, Hedenborg G, Hogberg M, Vesterberg O. Liver function tests and urinary albumin in house painters with previous heavy exposure to organic solvents. Occup Environ Med 1994; 51:347–53.

70. Chen JD, Wang JD, Jang, JP, Chen YY. Exposure to mixtures of solvents among paint workers and biochemical alternations of liver function. Br J Ind Med 1991; 48:696–701.

71. Sotaniemi EA, Sutinen S, Arranto AJ, Pelkonen RO. Liver injury in subjects exposed to chemicals in low doses. Acta Med Scand 1982; 212:207–15.

72. Dossing M. Noninvasive assessment of microsomal enzyme activity in occupational medicine: present state of knowledge and future perspectives. Int Arch Environ Health 1984; 53:205–18.

73. Charbonneau M, Couture J, Plaa GL. Inhalation versus oral administration of acetone: Effect of the vehicle on the potentiation of CCl_4-induced liver injury. Toxicol Lett 1991; 57:47–54.

74. Charbonneau M, Tuchweber B, Plaa GL. Acetone potentiation of chronic liver injury induced by repetitive administration of carbon tetrachloride. Hepatology 1986; 6:694–700.

75. Waldron HA, Cherry N, Johnston JD. The effects of ethanol on blood toluene concentrations. Int Arch Environ Health 1983; 51:365–9.

76. Wallen M, Naslund PH, Nordqvist MB. The effects of ethanol on the kinetics of toluene in man. Toxicol Appl Pharmacol 1984; 76:414–9.

77. Liira J, Riihimaki V, Engstrom K. Effects of ethanol on the kinetics of methyl ethyl ketone in man. Br J Ind Med 1990; 47:235–30.

78. Edling C. Anesthetic gases as an occupational hazards: a review. Scand J Work Environ Health 1980; 6:85–93.

79. Neuberger J, Vergani D, Mieli-Vergani G, Davis M, Williams R. Hepatic damage after exposure to halothane in medical personnel. Br J Anaesth 1981; 53:1173–7.

80. Dahlgren B-E. Hepatic and renal effects of low concentrations of methoxyflurane in exposed delivery ward personnel. J Occup Med 1980; 22:817–9.

81. Guzelian PS, Vranian G, Boylan JJ, et al. Liver structure and function in patients poisoned with chlordecone (kepone). Gastroenterology 1980; 78:206–13.

82. Cocco P, Blair A, Congia P, Saba G, Ecca AR, Palmas C. Long-term health effects of the occupational exposure to DDT. A preliminary report. Ann NY Acad Sci 1997; 837:246–56.

83. Tamburro CH. Chronic liver injury in phenoxy herbicide-exposed Vietnam veterans. Environ Res 1992; 59:175–88.

84. Neuberger M, Rappe C, Bergek S, et al. Persistent health effects of dioxin contamination in herbicide production. Environ Res Sect A 1999; 81:206–14.

85. Michalek JE, Ketchum NS, Longnecker MP. Serum dioxin and hepatic abnormalities in veterans of Operation Ranch Hand. Ann Epidemiol 2001; 11:304–11.

86. Brown DP, Jones M. Mortality and industrial hygiene study of workers exposed to PCBs. Arch Environ Health 1981; 36:120–9.

87. Sala M, Sunyer J, Otero R, Santiago-Silva M. Organochlorine in the serum of inhabitants living near an electrochemical factory. Occup Environ Med 1999; 56:152–8.

88. Fischbein A. Liver function tests in workers with occupational exposure to polychlorinated biphenyls (PCBs): comparison with Yusho and Yu-Cheng. Environ Health Perspect 1985; 60:145–50.

89. Pimentel JC, Menezes AP. Liver disease in vineyard sprayers. Gastroenterology 1977; 72:275–83.

90. Zimmerman HJ, Lewis JH. Chemical- and toxin-induced hepatotoxicity. Gastroenterol Clin North Am 1995; 24:1027–45.

91. Rahman MM, Chowdhury UK, Mukherjee SC, et al. Chronic arsenic toxicity in Bangladesh and West Bengal, India – a review and commentary. J Toxicol Clin Toxicol 2001; 39:683–700.

92. Hoet P, Graf ML, Bourdi M, et al. Epidemic of liver disease caused by hydro chlorofluorocarbons using ozone-sparing substitutes of chlorofluorocarbons. Lancet 1997; 350(9077):556–9.

93. Tamburro CH, Liss GM. Tests for hepatotoxicity: usefulness in screening workers. J Occup Med 1986; 28:1034–44.

94. Wright C, Rivera J, Baetz J. Liver function testing in a working population: three strategies to reduce false-positive results. J Occup Med 1988; 30:693–7.

95. Herip DS. Recommendations for the investigation of abnormal hepatic function in asymptomatic workers. Am J Ind Med 1992; 21:331–9.

96. Hodgson M, Goodman-Klein B, Van Thiel D. Evaluating the liver in hazardous waste workers. Occup Med State Art Rev 1990; 5:67–78.

97. Lee WM. Drug-induced hepatotoxicity. N Engl J Med 2003; 349:474–85.

98. Hay JE, Czaja AJ, Rakela J, Ludwig J. The nature of unexplained chronic aminotransferase elevations of a mild to moderate degree in asymptomatic patients. Hepatology 1989; 9:193–7.

26.2 **Disorders of the Gut and Pancreas**

Stan Lee, Lora E Fleming, Carl A Brodkin

INTRODUCTION AND APPROACH TO THE PATIENT

Occupational and environmental diseases of the gastrointestinal (GI) tract often are unrecognized. A variety of toxic exposures in the workplace may cause GI symptoms (see Table 26.2.1). Organic solvents may cause nausea and vomiting by acute solvent intoxication, presumably mediated through their effects on the central nervous system. In addition, exposure to a variety of toxins may cause non-specific GI symptoms, such as nausea among workers exposed to lead.

The prevalence of non-malignant GI diseases of occupational and environmental etiology is unknown. This is due in part to lack of clinical recognition: because GI symptoms are so common, clinicians often fail to consider workplace exposures in the differential diagnosis.

The clinical evaluation of GI disease of suspected environmental origin follows the same general principles as that in general medical practice. The history and physical examination should not be limited to the GI system. Toxins that cause GI symptoms, such as metals, solvents, and pesticides, often cause more direct effects on other systems such as the central nervous system or skin. Laboratory tests of GI system anatomy and function are rarely diagnostic of etiology. In contract to infectious diarrhea in an agricultural worker, with a finding of ova and parasites in the stool, organophosphate poisoning in the same worker would have no specific GI finding. As with the physical examination, the laboratory investigation should never be limited to tests of the GI system and should be directed by the history. Nevertheless, acute GI symptoms, such as vomiting, abdominal pain, and severe diarrhea, have to be ameliorated because these symptoms often are what brought the patient to medical attention, not the fact of a toxic exposure. The suspected or established causes of common GI disturbances are summarized in Table 26.2.2 and discussed in detail in the following section.

UPPER GASTROINTESTINAL DISORDERS

Esophagitis and gastritis

Occupational and environmental causes

Most cases of occupationally related esophagitis and gastritis are associated with corrosives and solvents. Accidental exposures to corrosives, which include strong acids (such as sulfuric and chromic acids), fixers (such as formaldehyde), and strong bases (such as lye) cause direct tissue injury. Ingestion injury is the classic route of exposure for the aforementioned toxins. However, alternative routes of exposure, including dermal absorption and inhalation of high concentrations of irritant vapors, may be important with other agents. Grade 2 esophagitis has been reported in a plastics industry worker accidentally exposed to dimethylacetamide and 1,2-ethanediamine.[1]

Occupationally related gastritis has also been reported without an ingestion exposure. Solvents often have excellent penetration through both dermal and inhalational routes; for example, up to 10% of topical and 2% of inhaled dimethylacetamide is absorbed into the blood stream.[2] Excessive exposure to solvents frequently causes nausea and anorexia, through the central nervous system (see Chapter 40). Solvents additionally exert direct irritational effects on gastric (as well as bowel) mucosae, contributing to symptoms. More severe or localized effects are most likely to occur following ingestion. Gastritis has been observed in worker populations exposed to the solvent dimethylformamide, another solvent with high skin penetration. Chronic gastritis has been reported in a laboratory technician using a solution containing 80% methylmethacrylate for tissue preparation; concomitant skin changes were also present, with contact dermatitis. Interestingly, GI symptoms were reproduced with positive skin patch testing with methylmethacrylate.[3] Chronic gastritis has also been observed in several workers following an industrial exposure to methylmethacrylate; the symptoms continued for several years despite withdrawal from exposure.

Clinical course, diagnosis and management

Except for a history of ingestion and/or inhalation, occupationally related esophagitis and gastritis present similarly to non-environmentally related cases. Symptoms of esophagitis may include throat pain and dysphagia. Symptoms of gastritis may include upper- to mid-epigastric abdominal pain, with or without food intolerance.

The diagnosis and treatment is also similar to non-occupational cases, but must emphasize elimination or protection from exposure. This can serve as a diagnostic trial as well as a therapeutic intervention.

Peptic ulcer disease (gastric and duodenal)

Occupational and environmental causes

Peptic ulcer disease, encompassing both gastric and duodenal ulcers, has been reported in higher prevalence among certain occupations, with increased risk observed in a number of epidemic studies. There is a controversial association between occupational stress (either physical or emotional) and an increased prevalence of peptic ulcers; it is a controversy partially due to inconsistent and non-specific definitions of stress.

Traditionally, a number of sedentary, professional jobs with high stress, such as air traffic controllers and executives, have been found to have a higher prevalence of ulcers among workers.[4] However, more recent work has shown an increased prevalence of peptic ulcers in unskilled workers as well. In particular, immigrants and manual labor workers

Symptom	Type of exposure (examples)
Nausea and vomiting	Central nervous system depressant (organic solvents with acute solvent intoxication) Cholinesterase inhibitors (organophosphates, carbamates)
	Metabolic Methemoglobin formers (organic nitrogen compounds)
	Caustic Irritants (epoxy resins, copper and tin fumes)
Constipation	Heavy metals (lead, barium, thallium)
Diarrhea	Infections (parasites, bacteria) Cholinesterase inhibitors (organophosphates) Metals (arsenic, phosphorus)
Jaundice	Hepatotoxins (organic solvents) Hemolytic agents (arsine, naphthalene, phenylhydrazine, stilbene)

Table 26.2.1 Major acute gastrointestinal symptoms and their common occupational and environmental causes

Disorder	Exposure or occupation (examples)
Upper GI tract disorders	
Esophagitis/gastritis	Dimethylformamide Methylmethacrylate Dimethylacetamide
Peptic ulcer disease	Shift work
Pancreatitis	Chlorinated naphthalenes Organophosphate pesticides Organic solvents Scorpion toxin
Lower GI tract disorders	
Infectious gastroenteritis	Hospital workers Laboratory workers Food producers Abbatoir workers Farm workers Sewage workers
Celiac disease	Allergens associated with hypersensitivity pneumonitis (see Chapter 19.6)
Pneumatosis cystoides intestinalis	Trichloroethylene
Non-specific toxic GI syndromes	Lead
	Other heavy metals Organophosphate pesticides

Table 26.2.2 Environmental agents/occupations associated with gastrointestinal disorders

have a higher prevalence and mortality from peptic ulcer disease (gastric rather than duodenal) than sedentary workers. Among some groups of miners, such as the copper miners in Chile, the incidence of peptic ulcer disease is much higher than in mine administrators or mechanics. Of note, the increases among manual and migrant workers parallel the increased mortality rate among lower socioeconomic classes, and may be a confounding factor in these studies.[5,6]

The role of physical work, energy expenditure, and other physical factors appears to be important in ulcer prevalence and mortality rates.[7] In a study in the metalworking indus-

try in Italy, an increased prevalence of peptic ulcer disease and chronic gastritis was noted, which correlated in a dose-related fashion with number of years worked, noise, temperature, vibration, workshift, and workload.[8]

Ulcer prevalence is higher in shift workers than in daytime workers;[9] this increased prevalence is believed to be due to sleep disturbance and altered eating patterns in the shift worker. A study from Denmark found that low socioeconomic status and non-daytime work were associated with an increased risk of gastric ulcer.[10] The authors hypothesized that shift workers experienced physiologic and psychologic stress from disruption in circadian rhythms, limitations in family and social life, and sleep difficulties. During deep (e.g., rapid eye movement [REM]) sleep, there is a decrease in gastric acid secretion and an increase in gastric motility. Disruption of sleep processes may, therefore, theoretically increase the risk of ulcer disease.[10]

In addition to stress, food and smoking may also play a role in peptic ulcer disease. A study in a Japanese plastic processing plant demonstrated an association between peptic ulcers and smoking, as well as family history.[5] In another study, fishermen and transportation workers in Norway had an increased prevalence of both gastric and duodenal ulcers compared with 11 other occupational groups. This prevalence was believed to be due to irregular meals, high coffee intake, and heavy smoking.[6] Similar findings in a Russian study of railroad workers found an increased prevalence of peptic ulcer disease that correlated with irregular hurried meals of both cold and fried foods.[11]

Clinical course, diagnosis, and management

The diagnosis and treatment do not differ from that in the general medical setting. Management of shift work may be challenging, but regular meals and sleep habits should be emphasized. Acid suppression should be prescribed to effect ulcer healing or symptom resolution. *Helicobater pylori* should be treated if present. Use of non-steroidal anti-inflammatory drugs and aspirin should be eliminated if possible. Behavioral changes such as smoking cessation and decreased coffee and alcohol consumption should be encouraged.

Pancreatitis

Occupational and environmental causes

Toxin-induced pancreatitis may be more common than is now recognized, especially given the high proportion of cases now considered to be idiopathic or drug related. Extremely high exposures to a variety of occupational toxins (such as the chlorinated naphthalenes), that are also associated with severe liver damage and systemic toxicity, have been associated with diffuse pancreatic damage.[12] Isolated islet cell injury has been reported with accidental ingestion of the rodenticide pyriminil (Vacor).

The organophosphate pesticides have been associated with pancreatitis and other pancreatic disorders. Accidental ingestion of the organophosphate pesticide *O*-ethyl-Sphenylethylphosphophenodithioate leads to pancreatitis, frequently with pancreatic pseudocyst formations, during the acute stages of organophosphate poisoning. A male farm worker exposed to the organophosphate Q Dimethoate developed pancreatitis with acute organophosphate poisoning.[13] Two out of nine patients who ingested parathion developed painless acute hemorrhagic pancreatitis.[14]

Acute and chronic pancreatitis have also been associated with occupational exposures to organic solvents.[15,16] Numerous cases have now been described in association with occupational exposure to perchloroethylene, trichloroethylene (TCE), mineral spirits, solvent-based paints, and diesel fuel. There have been at least two case reports of pancreatitis associated with occupational exposure to the solvent dimethylformamide (a known hepatotoxin) with no history of concurrent alcohol use; full recovery was apparent following removal from exposure.[17] Experimental animal evidence also indicates that this solvent causes pancreatic damage.

Acute pancreatitis has also been reported with scorpion bites (*Tityus trintatis*), both occupationally and environmentally, in Trinidad.

Pathogenesis

Experimental models of poisoning in pigs and dogs with organophosphates reveal increases in amylase levels and increased intraductal pressures within the pancreas. The postulated mechanism is the stimulation of parasympathetic pathways to the pancreas through cholinesterase inhibition, which, in turn, augments the secretory flow, increasing intraductal pressure. This response can be attenuated experimentally through pretreatment with atropine. Pancreatitis associated with scorpion toxin appears to be related to increased cholinergic stimulation, as well as a direct toxic effect.[18,19]

Clinical course, diagnosis, and management

Clinical features of pancreatitis of environmental or occupational etiology do not appear to differ from those of other established causes. The key difference in treatment is prevention of re-exposure to the suspected toxin. As with other occupational GI diseases, removal of the affected individual can be a useful diagnostic as well as therapeutic intervention.

LOWER GASTROINTESTINAL DISORDERS

Infectious gastroenteritis

Occupational and environmental causes

Occupationally related gastroenteritis has been reported in workers and their families from a number of occupations (Table 26.2.3). In particular, parasitic and bacterial forms of gastroenteritis have been noted in specific occupations (such as healthcare workers, laboratory technicians, and sewage workers) that involve contact with infected materials.[20–24] Zoonotic illness resulting in gastroenteritis has been reported among animal handlers and laboratory technicians; agricultural workers and other rural manual laborers (and their families) have been noted to have increased parasitic and bacterial infestations, probably due to infected water supplies, poor hygienic conditions, and the use of night soil (human waste) as a fertilizer.

Clinical course, diagnosis, and management

While the signs and symptoms, as well as the diagnosis and treatment, of occupationally related gastroenteritis are the same as for any gastroenteritis, management should emphasize examination of family members who may be infected from common sources.

Celiac disease

Occupational and environmental causes

Hypersensitivity pneumonitides such as farmer's lung and bird fancier's lung have been associated with celiac disease in some cases. Celiac disease involves a malabsorption syndrome, with duodenal or jejunal villous changes

Occupation	Pathogens	Reference
Occupations with infected materials		
Laboratory workers	Shigella	Kolavic et al., 1997[37]
Healthcare workers (patient care)	Brucellosis, typhoid	Pike, 1979[22]; Pike, 1976[23]
Food production	Tularemia, tuberculosis	
Sewage workers	*Salmonella typhimurium* enteritis	Steckelberg et al., 1988[38]; Standaert et al., 1994[39]
	Cryptosporidiosis	Koch et al., 1985[24]
	Campylobacter jejuni enteritis	Jones, 1979[40]
	Parasitic infections (*Entamoeba histolytica, Giardia lamblia*)	Clark et al., 1984[21]; Hays, 1977[41]
		Hickey, 1975[42]
	Unclassified	Khuder et al., 1998[20]
Occupations with animal contact		
Laboratory worker (working with coyotes)	*Campylobacter jejuni* enteritis	Fox et al., 1989[43]
Abattoir workers	Salmonella	Deseö & Engeli, 1979[44]
Agricultural and rural manual occupations		
Agricultural workers	Gastrointestinal parasitoses	Sterba et al., 1988[45]; Ungar et al., 1986[46]; Ortiz, 1980[47]
Road workers	Gastrointestinal parasitoses	Latham et al., 1983[48]

Table 26.2.3 Occupational gastroenteritis: occupations and pathogens

observed on biopsy; it can present clinically, prior to or concomitant with the pulmonary disease.[25]

There is still considerable controversy regarding the actual existence of this disease entity.[26] Berrill's investigation of 42 patients with bird fancier's lung (including exposure history, diffuse lung disease, and precipitins to bird serum) showed that eight persons had villous atrophy on jejunal biopsy.[25] In another large series, four of 57 patients with farmer's lung had celiac disease on biopsy; low red cell folate levels and multiple food antibodies were also observed.[27] Other investigations have failed to show celiac disease on biopsy of patients who had proven bird fancier's lung, and this may represent as infrequent complication.

Pathogenesis

This environmentally related enteropathy appears to be distinct from traditional celiac disease. There often are specific antibodies to birds or molds that are distinct from the avian antibodies seen with common celiac disease (these antibodies are believed to be antigens to hen's egg yolk).[28] Specific respiratory responses to provocation inhalation tests are observed with these patients that are not seen in patients with common celiac disease. In addition, although these patients have antibodies to gluten, often these are not antibodies to the gliadin fraction of gluten (seen with common celiac disease). Of interest, this enteropathy seems to respond to removal of the affected individual from exposure, in combination with a gluten-free diet. One etiologic theory posits that there may be a genetic predisposition that is triggered by exposure to specific antigens; notably, both celiac disease and some types of fibrosing alveolitis, including farmer's lung disease, are more common in persons of the HLA B8 genotype.

Clinical course, diagnosis, and management

The signs and symptoms of this disease entity are due to the concurrent involvement of the GI and respiratory systems, including mouth ulcers, food intolerance, abdominal pain, diarrhea, constipation, as well as weight loss, dyspnea, general malaise, and bronchospasm. These symptoms may coexist or can precede one another.

A history of occupational or heavy environmental exposure to hay, straw, or birds should raise clinical suspicion in an individual with lower GI symptoms. A duodenal or jejunal biopsy showing villous atrophy as well as antigen testing (e.g., avian precipitins [bird fancier's lung] or *Micropolyspora faeni* [farmer's lung]) are diagnostic. For diagnostic issues regarding the respiratory component, please refer to Chapter 19.6. In addition, there should be no evidence for malignancy or collagen vascular disease. Of note, there are reports of co-existing celiac disease in spouses, supporting a common source exposure.

Removal of the individual from exposure in combination with dietary restrictions (e.g., gluten free, egg free) appear to be key factors in management of the condition. Sometimes, more aggressive treatment, such as corticosteroids, is necessary, particularly for the lung disease. The prognosis is good, especially with removal of the individual from exposure.

Pneumatosis cystoides intestinalis

Occupational and environmental causes

Pneumatosis cystoides intestinalis (PCI) is a relatively rare, usually benign condition, characterized by the formation of multiple intramural gas-filled cysts along some portion of the GI tract involving most commonly, though not invariably, the lower gastrointestinal tract. Over 350 cases have been reported in Japan, many of them associated with occupational exposure to TCE.[29–31]

There appear to exist two etiologic groups of PCI. One is primary or idiopathic PCI, with no particular responsible or associated abnormalities; it is a relatively benign condition that occurs more frequently in women. The other group, so-called secondary PCI, is seen with a broad variety of associated lesions, including intestinal obstruction (with concurrent pyloric stenosis related to peptic ulcer disease), chronic obstructive pulmonary disease, and connective tissue diseases. Since 1952, when the first cases were reported, the majority of patients have fallen in the second group, with lesions predominantly in the small intestine. More recently, in Japan, there have been a series of reports of primary PCI, predominantly in the large intestine (especially the sigmoid colon); this condition also has been called pneumatosis cystoides coli (PCC). Many of these PCI (or PCC) patients have a history of occupational exposure to TCE, for degreasing metal parts and products.

In cases of TCE-associated PCI, TCE has been found in gas through endoscopic collection in the cystic spaces, and the metabolite trichloroacetic acid (TCA) has been found in the urine and bile of patients. However, the etiologic mechanism of TCE is not well understood.[32] Another possible mechanism is the inhibition of bacterial hydrogen consumption by alkyl halides such as TCE. This may lead to increased net hydrogen gas production, resulting in 'counterperfusion supersaturation' and formation of gas cysts.[33]

Clinical course, diagnosis, and management

The symptoms of PCI are non-specific and include abdominal fullness, tenderness, and pain; constipation; and a frothy mucous discharge from the rectum (described by patients as foamy tomato juice). Pneumoperitoneum occurs frequently, but because of the sterility of the gas collections, patients rarely have complications of peritonitis.[34] A period of up to 10 years may be required before symptoms develop. On barium enema, polypoid changes are noted, with multiple elevated lesions found on sigmoidoscopy. Needle aspiration of these areas reveals gas. No malignancy or other source for the pain and hematochezia is identified in the workup. Associated etiologic conditions should be sought to exclude secondary PCI.

Removal of the individual from exposure to TCE and, in some cases, oxygen therapy are the major forms of treatment for PCI.[35] Some studies have examined the use of metronidazole to decrease anaerobic bacteria and reduce production of luminal gas. Primary PCI often disappears spontaneously, with or without other interventions. For secondary PCI, treatment of the underlying disease process is generally necessary. With pneumatosis secondary to TCE exposure, removal of the individual from further exposure is associated with a good prognosis.

Non-specific toxic gastrointestinal syndromes

Lead poisoning

Lower gastrointestinal symptoms have been considered a hallmark of lead intoxication, both in children and in adults. Symptoms of colic with either constipation or diarrhea, sometimes severe enough to mimic an acute abdomen, are particularly dominant in acute poisoning, in which a rapid rise in tissue lead levels occurs. In more chronic cases, GI symptoms are less apparent. The effect on the GI tract is probably, in part, due to inhibition of autonomic function of intestinal smooth muscle. In its most extreme form, this condition may lead to toxic megacolon, which is well described in children.

Management of lead toxicity involves removal of the individual from exposure in every case, and careful evaluation to exclude other remediable GI lesions such as ulcers or malignancy. In acute lead poisoning, chelation therapy usually results in prompt relief of GI symptoms. Chelation may be accomplished by intravenous calcium disodium EDTA therapy or oral meso-2,3-dimercaptosuccinic acid (DMSA; Succimer) therapy.[36]

Other metals

Many other metals, including aluminum, arsenic, barium, copper, iron, mercury, and thallium, can cause gastroenteritis with anorexia, and a combination of upper GI (e.g., nausea, vomiting) and lower GI changes in bowel habits. In general, these toxicities are related to acute and subacute exposures, especially through the oral route, and less frequently with long-term exposures. The pathogenesis is not well understood in most cases, but, in general, it appears to involve some disruption of epithelial cell function, leading to cellular necrosis in severe cases.

Cholinesterase inhibitors

Methylcarbamates and organophosphates inhibit cholinesterase, and may cause anorexia, vomiting, cramps, and diarrhea owing to their cholinergic (muscarinic) effects on bowel function. Increased motility and intestinal secretion, and impaired salt and water reabsorption probably account for the major lower GI symptoms that may occur in acute poisoning. The treatment is removal of the individual from exposure; atropine inhibits the muscarinic effects acutely (see Chapter 48).

References

1. Marino G, Anastopoulos H, Woolf AD. Toxicity associated with severe inhalational and dermal exposure to dimethylacetamide and 1,2-ethanediamine. J Occup Med 1994; 36:637-41.
2. Kennedy GL, Pruett JW. Biologic monitoring for dimethyl acetamide: measurement for 4 consecutive weeks in a workplace. J Occup Med 1989; 31:47-50.
3. Mathias CGT, Caldwell TM, Maibach HI. Contact dermatitis and gastrointestinal symptoms from hydroxyethylmethacrylate. Br J Dermatol 1979; 100:447-9.
4. Dunn JP, Cobb S. Frequency of peptic ulcer among executives, craftsmen and foremen. J Occup Med 1962; 4:343-8.
5. Araki S, Goto Y. Peptic ulcer in male factory workers: a survey of prevalence, incidence and aetiological factors. J Epidemiol Community Health 1985; 39:82-5.
6. Ostensen H, Burhol PG, Stormer J, Bonnevie O. The incidence of peptic ulcer disease related to occupation in the northern part of Norway. Scand J Gastroenterol 1985; 20:79-82.
7. Sonnenberg A, Sonnenberg GS, Withers W. Historic changes of occupational work load and mortality from peptic ulcer in Germany. J Occup Med 1987; 28:756-61.
8. Magni G, Rizzardo R, De Leo D, Salmi A. Adverse environmental factors, peptic ulcer, and chronic gastritis in a metalworking industry. Med Lav 1984; 75:215-20.
9. Segawa K, Nakazawa S, Tsukamoto Y, et al. Peptic ulcer is prevalent among shift workers. Dig Dis Sci 1987; 32:449-53.
10. Tuchsen F, Jeppesen HJ, Bach E. Employment status, non-daytime work and gastric ulcer in men. Int J Epidemiol 1994; 23:365-70.
11. Zhangabylov AK, Bekisheva AS. [Analysis of the etiologic significance of nutrition factors in the occurrence of peptic ulcer in railroad workers.] Vopr Pitan 1989; (3):22-5 (article in Russian).
12. Braganza JM, Jolley JE, Lec WR. Occupational chemicals and pancreatitis. Int J Pancreatol 1986; 1:9-19.
13. Marsh WH, Vukov GA, Conradi EC. Acute pancreatitis after cutaneous exposure to an organophosphate insecticide. Am J Gastroenterol 1988; 83:1158-60.
14. Lankisch PG, Muller CH, Niederstadt H, Brand A. Painless acute pancreatitis subsequent to anticholinesterase insecticide (parathion) intoxication. Am J Gastroenterol 1990; 85:872-5.
15. McNamee R, Braganza JM, Hogg J, et al. Occupational exposure to hydrocarbons and chronic pancreatitis: a case-referent study. Occup Environ Med 1994; 51:631-7.
16. Hotz P, Pilliod J, Bourgeois R, Boillat MA. Hydrocarbon exposure, pancreatitis and bile acids. Br J Ind Med 1990; 47:833-7.
17. Chary S. Dimethylformamide: a cause of acute pancreatitis? Lancet 1974; ii:356 (letter).
18. Dressel TD, Goodale RL, Zweber B, et al. The effect of atropine and duct decompression on the evaluation of diazinon-induced acute canine pancreatitis. Ann Surg 1982; 195:424-34.
19. Gallagher S, Sankaran H, Williams J. Mechanism of scorpion toxin-induced enzyme secretion in rat pancreas. Gastroenterology 1981; 80:970-3.
20. Khuder SA, Arthur T, Bisesi MS, et al. Prevalence of infectious diseases and associated symptoms in waste water treatment workers. Am J Ind Med 1998; 33:571-7.
21. Clark CS, Linneman CC, Clark JG, Gartside PS. Enteric parasites in workers occupationally exposed to sewage. J Occup Med 1984; 26:273-5.
22. Pike RM. Laboratory-associated infections: incidence, fatalities, causes, and prevention. Ann Rev Microbiol 1979; 44:41-66.
23. Pike RM. Laboratory-associated infections: summary and analysis of 3,921 cases. Health Lab Sci 1976; 13:105-14.
24. Koch KL, Phillips DJ, Aber RC, Current WL. Cryptosporidiosis in hospital personnel. Ann Intern Med 1985; 102:593-6.
25. Berrill WT, Fitzpatrick PF, Macleod WM, et al. Bird fancier's lung and jejunal villous atrophy. Lancet 1975; 2:1006-8.
26. Hendrick DJ, Faux JA, Anand B, et al. Is bird fancier's lung associated with coeliac disease? Thorax 1978; 33:425-8.
27. Turton CW, Turner-Warwick M, Owens R, et al. Red cell folate levels, food antibodies and reticulin antibodies in farmer's lung – is there an association with coeliac disease? Br J Dis Chest 1983; 77:397-402.
28. Faux JA, Hendrick DJ, Anand B. Precipitins to different avian serum antigens in bird fancier's lung and coeliac disease. Clin Allergy 1978; 8:101-8.

29. Hosomi N, Yoshioka H, Kuroda C, et al. Pneumatosis cystoides intestinalis: CT findings. Abdom Imaging 1994; 19:137-9.

30. Ogata M, Kihara T, Kamoo R, et al. A report of a worker suffering from pneumatosis cystoides intestinalis following trichloroethylene exposure. Ind Health 1988; 26:179-82.

31. Yamaguchi K, Shirai T, Shimakura K, et al. Pneumatosis cystoides intestinalis and trichloroethylene exposure. Am J Gastroenterol 1985; 80:753-7.

32. Kaneko T, Saegusa M, Tasaka K, et al. Immunotoxicity of trichloroethylene: a study with MRL -1pr/1pr mice. J Appl Toxicol 2000; 20:471-5.

33. Florin THJ. Alkyl halides, super hydrogen production and the pathogenesis of pneumatosis cystoides coli. Gut 1997; 41:778-84.

34. Boerner RM, Fried DB, Warshauer DM, Isaacs K. Pneumatosis intestinalis: two case reports and a retrospective review of the literature from 1985 to 1995. Dig Dis Sci 1996; 41:2272-85.

35. Forgacs P, Wright PH, Wyatt AP. Pneumatosis cystoides intestinalis treated by oxygen breathing. Lancet 1979; i:579-82.

36. Levin SM, Goldberg M. Clinical evaluation and management of lead-exposed construction workers. Am J Ind Med 2000; 37:23-43.

37. Kolavic SA, Kimura A, Simons SL, et al. An outbreak of Shigella dysenteriae type 2 among laboratory workers due to intentional food contamination. JAMA 1997; 278:396-8.

38. Steckelberg JM, Terrell C, Edson RS. Laboratory-acquired Salmonella typhimurium enteritis: association with erythema nodosum and reactive arthritis. Am J Med 1988; 85:705-7.

39. Standaert SM, Hutcheson RH, Schaffner W. Nosocomial transmission of Salmonella gastroenteritis to laundry workers in a nursing home. Infect Control Hosp Epidemiol 1994; 15:22-6.

40. Jones A. Campylobacter enteritis in a food factory. Lancet 1979; i:618-9.

41. Hays BD. Potential for parasitic disease transmission with land application of sewage plant effluents and sludge, review paper. Water Res 1977; 11:583-95.

42. Hickey JL, Reist PC. Health significance of air-borne microorganisms from waste water treatment processes. J Water Pollut Control Fed 1975; 47:2741-57.

43. Fox JG, Taylor NS, Penner JL, et al. Investigation of zoonotically acquired Campylobacter jejuni enteritis with serotyping and restriction endonuclease DNA analysis. J Clin Microbiol 1989; 27:2423-5.

44. Deseö L, Engeli P. [Symptomless enteritis-salmonella excreta in an abbatoir.] Schweiz Med Wochenschr 1979; 109:1995-9 (article in German).

45. Sterba J, Ditrich O, Prokopic J, Kadlcik K. Gastrointestinal parasitoses discovered in agricultural workers in South Bohemia, Czechoslovakia. Folia Parasitol 1988; 35:169-73.

46. Ungar BLP, Iscoe MHS, Bartlett JG. Intestinal parasites in a migrant farmworker population. Arch Intern Med 1986; 146:513-15.

47. Ortiz JS. The prevalence of intestinal parasites in Puerto Rican farm workers in western Massachusetts. Am J Public Health 1980; 70:1103-5.

48. Latham MC, Wolgemuth JC, Hall A. Nutritional status, parasitic infections and health of roadworkers in 4 areas of Kenya: Part II Kirinyaga and Murang'a districts, the Highlands. East Afr Med J 1983; 60:75-81.

Chapter 27
Endocrine and Reproductive Disorders

27.1 Endocrine Disorders

Ulrike Luderer, Mark R Cullen

During the past decade, interest in the effects of environmental agents on the endocrine system has burgeoned. This is, in part, due to the concern that environmental contaminants, acting via hormonal mechanisms, may be responsible for a number of adverse health outcomes in humans and wildlife. It has been hypothesized that these environmental endocrine disrupters may be playing roles in the etiology of breast, testicular, and prostate cancer, decreased fertility, endometriosis, and abnormalities of male reproductive system development such as hypospadias and cryptorchidism.[1-3] Although much of the impetus has come from concern about the reproductive effects of these agents, new knowledge has also begun to accumulate regarding their impact on thyroid, adrenal, and pituitary function. At the same time, study of the effects of the environment on the endocrine functions of gastrointestinal organs, and bone and calcium metabolism has begun, albeit in a more limited way to date. Collectively, these aspects are the subjects of this chapter. Related discussions of the reproductive effects appear in Chapter 27.2, while the subject of neoplasms of the endocrine and reproductive organs is covered in Chapters 30.7 and 30.8.

Although understanding of this potentially enormous subject remains relatively limited compared with other targets of environmental factors, certain principles regarding non-reproductive endocrine disorders can be stated that simplify the practitioner's task. First, with the possible exception of the potent rodenticide Vacor, it appears that agents that affect endocrine functions other than reproduction tend to be ones with diffuse effects on other organs as well, such as heavy metals, pesticides, and solvents. In general, therefore, the search for environmental factors is most relevant to patients with medical problems in addition to those problems that might be attributable to endocrinopathy, such as central nervous system (CNS), hepatic, respiratory, dermal, and, importantly, reproductive disorders. In other words, it would be uncommon, given our present understanding, to find an endocrine disorder as the sole manifestation of environmental toxicity in adults. This is in marked contrast to agents with primary reproductive effects that may often dominate the clinical picture of toxicity, obscuring other less salient effects. Subclinical effects, however, could precede other measurable effects, because even subtle alterations may be potentially useful as biomarkers in exposed populations. The advantage they provide over merely measuring exposure levels is that changes in these endpoints indicate that sufficient absorption has occurred to cause a physiologic effect. Interventions to reduce exposure can then be instituted before the onset of clinically significant effects.

The corollary of the first principle is that environmental agents typically cause subtle, rather than profound disturbances of endocrine function, except in cases of massive exposures in adults. Classic presentations of organ failure or hyper-reactivity, such as myxedema, thyroid storm, pituitary apoplexy, and addisonian crisis (adrenal insufficiency) are not part of the spectrum of endocrinopathies described in human cases or predicted by dose–response testing in animals or cell cultures. Rather, the effects of environmental agents on endocrine functions other than reproduction tend to be subtle and easily masked, unless they are specifically considered and tested for. However, given our increasing understanding of the importance of endocrine balance for a wide range of crucial functions, such as growth and development, response to stress, and risk for longterm cardiovascular disease, these relatively subtle effects of the environment may be more important than previously appreciated, particularly on a population basis. Indeed, recent work suggests that even small disruptions of thyroid homeostasis in utero and during early postnatal development may have significant adverse effects on the developing brain. For example, it has been long known that infants with congenital hypothyroidism will develop mental retardation and severe motor abnormalities if not treated from birth with thyroxine; however, only recently has it begun to be appreciated that even with thyroxine replacement from birth, these children may manifest subtle, but measurable, deficits of IQ, motor function, and coordination.[4]

MECHANISMS OF ENDOCRINE TOXICITY

There are a variety of mechanisms by which toxicants can affect endocrine function (Table 27.1.1). Induction of cell death within an endocrine gland or tissue is used therapeutically in the treatment of Graves' disease by means of ablative therapy with radioactive iodine. Induction of apoptosis or programmed cell death in ovarian follicle cells also appears to be one mechanism by which the chemotherapeutic drug cyclophosphamide causes ovarian failure. Many diverse compounds have been shown to disrupt endocrine function by binding to hormone receptors, acting as receptor agonists or antagonists (see Chapter 45). The organochlorine insecticide methoxychlor is an estrogen receptor agonist, while

Mechanism	Example	References
Induction of cell death	Cyclophosphamide, radioactive iodine	69
Hormone receptor binding	Methoxychlor, p,p'-DDE*	70,71
Transport protein binding	Polychlorinated biphenyls	16
Altering hormone synthesis or secretion	Perchlorates, thiocyanates, styrene	38,47
Altering hormone metabolism	Heptachlor, chlordane	72
Altering hormone receptor levels	Gonadotropin-releasing hormone agonists	73
Modulating intracellular signaling pathways	Lithium	38

*1,1-dichloro-2,2'-bis(p-chlorophenyl) ethylene

Table 27.1.1 Mechanisms of endocrine toxicity

1,1-dichloro-2,2'-bis(p-chlorophenyl) ethylene (p,p'-DDE), a metabolite of another organochlorine insecticide, 1,1,1-trichloro-2,2'-bis(p-chlorophenyl) ethane (DDT), is a potent androgen receptor antagonist. Yet other compounds compete with endogenous ligands for non-receptor transport proteins. Hydroxylated metabolites of various polychlorinated biphenyls have been demonstrated to potentially bind transthyretin, disrupting thyroid homeostasis. Some endocrine toxicants act by altering hormone synthesis or secretion. For example, the aromatic solvent styrene increases pituitary prolactin secretion, and thiocyanates and perchlorates inhibit thyroid hormone synthesis by blocking iodine uptake into the thyroid.

Endocrine homeostasis can also be disturbed by compounds that alter hormone metabolism. The cyclodiene insecticides heptachlor and chlordane are potent inducers of hydroxylases that metabolize sex steroids, resulting in reduced circulating levels of these hormones. Additional mechanisms by which toxicants might disrupt endocrine function are by up- or down-regulating hormone receptor levels or by interfering with hormonal intracellular signaling pathways. For example, lithium suppresses thyroid hormone release by inhibiting cyclic AMP-mediated effects of thyroid-stimulating hormone (TSH).

A useful mechanistic distinction for understanding the developmental effects of endocrine toxicants is that of organizational versus activational effects of hormones.[5] Organizational effects occur early during development, usually before birth, and are permanent. In contrast, activational effects usually occur during adult life and are transient. Organizational effects of hormonally active toxicants usually require lower doses and shorter exposures during critical windows of development than do activational effects. Examples of organizational effects of hormones include the stimulation by androgens of male reproductive duct and gland development, and the masculinization of the CNS by exposure to estrogens in utero. Examples of activational effects include the stimulation of thyroid gland hyperplasia by TSH or of uterine endometrial proliferation by estrogens.

CLINICAL EVALUATION
History and physical examination

For the reasons outlined earlier, the typical historic and physical findings associated with primary endocrine diseases are not likely to be found in patients with endocrine effects resulting from environmental factors. In fact, where classic findings such as frontal bossing, lid lag, galactorrhea, and hyperpigmentation are uncovered, serious consideration must be given to non-environmental causes such as autoimmune disease or tumors. Nonetheless, any suspicion of endocrine dysfunction should prompt a thorough review of systems for each of the classic historic features of primary endocrine disturbance and a careful physical examination that includes a search for the well-known physical findings.

Far more relevant to uncovering endocrine effects of environmental agents are the subtle and less specific consequences of hormonal imbalances. The client's medical history should include information on each of the following topics:

- sleep disturbance or changes in energy level or mood;
- alterations in weight, appetite, and bowel function;
- sexual interest and function, and, in women, menstrual changes;
- changes in temperature perception, sweating, or flushing; and
- alterations of body habitus, hair growth, and skin texture.

In addition to these specific inquiries, the history should also include a careful search for other toxic effects of suspected causal agents, for the reasons mentioned earlier. Often, these effects may overlap with or obscure endocrine-related phenomena, especially those that involve the CNS, gastrointestinal, or reproductive symptoms. The presence of such symptoms, although initially confusing, should heighten rather than diminish suspicion of environmentally induced endocrinopathy. These non-specific symptoms mandate a search, usually requiring laboratory tests, to identify effects on each organ that may be contributing to the symptoms. It should not be presumed that identification of one possible disorder, such as mild encephalopathy, precludes the need to evaluate the integrity of endocrine function when exposure to a suspect agent has occurred.

The same general principle applies to the physical examination. Although careful examination may uncover a very revealing and localizing sign, such as a goiter or change in a secondary sexual characteristic, the greater usefulness of the examination is in identification of more typical, non-endocrine markers of toxicity from the environmental agent in question, such as Mees lines (skin lesions associated with heavy metal exposure) or neurologic changes due to solvents, organophosphates, organochlorine, or heavy metals. A second important role for the physical examination is to carefully evaluate evidence of non-environmental causes for endocrinopathy such as a tumor (e.g., if milk can be expressed from the breast of a non-lactating woman).

Laboratory evaluation

Given the subtle, non-specific nature of historic clues and physical findings for endocrinopathy of environmental origin, the appropriate use of laboratory tests is essential. There are four specific goals in the use of these tests:

- detection of mild, often subclinical alterations of function;
- localization of the injury within the hierarchy of endocrine regulation (e.g., hypothalamus or pituitary versus end organ);
- exclusion of tumor or other primary endocrine organ failure due to non-environmental causes; and
- establishment of markers of exposure to a causal agent or evidence of other organ system damage from the agent.

Satisfactory accomplishment of the first three goals requires a detailed understanding of the available strategies for testing and localizing endocrine lesions, which is beyond the scope of this text. Certain generalization is worth noting here regarding available tests.

Tests of end-organ function

The circulating levels of virtually every hormone can now be measured directly, including thyroid hormones, adrenal steroids and amines, anterior and posterior pituitary secretions, parathormone, and 1,25-dihydroxycholecalciferol. For some of these hormones, levels are sufficiently stable over time so that a single measurement accurately reflects organ function. Examples of these include thyroid hormones and cholecalciferols. For others, such as cortisol and insulin, blood levels fluctuate so rapidly that baseline function cannot be adequately assessed from a single or even from multiple random measures; instead, some integrated measure is needed, such as collection of steroid metabolites in a timed urine collection, or the hormone must be measured under specified conditions known to maximize or suppress glandular activity, such as fasting or glucose ingestion for insulin secretion. For some hormones, such as insulin, indirect measurements of hormonal function are often more readily available, such as blood glucose levels.

However baseline function of the end organs is assessed, it must be remembered that the endocrine system as a whole is finely balanced to ensure homeostasis even in the face of injury. For example, a partially diseased thyroid gland may still be capable of secreting an adequate (i.e., normal) level of thyroxine (T4) by stimulating the pituitary compensatory secretion of TSH. Thus, a subtle lesion in the thyroid axis would not necessarily be revealed by simple measurement of the end product, but would

become apparent if TSH were simultaneously measured. For other hormones, even simultaneous measurement of trophic hormone and its end product may mask a lesion. For example, mild adrenal insufficiency may not be apparent from cortisol levels or urinary excretion of adrenal metabolites under normal conditions, but they may be significant or even life threatening under stresses such as infection or bleeding.

An array of stress tests have been devised that can allow detection of more subtle lesions that are insufficient to alter function under normal conditions. The best known example of such is the glucose tolerance test, which indirectly assesses the adequacy of insulin regulation by measurement of timed glucose levels after a challenge. In the reverse direction, administration of insulin to induce mild hypoglycemia is an excellent way to assess whether the adrenal axis is intact, because lowering of blood sugar is a very potent stimulus for cortisol secretion. The same stress should also induce an outpouring of growth hormone, even if baseline levels are low. It is important to recognize, however, that many of these stresses are inherently dangerous, especially in patients with suspected defects of endocrine function. The tests should be performed under tightly controlled circumstances and always by individuals experienced in their administration and interpretation.

DISORDERS OF THYROID FUNCTION

The ability of environmental factors to affect the function of the thyroid gland has been appreciated for centuries because of the occurrence of endemic goiters. Although iodine deficiency was recognized as an important cause of goiter before the days of dietary supplementation, the presence of various goitrogens in medicines, food, and drinking water was also recognized. These compounds include perchlorates and thiocyanate, which inhibit iodine transport into the thyroid, and a number of compounds that inhibit organification of iodine, including the metal cobalt and several classes of cyclic organic compounds, such as substituted phenols. Particularly concerning are the developmental effects of such alterations, given the important role of T4 in CNS development. A recent study of electroplating workers with chronic cyanide exposure, which causes thiocyanate accumulation, demonstrated reduced serum T4 and tri-iodothyronine (T3), and elevated TSH concentrations relative to controls.[6] Perchlorate has historically been used to treat Graves' disease, effectively lowering T4 levels; however, it was discontinued due to a number of reports of aplastic anemia. Environmental perchlorate contamination of drinking water has been linked to reduced T4 and increased TSH in newborns.[7] While increased rates of congenital hypothyroidism have not been observed, this endpoint is not sensitive for detecting subclinical thyroid dysfunction.[8] Two studies of workers with inhalational perchlorate exposure, in contrast, did not find evidence of altered thyroid function,[9,10] although the applicability of these findings to pediatric populations is unclear. More recent investigations of orally administered perchlorate in human volunteers have documented inhibition of I-123 uptake by the thyroid at low doses (0.01–0.043 mg/kg/day).[11–13] These findings indicate inhibition of the sodium-iodide symporter, with mild changes in thyroid hormone levels at higher doses (0.5 mg/kg/day) in the short term.[3] Additional health concerns regarding perchlorate have focused on rodent models, demonstrating a lowest observable adverse effect level (LOAEL) of 0.01 mg/kg/day based on brain morphometric and thyroid hormonal changes in rat pups, with thyroid follicular epithelial cell hyperplasia observed at 0.1 mg/kg/day.[14] In aggregate, these investigations have led to recommendations for lowered reference doses, with proposed reference doses as low as 1 ppb for drinking water (Drinking Water Equivalent Level [DWEL]).[14]

The effect of ionizing radiation on the thyroid gland has also been appreciated for many years.[15] Low to moderate doses of local irradiation to the gland, either through an external X-ray study or by absorption of radioactive iodine, have been responsible for the development of benign and malignant tumors (see Chapter 30.7). High doses of ionizing radiation are ablative and are the basis for one of the standard treatments for Graves' disease. To date, clinical studies do not suggest that the low, carcinogenic doses are associated with functional changes; hypothyroidism has not been described as a relevant effect of radiation exposure except in the setting of very high therapeutic doses.

More recently, the effects of environmental contaminants such as heavy metals, solvents, pesticides, and related compounds have been recognized as causing functional thyroid effects either clinically or in experimental animals. In humans, depressed levels of thyroid function have been correlated with exposures to lead, carbon disulfide, polybrominated biphenyls (PBBs), polychlorinated biphenyls (PCBs), dioxins, and furans. These agents have been shown to act by a variety of mechanisms in laboratory studies, including enhancement of T4 glucuronidation, and thus excretion, by PCBs, DDT, and chloroacetanilides; binding to serum thyroid hormone transport proteins by PCBs;[16] and inhibition of peripheral T4 deiodination by methoxychlor.[17] As with the goitrogens discussed above, the effects of disruption of thyroid homeostasis by these compounds during prenatal and postnatal development have been of particular concern because of the importance of thyroid hormone to normal brain development.[18] During the first trimester of pregnancy, the developing embryo is totally dependent on maternal T4, and even subclinical decreases in the maternal free thyroxine index during early gestation have been associated with impaired psychomotor development and reduced IQ.[18] The fetus begins to synthesize T4 around week 10 to 12 of gestation, but some T4 is still transported from the mother throughout gestation. Thus, the severe sequelae of congenital hypothyroidism are seen after birth, with the withdrawal of the maternal source of T4.[4]

Thyroid function in lead workers has been studied quite extensively. Results suggest mild depression of function in chronically and heavily exposed adults,[19,20] without substantial effects at lower levels.[21] Challenge testing has suggested that the level of the lesion is at the hypothalamus, although neither pituitary nor direct thyroid effects, as predicted by animal studies, could be excluded. Significantly, a careful study of young inner-city children failed to reveal any relationship between lead exposure and thyroid function, although screening for such an effect in the face of childhood lead poisoning is recommended in view of the ramifications of even mild hypothyroidism on child development.[22]

Early reports of depressed thyroid function in carbon disulfide-exposed workers have been neither clinically studied nor confirmed in more recent cohorts.[23] As is generally true for endocrine effects, other clinical effects of carbon disulfide poisoning, including neuropathy and cardiovascular disease, tend to dominate the clinical picture in the only available reports.

The study of the agricultural communities in Michigan accidentally exposed to PBBs in the 1970s provides the only report of an outbreak of non-goitrogenic thyroid dysfunction attributable to environmental contamination by chemicals.[24] Although sophisticated testing of those with depressed T4 levels was not conducted to establish the level of injury in the thyroid–pituitary–hypothalamic axis, the report of increased antithyroid antibodies serves as indirect evidence of a primary effect on the thyroid gland itself.

Studies of adult humans exposed to relatively high levels of PCBs provide conflicting data about the effects of these compounds on thyroid function. In adults who 16 years earlier had consumed cooking oil ('Yusho rice oil') contaminated with PCBs, serum T3 and T4 were elevated, but TSH and antithyroid antibodies were not changed compared to controls.[25] Serum PCBs did not correlate with T4 or T3 in that study. In contrast, a history of current or former occupational PCB exposure among transformer repairmen was associated with a lower T4 and T4-RT3 index compared to unexposed controls.[26] In the same study, adipose or serum PCB concentrations were not significantly associated with exposure, suggesting that exposure history may have been spurious or that the relationship between PCB body burden and thyroid function is not a linear one. A recent study of employees in a former PCB plant found increased thyroid volumes and increased prevalence of antithyroid antibodies in the employees compared to controls, but no differences in T4 or TSH levels.[27] Unlike the conflicting human data, experimental studies in adult rats demonstrate suppression of serum T4 by PCBs.[16]

Exposure to another class of chlorinated polyaromatic hydrocarbons, the dioxins, has also been associated with subclinical changes in thyroid hormone secretion in some human studies. There was a positive relationship between serum 2,3,7,8-tetrachlorodibenzo-p-dioxin (TCDD) concentration and T4 and free T4 index, but not TSH or thyroid disease, in industrial workers exposed to TCDD contamination 15 years previously.[28] Similarly, another study of chemical workers also found a positive association between serum TCDD concentration and T4, but not TSH.[29] In contrast, free T4 index did not differ between Operation Ranch Hand Vietnam veterans exposed to TCDD in Agent Orange and controls.[28]

PCBs, like dioxins and furans, are highly persistent, lipophilic, organochlorine pollutants for which more than 90% of human exposure occurs via food intake, primarily meat, fish, and dairy products (see Chapter 45).[30] Breastfeeding can be an important source of exposure, accounting for 12% to 14% of the total PCB and dioxin intake in one study.[30] One recent study in children found a negative relationship between serum PCB levels and serum levels of free T3, and a positive correlation with TSH.[31] A study of breast-fed Japanese infants found significant negative correlations between total dioxin equivalents contributed by PCBs, dioxins, and furans in the breast milk, and serum T4 and T3 levels.[32] A Dutch study found a positive correlation between breast milk PCBs and dioxins and neonatal TSH, but no relationship with T4.[33] Another study of background level PCB exposure in the US, in contrast, found no significant correlation between maternal PCB levels and neonatal T4, T3, or TSH levels at birth.[34] The significance of small reductions in thyroid hormone levels observed in the former studies on the developing brain are not yet fully characterized. However, studies of human populations with prenatal and perinatal environmental PCB exposures demonstrate neurologic deficits that are consistent with a mechanism involving disruption of thyroid hormone homeostasis. These studies reported inverse relationships between various indices of PCB exposure and motor function, attention, IQ, and memory deficits.[4,35] Moreover, animal studies have shown that maternal PCB exposure causes reduced T4 and T3 levels in fetal brains, as well as motor deficits and impaired learning.[4,35]

Thyroid function has been studied in women exposed to cobalt-based paints.[36,37] Cross-sectional blood tests suggest that one effect is dose-related elevation of T4, free T4, and the T4-to-T3 ratio, without a change in TSH levels or pituitary function. The results suggest reduced peripheral deiodination of T4 to T3, but the clinical significance of this observation is unclear.

For none of the settings in which human effects have been observed and reported are there adequate longitudinal data on the natural history or response to any intervention. Lead workers removed from further exposure appear to have gradual amelioration of depressed T4 levels. The effects of chelation or thyroid supplementation are unknown. The potential reversibility of lesions due to other exposures described above is also unknown, but at a minimum, removal of the affected individual from any further exposure would seem advisable once non-environmental causes have been excluded.

In addition to the effects that have been reported in workers and communities, experimental studies in animals suggest that the thyroid is potentially susceptible to injury from widely used chemicals. These include insecticides such as organophosphates, carbamates and organochlorines, fungicides, food colorants, and mercury.[38] It is premature to

recommend that exposed individuals be screened or otherwise evaluated for these effects outside research protocols. Nonetheless, exposure to these agents should be considered as potentially causal in patients who are identified with thyroid functional abnormalities when other established factors have been excluded.

DISORDERS OF ADRENAL FUNCTION

Very little is known about the effects of environmental agents on adrenal cortical or medullary function in humans. Occupationally, only workers heavily exposed to lead and PCBs have been studied.

Results of studies of lead-exposed workers suggest that secretion of corticosteroids is depressed in response to insulin-induced hypoglycemia and vasopressin; baseline levels of 17-hydroxy (glucocorticoid) and 17-keto (androgenic) steroids were low normal. Because response to administration of adrenocorticotropic hormone (ACTH) was normal, it was presumed that the lesion was at the hypothalamic-pituitary level, but primary toxicity on the adrenal itself could not be excluded. Neither the clinical relevance nor the appropriate treatment for these lesions has been characterized. Importantly, all workers demonstrating these effects also had other evidence of lead toxicity, requiring all the workers to be removed from exposure and chelation therapy to be instituted in those more severely affected.

In a study of humans massively exposed to the pesticide gramoxone by ingestion, levels of adrenocortical hormones were measured and found to be markedly elevated in those who later died, but normal or low in survivors.[39] Whether this factor represents toxicity to the adrenal gland or axis or whether it is a non-specific response to systemic poisoning could not be ascertained; the effects of lower doses of this and related agents are unknown.

Current and former transformer repairmen exposed to PCBs were found to have lower urinary 17-hydroxycortisone excretion than controls.[26] Moreover, urinary 17-hydroxycortisone was negatively correlated with adipose tissue PCB concentration.[26] It is not known whether there was a concurrent effect on serum glucocorticoid concentrations, as they were not measured. Reduced urinary 17-hydroxycortisone may reflect a suppressive effect of PCBs on adrenal glucocorticoid secretion or synthesis, resulting in reduced serum levels of glucocorticoids.

Animal studies suggest that the adrenal gland may be more sensitive to environmental effects than the limited human data would suggest. A broad range of organochlorine, organophosphate, and carbamate pesticides has been tested, and evidence of histologic alterations in adrenocortical cells has been found; similar effects have been shown with ammonium sulfate fertilizer. The herbicide paraquat has been established to be a potent inhibitor of aldosterone synthesis in the adrenal gland, with action similar to the drugs spironolactone and metyrapone;[40] depression of aldosterone secretion has been demonstrated in animals. Several organophosphates, including malathion and diazinon, have been shown to interfere with adrenomedullary function, causing enhanced secretion of epinephrine and norepinephrine, with resulting hyperglycemia, glycogen deposition in the liver, and exhaustion of adrenal stores of these amines.[41,42] Mirex, toxaphene, and dioxin (2,3,7,8 TCDD) have been shown to cause direct suppression of glucocorticoid synthesis by the adrenal, with resultant hypoglycemia that could be reversed by cortisone administration.[43–45] The solvent 1,1,1-trichloroethane suppresses plasma corticosterone and ACTH concentrations, possibly via an effect on hypothalamic corticotropin-releasing hormone (CRH) in rodents.[46] High doses relative to likely human environmental exposures have been used in these studies, so the relevance to humans remains unclear.

DISORDERS OF THE PITUITARY GLAND

Lead, styrene, and beryllium have been demonstrated to affect the pituitary gland of occupationally exposed workers. The data on lead have already been summarized earlier in the sections on thyroid and adrenal function. There is further evidence for an effect on the pituitary–gonadal axis (see Chapter 27.2). However, sophisticated testing of these workers failed to demonstrate any effects on growth hormone or prolactin secretion from the anterior pituitary or any evidence of posterior pituitary dysfunction.

The effect of styrene on hypothalamic–pituitary function has been studied in several groups of exposed workers. Although thyroid and gonadotropic hormones appeared to be unaffected by the exposure, baseline prolactin and growth hormone levels were elevated in a dose-dependent fashion.[47] Significantly, there was a very marked and dose-dependent enhancement of the prolactin response to thyrotropin-releasing hormone (TRH), suggesting the possibility of a defect in the normal counter-regulation of prolactin, which is controlled by hypothalamic dopamine.[48] These results suggest the possibility that styrene specifically depletes dopamine from the tuberoinfundibular portion of the hypothalamus. Depletion of dopamine in this portion of the hypothalamus following styrene inhalation has been demonstrated in experimental studies in the rabbit.[49]

Notably, in occupational studies of pituitary function, workers experienced prominent, albeit vague, CNS complaints, suggesting that endocrine disturbance was not the first or sole toxicity resulting from the exposure. Although the clinical significance remains unclear, levels of prolactin observed in this condition could be a cause of galactorrhea, secondary infertility, or both in the appropriate exposure setting. Despite the hypothetical possibility of reduced fertility caused by hyperprolactinemia, a recent study found no effect of styrene exposure on time-to-pregnancy, an indicator of fertility, in men.[50]

Patients with chronic beryllium disease due to beryllium exposure may exhibit granulomas in the pituitary gland similar to those seen in sarcoidosis. However, functional disorders of the anterior and posterior pituitary gland similar to those seen occasionally in sarcoidosis have not been described in beryllium disease. Nonetheless, the occurrence of granulomas in this organ raises the possibility of functional defects that should be considered when they are clinically suggested.

In addition to the above-mentioned studies, limited human data suggest that pituitary secretion of the reproductive hormones luteinizing hormone (LH) and follicle-stimulating hormone (FSH) may be suppressed by occupational exposure to toluene[51,52] and herbicides[53] and enhanced by occupational exposure to carbon disulfide.[23]

Very little experimental work on pituitary responses to environmental agents has been conducted to date. Animal studies have demonstrated effects of the aromatic solvents toluene and xylene on pituitary hormone secretion; however, the results of these studies have been inconsistent. One study reported effects of toluene exposure on prolactin levels, but not on LH, FSH, TSH, or cortisosterone concentrations,[54] while another reported effects on LH and FSH levels.[55] Xylenes were found to suppress both serum prolactin and corticosterone in rats in the third study.[56]

DIABETES MELLITUS

It is evident from the above-mentioned effects of xenobiotics on the adrenal and pituitary glands that agents that enhance production or release of growth hormone or adrenomedullary amines could induce some degree of glucose intolerance. However, no human case nor animal model of diabetes that has developed via such a pathway has yet been described.

One single agent, the rodenticide Vacor (pyridyl N-p-nitrophenyl urea), has been implicated as a cause of diabetes mellitus after human ingestion.[57] Notably, glucose intolerance was the major clinical toxicity in reported cases, although autonomic and peripheral neuropathy with orthostatic hypotension were concomitantly observed. Animal studies have now documented the very strong binding of Vacor to pancreatic islet beta cells by a mechanism similar to that of the drug streptozocin. Whether this inhibition of insulin release may be reversible is unclear. Studied cases have demonstrated subsequent cytotoxic effects on the islet cells, and chronic insulin-dependent diabetes has resulted. Anti-islet cell antibodies have been measured in serum from some patients. It is unclear whether specific treatment early in toxicity, such as with the competitive binder streptozocin, may lead to a better outcome than supportive care alone.

Positive relationships have been observed between serum TCDD levels and both fasting serum glucose levels and risk of diabetes in workers exposed to chemicals contaminated with TCDD.[58] An association between TCDD levels and risk of diabetes mellitus has also been observed among US veterans of Operation Ranch Hand, who were exposed to TCDD in Agent Orange.[59] Interestingly, even among non-diabetic Ranch Hand veterans, there was a positive relationship between serum insulin and TCDD exposure category, suggesting hyperinsulinemia as a possible mechanism for the development of diabetes in dioxin-exposed individuals.[59] Increased rates of diabetes-related mortality have been reported in female TCDD-exposed individuals in one study,[60] but not in two other studies.[61,62] A large international study that combined 36 dioxin-exposed cohorts from 12 countries found an increased risk of mortalit from diabetes, but did not reach statistical significance.[63] However, because most people with diabetes mellitus now survive for years after diagnosis, one would not necessarily expect to see an association with diabetes-related mortality even if there were a true association between dioxin exposure and risk of diabetes.

DISORDERS OF CALCIUM AND BONE METABOLISM

Calcium homeostasis and bone metabolism are under the control of the parathyroid hormone and the hepatic and renal metabolites of vitamin D. As well, the gastrointestinal tract, bone, and kidney are important target organs that determine the systemic impact of these hormones.

Virtually no data are available regarding the effect of toxins on the function of the parathyroid gland; one study of lead-exposed workers showed no effect. Although a variety of chemicals and ionizing radiation are capable of inducing parathyroid adenomas under appropriate experimental conditions, the relevance to human exposure is questionable. Hypoparathyroid states due to toxins have not been described in either humans or animals.

Vitamin D metabolism has been investigated in cases involving childhood lead poisoning because of the clinical observation of poor growth and abnormal bone structure in affected children.[64] The best evidence currently suggests that lead directly interferes with renal metabolism of 25-hydroxycholecalciferol to the more active 1,25-dihydroxy derivative. Whether supplementation with this metabolite could reverse some of the adverse sequelae of lead poisoning in this population has not been established.

Beryllium disease has been associated with hypercalcemia in a small number of patients. Although reports of vitamin D metabolism in this specific setting have not yet been published, it is likely that the hypercalcemia is related to that seen in other granulomatous disorders – namely, increased conversion of 25-hydroxycholecalciferol to the active moiety by hydroxylase in the granulomas, leading effectively to hypervitaminosis D. The administration of corticosteroids generally is satisfactory treatment for this metabolic complication.

Another environmental and occupational disease state associated with abnormalities of calcium metabolism in humans is chronic cadmium intoxication. Osteopenia is frequently seen in advanced cases, and it is often the first clinical manifestation (i.e., pathologic fractures) which is responsible for the Japanese name *itai-itai* (literally meaning 'ouch-ouch') for this condition. It is presumed that the bone disease occurs as a consequence of the renal tubular defect induced by prolonged exposure to cadmium, with subsequent metabolic acidosis, calcium loss, and bony

demineralization.[65] Recently, lower levels of cadmium exposure have been associated with reduced bone mineral density and osteoporosis in manufacturers of heat exchangers and in battery workers.[66,67]

Recently, serum levels of p,p′-DDE, a metabolite of the organochlorine insecticide DDT, have been found to be negative predictors of bone mineral density in postmenopausal women.[68] The authors speculated that p,p′-DDE may affect bone density via its ability to potently antagonize androgen receptor binding.

Beyond these reports, there are few experimental data by which to predict which other classes of toxins may have effects on vitamin D metabolism short of widespread systemic toxicity.

References

1. Colborn T, vom Saal FS, Soto AM. Developmental effects of endocrine-disrupting chemicals in wildlife and humans. Environ Health Perspect 1993; 101:378-84.
2. Safe DH. Environmental and dietary estrogens and human health: is there a problem? Environ Health Perspect 1994; 103:346.
3. Toppari J, Larsen JC, Christiansen P, et al. Male reproductive health and environmental xenoestrogens. Environ Health Perspect 1996; 104(Suppl 4):741-803.
4. Sher ES, Xu XM, Adams PM, et al. The effects of thyroid hormone level and action in developing brain: are there targets for the actions of polychlorinated biphenyls and dioxins? Toxicol Ind Health 1998; 14:121-58.
5. Guillette LJJ, Crain DA, Rooney AA, et al. Organization versus activation: the role of endocrine-disrupting contaminants (EDCs) during embryonic development in wildlife. Environ Health Perspect 1995; 103(Suppl 7):157-64.
6. Banerjee KK, Bishayee A, Marimuthu P. Evaluation of cyanide exposure and its effects on thyroid function of workers in a cable industry. J Occup Environ Med 1997; 39:258-60.
7. Brechner RJ, Parkhurst GD, Humble WO, et al. Ammonium perchlorate contamination of Colorado river drinking water is associated with abnormal thyroid function in newborns in Arizona. J Occup Environ Med 2000; 42:777-82.
8. Lamm SH, Doemland M. Has perchlorate in drinking water increased the rate of congenital hypothyroidism? J Occup Environ Med 1999; 41:409-11.
9. Gibbs JP, Ahmad R, Crump KS, et al. Evaluation of a population with occupational exposure to air borne ammonium perchlorate for possible acute or chronic effects on thyroid function. J Occup Environ Med 1998; 40:1072-82.
10. Lamm SH, Braverman LE, Li FX, et al. Thyroid health status of ammonium perchlorate workers: a cross-sectional occupational health study. J Occup Environ Med 1999; 41:248-60.
11. Lawrence JE, Lamm SH, Pino K, Richman K, Braverman LE. The effect of short-term low-dose perchlorate on various aspects of thyroid function. Thyroid 2000; 10:659-63.
12. Lawrence JE, Lamm SH, Braverman LE. Low dose perchlorate (3 mg daily) and thyroid function. Thyroid 2001; 11:295.
13. Greer MA, Goodman G, Pleus RC, Greer SE. Health effects assessment for environmental perchlorate contamination: the dose-response for inhibition of thyroidal radioiodine uptake in humans. Environ Health Perspect 2002; 110:927-37.
14. US Environmental Protection Agency. Perchlorate environmental contamination: toxicologic review and risk characterization based on emerging information. NCEA-1-0503, January 16, 2002. Washington, DC: US Environmental Protection Agency.

15. Van Middlesworth L. Effects of radiation on the thyroid gland. Adv Intern Med 1989; 34:265-84.

16. Cheek AO, Kow K, Chen J, et al. Potential mechanisms of action of thyroid disruption in humans: interaction of organochlorine compounds with thyroid receptor, transthyretin, and thyroid-binding globulin. Environ Health Perspect 1999; 107:273-8.

17. Zhou L-X, Dehal SS, Kupfer D, et al. Cytochrome P450 catalyzed binding of methoxychlor to rat hepatic microsomal iodothyronine 5'-monodeiodinase, type 1: does exposure to methoxychlor disrupt thyroid hormone metabolism? Arch Biochem Biophys 1995; 322:390-4.

18. Vulsma T. Impact of exposure to maternal PCBs and dioxins on the neonate's thyroid hormone status. Epidemiology 2000; 11:239-41.

19. Cullen MR, Robins JM, Kayne RD. Endocrine and reproductive dysfunction in men associated with occupational inorganic lead intoxication. Arch Environ Health 1984; 39:431-40.

20. Robins JM, Cullen MR, Connors BB, et al. Depressed thyroid indices associated with occupational exposure to lead. Arch Intern Med 1983; 143:220-4.

21. Schumacher C, Brodkin CA, Alexander B, et al. Thyroid function in lead smelter workers: absence of subacute or cumulative effects with moderate lead burdens. Int Arch Occup Environ Health 1998; 71:453-8.

22. Siegel M, Forsyth B, Siegel L, et al. The effect of lead on thyroid function in children. Environ Res 1989; 49:190-6.

23. Wagar G, Tolonen M, Stenman UH, et al. Endocrinologic studies in men exposed occupationally to carbon disulfide. J Toxicol Environ Health 1981; 7:363-71.

24. Bahn AK, Mills JL, Snyder PJ, et al. Hypothyroidism in workers exposed to polybrominated biphenyls. N Engl J Med 1980; 302:31-3.

25. Murai K, Okamura K, Tsuji H, et al. Thyroid function in "yusho" patients exposed to polychlorinated biphenyls (PCB). Environ Res 1987; 44:179-87.

26. Emmett EA, Maroni M, Jefferys J, et al. Studies of transformer repair workers exposed to PCBs: II. Results of clinical laboratory investigations. Am J Ind Med 1988; 14:47-62.

27. Langer P, Tajtakova M, Fodor G, et al. Increased thyroid volume and prevalence of thyroid disorders in an area heavily polluted by polychlorinated biphenyls. Eur J Endocrinol 1998; 139:402-9.

28. Calvert GM, Sweeney MH, Deddens J, et al. Evaluation of diabetes mellitus, serum glucose, and thyroid function among United States workers exposed to 2,3,7,8-tetrachlorodibenzo-p-dioxin. Occup Environ Med 1999; 56:270-6.

29. Suskind RR, Hertzberg VS. Human health effects of 2,4,5-T and its toxic contaminants. JAMA 1984; 251:2372-80.

30. Patandin S, Dagnelie PC, Mulder PGH, et al. Dietary exposure to polychlorinated biphenyls and dioxins from infancy until adulthood: a comparison between breast-feeding, toddler, and long-term exposure. Environ Health Perspect 1999; 107:45-51.

31. Osius N, Karmaus W, Kruse H, et al. Exposure to polychlorinated biphenyls and levels of thyroid hormones in children. Environ Health Perspect 1999; 107:843-9.

32. Nagayama J, Okamura K, Iida T, et al. Postnatal exposure to chlorinated dioxins and related chemicals on thyroid hormone status in Japanese breast-fed infants. Chemosphere 1998; 37:1789-93.

33. Koopman-Esseboom C, Weisglas-Kuperus N, de Ridder MA, et al. Effects of polychlorinated biphenyl/dioxin exposure and feeding type on infants' mental and psychomotor development. Pediatrics 1996; 97:700-6.

34. Longnecker MP, Gladen BC, Patterson DG, et al. Polychlorinated biphenyl (PCB) exposure in relation to thyroid hormone levels in neonates. Epidemiology 2000; 11:249-54.

35. Porterfield SP, Hendry LB. Impact of PCBs on thyroid hormone directed brain development. Toxicol Ind Health 1998; 14:103-20.

36. Prescott E, Netterstrom B, Faber J, et al. Effect of occupational exposure to cobalt blue dyes on the thyroid volume and function of female plate painters. Scand J Work Environ Health 1992; 18:101-4.

37. Christensen JM, Poulsen OM. A 1982-1992 surveillance programme on Danish pottery painters. Biologic levels and health effects following exposure to soluble or insoluble cobalt compounds in cobalt blue dyes. Sci Total Environ 1994; 150:95-104.

38. Capen CC. Mechanisms of chemical injury to the thyroid gland. Prog Clin Biol Res 1994; 387:173-91.

39. Barsony J, Kertesz F. Investigation of adrenal steroids and 25-hydroxy-cholecalcipherol in human gramoxone poisoning. Arch Toxicol Suppl 1985; 8:280-3.

40. Blanchouin-Emeric N, Defaye G, Toury R, et al. The reoxidation of cytochrome P-450 by paraquat inhibits aldosterone biosynthesis from 18-hydroxycorticosterone. J Steroid Biochem 1988; 31:331-5.

41. Matin MA, Husain K, Khan SN. Modification of diazinon-induced changes in carbohydrate metabolism by adrenalectomy in rats. Biochem Pharmacol 1990; 39:1781-6.

42. Liu PS, Kao LS, Lin MK. Organophosphates inhibit catecholamine secretion and calcium influx in bovine adrenal chromaffin cells. Toxicology 1994; 90:81-91.

43. Bestervelt LL, Cai Y, Piper DW, et al. TCDD alters pituitary-adrenal function. I: adrenal responsiveness to exogenous ACTH. Neurotoxicol Teratol 1993; 15:365-7.

44. Jovanovich L, Levin S, Khan MA. Significance of mirex-caused hypoglycemia and hyperlipidemia in rats. J Biochem Toxicol 1987; 2:203-13.

45. Mohammed A, Hallberg E, Rydstrom J, et al. Toxaphene: accumulation in the adrenal cortex and effect on ACTH-stimulated corticosteroid synthesis in the rat. Toxicol Lett 1985; 24:137-43.

46. Pise VM, Reigle TG, Muralidhara S, et al. Effects of acute inhalation exposure to 1,1,1-trichloroethane on the hypothalamo-pituitary-adrenal axis in male Sprague-Dawley rats. J Toxicol Environ Health 1998; 54(Part A):193-208.

47. Mutti A, Vescovi PP, Falzoi M, et al. Neuroendocrine effects of styrene on occupationally exposed workers. Scand J Work Environ Health 1984; 10:225-8.

48. Arfini G, Mutti A, Vescovi P. Impaired dopaminergic modulation of pituitary secretion in workers occupationally exposed to styrene: further evidence from PRL response to TRH stimulation. J Occup Med 1987; 129:826-30.

49. Mutti A, Falzoi M, Romanelli A, et al. Regional alterations of brain catecholamines by styrene exposure in rabbits. Arch Toxicol 1984; 55:173-7.

50. Kolstad HA, Bisanti L, Roeleveld N, et al. Time to pregnancy for men occupationally exposed to styrene in several European reinforced plastics companies. Scand J Work Environ Health 1999; 25(Suppl 1):66-9.

51. Svensson B-G, Nise G, Erfurth EM, et al. Neuroendocrine effects in printing workers exposed to toluene. Br J Ind Med 1992; 49:402-8.

52. Svensson B-G, Nise G, Erfurth EM, et al. Hormone status in occupational toluene exposure. Am J Ind Med 1992; 22:99-107.

53. Garry VF, Burroughs B, Tarone R, et al. Herbicides and adjuvants: an evolving view. Toxicol Ind Health 1999; 15:159-67.

54. von Euler G, Fuxe K, Hansson T, et al. Effects of chronic toluene exposure on central monoamine and peptide receptors and their interactions in the adult male rat. Toxicology 1988; 52:103-26.

55. Andersson K, Fuxe K, Toftgard R, et al. Toluene-induced activation of certain hypothalamic and median eminence catecholamine nerve terminal systems of the male rat and its effects on anterior pituitary hormone secretion. Toxicol Lett 1980; 5:393-8.

56. Andersson K, Fuxe K, Nilsen OD, et al. Production of discrete changes in dopamine and noradrenaline levels and turnover

in various parts of the rat brain following exposure to xylene, ortho-, meta- and para-xylene and ethylbenzene. Toxicol Appl Pharmacol 1981; 60:535-48.

57. Karam JH, Lewitt PA, Young CW, et al. Insulinopenic diabetes after rodenticide (Vacor) ingestion. Diabetes 1980; 29:971-8.

58. Sweeney MH, Calvert GM, Egeland GA, et al. Review and update of the results of the NIOSH medical study of workers exposed to chemicals contaminated with 2,3,7,8-tetrachlorodibenzodioxin. Teratog Carcinog Mutagen 1997-98; 17:241-7.

59. Michalek JE, Akhtar FZ, Kiel JL. Serum dioxin, insulin, fasting glucose, and sex hormone-binding globulin in veterans of Operation Ranch Hand. J Clin Endocrinol Metab 1999; 84:1540-3.

60. Pesatori AC, Zocchetti C, Guercilena S, et al. Dioxin exposure and non-malignant health effects: a mortality study. Occup Environ Med 1998; 55:126-31.

61. Ott MG, Olson RA, Cook RR. Cohort mortality study of chemical workers with potential exposure to the higher chlorinated dioxins. J Occup Med 1987; 29:422-9.

62. Steenland K, Piacitelli L, Deddens J, et al. Cancer, heart disease, and diabetes in workers exposed to 2,3,7,8-tetrachlorodibenzo-p-dioxin. J Natl Cancer Inst 1999; 91:779-86.

63. Vena J, Boffetta P, Becher H, et al. Exposure to dioxin and non-neoplastic mortality in the expanded IARC International Cohort Study of Phenoxy Herbicide and Chlorophenol Production Workers and Sprayers. Environ Health Perspect 1998; 106(Suppl 2):645-53.

64. Osterloh JD. Observations on the effect of parathyroid hormone on environmental blood lead concentrations in humans. Environ Res 1991; 54:8-16.

65. Nogawa K, Tsuritwni I, Kido T, Honda R, Yamada Y, Ishizaki M. Mechanism for bone disease found in inhabitants environmentally exposed to cadmium: decreased serum 1-alpha 25 dihydroxy vitamin D levels. Int Arch Occup Environ Health 1987; 59:21-30.

66. Jarup L, Alfven T, Persson B, et al. Cadmium may be a risk factor for osteoporosis. Occup Environ Med 1998; 55:435-9.

67. Alfven T, Elinder CG, Carlsson MD, et al. Low-level cadmium exposure and osteoporosis. J Bone Miner Res 2000; 15:1579-86.

68. Beard J, Marshall S, Jong K, et al. 1,1,1-trichloro-2,2-bis(p-chlorophenyl)-ethane (DDT) and reduced bone mineral density. Arch Environ Health 2000; 55:177-80.

69. Davis BJ, Heindel JJ. Ovarian toxicants: multiple mechanisms of action. In: Korach KS, ed. Reproductive and developmental toxicology. New York: Marcel Dekker; 1998:373.

70. Gray LE Jr, Ostby J, Ferrell J, et al. A dose-response analysis of methoxychlor-induced alterations of reproductive development and function in the rat. Fundam Appl Toxicol 1989; 12:92-108.

71. Kelce WR, Stone CR, Laws SC, et al. Persistent DDT metabolite p,p'-DDE is a potent androgen receptor antagonist. Nature 1995; 375:581-5.

72. Haake J, Kelley M, Keys B, et al. The effects of organochlorine pesticides as inducers of benz[a]pyrene hydroxylases. Gen Pharmacol 1987; 18:165-9.

73. Han YG, Kang SS, Seong JY, et al. Negative regulation of gonadotropin-releasing hormone and gonadotropin-releasing hormone receptor gene expression by a gonadotrophin-releasing hormone agonist in the rat hypothalamus. J Neuroendocrinol 1999; 11:195-201.

27.2 **Disorders of Reproduction and Development**

Ulrike Luderer, Mark R Cullen, Donald R Mattison

Extraordinary awareness, interest, and concern have arisen in the past three decades regarding the effects of physical activity and occupational and environmental exposures on human reproductive and developmental health. These factors have paralleled increased interest in reproductive health, motivated in part by an explosion of technology to enhance fertility and minimize adverse pregnancy outcomes. At the same time, the focus on reproduction and development has followed increased concerns about the effects of chemical, biologic, and physical hazards on health generally.

Certain unique social, scientific, and medical circumstances have contributed further to these concerns. Most obvious has been the enormous shift of women into the workforces of developed countries. Most women now work before, during, and after their pregnancies. Furthermore, the range of occupations undertaken by women has expanded to include virtually all of those formerly limited to men. Not surprisingly, issues such as the safety of occupational exposure standards for women of reproductive age, pregnant women and their fetuses, and the appropriate modifications of work practices and the work environment for the pregnant woman have challenged traditional approaches to occupational safety, which were developed in an earlier era.

More recently, the concern has been raised that environmental pollutants, at levels to which the general public is exposed, may be having adverse effects on human reproduction and development. Exposure to chemical pollutants that disrupt endocrine function by mechanisms such as binding to intracellular steroid receptors has been associated with reproductive failure and abnormal sexual differentiation in wildlife and laboratory species.[1] Such observations led to hypotheses that similar abnormalities in humans, including declining sperm counts and increased incidence of abnormal urogenital development, breast cancer, and testicular cancer, may be caused by environmental exposures to endocrine-disrupting chemicals.[1-4] These hypotheses have generated considerable controversy,[5,6] and are currently under active investigation. Relevant research will be discussed in later sections of this chapter.

Unfortunately, these challenges uncovered a second aspect of the reproductive-environmental health problem, namely, the extraordinary paucity of useful information. Even today, information is available on reproductive and developmental effects for a relatively small number of physical, chemical, and biologic agents, and primarily for those effects that occur at high levels of exposure. Human epidemiologic studies are difficult to perform because of the sensitive nature of the information required, and the problems of classifying individuals based on their exposures during the often brief periods of biologic interest. Toxicologic studies are no less difficult to interpret given the differences between the reproductive biology of humans and experimental animals. The net effect is that even though the issue of reproductive and developmental health in the workplace has emerged as serious and promi-

nent, the availability of scientific and clinical data on which to make decisions remains limited.

In response to these realities, many employers, physicians, and regulators proposed that women who were pregnant or were capable of becoming pregnant should be removed from exposure to any hazard that could possibly affect fecundity, fertility, or the outcome of pregnancy. However, this approach was based on the mistaken premise that environmental agents would have their impacts only on fetuses in recognized pregnancies following exposure of the female. In fact, successful reproduction and development entails events in men and women that long precede recognized pregnancy as well as critical events in the fetus, placenta, and infant (Fig. 27.2.1).

Further, many harmful agents are known to have long half-lives in the body, whereas others, at least theoretically, could cause effects on target tissues that persist long after the agent itself has disappeared. Therefore, protection of reproductive and developmental health could not scientifically be viewed as a matter of limiting exposure to pregnant women alone, but must also include the infant after birth and men. Even if such policies could scientifically limit their focus to women, there remain the social issues raised by a health policy that overtly discriminates against the job rights of fecund or pregnant women, a view underscored by the United States Supreme Court in its 1991 decision of United Auto Workers versus Johnson Controls, Inc., in which the majority found that federal law prohibits job discrimination purely on the basis of pregnancy or the ability to become pregnant.

This chapter (1) defines adverse reproductive and developmental health outcomes, (2) summarizes non-environmental risk factors, (3) reviews sources of agent-specific data, (4) provides listings of agents for which reasonably good data exist, (5) outlines clinical approaches to common reproductive and developmental health concerns, and (6) discusses workforce or population-based prevention strategies.

ADVERSE REPRODUCTIVE AND DEVELOPMENTAL HEALTH OUTCOMES

Because of the complexity of reproduction and development, there are multiple adverse reproductive outcomes in humans (Fig. 27.2.1). Although knowledge of the biologic bases of these events remains limited, some information exists regarding their background distribution in populations of interest (Table 27.2.1) and the factors that predispose to their occurrence.

Infertility and subfertility

Because the concept of fertility often is discussed imprecisely, some definitions are presented here. *Fecundity* is the capability of the male, female, or couple to produce

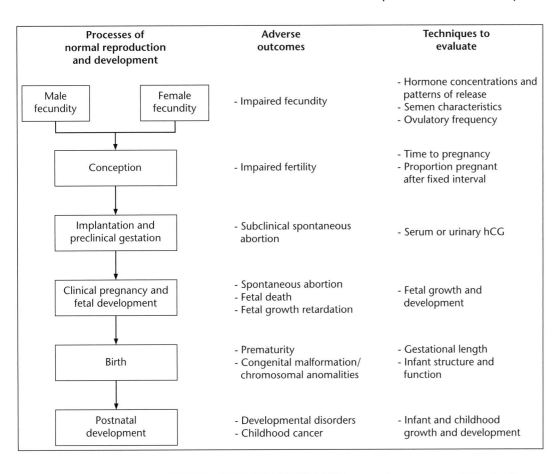

Processes of normal reproduction and development	Adverse outcomes	Techniques to evaluate
Male fecundity / Female fecundity	- Impaired fecundity	- Hormone concentrations and patterns of release - Semen characteristics - Ovulatory frequency
Conception	- Impaired fertility	- Time to pregnancy - Proportion pregnant after fixed interval
Implantation and preclinical gestation	- Subclinical spontaneous abortion	- Serum or urinary hCG
Clinical pregnancy and fetal development	- Spontaneous abortion - Fetal death - Fetal growth retardation	- Fetal growth and development
Birth	- Prematurity - Congenital malformation/ chromosomal anomalities	- Gestational length - Infant structure and function
Postnatal development	- Developmental disorders - Childhood cancer	- Infant and childhood growth and development

Figure 27.2.1: Normal processes of reproduction and development, representative adverse outcomes, and suggested techniques to evaluate the mechanism of the adverse outcome. For example, although subclinical spontaneous abortion may be initially manifest by increased time to pregnancy (impaired fertility), it is necessary to use urinary or serum measurement of the hCG to define early pregnancy and determine which conceptions failed to continue to develop.

Reproductive or developmental outcome	Percent
Infertility (of couples)	10–15
Preimplantation pregnancy loss	20–30
Spontaneous abortion (including clinically unrecognized)	15–50
Clinically recognized spontaneous abortion	10–15
Stillbirth (beyond 28 weeks)	<3
Premature, postmature, growth retardation	10
Birth defects	
identified at birth	3–5
identified over first year of life	5–15
Data from references 7, 8, 15–17.	

Table 27.2.1 Rates of adverse reproductive outcomes

offspring. It may be measured indirectly by such tests as a sperm count, ovulatory rate, endometrial biopsy; or more directly by measuring the conception rate of a couple followed over a fixed period of time. *Fertility* is the actual production of offspring by a couple. It is measured by recording live births over a particular time interval. *Subfertility* refers to a reduction in the expected birth rate due to factors other than choice, contraception use, or other clinical steps to diminish live births. It often is measured as a delay in the time that it takes to have a live birth during active attempts at pregnancy. *Infertility* is a couple's failure to achieve a clinically recognized pregnancy and usually is defined as one year of unsuccessful attempts. The basis for infertility or for subfertility may be the impairment of male or female fecundity, a problem with conception or implan-

tation, or some difficulty in carrying live births to term (see pathophysiology section). In practice, and for the purpose of this discussion, infertility usually is reserved for couples who have trouble conceiving (achieving a clinically recognized pregnancy); postconception problems are considered separately.

Six to fifteen percent of all couples are infertile.[7,8] The bases for failure to conceive within a year of trying are roughly due one-third to male factors, one-third to female factors, and one-third to couple and unexplained factors.

The known factors associated with impaired male fecundity include chromosomally determined sterility (e.g., Klinefelter's syndrome [47, XXY], male Turner's or Noonan's syndrome [mosaic 46XY, 45X]), congenital cryptorchidism, endocrinopathies (e.g., pituitary or testicular failure), testicular infections (e.g., mumps orchitis), gonadotoxic drugs (e.g., antineoplastics, potent vitamin A derivatives), urologic disorders and duct obstructions, retrograde ejaculation, and varicocele. Increasing age seems to be associated with decreased fecundity in men as well as women.[9]

Factors associated with impaired female fecundity also include chromosomal, endocrine, and anatomic disturbances, gonadotoxic drugs, and increasing age. In women, common endocrine problems are ovarian failure and disorders of hormonal imbalance, such as the amenorrhea-hirsutism disorders and prolactin-secreting pituitary adenomas. Congenital (e.g., abnormal uterus) and acquired (e.g., from pelvic inflammatory disease or endometriosis) anatomic disturbances resulting in fallopian tube blockage, or failure of the fertilized egg to implant, are also common.

Diagnosis of one of the above-mentioned factors that are known to impair male and female fecundity does not necessarily rule out an environmental or occupational cause. For example, environmental agents may be the cause of chromosomal damage, endocrine abnormalities, or endometriosis.

Although there are large differences in fertility rates among different ethnic and racial groups, it appears most likely that these differences are based more on cultural and social factors than on biologic factors. There are lifestyle factors that impair fecundity and fertility. Tobacco use decreases the number of morphologically normal motile sperm in the ejaculate, impairs ovulation, tubal transport, and implantation, and reduces fecundity in both men and women.[10,11] Alcohol and other substances that are abused may also impair fecundity or fertility. Two recent studies of the effect of moderate alcohol consumption demonstrated reduced fecundity in women, but not men.[12,13] Caffeine consumption may be associated with reduced fecundity in non-smoking women.[13,14] Starvation and very high levels of physical activity also reduce fecundity. The complexity of these exposures and other associated lifestyle factors complicates the characterization of causation.

Spontaneous abortion

The rate of spontaneous abortion in a population depends on the method of quantitation. About 10–15% of clinically recognized pregnancies are aborted, largely in the first trimester. Prospective studies using the specific and sensitive assays for human chorionic gonadotropin (hCG) for early pregnancy detection demonstrate that about 30–60% of implanted pregnancies end in spontaneous abortion.[15] At present no accurate data exist on *preimplantation* pregnancy losses in natural pregnancies because there is no clinically available test for preimplantation pregnancy; however, a protein termed early pregnancy factor (EPF) shows promise as such a marker.[16] Data are available from two prospective studies using daily measurements of EPF and hCG: in a study of natural pregnancies, 17% of EPF increases were not followed by hCG increases;[16] in a study of in-vitro fertilizations, 31% of EPF rises were not followed by hCG rises,[17] consistent with preimplantation loss. The significance of extremely early losses remains unclear, as does the range of factors that may influence their occurrence. Therefore, this discussion focuses on the factors that influence rates of clinically recognized spontaneous abortions.

Among the clinically recognized abortions, about half that come to pathologic evaluation are chromosomally abnormal, often remarkably so. This suggests that spontaneous abortion in these cases is biologically determined; the adverse health outcome is the fetal disorder, not its loss. There is little information on factors that determine the rate of these chromosomal abnormalities, nor is it known whether or not they are influenced by any of the factors that are associated with loss of apparently normal pregnancies.

The causes for loss in the first trimester of chromosomally normal fetuses are partially understood. There is a strong age dependency, with spontaneous abortion more common in very young women (i.e., younger than 18 years of age) and older women, especially those older than 35 years of age, at which point the rate is about double; the effects of paternal age, if they do occur, are slight. Prior spontaneous abortion is a comparable risk factor, supporting the impression that some women miscarry repeatedly. Tobacco also is an important risk factor for early spontaneous abortion, with about a 50% increase seen in those women who smoke during pregnancy compared with those who quit before conception.[18,19] The effect of moderate alcohol consumption is uncertain, with mixed results being generated from available studies once the effects of other known factors are accounted for.[20,21] Similarly, nutritional factors, other than extreme malnourishment early in pregnancy, do not appear to be associated with an increased risk for early pregnancy loss, demonstrated by the rather good record of women with weight loss associated with hyperemesis gravidarum.

Late spontaneous abortion and fetal death

After the first trimester, spontaneous pregnancy losses are less common. In the second trimester, they are associated with anatomic problems of the mother, such as an incompetent cervix, severe disease of mother or fetus, or infection, such as urinary tract infection, cervical infection, or parvovirus, the cause of epidemic fifth disease in young children. An in-depth analysis of maternal diseases is beyond the scope of this text. Fetal disorders associated with fetal death in mid- and late pregnancy are discussed later in the section on fetal growth retardation. Brain injury, often occurring late in gestation as a complication of development (such as umbilical cord strangulation or compression), is another explicable cause of fetal death.

Fetal growth retardation

Fetal or intrauterine growth retardation refers to impaired growth of the fetus during development, which is measured by comparing the size of the fetus or infant to ethnic-appropriate, gender-specific data based on gestational age. A fetus or infant below the 10th percentile for age may be considered growth retarded. Accurate determination of gestational age is essential for the appropriate diagnosis of growth retardation.

Although growth retardation may be due to an underlying disease of the fetus itself, such as a genetic or chromosomal abnormality, or the presence of multiple fetuses, many cases represent established conditions including severe maternal malnutrition or illness; maternal use or abuse of tobacco, alcohol, or drugs; and exposure to teratogenic drugs or infections. The role of socioeconomic status beyond these specific factors is less clear, although a prior history of a pregnancy complicated by fetal growth retardation is a strong independent predictor.

Because of the difficulty in some cases in distinguishing fetal growth retardation from either genetically small size (e.g., dwarfs, small parents) or prematurity, the precise incidence of fetal growth retardation is uncertain. Overall, about 1 in 16 live neonates in the United States weighs under 2500 g. Of these neonates, about 15–20% are believed to be term births with pure fetal growth retardation; the remainder are due to prematurity or a combination of prematurity and growth retardation.

Prematurity

Prematurity is defined as birth prior to 37 weeks' gestation; it is a clinical problem if the baby is small or significantly immature, especially in terms of lung development. Surprisingly little is known about the factors that precipitate premature delivery. Ascending urogenital infections are an important, largely preventable, cause of prematurity.[22] Other causes include premature rupture of the membranes, or other maternal or fetal injury or disease. Among lifestyle factors, smoking is most clearly associated with prematurity. Prematurity also occurs more commonly among women of low socioeconomic status, those with less prenatal care, and those who drink alcohol, or abuse drugs during pregnancy. As with many reproductive outcomes, a history of a prior premature delivery is predictive of another.

Congenital malformations and chromosomal abnormalities

Depending on the length of observation and the precision of diagnosis, 3–5% of all live births are recognized as having either a congenital malformation or a chromosomal disorder, with an increasing number recognized after the first year of life. Although a very small fraction of these conditions can be traced to heritable genetic disease of the parents, the vast majority are acquired in the reproductive process itself and, hence, are subject to environmental effects (Table 27.2.2).

A chemical, physical, or biologic agent that causes a birth defect, gross chromosomal alteration, or functional deficit with expression at some point after birth is termed a teratogen or developmental toxicant. In general, established causes of birth defects are associated with particular syndromes, malformations, functional deficits, or patterns of developmental toxicity. This is most striking for the first well-characterized group of developmental toxicants, the infectious agents, which include rubella, syphilis, toxoplasmosis, and cytomegalovirus. Thyroid insufficiency in pregnancy or the use of antithyroid medications may result in cretinism. Other drugs also have been found to cause congenital malformations since the outbreak of phocomelia was recognized to be associated with use of the sedative thalidomide during the first trimester of pregnancy. Those drugs with established or suspected teratogenicity are listed in Table 27.2.3.

There are increasing data suggesting that at least some birth defects may be related to nutritional factors. Diets low in folic acid have been associated with neural tube defects, and supplementation with folic acid during the periconception period has been demonstrated to reduce the risk of these defects by about 50%.[23] To date, trials with folic acid and other vitamin supplements have not reduced the frequency of other common defects. Iodine is another essential nutrient for normal development, as evidenced by high rates of cretinism in areas with endemic goiter. Although nutritional supplementation may improve reproductive or developmental outcomes, excess exposure to some vitamins, notably vitamin A and its derivatives, is

Cause	Percent
Unknown	65–75
Genetic	10–25
Environmental	
Maternal conditions	4
Infections	3
Mechanical	1–2
Developmental toxicants	1

Data from reference [150].

Table 27.2.2 Cause of human developmental abnormalities

Aminopterin
Androgens; testosterone
Aspirin; non-steroidal anti-inflammatory drugs†
Busulfan
Captopril and other angiotensin-converting enzyme inhibitors
Carbamazepine
Chlorambucil
Codeine, other opioids‡
Warfarin (Coumadin)
Cyclophosphamide
Cytarabine
Diazepam, other benzodiazepines‡
Estrogens; diethylstilbestrol#
Ethanol
Lithium
Mechlorethamine (nitrogen mustard)
Methimazole
Methotrexate
Misoprostal
Penicillamine
Phenytoin
Progestagens; medroxyprogesterone#
Propylthiouracil
Tetracycline and derivatives
Thalidomide
Trimethadione
Valproic acid
Vitamin A, isotretinoin, 13-cis-retinoic acid and etretinate
5-Fluorouracil

* Although this table lists drugs known or suspected to cause developmental toxicity, it is incomplete in several important ways: the adverse developmental effect is not defined; the risk for the adverse effect as a function of dose, duration of exposure, and timing of exposure with respect to pregnancy are not included; and the benefit of treatment of maternal, fetal, or pregnancy-related disease is not characterized. These and other factors need to be considered when counseling patients about the impact of these drugs on development. Adapted from references [24, 151].
† Late third trimester use is associated with constriction of the ductus arteriosus. Use during the first and second trimesters is considered safe.
‡ Use during late pregnancy is associated with withdrawal syndromes in the neonate.
# Combinations of estrogens and progestagens in oral contraceptive formulations have not been associated with increased risk of major malformations.

Table 27.2.3 Therapeutic drugs known or suspected to cause developmental toxicity*

associated with an increased risk for reproductive or developmental toxicity.[24] The importance (benefit and/or risk) of essential dietary minerals and overall protein and caloric intake has not been established.

Maternal disorders associated with an increased risk of congenital anomalies are diabetes mellitus, phenylketonuria, and hypothyroidism. Maternal age is also an important risk factor, especially for Down's syndrome and disorders of the CNS such as anencephaly and spina bifida. Alcoholism and substance abuse during pregnancy are associated with fetal developmental disorders that may be recognized as birth defects in extreme cases or as developmental disorders of childhood in more subtle presentations. At present, there are no compelling data to suggest that tobacco use is associated with birth defects.

Developmental delay and disability

A distressingly high proportion of children, perhaps up to 10%, experience some measurable delay in achievement of developmental milestones, as noted on routine well-baby checks or as determined by more specialized testing. These delays may be associated with evidence of structural neurologic damage, such as seizures, motor deficits, or systemic disorders, suggesting either metabolic or congenital disease. Most commonly, however, the delays are functional and are not easily classifiable into another disease category. When they are mild and compensated, the conditions are termed developmental delays. Persistent deficits are called developmental or learning disabilities.

When the losses are profound relative to age-specific standards, mental retardation is diagnosed. The cause of the vast majority of such cases is unknown. Clearly, children with prenatal disorders such as growth retardation and prematurity, exposure to known developmental toxicants, and traumas associated with labor and delivery that result in low Apgar scores are at higher risk. Intrauterine or postpartum infection may play a role in some cases. Because most of the normative standards for the developmental milestones are race and social class specific, poor and non-white children appear to have higher rates, but successes of early learning programs suggest these differences are likely artifactual. The roles of dietary and behavioral factors (i.e., nurture) remain speculative.

Childhood cancer

Acute leukemia occurs with an incidence of about 4 per 100,000 per year throughout the first 15 years of life. It occurs in very high frequency in children with Down's syndrome and other rare congenital disorders, including Fanconi's syndrome, Bloom's syndrome, and immunodeficiencies. Genetic factors are suggested by a high rate of concordance in identical twins early in life. Postpartum exposures to benzene, ionizing radiation, and other agents that injure the bone marrow also are established causes (see Chapter 30.3). Other causes, however, are not well defined; viral infections have been suggested but remain unproven.

Malignant brain tumors are slightly less common than leukemia after the first year of life. The causes of these tumors remain poorly understood. Other cancers of childhood are very rare, and little is known about causes other than genetic factors, which explain a high fraction of cases of Wilms' tumor of the kidney and retinoblastoma; both conditions may be transmitted by autosomal dominant suppressed genes with incomplete penetrance. The occurrence of cases with features of hereditary disease in the absence of positive family history suggests the occurrence of spontaneous mutation at the prezygotic phase, possibly due to environmental mutation.

PATHOPHYSIOLOGY: THE MECHANISTIC BASIS FOR REPRODUCTIVE AND DEVELOPMENTAL TOXICITY AND LABORATORY EVALUATION

The physiologic events that are responsible for normal reproductive and developmental events are summarized in Figure 27.2.1 and Table 27.2.1. A *reproductive toxicant* is a chemical, physical, or biologic agent that alters male or female fecundity or that affects couple-specific factors, resulting in an alteration in fertility. Such agents must act on the male, female, or couple at a stage that precedes clinically recognized pregnancy (Fig. 27.2.1). A *developmental toxicant* may act on male or female gametes before pregnancy, on the developing embryo/fetus during pregnancy, or on the developing infant/child after pregnancy.

Male fecundity

Three systems are required to function effectively to ensure normal male fecundity: (1) the hypothalamic-pituitary-gonadal (HPG) endocrine axis, (2) testicular spermatogenesis, and (3) the accessory gland and transport system of the genitalia. Each of these systems is potentially subject to injury by an environmental hazard, although far more is known about the potential vulnerability of the first two than the last one.

The endocrine axis includes the hypothalamic hormone, gonadotropin-releasing hormone (GnRH), the pituitary hormones, luteinizing hormone (LH), follicle-stimulating hormone (FSH), and testosterone, generated by the Leydig cells of the testes in response to LH. The system is controlled by a negative feedback loop. Testicular failure results in elevations of LH and FSH, whereas testosterone or other sex steroids, such as estrogens, or environmental agents that can mimic the effect of steroids on the pituitary can inappropriately turn off the production of these hormones, leading to decreased testosterone production.

Unlike the situation in females, the HPG axis in males functions more or less continuously, so that measurement of disruption usually can be determined by a small number of blood samples for these hormones. Measurement of LH concentrations and secretory patterns must be repeated several times because the secretion of LH is pulsatile. Testosterone must be measured along with its binding hormone to determine free as well as total circulating hormone, because only the circulating hormone is active. Measurement of interfering steroids, such as estrogens and androgens (and xenobiotics, which are steroid agonists or antagonists), can be undertaken in urine and blood.

In general, the most important clinical effect of disruption of the HPG endocrine axis on male reproductive function is a reduction in male fecundity, either as a result of altered reproductive behavior, impaired sperm production or function, or both. Other manifestations may include testicular atrophy and feminization, but these problems are uncommon with environmental effects.

The second major component of the male reproductive tract required for normal fecundity is spermatogenesis, which occurs exclusively in the seminiferous tubules of the testes. In a cycle that takes about 70 days in humans, the primordial germ cells, called spermatogonia, mature to sperm under the obligate influences of testosterone and FSH. This maturation process requires both multiple mitoses, increasing the numbers of progenitor germ cells, and meioses, producing the sperm with their haploid complement of chromosomes.

Interference with spermatogenesis can be detected in several ways. The most readily available method is semen analysis, with evaluation of the numbers, viability, morphology, and motility of sperm in an ejaculate studied immediately after production under defined conditions of abstinence (typically 48 hours). More precise information regarding lesions in spermatogenesis can be obtained by testicular biopsy, in which the stage of spermatogenesis affected may be identified. A variety of newer tests also have been developed, including in-vitro assays of sperm penetration of hamster eggs, and sperm attachment to and penetration of the zona pellucida, and the sperm chromatin structure assay (SCSA), which assesses the susceptibility of sperm chromatin to breakage.[25] The importance to male fecundity of defects noted on these tests remains unclear, although the tests are in use both experimentally and in the clinical evaluation of infertile couples.

Clinically, lesions in spermatogenesis may be expected to have an effect on male fecundity, although there is no requisite number of cells or other finding on analysis of semen that directly predicts fecundity; usually less than 20 million cells per mL is associated with a clinically recognized disturbance in fecundity (Fig. 27.2.2). Decreased percentages of motile and morphologically normal sperm are also associated with decreased male fecundity.[26] Although the natural history of injuries to spermatogenesis is agent and circumstance specific, serial studies of affected men have led to recognition that partial lesions or disruption in late meiotic stages are generally somewhat reversible after removal of the affected individual from exposure and passage of several full spermatogenic cycles (e.g., several 70-day periods), whereas destruction of spermatogonia or complete azoospermia often is irreversible.

It is also important to recognize that effects on spermatogenesis could have profound effects on the reproductive or

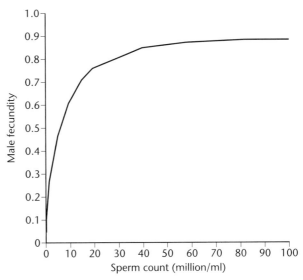

Figure 27.2.2: Relationship between sperm count and male fecundity. Data collected from human studies suggest that the sperm contribution to male fecundity is optimal at concentrations above 40 million/mL. When the sperm count falls below 20 million/mL, there is a rapid decline in male fecundity. Although the single parameter of sperm concentration in the ejaculate contributes to male fecundity, there are also other factors that play a role, including morphology and motility.[26,149]

developmental processes beyond male fecundity. The selection of chromosomes for passage to the oocyte occurs during this process so that mutations, chromosomal aberrations, or some chromosomal selection process could occur during this period that could be expressed later, with effects ranging from spontaneous abortion to developmental defects, or even childhood cancer. There are no established examples of such effects in humans, but male-induced early pregnancy loss (spontaneous abortion) has been shown with mutagens like dibromochloropropane in mice.

The final component of the male reproductive tract is the storage and transport of sperm in the male genitalia. This system begins with the Sertoli cells in the testis, where spermatogenesis begins; destruction of the Sertoli cells results in irreversible loss of fecundity. The epididymis stores sperm for 2 to 3 weeks, during which time the sperm become functionally mature. The vas deferens, accessory glands, prostate, and seminal vesicles each add components to semen and assist in its proper and timely delivery. Although less well characterized than testicular lesions, injury or functional modification of these post-testicular organs would be expected to result in reduced fecundity. Toxic injury to these components of the male reproductive system may be evaluated by assessment of the composition of the seminal fluid, including pH, volume and the specific products of each gland.

As with the process of spermatogenesis, the final stages of storage and transport of seminal fluid create, at least theoretically, opportunities for male-mediated effects on reproduction beyond fecundity. Heavy metals and organic compounds have been measured in seminal fluid. These agents could have an impact on sperm DNA during sperm maturation. Alternatively, contamination of the ejaculate with environmental toxicants could have an impact on early couple-specific factors, such as fertilization, or even affect the early zygote, resulting in disturbances of implantation or embryonic development. Further research is required to assess such effects and to date they have not been demonstrated in humans.

Female fecundity

As with males, female fecundity hinges on three systems: (1) the neuroendocrine gonadal axis, (2) oocyte development and release, and (3) the anatomic integrity of passages that allow sperm access to the oocyte and conceptus access to the uterus. Disorders of any component reduce female fecundity.

The human female neuroendocrine (hypothalamic-pituitary-ovary or HPO) axis is more complex than the male counterpart because of the added intricacy of temporal cycles. In order to facilitate the release of a mature oocyte (ovulation), LH and FSH concentrations must cycle, with suppression during menses, followed by a surge approximately 2 weeks later. Feedback by two ovarian hormones, estrogen and progesterone, produced by the supporting granulosa and thecal cells of the ovulatory follicle, are crucial to this orchestrated sequence. Also, the influence of hormones less consequential in males, such as prolactin, may sufficiently disturb this balance to disrupt the cycle. As in the male, LH, FSH, and sex steroid concentrations can be measured in the blood; however, in women, the concentrations must be assessed relative to the phase of the menstrual cycle in which the specimens were obtained.

Although the details of female reproductive physiology are beyond the scope of this text, the ramifications for evaluation of female fecundity can be summarized as follows. First, detection of a gross lesion in female fecundity is not difficult; anovulatory cycles may be recognized by the impact of hormones on the uterine endometrium, which is detectable by biopsy or by sequential hormonal analysis using repeated blood or urine specimens. On the other hand, localization of the lesions may be complex unless trophic hormones are persistently elevated, indicating ovarian failure. Another important ramification is the likelihood that many different types of toxicants, acting in diverse ways, would be predicted to upset normal function of this endocrine axis. In animals, a host of heavy metals and halogenated hydrocarbons are established causes of diminished female fecundity. In humans, only pharmacologic agents such as steroid hormones and antineoplastic drugs have been adequately studied, although other exposures, such as tobacco use, are known to impair female fecundity. Whatever the cause or locus of interference, females with abnormal neuroendocrine cycles have impaired fecundity; they also may have abnormal menses and disturbances in secondary sex characteristics.

The processes leading to the release of a mature oocyte prepared for fertilization also are complex. Unlike the male (who has an essentially unlimited supply of gametes), the female develops a finite set of oocytes in utero, supported by primordial follicles. At puberty, under the influence of trophic stimulation, these follicles develop in small numbers, sequentially becoming antral or preovulatory. The time span from emergence of a follicle as preovulatory to actual ovulation is about 3 months. From this distinction, it becomes clear that agents that may injure primordial follicles, such as the drug cyclophosphamide or tobacco use, can shorten the female's reproductive life span (i.e., produce premature menopause), whereas agents that may affect preovulatory follicles may cause short-term infertility that may reverse when exposure ends.

The role of anatomic lesions in female fecundity is straightforward. Such lesions, either congenital (e.g., abnormal uterus) or acquired (e.g., postinfectious occlusion of fallopian tubes), prevent the sperm from fertilizing the oocyte. Generally, these lesions are identifiable with available imaging techniques and may be corrected surgically.

Conception and couple-specific factors

Up to one-third of all couples seeking consultation for infertility are found to have normal male and female fecundity; the problem may be attributable to couple-specific factors. The most common of these factors are behavioral, involving frequency, timing, and technique of intercourse and contraceptive use. Occupational stressors, such as shift work, overtime work, and factors affecting libido, may also be important.

Biologic factors may explain some portion of the couple-specific cases of infertility as well. An example is incompatibility of the seminal fluid with the female reproductive tract due to the presence of antibodies or some other spermicidal action. Techniques for detection of such conditions are highly specialized. At present, the role of occupational or environmental factors in such disorders has not been established.

Implantation and early gestation

Before even a single menstrual period has been missed, the conceptus enters the earliest stages of embryogenesis. The mechanisms that facilitate the cellular division, differentiation, cell migration, and programmed cell death during this period are only beginning to be understood; they are discussed together with fetal development in the next section. Unique to this very early stage is the need for continued support of the new embryo by the ovary, in its luteal phase postfertilization, and by the uterus, which must respond to hormone stimulation (for endometrial development and myometrial quiescence) to allow embryonic implantation. The conceptus itself, through production of hCG and other factors, shares biologic responsibility for the success of implantation and its survival in the earliest stages as well.

Because these events occur before recognition of pregnancy, little opportunity for study in humans has been available. Animal studies have elucidated the timing and endocrinologic aspects of the period immediately after conception, and recently the possible role of toxicants has begun to be studied. These studies demonstrate that toxicant exposure during this window of development does not necessarily have an 'all or none' effect (death or no adverse effect), as previously assumed. They demonstrate that in addition to immediate death of the conceptus, exposures during this period can also cause a unique pattern of anatomical defects.[27] These results suggest that some previously unexplained human birth defects may be caused by exposures to toxicants or other stressors occurring prior to implantation. New techniques, such as the prospective monitoring of women with daily collections of urine, and sensitive and specific hormone assays, such as the newer assays for β-hCG, have also begun to shed light on the interval immediately after implantation in humans. For example, the longstanding prediction that a high proportion of embryos are lost during this period has proved to be true, perhaps as high as a half or more in some populations (see Table 27.2.1). It has also been learned that many women have normal pregnancies in the cycles immediately following such early losses, raising the question as to whether these are clinically important adverse reproductive outcomes.

Clinical pregnancy and fetal development

The remarkable sequence of events by which a single fertilized ovum develops into a well-differentiated fetus has been studied by embryologists for decades. Although the morphologic sequence has been clear for a long time, the cellular and molecular mechanisms that underlie the process are only just becoming clear, along with the myriad possibilities for disruption by endogenous and exogenous factors.

The major organ systems and anatomic structures are formed largely during the first trimester. Some landmark events and their approximate timing in human development are summarized in Table 27.2.4. A variety of biologic events appear to be crucial for normal development, including:
1. The presence of appropriate regulatory and structural genes.

Days from ovulation	Biologic event
1	Conception
5–7	Implantation begins
15	First missed menstrual period
18–19	Neural plate forms
20–21	First somite
23	Primordia of eye and ear
24–27	Neuropores close
27–30	Limb buds develop
29–32	Optic cup, lens form
33	Crown–rump length about 7 mm
37	Crown–rump length about 9 mm
38–42	Critical period for upper limb development
46–47	Cardiac chambers form
56–58	Palate closes
60–70	Fusion of urogenital folds, formation of external genitalia
84	Second trimester begins

Table 27.2.4 Early developmental milestones for the human fetus

2. Effective cell–cell communication via gap junctions and other surface molecules.
3. Appropriate exogenous stimuli by physiologic morphogens allowing specific cells to move, differentiate, and die based on their relative locations.
4. Adequate nutritional support allowing growth and survival.

It is obvious, therefore, that a wide range of possibilities exist for interference with development, and further, that the importance of these factors is time dependent. In other words, agents that may disrupt development at one stage may not have an impact earlier or later. Moreover, disruption of one of these vital elements may have very different clinical expressions depending on timing.

Although a detailed discussion of the mechanisms of developmental toxicity is beyond the scope of this text, some examples are illuminating. First, it is clear that major chromosomal anomalies, of whatever cause, could devastate the process of development if the genes that program the sequences of cell growth, differentiation, movement, and death are missing or abnormal. These problems would be expected to be lethal in a high proportion of cases, explaining why a high fraction of early spontaneous abortions are chromosomally abnormal. It also explains the multiple defects in those fetuses that survive, as well as the lethal or teratogenic effects of antimetabolites, such as antineoplastic drugs or other potent mutagens. Agents that interfere with regulatory genes, which determine the proper sequence for cellular events, also may be developmental toxicants. Transgenic experiments have proved the importance of these sequences, as well as the integrity of the genetic expression. Developmental toxicants, like vitamin A derivatives and the synthetic estrogen diethylstilbestrol (DES), act in part by altering normal regulatory gene expression or the effect of regulatory gene products.

Interference with cellular communication also may result in developmental toxicity. This problem may explain the action of certain teratogenic drugs, such as hydantoin and warfarin. Interestingly, in-vitro data suggest that certain environmental toxicants of interest, such as the ethylene glycol ethers, may disrupt cellular gap junctions.[28]

Interference with physiologic signals for cell behavior is another mechanism for effects produced by occupational and environmental hazards. Important physiologic agents in this regard include retinoic acid and thyroid hormone, likely explaining the important effects of agonists or antagonists of these endogenous compounds.

Disruption of nutritional support also may explain developmental toxicity, as well as growth retardation, during later stages of development. The crucial need for sources of energy in all cells, as well as appropriate maintenance of tissue osmolarity and pH, may explain why certain inborn errors of carbohydrate metabolism are devastating, as well as why deprivation of B vitamins, such as folic acid or riboflavin, may be teratogenic.

After essential organogenesis is complete, largely during the first trimester, the possibilities for environmental factors to affect the gross structure of the fetus are reduced. At this stage, the fetus is subject to many influences, requiring continuous delivery of nutrients by the placenta, and avoidance of toxicants that may cause systemic or specific organ system dysfunction. The central nervous system, which is continuing to develop and establish new cell–cell interactions (and will for many years postpartum), and the external genitalia, which are also continuing to develop during this period, are especially vulnerable to intoxication at this stage. Further, from this period through delivery, the fetus is dependent on preservation of its status in utero to allow the fullest maturation of its organs, such as the lungs and gastrointestinal tract, which would be vulnerable to the outside environment should premature delivery occur.

Sources of fetal susceptibility during the second and third trimesters include: (1) the placental supply of nutrients; (2) toxicants that may enter the fetus through the placenta, especially neurotoxicants; and (3) factors that may lead to prematurity. The first two susceptibility factors are reasonably well understood. The human placenta allows passage of a wide range of materials at rates determined by their molecular weights, lipid solubility, and other characteristics. These materials include drugs and chemicals to which women may be exposed during pregnancy. These may, on the one hand, interfere with delivery of necessary nutrients, as with asphyxiants or placental toxicants such as cadmium, or they may cause fetal toxicity directly, as with lead and organic mercury. It should also be noted that the fetus may be exposed by means other than the placental blood supply to certain hazards, especially physical hazards such as radiation, noise, heat, and injury, but the effects are comparable to transplacental sources of harm during this period.

The clinical effects of transplacental injury during the second and third trimesters may be varied and may not be apparent, either in utero or at birth. Unless a devastating insult occurs, such as fetal alcohol syndrome, the outcomes include growth retardation and developmental disruptions. Although evidence of transplacental exposure can be documented via cord blood analysis if the exposure is persistent or ongoing, such analysis is not recommended for routine clinical purposes. The placenta and body fluids of the newborn are other areas where such exposure could be confirmed, if desired.

Childbirth

A variety of adverse events may occur at or near the time of delivery, including stillbirth, fetal injury, or perinatal death. As noted, the most common reasons for these complications are pre-existing disease in the mother or the fetus or an obstetric catastrophe, as occurs with placental anomalies, multiple fetuses, gross prematurity, and cord strangulation. Rarely, extrinsic events or hazards such as overwhelming injury to the mother or near-lethal intoxication may be implicated.

Postnatal development

After birth, the infant is directly vulnerable to environmental exposures, such as inhalation or ingestion of contaminants brought home by the parents; ingestion of household poisons, such as lead or mercury in paints; and exposure to indoor and outdoor pollutants. As discussed in Chapter 10, the newborn and infant may have both unique exposures and sensitivity to some of these agents. The present discussion is limited to effects that result from the reproductive process itself, i.e., exposures that have occurred in utero or before conception. One unique and important source of postpartum exposure and risk that is related to reproduction, ingestion of breast milk during lactation, is discussed subsequently.

It has been noted that many effects of hazardous exposures during reproduction or development may not be recognized until after birth. For most cases, this is because the effect is sufficiently subtle or preclinical that it was not noticed at birth. In contrast, the manifestation of abnormal neurologic development and the occurrence of childhood cancer may require additional biologic events after birth. Each of these conditions has become the subject of serious inquiry.

The possibility that exposures during pregnancy could have an impact on development of the CNS long after birth is suggested by two factors. First, many CNS toxicants are long lived in the body; hence, they are likely to persist after prenatal exposures. Second, unlike other major organs that mature largely before birth, the CNS continues active development over a period of years. Although little is known about how agents may disrupt this process at the cellular level (as opposed to causing cell injury), or even whether the effects that emerge after birth represent a true de novo injury or merely inadequate repair of prior effects, at least two important agents, lead and polychlorinated biphenyls (PCBs), have been demonstrated to result in ongoing dysfunction in humans, measurable at 5–10 years of age. Unfortunately, there is no way to distinguish these causes of impairment from the myriad other causes for learning deficits unless other indications of poisoning by the same agents are apparent.

The fact that prenatal environmental factors could be causes of childhood or early adulthood cancer was recognized two decades ago, when females exposed in utero to DES had an increased risk of vaginal adenocarcinoma. Knowledge of the mechanisms of carcinogenesis has further enhanced interest, because two cancers of childhood, Wilms' tumor of the kidney and retinoblastoma, are often associated with the presence of a mutation of tumor suppressor genes. The possible mechanisms for reproductively or developmentally mediated carcinogenesis include:

1. Mutations of male or female gametes due to preconception exposures.
2. Somatic mutation occurring shortly after fertilization due to male or female parental exposures.
3. Transplacental or direct in utero exposure to mutagens or carcinogens from maternal exposure.
4. Transplacental injury to target tissue, changing its postpartum susceptibility to transformation.

While the fourth mechanism has been associated with an established human environmental exemplar, namely DES, epidemiologic studies implicating parental exposures suggest that the other mechanisms may also be relevant.

Lactation

Breast feeding has been extolled in both developed and developing countries as the most healthful way to nourish newborns and infants. Unfortunately, breast milk also may be a source of harmful substances to which the mother has been exposed before, during, and after pregnancy.

Knowledge of the physiology of lactation allows some reasonable prediction of what types of materials will be concentrated in milk. Factors that enhance concentration include low molecular weight, high pK (i.e., basic), low polarity (i.e., neutral), and fat solubility. The most significant predictor of a substance's milk content is the maternal blood or fat level of the substance, but for a given toxicant, milk may have as little as 1% or as much as 100-fold the level in the mother's plasma.

The most significant concerns regarding environmental exposures from breast milk have been heavy metals, halogenated solvents, pesticides, PCBs and dioxin (Table 27.2.5).[29-31] Not only are these materials highly concentrated in milk, as would be predicted, they also are long lived in maternal tissues and potentially very toxic.

Studies of large populations (Table 27.2.5) have not suggested that typical levels in milk approach those known to be associated with harm from these agents, even in the very vulnerable newborn age group, who have no other source of nutrition. Obviously, this is not the case in areas where there is significant past, ongoing, or other excessive maternal exposure or endemic contamination. In such cases, the level of the potential toxicant and ongoing exposure to the mother can be quantified, ideally before neona-

tal exposure occurs. If necessary, levels in the mother's milk itself can be measured, although these measurements are expensive and not widely available. Once exposure through milk has occurred, the most important information, i.e., the dose transmitted to the infant, can be obtained by sampling the baby's blood or other relevant tissue.

DATABASES FOR EVALUATING ENVIRONMENTAL AND OCCUPATIONAL REPRODUCTIVE AND DEVELOPMENTAL HAZARDS

In order to develop rational occupational health policies to reduce reproductive and developmental toxicity, information on effects in animals and human responses to exposure is essential. Unfortunately, there are substantial gaps in these important data.

Human epidemiology and clinical studies

Despite the fact that adverse reproductive events are extremely frequent in the population (see Table 27.2.1), the study of the effects of occupational and environmental factors has been very difficult. At the most conspicuous level, vital records of the kind that have been crucial for the study of mortality and cancer are not well maintained; early reproductive failures such as infertility and spontaneous abortions are not documented in any consistent fashion, nor are they even recognized with any uniformity. Later and less common adverse outcomes are documented but are rarely systematically available for analysis, although some birth defect registries have recently been developed to facilitate research. In the meantime, studies of events such as fetal deaths, growth retardation, and birth defects are difficult to perform, because the numbers of such events in any defined exposed population are small; case-control studies are hampered by a lack of knowledge of exposures within the larger population to all but the most conspicuous hazards, such as physical stressors.

Even if the events could be easily and consistently identified and verified, establishing exposure status is a formidable barrier. Not only the nature of exposure but its timing are crucial in classifying risk for any given outcome of interest. Further, for practical reasons, most studies have been retrospective, relying on recall of past exposures and confounding risk factors, with the potential for recall bias. Combined with the very sensitive nature of the information being gathered, it is not surprising that the performance of such studies has been limited.

In order to circumvent some of these difficulties, more recent epidemiologic studies have sought subtler endpoints that might be more readily discernible in exposed populations, with use of biomarkers of exposed effect. The best established and most straightforward methods are semen analysis and serum hormone measurements. More recent studies have prospectively collected daily urine samples

Compound	Per cent quantifiable‡	Range of means reported (ppm milk fat)
All DDT	70–100	
p,p'-DDT		0.2–4.3
p,p'-DDE		1.2–14.7
Dieldrin	0.04–100	0.05–0.24
Lindane and isomers	4–68	
γ-HCH		0.008–0.08
α-HCH		0.003–0.02
β-HCH		0.27–0.53
HCB		0.04
Heptachlor and heptachlor epoxide	25–100	0.035–0.13
Oxychlordane and chlordane	46–100	0.05–0.12
PCBs	20–100	0.8–1.5

* These data represent pesticide concentrations in breast milk that have been gathered by a range of analytic approaches over a period of 4 decades.
‡ The per cent of samples in which quantifiable levels of the indicated pesticide were observable. Note that these percentages are likely to vary with the analytical method used.
DDE = 1,1-Dichloro-2,2-bis (p = chlorophenyl ethylene); HCB = hexachlorobenzene; HCH = hexachlorocyclohexane; PCB = polychlorinated biphenyls.

Table 27.2.5 Breast milk pesticide concentrations reported in the United States*

from cohorts of women exposed to various hazards, for analysis of preclinical spontaneous abortions and menstrual cycle abnormalities. Endpoints for human epidemiologic studies that are currently considered relevant for assessing reproductive and developmental effects are summarized in Table 27.2.6, along with some endpoints that are being evaluated in more recent studies.

Application to clinical practice of the existing limited body of epidemiologic data should be carried out cautiously. Although relevance to humans is obviously not an issue, quality, in terms of classification of exposure, control of confounding bias, and occurrence of biases are important. Further, the direct relationship between the populations studied and the individual or group for whom the data are applied must also be considered before the results are interpreted by the practitioner.

Experimental studies in animals

As with other effects of environmental hazards, animal studies form a major portion of our knowledge base about which

---

Endpoints that are evidence of a human hazard
Couple specific
  Infertility: absence of pregnancies
  Subfertility: increased time to pregnancy or decreased standardized fertility ratio (lower birth rate)
Female specific
  Decreased reproductive life span: delay in puberty or premature menopause
  Menstrual dysfunction: anovulatory cycles or dysfunctional cycles
  Abnormal reproductive hormone concentrations
Male specific
  Abnormal semen analysis: decreased sperm count or abnormal sperm viability or morphology
  Abnormal reproductive hormone concentrations
Fetal/developmental
  Increased spontaneous abortion rate (clinical or preclinical pregnancies)
  Increased rate of fetal death
  Prematurity/growth retardation: smaller live births
  Increase in rate of birth defects or congenital anomalies
  Decreased age-specific function of offspring, e.g., childhood neuropsychologic performance
  Increased rate of childhood disease, e.g., cancer

Endpoints suggestive of human hazard
Couple specific
  Decreased coital frequency
  Increase in antisperm antibodies
  Abnormal postcoital test for sperm motility
Female specific
  Decreased libido
  Abnormal menstrual cycle lengths
  Changes in reproductive hormone levels within the normal ranges
Male specific
  Decreased libido
  Minor changes in sperm morphology or viability
  Decrease in sperm function on in vitro tests
  Changes in reproductive hormone levels within the normal ranges
Fetal/developmental
  Increased rate of disorders of pregnancy, e.g., pre-eclampsia

Table 27.2.6 Endpoints of human epidemiologic studies that support or suggest evidence of a reproductive or developmental toxicant

---

agents may be harmful to humans, at what doses, and by what mechanisms. Because of the difficulty of studying reproductive and developmental hazards in humans, animal experiments are crucial to our ability to predict effects.[32]

Unfortunately, there are serious limitations to animal experimentation in this arena as well. The most important issues are the following.

1. The timing of exposure relative to the timing of vulnerable reproductive or developmental processes is extremely important (see Table 27.2.4). Large doses of a toxicant could be harmless if delivered before or after a crucial event, like the formation of a body part or organ, whereas very small doses could be devastating if delivered at a crucial moment. For this reason, no single experiment can, in and of itself, exclude the possibility of a harmful effect for many agents that are short-lived in the body. Reproductive and developmental effects are likely to differ, depending on the timing of the exposure.

2. The central concept of a progressive, continuous dose–response relationship, which underlies all of toxicology (see Chapter 5), does not apply directly or simply to many situations in reproductive and developmental toxicology. Not only does timing alter responsiveness but the interactions between the parent and offspring also may alter dose–response relations. For example, at a very high dose, the primary effect of a toxicant may be maternal harm, with possible fetal death. At a lower dose, sublethal but possibly more relevant effects, such as teratogenesis, may be seen; further, only at doses below those that directly impair development of the fetus might effects such as mutagenesis or carcinogenesis become evident. Thus, interpretation of animal studies requires evaluation of different dose ranges, which cause different effects at different points in time.

3. Extrapolation from various animal species to humans presents challenges. In addition to the differences between species that affect all studies in toxicology (e.g., absorption, distribution, metabolism, elimination), reproductive patterns differ among the mammalian species; only primates simulate the human pattern very closely. For this reason, many relevant endpoints in animals, such as fetal resorptions, have no clear human counterpart, and many phases of human reproduction, such as menstrual cycle length, have no obvious animal analog in the species most available for study. Extrapolation of effects from one species to another, therefore, has limitations, despite being crucial for predicting human responses and protecting public health. A comparison between human and animal responses to pharmacologic agents (for which there are far better human data than for environmental agents) is instructive.[32] A total of 203 drugs were evaluated, of which 38 were known to cause birth defects or other developmental disturbances in humans, whereas 165 were deemed safe. Of the 38 harmful drugs, 37 had been proved to have positive responses in some experimental model. On the other hand, 118 of the 165 safe drugs also had positive responses in some animal experiments. The high negative predictive value of animal tests is demonstrated by the fact that of 48 negative results in animals all but one proved

safe. On the other hand, the tests have limited positive predictive value; of 155 drugs that tested positive, only 37 were truly teratogenic for humans.

This is not to imply that animals are uniformly, or even consistently, more sensitive to reproductive hazards than humans. For example, mice and rats proved very insensitive to the notorious drug thalidomide, although rabbits are sensitive to the agent. Conversely, the widely distributed polycyclic aromatic hydrocarbons are potent ovarian toxicants in many species, but humans appear relatively insensitive by comparison. Because of such interspecies and interindividual variability in sensitivity to toxicants, risk assessors often apply 'uncertainty factors' or 'safety factors' when extrapolating from animal data to humans. Frequently, two factors of 10 are applied, one to account for interindividual variability and the other for interspecies variability. For example, if the dose level at which no reproductive toxicity occurs in animals (no observed adverse effect level, NOAEL) for a compound is 5 mg/kg, the estimated human NOAEL for reproductive toxicity might be interpreted as 0.05 mg/kg. If animal studies do not provide a dose level at which no effects occur, an additional uncertainty factor of 10 is often applied to the lowest dose level studied (lowest observed adverse effect level, LOAEL).

4. Perhaps the most serious limitation of toxicology for the practitioner remains the dearth of testing altogether. Analyses performed for the State of California in its attempt to develop a prospective control policy for reproductive and developmental toxicants ('Proposition 65') revealed that only a small fraction of even the highest volume chemicals and other environmental pollutants had undergone sufficient toxicologic study to allow inference to human risk;[33,34] similar observations have more recently been made by the US Environmental Protection Agency's Endocrine Disrupters Screening and Testing Advisory Committee.[35]

Despite these problems, data from animal experiments remain central to the practitioner's task of clinical evaluation and prevention because they form the bulk of the available information. Because most practitioners have little experience in the design and conduct of such experiments, two issues should guide judgment when these elements are reviewed in relation to a particular case or problem. First, the study should be of reasonable design. Doses large enough to demonstrate an effect, as well as doses comparable to those humans could receive, should have been delivered at times that make sense relative to the endpoints evaluated, and the study's statistical power should be sufficient to reasonably exclude chance as an explanation for results. For developmental effects, greater weight should be given to studies in which the developmental endpoints are affected selectively.

Equally important in the interpretation of experimental animal data for evaluation of human risk is the particular endpoint chosen. As noted earlier, many consequences that may occur in animals have no obvious counterpart in humans, or none that can be easily interpreted. Table 27.2.7 lists those endpoints in animal studies that are

---

Endpoints considered to have predictive value for identifying human reproductive and developmental toxicants

Breeding studies
    Reduced mating indices (proportion of males or females exposed who mated)
    Reduced fertility indices (proportion of males or females exposed who succeeded in producing pregnancy or becoming pregnant)
    Reduced gestation index (proportion of pregnant females producing live offspring)
    Lower number of implantations
    Higher number of preimplantation and postimplantation losses
    Lower litter size at birth
    Reduced live birth index (proportion of all fetuses born live)
    Reduced survival indices (proportion live at one point in time after birth compared with an earlier time after birth)
    Decreased reproductive capacity of offspring (rebred for a second generation)
    Increased malformations or disease in offspring (see fetal studies, later)

Male studies
    Azoospermia
    Oligospermia
    Disruption of sperm motility or morphology

Female studies
    Estrous cycle disruption
    Decreased numbers of ovarian follicles or oocytes
    Decreased reproductive period (delay in puberty, early menopause)
    Uterine disruption histologically

Fetal studies
    Fetal deaths
    Fetal malformations

Endpoints suggestive of possible human reproductive or developmental toxicants

Breeding studies
    Decreased weight of offspring

Male/female studies
    Histologic change in gonads without germ cell loss
    Decreased gonadal, uterine or accessory organ weight
    Altered endocrine function

Fetal studies
    Growth retardation
    Developmental variations
    Functional deficits

Table 27.2.7 Endpoints of animal experiments with predictive value for human reproductive and developmental toxicity

considered highly predictive and those that are considered potentially predictive of human reproductive or developmental effects. These endpoints are listed according to whether they are detected in breeding studies (in which the male, female or both have been exposed), female exposure and female endpoints, or male exposure and male endpoint studies. Although there may be some specificity of the outcome of these studies for particular human effects, the reader is cautioned to remember that agents with reproductive or developmental toxicity may have different effects in humans than in animals and may, in fact, have more than one effect depending on dose and timing of exposure.

Other tools

Because the combined data from human and animal reproductive and developmental toxicity studies are so limited, the practitioner often must consider other forms of information in clinical decision making. In general, these sources involve drawing inferences about hazards for which there is some non-reproductive animal or in-vitro data suggesting a mechanism of action that may be relevant to a reproductive or developmental endpoint. For example, in-vitro data may suggest that a compound is highly mutagenic, which would make it a suspect reproductive or developmental hazard by inference. Similarly, a new compound with affinity to steroid receptors, either before or after metabolism, would merit suspicion even prior to any reproductive or developmental toxicity testing. Recognition of the usefulness of in-vitro data for screening large numbers of compounds for their potential to disrupt endocrine and reproductive function recently led the Endocrine Disrupters Screening and Testing Advisory Committee to recommend a battery of screening tests that include in-vitro assays of receptor binding, gene expression, and steroidogenesis.[35] Generic knowledge about the chemistry of a possible hazard, such as knowledge that it is highly fat soluble and of low molecular weight, hence highly likely to be transmitted to an infant in breast milk, also could be of interest.

CLASSIFICATION OF HUMAN DISORDERS OF REPRODUCTION AND DEVELOPMENT

The following sections discuss the established and suspected occupational and environmental causes of the major disturbances of reproduction and development. For each disorder, male and female exposure risks associated with the outcome are discussed separately. Also for each disorder, emphasis is placed on the timing and dose of exposure of the parent relative to that outcome, to the extent that it is known.

Infertility and subfertility

Male exposures

Several chemical and physical factors in widespread use have been determined to decrease male fecundity in humans through occupational or environmental exposure. These factors are summarized in Table 27.2.8.

Although the potential for radiation injury and medicinal use of drugs to cause reduced fecundity had been appreciated for years, the occurrence of epidemic infertility among men manufacturing DBCP in California in the early 1970s demonstrated that male reproductive effects might be the only manifestation of a workplace hazard. Although other clinical effects from the hazards listed in Table 27.2.8 may coexist with fertility loss, each agent has the potential to impair fecundity with no other overt evidence of toxicity.

Review of Table 27.2.8 also demonstrates that the exposures that have been demonstrated to impair male fecundity are relatively high levels associated with manufacturing or occupational use of the chemical. Low-dose exposures that may occur from environmental contact

Hazard	Setting of established risk
Metals	
Lead	Occupational uses
Pesticides	
DBCP	Chemical manufacture and pesticide application
EDB	Chemical manufacture
Chlordecone	Chemical manufacture
Solvents	
Ethylene glycol ethers	Occupational uses
Carbon disulfide	Occupational uses
2-bromopropane	Electronics industry
Pharmaceuticals	
Estrogens	Drug manufacture
Physical agents	
Ionizing radiation	Occupational accidents
Heat	Occupational exposures

DBCP = Dibromochloropropane; EDB = Ethylenedibromide.

Table 27.2.8 Hazards that have been determined to reduce human male fecundity

through food or water have not generally been shown to be significant. A report of declining sperm counts over the past half century in humans, which was later hypothesized to be caused by exposure to estrogenic pollutants at levels present in the general environment, has raised the possibility of more widespread effects of toxicants on male fecundity.[3,36] The study was criticized for its statistical methods and the fact that it combined sperm count data obtained in different laboratories using different methodologies.[6,37] More recent studies have demonstrated declining sperm counts in some parts of the world, but not others (reviewed by Daston et al.[6]), suggesting that environmental factors likely do affect sperm counts, but that there is not one overriding environmental factor affecting them worldwide.

Mechanisms for injury by each of the various hazards are incompletely known in general, and likely differ, but in each case, they are associated with a reduction in the numbers or quality, or both, of sperm produced. Lead appears to have effects on both the HPG endocrine axis and directly on the germinal epithelium of the testis.[38] DBCP and the structurally related solvent, 2-bromopropane, are directly toxic to spermatogonia, with secondary increases in the levels of the trophic hormones.[39-42] Complete destruction of the spermatogonia would be expected to result in irreversible azoospermia, and this has indeed been observed in the most severely intoxicated DBCP workers. Glycol ether solvents,[43,44] in contrast, appear to affect the more mature spermatids, and therefore the effects are reversible after exposure cessation. Heat[45] and ionizing radiation[46,47] also appear to have effects limited to spermatogenesis, with well-preserved HPG endocrine axis function. Exposure to estrogens in oral contraceptive manufacture[48] suppresses the HPG axis, resulting in suppression of gonadal function in male workers. Ethylene dibromide appears to affect semen quality in men primarily by actions downstream from the testis, in the accessory sex glands.[49,50]

The widely used aromatic solvents have received much attention as possible reproductive toxicants.[51] Two epidemiological studies suggest that the solvent toluene may act on the HPG axis in exposed workers to suppress LH and FSH secretion, with secondary testosterone suppression.[52,53] Acute controlled exposures to toluene had minimal effects on LH mean levels and no effect on FSH, suggesting that the occupational effects are related to chronic exposure.[54] The effects on the HPG axis observed in these studies were within the normal ranges, so perhaps it is not surprising that time-to-pregnancy in toluene-exposed workers did not differ from that of unexposed workers.[55] Occupational exposure to another aromatic solvent, styrene, also did not affect fecundity in workers in the reinforced plastics industry.[56]

Although the number of agents with well-characterized effects on male fecundity is small, there are several important hazards that are suspected to affect spermatogenesis based on animal experiments and some human reports. Important agents include organophosphate insecticides,[57,58] metals (boron, cadmium, mercury, chromium), anesthetic agents (nitrous oxide, halothane), the solvent n-hexane,[59] ethylene oxide,[60] chloroprene, and epichlorhydrin. Of note, a recent study found no effects of occupational metal exposure in the form of welding on male fecundity.[61] Based on animal studies, postspermatogenic effects on the excurrent ducts appear to be involved in the mechanisms by which agents like ethane dimethanesulfonate,[62] alpha-chlorohydrin, epichlorohydrin, methyl chloride, sulfasalazines, and the imidazoles interfere with male fecundity.[63] Many pharmacologic agents, such as adrenergic and cholinergic antagonists, interfere with the transport function of the male urogenital tract and, thus, have an indirect impact on fecundity.

Much recent work has focused on the effects of in-utero exposure to toxicants on the development of the reproductive system and subsequent reproductive function during adulthood. DES is currently the only agent proved to adversely affect human reproductive system development with in-utero exposure. However, animal studies demonstrate adverse effects of in-utero exposure to a variety of chemicals on male reproductive system development and adult function at lower doses than are toxic to the adult male. These include phthalate ester plasticizers,[64] dioxins,[65] the fungicide vinclozolin,[66] p,p'-DDE, a metabolite of the insecticide DDT,[66] and the insecticide methoxychlor.[67] Several of these compounds act as antiandrogens (p,p'-DDE, vinclozolin, phthalates), exerting significant adverse effects on accessory sex gland development.

Female exposure

Historically, the female reproductive system has been more difficult than the male reproductive system to investigate in humans because there is no counterpart single assay to semen analysis that can be obtained non-invasively. During the last 10 years, this imbalance has begun to be remedied through the use of new epidemiological techniques such as studies of time-to-pregnancy. Using this methodology, dental hygienists exposed to nitrous oxide were found to have a dose-related decrement in fecundity.[68] Since that study, nitrous oxide exposure and shift

Hazard	Setting of established risk
Solvents	
Toluene	Occupational uses
2-bromopropane	Electronics industry
Nitrous oxide	Hospital work
Antineoplastic drugs	Therapeutic uses
Physical agents	
Ionizing radiation	Occupational accidents
	Therapeutic uses
Shift work	Occupational exposures

Table 27.2.9 Hazards associated with reduced human female fecundity

work in midwives,[69] and exposure to formaldehyde,[70] toluene,[55] and high occupational energy expenditure (physical activity) combined with night work[71] were also associated with reduced fecundity in women. In contrast, exposures to antineoplastic drugs and anesthetic gases[71] were not found to reduce fecundity in hospital workers. Agents which have been associated with reduced female fecundity are summarized in Table 27.2.9.

In 1996, Korean researchers reported female reproductive dysfunction (amenorrhea, low estradiol and high FSH and LH levels) in electronics workers exposed to 2-bromopropane (2-BP), a solvent structurally related to DBCP, that had been introduced to replace ozone-depleting chlorofluorocarbons.[42] Subsequently, 2-BP was shown to reduce estrous cycling and fertility in rats.[72] In experimental animals, including primates, lead suppresses fecundity, probably by a combined effect on HPO axis endocrine function and direct ovarian or oocyte toxicity. However, this process has never been demonstrated in a human population. Similarly, animal data have suggested that ionizing radiation in high doses destroys primordial oocytes. Although premature menopause has been documented in women receiving therapeutic doses (i.e., >2.5 Gy), few studies have been conducted to explore the effect.[47]

The reproductive effects of many members of the large class of organochlorine chemicals have been extensively studied. PCBs and estrogenic organochlorine compounds appear capable of disrupting female fecundity based on endocrine effects on the timing of HPO axis hormonal function, but infertility, per se, has not been documented among women who have been exposed. Taiwanese and Japanese women who consumed cooking oil contaminated with PCBs and furans have more menstrual abnormalities, but not higher rates of infertility, than control women.[73] A recent large retrospective study of women exposed to PCBs, heavy metals, and other contaminants by consuming Great Lakes fish, found no effect on fecundity.[74] Limited data have linked exposure to dioxins in monkeys and in a nude-mouse model to endometriosis, a disease frequently associated with infertility in women.[75,76]

As in males, animal studies have demonstrated effects of in-utero exposures to toxicants on reproductive system function in adulthood in females as well. Gestational exposure to the insecticide methoxychlor[67] and to dioxin[77] are the most well-studied examples.

Spontaneous abortions

Female exposures

Despite the methodologic problems in studying spontaneous abortions (SAB), a variety of hazards and occupations have been associated with an increased risk for this complication in human populations. Although there remain uncertainties, the associations that are presently accepted as most likely to cause SAB are summarized in Table 27.2.10.

Healthcare workers have been extensively studied, and increase SAB risk has been associated with exposure to antineoplastic agents,[78] anesthetic gases, and ethylene oxide. Although the preponderance of evidence supports these associations, not all studies have yielded consistent results. One interpretation is that only high levels of exposure enhance the risk for SAB, with lesser exposures showing no effects. Ethylene oxide studies support this interpretation. Women who were engaged in sterilizing instruments using ethylene oxide during pregnancy had elevated risks of SAB in two studies,[79,80] whereas women who handled instruments after sterilization did not.[81] Similarly, exposure to anesthetic gases was significantly associated with SAB in older studies performed prior to use of scavenging equipment of waste gas, but not in more recent studies performed after the introduction of scavenging equipment. A recent study directly compared SAB risks in dental assistants exposed to the anesthetic gas nitrous oxide in the presence or absence of scavenging systems. Women in the unscavenged group had elevated risk, whereas the risk for the women in the scavenged group was not distinguishable from the unexposed women.[82] It is also possible that other exposures of these women, such as the physical and other stresses of their jobs, also may account for some differences among studies.

The data for metals are surprisingly limited given their ubiquitous nature in the workplace and environment. Many older descriptive studies documented that women exposed to lead at work experienced SABs frequently,

but classification of exposures was limited and confounded by other lead effects that were difficult to evaluate; studies of environmentally exposed women have not been impressive regarding the risk for spontaneous abortion. The findings regarding mercury, a reproductive toxicant in animals, have not been consistent. The study described above, that identified waste nitrous oxide as a cause of increased spontaneous abortion, did not find an elevated risk for mercury exposure in dental assistants.[82]

Extensive epidemiologic literature exists on solvents, with the weight of the evidence suggesting that occupational solvent exposure in general is associated with increased risk of spontaneous abortion.[83,84] Identifying which specific solvents or classes of solvents are the culprits has proven more difficult, with the possible exception of the ethylene glycol ethers, which are potent reproductive toxicants in animals, and the aromatic solvents toluene and benzene. Multiple studies of the semiconductor industry have all found excesses of spontaneous abortions among women exposed to ethylene glycol ethers in computer chip production.[85-88] However, these data must be interpreted cautiously because the solvent exposures in this setting are generally low and the environment is replete with other physical and chemical hazards that may confound the association of up to a doubled risk for first trimester spontaneous abortion. Studies of laboratory workers,[89] electronics workers,[90] and petrochemical workers[91] have implicated aromatic solvents as potential causes of SAB. The solvent perchloroethylene has also been associated with increased risk of SAB in a study of dry-cleaning workers.[92]

The associations between spontaneous fetal loss and both PCBs and pesticides are based on studies of women who have been very heavily exposed. Increased spontaneous abortion was one of the outcomes noted among women poisoned by PCBs in the infamous rice-oil contamination episodes in Japan and Taiwan (see Chapters 44 and 45). Fetal loss after pesticide poisoning has been widely described in case reports, but usually after the mother herself is poisoned. There are few human studies that incriminate either occupational or ambient environmental levels of exposures in humans for this endpoint, although many widely used compounds are suspected based on animal effects. A recent study in Turkey found that the rate of self-reported SAB increased with increasing serum levels of the fungicide hexachlorobenzene in women who had been intoxicated with the pesticide during the 1950s and in control women.[93] A relationship between occupational exposure to pesticides and SAB is also suggested by a recent case-control study which found that women who worked in agriculture or lived on farms were at increased risk for infertility.[94]

The data on physical activity are extensive and controversial. The evidence is strongest for shiftwork (night shifts or rotating shifts), which was associated with elevated risk of SAB in six of nine studies.[95] Some, but not all, studies have shown that heavy lifting, standing 8 or more hours per day, and physically heavy work increased the risk for spontaneous abortion.[96] In contrast, many studies of leisure time exercise did not find an increase in SAB rate,

Hazard	Setting of established risk
Medical hazards	
Antineoplastic drugs	Oncology nurses
Anesthetic gases	Operating room personnel
Nitrous oxide	Dental assistants
Ethylene oxide	Sterilizer operators
Metals	
Lead	Occupational uses
Solvents	
Ethylene glycol ethers	Semiconductor manufacture
Aromatic solvents	Occupational use
Mixed organic solvents	Occupational use
Other chemicals	
PCBs	Heavy food contamination
Pesticides	Accidental poisoning
Physical agents	
Heavy labor	
Shift work	

Table 27.2.10 Hazards associated with increased risk for spontaneous abortion or fetal death after female exposure

and some even found protective effects.[96] This apparent contradiction may be explained by various factors, including the much longer duration of occupational exposures compared to leisure exposures, and differences in the fitness levels and socioeconomic status of the women in the two kinds of studies. Few data exist on exposure to noise, vibration, heat, and cold and rates of SAB.

Several widespread physical factors are less likely to be important causes of spontaneous abortion at typical exposures found in occupational or environmental settings, including background ionizing radiation, non-ionizing radiation, and the use of video display terminals. While high doses of radiation during the first 8 weeks of pregnancy, as experienced by victims of the atomic bomb blast in Japan, clearly cause SAB, lower occupational and environmental doses do not.[97] Non-ionizing, electromagnetic radiation from occupational exposure to video display terminals[98,99] and magnetic resonance imaging machines,[7] and residence in houses with high current configurations (wire codes)[100] have not been found to increase risk of SAB. A few exposures, such as use of electric blankets during the first trimester of pregnancy and occupational exposure to microwave radiation, have been associated with increased SAB risk,[100,101] and reproductive effects of non-ionizing radiation remain under intensive investigation.

Psychological stress has received increasing attention as a cause of adverse pregnancy outcomes. In the only study to look at the effect of stress on spontaneous abortion rates, major negative life events were associated with increased risk of chromosomally normal SABs compared to chromosomally abnormal SABs.[102]

Male exposures

As noted earlier, there are some theoretical ways in which male exposure could enhance risk for spontaneous abortion. It is important to note that animal studies have demonstrated these effects, predominantly for those chemicals that produce mutations or other types of sperm and somatic cell DNA damage. Several studies have noted increased spontaneous abortions in spouses of men exposed to various suspect agents, such as lead, solvents,[103] and mercury. However, none has been confirmed or further elucidated mechanistically at this time. A recent large study of male welders did not confirm previous findings that this common paternal exposure causes SAB in wives of exposed men.[104]

Fetal growth retardation and prematurity

Female exposures

Given the rising awareness of the associations between these developmental endpoints and infant and childhood morbidity and mortality, there is great interest in identifying preventable environmental causes. Unfortunately, few have been found to date.

Lead is probably the best appreciated preventable exposure. Women exposed occupationally during gestation have had documented smaller and often premature offspring.[105] In addition, the same exposures are associated with various birth defects and childhood developmental abnormalities consistent with direct fetal exposure in utero and associated tissue disruption. Lead exposure in utero has also been associated with reduced postnatal growth rates.[106]

Children born to women exposed to PCBs during food-borne outbreaks also had smaller offspring, although the infants were not obviously premature. Other stigmata of exposure in these children included skin discoloration and other evidence of ectodermal dysplasia. Small dose-related effects on birth weight also have been documented in areas of heavier environmental exposure via contaminated fish.[107]

Another well-defined cause of fetal growth retardation is external (gamma or x-ray) ionizing radiation, which also is a cause of birth defects. The fetus is especially sensitive in the second part of the first trimester and early second trimester. Although the dose–response for this effect is not well established, it is a clear risk after accidental exposures in the range of 0.05–0.5 Gy (5–50 rad). What is less clear is the risk at levels just below this limit, which are most likely to be found in the workplace. Since 5 rads is the allowable dose per year for non-pregnant workers in many places, exposures in this range are not rare. Radionuclide exposures that might occur in the workplace or environmentally have not generally shown potential for causing growth retardation. Only radioactive iodide has been well established as a cause of fetal injury and then only after large (i.e., therapeutic) exposure doses.

Exposures among healthcare workers have recently been associated with low birth weight and prematurity. Midwives with nitrous oxide exposure during pregnancy were found to have higher rates of low birth weight.[69] Dental assistants exposed to the sterilant ethylene oxide had non-significantly elevated risk of preterm birth.[80]

Knowledge of the effects of alcohol on fetal growth has raised many concerns about solvent exposures, especially those occurring occupationally. Although these are biologically realistic concerns, data gathered to date suggest only an increased risk for maternal pre-eclampsia by an unknown mechanism.[108] In mothers who develop this complication, growth retardation and prematurity are probably more likely.

Similarly, knowledge of the risks to fetal growth of cigarette smoking in pregnancy have raised concerns about exposures to carbon monoxide and other asphyxiants. However, evidence of fetal injury, including growth retardation, has been shown only after episodes of maternal intoxication.

On the other hand, the very much lower levels of ambient oxygen associated with high altitude do result in babies of smaller weight, which is of unclear consequence. Further, fetal toxicity has been documented anecdotally in women who experience pressure changes associated with deep sea diving, and increased fetal mortality was demonstrated in a sheep model for maternal-fetal bends.[109]

As with spontaneous abortions, there is an extensive amount of literature evaluating physical activity late in pregnancy and the risk for delivery of small or premature babies. Taken together, the weight of the evidence does not support a large effect of physical activity on birth weight.[110-113] While physical activity per se does not appear to increase risk of prematurity,[112,113] high energy expenditure combined with high work speed,[111] prolonged standing, and long working hours[110] were more consistently associated with preterm birth.

Male exposures

There are no established factors that relate these outcomes to male exposures. There are suggestions that the spouses of male workers exposed to lead may have smaller offspring than others, but the possibility that these women were also exposed, either at the worksite or by indirect exposure via contaminated clothing, is difficult to exclude.

Birth defects

Female exposures

Possibly the most dreaded concern about environmental exposure is the likelihood of risk for birth defects. Thus far, only a few hazards have been associated definitively with birth defects. Known associations are summarized in Table 27.2.11.

Most of the well-described human environmental developmental toxicants have been recognized after an environmental disaster or epidemic, with presumably high levels of exposure to the causal agent, often with associated maternal morbidity as well. Although in each case there is incontrovertible evidence of effects on humans at high doses and a parallel animal model, the dose–response relationship at low exposure levels remains uncertain, which may be important in counseling pregnant women who seek advice after an exposure has occurred. Historic reports and isolated descriptions of babies born to women occupationally exposed to lead document frequent occurrences of various defects including CNS disorders and urorectal malformations similar to patterns seen in some experimental models of lead-induced teratogenesis.[114] The effects at doses that would be expected to occur in working women under current lead standards are less certain. At least one large study found an overall excess of minor anomalies of various kinds, whereas other studies have not identified such excesses.

Methyl mercury developmental toxicity was first described during the 1950s after residents around Minamata Bay in Japan consumed fish contaminated with methyl mercury that formed from industrial discharge of mercury into the water. Affected offspring had microcephaly, limb deformities, cerebral palsy, mental retardation, and other defects.[115] Similar outcomes have been seen following other mass poisoning episodes. During the past decade, concern has emerged that levels of methyl mercury found in large, predatory fish such as tuna may pose a developmental hazard in populations who regularly consume large quantities of fish. These studies have focused mainly on neurodevelopmental deficits that are not apparent at birth, and are discussed in the subsequent section.

Similar to the situation with methyl mercury, the risk of birth defects in humans following PCB exposure was first appreciated after two mass poisoning episodes in which cooking oil was contaminated with PCBs.[116] Also similar to the situation with methyl mercury, much attention has focused on possible developmental effects of lower levels of PCB exposure due to consumption of contaminated fish. These studies are also discussed below.

The well-known adverse developmental effects of ethanol and toluene abuse[117] have generated concern that occupational exposure to these and other solvents may also increase risk for birth defects. Thus far, occupational exposures to either of these solvents, which tend to be orders of magnitude lower than with abuse, have not been associated with birth defects. Although many other solvents are developmental toxicants in animals, few human studies have demonstrated increased rates of malformations with occupational solvent exposure. This is likely due both to the rarity of major malformations and to the relatively lower doses to which humans are exposed. Recently, a large multicenter European group reported increased risk for congenital malformations among women exposed to glycol ether solvents during the first trimester of pregnancy.[118] A significantly elevated odds ratio for major malformations and solvent exposure was reported in a meta-analysis of studies on solvent exposure.[83]

Over the past decade, much attention has been paid to the effects of low-level environmental exposures to agents that act by disrupting endocrine function on in-utero development. Compounds that act as antiandrogens or estrogen agonists have been shown to cause malformations of the urogenital system in laboratory animals, and the hypothesis has been put forward that in-utero exposure to environmental pollutants may be responsible for the increasing incidence of abnormalities of human male urogenital development, such as cryptorchidism and

Hazard	Identified defects	Reported setting
Metals		
Lead	Various patterns	Occupational, environmental
Methyl mercury	Psychomotor retardation (seizures, paresis, mental retardation)	Food-borne contamination
Solvents		
Toluene	Microcephaly, craniofacial anomalies	Glue sniffing
Ethanol	Microcephaly, craniofacial anomalies	Abuse
Glycol ethers	Various patterns	Occupational
Other chemicals		
PCBs	Ectodermal dysplasia (dermal pigmentation, dystrophic nails, mucosal dysplasia, mental retardation)	Food-borne contamination
Physical hazards		
Ionizing radiation	Microcephaly	Atomic blast
Heat	Neural tube defects	

Table 27.2.11 Hazards that cause developmental toxicity after maternal exposure

hypospadias.[4] Only a few epidemiological studies have been completed so far. One demonstrated an increased risk of cryptorchidism, but not hypospadias, in the sons of female gardeners.[119] An ecological study found high rates of surgery to correct cryptorchidism in municipalities with high rates of pesticide use.[120]

Male exposures

Female spouses of workers exposed to lead, solvents, and anesthetic gases have all been reported to have excesses of birth defects in isolated studies. However, none of these observations has been duplicated, nor has a clear model emerged, so at present there are no established or highly suspect male-mediated teratogenic hazards. However, it should be borne in mind that this possibility has not been readily evaluable in the environmental disaster situations in which most female-mediated causes were discovered because men and women were, in general, both exposed simultaneously.

Impaired postpartum development

Female exposures, including breast milk

Four important developmental toxicants are associated with delays in CNS development: lead,[121] PCBs,[116,122] methyl mercury,[115] and ionizing radiation.[97,123] Controversy exists over whether environmental exposures to the general population, such as from eating fish that contain low levels of PCBs or methyl mercury, pose a measurable risk to CNS development. Carefully conducted longitudinal studies suggest that subtle changes in outcomes such as intelligence quotient, learning, and behavior may be detectable following these exposures on a population basis, though not on an individual basis. Children whose mothers consumed Lake Michigan fish during pregnancy continued to have cognitive deficits through 11 years of age that correlated with cord blood PCB concentrations.[124,125] Data from studies of two populations of women that consumed ocean fish, containing background levels of methyl mercury, daily during pregnancy have produced conflicting results. Reports from the Faroe Islands study demonstrated subtle dose-related effects on motor function, language, and memory even at 7 years of age,[126,127] whereas the Seychelles Islands study did not report adverse effects through 5.5 years of age.[128] One caveat with these studies, as with any epidemiological study of environmental exposures, is that the measured exposure (PCB or mercury concentrations) represents one of numerous potential exposures. It is possible that the observed effects are due to an unmeasured exposure that is present in similar proportions to the measured exposure.

With ionizing radiation exposure, typically delivered between weeks 7–16 in utero, the cause of persistent deficits is likely inability to compensate for early diffuse injury. With chemical causes, the pathogenesis is more complicated because the toxicants themselves persist for long periods in the fetus and child and in the target CNS tissue, suggesting that ongoing neurologic injury may occur through early childhood. Of clear therapeutic importance in this regard is the possibility of further postpartum exposures to the causal agent. For lead, the source generally is the home environment, including drinking water, paint, and dust. For methyl mercury and PCBs, breast milk is also a source of concern, because each agent is well concentrated in milk. In fact, anecdotal evidence suggests that postpartum exposures to mercury and PCBs in breast milk alone may cause CNS deficits, but few cases have been available for study in which exposure to the mother began, de novo, postpartum.

Of interest, organic solvents, except in the setting of glue sniffing, have not been shown to cause chronic neurologic or developmental impairment in children when mothers have been exposed during pregnancy or breast feeding.[129] Evidence for other neurotoxicants, such as various pesticides, is too limited to judge risk.

Male exposures

Presently no model for male transmission of a developmental lesion has been demonstrated involving exposure prior to birth. Of course, the possibility of contamination of children from paternal work materials, such as indirect para-occupational exposures from clothing remains of concern for such hazards as lead and pesticides, and other toxicants.

Childhood cancer

Female exposures

Although in-utero exposure to carcinogenic or mutagenic agents may be substantial when pregnant women are occupationally or environmentally exposed, there is very little data documenting increased risks for childhood cancer as a result. The single situation for which transplacental carcinogenesis has been unequivocally proved is for DES. Taken medicinally by mouth, this agent confers a substantial risk of a rare vaginal adenocarcinoma in female offspring after puberty.[130] No counterpart has been shown in women exposed to estrogens at work, although this is clearly a concern.

Several studies also have demonstrated risk for childhood leukemia in offspring of women exposed medically to ionizing radiation. Surprisingly, however, follow-up studies of atomic blast victims have not demonstrated a high rate of leukemia in children exposed to very high doses of radiation in utero, although increased risks of several cancers have been reported among individuals exposed to high doses of radiation in utero or during childhood compared to individuals exposed as adults.[152]

Increased risk of childhood brain tumor has been associated with nitrosamine exposure due to maternal consumption of cured meats during pregnancy in some studies,[131,132] but not in others.[133] Elevated risk of brain tumors has also been observed in children whose mothers were exposed to farm animals during pregnancy.[134] Of note, two recent studies have *not* substantiated an association between maternal exposure to electromagnetic fields during gestation and childhood brain tumor risk.[135,136]

Beyond these examples, other evidences of childhood cancer risk from maternal exposures before or during pregnancy have not been demonstrated, although some epidemiologic studies have reported higher rates of solvent exposures during pregnancy in mothers of children with brain tumors and an association between agricultural work and childhood leukemia.[137]

Male exposures

The availability of cancer registries that provide information on parental occupations has led to the investigation of the relationship between paternal occupation and rates of the common childhood cancers. Employment in occupations with exposures to motor vehicle exhaust and pesticides have been linked to childhood leukemia, albeit inconsistently. A highly publicized study found a similar link with paternal exposure to ionizing radiation at an English nuclear power plant; however, subsequent studies have not substantiated this association, and it is at odds with the experience of atomic blast victims.[97]

In several studies, brain tumors have been associated with paternal work in agriculture and aircraft industries and with painting. A previous association between preconception paternal exposure to electromagnetic fields and childhood brain tumor risk has not been substantiated.[138] Somewhat more consistently, several studies have found metal work, especially auto body and auto mechanic work, and welding, to be more common among fathers of children with Wilms' tumor and other brain tumors.[138,139] Similar associations have been noted with retinoblastoma and hepatoblastoma.

At present, none of these associations can yet be considered causal. Nonetheless, some consistency in pattern and a biologic basis for plausibility make this a fruitful area for future preventive investigations and underscore the importance of male factors in healthful reproduction.

CLINICAL EVALUATION OF PATIENTS WITH REPRODUCTIVE AND DEVELOPMENTAL RISKS AND DISORDERS

There are four clinical contexts in which individuals or couples typically seek medical advice regarding environmental and occupational effects on reproduction or development, or in which the practitioner should consider the possibility of such effects. These are: (1) infertile couples, (2) couples or women planning pregnancy or who are newly conceiving, (3) pregnant women or their partners who have had an exposure to an environmental hazard of concern before or during pregnancy, and (4) couples or women who have experienced an adverse reproductive or developmental outcome.

For each of these clinical situations, the practitioner will want to consult additional sources of information about the possible reproductive hazards that are identified. These

include books[7,140-142] electronic databases,[143-145] and articles, including those referenced in this chapter.

Infertile couples

The standard approach to the evaluation and management of infertility involves a detailed medical and reproductive history of both parents and the use of laboratory tests, such as semen analysis and evaluation of female hormonal cycling and anatomy as appropriate to identify the physiologic basis for reproductive failure. Prior to identifying the apparent problem, it is difficult to evaluate or manipulate environmental or occupational factors meaningfully.

When the male partner has been demonstrated to have a low sperm count or otherwise abnormal sperm, it is appropriate to consider the common causes of testicular dysfunction and to review the male exposure history in detail, with emphasis on exposures within the past year, especially current ones. Any possible exposure to the hazards reviewed in Table 27.2.8 should form the basis for further consideration, irrespective of the possibility of another non-environmental risk. Furthermore, if no other risk factors are identified, suspect agents of interest, such as those mentioned in the section on hazards to male fertility, should be considered.

If an established or possible suspect exposure is identified, it is reasonable to attempt to further qualify, and if possible, quantify the intensity of exposure (e.g., by blood or urine testing where applicable) before establishing an intervention plan. The choice of how to proceed depends on this investigation, with the clinician establishing some estimate of the likelihood that the environmental factor is important based on the agent, the intensity of exposure, and the coexistence of other risks.

Having established some reasonable likelihood of effect, the next step is an intervention trial, removing the man from further exposure. Before such a plan is undertaken, at least two preintervention semen specimens should be obtained for analysis because of intrinsic variability. If azoospermia is demonstrated twice, a trial still is reasonable but the prognosis for recovery is poor, which should be considered in further planning; assessment of the role of prior exposures is a separate task, which is discussed later. After discussing the economic and personal ramifications with the patient, the therapeutic trial of removal should be continued for 6–12 months (2–5 cycles of spermatogenesis) before any judgment is made, with repeat semen analysis performed bimonthly. The choice as to whether to continue attempting pregnancy during this interval depends on other properties of the hazard, such as the potential for other male-mediated effects. In the case of lead, at least, deferral may be the conservative choice.

If there is no improvement after a year, a period of continued removal may be scientifically reasonable (depending on, for example, body burden and disposition) but, practically speaking, is far less likely to be successful. At this stage, other factors should be given greater weight and the likelihood of trial failure added to the therapeutic equation.

Infertility of the female is far less readily evaluated, in part because so little is known about factors that may cause it, and in part because there is no counterpart to semen for ready analysis. Further, not only are few factors studied but the physiologic basis for possible environmental effects remains unclear, such as whether hazards act only by disrupting ovulation or may cause loss of fecundity at a later stage, such as during tubal transport or implantation.

The approach for women, therefore, is based on a more global perspective of the situation. If other female or couple-specific factors are not identified, it is reasonable to consider removing the woman from any environmental exposure that has been strongly associated with adverse outcomes (Table 27.2.9); indeed, this would be appropriate advice for the fertile couple as well. For agents less strongly associated with reproductive risk, the choice is more difficult and depends on the availability of other therapeutic options and the informed choice of the woman. In every case, it is very important that the patient appreciate how little is known about occupational risks to female fecundity and, therefore, that removal from the workplace or affected environment has only a small likelihood of remedy. On the other hand, it is not unreasonable to emphasize the risks to the pregnancy or offspring if conception is successful within the exposed environment.

If a therapeutic trial of removal of the individual from the workplace is undertaken, the duration and endpoint should also be considered. If cycles are anovulatory, it is reasonable to wait for at least 6–12 months, because the preovulatory maturation of the corpus luteum takes about 3 months. If the trial is based on anovulation, direct or indirect hormonal evaluation is essential to establish the basis for success or failure. For women who are infertile despite normal ovulation, the only reasonable endpoint is conception.

Couples or women planning conception or who are newly pregnant

Advising prospective parents about environmental risks begins by establishing a detailed profile of non-environmental factors that may be relevant and understanding the concerns and questions of the couple or woman patient. Has there been a prior adverse outcome in the history of the patient or a coworker or colleague? Has there been a specific exposure or risk of concern? Are there hidden fears about pregnancy that may be focused on the environment or workplace? If the answer to any of these is yes, the specific issues and circumstances should be directly addressed and resolved.

If there is no extraordinary basis for concern, the general principles of preventive care are appropriate. Occupational, avocational, and other ambient environmental exposures should be noted, with special attention to factors summarized in Tables 27.2.10 and 27.2.11, and suspected agents described in the sections on effects of exposures during pregnancy. If there is potential exposure to any of these hazards, opportunities for prevention should be reviewed, which may be as simple as modifying a normal or chosen activity, such

as a hobby involving pesticides, metals, or solvents, or as complex as planning a job modification. The need for developing a detailed or expansive database is often inverse to the patient's willingness or ability to modify or discontinue exposure. For example, it may be reasonable to recommend that a pregnant woman suspend use of garden chemicals during the period of pregnancy and breast feeding without much investigation, whereas considerable information might be necessary before advising an agricultural worker or horticulturist in the same situation.

For exposures whose elimination or control is not easily accomplished, a more formal investigation including risk assessment and control strategy is indicated. Each potential exposure of interest and its dose should be identified to the greatest extent possible, because high or uncontrolled occupational exposures merit steps very different from trace environmental contamination, a point that is crucial for the patient to understand as well. Also, the potential for postpartum exposure to the agent in breast milk should be evaluated based on the principles listed earlier.

Next, the database for each hazard should be reviewed, starting with the discussions in the preceding sections. The clinician may need to consult more detailed sources referenced above. With that information in hand, physician and patient together can proceed to establish the third element of the equation, the options for control. In this setting, these options include not only the factors normally considered in occupational and environmental health practice, such as a job change or use of personal protective equipment, but also certain alternatives, such as considering bottle feeding rather than breast feeding, or a choice to modify exposures for a specific limited period of time. For each control strategy, the two important aspects of concern are the effectiveness of the approach to reduce exposure and the acceptability of the approach to the patient, employer, or both.

Once the relevant exposures are deciphered, databases obtained, and control options ranked, the choices for preventive management of a pregnancy may be undertaken. There are no definite rules, although elimination or strict and rigid control of the known and suspected factors is highly desirable. Similarly, because maternal illness itself is a risk factor for the fetus, occupational or environmental risks of sufficient magnitude to make the mother systemically ill, such as with solvent intoxication or metal fumes, are best completely avoided or rigidly controlled. Management of physical stresses, although included in the tables, are less straightforward because we presently lack adequate dose–response information; strenuous labor, cold, noise, vibration, and shift work are best curtailed, if possible, after the second trimester.

Beyond these basic principles, there is wide latitude for choice, depending on the preferences of the patient. Although it is appropriate for the clinician to be conservative and generally risk averse, strong or sweeping generalizations to avoid everything, which may be reasonable when advising about use of medications that are not important in the treatment of life-threatening disease, are not easily adopted to environmental and occupational factors. Rather, more hazard-specific and balanced information is likely to be of most use to the patient, although gathering this information is far more demanding of the time and thoughtfulness of the clinician.

Pregnant women who have been exposed to a hazard

Sometimes, women or couples consider the possibility of adverse effects from the environment *after* there has been an exposure of concern. Unlike the preventive setting described earlier, this situation demands a very specific and goal-directed role for the clinician, centered on a single specific task of risk assessment. At the outset, it must be appreciated that there will ultimately be only three options for subsequent action: reassurance, cessation of exposure, or recommendation for therapeutic termination of pregnancy.

After establishing the basis for concern, the first challenge is determining the risk of an adverse outcome based on knowledge of the exposure. As always, this begins with the determination of what actual hazard was involved, the timing of exposure with respect to the pregnancy, some estimate of dose, and a characterization of other factors that may modify risk. Almost invariably, these facts must be reconstructed from the patient's history; occasionally, a toxicant or its metabolites can be measured directly in the parent.

Once an exposure is verified and an estimate of dose and timing with respect to pregnancy is made, the possibility of a measurable effect on the pregnancy must be determined using the available databases. Given the gravity of the situation, it is advisable to obtain the most complete and current information available for that toxicant. The information in this text may serve as a guide, but it should be supplemented by the most current animal and human data available, except in a case of gross overexposure to a well-characterized hazard such as lead or methyl mercury.

If it appears possible that the exposure at its estimated dose may have an impact on the outcome of the pregnancy, then the timing of exposure should be assessed. Similarly, exposures that occur in the second trimester and beyond are unlikely to cause fetal malformations, although growth and development of the fetus remain at risk.

If after review of exposure, dose, and timing there is still basis for concern about the outcome of the pregnancy, then it becomes important to quantify the concern. For example, exposures that occur in the second trimester and beyond are unlikely to cause gross fetal malformations, although growth and development of the fetus remain at risk. Using conservative estimates from the available data, how likely is the outcome of concern to occur? For childhood cancers or fetal malformations, these are best expressed as straight probabilities of an all-or-nothing outcome. For developmental or growth effects, these possibilities may be conceptualized on a continuous scale from minimal to severe; however, inherent uncertainties often limit specific characterization.

As noted, the real challenge in this situation is that, at the end, the choices for action are extremely limited. Although there may be some small room for action, such as taking steps to hasten removal of a toxicant or reduce later exposures, the basic choice comes down to therapeutic abortion versus reassurance. Because there is almost always some degree of uncertainty regarding the risk of an adverse developmental outcome and because many people have very strong pre-existing feelings towards therapeutic abortion, the clinician in these situations must present choices in the clearest and most distinct way possible. It is best for the clinician to very clearly delineate the risks and associated uncertainties, to present pregnancy termination as an option in cases with very high risks of developmental effects, to provide reassurance for continuation of pregnancy in the majority of cases in which the risk is small, and, perhaps most importantly, to be supportive of what ultimately must be the patient's choice.

Patients who have had adverse outcomes

Evaluation of a couple who has experienced an adverse reproductive outcome in the past may be important for two reasons: (1) concern about future pregnancies; and (2) attribution for medical-legal purposes. When the medical-legal issues are involved, the approaches are similar to those used to evaluate any environmental or occupational injury or illness, using the principles outlined in Chapter 3 of this text and the data provided earlier, as supplemented by other detailed and updated sources of information.

Evaluation of a prior event for the purpose of subsequent reproductive planning requires a somewhat different formulation. In general, patients who have had a prior adverse outcome, such as a developmentally abnormal child, fear a recurrence based on some underlying, immutable risk factor such as genetics. Recognition of a preventable or remediable basis for prior risk could provide a basis for reassurance and optimism about future pregnancies. However, depending on the circumstances surrounding exposure with the previous pregnancy, issues of self-blame and regret may complicate the benefit of this message.

Although it is important to decipher the patient's actual agenda in seeking consultation around an adverse event, it is best to separate the past and the future. First, one can evaluate the likelihood that a defined exposure may have been responsible for a prior adverse outcome. Second, based on this calculation and all other available information about the couple, such as current environment, persistence of prior exposures in the body, and results of genetic or other evaluations that have occurred, the prospects for the future can be estimated. The possibility of an immutable risk needs to be specifically considered in the patient's interest, so that referral for genetic or other appropriate counseling can be undertaken.

After these steps are complete, the general preventive approach for future pregnancies can be laid out as described earlier, modified by the special knowledge about the past and the unique perspective the patient will undoubtedly have because of it. Importantly, the recommendation for the future may appear to contradict the verdict on the past, a paradox the clinician must anticipate and be prepared to explain. For example, a couple may have just lost a 2-year-old child to leukemia, which they might attribute to low-level ionizing radiation exposure to the father in the year prior to conception. Although support for this possibility in the current literature is small, advising the couple to reduce or eliminate such exposures prior to the next conception would not be unreasonably risk averse. In such a case, however, it would also be very important to be certain that an underlying heritable risk, such as Fanconi's syndrome, is not a factor.

PREVENTION OF REPRODUCTIVE AND DEVELOPMENTAL RISKS IN AN OCCUPATIONAL SETTING

One of the foremost challenges for corporations in the United States and other developed countries has been the development of reproductive and developmental health policies consistent with good preventive principles, existing exposure regulations, and the law. Although our knowledge of reproductive and developmental effects of hazards suggest possibly differential effects on each parent and fetus, United States law, subsequent to the case of Johnson Controls, requires women be given the right to work in any place where men may work, as long as they are adequately informed about possible fetal risks should they get pregnant. In other words, gender-specific administrative controls may not be used to prevent reproductive or developmental harm.[146] In this section, we outline some approaches that may accomplish the goals of preventive reproductive health while adhering to these social mandates (Fig. 27.2.3). There are four key components that we recommend for institution in all workplaces and other defined organizations.

1. *Primary control of hazards to levels safe for men and non-pregnant and pregnant women.* Although existing occupational standards have not, in general, required exposures be reduced to levels believed to minimize risks to reproduction and development, such levels are definable and achievable in many, if not most, workplaces by engineering controls; they may be achievable in all, with the addition of personal protective equipment and administrative controls.[147] The adherence to such strict standards, which are gender neutral and as safe as possible for reproduction and development, is the cornerstone of an effective plan.

2. *Hazard identification.* All agents known or suspected to present a risk for reproduction or development should be identified clearly as such and well marked within the work environment, so that inadvertent exposures become far less likely.

3. *Reproductive and developmental health education.* Because the existing standards have not been calculated to

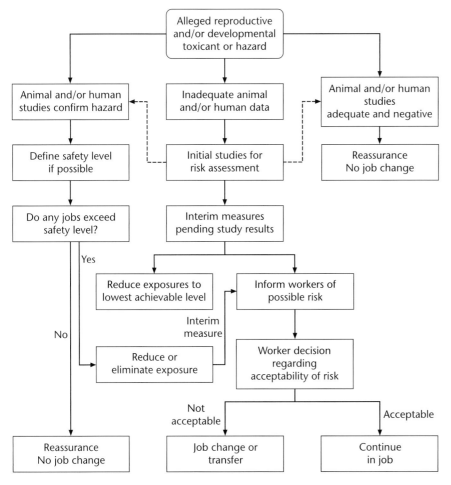

Figure 27.2.3: Proposed scheme for management of reproductive and developmental toxicants in the occupational setting. Many occupational exposures fall in the category identified as 'inadequate animal and/or human data'. In this case, it will be necessary to gather additional information as well as put interim measures in place to both inform and protect the workers. Exposures should be reduced to the lowest level achievable using engineering controls and personal protective equipment. The workers also must be informed that the exposure may pose a hazard to reproduction or development. In this setting, the workers should be allowed to determine whether or not the potential for effect is sufficient for concern. If not, the worker may reasonably decide to continue on the job. If there is concern, the worker should be provided with a choice of alternative jobs, without professional disincentives, that carry a minimal reproductive or development risk.

provide a margin of safety for reproductive and developmental health, and because the basis for personal decisions must be made with adequate information, broad-based and unbiased education of all potentially exposed workers of both sexes is crucial.

4. *A flexible work-modification plan.* Despite the institution of controls to minimize risk in a gender neutral fashion, some workers are likely to choose a greater level of risk aversion when planning pregnancy, after conception, or while breast feeding. There are many excellent medical reasons and other understandable personal reasons for this choice. Ideally, these choices should be available to individual employees of either sex without undue company scrutiny, interference, or disincentives, such as loss of wage, job security, or career path. Although the experience in most companies is that few employees actually use these options, their availability is widely appreciated by employees as a benefit. More important, such flexibility facilitates the practice of the highest quality preventive medicine.[148]

CONCLUSIONS

Physicians and other healthcare professionals are increasingly called on to counsel patients, unions, corporations, and public health agencies concerning the impact of occupational exposures on reproductive and developmental health. It is important to recognize certain fundamental principles in responding to these concerns: (1) the available data on human reproductive and developmental hazards are deficient; (2) because human data are lacking, it is essential to extrapolate information from animal data (this is also a central component of the protection of public reproductive and developmental health); (3) the criteria or stringency of data analysis for assigning causation are substantially different from those required for the protection of the public health; (4) our knowledge of reproductive and developmental toxicity is developing rapidly and is expected to change substantially in the future; and (5) finally, men and women must be treated equally so that reproductive and developmental health are protected.

References

1. Colborn T, vom Saal FS, Soto AM. Developmental effects of endocrine-disrupting chemicals in wildlife and humans. Environ Health Perspect 1993; 101:378–84.
2. Colborn T, Dumanoski D, Myers JP. Our stolen future: are we threatening our fertility, intelligence, and survival? A scientific detective story. New York: Dutton, 1996
3. Sharpe RM, Skakkebaek NE. Are oestrogens involved in falling sperm counts and disorders of the male reproductive tract? Lancet 1993; 341:1392–5.
4. Toppari J, Larsen JC, Christiansen P, et al. Male reproductive health and environmental xenoestrogens. Environ Health Perspect 1996; 104(Suppl 4):741–803.
5. Safe DH. Environmental and dietary estrogens and human health: is there a problem? Environ Health Perspect 1994; 103:346–51.
6. Daston GP, Gooch JW, Breslin WJ, et al. Environmental estrogens and reproductive health: a discussion of the human and environmental data. Reprod Toxicol 1997; 11:465–81.
7. Frazier LM, Hage ML, eds. Reproductive hazards of the workplace, 1st edn. New York: John Wiley and Sons, 1998.
8. Abma J, Chandra A, Mosher W, Peterson L, Piccinino L. Fertility, family planning and women's health: new data from the 1995 National Survey of Family Growth. National Center for Health Statistics. Vital Health Stats 1997; 23.
9. Ford WC, North K, Taylor H, Farrow A, Hull MG, Golding J. Increasing paternal age is associated with delayed conception in a large population of fertile couples: evidence for declining fecundity in older men. The ALSPAC Study Team (Avon Longitudinal Study of Pregnancy and Childhood). Hum Reprod 2000; 15:1703–8.
10. Jensen TK, Henriksen TB, Hjollund NH, et al. Adult and prenatal exposures to tobacco smoke as risk indicators of fertility among 430 Danish couples. Am J Epidemiol 1998; 148:992–7.
11. Alderete E, Eskenazi B, Sholtz R. Effect of cigarette smoking and coffee drinking on time to conception. Epidemiology 1995; 6:403–8.
12. Jensen TK, Hjollund NH, Henriksen TB, et al. Does moderate alcohol consumption affect fertility? Follow up study among couples planning first pregnancy. Br Med J 1998; 317:505–10.
13. Hakim RB, Gray RH, Zacur H. Alcohol and caffeine consumption and decreased fertility. Fertil Steril 1998; 70:632–7.
14. Jensen TK, Henriksen TB, Hjollund NH, et al. Caffeine intake and fecundability: a follow-up study among 430 Danish couples planning their first pregnancy. Reprod Toxicol 1998; 12:289–95.
15. Wilcox AJ, Weinberg CR, O'Connor JF, et al. Incidence of early loss of pregnancy. N Engl J Med 1988; 319:189–94.
16. Fan XG, Zheng ZQ. A study of early pregnancy factor activity in preimplantation. Am J Reprod Immunol 1997; 37:359–64.
17. Mesrogli M, Dieterle S. Embryonic losses after in vitro fertilization and embryo transfer. Acta Obstet Gynecol Scand 1993; 72:36–8.
18. Ness RB, Grisso JA, Hirschinger N, et al. Cocaine and tobacco use and the risk of spontaneous abortion. N Engl J Med 1999; 340:333–9.
19. Chatenoud L, Parazzini F, di Cintio E, et al. Paternal and maternal smoking habits before conception and during the first trimester: relation to spontaneous abortion. Ann Epidemiol 1998; 8:520–6.
20. Abel EL. Maternal alcohol consumption and spontaneous abortion. Alcohol Alcoholism 1997; 32:211–9.
21. Windham GC, Von Behren J, Fenster L, Schaefer C, Swan SH. Moderate maternal alcohol consumption and risk of spontaneous abortion. Epidemiology 1997; 8:509–14.
22. Saling E. Basic aspects of prematurity prevention and results achieved by a suitable, simple program. J Perinatal Med 1998; 26:466–8.
23. MMWR. Use of folic acid-containing supplements among women of childbearing age –United States, 1997. MMWR 1997; 47:131–4.
24. Koren G, Pastuszak A, Ito S. Drugs in pregnancy. N Engl J Med 1998; 338:1128–37.
25. Evenson D, Jost L. Sperm chromatin structure assay: DNA denaturability. Methods Cell Biol 1994; 42(B):159–76.
26. Bonde JPE, Ernst E, Jensen TK, et al. Relation between semen quality and fertility: a population-based study of 430 first-pregnancy planners. Lancet 1998; 352:1172–7.
27. Rutledge JC, Generoso WM. Malformations in pregastrulation developmental toxicology. In: Korach KS, ed. Reproductive and developmental toxicology. New York: Marcel Dekker, 1998;73–86.
28. Welsch F, Stedman DB. Inhibition of intercellular communication between normal human embryonal palatal mesenchyme cells by teratogenic glycol ethers. Environ Health Perspect 1984; 57:125–33.
29. Wolff MS. Occupationally derived chemicals in breast milk. Am J Ind Med 1983; 4:259–81.
30. Mattison DR, Wohlleb J, To T, et al. Pesticide concentrations in Arkansas breast milk. J Ark Med Soc 1992; 88:553–7.
31. Jensen AA, Slovak SA. Chemical contaminants in human milk. Boca Raton: CRC Press, 1991.

32. Jelovsek FR, Mattison DR, Chen J. Prediction of risk for human development toxicity: how important are animal studies? Obstet Gynecol 1989; 74:624–36.

33. Mattison DR, Working PK, Blazak WF, et al. Criteria for identifying and listing substances known to cause reproductive toxicity under California's Proposition 65. Reprod Toxicol 1990; 4:163–75.

34. Mattison DR, Hanson J, Kochhar DM, Rao KS. Criteria for identifying and listing substances known to cause developmental toxicity under California's Proposition 65. Reprod Toxicol 1989; 3:3.

35. Gray LEJ. Tiered screening and testing strategy for xenoestrogens and antiandrogens. Toxicol Lett 1998; 102-103:677–80.

36. Carlsen E, Giwercman A, Keiding N, Skakkebaek NE. Evidence for decreasing quality of semen during past 50 years. Br Med J 1992; 305:609–13.

37. Bromwich P, Cohen J, Stewart I, Walker A. Decline in sperm counts: an artefact of changed reference range of 'normal'? Br Med J 1994; 309:19–22.

38. Apostoli P, Kiss P, Porru S, Bonde JP, Vanhoorne M. Male reproductive toxicity of lead in animals and humans. ASCLEPIOS Study Group. Occup Environ Med 1998; 55:364–74.

39. Whorton D, Krauss RM, Marshall S, Milby TH. Infertility in male pesticide workers. Lancet 1977; 2:1259–61.

40. Whorton MD, Foliart DE. Mutagenicity, carcinogenicity, and reproductive effects of dibromochloropropane (DBCP). Mutat Res 1983; 123:13–30.

41. Potashnik G, Porath A. Dibromochloropropane (DBCP): a 17-year reassessment of testicular function and reproductive performance. J Occup Environ Med 1995; 37:1287–92.

42. Kim Y, Jung K, Hwang T, et al. Hematopoietic and reproductive hazards of Korean electronic workers exposed to solvents containing 2-bromopropane. Scand J Work Environ Health 1996; 22:387–91.

43. Welch LS, Schrader SM, Turner TW, Cullen MR. Effects of exposure to ethylene glycol ethers on shipyard painters: II. Male reproduction. Am J Ind Med 1988; 14:509–26.

44. Gray TJB, Moss EJ, Creasy DM, Gangolli SD. Studies on the toxicity of some glycol ethers and alkoxyacetic acids in primary testicular cell cultures. Toxicol Appl Pharmacol 1985; 79:490–501.

45. Mieusset R, Bujan L. Testicular heating and its possible contributions to male infertility: a review. Int J Androl 1995; 18:169–84.

46. Jordan S, Hasegawa CM, Keehn RJ. Testicular changes in atomic bomb survivors. Arch Pathol 1966; 82:542–54.

47. Ash P. The influence of radiation on fertility in man. Br J Radiol 1980; 53:271.

48. Harrington JM, Stein GF, Rivera RO, de Morales AV. The occupational hazards of formulating oral contraceptives: a survey of plant employees. Arch Environ Health 1978; 33:12–5.

49. Schrader SM, Turner TW, Ratcliffe JM. The effects of ethylene dibromide on semen quality: a comparison of short-term and chronic exposure. Reprod Toxicol 1988; 2:191–8.

50. Ratcliffe JM, Schraeder SM, Steenland K, Clapp DE, Turner T, Hornung RW. Semen quality in papaya workers with long-term exposure to ethylene dibromide. Br J Ind Med 1987; 44:317–26.

51. De Celis R, Feria-Velasco A, González-Unzaga M, Torres-Calleja J, Pedrón-Nuevo N. Semen quality of workers occupationally exposed to hydrocarbons. Fertil Steril 2000; 73:221–8.

52. Svensson B-G, Nise G, Erfurth E-M, Nilsson A, Skerfving S. Hormone status in occupational toluene exposure. Am J Ind Med 1992; 22:99–107.

53. Svensson B-G, Nise G, Erfurth EM, Olsson, H. Neuroendocrine effects in printing workers exposed to toluene. Br J Ind Med 1992; 49:402–8.

54. Luderer U, Morgan MS, Brodkin CA, Kalman DA, Faustman EM. Reproductive endocrine effects of acute exposure to toluene in men and women. Occup Environ Med 1999; 56:657–66.

55. Plenge-Bönig A, Karmaus W. Exposure to toluene in the printing industry is associated with subfecundity in women but not in men. Occup Environ Med 1998; 56:443–8.

56. Kolstad HA, Bisanti L, Roeleveld N, Baldi R, Bonde JP, Joffe M. Time to pregnancy among male workers of the reinforced plastics industry in Denmark, Italy and The Netherlands. Scand J Work Environ Health 2000; 26:353–8.

57. Padungtod C, Lasley BT, Christiani DC, Ryan LM, Xu X. Reproductive hormone profiles among pesticide factory workers. J Occup Environ Med 1998; 40:1038–47.

58. Padungtod C, Savitz DA, Overstreet JW, Christiani DC, Ryan LM, Xu X. Occupational pesticide exposure and semen quality among Chinese workers. J Occup Environ Med 2000; 42:982–92.

59. Boekelheide K. 2,5-Hexanedione alters microtubule assembly: I. Testicular atrophy, but not nervous system toxicity correlates with enhanced tubulin polymerization. Toxicol Appl Pharmacol 1987; 88:370–82.

60. Mori K, Kaido M, Fujishiro K, et al. Dose dependent effects of inhaled ethylene oxide on spermatogenesis in rats. Br J Ind Med 1991; 48:270–4.

61. Hjollund NHI, Bonde JPE, Jensen TK, et al. A follow-up study of male exposure to welding and time to pregnancy. Reprod Toxicol 1998; 12:29–37.

62. Klinefelter GR, Laskey JW, Perreault SD, et al. The ethane dimethylsulfonate-induced decrease in the fertilizing ability of cauda epididymal sperm is independent of the testis. J Androl 1994; 15:318–27.

63. Klinefelter GR, Hess RA. Toxicology of male excurrent ducts and accessory sex glands. In: Korach KS, ed. Reproductive and developmental toxicology. New York: Marcel Dekker, 1998;553–91.

64. Mylchreest E, Sar M, Cattley RC, Foster PM. Disruption of androgen-regulated male reproductive development by di(n-butyl) phthalate during late gestation in rats is different from flutamide. Toxicol Appl Pharmacol 1999; 156:81–95.

65. Gray LE, Kelce WR, Monosson E, Ostby JS, Birnbaum LS. Exposure to TCDD during development permanently alters reproductive function in male long Evans rats and hamsters: reduced ejaculated and epididymal sperm numbers and sex accessory gland weights in offspring with normal androgenic status. Toxicol Appl Pharmacol 1995; 131:108–18.

66. Kelce WR, Lambright CR, Gray LE Jr, Roberts KP. Vinclozolin and p,p'-DDE alter androgen-dependent gene expression: in vivo confirmation of an androgen receptor-mediated mechanism. Toxicol Appl Pharmacol 1997; 142:192–200.

67. Gray LE Jr, Ostby J, Ferrell J, et al. A dose–response analysis of methoxychlor-induced alterations of reproductive development and function in the rat. Fundamental Appl Toxicol 1989; 12:92–108.

68. Rowland AS, Baird DD, Weinberg CR, Shore DL, Shy CM, Wilcox AJ. Reduced fertility among women employed as dental assistants exposed to high levels of nitrous oxide. N Engl J Med 1992; 327:993–7.

69. Bodin L, Axelsson G, Ahlborg GJ. The association of shift work and nitrous oxide exposure in pregnancy with birth weight and gestational age. Epidemiology 1999; 10:429–36.

70. Taskinen HK, Kyyrönen P, Sallmén M, et al. Reduced fertility among women wood workers exposed to formaldehyde. Am J Ind Med 1999; 36:206–12.

71. Zielhuis G, Peelen SJM, Florack EIM, Roeleveld N. Hospital work and fecundability. Scand J Work Environ Health 1999; 25(Suppl 1):47–8.

72. Lim CH, Maeng SH, Lee JY, et al. Effects of 2-bromopropane on the female reproductive function in Sprague-Dawley rats. Ind Health 1997; 35:278–84.

73. Yu M-L, Guo YL, Hsu C-C, Rogan WJ. Menstruation and reproduction in women with polychlorinated biphenyl (PCB) poisoning: long-term follow-up interviews of the women

from the Taiwan Yucheng Cohort. Int J Epidemiol 2000; 29:672–7.

74. Buck GM, Sever LE, Mendola P, Zielezny M, Vena JE. Consumption of contaminated sport fish from Lake Ontario and time-to-pregnancy. Am J Epidemiol 1997; 146:949–54.

75. Rier SE, Martin DC, Bowman RE, Becker JL. Immunoresponsiveness in endometriosis: implications of estrogenic toxicants. Environ Health Perspect 1995; 103(Suppl 7):151–6.

76. Bruner-Tran KL, Rier SE, Eisenberg E, Osteen KG. The potential role of environmental toxins in the pathophysiology of endometriosis. Gynecol Obstet Invest 1999; 48(Suppl 1):45–56.

77. Gray LE, Ostby JS. In utero 2,3,7,8-tetrachlorodibenzo-p-dioxin (TCDD) alters reproductive morphology and function in female rat offspring. Toxicol Appl Pharmacol 1995; 133:285–94.

78. Selvan SG, Lindbohm M-L, Hornung RW, Hemminki K. A study of occupational exposure to antineoplastic drugs and fetal loss in nurses. N Engl J Med 1985; 313:1173–8.

79. Hemminki K, Mutanen P, Saloniemi I, Niemi ML, Vaino H. Spontaneous abortions in hospital staff engaged in sterilising instruments with chemical agents. Br Med J 1982; 285:1461–3.

80. Rowland AS, Baird DD, Shore DL, Darden B, Wilcox AJ. Ethylene oxide exposure may increase the risk of spontaneous abortion, preterm birth, and postterm birth. Epidemiology 1996; 7:363–8.

81. Hemminki K, Kyyronen P, Lindbohm M. Spontaneous abortions and malformations in the offspring of nurses exposed to anesthetic gases, cytostatic drugs, and other potential hazards in hospitals, based on registered information of outcome. J Epidemiol Commun Health 1985; 39:141–7.

82. Rowland AS, Baird DD, Shore DL, Weinberg CR, Savitz DA, Wilcox AJ. Nitrous oxide and spontaneous abortion in female dental assistants. Am J Epidemiol 1995; 141:531–8.

83. McMartin KI, Chu M, Kopecky E, Einarson TR, Koren G. Pregnancy outcome following maternal organic solvent exposure: a meta-analysis of epidemiologic studies. Am J Ind Med 1998; 34:288–92.

84. Gold EB, Tomich E. Occupational hazards to fertility and pregnancy outcome. Occup Med State Art Rev 1994; 9:435–69.

85. Pastides H, Calabrese EJ, Hosmer DW Jr, Harris DR Jr. Spontaneous abortion and general illness symptoms among semiconductor manufacturers. J Occup Med 1988; 30:543–51.

86. Huel G, Mergler D, Bowler R. Evidence for adverse reproductive outcomes among women microelectronics assembly workers. Br J Ind Med 1990; 47:400–4.

87. Lipscomb JA, Fenster L, Wrensch M, Shusterman D, Swan S. Pregnancy outcomes in women potentially exposed to occupational solvents and women working in the electronics industry. J Occup Med 1991; 33:597–604.

88. Schenker MB, Gold EB, Beaumont JJ, et al. Association of spontaneous abortion and other reproductive effects with work in the semiconductor industry. Am J Ind Med 1995; 28:639–59.

89. Taskinen H, Kyyronen P, Hemminki K, Hoikkala M, Lajunen K, Lindbohm M-L. Laboratory work and pregnancy outcome. J Occup Med 1994; 36:311–9.

90. Ng TP, Foo SC, Yoong T. Risk of spontaneous abortion in workers exposed to toluene. Br J Ind Med 1992; 49:804–8.

91. Xu X, Cho S-I, Sammel M, et al. Association of petrochemical exposure with spontaneous abortion. Occup Environ Med 1998; 55:31–6.

92. Doyle P, Roman E, Beral V, Brookes M. Spontaneous abortion in dry cleaning workers potentially exposed to perchloroethylene. Occup Environ Med 1997; 54:848–53.

93. Jarrell J, Gocmen A, Foster W, Brant R, Chan S, Sevcik M. Evaluation of reproductive outcomes in women inadvertently exposed to hexachlorobenzene in Southeastern Turkey in the 1950s. Reprod Toxicol 1998; 12:469–76.

94. Fuortes L, Clark MK, Kirchner HL, Smith EM. Association between female infertility and agricultural history. Am J Ind Med 1997; 31:445–51.

95. Nurminen T. Shift work and reproductive health. Scand J Work Environ Health 1998; 24(Suppl 3):28–34.

96. Nesbitt T. Ergonomic exposures. In: Frazier LM, Hage, ML, eds. Reproductive hazards of the workplace. New York: John Wiley and Sons, 1998;431–62.

97. Suruda AJ. Radiation. In: Frazier LM, Hage, ML, eds. Reproductive hazards of the workplace. New York: John Wiley and Sons, 1998;367–90.

98. Schnorr TM, Grajewski BA, Thun MJ, et al. Video display terminals and the risk of spontaneous abortion. N Engl J Med 1991; 324:727–33.

99. Delpizzo V. Epidemiological studies of work with video display terminals and adverse pregnancy outcomes (1984–1992). Am J Ind Med 1994; 26:465–80.

100. Belanger K, Leaderer B, Hellenbrand K, et al. Spontaneous abortion and exposure to electric blankets and heated water beds. Epidemiology 1998; 9:36–42.

101. Ouellet-Hellstrom R, Stewart WF. Miscarriages among female physical therapists who report using radio- and microwave-frequency electromagnetic radiation. Am J Epidemiol 1993; 138:775–86.

102. Neugebauer R, Kline J, Stein Z, Shrout P, Warburton D, Susser M. Association of stressful life events with chromosomally normal spontaneous abortion. Am J Epidemiol 1996; 143:588–96.

103. Taskinen H, Anttila A, Lindbohm M-L, Salimen M, Himminki K. Spontaneous abortions and congenital malformations among the wives of men occupationally exposed to organic solvents. Scand J Work Environ Health 1989; 15:354–62.

104. Hjollund NHI, Bonde JPE, Hansen KS. Male-mediated risk of spontaneous abortion with reference to stainless steel welding. Scand J Work Environ Health 1995; 21:272–6.

105. Sokas RK. Metals. In: Frazier LM, Hage, ML, eds. Reproductive hazards of the workplace. New York: John Wiley and Sons, 1998;123–61.

106. Shukla R, Bornschein R, Dietrich K, et al. Fetal and infant lead exposure: effects on growth in stature. Pediatrics 1989; 84:604–12.

107. Jacobson JL, Jacobson SW, Humphrey HE. Effects of exposure to PCBs and related compounds on growth and activity in children. Neurotoxicol Teratol 1990; 12:319–26.

108. Eskenazi B, Bracken MB, Holford TR, Grady J. Exposure to organic solvents and hypertensive disorders of pregnancy. Am J Ind Med 1988; 14: 177–88.

109. Mitchell LV, DeHart RL. Temperature, hypoxia, and atmospheric pressure. In: Frazier LM, Hage, ML, eds. Reproductive hazards of the workplace. New York: John Wiley and Sons, 1998;415–28.

110. Berkowitz GS. Employment-related physical activity and pregnancy outcome. J Am Med Women Assoc 1995; 50:16–9.

111. Florack EIM, Pellegrino AEMC, Zielhuis GA, Rolland R. Influence of occupational physical activity on pregnancy duration and birthweight. Scand J Work Environ Health 1995; 21:199–207.

112. Alderman BW, Zhao H, Holt VL, Watts DH, Beresford SAA. Maternal physical activity in pregnancy and infant size for gestational age. Ann Epidemiol 1998; 8:513–9.

113. Magann EF, Evans SF, Newnham JP. Employment, exertion, and pregnancy outcome: assessment by kilocalories expended each day. Am J Obstet Gynecol 1996; 175:182–7.

114. Gerber G, Leonard A, Jacquet P. Toxicity, mutagenicity and teratogenicity of lead. Mutat Res 1980; 76:115–41.

115. Burbacher T, Rodier R, Weiss B. Methyl mercury developmental neurotoxicity: a comparison of effects in humans and animals. Neurotoxicol Teratol 1990; 12:191–202.

116. Chen YCJ, Guo YO, Hsu CC, Rogan WJ. Cognitive development of Uu-Chen (oil disease) children prenatally exposed to heat degraded PCBs. JAMA 1992; 268:3213–8.

117. Wilkins-Haug L, Gabow P. Toluene abuse during pregnancy; obstetric complications and perinatal outcomes. Obstet Gynecol 1991; 4:504–9.

118. Cordier S, Bergeret A, Goujard J, et al. Congenital malformations and maternal occupational exposure to glycol ethers. Epidemiology 1997; 8:355–63.

119. Weidner ID, Moller H, Jensen TK, Skakkebaek NE. Cryptorchidism and hypospadias in sons of gardeners and farmers. Environ Health Perspect 1998; 106:793–6.

120. García-Rodríguez J, García-Martín M, Nogueras-Ocaña M, et al. Exposure to pesticides and cryptorchidism: geographical evidence of a possible association. Environ Health Perspect 1996; 104:1090–5.

121. Bellinger D, Needleman H. Prenatal and early postnatal exposure to lead: developmental effects, correlates, and implications. Int J Mental Health 1985; 14:78–111.

122. Yu M-L, Hsu C-C, Gladen BC, Rogan WJ. In utero PCB/PCDF exposure: relation of developmental delay to dysmorphology and dose. Neurotoxicol Teratol 1991; 13:195–202.

123. Wood JW, Johnson KG, Omri Y. In utero exposure to Hiroshima atomic bomb. An evaluation of head size and mental retardation: twenty years later. Pediatrics 1967; 39:385–92.

124. Jacobson JL, Jacobson SW, Humphrey HE. Effects of in utero exposure to polychlorinated biphenyls and related contaminants on cognitive functioning in young children. J Pediatrics 1990; 116:38–45.

125. Jacobson JL, Jacobson SW. Evidence for PCBs as neurodevelopmental toxicants in humans. Neurotoxicology 1997; 18:415–24.

126. Grandjean P, Weihe P, White R, Debes F. Cognitive performance of children prenatally exposed to 'safe' levels of methylmercury. Environ Res 1998; 77:165–72.

127. Grandjean P, Budtz-Jorgensen E, White RF, et al. Methylmercury exposure biomarkers as indicators of neurotoxicity in children aged 7 years. Am J Epidemiol 1999; 150:301–5.

128. Davidson PW, Myers GJ, Cox C, et al. Effects of prenatal and postnatal methylmercury exposure from fish consumption on neurodevelopment: outcomes at 66 months of age in the Seychelles child development study. JAMA 1998; 280:701–7.

129. Eskenazi B, Gaylord L, Bracken MB, Brown D. In utero exposure to organic solvents and human neurodevelopment. Develop Med Child Neurol 1988; 30:492–501.

130. Herbst AL, Ulfelder H, Poskanzer DC. Adenocarcinoma of the vagina: association of maternal stilbestrol therapy with tumor appearance in young women. N Engl J Med 1971; 284:878–81.

131. Bunin GR, Kuijten RR, Boesel CP, Buckley JD, Meadows AT. Maternal diet and risk of astrocytic glioma in children: a report from the childrens cancer group (United States and Canada). Cancer Causes Control 1994; 5:177–87.

132. Preston-Martin S, Pogoda JM, Mueller BA, Holly EA, Lijinsky W, Davis RL. Maternal consumption of cured meats and vitamins in relation to pediatric brain tumors. Cancer Epidemiol Biomark Prev 1996; 5:599–605.

133. Lubin F, Farbstein H, Chetrit A, et al. The role of nutritional habits during gestation and child life in pediatric brain tumor etiology. Int J Cancer 2000; 86:139–43.

134. Holly EA, Bracci PM, Mueller BA, Preston-Martin S. Farm and animal exposures and pediatric brain tumors: results from the United States West Coast Childhood Brain Tumor Study. Cancer Epidemiol Biomark Prev 1998; 7:797–802.

135. Preston-Martin S, Gurney JG, Pogoda JM, Holly EA, Mueller BA. Brain tumor risk in children in relation to use of electric blankets and water bed heaters. Results from the United States West Coast Childhood Brain Tumor Study. Am J Epidemiol 1996; 143:1116–22.

136. Gurney JG, Mueller BA, Davis S, Schwartz SM, Stevens RG, Kopecky KJ. Childhood brain tumor occurrence in relation to residential power line configurations, electric heating sources, and electric appliance use. Am J Epidemiol 1996; 143:120–28.

137. Savitz, DA, Chen J. Prenatal occupation and childhood cancer: review of epidemiologic studies. Environ Health Perspect 1990; 88:325–37.

138. Wilkins JR, Wellage LC. Brain tumor risk in offspring of men occupationally exposed to electric and magnetic fields. Scand J Work Environ Health 1996; 22:339–45.

139. Olshan AF, Breslow NE, Daling JR, et al. Wilms' tumor and paternal occupation. Cancer Res 1990; 50:3212–7.

140. Paul M, ed. Occupational and environmental reproductive hazards. Baltimore: Williams & Wilkins, 1993.

141. Korach KS, ed. Reproductive and developmental toxicology. New York: Marcel Dekker, 1998.

142. Schettler T, Solomon G. Generations at risk: reproductive health and the environment. Cambridge: MIT Press, 1999.

143. REPRORISK. Micromedex Healthcare Series Databases. Micromedex Inc., Englewood, CO. (12/00).

144. TOXNET. Toxicology Data Network. Toxicology and environmental health information program, National Library of Medicine, 2000. http://toxnet.nlm.nih.gov//.

145. MEDLINE. PUBMED. National Library of Medicine, 2000. http://www.ncbi.nlm.nih.gov/PubMed//.

146. Mattison DR. Exclusion of fertile women from the workplace: bad medicine, worse law. J Ark Med Soc 1990; 86:491–2.

147. Stijkel A, van Dijk FJH. Developments in reproductive risk management. Occup Environ Med 1995; 52:294–303.

148. Brooks L, Merkel SF, Glowatz MJ, Comstock ML, Shoner LG. A comprehensive reproductive health program in the workplace. Am Ind Hyg Assoc J 1994; 55:352–7.

149. Mattison DR. An overview of biologic markers in reproductive and developmental toxicology: concepts, definitions and use in risk assessment. Biomed Environ Sci 1991; 4:8–34.

150. Brent RL, Beckman DA. Principles of teratology. In: Evans MI, ed. Reproductive risks and prenatal diagnosis. Norwalk: Appleton and Lange, 1992.

151. Rayburn WF, Zuspan FZ, eds. Drug therapy in obstetrics and gynecology, 3rd edn. St Louis: Mosby Year Book, 1992.

152. UNSCEAR (United Nations Scientific Committee on the Effects of Atomic Radiation) 2000. Sources and effects of ionizing radiation. Report to the General Assembly, with scientific annexes. New York: United Nations, 2000.

Chapter 28
Neurologic and Psychiatric Disorders

28.1 Central Nervous System Diseases
Jordan A Firestone, William T Longstreth Jr

Chemical agents capable of damaging the central nervous system (CNS) are ubiquitous in the environment. Industrial processes are notorious sources for some of the most well known of these neurotoxins, which contaminate both the worksite and the surrounding environment. The United States Environmental Protection Agency lists over 65,000 chemicals currently used in the US for commercial purposes, adding 2000–3000 new ones each year.[1] Reflecting the growing public concern about chemical exposures, the Environmental Protection Agency[2] and the Food and Drug Administration[3] have issued revised guidelines for risk assessment, including specific test batteries for neurotoxicity and developmental neurotoxicity. Unfortunately, only a few chemicals have been thoroughly tested, and the guidelines have been criticized for being ineffective at identifying potential neurotoxins.[4] Although neurotoxicity is apparent when intense high-level exposures result in acute illness, there is increasing evidence linking chronic low-level exposures with neurodegenerative diseases.[5] Given the frequency with which potentially neurotoxic exposures occur, clinicians may be missing these causal factors in many patients presenting with central neurologic symptoms.

The effects of toxins on the nervous system are protean. The nervous system is uniquely susceptible to intoxication for several reasons (Table 28.1.1). When the peripheral nervous system is affected, characteristic symptoms and signs develop (see Chapter 28.2). In these cases, much can be done to specifiy the degree and type of dysfunction, including a histologic examination of a peripheral nerve biopsy specimen. On the other hand, the effects of toxins on the CNS – the brain and spinal cord – are more complex than on the peripheral nervous system. Clinical disorders of the CNS are variable in their presentation and difficult to classify, often involving a host of non-specific symptoms. Typically, the brain and spinal cord cannot undergo biopsy for histologic examination. Thus, clinicians often focus on describing neurologic function and excluding other neurologic conditions, rather than on diagnosing a specific neurotoxic disease. This chapter will review the challenges in diagnosis, organize an approach to patients with CNS dysfunction as the result of a neurotoxic exposure, and present a scheme for classifying diseases related to neurotoxins.

CLINICAL EVALUATION

In order to facilitate an accurate diagnosis, a clinical evaluation must include a detailed account of the patient's initial presentation. The most important elements of this evaluation are a comprehensive history and detailed neurologic examination, which together yield the most relevant diagnostic information. Because neurotoxic diseases may be evanescent, documentation of a thorough baseline neurologic examination is crucial, and close follow-up is important. The differential diagnosis can be further refined by review of relevant exposure documents, such as Material Safety Data Sheets (MSDS) and duty logs, as well as literature searches for reported associations. Consultation with a neurologist may be needed to define subtle features of the neurologic examination and help decide what ancillary testing is appropriate to clarify the disease process and exclude other causes for the patient's problems.

History

The first challenge facing the clinician is to determine if the patient's condition is related to a neurotoxic exposure; the cornerstone for this evaluation is a detailed history.

The manner in which a patient with a potential neurotoxic exposure presents for medical evaluation is related in part to the level of the exposure and potency of the toxin. The most straightforward presentation is when the patient is aware of a specific chemical exposure. The person may have learned that exposure to some substance is potentially hazardous and is worried about possible injury. The concern is augmented when the organ targeted for injury is the brain. In this situation, determining the level of exposure represents the challenge. At one extreme, the exposure may be extremely small, and the risk of detectable disease equally small; for example, the patient who is otherwise healthy and is concerned because of an exposure to aluminum while using aluminum cookware and soft-drink cans. For such cases, a history and physical examination are generally adequate to convince the clinician whether a serious problem exists. At the other extreme, a patient may present with obvious dysfunction of the CNS related to a massive neurotoxic exposure. Many times, such large exposures are accidental, but other times, they are intentional, as occurs with homicide, suicide, and substance abuse. Examples would include the accidental exposure of a worker to carbon monoxide, the use of cyanide for homicide, and the sniffing of glue in search of euphoria.

When the patient has symptoms but does not immediately associate them with some exposure, the clinician must question the patient about environmental exposures,

- Neurons and their processes have a high surface area, increasing their effective exposure to chemicals
- The high lipid content of neuronal structures results in accumulation and retention of lipophilic chemicals
- Metabolic demands are high, so neurons are strongly affected by energy or nutrient depletion
- High blood flow, for high metabolic demands, increases the effective exposure to circulating chemicals
- Chemical toxins interfere with normal neurotransmission by mimicking the structures of endogenous molecules
- Following chemical injury, recovery of the normal, complex interneuronal connections is imperfect
- Neurons cannot regenerate once killed by chemical exposures

Table 28.1.1 Factors contributing to the susceptibility of the nervous system to chemical injury

particularly those occurring at work. Questions to identify neurotoxic exposures should include a detailed occupational and environmental health history (see Chapter 3). An exposure may have resulted in a disease that has forced the patient to retire; in this case, the key will lie in questioning the patient or the patient's family about exposures that have occurred in the past. It may also be necessary to explore past exposures in cases of chronic neurodegenerative diseases, for which the clinician may not have a ready explanation and may therefore erroneously attribute to aging alone.

If a worker has neurologic symptoms that he or she believes are related to a particular neurotoxin, then the clinician needs to document the symptoms and determine whether they are consistent with the known effects of the neurotoxin at that level of exposure. For example, a worker spills an insecticide, such as malathion, and develops transient confusion, agitation, flushing, blurred vision, dry skin, and dry mouth. Here, the neurotoxic effects of an organophosphate resulting in cholinergic excess are readily apparent (see Chapter 48). Unfortunately, most clinical situations are not as straightforward. If after consulting with appropriate sources there is no apparent link between the symptoms and exposure, then the condition is either not related to the exposure or represents a newly recognized manifestation of a neurotoxin. In such cases, principles of causation must be applied (see Chapter 1).

The pattern of associated symptoms is useful in recognizing and identifying a particular neurotoxic syndrome, and certain neurologic complaints should alert a clinician to explore the occupational health history thoroughly (Table 28.1.2). Higher cortical functions can be extremely sensitive to various brain insults, including neurotoxins. Complaints of changes in cognition, behavior, and mood should always prompt questions about exposure to neurotoxins. In addition, many parts of the nervous system

- Demonstrable exposure
- Temporal connection
- Cognitive or behavioral changes
- Incoordination
- Non-focal dysfunction

Table 28.1.2 Pattern recognition for neurotoxicity

must be operating normally for coordination to be intact, so complaints about incoordination should also raise suspicion about neurotoxins. Such complaints can take many forms, including dizziness, unsteadiness of gait, or difficulty with fine finger movements. The patient is usually aware of problems with coordination, although they may be difficult to characterize. The patient may not necessarily be as aware of problems with cognition. These complaints may come from friends and family members instead of the patient.

A key element in recognizing a pattern consistent with neurotoxicity is the distinction between focal and more diffuse involvement of the CNS. Typically, evidence of focal involvement weighs against the problem being related to a neurotoxin. In this context, focal changes need to be distinguished from system-specific involvement. A focal lesion generally refers to a specific site of injury, such as a tumor or stroke, which is anatomically localized but has a broader functional impact. Thus, the patient with temporary hemiparesis and aphasia may have had an ischemic injury in the middle cerebral artery distribution due to vascular disease, rather than a neurotoxic cause. In contrast, system-specific injury often reflects that system's inherent metabolic or physiologic susceptibility to intoxication rather than its anatomic localization. A recent example that has revolutionized thinking about neurotoxins involves the effects of a meperidine derivative, 1-methyl-4-phenyl-1,2,3,6-tetrahydropyridine (MPTP), that selectively damages the dopaminergic motor system of the brain. The resulting clinical picture is indistinguishable from Parkinson's disease. This system-specific neurotoxin will be discussed in more detail later in this chapter.

Another element to be considered is the temporal sequence of events. Key distinctions include acute versus insidious onset, constant versus intermittent dysfunction, and progression versus stabilization or improvement. A consistent temporal association between symptoms and exposures is an important aspect in assessing a likely toxic etiology. Little doubt exists when acute symptoms are associated with accidental overexposures, as in organophosphate poisoning. Intermittent complaints may be associated with non-continuous exposures, such as with a rotating duty roster. Perhaps the most challenging time course is one of insidious onset with progressive deterioration. In this case, other clues may be useful, such as anatomic or functional localization. For example, a progressive hemiparesis may suggest a focal neoplasm, whereas progressive gait instability may reflect a system-specific cerebellar effect of chronic solvent toxicity.

By combining facts about the exposure scenario with the symptom complex and temporal sequence, a pattern of CNS dysfunction consistent with neurotoxicity may emerge. Recognition of this pattern is essential to diagnosis. The information gleaned from the initial history further guides the clinician in the subsequent physical examination and later selection of ancillary tests.

Test areas	Maximum score	Score
Orientation		
What is the (year) (season) (date) (day) (month)?	5	_____
Where are we: (state) (county) (town) (hospital) (floor)?	5	_____
Registration		
Name three objects: 1 second to say each. Then ask the patient all three after you have said them. Give 1 point for each correct answer. Then repeat them until he or she learns all three.	3	_____
Attention and calculation		
Serial 7s. 1 point for each correct. Stop after five answers. Alternatively spell 'world' backward.	5	_____
Recall		
Ask for the three objects repeated above. Give 1 point for each correct response.	5	_____
Language		
Name a pencil and watch.	2	_____
Repeat the following 'No ifs, ands, or buts.'	1	_____
Follow a three-stage command: 'Take a paper in your right hand, fold it in half, and put it on the floor.'	3	_____
Read and obey the following: Close your eyes. Score 1 point only if he or she actually closes his or her eyes.	1	_____
Write a sentence. Do not dictate a sentence; it is to be written spontaneously. It must contain a subject and verb and be sensible. Correct grammar and punctuation are not necessary.	1	_____
Copy design. On a clean piece of paper, draw intersecting pentagons, each side about 1 inch, and ask the patient to copy it exactly as it is. All 10 angles must be present and 2 must intersect to score 1 point. Tremor and rotation are ignored.	1	_____

* Modified from Folstein MF, Folstein SE, McHugh PR. "Mini-Mental State." A practical method for grading the cognitive state of patients for the clinician. J Psychiatr Res 1975; 12:189–198. Copyright 1975, with kind permission from Pergamon Press Ltd, Headington Hill Hall, Oxford OX3 OBW, UK; and Bleecker ML, Bolla-Wilson K, Kawas G, Agnew J. Age-specific norms for the Mini-Mental State Exam. Neurology 1988; 38:1565–8.

Table 28.1.3 Mini Mental State Examination*

Physical examination

By the time the history is completed, the clinician should have strong suspicions about what the neurologic examination will show. The examination thus provides an opportunity to test hypotheses generated from the history by either confirming expected findings or eliminating alternative explanations. Although the general medical examination may supply clues that the patient has been exposed to a neurotoxin – for instance, gingivitis can occur with chronic mercury poisoning and transverse white lines in the fingernails (Mees' lines) can be seen with arsenic poisoning – such pathognomonic findings are often not present. Therefore, the neurologic examination is essential to document the localization, the type, and the degree of neurologic impairment. There are six broad areas that should be screened in a routine neurologic examination:

- mental status;
- cranial nerves;
- motor system;
- reflexes;
- sensation; and
- coordination and gait.

A structured approach to these six areas helps ensure completeness and reproducibility.[6]

Testing the mental status and higher cortical functions begins with an assessment of the form and content of communication with the patient during the clinical interview. More formal, structured neuropsychologic screens provide advantages of reproducibility and reliability.[7] One commonly used screen that can be easily performed in the clinic is the Mini Mental State Examination (MMSE; Table 28.1.3). Age-adjusted norms have been established, with 29 or 30 being a normal score for persons under age 65 years.[8] Although a normal score cannot rule out subtle cognitive problems, an abnormal score is concerning. Bedside neuropsychologic testing is insensitive to subtle abnormalities that the patient, family members, or friends may readily recognize. In these situations, more detailed neuropsychologic testing is indicated. Certain abnormalities of higher brain function, such as aphasias or apraxias, may suggest focal cortical involvement. The finding of such focal signs on detailed testing makes it unlikely that neurotoxicity is the sole explanation for the patient's complaints.

The 12 cranial nerves should be screened to search for evidence as much to refute as to support the hypothesis that a patient's complaints are related to a neurotoxin. For instance, the finding of a bilateral intranuclear ophthalmoplegia would push the clinician strongly toward a diagnosis of multiple sclerosis. Multiple sclerosis is frequently a consideration in patients suspected of having a neurotoxin-related disease, given the various symptoms and signs with which multiple sclerosis can present and that it affects young men and women who may try to relate their symptoms to something in the workplace.

The first cranial nerve serves olfaction. While not easy to test in a reliable fashion, impairment of olfaction as an early finding is noteworthy. An area of controversy has been the hypothesis proposed by some investigators that certain neurotoxins gain access to the brain via the olfactory system, thence spreading to the neighboring hippocampal systems, affecting memory, or the basal ganglia, affecting motor function. Olfactory impairment is a common finding in patients with neurodegenerative diseases,[9,10] as well as chronic rhinosinusitis. Various substances can be used to test olfaction, and kits are available for formal assessment.[11]

The second cranial nerve, serving vision, is susceptible to neurotoxic injury. Bilateral findings can suggest a diffuse neurotoxic process, and bilateral optic neuropathy has been described with exposures to heavy metals, solvents, and insecticides. However, unilateral dysfunction suggests other disease processes. Physical findings include diminished visual acuity, a relative afferent pupillary defect to a swinging light, and a pale optic disc. Testing of the visual field is an important screen for focal brain disease, and therefore most visual field defects suggest an alternative cause for the patient's complaints. Bilateral field defects can rarely result from toxins. Blindness with unreactive pupils points to a problem anterior to the optic chiasm, as can occur with methanol intoxication. On the other hand, preservation of the pupillary light response indicates that the problem is in the brain, not in the eyes, termed cortical blindness. Poisoning with organic mercury can produce this syndrome, with constricted visual fields and eventual loss of vision. Neuropathologic examination in such patients confirms damage to the cerebral cortex serving vision.

Several aspects of the second cranial nerve can be tested. Visual acuity, visual fields, pupillary light response, and fundoscopy should be checked (see Chapter 20.1). Tests of color vision can be easily administered in the clinical setting and serve as sensitive screens of optic nerve function. For this reason, they have also been advocated for inclusion as a standard element in epidemiologic field studies.[12]

Examination of extraocular movements – cranial nerves III, IV, and VI – can give evidence to support a neurotoxic exposure. Certain types of gaze-evoked nystagmus can be seen with acute intoxications affecting the cerebellar system. Diplopia resulting from extraocular muscle paresis can occur with a number of neurotoxins, but this typically reflects dysfunction of the peripheral, not the central nervous system. Many degenerative diseases of the brain, including those related to toxins, can be associated with slowing of the saccadic, or normally lightning-like, eye movements.

The remaining cranial nerves are less frequently affected by neurotoxins acting on the brain. The fifth and seventh cranial nerves serve facial sensation and strength. The eighth cranial nerve serves hearing and balance. The ninth and tenth cranial nerves serve the function of swallowing. These cranial nerves are more frequently affected in their peripheral portion by neurotoxins; CNS involvement typically suggests a vascular, neoplastic, inflammatory, or demyelinating etiology.

The cranial nerves serving motor function, including V, VII, XI, and XII, can be involved in processes such as

	Upper motor neuron	Lower motor neuron
Atrophy	Moderate	Marked
Tone	Increased	Decreased
Reflexes	Increased	Decreased
Plantar response	Extensor	Flexor
Fasciculations	Absent	Present

Table 28.1.4 Localizing weakness based on examination

amyotrophic lateral sclerosis, that affect alpha motor neurons in the anterior horn of the spinal cord. Some associations between motor neuron disease and environmental exposures, including exposures to specific solvents and heavy metals, have been observed.[13,14] The tongue, served by cranial nerve XII, can be a good place to detect the resulting weakness and atrophy. Fasciculations can also be seen, though they can be difficult to distinguish from other movements. The task is made easier by examining the tongue while it is resting in the mouth, rather than protruded. For unclear reasons, muscles that serve eye movements are typically spared.

Examination of the motor system should include assessments of the strength, bulk, and tone of the muscles. All three elements must be considered, because although weakness suggests a problem in the motor system, it may reflect dysfunction of the muscle itself, the neuromuscular junction, the peripheral nerve, the anterior horn cell, or the so-called upper motor neuron. Localization within this pathway strongly influences diagnostic considerations and the ordering of ancillary tests.

Although the lower (alpha) motor neuron is influenced by many higher centers and descending systems, the simplified model distinguishing between upper and lower motor neuron lesions is useful clinically. Findings on the examination often suggest localization to the upper or lower motor neuron (Table 28.1.4). Both categories involve weakness. Diminished bulk, or atrophy, can also occur with either type of lesion, although it is usually more marked with a lower motor neuron lesion. In addition to reflex abnormalities (discussed later), the most useful feature in separating the two categories is a change in muscle tone. Tone is best assessed with passive movements of the limb, usually the upper extremity. It is important for the patient to be fully co-operative to avoid a superimposed component of volitional tone, which can confound interpretation. Lower motor neuron lesions, involving the motor system from the anterior horn cell to the muscle proper, produce decreased muscle tone, or hypotonia. Upper motor neuron lesions, involving higher centers and descending systems that modulate activity of the anterior horn cell, produce increased tone, or hypertonia. Two exceptions are those related to cerebellar dysfunction and to certain lesions of the basal ganglia, which can produce hypotonia.

The increased tone seen with involvement of the descending motor tracts is called spasticity. It is characterized by a resistance to passive movement, which is variable throughout the range of movement and depends on the speed of movement. Unlike spasticity, rigidity is characterized by increased tone that does not vary throughout the range of movement or with the speed of movement. Rigidity usually results from basal ganglion dysfunction.

Spasticity may reflect a toxin-related dysfunction of the descending tracts that directly influences the lower motor neuron, producing a clinical myelopathy. These tracts contain some of the longest axons in the nervous system, and are thus vulnerable to some of the same agents that cause length-dependent peripheral axonopathy, such as tri-ortho-cresyl-phosphate.[15,16] Nitrous oxide is another agent that can damage central tracts, giving a clinical picture similar to that seen with vitamin B_{12} deficiency,[17] though this typically occurs only after repeated exposures, such as with substance abuse. Early after an exposure to such toxins, the signs and symptoms related to the peripheral nervous system injury may predominate, while only later does the injury to the CNS become evident.

Rigidity, reflecting dysfunction in central motor systems that do not directly influence the lower motor neuron, can also be related to neurotoxins. Rigidity is one of the cardinal manifestations of parkinsonism, reflecting dysfunction of the basal ganglion. The other features of this syndrome are bradykinesia with a paucity and slowness of movements, resting tremor with a typical frequency of 3–7 Hz, and postural instability with the potential for frequent falls. The diagnosis of parkinsonism is based on clinical assessment; ancillary tests are not helpful. Several neurotoxins can damage the neural inputs or outputs of the basal ganglion and result in this syndrome. Such selective neurotoxins include carbon monoxide, carbon disulfide, manganese, rotenone, and MPTP. The marked similarities between toxin-induced movement disorders and idiopathic Parkinson's disease have raised concerns that the two conditions may be related,[5,18] as discussed in more detail later.

Rather than manifesting with rigidity and bradykinesia, injury to certain regions of the basal ganglion can manifest with the opposite picture: reduced tone and hyperkinesias. The hyperkinesias can manifest as a variety of involuntary movements involving the face, trunk, and limbs. Careful observation during the history and physical examination is usually enough to suspect such a movement disorder. The causes of such disorders are numerous, including genetic diseases such as Huntington's or Wilson's disease. Neurotoxic exposures can also produce this picture; for example, as an acute effect of a drug such as cocaine, or as a delayed effect of a drug such as haloperidol.[19–21]

Tendon reflexes provide a quick screen, reflecting balance between the function of the upper and lower motor neuron. Increased tendon reflexes, especially in the setting of other findings of upper motor neuron dysfunction, strongly suggest a problem in the CNS. Initially reduced or absent tendon reflexes cannot rule out CNS involvement, because the injury to the peripheral nervous system that produces hyporeflexia may initially mask the manifestations of the concomitant CNS injury, as in the case of tri-ortho-cresyl-phosphate poisoning. Examination of the tendon reflexes can also suggest an injury to the cerebellum. In these situations, pendular reflexes are present: the limb keeps swinging longer than usual following elicitation of the reflex. A reflex that gives strong evidence in favor of an upper motor neuron lesion is the extensor plantar response or the so-called Babinski sign.

Examination of sensation can help localize dysfunction to the peripheral as opposed to the central nervous system. Screening involves checking the patient's sensitivity to several modalities in several locations, including vibration in the distal lower extremities. Most patients with a normal sensory system can appreciate vibration in the great toe from a vigorously thumped 128-Hz frequency tuning fork for more than 10 seconds. Typically, findings on the sensory examination that point to a problem in the CNS do not suggest a neurotoxic lesion. Thus, the dissociated sensory loss of a spinal cord syrinx or the crossed sensory changes of a brainstem stroke exclude an etiology related to a neurotoxin. In patients in whom the sensory examination shows a stocking–glove type of reduced sensation, a diffuse peripheral polyneuropathy should be suspected, which can be metabolic or toxin induced.

The presence of incoordination on the physical examination is non-specific. For coordination to be normal, many of the aspects of the motor and sensory function already discussed must be intact. Incoordination could indicate a problem in the CNS, the peripheral nervous system, or both. It could indicate a problem in the motor systems, sensory systems, or both. Incoordination can result from either acute or chronic intoxication. Despite its lack of specificity, incoordination is a sensitive screen for evidence of neurotoxic effects on the nervous system, because coordination testing reflects broadly the function of the nervous system.

Evaluation of coordination should include both the upper and lower extremities. Tasks should be carefully observed for speed, smoothness, and agility. For the upper extremities, the patient should move quickly from one target to another, e.g., finger to nose. For the lower extremities, the heel should be moved up and down the shin of the opposite leg. Rapid alternating movements, such as finger and toe tapping, or clapping first the front and then the back of one hand on another, should be evaluated. Gait should be observed first with the patient walking naturally and then with increasing difficulty by having the patient walk on heels and toes, tandem walk forward and in reverse, and in a semi-squat while holding a tandem position. Though computerized posturography has progressed as a tool for clinical assessment,[22,23] incoordination is not easily quantified, and the decision about its presence or absence ultimately relies on clinical judgment.

Ancillary testing

Ancillary tests of CNS function can serve several purposes in the evaluation of patients suspected of having a neurotoxin-related disease. Most importantly, these tests can exclude other diseases. For example, imaging studies may show focal abnormalities such as neoplasm or stroke that account for a patient's complaints. Tests can be used to help clarify uncertainties in the clinical presentation by demonstrating objective abnormalities underlying the patient's subjective descriptions. For example, a substantially elevated carboxyhemoglobin level may explain vague complaints of headache and decreased concentration resulting from occult carbon monoxide exposure. Ancillary tests can also be used as more sensitive screens for the effects of neurotoxins on the CNS than the routine history and physical examination. This benefit is particularly apparent in the evaluation of cognitive function, which can be rigorously assessed with neuropsychologic testing, to follow up screening findings on the MMSE. Finally, ancillary testing can be used to quantify neurologic deficits. Such measurements may be used to gauge the degree of impairment for compensation purposes, to assist with vocational counseling by providing a guide for what a patient may be able to accomplish with such deficits, and to provide a baseline from which to judge the clinical course of the illness or response to treatment. Ancillary tests will be considered in a few broad groups as follows:

- anatomic studies, such as computed tomographic (CT) scanning and magnetic resonance imaging (MRI) of the head;
- physiologic tests, such as elicitation and averaging of sensory-evoked potentials;
- functional assessments, such as neuropsychologic testing;
- bioassays, such as cholinesterase levels; and
- miscellaneous tests, such as positron emission tomography (PET).

Anatomic studies

Most neurotoxins do not produce injuries that can be detected by imaging studies that detail the anatomy of the brain and spinal cord. An exception is the group of toxins that can injure the basal ganglion and may result in bilateral abnormalities in the globus pallidus. In most circumstances, the clinician will use imaging studies to exclude other, non-neurotoxic diseases. CT scanning is an excellent screen for mass lesions, such as brain tumors, which will usually lead to symptoms or signs indicating a focal dysfunction of the brain. If the history and physical examination lack such findings, then the yield from CT scanning is low. As a screening test, MRI has proven to be more sensitive than CT scanning for most conditions.[24] MRI supplies more anatomic detail than does CT scanning: contrast agents can increase the sensitivity of both techniques. One situation in which MRI is particularly good is in detecting abnormalities of the white matter, so-called leukoencephalopathy.[25] Multiple sclerosis has many clinical presentations, and although most suggest focal or multifocal involvement of the brain or spinal cord, some could be confused with neurotoxin-related disease. Confusion is most apt to occur in distinguishing the chronic progressive forms of multiple sclerosis from a disease caused by a neurotoxin. In such cases, the presence of characteristic periventricular white matter hyperintensities may support

the diagnosis of multiple sclerosis. It is imperative that the medical history correlates with the imaging results, because in many cases the MRI may also be non-specific, showing abnormalities that are of uncertain significance. For instance, the finding of unidentified bright objects (UBOs) is common in otherwise normal people.

Toxins are often suspected in the differential diagnosis of cognitive decline or dementia. Imaging may be used to evaluate such patients, though it most commonly does not yield a specific diagnosis and cannot help distinguish whether or not dementia is related to a neurotoxin. Cerebral cortical atrophy, often demonstrated in such cases, does not correlate well with cognitive performance.[26] Atrophy is a non-specific finding that may look the same in Alzheimer's disease, Huntington's disease, or a solvent-related dementia.

One finding on imaging studies that suggests a neurotoxic etiology is bilateral and symmetric damage to the basal ganglion, most commonly involving the globus pallidus. These findings are of particular interest when the patient has clinical evidence of parkinsonism. Carbon monoxide, carbon disulfide, and manganese are examples of agents that can produce these lesions. The case of a 27-year-old man found unconscious in a parked recreational vehicle is illustrative. He had been using a small charcoal burner to keep warm and had suffered severe, acute carbon monoxide poisoning. The patient eventually regained consciousness but had parkinsonism, with bradykinesia, rigidity, and resting tremor. MRI showed bilateral symmetric hyperintensities in the globus pallidus, typical of what can be seen in such cases (Fig. 28.1.1).

Although CT scanning can demonstrate the bilateral abnormalities of the globus pallidus, MRI is the preferred method in these circumstances. However, there are some caveats to interpretation. First, the finding of bilateral basal ganglia abnormalities on imaging is not specific to a neurotoxic etiology: Wilson's disease and certain inherited mitochondrial disorders can have a similar appearance. Next, if the neurotoxin causes parkinsonism by selective damage to the substantia nigra, as occurs with MPTP, in contrast to widespread damage to the basal ganglia, such as with carbon monoxide, then the imaging may be unremarkable. Finally, although MRI abnormalities may be seen early in the course of disease, the findings may normalize over time, even when symptoms persist.

To summarize, the clinician suspecting that a patient whose history or physical examination findings suggest neurotoxic involvement of the brain or spinal cord should have low expectations about the imaging results. Nonetheless, given the broad differential diagnosis, which includes diseases like multiple sclerosis whose presentations can be non-specific, imaging is often necessary. Screening should be done with the most sensitive test, which is MRI. The clinician must be cautious not to overinterpret non-specific findings.

Physiologic tests

Physiologic dysfunction of the CNS may not be manifest by imaging tests. Tests that reflect physiologic rather than

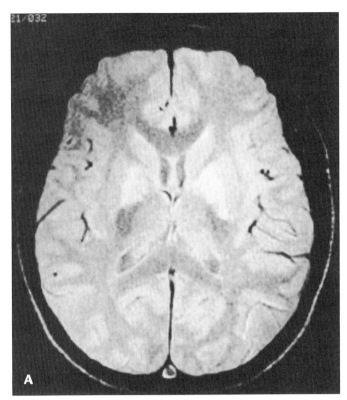 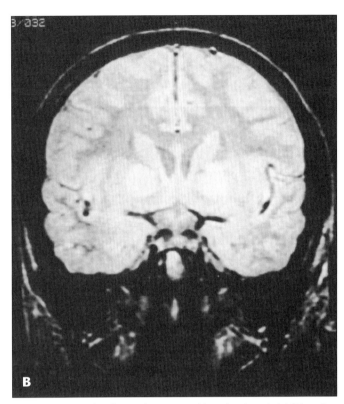

Figure 28.1.1: Magnetic resonance imaging scan of a 27-year-old man with parkinsonism related to carbon monoxide poisoning. Axial (A) and coronal (B) spin density images of the brain, including basal ganglia, are shown. Hyperintensities are present in the lentiform, or lens-shaped, nucleus of the basal ganglion. The lentiform nucleus has two parts: (1) the more medial globus pallidus and (2) the more lateral putamen. Note involvement of the globus pallidus, with relative sparing of the putamen.

anatomic changes are useful in the evaluation of many diseases related to a neurotoxic exposure.

The electroencephalogram (EEG) is used to record the electrical activity of the brain. Many things can affect the EEG tracing, so changes rarely point to a specific cause. The EEG is also difficult to quantify, and subtle intoxication can lead to EEG changes that can be difficult to interpret. Spectral analysis techniques have been developed,[27] but although they have been used in epidemiologic studies, there remain considerable barriers to their effective application in most clinical situations.[28] Many toxins that affect brain function, such as organic solvents and heavy metals, will affect the appearance of the EEG diffusely. The changes that are most obvious on the EEG, such as diffuse slowing, are often associated with evidence of toxic encephalopathy on the neurologic examination, with alteration of cognition, coordination, or both. These diffuse findings can be contrasted with EEG evidence of focal brain dysfunction, which is typically not related to neurotoxins.

A common application of EEG testing is in the evaluation of seizures. Epilepsy can be diagnosed when the EEG tracing shows characteristic epileptiform discharges in the appropriate clinical setting. Generalized convulsions can be a manifestation of a neurotoxic exposure, such as to an organochlorine insecticide. However, the convulsions themselves do not necessarily indicate a diagnosis of epilepsy, which is defined by the recurrence of unprovoked seizures. Unless the EEG is done around the time of a toxin-induced seizure, the tracing should be free of epileptiform activity.

Whereas quantitative information is difficult to obtain from a routine EEG, it is more readily obtained from evoked potentials. In these tests, a sensory stimulus is used to trigger a neural response. By averaging the response to many discrete stimuli, a time-linked sensory-evoked response can be detected. Although evoked potentials can provide quantitative information, many variables can confound interpretation and results are not specific. As always, the entire clinical scenario must be considered. Nonetheless, event-related potentials have shown great promise as sensitive indicators of brain dysfunction in population studies.[22]

Functional information about the visual pathways can be obtained from visual-evoked potentials. Providing retinal function is normal, the results can provide an indication of dysfunction in the optic nerves. Although such optic nerve dysfunction could result from a neurotoxin, it may also result from a vitamin deficiency, a tumor, or a demyelinating disease. As in other parts of the nervous system, asymmetric involvement tends to favor etiologies other than those related to neurotoxins.

The brainstem auditory-evoked response (BAER) screens auditory pathways that are both peripheral and central, from the cochlea of the inner ear to the medial geniculate nucleus of the diencephalon. The most common abnormalities related to toxic exposures involve injuries to the peripheral portions of this system.

Somatosensory-evoked potentials can be elicited by stimulation of peripheral nerves in the upper and lower extremities. Like the BAER, this test indicates the function of not only the peripheral, but also the centrally projecting sensory pathways. If the peripheral system is capable of carrying a signal, then the coexistence of central and peripheral involvement, as with tri-ortho-cresyl-phosphate poisoning, can be demonstrated with this test.

Functional assessments

The ultimate impact of neurologic disease is in terms of functional limitations. The neurologic examination itself is purposely organized into functional components. These basic maneuvers have been extended through a variety of functional assessments developed to recognize, characterize, and quantify functional deficits. In certain cases, tests of sensory threshold and posturography may be useful, though a detailed examination is generally adequate to detect clinically significant functional limitations. By far the most important for evaluating global cerebral changes within the CNS are assessments of neuropsychologic functioning.

Neuropsychologic testing is the best method to assess subtle abnormalities of cognitive function. The spectrum of neuropsychologic tests is great, and selection must be tailored to the particular situation. For instance, the tests administered to an individual with complaints of chronic memory problems may differ substantially from the tests used to screen a large number of workers in an epidemiologic study or from that used to monitor acutely exposed workers. When screening large numbers of persons, the test battery must be short. Some tests are hand administered, such as the Neurobehavioral Core Test Battery of the World Health Organization;[29] others are administered via a microcomputer, such as the Neurobehavioral Evaluation System.[30] These screens can typically be administered in 40 to 90 minutes. Although such screens may perform well for assessing and comparing groups of exposed persons, more extensive testing (typically lasting many hours) is performed for clinical evaluation of an individual patient.

Extensive neuropsychologic testing provides the most sensitive assessment of brain dysfunction. When dysfunction is identified, the testing can also indicate the degree of impairment, and where rehabilitation efforts should be focused. A baseline is also useful for comparison in subsequent testing: neurotoxic injury should stabilize following cessation of an exposure without further deterioration and with possible variable improvement, whereas problems related to neurodegenerative disorders, such as Alzheimer's disease, may be expected to worsen. Thus, repeated testing over time may be indicated depending on the disease course.

Many tests are available to evaluate the areas of memory, intelligence, executive function, personality, mood, and coordination. Two of the most widely used comprehensive sets of tests are the Halstead–Reitan Battery and the Luria Nebraska Neuropsychological Battery. Although the latter has some advantages when dealing with patients who have minimal education or severe brain damage, the former may be a more sensitive screen for the subtle effects of a neurotoxin. Tests evaluating verbal memory, attention, visual tracking, and visual memory are particularly important for assessing neurotoxic injury. Many screens of personality and mood are available, but the most commonly used is the Minnesota Multiphasic Personality Inventory (MMPI). Several tests of coordination are available that assess motor speed, reaction time, dexterity, and balance. Some of the available tests are old and have well-established norms. Others, more recently developed, have the advantage of evaluating different functions in different ways, but are limited by a lack of established normative values.

Neuropsychologic testing should be performed by or under the supervision of a qualified neuropsychologist. The interpretation of the tests must be in the context of the patient's past education. Verbal performance is thought to be relatively resistant to the effect of neurotoxins on brain function, and it is often used as an estimate of pre-exposure function. Therefore, with an important neurotoxic exposure, evaluation of memory could elicit scores much lower than would be expected based on verbal performance. Psychologic factors can also affect test results, as can alcohol and drug abuse. Concurrent depression or anxiety can adversely affect test performance, and should be considered in the assessment of cognitive impairment. Such a situation could still be related to a workplace exposure as a secondary effect, if the exposure is the proximate cause of the psychologic condition.[7,31]

Bioassays

Many clinical laboratory tests can be performed to evaluate the possibility that a patient has an illness related to a neurotoxin. The body's burden of some neurotoxins, such as lead or other metals, can be estimated based on levels in the blood or urine. For other neurotoxins, indirect measures are available, such as red blood cell cholinesterase activity in cases of organophosphate exposure or carboxyhemoglobin level in cases of active carbon monoxide exposure. For most neurotoxins, however, direct or indirect monitoring is not readily available. Most other tests of the blood, urine, or spinal fluid are aimed at evaluating other diagnostic possibilities. Multiple sclerosis and spirochetal diseases, such as syphilis and Lyme disease, can mimic almost any disease of the CNS, including those related to neurotoxins. Thus, developing and refining bioassays is an area of ongoing research interest.[32]

Genetic screening represents the latest challenge in the application and interpretation of new bioassays. With the technologic innovations that have accompanied the human genome project have come an explosion of data regarding human genetic variability. Genetic polymorphisms are now thought to hold one of the keys to understanding differences between individuals in susceptibility to toxin-related diseases.[33] Candidate genes include the enzyme systems responsible for bioactivation and detoxification of xenobiotics and the receptor and transporter systems involved in neurotransmission.[5] The sheer quantity of data and its rapid rate of acquisition have produced significant pragmatic challenges for data storage and manipulation as well as statistical assessment, spurring development of the related field of bioinformatics. One early conclusion from this work is that the vast majority of diseases are multifactorial, involving the combined effects of several processes.

Miscellaneous tests

New technology is constantly evolving. Some applications, such as transcranial Doppler (TCD), will probably never be of much help in diagnosing neurotoxic diseases. Others, such as PET, single-photon emission computed tomography (SPECT), and functional magnetic resonance imaging (fMRI), may find a use in allowing direct assessment of the effects of specific neurotoxins on brain function. Still others, such as magnetic resonance spectroscopy[34] and magnetic resonance microscopy,[35] may help define the pharmacokinetic and pathologic effects of toxic exposures. Whether any of these new tests will have enough specificity to be useful for clinical diagnosis remains open to question.[36] Currently these tests are primarily useful as research tools.

CLASSIFICATION OF DISEASES OF THE CENTRAL NERVOUS SYSTEM RELATED TO NEUROTOXINS

Diffuse toxic encephalopathy
• Acute
• Chronic
Selective toxic encephalopathy
• Cell bodies
• Ion channels
• Neurotransmitter systems

The classification scheme presented here primarily emphasizes the clinical manifestations of toxic exposures to the CNS. While it would be most desirable to develop a concise scheme based entirely on each individual toxin's mechanism of action,[37] the multiplicity of known mechanisms for selected toxins, coupled with a limited database for most others, makes such an approach clinically impractical.[38] Although some selective toxins produce characteristic clinical syndromes, it remains more useful for diagnostic purposes to rely on a classification based on two features of the toxin's effects: anatomic distribution and time course.

The clinical manifestations of a toxin are related to which anatomic areas of the brain or spinal cord are compromised. Toxic encephalopathy is the phrase used to indicate a dysfunction of the brain caused by a toxic exposure. Toxic myelopathy is the phrase used to indicate toxin-related dysfunction of the spinal cord. For encephalopathies, the effects of toxins that are diffuse and lead to non-specific clinical syndromes are distinguished from those that are selective and lead to specific clinical syndromes. The time course of neurotoxic injury often impacts on the reversibility of the effect. The nervous system is noted for its plasticity, or ability to compensate for subtle alterations of function. However, when tolerances are exceeded, more sustained or irreversible damage to the CNS may occur. This is very important, because under most circumstances, the brain and spinal cord lack the capacity to regenerate neurons.

While it would be possible to draw distinctions between the acute and chronic forms of both diffuse and selective encephalopathies, these distinctions will only be discussed in detail in the context of diffuse encephalopathy. The selective encephalopathies are instead categorized by toxic effects involving clearly established cellular mechanisms.

Diffuse toxic encephalopathy–acute

Acute diffuse toxic encephalopathy reflects a global cerebral dysfunction of rapid onset (typically days or weeks). It is a condition that many have experienced when they have felt the effects of an alcoholic beverage. There is nothing specific about these encephalopathies; virtually any organic solvent has the potential to produce such effects (see Chapter 40). The effects typically resolve completely, but if overwhelming can result in a non-specific chronic encephalopathy, as discussed in a later section.

Pathogenesis

Toxins producing an acute encephalopathy interfere with basic cell functions in the brain, although the exact mechanisms remain obscure for some agents. Typically, such toxins gain easy access to the brain, and thus have the ability to alter brain function rapidly. Although active transport systems exist to convey many compounds into the CNS, most of these agents gain entry because they are highly lipid soluble and can readily diffuse across membranes. Besides organic solvents, which can alter cellular membrane function, several gases can also affect brain function diffusely, including the gas anesthetics, carbon monoxide, hydrogen sulfide, and cyanide. Heavy metals can also cause acute encephalopathies, but this is more commonly associated with the organic metals (e.g., methyl mercury or tetraethyl lead) than with the inorganic ones (e.g., lead, arsenic, mercury, or thallium).

Clinical and diagnostic approach

The clinical manifestations of an acute diffuse toxic encephalopathy depend on the intensity of exposure. The symptoms and signs can range from mild euphoria with a normal examination, to stupor, coma, and death. The earliest manifestations are behavioral, with some alteration in mood typically reflecting disinhibition. Headache and seizures may also be relatively early manifestations. In general, the greater the exposure, the more severe the impairment of cerebral function, and suppression of level of consciousness. With moderate exposures, the physical examination shows evidence of the intoxication, such as lateral gaze-evoked nystagmus and incoordination, with sloppy fine finger movements and gait ataxia. The cerebral cortex is more sensitive to these toxins than the brainstem; typically, even when consciousness is lost, brainstem function remains intact. Thus, the pupillary light responses, corneal reflexes, oculocephalic reflex, gag reflex, and spontaneous respiration are preserved until late in the clinical course, unless some complication occurs. In the absence of asymmetric signs suggesting a focal brain injury, the combination of unconsciousness with intact brainstem function suggests a toxic or metabolic etiology. Aspiration with respiratory arrest or cardiotoxicity with hypotension may lead to further loss of function and death.

Diagnosis does not generally present a challenge for acute syndromes, because the exposure and clinical manifestations are closely linked in time. An accurate history, if it can be obtained, will usually indicate the diagnosis. However, because toxic and metabolic encephalopathies can be indistinguishable, blood should be sent for electrolyte and glucose levels, renal function tests, liver function tests, and, when appropriate, endocrinologic screens. Arterial blood gases may also be indicated, both to evaluate acid–base disturbances and to assess hypoxia or hypercarbia in order to guide decisions regarding ventilatory support.

If the patient presents at the time of maximal symptomatology, the toxin is most likely to be present systematically, with the greatest likelihood of detection. Because a detailed history is not always initially available, a high index of clinical suspicion should guide the selection of ancillary tests. Blood and urine toxicologic screens will detect most substances of abuse. Screens are more difficult for the types of exposures that would occur in the workplace. Most heavy metals can be detected, but most solvents cannot be detected using readily available tests. The presence of a solvent may be suggested by an elevated serum osmolality that is not explained by abnormal sodium, glucose, urea or ethanol levels, or by measuring metabolic levels. A carboxyhemoglobin level may be useful in detecting occult carbon monoxide, if the specimen is obtained at, or very soon following, the period of active exposure. Acute and convalescent cholinesterase activity levels are useful in documenting organophosphate exposure. While such confirmatory testing is desirable, a complete history is often adequate to establish a causal link between a toxic exposure and an acute clinical syndrome severe enough to require medical attention.

The postictal confusional state, following a generalized seizure or ongoing partial complex status epilepticus, can present with symptoms such as delirium that might be confused with toxic encephalopathy. In such situations, an EEG may be useful in establishing the proper diagnosis. The most difficult situation to interpret is when a neurotoxin lowers the seizure threshold in an individual with an underlying susceptibility for seizures. Thus, for some individuals, provoked seizures occur only in the setting of exposure to a neurotoxin, though the toxin may not be the only causal factor.

With a suggestive history and a physical examination that does not reveal focal brain dysfunction, further ancillary testing is typically not needed. However, if questions exist about the history or physical examination, then imaging may be necessary. Other conditions can mimic a toxic-metabolic encephalopathy, including psychosis, meningitis, subarachnoid hemorrhage, head trauma, early central herniation syndrome, and multiple small cerebral emboli. For any of these conditions, brain imaging followed by sampling of the cerebrospinal fluid may be necessary.

Treatment and prognosis

As with most overdoses, treatment of an acute diffuse toxic encephalopathy is primarily supportive. The patient should be physically removed from the source of exposure, including removal of contaminated clothing and thorough cleansing of exposed skin. Vital functions, such as respiration and circulation, are supported until the toxin is cleared. Because most toxins causing these conditions act diffusely on the brain, specific antidotes are typically not available. Specific treatments are indicated for certain exposures, such as ethanol for methanol intoxication, induced methemoglobinemia for cyanide or hydrogen sulfide exposure, chelation for heavy-metal toxicity and high-dose oxygen (including possible hyperbaric therapy) for acute carbon monoxide poisoning.

For most of the toxins that act diffusely on the brain, recovery from a single or limited number of exposures is complete. The process of recovery is a reversal of the sequence described previously, with the level of consciousness gradually returning to normal. Withdrawal syndromes involving severe agitation and seizures are uncommon without repeated exposures. In severe cases the brain is damaged from a single exposure, when a chronic encephalopathy ensues. More often, the prognosis is a function of the cardiac and pulmonary decompensation that can complicate an acute diffuse toxic encephalopathy.

Specific agents

The syndrome of acute diffuse toxic encephalopathy is not specific. It may be caused by any neurotoxin that can gain ready access to the CNS. Such agents include solvents, metals, and gases (see Table 28.1.5). As the acute

Neurotoxin	Target	Clinical syndrome
Tetrodotoxin	Ion channel	Paralysis
Organochlorines	Ion channel	Paralysis
Organophosphate	Acetylcholinesterase	Cholinergic excess
MPTP*	Dopaminergic cells	Parkinsonism
Carbon monoxide	Globus pallidus	Parkinsonism
Carbon disulfide	Globus pallidus	Parkinsonism
Manganese	Globus pallidus	Parkinsonism
3-Nitropropionic acid	Basal ganglion	Dystonia
Domoic acid	Glutaminergic system	Amnesia
BOAA†	Glutaminergic system	Lathyrism
Organic mercury	Occipital cortex	Cortical blindness
Nitrous oxide	Spinal cord	Spastic paraparesis
Fluoroethyl acetate	Cerebellum	Ataxia
Rotenone	Mitochondrion	Parkinsonism

*1-Methyl-4-phenyl-1,2,3,6-tetrahydropyridine.
†Beta-N-oxalylamino-L-alanine.

Table 28.1.5 Examples of selective neurotoxins

encephalopathy clears, evidence may emerge of a residual chronic encephalopathy, which is discussed in the next section.

Diffuse toxic encephalopathy–chronic

Chronic diffuse toxic encephalopathy represents persistent injury to the brain, as a result of cumulative or multiple repeated exposures (often over a period of months or years) or, rarely, a single massive exposure to a toxic that causes severe acute diffuse encephalopathy. Evidence exists to implicate numerous toxins causing acute toxin encephalopathy, such as solvents and metals, in producing a chronic diffuse toxic encephalopathy. With repeated episodes of acute encephalopathy, often over many months or years, persistent impairment can occur.

Pathogenesis

Although the mechanisms are not completely understood, continuous or repeated exposures can lead to an encephalopathic condition that can no longer be completely reversed, even though the toxin itself has cleared. This process is thought to reflect the fact that typical protective mechanisms have been damaged or overwhelmed. The resulting irreversible brain damage produces persistent neurologic dysfunction. It is likely that metabolic pathways for detoxifying and excreting exogenous toxins are involved.[39] These systems are known to be in a dynamic balance, responding to external factors through complex interactions that may result in relative excesses of toxic metabolites. Extensive evidence has accumulated regarding the mechanisms of oxidative stress and apoptosis in neurodegeneration.[40] These mechanisms may provide common final pathways for injury when activated by a variety of toxic exposures.

Clinical and diagnostic approach

The clinical manifestations of chronic diffuse toxic encephalopathy usually involve varying degrees of cognitive impairment. The earliest problems are often subtle, and include changes in behavior and mood. Alternatively, a toxin may produce cognitive dysfunction to which the patient responds emotionally. The clinician may recognize the emotional change, rather than cognitive difficulties, and consider psychiatric referral. In either case, the organic nature of the complaints must be recognized. Some agents have been considered to alter mood more commonly. For example, inorganic mercury (historically used in hat manufacture) has been associated with mania, typified by the Mad Hatter in *Alice in Wonderland*, while carbon disulfide has been associated with depression. Generalizations regarding mood effects are probably not justified; psychosocial factors unique to the exposed individual are likely more important in determining that individual's response.

With progressive dysfunction, cognitive impairment becomes more readily apparent in the history and physical examination. Complaints and examples of declining skills include trouble balancing a checkbook, difficulty remembering appointments, and getting lost in conversations or while traveling. Unfortunately, the condition can remain unrecognized or attributed to other causes until it has advanced to the stage of frank dementia.

Much of the laboratory evaluation is devoted to excluding the rare, treatable causes of dementia. Exactly what constitutes an appropriate panel of screening tests has been debated.[41] In the appropriate exposure scenario, a broader battery of testing is indicated. For example, evidence of exposure to heavy metals can be assessed directly by measuring levels in the blood or urine. Because these levels are more reflective of recent exposures, they may not adequately assess relevant past exposures or the body's accumulation of the metal (see Chapter 39). When the index of suspicion is high, a chelation challenge can be performed to exclude more completely the possibility of previous exposures, such as with lead. Unfortunately, such measurements are variable, making it crucial that clinical correlation guide appropriate treatment.[42] The differential diagnosis of presenile or senile dementia of the Alzheimer's type should also be considered.

Treatment and prognosis

Specific therapies for chronic diffuse toxic encephalopathies are limited, as would be predicted with diffuse destruction of brain tissue that generally lacks the capacity to regenerate. The patient should be separated as soon as possible from the neurotoxic exposure, and, in the case of certain metals, chelation therapy can be considered in an attempt to reduce the body's accumulated burden of the toxin. Other agents that can further injure the brain should be strictly avoided, as it does not make sense to avoid one neurotoxin but to continue being exposed to others – e.g., alcohol use. Medications prescribed by physicians should be reviewed carefully to exclude those drugs whose effects might adversely impact cognitive function.

The prognosis for a return of cognitive function is poor. Even in the absence of further exposure, cognitive function may continue to decline with aging. On the other hand, changes in behavior and mood may be more amenable to treatment; consultation with a psychiatrist may be helpful, in this regard. Anxiety or depression can aggravate cognitive impairment, and treatment of psychologic factors may result in significant improvement. Cognitive therapy and strategies to improve organizational skills may be appropriate, and should be supervised by a trained neuropsychologist.

Specific agents

Similar to the acute diffuse toxic encephalopathy, clinical symptoms and signs of the chronic diffuse toxic encephalopathy are non-specific and are not associated exclusively with a particular exposure. Thus, the clinical appearance may be the same whether the exposure has been a solvent, such as toluene, or a metal, such as inorganic lead. Of note, such non-specific encephalopathies can also follow exposures to agents that have the potential to yield selective injuries with specific syndromes. For example, in some patients, exposure to carbon monoxide

656 Central Nervous System Diseases

results in a chronic diffuse toxic encephalopathy instead of the selective injury to the basal ganglia, discussed in the next section.

Selective toxic encephalopathy

Why some neurotoxins exert selective effects, injuring a particular part of the nervous system, remains uncertain in most cases. For instance, the globus pallidus is particularly sensitive to carbon monoxide, and the occipital cortex to mercury. For some of these toxins, selective effects reflect pathophysiologic actions through specific cellular mechanisms.[38] The resulting clinical syndromes can reflect either reduced function within the injured neurotransmitter system or a relative imbalance between the functions of remaining neurotransmitter systems. Although it is likely that selective encephalopathies reflect both nervous system-related and exposure-related factors, the reasons for selective vulnerability of specific brain regions are largely unknown.

One factor that may explain some of the variation in susceptibility is the timing of exposures relative to critical periods of nervous system development. The nervous system's many discrete neuronal populations and interacting systems continue to develop at variable rates throughout the first three decades of life. Toxic exposures may exert their most profound effects when the organism is in a particularly vulnerable stage, leading to problems that would not occur with exposures at other stages of life.[43] The most prominent example of this phenomenon is the susceptibility of infants to lead encephalopathy, which underscores the importance of thorough neurodevelopmental toxicology testing.[4]

Most of the toxins capable of producing an acute selective toxic encephalopathy act on neurons. While it is possible for any constituent of the CNS to be the target of a selective toxin, clinical examples of damage to the CNS's glial cells, myelin, or vasculature are uncommon and will not be discussed here. Rather, the discussion will concentrate on the toxins directed at the neuron itself, considering those acting on the neuron cell body, ion channels, neurotransmitter systems, or structural integrity. As opposed to the toxins leading to the non-specific encephalopathies described in the previous section, many of these toxins produce characteristic syndromes. Examples of some selective neurotoxins (Table 28.1.5) are discussed in the following section.

Cell bodies

Some neurologic diseases are characterized by pathologic findings involving loss of a particular population of neuronal cell bodies. For example, pigmented cells of the substantia nigra are lost in Parkinson's disease, anterior horn cells in amyotrophic lateral sclerosis, and pyramidal cells of the hippocampal formation in Alzheimer's disease. Although the initiating factors may not necessarily involve attack directly at the cell body, the loss of cell bodies is what distinguishes these diseases from others in which the pathophysiology primarily involves cellular dysfunction

rather than cellular death. The mechanisms of cell death activated in these diseases remain uncertain, but evidence implicating the related mechanisms of mitochondrial dysfunction, energy depletion, oxidative stress, and apoptosis continues to accumulate.[40,44]

Perhaps the most prominent example of a selective neurotoxin is MPTP. Research on the effects of MPTP has revitalized interest in the basic mechanisms activated by selective neurotoxins in producing neurologic disease. These findings have raised substantial concerns regarding the contribution of toxins to degenerative diseases of the CNS. The distinct possibility exists that devastating illnesses such as Parkinson's disease, amyotrophic lateral sclerosis, Alzheimer's disease, and many others, whose causes have been considered idiopathic, are actually related to environmental toxins. The strength of these arguments is largely related to what has been learned from the MPTP model of Parkinson's disease.

MPTP became infamous as a meperidine derivative that some intravenous drug abusers mistakenly injected in the hope of achieving narcotic effects.[45] These individuals rapidly developed a condition virtually indistinguishable from idiopathic Parkinson's disease. MPTP was later shown to produce similar effects when given to certain animal species, and using those models, the mechanism of action of MPTP has been identified.[46] A key step involves its conversion by glial monoamine oxidase B to 1-methyl-4-phenylpyridium ion (MPP+). Support for the concept of MPTP being a toxic precursor, or protoxin, is that inhibition of monoamine oxidase B can prevent the effects of MPTP. MPP+ has avid affinity for the dopamine transporter located at the terminal axons of dopaminergic neurons. It is thereby concentrated selectively in dopaminergic cells of the substantia nigra, activating a lethal biochemical cascade. Most intriguing from an occupational and environmental perspective is that MPP+ is a substance called cyperquat, used in the past as an herbicide and chemically related to paraquat, an herbicide that remains in common use. Even more compelling is a recent report describing the effects of rotenone, a common pesticide and mitochondrial complex I inhibitor.[47] With chronic, systemic exposures to rotenone, rats developed a neurodegenerative disease with pathologic findings comparable to human Parkinson's disease patients.[48]

Elucidation of the mechanism for neurotoxic injury related to MPTP raises the possibility that other neurotoxins could affect selective neuronal populations, resulting in clinical manifestations of neurodegenerative diseases. An apparent inconsistency is that these diseases usually manifest as progressive disorders in later life, whereas the most intense chemical exposures proposed to cause them probably occur over a limited period, at an earlier age. This inconsistency may be explained through the combined effects of aging and exposure to a selective toxin (Fig. 28.1.2). Later in life, neurons begin to die, presumably as a part of natural aging. Normally, the excess of neurons in the brain protects against the development of symptoms. However, the loss of neurons may be more important if a proportion of the available cells have been eliminated by an earlier exposure. In

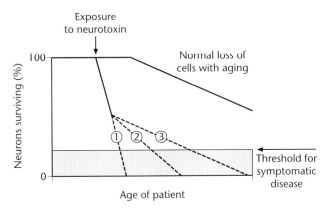

Figure 28.1.2: Hypothetical loss of neurons with exposure to a selective neurotoxin. The loss may be so great that the threshold for symptomatic disease is crossed at the time of an acute exposure (option 1). Alternatively, not enough neurons may be destroyed to produce symptomatic disease acutely. But with further loss due to increased vulnerability (option 2) or to aging alone (option 3), the threshold for symptomatic disease may be crossed. (Modified from Langston JW. Predicting Parkinson's disease. Neurology 1990; 40(Suppl 3):70-74.)

this case, the subsequent age-related loss of cells may lead to a point where a threshold is passed. Beyond this threshold, the loss of cells leads to clinically apparent disease that slowly progresses as the aging process continues. Alternatively, the toxin may have made the cells more vulnerable to the effects of aging, resulting in accelerated senescence. Such hypotheses have generated interest in many idiopathic degenerative diseases of the brain and spinal cord, as conditions that are potentially related to environmental toxins, and prompted a search for a multifactorial model to explain why some individuals are more susceptible to neurotoxic effects.

Ion channels

Normal nervous system function depends intimately on membrane-associated ion channels. Consequently, brain function can be severely disrupted when ion channels are affected by a neurotoxin. Some of the most potent biologic toxins have ion channels as their target.[49–52] Some of these channel blockers include tetrodotoxin from puffer fish and saxitoxin from shellfish contaminated by a red tide. Other toxins potentiate channel function by increasing either the frequency or duration of channel openings, thereby increasing ionic permeability. Examples include ciguatoxin from certain marine fish, and some insecticides, including organochlorines and pyrethrins.

Biologic toxins are typically found in specific geographic areas, and although the clinical syndrome may suggest the diagnosis, these conditions are so rare that a high index of suspicion and thorough history are the keys to diagnosis. A greater threat is probably associated with insecticides, because of their widespread use. With any toxin that affects membrane channels, sensory symptoms around the mouth and face can be the earliest manifestations. With higher exposures, sensory symptoms become more widespread and motor signs of intoxication develop.

Seizures can also occur, especially with organochlorine pesticides. With severe poisoning, paralysis and respiratory arrest may intervene, resulting in death. Treatment is usually supportive, and, assuming no complication such as cardiopulmonary arrest has occurred, recovery may be complete.

Neurotransmitter systems

The number and diversity of known neurotransmitter systems have steadily increased. These systems provide a direct means by which a toxin can produce selective dysfunction of the CNS. Regulation of synaptic neurotransmission is complex, and any aspect can become the target of a toxin. Thus, a toxin can act to block or stimulate a postsynaptic receptor, block or be taken up by a synaptic transport system, or block transmitter degradation enzymes. Many of these effects occur with pharmaceutical agents commonly used in clinical practice. More relevant to the current discussion are the effects of naturally occurring biologic toxins and synthetic chemicals encountered in occupational settings and as environmental contaminants.

Cholinergic system   One of the most well-characterized neurotransmitter systems is the cholinergic system. Acute cholinergic dysfunction produces a set of distinct clinical syndromes, characterized by relative excess or deficiency of cholinergic activity. A number of toxins can produce excess activation of the cholinergic system. The hyperactivity can occur directly with toxins acting as receptor agonists, such as those found in certain species of mushrooms (e.g. *Amanita muscaria*, for which a whole class of cholinergic receptors is named). Alternatively, activation may occur indirectly with toxins that inhibit acetylcholinesterase and thereby increase the availability of acetylcholine at the synapse. This is the mechanism of the organophosphate pesticides and organophosphorus chemical warfare agents (see Chapter 48). Still other toxins can inhibit the cholinergic system by acting as receptor blockers, such as in the plant species used in mystical rituals (e.g. *Datura stramonium*). Regardless of whether the toxin gains access to the CNS, effects on the autonomic nervous system and neuromuscular junction are common and can be used to define the severity of the poisoning.

The syndrome of cholinergic excess variably includes nausea, vomiting, diaphoresis, sialorrhea, lacrimation, abdominal cramps, diarrhea, bradycardia, miosis, and muscle fasciculations with weakness. The specific constellation of symptoms can vary between individuals. If the toxin gains access to the CNS, symptoms may include confusion, agitation, ataxia, tremor, and seizures. In some cases, the relative preponderance of peripheral symptoms can mask injury to the CNS. For example, the early course of poisoning with tri-ortho-cresyl-phosphate may be dominated by signs of lower motor neuron hypotonic weakness, later replaced by signs of upper motor neuron spasticity and incoordination.

Given the characteristic symptoms and signs, the diagnosis of cholinergic excess should be suspected and empiric treatment initiated even in the absence of a detailed history. Atropine will block the muscarinic effects of excess acetylcholine but not the nicotinic effects. Certain oxime compounds, such as pralidoxime, can facilitate acetylcholinesterase reactivation, and should be used for poisoning involving prominent nicotinic symptoms. Although these treatments may reverse the acute manifestations of cholinergic excess, with severe poisoning some cognitive and behavioral symptoms may persist and new problems may arise at the neuromuscular junction.

With toxins that produce cholinergic inhibition, hallucinatory effects are common, and for some agents are the motivation to consume the toxin. Many of the other CNS manifestations are similar to cholinergic excess, including confusion, agitation, and seizures. On the other hand, systemic symptoms are in many ways opposite to those described earlier, and include atropine-like symptoms of flushing, dry skin, tachycardia, and mydriasis. Cholinergic drugs can be administered, but usually the altered state will clear with supportive therapy alone.

Catecholaminergic systems and parkinsonism The catecholaminergic neurotransmitter systems are common targets for selective agents. This makes them some of the most important systems for pharmaceutical drug actions. The systems can become hypoactive, as with dopamine receptor blockade by antipsychotic agents, or hyperactive, as when release of endogenous stores of norepinephrine is potentiated by amphetamines. Catecholamine transporters may also be targeted, as with serotonin selective reuptake inhibitors, providing another mechanism for increasing synaptic transmission. Although many other examples exist relevant to clinical pharmaceutics and drug dependence, or occupational diseases, the most pertinent effects relate to diminished dopaminergic activity in the basal ganglia resulting in a parkinsonian syndrome.

The best understood toxin that produces parkinsonism is MPTP. As described earlier, its metabolite, MPP+, accesses neurons through a selective dopamine transporter. However, its ultimate effect is to decrease dopaminergic activity by killing cells in the substantia nigra. Other toxins that can lead to parkinsonism are carbon monoxide, carbon disulfide, and manganese.[53] Although this occurs more commonly following chronic exposures, the syndrome has been reported following a single severe exposure. Often, a diffuse encephalopathy occurs initially, with the more selective injury to the basal ganglia recognized later. For example, this has been described in patients from China with acute poisoning from ingesting mildewed sugar cane, in which the toxic agent has been identified as 3-nitropropionic acid.[54] While the severe poisoning initially produced a diffuse toxic encephalopathy, a fourth of survivors later demonstrated persistent dystonia, and MRI of these patients revealed hypodensities in the basal ganglia. In contrast to MPTP, the mechanism by which these agents induce parkinsonism involves a selective insult to the output cells of the basal ganglia located in the globus pallidus. Despite mechanistic differences, the clinical syndrome of parkinsonism is similar.

Regardless of the cause, a trial of dopaminergic drugs for bradykinesia and rigidity, or anticholinergic drugs for tremors, may be efficacious.

Glutamatergic system Another neurotransmitter system that has been studied extensively in recent years is the excitatory glutamatergic system. Excessive activation of glutamate receptors results in toxic levels of calcium influx, thereby mediating so-called excitatory neurotoxicity.[55] The complex intracellular events leading to cell death are not yet entirely clear, but the process may be involved in a variety of toxic, ischemic, and traumatic injuries to the CNS. This has motivated extensive research in the hope that modulation of such processes could provide therapeutic benefit. So far, though, clinical applications remain elusive.

Several neurotoxins are now recognized to act through hyperactivity of the glutamatergic system. One clinical syndrome was first reported in a group of patients from Canada who became acutely ill following ingestion of contaminated mussels.[56] The acute illness was characterized by headaches, seizures, hemiparesis, ophthalmoplegia, and alterations in the level of consciousness. In patients who recovered from the acute illness, chronic memory problems and peripheral polyneuropathy persisted. Neuropathologic examination in four patients who died demonstrated necrosis in the hippocampus, similar to that demonstrated in experimental animals given excitatory amino acid neurotransmitters. The offending agent has been identified as domoic acid, a potent excitotoxin.

Lathyrism is another disease related to a neurotoxin acting through the glutamatergic system. In times of famine, excessive consumption of the grass pea, *Lathyrus sativus* and related species, has led to a neurologic condition characterized by spastic paraparesis. The offending agent in the pea is thought to be beta-N-oxalylamino-L-alanine (BOAA). Like domoic acid, BOAA is proposed to mimic an excitatory neurotransmitter,[57] producing damage to the brain and spinal cord.

Amyotrophic lateral sclerosis shares some clinical features of lathyrism, suggesting that it might result from exposure to a substance that could kill or injure anterior horn cells. The increased incidence of motor neuron disease that occurs on Guam has been a mystery for years, and consumption of the cycad nut has been proposed as a cause of the condition. The cycad nut has a BOAA-like constituent, beta-N-methylamino-L-alanine. Although many uncertainties remain, the idea that an environmental excitotoxin contributes to this and other neurodegenerative diseases has gained wide acceptance.[58]

Other systems Many other neurotransmitter systems exist, including those served by small molecules, such as gamma-aminobutyric acid (GABA) and adenosine; peptides, such as the endogenous opiates; and the recently recognized atypical transmitters, such as nitric oxide and D-lysine.[59] The roles for these systems in normal neurologic function are incompletely understood. Thus, while tempting, it seems premature to speculate about the potential role for these transmitters in disease processes. Nonetheless, many drugs and toxins are known to affect these systems, and many more undoubtedly exist that are not yet recognized. History suggests that as basic information about these systems continues to accumulate, evidence for their involvement in neurotoxic processes will be forthcoming.

SUMMARY

Diseases affecting the CNS are challenging to diagnose and to treat, and those related to neurotoxins are no exception. The history and physical examination should allow the clinician to form and test hypotheses about the existence of neurotoxin-related disease. Problems of cognition and coordination should always prompt the clinician to question the patient about exposure to potential neurotoxins. Diagnostic hypotheses can be refined with judicious use of ancillary tests; however, these are frequently limited by lack of either sensitivity or specificity. Consultation with a neurologist may be useful in ruling out specific diagnoses.

A classification scheme that may be useful to a clinician involves a distinction between diffuse and selective effects, characterized further by time course and specific mechanism of toxic effect, where known. This scheme will need to be revised as more is learned about the detailed mechanism of action of neurotoxins and the interactions of the toxin with host factors, including age and genetic susceptibility. As this knowledge increases, it is likely that more and more diseases will be linked to neurotoxic exposures. Some may be previously unrecognized diseases, but more promising are the well-recognized degenerative diseases for which the cause is currently unknown and for which environmental exposures may play a role. Identification of such exposures may allow the opportunity for prevention of these often disabling and sometimes fatal degenerative diseases.

References

1. US Government, EPA. Toxic Substances Control Act (TSCA). Chemical substances inventory – revised inventory synonym and preferred name file. Washington, DC: Office of Pollution, Prevention, and Toxics; 2000.
2. US Government, EPA. Health Effects Test Guidelines. OPPTS 870 Series. Washington, DC: Office of Prevention, Pesticides, and Toxic Substances (OPPTS); 1998.
3. US Government, FaDA. Neurotoxicity studies. In: Redbook 2000 – Toxicological Principles for the Safety of Food Ingredients. Washington, DC: Center for Food Safety & Applied Nutrition, Office of Premarket Approval; 2000.
4. Claudio L, Kwa WC, Russell AL, Wallinga D. Testing methods for developmental neurotoxicity of environmental chemicals. Toxicol Appl Pharmacol 2000; 164:1-14.
5. Feldman RG, Ratner MH. The pathogenesis of neurodegenerative disease: neurotoxic mechanisms of action and genetics. Curr Opin Neurol 1999; 12:725-31.
6. Swanson PD, ed. Signs and symptoms in neurology. Philadelphia, PA: JB Lippincott; 1984.
7. Feldman RG. Occupational and environmental neurotoxicology. Philadelphia, PA: Lippincott-Raven; 1999.
8. Bleecker ML, Bolla-Wilson K, Kawas C, Agnew J. Age-specific norms for the Mini-Mental State Exam. Neurology 1988; 38:1565-8.
9. Mesholam RI, Moberg PJ, Mahr RN, Doty RL. Olfaction in neurodegenerative disease: a meta-analysis of olfactory

10. functioning in Alzheimer's and Parkinson's diseases. Arch Neurol 1998; 55:84-90.
10. Wszolek ZK, Markopoulou K. Olfactory dysfunction in Parkinson's disease. Clin Neurosci 1998; 5:94-101.
11. Smith DV. Assessment of patients with taste and smell disorders. Acta Otolaryngol Suppl 1988; 458:129-33.
12. Kulig BM. Comprehensive neurotoxicity assessment. Environ Health Perspect 1996; 104(Suppl 2):317-22.
13. Olanow CW, Arendash GW. Metals and free radicals in neurodegeneration. Curr Opin Neurol 1994; 7:548-58.
14. McGuire V, Longstreth WT Jr, Nelson LM, et al. Occupational exposures and amyotrophic lateral sclerosis. A population-based case-control study. Am J Epidemiol 1997; 145:1076-88.
15. Woolf AD. Ginger Jake and the blues: a tragic song of poisoning. Vet Hum Toxicol 1995; 37:252-4.
16. Glynn P. Neuropathy target esterase. Biochem J 1999; 344(Pt 3):625-31.
17. Louis-Ferdinand RT. Myelotoxic, neurotoxic and reproductive adverse effects of nitrous oxide. Adverse Drug React Toxicol Rev 1994; 13:193-206.
18. Riess O, Kruger R. Parkinson's disease – a multifactorial neurodegenerative disorder. J Neural Transm Suppl 1999; 56:113-25.
19. Cardoso F, Jankovic J. Movement disorders. Neurol Clin 1993; 11:625-38.
20. Montastruc JL, Llau ME, Rascol O, Senard JM. Drug-induced parkinsonism: a review. Fundam Clin Pharmacol 1994; 8:293-306.
21. Howard JS III. Cocaine, neuroleptics, and tardive dyskinesia as paleocortical escape. Integr Physiol Behav Sci 1996; 31:306-14.
22. Araki S, Yokoyama K, Murata K. Neurophysiological methods in occupational and environmental health: methodology and recent findings. Environ Res 1997; 73(1-2):42-51.
23. Allum JH, Shepard NT. An overview of the clinical use of dynamic posturography in differential diagnosis of balance disorders. J Vestib Res 1999; 9:223-52.
24. Forsting M. MR imaging of the brain: metabolic and toxic white matter diseases. Eur Radiol 1999; 9:1061-5.
25. Filley CM. Toxic leukoencephalopathy. Clin Neuropharmacol 1999; 22:249-60.
26. Triebig G, Lang C. Brain imaging techniques applied to chronically solvent-exposed workers: current results and clinical evaluation. Environ Res 1993; 61:239-50.
27. Lin Z, Chen JD. Advances in time-frequency analysis of biochemical signals. Crit Rev Biomed Eng 1996; 24:1-72.
28. Duffy FH, Hughes JR, Miranda F, Bernad P, Cook P. Status of quantitative EEG (QEEG) in clinical practice, 1994. Clin Electroencephalogr 1994; 25:VI-XXII.
29. Anger WK, Cassitto MG. Individual-administered human behavioral test batteries to identify neurotoxic chemicals. Environ Res 1993; 61:93-106.
30. Anger WK, Otto DA, Letz R. Symposium on computerized behavioral testing of humans in neurotoxicology research: overview of the proceedings. Neurotoxicol Teratol 1996; 18:347-50.
31. Bleecker ML, Hansen JA. Occupational neurology and clinical neurotoxicology. Baltimore, MD: Williams & Wilkins; 1994.
32. Manzo L, Artigas F, Martinez E, et al. Biochemical markers of neurotoxicity. A review of mechanistic studies and applications. Hum Exp Toxicol 1996; 15(Suppl 1):S20-35.
33. Brookes AJ. The essence of SNPs. Gene 1999; 234:177-86.
34. Van Zijl PC, Barker PB. Magnetic resonance spectroscopy and spectroscopic imaging for the study of brain metabolism. Ann N Y Acad Sci 1997; 820:75-96.
35. Lester DS, Pine DS, Delnomdedieu M, Johannessen JN, Johnson GA. Virtual neuropathology: three-dimensional visualization of lesions due to toxic insult. Toxicol Pathol 2000; 28:100-4.
36. Imaging Brain Structure and Function: Emerging Technologies in the Neurosciences. Proceedings of a conference. Bethesda, MD, March 28-29, 1996. Ann N Y Acad Sci 1997; 820:1-315.

37. Philbert MA, Billingsley ML, Reuhl KR. Mechanisms of injury in the central nervous system. Toxicol Pathol 2000; 28:43-53.

38. Spencer PS, Schaumburg HH, Ludolph AC. Experimental and clinical neurotoxicology, 2nd edn. New York: Oxford University Press; 2000.

39. Costa LG. The emerging field of ecogenetics. Neurotoxicology 2000; 21:85-9.

40. Cassarino DS, Bennett JP Jr. An evaluation of the role of mitochondria in neurodegenerative diseases: mitochondrial mutations and oxidative pathology, protective nuclear responses, and cell death in neurodegeneration. Brain Res Brain Res Rev 1999; 29:1-25.

41. Fleming KC, Adams, AC, Petersen RC. Dementia: diagnosis and evaluation. Mayo Clin Proc 1995; 70:1093-107.

42. Porru S, Alessio L. The use of chelating agents in occupational lead poisoning. Occup Med (Lond) 1996; 46:41-8.

43. Weiss B, Landrigan PJ. The developing brain and the environment: an introduction. Environ Health Perspect 2000; 108(Suppl 3):373-4.

44. Beal MF. Mitochondrial dysfunction in neurodegenerative diseases. Biochim Biophys Acta 1998; 1366:211-23.

45. Langston JW, Ballard P, Tetrud JW, Irwin I. Chronic parkinsonism in humans due to a product of meperidine-analog synthesis. Science 1983; 219:979-80.

46. Kopin IJ. Parkinson's disease: past, present, and future. Neuropsychopharmacology 1993; 9:1-12.

47. Degli Esposti M. Inhibitors of NADH-ubiquinone reductase: an overview. Biochim Biophys Acta 1998; 1364:222-35.

48. Betarbet R, Sherer TB, MacKenzie G, Garcia-Osuna M, Panov AV, Greenamyre JT. Chronic systemic pesticide exposure reproduces features of Parkinson's disease. Nat Neurosci 2000; 3:1301-6.

49. Watters MR. Organic neurotoxins in seafoods. Clin Neurol Neurosurg 1995; 97:119-24.

50. Grishin E. Polypeptide neurotoxins from spider venoms. Eur J Biochem 1999; 264:276-80.

51. Possani LD, Becerril B, Delepierre M, Tytgat J. Scorpion toxins specific for Na+-channels. Eur J Biochem 1999; 264:287-300.

52. Jones RM, Bulaj G. Conotoxins – new vistas for peptide therapeutics. Curr Pharm Des 2000; 6:1249-85.

53. Albin RL. Basal ganglia neurotoxins. Neurol Clin 2000; 18:665-80.

54. Ming L. Moldy sugarcane poisoning – a case report with a brief review. J Toxicol Clin Toxicol 1995; 33:363-7.

55. Dawson R Jr, Beal MF, Bondy SC, Di Monte DA, Isom GE. Excitotoxins, aging, and environmental neurotoxins: implications for understanding human neurodegenerative diseases. Toxicol Appl Pharmacol 1995; 134:1-17.

56. Teitelbaum JS, Zatorre RJ, Carpenter S et al. Neurologic sequelae of domoic acid intoxication due to the ingestion of contaminated mussels. N Engl J Med 1990; 322:1781-7.

57. Vecsei L, Dibo G, Kiss C. Neurotoxins and neurodegenerative disorders. Neurotoxicology 1998; 19:511-4.

58. Spencer PS, Ludolph AC, Kisby GE. Are human neurodegenerative disorders linked to environmental chemicals with excitotoxic properties? Ann N Y Acad Sci 1992; 648:154-60.

59. Snyder SH, Ferris CD. Novel neurotransmitters and their neuropsychiatric relevance. Am J Psychiatry 2000; 157:1738-51.

28.2 **Disorders of the Peripheral Nervous System**
Michael Pulley, Alan R Berger

The peripheral nervous system (PNS) is vulnerable to toxic and occupational injuries that may result in generalized polyneuropathies, focal compressive mononeuropathies, impaired neuromuscular transmission, or myopathy. Neurologic dysfunction may occur in isolation or in concert with other organ system involvement. Occasionally, the latter type of dysfunction suggests a toxic etiology (e.g., gastrointestinal symptoms in acute lead poisoning or alopecia and hyperkeratosis with subacute thallium poisoning). Most often, nervous system dysfunction occurs in isolation, its clinical manifestations being indistinguishable from naturally occurring disorders.

A detailed social and occupational history, and determination of the disease's course relative to the toxin exposure, is vital in establishing a link between the nervous system damage and an occupational or toxic insult. For these reasons, it is imperative that physicians caring for patients with potential occupational and environmental diseases have extensive knowledge of the way in which naturally occurring PNS diseases present, progress, and differ from those of occupational and toxic origin.

The peripheral neuropathies are a heterogeneous group of disorders; although much is known about the frequency of the different varieties of diabetic and hereditary neuropathies, there is little data concerning the overall frequency of PNS disease in the general population. A Centers for Disease Control survey of 5000 veterans, utilizing electrodiagnostic and strict clinical criteria, observed a 5% incidence of peripheral nerve dysfunction. A recent survey of 200 workers in a petrochemical facility, utilizing similar criteria, discovered 18% to have evidence of clinical or subclinical neuropathy; the overwhelming majority were traumatic-compressive. Others represented diabetic, alcoholic, and hereditary neuropathy seen in the general population. While symptomatic occupationally induced toxic neuropathy is relatively rare in North America, incidence has not been well characterized; asymptomatic toxic neuropathy may be more common, especially among exposed groups, e.g., exterminators and grouters.

CLINICAL EVALUATION
History

A focused neurologic, toxicologic, and occupational history is the cornerstone of the clinical evaluation. Because the clinical signs are usually insufficient to establish the etiology, specific elements of the history may be the only clue that suggests toxic or occupational causes. The examiner should inquire about both positive and negative symptoms relevant to motor, sensory, and autonomic function. A complete list of medications and family illnesses should be obtained. Attention should be paid to the following symptoms: (1) motor symptoms and signs, e.g., cramps, fasciculations, myokymia (undulating muscle movements), weakness, easy fatigability, and muscle wasting; (2) sensory symptoms and signs, e.g., paresthesias (tingling or burning), dysesthesias (distorted sensations elicited by tactile stimuli), pain, numbness, anesthesia, and ataxia; and (3) autonomic symptoms, e.g., gustatory sweating, postural hypotension, gastrointestinal and genitourinary dysfunction and anhidrosis.

In patients suspected of having a peripheral neuropathy, the medical history may suggest not only the presence of neuropathy but also a pre-existing medical condition that could predispose the patient to either focal nerve entrapments or a generalized peripheral neuropathy (e.g. diabetes mellitus), that may suggest the underlying physiologic nature of the neuropathy. The clinical history may also indicate whether the process is generalized (as might be caused by toxins) or focal (as seen with occupationally related nerve lesions). The history may also disclose specific items that definitively identify a specific toxin or occupational insult.

Myopathic and neuromuscular junction dysfunction are manifested by weakness without sensory loss. Weakness is most prominent in the shoulder and pelvic girdle muscles and may be reported as difficulty climbing stairs or arising from a low chair. Getting out of a car is often difficult for patients with proximal weakness. Fatigability may result from impaired neuromuscular transmission. The historian should specifically inquire about the distribution of weakness (e.g., proximal versus distal and pelvic girdle versus shoulder), the presence or absence of pain and tenderness, sensory loss, and involvement of the extraocular muscles (manifested as ptosis or diplopia). The temporal profile should be determined, specifically the acuteness of onset, chronicity, and rapidity of progression. Almost all toxic neuropathies have their onset temporally related to exposure. It is a general rule in neurotoxicology that nerve dysfunction should begin around the time of ongoing or recent exposure and should eventually stabilize after exposure is terminated.

In some cases, prolonged low-level exposure to toxins may damage the PNS so insidiously that the patient either does not recognize the dysfunction or is not able to establish a temporal relationship between exposure and disease. Therefore, the history must carefully explore all possible exposures or inciting conditions, both by the compound's formal and common name and source (e.g., mercury and its lay term, 'thermometer tubes', or nitrous oxide and its common reference, 'sniffing the blue tank').

The occupational history should focus on habits that potentially predispose the patient to occupationally related nervous system disease (e.g., does the patient wear protective devices and change clothing before coming home; whether there is eating in the workplace). The health of coworkers, family members, and household pets should be inquired about; a similar illness might indicate a common exposure. Improvement of symptoms during time away from potential exposure (e.g., weekends or holidays away from the job) and the condition of the workplace (ventilation and drainage) are important items to be determined. In addition, a complete list of occupational exposures should be obtained because, occasionally, a combination of toxins may be responsible. In some instances, a visit to the workplace is crucial in identifying a specific toxic or responsible environmental condition. In suspected iatrogenic or domestic toxicants, family members and friends should be questioned. A visit to the home may also be helpful. Specific questions regarding hobbies, food and water sources and recent pesticide applications or other chemical often yield crucial information.

Physical examination

The scope and depth of the physical examination are shaped by the information and differential diagnosis generated by the history. As an example, a history of occupational trauma suggests that a focal compressive neuropathy is likely and focuses the examination on potentially vulnerable nerves. Alternatively, a history indicating generalized nerve dysfunction directs the clinician towards probable polyneuropathy. Motor symptoms, without sensory loss, suggest muscle or neuromuscular junction dysfunction and mandate specific attention to proximal muscle strength and examination of extraocular muscles.

The neurologic examination is performed in the conventional manner; a determination should be made regarding the predominant modalities affected (motor, sensory, autonomic, or mixed) and the overall pattern, distribution, and severity of the deficits. Specific topographic patterns of peripheral nerve dysfunction include focal or multifocal, bilaterally symmetric, proximal versus distal, and upper versus lower extremity.

A brief bedside examination of mental status usually suffices when assessing patients suspected of having PNS disease. Questions should be included that examine orientation, short- and long-term memory, abstract thinking, calculation, and attention. An overall sense of the patient's mental status can often be obtained by the manner and attentiveness with which the patient relates the neurologic history. More subtle cognitive abnormalities are best identified by formal neuropsychologic testing (see Chapter 28.1).

The cranial nerve examination should especially focus on facial sensation and the strength of facial musculature. Because most neuropathic toxins produce a length-dependent distal axonopathy, facial sensation and muscle strength are spared until late in the disease course. Although facial numbness is a feature of trichlorethylene (TCE) intoxication, its presence may be related to a naturally occurring condition, such as Sjogren's syndrome or scleroderma, rather than a toxic neuropathy.

The motor examination should determine the topographic distribution of the deficit (e.g., multiple distal nerve segments, radicular or segmental, or limited to a few specific nerves). Most toxic insults produce generalized distal axonopathies; as such, weakness initially involves the distal legs with subsequent progression to the proximal leg muscles and hands. Findings that substantially differ from this, such as early proximal muscle weakness or hand involvement occurring prior to distal leg weakness, are less consistent with most toxic neuropathies and suggest another diagnosis.

Weakness and/or atrophy in a single nerve distribution usually indicates a focal peripheral nerve lesion. The examination should determine whether all muscles of that nerve are affected or only those distal to potential entrapment sites. Aside from lead and TCE, most toxins do not cause focal nerve damage; such findings most often result from focal compression, which may or may not be caused by occupationally related trauma. Muscle atrophy suggests a chronic problem. Fasciculations are clinically obvious muscle twitchings, which, aside from suggesting a lower motor neuron process, may occur with lesions anywhere from the anterior horn cell to the distal nerve terminal.

The sensory examination should attempt to identify the predominant modality (and fiber size) affected. Large-fiber dysfunction involves loss of joint position sense, vibration, touch-pressure sensitivity, areflexia, sensory ataxia, and pseudoathetosis. Small-fiber dysfunction is characterized by a loss of pain and temperature sense, retained reflexes, and occasionally, autonomic dysfunction. In general, sensory abnormalities are most reliable when they correspond to appropriate patient complaints. Unfortunately, the sensory examination findings may be inconsistent or variable. Too much diagnostic emphasis should not be placed on inconsistent or neurologically inappropriate sensory findings. The presence of hyperesthesia (exaggerated response to sensory stimuli) or dysesthesia (unpleasant response to a normal non-noxious stimulus) should be noted. Mild sensory deficits are best appreciated when sensory stimuli are initially applied to areas of lesser sensitivity, and then the results are compared with those in corresponding normal areas.

Patterns of sensory deficits include a distal stocking–glove distribution (which would be most common in generalized neuropathies), segmental or dermatomal sensory loss (as occurs with radicular disease), or sensory loss in the distribution of one or more peripheral nerves. Most toxic polyneuropathies are of a mixed nature with all sensory modalities affected. The sensory examination should be correlated with the motor findings to determine whether a generalized or focal problem exists and to localize it topographically (e.g., anterior horn cell, ventral root, dorsal root ganglia, or peripheral nerve).

Tendon reflex testing should include the biceps (C5 and C6), brachioradialis (C5 and C6), triceps (C7), patella (L3 and L4), and Achilles (S1) reflexes. Reflex loss usually localizes the process to the PNS; in contrast, hyper-reflexia usually results from upper motor neuron lesions. In generalized axonal neuropathies, the initial tendon reflex to be diminished is the Achilles, followed by the patella and upper limb reflexes. Focal or asymmetric reflex loss suggests radicular or focal peripheral nerve disease. The presence or absence of a reflex, and its intensity, are poor indicators of disease severity, progression, or recovery. Patients often substantially recover sensory and motor function, yet have a poor return of tendon reflexes.

Examination of gait and stance is of critical importance in neurologic diagnosis. Patients with weakness of distal leg muscles may walk with a steppage gait as a result of bilateral weakness of the ankle dorsiflexors. A waddling gait occurs in patients with proximal weakness. Severe large-fiber sensory loss may be initially manifested as gait instability, resulting in a wide-based stance and instability on standing with the eyes closed but not with eyes open (positive Romberg's test). Painful neuropathies may preclude the patient from walking; such individuals often walk on their toes to avoid tactile stimulation to their soles or have a slow, hesitant gait because of painful movements (antalgic gait). Tests of coordination are generally normal in patients with peripheral nerve disease. Severe sensory loss resulting in limb and gait ataxia should not be confused with cerebellar disease.

LABORATORY EVALUATION
Electrodiagnostic studies

The most critical laboratory investigation in evaluating peripheral neuropathies is the electrodiagnostic examination. Commonly referred to as nerve conduction velocity (NCV) and electromyography (EMG), the study consists of a nerve conduction portion, in which electrical stimulation is externally applied to the nerves to determine their conductive properties, and a needle EMG portion, which utilizes a sterile needle electrode, inserted directly into the muscle. Needle EMG assesses the electrical activity of a muscle and provides information regarding muscle function and motor unit integrity. Taken in concert, nerve conduction and needle EMG studies provide objective measurements of muscle, neuromuscular junction, and peripheral nerve function and are invaluable in diagnosing diseases of the PNS.

Techniques employed

Sensory conduction studies. The most sensitive electrophysiologic technique in evaluating peripheral neuropathies is the determination of sensory and mixed nerve conduction velocities and sensory potential amplitudes. Sensory conduction studies are performed by electrically stimulating either the pure sensory nerve or the mixed sensorimotor nerve. The recordings are made over the respective nerves, either distal (antidromic recording) or proximal (orthodromic recording) to the site of stimulation. Stimulation must always be supramaximal to ensure activation of all available sensory axons, and strict attention must be paid to limb temperature and proper positioning of recording and stimulating electrodes.

Sensory potentials may be difficult to obtain in elderly patients or those with peripheral nerve disease and usually require computer averaging to increase the signal-to-noise ratio. Information obtained from conventional nerve conduction studies predominantly reflects conduction within large-diameter sensory fibers. Degeneration of sensory axons is directly reflected by a diminution of sensory potential amplitudes. As such, amplitude abnormalities, rather than conduction velocities, tend to be the most sensitive indicator of an axonal peripheral neuropathy.

Segmental demyelination results in prolongation of distal latencies and slowed conduction velocity. Sensory

potentials are often temporally dispersed, resulting in complex polyphasic (serrated) potentials. Unlike neuropathies, preganglionic lesions (at or proximal to the root level) do not affect the distal sensory potential. Sensory conduction studies are therefore useful in distinguishing radicular disease from peripheral neuropathy.

Motor conduction studies. Motor conduction studies are performed by supramaximally stimulating mixed or motor nerves and recording the compound muscle action potential (CMAP) over the muscle's endplate region. Stimulation is at a proximal and distal site, and conduction velocity is determined for the intervening nerve segment. The amplitude of the CMAP represents the surface-recorded summation of multiple muscle fiber potentials, and as such, it parallels but does not directly correlate with the number of available motor axons. Because CMAPs are in the millivolt rather than the microvolt range (like sensory potentials), they are usually easier to obtain and do not require averaging techniques. Motor conduction velocities can be determined for any accessible nerve by varying the site of stimulation. Similar to sensory conduction, motor conduction studies generally reflect large-fiber function; the distal latency and conduction velocity reflect conduction in the fastest fibers.

All neuropathic lesions, including peripheral neuropathies, which result in axonal degeneration, will diminish CMAP amplitude. In most axonal sensorimotor neuropathies, changes in motor potential amplitudes lag behind those of sensory potentials. In axonal neuropathies, distal latencies and motor conduction velocities tend to remain unchanged until the loss of large-diameter, fast-conducting fibers necessitates conduction through only small-diameter fibers. In contrast, demyelinating neuropathies result in distal motor latency prolongation, slowed motor conduction velocities, and CMAP temporal dispersion; this is especially evident with proximal stimulation. Low-amplitude CMAPs with intact corresponding sensory potentials strongly suggest pathologic changes at or proximal to the root level. When motor or sensory conduction is focally slowed across a potential entrapment site, a compressive lesion should be suspected.

Needle EMG. Needle electrode recordings from normal and injured muscle provides crucial information regarding motor unit function. Resting normal muscle has little or no electrical activity aside from brief insertional discharges. Separation of the muscle fiber from its innervating nerve fiber (denervation) results in abnormal electrical activity, termed spontaneous activity (fibrillation or positive sharp wave potentials that occur with the needle at rest). The degree of spontaneous activity is only a rough guide to the extent of motor unit degeneration. Spontaneous activity is usually indicative of a neuropathic process, although it can also be seen in certain myopathies and, occasionally, in normal muscles.

Fasciculation potentials may be evident clinically and by needle EMG. They represent the involuntary and random firing of single motor units. They have little localizing value because they may occur with anterior horn cell disease, radiculopathies, peripheral neuropathies, and a number of benign conditions.

Quantitative analysis of voluntary motor units (amplitude, duration, and degree of polyphasia) provides information regarding the chronicity of the neuropathic lesion or may suggest the presence of a myopathic process. Chronic motor unit reinnervation results in motor unit potentials (MUPs) that are increased in amplitude and prolonged in duration and may be polyphasic compared with those of normal units. This is in contrast to the small-amplitude, short-duration MUPs evident in many myopathies. Needle EMG also provides information regarding voluntary motor unit recruitment. Reduced recruitment is characteristic of most neuropathic conditions; myopathies tend to have normal motor unit recruitment despite clinical weakness. Because needle EMG analysis can be performed on multiple proximal and distal muscles, it is useful in determining the distribution and severity of a neuropathic process.

Quantitative sensory testing. Quantitative sensory testing (QST) is a non-invasive, painless technique to quantify vibration, temperature, and pain appreciation. It uses precisely measured and repeatable sensory stimuli to determine the absolute threshold of sensory appreciation. Several commercially available QST devices exist for each sensory modality to be quantified. QST is simple and can be administered by technicians. Accurate, age-controlled mean and standard deviation values are available. QST is especially recommended for rapid screening of large populations (e.g., workers at risk for toxic neuropathy) and/or longitudinal evaluations of patients at risk for subtle sensory dysfunction (e.g., cumulative trauma disorders). QST abnormalities may predate nerve conduction abnormalities in generalized peripheral neuropathies.

Nerve biopsy. The utility of nerve biopsy has been exaggerated. It has limited use in patients with generalized axonal toxic neuropathies and should be reserved for centers that have the expertise to examine and quantify the specimen fully. Nerve biopsy is usually performed on the sural nerve at the ankle and calf level. It is most helpful in identifying the etiology of multifocal neuropathies, such as amyloidosis, sarcoidosis, leprosy, and vasculitis. In general, nerve biopsy has little or no role in the evaluation of the patient with suspected toxic neuropathy because most of these entities result in axonal degeneration without specific diagnostic findings distinct from endocrine, metabolic, or nutritional neuropathies. Specific exceptions, such as suspected exposures resulting in giant axonal neuropathy, are discussed in the section on specific toxic neuropathy below.

PATHOPHYSIOLOGY OF PNS DISORDERS

Neurotoxic and occupational insults to the PNS usually produce syndromes that clinically mimic naturally occurring disorders. The PNS is relatively limited in the ways it manifests injury. Certain insults tend to produce stereotypical disease manifestations; their recognition helps establish the nature of the neuropathic lesion.

Classification involves identifying the main site of neuropathic dysfunction (e.g., muscle, neuromuscular junction, or peripheral nerve, with differentiation between cell body, axon, and myelin) and the distribution of such lesions (e.g., proximal, distal symmetric, focal, multifocal, or segmental). The following is a brief summary of the generic types of peripheral nerve dysfunction, each of which may be caused by a number of metabolic, nutritional, infectious, and ischemic causes, as well as by toxins and trauma.

Symmetric generalized neuropathies

Distal axonopathies (central-peripheral axonopathy and dying back neuropathy)

The most common peripheral neuropathy that results from PNS insults, particularly toxin-induced injuries, is a symmetric distal axonopathy (Fig. 28.2.1). In many cases, the biochemical and pathophysiologic mechanisms are poorly understood. These neuropathies probably reflect failure of axonal transport, with resultant degeneration of vulnerable distal nerve segments, predominantly affecting large-diameter axons. Degeneration subsequently proceeds proximally toward the nerve cell body, both in the PNS and in central projections within the spinal cord.

Most distal symmetric axonopathies have a subacute onset with gradual progression. Neuropathies resulting from low-level toxin exposure may be relatively asymptomatic, with deficits apparent only to the physician on careful neurologic examination. Because the longest, largest diameter fibers are usually the most clinically affected, motor and sensory findings initially appear in the feet, only later moving proximally (length-dependent relationship). Sensory loss is initially in a stocking, and later glove, distribution. As the neuropathy worsens, the distal ends of intercostal nerves are affected, producing a cuirass, or shield, over the midthorax and abdomen. With extreme progression, the vertex of the head is affected. There is usually an early and symmetric loss of ankle reflexes; the more proximal reflexes may be spared until late in the disease. In most toxic neuropathies, sensory symptoms and signs initially predominate over motor deficits. Muscle wasting may occur in chronic cases, and trophic changes may be present, including loss of hair over the distal leg, skin ulceration, and loss of sweating in the feet.

Because recovery depends on axonal regrowth, complete recovery is often prolonged and slow. Axonal regeneration occurs at a rate of, on average, 2–3 mm/day. Even after removal from exposure, recovery may take months to years as the recovering nerves regenerate to their muscle end-organs through intact Schwann cell tubes, or uninjured motor axons supply collateral sprouts that innervate denervated muscle fibers. Function is restored in the reverse order to that lost; proximal muscles recover before distal muscles, and sensory loss recedes from proximal to distal levels. The clinical manifestations of concur-

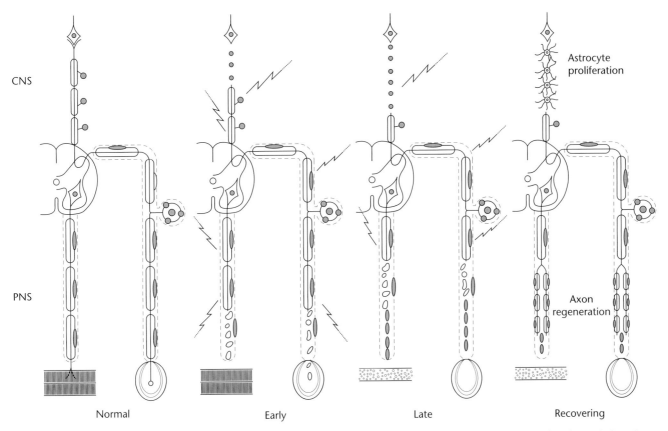

Figure 28.2.1: The cardinal pathologic features of toxic distal axonopathy. The jagged lines (lightning bolts) indicate that the toxin is acting at multiple sites along motor and sensory axons in the peripheral nervous system (PNS) and central nervous system (CNS). Axon degeneration has moved proximally (dying-back) by the late stage. Recovery in the CNS is impeded by astroglial proliferation. (Adapted from Schaumburg HH, Spencer PS, Thomas PK, eds. Disorders of peripheral nerves. Philadelphia: FA Davis, 1983.)

rent degeneration of central axons may be initially masked by the lower motor neuron dysfunction but become clinically evident as peripheral nerve function recovers. The sequential manifestation of early PNS dysfunction, followed by central nervous system (CNS) symptoms as PNS function improves, is especially characteristic of some toxic neuropathies (e.g., organophosphates). Symptoms of CNS dysfunction include hyper-reflexia, Babinski's signs, and spastic tone.

Demyelinating neuropathies

Acquired demyelinating neuropathies (myelinopathies) are conditions in which the predominant lesions occur in the myelin sheath or Schwann cells (Fig. 28.2.2). Various degrees of associated axonal degeneration may accompany them. The most common example of an acquired demyelinating neuropathy is the Guillain–Barré syndrome (acute inflammatory demyelinating neuropathy, AIDP). Almost all toxins result in axonal rather than demyelinating neuropathies, with the notable exceptions of buckthorn toxin, diphtheria toxin, and perhexiline (Pexid).

Acquired demyelinating neuropathies usually have a subacute onset. Although initial clinical deficits usually involve the distal limbs, similar to axonopathies, the demyelinating neuropathies may be patchy, resulting in early proximal weakness, arm involvement before legs, and facial numbness. Early and diffuse areflexia is charac-

teristic. Unlike axonopathies, in which sensory symptoms predominate, myelinopathies may be predominantly motor. Sensory symptoms may be transient, mild, or inapparent. Large- rather than small-fiber modalities tend to be most severely affected. Occasionally, this large-fiber sensory loss results in limb and gait ataxia. Muscle wasting is usually minimal unless substantial axonal degeneration has occurred. Recovery not only begins earlier than with axonopathies but is usually more complete, owing to the greater number of intact axons. Signs of CNS dysfunction are only rarely present, resulting from concurrent demyelination within the CNS.

Neuronopathies

Injury to the cell body is termed neuronopathy; the clinical manifestations reflect dysfunction restricted to the segments innervated by the affected cell bodies. Neuronopathies are rarely caused by toxic insults. Motor, sensory, and autonomic neurons may be affected. Toxic neuronopathies, such as those from mercury, may affect the CNS or PNS, and neurons (Fig. 28.2.3); other causes of toxic neuronopathies include pyridoxine, megavitaminosis and doxorubicin (Adriamycin).

The pathologic basis is heterogeneous and, in most cases, poorly understood. Toxic neuronopathies, such as that from doxorubicin, probably result from disruption of sensory neuron nucleic acid metabolism with subsequent

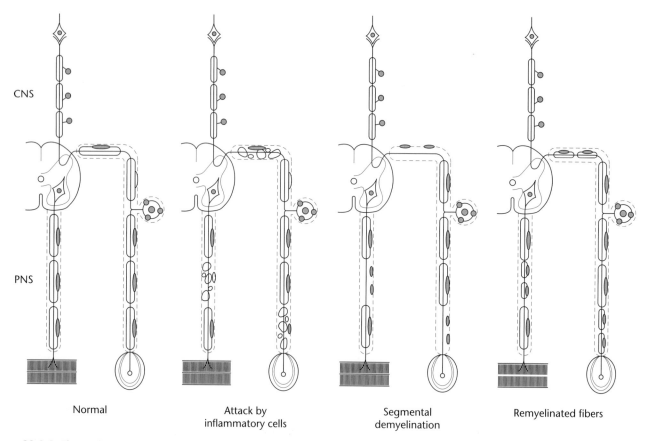

CNS

PNS

Normal

Attack by
inflammatory cells

Segmental
demyelination

Remyelinated fibers

Figure 28.2.2: The cardinal pathologic features of an inflammatory PNS myelinopathy. Axons are spared, as is CNS myelin. (Adapted from Schaumburg HH, Spencer PS, Thomas PK, eds. Disorders of peripheral nerves. Philadelphia: FA Davis, 1983.)

sensory axon degeneration. Dorsal root ganglia may be vulnerable to high molecular weight toxins because of a poorly formed blood–nerve barrier. The presence of fenestrated blood vessels in dorsal root ganglia increases vascular permeability and therefore toxin exposure.

Most neuronopathies are characterized by rapid or subacute onset of motor or sensory deficits that do not obey the length-dependent relationships seen with distal axonopathies. Initial sensory loss can occur anywhere; facial numbness occurring concurrently with sensory loss in the limbs is characteristic and reflects simultaneous involvement of cranial nerve and spinal dorsal root ganglia. Sensory loss is usually widespread, but strength is preserved. Although all sensory modalities are affected, vibration and position sense are the most severely impaired. Generalized areflexia is common and reflects loss of large-fiber function. Recovery is variable and often incomplete because of sensory neuron degeneration. Ganglion cells that are damaged but not killed may recover. Clinical recovery depends on the return of function within surviving neurons and collateral sprouting from intact sensory axons. Although CNS signs are not invariable, they may be present.

Focal (mononeuropathy) and multifocal neuropathies

Focal neuropathies may be caused by traumatic compression, chronic entrapment in fibro-osseous tunnels, traction

injuries, or ischemic injury, usually caused by small-vessel angiopathy (such as diabetes or necrotizing arteritis). Focal neuropathies are rare in toxic disease (exceptions are lead-related neuropathy, initially producing wrist drop, and TCE, producing trigeminal neuropathy). The most common focal neuropathies include:
1. Median nerve entrapment at the wrist or elbow.
2. Ulnar nerve entrapment at the elbow or wrist.
3. Radial nerve compression in the upper arm or forearm.

Focal nerve lesions can be classified by the degree of myelin and axonal injury. Various nomenclature systems have been proposed; regardless of which is used, each specifies the nature of the nerve injury as follows.
1. Mild injury in which myelin is damaged but the axon cylinders remain unaffected (Class I, neurapraxia).
2. More severe injury in which axonal continuity is lost but the nerve's connective tissue framework is maintained (Class II, axonotmesis).
3. Injury in which both nerve fibers and the connective tissue framework with varying degrees of damage (Class III, neurotmesis).

Aside from severe industrial accidents with open wounds, most occupationally related focal neuropathies are Class I and II. Some entrapments may be predisposed by an underlying, baseline condition. As an example, some patients with carpal tunnel syndrome (CTS) have congenitally small diameters of the carpal tunnel, a condition predisposing to median nerve entrapment. Focal neuropathies are charac-

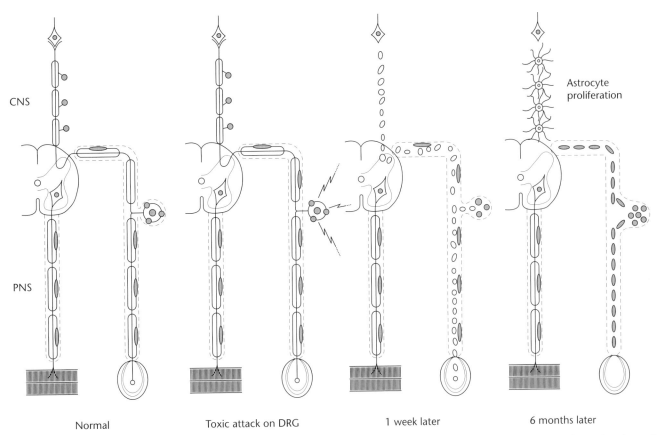

CNS

PNS

Astrocyte
proliferation

Normal   Toxic attack on DRG   1 week later   6 months later

Figure 28.2.3: The cardinal features of a rapidly involving toxic sensory neuronopathy. The jagged lines (lightning bolts) indicate that the toxin is directed at neurons in the dorsal root ganglion (DRG). Degeneration of these cells is accompanied by fragmentation and phagocytosis of their peripheral-central processes. The Schwann cells remain; there is no axonal regeneration. (Adapted from Schaumburg HH, Spencer PS, Thomas PK, eds. Disorders of peripheral nerves. Philadelphia: FA Davis, 1983.)

terized by sensory and motor deficits within the distribution of the involved nerve or nerves. Many entrapments, such as CTS, are associated with pain, which may bring the patient to medical attention. In some instances, the mononeuropathy may be symptomatic only during, or after, repeated movement or work-related activities.

Other entrapments, such as ulnar nerve lesions at the elbow or wrist, may be painless and present with weakness more than with sensory loss. Such cases may initially display advanced degrees of muscle atrophy because of the long delay in seeking medical attention. In focal neuropathies, only the segmental reflexes subserved by the involved nerve are affected. The degree of recovery generally depends on the underlying etiology (overuse, ganglion, fibrous band, hypertrophied muscle, or inflammation), the ability to avoid aggravating activities, and the degree of motor axon degeneration.

TOXIC AND OCCUPATIONAL PNS DISORDERS
Toxic peripheral neuropathies

Toxic polyneuropathies (TxPN) are relatively infrequent in North America. Most toxic polyneuropathies encountered in routine clinical practice are due to iatrogenic pharmaceutical intoxications, with occupational exposures less common. The majority, and unfortunately the most difficult, cases of TxPN are individual intoxications due to small-scale occupational exposures, or intentional and homicidal ingestions.

The identification that a sporadic peripheral neuropathy results from toxin exposure in the occupational setting is often made difficult by an unclear exposure history. TxPN are usually distal axonopathies and thus clinically and electrophysiologically resemble neuropathies from metabolic abnormalities, nutritional deficiencies, or systemic illness. Clinically relevant and reliable toxicologic tests are often unavailable or unhelpful, either because the necessary laboratory tests are not available, or the substance is undetectable because of the delay between exposure and examination. When a naturally occurring medical cause is not *readily* apparent, diagnosis of a TxPN must be made with caution based on the principles discussed below (see following section).

The underlying pathology of many TxPN is a central-peripheral axonopathy.[1,2] Our limited knowledge of the biochemical and pathophysiologic mechanisms of most neurotoxins has led to an overly simplified classification system according to compound class (e.g., solvents, metals). Such a classification is of limited clinical utility. A compound should not be presumed to be neurotoxic because of a superficial resemblance to a related known toxin of similar class; all compounds within the same class are not necessarily neurotoxic (e.g., acrylamide monomer is capable of producing a devastating peripheral neuropathy, while the polymer does not). Structure–toxicity relationships are clear for some classes of substances, such as organophosphates and hydrocarbons.

Cardinal tenets of neurotoxic illness affecting the peripheral nervous system

The identification of a neurotoxic illness should satisfy, or at least not be inconsistent with, the following basic principles of neurotoxic disease.[3] The key to correctly recognizing the presence of a TxPN does not depend on remembering the specific characteristics of the many potential neurotoxins, as much as understanding and applying these basic tenets.

Strong dose–response relationship. Most neurotoxins produce a consistent pattern of disease, commensurate with the dose and duration of exposure. Neurotoxins rarely cause focal or asymmetric deficits. Since most neurotoxins cause diffuse myelin and/or neuronal dysfunction, their related symptoms and signs are usually widespread and symmetric. In the case of TxPN, this usually means a relatively symmetric distal axonopathy with initial symptoms in the feet and proximal progression, with continued exposure. Less frequently does an occasional toxin cause strikingly asymmetric or focal dysfunction (e.g., lead and trichloroethylene).

Consistency of response. Although the same toxin may produce strikingly different clinical syndromes if the exposure dose or duration is different, a similar and consistent illness typically results in patients with similar exposures (though individual variation may occur). Neurotoxicity should be suspected when similar clinical manifestations occur in a group of individuals with a common chemical exposure.

Proximity of symptoms to exposure. Neurotoxic illness usually occurs concurrent with exposure or following a short latency. Neurologic symptoms do not generally begin months to years after exposure. The two most common exceptions are the 2–6-week delay following exposure to organophosphates and the occasional 2-month latency between cisplatin intoxication and onset of neuropathic symptoms.

In addition, the extent and severity of neuropathy are usually commensurate with the degree of toxin exposure. Thus, it is unlikely that a single, brief, low-level exposure will result in a devastating peripheral neuropathy.

Some lipid stored agents (e.g., chlorinated hydrocarbons) are detectable in fat biopsies years following exposure. Although this provides a valuable marker of previous exposure, there is no evidence that this state is associated with risk for future neurotoxicity, and attempts at removal or mobilizing the body burden are unnecessary.

Improvement usually follows cessation of exposure. Toxic polyneuropathies generally plateau and then gradually improve after removal of the neurotoxic agent. Some

degree of recovery is the rule, except in the most severely affected cases. A neuropathy that shows no improvement or continues to deteriorate, despite the cessation of exposure to a suspected neurotoxin, is less likely to be neurotoxic in nature. The clinical picture may become somewhat murky, however, in certain toxic axonopathies in which cessation of exposure may be followed by worsening of symptoms (coasting) for several weeks before recovery commences.

Confusing aspects of neurotoxic illness

Multiple clinical syndromes may result from different levels of exposure to a single toxin. Different exposure levels to the same substance may produce dramatically different syndromes. Most confusing is the bizarre constellation of symptoms that may arise from intoxication with intermediate levels of a neurotoxin. Examples include the different clinical syndromes produced by acute high-level and intermediate-level exposure, and prolonged low-level acrylamide intoxication. Exposures to high-level acrylamide causes early CNS dysfunction with drowsiness, disorientation, hallucinations, seizures, and severe truncal ataxia, followed by neuropathy of variable severity. In contrast, prolonged, lower-level exposure causes minimal CNS dysfunction but a marked peripheral neuropathy. Exposure to intermediate levels of acrylamide causes hallucinations, mental confusion and cognitive dysfunction, followed by sensory complaints affecting the distal limbs.

Another example is organophosphate poisoning in which there may be early, severe cholinergic symptoms resulting from excessive muscarinic receptor stimulation. Within 2 weeks generalized paralysis may occur with respiratory distress owing to nicotinic receptor blockade. After a few weeks, a distal axonopathy may be evident.

In some instances, a single compound may produce similar clinical symptoms at both high-level and low-level exposure, although different anatomic structures are affected. High-dose pyridoxine intoxication produces widespread sensory loss due to dorsal root ganglion dysfunction; low-level exposure produces similar symptoms but due to a distal axonopathy.

Asymptomatic disease. Prolonged, low-level exposure may occasionally produce widespread subclinical dysfunction. Clinical deficits may go unnoticed by the patient unless they perform a skilled job that requires fine-motor control or intact sensibility. Insidiously developing subclinical TxPN may occur in individuals who deny any disability.

Enhancement by chemical interaction. An agent without known neurotoxic activity may enhance the toxicity of a known neurotoxin that is present at a generally subtoxic level, a phenomenon sometimes termed the 'bystander effect'. This phenomenon has raised the general public's concern that the combined effects of multiple chemicals in hazardous waste disposal sites may be more toxic than their separate effects. Such sites may contain low, levels of neurotoxic solvents, metals or pesticides, whose neurotoxicity may be potentiated by one or other of the chemicals present. Neurotoxic potentiation is illustrated by the epidemic of peripheral neuropathy which occurred in German youths who abused paint thinner containing n-hexane. Initially there were no instances of neuropathy, but when the paint thinner was reformulated by lowering the concentration of n-hexane and adding methyl ethyl ketone (MEK), there resulted an epidemic of severe distal axonopathy. Experimental evidence subsequently showed that while MEK by itself was not a significant neurotoxin, the compound dramatically potentiated the neurotoxic effects of n-hexane.

Chemical formula may not predict toxicity.   The neurotoxic potential of a compound cannot be accurately predicted by its chemical formula. This is especially important to consider when evaluating cases of potential occupational exposure to chemicals that superficially resemble a known neurotoxin. An example is workers exposed to acrylamide polymer, a substance without associated neurotoxicity, who have been alarmed by healthcare providers familiar only with the effects of acrylamide monomer, a potent neurotoxin. Unpredictability exists because the underlying biochemical mechanisms and active metabolites of most neurotoxins are unknown.

Identification of toxic peripheral neuropathy
The presence of a toxic peripheral neuropathy is suggested by the following:
1. clinical suspicion raised by history and reinforced by compatible findings on physical exam;
2. lack of naturally occurring alternative explanations;
3. consistency with basic principles of neurotoxic disease (see above);
4. compatible laboratory findings (e.g., electrodiagnostic studies);
5. demonstration of elevated body burdens for a neurotoxic agent, (usually available only for active or recent exposures) or resolution of condition with removal from exposure.

The initial step is a suspicion raised by a thorough occupational history. Unfortunately, most toxic polyneuropathies are insidious in onset, and many patents are unable to discern a relationship between their symptoms and chronic, low-level, toxin exposure. Inquiry should focus on potential occupational, environmental, and iatrogenic exposures. The nature of the suspected toxin should focus the physical examination towards relevant deficits. Thus a suspicion of mercury poisoning should prompt a careful examination for tremor and mild cerebellar dysfunction. The role of the neurologic exam is to demonstrate that neurologic deficits are in a pattern and of a severity that is consistent with neurotoxic illness. Since the clinical deficits resulting from a TxPN are generally symmetric in distribution, the presence of multifocal deficits should suggest a diagnosis other than neurotoxic disease. In addition, since most TxPN affect mixed nerve function, finding a purely small-fiber neuropathy makes neurotoxic disease less likely.

Determination of body burdens
Several factors potentially limit the interpretation of screening levels for heavy metals. The toxin exposure may be too remote, allowing time for the offending agent to be cleared from the blood or other biologic specimen. In cases of prolonged exposure, the neurotoxin may be sequestered in various tissues and therefore not available to laboratory identification. With some chemicals, reliable reference ranges have not been established. In some cases, identification of the toxic form of a metal is required. Caution must thus be exercised when interpreting body burden results. An example is arsenic levels, which may be raised by recent shell food ingestion due to non-toxic organic forms. In such cases special testing may be required to assess the level of toxic inorganic arsenic. In some cases prolonged exposure (e.g., lead), or elevated levels in urine or serum after chelation, may increase the sensitivity of testing.

Electrodiagnostic assessment
Electrophysiologic findings should be consistent with a distal axonopathy or mixed axonal, demyelinating neuropathy. Only a few rare neuropathies, such as n-hexane, perihexiline, amiodarone, and early arsenic poisoning, have predominant slowing of conduction velocities.

Quantitative sensory testing
Quantitative thresholds for thermal and vibration appreciation have proven useful in documenting objective evidence of sensory impairment and monitoring the course of recovery or deterioration. These procedures are non-invasive and reproducible, and can be performed by a trained technician.

Systemic features suggestive of neurotoxic disease
The neuropathies resulting from most neurotoxins are remarkably similar in both their clinical and electrophysiologic characteristics. Occasionally, there may be systemic complaints or signs which suggest the nature of the neurotoxic insult. Usually these symptoms/signs are apparent with either acute high-level, or chronic low-level intoxication. The following clinical characteristics may be the identifying feature that suggests a TxPN.
* *Acrylamide*: dermal contact associated with contact dermatitis and/or excessive sweating of hands and feet.
* *Carbon disulfide*: chronic low-level exposure associated with a variety of behavioral and psychiatric abnormalities, along with peripheral neuropathy.
* *Ethylene oxide*: cognitive impairment and neuropathy with prolonged low-level exposure.
* *Hexacarbons*: acute, high-level exposure may mimic AIDP with prominent autonomic dysfunction.
* *Lead*: Mee's lines, blood abnormalities (basophilic stippling, anemia), gastrointestinal abnormalities, and predominantly a motor neuropathy.
* *Mercury*: tremor and ataxia with a predominantly sensory neuropathy.
* *Ethyl bromide*: corticospinal and cerebellar dysfunction along with an axonal neuropathy.

- *Organophosphate intoxication*: early cholinergic symptoms, with possible intermediate syndrome preceding neuropathy and late emergence of corticospinal tract dysfunction as the peripheral neuropathy resolves.
- *Polychlorinated biphenyls*: symmetric sensory neuropathy associated with brown acneiform skin eruptions (chloracne) and brown pigmented nails.
- *Thallium*: prominent GI distress with high-level exposure, alopecia, Mee's lines, hyperkeratosis with prolonged exposure, and sensory greater than motor neuropathy.

Specific toxic neuropathies

Metals

Excessive exposure to specific inorganic and organic metal compounds may cause peripheral nerve disease. Heavy metals are commonplace in industrial and agricultural settings. Exposure may be through inadvertent contamination or through voluntary ingestion, e.g., suicide attempts with arsenic or thallium. Two properties of metals are important in regard to the peripheral neuropathies they produce. The first is that metal compounds tend to be stored in a number of body organs (e.g., lead in bones). Delayed and gradual release of the toxin back into the circulation from these tissues even after cessation of exposure, may delay the time to recovery. The second property of metals is that, when present in sufficient quantity, they rarely affect the PNS in isolation. As such, systemic symptoms and signs related to hematopoietic, renal, and gastrointestinal dysfunction may accompany the peripheral neuropathy.

Arsenic

Acute arsenic poisoning classically occurred as a homicide or suicide, where a massive exposure was the usual case. However, chronic low-grade exposure, as well as occasional acute exposures, in the occupational setting also occur. Arsenic toxicity has been described in the smelting of lead and copper ore, mining, and the manufacture of integrated circuits or microchips. Non-occupational exposure may occur through contaminated well water, tainted illicit drugs, and the use of treated lumber (e.g., CCA). Arsenic gains entry to the body by inhalation, GI absorption and via dermal contact. The toxicity of arsenic may be related to its affinity for thiol groups. This affinity leads to binding with lipoic acid, which interferes with the conversion of pyruvate to acetyl CoA, and thus energy metabolism.[4]

Clinical considerations. The manifestations of arsenic toxicity depend on the level of exposure. Acute high-level exposure results in rapid onset of severe abdominal pain, vomiting and diarrhea. Cardiovascular effects include tachycardia, hypotension and vasomotor collapse with possible death. Poisoning may also cause CNS dysfunction that may be transient (psychosis, somnolence or stupor) or prolonged (behavioral and cognitive problems).[5] If an individual survives acute high-level exposure, a neuropathy

manifests within about a week. Painful paresthesias and numbness are the predominant early symptoms beginning in the feet and then affecting the hands. Weakness soon follows and is also expressed in a length-dependent pattern, starting with the feet and later involving the hands.[6] With high-dose exposure or inadequate treatment, the weakness may become severe and involve the respiratory muscles, mimicking Guillain–Barré syndrome. The deep tendon reflexes are depressed or absent early in the process.

Chronic low-level arsenic exposure results in dermatologic manifestations prior to overt clinical neuropathy. Patients may complain of non-specific symptoms such as anorexia, malaise, generalized weakness and vomiting. The dermatologic changes that follow include white transverse lines in the nails (Mee's lines), hyperkeratosis, hyperpigmentation of the skin, and irritation of the mucous membranes. Although the neuropathy is asymptomatic at this point, careful examination or electrophysiologic testing may reveal its presence. Continued exposure leads to development of symptomatic neuropathy. As with that caused by acute exposure, this is characterized by prominent sensory burning and numbness of the feet and later the hands.

Small and large sensory fibers are affected with resultant difficulties with proprioception in addition to the dysesthesias. Weakness tends to be mild and limited to the most distal muscles. Hematologic disturbances including symptoms of anemia and pancytopenia may also result from chronic arsenic exposure. Recovery is variable, often with mild persistent neuropathy. The neuropathy may continue to worsen for a period of weeks after removal from exposure (coasting) in both the acute and chronic neuropathies, and may result in significant residua.

Diagnostic considerations. Arsenic levels may be measured in the urine, and less effectively in the hair and nails. Urine arsenic levels may remain elevated for weeks after exposure. Levels greater than 25 µg per 24 hour urine specimen are abnormal unless there was recent seafood ingestion (a source of organic arsenic). Low-level long-term exposure, or exposure that has since ceased, may only be detected by measuring levels in the hair and nails, with limited reliability. Arsenic accumulates in these tissues due to binding with keratin. Blood arsenic levels are usually not helpful unless there is active exposure.

Nerve conduction studies reveal low amplitude or absent sensory responses. There is mild slowing of motor conduction velocities indicating loss of large, fast-conducting myelinated axons. EMG reveals active and chronic denervation in distal muscles.[7]

Treatment. Acute arsenic toxicity may be life threatening and treatment in an intensive care setting with aggressive fluid and electrolyte resuscitation is indicated with cardiovascular compromise. The primary consideration in chronic arsenic toxicity is terminating exposure. Removal of arsenic from the body is facilitated by chelation therapy. The agents used are British antilewisite (BAL or dimercaprol) and dimercaptosuccinic acid (DMSA). BAL is a dithiol and allows excretion of arsenic by formation of a non-toxic ring. The treatment should be started as soon as possible after poisoning and continued for several months. Unfortunately, the fully developed neuropathy is unlikely to respond to therapy.[8]

Lead

Lead toxicity has been a common problem in the past. Although elimination of lead-based paints and other environmental sources of contamination has reduced the frequency of lead intoxication, exposure may still occur, especially in the industrial setting. Occupational exposure has been reported in battery manufacturing, smelting plants, demolition, automobile radiator repair and working in indoor gun firing ranges. Paint ingestion is still a source of lead toxicity as is drinking 'moonshine' whiskey and burning batteries for heat. Both organic and inorganic lead causes toxicity. Lead gains access to the tissues via ingestion, inhalation or dermal contact. Lead interacts with carboxyl, sulfhydryl, amino and phosphate groups.[9] This leads to disruption of the heme biosynthetic pathway and deficient activity of cytochromes, which are important for detoxification of harmful free radicals. Inorganic lead displaces calcium ions, disrupts ion transport through calcium channels, inhibits calcium adenosine triphosphatasae activity, and results in accumulation of intracellular calcium. These factors likely play a role in the neurologic toxicity of lead.

Clinical considerations. Children most commonly display CNS dysfunction from lead intoxication. This may present as chronic cognitive dysfunction (developmental delay or loss of milestones) or an acute encephalopathy (see Chapter 28.1). Encephalopathy is also seen with acute, high-level exposure in adults; in both age groups dysfunction can progress to seizures, coma, or death.[10] Although there may be some cognitive and behavioral dysfunction in adults with chronic, low-level, lead exposure, this is uncommon.

Peripheral neuropathy resulting from chronic lead exposure is most commonly seen in adults and rarely occurs in children. Lead neuropathy develops insidiously with chronic exposure. The manifestations are unusual in that motor dysfunction predominates and there may be few, if any, sensory symptoms or signs. The pattern is distal, symmetric weakness with atrophy and loss of deep tendon reflexes and occasionally fasciculations. The arms are involved preferentially in many cases and in generalized cases become affected relatively early. Although the older literature contained reports of focal neurologic deficits such as wrist drop, manifestations such as these are less common. It is thought that these may be due to secondary compression neuropathies. Although lower motor neuron damage is associated with lead exposure, no causal relationship has been demonstrated between lead exposure and development of idiopathic motor neuron syndromes such as amyotrophic lateral sclerosis.[11] Chronic lead exposure causes systemic toxicity in addition to neuropathy. Microcytic, hypochromic anemia is often seen, as are GI disturbances including constipation and abdominal pain. Other less common manifestations include renal dysfunction, fatigue, weight loss, and occasionally gout.

Diagnostic considerations. The electrophysiologic findings in lead neuropathy are controversial. In animal models, demyelination has been demonstrated, while in humans the physiology is generally axonal. Electromyographic evidence of active denervation and chronic motor unit reinnervation in distal muscles reflect the presence of axonal degeneration. Nerve conduction studies show evidence of sensory axon loss, even though sensory symptoms are minimal or absent. Compound motor action potential amplitudes are reduced in more severe cases. Nerve conduction studies may be abnormal before the appearance of symptoms.[12] The degree of abnormality correlates with the lead burden in the body.[13] Somatosensory evoked potential (SSEP) amplitudes are correlated with blood lead levels. SSEP latencies have been reported to be prolonged in both central and peripheral nerve segments. Neuropsychologic testing reveals abnormalities in memory, attention and visuospatial functioning. Confirmation of current or past lead exposure is usually possible.

Laboratory evaluation reveals a microcytic, hypochromic anemia with basophilic stippling of erythrocytes. Urinary lead levels can be measured. Chelating agents that draw lead from soft tissues and allow for its excretion may increase the diagnostic senstivity; however, they are not usually necessary for diagnosis. The ratio of the micrograms of lead excreted to milligrams of calcium ethylenediamine tetra-acetic acid (CaEDTA) administered should not exceed 0.6 and the 24-hour urinary lead level after chelation therapy (usually with CaEDTA) should not be greater than 1 mg.[14]

Treatment. The initial step is removal of the affected individual from further exposure. Treatment of lead intoxication is based on chelation. The goal is the mobilization of lead from the bone to allow elimination. Penicillamine, succimer, CaEDTA and BAL administered in short course are all effective chelating agents and improvement usually begins within 2 weeks (see Chapter 39.8). Oral agents (e.g., succimer) are usually adequate for milder cases, while combination therapy with EDTA and sometimes in combination with BAL is recommended for more severe intoxication that includes encephalopathy. Diazepam should be provided for treatment of seizures associated with lead toxicity although they are often refractory. In those cases that involve brain edema, mannitol, hyperventilation and fluid restriction should all be utilized to lower intracranial pressure. The mortality rate is high in those presenting with seizures and encephalopathy. Complete recovery from neuropathy is usual except in severe cases. The improvement typically begins 2 weeks after initiation of chelation therapy.

Mercury

Elemental mercury is used in thermometers, barometers and other gauges. Organic mercurial compounds have been used as a preservative in latex paints, in various disinfectants and are also used as industrial catalysts. Inorganic mercurial salts and elemental mercury are present in the manufacture of chlorine, in dental amalgams, and in the natural gas industry. Outbreaks of mercury toxicity have been reported due to contaminated fish in Minamata Bay, Japan[15] and in Iraq related to application of an organic mercury-containing fungicide to grain.[16] Elemental mercury vapor is absorbed by inhalation. Mercury salts are absorbed through the skin and GI tract, and organic mercury is usually absorbed through the GI tract. While there is evidence that inhalation of low levels of mercury vapor occurs with mercury amalgam dental fillings, raising health concerns, no causal relationship between the presence of mercury amalgam dental fillings and clinical toxicity has been established to date.[17]

Clinical considerations. The form of mercury that one is exposed to determines the pattern of nervous system involvement and whether there are associated systemic symptoms. Although CNS dysfunction dominates, there are some reports of PNS effects. Elemental mercury is very lipid soluble and tends to cause more CNS involvement with little or no systemic signs. Low-level toxicity due to elemental mercury, known as micromercurialism, causes tremor, fatigue, GI dysfunction, anorexia and weight loss. Continued exposure leads to more prominent tremor that may involve the head, face and even the eyelids. Personality change, hyperexcitability and insomnia are other possible effects of chronic elemental mercury exposure. Mercury salts also cause systemic toxicity including GI symptoms and nephrotic syndrome. PNS involvement has been reported with exposure to all forms of mercury.

The relationship of mercury exposure to neuropathy is better established with mercury vapor than with organic mercury compounds. Mercury vapor exposure is associated with a subacute, motor neuropathy that may be confused with Guillain–Barré syndrome. However, electrophysiology reveals damage to motor axons rather than demyelination. There is usually a preceding irritation of the upper respiratory tract that may be mistaken for an infection. As with other forms of mercury exposure, mercury vapor may also cause neuropsychologic dysfunction. Organic mercury compounds such as methyl mercury cause tremor, hearing loss, constriction of visual fields, mental impairment and dysarthria with prolonged exposure. The other prominent symptom seen more often with organic mercury toxicity is sensory ataxia. This is thought to be due to damage of dorsal root ganglion neurons. Sensory neuron damage may be heralded by distal paresthesias, which progress more proximally and may involve the tongue.[18] Complex organic mercurials are also associated with nephrotoxicty.

Diagnostic considerations. Diagnosis of mercury intoxication is based on eliciting the appropriate exposure history in the setting of a neurologic syndrome as described above. Mercury levels can be measured in urine, blood and hair with limited reliability in the latter. Blood mercury level is a good indicator of recent exposure while urine measurements including serial measurements (after administering penicillamine) are better for chronic exposure.[19] Electrodiagnostic testing in cases of mercury intox-

ication has been reported to show a motor greater than sensory axonal neuropathy.[20] Nerve conduction studies may reveal evidence of a developing neuropathy in exposed workers prior to symptom onset.[19]

Treatment. Mercury intoxication is primarily treated by removal from exposure. Although excretion of mercury in the urine is increased by chelation with agents such as penicillamine or dimercaprol,[21] it is not clear that this speeds recovery from the toxic effects. The prognosis is good for complete recovery in most cases, depending on severity of illness.

Thallium

Thallous salts were commonly used as pesticides and rodenticides in the past. Although rarely used now, accidental (mostly children) or homicidal poisoning continues to occur. Occupational thallium exposure is usually low-level and chronic, rather than acute and high level. Occupations that pose some risk include smelting plants, mines and cement factories. Consumption of contaminated food and water may also be a source of intoxication. Thallium is absorbed through the GI tract, by dermal contact or by inhalation. Thallium is distributed throughout the body as potassium would be and substitutes for it in reactions.[22,23] However, the mechanism of toxicity has not been clearly elicited.

Clinical considerations. Thallium intoxication causes a distal, symmetric sensory greater than motor peripheral neuropathy. Pain is a prominent feature. Degeneration affects the distal portion of the longest axons initially and the large diameter sensory fibers are most susceptible. Involvement of small unmyelinated fibers may lead to a delayed autonomic neuropathy.[24]

The manifestation of thallium neuropathy depends on the temporal course and intensity of exposure. The most common scenario is a massive, acute ingestion. Vomiting, abdominal pain and diarrhea occur within hours but may be delayed up to a day. Severe, burning distal paresthesias in the legs develop within 2–5 days and are accompanied by intense joint pains. Large and small fiber sensory modalities are affected and the sensory abnormalities include the hands and trunk relatively early. Although weakness is not usually a prominent complaint, it is frequently present on examination. Surprisingly, deep tendon reflexes tend to be preserved early in the disease process in spite of large fiber sensory loss. Cardiac and respiratory failure leading to death may also occur with massive ingestion. The mental status may decline to lethargy or coma. Although alopecia is the classic sign of thallium intoxication, it does not appear until approximately 15–39 days after ingestion and is not helpful in the acute setting. Alopecia is not specific for thallium poisoning and does not always occur. Renal insufficiency and paralytic ileus are other systemic manifestations sometimes seen with acute thallium poisoning. The presentation of an acute neuropathy with abdominal pain needs to be distinguished from acute intermittent porphyria and other metal poisonings (e.g., arsenic and lead). The recovery in acute thallium poisoning tends to be incomplete. There is often residual CNS dysfunction. The recovery of the peripheral nerves is slow and there is often persistent sensory loss. In those with severe motor axon damage, weakness may also persist.

With a smaller initial ingestion, thallium neuropathy may present subacutely. Subacute thallium neuropathy evolves more slowly, beginning more than a week after exposure. Alopecia, hyperkeratosis and Mee's lines are more common. Other neurologic features reported with subacute thallium intoxication include cranial neuropathies, chorea and ataxia.[22] The neuropathy is characterized by defects in all sensory modalities. Walking may be affected early on because of painful paresthesias in the feet. Although distal weakness is usually detected, the patient does not often complain of it and it is usually not severe. The deep tendon reflexes are slightly reduced or normal. Autonomic dysfunction may lead to hypertension and tachycardia. Subacute neuropathy tends to have a much better prognosis. With termination of exposure, most patients recover within 6 months. Hair regrowth begins earlier at about 10 weeks after withdrawal.

Diagnostic considerations. Thallium levels can be measured in urine, blood or body tissues. Sensitive methods capable of detecting microgram quantities are available. Although established blood levels that indicate toxicity are available, they do not reflect the total body burden, as thallium is sequestered in tissue. In cases without alopecia, a potassium chloride challenge will cause the urinary excretion of thallium to rise even when the baseline level in blood and urine is normal. Cerebrospinal fluid protein is normal in cases of thallium neuropathy. Nerve conduction studies demonstrate reduced sensory potential amplitudes with conduction velocity slowing. EMG shows evidence of acute and chronic motor axon degeneration. The electrophysiologic abnormalities can be used to follow the degree of peripheral nerve damage.[25]

Treatment. GI elimination is enhanced by administration of Prussian blue or activated charcoal, which bind thallium in the gut.[26,27] Laxatives are also helpful since constipation and paralytic ileus are frequently present. Forced diuresis or administration of potassium chloride enhances urinary excretion. Thallium has a half-life of 30 days in the body if no measures are taken to promote excretion.

Pesticides, herbicides and rodenticides

Organophosphates

Organophosphorous (OP) compounds are used as insecticides, antioxidants, petroleum additives, flame retardants, lubricants and plastic modifiers. The best characterized peripheral neuropathy caused by these compounds in humans is that due to triorthocresylphosphate (TOCP), although exposure to other OP such as parathion, chlorpyrifos, mipafox, trichlorfon and leptophos may cause a similar neuropathy. Intoxication is usually due to accidental exposure from agricultural pesticide spraying. Individuals affected may be those mixing or applying the pesticide or those working in the fields shortly after spraying. OPs are absorbed through the respiratory and GI tracts as well as through the skin.[28] The action of OP is to irreversibly inhibit acetyl cholinesterase (AChE) in erythrocytes and nervous tissue by phosphorylation. Acetylcholine accumulates due to lack of degradation, leading to excessive stimulation of both muscarinic and nicotinic receptors. Most OP esters are quickly degraded in the environment. Pesticides containing OP are also intentionally ingested in suicide attempts.

Clinical considerations. The acute or type I OP syndrome is primarily due to excessive muscarinic cholinergic stimulation.[29] The effects are frequently seen within hours of exposure and are always present within one day. The specific OP and the degree of exposure determine the intensity of the acute syndrome. Characteristic symptoms include nausea, vomiting, diarrhea, bronchospasm, bradycardia, sweating, salivation, and micturition (see Chapter 48) . Extreme intoxication leads to CNS involvement with fatigue, nervousness, emotional lability, decreased alertness, cognitive impairment, convulsions and coma (see Chapter 28.1). Prior OP exposure may increase susceptibility to developing the acute syndrome on subsequent exposure because of a decrease in functional AChE. The acute syndrome may have prominent mental status changes and other drug or toxin ingestion needs to be considered.

The type II or intermediate OP syndrome is the result of overstimulation of nicotinic ACh receptors in skeletal muscle.[30] The onset occurs within 12–96 hours of exposure. There may be a symptom-free interval of 1–4 days between the acute and intermediate syndromes. The initial feature is usually respiratory insufficiency. Proximal muscle and neck flexor weakness follow and distal extremity strength is usually preserved. Cranial muscles, including extraocular muscles, may be involved. Sensory function is unaffected. Dystonic posturing is occasionally seen. Recovery begins in the cranial muscles 5–15 days after exposure. It then proceeds from the respiratory muscles to the proximal muscles and lastly the neck flexors. Since atropine is specific for muscarinic receptors, it does not prevent or treat the intermediate syndrome. The differential diagnosis of the intermediate syndrome includes Guillain–Barré syndrome, periodic paralysis or a severe attack of myasthenia gravis.

Regardless of whether exposure has caused the type I or type II syndromes, a central-peripheral axonopathy may develop with exposure to some OPs. Central-peripheral axonopathy refers to a process that affects the distal portions of peripheral axons initially, but, with continued exposure, leads to damage of the distal portions of central axons. The delayed appearance of this neuropathy, 7–21 days after exposure, led to the phrase organophosphate-induced delayed polyneuropathy (OPIDP). This neuropathy is not related to the inhibition of AChE but rather to a distinct esterase localized to nervous tissue, termed neuropathy target esterase. Although the OPIDP is less frequent than the cholinergic syndromes, it causes significant morbidity. Most agricultural OPs do not cause the OPIDP and those that cause subtle cholinergic symptoms seem more likely to cause delayed neuropathy. OPIDP frequently occurs in the setting of low-level, chronic exposure.

Although most toxic central-peripheral axonopathies are chronic, OPIDP is subacute. Symptoms are usually maximal within two weeks after onset. Initial manifestations include painful paresthesias in the feet and cramping pain in the calf muscles. Motor symptoms and signs are prominent and there is early weakness of the leg muscles including foot drop. The intrinsic hand muscles become involved next and the proximal muscles are spared until later in the course. Sensory loss can usually be detected with careful examination. Ataxia may be present, that is more severe than expected based on the degree of sensory loss and weakness. Although the ankle reflex is typically absent, the activity of the other reflexes is variable. The OPIDP needs to be distinguished from other toxic causes of a central-peripheral distal axonopathy.

Diagnostic considerations. Electrophysiologic testing is a very sensitive indicator of OP peripheral neurologic effects.[31] Shortly after OP exposure, a single stimulus produces spontaneous repetitive motor action potentials (SRMAPs) following the initial compound motor action potential.[32] While the ability to elicit SRMAPs is a sensitive marker of OP exposure, there is no correlation with the degree of intoxication. Once muscle weakness becomes evident, repetitive nerve stimulation produces decremental responses. In contrast to myasthenia gravis where the decrement is usually maximal by the fourth response, here it is most prominent by the second. With mild OP intoxication, rapid rates of stimulation may be necessary to demonstrate decrement, and there may be a subsequent incremental response. With high-level exposure, decrement is evident with slow rates of stimulation and SRMAPs may be absent.[31]

OPIDP is characterized electrophysiologically as a sensorimotor axonal neuropathy. Sensory nerve conduction abnormalities appear earlier and more prominently than motor nerve abnormalities, despite clinical motor symptoms. Sensory nerve action potentials are reduced in amplitude or absent, while motor conduction studies are normal or reveal minimal slowing of conduction velocity.[33] Needle EMG reveals evidence for acute and chronic denervation in the distal limb muscles. In the intermediate syndrome, EMG is normal, despite prominent muscle weakness.

Routine clinical laboratory findings are usually normal. Recent exposure to OP causes reduction in erythrocyte AChE levels. AChE levels less than 20% of baseline values are frequently associated with severe weakness. The wide range of normal erythrocyte AChE levels makes a single determination difficult to interpret. Serial measurements showing progressive decline in activity are more useful. The CSF protein level in OPIDP is normal or only mildly elevated.

Treatment. The acute and intermediate OP syndromes have a good prognosis as long as there is adequate supportive care. Although only 40–60% of AChE content is regenerated by 1 week after exposure, this is usually sufficient for functional recovery. Cognitive and behavioral abnormalities may persist after recovery from the acute syndrome.

Patients with mild OPIDP usually have excellent recovery. With more severe initial deficits, residual deficits such as claw hand deformity, foot drop or atrophy may persist. Damage of central axons may only become apparent after recovery from the peripheral neuropathy. Injury of distal portions of the corticospinal and spinocerebellar tracts may lead to spasticity or ataxia.

Vacor

N-3-pyridylmethyl-N-p-nitrophenyl urea (PNU) or vacor is a rodenticide that is structurally related to nicotinamide. Accidental or intentional ingestion is the most common form of exposure. This leads to a severe acute distal axonopathy with significant autonomic involvement. Vacor also damages the beta cells of the pancreas leading to acute diabetes mellitus. Massive ingestion leads to limb weakness and impairment of postural reflexes within the first hour. This rapidly progresses to severe generalized weakness including the cranial nerve innervated muscles, urinary retention and diabetic ketoacidosis. Those that survive the acute ingestion frequently continue to have endocrine and autonomic dysfunction. Motor weakness improves gradually over the course of months. The few autopsy studies reported have demonstrated wallerian-like degeneration in the peripheral nerves, roots and dorsal root ganglia.[34] Animal studies of vacor-induced neuropathy indicate defects of fast axonal transport in distal nerves.[35] There is also abnormal morphology of the neuromuscular junction. This impairment may explain the rapid onset of weakness. Although the precise biologic mechanism of vacor neuropathy is unclear, it can be prevented experimentally by administering nicotinamide.

Solvents

Carbon disulfide

Carbon disulfide is a clear liquid, which is a vapor at room temperature. Carbon disulfide is absorbed by inhalation, dermal contact and, although less common, can also be absorbed through the GI tract. It is used in the production of cellophane films and viscose rayon fibers (see Chapter 40). It is also a major metabolite in the breakdown of the drug disulfiram (antabuse), which is used as a deterrent for alcohol abuse. The toxicity of this compound is most likely related to its reactivity with amine, sulfhydryl and hydroxyl groups, which results in the formation of reactive sulfur atoms. Isothiocyanates are produced, which can covalently bind to and cross-link cytoskeletal proteins such as neurofilaments. This may be related to the formation of giant axonal swellings seen in experimental studies performed in rats. These are similar morphologically to those seen in hexacarbon and acrylamide neuropathies.

Clinical considerations. Acute or subacute high-level exposure results primarily in CNS dysfunction including confusion, hallucinations, memory impairment, and emotional lability (see Chapter 28.1).[36] Chronic, low-level exposure causes a combination of peripheral neuropathy and CNS abnormalities. The neuropathy may be asymptomatic and only detected by electrophysiologic testing when exposure is low but, as the concentration increases, a progressive sensorimotor distal polyneuropathy emerges. This neuropathy produces distal numbness and weakness along with painful cramping in the legs. The knee and ankle reflexes are often absent. Continued exposure leads to involvement of the arms. CNS manifestations of prolonged exposure include headache, dizziness, depression, memory impairment and impaired sexual arousal. Exposed persons may also have extrapyramidal signs of tremor, bradykinesia, and cogwheel rigidity, as well as hemiparesis or spasticity.

Diagnostic considerations. Although CS_2 is difficult to measure, urinary levels of its metabolite, 2-triothiazoli-dine-4-carboxylic acid, have proved to be a sensitive measure of exposure. Nerve conduction studies reveal slowing of conduction velocities and prolongation of motor and sensory latencies. Needle electromyography reveals active and chronic denervation in distal leg muscles, reflecting axonal degeneration and chronic motor unit reinnervation.[37,38] The spinal fluid profile is unremarkable.

Treatment. Early cessation of exposure is the key to prevent further decline. There may be a role for the use of pyridoxine to treat the neuropathy. The effects may be related to the reactivity of CS_2 with pyridoxine. The degree of recovery depends on the severity of dysfunction at the time of removal from exposure. In mild cases almost complete recovery from neuropathy and most of the CNS abnormalities can be expected. Occasionally, CNS recovery is incomplete, probably due to residual spinal cord damage. Severe neuropathy may not completely recover, and as many as a third may have symptoms and signs of neuropathy 10 years later.[38]

n-Hexane and methyl-n-butyl ketone

These compounds are clear, colorless, volatile liquids used as solvents (see Chapter 40). They are metabolized to the toxic compound 2,5 hexanedione.[39] Hexacarbons gain entry to the body via inhalation, dermal contact and, rarely, ingestion. Exposure occurs in the petroleum production and refining industries. They are also components of lacquers and glues, which are widely used in the shoe and cabinet making industries. Methyl-n-butyl ketone (MnBK) use in the manufacturing of plastic-coated and color-coated fabrics prompted an epidemic of peripheral neuropathy.[40] Intentional inhalation (glue sniffing) is also a cause of high-level hexacarbon exposure. Methyl ethyl ketone (MEK) is not significantly neurotoxic by itself, but is present in many solvent mixtures with n-hexane and MnBK, and may potentiate their neurotoxicity.

Clinical considerations. Isolated high-level acute exposure causes CNS depression and narcosis. However, repeated massive exposure such as glue sniffing leads to a subacute, predominantly motor neuropathy with cranial nerve dysfunction.[41] This neuropathy may be associated with autonomic dysfunction including impotence, hyper- or anhidrosis, and vasomotor instability. Chronic exposure to lower levels results in a slowly developing central-peripheral axonopathy that affects the sensory and motor systems in a length dependent fashion.[42] Nerve fiber degeneration affects the distal portions of peripheral axons first, but with continued exposure leads to damage of distal corticospinal, dorsal column, and other central pathways. All sensory modalities are affected, beginning in the feet with dysfunction gradually progressing proximally with continued exposure. Numbness rarely progresses higher than the knee in spite of the eventual involvement of the hands, and pain is not a complaint. Although ankle reflexes are lost early in the course, the other reflexes are usually spared. Distal leg and arm weakness and atrophy occur with continued exposure. In severe cases, the neuropathy is complicated by malaise, weight loss, abdominal pain, and leg cramps. Worsening of symptoms after removal from exposure, a phenomenon described as 'coasting,' is common.

Diagnostic considerations. Electrophysiologic testing demonstrates a sensorimotor axonal neuropathy.[43] Active denervation is detected in distal muscles often before nerve conduction studies become abnormal. In severe cases, nerve conduction studies reveal marked slowing of distal motor conduction velocities, which is an unusual finding in other toxic neuropathies. Asymptomatic workers employed in factories where cases of solvent polyneuropathy have occurred have been demonstrated to have slowing of conduction velocities. The nerve biopsy reveals a very characteristic morphologic abnormality known as giant axonal swelling. This arises as a result of the accumulation of neurofilaments.[44] Giant axonal swellings are also seen with acrylamide and carbon disulfide exposure, and in the genetic giant axonal neuropathy.

The accumulation of neurofilamentous material is most prominent at the paranodal region, and is likely related to cross-linking and disruption of axonal transport. Spinal fluid protein is usually normal unless the nerve roots become involved, in which case CSF protein may be elevated. Because of the subacute presentation and the presence of conduction slowing, the neuropathy associated with repeated high-level hexacarbon exposure needs to be differentiated from Guillain–Barré syndrome.

Treatment. The only treatment is cessation of exposure to allow recovery. As mentioned above, symptoms frequently continue to worsen for 1–4 months after cessation of exposure. The 'coasting' phenomenon is possibly due to the lipid solubility of hexacarbons, which delays their elimination from the body. Measurement of 2,5-hexanedione in the urine can help detect exposure before significant toxicity occurs. Recovery depends on the severity of neuropathy. Patients with mild neuropathy usually make a complete recovery in less than a year. Residual distal atrophy, weakness and sensory loss are not uncommon with severe neuropathies. The effects of central damage (spasticity, long-tract weakness) may only become evident after resolution of the neuropathy.

Trichloroethylene

The solvent trichloroethylene (TCE) is used as a degreasing agent, a cleaner for photographic equipment and lenses, and in the extraction of fats and oils from vegetables (see Chapter 40). It is also used in the dry cleaning and rubber production industries, and previously was used as an anesthetic agent. Toxicity may be related to a breakdown product, dichloroacetylene (DCA), rather than TCE itself. TCE is usually absorbed by inhalation and is very lipid soluble.

Clinical considerations. Acute exposure is the most common scenario and trigeminal nerve dysfunction is a frequent manifestation. The sensory loss is usually in the distribution of all three trigeminal divisions and there may be weakness of mastication. Other cranial neuropathies affecting the facial, optic, oculomotor and glossopharyngeal nerves have been reported. There is a questionable relationship to a distal sensorimotor peripheral neuropathy. Acute exposure to TCE also causes CNS dysfunction with altered mental status and ataxia. Chronic exposure has also been reported to cause cognitive dysfunction and peripheral neuropathy.

Diagnostic considerations. Trigeminal somatosensory evoked potentials have been used to measure the effects of TCE exposure. Abnormalities are reported in asymptomatic individuals exposed to TCE. Slowing of nerve conduction velocity in facial, trigeminal (blink) and extremity peripheral nerves has been reported. Pathologically, axon degeneration, cell loss in the cranial nerve nuclei, and myelin degeneration have been reported in autopsy studies.

Treatment. Removal of the individual from the exposure source is the first step. If ingested, lavage should be performed. The mental status changes usually resolve rapidly but facial numbness tends to persist. In one case, long-term follow-up 18 years later revealed continued facial sensory disturbance.

Allyl chloride

Allyl chloride is a reactive halogenated hydrocarbon that is used in the manufacture of glycerin and epoxy resin. Exposure to high levels for long duration results in a distal symmetric neuropathy. This is gradual in onset and presents with distal numbness and weakness along with reduced ankle reflexes.[45] Nerve conduction studies reveal prolonged distal latencies. EMG demonstrates active and chronic denervation in distal muscles. Cessation of exposure usually results in good recovery. Animal studies reveal abnormal accumulation of neurofilaments. There is also degeneration in the distal terminals of both peripheral and central axons.

Mixed solvents

A variety of solvent mixtures, including toluene, have been associated with electrophysiologic changes in peripheral (particularly autonomic) nerve function. Further research is require to assess the clinical and pathological impact of solvents on the peripheral nervous system. Electrophysiologic studies and trial removal from exposure should be considered in exposed individuals with persistent neuropathic symptoms.

Plastics

Acrylamide

Acrylamide is used in grouting agents for soil and sealing applications, and polyacrylamide is used as a flocculator in waste water treatment plants. Although acrylamide monomer is the toxic form, polyacrylamide (which is innocuous) may be contaminated by up to 2% monomer and therefore may be a source of toxicity. Absorption takes place by dermal contact, inhalation or ingestion. Acrylamide neuropathy is a popular experimental animal model for studying the processes of axonal transport, dying-back neuropathy and axonal swelling. Acrylamide appears to interfere with axonal transport[46,47] resulting in an accumulation of neurofilaments and axonal swelling.[48,49] The swelling is most prominent in the paranodal region, possibly due to the constriction of the axon at that point.

Clinical considerations. The manifestations of acrylamide toxicity depend on the degree and duration of exposure. The usual route of exposure is through the skin and thus a contact dermatitis is usually present prior to the clinical symptoms of neuropathy. In the setting of acute exposure, malaise, dizziness, anorexia and headache are often present. With high-level acute exposure, the neurologic picture includes encephalopathy with seizures and truncal ataxia followed by peripheral neuropathy. Early behavioral changes may be less apparent to the patient than others. In chronic, low-level exposure, the dermatitis persists but the CNS effects are not as prominent.

The neuropathy resulting from acrylamide is a classic example of a central-peripheral distal axonopathy.[50] Initial clinical manifestations include toe numbness and widespread hyporeflexia. Large fiber sensory dysfunction with loss of vibration and proprioception is common while pain and paresthesias are rare. Acute, high-level exposure often results in widespread autonomic dysfunction such as impairment of reflex changes in heart rate and blood pressure, vasomotor changes in fingers and toes, and excessive sweating. Overt autonomic dysfunction rarely occurs in chronic exposure and may be limited to excessive sweating of the hands and feet. Although sensory complaints dominate, motor and cerebellar deficits may be evident on physical examination. Cranial nerve function is unaffected.

Diagnostic considerations. Neurophysiologic testing reveals reduced amplitude sensory responses with preservation of motor amplitude and conduction velocity.[51]

These findings are characteristic of a distal axonopathy and in some instances the electrophysiologic abnormalities may precede the development of symptoms. The sural nerve biopsy correlates with the physiologic and clinical manifestations, showing reduced numbers of large diameter, thickly myelinated fibers.

Treatment. Preventing further exposure to acrylamide is the primary treatment modality. Acute ingestion should prompt gastric lavage to reduce levels of intoxication. Liver and renal failure may complicate recovery. Removal from exposure usually results in recovery if the neuropathy is mild. Some residual loss of vibratory sensation may be apparent. However, in the case of severe neuropathy, spasticity, ataxia, more profound sensory dysfunction and memory problems may remain. Central nervous system dysfunction, such as spasticity and upper motor neuron weakness may be obscured initially by peripheral nerve dysfunction. As nerve recovery ensues, clinical dysfunction may remain due to unresolved central nervous system dysfunction. Coasting, the worsening of symptoms after termination of exposure, may occur.

Dimethylaminoproprionitrile (DMAPN)

DMAPN had been used as a catalyst in polymerization reactions until 1978. It was found to be responsible for an outbreak of toxic axonopathy in the production of polyurethane foams. Since that time, it is no longer used and no additional cases have been reported.

Clinical considerations. The peripheral neuropathy associated with DMAPN is very distinct in that there are prominent urinary symptoms that manifest prior to the onset of sensory or motor complaints.[52] The degree of exposure determines the rapidity of onset of symptoms. The exposed individual often complains initially of urinary hesitancy and abdominal pain. This progresses to reduced frequency of urination, decreased urinary stream and incontinence. Sexual dysfunction follows with partial or complete impotence. About the same time, sensory symptoms develop in the feet. The sensory symptoms progress to involve the proximal legs and the hands while weakness develops in the distal legs. Abnormality of sensation to pain, temperature and touch in the sacral dermatomes is characteristic of DMAPN neuropathy. There is also loss of distal vibratory sensation but the reflexes are surprisingly well preserved. The preservation of reflexes, autonomic features and preferential loss of pain and temperature sensation suggest more prominent involvement of the small nerve fibers. However, the available morphologic data have not borne this out. Other than bladder and sexual abnormalities, other autonomic function is preserved. The cranial nerves are not affected. The differential diagnosis is primarily that of diabetic small-fiber neuropathy or amyloid neuropathy.

Diagnostic considerations. Urodynamic studies reveal hypocontractility of the bladder, consistent with autonomic nerve dysfunction. In mild cases of DMAPN neuropathy, electrodiagnostic testing may be normal. In most cases, the sensory potential amplitudes are reduced in the lower extremities. Severe cases may demonstrate slowing of motor conduction velocity.

Treatment. Removal from exposure is the only form of treatment. The prognosis for recovery is good in young patients. Older individuals tend to have more persistent bladder and sexual dysfunction.

Gases

Methyl bromide

Methyl bromide is used in insecticides, fire extinguishers, refrigerants and fumigants. Acute, high-level exposure may be fatal. Chronic, high-level exposure to methyl bromide causes multifocal neurologic dysfunction involving the peripheral nerves, pyramidal tracts and cerebellum. The neuropathy usually appears after 3–7 months of exposure and is a distal sensorimotor polyneuropathy. Paresthesias in the distal extremities are the first symptoms. Pain and ataxia develop later. The optic nerves may be involved and color vision loss may reveal toxic exposure to methyl bromide at an early stage. Electrophysiologic testing reveals a distal, motor predominant neuropathy.[53] Sural nerve biopsy reveals loss of large myelinated axons. The cerebrospinal fluid is normal. The prognosis appears to be good in most cases, although recovery may take 6–8 months.

Ethylene oxide (EtO)

EtO is used in the sterilization of medical equipment, particularly that which is heat sensitive. After sterilization, the object must be allowed to aerate or residual EtO may be present. EtO is used in the production of ethylene glycol (antifreeze) and other chemical compounds, as well as the production of polyester fibers and polyethylene films. As this is a gaseous compound, the primary route of exposure is via inhalation.

Clinical considerations. Acute exposure causes respiratory tract and mucous membrane irritation as well as nausea, vomiting, headache, dizziness and anorexia. EtO exposure results in a distal sensorimotor axonopathy.[54] This may be seen after long duration, low-level exposure or with subacute, higher level exposure. Clinical symptoms include distal numbness and weakness, incoordination and ataxia. Sensory loss begins in the feet and, with continued exposure, begins to involve the hands. Weakness also begins distally and there is diffuse reduction of reflexes with the ankle jerks usually absent. Chronic exposure also causes CNS dysfunction including memory and concentration problems, as well as dysarthria and increased tone. Removal from exposure is the only therapy. There is usually a gradual recovery from the neuropathy once exposure is terminated.

Diagnostic considerations. Electrophysiologic testing is consistent with a distal axonopathy. EMG reveals active and chronic denervation changes in distal muscles. Nerve conduction studies demonstrate reduced amplitude sensory and motor potentials with normal conduction velocity or only mild slowing. Nerve conduction abnormalities may appear prior to the onset of symptoms in exposed individuals. Sural nerve biopsy shows evidence of axon degeneration.

Polychlorinated biphenyls (PCBs)

PCBs have previously been used in electrical insulation as well as plasticizers (see Chapter 45). Although there is a lot of discussion about the toxicity of PCBs, neurotoxicity associated with specific congeners has not been well characterized. The use of PCBs was banned in the 1970s but contaminated products remain. Although PCB contamination of waterways and marine life is the most common source of exposure, there are no reported cases of toxicity as a result. Neuropathy caused by PCBs has been reported in an outbreak caused by contaminated cooking oil in Taiwan. Most cases reported more recently have been electrical workers involved in the removal of PCB contaminated transformers. PCBs are very lipid soluble and may remain in the tissues long after removal from exposure.

Clinical considerations. The peripheral neuropathy associated with PCB exposure is a distal symmetric sensorimotor neuropathy.[55] Encephalopathy is usually coexistent with neuropathy. Worsening of symptoms after termination of exposure has been described. Removal from exposure usually results in improvement. Most patients have some persistent deficit several years later.

Diagnostic considerations. Nerve conduction studies demonstrate significant slowing of sensory and motor nerves. Although PCB levels in the blood can be obtained, they do not correlate with the presence of neurologic symptoms.

FOCAL NERVE INJURIES

(See also Chapter 23.3)

Radial nerve

Source of injury

Most radial nerve injuries result from external trauma. The radial nerve may be damaged in the axilla by lacerations, crutch use, missile wounds, or pressure from the head of a sleeping person ('lover's Saturday night palsy'). Proximal nerve injury affects the triceps muscle and weakens forearm extension. The most frequent radial nerve lesion is compression of the nerve against the middle third of the humerus. These are usually Class I lesions with predominantly conduction block. Severe weakness with total paralysis of wrist and finger extensors may occur.

Radial nerve entrapment may result from a fibrous band derived from the lateral head of the triceps. This usually occurs in heavily muscled individuals involved in activities requiring prolonged and vigorous elbow extension.

Entrapment may also occur in the region of the supinator muscle by fibrous bands on the surface of the muscle (arcade of Frohse) or within the muscle itself by tumors, ganglia, or inflammatory conditions. A painful elbow may result from entrapment of the posterior interosseous nerve. The superficial radial nerve is vulnerable to a host of injuries, including lacerations or compression from tight wristwatches, handcuffs, or plaster casts, owing to its superficial position at the wrist.

Posterior interosseous nerve compression

The posterior interosseous nerve may be compressed as it enters the supinator muscle under a fibrous arch (arcade of Frohse) or within the substance of the muscle.[56] Common causes of injury include ganglia, tumors (especially lipomas), fibrous bands, fractures or dislocations of the radius. The condition may occur spontaneously without an identifiable cause. Many so-called idiopathic cases have been found to be the result of entrapment at the arcade of Frohse. The clinical syndrome of 'resistant' tennis elbow is, in many cases, a result of posterior interosseous nerve entrapment, most often by the arcade of Frohse. It often is misdiagnosed as tennis elbow caused by lateral epicondylitis because both conditions result in lateral elbow pain. Posterior interosseous nerve entrapment is characterized by pain on firm palpation of the extensor muscle mass distal to the radial head; in contrast, lateral epicondylitis has marked tenderness with palpation of the lateral epicondyle.

Posterior interosseous nerve lesions result in an inability to extend the fingers and abduct the thumb; wrist extension is usually less affected as a result of sparing of the extensor carpi radialis. Radial deviation may occur with wrist extension because of extensor carpi ulnaris weakness. Sensation is spared over the dorsum of the hand. The degree of weakness is variable and may not affect all distal radial muscles to the same extent. In patients with rheumatoid arthritis, posterior interosseous nerve lesions must be distinguished from rupture of the extensor tendons to the thumb and fingers.

Treatment and prognosis of specific radial nerve injuries

Radial nerve injuries in the upper arm. Most radial nerve lesions resulting in wrist drop should be treated with a cock-up wrist splint, described later, that maintains mild wrist extension. Mild cases, in which weakness is not complete, may need no specific therapy. Complete recovery, over weeks to a few months, generally occurs in most radial nerve lesions resulting from compression. The ultimate degree of recovery depends on the severity and duration of compression.

Patients with radial nerve entrapment within the triceps muscle usually recover spontaneously. Rarely, exploration and decompression may be needed in cases of progressive weakness or poor recovery.[57] Radial nerve injury secondary to fractures of the humerus have an excellent prognosis for spontaneous recovery. Mild cases of posterior interosseous nerve entrapment often recover spontaneously. A period of observation ranging from 3 to 6 months is generally prescribed to allow spontaneous recovery. More severe cases, in which weakness is present or with poor recovery, may require surgical exploration and removal of identified masses (tumors, lipomas, or ganglia) or constricting bands. Entrapment under the arcade of Frohse, if present, is released. Nerve compression caused by radial fractures should be observed initially for 2–3 months.

Regardless of the cause of the radial nerve palsy, most cases of wrist and finger drop require a proper splint to protect against hyperextension of the paralyzed wrist extensor muscles and shortening of the flexor muscles.[58] A static cock-up splint, maintaining the wrist at about 15–30 degrees of extension, is usually all that is required in cases with mild wrist extensor muscle weakness. Palmar sensation should not be obscured by a palmar pad. The metacarpophalangeal (MCP) joints may need to be supported in extension, with the thumb extended and radially abducted. Finger joints must be regularly exercised because they rapidly become stiff when immobilized for even a short time. This type of splint supports the hand in a position of function, thereby encouraging continued use. If the hand is able to be opened sufficiently by interphalangeal (IP) joint extension, MCP joint support may be unnecessary. In more severe cases, dynamic splints are useful. Such splints utilize a finger slip around the proximal IP joint to support the MCP joints in slight extension, thereby allowing active finger flexion while offering protective positioning at rest.

During the stage of paralysis, daily passive exercises should be used to maintain adequate range of joint movement, including large arm excursion. After voluntary activity returns, specific exercises are employed to strengthen the wrist and finger extensors. Intrinsic hand muscles become weak and inefficient, owing to dependence on the synergistic action of the wrist extensors, and may need strengthening to restore adequate hand function.

Median nerve

Source of injury

The superficial position of the median nerve in the upper arm renders it vulnerable to missile wounds and lacerations. It is better protected in the forearm where it lies deep within the pronator teres muscle. Median nerve compression has been attributed to crutches pressing on the axilla, tourniquets, rifle sling palsy, and pressure from the head of a sleeping partner on the brachioaxillary angle or medial aspect of the arm.

Median nerve damage secondary to bony fracture is less common than with other upper limb nerves because it is protected by overlying arm muscles. Fractures of the elbow occasionally result in median nerve damage. The anterior interosseous nerve may be damaged by forearm fractures because the nerve is closely related to the radius and ulna as it descends on the interosseous membrane.

Chronic median nerve entrapment may result from chronic compression in well-defined fibro-osseous tunnels or following repeated episodes of strenuous muscle activity.[59] The most common nerve entrapment in the upper limb is median nerve compression under the transverse carpal ligament (CTS). Other median nerve entrapments include the pronator syndrome, the anterior interosseous syndrome, and entrapment by the supracondylar ligament.

Carpal tunnel syndrome

CTS is by far the most common entrapment neuropathy in the arm. The usual presentation is with acroparesthesias, numbness, tingling, and burning sensations, usually in the lateral three fingers. Nocturnal exacerbation of pain and paresthesias is characteristic and may either wake the patient from sleep or be prominent on awakening in the morning. Although pain may involve the forearm and shoulder region, it is rare for patients to describe numbness or paresthesias radiating proximal to the wrist. Shaking the hand frequently relieves pain. Repetitive tasks, be they occupationally related or hobbies, such as knitting and sewing, often precipitate or aggravate symptoms.

Objective sensory loss most consistently involves the second and third fingers, occasionally there is splitting of the fourth finger with sensory loss on the lateral but not the medial aspect. The palm is usually spared. Raynaud's phenomenon may occasionally be present. If the condition is left untreated, weakness and wasting of median innervated thenar muscles eventually develops, particularly thumb abduction and opposition. Eventually, the thumb is unable to be maintained in the opposed and abducted position (post position). As a result, the thumb is restricted to the plane of the palm, precluding it from acting as a post against which the other fingers can push. Thenar atrophy may occasionally precede weakness. Percussion of the median nerve at the wrist may reproduce sensory symptoms in the median nerve distribution (Tinel's sign). Forced hand flexion (Phalen's test) or extension (reverse Phalen's test) may reproduce the sensory symptoms. Asymptomatic motor and sensory signs may rarely be discovered, particularly in older individuals.

A discussion of work-related factors, including forceful and repetitive hand use, in the development of CTS is provided in Chapter 23.3. CTS may develop acutely after a prolonged episode of unaccustomed hand use, such as house-painting. In patients with pre-existing CTS, vigorous hand activity can aggravate symptoms. Much of the original support for CTS as a repetitive movement injury can be traced to studies using poor case definition or workers' compensation claims, and the specific role of chronic repetitive hand use in CTS remains unsettled.[60] Two longitudinal studies of median nerve conductivity in workers engaged in a variety of industrial activities[61,62] failed to demonstrate any deterioration of median nerve function over a period of greater than 5–10 years.

It has been suggested that a substantial increase in intracarpal pressure results from wrist flexion and extension. In addition, there is some evidence to suggest that patients with reduced cross-sectional diameters of their carpal bones may be at increased risk of CTS. However, in at least one study, routine measurements of carpal tunnel dimensions did not predict the likelihood of developing CTS in an occupational setting. Although CTS most commonly involves the dominant hand, bilateral involvement is extremely common. In many cases, only one side is symptomatic, the asymptomatic lesion evident only by electrodiagnostic studies. Most cases of CTS are probably the result of non-specific tenosynovitis of the flexor tendons. Other causes include tuberculous tenosynovitis, rheumatoid arthritis, osteoarthritis of the carpus, pregnancy, hemodialysis, myxedema, acromegaly, and infiltration of the transverse carpal ligament in primary amyloidosis. CTS is common in patients with generalized peripheral neuropathies, such as uremia and diabetes. In such patients, it is believed that the generalized neuropathy predisposes the median nerve to compression. Acute CTS can be caused by hemorrhage or infection in the carpal tunnel and constitutes a medical emergency. CTS should be considered for any unexplained pain or sensory disturbance in the hand.

Electrodiagnostic studies. In many cases, the diagnosis is obvious from the clinical signs and symptoms. Diagnostic confirmation in atypical cases and an estimate of severity can be obtained by nerve conduction studies. Confirmatory electrodiagnostic studies should be obtained in all patients undergoing surgery. The most sensitive physiologic parameter is sensory and mixed nerve conduction across the carpal ligament. Median motor conduction is less often abnormal than sensory conduction, but may show prolonged distal latencies and reduced compound motor action potential amplitudes, the latter usually reflecting axonal degeneration. Comparison of distal motor latencies between the median innervated second lumbrical muscle and the ulnar interosseous muscle has proven to be sensitive and specific for mild CTS.

Treatment and prognosis. Conservative medical therapy is appropriate when there are mild sensory symptoms without weakness or atrophy, intermittent symptoms, or acute CTS related to a specific injury or overactivity.[58] Occupationally related symptoms often respond to a switch in jobs to one not requiring repetitive hand movements. Nocturnal immobilization, using a volar wrist splint that maintains the wrist in the neutral position, is usually the initial treatment. Splinting is most useful when symptoms are intermittent and nocturnally exacerbated. The splint should be worn for as long as it is effective; if symptoms recur, further splinting is usually not helpful. Occasionally, the splint may be worn during the day at work to prevent the wrist from assuming a potentially aggravating position. If possible, repetitive actions that aggravate symptoms should be avoided.

Splinting, in general, usually offers only temporary or minimal relief. In patients without marked sensory loss, thenar weakness, or muscle wasting, a local injection of a mixture of lidocaine (Xylocaine) and methylprednisolone (Solu-Mediol) can be tried. Low-dose oral prednisone or diuretics (especially in cases complicating pregnancy) may occasionally be effective. Eventually, however, many patients require surgical release.

Carpal tunnel surgery is indicated when conservative therapy fails to alleviate abnormal sensations or when thenar weakness or atrophy (evidence of axonal injury) is present. Surgery may also be needed in patients with occupations that chronically aggravate the symptoms. In such cases, the patient is often faced with a surgical option or the necessity to find an alternative form of work. Surgery is usually effective in relieving pain and stopping the progression of weakness in almost all cases. The long-term prognosis on returning to the same exposure setting is guarded, and may result in aggravation of the condition.

Surgery is almost always successful in halting the progression of weakness. If the lesion is not too advanced, recovery of strength usually occurs. Most cases of failed carpal tunnel release result from either incomplete transection of the transverse carpal ligament or faulty initial diagnosis. As indicated previously, preoperative electrodiagnosis is essential to avoid this latter mistake. Reported complications of surgery include neuroma formation, a tender dysesthetic scar, transection of the palmar cutaneous branch, infection, incomplete release, development of a complex regional pain syndrome, and damage to the superficial palmar arch.

Median nerve entrapment at the elbow (pronator syndrome and anterior interosseous syndrome)

The pronator syndrome results from compression of the median nerve as it passes between the two heads of the pronator teres muscle and under the fibrous arch of the flexor digitorum superficialis muscle.[56,59] The most frequent cause of entrapment is fibrous bands in the substance of the muscle or passage through a tight flexor superficialis arch. Repeated pronation-supination activity may precipitate symptoms in patients with hypertrophied volar forearm muscles. The nerve may occasionally be compressed under the lacertus fibrosus, a fascial band extending from the biceps tendon to the forearm fascia. The pronator syndrome is characterized by diffuse forearm aching and paresthesias in the median nerve distribution over the hand. The degree of weakness varies, ranging from no weakness, to mild involvement of thenar and forearm musculature.

Various tests have been advocated to localize the level of nerve entrapment within the pronator muscle mass. Pain in the proximal forearm induced by forced wrist supination and wrist extension suggests compression within the pronator teres. Pain with forced forearm pronation of the fully supinated and flexed forearm suggests entrapment under the lacertus fibrosus. Compression of the median nerve under the flexor superficialis arch is suggested by pain on forced flexion of the proximal interphalangeal joint of the middle finger.

Anterior interosseous nerve compression causes weakness of the flexor pollicis longus, pronator quadratus, and the median innervated flexor digitorum profundus muscles. The resulting clinical deficit is impaired flexion of the terminal phalanx of the thumb and index finger. There is no associated sensory loss. The anterior interosseous nerve may be damaged by forearm lacerations or fractures, fibrous bands within the pronator teres, entrapment by the fibrous arch of the flexor superficialis, and as a manifestation of acute brachial neuritis. Occasionally, anterior interosseous nerve dysfunction may occur without precipitating events or follow vigorous forearm muscular activity.

Median nerve entrapment at the elbow may infrequently occur from an anomalous fibrous band that extends from the medial epicondyle to a bony spur on the anteromedial surface of the humerus (ligament of Struthers). The resultant weakness involves all median innervated muscles, including the pronator teres, and is accompanied by loss of the radial pulse when the arm is extended. Radiographs often demonstrate the anomalous bony spur.

Electrophysiologic studies. Nerve conduction studies in proximal median nerve compression syndromes are frequently normal. In more severe cases, the amplitudes of distal motor and sensory potentials may be reduced. Distal motor latencies may occasionally be prolonged with stimulation proximal to the elbow, but forearm median motor conduction velocities are usually normal. The most consistent and sensitive physiologic findings are neurogenic changes in median nerve innervated forearm and hand median muscles on needle EMG. In mild cases in which pain but not weakness is present, all electrophysiologic studies may be normal.

Treatment and prognosis. Conservative treatment of the pronator syndrome and spontaneous anterior interosseous nerve entrapment initially involves resting the arm by avoiding elbow flexion and pronation.[58] Gentle splinting of the arm in supination occasionally relieves symptoms but may also aggravate the condition. Corticosteroid injections into the pronator teres muscle may be of temporary benefit. In mild cases, non-steroidal anti-inflammatory medications may be useful. In both syndromes, persistent or progressive symptoms require exploratory surgery. Occasional cases are the result of schwannomas or other nerve tumors, which can sometimes be visualized by MRI imaging. Surgical excision of the spur and ligament in median nerve compression by the ligament of Struthers is usually successful.

Most entrapment injuries to the median nerve do not require splinting. Traumatic injury, however, frequently results in extensive and severe hand weakness for extended periods. In such cases, proper splinting of the thumb is essential to prevent deformity and preserve hand function. Regardless of the site of median nerve injury, thumb movement will be impaired. Loss of thumb abduction leaves it lying adjacent to the index finger, which predisposes to thumb web adductor contractures. A C-bar or wooden dowel, inserted between the thumb and second metacarpal, maintains thumb abduction, while an opponens bar on the proximal phalanx of the thumb stabilizes it in opposition to the index and middle fingers, thereby allowing full wrist movement and posting of the thumb.

Ulnar nerve

Source of injury[56,59]
Ulnar nerve entrapment is second to CTS as the most common nerve entrapment in the arm. Ulnar compression may occur in the axilla or upper arm, elbow region (either ulnar groove or cubital tunnel), or distally at the wrist or hand. The nerve is relatively exposed as it passes around the elbow and at the wrist, making it vulnerable to mild compressive or penetrating injuries. In the forearm, the muscle mass of the flexor carpi ulnaris affords the nerve relatively safety, save for severe penetrating wounds. Most compression injuries of the ulnar nerve are Class I and II. Improper positioning during anesthesia may result in an ulnar palsy. Occasionally, forceful, repetitive, flexion-extension movements of the arm may precipitate symptoms of ulnar nerve dysfunction. It is not clear whether ulnar neuropathy can be caused by repetitive arm movements. The relative infrequency of occurrence, in contrast to CTS, has prevented there being a sufficient number of prospective studies, with electrophysiologic verification, to examine this issue.

Dislocations or fractures of the elbow or chronic compression resulting from habitual leaning against the elbows may damage the ulnar nerve. Entrapment may occur in the cubital tunnel, where the nerve lies under the aponeurotic band between the two heads of the flexor carpi ulnaris. Occasionally, ulnar nerve dysfunction becomes evident many years after a supracondylar fracture of the humerus, leading to an increased carrying angle at the elbows (tardy ulnar palsy).

Ulnar entrapment at the elbow
The exposed position of the ulnar nerve at the medial epicondyle leaves the nerve susceptible to minor trauma or chronic compression. The nerve enters the forearm through a narrow opening (cubital tunnel) formed by the epicondyle, the medial collateral ligament of the joint, and the firm aponeurotic band to which the flexor carpi ulnaris is attached. This entire structure, formerly known as the cubital tunnel, has recently been renamed the humero-ulnar aponeurotic arcade (HUA). It is estimated that up to one-half of normal individuals have thickened and enlarged ulnar nerves, predisposing to compression either in the ulnar groove or HUA. Elbow flexion reduces the size of the opening under the aponeurotic band while extension widens it. Ulnar nerve dysfunction may therefore occur secondary to HUA narrowing during elbow flexion, without additional external trauma or local pathologic changes, or may be the result of any condition that increases nerve size or reduces the space available for the nerve. Some patients give no history of recent ulnar injury but report a previous elbow fracture or traumatic injury. This tardy ulnar palsy is frequently insidious in onset and probably results from narrowing of the HUA secondary to osteoarthritis or an increased carrying angle at the elbow.

The clinical deficits resulting from ulnar nerve lesions at the elbow are variable. Sensory symptoms usually precede weakness. Numbness, paresthesias, or pain in the fourth and fifth fingers are most common. Symptoms are occasionally positionally provoked, especially by prolonged elbow flexion, as during sleep or while talking on the phone. Although a chronic ache in the elbow is common, it is unusual for sensory symptoms and signs to extend proximal to the wrist. Cutaneous sensory appreciation is impaired in the fifth finger with occasional splitting of the fourth finger. Objective sensory impairment may involve the dorsum of the hand but does not extend proximal to the wrist crease. Because patients with ulnar neuropathies may not be bothered by paresthesias and pain, they may present with an advanced degree of weakness and wasting.

The first dorsal interossei are usually the earliest and most severely affected muscles; weakness and wasting of other ulnar hand and forearm muscles may follow. Severe weakness results in a claw hand deformity with variable flexion of the distal digits, depending on the degree of profundus muscle weakness. Ulnar neuropathy results in the loss of power grip and impaired precision movements.

Electrodiagnostic studies. Slowed motor or sensory nerve conduction across the elbow, relative to the forearm segment, is a clear localizing sign. Unfortunately, focal slowing of motor conduction is present in only 50–60% of cases. Absolute slowing of motor conduction across the elbow segment, regardless of forearm conduction, has been reported in 65–85% of patients with motor and sensory signs and about 50% of patients with only sensory impairment. Sensory potentials are frequently reduced in amplitude, including the dorsal cutaneous branch. Motor potential amplitudes are diminished in lesions resulting in motor axon degeneration. Nerve conduction studies may be normal in mild cases without weakness, but if axonal degeneration is present, needle EMG will demonstrate active and/or chronic denervation in ulnar-innervated muscles.

Treatment and prognosis.[58] Conservative therapy is reserved for three groups of patients: (1) those in whom symptoms are only posturally precipitated, (2) those mild cases in whom symptoms are aggravated by job-related activity, and (3) those who demonstrate only sensory symptoms without substantial progression. Therapy consists of avoiding aggravating movements, such as repeated elbow flexion and extension or habitually resting on the elbows. Splinting the elbow in extension for prolonged periods, especially during sleep, may occasionally be helpful. Elbow pads can be used in those who habitually rest on their elbows. Conservative therapy should be continued for at least 2–3 months or for as long as symptoms remain intermittent or mild, and weakness is absent. Careful follow-up is important to detect a progressive lesion that may result in substantial axonal degeneration. Non-steroidal anti-inflammatory agents are occasionally helpful.

Progressive sensory symptoms, new weakness, or worsening electrophysiologic deterioration dictates surgical inter-vention. Most surgeons now recommend either simple decompression within the HUA, or anterior transposition of the ulnar nerve, deep to the flexor forearm muscle mass. Clinical improvement can be expected in about 75% of cases. The severity of the preoperative lesion is important in predicting recovery; earlier intervention results in better recovery than waiting until severe wasting has occurred. Complications include neuroma formation, recurrent scarring around the nerve, and persistent pain, possibly caused by interruption of the nerve's blood supply.

Splints for ulnar lesions are designed to prevent hyper-extension of the ring and little finger's metacarpophalangeal (MCP) joints. A restraint on the dorsum of the proximal phalanx supports the MCP joint. Should IP joint flexion persist, a dynamic splint may be used to extend the distal IP joint.

Ulnar nerve lesion at the wrist

The ulnar nerve may be lacerated at the wrist or compressed either within Guyon's canal or more distally within the palm. The most common cause of distal ulnar compression is chronic repeated trauma to the palmar area, such as that which occurs among heavy laborers or cyclists. Other etiologies include ganglions that compress the nerve, either within Guyon's canal or distally along the deep terminal motor branch, fractures of the carpal bones, lipomas and other tumors, and rheumatoid arthritis. Acute trauma, such as a fall on the outstretched hand, may damage the nerve as it passes between the pisiform bone and the hook of the hamate.

Compression within Guyon's canal may result in any combination of weakness in hypothenar and thenar ulnar innervated muscles and sensory loss in the medial two fingers. Sensory innervation to the palmar and dorsal surfaces of the hand is spared. Distal ulnar compression should be suspected when ulnar innervated thenar muscles are weaker than hypothenar muscles. Other clinical scenarios include selective weakness of the hypothenar muscles and isolated sensory loss of the medial two fingers. Rarely, a more proximal wrist lesion may additionally affect the palmar sensory branch.

Electrodiagnostic studies. The most specific electrodiagnostic finding is a prolonged distal motor latency to the first dorsal interosseous muscle compared with the abductor digiti minimi muscle. The digital sensory potential to the fifth finger is of low amplitude or absent; dorsal cutaneous sensory potential is spared. Depending on the site of lesion, needle EMG may demonstrate active or chronic denervation in either hypothenar or thenar muscles with sparing of ulnar-innervated forearm muscles.

Treatment and prognosis. Conservative therapy is indicated when there are sensory symptoms alone. Maneuvers responsible for or aggravating the injury should be corrected. Surgery is indicated when conservative therapy has failed to relieve discomfort, when motor or sensory dysfunction progresses, or when the deficit has no clear cause and may be the result of a mass.

TOXIC NEUROMUSCULAR DISORDERS

The incidence of clinical neuromuscular transmission dysfunction resulting from toxins is infrequent compared with that of peripheral neuropathy. Recognition of a toxic etiology is vital, however, because complete function is usually returned after the offending agent(s) is(are) identified and eliminated. A discussion of the physiology of neuromuscular transmission is beyond the scope of this chapter, and the reader is referred to one of the many excellent texts dealing with this subject. The following is a brief description of the various toxins that have been identified to disrupt neuromuscular transmission.

Snake envenomation

The venom of certain poisonous snakes may produce acute, widespread weakness that clinically resembles a myasthenic crisis.[63] Two families of snakes have venom with a predilection for the neuromuscular junction, i.e., the Elapidae (coral snakes, cobras, mambas, and kraits) and the Hydrophiidae (sea snakes). Envenomation with cobra venom causes symptoms and signs within minutes to hours. The symptoms include ptosis, oculomotor paralysis, lower bulbar nerve dysfunction (resulting in lingual, laryngeal, and pharyngeal dysfunction), diffuse weakness, and eventually, respiratory compromise. In addition to neuromuscular blockage, local muscle necrosis may result. Impaired neuromuscular transmission from snake venom results from: (1) postsynaptic acetylcholine receptor blockade, which may be irreversible or partially reversible, and (2) presynaptic inhibition of acetylcholine release. Treatment of snake envenomation includes administration of anticholinesterases to antagonize postsynaptic receptor blockade, specific antivenom, debridement of necrotic muscle tissue, and mechanical respiration, when needed.

Arthropod envenomation

Impaired neuromuscular transmission may result from the toxins of black widow spiders, scorpions, female ticks, and wasps.[64] Black widow venom increases acetylcholine release and, probably, also prevents endocytosis of acetylcholine vesicles to nerve terminal membranes. The eventual result is depletion of such vesicles and impaired neuromuscular transmission. Clinical symptoms begin within 15–60 minutes of toxin injection and predominantly involve severe muscle cramps of the abdomen and limbs. Treatment is aimed at reducing muscle cramping by warming, infusing calcium gluconate, and administering magnesium sulfate to antagonize acetylcholine release. Atropine may help antagonize the cholinergic symptoms, and the administration of 2.5 mL of reconstituted antiserum is recommended.

Acute weakness may also be caused by the toxin from North American ticks (*Dermacentor andersoni* and *D. variabilis*). Tick paralysis may clinically resemble acute inflammatory demyelinating neuropathy (AIDP) and may result in respiratory paralysis.[65] The exact site of the pathologic change remains uncertain; terminal motor nerve endings and neuromuscular junctions have both been implicated. Removal of the tick is curative, often leading to rapid clinical recovery. Anticholinesterase therapy is usually ineffective.

Scorpion toxin indirectly affects the neuromuscular junction by inducing AChE release, caused by repetitive nerve terminal impulses.[66] These repetitive action potentials are believed to result from a toxin-induced delay in the normal sodium channel inactivation, thereby prolonging the nerve action potential. Clinical neuromuscular junction dysfunction is usually minimal.

Weakness simulating ocular myasthenia may result from the stings of wasps, bees, and hornets. Ocular symptoms may persist for weeks and are responsive to anticholinesterases and prednisone. Generalized weakness is rare.

Toxic myopathies

A number of toxic chemicals may primarily affect muscle.[67] The most common is alcohol, which produces a number of clinical scenarios, resulting from a combination of a primary toxic effect on muscle, related nerve disease, and metabolite disturbances, especially potassium. Most other toxic myopathies result from pharmaceutical agents, rather than industrial or occupational exposure. In many cases, the relationship between toxin and muscle weakness is not initially apparent. Most toxic myopathies are generalized and symmetric in nature, affecting proximal muscles most severely. Cranial nerve musculature is usually spared. Focal myopathies are usually caused by the local injection of toxic agents.

Focal myopathies

Focal muscle dysfunction, secondary to toxins, usually results from intramuscular injections, either from a local effect of the needle or the administered drug. Drugs with a known local toxic effect include diazepam (Valium), lidocaine, digoxin (Lanoxin), chloroquine (Aralen), opiates, and chlorpromazine (Thorazine). Paraldehyde and cephalothin sodium (Keflin) produce local irritation and abscess formation. Clinical weakness is usually minimal. The most common manifestation is an elevated creatine kinase (CK) level. Occasionally, severe induration and contractures may result. This is especially common with intramuscular injections of antibiotics in children or with meperidine (Demerol) or pentazocine (Talwin).

Acute/subacute myopathies

Many drugs can cause rapid-onset, symmetric, proximal muscle weakness, which is often painful.[67] The underlying mechanism is usually related to either potassium deficiency or an inflammatory myopathy. Occasionally, as with L-tryptophan, inflammation may predominate in the fascial tissue rather than the muscle itself. The serum CK concentration is usually markedly elevated, and myoglobinuria may be present. Drugs implicated in such myopathies include clofibrate (Atromid-S), epsilon-aminocaproic acid (Amicar), emetine hydrochloride, and vincristine (Oncoven). Clear inflammatory myopathies have been reported in patients taking procainamide (Provestyl), levodopa (Larodopa), and D-penicillamine. Patients ingesting certain brands of the amino acid L-tryptophan have developed severe myalgias and occasionally weakness. Pathologic changes have included a marked perimysial and perivascular inflammatory response with varying degrees of muscle necrosis. Recovery was often exceedingly prolonged and far outlasted the period of exposure. In most of these inflammatory myopathies, spontaneous recovery often accompanies removal of the drug, but steroids additionally may be needed.

Acute muscle weakness caused by hypokalemia is usually generalized and often painful. Frank muscle necrosis may result, and elevated CK levels and myoglobinuria may be present. Hypokalemia may result from diuretics, purgatives, amphotericin B (Fungizone), and carbenoxolone. Amphotericin B and carbenoxolone, along with amphetamines, have been implicated in producing a severe necrotizing myopathy with rhabdomyolysis.

Chronic myopathies

Many drugs produce a chronic painless myopathy presenting with limb-girdle weakness. Proximal leg and pelvic muscles are usually affected to a greater degree than are arm muscles. CK levels may be normal. The most commonly implicated drugs are corticosteroids, which produce weakness through their interference with oxidative metabolism and inhibition of protein synthesis. Other drugs include chloroquine, which can produce a clinical picture identical to that from steroids, heroin, and chronic hypokalemia. Muscle weakness has also been ascribed to perhexiline, colchicine, and rifampin (Rimectane).

Alcoholic myopathy

The deleterious effect of alcohol on muscle may be through a direct toxic effect or associated malnutrition and electrolyte disturbance. Alcohol may produce acute, subacute, and chronic weakness.[67] The acute variety usually follows binge drinking and is associated with painful swollen muscles and myoglobinuria. An acute but painless variety of muscle weakness may also occur, associated with marked hypokalemia, elevated CK levels, and muscle necrosis. Recovery proceeds over several weeks to months, but the problem may recur with subsequent drinking bouts.

References

1. Schaumburg HH, Wisniewski HM, Spencer PS. Ultrastructural studies of the dying-back process. I. Peripheral nerve terminal and axon degeneration in systemic acrylamide intoxication. J Neuropathol Exper Neurol 1974; 33:260.
2. Spencer PS, Schaumburg HH. Central-peripheral distal axonopathy – the pathogenesis of dying-back polyneuropathies. In: Zimmerman H, ed. Progress in neuropathology, vol. 3. New York: Grune and Stratton, 1976;253.
3. Schaumburg HH, Spencer PS. Recognizing neurotoxic disease. Neurology 1987; 37:276.
4. Klassen C. Heavy metals and heavy metal antagonists. In: Goodman, Gilman A, Rall TW, Nies AS, Taylor P, eds.
5. O'Shaughnessy E, Kraft GK. Arsenic poisoning: long-term follow-up of a non-fatal case. Arch Phys Med Rehab 1976; 57:403.
6. Windebank AJ, McCall JT, Dyck PJ. Metal neuropathy. In: Dyck PJ, Thomas PK, Lambert EH, Bunge RP, eds. Peripheral neuropathy, 2nd edn. Philadelphia: WB Saunders, 1984;2133.
7. Oh SJ. Electrophysiologic profile in arsenic neuropathy. J Neurol Neurosurg Psych 1991; 54:1103.
8. Heyman A, Pfeiffer JB, Taylor HM. Peripheral neuropathy caused by arsenical intoxication: a study of 41 cases with observation on the effects of BAL (2,3-dimercapto-propanol). N Engl J Med 1956; 254:401.
9. Feldman RG. Occupational and environmental toxicology. Philadelphia: Lippincott-Raven Publishers, 1999;30.
10. Whitfield CL, Ch'ien LT, Whitehead JD. Lead encephalopathy in adults. Am J Med 1972; 52:289.
11. Chancellor AM, Slattery JM, Fraser H, Warlow CP. Risk factors for motor neuron disease: a case-control study based on patients from the Scottish Motor Disease registry. J Neurol Neurosurg Psych 1993; 56:1200.
12. Seppalainen AM, Hernberg S. Sensitive technique for detecting subclinical lead neuropathy. Br J Ind Med 1972; 29:443.
13. Seppalainen AM, Tola S, Hernberg S, Kock B. Subclinical neuropathy at 'safe' levels of lead exposure. Arch Environ Health 1975; 30:180.
14. Markowitz ME , Rosen JF. Need for the lead mobilization test in children with lead poisoning. J Pediatr 1991; 119:305.
15. Kyrland LT, Faro SN, Siedler H. Minamata disease. The outbreak of a neurologic disorder in Minamata, Japan and its relationship to the ingestion of seafood contaminated by mercuric compounds. World Neurol 1967; 1:370.
16. Bakir F, Damluji SF, Amin-Zaki L, et al. Methylmercury poisoning in Iraq. Science 1973; 181:230.
17. Brune D, Evje DM. Man's mercury loading from a dental amalgam. Sci Total Environ 1985; 44:51.
18. Takeuchi T. Pathology of Minamata disease. In: Kutsuma M, ed. Minamata Disease. Kumamoto: Study Group of Minamata Disease, Kumamoto University, Japan, 1968;141.
19. Albers JW, Kallenbach LR, Fine LJ, et al. and the Mercury Studies Group. Neurological abnormalities associated with remote occupational elementary mercury exposure. Ann Neurol 1988; 24:651.
20. Singer R, Valciukas JA, Rosenman KD. Peripheral nerve toxicity in workers exposed to inorganic mercury compounds. Arch Environ Health 1987; 42:181.
21. Campbell D, Gonzales M, Sullivan JB Jr. Mercury. In: Sullivan JB Jr, Kreiger GR, eds. Hazardous materials toxicology: clinical principles of environmental health. Baltimore: Williams and Wilkins, 1992;824.
22. Davis LE, Stadefr JC, Kornfeld M, Abercrombie DM, Butler C. Acute thallium poisoning: toxicological and morphological studies of the nervous system. Ann Neurol 1981; 10:38.
23. Douglas KT, Bunni MA, Baindur SR. Minireview: thallium in biochemistry. Int J Biochem 1990; 22:429.
24. Nordentoft T, Anderson EB, Morgensen PH. Initial sensorimotor and delayed autonomic neuropathy in acute thallium poisoning. Neurotoxicol 1998; 19:421.
25. Dumitru D, Kalantri A. Electrophysiologic investigation of thallium poisoning. Muscle Nerve 1990; 13:433.
26. Moore D, House I, Dixon A. Thallium poisoning: diagnosis may be elusive but alopecia is the clue. BMJ 1993; 306(6891):1527.
27. Stevens W, van Peteghem C, Heyndricks A et al. Eleven cases of thallium intoxication treated with Prussian blue. Int J Clin Pharmacol 1974; 10:1.
28. Metcalf DR, Holmes JH. EEG, psychological and neurological alterations in humans with organophosphorous exposure. Ann NY Acad Sci 1969; 160:357.

Goodman and Gilman's the pharmacological basis of therapeutics. Elmsford, New York: Pergamon Press, 1990;1602.

29. Wadia RS, Sadagtopan C, Amin RB, Sardesai HV. Neurological manifestations of organophosphorous insecticide poisoning. J Neurol Neurosurg Psych 1974; 37:841.

30. DeBleeker J. The intermediate syndrome in organophosphate poisoning: an overview of experimental and clinical observations. Clin Toxicol 1995; 33:683.

31. Wadia RS, Chitra S, Amin RB, Kiwalkar RS, Sardesai HV. Electrophysiologic studies in acute organophosphate poisoning. J Neurol Neurosurg Psych 1987; 50:1442.

32. Besser R, Gutman I, Dillmann U, Weilemann LS, Hopf HC. End-plate dysfunction in acute organophosphate intoxication. Neurology 1989; 39:561.

33. Misra UK, Nag D, Khan WA, Ray PK. A study of nerve conduction velocity, late responses and neuromuscular synapse function in organophosphate workers in India. Arch Toxicol 1988; 61:496.

34. LeWitt P. The neurotoxicity of the rat poison vacor. N Engl J Med 1980; 302:73.

35. Watson DF, Griffin JW. Vacor neuropathy: ultrastructural and axonal transport studies. J Neuropathol Exp Neurol 1987; 46:96.

36. Gordy ST, Trumper M. Carbon disulfide poisoning with a report of six cases. JAMA 1938; 110:1543.

37. Chu C-C, Huang C-C, Chen R-S, Shih T-S. Polyneuropathy induced by carbon disulfide in viscose rayon workers. Occup Environ Med 1995; 52:404.

38. Seppalainen AM, Tolonen M. Neurotoxicity of long term exposure to carbon disulfide in the viscose rayon industry. A neurophysiologic study. Work Environ Health 1974; 11:145.

39. O'Donoghue JL, Krasavage WJ. Hexacarbon neuropathy: a gamma-diketone neuropathy? J Neuropath Exp Neurol 1979; 38:333(abst).

40. Mendell JR, Saida K, Ganansia MG, et al. Toxic polyneuropathy produced by methyl n-butyl ketone. Science 1974; 185:787.

41. Schaumburg HH, Spencer PS. Environmental hydrocarbons produce degeneration in cat hypothalamus and optic tract. Science 1978; 199:199.

42. Korobkin R, Asbury AK, Sumner AJ, Nielsen SL. Glue sniffing neuropathy. Arch Neurol 1975; 32:158.

43. Davenport JG, Farrell DF, Sumi SM. 'Giant axonal neuropathy' caused by industrial chemicals: neurofilamentous masses in man. Neurology 1976; 26:919.

44. Asbury AK, Gale MK, Cox SC, Baringer JR, Berg BO. Giant axonal neuropathy: a unique case with segmental neurofilamentous masses. Acta Neuropathol 1972; 20:237.

45. He F, Zahng S. Effects of allyl chloride on occupationally exposed subjects. Scand J Work Environ Health 1985; 11:43.

46. Gold BG, Griffin JW, Price DL. Slow axonal transport in acrylamide neuropathy: different abnormalities produced by single-dose and continuous administration. J Neurosci 1985; 5:1755.

47. Miller MS, Spencer PS. Single dose of acrylamide reduce retrograde transport velocity. J Neurochem 1984; 43:1401.

48. Schaumburg HH, Arezzo JC, Spencer PS. Delayed onset of axonal neuropathy in primates after prolonged low-level administration of a neurotoxin. Ann Neurol 1989; 26:576.

49. Spencer PS, Schaumburg HH. Ultrastructural studies of the dying back process. III. The evolution of experimental peripheral giant axonal degeneration. J Neuropathol Exp Neurol 1977; 36:276.

50. Schaumburg HH, Wisniewski HM, Spencer PS. Ultrastructural studies of the dying back process. Peripheral nerve terminal and axon degeneration in systemic acrylamide intoxication. J Neuropathol Exp Neurol 1974; 33:260.

51. Fullerton PM. Electrophysiologic and histologic observations on the peripheral nerves in acrylamide poisoning. J Neurol Neurosurg Psych 1969; 32:186.

52. Pestronk A, Keogh J, Griffin JG. Dimethylaminopropionitrile intoxication: a new industrial neuropathy. Neurology 1979; 29:540.

53. Cavalleri F, Galassi G, Ferrari S. Methyl bromide induced neuropathy: a clinical, neurophysiological and morphological study. J Neurol Neurosurg Psychiat 1995; 58:383.

54. Gross JA, Haas ML, Swift TR. Ethylene oxide neurotoxicity: report of four cases and review of the literature. Neurology 1979; 29:978.

55. Murai Y, Kuroiwa Y. Peripheral neuropathy in chlorobiphenyl poisoning. Neurology 1971; 21:1173.

56. Stewart JD, ed. Focal peripheral neuropathies. Philadelphia; Lippincott, Williams and Wilkins, 2000.

57. Mitsunage MM, Nakano K. High radial nerve palsy following strenuous muscular activity. Clin Orthop 1988; 234:39.

58. Berger AR, Schaumburg HH. Rehabilitation of focal nerve injuries. J Neurol Rehab 1988; 2:65.

59. Dawson DM, Hallett M, Wilbourne AJ, eds. Entrapment neuropathies. Philadelphia; Lippincott, Williams and Wilkins, 1999.

60. Berger AR, Herskovitz S. Cumulative trauma disorder. In: Rosenberg NL, ed. Occupational and enviromental neurology. Boston: Butterworth-Heinemann, 1995;235.

61. Nathan PA, Keniston RC, Myers LD, Meadows KD, Lockwood RS. Natural history of median nerve sensory conduction in industry: relationship to symptoms and carpal tunnel syndrome in 558 hands over 11 years. Muscle Nerve 1998; 21:711.

62. Nilsson T, Hagberg M, Berstrom L, Lundstrom R. A five-year follow-up of nerve conduction over the carpal tunnel. Stockholm workshop 94. Hand-arm vibration syndrome. Arbete Och Halsa Vetenskaplig skriftserie 1995; 5:117.

63. Campbell CH. The effects of snake venoms and their neurotoxins on the nervous system of man and animals. In: Hornabrook RW, ed. Topics in tropical neurology. Philadelphia: FA Davis, 1975;259.

64. Gilbert EW, Stewart CM. Effective treatment of arachnoidism by calcium salts. Am J Med Sci 1935; 189:532.

65. Cherington M. Botulism: ten-year experience. Arch Neurol 1974; 30:432.

66. Warnick JE, Albuquerque EX, Diniz CR. Electrophysiologic observations on the action of the purified scorpion venom, Tityustoxin, on nerve and skeletal muscle of the rat. J Pharmacol Exp Ther 1976; 198:155.

67. Griggs RC, Mendell JR, Miller RG, eds. Evaluation and treatment of myopathies. Philadelphia: FA Davis, 1995.

28.3 Psychosocial Stressors and Psychiatric Disorders in the Workplace

Nancy Fiedler, Lawrence B Stein

Most adults spend a significant part of their daily life in the workplace and research has demonstrated that a stimulating job contributes to a more meaningful life, higher self-esteem, and opportunities to increase socioeconomic status. However, psychosocial and physical work stressors also contribute to a decrease in work function and to psychologic disturbances ranging from stress reactions to diagnosable psychiatric illnesses. For example, some occupations such as emergency workers may be more prone to stress-related illnesses due to the unrelenting demands that are a routine part of their occupation.

Psychiatric illness (e.g., depression and anxiety) is recognized as a leading occupational health problem by the National Institute of Occupational Safety and Health[1] and often occurs from the interaction of work and non-work related environmental stressors and individual predispositions. Therefore, to the extent that the occupational practitioner can identify work-related factors contributing to psychiatric illness and develop appropriate intervention strategies, the impact on the individual and the organization can be mitigated. This chapter offers an overview of the literature on work-related psychosocial and physical stressors and individual susceptibilities associated with psychiatric symptoms and illness. Following this overview and in the context of a public health prevention model, methods for identifying risks within the workplace and preventing the effects of psychiatric illness on the individual and the organization are presented.

OCCUPATIONS, PSYCHIATRIC DISORDERS, AND PRODUCTIVITY

Psychiatric disorders impair productivity through several avenues that include reduced labor supply, absenteeism, poor morale, and reduced quality of work. Statistics validating the overall economic impact of psychiatric disorders within the United States abound; depression is estimate to cost $43.7 billion, while alcoholism costs approximately $89 billion per year.[2] This amount includes costs of lost productivity, as well as healthcare. Aside from alcoholism, drinking behavior of undiagnosed employees, such as coming to work 'hung over', has also been associated with problems at work.[3,4] In short, the costs of behavioral problems and psychiatric disorders affect not only workers and their families, but also managers, coworkers, employers and insurance companies.

As an initial step toward understanding occupational risk factors that contribute to psychiatric disorders, epidemiologic studies have compared prevalence rates across occupations. For example, the Epidemiologic Catchment Area (ECA) community survey of psychiatric disorders found, after controlling for demographic differences among 104

occupations, that lawyers, teachers, counselors (not college), and secretaries had elevated rates of major depression compared to the overall rate for employed individuals; movers (freight, stock, and material), transport and material moving occupations, handlers, equipment cleaners and laborers, janitors and cleaners, and waiters and waitresses had elevated rates of alcoholism.[5] The ECA study also found, however, that the risk for a diagnosis of alcoholism increased for managers and construction laborers when they were unemployed, confirming the overall protective nature of being employed.

Comparisons of psychiatric disorders across occupations, while intriguing and heuristically valuable, do not specify what factors within these occupations contribute to risk. Thus, a significant literature has developed in which the behavioral consequences of psychosocial and physical risk factors have been explored.

WORK-RELATED PSYCHOSOCIAL RISKS FOR PSYCHIATRIC DISORDER

The mechanism for higher rates of psychiatric disorder among occupations varies with both health-enhancing and deleterious characteristics of the job and individual susceptibilities. Moreover, job characteristics may contribute to the type of psychiatric disorder. With regard to job qualities, evidence appears to be converging to support the significance of job demands and control over decisions as proposed by Karasek.[6] For example, employees in lower status positions, who often experience little control over decisions, also have higher rates of psychiatric disorders than those in higher positions (i.e., more depression and anxiety). Although common sense suggests that high demands would cause increased illness, both Mandell et al.[5] and Hemmingson & Lundberg[7] reported greater risk of alcoholism with lower or no workload.

The latter is also consistent with the reported higher rates of alcoholism among unemployed workers and suggests that the relationship between job demands and psychiatric disorder may be curvilinear. That is, low work load (or unemployment) or working in an environment with strenuous demands and little or no control may have serious implications for an individual. In addition, moderators mitigate the negative effects of job demands. Stansfeld et al.[8] reported that high social support and skill discretion were protective against absence due to psychiatric illness. Social support consisted of a high level of support from colleagues and supervisors coupled with clear and consistent information from supervisors, and skill discretion referred to job variety and the opportunity to use skills at work.

More recently, a nationwide study of Swedish males found that a combination of low work control, low work demands, and low work social support was related to later alcoholism after controlling for other risk factors.[7] This finding further supports the association between low work demands and alcoholism and incorporates other important psychosocial moderators. In a follow-up interview for the ECA study, Mausner-Dorsch & Eaton[9] found support for the association between major depressive episode, depressive syndrome, and dysphoria and job strain defined as a combination of high demands and low control over decisions. Moreover, they found that women were at greater risk both because they were more susceptible to job strain and were probably more exposed to it in their work environment. The latter illustrates the interactive effect of individual susceptibility and work-related stressors on eventual psychiatric illness.

In summary, the relationship between job demands and psychiatric illness is moderated, particularly when demands are high, by perception of control over decisions. That is, if the individual has control, demands may not have the same negative impact on psychiatric function.

Work–family conflict

In addition to work stressors, pressures external to work also impact the incidence of psychiatric illness. For example, work–family conflicts, defined as the incompatibility between the role demands of a career and family (e.g., long work hours preventing time with spouse or other family members), have been associated with lower job, marital, and life satisfaction.[7] More specific to the workplace, individuals who are experiencing high work–family conflict are more prone to job turnover and decreased job productivity. Some gender differences have been found; women show elevated risk of disability when they report both work and marital interpersonal conflict, whereas interpersonal conflict was not predictive of work disability for men.[10] Instead, life dissatisfaction, neuroticism, monotonous work, and stress of daily activities predicted work disability for men. Duxbury & Higgins[11] report that men experience work–family conflict due to work expectations, while women experience more work–family conflicts due to family expectations.

This overview suggests that greater risk for psychiatric disorder occurs when the following work and non-work related conditions converge: (1) the employee is either insufficiently challenged (low job demands) or has too many demands with little control, (2) social support is low

at work, (3) work and family roles conflict, (4) the employee is female. Since women are more often in occupations with less control and simultaneously have more family responsibilities,[12] gender may be a surrogate for differences in exposure to stressors at work and in the home. Table 28.3.1 summarizes the work-related psychosocial risk factors and associated psychiatric symptoms.

PHYSICAL RISK FACTORS

Physical aspects of the work environment also contribute to the occurrence of stress and psychiatric disturbance. Exposure to toxic chemicals, poor indoor air quality, noise, shiftwork, and trauma are some of the physical stressors associated with psychiatric illness.

Neurotoxicant exposure

Numerous studies document psychiatric symptoms associated with exposure to lead, organic solvents, carbon monoxide, and mercury. Lead exposure, whether acute or chronic, may result in non-specific symptoms often found in psychiatric disorders, such as fatigue, decreased libido, restlessness and depression.[13,14] Organic solvent exposure is well known to produce a variety of psychiatric symptoms ranging from mild mood disturbances to severe psychoses. Acute solvent exposure is most often followed by mood changes, transient euphoric reactions, or complaints of mental confusion.[15] The organic affective syndrome, identified by the World Health Organization and by NIOSH, is associated with chronic solvent exposure and is characterized by symptoms such as irritability, poor concentration, and loss of interest, symptoms also seen in several psychiatric disorders.[16,17] Post-traumatic stress disorder,[18] somatoform disorder,[19] schizophreniform disorder,[20] and panic disorder[21] have been documented to occur following long-term exposure to organic solvents.

Similarly, carbon monoxide (CO) exposure from motor vehicle exhaust or malfunctioning heating systems can produce symptoms such as fatigue, apathy, emotional lability, lowered frustration tolerance, impulsivity, irritability, and at times, psychosis.[22-25] The symptoms of CO exposure may be delayed and may occur from 3 to 240 days after recovery from acute intoxication;[26] 50–75% of exposed patients recover from this delayed syndrome within one

Psychosocial risk factors	Symptoms	Possible psychiatric illness
High job demands with low decision latitude[7,48]	Feelings of helplessness and hopelessness in both home and work environments; lack of sense of personal accomplishment; and irritability; emotional exhaustion; feelings of depersonalization	Depression and anxiety
Lack of social support[53]	Increased conflict at home; decreased feelings of self-efficacy in decision making; decreased commitment to organization; increased absenteeism	Depression and anxiety
Work–family conflict[9-11]	Decreased marital satisfaction; decreased job productivity; increased sense of guilt	Depression; anxiety; and heavy alcohol consumption
Interpersonal conflicts with coworkers and supervisors[48]	Increased use of sick leave time; decreased self-esteem; emotional exhaustion; feelings of depersonalization	Depression; anxiety; somatic symptoms

Table 28.3.1 Psychosocial risk factors, symptoms associated with these factors, and possible psychiatric illness that may result from prolonged exposure to stressors

year.[27] Exposure to mercury, which occurred when hatmakers used mercury to process felt (hence the phrase, 'mad as a hatter'), has been found to result in both mania and chronic depressed mood with apathy and extreme shyness and withdrawal.[28] Chronic mild exposure may cause irritability, nervousness, fatigue, and depression.[29]

Because the clinical presentation of neurotoxicant exposure has significant overlap with symptoms arising from many other factors to include work and non-work related psychosocial stressors, a good exposure history is essential to develop appropriate intervention. For example, if the health practitioner is presented with psychiatric symptoms without exploration of neurotoxicant exposures, behavioral therapy and psychotropic medications may be prescribed when removal or reduction of exposure is the appropriate intervention. Thus, inquiry about the chemicals used at work and at home is an important part of an evaluation for psychiatric disorder.

Indoor air quality

Sick building syndrome or non-specific building-related illness (NSBRI) presents as a constellation of symptoms that overlap to some extent with symptoms of stress and psychiatric illness. Symptoms include mucous membrane irritation, headache, fatigue, shortness of breath, rash and abnormal odor perception.[30,31] In at least one cross-sectional study, workers in a sick versus control building reported an increased number of psychologic symptoms which did not account for NSBRI but appeared to be independent consequences of poor indoor air quality.[32] Several work-site factors are hypothesized to account for the symptoms associated with poor indoor air quality to include direct toxic effects of the chemical mixtures, psychosocial job stress (e.g., poor supervision, high job demands) and noxious odors. Most studies suggest that symptoms likely result from an interaction of these chemical and psychosocial stressors, with each workplace presenting a unique combination of factors.

Noise and shiftwork

It has been noted that factory and construction workers exposed to high levels of noise have demonstrated a wide variety of complaints beyond hearing.[33] For example, individuals exposed to excessive noise have reported symptoms of depression, anxiety, insomnia, and weight loss.[34] Exposure to loud and unsystematic noise has also been demonstrated to create an uncomfortable workplace, decrease worker production, and is viewed by the worker as a significant physical, social, and cognitive stressor.[35] Shiftwork represents another source of physical and psychological stress for employees. Little evidence exists regarding a causal relationship between shiftwork and psychiatric disorders, with the exception of individuals with shift maladaptation syndrome (see Chapter 38).

Nonetheless, shiftworkers report lower subjective levels of physical health and wellbeing.[36-38] In addition, they have higher rates of alcohol and substance abuse[39] as compared to daytime workers and high rates of neuroticism.[40,41] It has

also been noted that the 'graveyard' shift (e.g., midnight to 8:00 am) is associated with the most problems (e.g., higher accident rates, lower performance quality); however, the swing shift has the most negative impact on social patterns and interpersonal interactions.[42] At present, studies investigating the prevalence of depression in shiftworkers are contradictory and inconsistent, which reflects the necessity for further research to determine more thoroughly the potential psychological consequences of the worker's schedules on psychological functioning.

Workplace trauma

Workplace trauma can occur under several conditions: (1) physically hazardous working conditions where safety procedures are inadequate or not practiced, (2) the nature of the work is inherently traumatic (e.g., emergency response teams), and (3) work settings with risk for violence. The construction trades have a higher rate of injury and death than many other trades[43] and workers who are injured or who witness the injury or death of a coworker are at risk for post-traumatic stress disorder. Similarly, emergency response workers such as police, firefighters, and emergency medical technicians, by the nature of their work, encounter and manage violence, death, and injury on a routine basis.[44]

Finally, employees in service positions may encounter violence under the following conditions: exchanging money, interacting with the public, working at night or in the early morning, delivering goods, and working alone. In work settings where trauma is likely to occur, preventive measures should be emphasized, and emergency procedures need to be implemented following a trauma to prevent psychiatric disorder and disability.

INDIVIDUAL SUSCEPTIBILITY

Risk factors for psychiatric disorders do not confine themselves to work stressors but also lie within the individual. Many of these factors may be psychosocial while others may be biologic or genetic. For example, compared to men, women are exposed to more job strain[9] and may also be more sensitive to it and to interpersonal conflict than men.[10] Gender is another well-known risk factor for specific psychiatric disturbance, with women being more vulnerable to depression and men abusing alcohol more than women.[45] Individuals who have a history of previous psychiatric disturbance or trauma are also at greater risk either for exacerbation of current psychiatric illness or recurrence with exposure to work-related stressors.

Similarly, individuals with lower socioeconomic status and those who are unemployed are more at risk for a wide variety of psychopathology including depression, anxiety, substance abuse, and schizophrenia. On the other hand, being employed in a job that is satisfying and productive may act as a buffer against these types of problems. Although in the early stages of investigation, genetic factors may contribute to risk particularly for susceptibility to neurotoxicant exposures.[46,47]

RECOGNIZING AND ASSESSING STRESS, BURNOUT, AND PSYCHIATRIC ILLNESS IN THE WORKPLACE

Prevention of psychiatric disorder requires assessment of the job characteristics that contribute to symptoms and early diagnosis to reduce individual and organizational disabilities. The following section provides an overview of psychiatric disorders most frequently seen in the workplace and measures to screen for these symptoms (Table 28.3.2).

Stress symptoms and burnout

Stress-related problems often present as physical symptoms such as gastrointestinal distress, chronic headache, low back pain, and fatigue. Symptoms of anxiety and depressed mood that fall short of diagnostic criteria for depression and anxiety disorders, manifest themselves as stress syndromes. Job dissatisfaction and poor morale are organizational manifestations of stress. For example, machine-paced assembly work has been associated with somatic complaints, job dissatisfaction, anxiety, irritability, and depression.[35] Stress symptoms, while overlapping, can be distinguished from psychiatric disorders based on three criteria: number of symptoms, chronicity of symptoms, and effects on function.

Typically, to meet criteria for a psychiatric disorder, the individual must report a specified number and type of symptoms that have persisted over a given time period (e.g., 2 weeks) and that interfere in the performance of significant life functions at home and/or work. For example, feeling depressed and worried yet not reporting significant effects on interpersonal or work function such as conflicts with coworkers or impaired work performance would probably not meet criteria for a psychiatric disorder.

However, within the work environment, if these symptoms occur in several individuals, a net effect on productivity and morale may be observed. Thus, assessing job-related stress and intervening can prevent more serious individual and organizational disorder if these symptoms persist.

Job burnout is probably the extreme example of a stress-related syndrome. Although it is not an official medical or psychiatric diagnosis, it is often thought of as a precursor to psychiatric disorder. Maslach[48] proposed a tripartite model of burnout that encompasses both job and personal characteristics. Included in this model are emotional exhaustion, cynicism, and a lack of sense of personal accomplishment. It has been duly noted that increased levels of emotional exhaustion, which refers to feelings of 'being overextended, drained, or used up', is correlated with physical symptoms such as gastrointestinal disorders, chronic fatigue, hypertension, headaches, sleep disturbances, and flu/cold symptoms. On the other hand, chronic feelings of cynicism (i.e., negative or detached feelings concerning job and work-related behaviors) and ineffectiveness (i.e., decreased feelings of competency) are thought to contribute to other problems such as despondency, hopelessness, and, in extreme cases, depression and anxiety.

Workers experiencing high levels of burnout in any one of these three domains tend to have a higher rate of job turnover, higher rates of absenteeism, are more inflexible about work-related rules and procedures, and are more dissatisfied with their job when compared to their more engaged counterparts. Although burnout is seen across jobs and work settings, it is more likely when the job involves frequent contact with people who are in need of help (e.g., health and service fields) and when a job supervisor is perceived as being unresponsive to employee needs. When either the type of work or the supervisory climate promote burnout, assessment for burnout is the first step to prevent disability and high worker turnover (Table 28.3.2).

Measures	Description of measure	Administration time (minutes)	Psychometric properties
Stressors			
Job content questionnaire[76]	Assesses psychologic demands, decision latitude, social support and job insecurity.	30	Test-retest reliabilities ranging from .84 to .87
Hassles and uplifts scales[74]	Global measure of stressful life events. Helps to identify work and non-work related stressors along with positive aspects of work and personal life.	30	Test-retest reliabilities are .79 for frequency of uplifts and .60 for intensity of hassles
Stress symptoms			
Maslach burnout inventory[48]	Measures three aspects of burnout: (1) emotional exhaustion; (2) lack of sense of personal accomplishment; and (3) depersonalization.	30	Test-retest reliability ranging from .79 to .89
Symptom checklist-90-R[73]	A multidimensional measure of symptoms associated with psychologic distress and a wide variety of psychiatric disorders.	15	Internal consistency ranges from .77 to .90; test-retest reliability is .78 to .90
Beck depression inventory[72]	A unidimensional scale that measures severity of depression.	15	Test-retest reliability of .90, internal consistency of .86, and coefficient alpha of .94
Impact of event scale[75]	A multidimensional scale used to assess symptoms associated with post-traumatic stress disorder.	15	Coefficient alpha of .42 to .82
Michigan alcohol screening test[77]	A scale that measures past and present alcohol consumption.	15	Coefficient alpha of .95
Beck anxiety inventory[71]	A unidimensional scale that measures severity of anxiety.	15	Test-retest reliability of .89, internal consistency of .85, and coefficient alpha of .87

Table 28.3.2 Instruments used to screen for stressors and psychiatric symptoms in the workplace

Psychiatric disorders

Depressive and anxiety disorders

Comparisons across occupations show that depressive disorders, in particular, are prevalent in the workplace. Diagnostic criteria common to all of the depressive disorders (major depression, dysthymia) include depressed mood and a loss of interest or pleasure in usual activities with symptoms of decreased or increased appetite, sleep disturbance, poor concentration, fatigue, and thoughts of death. Anxiety disorders include generalized anxiety disorder, panic disorder, and phobias and are characterized by excessive worry and a number of psychologic and physical symptoms such as shortness of breath, heart pounding, sweating, chest pain, nausea, and fear of losing control. Phobias can range from those that are specific to situations or things to a fear of being outside of the home (i.e., agoraphobia). The same screening tools suggested under stress disorders can also be useful to screen for depression and anxiety disorders with severity greater in the individual who has a diagnosable psychiatric disorder.

Post-traumatic stress disorder (PTSD) is an anxiety disorder specifically related to traumatic exposures. In the workplace, traumatic events include death or serious injury to self or others and workplace violence. For example, NIOSH data reveal that homicide is the second leading cause of occupational death, following work-related motor vehicle accidents, and surpassing machine-related deaths.[49] The individual's response to a traumatic event such as seeing a coworker seriously injured or killed involves intense fear, helplessness, and horror. Symptoms of PTSD include intrusive thoughts/dreams and recollections of the trauma, re-experiencing the trauma, and avoidance of stimuli that arouse recollection of the trauma. PTSD is not inevitable following a traumatic experience and can be prevented with debriefing and counseling immediately following an event.[50]

Substance abuse and dependence

A vast literature documents the occurrence and deleterious effects of substance abuse in the workplace. Workers showing a pattern of poor performance that includes absenteeism, lateness, conflicts with coworkers, and frequent illness may alert the occupational health professional to a substance abuse problem. However, as is evident from the list, these work-related symptoms are not unique to substance abuse and may have numerous causes. Thus, diagnosing a substance abuse problem as a non-mental health professional, and in the absence of information about the individual's pattern of substance use, is difficult and potentially harmful. Denial is a major psychologic dimension of substance abuse and therefore, if the diagnosis is suggested to the individual with inadequate documentation, it may serve to reinforce denial.

Diagnosis of substance abuse includes an inability to control the use of a mood-altering substance and is not confined to alcohol or illicit drugs but also includes prescription and non-prescription medications. Abuse is not determined by quantity of use but rather by the fact that the individual continues to use the substance despite adverse medical, social, family, or occupational consequences. Thus, the diagnosis is behavioral and does not depend on the amount or type of substance used. To make this point more clearly, virtually the same criteria are applied to diagnose pathologic gambling.[45]

Psychoses

Psychotic disorders are characterized by delusions, hallucinations, incoherent speech, disorganized behavior, and flat or inappropriate affect. Since psychoses are frequently diagnosed in young adulthood, some individuals may have their first episode while employed. Psychotic individuals are often not employed, but with medication may be returned to a workplace with proper accommodations.

STRATEGIES FOR PREVENTION
Primary prevention

What can we do to make work less stressful and individuals less vulnerable to what may, to some extent, be an inevitable part of work? Jobs where workers have little control over decisions seem to produce greater risk for psychiatric disorder. Therefore, programs to enhance employee participation in decisions are interventions that may prove to reduce psychiatric morbidity. For example, Karasek recommended that specific Quality of Work Life programs (QWL) be used by organizations to ensure that employees feel a sense of empowerment. More specifically, this process enables workers to set their own goals, make decisions, and solve problems within their sphere of responsibility. Although QWL interventions have focused primarily on lower-level employees, Quality Circles (QC), which are often found within various organizational strata (e.g., middle management, blue-collar workers), include groups of volunteers who work together on a particular job, meet regularly, and discuss job-related problems and possible solutions. Porras and Silvers[51] have noted that QCs have a positive impact on employee attitudes, which may decrease job strain and burnout. However, the effect of QCs on job productivity is more equivocal.[52]

On an individual basis, wellness programs that enhance resilience through better diet, exercise, and relaxation may also improve mental health. These programs typically include stress management workshops, health risk assessments, exercise facilities, subsidized cafeterias, individual counseling, and seminars and lectures. Programs that reduce work–family conflict can also reduce the incidence of psychiatric disorder. For example, employee-sponsored daycare centers have been demonstrated to increase job satisfaction and decrease work-related stress on working mothers.[53]

Other factors such as flexible work hours[54] and parental leave programs[55] have observed similar findings. Perhaps the existence of these programs helps the employer or organization to acknowledge and support the challenges that employees often face. Also, these programs help employees feel more empowered and valued as individuals who make significant contributions at the workplace. Some preliminary research indicates that when upper level managers support wellness programs, and when employees have easy access to these services, notable decreases in medical expenses and increases in productivity[56] are typically seen.

Accurately assessing physical and psychosocial hazards within the workplace is an important step toward preventing psychiatric disorders. Reducing exposure to neurotoxicants and to hazardous working conditions need to be considered when increased rates of symptoms and psychiatric disturbance are noted. For example, reducing exposure to neurotoxicants through engineering controls and programs to train employees in the use of protective equipment will reduce exposure and disability. NIOSH has provided specific recommendations for shift workers to reduce the health effects of working non-daytime hours. Also, debriefing programs are standard operating procedures for emergency workers such as police following traumatic exposures. Such prevention programs are examples of proactive efforts to reduce psychiatric morbidity based on knowledge of the inherent risks of the work.

Secondary prevention

Employee Assistance Programs (EAP) are offered in over 20,000 US companies. The purpose of these programs is to detect and treat individuals with psychiatric disorders.[57] Initially, EAPs were developed in recognition of the impact substance abuse has on work productivity. However, it became apparent that other psychiatric disorders and psychosocial problems such as elder care, child care, and financial management also significantly impact work function. Therefore, EAPs broadened their scope to include evaluation and referral services for any personal problem. These 'broad brush' programs encourage employees to seek services on their own or as 'self-referrals' rather than wait until job performance suffers. Some investigators have reported significant improvement in absenteeism, lost time, warnings and supervisors ratings of performance[58-62] when comparing these indicators before and after EAP counseling. However, despite the proliferation of EAPs and widespread claims of their cost-effectiveness, more evaluation is needed.

Although EAPs have increased access to psychiatric services, there is a paucity of literature to document the effects of psychiatric treatment on work-related variables. Mintz et al.[63] reviewed the literature addressing the effect of psychiatric treatment on the capacity to work for those diagnosed with drug addiction, alcoholism, anxiety and affective disorders, gambling, and schizophrenia, and concluded that most attention has been given to work outcomes for substance abusers. The authors found that long-term treatment was not more beneficial than standard alcohol treatment regimens and that successful treatment aimed at reducing abusive drinking increased productivity.

In a separate review, data on occupational outcomes from 10 treatment studies for depression were analyzed.

Symptom improvements occurred more rapidly than improvements in work-related variables, such as missed time, lower productivity, and interpersonal problems, and were not affected by treatment duration. Work outcomes improved, however, as treatment duration increased, with maximum benefits achieved at 4–6 months. For schizophrenia, neuroleptic drugs reduce symptoms, but some studies suggest that they may also adversely affect work capacity by interfering with the learning process.[64] Overall, the most striking finding was the lack of attention in the psychiatric outcome research to the effects of treatment on functional work capacity, despite the stated importance of occupational impairment inherent in the DSM-IV criteria for most psychiatric disorders.[45]

In sum, psychiatric disorders and associated behavioral problems, such as alcohol consumption, significantly impact productivity – regardless of their cause or relationship to worksite factors and stressors. From the data available, either through program evaluation of EAPs or in the general treatment outcome literature, it appears that when employed individuals are treated, their work improves. This finding is encouraging and further supports the importance of health insurance benefits that include psychiatric treatment.

Tertiary prevention – fitness for duty

When an employee has been out of work for psychiatric treatment (e.g., depression or anxiety) or a question arises about the employee's ability to function on the job, a fitness for duty evaluation may be requested. Fitness for duty is defined as the individual's ability to perform a job based on the specific job requirements. Therefore, this evaluation requires a detailed understanding of the job duties. Often this can be problematic since job descriptions are not necessarily informative or sufficiently behavioral in their descriptions (see Table 28.3.3 for guidelines). Ancillary materials such as interviews with workers in similar positions or with supervisors may be needed to understand the essential behaviors expected to perform the job.

Fitness for duty can never be based solely on psychiatric diagnosis but rather must be based on a behavioral analysis of the employee's abilities. Past job performance is the best predictor of future job performance. Further, determining a global assessment of functioning can be useful as a behavioral guide for the individual's current level of function and ability to perform daily tasks related to work.[65] Overall, matching an assessment of the employee's current behavioral function with the essential functions required to perform a job, along with consideration of the employee's premorbid level of function on the job, will give the best prediction of an employee's fitness for return to a job.

Accommodation in the workplace

Since the Americans with Disabilities Act of 1990 (ADA) was passed, employers have been under pressure to employ

Steps involved in constructing an observational and behavioral based performance analysis	Sample occupation: Executive Assistant	Sample occupation: Baker
Step 1: Observation: observe a worker complete job tasks from preparation to finish	Watch a sample of administrative assistants perform daily work duties	Watch a sample of bakers perform the duties involved in the production of bread
Step 2: Describe: develop a description of job tasks in observable and behaviorally oriented terms	Verbal fluency skills to communicate effectively on phone and face-to-face with coworkers; attention and concentration to organize complex schedule; motor skills needed to type, learn and remember software programs (e.g., word processors. spreadsheets, etc.)	Read recipe card; motor skills and coordination to handle oven and mixing; psychomotor speed to safely retrieve finished product from oven
Step 3: Rank-order: by consulting supervisors and workers, rank-order from highest to lowest the tasks that are most crucial to a job	Through both direct observation and through interviews with present workers and supervisors, determine the most important aspects of the job; determine if others are available to help if parts of job cannot be completed	Through both direct observation and interviews with present workers and supervisors, determine the most important aspects of the job; determine if others are available to help if parts of job cannot be completed
Step 4: Develop worksheet: construct a worksheet to be given to individuals conducting fitness for duty evaluations which include key components of performance analysis	Give list to the individual conducting the assessment to ensure that they have an understanding of duties required to work effectively as an administrative assistant	Give list to the individual conducting the assessment to ensure that they have an understanding of duties required to work effectively as a baker

Table 28.3.3 Observationally and behaviorally based performance

and accommodate individuals with disabilities, including psychiatric illness. The number of discrimination claims against employers based on emotional/psychiatric impairment has also increased since the passage of this legislation. For example, in 1997 the Equal Employment Opportunity Commission (EEOC) reported that 15% of discrimination claims were due to emotional/psychiatric impairment, which represented the largest category of claims in that year.

The ADA prohibits discrimination based on disability and provides that employers must make 'reasonable accommodations' to the disabilities of 'qualified' applicants so long as this does not impose 'undue hardship'. 'Qualified' means that the individual can perform the essential functions of the job, except for the disability. 'Reasonable accommodation' refers to any modification or adjustment to a job or work environment that will allow the qualified employee with the disability to perform the job functions. 'Undue hardship' refers to an action requiring significant difficulty or expense.[66] Employers are not allowed to inquire about a disability prior to employment, and the applicant does not have to reveal a psychiatric history at time of hire. Moreover, if a long-term employee who was previously performing the job develops a psychiatric disorder, the employer is obligated to make accommodations.[67]

For people who are hospitalized for psychiatric diagnoses such as schizophrenia, employment rates have traditionally been low, with less than 20% of this group employed.[67] The best predictors of future work performance among the chronically mentally ill seem to be ratings of the individual's work adjustment in a sheltered job site, the ability to function socially with others, and prior employment history.[68,69] Thus, diagnosis alone (e.g., psychotic vs. non-psychotic) is not as predictive of work capacity as is objective behavioral performance. While these findings apply

---

Management strategies
Review strengths and weaknesses with employees
Set behavioral goals for job performance
Deliver positive feedback and criticism in constructive manner
Meet regularly with employees
Be flexible in administrative policies (e.g., allow relaxation breaks for anxiety)
Accommodations for workers with psychiatric disabilities
Utilize flextime when needed
Consider job sharing
Arrange environment to reduce excess noise or visual distractions
Extend leave time
Allow workers to call supportive individual during day (e.g., family, friends)
Join meetings between employer, supervisor and employment service

* As noted at http://janweb.icdi.wvu.edu/kinder/pages/psychiatric.html

Table 28.3.4 Employing and accommodating workers with psychiatric disabilities*

specifically to the psychoses, the same guidelines are applicable for any physical or psychiatric illness.

The Mental Health Law Project's guidebook[70] on the ADA provides a helpful document outlining reasonable accommodations for individuals with psychiatric disabilities. Accommodations include analysis of the individual employee's behavioral problems, such as anxiety, and sensitivity to criticism, followed by the development of accommodations based on individual needs (see Table 28.3.4 for guidelines).

SUMMARY AND CONCLUSIONS

With increasing attention to psychiatric disorders in the workplace and growing concerns about how working conditions contribute to psychiatric illness, the occupational health practitioner will be called upon to prevent, identify, and manage psychiatric disorders. Developing effective screening programs to identify stressful working conditions and early signs of psychiatric symptoms can help reduce lost productivity and disability. As for most occupational health programs, these efforts will require close coordination between the occupational health professional, management, and employees to develop meaningful programs that will succeed in reducing psychiatric disability. Although sometimes less apparent to the observer, the disabilities associated with psychiatric illness deserve accommodation and will require creative approaches to help managers overcome the biases toward mental illness that still exist in the greater community and the workplace.

References

1. Millar JD. Mental health and the workplace: an interchangeable partnership. Am Psychol 1990; 45:1165–6.
2. Hurley J, Horowitz J. Alcohol and health. New York: Sphere Publishing, 1990.
3. Harwood JJ, Kristiansen P, Rachal JV. Social and economic costs of alcohol abuse and alcoholism. Issue Report No. 2. Research Triangle Park, NC: Research Triangle Institute, 1985.
4. Ames GM, Grube JW, Moore RS. The relationship of drinking and hangovers to workplace problems: an empirical study. J Stud Alcohol 1997; 58:37–47.
5. Mandell W, Eaton WW, Anthony JC, et al. Alcoholism and occupations: a review and analysis of 104 occupations. Alcohol Clin Exp Res 1992; 16:734–46.
6. Karasek RA. Job demands, job decision latitude, and mental strain: implications for job redesign. Adm Sci Q 1979; 24:285–308.
7. Hemmingsson T, Lundberg I. Work control, work demands, and work social support in relation to alcoholism among young men. Alcohol Clin Exp Res 1998; 22:921–7.
8. Stansfeld SA, Fuhrer R, Head J, et al. Work and psychiatric disorder in the Whitehall II Study. J Psychosom Res 1997; 43:73–81.
9. Mausner-Dorsch H, Easton WW. Psychosocial work environment and depression: epidemiologic assessment of the demand–control model. Am J Public Health 2000; 90:1765–70.
10. Appelberg K, Romanov K, Heikkila K, et al. Interpersonal conflict as a predictor of work disability: a follow-up study of 15,348 Finnish employees. J Psychosom Res 1996; 40:157–67.
11. Duxbury LE, Higgins CA. Gender differences in work–family conflict. J Appl Psychol 1991; 76:60–74.
12. Hochschild A, MacHung A. The second shift. New York: Avon Books, 1990.
13. Eskanazi B, Maizlish N. Effects of occupational exposure to chemicals on neurobehavioural functioning. In: Tarter RE, VanThiel DH, Edward KL, eds. Medical neuropsychology, the impact of disease on behavior. New York: Plenum, 1988;223–63.
14. Schottenfeld RS, Cullen MR. Organic affective illness associated with lead intoxication. Am J Psychiatry 1984; 141:1423–6.
15. Johnson BL, Baker EL, El Batawi M, et al. Prevention of neurotoxic illness in working populations. New York: John Wiley and Sons, 1987.
16. NIOSH. Bulletin 48. Organic solvent neurotoxicity. Washington DC: National Institute for Occupational Safety and Health, 1987.
17. World Health Organization. Chronic effects of organic solvents on the central nervous system and diagnostic criteria. Copenhagen: WHO Regional Office for Europe, 1985.
18. Morrow LA, Ryan CM, Goldstein G, et al. A distinct pattern of personality disturbance following exposure to mixtures of organic solvents. J Occup Med 1989; 31:743–6.
19. Schottenfeld RS, Cullen MR. Recognition of occupation-induced post traumatic stress disorders. J Occup Med 1986; 28:365–9.
20. Goldblum D, Chouinard G. Schizophrenia psychosis associated with chronic industrial toluene exposure: case report. J Clin Psychiatry 1985; 46:350–1.
21. Dager SR, Holland JP, Cowley DS, et al. Panic disorder precipitated by exposure to organic solvents in the work place. Am J Psychiatry 1987; 144:1056–8.
22. Ely EW, Moorehead B, Haponik EF. Warehouse workers' headache: emergency evaluation and management of 30 patients with carbon monoxide poisoning. Am J Med 1995; 98:145–55.
23. Lezak MD. Neuropsychological assessment. New York: Oxford University Press, 1995
24. Meredith T, Vale A. Carbon monoxide poisoning. Br Med J 1988; 296:77–9.
25. Min SK. A brain syndrome associated with delayed neuropsychiatric sequelae following acute carbon monoxide intoxication. Acta Psychiatr Scand 1986; 73:80–6.
26. Ernst A, Zibrak JD. Carbon monoxide poisoning. N Engl J Med 1998; 339:1603–8.
27. Choi IS. Delayed neurologic sequelae in carbon monoxide intoxication. Arch Neurol 1983; 40:433–5.
28. Maghazaji HI. Psychiatric aspects of methylmercury poisoning. J Neurol Neurosurg Psychiatry 1974; 37:954–8.
29. Gross LS, Nagy RM. Neuropsychiatric aspects of poisonous and toxic disorders. In: Yudofsky SC, Hales RE, eds. American Psychiatric Press textbook of psychiatry, 2nd edn. Washington DC: American Psychiatric Press, 1992.
30. Menzies D, Bourbeau J. Building-related illnesses. N Engl J Med 1997; 337:1524–31.
31. Redlich CA, Sparer J, Cullen MR. Sick-building syndrome. Lancet 1997; 349:1013–6.
32. Bauer RM, Greve KW, Besch EL, et al. The role of psychological factors in the report of building-related symptoms in sick building syndrome. J Consult Clin Psychol 1992; 60:213–9.
33. Loewen L, Suedfeld P. Cognitive and arousal effects of masking office noise. Environ Behav 1992; 24:381–95.
34. Bing-shuang H, Yue-lin Y, Ren-yi W, et al. Evaluation of depressive symptoms in workers exposed to industrial noise. Homeostasis Health Dis 1997; 38:123–5.
35. Dejoy DM. Information input rate, control over task pacing, and performance during and after noise exposure. J Gen Psychol 1985; 11:229–42.
36. Akerstedt T. Psychological and psychophysiologic effects of shift work. Scand J Work Environ Health 1990; 16:67–73.
37. Frese M, Semmer N. Shiftwork, stress, and psychosomatic complaints: a comparison between workers in different shiftwork schedules, non-shiftworkers, and former shiftworkers. Ergonomics 1986; 29:99–114.
38. Verhaegen P, Dirkx J, Maasen A, et al. Subjective health after twelve years of shift work. In: Haider M, ed. Night and shiftwork: longterm effects and their prevention. Frankfurt Am Main: Verlag Peter Lang, 1986;67–74.
39. Costa G, Apostali P, D'Andrea F, et al. Gastrointestinal and neurotic disorders in textile shift workers. In: Reinberg A, Vieux N, Andlauer P, eds. Night and shift work: biologic and social aspects. Oxford: Pergamon Press, 1981;187–96.
40. Harma M, Illmarinen J, Knauth P. Physical fitness and other individual factors relating to the shiftwork tolerance of women. Chronobiol Int 1988; 5:417–24.
41. Tasto DL, Colligan MJ, Skjel EW, et al. Health consequences of shift work (SRI Project URU-4426). Washington DC: US Department of Health, Education and Welfare, NIOSH, 1978.
42. Cole R, Loving R, Kripke D. Psychiatric aspects of shiftwork. In: Scott A, ed. Occupational medicine: state of the art reviews. Philadelphia: Hanley & Belfus, 1990.

43. Keyserling WM. Occupational safety preventing accidents and overt trauma. In: Levy BS, Wegman DH, eds. Occupational health: recognizing and preventing work-related disease and injury, 4th edn. Philadelphia: Lippincott Williams & Wilkins, 2000;181–94.

44. Regehr C, Hill J, Glancy G. Individual predictors of traumatic reactions in firefighters. J Nerv Ment Dis 2000; 188:333–9.

45. American Psychiatric Association. Diagnostic and statistical manual of mental disorders, 4th edn. Washington DC: APA, 1994.

46. Kawamoto T, Koga M, Murata K, et al. Effects of ALDH2, CYP1A1, and CYP2E1 genetic polymorphisms and smoking and drinking habits on toluene metabolism in humans. Toxicol Appl Pharmacol 1995; 133:295–304.

47. Soderkvist P, Ahmadi A, Akerback A, et al. Glutathione S-transferase M1 null genotype as a risk modifier for solvent-induced chronic toxic encephalopathy. Scand J Work Environ Health 1996; 22:360–3.

48. Maslach C, Jackson SE, Lieter MP. Maslach burnout inventory manual. Palo Alto: Consulting Psychologists Press, 1996

49. NIOSH. Bulletin 57. Violence in the workplace: risk factors and prevention strategies. Washington DC: National Institute of Occupational Safety and Health, 1996.

50. Tucker P, Trautman R. Understanding and treating PTSD: past, present, and future. Bull Menninger Clin 2000; 64:37–51.

51. Porras JL, Silvers RC. Organizational development and transformation. Ann Rev Psychol 1991; 42:51–78.

52. Cordery KL, Mueller WS, Smith LM. Attitudinal and behavioral effects of autonomous group work: a longitudinal field study. Acad Manage J 1991; 34:464–76.

53. Warren J, Johnson P. The impact of workplace support on work–family role strain in family relations. J Appl Fam Child Stud 1995; 44:163–9.

54. Barling J, Barenbug A. Some personal consequences of 'flextime' work schedules. J Soc Psychol 1984; 123:137–8.

55. McGovern P, Dowd B, Gherdingen D, et al. Time off work and the postpartum health of employed women. Med Care 1997; 35:507–21.

56. Caudron S. The wellness payoff. Pers J 1990; 69:54–60.

57. Adamson DW, Gardner MD. Employee assistance programs and managed care: merge and converge. In: Sauber SR, ed. Managed mental healthcare: major diagnostic and treatment approaches. Bristol: Brunner/Mazel, Inc., 1997;67–82.

58. Cooper CL, Sadri G. The impact of stress counselling at work. J Soc Behav Pers 1991; 6:411–23.

59. Guppy A, Marsden J. Assisting employees with drinking problems: changes in mental health, job perceptions and work performance. Work Stress 1997; 11:341–50.

60. Mitchie S. Reducing absenteeism by stress management: valuation of a stress counselling service. Work Stress 1996;10:367–72.

61. Ramanathan CS. EAP's response to personal stress and productivity: implications for occupational social work. Soc Work 1992; 37:234–9.

62. Walsh DC, Hingson RW, Merrigan DM, et al. A randomized trial of treatment options for alcohol-abusing workers. N Engl J Med 1991; 325:775–82.

63. Mintz J, Mintz LI, Arruda MJ, et al. Treatments of depression and the functional capacity to work. Arch Gen Psychiatry 1992; 49:761–8.

64. Hogarty GE, McEvoy JP, Munetz M, et al. Dose of fluphenazine, familial expressed emotion, and outcome in schizophrenia: results of a two-year controlled study. Arch Gen Psychiatry 1988; 45:797–805.

65. Sperry L. Psychiatric consultations in the workplace. Washington DC: American Psychiatric Press, 1993.

66. United States Department of Justice. The Americans with Disabilities Act: Questions and Answers. Washington DC: Civil Rights Division, US Department of Justice, 1991.

67. Carling PJ. Reasonable accommodations in the workplace for individuals with psychiatric disabilities. Consult Psychol J 1993; 46–62.

68. Anthony WA, Jansen MA. Predicting the vocational capacity of the chronically mentally ill. Am Psychol 1984; 39:537–44.

69. Massel HK, Liberman RP, Mintz J, et al. Evaluating the capacity to work of the mentally ill. Psychiatry 1990; 53:31–43.

70. Mental Health Law Project. Mental health consumers in the work place: how the Americans with Disabilities Act protects you against employment discrimination. Washington DC: Mental Health Law Project, 1992.

71. Beck AT. Beck anxiety inventory. San Antonio: The Psychological Corporation, 1993.

72. Beck AT. Beck depression inventory. San Antonio: The Psychological Corporation, 1978

73. Derogatis LR. SCL-90-R administration, scoring and procedures manual-III. Towson: Clinical Psychometric Research, 1983.

74. Dohrenwend BS, Krasnoff L, Askenasy AR, et al. Exemplification of a method for scaling life events: the peri life events scale. J Health Soc Behav 1978; 19:205–29.

75. Horowitz M, Wilner N, Alvarez W. Impact of event scale: a measure of subjective stress. Psychosom Med 1979; 41:209–18.

76. Karasek R, Theorell T. Healthy work. New York: Basic Books, 1990

77. Selzer ML, Vinokur A, Van Rooijen L. A self-administered short Michigan screening test. J Stud Alcohol 1975; 36:117–26.

Chapter 29
Dermatologic Diseases

29.1 Contact Dermatitis

Kalman L Watsky, Christina A Herrick, Elizabeth F Sherertz, Frances J Storrs

The types of contact dermatitis that may be associated with the workplace are listed in Table 29.1.1 and are the focus of this chapter. By far the most common type is irritant contact dermatitis (ICD), representing approximately 80% of occupational contact dermatitis, with the remaining 20% being allergic. Other occupational skin diseases are discussed in Chapters 20.2 and 21.9. The patient does not walk in with an established diagnosis, however, and one needs to start with a systematic approach to evaluate the individual with skin disease.

APPROACH TO THE WORKER WITH SKIN DISEASE

The key elements to consider in evaluating a patient with skin disease are summarized in Table 29.1.2. It is most useful to see the patient at a time when the dermatitis is active, but this is not always possible. Speaking directly to the patient rather than relying on the history gathered by the nurse, the physician, or the supervisor is helpful.

History of dermatitis

The patient's description of events at the onset of the skin problem can be very important to the ensuing investigation. The date of onset generally should be during employment at the job in question. However, a person may have worked at a previous job with similar tasks and exposures, and developed contact allergy or irritation that could recur or be aggravated by the current job. If the person had a previous dermatologic disease (e.g., atopic dermatitis, psoriasis), a history of the time course of worsening of the dermatitis should be sought. The rapidity with which symptoms and signs occurred can give important clues. Immediate (or within hours) onset of itching and swelling with hive-like lesions suggests contact urticaria. Burning, stinging, and a red, dried appearance at the time of an exposure suggest an acute irritant reaction. Chronic irritant dermatitis can take much longer to develop. Approximately 3 months of constant wetting and drying is the typical time course in wet-work jobs.[1] Allergic contact dermatitis (ACD) may occur in a less predictable manner; it may occur within weeks of exposure to a new material, or it may develop after months or years. Itching, blistering, and spreading of lesions are common at some time in the course of contact allergic dermatitis (see later).

The anatomic site of the lesions at the onset of dermatitis also is important. The hands are the most likely site, and it should be noted which hand and which site on the hand (dorsum, fingers, palm) was first involved. In general, the *initial site* of involvement should correspond to sites exposed during a job task to provide evidence for occupational dermatitis. Later in the course of the condition, other body sites may become involved that may not clearly be related to direct exposure.

The course of the dermatitis related to time away from work is important in trying to establish evidence for work-relatedness. Documenting improvement away from the initial worksite is supportive evidence that work exposures are playing a role. It is important to note treatments undertaken during the time away from work, because some treatments (e.g., systemic corticosteroids) may suppress an ongoing problem and thus confuse the temporal relationship. Lack of improvement away from work is more difficult to assess: some chronic dermatoses may be very slow to improve even with time off from work, therapy, and protection. Activities undertaken away from work (household chores, hobbies) also may cloud the issue. At times, workers are moved to light duty or modified type of work after a skin problem develops. It is important to try to determine what differences there are between initial and modified duties, particularly with regard to the type and frequency of materials contacted, hand washing, and protective equipment. These differences also can give clues to which procedure may be contributing to the dermatitis.

The time course of recognition and treatment of the dermatitis also is important, as this may modify the appearance of the dermatitis even before a physician has seen the patient. Depending on the initial severity of a dermatitis, an employee may treat himself or herself for weeks or promptly seek medical evaluation. Encourage the patient to bring pharmacy printouts, bags of medications, notes from other physicians, or any other information to try to compile a history of topical and systemic medications. Topical treatments are of particular importance, because sometimes ingredients in these products can cause irritation or allergic reactions themselves, thus perpetuating what may have been a self-limited problem. Treatment with systemic corticosteroids that leads to clearing of the dermatitis and is followed by a subsequent flare of the dermatitis despite continued absence from work suggests that non-work factors may be playing a role. These issues further complicate assessment of the patient.

Occupational history

General principles for taking an occupational history are discussed in Chapter 1. When considering patients with

Irritant contact dermatitis
Single exposure dermatitis
Cumulative irritant dermatitis
Frictional irritant dermatitis
Psoriasiform dermatitis
Fiberglass dermatitis
Low humidity dermatitis
Post-traumatic eczema
Allergic contact dermatitis
Contact urticaria*
Contact photodermatitis
Phototoxic
Photoallergic

*Urticaria appears on the list as it may eventuate into dermatitis (see text).

Table 29.1.1 Occupational contact dermatitis

I. **History**
  A. *Present illness*
    Date of onset
    Body site at onset
    Patient description
      Onset – abrupt or gradual
      Appearance, spread
      Frequency
      Effect of treatment
    Course of disease
      Effect of weekend, vacation
      Work procedure change
    Treatment and effect on dermatitis
  B. *Occupational information*
    Current employer
    Employment dates
    Job title
      At time of onset
      Description of job tasks
      Materials contacted
      Protection
      Water exposure
      Hand washing
    Clothing/equipment
      Protective creams/cleansers
      Skin cleaning
      Method and frequency
    Other workers affected
    Job since dermatitis
    Previous job tasks or jobs
      Episodes of dermatitis
    Second job
    Dates of disability
    Date of job changes
  C. *Personal history*
    Other exposures
      Animals
      Foods
      Plants
      Clothing
      Personal care products
      Hobbies
    Past history of skin disease
      Plant dermatitis
      Hand dermatitis
      Psoriasis
      Athlete's foot
    History of atopy
    Personal/family
      Atopic dermatitis
      Hay fever
      Asthma
    Medical problems
    Medications

      Prescribed
      Over-the-counter
II. **Physical examination**
    Lesion type
    Secondary changes
    Distribution
    Other skin disease
    Photographic documentation
III. **Diagnostic techniques**
    Skin scrapings
    Fungus
    Fibers
    Culture
    Skin biopsy
    Patch test
    Contact urticaria test
    Photopatch test
IV. **Supplemental information**
    Material safety data sheets
    Medical records
    Workplace
    Other physician

Table 29.1.2 Clinical evaluation of the worker with skin disease

skin problems, it is useful to *have patients explain their routine*, having them use their hands to demonstrate how they handle materials. Ask specifically about the amount of time spent each day with *wet exposure*, wearing protective clothing, and frequency of contact with *irritating chemicals*. If items or material safety data sheets (MSDS) are brought from the workplace, go over each item with the patient to determine the type of contact and the frequency of exposure. Repetitive motion tasks or handling materials that could cause *friction or trauma* to the skin should be noted. Information about the *physical environment* in the workplace, such as temperature, humidity, patterns of airflow, and exposure to ultraviolet light, should be sought.

It also is important to ask about other *intermittent job tasks* that may have a relationship to the onset of dermatitis, such as periodic cleaning routines, machinery maintenance, changing cutting oils, and overtime work. There may be a discrepancy between the specific type of protective clothing (e.g., gloves) recommended and the actual use of these items in the workplace. Does the worker follow the recommended use, is protection optional, or does the worker have problems with consistent usage because he or she perceives the protection as inadequate (e.g., gloves tear, get saturated, or hamper dexterity)?

Asking whether *other workers are affected* who work at the same job can be helpful, although a site visit or examination of the other workers, when feasible, is more valuable. The sudden development of dermatitis by many workers suggests a breakdown in housekeeping or the recent introduction of an irritant into the industrial process. It also is helpful to ask the worker what he or she believes is the cause. The question may narrow down the relevant part of the job task. Inquiring whether or not the patient likes the job and wants to continue (if the dermatitis can be improved) may be significant, because motivation may be a helpful factor in predicting prognosis, depending on the type of dermatitis involved. This question also may help uncover the rare malingerer. For example, if a diagnosis of

ICD is made and a specific glove is recommended, the motivated employee may be more likely to *use* the protective glove to reduce the dermatitis and stay on the job.

With regard to skin disease, it also is important to inquire about previous work descriptions, exposures, and episodes of dermatitis, as well as second jobs or combined schooling with a job. One of our patients was concerned that her hand dermatitis was due to her office job. She also was going to school to become a hairdresser, and the wet-work exposures in this setting were much more likely to be the cause of her dermatitis.

Personal history

Obtaining *a history of previous skin disease* should be a focal point in talking with the patient. This history may provide clues to the current skin problem and may have prognostic implications.

Atopic history

Childhood atopic dermatitis (atopic eczema) is fairly common (greater than 10% of children in the United States), and is characterized by dry, pruritic skin, usually appearing in flexural areas. The skin in an atopic individual is more susceptible to irritants, such as rough fibers, and to changes in the environment, such as wet–dry and hot–cold changes. Determining an atopic background most often is done by eliciting a personal and/or family history (in first-degree relatives) of atopic dermatitis (eczema), hay fever and allergic rhinitis, or childhood asthma. A history of one or more of these conditions may be elicited in up to 25% of individuals, indicating that atopy is common. A history of childhood eczema is a common factor in adults who develop hand dermatitis. In his study of compensated skin disease in South Carolina, Shmunes found that the relative odds of developing work-related skin disease were 13.5 times greater for an individual with a history of atopic skin disease.[2] Further, the course of work-related dermatitis may be more prolonged in an atopic patient.

Psoriasis is a common skin disorder that may have potential for aggravation or development of new lesions in response to occupational factors, especially friction or repeated trauma involving the hands. Psoriasis on the hands as a result of work-related trauma may appear to be dermatitis at first glance. The presence of psoriasis should not fool the physician because ACD may coexist with psoriasis.[3] A history of *skin contact allergy* to jewelry, rubber articles, plants such as poison ivy, or other materials may provide a clue to the current dermatitis.

Other information in the personal history that should be sought is listed in Table 29.1.2. The patient's personal hygiene routine may give hints of other potential contact allergen exposure. Oral medications may predispose the person to special problems. For example, use of a medication that is potentially phototoxic (e.g., tetracycline) while continuing to work at a job with significant ultraviolet exposure could lead to severe sunburn. Hobbies are often sources of contact with potential allergens and irritants. Emphasis on pre-existing skin diseases as well as non-work exposures is essential in that surveys of skin diseases occurring in the workplace have shown that a minority of them are fully related to the patient's work.[4]

Physical examination

The physical examination should encompass not only the affected area of skin but also hair, nails, and sites not directly affected by workplace exposure. Evidence of other skin disease, especially flexural eczema, psoriasis, dermatophyte fungal infection, acne, and acute or chronic sun damage, should be noted. The size, color, and type of primary lesion (macule, papule, vesicle, wheal, pustule), as well as the presence of secondary lesions, such as scales, crusts, fissures, erosions, or ulcerations, should be noted. The configuration of lesions, linear grouping, or cut-off at sun-exposed sites or sites of protective equipment such as gloves or facemasks should be noted. Patterns of localization of dermatitis on the hands can occasionally be useful. Primary web space involvement is usually, but not always, irritant. Vesicles localized on the fingertips often are associated with allergy. Note whether both dorsal and palmar surfaces are involved. Nail changes may indicate chronicity of lesions. See the discussion about specific disorders for more detail on clinical clues. Often, however, it is not possible to distinguish clinically the type of dermatitis without further diagnostic testing. Recording the distribution of lesions on a drawing of the body or hands is helpful.

Diagnostic techniques

A number of techniques can be helpful in the evaluation of a patient with possible occupational dermatitis. In general, an experienced physician (e.g., dermatologist) should perform and interpret these tests. If scaling is present, a *skin scraping* to which 10–20% *potassium hydroxide* (KOH) is applied may be examined under a microscope for evidence of fungal hyphal elements. The same technique may be used to look for irritating fibers (e.g., fiberglass).

Cultures should be considered if a primary or secondary infection is suspected. Bacterial superinfection (impetigo) is common in crusted eczematous dermatoses, and a cotton swab sample taken from beneath a crust or a ruptured pustule may be submitted for bacterial culture, in the search for *Staphylococcus aureus* or group A β-hemolytic *Streptococcus* in particular. Marginated scaling lesions that are suspected to be the result of dermatophyte or Candida infection may be cultured from scrapings of scale using fungal media. If herpetic viral infection is suspected, cultures can be obtained from vesicular lesions if the appropriate medium is available. Culture or typing for other viral infection, such as wart papilloma virus, can only be performed if special facilities are available.

At times, a *skin biopsy* may be helpful to characterize the microscopic inflammatory pattern, confirm the presence of neoplastic lesion, or establish a cutaneous diagnosis of a non-dermatitis type. Skin biopsy of dermatitis and eczema may be non-specific. The biopsy technique usually is performed with local anesthesia, a small punch biopsy, and suture closure.

The following diagnostic techniques can be especially useful in evaluating skin disease that may be wholly or partially occupational in origin. These techniques in particular should be reserved for physicians trained in their usefulness, pitfalls, methodology, and interpretation.

Patch testing

Diagnostic epicutaneous patch tests can help establish contact *allergy* (delayed contact hypersensitivity) to a given material. The concentration of the material to be tested should be standardized. Physicians with little experience in patch testing should only test with *known* substances in concentrations that will not give an irritant reaction when applied to the skin. Commercially available patch tests that have been developed under Food and Drug Administration (FDA) guidelines are available in the United States for common cutaneous allergens such as rubber additives, formaldehyde and related preservatives, nickel, and neomycin. In Canada and Europe, a wider selection of allergens can be purchased. Common allergens in occupational ACD are listed in Table 29.1.3. Many of these allergens also are common outside the workplace. There

Allergen	Patch testing concentration**	Source examples
Acrylates	1–5%	Glues; paints, cosmetics (nails), dental appliances, artificial hips
Balsam of Peru	25%	Perfume screen, plastics, medications
Benzocaine‡	5%	Topical anesthetics, para-amino chemical cross-reactions
Benzoyl peroxide medication	1%	Catalyst for acrylic resins, bleaching agent foods, topical
Black rubber chemicals‡	0.6%	Mixture of *P*-phenylenediamine related chemicals used in black rubber
2-Bromo-2-nitropropane-1,3-diol (Bronopol)*†	0.5%	Cosmetic and industrial preservative
Carbamates‡	1%	Rubber, fungicides
Chloroxylenol (*P*-chloro-) m-xylenol	1%	Photography, rubber, glues, photocopy, cosmetic and industrial preservative
Cinnamic aldehyde‡	1%	Plastics, flavoring, perfumes
Cobalt chloride‡	1%	Nickel co-reactor, animal feeds, photography, acrylates, paints, glazes
Diaminodiphenylmethane	0.5%	Epoxy and polyurethane curing agent, para-amino chemical cross-reactions
Diazolidinyl urea (Germall II)*†	1% petrolatum or water	Cosmetic and industrial preservative
Disperse yellow 3	1%	Nylon dyes
Epoxy resin‡	1%	Plastics, paints, glues
Ethylenediamine dihydrochloride‡	1%	Fluxes, stabilizer in topical medications
Formaldehyde‡	1% water	Preservative, fabric finishes, plastics
Fragrance mix	8%	Additive in many personal care products
Glutaraldehyde	1% water	Medical and dental sterilizing solutions, leather fixatives
Glyceryl monothioglycolate	1%	Permanent waving solutions
Imidazolidinyl urea*†‡	2% petrolatum or water	Cosmetic and industrial preservative
5-Chloro-2-methyl-4-isothiazolin-3-one and 2-methyl-4-isothiazolin-3-one (Kathon CG)*	0.1% water or petrolatum	Cosmetic and industrial preservative
Lanolin (wool wax alcohol)*	30%	Topical medications
Mercaptobenzothiazole‡	1%	Rubber accelerator (especially gloves), fungicide (veterinarians), anticorrosive
P-Methylaminophenol sulfate (Metol)	1%	Black and white photo developer
Neomycin‡	20%	Topical antibiotic preparations
Nickel sulfate‡	2.5%	Metal tools and devices, jewelry
Para-tertiary-butylphenol formaldehyde resin‡	1%	Neoprene plastics and glues (e.g., shoes)
Phenol formaldehyde resin	5%	Plastics, glues (e.g., plywood)
Para-phenylenediamine‡	1%	Hair dye (humans and animals), para-amino chemical cross-reactor
Potassium dichromate‡	0.25%	Leather fixative, anticorrosion chemical, paints
Propylene glycol	10% water	Topical medicaments, tattoos, foods, brake fluids, antifreeze, plastics
Quaternium 15*†‡ (Dowicil 200)	2%	Cosmetic and industrial preservative
Rosin (colophony)*‡	20%	Cosmetics, glues, soldering flux, anti-skid (violinists, athletes)
Sesquiterpene lactone mix	0.1%	Allergen in chrysanthemum and other weeds
Thimerosal (merthiolate)	0.1%	Preservative (e.g., vaccines), cross-reacts with some mercury compounds
Tetramethylthiuram disulfide‡	1%	Rubber accelerator (especially shoes and gloves), fungicides
Thioureas	1%	Rubber accelerator
Tixocortol-21-pivalate	1%	Marker for corticosteroid allergy

*CTFA (Cosmetic, Toiletry and Fragrance Association) name, appears on cosmetic labels. ( ) is trade name and may be used in other industries.
†Formaldehyde-releasing preservatives.
‡Commercial allergens commonly available in the United States.
**Diluted in petrolatum unless otherwise designated.

Table 29.1.3 Common contact allergens

are several reference textbooks which discuss common allergens and irritants related to specific occupations.[5-7] The tests usually are applied to the upper back on aluminum disc chambers or plastic chambers held in place with non-sensitizing tape. The tests are left in place for 2 days, and then removed and read. A second reading at 3, 4, or 7 days after patch test application is important for a final interpretation. An erythematous, spreading, indurated or vesicular response at an allergen site indicates a positive allergic response. At times, irritant and allergic reactions are indistinguishable.

Patch tests should be considered as a confirmatory test when an individual is exposed to a potential allergen or when the clinical presentation suggests that contact allergy is playing a role in the dermatitis. Test results require careful interpretation to discern allergic from irritant responses, as well as to determine the relevance of a positive result to the patient's dermatitis and exposures. There are nuances to the technique, including timing of testing related to systemic corticosteroid therapy, that dictate that patch testing should be performed only by physicians experienced in the method. These tests are used only to diagnose *allergy* and are one component of the total evaluation. False-negative and false-positive results can occur. Patch tests often are negative in occupational contact dermatitis. Standard textbooks offer details of patch testing methods.[6,7] For many substances that have not been standardized, De Groot's book provides suggested concentrations and vehicles of patch testing.[8]

Contact urticaria testing

Contact urticaria should be considered when an immediate itching, edematous urticarial eruption or angioedema occurs at the site of contact with a substance. Occupationally, this has been seen mostly with food handlers, particularly meat and fish processors. With increasing use of latex gloves, contact urticarial reactions to latex gloves and other medical devices has been seen more commonly in medical and related personnel and certain patient populations. This has prompted a move to non-latex alternatives, especially in hospitals.[9] General guidelines for this type of testing are available in reference texts,[6,7] and Hausen and Hjorth give specific suggestions for testing foods.[10]

Testing for contact urticaria involves applying the substance in question (e.g., saline in which a piece of a latex glove or the glove itself has been soaked, or a piece of meat or fish flesh) to normal skin, previously affected skin, or skin adjacent to active dermatitis. Signs of itching, redness, and swelling should be sought within $\frac{1}{2}$ to 2 hours of application. If no reaction is seen, a small scratch or prick that draws no blood with a sterile needle is induced on normal skin, and the substance is applied to this site, followed by observation. It is important that this testing be performed with positive (histamine) and negative (saline) controls and in an environment where resuscitation equipment is readily available because life-threatening anaphylaxis may occur. Delayed contact urticaria may occur, so patients should be followed up 1–2 days after testing.

Photopatch testing

When allergy to a substance in combination with ultraviolet exposure is being considered, phototesting and photopatch testing are indicated. Phototesting involves exposure of the patient's skin to measured doses of ultraviolet A (UVA), ultraviolet B (UVB), or both to determine whether or not a sunburn reaction occurs at less than the predicted dose of ultraviolet light. Photopatch tests are performed by applying two sets of allergens to a patient's back. After 1 day, one set is exposed to a measured dose (usually 10 joules) of ultraviolet A, and final readings are taken at 2 and 3 days to determine whether there is a reaction to any allergen, with or without the ultraviolet exposure.[11]

Supplemental information and diagnostic criteria

The uses and limitations of MSDS are summarized elsewhere in this text. Medical records from the workplace and private physician can help with details of clinical description of the acute events, chronology of medication use, and diagnostic work-up previously performed. Combining the history, physical findings, and results of the diagnostic evaluation can be complicated. Criteria for determining occupational causation and aggravation for contact dermatitis are summarized in Table 29.1.4. An affirmative answer to at least four criteria strengthens the case for workplace exposure substantially contributing to the dermatitis. The level of diagnostic certainty required, as with any occupational illness, depends on the circumstances, the standard for most compensation systems being 'more probable than not'.

IRRITANT CONTACT DERMATITIS

Irritant contact dermatitis (ICD), an inflammatory disease caused by skin contact with material that inflicts damage through a non-immunologic mechanism, is the most common occupational skin disease. The material that

---

Questions*

1. Is the clinical appearance consistent with contact dermatitis?
2. Are there workplace exposures to potential cutaneous irritants or allergens?
3. Is the anatomic distribution of dermatitis consistent with cutaneous exposure during the job task?
4. Is the temporal relationship between exposure and onset consistent with contact dermatitis?
5. Are non-occupational exposures excluded as possible causes?
6. Does dermatitis improve away from work exposure to the suspected irritant or allergen?
7. Do patch or provocation tests identify a probable causal agent?

*Answering yes to at least four questions may provide adequate probability for workplace exposure.
From Mathias CGT. Contact dermatitis and workers' compensation: criteria for establishing occupational causation and aggravation. J Am Acad Dermatol 1989; 20:842–8, with permission from The Association for Professionals in Infection Control and Epidemiology.

Table 29.1.4 Contact dermatitis: Mathias criteria for probable occupational causation

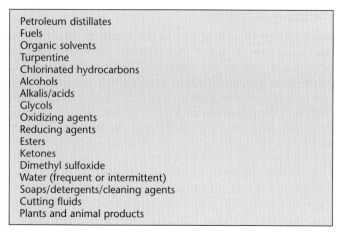

Petroleum distillates
Fuels
Organic solvents
Turpentine
Chlorinated hydrocarbons
Alcohols
Alkalis/acids
Glycols
Oxidizing agents
Reducing agents
Esters
Ketones
Dimethyl sulfoxide
Water (frequent or intermittent)
Soaps/detergents/cleaning agents
Cutting fluids
Plants and animal products

Table 29.1.5 Examples of industrial materials that can cause skin irritation

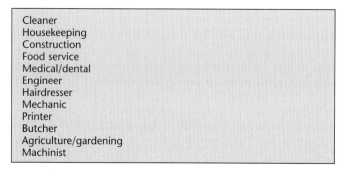

Cleaner
Housekeeping
Construction
Food service
Medical/dental
Engineer
Hairdresser
Mechanic
Printer
Butcher
Agriculture/gardening
Machinist

Table 29.1.6 Occupations at high risk for irritant contact dermatitis

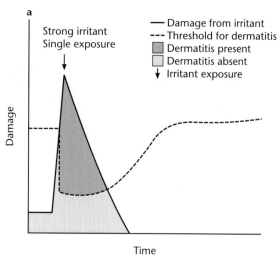

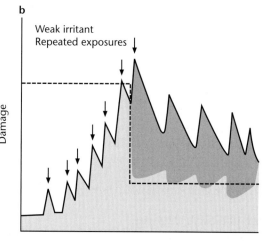

Figure 29.1.1: (a) Schematic for the time course of dermatitis with a single strong irritant exposure. Note rapid healing and recovery of threshold expected when exposure is stopped. (b) Time course of repeated insult with a weak irritant leading to dermatitis. The lowered threshold for dermatitis that results leads to perpetuation of dermatitis, even with less frequent damaging individual exposures. (Adapted from Malten KE. Thoughts on irritant contact dermatitis. Contact Derm 1981; 7:238–47; and from Dahl MV. Chronic irritant dermatitis: mechanisms, variables, and differentiation from other forms of contact dermatitis. Adv Dermatol 1988; 3:261–76. © 1988 Munksgaard International Publishers Ltd, Copenhagen, Denmark.)

contacts the skin usually is a chemical that is toxic to the skin in single or in cumulative (repetitive or frequent) exposure. Examples of industrial irritants are listed in Table 29.1.5, and occupations at high risk for ICD are listed in Table 29.1.6. Lists of irritants associated with specific jobs are available from several sources.[1,5] Physical factors such as mechanical forces (friction, repetitive motion) and ambient environment (heat, cold, humidity) also can lead to ICD.

Pathogenesis

The pathophysiology is not well understood. There is evidence that both external environmental factors and host-related factors contribute to the likelihood that an irritant skin reaction may occur, particularly when exposure to weak irritants is being considered.

Strong irritants elicit symptoms of burning and stinging as well as signs of redness and swelling in most exposed individuals within a short time period. The progression to blistering dermatitis or chemical burn depends on the concentration of the irritant and the duration of skin contact. Healing begins to occur after the irritant is removed from the skin, but during this healing phase there is a reduced threshold for developing dermatitis from the same or weaker irritants. *Weak irritants* tend to cause damage in a subtler manner. The stinging or burning sensation may not occur; thus, there may be no subjective signal that damage is being done. Repeated exposure to a weak

irritant may be necessary to produce clinical evidence of dermatitis, so-called *cumulative insult* damage. The latency period for development of ICD of this type may vary from days, if contact with the weak irritant is constant, to years if contact is intermittent. Further complicating the picture is the fact that additional weak irritants, even water and soap, add further insult and contribute to the prolonged healing times necessary for dermatitis of this type. The schematic diagrams shown in Figure 29.1.1 contrast the time course of skin damage and dermatitis from strong versus weak irritants, and the effect on the threshold for developing dermatitis.[12,13]

Environmental or exogenous factors that may predispose a person to the development of cutaneous irritation from a given material include the type of irritant and the amount that penetrates the skin (which may depend on the concentration and vehicle for the irritant and time of contact with skin). The body site where contact occurs also makes a difference: eyelid skin is more prone to air-borne irritants than is palmar skin. Percutaneous penetration also varies with anatomic site; for example, the dorsal surfaces of the hands may be more likely to develop dermatitis than the palms due to differences in stratum corneum penetration by the irritant. Temperature and humidity also may be important. Working in a hot or cold, dry environment may cause chapping and water loss from the skin that could predispose the skin to penetration by some irritants, whereas heat, sweat, and occlusive clothing also could contribute to irritant effects of a material on skin.

Perhaps the single most important environmental factor in ICD is the role of water or *wet work*.[14,15] Hydration of the skin increases the potential for the penetration of many substances. Intermittent wet and dry exposure leads to water loss, which can generate breaks in the skin barrier that solvents can traverse. The addition of soap or detergent to the water exposure, either in the hygiene routine or the industrial process itself, can lead to loss of superficial skin lipids, alkaline damage to the skin, or abrasive action on the stratum corneum that also contributes to irritant skin damage.[16] Water exposure itself, or in combination with soap, can act as a weak irritant that lowers the threshold for dermatitis from other substances that might be otherwise tolerated, as shown in Figure 29.1.1(b).[17,18] For this reason, avoidance of wet work is often recommended during the healing phase of contact dermatitis of any cause, and it also is recommended for individuals with endogenous factors (see later) that might make them more likely to develop ICD.

Atopic dermatitis has a strong association with the development of occupational ICD, as noted earlier. Individuals with atopic dermatitis have a low threshold for irritation and require a long time to heal. Individuals with a positive atopic history but no apparent dermatitis also may have a higher risk of hand dermatitis.[17,19] Separating the endogenous atopic dermatitis from the relative importance of external irritants may be difficult. A history of new dermatitis at sites not previously involved but compatible with job-related exposure or a history of significantly more severe involvement (aggravation) at sites of pre-existent dermatitis suggests that the exogenous exposures are contributing to an ICD flare of atopic dermatitis. The link between atopy and potential for ICD is a powerful case for preplacement evaluation and job modifications, because preventative measures could have a significant impact on reducing the number of cases of occupational skin disease. Other host factors for ICD include skin care regimen and skin types.

The point of injury by irritants at the cellular level is variable. The stratum corneum barrier may be compromised or cell membranes may be disrupted, particularly by detergents. Damage to the epidermis can trigger the release of various cytokines and inflammatory mediators that potentiate the damage and inflammation. Some irritants have direct effects on blood vessels, causing vasodilatation,

and others may directly stimulate polymorphonuclear leukocyte chemotaxis or mast cell degranulation. The degree of inflammation seen clinically or histologically depends on the specific irritant involved, its concentration, and the type of exposure.[20]

Clinical course

The clinical manifestations of ICD usually reflect the epidermal damage: a glazed look to the skin, with dryness of the surface ranging from a chapped scaling appearance to cracking or fissuring (Fig. 29.1.2). Erythema is variable and may be very faint when it is caused by weak irritants. Burning and stinging may be more prominent than itching. The web spaces of the fingers may be affected first, especially in ICD associated with wet work. In general, the presence of multiple small vesicles, especially around the nail fold, is not common in ICD and its presence should suggest the possibility of concomitant contact allergy to

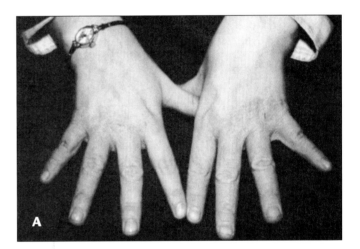

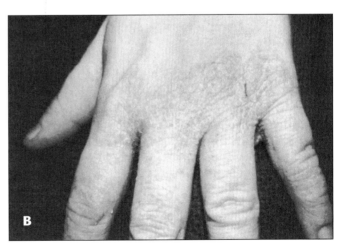

Figure 29.1.2: Contact irritant dermatitis. Irritant contact dermatitis usually begins in the web spaces of the fingers and than spreads to involve the adjacent skin. The dorsum of the hand may be involved more than the palm. Redness, scaling, and itching without obvious vesiculation are most characteristic. This sort of dermatitis is common in people who do wet work, and is especially common in people who have a history of childhood eczema and who also do wet work.

the same or another offending agent.[21] Large blisters of acute onset may occur with a strong irritant, causing the equivalent of a chemical burn, but these blisters usually resolve rapidly with removal of the irritant and wound care. With epidermal disruption, secondary infection may occur and lead to amber-colored crusting of the involved sites. With cumulative irritant dermatitis or chronic irritant exposure, the skin becomes hyperkeratotic. At sites like the hands, this thickened skin is prone to fissures.

Diagnosis

The major considerations in the differential diagnosis of ICD are atopic dermatitis (Fig. 29.1.3) and ACD, and it may be extremely difficult to distinguish among these conditions clinically. Table 29.1.7 contrasts features of irritant and ACD. In chronic cases, other disorders such as psoria-

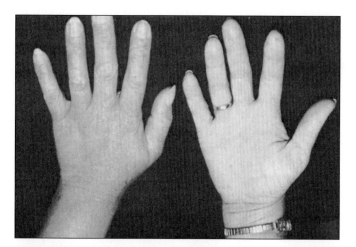

Figure 29.1.3: Atopic hand eczema. This hairdresser is not allergic to anything in her workplace on patch testing. The frequent wetting and drying of her hands in her work has given her chronic dermatitis on both her palms and her dorsal hands. Notice the distal distribution, which is characteristic of irritant dermatitis caused by wet work exposures in atopics.

sis and acquired keratoderma also should be considered. There is no routine laboratory test to confirm a diagnosis of ICD: skin biopsy results are non-specific, and patch tests are used to confirm or exclude contact allergy. The history of exposures, job description, and clinical presentation lead to a clinical diagnosis of ICD.

Treatment and prognosis

Avoidance of strong irritants usually leads to prompt improvement of an acute case of ICD. Oral antibiotic treatment of secondary infection, soaks and debridement of crusts or bullae, and topical emollients often are adequate in this setting. If a chemical burn has occurred, specific emergency treatment should be instituted depending on the nature of the irritant chemical involved. For dermatitis due to weaker irritants or cumulative or multiple exposures, it is helpful to move the patient away from the job task associated with those or other irritants. As mentioned earlier, the threshold for further irritation is lowered, so that ideally all irritant exposures (occupational, domestic and hobby, and therapeutic) should be minimized. In the workplace, reducing exposure to the irritant through job modification or appropriate protective clothing may be helpful. If a similar problem has been seen among a number of workers at a given job, consideration should be given to replacement of the offending agent with a less irritating material. The proper glove may be helpful but barrier creams generally are not beneficial.[22,23]

Skin cleaning should be performed as gently as possible, and abrasives, solvents, or harsh detergents should be avoided. If there is a marked inflammatory reaction, a topical corticosteroid in a simple ointment base (e.g., petrolatum) may be of benefit. Corticosteroid creams contain preservatives that can sensitize the skin. Ointments do not contain these additives or water in the base, which can be drying. Lack of response or worsening of symptoms with use of a topical corticosteroid may rarely indicate contact allergy to the steroid moiety itself.[24] Bland emollients such

Variables	Irritant	Allergic
Who	Many people	Few people
Where	Localized	Spreads
When	Soon with strong irritants (minutes to hours) Late with weak irritants (months)	24–72 hours
Job-relatedness	Improves with long (3 weeks) vacations	May improve even on weekends
Atopy	Predisposes	No predisposition
Morphology	Erythema, scale, fissures	Vesicles or inseparable from irritant
Distribution	Hands 90%	Hands 90%
Intermittent and frequent water exposure	May cause and perpetuate	May perpetuate
Immunology	Not known to be relevant (1991)	Type IV (cell-mediated immunity, delayed hypersensitivity)
Histology	Spongiosis or upper epidermal damage, some lymphocytes	Spongiosis with lymphocytic cellular infiltrate or inseparable from irritant
Chronicity	Often	If diagnosed early clears, can be chronic
Diagnosis	History and physical observation	History, physical, and patch testing
Examples	Hairdressers and machinists chronic hand dermatitis	Poison oak/ivy, nickel, chrome

Table 29.1.7 Generalizations about irritant versus allergic contact dermatitis

as white petrolatum are preferable to popular commercial moisturizing lotions, which can occasionally lead to further irritation.[25] Systemic corticosteroids may alleviate symptoms of inflamed ICD, but they should be reserved for short-term therapy of more severe cases. Oral antibiotics to cover *Staphylococcus aureus* and group A β-hemolytic streptococcal infection, in particular, should be used if crusted fissures are evident.

As the dermatitis improves, the strength and dosage interval of the topical corticosteroid should be tapered. The time course to improvement can be variable. As a general rule, the longer the duration of dermatitis, the longer the recovery time. The presence of atopy also prolongs healing time. The recommended length of time away from exposures or with modified duties is variable. Photographs of the dermatitis at the beginning and end of the time-off period may be of great value. If the dermatitis does not improve with the avoidance and treatment outlined, then other diagnoses should be considered and the therapeutic regimen should be scrutinized.

The prognosis of ICD depends on exogenous factors, such as the ability of the person to avoid irritants, and endogenous factors, such as the presence of atopy. For an isolated episode of an acute case of ICD to a strong irritant, the prognosis for recovery is good. Chronic ICD may not have such an optimistic prognosis. In fact, occupational contact dermatitis in general carries a poor prognosis, which is frustrating to the patient, employer, physicians, and insurance carriers.[26] For example, a follow-up study of patients with soluble-oil dermatitis (metal-working industry) indicated that the patients who experienced the resolution of their dermatitis after discontinuing oil contact did so within 3 months.[27] If there was no improvement within that time, the patients were not likely to improve whether they avoided soluble-oil contact or not. Overall, approximately 70% of these patients had not healed 2 years after being diagnosed.[27]

Strides made in industrial hygiene and dermatologic diagnosis and treatment in the last 20 years have not led to an improvement of the prognosis. In long-term follow-up investigations of patients diagnosed with occupational contact dermatitis, 25% of patients have persistent dermatitis, 50% of patients had periodic flares of dermatitis, and only 25% completely healed. These percentages are similar for patients who change or leave their jobs owing to their skin disease; the majority continues to have dermatitis.[28] Factors to be considered in persistent occupational dermatitis are summarized in Table 29.1.8. Perhaps the most difficult of these factors to determine is the development of secondary dermatoses due to a lowered irritant threshold or other factors, or the concept that dermatitis begets dermatitis. It may not be possible to predict when and how much improvement will occur for a given patient with contact dermatitis.

Prevention

Given the poor prognosis of ICD, improved preventive strategies are essential.[29,30] Prophylactic strategies should

Incorrect dermatologic diagnosis
Proper diagnosis of occupational contact dermatitis, but
    Failure to establish specific cause
    Failure to eliminate exposure to causative agent(s)
Improper therapeutic intervention
Development of secondary dermatoses
    Infection
    Neurodermatitis/Lichen simplex chronicus
    Reactivation of atopic dermatitis
Improper job modification or change
Improper cleansing routines
Development of
    Cross-sensitivities
    Multiple sensitivities
    New sensitivities
Malingering

From Birmingham DJ. Prolonged and recurrent occupational dermatitis: some whys and wherefores. In Adams RM ed. Occup Med State Rev 1986; 1:349–56; and Hogan DJ, Dannaker CJ, Maibach HI. The prognosis of contact dermatitis. J Am Acad Dermatol 1990; 23:300–7, with permission from American Academy of Dermatology.

Table 29.1.8 Some reasons for poor outcome of occupational contact dermatitis

Individuals
  Vocational counseling/pre-placement screening
    Atopic dermatitis
    Family history of atopy
    History of contact dermatitis
    Leisure activities/hobby exposures
Identification of irritants
  Literature sources
    Material safety data sheets
  Predictive tests of skin irritancy and allergenicity
    Draize test (animals)
    Cumulative irritation test (human/animals)
Work environment
  General
    Ventilation
    Temperature
    Humidity
    General housekeeping
    Airflow patterns
  Industrial process
    Reduce skin contact (automation, enclosure)
    Substitute less irritating chemicals
    Appropriate protective clothing/gloves
    Label hazardous materials/work sites
    Reduce mechanical irritation
  Education
    Workers and management
      Exposures
      Job procedures/technique training
      Emergency measures
      Information on patient's job exposures
      Healthcare providers
      Recognition and treatment of skin disease
  Skin care program
    Choice of soap, detergent, cleanser
    Soft towels
    Moisturizing creams
  Assess hand washing routine (avoid excess hand washing)
    Protective clothing
    Simple lubricants (e.g., petrolatum)

Table 29.1.9 Prevention of contact dermatitis

include those outlined in Table 29.1.9. Identification of workplace irritants, modification of work practices and industrial processes, and worker education can reduce irritant exposures and incidence and severity of ICD. Early recognition and appropriate treatment are also essential. Workers with atopic dermatitis should be counseled as to the risks of wet-work careers such as housekeeping, medical fields, and hairdressing. Intermittent wetting and drying is particularly damaging (e.g., hand washing). Preplacement screening for atopy for wet-work or other high-risk occupations might reduce risk but is of unproven value and is ethically and legally problematic. Educational programs should also address possible irritant exposures outside the workplace, as in domestic chores or hobbies, because an accumulation of irritant insults may lead to dermatitis.

In the context of the job description, it is important to know which chemicals or other materials are irritating to human skin. Strong irritants may be identified on material safety data sheets, but weak irritants or those that may result in dermatitis from cumulative exposure may not be identified as such. Other sources of information on potential irritancy should be sought in the industrial literature. For new products likely to have significant exposure to human skin, predictive testing of irritant potential can be performed. There are a number of methods advocated for use in experimental animals or humans. These methods are widely used to evaluate skin care products and topical medications, but they could be adapted for evaluation of industrial compounds, if necessary. Further preventive strategies are similar to those discussed later under ACD and are summarized in Table 29.1.9.

LOW HUMIDITY DERMATOSES
Pathophysiology

At humidities of 50% and higher, the stratum corneum is at a steady state and remains pliable. In situations that are hot and dry and in which there is flowing air, the stratum corneum dries out and fissures, resulting in chapped skin.[31] This mechanism plays a role in the development of some cases of allergic contact dermatitis and most irritant dermatitis associated with intermittent wetting and drying.[32] It plays a primary role in explaining a dermatitis that is common in hot, dry, well-ventilated workplaces. As with most types of irritant dermatitis, this problem can affect many workers (Table 29.1.7).

Clinical course

Patients working in these environments, and especially those sitting exactly at points of maximum airflow, note itching on their exposed skin surfaces (especially the face and neck). This problem is followed by scaling and, finally, by the development of patches of asteatotic eczema (xerosis, erythema craquele, chapping). Although exposed surfaces are involved most often, covered skin may be included as well. Erythema or flushing and even urticaria (perhaps as a result of rubbing and scratching) also may be part of the syndrome. Individuals with a personal history

of atopic dermatitis are particularly vulnerable, and those who already have some sort of dermatitis will note that it worsens. Persons in whom this problem is likely to be prevalent include any workers in low humidity environments, which are common with current heating and air-conditioning systems.

Diagnosis

History and suspicion are most helpful initially, but inspection of the workplace, with documentation of low humidity and high temperature and airflow, as well as correction of the skin complaints after remediation of these factors, is diagnostic. Air-borne gaseous and particulate substances and other causes of dermatitis (allergic, contact, seborrheic) may complicate the diagnosis, and they should be sought as well.

Low humidity dermatitis may be the actual explanation for some skin diseases that have been attributed to visual display terminals, carbonless paper, and even the sick building syndrome (see Chapters 38 and 23.2), and thus its diagnosis and correction can improve the morale of an entire workforce.[33]

Treatment and prognosis

Raising the humidity and lowering the temperature, when possible, solves most complaints. Moving a worker away from under or beside an air duct helps even more. Simple lubricants, devoid of common sensitizers that can complicate the problem, hasten the recovery of the xerotic skin. In some instances, topical corticosteroids are required briefly.

IRRITANT CONTACT DERMATITIS DUE TO FIBERGLASS
Pathophysiology

Fiberglass dermatitis is a specific type of ICD in which the mechanical effect of the sharp fiber spicules causes a sensation of itching and, at times, an inflammatory reaction.[34] The fiber size (>4.5 μm) is important in determining the likelihood of skin irritation. Textile glass and wool fibers that are used for insulation are the types most often implicated in skin irritation.

Clinical course

The skin lesions are small papules that are often crusted due to scratching. Hive-like lesions and linear excoriations may occur, and lesions have a predilection for exposed surfaces as well as areas of the skin where clothing is close to the skin (e.g., the waistline). Intense pruritus may be the chief complaint, and clinically apparent lesions may be absent. Fibers may be found on tape strippings of the skin or skin scrapings examined with potassium hydroxide preparation.

Diagnosis

The differential diagnosis includes infestations by scabies or body lice, irritation from dust exposure, neurodermatitis, and other types of contact dermatitis. A history of exposure such as working with fiberglass insulation or in indoor environments undergoing renovation should be sought.

Treatment and prognosis

In fiberglass workers, the symptoms of irritation often are relieved with gentle washing of exposed sites with non-abrasive soap and water. New workers tend to be more affected, and work hardening can occur over time in some workers. Topical corticosteroids are of limited benefit.

Prevention

To prevent fiberglass dermatitis, it is helpful for workers to wear loose clothing with long sleeves and pants, avoid rubbing the skin, and wash work clothes separately. Careful skin cleaning after working with fiberglass and use of skin emollients also may help.

POST-TRAUMATIC ECZEMA
Pathophysiology and clinical course

Post-traumatic eczema is a term used for the occurrence of dermatitis at a site of previous injury to the skin. The pathophysiology is not well understood and may be related to the lowered threshold for irritant dermatitis at sites of skin damage. Mathias has described an idiopathic type and an isomorphic reaction (i.e., the occurrence of a cutaneous lesion of a recognizable skin disease at a trauma site).[35] Patients with typical lesions of psoriasis, vitiligo, and lichen planus at other sites may develop new lesions at sites of trauma through the isomorphic reaction. Idiopathic post-traumatic eczema is an inflammatory, scaling reaction limited to the previous trauma site. The eruption usually begins within weeks of the injury and may persist for months to years after the initial injury.

Diagnosis

It is essential to exclude infection (bacterial, herpetic, fungal) at the injury site through appropriate laboratory techniques and culture. Contact dermatitis resulting from medications used to treat the wound (e.g., neomycin, adhesive, benzocaine) also should be excluded.

Treatment and prognosis

Topical corticosteroids may be helpful in the treatment of post-traumatic eczema, but patients may have intermittent active dermatitis at the trauma site. If the initial injury was occupational, this prolonged dermatitis at the injury site may be considered work related.

FRICTIONAL CONTACT DERMATITIS
Pathophysiology and clinical course

Frictional dermatitis results at points of chronic irritation and trauma. It is most easily recognized as calluses, and some occupations have distinctively distributed calluses.[36]

Skin diseases that koebnerize (develop lesions typically at trauma sites [isomorphic phenomenon]) such as psoriasis or lichen planus may involve the palms and present a clinical picture that, at first glance, looks like frictional contact dermatitis and even may have foci of spongiosis histologically. Some people develop similar lesions clinically and histologically, although they do not have psoriasis or a family history. Clinicians may call frictional contact dermatitis psoriasiform dermatitis or hyperkeratotic dermatitis of the palms.[37] This entity does not vesiculate, seldom itches, and may involve the weight-bearing portions of the feet if heavy shoes are worn and if the patient is obese. The condition improves dramatically when the mechanical trauma is withdrawn, but it may take a month or longer to do so. Workers with impressive mechanical hand trauma are at greatest risk (e.g., construction workers, machinists, forest industry workers, and baggage handlers).

A more subtle but equally distinctive frictional dermatitis can occur in office workers who handle large volumes of papers, and especially carbonless copy paper. This dermatitis is found on the fingertips, where maximum paper contact occurs. It does not vesiculate or itch but rather is characterized by areas of redness, scaling, and painful fissuring. These patients may have no previous history of hand dermatitis and often are not atopic.[33]

Diagnosis

This entity receives little mention in most comprehensive reviews of hand dermatitis. Exclusion of other entities such as irritant and allergic dermatitis, genuine psoriasis, and dermatophyte infection is important.

A biopsy can be of great help but will not absolutely exclude genuine psoriasis, which can be similar to frictional dermatitis histologically. Psoriasis may first begin on the palms in the setting of occupational trauma and only with the spread of the disease to distant sites can it be differentiated with confidence from the more nebulous frictional dermatoses. Clearing of the dermatitis with trauma avoidance is of the greatest diagnostic help.

Treatment and prognosis

Trauma avoidance, simple lubricants, and phototherapy are helpful.[38] Topical corticosteroids are of little help. Chronicity occurs, but clearing with a job change is more common.

Industry	Possible sensitizing agents
Textile	Azo dyes, formaldehyde, resins
Painting	Epoxy, acrylates
Printing	Acrylates, epoxy resins
Agriculture	Pesticides, plants, rubber
Food preparation	Flavorings and preservatives
Medical/dental/veterinary	Rubber, acrylates, medications
Hairdressers	Paraphenylenediamine, nickel, glyceryl monothioglycolate, rubber
Metal workers	Biocides in cutting fluids, metals
Rubber manufacture	Thiuram, carbamates, mercaptobenzothiazole
Leather tanning	Chromate, formaldehyde
Plastics manufacture	Formaldehyde, phenolic resins, epoxy resins

Table 29.1.10 Examples of occupations at risk for contact allergy

ALLERGIC CONTACT DERMATITIS

ACD is caused by skin contact with material that triggers an immunologic reaction, leading to inflammatory skin lesions. Approximately 20–25% of cases of occupational contact dermatitis are found to be allergic in origin, although some studies have reported up to 50%.[39] Certain occupational groups are at greater risk for developing contact allergy due to occupational exposure to common allergens (Table 29.1.10), with agricultural and manufacturing jobs being most often cited. In California and Oregon, for example, poison oak dermatitis is among the most commonly reported job-related illnesses. Common allergens in occupational ACD are summarized in Table 29.1.3, but these allergens represent only a small portion of known industrial allergens.

Pathophysiology

ACD is a type of delayed hypersensitivity reaction. A hapten for contact hypersensitivity usually is a low-molecular-weight, lipid-soluble material (to allow penetration through the stratum corneum to viable epidermis). The hapten then binds or complexes with cell surface or structural proteins on various cells, including Langerhans' cells (epidermal antigen-presenting cells) and keratinocytes. It appears that the Langerhans' cell processes and presents the antigen to T lymphocytes, and a cascade of events follows involving a number of interleukins and chemotactic factors that leads to a clonal proliferation of sensitized lymphocytes and to the inflammatory reaction seen clinically. There are several recent reviews of the mechanisms of ACD, and our understanding of the intricacies of the processes is still evolving.[40–42] Recent data support the role of cutaneous irritancy as a necessary factor in the development of allergic contact dermatitis.[43,44]

Clinical course

The clinical appearance of *acute ACD* usually is an erythematous, vesicular, edematous eruption at the sites of contact with the allergenic substance (Table 29.1.7). The eruption is worse at sites with the most concentrated allergen exposure, and it may be milder (scattered erythematous papules) on areas where there was minimal exposure or where the allergen was washed off. The distribution of lesions may offer clues to the source of the allergen (e.g., gloves, clothing, air-borne) (Fig. 29.1.4). In severe, acute cases, the lesions may extend beyond sites of direct exposure because of the intensity of the inflammatory reaction and a phenomenon known as an auto-sensitization, or id, reaction. Because id reactions on the hands also are associated with fungal infections, the feet should be carefully examined. Inspecting the feet may provide clues to ACD because exposure may be originating from the person's

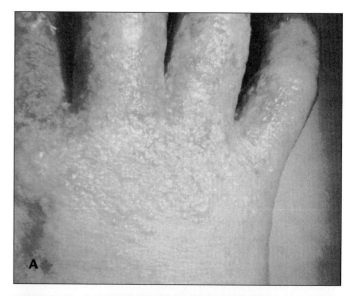

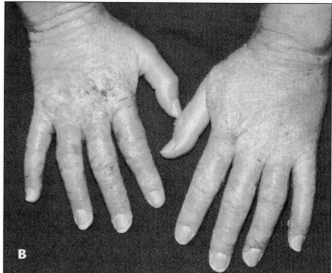

Figure 29.1.4: (a) and (b) Allergic contact dermatitis. Allergic contact dermatitis is characterized in its acute phase by vesicles with crusting and scaling. Erythema and edema are also features of this condition. The patient in (a) used neomycin-containing ointment on irritant dermatitis. The patient in (b) was a hairdresser who became allergic to the rubber gloves she was using to protect her hands from wet work.

footwear (e.g., rubber chemical). The lesions in acute ACD often occur 1–2 days after exposure, and may take 2 weeks to resolve. Thus, this time course differs from acute irritant exposure.

With repeated exposure to an allergen *chronic ACD* can develop. The clinical picture is variable, depending on the time interval between exposures (daily, weekly), and whether concomitant irritation is occurring with the same or other materials. In chronic ACD, the lesions generally are erythematous, scaling, and thickened. Vesicles may or may not be present, but they should be looked for very carefully. The hands are the most frequent site of involvement in ACD as well as in ICD. The dorsal surfaces may be more involved than the palms. However, the pattern of lesions on the hands cannot be reliably used to clinically distinguish ACD from ICD.[45]

Diagnosis

The diagnosis of ACD is based on the occupational history and results of skin patch testing. A clinical impression alone can be incorrect, particularly with regard to the offending agent. Patch testing is summarized above, and as noted, there are several limitations to patch testing. There are limited commercially available allergens in the United States (Table 29.1.3), and both false-negative and false-positive results can occur. Adams' *Occupational skin disease*[5] and other reviews[39,46] offer valuable information about patch testing.

If patch testing gives a positive result, a determination should be made as to whether or not the allergen is present in the work environment. If so, avoidance of this allergen by the patient should be attempted by wearing adequate protective clothing, changing the industrial process to reduce worker exposure, or substituting a less allergenic material. If these measures are not feasible, then the worker may need to be removed from the job.

If patch testing is negative, the person's clinical history, examination, and exposures should be reviewed. If ACD is still suspected, one must question whether the proper allergens were tested and, if so, were they tested with the proper concentration and vehicle. A visit to the workplace to observe the patient performing his or her job may result in increasing the pool of suspected allergens. After an interval of several weeks, repeat patch testing might be performed with the same and additional allergens. It is preferable to have the patient tested when no systemic corticosteroids are being taken. Ultraviolet light can alter immune responsive cells in the skin; therefore it is best to avoid testing in the setting of recent ultraviolet exposure at the test site.[47] If contact allergy is suspected in such an individual (e.g., a brick mason who works shirtless in the summer), it may be worthwhile to repeat patch tests in the winter.

Other possibilities to be considered when faced with unexpected negative patch tests are contact urticaria or photocontact dermatitis. Eczematous dermatitis, for example, may result from scratching the area affected by contact urticaria induced by rubber gloves.

Treatment and prognosis

Avoidance of the allergen by one of the methods noted earlier is the first step in the management of ACD.[48] Unfortunately, these measures alone often do not solve the problem for several reasons. (1) The allergen (e.g., nickel) may be commonplace in both the workplace and the domestic environment, thereby making avoidance extremely difficult. (2) The allergen (e.g., glyceryl monothioglycolate in hairdressing) may be very common in the work environment, not only in direct contact in an industrial step but as residual in other steps of a process. In the example of glyceryl monothioglycolate, even if the affected hairdresser stops using the offending permanent wave solutions on his or her clients, there is still potential for the hairdresser to react to the product on other clients. Further, routine use of gloves may not protect the worker because the allergen can penetrate the gloves.[49] (3) In addition, ICD, atopic dermatitis, psoriasis, and another dermatosis may be part of a given patient's diagnosis, so that avoidance of the allergen alone does not solve the problem. When there is a reduced threshold for irritation, a recovery phase also may occur with ACD. Thus, general protective measures outlined for ICD are useful in treating ACD as well.

For acute ACD, removal of the affected individual from work and irritant exposures is indicated. Cool water or astringent agents such as aluminum acetate (Burow's solution) used as compresses are helpful in the treatment of weeping vesicular dermatitis. Topical corticosteroids applied once or twice daily also are useful. The strength of the corticosteroid chosen should depend on the body site involved and the severity of the reaction. Potent topical corticosteroids generally should not be used on the face or intertriginous sites, such as the groin, for prolonged periods (> 1 week). If medical treatment is sought early in the presentation of severe, acute ACD, systemic corticosteroids may be useful. A 2–3-week course of prednisone (0.5–0.75 mg/kg/day, with optional tapering) often is helpful. Shorter courses, or dose-packs, may result in rebound of signs and symptoms. Patch testing should be deferred until the systemic corticosteroids dose is lowered or completed. With vesicular dermatitis, secondary infection should be suspected and treated systemically, if present. It is prudent to avoid potentially complicating topical therapy of ACD with treatments such as neomycin-containing antibiotic ointments, medicated petroleum jelly, or even rubber gloves as such treatment could become part of the allergic problem if the patient also develops an allergy to one of these materials. Multiple contact allergies can develop. Systemic antihistamines can be useful for symptoms of ACD. Because most antihistamines are potentially sedating, caution should be used in prescribing them to workers who remain on the job. Newer low-sedating antihistamines may be potential alternatives that may not interfere with safety or job performance.

For chronic ACD, treatment measures are similar. Phototherapy with psoralens plus ultraviolet A (PUVA) may also be beneficial.[50]

Prevention

Many of the preventive measures discussed under ICD are applicable to ACD as well (Table 29.1.9). With regard to *preplacement evaluation, eliciting a history of contact allergy* to nickel, gloves, or other allergens relevant to a specific job situation can be useful. For example, an individual may have a past history of nickel allergy that had manifested as a jewelry reaction. The associated rash may have long since resolved with avoidance of the offending jewelry. That individual could develop a new eruption if the new job involved frequent handling of nickel-plated metal parts. *Educating the potential worker about* the nature of the job and *potential allergen exposures* (e.g., poison ivy or oak in an outdoor job) also is useful in that this information may help an individual recall a past problem with that allergen. To educate the person effectively, however, the potential allergens in the workplace need to be identified. There are methods of predictive testing available to determine the sensitizing potential of chemicals in contact with human skin.

If a situation arises in which a potentially allergenic substance is to be introduced into the workplace, the question may arise regarding testing of employees to determine whether an individual is already allergic to that substance.[51] This generally is not recommended for several reasons. An allergy may develop later even if the test is currently negative, and screening patch tests will not predict this possibility. Also, there is a risk of sensitizing the individual to the substance through the 2-day occlusive patch test, which may be a different exposure than might be encountered in the routine job activity. Predictive patch testing generally is limited to pre-marketing product evaluation and involves special techniques.

Protective clothing can be useful in minimizing skin contact with an allergen *if* (1) the clothing (such as gloves) is properly worn and (2) the clothing has been chosen so that it prevents penetration of the offending agent.[52] Choosing specific gloves so that a hairdresser avoids contact with glyceryl monothioglycolate is a good example. Reference texts are available that detail penetration times for various gloves and chemicals.[53]

In general, *barrier creams* have limited usefulness, but more recently, creams have been developed that aim at specific allergens. Products applied by outdoor workers prior to exposure to poison oak and ivy have been found to be effective in preventing or decreasing the occurrence of poison oak and ivy allergic dermatitis.[54,55] Other barrier creams have been developed in an attempt to inactivate an allergen (e.g., chemical reduction of chromium) or to chelate metal allergens.[56]

CONTACT URTICARIA

Immediate urticarial reactions to topical materials in the workplace, or so-called *contact urticaria,* has been recognized for many years, particularly in workers in the fish and meat industries. There is heightened awareness of contact urticaria in recent years due to the increased recognition of immediate reactions to latex gloves and products in the healthcare field.[9,57]

Pathogenesis

The wheal and flare reaction of contact urticaria can occur through either allergic (immunologic) or non-allergic (non-immunologic) mechanisms. Allergic contact urticaria usually is mediated by an IgE mechanism, and it is more common in atopic individuals (e.g., latex contact urticaria). As with delayed contact allergy, there may be a history of frequent exposure to an agent over time before symptoms occur, and a low proportion of individuals exposed to the agent develop an allergic reaction. In the non-immunologic type, many exposed individuals may be affected by the offending agent despite no prior exposure, paralleling what can occur with strong irritants. Atopic individuals are not predisposed to non-immunologic contact urticaria. There appears to be a direct effect on blood vessel walls through the release of vasoactive substances, leading to the wheal and flare.

Clinical course

The mechanism of contact urticaria (allergic versus non-allergic) may not be distinguished by the clinical presentation. There may be the onset of itching, stinging, or burning immediately or within minutes of contact with the agent. Preservatives (e.g., sorbic acid) or perfume ingredients (e.g., aldehydes) may explain the burning some people experience with cosmetics. This urticarial-like reaction is non-immunologic. The clinical lesions of contact urticaria may range from erythema to urticaria or angioedema, or all three (Fig. 29.1.5). Lesions usually are limited to sites of exposure, and again, the hands and forearms are the sites affected most often. Examples of materials that can cause contact urticaria in the occupational setting are listed in Table 29.1.11. Fish, foods, animal proteins, flavorings, and perfume ingredients are among the agents associated most often with contact urticaria.

With the institution of universal precautions in all allied health fields, contact urticaria is important to recognize because life-threatening anaphylactic reactions have occurred in healthcare workers (as well as in patients) exposed to latex products. Contact urticaria to latex (also called latex hypersensitivity) may present as asthma, hand dermatitis, or anaphylaxis depending on the source of exposure, e.g. air-borne latex protein in glove powder, gloves themselves, or mucosal contact with latex products. Groups at greatest risk include healthcare workers, patients with meningomyelocele, and those with atopic dermatitis.[9,57]

A curious aspect of contact urticaria is that symptoms and signs may not occur with every exposure. In some cases, the reaction occurs only when the material is in contact with previously damaged skin (e.g., irritant dermatitis, atopic eczema), and if contact occurs when the underlying dermatitis is in remission, no urticaria or pruritus may be evident. Further, the clinical lesions of contact urticaria (erythematous wheals) may evolve into a vesicular

Foods	Medications	Flavorings/preservatives*	Miscellaneous
Apple	Bacitracin	Balsam of Peru	Acrylic monomer
Beer	Benzocaine	Benzoic acid	Alcohol
Carrot	Chloramphenicol	Cinnamic acid/aldehyde	Aliphatic polyamine
Egg	Neomycin	Sodium benzoate	Diethyltoluamide
Fish	Penicillin	Sorbic acid	Formaldehyde
Lettuce	Promethazine		Lindane
Meat (poultry, beef)	Streptomycin		Latex
Milk			Metals: nickel
Potato			Platinum
Spices			Xylene
* Usually cause non-immunologic contact urticaria.			

Table 29.1.11 Sources of contact urticaria in the workplace

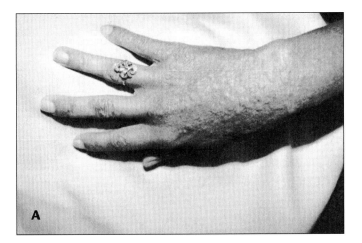

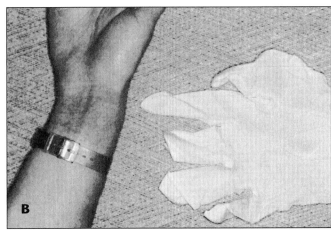

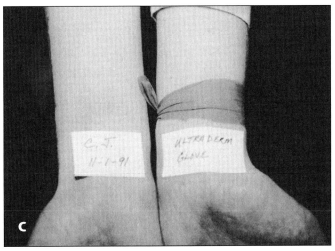

Figure 29.1.5: (a)–(c) Contact urticaria to latex. Wearing a latex glove, especially a wet one, for as short a time as 10 minutes can produce urticaria on the skin underneath the glove (a). Sometimes the urticaria is more conspicuous on the wrist than it is on the hand (b). An alternative way of producing contact urticaria is by tying a piece of the suspect glove onto the normal skin for 10–30 minutes and then observing the area of skin where the glove fabric has had contact (c).

dermatitis resembling typical ACD. For this reason, the time course of symptoms – itching at the time of or soon after contact – is a key point in suspecting the diagnosis of contact urticaria as the triggering factor for the subsequent evolution of the condition into eczematous dermatitis.

Diagnosis and differential diagnosis

Idiopathic urticaria usually can be distinguished from contact urticaria by its distribution. Physical urticarias, such as pressure or cold urticaria, may be more difficult to distinguish without contact urticaria testing or other test-ing for physical urticarias. Dermographism, the most common physical urticaria, can be mistaken for type I allergy.[58] For example, a worker who cleans and packs fish on ice is exposed to the fish, the cold environment, rubber gloves, and the mechanical pressure of grasping the knife, any one of which could trigger urticarial lesions. Testing to demonstrate that the fish caused urticarial lesions could lead to intervention with protective vinyl gloves that might allow the worker to continue on the job. Irritants can cause immediate symptoms, usually burning more than itching, but there can be an overlap of irritant, aller-gic, and urticarial reactions triggered by certain agents (e.g., formaldehyde, acrylates, ammonium persulfate in hair bleaches).

Testing for immediate reactions to latex proteins begins with a RAST (radio-allergosorbent test) for latex. If this is negative, having the patient wear a latex glove (or portion of glove) on a moistened hand is the next step. The risk of anaphylaxis is lower with this approach than with the skin prick test, still considered the gold standard.[57]

ACD can be difficult to distinguish in the case of an eczematous reaction developing after immediate symptoms. Contact urticaria testing with a delayed eczematous reaction at the test site occasionally can demonstrate the problem, or performing both contact urticaria testing and standard patch testing at times may be useful. Latex protein can cause a type 4 delayed-type response as well as a type 1 reaction.[59,60]

Treatment and prognosis

As with other types of contact dermatitis, avoidance of contact of the allergen with the skin is important. Oral antihistamines are useful to relieve itching. Systemic corticosteroids or epinephrine should be held in reserve for severe cases. Topical corticosteroids may be useful when eczematous lesions evolve. Protective gloves or sleeves can be useful if they are chosen carefully. As noted, the gloves themselves may be causing the problem. If glove-induced contact urticaria is suspected, it is most often due to the latex component, but immediate reactions to other components such as cornstarch or rubber additives have been reported. It may be important to analyze the situation before trying to recommend a substitute glove.

Prevention

Recognition that there are materials in the workplace that could cause both non-immunologic and immunologic contact urticaria is the first step. *Worker education* and *personal protection* are important. Because atopic individuals are more likely to develop immunologic contact urticaria, medical surveillance for early diagnosis and exposure modification may be helpful.

CONTACT PHOTODERMATITIS
Pathogenesis

Some naturally occurring and synthetic chemicals may cause contact dermatitis only in the presence of light, which may be sunlight or artificial light sources that emit specific wavelengths. This general reaction is known as contact photodermatitis, and there are two categories of reaction: phototoxic and photoallergic. Phototoxic reactions have non-immunologic mechanisms, in which a chemical, by the nature of its structure, absorbs a specific wavelength of light and produces a product that causes cellular damage. The mechanism may or may not involve production of reactive oxygen species. Photoallergic reactions involve conversion, by exposure to light, of a chem-

ical into an immunologically reactive hapten that leads to a delayed allergic hypersensitivity reaction. A recent review covers the spectrum of photosensitivity disorders.[61]

Clinical course

It can be difficult to distinguish clinically phototoxic from photo-ACD. In both, exposed areas of the skin such as the face, anterior V of the neck, backs of the hands, and uncovered sites on the arm (to the shirt sleeves) and legs frequently are involved. Hairy areas, upper eyelids, and below the chin may be spared. Phototoxic reactions may appear as a painful, exaggerated sunburn that may develop bullae and subsequent pigmentation. When the offending agent is avoided, the dermatitis usually disappears promptly. Photo-ACD may have many of the features outlined under ACD (itching, vesiculation).

Diagnosis and differential diagnosis

The distribution (on sun-exposed surfaces) of the reaction is an important clinical feature in suspecting the diagnosis, and the condition sometimes is difficult to distinguish from air-borne contact exposure. The method for photopatch testing is outlined in a previous section. Examples of substances that can cause contact photodermatitis with topical exposure and occupations at risk are given in Table 29.1.12.

Topical agent	Occupational example
Phototoxic	
Coal-tar derivatives	
Pitch, creosote	Railroad, construction
Acridine	Chemical/laboratory
Anthracene	
Dyes	
Anthraquinone	Textile, laboratory
Eosin	
Methylene blue	
Drugs	
Phenothiazines	Medical, pharmaceutical
Sulfonamides	
Plants and derivatives	
Compositae (yarrow)	Agricultural
Umbelliferae (celery, parsnip)	Vegetable workers
Rutaceae (lime, lemon)	Bartenders
Psoralen	Medical workers
8-Methoxypsoralen	
Photoallergic	
Antifungal agents	
Fentichlor	
Fragrances	Perfume/cosmetic industry
Methyl coumarin	
Musk ambrette	
Halogenated salicylanilide	Soap, cosmetic industry
Soap, deodorants	Usage exposure
Phenothiazines	Medical
Agricultural	
Sunscreens	Outdoor workers
PABA esters	
Benzophenones	
Whiteners	Textile workers

Table 29.1.12 Contact photodermatitis

Treatment and prognosis

Avoidance of contact with the offending agent is the most important measure in prevention and treatment. Protective measures such as clothing and topical sunscreens may be helpful, but it is important to be sure that the individual is not experiencing photodermatitis resulting from a chemical sunscreen ingredient (e.g., benzophenone). Other treatment measures are the same as those outlined under ACD. Prognostically, phototoxic eruptions usually resolve fairly quickly. Chronic photo-ACD may rarely eventuate into a marked and persistent photosensitivity reaction that continues despite avoidance of the triggering agent. Such persistent light reactivity (chronic actinic dermatitis) is difficult to manage and may require immunosuppressive agents.

References

1. Bruze M, Emmett EA. Occupational exposures to irritants. In: Jackson EM, Goldner R, eds. Irritant contact dermatitis. New York: Marcel Dekker, Inc., 1990:81–106.
2. Shmunes E. Predisposing factors in occupational skin diseases. Dermatol Clin 1988; 6:7–13.
3. Sherertz EF, Zanolli MD. Occupational allergic contact and frictional dermatitis leading to plaques of psoriasis: a challenge in diagnosis. Am J Contact Derm 1991; 2:52–55.
4. Meding B. Epidemiology of hand eczema in an industrial city. Acta Derm Venereol Suppl (Stockh) 1990; 153:1–43.
5. Adams RM, ed. Occupational skin disease, 2nd edn. Philadelphia: WB Saunders, 1990.
6. Rietschel RL, Fowler JF. Fisher's contact dermatitis, 4th edn. Baltimore: Williams and Wilkins, 1995.
7. Rycroft RJG, Menne T, Frosch PJ, Benezra C. Textbook of contact dermatitis, 1st edn. Berlin: Springer-Verlag, 1992.
8. De Groot AC. Patch testing: test concentrations and vehicles for 2800 allergens. Elsevier: New York, 1986.
9. Warshaw E. Latex allergy. J Am Acad Dermatol 1998; 39:1–25.
10. Hausen BM, Hjorth N. Skin reactions to topical food exposure. Dermatol Clin 1984; 2:567–78.
11. DeLeo V, Gonzalez E, Kim J, Lim H. Phototesting and photopatch testing: when to do it and when not to do it. Am J Contact Derm 2000; 11:57–61.
12. Malten KE. Thoughts on irritant contact dermatitis. Contact Derm 1981; 7:238–47.
13. Dahl MV. Chronic irritant contact dermatitis: mechanisms, variables, and differentiation from other forms of contact dermatitis. Adv Dermatol 1988; 3:261–76.
14. Duarte I, Terumi Nakano J, Lazzarini R. Hand eczema: evaluation of 250 patients. Am J Contact Derm 1998; 9:216–23.
15. Smith HR, Armstrong DK, Wakelin SH, Rycroft RJ, White IR, McFadden JP. Descriptive epidemiology of hand dermatitis at the St. John's contact dermatitis clinic 1983–97. Br J Dermatol 2000; 142:284–7.
16. Mathias CGT. Contact dermatitis from use or misuse of soaps, detergents, and cleansers in the workplace. Occup Med State Art Rev 1986; 1:205–18.
17. Majoie IM, von Blomberg BM, Bruynzeel DP. Development of hand eczema in junior hairdressers: an 8-year follow-up study. Contact Derm 1996; 34:243–7.
18. Warren R, Ertel KD, Bartolo RG, Levine MJ, Bryant PB, Wong LF. The influence of hard water (calcium) and surfactants on irritant contact dermatitis. Contact Derm 1996; 35:337–43.
19. Meding B. Prevention of hand eczema in atopics. Curr Prob Dermatol 1996; 25:116–22.
20. Nickoloff BJ. Immunologic reaction triggered during irritant contact dermatitis. Am J Contact Derm 1998; 9:107–10.
21. Sun CC, Guo YL, Lin RS. Occupational hand dermatitis in a tertiary referral dermatology clinic in Taipei. Contact Derm 1995; 33:414–8.
22. Wigger-Alberti W, Elsner P. Do barrier creams and gloves prevent or provoke contact dermatitis? Am J Contact Derm 1998; 9:100–6.
23. Berndt U, Wigger-Alberti W, Gabard B, Elsner P. Efficacy of a barrier cream and its vehicle as protective measures against occupational irritant contact dermatitis. Contact Derm 2000; 42:77–80.
24. Boffa MJ, Wilkinson SM, Beck MH. Screening for corticosteroid contact hypersensitivity. Contact Derm 1995; 33:149–51.
25. Hannuksela M. Moisturizers in the prevention of contact dermatitis. Curr Prob Dermatol 1996; 25:214–20.
26. Holness DL, Nethercott JR. Work outcome in workers with occupational skin disease. Am J Ind Med 1995; 27:807–15.
27. Pryce DW, Irvine D, English JSC, Rycroft RJG. Soluble oil dermatitis: a follow-up study. Contact Derm 1989; 21:28–35.
28. Lushniak BD. The epidemiology of occupational contact dermatitis. Dermatol Clin 1995; 13: 671–9.
29. Mathias CG. Prevention of occupational contact dermatitis. J Am Acad Dermatol 1990; 23:742–8.
30. Halkier-Sorensen L. Occupational skin diseases. Contact Derm 1996; 35(suppl):1–120
31. Rycroft RJG. Low humidity and microtrauma. Am J Ind Med 1985; 8:371–3.
32. Hosoi J, Hariya T, Denda M, Tsuchiya T. Regulation of the cutaneous allergic reaction by humidity. Contact Derm 2000; 42:81–4.
33. Buring JE, Hennekens CH. Carbonless copy paper: a review of published epidemiologic studies. J Occup Med 1991; 33:486–95.
34. Konzen JK. Fiberglass and the skin. In: Maibach HI, Gellin GA, eds. Occupational and industrial dermatology. Chicago: Year Book Medical Publishers Inc., 1982.
35. Mathias CGT. Post-traumatic eczema. Dermatol Clin 1988; 6:35–42.
36. Ronchese F. Calluses, cicatrices, and other stigma as an aid to personal identification. JAMA 1945; 128:925–32.
37. Hersle K, Mobacken H. Hyperkeratotic dermatitis of the palms. Br J Dermatol 1982; 107:195–202.
38. Schempp CM, Muller H, Czech W, Schopf E, Simon JC. Treatment of chronic palmoplantar eczema with local bath-PUVA therapy. J Am Acad Dermatol 1997; 36:733–7.
39. Nethercott VR, Holness DL, Adam RM, et al. Patch testing with routine screening tray in North America, 1985 through 1989: frequency of response. Am J Contact Derm 1991; 2:122–9.
40. Belsito DV. The rise and fall of allergic contact dermatitis. Am J Contact Derm 1997; 8:193–201.
41. Grabbe S, Schwarz T. Immunoregulatory mechanism involved in elicitation of allergic contact hypersensitivity. Immunol Today 1998; 19:37–44.
42. Krasteva M, Kehren J, Ducluzeau MT, et al. Contact dermatitis I. Pathophysiology of contact sensitivity. Eur J Dermatol 1999; 9:65–77.
43. McFadden JP, Basketter DA. Contact allergy, irritancy and 'danger.' Contact Derm 2000; 42:123–7.
44. Zhang L, Tinkle SS. Chemical activation of innate and specific immunity in contact dermatitis. J Invest Dermatol 2000; 115:168–76.
45. Cronin E. Clinical patterns of hand eczema in women. Contact Derm 1985; 13:153–61.
46. Storrs FJ, Rosenthal LE, Adams RM, et al. Prevalence and relevance of allergic reactions to patients patch tested in North America, 1984–1985. J Am Acad Dermatol 1989; 20:1038–45.
47. Bergstresser PR. Ultraviolet immunosuppression 2000. Prog Dermatol 2000; 34(3).
48. Woolner D, Soltani K. Management of hand dermatitis. Comprehensive Ther 1994; 20:422–6

49. Storrs FJ. Permanent wave contact dermatitis: contact allergy to glyceryl monothioglycolate. J Am Acad Dermatol 1984; 11:74–85.

50. Zemstov A. Treatment of palmoplantar eczema with bath-PUVA therapy. J Am Acad Dermatol 1998; 38:505–6

51. Milkovic-Kraus S, Marcan J. Can pre-employment patch testing help to prevent occupational contact allergy? Contact Derm 1996; 35:226–8

52. Mellstrom GA, Wrangsjo K, Wahlberg JE, Fryklund B. The value and limitations of protective gloves in medical health service: part II. Dermatol Nurs 1996; 8:287–95

53. Forsberg K, Keith LH. Chemical protective clothing performance index book. New York: John Wiley & Sons, 1989.

54. Orchard S, Fellman JH, Storrs FJ. Poison ivy/oak dermatitis. Use of polyamine salts of linoleic acid dimer for topical prophylaxis. Arch Dermatol 1986; 122:783–9.

55. Marks JG, Fowler JF, Sherertz EF, Rietschel RL. Prevention of poison ivy and poison oak allergic contact dermatitis by quaternium-18 bentonite. J Am Acad Dermatol 1995; 33:212–6.

56. Gawkrodger DJ, Healy J, Howe AM. The prevention of nickel contact dermatitis. A review of the use of binding agents and barrier creams. Contact Derm 1995; 32:257–65.

57. Cohen DE, Scheman A, Stewart L, et al. American Academy of Dermatology's position paper on latex allergy. J Am Acad Dermatol 1998; 39:98–106.

58. Armstrong DKB, Smith HR, Rycroft RJG. Glove-related hand urticaria in the absence of type 1 latex allergy. Contact Derm 1999;41:42.

59. de Groot H, de Jong NW, Duijster E, et al. Prevalence of natural rubber latex allergy (type I and type IV) in laboratory workers in The Netherlands. Contact Derm 1998; 38:159–63.

60. Wilkinson SM, Burd R. Latex: a cause of allergic contact eczema in users of natural rubber gloves. J Am Acad Dermatol 1998; 38:36–42.

61. Gould JW, Mercurio MG, Elmets CA. Cutaneous photosensitivity diseases induced by exogenous agents. J Am Acad Dermatol 1995; 33:551–73.

29.2 **Other Dermatoses**

Christina A Herrick, Kalman L Watsky

The spectrum of occupational and environmental skin disease includes numerous other dermatoses in addition to the various forms of contact dermatitis. In this section of the chapter, we deal with non-malignant skin reactions to chemical, physical, and biologic agents. Skin cancer, the first recognized form of occupational skin disease, is discussed in Chapter 30.10. Acute skin injuries, including lacerations and punctures, account for a large proportion of all occupational injuries, but they are outside the scope of this chapter.

Skin disease continues to be the second most common form of occupational illness, with only repetitive trauma disorders accounting for more cases each year.[1] Data from the 2001 Bureau of Labor Statistics (BLS) annual survey shows that 12% of non-fatal occupational illnesses reported in 2000 in private industry were diseases of the skin. This represents an incidence of 46 cases per 100,000 full-time workers, although the true magnitude of occupational skin disease may be 10- to 50-fold higher than the annual survey suggests due to under-reporting and misclassification. Data from the United States and elsewhere estimate that contact dermatitis accounts for greater than 90% of cases of occupational skin disease.[2,3] The remaining disorders represent a wide variety of cutaneous diseases whose prevalence is not well known. This section discusses the manifestations, pathogenesis, diagnosis, treatment, and prognosis of these dermatoses, organized by their causal agents.

    CHEMICAL
    Acne and folliculitis
    Chloracne
    Disorders of pigmentation
    PHYSICAL
    Radiodermatitis
    Urticaria
    Photodermatoses
    Erythema ab igne
    Miliaria
    Frostbite and chilblains
    Vibration-induced white finger disease
    Occupational acro-osteolysis and scleroderma
    Foreign body reactions
    Blisters and calluses
    BIOLOGIC
    Bacteria
    Fungi
    Viruses
    Parasites

OCCUPATIONAL ACNE

Acne is a disorder of the pilosebaceous unit. Environmental and occupational acne can be divided into three types: oil folliculitis, acne vulgaris induced or exacerbated by environmental exposures, and chloracne. In each instance, work-related acne is due to the action of chemical and mechanical factors on the follicular wall.

Oil acne (folliculitis)

Workers at risk include machinists; oil field workers; oil refiners; auto, truck, aircraft, and boat mechanics; rubber workers; roofers; and road maintenance workers.

Pathogenesis
The hair follicle is particularly susceptible to irritation from lipids, which disperse into sebum. Petroleum distillates such as non-synthetic cutting oils, pitch, and tar may alter the keratinization of the wall of the follicle, causing plugging of the follicle (comedo formation) or induce an inflammatory reaction by rupture of the follicular wall (folliculitis).

Clinical course
Oil acne presents as acneiform (follicular) lesions at the location of exposure, most commonly on the dorsae of the hands and forearms. Comedones as well as inflammatory folliculitis may occur in exposed sites. Covered areas of the body also may be involved due to saturation of clothing with oils. Pitch or coal tar acne is associated primarily with comedones across the malar area and periorbitally, with few inflammatory lesions.[4]

Diagnosis
The areas of involvement in oil acne are different from those seen in either acne vulgaris or chloracne (Table 29.2.1). The history usually is adequate to confirm the diagnosis.

Prevention
Protective clothing should be used, particularly aprons and arm shields. Mandatory daily laundering of work clothes and end-of-shift showers are helpful. If exposure cannot be prevented, then dilute synthetic water-based cutting fluids should be substituted for neat (i.e., straight petroleum-derived) oils.

Treatment and prognosis
Approaches to treatment are similar to those for routine acne.[5] Oral antibiotics, especially tetracycline and erythromycin, reduce inflammation and treat secondary infection. Topical antibiotics (clindamycin; erythromycin) can also be useful. Comedones are more refractory to treatment but may respond to long-term topical retinoids (tretinoin; adapalene). Once the exposure has ended, the eruption gradually subsides.

Acne vulgaris

Persons at risk include workers in fast food restaurants, actors, actresses, models, and cosmeticians.

	Age	Distribution	Clinical features	Associated conditions
Oil acne (folliculitis)	Any age	Exposed sites	Open comedones, pustules	None
Acne vulgaris	Peak incidence, ages 11 to 20	Face, neck, chest	Open and closed back comedones, papules, pustules, cysts, scar	None
Chloracne	Any age	Face, especially the malar crescent and auricular creases, axillae, groin; nose spared	Open and closed comedones, straw-colored cysts	Xerosis, conjunctivitis, actinic elastosis, peripheral neuritis, liver abnormalities

Table 29.2.1 Differential features of acne

Pathogenesis

Acne vulgaris can be induced or exacerbated by numerous environmental stimuli in addition to oil. Friction, heat, and sweating also play a role in the development of acne lesions.

Clinical course and diagnosis

The lesions typically involve the face, neck, upper chest and back (see Table 29.2.1). The history of exposure to oils and grease, oil-based make-up, or friction (e.g., from a headband) usually is adequate to arrive at the diagnosis.

Prevention

Avoiding contact with the offending substance and adequate hygiene usually are helpful in preventing the condition.

Treatment and prognosis

Oral antibiotics, especially tetracycline and erythromycin, reduce inflammation and treat secondary infection. Topical antibiotics (clindamycin; erythromycin) can also be useful. Comedones are more refractory to treatment but may respond to long-term topical retinoids (tretinoin; adapalene).

Chloracne

Although originally described approximately 100 years ago by Von Bettman,[6] chloracne more recently has entered the world's lexicon as a consequence of Agent Orange use during the Vietnam War and industrial accidents with dioxin and its related compounds.[7] Chloracne is believed to be a sensitive indicator of systemic exposure to specific polyaromatic hydrocarbons. Persons at risk include workers in production of halogenated aromatic hydrocarbon-based pesticides and herbicides, electrical workers exposed to older polychlorinated biphenyl (PCB)-type transformer oils, and environmental workers engaged in cleaning up or disposing of previously produced agents. Table 29.2.2 lists the major chemicals that have been incriminated.

Pathogenesis

To a much greater extent than other petroleum products, agents that cause chloracne induce a marked dyskeratosis of the follicular epidermis, which causes a non-inflammatory keratin build-up in the follicle referred to as a comedo (Fig. 29.2.1). Comedo formation often progresses to a character-

Polyhalogenated naphthalenes*
　Polychloronaphthalenes
　Polybromonaphthalenes
Polyhalogenated biphenyls
　Polychlorinated biphenyls (PCBs)
　Polybrominated biphenyls (PBBs)†
Polyhalogenated dibenzofurans*
　Polychlorodibenzofurans, especially tri-, tetra-, penta-, and hexachlorodibenzofuran
　Polybromodibenzofuran, especially tetrabromodibenzofuran
Contaminants of polychlorophenol compounds, especially herbicides (2,4,5-T and pentachlorophenol) and herbicide intermediates (2,3,5-trichlorophenol)
　2,3,7,8-Tetrachlorodibenzo-*p*-dioxin (TCDD)
　Hexachlorodibenzo-*p*-dioxin
　Tetrachlorodibenzofuran
Contaminants of 3,4-dichloroaniline and related herbicides (Propanil, Methazole)
　3,4,3',4'-Tetrachloroazoxybenzene
　3,3,3'4'-Tetrachloroazobenzene
Others‡
　1,2,3,4'-Tetrachlorobenzene (experimental)
　Dichlobenil (Casoron)–a herbicide (clinical only)
　DDT (crude trichlorobenzene)

* Polychlorodibenzofurans and hexachloronaphthalenes may occur as contaminants in some PCBs.
† Polybromonaphthalenes may occur as contaminants in some PBBs.
‡ Not confirmed as chloracne-producing agents.
With permission from Taylor JS. Environmental chloracne: update and overview. Ann NY Acad Sci 1979; 320: 295–307. ©1979 New York Academy of Sciences, USA.

Table 29.2.2 Chloracne-producing chemicals.

istic straw-colored cystic lesion, the chloracne cyst. The development of chloracne can be generally correlated with serum levels of the chloracne-inducing agent, particularly with tetrachlorodibenzodioxin (TCDD).[8] The experience with PCBs and pesticides has been less clear because the specific causal metabolite may differ from what is measured (see Chapters 45 and 48). Individual variation in follicles is clearly evident, with some individuals showing higher serum levels of TCDD without chloracne than others who have the cutaneous disease. The follicular level of the agent may be of greatest importance in producing clinical change.

Clinical course

Several clinical features distinguish chloracne from acne vulgaris (Table 29.2.1).[3,7] The onset of chloracne is seen within 2–8 weeks of exposure to a chloracne-producing

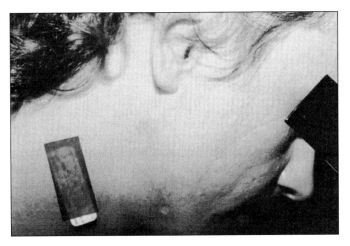

Figure 29.2.1: Chloracne: comedones and scarring on the cheek and neck.

agent. The disease will continue to progress and subsequently regress over a 4–6-month period, presuming that there is no further exposure to the chloracne-producing agent. If the exposure has been intense, clinical lesions of chloracne may continue to appear many years after the exposure has ended. The primary lesion of chloracne is the comedo as well as the straw-colored cyst. The inflammatory papules and pustules of acne vulgaris are not evident. The distribution of lesions is also of primary importance (see Table 29.2.1). The most uniquely involved areas are the postauricular folds, the malar crescent, and the genitalia. The nose typically is spared. Associated cutaneous features include xerosis, pigmentation, conjunctivitis, and scarring.

Non-cutaneous findings are varied following exposure to the chemicals that cause chloracne.[3,7] Hepatomegaly may occur, as may liver damage. Liver damage is associated more commonly with chloronaphthalenes than with PCBs. Porphyria cutanea tarda has been associated with exposure to chloracne-producing agents in some cases, but the causal link remains weak. Hepatic porphyria has been attributed to TCDD exposure. Peripheral neuropathy also has been reported.

The chloracne-causing agents (Table 29.2.2) vary in their potency, with TCDD causing chloracne at the lowest concentrations. Microgram concentrations of TCDD applied directly to the skin over a period of time induce chloracne.

Diagnosis
A history of exposure to a chloracne-producing agent and lesions consistent with chloracne suggest the diagnosis. Serum lipid and adipose levels of suspect compounds and metabolites should be obtained for confirmation of exposure; this measurement must be performed by an experienced laboratory with gas chromatography/mass spectroscopy (GC/MS) capabilities and carefully controlled comparisons. Biopsy may be useful for diagnosis because chloracne-producing agents cause loss of follicular sebaceous glands. It may be difficult to distinguish actinic elastotic comedones from mild cases of chloracne.

Treatment
The treatment of chloracne is difficult, although some success has been seen with oral antibiotics, topical retinoic acid, and oral isotretinoin.[9] Cyst formation may be prevented by early institution of retinoid therapy.

Prevention
Chloracne-producing agents are unwanted byproducts of industrial processes. Even minute exposures must be avoided. Therefore, the following guidelines should be followed at any plant where chloracne-causing agents are produced or used: (1) clean locker room and shower facilities, (2) use disposable impervious clothing for workers with potential for direct contact, (3) routinely monitor for plant contamination using wipe samples, and (4) routinely educate and monitor workers.

PIGMENTARY DISORDERS

Occupational and environmental causes of cutaneous dyspigmentation are varied and may be exhibited as hyperpigmentation or hypopigmentation. The differential diagnosis should always include inherited or idiopathic conditions, and thus, a thorough investigation should be undertaken in each case.

Hyperpigmentation

Workers at risk include those exposed to heavy metals and those working with organic nitrogen compounds and dyes. Compounds that may cause hyperpigmentation are listed in Tables 29.2.3 and 29.2.4.

Pathogenesis
Mechanisms of hyperpigmentation include: (1) exogenous pigment deposition, (2) deposition in skin systemically, (3)

Chemical	Color
Aniline dyes	Pigmented contact dermatitis
Azo dyes	Pigmented contact dermatitis
Danthron	Red-brown
Dihydroxyacetone	Yellow-orange
2,4-Dinitrophenol	Yellow
Dinitrosalicylic acid	Yellow
Henna (2,4-dihydroxynaphthoquinone)	Reddish orange
Nitrazepam	Yellow
Phenazopyridine (Pyridium)	Yellow
Picric acid	Jaundiced appearance
Sodium nitrite	Yellow
Tetryl (Tetra-nitromethylaniline)	Canary yellow

Adapted from Lerner EA, Sober AJ. Chemical and pharmacologic agents which cause hyperpigmentation of the skin. In: Fitzpatrick TB, Wick MM, Toda K, eds. Brown melanoderma: biology and disease of epidural pigmentation. Tokyo: University of Tokyo Press, 1986: 215–227.

Table 29.2.3 Hyperpigmentation: nitro compounds and dyes that stain skin

Substance	Color	Location
Arsenic	Bronze	Diffuse, especially trunk and proximal extremities
Bismuth (chromium)	Blue-gray	Diffuse
Copper	Greenish	Hair
Gold (chrysiasis)	Blue-gray	Sun-exposed areas, especially periorbitally
Iron	Brown	Tattoo
Lead	Pallor and vividity	Generalized, gingival leadline
Mercury	Slate gray	Skin folds
Silver (argyria)	Slate gray	Sun-exposed areas

Adapted from Lerner EA, Sober AJ. Chemical and pharmacologic agents which cause hyperpigmentation of the skin. In Fitzpatrick TB, Wick MM, Toda K, eds. *Brown Melanoderma: Biology and Disease of Epidural Pigmentation.* Tokyo, University of Tokyo Press, 1986 pp 215–227.

Table 29.2.4 Hyperpigmentation: metals that may be systemically or locally deposited in skin

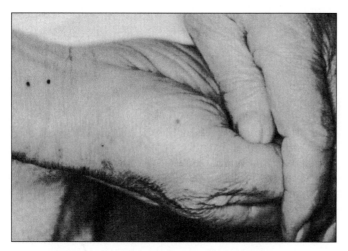

Figure 29.2.2: Argyria: silver tattoos in a silver worker.

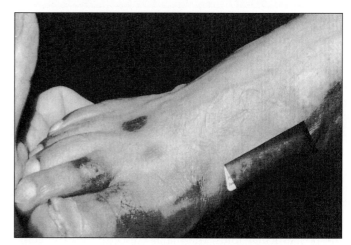

Figure 29.2.3: Postinflammatory hyperpigmentation and hypopigmentation following irritant contact dermatitis.

photoeruptions, and (4) postinflammatory hyperpigmentation.[10] Exogenous pigment deposition is typically due to a tattoo (e.g., silver shavings in a jewelry worker) or superficial staining by dye-like compounds. The most important of these factors are listed in Tables 29.2.3 and 29.2.4. Systemic toxicity with a variety of heavy metals can lead to cutaneous dyspigmentation. The most striking form of dyspigmentation is argyria due to systemic deposition of silver (Fig. 29.2.2).

The most common forms of occupational and environmental hyperpigmentation are photoeruption and postinflammatory hyperpigmentation (Fig. 29.2.3). Photoeruptions include sunburn as well as the exacerbated sunburn response (phototoxic dermatosis) that results from exposure of the skin to furocoumarins and light in the UVA spectrum.[11] Postinflammatory hyperpigmentation is typically dermal and can follow any skin injury. Dermal pigment results from deposition of melanin, hemosiderin, or both.

Clinical course

The pattern of pigmentation varies depending on the etiology (Tables 29.2.3 and 29.2.4). With photodermatoses, the pigmentary changes are usually noted in sun-exposed sites: the face, the V of the neck, and the dorsa of the hands. Pigmentation resulting from heavy metal toxicity may be exacerbated by exposure to the sun. Postinflammatory hyperpigmentation occurs at the sites of skin injury. Hyperpigmentation may be epidermal, dermal, or mixed. The type often can be distinguished by a Wood's lamp examination, which shows epidermal hyperpigmentation to be accentuated and dermal pigmentation to be diminished.

Diagnosis

The pattern of pigmentary change often suggests the diagnosis. Wood's lamp examination may be helpful. Biopsy may give important information in cases of dermal tattoos or systemic toxicity from heavy metals (Tables 29.2.3 and 29.2.4).

Prevention

Sunscreens can be effective in limiting photoeruptions. Protective clothing is needed to prevent exogenous pigment deposition. This protection is doubly important in working with organic dye-like compounds because many of these compounds are toxic and are absorbed through intact skin (see Chapter 42). Prevention of systemic absorption of metals requires the range of industrial hygiene practices.

Treatment and prognosis

The hyperpigmentation that results from tattoos and systemic heavy metal toxicity may be irreversible. Exogenous staining of the stratum corneum resolves without treatment within a period of a few weeks. Postinflammatory hyperpigmentation may persist for months, especially in those who are more darkly pigmented. Epidermal hyperpigmentation may respond to treatment with agents containing hydroquinone and retinoic acid. Side effects of hydroquinone include contact dermatitis as well as exogenous ochronosis. Dermal pigmentation has no effective therapy.

Hypopigmentation

Hypopigmentation of the skin due to occupational or environmental causes has two principal etiologies: chemical leukoderma and postinflammatory hypopigmentation (Figs 29.2.4 and 29.2.5). Chemical leukoderma can result from skin contact with substances containing hydroquinone or derivatives of alkyl phenols and catechols (Table 29.2.5). Those at risk include rubber workers, photographic developers, hospital housekeepers, printers, and workers in the oil, paint and plastics industries.[3] Cutaneous injury, from inflammation or trauma, may also produce a focal loss of skin pigment (Fig. 29.2.5).

Clinical course

Chemical leukoderma was first described in 1939 as an epidemic of depigmentation at a tannery due to the use of rubber gloves containing monobenzyl ether of hydroquinone.[12,13] Pigment was lost in areas exposed to the compound but also at sites distant from exposed skin. This pattern of pigment loss may be difficult to distinguish clinically from idiopathic vitiligo. Postinflammatory hypopigmentation occurs at the location of previous skin injury, either from trauma or dermatitis.

Pathogenesis

The compounds known to cause chemical leukoderma are very similar in structure to that of melanin and its precursors, and they are known to have a direct cytotoxic effect

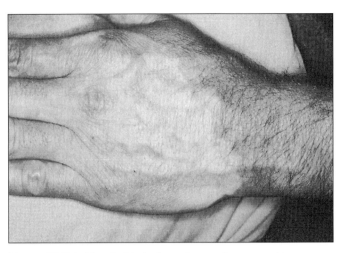

Figure 29.2.4: Chemical leukoderma in a worker exposed to phenolic compounds.

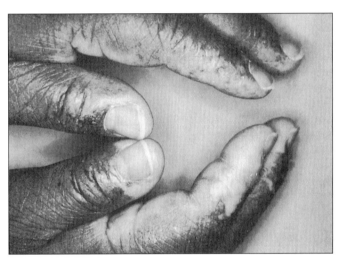

Figure 29.2.5: Postinflammatory hypopigmentation following a chemical burn due to ethylene oxide.

on melanocytes. The effects possibly are due to the formation of free radicals, leading to damage of cellular membranes and formation of antigens, which activate lymphocytes.[14] This theory would explain why the loss of pigment cells may occur at sites distant from the sites of exposure. Postinflammatory hypopigmentation likely is due to a defect in the transfer of pigment from melanocytes to keratinocytes.

Diagnosis

Wood's lamp examination is helpful in distinguishing postinflammatory hypopigmentation from chemical leukoderma. Chemical leukoderma typically demonstrates complete depigmentation. Skin biopsy with special stains for melanocytes also may be helpful. It can be difficult to distinguish idiopathic vitiligo from chemical leukoderma, and therefore, a complete history of chemical exposures needs to be obtained in all instances.

Hydroquinone
Monobenzyl ether of hydroquinone
Monoethyl ether of hydroquinone (hydroxyanisole)
p-Isopropylcatechol
p-Methylcatechol
p-tert-Butylcatechol
p-tert-Butylphenol
p-tert-Butylphenol
p-tert-Amylphenol
Mercaptoamines
    N-(2-Mercaptoethyl)-dimethylamine hydrochloride
    2-Mercaptoethylamine hydrochloride
N, N', N"-Triethylenethiophosphoramide (thiotepa)

Reprinted from Bolognia JL, Pawelek JM. Biology of hypopigmentation. J Am Acad Dermatol 1988; 19:217–255, with permission from the American Academy of Dermatology, Inc.

Table 29.2.5 Compounds known to produce chemical leukoderma.

Prevention

Melanocytotoxic agents should be used only with caution and with strict adherence to protective safety measures. Worker education regarding the effects of these chemicals is essential.

Treatment

Chemical leukoderma can respond to long-term treatment with psoralen plus UVA light (PUVA).[15] Localized areas of pigment loss also may be treated with epidermal allografts.[16] Postinflammatory hypopigmentation usually resolves over time. Permanent postinflammatory pigment loss may require cosmetic cover-up.

RADIODERMATITIS

Workers at risk are numerous and include all those involved with radioactive substances. Medical and industrial workers exposed to x-ray-emitting devices and isotopes, workers in uranium mining in the field of nuclear energy, and nuclear waste management personnel are particularly at risk.

Clinical course

Cutaneous findings of acute, intense radiation damage include early blistering, with eventual loss of skin and skin appendages in the exposed area. Chronic radiation damage results in epidermal atrophy, enlarged blood vessels, and pigmentary changes (poikiloderma). The clinical appearance is that of a burn scar. Cutaneous carcinoma may develop in radiated skin many years later.

Other effects include dryness and cracking of irradiated skin, alopecia, and chronic skin ulcers. If extensive areas of the body are exposed, the skin changes become a small part of the acute radiation syndrome, with its three phases of early nausea and prostration, followed in 1–2 days by a general feeling of wellbeing, and a third phase in about a week of fever, weight loss, gastrointestinal symptoms, and possible death from bone marrow suppression and infection (see Chapter 33.1).

Pathogenesis

Radiodermatitis commonly refers to alterations in the skin produced by ionizing radiation. Radioactive particles pass through and damage cell structures, including chromosomes, particularly in rapidly dividing tissue layers. Lethal damage to basal cells results in initiation of a classic inflammatory response. Death of melanosomes may result in subsequent pigmentary alteration. Non-lethal damage enhances the possibility of cell transformation and subsequent neoplasia (see Chapter 30.10).

Diagnosis

A history of radiation exposure and a compatible clinical picture are suggestive. A biopsy may be useful to confirm the diagnosis.

Prevention

Radiation can be measured, and routine monitoring is needed for any worker with potential exposure. Protective shielding, based on the form of exposure, should prevent radiation damage and should be required for workers with radiation exposures.

Treatment and prognosis

Treatment of acute radiation exposure is supportive. Because radiation exposure is irreversible and produces effects many years later, monitoring of exposed individuals for the development of cutaneous malignancies and premalignancies is needed; early diagnosis and treatment may alter the natural history of the condition. Routine use of sunscreens may prevent augmentation of x-ray-induced sequelae by radiation with the longer wavelengths of ultraviolet light.

PHYSICAL URTICARIA

Urticaria, also known as hives, is a common condition that may affect up to 20% of the population at some time during the course of their lives. Urticaria may result from occupational or environmental exposures. Contact urticaria (see Chapter 29.1) has been increasingly recognized as an important and potentially serious entity. The physical urticarias may be exacerbated by environmental exposures.

Clinical course

Physical urticarias have been divided into several subgroupings.[17] Dermographism usually presents as hives, which are elicited by stroking or scratching. Pressure urticaria may be seen at localized points of skin pressure. Cholinergic urticaria presents as small wheals surrounded by wide areas of erythema in response to heat and sweating. Cold urticaria develops at sites of contact with cold and may be familial. Solar urticaria develops in response to light of varying wavelengths. All of these physical forms of urticaria may be accompanied by systemic complaints such as headache, wheezing, or syncope. Rare forms of physical urticarias include heat contact urticaria, aquagenic urticaria, vibratory angioedema, and exercise anaphylaxis.[18,19]

Pathogenesis

Urticaria can represent an IgE-mediated response to a variety of stimuli. Acute urticaria usually is due to exposure to various foods or medications. A specific cause of chronic urticaria, arbitrarily defined as urticaria lasting more than 6 weeks, is rarely discovered. Many of these cases may represent patients with autoreactive anti-IgE receptor antibodies.[20] In evaluating any patient with urticaria, it is important to exclude physical urticarias as a possible cause to avoid unnecessary testing.

Diagnosis

Clinical history and appearance usually are adequate to make a diagnosis of physical urticaria. Firm stroking of the skin leads to hives in patients with dermographism. Cholinergic urticaria may be induced by physical exercise or a hot shower. The diagnosis of cold urticaria may be made by using a 3–5-minute skin exposure to ice, a

5–15-minute exposure to cold water, or a 5–10-minute exposure to cold air. Solar urticaria may be induced by phototesting the skin at the appropriate wavelengths, whereas pressure urticaria requires local application of weights.

Prevention
The various forms of physical urticaria require specific preventive measures according to the nature of the eliciting stimulus. Job reassignment may be necessary.

Treatment and prognosis
The treatment of physical urticaria primarily is preventive, although antihistamines and mast cell stabilizers also are used.[21] Accurate diagnosis in the workplace setting is critical to avoid unnecessary evaluation. The prognosis for the various forms of physical urticarias is variable, although most patients improve over a period of months to years. A recent study showed that only 16% of patients with physical urticaria were symptom free one year after diagnosis, compared with 47% of those with other forms of chronic urticaria.[22]

PHOTODERMATOSES

Photoeruptions related to occupational and environmental exposures are of several types. Excessive exposure to the sun is a risk for a number of outdoor occupations. Phototoxic reactions are an exaggerated sunburn response and occur in association with a variety of chemical exposures. Photoallergic eruptions require light and a photoallergen in order to fully develop. This last topic is discussed at greater length in Chapter 29.1. Persons at risk include farm workers, roofers, commercial fisherman, and other outdoor workers.

Clinical course
Sunburn typically presents as a first-degree burn, characterized by erythema in sun-exposed sites followed in 1–2 days by desquamation. Phototoxic dermatoses represent an exaggerated sunburn response that occurs at sites that are exposed to both the sun's rays and photoactive agents. Second-degree burns may result, characterized by intense erythema and bullae formation. The postinflammatory hyperpigmentation that results may persist for several weeks.

Pathogenesis
Sunburn is primarily due to light in the UVB spectrum. Occupational phototoxic dermatoses are principally the result of exposure to light in the UVA spectrum in combination with furocoumarins (Table 29.2.6) and tar products.[11,23] UVA is believed to be the wavelength of light primarily responsible for skin aging, although both UVA and UVB have been implicated in photocarcinogenesis.

Diagnosis
A history of sun exposure, combined with a typical photodistribution, usually is adequate to make the diagno-

Bergamot	Giant hogweed
Bitter orange	Lemon
Carrot	Lime
Celery	Masterwort
Citron	Parsnip
Cow parsley	Persian lime
Dill	Rue

Adapted from Fisher AA. Contact dermatitis, 3rd edn. Philadelphia: Lea and Febiger, 1986.

Table 29.2.6 Some common plants containing furocoumarins

sis. Exposure to photoactive substances is further evidence in support of the diagnosis. A biopsy may be helpful. It is important to exclude other causes of photosensitivity (e.g., lupus erythematosus, medications) in the evaluation of a patient with a photodermatosis.

Prevention
Sunscreens are helpful in the prevention of sunburn. It is important to use those with a sun protection factor (SPF) rating of #15 or better. These compounds are less effective in preventing damage from UVA, and therefore, physical sunblocks are more useful in these cases. Use of protective clothing when working with photoactive substances is important in the prevention of phototoxic dermatoses.

Treatment and prognosis
Treatment of photoeruptions includes open-wet dressings and bland emollients. Rarely, a course of systemic steroids is necessary for severe cases. Postinflammatory hyperpigmentation resolves over a period of several months. Workers with clinical signs of chronic sun exposure are at risk for cutaneous malignancies and should be followed closely.

ERYTHEMA AB IGNE

This condition may occur in workers exposed to furnaces, such as cooks, stokers, glass blowers, and kiln operators. In addition, long-term exposure to a heating pad, stove, or heater is a risk factor.

Clinical course
The early changes are an asymptomatic reticulated pattern of the cutaneous blood vessels (livedo reticularis), which proceeds to reticulated pigmentation. Localized poikiloderma (epidermal atrophy, telangiectasia, and pigment alteration) develops later. The area usually is regional, corresponding to the site of repeated applications of heat. Both squamous cell and Merkel cell carcinomas have been reported to occur in the poikilodermatous area.[24,25]

Pathogenesis
Radiant energy applied to the same area over time produces this change. Persistent vasodilation of the dermal-subcutaneous vasculature is the likely cause of the early changes (Fig. 29.2.6).

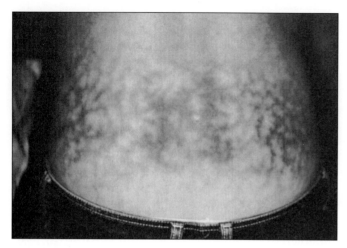

Figure 29.2.6: Erythema ab igne due to prolonged use of a heating pad for a back injury.

Diagnosis

The local nature of the condition, along with a history of exposure to heat, is suggestive. A biopsy of the affected area may be useful to exclude other conditions associated with livedo reticularis.

Prevention

Repeated exposure to intense radiant energy must be avoided. Education of workers at risk is the key to prevention.

Treatment

Cessation of exposure may bring regression of early changes. Once permanent change has occurred, the area must be monitored for future development of skin carcinoma, similar to the monitoring of skin damaged by ionizing radiation.

MILIARIA

Bakers, foundry workers, cooks, coke oven operators, and workers with similar exposure to excessive heat that causes sweating are at particular risk for developing this condition.

Clinical course

This condition results from blockage of the sweat ducts. Clinical lesions are on a spectrum encompasssing clear vesicles if the blockage is in the superficial epidermis (miliaria crystallina), macules or papules if the blockage is in the lower epidermis (miliaria rubra), or flesh-colored to pale white papules if the obstruction is in the dermis (miliaria profunda). The trunk is the most commonly affected location, especially the chest, back, submammary, and axillary areas. The palms and groin also may be involved. Symptoms usually are absent with miliaria crystallina, while miliaria rubra and miliaria profunda may be pruritic or painful.

Scaling results from the superficial vesicles, whereas deeper plugging, if extensive, may lead to inadequate body thermoregulation with accompanying heat exhaustion. If the condition progresses due to continued heat exposure, the lesions of miliaria profunda, which are indicative of loss of sweating mechanisms, may result in extreme susceptibility to systemic illness resulting from heat stress (see Chapter 34).

Pathogenesis

Sweating and maceration cause plugging of the eccrine sweat duct with ductal keratin. Microbial organisms may invade the macerated keratin and cause further plugging of the duct.

Diagnosis

Diagnosis is made by the clinical picture, symptoms, and the history of onset after excessive heat exposure and sweating. Excessive sweating also may exacerbate an underlying skin disease.

Prevention

Repeated heat exposures should be avoided in workers prone to miliaria. Hexachlorophene soap may be useful to decrease the skin's bacterial population. Maceration of the skin should be avoided by frequent clothing changes when sweating is profuse.

Treatment and prognosis

Removal of the worker from the hot working environment cures the disease, although the lesions and symptoms may persist for several days. A period of a week or more should elapse before re-exposure of the individual to the hot environment is attempted, particularly if the eruption is severe enough to cause a decrease in systemic heat tolerance. Some individuals are very susceptible to this condition and may need to avoid occupational heat stress altogether.

FROSTBITE, IMMERSION FOOT, AND CHILBLAINS

These conditions caused by local tissue exposure to cold may affect a wide range of workers (see also Chapter 34). Persons at risk for frostbite include those who work in refrigerated environments, fire fighters, sailors, pipeline maintenance workers, and military personnel in frigid northern areas. Sewer and construction workers, as well as military personnel working in extremely cold weather, are at risk for immersion foot. Chilblains affect primarily northern European workers exposed to cold, damp conditions.

Clinical course

Frostbite results from exposure to extreme cold, which initially causes blanching of exposed skin, especially on acral areas (Fig. 29.2.7). Dysesthesia accompanies this early cutaneous alteration. As exposure continues, the skin becomes frozen and appears white or waxy and becomes anesthetic. On rewarming, the extent of injury emerges over several days with an initial bluish appearance, then redness, edema, and blistering. Severe pain accompanies

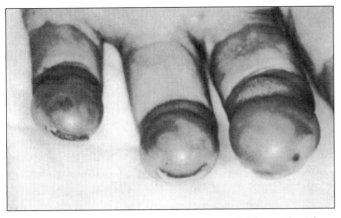

Figure 29.2.7: Frostbite of the distal fingers in a bridge worker. The yellow discoloration is due to povidone-iodine (Betadine).

the rewarming. Lines of necrosis develop, and recovery is often prolonged.

Immersion foot is cold injury in conjunction with water.[26] Continuous exposure for as few as 19 hours may cause an extremity to become pale bluish, edematous, and numb. The clinical course then progresses to erythema, further swelling, and extreme pain as the foot is warmed. This phase may last for weeks to months. Paresthesias, vasomotor instability, and joint stiffness may persist for years.

Chilblains are characterized by red to bluish plaques accompanied by burning or itching, with an occasional vesicular component that may occur within 24 hours of exposure to a cold damp climate. Pressure eliminates the color of the plaque, which may progress to swelling and ulceration. These plaques may become chronic nodules, which tend to develop bullae and ulcerate, leading to fibrosis. They may disappear in warm weather and reappear in cold weather. Children frequently are affected.

Pathogenesis

During intense cold exposure, there is channeling of blood from superficial vessels to conserve core body heat. Skin tissue can become cold enough for ice crystals to form in cells, leading to tissue death. Immersion foot results from constriction of cutaneous blood vessels by footwear and prolonged low temperatures of the skin not sufficient to cause freezing of the cells. Chilblains result from localized vascular injury due to exposure of the skin to cold and damp areas. Genetic factors that allow vasomotor instability in this type of environment are probably relevant.

Diagnosis

Characteristic signs and symptoms following extreme cold exposure are diagnostic of frostbite, although the extent of tissue injury may not be known for days to weeks.

Chilblains and immersion foot also have characteristic histories of cold exposure preceding the cutaneous findings. However, the cold exposure is less severe with these conditions, the clinical appearance is different, and a wet-work environment is essential in the diagnosis of immersion foot. A skin biopsy may be needed to differentiate chilblains from vasculitis, connective tissue disease, and cryoglobulinemia.

Treatment and prognosis

Immediate and rapid rewarming of the affected area, usually by immersion in warm water, is recommended for frostbite and immersion foot. Warm drinks and warm food raise core body temperature, increasing cutaneous blood flow. Analgesics for pain and vigorous surveillance for and treatment of infection are required.

For frostbite, the depth and extent of tissue necrosis dictate the long-term prognosis. Surgical debridement or amputation of gangrenous tissue may be required. Infection can greatly increase the damage from frostbite. Even when gangrene is absent, long-term effects may include vascular and neurologic alterations of the affected area such as episodic vasoconstriction, increased sweating, and paresthesias of the injured part.

Long-term sequelae from immersion foot are similar to those of frostbite and may persist for years.

Chilblains are treated symptomatically and do not require rapid rewarming. Vasodilating agents (e.g., calcium channel blockers) have proved effective when symptoms resist or recur.[27] Moving to a warm climate is helpful in some instances, but some cases become progressive and chronic despite the use of therapeutic measures.

Prevention

Cold injury may be prevented by using protective clothing, which prevents chilling of skin tissues. It is important that the clothing is not tight fitting, so as not to compromise cutaneous circulation. Education of workers regarding the early changes of these conditions and potential problems associated with prolonged cold exposure is essential.

VIBRATION-INDUCED WHITE FINGER DISEASE (HAND-ARM VIBRATION SYNDROME)

Workers at risk for vibration-induced white finger disease, or hand-arm vibration syndrome (HAVS), include operators of vibrating tools, piston-operated compressed air tools, and tools that are turned by electric motors or air-driven turbines. Most recently, HAVS has been reported in workers operating high pressure hoses.[28] This condition may be exacerbated by occupational activities in cold weather.

Clinical course

HAVS, characterized by blanching of the fingers when operating vibrating tools, is accompanied in its early stages by mild numbness and tingling. With continued operation, the fingers may develop loss of sensation and decreased dexterity. The blanching may be followed by cyanosis and hyperemia as in classic Raynaud's phenomenon, although it tends to be asymmetric. Vascular changes are more prominent when vibrating tools are handled in cold weather. The number of occurrences and the severity of symptoms may be exacerbated by continued work with vibrating tools. Although at first a single digit may be affected, the condition eventually may involve all the fingers on both hands, although the thumbs often are spared (see also Chapter 23.3).

Cold exposure or emotional stimuli leading to pallor of the fingers followed by bluish cyanosis and subsequently erythematous hyperemia, known as Raynaud's phenomenon, may be idiopathic or familial, but it also may be a cutaneous sign of an underlying connective tissue disease.

Pathogenesis

Skin, vascular and nerve changes are seen in skin biopsies of patients with vibration-induced white finger disease.[29] Vascular abnormalities in these patients include microangiopathic, vasospastic and thrombotic changes. HAVS has been associated with vibrating frequencies between 30 and 300 Hz. The effects of vibration are probably exacerbated by the pressure required to hold and guide a vibrating tool, which leads to vasoconstriction.

Diagnosis

A history of exposure to vibrating tools is necessary to make a diagnosis of HAVS. A thorough investigation for possible underlying connective tissue disease should be undertaken in every case.

Prevention

Insulation from vibrations, combined with tools designed to decrease the pressure needed for tool guidance, is useful. Operators of vibrating tools should be made aware of the risk of vibration injury to the hand and instructed to report the early changes. All workers with Raynaud's phenomenon, whether or not the condition is job related, should have protection of their hands from cold weather to avoid exacerbation of the disorder.

Treatment and prognosis

Treatment of Raynaud's phenomenon involves both physical and pharmacologic therapies that are beyond the scope of this text. Avoidance of vibrating tools and protection from cold are important factors. The prognosis depends on the cause and extent of vascular injury. In general, early vibration changes will stabilize or revert if the trauma is discontinued.

OCCUPATIONAL ACRO-OSTEOLYSIS AND SCLERODERMA

Cleaners of vinyl chloride polymerization reactor tanks have been reported to develop Raynaud's phenomenon in association with osteolytic bone changes.[30] This association, however, has more recently come under question.[31] Likewise, workers exposed to silica dust have been reported to be at risk for developing Raynaud's phenomenon and scleroderma, with the simultaneous use of vibrating tools apparently contributing to development of disease.[32] Exposure to organic solvents has also been associated with development of systemic sclerosis.[33]

Clinical course

Occupational acro-osteolysis is the term used to define the triad of Raynaud's phenomenon, sclerodermatous skin changes, and lytic bone lesions reported in workers exposed to vinyl chloride.[34] Progressive systemic sclerosis associated with exposure to silica is difficult to distinguish from the idiopathic form of scleroderma. Prominent cutaneous features of this disorder include sclerodactyly, Raynaud's phenomenon, and digital necrosis.

Diagnosis

Patients presenting with Raynaud's phenomenon without a history of vibration exposure should be questioned regarding exposure to vinyl chloride, silica, organic solvents, and epoxy resins. A thorough investigation for possible underlying connective tissue disease should be undertaken in every case.

Prevention

Workers cleaning polymerization reactor tanks of vinyl chloride need complete skin and respiratory protection. Respiratory protection also is critical in those workers exposed to silica. All workers with Raynaud's phenomenon, whether or not the condition is job related, should have protection of their hands from cold weather to avoid exacerbation of the disorder.

Treatment and prognosis

Acro-osteolysis tends to stabilize after withdrawal from vinyl chloride monomer exposure. Scleroderma of any cause, however, tends to be progressive.

FOREIGN BODY REACTIONS

Workers in construction, electronics, metal working, and mining are at greatest risk for foreign body reactions, but these reactions occur throughout the workplace.

Clinical course

Foreign body reactions occur when the epidermal barrier is broken by various substances. The appearance of the reaction varies depending on whether it is acute or chronic. Acute reactions resemble irritant dermatitis. Chronic reactions typically are more papulonodular. Secondary bacterial infection may complicate the clinical picture. Common examples include reactions to metal filings and wood splinters. Fiberglass may cause an acute reaction that is extremely pruritic (see Chapter 29.1). Other specific causes of foreign body reactions in the occupational setting include beryllium and silica.[35,36] An unusual occupational form of foreign body reaction is seen in the exposed skin of clam diggers as a result of exposure to avian schistosomes, so-called swimmer's itch.[37] Hairdressers may develop trichogranulomas following penetration of short hairs into the skin.[38]

Pathogenesis

A granulomatous response is the consequence of a chronic foreign body reaction. This is typically a non-allergic response, but in the case of beryllium, the granulomatous response is due to delayed hypersensitivity. Acute reactions are eczematous and represent a form of irritant contact dermatitis.

Diagnosis

Biopsy may be helpful in arriving at a diagnosis of chronic foreign body reaction. In the case of systemic berylliosis with cutaneous granulomas, the lesions may be indistinguishable from sarcoidosis. In-vitro lymphocyte transformation testing with beryllium often is helpful (see Chapter 39.3).

Prevention

Awareness of the risks of foreign body reaction and protective clothing are the two most important factors in prevention.

Treatment and prognosis

Systemic berylliosis is only rarely a cause of cutaneous granulomas. Localized granulomas of any cause may be treated surgically. Topical therapies including open wet dressings and topical steroids are useful in the treatment of acute foreign body reactions. Fiberglass may be removed by using tape stripping of the skin.

BLISTERS AND CALLUSES

Repetitive tasks often lead to marks on the skin of workers in various industries. The most common of these are blisters and calluses.

Clinical course

Calluses appear over areas of trauma, especially on the hands and bony prominences. They are distinguished from warts by preservation of the skin markings throughout the lesion. They also may be associated with lichenification and fissures. Acute trauma to the skin, whether from friction or extremes of temperature, results in blisters. On thin skin, the overlying epidermis may be lost, resulting in an erosion.

Pathogenesis

The epidermal response to chronic trauma is thickening, resulting in calluses and lichenification. In patients who are prone to various skin disorders (e.g., psoriasis) trauma can lead to the development of new skin lesions (Koebner phenomenon) (Fig. 29.2.8). Blisters are created when the epidermis separates from the dermis.

Diagnosis

Collection of a patient history is essential. The Koebner phenomenon may complicate the diagnosis.

Prevention

Because calluses and lichenification are an adaptive response to chronic trauma, prevention is not necessarily

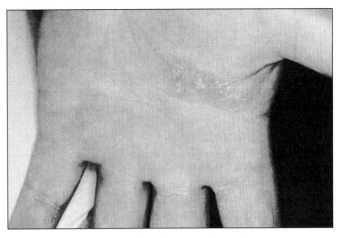

Figure 29.2.8: Psoriasis of the palm in a train conductor demonstrating the Koebner phenomenon due to friction from a ticket punch. Patch testing was negative.

desired. However, thickened lesions may fissure and become secondarily infected. Protective clothing often is useful in these cases, as is skin lubrication.

Treatment and prognosis

Calluses may be treated surgically, by paring, or chemically, by using keratolytics (e.g., salicylic acid, urea). Prevention of further trauma is necessary to allow healing. Blisters are best left intact to allow re-epithelialization, unless they are painful or secondarily infected. Erosions should be treated with an occlusive dressing because this approach enhances re-epithelialization.

BIOLOGIC CAUSES OF OCCUPATIONAL DISEASES

Occupational exposures are responsible for a wide variety of infectious skin diseases.[2] These can occur through direct skin contact, inoculation or inhalation. Up to 5% of all workers' compensation claims for skin diseases are due to infection, but data are not available to correlate the various agents with given occupations (see also Chapter 22).

It is important to recognize any potential case of infectious occupational skin disease as a sentinel health event.[39,40] Action by the physician in consultation with public health authorities could prevent disease in other workers.

Bacterial diseases

Table 29.2.7 details the most common causes of occupational skin disease due to bacteria. In general, workers at greatest risk are those who work with animals (Fig. 29.2.9) and those in the construction trades.

Bacterial infections require identification of the pathogenic organism by a variety of techniques: culture, histology, and immunologic methods. Treatment is based on the definitive identification of a causative agent, and prognosis depends on early and effective treatment. Work-related

Disease	Causative agent	Workers at risk	Clinical findings
Anthrax	*Bacillus anthracis*	Abattoir workers, dock workers, hunters, workers with animal skin or hair	Ulcerated or bullous dark raised nodule; systemic signs of infection
Furuncles	*Staphylococcus aureus*	Military personnel, athletes, butchers	Red, tender fluctuant nodule; local symptoms unless severe
Brucellosis	*Brucella abortus, B. suis, B. melitensis*	Veterinarians, meat packers, abattoir workers	Maculopapular or petechial rash or skin ulcer, severe systemic signs of infection
Erysipeloid	*Erysipelothrix insidiosa*	Fishermen, butchers, workers with poultry, rabbits or pigs	Painful, erythematous plaques; lymphangitis
Mycobacterial infections, swimming pool granuloma	*Mycobacterium marinum*	Gulf fishermen, butchers, fish tank workers	Ulcerating papules and nodules along lympathic drainage
Prosector's wart	*Mycobacterium tuberculosis*	Pathologists, morgue attendants, veterinarians, farmers	Warty nodular lesion
Tularemia	*Francisella tularensis*	Hunters, veterinarians, abattoir workers	Ulcer with deep eschar; systemic symptoms accompanied by maculopapular rash with purpura
Lyme disease	*Borrelia burgdorferi*	Outdoor workers in endemic areas	Erythema migrans
Impetigo	Group A streptococci, *S. aureus*	Construction workers, farmers	Crusted erosions

Table 29.2.7 Bacterial diseases

	Causative agent	Workers at risk	Clinical findings
Candidiasis	*C. albicans*	Bartenders, dishwashers	Chronic paronychia, intertrigo
Dermatophytes	Epidermophyton, Microsporum, and Trichophyton species	Veterinarians, agricultural workers	Tinea pedis, manum, corporis
Sporotrichosis	*Sporothrix schenckii*	Agricultural and forestry workers	Ulcerating papule with nodules following lymphatics
Mycetoma	Actinomycetes, *Pseudoallescheria boydii*	Agricultural workers	Chronic, indurated swelling with sinus tracts, usually on hands or feet
Chromomycosis	*Fonsecaea pedrosoi*	Agricultural workers	Verrucous plaques with scarring
T. versicolor	*Pityrosporum orbiculare*	Workers in hot, humid environments	Scaling hypopigmented or hyperpigmented macules in a shawl-like distribution

Table 29.2.8 Fungal diseases

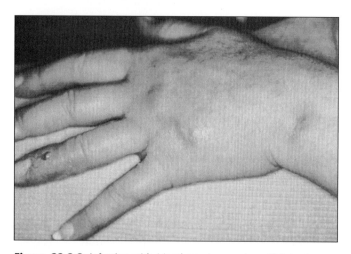

Figure 29.2.9: Infection with *Mycobacterium marinum* (fish tank granuloma), which demonstrates sporotrichoid spread in pet shop worker.

bacterial infections can be prevented by protective gear and awareness of the risks. Education of workers regarding the potential infectious agents in their work environment is an essential part of prevention.

Fungal diseases

A variety of superficial fungi are responsible for occupational disease. The most common of these are detailed in Table 29.2.8. In general, workers at greatest risk are those in the agricultural trades. Candida and dermatophyte infections are the most common superficial fungal infections seen in the occupational setting. Candida infection commonly presents as a chronic paronychia due to wet work (Fig. 29.2.10). Dermatophytosis may be acquired by exposure to species that are anthropophilic, zoophilic, or geophilic. An unusual variant of tinea pedis (one hand–two feet tinea) needs to be considered in the differential diagnosis of hand dermatitis (see Chapter 29.1). The specific diagnosis of Candida infection and dermatophytosis may be made by potassium hydroxide examination of scale and by fungal culture. Topical antifungal agents usually are adequate for treatment, although occasionally administration of oral antifungals (griseofulvin, ketoconazole, itraconazole, terbinafine) is necessary. As with other occupationally acquired infections, work-related fungal diseases may be prevented primarily through the use of protective gear and awareness of risks.

	Causative agent	Workers at risk	Clinical findings
Herpetic whitlow	Herpes simplex type 1 > type 2	Hospital workers	Vesicles on an erythematous base
Farmyard pox	Orf–sheep, goats, milker's nodules–cows (paravaccinia viruses)	Farm workers	Painless papulovesicle, evolves over 6 weeks
Butcher's warts	Human papillomavirus, type 7	Meat handlers	Verrucous papules on the hands

Table 29.2.9 Viral diseases

	Causative agent	Workers at risk	Clinical finding
Leishmaniasis	*L. tropica, L. brasiliensis*	Tropical forest workers	Mucocutaneous ulcers
Swimmer's itch	Avian schistosomes	Skin divers, dock workers	Urticarial papules on exposed skin
Larva migrans	*Ancylostoma braziliense*	Workers in subtropical and tropical beaches	Mobile, serpiginous plaque, especially on the feet

Table 29.2.10 Parasitic diseases

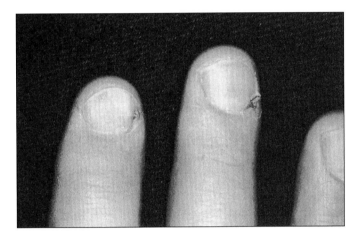

Figure 29.2.10: Chronic paronychia due to *Candida albicans* in a bartender, also known as bar rot.

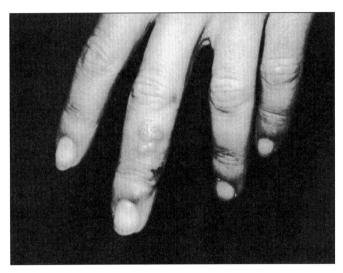

Figure 29.2.11: Herpetic whitlow due to herpes simplex virus type 1 in a healthcare worker.

Viral diseases

The most significant occupationally acquired viral infection is herpes simplex infection of the finger (herpetic whitlow), which is usually seen in healthcare workers. Farm workers and meat handlers also are at risk for occupational viral diseases, as indicated in Table 29.2.9.

Herpetic whitlow can be due to herpes simplex virus type 1 or type 2. It presents as a recurrent, often painful vesicular eruption on an erythematous base (Fig. 29.2.11). Lesions occur at the site of contact, generally on a finger. Untreated infections last for 1 to 2 weeks, though therapy with oral antivirals (acyclovir, valacyclovir, famciclovir) is helpful in shortening the course. Diagnosis is made by a Tzanck smear, showing multinucleated giant cells, or by viral culture. Prevention is through use of adequate barrier methods.

Human immunodeficiency virus (HIV) may be transmitted in the occupational setting as well. The risk of percutaneous infection has led to the increased use of gloves, which, in turn, has led to an increased incidence of reactions to gloves in healthcare workers (see Chapter 29.1).

Parasitic diseases

Parasites are unusual causes of occupational disease in temperate climates. However, workers in developing countries are at particular risk. Several of the parasitic diseases reported in the occupational setting are included in Table 29.2.10.

References

1. Bureau of Labor Statistics, US Department of Labor, 2001.
2. Lushniak BD. Occupational skin diseases. Prim Care 2000; 27:895–916.
3. Fowler JF. Occupational dermatology. Curr Prob Dermatol 1998; 10:211–46.
4. Adams BB, Chetty VB, Mutasim DF. Periorbital comedones and their relationship to pitch tar: a cross-sectional analysis and a review of the literature. J Am Acad Dermatol 2000; 42:624–7.
5. White GM. Acne therapy. Adv Dermatol 1999; 14:29–58.
6. Von Bettman S. Chlorakne ein besondere Form von professioneller Hauterkrankung. Dtsch Med Wochenschr 1901; 27:437.
7. Tindall JP. Chloracne + chloracnegens. J Am Acad Dermatol 1985; 13:539–58.

8. Coenraads PJ, Olie K, Tang NJ. Blood lipid concentrations of dioxins and dibenzofurans causing chloracne. Br J Dermatol 1999; 141:694–7.

9. Zugerman C. Chloracne: clinical manifestations and etiology. Dermatol Clin 1990; 8:209–13.

10. Mosher DB, Fitzpatrick TB, Ortonne J-P, et al. Hypomelanoses and hypermelanoses. In: Freedberg IM, Eisen AZ, Wolff K, et al, eds. Fitzpatrick's dermatology in general medicine. New York: McGraw-Hill, 1999;945–1017.

11. Seligman PJ, Mathias CG, O'Malley MA, et al. Phytophotodermatitis from celery among grocery store workers. Arch Dermatol 1987; 123:1478–82.

12. McNally WD. A depigmentation of the skin by rubber gloves. Ind Med 1939; 8:405–10.

13. Oliver EA, Schwartz L, Warren LH. Occupational leukoderma: preliminary report. JAMA 1939; 113:927–8.

14. Bolognia JL, Pawelek JM. Biology of hypopigmentation. J Am Acad Dermatol 1988; 19:217–55.

15. Iliev D, Elsner P. An unusual hypopigmentation in occupational dermatology: presentation of a case and review of the literature. Dermatology 1998; 196:248–50.

16. Orentreich N, Selmanowitz VJ. Autograft repigmentation of leukoderma. Arch Dermatol 1972; 105:734–6.

17. Mahmood T. Physical urticarias. Am Fam Phys 1994; 49:1411–4.

18. Shadick NA, Liang MH, Partridge AJ, et al. The natural history of exercise-induced anaphylaxis: survey results from a 10-year follow-up study. J Allergy Clin Immunol 1999; 104:123–7.

19. Luong KV, Nguyen LT. Aquagenic urticaria: report of a case and review of the literature. Ann Allergy Asthma Immunol 1998; 80:483–5.

20. Greaves MW, O'Donnell BF. Not all chronic urticaria is 'idiopathic'! Exp Dermatol 1998; 7:11–13.

21. Lee EE, Maibach HI. Treatment of urticaria. An evidence-based evaluation of antihistamines. Am J Clin Dermatol 2001; 2:27–32.

22. Kozel MM, Mekkes JR, Bossuyt PM, et al. Natural course of physical and chronic urticaria and angioedema in 220 patients. J Am Acad Dermatol 2001; 45:387–91.

23. McKee RH, Maibach HI. The phototoxic and allergenic potential of EDS liquids. Contact Derm 1985; 13:72–9.

24. Hewitt JB, Sherif A, Kerr KM, et al. Merkel cell and squamous cell carcinomas arising in erythema ab igne. Br J Dermatol 1993; 128:591–2.

25. Iacocca MV, Abernethy JL, Stefanato CM, et al. Mixed Merkel cell carcinoma and squamous cell carcinoma of the skin. J Am Acad Dermatol 1998; 39:882–7.

26. Chow S, Westfried M, Lynfield Y. Immersion foot: an occupational disease. Cutis 1980; 25:662.

27. Rustin MH, Newton JA, Smith NP, et al. The treatment of chilblains with nifedipine: the results of a pilot study, a double-blind placebo-controlled randomized study and a long-term open trial. Br J Dermatol 1989; 120:267–75.

28. Cooke R, House R, Lawson IJ, et al. Hand-arm vibration syndrome from exposure to high-pressure hoses. Occup Med (Lond) 2001; 51:401–9.

29. Noel B. Pathophysiology and classification of the vibration white finger. Int Arch Occup Environ Health 2000; 73:150–5.

30. Dinman BD, Cook WA, Whitehouse WM, et al. Occupational acroosteolysis. I. An epidemiological study. Arch Environ Health 1971; 22:61–73.

31. McLaughlin JK, Lipworth L. A critical review of the epidemiologic literature on health effects of occupational exposure to vinyl chloride. J Epidemiol Biostat 1999; 4:253–75.

32. Haustein UF, Anderegg U. Silica induced scleroderma – clinical and experimental aspects. J Rheumatol 1998; 25:1917–26.

33. Aryal BK, Khuder SA, Schaub EA. Meta-analysis of systemic sclerosis and exposure to solvents. Am J Ind Med 2001; 40:271–4.

34. Markowitz SS, McDonald CJ, Fethiere W, et al. Occupational acroosteolysis. Arch Dermatol 1972; 106:219–23.

35. Rossman MD. Chronic beryllium disease: diagnosis and management. Environ Health Perspect 1996; 104(Suppl 5):945–7.

36. Mowry RG, Sams WM, Jr, Caulfield JB. Cutaneous silica granuloma. A rare entity or rarely diagnosed? Report of two cases with review of the literature. Arch Dermatol 1991; 127:692–4.

37. Osment LS. Update: seabather's eruption and swimmer's itch. Cutis 1976; 18:545–7.

38. Hogan DJ. Subungual trichogranuloma in a hairdresser. Cutis 1988; 42:105–6.

39. Newman LS. Occupational illness. N Engl J Med 1995; 333:1128–34.

40. Rutstein DD, Mullan RJ, Frazier TM, et al. Sentinel Health Events (occupational): a basis for physician recognition and public health surveillance. Am J Public Health 1983; 73:1054–62.

Chapter 30
Cancer

30.1 Malignancies of the Respiratory Tract and Pleura
Mark B Russi

LUNG CANCER

Epidemiology

Lung cancer, a virtually unknown disease 100 years ago, now kills more American men and women than any other tumor. Although cigarette smoking represents the most important risk factor for lung cancer, occupational and environmental exposures, both singly and in conjunction with tobacco, are responsible for a substantial burden of preventable disease. This chapter addresses current estimates of the proportion of lung cancer attributable to occupation, provides a framework for the occupational medicine practitioner to make etiologic judgments, and discusses specific exposures associated with lung cancer.

Estimates during the 1960s and 1970s regarding the percentage of lung cancer attributable to occupation varied from 1% to greater than 60%. More recent studies suggest a narrower range of risk. Doll and Peto in the early 1980s proposed that 15% of male lung cancer cases and 5% of female lung cancer cases in the US resulted from occupational exposures.[1] The combined data from five American case–control studies spanning a wide range of industrial activities suggested that between 3% and 17% of lung cancers were due to well-recognized occupational carcinogens.[2] Another multicenter case–control study suggested that 9% of lung cancers were due to work in occupations with excess lung cancer risk.[3] A recent review has suggested that occupational exposures are responsible for 9% of lung cancer among men and 2% among women.[4] Much of the burden of lung cancer morbidity among working populations has been attributed to heavy exposures in the past.

There may be numerous complex interactions between the risk factors for lung cancer. Studies illustrating the combined effect of cigarette smoking with asbestos, arsenic, and radon exposure provide illustrative examples. When interactions exist between occupational or environmental exposure and any other risk factor, such as cigarette smoking, the percentage of lung cancer associated with the exposure reveals only what percentage of lung cancer could be eliminated through elimination of the exposure. The percentage itself does not reveal whether another exposure or several other exposures must be present to induce disease, only what percentage of disease would be eliminated if the exposure did not exist.

Assigning the proportion of lung cancer attributable to specific occupational or environmental exposures has been challenging due to the difficulty of both estimating accurate exposure levels in the workplace and extending the results of studies in highly exposed groups to the population at large. Estimates of risk may vary considerably due to wide ranges of exposure among different occupational groups to agents of importance, such as asbestos. Further, reconstructing an accurate exposure history for cohorts of workers over several decades is difficult. Once data exist for a highly exposed population, extension to the general population requires accurate exposure estimates for all occupations, as well as domestic and environmental exposure settings. An alternative method extends job category-based risk estimates for specific occupations to the total number of workers employed in such occupations based on census data. While such studies provide a simpler extrapolation method, they do not consider exposures outside the workplace, and job category-based risk estimates themselves may be subject to a number of biases. Better data regarding interacting risk factors, occupational carcinogen doses, and exposures of the population at large may lead in the future to more precise estimates of the percentage of lung cancer due to occupational or environmental exposures.

Clinical evaluation

In individuals exposed to one or more carcinogens, a determination of etiology may be difficult. Although a few occupational lung carcinogens predispose more persons to one histologic type or location than others, lung cancers caused by occupational exposures do not differ from cancer induced by other causes in a way that allows pathologic, anatomic, or clinical distinction. From a public health standpoint, recognition of the cause of an individual worker's lung cancer may serve to identify excess risk at the group level, an indication for action to reduce exposure. Although individual etiologic diagnosis does not have an impact on selection of therapy, the occupational and environmental medicine physician may be called on to decide whether or not an individual's cancer is work related, often for purposes of workers' compensation.

A legal solution to this issue, as seen in the case of specific exposures in certain countries and specific occupations in the US, has been to establish a legal presumption that the cancer was caused by workplace exposures if an agreed-upon degree of exposure in the specified settings can be proved. However, such approaches currently are limited, and include asbestos-associated cancers, and some radiation-associated lung cancers in certain settings. Most individual cases arise in industries or exposure groups not formally recognized to have presumptive exposure under the workers' compensation laws.

An alternative approach bases individualized etiologic diagnosis of occupational lung cancer on the *probability* that a given cancer is occupational. This does not imply medical certainty but only that the exposure most likely caused or contributed to the development of the cancer. In the case of lung cancer due to uranium mining, various formulas have been developed to rate factors influencing the assessment of probability, including dose (average amount of exposure multiplied by years of exposure), amount of cigarette smoking, age, latency (years since first exposure), and histologic type of lung cancer. Similar formulas have been attempted for asbestos-related cancer.

Typically, however, the clinician must use quantitative or semiquantitative reasoning without a simple or legally sanctioned formula. The first step is to determine whether or not the patient was exposed to a factor causally related to lung cancer or that he or she worked in an industry with known increased risk. A complete occupational and environmental history, including a thorough review of all potential workplace carcinogens, is a prerequisite. Although workers may have histories of lifelong employment in well-established risky industries such as shipbuilding, insulating, or smelting, more often than not, a complicated history of numerous potential work exposures must be pieced together carefully.

Assessment of dose is the next step. Most epidemiologic studies of occupational lung cancer have used surrogates for dose, such as job description, or attempted rough reconstructions based on worker interviews. Quantitative information is rarely available, and dosages are often listed as only low, medium, or high. In assessing an individual's exposure, one may access certain information by interview and review of industrial hygiene data, but historical estimates of exposure for the industry or occupation in question must often suffice. Often, dose cannot be determined because the suspect exposure is not fully characterized. Work in the vicinity of coke ovens provides an example in which the specific carcinogen is unknown but the association between occupation and lung cancer is strong. Dose in such cases must be estimated by the individual's proximity to the coke oven and length of employment.

Latency must also be taken into consideration because many cancers do not appear until 30 to 40 years after exposure has occurred. Latency is dependent on whether a substance acts early in the carcinogenic process or at a later stage. A simplified initiator and promoter model of carcinogenesis may apply to cigarette smoking and asbestos exposure, but not to some other etiologies, including radiation. Asbestos probably acts as a tumor promoter, albeit with a long latency. Arsenic may be an example of a lung carcinogen that acts late in the transformation process.

Finally, a thorough smoking history – including passive smoke exposure – must be gathered from any patient with lung cancer. The individual's smoking history deserves special attention in cases in which the relative risk associated with the occupational or environmental exposure of interest is small. Domestic radon exposure should also be considered, though most individuals with radon-induced lung cancer will have been exposed to relatively average dose levels.

Substance	Major exposure settings
Asbestos	Insulation workers, shipyard workers
Arsenic	Smelting of copper, zinc, lead; arsenical pesticide processing
Chloromethyl ethers	Chemical production workers
Chromium	Chromate production, pigment manufacture, electroplating
Crystalline silica	Mining, sandblasting, stonework, foundry work
Mustard gas	Mustard gas production workers
Nickel	Nickel mining, refining, plating
Polyaromatic hydrocarbons	Coke oven workers, rubber workers, aluminum reduction workers, roofers
Radon	Uranium mining, hard rock mining, widespread domestic exposure
Environmental tobacco smoke	Environments with active smokers

Table 30.1.1 Known lung carcinogens

Substance	Exposure settings
Beryllium	Beryllium production/processing
Cadmium	Smelting, battery production
Man-made vitreous fibers (MMVF)	Insulating, rock slag, wool production
Ambient air pollution	Indoor and outdoor environments

Table 30.1.2 Probable lung carcinogens

In the end, rational judgment as to the work-relatedness of a case of lung cancer demands careful consideration of a patient's exposure history and a working knowledge of the epidemiology of occupational or environmental carcinogens. The following section addresses known and probable agents, summarized in Tables 30.1.1 and 30.1.2, respectively.

KNOWN LUNG CARCINOGENS
Asbestos (see Chapter 46)

The earliest recognition of asbestos as a possible lung carcinogen occurred in a case report by Kenneth Lynch and Atmar Smith in 1935.[5] Subsequent work by Merewether in 1949[6] and Gloyne in 1951[7] revealed an increased frequency of lung cancer at necropsy in patients with asbestosis when compared with patients with silicosis. A proven or highly probable causal relationship between asbestos and lung cancer was agreed upon in 1953 at the International Symposium on the Epidemiology of Lung Cancer (Council of the International Organizations of Medical Sciences). In 1955, a careful study by Sir Richard Doll based on necropsy data from 105 asbestos textile workers revealed a 10-fold increased rate of lung cancer in workers employed over 20 years in the trade, firmly establishing asbestos as a major lung carcinogen.[8] Further support was lent by Selikoff's study of 632 insulation workers in 1964, which revealed a sevenfold increase in the rate of lung and pleural tumors over that of the general population.[9] Numerous studies have since confirmed the carcinogenic potential of asbestos.[10–14]

As epidemiologic and basic scientific research of asbestos exposure has progressed, a number of secondary issues have arisen.[15] The interaction between cigarette smoking and asbestos exposure in producing lung cancer remains to be precisely quantified. The question of whether lung cancer arises from asbestos exposure itself or merely from lung fibrosis induced by asbestos is also a topic of some debate. Markedly different dose–response relationships in different trades and industries are still unexplained, and controversy exists regarding the carcinogenic potential of various asbestos fiber types. Finally, the concept of a threshold effect and its implications for the risk of very low-level asbestos exposure remain unresolved.

Although various models have been proposed for the interaction of cigarette smoking and asbestos exposure, the bulk of epidemiologic evidence implicates asbestos as a carcinogen by itself, whose effect is augmented by cigarette smoking. A synergistic relationship between the two carcinogens is commonly accepted, and a recent review of 23 studies addressing smoking and asbestos exposure lends support to a multiplicative interaction.[16] Asbestos exposure appears to multiply lung cancer risk by a similar factor in smokers and non-smokers. Because smoking impedes clearance of inhaled fibers, smokers may suffer increased penetration of fibers into airway walls.[17,18] Carcinogenic polycyclic aromatic hydrocarbons (PAHs) in cigarette smoke may also adsorb onto asbestos fibers, enhancing their transport into cells.[19]

The question of whether asbestos itself or asbestosis is the true risk factor for lung cancer has implications for present surveillance practices as well as compensation issues. If the development of asbestosis is not a necessary intervening step in carcinogenesis, the current practice of close radiologic monitoring of asbestotics also may be appropriate for significantly exposed persons without asbestosis. Clearly, most lung cancers arising in persons with significant asbestos exposure occur in the setting of radiologically documentable asbestosis, and cohort studies of asbestotics have revealed some of the highest rates of lung cancer mortality.[20–22] Correlations between asbestosis and lung cancer also have been shown to be stronger than those between cumulative asbestos exposure and lung cancer.[23] The finding in some studies that asbestos-related cancers frequent the lower lobes where fibrosis is maximal, as well as the occurrence in some series of a disproportionate number of adenocarcinomas, a cancer that may arise in areas of scar formation, is cited as evidence that fibrosis is a prerequisite for asbestos-related lung cancer. On the other hand, lung cancers do appear in heavily exposed individuals without clinical, radiologic, or pathologic evidence of asbestosis;[24–26] many studies reveal no predominance of adenocarcinoma among asbestos-related lung cancer cases; some studies reveal no lower lobe predominance of asbestos-related tumors;[27,28] and in-vitro experimental models have demonstrated a tumor-promoting effect of asbestos.[15] Because a clear understanding of the pathophysiologic mechanisms underlying both asbestosis and cancer remains elusive at present, resolution of these issues likely will come only with continued study of host-related and exogenous mechanisms of disease, as well as epidemiologic investigation of heavily exposed subgroups without evidence of asbestosis.

Cohort mortality studies conducted to date have revealed that the dose response for asbestos and lung cancer may be 50-fold higher in occupations involving insulation products and chrysotile textiles than it is in the lower-risk occupations of chrysotile mining and friction products work. Although in some cases the discrepancy has been attributed to inadequate historical dose estimates, many claim that examining the fiber types and sizes most commonly used in these industries may yield a more complete explanation of the phenomenon. Asbestos minerals are divided into two classes: (1) the amphiboles, including amosite, crocidolite, anthophylite, actinolite, and tremolite; and (2) the serpentine class, of which the only member is chrysotile. Ninety percent of all asbestos used in the US is chrysotile. Although some of the lowest rates of lung cancer have been reported in miners, cement manufacturers, and friction products workers, whose sole exposures are to chrysotile, some of the highest rates have been found in the asbestos textile industry, where chrysotile is used exclusively. And although autopsy studies have revealed low levels of chrysotile asbestos in heavily exposed persons, suggesting greater clearance of chrysotile from the lung relative to other fibers and possibly reduced overall toxicity, animal studies of asbestos-related lung cancer reveal chrysotile to be a potent carcinogen.[29]

One explanation for the paradoxically high rates of lung cancer in chrysotile asbestos textile workers is that low-level contamination of the textile with other forms of asbestos such as tremolite is responsible. Although tremolite fibers are seen at autopsy in the lungs of chrysotile workers, this explanation would imply an inordinately high toxicity of tremolite given the relatively low exposure doses. Studies of populations exposed solely to chrysotile also reveal elevated lung cancer risk.[30] Another proposed resolution to the controversy derives from fiber length measurements. It may be that carcinogenicity is more directly a function of exposure to very long asbestos fibers (exceeding 10 to 20 μm) than merely to all fibers greater than 5 μm.[31] Because chrysotile textile contains higher proportions of very long fibers than does the chrysotile to which miners and other lower-risk groups are exposed, lung cancer rates may be elevated on that basis alone. As more detailed environmental exposure data, including mineralogic analysis and fiber length distributions, are combined with careful reconstructions of historical exposure settings, much of the present paradox may clarify itself.[15]

A final issue that has arisen out of asbestos research is the degree to which very low-level exposures pose risk to the general population. The manner in which this issue is resolved carries important implications for the allocation of public health and economic resources for asbestos abatement in public buildings. In favor of a threshold level, below which cancer risk is not elevated above that of the general population, stand the majority of cohort mortality studies, animal studies of low-dose laboratory exposures, negative autopsy-derived asbestos fiber counts in lung cancers drawn from the general population, and the lack of elevated cancer rates among a well-studied population of non-miner residents of Quebec asbestos mining regions with higher than normal background asbestos exposure.[32,33]

Arguments against the existence of a safe level of asbestos exposure include the linearity of dose response to asbestos at higher levels in both cohort mortality studies and animal inhalation studies, as well as the results of two cohort mortality studies in which exposure to low levels for brief periods has been associated with increased lung cancer risk.[15] Some have suggested that the assumption of linear dose response with no threshold is conservative and appropriate for public and individual health practice. Nonetheless, given the quality of present data, decisions to allocate resources to asbestos abatement in public buildings with negligible potential for exposure should be made with serious consideration of the relative reduction in risk compared with that obtainable through alleviation of other, possibly more pressing, public health hazards. Removal of asbestos already in place also raises the possibility of increased rather than decreased total exposure under conditions of substandard abatement practices.

Arsenic (see Chapter 39.2)

The first cases of arsenic-induced lung cancer were reported by Saupe in 1930.[34] Subsequent studies have revealed lung cancer risk elevations associated with arsenic exposure in the settings of copper smelting,[35–38] tin mining,[39] and the manufacture of arsenical pesticides.[40] A recent study reported elevation of lung cancer risk among lead smelter workers also exposed to arsenic.[41]

Arsenic is considered a late-stage promoter of cancer and may act by interfering with DNA repair and by modulating cell growth signaling pathways.[42] Arsenic-induced lung cancer was found to have a predilection for the upper lobes in one study. Another study of copper smelter workers suggested a higher percentage of adenocarcinomas when compared with controls. A clear dose–response relationship has emerged from studies of arsenic-exposed workers, and the risk of lung cancer may be increased by as much as ninefold in heavily exposed workers. There appears to be synergism between arsenic exposure and smoking in the induction of lung cancer.[43]

Chloromethyl ethers

Bis-chloromethyl ether (BCME) and chloromethyl methyl ether (CMME) were first suspected as lung carcinogens in 1962, when cases of small-cell carcinoma of the lung were noted in a chemical manufacturing plant in Philadelphia. Subsequent institution of a screening program documented additional cases, and in 1973, a report associating lung cancer with CMME was published by Figueroa and colleagues.[44]

The chloromethyl ethers are associated primarily with the ion exchange resin industry. They also may form when chloride reacts with formaldehyde under appropriate conditions in textile manufacturing plants. BCME is the more potent of the two carcinogens, and both are highly reactive as alkylating agents in vivo. They are associated primarily with the induction of small-cell lung carcinoma.

Numerous studies have documented the association of chloromethyl ethers with lung cancer, including an industry-wide cohort study sponsored by the National Institute for Occupational Safety and Health (NIOSH).[45] The relative risk of lung cancer may be quite elevated, and long-term exposure does not appear to be an absolute prerequisite for disease. Standardized mortality ratios (SMR) from 2.8 to 5.0 have been reported in exposed populations, with relative risks as high as 7.0 to 18.0 within the highest exposure categories.[46] Risk appears to peak at less than 20 years following exposure, and several authors have documented a decline in risk following cessation of exposure.

Chromium (see Chapter 39.5)

In 1935, two cases of lung cancer that had occurred more than 20 years previously were reported in a German chromium manufacturing facility. A subsequent report by Machle in 1948 detailed respiratory cancers occurring in the chromate-producing industry in the US.[47] Chromium has since proved to be a human carcinogen, with increased incidences of lung cancer in the chrome plating, chrome alloy, chromate pigment, chromate production, and ferrochromium industries. Highest risks of lung cancer are in the chromate production industry, and may persist at 20 years following cessation of exposure.[48] Risks in the pigment industry are lower and generally associated only with zinc chromate exposure. Although chromium exposure in electroplating facilities is a risk factor for lung cancer,[49,50] exposures to other lung carcinogens such as nickel may confound this relationship. Risk is not as well established in the ferrochromium industry, in which study results are conflicting, and concomitant exposures to PAHs and asbestos may play a more important role. Similarly, elevated rates of lung cancer among chromium-exposed welders in some studies may be confounded by nickel and asbestos exposures.[51–54] Conflicting results exist regarding the role of chromium as a carcinogen in the leather tanning industry. Several studies suggest that industries with improved controls over chromium exposures are not associated with elevated lung cancer risks, though statistical power to detect marginal risk elevations has been limited by cohort sizes.[55–59]

Chromium exposure appears to be a risk factor for all lung cancer cell types, and hexavalent chromium is listed by the International Agency for Research on Cancer (IARC) as a known human carcinogen.[60] The evidence implicating trivalent chromium as a human carcinogen is less compelling. While some studies suggest elevated risk among trivalent chromium-exposed workers,[61] concomitant exposures to hexavalent chromium have made dose reconstructions challenging. A recent study combined historical air sampling data with analysis of settled dust samples to estimate trivalent and hexavalent exposures. Cumulative hexavalent exposure was associated with an increased lung cancer risk, while cumulative trivalent exposure was not.[62]

Crystalline silica (see Chapter 46)

Crystalline silica exposures occur in mining, sandblasting, construction, and foundry work. In 1996, the IARC upgraded its classification of crystalline silica from a probable human carcinogen (Group 2A) to a definite human carcinogen (Group 1).[63] The strongest evidence implicating crystalline silica as a human lung carcinogen derives from studies of individuals with silicosis. Steenland and Stayner have reported a lung cancer summary relative risk from 19 cohort and case–control studies of silicotics as 2.3 (95% confidence interval [CI], 2.2–2.6).[64] Both smoking and non-smoking silicotics have been shown to have elevated lung cancer risks. The same authors reported a lung cancer summary relative risk based on 16 large studies of silica-exposed workers as 1.3 (95% CI, 1.2–1.4).[64]

More recent studies have largely corroborated the combined relative risks reported by Steenland and Stayner. A recent mortality study of silicotic patients in Sardinia revealed a SMR for lung cancer of 1.37 (95% CI, 0.98–1.91), though the correlation with severity of silicosis based on the International Labour Organization (ILO) category of the chest radiograph was weak.[65] A study of 4626 industrial sand workers found a lung cancer SMR of 1.60 (95% CI, 1.31–1.93) and revealed a significant dose response based on average exposure.[66] An important recent study pooled 10 cohorts comprising 65,980 workers and 1072 lung cancer deaths and produced quantitative exposure estimates comparable across the cohorts. The study revealed that the log of cumulative silica exposure, with a 15-year lag, was a strong predictor of lung cancer ($P = 0.0001$).[67]

Mustard gas

The first association between mustard gas (bis [β-chloroethyl] sulfide) exposure during World War I and lung cancer was made by Case and Lea in 1955.[68] Subsequent studies of Japanese workers involved in the production of mustard gas during World War II revealed substantial lung cancer risk elevations.[69] British production workers during World War II exhibited much less pronounced elevations of risk.[70] Latency has been estimated at 20 years, and there appears to be a higher rate of squamous cell carcinomas among those exposed.

Nickel (see Chapter 39.6)

The first mention in the literature of respiratory cancers associated with nickel was a report of nasal cancer cases in a nickel refinery in 1933 by Bridge.[71] Subsequent studies of workers in nickel mining, nickel refining, and nickel subsulfide roasting facilities have revealed high rates of lung cancer and nasal cancers. Nickel carbonyl, nickel subsulfide, nickel oxides, nickel acetate, nickel hydroxide, nickel fluoride, soluble nickel dusts, and nickel itself are animal carcinogens, but the specific forms of nickel carcinogenic to man remain the subject of ongoing investigation. Results of a collaborative investigation of nine cohorts of nickel workers and one case–control study attribute most respiratory cancers to oxidic and sulfitic nickel.[72] Soluble forms of nickel appear to induce cancers at lower doses than do less soluble forms. Nickel-associated lung cancers have been noted more frequently in the large airways.

Exposure to metallic nickel has not been associated with increased lung cancer risk in humans.[73] Studies of workers exposed to nickel alloys and pure nickel dust have not revealed an elevated rate of lung cancer, and elevated rates of lung cancer among nickel-exposed welders may be attributable to chromium or asbestos exposures.[52–54] Similarly, confounding by chromium may be responsible for elevations of lung cancer risk among nickel/chromium plating workers.[49]

Polycyclic aromatic hydrocarbons (see Chapter 44)

The link between human cancer and the PAHs was first forged by Sir Percivall Pott when he reported the development of scrotal cancer among English chimney sweeps in 1775.[74] In the early part of the 20th century, many investigators suggested that increasing rates of lung cancer in the general population might be due to the use of tar and tar products. The first formal study of PAHs and lung cancer was carried out at a coal carbonization facility in Japan in 1936. Of the malignant neoplasms occurring in men at this facility, 80% (12 of 15 cases) were lung cancer – this at a time when lung cancer accounted for only 3% of all cancers in Japan.

PAHs occur as large mixes of substances formed through the incomplete combustion of coal tar, pitch, coke, and oil. Each compound is made up of at least three aromatic rings and contains only carbon and hydrogen. Occupational exposure to the PAHs of coal tar occurs in coal gasification facilities, gas and coke works, iron and steel foundries, aluminum reduction plants, tar distillation facilities, shale oil extraction operations, wood impregnation facilities, and in the roofing and transportation industries. Other sources of PAHs include carbon black (a pyrolysis product of petroleum or natural gas), petroleum distillates, soot, and diesel exhaust.

Increased risk of lung cancer has been found in coke oven workers,[75,76] tar distillation workers,[77] roofers,[78] chimney sweeps,[79] truckers,[80,81] and persons employed in coal gasification facilities[82] and aluminum reduction plants.[83–85] Coke oven workers have been well studied, and a dose response based on proximity to the coke oven is firmly established. Risk among tar distillation workers is less well documented, and not all studies have revealed correlations between exposure and disease. Elevations of lung cancer risk among roofers and asphalt workers are likely due to coal tar and bitumen fume exposure. A long-term cohort study among Swedish chimney sweeps reported a doubling of lung cancer risk, and several smaller studies have revealed similar findings. Excess lung cancer risk has been reported among truckers and attributed to diesel exhaust, which contains variable amounts of PAHs. Estimation of dose in many such studies has been challenging, and dose responses have not been consistent.[86,87] Coal gasification has been long associated with increased risk of lung cancer. Among aluminum reduction workers, those exposed to Soederberg electrolysis typically experience both higher PAH exposure and greater risk of lung cancer than those employed in plants using the prebake process. Although many studies of aluminum reduction workers have revealed no excesses of lung cancer nor clear dose–response relationships,[88,89] a nested case–control study of workers from two Soederberg plants showed a dose–response relationship based on years of exposure as well as measured benzene soluble fraction and benzo[a]pyrene.[85] Exposure to PAHs appears to elevate the risk for all cell types of lung cancer.

Exposure to PAHs is also widespread in the environment, deriving from tobacco smoke, fire fumes, ambient air pollution, and cooked food. Several studies have demonstrated increased lung cancer mortality associated with urban air pollution, but it is uncertain to what degree such excesses can be attributed to PAH contamination. There is evidence implicating environmental PAH as a lung cancer risk factor from studies in China of women heavily exposed to cooking and/or heating fumes.[90–92]

Radon (see Chapter 33.1)

In 1597, Georgius Agricola wrote of a characteristic wasting disease observed in central European miners.[93] Nearly 300 years later, Harting and Hesse identified 'mountain illness' as lung cancer and associated it with underground mining.[94] Ongoing studies in the early 20th century supported the link between radon and lung cancer at the mines of Schneeberg in Germany and Joachimsthal in Czechoslovakia. By the late 1950s, a study of uranium miners on the Colorado plateau demonstrated elevated rates of lung cancer in heavily exposed workers, and numerous subsequent studies have confirmed that risk in other mining populations. With the discovery of high radon levels in homes built on the Reading Prong geologic formation in Pennsylvania in the 1980s, considerable attention turned to the hazard of low-level radon exposure in the general population.

Radon 222 is an inert gas released in the radioactive decay of uranium 238. It has a half-life of 3.8 days and decays with alpha-particle emission through the short-lived radon daughters of polonium 218, lead 214, bismuth 214, and polonium 214 to lead 210. Polonium 218 and polonium 214 are themselves alpha-particle emitters. The radioactive particles may attach to aerosols or inhaled particles, gain access to cells lining the airways, and irradiate those cells at close range, causing chromosomal damage. Radon is an established carcinogen only in the respiratory tract.

Units of radiation most commonly used for occupational and domestic exposures are the working level (WL), the working level month (WLM), and the concentrations of picocuries per liter (pCi/L) or becquerels per cubic meter (Bq/m^3). One WL is any combination of radon progeny in 1 liter of air that ultimately releases 130,000 MeV of alpha energy during decay. Exposure to 1 WL for 170 hours equals 1 WLM. A radon concentration in the domestic setting of 1 pCi/L (2.2 radioactive decays per minute per liter of air) is approximately equal to 0.005 WL. One pCi/L is approximately equal to 37.5 Bq/m^3. A typical domestic indoor radon exposure of 0.8 pCi/L is roughly equivalent to 0.2 WLM/year, which translates into an approximately 15 WLM exposure over a lifetime. The present occupational standard for exposure in mines is 4 WLM per year.

A high lung cancer mortality rate has been recognized among underground miners. Most studies have focused on uranium and iron miners, but elevated rates of lung cancer in miners of tin, zinc and lead, magnetite, fluorspar, metal ores, and niobium have been revealed as well. A pooled analysis of data from 11 mining cohorts determined that 40% of lung cancer among miners was due to radon.[95] The study, which comprised over 65,000 men and more than 2700 lung cancer deaths, found that the association between estimated radon exposure and risk of lung cancer remained linear throughout the dose range examined. Overall excess relative risk was 0.0049 per WLM. Risk tended to decline with increasing age and time since last exposure. Consistent with other studies,[96] it increased with duration of exposure, suggesting that for a given cumulative dose, longer duration exposures to lower radon levels are more harmful than short-term exposures to higher levels.

The interaction of smoking with radon exposure has been addressed in a number of studies. Analyses of non-smoking miners as well as a case–control study in Navajo men in whom smoking rates were very low have confirmed radon's status as an independent carcinogen.[97,98] The interaction of smoking and radon exposure contributes to the difficulty of assigning radon-related relative risks for the various tumor histologies. Early reports suggested relatively high rates of small-cell carcinoma, but more recent studies reveal a distribution of cell types that does not differ from that of the general population. In the combined analysis of 11 mining cohorts, it was estimated that radon accounted for 70% of lung cancer among non-smoking miners and 39% among miners who smoked. An extrapolation based on these data suggested that 30% of lung cancer deaths among non-smokers in the general population may be due to radon, while radon may account for as much as 11% of lung cancer deaths among smokers.[95]

With the investigation of indoor air quality in the 1970s, it became apparent that radon was invariably present in homes and other indoor spaces. Little attention was directed at the problem, however, until the mid 1980s, when a home located on the Reading Prong in Pennsylvania was found to have extremely high radon levels. Subsequent investigation of other dwellings located on the same geologic formation revealed radon concentrations in excess of 110 pCi/L. The lifetime dose for an individual living in such a dwelling would exceed 1500 WLM and would lie well within the dose range of heavily exposed miners. Subsequent surveys have revealed other areas with unusually high radon levels, including a region in the Tyrolean Alps, where indoor radon levels exceeding 6000 pCi/L have been measured.[99]

Surveys suggest that average domestic exposures in the US range from 0.8 to1.5 pCi/L. Primary sources of domestic radon are rock, soil, building material, and drinking water. Domestic radon levels are determined by the ease with which air can pass from soil or rock into the dwelling and the adequacy of ventilation; older dwellings are somewhat more prone to elevated levels. Most domestic radon measurements are made under conditions intended to maximize instrument readings – namely, basement sampling with windows closed. Such levels may differ by as much as fivefold from the average radon exposure in lived-in areas over the course of a year. Estimates that one in three homes have unacceptably high radon levels (greater than 4 pCi/L) are based largely on basement sampling and may not accurately reflect actual domestic exposures.

Three principal study types have been used to evaluate the lung cancer risk of domestic radon exposure: ecologic surveys, case–control studies utilizing geologic and construction characteristics to estimate dose, and case–control studies utilizing measured radon levels. Ecologic surveys carried out in the US, Canada, Europe, and China have related estimates of prevailing radon exposure to lung cancer trends within specific geographic areas. Some such studies have shown higher rates of lung cancer in regions with greater average radon exposures, while others have not. Case–control studies, in which domestic radon levels have been estimated based on the geologic and construction characteristics of houses and neighborhoods, have been carried out in Sweden, the US, and Canada. Study results are mixed and suffer from small numbers of cases and controls. Surrogate exposure indices also do not consistently parallel measured levels of radon exposure. One study revealed that only 5% of the variance among domestic radon levels could be accounted for by geologic variables, and that geologic and housing-related variables combined accounted for only 15%–18% of the variance.[100]

The most reliable data regarding an association between domestic radon exposure and lung cancer come from a series of case–control studies in which actual radon measurements have been made in dwellings inhabited by subjects. More than 20 such studies have been undertaken. A meta-analysis of eight studies, each of which examined at least 200 lung cancer cases, has revealed a statistically significant summary odds ratio of 1.14 (95% CI, 1.0–1.3) associated with exposures of 4 pCi/L.[101] The meta-analysis, which included more than 4200 lung cancer cases and over 6600 controls, concluded that actual risk in the general population from radon exposure is not likely to be higher than mining study-derived estimates. Several studies published subsequent to the meta-analysis have produced corroborating results.[102–104] Domestic radon studies of non-smokers have revealed similar risk elevations.[105,106]

Based on the accumulated evidence, it is reasonable to estimate that 15,000 lung cancer deaths per year in the US population are attributable to radon exposure. Because most individuals are exposed to low levels of radon, it has been estimated that mitigation of all dwellings to below 4 pCi/L would result only in a 2%–4% drop in lung cancer mortality.[95] Due to the mobility of the US population, only a small percentage of radon-related lung cancers will occur in individuals currently living in dwellings with radon levels above 4 pCi/L. Still, radon levels in certain dwellings yield cumulative lifetime exposures comparable to those of miners. Although the use of radon mitigation systems in

such dwellings is clearly desirable, disagreement exists both as to how such high-risk dwellings should be identified, and whether or not radon mitigation should be instituted in dwellings with levels only marginally above the Environmental Protection Agency (EPA) action level of 4 pCi/L. Unfortunately, there is little that can be done to reduce background low-level lung cancer risk within the large segment of the population with low or average lifetime radon exposure.

Environmental tobacco smoke

Environmental tobacco smoke (ETS) contains over 5000 chemicals, of which 43 are listed as known human or animal carcinogens by the IARC.[107,108] ETS consists of side-stream smoke from the burning tip of a cigarette, as well as mainstream smoke inhaled and exhaled by the smoker. Most vapor phase contaminants and more than half of the air-borne particulates derive from the sidestream component.[109]

A meta-analysis carried out by the US EPA examined more than 30 studies, generating country-specific summary relative risks. Most studies enrolled female non-smokers, with exposure tagged to the spouse's smoking habits. The summary relative risk for the US based on eight studies was 1.22 (90% CI, 1.04–1.42). To date there have been more than 75 epidemiologic studies which have examined ETS and lung cancer, and 20 meta-analyses.[110] One meta-analysis of 37 published studies involving more than 4600 cases of lung cancer reported a 26% (95% CI, 7%–47%) adjusted excess lung cancer risk among non-smokers who lived with a smoker.[111] Dose response based on both number of cigarettes smoked by the spouse and duration of exposure was statistically significant. A more recent meta-analysis examining 35 case–control studies and five cohort studies generated a pooled relative risk associated with exposure to husbands' smoking of 1.19 (95% CI, 1.10–1.29) for case–control studies and 1.29 (95% CI, 1.04–1.62) for cohort studies.

Because workplace exposure to ETS continues to be prevalent in many industries, ETS is also an important occupational risk factor for lung cancer. Based on the pooled results of five ETS studies, it has been estimated that non-smoking women exposed to smoking in the workplace have a 25% increased risk (95% CI, 8%–41%) over their baseline lung cancer risk.[112] Studies which have directly assessed workplace exposures to ETS generate risk estimates similar to those from studies of domestic exposures to spousal smoking.[113] Compared with mean nicotine concentrations from 1 to 3 $\mu g/m^3$ in the homes of smokers, mean concentrations in workplaces which permit smoking range from 2 to 6 $\mu g/m^3$ in offices, from 3 to 8 $\mu g/m^3$ in restaurants, from 1 to 6 $\mu g/m^3$ in the workplaces of blue-collar workers, and from 10 to 40 $\mu g/m^3$ in bars.[114] According to the NHANES III study, nearly 40% of US workers report being exposed to ETS in the workplace.[115]

Accumulated epidemiologic evidence strongly implicates ETS as a significant lung cancer risk factor. The US

EPA has estimated that ETS accounts for approximately 3000 lung cancer deaths per year in non-smokers.[109]

PROBABLE LUNG CARCINOGENS

Exposures considered as probable lung carcinogens are summarized in Table 30.1.2.

Beryllium (see Chapter 39.3)

The primary occupational groups exposed to beryllium are miners, beryllium production workers, workers in the production and fabrication of beryllium alloys, and workers in the electronics industries. Data supporting the association between beryllium exposure and lung cancer are derived from cohorts of workers at beryllium production facilities in Ohio and Pennsylvania and from the US Beryllium Case Registry, a database which has tracked clinical outcomes among individuals with acute and chronic beryllium disease. Follow-up of men and women enrolled in the Beryllium Case Registry has revealed a doubling of lung cancer risk based on 28 observed lung cancer deaths,[116] while a cohort study of over 9000 workers employed in seven beryllium processing facilities reported an SMR of 1.26 (95% CI, 1.12–1.42).[117] Significantly elevated SMRs were found at two of the seven plants, and the highest rates of lung cancer were seen among employees with a history of acute beryllium disease at a Lorain, Ohio, facility. A recent nested case–control study from one of seven production facilities found that lung cancer cases had shorter work tenures and lower lifetime cumulative beryllium exposures than controls, but higher average and maximum exposures.[118]

Some controversy surrounds the association between beryllium exposure and human lung cancer.[119–121] Cancer excesses were primarily associated with work during early production years, when exposures were greatest, and questions persist regarding why certain processing facilities had greater excesses than others. Concern has been raised regarding a possible contribution to lung cancer mortality from acid mists at certain facilities and from residual confounding due to cigarette smoking. The IARC has concluded that there is sufficient evidence that beryllium is carcinogenic to humans.[122]

Cadmium (see Chapter 39.4)

Primary occupational exposures to cadmium occur in the smelting and refining of copper, zinc, and lead, as well as in electroplating, welding, and the manufacture of batteries, plastics, and paints. Human epidemiologic study results have been mixed regarding the potential of cadmium exposure to cause lung cancer in humans. Elevated risk has been observed among US cadmium-exposed production workers,[123,124] and a study of cadmium recovery workers found elevated lung cancer risk among those exposed to both cadmium and arsenic.[125] However, the same study did not show elevated lung cancer risk among workers exposed solely to cadmium, and a study of copper cadmium alloy workers did not reveal a positive correlation between cadmium exposure and lung cancer risk.[126] Swedish nickel-cadmium battery workers were shown to have an elevated lung cancer risk, with an SMR of 176 (95% CI, 101–287), but there was no apparent dose response between cadmium or nickel and lung cancer risk.[127] The IARC concluded in 1993 that there was sufficient evidence that cadmium is carcinogenic to humans.[122]

Man-made vitreous fibers (MMVF) (see Chapter 46)

MMVF include rock wool, slag wool, glass fibers, and ceramic fibers. These materials are used primarily for insulation and have received particular scrutiny because the occupational groups exposed to them are those that have borne the legacy of past widespread asbestos use. There are two large study populations of MMVF-exposed workers: an American cohort of over 16,000 male workers at 17 US production plants[128] and a European cohort of over 22,000 workers in 14 plants.[129] Only one cohort study has examined workers exposed to refractory ceramic fibers (RCF).[64,130]

In the large American cohort, the overall lung cancer SMR was 1.13 (95% CI, 1.03–1.23). Glass wool workers had an SMR of 1.12 (95% CI, 1.00–1.24), while rock/slag wool workers had an SMR of 1.36 (95% CI, 1.06–1.71).[128] In the large European cohort, overall SMR for workers with 1 year or more of employment was 1.05 (95% CI, 1.02–1.09). Glass wool workers had an SMR of 1.27 (95% CI, 1.07–1.50), while rock/slag wool workers had an SMR of 1.34 (95% CI, 1.08–1.63).[129] A recent study of over 32,000 workers employed for 1 year or more at any of 10 US fiberglass manufacturing facilities found a 6% excess mortality from respiratory cancer ($P = 0.05$). There was a statistically non-significant 3% excess mortality among longer-term (>5 years) workers. Duration of exposure and cumulative exposure did not appear to be associated with increased risk of respiratory cancer.[131] Several nested case–control studies examining glass wool and rock/slag wool exposures have allowed more detailed exposure and dose–response assessments, and have shown mixed results.[132–134]

RCF, potent carcinogens in animal models, have not been shown to be carcinogenic in human studies.[130] However, the limited size of the exposed cohort and its relatively young age do not allow one to conclude that such fibers are without risk. A recent risk analysis has concluded that deaths in the RCF cohort are significantly below that which would be expected if RCF had the potency of either crocidolite or amosite. Mortality was also reported to be lower than would be expected if RCF had the potency of chrysotile, but the difference was not statistically significant.[135]

The current human epidemiologic evidence regarding lung cancer risk is strongest for rock wool and slag wool. Results regarding glass wool are mixed. Though recent follow-up data on exposed workers suggest a small risk, dose–response relationships have not been consistent. It is not possible to draw positive or negative conclusions from the limited epidemiologic study of RCF. The IARC considers MMVF to be possible human carcinogens (Group 2B).[136]

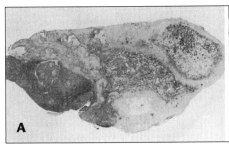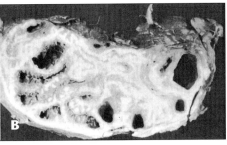

Figure 30.1.1: Gross anatomy of malignant mesothelioma. A: Right lung encased with malignant pleural tumor. B: Peritoneal tumor.

Ambient air pollution (see Chapter 51)

Considerable evidence has accumulated to suggest that exposure to ambient air pollution may increase lung cancer risk. Studies addressing the issue are extremely challenging due to a number of issues: pollution levels are difficult to characterize over the long periods of time which must be considered when evaluating lung cancer incidence; factors which affect exposure levels to the individual are challenging to measure, as are confounding exposures over large population groups; the air pollutants measured may themselves not impart cancer risk, and may or may not correlate well with potentially carcinogenic agents; and most measurement data represent average levels over large areas.

Still, compelling results have accumulated from case–control and cohort studies, which suggest relative risks for lung cancer in the range of 1.5.[137] In general, more recent studies have better controlled for differences in smoking among subjects, and some have tagged increased lung cancer risk to elevations of specific pollutants, such as fine or sulfate particulates.[138,139] Pope et al have recently reported on the lung cancer mortality in a prospective cohort of approximately 1.2 million adults enrolled in 1982.[140] Fine particulate and sulfur oxide-related pollution were associated with all-cause, lung cancer, and cardiopulmonary mortality. Each 10 µg/m³ elevation in fine particulate air pollution was associated with an approximately 8% increased risk of lung cancer mortality. The authors reported no associations with coarse particle fraction or total suspended particles.

OTHER RESPIRATORY TRACT CANCERS

Mesothelioma

The link between malignant mesothelioma and asbestos exposure was first suggested in case reports from the 1940s. Further evidence was gathered by Wagner and associates in 1960 in a study of diffuse pleural mesotheliomas associated with asbestos mining in South Africa.[141] In 1964, Selikoff and colleagues reported a surprisingly high incidence of death from mesothelioma in a cohort of 632 insulation workers.[9] In a larger cohort of 17,800 asbestos insulation workers followed from 1967 to 1976, nearly 8% of deaths were due to the tumor.[142] Subsequent studies have found consistently elevated rates of mesothelioma in asbestos workers.

Diffuse malignant mesothelioma is a rare tumor of the serosal membranes of the lung and abdomen (Fig. 30.1.1). Incidence rates in American men range from four to 11 cases per million per year, and in American women, from one to four cases per million per year. Between 50% and 100% of all malignant mesotheliomas in North America and South Africa are attributable to asbestos exposure. In Turkey, the fibrous mineral zeolite has also been associated with a large epidemic of cases. Pleural mesotheliomas are more common than peritoneal mesotheliomas and account for nearly 90% of cases. Studies demonstrate an average latency period from first exposure to onset of disease of 30 to 35 years. Although higher cumulative exposures to asbestos generally correlate with a greater risk of malignant mesothelioma, studies have revealed that the tumor may occur with short-term (1 to 2 years) exposures and lower exposure levels. Household contacts of asbestos workers who may have washed asbestos-contaminated clothing, for example, are a recognized risk group.[143] Smoking does not appear to increase the risk of mesothelioma. There is no evidence that asbestos increases the risk of solitary benign mesothelioma.

Asbestos fiber type may influence the incidence of malignant mesothelioma. Lower rates have been reported in those exposed only to chrysotile, and some studies of chrysotile miners have not revealed elevated risk of mesothelioma.[144,145] Malignant mesothelioma may be more common with exposure to the longer crocidolite fibers than with exposure to amosite and anthophylite. A recent autopsy study employing analysis of retained asbestos fibers in young people who died of mesothelioma has estimated that 80% of the disease is due to amosite and crocidolite.[146] Others have suggested that chrysotile asbestos is the main cause of pleural mesothelioma, citing the necessity to consider longer follow-up periods for exposed cohorts, limited data regarding mesotheliomas among exposed household members, and more widespread exposure to chrysotile.[147] A reasonable synthesis of the current data is that chrysotile imparts a lower risk of mesothelioma than do the amphiboles, but that chrysotile-exposed workers are at risk for mesothelioma.[148] Peritoneal mesothelioma has not been associated with chrysotile exposure alone.

There is concern that other fibrous substances may induce mesothelioma. Erionite exposure appears to profoundly increase risk of mesothelioma, while MMVF do not. A recent study examined a cohort of 162 immigrants to Sweden from Karain, a Turkish village in which there is low-level environmental exposure to erionite, a fibrous zeolite. Of 18 deaths which occurred in the cohort, 14 (78%) were due to malignant pleural mesothelioma. In addition, there were five patients with mesothelioma who were still alive. Risks of mesothelioma were elevated 135-fold and 1336-fold, respectively, in men and women, compared with an age-matched Swedish population.[149] In contrast, no excesses of mesothelioma have been detected in the American cohort of MMVF production workers.[150] A recent German case–control study could neither detect nor exclude an association between MMVF and mesothelioma.[151]

Clinical features

Typical symptoms of malignant mesothelioma include chest pain, dyspnea, weight loss, and cough. Fever also may be present. Chest pain of a dull gnawing quality is the most common symptom and tends to localize over the involved side, although radiation to the arm or shoulder may occur. Cough is usually not a prominent symptom until the tumor has invaded the mediastinum.

Pleural effusion is the most common physical finding, and chest radiographs usually reveal unilateral fluid with persistent pleural thickening and nodularity following fluid removal. Early on, thoracic structures often are drawn towards the tumor by its dense desmoplastic growth (Fig. 30.1.2). In advanced disease, there may be enlargement of the affected hemithorax, bulging of intercostal spaces, and displacement of the trachea and mediastinum to the unaffected side. Local tumor growth also may depress the diaphragm, giving the impression of splenomegaly or hepatomegaly. Supraclavicular and axillary lymph node enlargement, subcutaneous nodules in the chest wall, and rib tenderness also may be seen in advanced disease.

Diagnosis

Diagnosis often is delayed due to the indistinct clinical features of early disease. Despite the fact that the overwhelming majority of cases of malignant mesothelioma are caused by asbestos exposure, asbestosis or other non-malignant effects are present in only about 20% of individuals diagnosed with the tumor. Pleural or peritoneal fluid is always exudative but of variable cellularity. Cytologic distinction of malignant cells from reactive mesothelial cells is often difficult. The presence of hyaluronic acid in fluid may be useful.

Ultimately, the diagnosis depends on defining the anatomy of the tumor and obtaining definitive tissue. In cases in which plain X-ray studies of chest and abdomen may be non-diagnostic, computed tomography (CT) scans are often very revealing (Fig. 30.1.3). Biopsy is definitive but may be difficult to interpret, even by experienced readers. The spindle cell types (Fig. 30.1.4) are generally differentiable from benign lesions and other tumors, but some mesotheliomas have striking adenomatous features, making them difficult to differentiate from metastatic adenocarcinoma. Immunohistochemical stains to exclude GI or GU cell origin and confirm mesenchymal surface markers are now widely employed to differentiate the two.

Treatment

No effective therapy exists for malignant mesothelioma. Also, there is no demonstrated benefit of early diagnosis beyond the timely acquisition of compensation benefits for the occupationally exposed. Average survival is 12 to 15 months from onset of symptoms, and most patients die within 1 year of diagnosis; there are a few long-term survivors, however, for unclear reasons. Death usually occurs from extension of the tumor into adjacent struc-

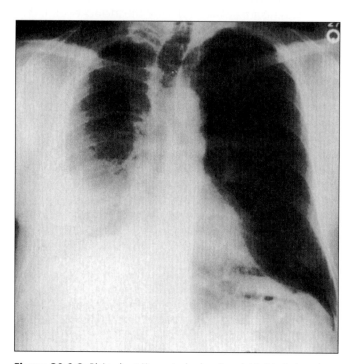

Figure 30.1.2: Plain chest X-ray study showing right-sided pleural malignant mesothelioma, with shift of thoracic contents.

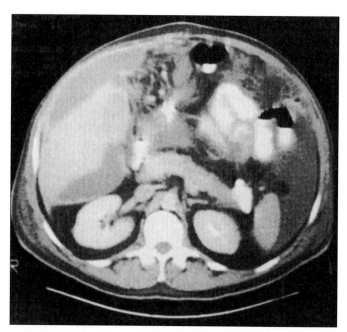

Figure 30.1.3: Malignant peritoneal mesothelioma encasing abdominal organs on CT scan.

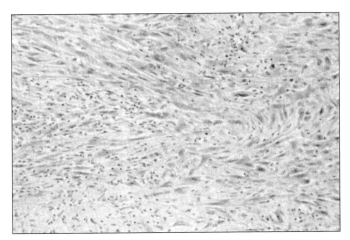

Figure 30.1.4: Histology of spindle cell malignant mesothelioma (H & E stain, high power).

tures in the chest or the abdomen; metastases occur uncommonly. Hypoglycemia and hemolytic anemia have been reported as paraneoplastic complications. In general, palliative care should be emphasized, although surgery, chemotherapy, and radiotherapy have potential value in individual cases.

Upper respiratory cancer

Known and probable carcinogenic agents are summarized in Table 30.1.3.

Sinonasal and nasopharyngeal cancers

The first recognized cases of occupational sinonasal cancer were reported in a Welsh nickel refinery in 1932. Since that time a number of industrial processes and specific exposures have been associated with the tumor. Sinonasal cancers are rare, occurring at a rate of less than 10 cases per million per year in the US. Squamous cell cancers, which make up about half of all sinonasal tumors, and adenocarcinomas have been linked with occupational exposures. Adenomas, lymphomas, melanomas, and adenoid cystic carcinomas make up the remainder of sinonasal cancers.

The primary exposures linked to sinonasal cancer are nickel, wood dust, formaldehyde, cutting oils, and chro-

mium. Cancers in nickel workers have occurred most frequently in the nose and ethmoid sinuses, and usually are of squamous histology.[152] Most epidemiologic studies were carried out in nickel refineries where exposures occurred to nickel oxides, nickel sulfide dust, soluble nickel compounds, and nickel carbonyl. Wood dust has been recognized as a sinonasal carcinogen since 1965, when a strikingly high incidence of the tumor occurred in an English furniture factory, and several case–control studies have documented increased risk among wood dust-exposed occupations since then.[153,154] The most frequently occurring tumor histology following wood dust exposure is adenocarcinoma. Wood dusts contain a number of biologically active substances as well as preservatives, pesticides, and fungal proteins. The active carcinogen in wood dust is unknown, although PAHs may play a role because wood often is charred in the furniture-manufacturing process.

A number of case–control studies have evaluated risk of sinonasal cancer among formaldehyde-exposed workers.[155-157] Pooled analyses suggest that risk of both adenocarcinoma and squamous cell carcinoma is increased. Risk of nasopharyngeal cancer has also been shown to be significantly elevated. Formaldehyde may potentiate the carcinogenic potential of wood dust exposure. An association between cutting oils and sinonasal cancer has been demonstrated in a small number of case–control studies, though a recent investigation found a significant association with nasopharyngeal cancer only.[158]

Occupations in which an increased risk of sinonasal tumors have been reported include shoe manufacturing and repair, textile and clothing manufacture, agricultural work, and food preparation. Leather dusts, natural fibers, pesticides, and PAHs have been suggested as possible etiologic agents. Exposure to wood smoke under poorly ventilated conditions in the home has been proposed as an environmental etiology, which may explain higher rates of nasopharyngeal carcinoma among Chinese, other Asians, and natives of Alaska. Cigarette smoking has not been implicated as a major cause of sinonasal cancer.

Although it is a rare tumor, sinonasal cancer should be suspected in a patient with significant exposures who complains of chronic nasal discharge, obstruction, fullness, intermittent bleeding, sinus pain, or pain in the upper teeth. The persistence of such symptoms despite usual clinical interventions for more typical sinus problems is cause for referral to an otorhinolaryngologist for further evaluation. The diagnostic evaluation, natural history, and treatments of occupational sinonasal cancer do not differ from non-occupationally related disease.

Laryngeal cancer

Laryngeal cancer is considerably more common than sinonasal cancer, making up about 2% of the annual cancer incidence in the US. The primary risk factor is cigarette smoking, with some additional risk imparted by alcohol consumption. Occupational risk factors may include exposure to asbestos, cutting oils, acid mists, and nickel. Nearly all tumors are of squamous histology.

Agents	Exposure settings
Sinonasal cancer	
Known carcinogens:	
Nickel	Nickel refining
Wood dust	Furniture making
Probable carcinogens:	
Chromium	Chromium pigment production
Cutting oils	Machinists
Formaldehyde	Production of formaldehyde resins, particle board, apparel
Laryngeal cancer	
Probable carcinogens:	
Asbestos	Insulating, shipyard work
Cutting oils	Machinists

Table 30.1.3 Upper respiratory tract carcinogens

Increased rates of laryngeal cancer linked to asbestos exposure have been observed in miners, insulators, shipyard workers, and manufacturers of asbestos products. A recent meta-analysis of 69 asbestos-exposed occupational cohorts yielded SMRs for asbestos of 157 and 133 with and without latency, respectively.[159] Greater risks have generally been found in older studies with less rigorous control for tobacco exposure.[160] Results have been mixed with regard to a dose response between asbestos exposure and elevation of laryngeal cancer risk.[161,162] Machinists have been shown to have an elevated risk of laryngeal cancer in several studies.[163–165] Risk appears to be attributable to straight mineral oil exposure and may be enhanced during processes likely to produce PAHs. Acid mists also have been associated with laryngeal cancer in some, but not all, studies.[166–168] Long-duration, high-level exposures appear to impart greater risk than do short-term exposures to lower levels. Rates of laryngeal cancer among nickel workers have been elevated in some studies based on small numbers, but others have reported no significant increases.[169–171] As with other respiratory tract cancers, occupationally related laryngeal cancer does not differ from non-occupational disease in its clinical presentation, natural history, or recommended therapy.

PREVENTION OF RESPIRATORY CANCER

Given the lack of effective treatment for most respiratory cancers, the most effective method to reduce their considerable mortality rate is primary prevention. Identification of etiologic agents in the workplace is an ongoing task that requires physicians, industrial hygienists, epidemiologists, and policy makers to be sensitive to patterns of exposure and disease and to act prudently even when information is incomplete. Adherence to workplace standards is likely to yield decreasing rates of occupational respiratory cancer over the next several decades because many cancers today reflect exposures prior to the implementation of current standards. Still, standards must be continually reassessed as better epidemiologic studies yield new information. Smoking cessation efforts in the workplace also are vitally important.

Secondary prevention in the form of mandated medical monitoring is an adjunctive approach to occupational disease prevention. The efficacy of lung cancer screening in high-risk populations and choice of diagnostic tools to use remains an area of controversy. Presently, the Occupational Safety and Health Administration (OSHA) mandates medical monitoring for workers exposed to the following carcinogens: asbestos, acrylonitrile, arsenic, bis-chloromethyl ether, cadmium, coke oven emissions, silica, and vinyl chloride. Medical monitoring in each case involves physical examination, chest radiograph, and ILO rating. Sputum cytology examination is required for some workers, including those exposed to arsenic or coke oven emissions. The asbestos standard requires chest radiographs every 5 years for the first 10 years after the initial exposure, and, after 10 years of latency, every 2 years

between the ages of 35 and 45 years and annually after age 45.

NIOSH recommends medical monitoring in addition for workers exposed to beryllium, carbon black, chromium VI, coal tar products, inorganic nickel, chrysene, and coal gasification processes. Recommended monitoring includes history, chest examination, chest radiograph, and, in some cases, sputum cytology.

Several studies have been performed to evaluate current tools for medical monitoring of lung cancer in the workplace. The value of the screening chest radiograph, even in workers with considerably elevated lung cancer risk, has yet to be firmly established, though re-analyzed results of clinical trials suggest that screening may improve clinical outcomes in detected cases.[172,173] One study has shown that lung cancer cases detected through chest X-ray screening have a 5-year survival rate of 19% versus 10% among cases detected through conventional healthcare.[174] Sputum cytology monitoring has been proposed as an alternative or supplemental monitoring tool. Lung cancers detected by sputum cytology tend to be squamous cell carcinomas of the major or segmental bronchus, whereas peripheral adenocarcinomas and large- and small-cell carcinomas more often are detected by X-rays. The addition of sputum cytology examination to radiographic screening has not brought about a decreased mortality from primary lung carcinoma. Sputum cytology results, however, may reveal mucosal changes that can identify individuals at increased risk.

Low-dose spiral CT has been proposed as a more effective means of screening high-risk populations for lung cancer.[175] In one study, 62 lung cancers were detected among 6341 participants. For single CT examinations, the mean detection rate (0.36%) was nearly 10 times greater than that achieved through chest X-ray screening.[176,177] Of the lung cancer cases detected, 83% were pathologic state IA, and 66% were less than 15 mm in diameter. Conventional radiography did not detect 63% of the cancers detected by spiral CT. The reported sensitivity and specificity were 57% and 95%, respectively. Another study evaluated spiral CT screening of 1000 smokers 60 years of age and over, of whom 14% reported asbestos exposure. Screening initially identified 233 individuals with non-calcified nodules, among whom 27 lung cancers were ultimately resected. Malignant disease was detected four times more frequently with spiral CT than with chest radiography (2.7% versus 0.7%), and stage I tumors were detected six times more frequently (2.3% versus 0.4%).[175,178,179] A screening program for 602 asbestos-exposed Finnish construction workers found abnormalities in 65 workers, among whom five lung cancers and one mesothelioma were detected. Sensitivity and specificity were estimated at 100% and 90%, respectively, with a positive predictive value of 8% in the studied population.[180]

The search for chemopreventive agents which might be administered to populations at high risk for lung cancer, such as heavy smokers or asbestotics, has not proven fruitful to date. Primary prevention trials with alpha-tocopherol with or without beta-carotene in the

Alpha-Tocopherol, Beta-Carotene (ATBC) Trial in 29,133 smokers in Finland, and with beta-carotene and retinyl palmitate in the Beta-Carotene and Retinol Efficacy Trial (CARET) in 18,254 smokers, former smokers, and asbestos-exposed workers in the US, have shown increases in lung cancer incidence, suggesting that beta-carotene itself or retinol might have carcinogenic properties.[181–183] A randomized trial in a population of 22,071 male physicians, of whom 11% were current smokers and 39% former smokers, showed no significant difference in the number of lung cancer cases between those receiving placebo and those receiving supplemental beta-carotene.[184] Despite the failures of such trials, epidemiologic evidence suggests that diets rich in fruits and vegetables confer some protection against respiratory and other cancers.[185] Beta-carotene may also affect different epithelial tissues differently, as evidenced by its apparent protective effect against precancerous oral lesions and a statistically non-significant reduction in secondary head and neck cancers.[186,187] Clearly, successes with chemoprevention, if they are to come, await a better understanding of the mechanisms underlying lower cancer rates among populations with apparently protective dietary habits.

References

1. Doll R, Peto R. The causes of cancer: quantitative estimates of avoidable risks of cancer in the U.S. today. J Natl Cancer Inst 1981; 66:1191-308.
2. Vineis P, Thomas T, Hayes R, et al. Proportion of lung cancers in males due to occupation in different areas of the US. Int J Cancer 1988; 42:851-6.
3. Morabia A, Markowitz S, Garibaldi K, Wunder E. Lung cancer and occupation: results of a multicentre case-control study. Br J Ind Med 1992; 49:721-7.
4. Steenland K, Loomis D, Shy C, Simonsen N. Review of occupational lung carcinogens. Am J Ind Med 1996; 29:474-90.
5. Lynch KM, Smith WA. Pulmonary asbestosis. III: Carcinoma of lung in asbesto-silicosis. Am J Cancer 1935; 56-64.
6. Merewether E. Chief Inspector of Factories. Annual Report for 1947. London: HMSO; 1949:79-81.
7. Gloyne SR. Pneumoconiosis. A historical survey of necropsy material in 1205 cases. Lancet 1951; 1:810.
8. Doll R. Mortality from lung cancer in asbestos workers. Br J Ind Med 1955; 12:81-6.
9. Selikoff IJ, Churg J, Hammond EC. Asbestos exposure and neoplasia. JAMA 1964; 188:22-6.
10. Armstrong B, DeKlerk N, Musk A, Hobbs M. Mortality in miners and millers in Western Australia. Br J Ind Med 1988; 45:5-13.
11. Dement J, Brown D, Okuin A. Lung cancer mortality among asbestos textile workers: a review and update. Ann Occup Hyg 1994; 38:525-32.
12. Gardner M, Powell C, Gardner A, Winter P, Fletcher A. Continuing high lung cancer mortality among ex-amosite factory workers and a pilot study of individual anti-smoking advice. J Soc Occup Med 1988; 38:69-72.
13. Raffn E, Lynge E, Korsgaard B. Incidence of lung cancer by histological type among asbestos cement workers in Denmark. Br J Ind Med 1993; 50:85-9.
14. Sluis-Cremer GK, Liddell F, Logan W, Bezuidenhout B. The mortality of amphibole miners in S. Africa. Br J Ind Med 1992; 49:566-75.
15. Cullen MR. Controversies in asbestos-related lung cancer. Occup Med 1987; 2:259-73
16. Lee PN. Relation between exposure to asbestos and smoking jointly and the risk of lung cancer. Occup Environ Med 2001; 58:145.
17. McFadden D, Wright JL, Wiggs B, et al. Smoking inhibits asbestos clearance. Am Rev Respir Dis 1986; 133:372-4.
18. Tron V, Wright JL, Harrison N, et al. Cigarette smoke makes airway and early parenchymal asbestos-induced lung disease worse in the guinea pig. Am Rev Respir Dis 1987; 136:271-5.
19. Gerde P, Scholander P. Adsorption of benzo(a)pyrene on to asbestos and manmade mineral fibres in an aqueous solution and in a biologic model solution. Br J Ind Med 1988; 45:682-8.
20. Berry G. Mortality of workers certified by pneumoconiosis medical panels as having asbestosis. Br J Ind Med 1981; 38:130-7.
21. Cookson W, Musk A, Glancy J, et al. Compensation, radiographic changes, and survival in applicants for asbestosis compensation. Br J Ind Med 1985; 42:461-8.
22. Hughes J, Weill H. Asbestosis as a precursor of asbestos-related cancer: results of a prospective study. Br J Ind Med 1991; 48:229-33.
23. Weiss W. Asbestosis: a marker for the increased risk of lung cancer among workers exposed to asbestos. Chest 1999; 115:536-49.
24. Finkelstein MM. Radiographic asbestosis is not a prerequisite for asbestos-associated lung cancer in Ontario asbestos-cement workers. Am J Ind Med 1997; 32:341-8.
25. Wilkinson P, Hansell DM, Janssenns J, et al. Is lung cancer associated with asbestos exposure when there are no small opacities on the chest radiograph? Lancet 1995; 345:1074-8.
26. Hillerdal G, Henderson DW. Asbestos, asbestosis, pleural plaques and lung cancer. Scand J Work Environ Health 1997; 23:93-103.
27. Weiss W. Asbestos and lobar site of lung cancer. Occup Environ Med 2000; 57:358.
28. Lee BW, Wain JC, Kelsey KT, et al. Association of cigarette smoking and asbestos exposure with location and histology of lung cancer. Am J Respir Crit Care Med 1998; 157:748-55.
29. Davis JMG, Addison J, Bolton RE, et al. Inhalation and injection studies in rats using dust samples from chrysotile asbestos prepared by a wet dispersion process. Exp Pathol 1986; 67:113-29
30. Yano E, Wang ZM, Wang XR, Wang MZ, Lan YJ. Cancer mortality among workers exposed to amphibole-free chrysotile asbestos. Am J Epidemiol 2001; 154:538-43.
31. Stanton MF, Layard M, Tegeris A, et al. Relation of particle dimension to carcinogenicity in amphibole asbestoses and other fibrous minerals. J Natl Cancer Inst 1981; 67:965-75.
32. Browne K. Is asbestos or asbestosis the cause of the increased risk of lung cancer in asbestos workers? Br J Ind Med 1986; 43:145-9.
33. Camus M, Siemiatycki J, Meek B. Nonoccupational exposure to chrysotile asbestos and the risk of lung cancer. N Engl J Med 1998; 338:1556-71.
34. Saupe E. Carcinoma of the lung in arsenic miners. Gewerbpathol 1930; 1:582.
35. Welch K, Higgins I, Oh M, Burchfiel C. Arsenic exposure, smoking, and respiratory cancer in copper smelter workers. Arch Environ Health 1982; 37:325-35.
36. Lee-Feldstein A. Cumulative exposure to arsenic and its relationship to respiratory cancer among copper smelter employees. J Occup Med 1986; 28:296-302.
37. Jarup L, Pershagen G, Wall S. Cumulative arsenic exposure and lung cancer in smelter workers: a dose-response study. Am J Ind Med 1989; 15:31-41.
38. Jarup L, Pershagen G. Arsenic exposure, smoking and lung cancer in smelter workers – a case-control study. Am J Epidemiol 1991; 134:545-51.
39. Taylor P, Qiao Y, Schatzkin A, et al. Relation of arsenic exposure to lung cancer among tin miners in Yunnan Province, China. Br J Ind Med 1989; 46:881-6.

40. Ott M, Holder B, Gordon H. Respiratory cancer and occupational exposure to arsenicals. Arch Environ Health 1974; 29:250-5.
41. Englyst V, Lundstrom NG, Gerharsson L, Rylander L, Nordberg G. Lung cancer risks among lead smelter workers also exposed to arsenic. Sci Total Environ 2001; 273:77-82.
42. Simeonova PP, Luster MI. Mechanisms of arsenic carcinogenicity: genetic or epigenetic mechanisms? J Environ Pathol Toxicol Oncol 2000; 19:281-6.
43. Hertz-Piccotto I, Smith AH, Holzman D, Lipsett M, Alexeeff G. Synergism between occupational arsenic exposure and smoking in the induction of lung cancer. Epidemiology 1992; 3:23-31.
44. Figueroa WG, Raszkowski R, Weiss W. Lung cancer in chloromethyl methy ether workers. N Engl J Med 1973; 288:1096-7.
45. Collingwood KW, Pasternack BS, Shore RE. An industrywide study of respiratory cancer in chemical workers exposed to chloromethyl ethers. J Natl Cancer Inst 1987; 78:1127-36.
46. Blair A, Kazerouni N. Reactive chemicals and cancer. Cancer Causes Control 1997; 8:473-90.
47. Machle W, Gregorio F. Cancer of the respiratory tract in the US chromate producing industry. Public Health Rep 1948: 63:1114-27.
48. Rosenman KD, Stanbury M. Risk of lung cancer among former chromium smelter workers. Am J Ind Med 1996; 29:491-500.
49. Sorahan T, Burges DC, Hamilton L, Harrington JM. Lung cancer mortality in nickel/chromium platers, 1946-1965. Occup Environ Med 1998; 55:236-42.
50. Itoh T, Takahashi K, Okubo T. Mortality of chromium plating workers in Japan – a 16-year follow-up study. J UOEH 1996; 18:7-18.
51. Sjogren B, Hansen KS, Kjuus H, Persson PG. Exposure to stainless steel welding fumes and lung cancer: a meta-analysis. Occup Environ Med 1994; 51:335-6.
52. Langard S. Nickel-related cancer in welders. Sci Total Environ 1994; 148:303-9.
53. Moulin JJ. A meta-analysis of epidemiologic studies of lung cancer in welders. Scand J Work Environ Health 1997; 23:104-13.
54. Becker N. Cancer mortality among arc welders exposed to fumes containing chromium and nickel. Results of a third follow-up: 1989-1995. J Occup Environ Med 1999; 41:294-303.
55. Paddle GM. Metaanalysis as an epidemiological tool and its application to studies of chromium. Regul Toxicol Phamacol 1997; 26:S42-S50.
56. Pastides H, Austin R, Lemeshow S, Klar J, Mundt KA. A retrospective-cohort study of occupational exposure to hexavalent chromium. Am J Ind Med 1994; 25:663-75.
57. Korallus U, Ulm K, Steinmann-Steiner-Haldenstaett W. Bronchial carcinoma mortality in the German chromate-producing industry: the effects of process modification. Int Arch Occup Environ Health 1993; 65:171-8.
58. Davies JM, Easton DF, Bidstrup PL. Mortality from respiratory cancers and other causes in United Kingdom chromate production workers. Br J Ind Med 1991; 48:299-313.
59. Alexander BH, Checkoway H, Wechsler L, Heyer NJ, Muhm JM, O'Keeffe TP. Lung cancer in chromate-exposed aerospace workers. J Occup Environ Med 1996; 38:1253-8.
60. IARC. IARC Monogr Eval Carcinog Risks Hum 1987, Supplement 7.
61. Mancuso TF. Chromium as an industrial carcinogen: Part I. Am J Ind Med 1997; 31:129-39.
62. Gibb HJ, Lees PSJ, Pinsky PF, Rooney BC. Lung cancer among workers in chromium chemical production. Am J Ind Med 2000; 38:115-26.
63. IARC Working Group on the Evaluation of Carcinogenic Risks to Humans: Silica, Some Silicates, Coal Dust and Para-Aramid Fibrils. Lyon, 15-22 October 1996. IARC Monogr Eval Carcinog Risks Hum 1997; 68:1-475.

64. Steenland K, Stayner L. Silica, asbestos, man-made mineral fibers, and cancer. Cancer Causes Control 1997; 8:491-503.
65. Carta P, Aru G, Manca P. Mortality from lung cancer among silicotic patients in Sardinia: an update study with 10 more years of follow up. Occup Environ Med 2001; 58:786-93.
66. Steenland K, Sanderson W. Lung cancer among industrial sand workers exposed to crystalline silica. Am J Epidemiol 2001; 153:695-703.
67. Steenland K, Mannetje A, Boffetta P, et al. Pooled exposure-response analyses and risk assessment for lung cancer in 10 cohorts of silica-exposed workers: an IARC multicentre study. Cancer Causes Control 2001; 12:773-84.
68. Case RA, Lea AJ. Mustard-gas poisoning, chronic bronchitis and lung cancer: investigation into possibility that poisoning by mustard gas in 1914-18 war might be factor in production of neoplasia. Br J Prev Soc Med 1955; 9:62-72.
69. Nishimoto Y, Yamakido M, Ishioka S, Shigenobu T, Yukutake M. Epidemiologic studies of lung cancer in Japanese mustard gas workers. In: Miller RW, ed. Unusual occurrences as clues to cancer etiology. Tokyo: Taylor & Francis; 1988:95-101.
70. Easton DF, Peto J, Doll R. Cancers of the respiratory tract in mustard gas workers. Br J Ind Med 1988; 45:652-9.
71. Bridge JC. Annual Report of the Chief Inspector of Factories and Workshops for 1932. London: HMSO; 1933:103-4.
72. ICNCM (International Committee on Nickel Carcinogenesis in Man). Report of the International Committee on Nickel Carcinogenesis in Man. Scand J Work Environ Health 1990; 16:1-84.
73. IARC. Chromium, nickel and welding. Monograph 49. Lyon: IARC; 1990.
74. Pott P. Chirurgical observations relative to the cataract, the polypus of the nose, the cancer of the scrotum, the different kinds of ruptures, and the mortification of the toes and feet. London: Hawes, Clark & Collins; 1775.
75. Lloyd JW, Lundin FE Jr, Redmond CK, Geiser PB. Longterm mortality study of steelworkers. IV. Mortality by work area. J Occup Med 1970; 12:151-7.
76. Costantino JP, Redmond CK, Bearden A. Occupationally related cancer risk among coke oven workers: 30 years of follow-up. J Occup Environ Med 1995; 37:597-604.
77. Maclaren WM, Hurley JF. Mortality of tar distillation workers. Scand J Work Environ Health 1987; 13:404-11.
78. Partanen T, Boffetta P. Cancer risk in asphalt workers and roofers: review and meta-analysis of epidemiologic studies. Am J Ind Med 1994; 26:721-40.
79. Evanoff BA, Gustavsson P, Hogstedt C. Mortality and incidence of cancer in a cohort of Swedish chimney sweeps: an extended follow up study. Br J Ind Med 1993; 50:450-9.
80. Steenland NK, Silverman DT, Hornung RW. Case-control study of lung cancer and truck driving in the Teamsters Union. Am J Public Health 1990; 80:670-4.
81. Steenland K, Deddens J, Stayner L. Diesel exhaust and lung cancer in the trucking industry: exposure-response analyses and risk assessment. Am J Ind Med 1998; 34:220-8.
82. Doll R, Vessey MP, Beasley RWR, et al. Mortality of gasworkers – final report of a prospective study. Br J Ind Med 1972; 29:394-406.
83. Andersen A, Dahlberg BE, Magnus K, Wannag A. Risk of cancer in the Norwegian aluminium industry. Int J Cancer 1982; 29:295-8.
84. Gibbs GW. Mortality of aluminum reduction plant workers, 1950 through 1977. J Occup Med 1985; 27:761-70.
85. Armstrong B, Tremblay C, Baris D, Theriault G. Lung cancer mortality and polynuclear aromatic hydrocarbons: a case-cohort study of aluminum production workers in Arvida, Quebec, Canada. Am J Epidemiol 1994; 139:250-62.
86. Gustavsson P, Plato N, Lidstrom EB, et al. Lung cancer and exposure to diesel exhaust among bus garage workers. Scand J Work Environ Health 1990; 16:348-54.
87. Health Effects Institute Diesel Epidemiology Expert Panel. Diesel emissions and lung cancer: epidemiology and

quantitative risk assessment. Cambridge, MA: Health Effects Institute; 1999.

88. Romundstad P, Haldorsen T, Andersen A. Cancer incidence and cause specific mortality among workers in two Norwegian aluminium reduction plants. Am J Ind Med 2000; 37:175-83.

89. Ronneberg A, Langmark F. Epidemiologic evidence of cancer in aluminum reduction plant workers. Am J Ind Med 1992; 22:573-90.

90. Zhou BS, Wang TJ, Guan P, Wu JM. Indoor air pollution and pulmonary adenocarcinoma among females: a case-control study in Shenyang, China. Oncol Rep 2000; 7:1253-9.

91. Seow A, Poh WT, The M, et al. Fumes from meat cooking and lung cancer risk in Chinese women. Cancer Epidemiol Biomarkers Prev 2000; 9:1215-21.

92. Mumford JL, He XZ, Chapman RS, et al. Lung cancer and indoor air pollution in Xuan Wei, China. Science 1987; 235:217-20.

93. Agricola G. De re metallica. Translated by Hoover H, Hoover L. New York: Dover; 1950.

94. Harting FH, Hesse W. Der Lungenkrebs, die Bergkrankheit in der Schneeberger Gruben. Vgschr Med Gerish Off Sanit 1879; 30:296-309 and 31:102-32, 313-37.

95. Lubin JH, Boice JD Jr, Edling C, et al. Lung cancer in radon-exposed miners and estimation of risk from indoor exposure. J Natl Cancer Inst 1995; 87:817-27.

96. Lubin JH, Qiao YQ, Taylor PR, et al. Quantitative evaluation of the radon and lung cancer association: a case-control study of Chinese tin miners. Cancer Res 1990; 50:174-80.

97. Samet JM, Kutvirt DM, Waxweiler RJ, Key CR. Uranium mining and lung cancer in Navajo men. N Engl J Med 1984; 310:1481-4.

98. Roscoe RJ, Steenland K, Halperin WE, et al. Lung cancer mortality among nonsmoking uranium miners exposed to radon daughters. JAMA 1989; 262:629-33.

99. Ennemoser O, Oberdorfer E, Brunner P, et al. Mitigation of indoor radon in an area with unusually high radon concentrations. Health Phys 1995; 69:227-32.

100. Levesque B, Gauvin D, McGrego RG, et al. Radon in residences: influences of geological and housing characteristics. Health Phys 1997; 72:907-14.

101. Lubin JH, Boice JD Jr. Lung cancer risk from residential radon: meta analysis of eight epidemiologic studies. J Natl Cancer Inst 1997; 89:49-57.

102. Field RW, Steck DJ, Smith BJ, et al. The Iowa radon lung cancer study – phase I: Residential radon gas exposure and lung cancer. Sci Total Environ 2001; 272:67-72.

103. Kreienbrock L, Kreuzer M, Gerken M, et al. Case-control study on lung cancer and residential radon in western Germany. Am J Epidemiol 2001; 153:42-52.

104. Alavanja MC, Lubin JH, Mahaffey JA, Brownson RC. Residential radon exposure and risk of lung cancer in Missouri. Am J Public Health 1999; 89:1042-8.

105. Kreuzer M, Gerken M, Kreienbrock L, Wellmann J, Wichmann HE. Lung cancer in lifetime nonsmoking men – results of a case-control study in Germany. Br J Cancer 2001; 84:134-40.

106. Lagarde F, Axelsson G, Damber L, Mellander H, Nyberg F, Pershagen G. Residential radon and lung cancer among never-smokers in Sweden. Epidemiology 2001; 12:396-404.

107. O'Neill IK, Brunnemann KD, Dodet B, et al., eds. Environmental carcinogens: methods of analysis and exposure measurement. Volume 9 – Passive smoking. Lyon: IARC; 1987. (IARC scientific publications no. 81.)

108. Brownson RC, Alavanja MC, Caporaso N, Somoes EJ, Chang JC. Epidemiology and prevention of lung cancer in nonsmokers. Epidemiol Rev 1998; 20:218-36.

109. Respiratory health effects of passive smoking: lung cancer and other disorders. Washington, DC: Office of Health and Environment, Office of Research and Development, US Environmental Protection Agency; 1992. (Publication no. EPA/600/6-90/006F.)

110. Taylor R, Cumming R, Woodward A, Black M. Passive smoking and lung cancer: a cumulative meta-analysis. Aust NZ J Public Health 2001; 25:203-11.

111. Hackshaw AK, Law MR, Wald NJ. The accumulated evidence on lung cancer and environmental tobacco smoke. BMJ 1997; 315:980-8.

112. Brown KG. Lung cancer and environmental tobacco smoke: occupational risk to nonsmokers. Environ Health Perspect 1999; 107(Suppl 6):885-90.

113. Reynolds P. Epidemiologic evidence for workplace ETS as a risk factor for lung cancer among nonsmokers: specific risk estimates. Environ Health Perspect 1999; 107(Suppl 6):865-72.

114. Hammond SK. Exposure of US workers to environmental tobacco smoke. Environ Health Perspect 1999; 107(Suppl 2):329-40.

115. Pirkle JL, Flegal KM, Bernert JT, et al. Exposure of the US population to environmental tobacco smoke. The Third National Health and Nutrition Examination Survey, 1988 to 1991. JAMA 1996; 275:1233-40.

116. Steenland K, Ward E. Lung cancer incidence among patients with beryllium disease: a cohort mortality study. J Natl Cancer Inst 1991; 83:1380-5.

117. Ward E, Okun A, Ruder A, Fingerhut M, Steenland K. A mortality study of workers at seven beryllium processing plants. Am J Ind Med 1992; 22:885-904.

118. Sanderson WT, Ward EM, Steenland K, Petersen MR. Lung cancer case-control study of beryllium workers. Am J Ind Med 2001; 39:133-44.

119. Deubner DC, Lockey JL, Kotin P, et al. Re: Lung cancer case-control study of beryllium workers. Am J Ind Med 2001; 40:284-5.

120. Sanderson WT, Ward EM, Steenland K, et al. Re: Response to criticisms of "Lung cancer case-control study of beryllium workers". Am J Ind Med 2001; 40:286-8.

121. MacMahon B. The epidemiological evidence on the carcinogenicity of beryllium in humans. J Occup Med 1994; 36:15-24.

122. IARC. Beryllium, cadmium, mercury and exposures in the glass manufacturing industry. Monograph 58. Lyon: IARC; 1993.

123. Thun MT, Schnorr TM, Smith AB, Halperin W. Mortality among a cohort of US cadmium production workers – an update. J Natl Cancer Inst 1985; 74:325-33.

124. Stayner L, Smith R, Thun M, Schnorr T, Lemen R. A dose-response analysis and quantitative assessment of lung cancer risk and occupational cadmium exposure. Ann Epidemiol 1992; 2:177-94.

125. Sorahan T, Lancashire RJ. Lung cancer mortality in a cohort of workers employed at a cadmium recovery plant in the United States: an analysis with detailed job histories. Occup Environ Med 1997; 54:194-201.

126. Sorahan T, Lister A, Gilthorpe MS, Harrington JM. Mortality of copper cadmium alloy workers with special reference to lung cancer and non-malignant diseases of the respiratory system, 1946-92. Occup Environ Med 1995; 52:804-12.

127. Jarup L, Bellander T, Hogstedt C, Spang G. Mortality and cancer incidence in Swedish battery workers exposed to cadmium and nickel. Occup Environ Med 1998; 55:755-9.

128. Marsh G, Enterline P, Stone R, Henderson V. Mortality among a cohort of US man-made mineral fiber workers: 1985 follow-up. J Occup Med 1990; 32:594-604.

129. Boffetta P, Saracci R, Andersen A, et al. Cancer mortality among man-made vitreous fiber production workers. Epidemiology 1997; 8:259-68.

130. Lockey J, Lemasters G, Rice C, McKay R, Gartside P. A retrospective morbidity, mortality and nested case-control study of the respiratory health of individuals manufacturing refractory ceramic fiber and RCF products. Submitted to the

Refractory Ceramic Fiber Coalition (RCFC), Washington DC, 1993.

131. Marsh GM, Youk AO, Stone RA, et al. Historical cohort study of US man-made vitreous fiber production workers: I. 1992 fiberglass cohort follow-up: initial findings. J Occup Environ Med 2001; 43:741-56.

132. Marsh G, Stone R, Youk A, et al. Mortality among US rock wool and slag wool workers: 1989 update. J Occup Safety Health Aust NZ 1996; 12:297-312.

133. Wong O, Foliart D, Tent L. A case-control study of lung cancer in a cohort of workers potentially exposed to slag wool fibers. Br J Ind Med 1991; 48:818-24.

134. Chiazze L, Watkins D, Fryar C, Kozone J. A case-control study of malignant and non-malignant respiratory disease among employees of a fibreglass manufacturing facility II: exposure assessment. Br J Ind Med 1993; 50:717-25.

135. Walker AM, Maxim LD, Utell M. Risk analysis for mortality from respiratory tumors in a cohort of refractory ceramic fiber workers. Regul Toxicol Pharmacol 2002; 35:95-104.

136. International Agency for Research on Cancer. Man-made mineral fibres and radon. IARC Monogr Eval Carcinog Risks Hum 1988; Vol. 43.

137. Katsouyanni K, Pershagen G. Ambient air pollution exposure and cancer. Cancer Causes Control 1997; 8:284-91.

138. Dockery DW, Pope CA 3rd, Xu X, et al. An association between air pollution and mortality in six US cities. N Engl J Med 1993; 329:1753-9.

139. Pope CA 3rd, Thun MJ, Namboodiri MM, et al. Particulate air pollution as a predictor of mortality in a prospective study of US adults. Am J Respir Crit Care Med 1995; 151:669-74.

140. Pope CA 3rd, Burnett RT, Thun MJ, et al. Lung cancer, cardiopulmonary mortality, and long-term exposure to fine particulate air pollution. JAMA 2002; 287:1132-41.

141. Wagner JC, Sleggs CA, Marchand P. Diffuse pleural mesothelioma and asbestos exposure in the North Western Cape Province. Br J Ind Med 1960; 17:260-71.

142. Selikoff I, Hammond E, Seidman H. Mortality experience of insulation workers in the US and Canada, 1943-1976. Ann N Y Acad Sci 1979; 330:91-116.

143. Anderson HA, Lillis R, Daum SM, Selifoll IJ. Asbestosis among household contacts of asbestos factory workers. Ann N Y Acad Sci 1979; 330:387-99.

144. Rees D, Myers J, Goodman E, et al. Case-control study of mesothelioma in South Africa. Am J Ind Med 1999; 35:213-22.

145. Hodgson JT, Darnton A. The quantitative risks of mesothelioma and lung cancer in relation to asbestos exposure. Ann Occup Hyg 2000; 44:565-601.

146. McDonald JC, Armstrong BG, Edwards CW, et al. Case-referent survey of young adults with mesothelioma: I. Lung fibre analysis. Ann Occup Hyg 2001; 45:513-18.

147. Smith AH, Wright CC. Chrysotile asbestos is the main cause of pleural mesothelioma. Am J Ind Med 1996; 30:252-66.

148. Stayner L, Dankovic D, Lemen R. Occupational exposure to chyrsotile asbestos and cancer risk: a review of the amphibole hypothesis. Am J Pub Health 1995; 86:179-86.

149. Metintas M, Hillerdal G, Metintas S. Malignant mesothelioma due to environmental exposure to erionite: follow-up of a Turkish emigrant cohort. Eur Respir J 1999; 13:523-6.

150. Marsh GM, Gula MJ, Youk AO, et al. Historical cohort study of US man-made vitreous fiber production workers: II. Mortality from mesothelioma. J Occup Environ Med 2001; 43:757-66.

151. Rodelsperger K, Jockel KH, Pohlabeln H, Romer W, Woitowitz HJ. Asbestos and man-made vitreous fibers as risk factors for diffuse malignant mesothelioma: results from a German hospital-based case-control study. Am J Ind Med 2001; 39:262-75.

152. Sunderman FW Jr, Morgan LG, Andersen A, Ashley D, Forouhar FA. Histopathology of sinonasal and lung cancers in nickel refinery workers. Ann Clin Lab Sci 1989; 19:44-50.

153. Gordon I, Boffetta P, Demers PA. A case study comparing a meta-analysis and a pooled analysis of studies of sinonasal cancer among wood workers. Epidemiology 1998; 9:518-24.

154. Mannetje A, Kogevinas M, Luce D, et al. Sinonasal cancer, occupation, and tobacco smoking in European women and men. Am J Ind Med 1999; 36:101-7.

155. Luce D, Gerin M, Leclerc A. Sinonasal cancer and occupational exposure to formaldehyde and other substances. Int J Cancer 1993; 53:224-31.

156. Partanen T. Formaldehyde exposure and respiratory cancer – a meta-analysis of the epidemiologic evidence. Scand J Work Environ Health 1993; 19:8-15.

157. Luc D, Leclerc A, Begin D. Sinonasal cancer and occupational exposures: a pooled analysis of 12 case-control studies. Cancer Causes Control 2002; 13:147-57.

158. Zhu K, Levine RS, Brann EA, Hall HI, Caplan LS, Gnepp DR. Case-control study evaluating the homogeneity and heterogeneity of risk factors between sinonasal and nasopharyngeal cancers. Int J Cancer 2002; 99:119-23.

159. Goodman M, Morgan RW, Ray R, Malloy CD, Zhao K. Cancer in asbestos-exposed occupational cohorts: a meta-analysis. Cancer Causes Control 1999; 10:453-65.

160. Kraus T, Drexler H, Weber A, Raithel HJ. The association of occupational asbestos dust exposure and laryngeal carcinoma. Isr J Med Sci 1995; 31:540-8.

161. Imbernon E, Goldberg M, Bonenfant S. Occupational respiratory cancer and exposure to asbestos: a case-control study in a cohort of workers in the electricity and gas industry. Am J Ind Med 1995; 28:339-52.

162. Gustavsson P, Jakobsson R, Johansson H. Occupational exposures and squamous cell carcinoma of the oral cavity, pharynx, larynx, and oesophagus: a case-control study in Sweden. Occup Environ Med 1998; 55:393-400.

163. Eisen EA, Tolbert PE, Hallockj MF, Monson RR, Smith TJ, Woskie SR. Mortality studies of machining fluid exposure in the automobile industry. III: A case-control study of larynx cancer. Am J Ind Med 1994; 26:185-202.

164. Wortley P, Vaughan TL, Davis S, Morgan MS, Thomas DB. A case-control study of occupational risk factors for laryngeal cancer. Br J Ind Med 1992; 49:837-44.

165. Russi M, Dubrow R, Flannery JT, Cullen MR, Mayne ST. Occupational exposure to machining fluids and laryngeal cancer risk: contrasting results using two separate control groups. Am J Ind Med 1997; 31:166-71.

166. Checkoway H, Heyer NJ, Demers PA. An updated mortality follow-up study of Florida phosphate industry workers. Am J Ind Med 1996; 30:452-60.

167. Steenland K. Laryngeal cancer incidence among workers exposed to acid mists (United States). Cancer Causes Control 1997; 8:34-8.

168. Soskolne CL, Jhangri GS, Siemiatycki J, et al. Occupational exposure to sulfuric acid in southern Ontario, Canada, in association with laryngeal cancer. Scand J Work Environ Health 1992; 18:225-32.

169. Burch JD, Howe GR, Miller AB, Semenciw R. Tobacco, alcohol, asbestos, and nickel in the etiology of cancer of the larynx: a case-control study. J Natl Cancer Inst 1981; 67:1219-224.

170. Shannon HS, Julian JA, Roberts RS. A mortality study of 11,500 nickel workers. J Natl Cancer Inst 1984; 73:1251-8.

171. Roberts RS, Julian JA, Muir DC, Shannon HS. A study of mortality in workers engaged in the mining, smelting, and refining of nickel. II: Mortality from cancer of the respiratory tract and kidney. Toxicol Ind Health 1989; 5:975-93.

172. Strauss G, Gleason R, Sugarbaker D. Chest X-ray screening improves outcome in lung cancer: a reappraisal of randomized trials on lung cancer screening. Chest 1995; 107(Suppl):270-9.

173. Strauss GM, Gleason RE, Sugarbaker DJ. Screening for lung cancer. Another look; a different view. Chest 1997; 111:754-68.

174. Salomaa E, Liippo K, Taylor P, et al. Prognosis of patients with lung cancer found in a single chest radiograph screening. Chest 1998; 114:1514-18.

175. Tossavainen A. International expert meeting on new advances in the radiology and screening of asbestos-related diseases. Scand J Work Environ Health 2000; 26:449-54.

176. Sone S, Takashima S, Li F, et al. Mass screening for lung cancer with mobile spiral computed tomography scanner. Lancet 1998; 351:1242-5.

177. Sone S. Lung cancer screening using mobile low-dose computed tomography: results from Nagano project in Japan. In: Proceedings of an international expert meeting on new advances in radiology and screening of asbestos-related diseases. Helsinki: Finnish Institute of Occupational Health; 2000:33-46. People and Work Research Reports, no 36.

178. Henschke C, McCauley D, Uankelevitz D, et al. Early lung cancer action project: overall design and finding from baseline screening. Lancet 1999; 354:99-105.

179. Henschke C. Early lung cancer action project: findings on baseline and annual repeat screening CT. In: Proceedings of an international expert meeting on new advances in radiology and screening of asbestos-related diseases. Helsinki: Finnish Institute of Occupational Health; 2000:31-2. People and Work Research Reports, no. 36.

180. Vehmas T, Kivisaari L, Zitting A, et al. Computed tomography (CT) and high resolution CT for the early diagnosis of lung and pleural disease in workers exposed to asbestos: Finnish experiences. In: Proceedings of an international expert meeting on new advances in radiology and screening of asbestos-related diseases. Helsinki: Finnish Institute of Occupational Health; 2000:53-6. People and Work Research Reports, no 36.

181. The Alpha-Tocopherol, Beta-Carotene Cancer Prevention Study Group. The effect of vitamin E and beta carotene on the incidence of lung cancer and other cancers in male smokers. N Engl J Med 1994; 330:1029-35.

182. Omenn GS, Goodman GE, Thornquist MD, et al. Risk factors for lung cancer and for intervention effects in CARET, the Beta-Carotene and Retinol Efficacy Trial. J Natl Cancer Inst 1996; 88:1550-9.

183. Omenn GS. Chemoprevention of lung cancer is proving difficult and frustrating, requiring new approaches. J Natl Cancer Inst 2000; 92:959-60.

184. Hennekens CH, Buring JE, Manson JE, et al. Lack of effect of long-term supplementation with beta carotene on the incidence of malignant neoplasms and cardiovascular disease. N Engl J Med 1996; 334:1145-9.

185. Ziegler RG, Mayne ST, Swanson CA. Nutrition and lung cancer. Cancer Causes Control 1996; 7:157-77.

186. Mayne ST, Cartmel B, Baum M, et al. Randomized trial of supplemental beta-carotene to prevent second head and neck cancer. Cancer Res 2001; 61:1457-63.

187. Garewal HS, Katz RV, Meyskens F, et al. Beta-carotene produces sustained remissions in patients with oral leukoplakia: results of a multicenter prospective trial. Arch Otolaryngol Head Neck Surg 1999; 125:1305-10.

30.2 Lymphohematopoietic Malignancies

Howard M Kipen, Daniel Wartenberg

Lymphohematopoietic (LH) malignancies are a heterogeneous group of neoplasms that arise from the clonal malignant transformation of various cell lines of the blood and lymphoid tissues. The transformed cell lines proliferate initially in the lymphoid tissues or bone marrow, where they may disturb normal immune function and hematopoiesis. Eventually, malignant cells spill over into the peripheral blood and other tissues, where traditional clinical syndromes become apparent. All LH neoplasms combined account for about 8% of the 1,300,000 new malignancies expected annually in the US. A 15% to 25% male predominance is evident for all subgroups (see Table 30.2.1).

Leukemic clones are characterized by an arrest in maturation of the multipotent stem cell, which is now believed to be the effect of a prior genetic or chromosomal alteration. Although the malignant clone is not truly hyperplastic, its growth is unregulated and becomes independent of homeostatic feedback controls. The particular LH neoplasm that affects a given individual depends on the level of stem cell development at which the maturation block has occurred. For example, developmental blockade at the pluripotent stem cell level causes aplastic anemia (see Chapter 21). If the block occurs a stage later, acute myelogenous leukemia (AML) results. Later stages of maturation arrest result in progressively more differentiated cells up through acute megakaryocytic leukemia. In chronic myelogenous leukemia (CML), relatively mature, although dysfunctional, cells are produced by an incomplete maturation block; however, the cells from this line typically become unstable due to subsequent development of an earlier block, with eventual proliferation of promyelocytes and blasts, leading to crisis.

Acute and chronic lymphocytic leukemias (ALL, CLL) are disorders of committed lymphopoietic stem cells, originating in lymphoid precursors of bone marrow, thymus, and lymph nodes. The solid tumors of the LH system, sometimes known as B-cell immunoproliferative disorders, include multiple myeloma (MM), Hodgkin's disease (HD), and non-Hodgkin's lymphoma (NHL).

LH neoplasms are often regarded as sentinel health events, but as with all occupational and environmental disease, the exposure and risk factor history are of paramount importance because none of these conditions, nor their associated markers such as cytogenetic aberrations, is regarded as pathognomonic for a particular cause. Genetic abnormalities, both inherited and acquired, and environmental factors have been shown to be etiologically important.[1,2] Families with increased incidence have been described, although in some cases, shared environmental influences have been present and certainly should always be sought. Identical twins have a high concordance for leukemia in the first year of life, but this concordance is not known to persist in later life, suggesting predominance of environmental factors. Individuals with some congenital disorders, such as Down's, Bloom's, Wiscott–Aldrich,

Fanconi's, and Klinefelter's syndromes, have an increased incidence of leukemia. Acquired genetic factors are discussed later. Variations by sex and race of the major LH neoplasms are shown in Table 30.2.1. Aplastic anemia from any cause is associated with a markedly increased risk for the development of acute leukemia. Previous treatment with alkylating agents, radiotherapy, or both, also predisposes an individual to various LH disorders, and therapeutic immunosuppression such as that accompanying transplantation produces an exceedingly high relative risk of NHL, over 40-fold within 2 years, with a latency as short as a few months.[3]

CLASSIFICATION

The study of the distribution and causes of the LH neoplasms, as with all diseases, is limited by accurate nosology. As a unit, the LH disorders are a fairly well-delineated group of cancers comprising the following conditions.

THE ACUTE LEUKEMIAS
Acute myelogenous leukemia
Acute lymphocytic leukemia

THE LYMPHOMAS
Hodgkin's disease
Non-Hodgkin's lymphoma
T-cell lymphoma (mycoses fungoides)

OTHER
Multiple myeloma
Myeloproliferative disorders (including chronic
    myelogenous leukemia, myelofibrosis with myeloid
    metaplasia, and polycythemia vera)
Chronic lymphocytic leukemia

A number of caveats are important. Nomenclatures within the LH neoplasms have changed frequently over the last three decades. The International Classification of Diseases (ICD) and clinical coding practices are not well synchronized with one another nor with trends in clinical diagnostic practice.[1,4–6] Thus, deaths due to myelodysplastic syndrome (see Chapter 21) are sometimes classified as a type of AML and sometimes separately, and within the NHLs there have been numerous shifts in nomenclature, whereas the ICD has retained older terminology.[2,7] Because in any population LH neoplasms are relatively rare, such inconsistency influences the relative incidence of specific LH cancers, and thus impedes epidemiologic recognition and investigation of etiologic associations. Consequently, the total number of LH neoplasms or leukemias based on death certificates usually is reliable, because LH tumors rarely are classified outside the overall leukemia and lymphoma rubric, but specific cell types still cannot be reliably ascertained from death certificates.

	Males		Females	
	White	*Black*	*White*	*Black*
Leukemia	13.8	10.3	8.4	6.2
Lymphocytic	6.3	4.4	3.7	2.3
Acute	1.9	1.2	1.4	0.8
Chronic	4.3	3.1	2.2	1.4
Myelogenous	5.5	4.6	3.7	3.2
Acute	3.4	2.6	2.4	2.0
Chronic	1.8	1.9	1.1	1.0
Lymphomas	23.5	19.6	16.2	10.9
Hodgkin's	3.2	2.5	2.7	1.9
Non-Hogkin's	20.3	17.1	13.5	8.9

Table 30.2.1 Rates (per 100,000) of the major lymphohematopoietic malignancies, 1994–1998, based on nine registries, adjusted to 1970 US standard populations. (Data from Ries et al.[86])

For practical reasons, in many epidemiologic analyses, the leukemias are considered as one. But the various LHs are a diverse group of conditions, both hematologically and etiologically. The emergence of various unifying understandings of pathogenesis such as oncogene activation adds some coherence to lumping together conditions whose distinguishing characteristics may be limited to subtle aspects of morphologic and functional cellular phenotype. Whereas virtually all LH tumors share the mechanistic similarity of one or more genes of lymphoid cellular origin having been abnormally activated and expressed, the mechanism may be a mutation, a translocation, a chromosome aberration, or acquisition of new viral DNA. Some have even hypothesized that a non-specific stimulus such as clonal hyperstimulation of B cells could eventuate in malignancy such as lymphoma or MM. The use of the broader term B-cell immunoproliferative disorders has been proposed for a combination of CLL, NHL, HD, and MM. The paradox is that, to the extent that the tumors are distinct entities with distinct sets of causes, imprecision in classification makes etiologic associations more difficult to observe with consistency, whereas to the extent that one cause may result in multiple distinct histologic abnormalities, splitting arbitrarily reduces epidemiologic power and the opportunity to observe statistically significant associations.

LABORATORY EVALUATION IN THE DIAGNOSIS OF LYMPHOHEMATOPOIETIC MALIGNANCIES OF OCCUPATIONAL OR ENVIRONMENTAL ORIGIN

Leukemias usually are recognized when a white blood cell count is elevated in the presence of circulating blast cells in a symptomatic individual, although presentations with normal white blood cell counts or with cytopenias are not uncommon. Diagnosis is based on a finding of leukemic cells in either peripheral blood, bone marrow, or

extramedullary tissue. Examination of marrow classically shows an infiltrate of uniformly appearing blast cells, causing an overall hypercellular appearance with a reduction in normal formed elements. The therapeutically important distinction between AML and ALL is made by a combination of morphology (e.g., Auer's rods in AML), reactions with cytochemical stains (e.g., TdT positive in ALL; lysosomal enzyme positive in AML), and cell surface immunophenotypic markers. CLL usually is associated with elevated numbers of apparently mature B lymphocytes in peripheral blood, although 5% have T-cell surface markers. Cytogenetic (karyotypic) characteristics are used to define subsets of therapeutic and prognostic significance within the major leukemic groups, and they also can be used to make etiologic inferences.

Lymphomas are diagnosed and classified by histopathologic examination of resected tissue, because reliance on aspirates is associated with an unacceptably high error rate. Disagreements in classification between experienced pathologists using biopsy material is reported to be higher than for most types of solid tumors, although immunologic markers are increasingly applied. Immunophenotyping through use of monoclonal antibodies has shown that 60% of NHL is B-cell derived and 30% to 40% is of T-cell origin. Cytogenetic evaluation commonly reveals abnormalities, including translocations in proximity to known oncogenes such as c-*myc*, and such data are becoming more incorporated into diagnosis and classification.

A number of studies have reported a statistically significant relationship between certain chromosome changes in AML and NHL and exposure to broad categories of occupational agents such as pesticides, solvents, petrochemicals, combustion products, and asbestos. This finding is consistent with the abnormal cytologic characteristics of secondary leukemia after cytotoxic and radiation therapy (see later), although such associations have been variably noted, with positive findings in Scandinavia and relatively more negative findings in the US and Canada. The most frequently implicated abnormalities are -5 and -7, which have been associated previously with leukemia occurring after prior administration of chemotherapy.[8–12] This work is enabled and complicated by rapid advances in chromosome banding techniques, which now demonstrate some sort of visible chromosome rearrangement in nearly all cases of AML, in contrast to much lower rates in earlier years. The stage of the leukemia at the time of analysis also complicates the picture because the karyotype is known to evolve during the natural history of AML and other leukemias.

Although these types of epidemiologic investigations are relatively new, they offer a tantalizing approach to the exploration and clarification of the relationship between endogenous carcinogenic factors such as oncogenes and activation by environmental factors. This approach assumes one can distinguish the chromosome changes due to the environment factor from those due to progression and transformation of the disease, and has not yet been widely applied to resolution of environmental etiology problems. A slightly different use of laboratory abnormalities relies on the possibility that chromosome changes such as sister chromatid exchange (SCE) may be predictive of neoplasms. Ethylene oxide, an animal carcinogen and probable human leukemogen, has been shown to cause increases in SCE in exposed workers,[13] although not all studies have been positive.[14–16] Benzene, a known human leukemogen, causes chromosomal abnormalities in exposed individuals.[7,17] Of course, all of these chromosomal markers may be thought of as exposure indices, but much work remains to be performed to improve their specificity, and they must be interpreted with care in clinical settings.

ACUTE MYELOGENOUS LEUKEMIA OR ACUTE NON-LYMPHOCYTIC LEUKEMIA
Epidemiology

The 31,500 annual incident leukemias in the US comprise about 3% of all malignant neoplasms. Of these, myeloid types represent about 45%, with lymphoid types about 37%, and the remainder other and unspecified.

Ionizing radiation, benzene, and cytotoxic drugs are well-established acute leukemogens. Each is discussed in detail later in the chapter. In all three cases, investigations have progressed from whether they are leukemogens to questions of dose–response, mechanism of action, and risks posed by lower-dose environmental exposure. Ethylene oxide is now classified as a human carcinogen, and suspected to cause AML in addition to other LH neoplasms (see Chapter 40); styrene, 1,3-butadiene, vinyl chloride, paints, and nitrites have been reported causes. Industries that have used any of these agents (e.g., printing, rubber manufacturing, and painting) may be implicated, although benzene exposure is often implicated as the most potent among the mixtures. A recent case–control study confirmed well-known risks and raised new questions.[18]

It is an accepted generalization that the leukemias have much shorter latencies than the 10- to 30-year periods accepted for solid tumors. Acute leukemia risk in atomic bomb radiation survivors peaked at 2 to 5 years after detonation and declined after 10 years. After chemotherapy, the peak incidence is at 5 to 8 years and there appears to be a decline in risk by 10 to 15 years (as opposed to the persistent and progressively higher increased risk for solid tumors). Based on these high-dose, high-intensity exposure situations, some investigators have inferred that risks from environmental exposures to benzene, ionizing radiation, and perhaps other leukemogens diminish after a certain latency has been achieved. There are no clear epidemiologic data to support this.

Dose–response relations for acute leukemogens remain controversial as well. It is possible that the pattern and rate of exposure, as well as simple cumulative dose according to Haber's law, influence the risk of leukemia from ionizing radiation, the risk increasing as exposure is concentrated in time. This finding has not been clearly demonstrated for chemical leukemogens, and appropriate models of carcinogenesis remain an area of scientific ferment. The very high risk of AML after high-dose benzene-induced aplastic anemia may be an example of the influence of the exposure rate, but there is no clear indication that the leukemogenic properties of benzene require clinical marrow injury. Study of US and Chinese cohorts has led to some convergence of the dose–response relationships between benzene exposure and AML, extending evidence for causal relationships to exposures reported to be below 40 parts per million-years (ppm-years) of cumulative exposure.[7]

Clinical features

Of potentially great mechanistic significance for epidemiologic studies of occupational and environmental agents is the marked increase in clonal cytogenetic abnormalities, with 7q- or 5q- detectable in 70% of AMLs secondary to chemotherapy versus 10% of de-novo AMLs.[9] These leukemias secondary to alkylating agents or radiotherapy are usually characterized by a latency period of 5–10 years which may be preceded by a myelodysplastic phase. These particular chromosomal markers are also associated with particularly poor prognoses. The converse finding that the aberrations most common in de-novo AML are rare in the secondary cases lends credence to the potential causal mechanistic specificity of cytogenetic evaluation. Interestingly, some feel that de-novo AML in older adults bears cytogenetic similarities to secondary AMLs, leading to the hypothesis that AML and myelodysplastic syndrome developing in the elderly may reflect cumulative mutagenic environmental exposures in genetically susceptible individuals.[19] As stated earlier, field epidemiologic studies so far have yielded inconsistent results with respect to environmental and occupational agents and their specific associations with characteristic cytogenetic markers.[10–12,20]

Diagnosis, prognosis, and treatment

Cytotoxic chemotherapy with transfusion support has led to increasing numbers of initial remissions, currently 60% to 80%. Maintenance therapy is needed for some months. Between 10% and 30% of patients are free of disease at 5 years and apparently are cured. Secondary leukemias are becoming an increasingly prominent issue as survival rates increase.[9]

Screening

There is no practical approach to screening or early diagnosis for either prevention or reduction of morbidity. Screening based on cytogenetic abnormalities in peripheral blood lymphocytes or DNA adducts has been suggested but is not validated and should be considered only in experimental settings.[21] Routine complete blood counts (CBCs) to detect benzene-induced marrow depression, and urinary phenols to detect excessive benzene exposure are not likely to be sensitive enough to be useful at current levels of exposure in the developed world, except for indicating serious breaches of industrial hygiene, leading to overexposures greater than 10-fold the permissible exposure limit (PEL).

ACUTE LYMPHOCYTIC LEUKEMIA
Epidemiology

ALL is primarily a disease limited to the first two decades of life, with peak incidence at ages 2 to 9 years, although there is a smaller late peak in incidence after age 60. It is the type of leukemia most closely associated with several congenital disorders characterized by chromosomal abnormalities. However, because ALL does not affect the majority of patients with Down's, Fanconi's, Bloom's, and Klinefelter's syndromes, an environmental contribution to cause is still strongly implied. Studies of the effect of paternal and maternal occupations on childhood leukemia risk usually have not been cell-type specific (30% of childhood leukemias are ANLL) and, in fact, usually combine leukemias and lymphomas. Paternal occupations linked to the combined tumor types include nuclear industry workers, motor vehicle mechanics, hydrocarbon-exposed occupations, and medical and social service workers. In mothers, leukemia is linked to employment as a pharmacist, textile worker, chemical-exposed worker, hydrocarbon-exposed worker, and work in a domestic, hotel, or catering job (for a review, see Colt & Blair[22]). Solvent exposures at home have also been implicated.[23] The data for the nuclear industry have the most biologic plausibility and consistency with worker outcomes. Although some studies have suggested that paternal exposure through employment at nuclear facilities increases childhood leukemia risk, alternative hypotheses have also been offered for the observed cluster of childhood leukemias around the Seascale nuclear facility in England (see below).

Clinical features

ALL typically is exhibited by constitutional symptoms, easy bruising, and lymphadenopathy due to infiltration and replacement of bone marrow and lymphatic tissue by an abnormal lymphoid precursor. This usually is a null cell but occasionally has T-cell or, very rarely, B-cell markers.

Diagnosis, prognosis, and therapy

Diagnosis is arrived at by examination of peripheral blood and bone marrow for excessive lymphoblasts. Combination chemotherapy currently results in a 4- to 5-year disease-free survival with a significant long-term cure rate.

Screening

No screening is indicated.

HODGKIN'S DISEASE
Epidemiology

HD (lymphoma) is a tumor of histiocytic or reticulum cells, which is pathologically distinguished by the presence of Reed–Sternberg cells, as well as the somewhat atypical clinical features of an infection. There are about 7400 new cases annually in the US, with an average age at diagnosis of 32 years. It has the unusual epidemiologic feature of a pronounced bimodal age distribution with peaks around age 20 and age 70 in developed countries. In contrast to NHL and MM, the incidence is not linearly increased with age. Although disease presentation patterns in young adults still suggest an infectious pattern, this is not suggested in older patients, and some occupational associations have been discovered, although not with consistency. The roles of ionizing radiation, benzene, and other environmental agents are considered later; however, a recent review emphasized the paucity of confirmed association with environmental agents.[24]

Clinical presentation

HD usually is characterized by lymph node enlargement, either asymptomatic or associated with constitutional symptoms. Staging is performed based on the extent of nodal and extranodal involvement, and whether or not disease is present on both sides of the diaphragm. A functional T-lymphocyte defect usually is present, and normochromic-normocytic anemia is often present.

Diagnosis and treatment

Accurate diagnosis usually requires a surgical biopsy because aspiration rarely is adequate. Thorough exploration using physical examination, radiologic, and nuclear medicine modalities to detect all possible areas of involvement is required for accurate staging. Although radiotherapy is difficult and demanding owing to shielding requirements to reduce acute complications as well as risk of secondary malignancies and hypogonadism, over 70% of patients are now considered curable by radiotherapy, with or without combination chemotherapy.

Screening

There is no applicable screening for HD.

NON-HODGKIN'S LYMPHOMA
Classification

NHL is characterized by monoclonal neoplasms associated with proliferation of lymphocytes, macrophages, and their precursor and derivative cells. They are dominantly of B-cell phenotypic lineage, although some may have mixed B and T markers, and T-cell types may be particularly malignant.

Classification has rapidly and competitively evolved in this field from the histologically based Rappaport

Classification of 1966 to the immunologically based Lukes–Collins Classification of 1973 to 1974 and, in 1982, to the more clinically and prognostically based Working Formulation of NHLs for Clinical Usage. Further classifications have been proposed in an attempt to delineate individual diseases likely to have distinct etiologies.[5,25] The implications for studies of etiology are difficult to specify but will surely complicate assessment of causal factors for a tumor observed today in light of epidemiologic information collected based on earlier nomenclatures, including the pre-Rappaport data, on which much of current epidemiologic understanding is based.

Epidemiology

NHL accounts for approximately 3% of new cancer cases annually in the US and has an annual incidence rate of about 16/100,000 based on 1994 to 1998 Surveillance, Epidemiology, and End Results (SEER) tumor registry estimates. The incidence of NHL is 50% higher in males than in females, and it is much higher in persons beyond the fifth decade. These characteristics plus a steep secular rise have been used to argue for etiologic attribution to occupational and chemical exposures, although detailed analysis does not yield a completely satisfactory explanation.[26] Except for Burkitt's lymphoma, which is highly prevalent in equatorial Africa, rates are higher in whites than in blacks, and they also increase with socioeconomic status in most studies. Clusters of T-cell lymphoma in southwestern Japan and the Caribbean, where 10% to 15% of the population is seropositive, are strongly associated with endemic human T-cell lymphocytic virus (HTLV-1) infection.[27,28] Burkitt's is strongly associated with EB virus.

Known risks apart from socioeconomic status include hydantoin therapy and immune suppression. The latter may be either a primary (genetic) defect, secondary to drug therapy (e.g., prophylaxis for transplant rejection), or acquired from infection (HIV, HTLVs), autoimmune disorders, or therapeutic irradiation. Although impaired immune surveillance has been proposed to explain the increased incidence associated with the above-mentioned factors (up to 40- to 100-fold in the case of immunosuppressive therapy), there are other hypotheses of the origin of B-cell neoplasms that may be more germane to the role played by occupational and environmental chemical exposures. This line of reasoning maintains that lymphomas may develop as a result of imbalanced immunoregulation rather than deficient immune surveillance. Whereas the immune impairment is clinically apparent in the congenital or therapeutic immunodeficiencies, the impairments associated with NHL developing in the general population are hypothesized to be much more subtle. It is hypothesized that individual and, perhaps, idiosyncratic reactions to common physical, chemical, and viral agents may lead to lymphoma, without frank immune deficiency. Oncogene activation or immune gene dysregulation due to mutagens and clastogens also may play a role. Occupations for which the risk of NHL has been reported to be elevated include rubber workers, veterinarians, uranium miners, asbestos-exposed workers, lumberjacks, metal workers, female textile workers, chemists, benzene-exposed workers, and farmers (see discussion later).[29,30]

Clinical presentation

The clinical presentation of occupation-related NHL is not known to be different from de-novo cases.

Diagnosis, prognosis, and therapy

Examination of lymph node material usually is preferable to examination of involved extranodal tissue. Selection of therapy is more dependent on histologic type (Burkett's, follicular, diffuse) than on staging, in contrast to the dominant importance of staging for HD. The dominant favorable prognostic indicator is the presence of a follicular pattern in the nodal architecture, because patients with this characteristic finding follow a more indolent course than do those with a diffuse pattern of equivalent cytologic characteristics.

Screening

No screening techniques are clinically applicable to this disease.

MYCOSIS FUNGOIDES (see Chapter 30.9)

This rare cutaneous T-cell lymphoma has been linked to metals, solvents, arsenic, and bismuth in case reports. Industries such as petrochemical, rubber, metals, machinery production, printing, and textiles also have been suggested to have an association. The construction industry, too, was implicated in one study, which showed a particularly high risk among machinists. Viral etiologies have also been considered.[31]

Clinical presentation, diagnosis, prognosis, and treatment

The clinical presentation, diagnosis, prognosis, and treatment of occupation-related mycosis fungoides are not known to be any different from those of de-novo cases.

Screening

Although, in general, skin cancer screening may be indicated, especially for outdoor workers, mycosis fungoides is too rare to warrant special attention.

MULTIPLE MYELOMA
Epidemiology

MM, with 15,000 new cases annually in the US, accounts for 1% of all malignant diseases and 15% of the LH malignancies that are relevant to this chapter. Its annual incidence is about twice that for HD. Less than 2% of MM occurs in patients younger than 40 years old, and the peak incidence occurs in patients 70 to 80 years old. Rates in non-whites are twice those of whites. Prior to 1949, it was classified as a bone tumor. In the US and other industrialized countries, there has been a striking increase in the age-standardized incidence over the past three to four decades.[32] Although some investigators maintain that this increase is attributable to diagnostic bias, it also is compatible with and suggestive of environmental and occupational factors as etiologic agents for MM. Ionizing radiation and occupational benzene exposure are well linked to increased myeloma risk and are discussed later. Excess risks, mostly less than twofold, also have been reported for petroleum refinery and petrochemical workers, farmers, woodworkers, food workers, printers, and those exposed to arsenic, lead, cutting oils, pesticides, and paint-related compounds.[31]

Clinical presentation

The clinical presentation of patients with occupation-related MM is no different than in de-novo cases.

Diagnosis, prognosis, and treatment

The classic diagnostic triad is marrow plasmacytosis (>10%), lytic bone lesions, and a monoclonal immunoglobulin spike in serum or urine.

Although 10% of patients have an indolent and very slowly progressive course, the vast majority require both chemotherapy for the myeloma and supportive care for complications such as hypercalcemia, renal failure, infections, and anemia.

Fifteen percent of patients die within 3 months of diagnosis, with a subsequent death rate of about 15% per year. Typically, there is a 2- to 5-year chronic course before refractory cytopenias and associated complications develop. Five percent of patients die with acute leukemia; whether this finding might represent an interaction with some of the common (leukemogenic) etiologic agents is unknown.

Screening

There is no screening relevant to the occupational setting.

MYELOPROLIFERATIVE DISORDERS

Myeloproliferative disorders are neoplastic disorders of the multipotent hematopoietic stem cell. Included are CML, polycythemia vera, essential thrombocytosis, agnogenic myeloid metaplasia with myelofibrosis, paroxysmal nocturnal hemoglobinuria (PNH), and, for purposes of this discussion, myelodysplastic syndrome, frequently called preleukemia or smoldering leukemia. Other than CML and myelodysplastic syndrome, the diseases run a prolonged

course over many years. We discuss CML, myelofibrosis, and polycythemia vera in detail because of relatively stronger links to environmental agents, although environmental and occupational causes of these disorders are not well studied. Myelodysplastic syndrome may be considered to have the same etiologic risk factors as AML (see also Chapter 21).

Chronic myelogenous leukemia

Epidemiology

Ionizing radiation exposure is clearly linked to the development of CML[33] and benzene is linked to CML but slightly less clearly than it is to AML.[34] Rubber workers and electrical workers have been found to be at increased risk for this particular malignant phenotype,[35-37] electrical workers perhaps due to non-ionizing radiation exposure. The incidence of CML is roughly comparable to that for AML during the first five decades (about 50/100,000) and then doubles after age 60, as opposed to AML, which increases over sixfold.[38]

Clinical features

CML is clinically characterized by an accumulation of both immature and mature granulocytic cells, leading to suppression of normal myelopoiesis and erythropoiesis. Twenty percent of cases are diagnosed by an elevated white blood cell (WBC) count in the absence of symptoms. Lymphadenopathy is rare. CML is characterized in 90% of cases by the well-known cytogenetic marker, the Philadelphia chromosome, resulting from a reciprocal translocation between the long arms of chromosomes 22 and 9. The breakpoints are near the proto-oncogenes, c-*sis* on 22 and c-*abl* on 9. Although this abnormality persists in all phases of the illness, the blastic phase usually is characterized by additional chromosome abnormalities, including aneuploidy, reflecting the more malignant character of this phase.[39]

Diagnosis, prognosis, and treatment

The high WBC count, marrow aspirate with a Philadelphia chromosome, and depressed leukocyte alkaline phosphatase activity are all considered diagnostic hallmarks of CML. Therapy for the chronic phase usually includes moderate doses of alkylating agents, most commonly busulfan, whose most serious complication is prolonged myelosuppression. Transplant approaches have been added over the past decade.[40]

Screening

No screening measures are applicable.

Myelofibrosis with myeloid metaplasia

Epidemiology

Myelofibrosis with myeloid metaplasia (agnogenic myeloid metaplasia) is another clonal stem cell disorder resulting in marrow fibrosis in association with proliferation of granulocytes, erythrocyte precursors, and megakaryocytes in extramedullary sites. The incidence appears to increase in individuals with prior ionizing radiation exposure (including radioactive phosphorus [^{32}P]-treated polycythemia vera) and has been reported to occur with benzene exposure[41]

Clinical features

Myelofibrosis usually is associated with constitutional symptoms and anemia (over 50% of patients are anemic at diagnosis), with virtually all patients developing anemia at some time during the course of the disease, due to decreased erythropoiesis, splenic pooling, and shortened red blood cell survival. High WBC counts are common, leading to a difficulty in differentiating this condition from CML, in which 10% to 15% of patients also may have marrow fibrosis.

Diagnosis, treatment, and prognosis

Bone marrow biopsy is required. Polycythemia vera and CML are the major considerations in the differential diagnosis. No therapy has been demonstrated to prolong life, but androgens have been used for anemia, myelosuppressive therapy for marked splenomegaly or thrombocytosis, and allopurinol to control hyperuricemia from tissue breakdown. The natural history is prolonged, with a median survival rate of 5 years from diagnosis. One-quarter of patients live 15 years after diagnosis.[42]

Polycythemia vera

Epidemiology

Polycythemia vera is characterized by elevated hemoglobin levels in a setting of increased production of all marrow cell lines. Splenomegaly is common. It is a disease of adults, with a slight male predominance and no known familial aggregation. Information on occupational or environmental etiology is lacking. However, because this is a clonal myeloproliferative disorder, often associated with chromosomal abnormalities, myelotoxic factors may well be operative.

Clinical features

No differences have been found in cases suspected to be caused by environmental factors versus those arising de novo.

Diagnosis, prognosis, and treatment

The diagnosis, prognosis, and treatment are independent of etiologic consideration. In cases treated with myelosuppressive agents or ^{32}P, cytogenetic abnormalities may increase from the approximately 10% rate reported for untreated patients.

Screening

No screening measures are applicable.

CHRONIC LYMPHOCYTIC LEUKEMIA

This disease of later life, characterized by high circulating levels of mature-looking lymphocytes, is actually a variant of well-differentiated NHL. Generally, it has a favorable prognosis and often requires no specific therapy. Although some environmental associations have been noted, this disorder has not been convincingly linked to any myelotoxic agent. Notably, sufficient data exist to rule out an association with ionizing radiation, at least in Japanese and perhaps other Asian populations, based on data from the atomic bomb.

OCCUPATIONAL AND ENVIRONMENTAL RISK FACTORS FOR LYMPHOHEMATOPOIETIC MALIGNANCIES

There are four well-accepted risk factors for LH malignancies:
- ionizing radiation;
- benzene inhalation;
- agricultural work; and
- cytotoxic and immunosuppressive drugs.

Less clear-cut evidence is suggestive of an association between LH malignancies and certain non-agricultural occupations, exposure to electromagnetic fields (one type of non-ionizing radiation), and exposure to solvents, notably trichloroethylene (TCE) in drinking water. We consider each in turn.

Known causes

Ionizing radiation (Table 30.2.2)

The importance of ionizing radiation as an etiologic agent for LH malignancies has been known since the early part of this century from studies of radiologists. The most compelling evidence for this association has come from studies of survivors of the atomic bomb blasts in Hiroshima and Nagasaki and patients treated for ankylosing spondylitis. For both of these types of exposures, leukemias (other than CLL) were noted as early as 3 years after exposure, with peak incidence occurring 5 to 10 years after exposure, and additional excess cases were still being diagnosed for three decades after.

There also is limited evidence for leukemia risk for occupational exposure to ionizing radiation. Studies of military personnel on maneuvers at a nuclear bomb test showed statistically elevated leukemia incidence and mortality, as do the most recent studies of workers at nuclear facilities. A review and pooled analysis of nuclear worker studies conducted by the International Agency for Research on Cancer[43] found statistically significant excesses for leukemia and MM in more than one study of individual facilities. Their pooled analysis found statistically significant excess relative risks for leukemia excluding CLL and

Risk factor	Specific exposure	Comments	Reference
Ionizing radiation	Radiologists	Radiologist RR ~ 10 for leukemias, relative to other physicians	March, 1944[83]
	Atomic bomb blasts	Noted a positive response for leukemias	Beebe et al., 1978[87]
	Treatment for ankylosing spondylitis	Peak leukemia incidence 5 years after first course of treatment	Court Brown & Doll, 1965[68]
	Nuclear bomb test workers	RR ~ 2.5 for leukemias	Caldwell et al., 1983[88]
	Nuclear facility workers	SMR ~ 1.6 for leukemias	Cardis et al., 1995[43]
	Naval shipyard workers	RR ~ 2–6 for leukemias	Stern et al., 1986[89]
	Bomb test fallout	RR < 2; children's OR elevated for ALL	Stevens et al., 1990[90]; Archer, 1987[91]
	Ingestion of radium-containing water	Local ecologic study; SIR ~ 1.5 for leukemias	Lyman et al., 1985[48]; O'Brien et al., 1987[92]
	Ingestion of radium-containing water	Broad ecologic study; no association found	Cohen, 1991[93]
	Paternal occupation in nuclear facility	RR ~ 2–6	Gardner et al., 1990[52]
Non-ionizing radiation	Residential magnetic fields	RR ~ 2–3	Wartenberg, 2001[76]; Ahlbom et al., 2000[77]; Greenland et al., 2000[78]
	Occupational magnetic fields	Risk varies by occupation	Savitz & Loomis, 1995[71]; Floderus et al., 1993[72]; Theriault et al., 1994[15]

RR, relative risk; SIR, standardized incidence ratio; SMR, standardized mortality ratio.

Table 30.2.2 Selected studies demonstrating the association between radiation exposure and lymphohematopoietic malignancies

for MM. The leukemia effect was consistent with, but smaller than, values estimated from the studies of atomic bomb survivors reported in the BEIR V report from the National Research Council.[44] All LH neoplasms studied in this Japanese population reveal a high incidence following radiation exposure, with the notable exception of CLL. The absence of positive data on this neoplasm from the atomic bomb data makes it one of the rare proven negative findings that can be asserted in environmental epidemiologic causation, or perhaps an indication that Japanese individuals are not susceptible for presumably genetic reasons.

No safe threshold has been demonstrated, but direct evidence for radiation carcinogenesis has been derived almost entirely from studies of single high doses in excess of 50 rads. The case–control study with the best dosimetry for diagnostic X-ray exposure showed no increased risk for leukemia at highly fractionated doses up to 300 rads,[45] although two earlier questionnaire studies did show an increased risk.[46,47]

Another suggested environmental cause of leukemia is ingestion of radium-containing groun dwater. One study that generated this hypothesis noted the geographic overlap of counties in Florida with both relatively high radium concentrations in the groun dwater and relatively high leukemia incidence rates.[48] This observation is ecologic and particularly subject to confounding, which could explain the findings. Suggestive but not clear-cut results have followed in subsequent studies.[49,50]

Several studies have investigated the possible association between inhaled radon exposure and leukemia. The suggested mechanism is that radon inhalation may result in a small amount of irradiation to the bone marrow that could lead to leukemia. A recent weight-of-evidence review of 19 ecologic studies, six miner cohort studies, and eight

case–control studies concluded that while an ecologic association exists, it is not supported by the other studies and is unlikely to be etiologic.[51]

One unanticipated occupational risk for leukemia has been suggested by studies of a local cancer excess (cluster) near a nuclear plant in England. After adjusting for antenatal X-ray exposure, Gardner and associates found an association between childhood leukemia risk and paternal occupation in the nuclear plant, the risk increasing with larger cumulative paternal exposure.[52] Although no such preconception risk was noted for survivors of the Hiroshima and Nagasaki atomic bomb blasts, the authors note that exposure to radiation from these atomic bombs was instantaneous, whereas that for workers is accumulated over many years. Laboratory studies of mice show similar paternal heritability of increased tumor risk, including tumors of the lung and lymphocytic leukemia.

An alternative explanation involving an infectious etiology has been proposed for this and related clusters. Kinlen and colleagues have suggested that the children in this community might have been at higher than normal risk because they were resident in an isolated, rural town without frequent exposure to infectious agents that are common among children in less isolated locales, impeding the establishment of herd immunity.[53–55] Mixing with populations from more urban areas, with wider exposure to viral agents, resulted in increased contacts between susceptible and infected individuals, promoting epidemics of underlying infections. Then, if the populations were large enough, these infectious epidemics could have resulted in extra cases of leukemia, an extremely rare response to a common and widespread infection. Regions with high population densities would be more likely to have established herd immunity, thereby preventing the infectious epidemics and subsequent leukemias. Many subsequent ecologic studies in other communities are consistent with this hypothesis.

Greaves developed a related hypothesis proposing an infectious etiology for childhood ALL, suggesting that children were at greater risk if they lived in more affluent areas because with greater affluence came more effective hygiene and thus reduced exposure to infectious agents in earliest childhood.[56–58] Like Kinlen, he argued that for susceptible children, in this case affluent, early childhood exposure to infectious agents underlay a substantial number of childhood leukemia cases. The Greaves hypothesis suggests that the increased risk is due to decreased immune responsiveness and thus exposure to any or many infectious agents would confer similar risk.[56–58] More detailed studies and identification of specific infectious agents are needed for confirmation of any of these competing hypotheses.

Benzene (Table 30.2.3)

Benzene is the best-recognized chemical leukemogen in the workplace and environment. Benzene's profound abilities to depress marrow function were recognized around the turn of the last century and actually led to its unsuccessful use as an antileukemic agent, persisting into the 1930s.

Based on series of cases observed from the 1940s through the 1960s, Italian and Turkish hematologists suggested that there may be a relationship between acute leukemia and occupational exposure to benzene-based inks and glues in the rotogravure printing and shoemaking industries, respectively.[59–61] Exposures were not well quantified, but both industries are known to have resulted in substantial numbers of cases of marrow depression as well, implying substantial exposure.

In the late 1970s and 1980s, cohort studies began to emerge, focusing on industrial rubber workers, refinery workers, and chemical workers. The most convincing and widely cited study involves a cohort of about 1200 rubber workers,[62] who at the most recent follow-up had nine cases of myelogenous leukemia, compared with 2.7 expected.[7] Clearly, the issue concerning the use of benzene now is not

whether it is a cause of leukemia but rather what level of risk accompanies a given level of exposure.

Under a US Supreme Court requirement to show the magnitude of the effect of a reduction in the Occupational Safety and Health Administration (OSHA) benzene PEL from 10 ppm to 1 ppm, the National Institute for Occupational Safety and Health (NIOSH) performed a quantitative risk assessment on the previously described group of rubber workers.[63] A dose–response was noted, including the projection that even 1 ppm of exposure for 40 years would lead to a 70% increase in leukemia risk (95% confidence interval [CI], 1.1–2.5). More recent observations of a large benzene-exposed cohort of Chinese workers from multiple industries seems to confirm this projection and suggests increased risk even below the 40 ppm-year cumulative level.[7] Epidemiologic evidence from relatively low-dose occupations, such as service station attendants and auto mechanics, has suggested a relationship of benzene with leukemia, but the evidence is not regarded as conclusive.[64] Beyond aplastic anemia and AML, there are varying levels of evidence supporting a role for benzene in the causation of numerous other LH malignancies, which are summarized in Table 30.2.3.

Agricultural exposures

A large amount of epidemiologic literature addresses the incidence of LH neoplasms in farmers and in children exposed to pesticides.[65,66] These studies partially overlap those of other agricultural workers, such as lumberjacks, forestry workers, wood mill workers, meat packers, and ranchers of poultry and cattle. Although various studies report excesses of leukemias, myelomas, HD, and NHL, there are discrepancies between well-studied geographic areas.[67] Technically rigorous studies have reported high rates of NHL in agricultural workers exposed to phenoxyacetic acid herbicides, chlorophenols (e.g., 2,4,5-T and 2,4-D), or both in the US, Canada, and Sweden since 1977. However, other reliable studies from New Zealand have repeatedly failed to find these associations. A possible interpretation of the discrepancy is the role of various confounding factors such as co-carcinogens and oncogenes in the various populations, although no specific explanation has been documented. A reasonable conclusion at this time is that NHL is probably causally associated with exposure to the herbicides listed above; HD, MM, and leukemias cannot be linked specifically to herbicides, although the higher occupational incidence among agricultural workers as a whole is clear. Hopefully unresolved questions will emerge from ongoing NCI/NIOSH studies of agricultural health.

Medical exposures

Although not strictly occupational or environmental, LH malignancies due to medical therapy provide a critical context for consideration of broader causes, both epidemiologically and mechanistically. CLL is the only LH malignancy (and one of only a handful of cancers) whose risk is not increased by therapeutic levels of ionizing radiation, at least not in the Japanese population.

Known

Pancytopenia: aplastic anemia[94]
Acute myelogenous leukemia and variants[7,63,95]

Suspected

Chronic myelogenous leukemia[7,61]
Chronic lymphocytic leukemia[7,36,37,60,80]
Paroxysmal nocturnal hemoglobinuria[60]
Multiple myeloma[7,96]

Reported

Acute lymphoblastic leukemia[59]
Myelofibrosis and myeloid metaplasia[97]
Non-Hodgkin's disease[98]
Thrombocythemia[97]

Table 30.2.3 Causal relation between benzene exposure and various hematologic disorders

The classic cohort[68] of 14,558 young men who were therapeutically irradiated for ankylosing spondylitis in the 1930s showed 52 leukemias versus 5.5 expected, with the risk cresting at 4 to 5 years and diminishing 8 to 9 years after exposure.

Cytotoxic drugs Alkylating agents and, to a lesser extent, antimetabolite therapy significantly increase the risk for AML, often with the identifiable 5q- or 7q- markers, and myelodysplastic syndrome. More specific immunosuppressive therapies preferentially promote NHL, with the relative risk (RR) estimated at 40- to 100-fold.[29] There is substantial cross-over of LH malignancy phenotype between the different classes of agents in spite of the useful distinction. Although there has been interest in the effects of cytotoxic agents on nurses, pharmacists, and others who are occupationally exposed, evidence of biologic effects has not been proved.[69] Nonetheless, rigid precautions to limit exposures are well justified by the risk in medically exposed individuals.[70]

Suspect causes

Non-ionizing radiation

Concern also has been raised over the leukemia incidence among workers exposed to electric and magnetic fields (EMF).[15,71,72] The risk was first documented in a case–control study of children living in homes with high magnetic fields, but, as yet, no mechanism for this risk has been established. Prompted by population-based studies, a series of occupational mortality studies have shown that workers in electrical, electronic, and telecommunications occupations and ham radio operators are at increased risk for ALL, AML, CML, and CLL. Because no viable mechanism has been postulated, there is much controversy over the definition of relevant exposure, although magnetic fields rather than electrical fields are implicated. Exposure metrics under consideration include peak, average, time-weighted average, and variability measures, although the data from different studies are contradictory (see Chapter 33.2).

Two recent expert panel reviews of the EMF issue were conducted in the US.[73,74] The first,[73] under the sponsorship of the National Academy of Sciences, using a consensus process, reported that 'no conclusive and consistent evidence shows that exposures to residential electric and magnetic fields produce cancer', but also asserted that 'an association between residential wiring configurations... and childhood leukemia persists in multiple studies...'. Interpretations of these statements varied. The second panel,[74] convened by the National Institute of Environmental Health Sciences, using a majority rule process, concluded that 'Extremely low frequency (ELF) EMF are possibly carcinogenic to humans (Group 2B)'. This was based principally on 'the results of studies on childhood leukemia in residential environments and on CLL [chronic lymphocytic leukemia] in adults in occupational settings'. In addition, the participants

stated that the in-vitro and mechanistic data provide weak support based on studies at very high levels of exposures (>100 uT).

To summarize this body of literature analytically, a variety of meta-analyses and pooled analyses were conducted. The most recent meta-analyses[75,76] reported that the risk for childhood brain tumors was elevated, although not statistically significant, while the risk for leukemia was elevated and marginally statistically significant, particularly at the higher exposure cut points. There was some evidence that supported an exposure–response gradient. The two pooled analyses of childhood leukemia[77,78] reported no overall effect but, again, elevated risks at the highest exposure categories.

In sum, there still is much controversy over whether exposure to EMFs causes cancer. The strongest and most consistent adverse effect data from EMF exposure are found for childhood leukemia. Although the most common childhood cancer, this is a very rare disease, with an incidence rate of approximately 1.5/100,000. If EMFs are carcinogenic, the excess risk suggested by the combined studies for exposures four times greater than background are in the range 50%–100%. However, there is added concern because exposures are ubiquitous, and rare high residential exposures can be greater than 50 times background while rare high occupational exposures, although typically only short term, can reach 1000 to 40,000 times background.

Asbestos

Beginning in the 1960s, case reports and case series have linked individuals with asbestosis to various immune disorders, both malignant and non-malignant. Clinical epidemiologic studies have linked asbestos exposure and asbestosis to increased prevalences of rheumatoid factor and other indices of immune activation and regulation. Exposure has been linked to NHL, CLL, and acute leukemias, although data are inconsistent and limited (for a review, see Becker et al.[79]). This remains an intriguing area for further investigation, possibly directed at co-factors necessary for an effect to emerge.

Rubber industry and other occupations

Rubber industry workers have been reported to have increased risks for AML, CML, and MM.[80] The extent to which this factor is independent of benzene exposure has not been definitively worked out due to the complexities of characterization of lifelong retrospective exposure. In this regard, the carcinogenic monomer 1,3 butadiene (see Chapter 41) may be an independent risk factor, although this is not clearly demonstrated.[81,82]

Chemical workers, machinists, and painters have been reported to have an increased incidence of LH malignancies and, in some cases, to have increased chromosomal abnormalities.[18,83,84] Especially noteworthy is the suspected relationship between ethylene oxide and AML (see Chapter 40 and Steenland and associates[85]). Although the evidence is not as clear cut as for benzene or radiation exposure, risks have been demonstrated in various settings and some of the inconsistencies could be explained by exposure misclassification as well as by the more commonly posited causal relationships. Confounding benzene exposures are frequently a problem in the interpretation of this literature based on historical chemical exposures.

Trichloroethylene and other solvent exposures

Several solvents have been investigated for possible carcinogenicity. TCE is an organic chemical that has been used in dry cleaning, for metal degreasing, and as a solvent for oils and resins. It has been shown to cause liver and kidney cancer in experimental animals. Evidence of excess cancer rates among occupational cohorts with the most rigorous exposure assessment is found for kidney cancer (relative risk [RR] = 1.7; 95% CI, 1.1–2.7), liver cancer (RR = 1.9; 95% CI, 1.0–3.4), and NHL (RR = 1.5; 95% CI, 0.9–2.3), as well as for cervical cancer, HD, and MM.[65] However, since few studies isolate TCE exposure, results are likely confounded by exposure to other solvents and other risk factors. Several studies of communities whose drinking water is contaminated with solvents including TCE show excess rates of leukemia and a few show excess NHL.

References

1. Linet MS. The leukemias: epidemiologic aspects. New York: Oxford University Press; 1985.
2. Tsongas TA. Occupational factors in the epidemiology of chemically induced lymphoid and hemopoietic cancers. In: Irons RD, ed. Toxicology of the blood and bone marrow. New York: Raven Press; 1985:149-77.
3. Goldstein BD, Kipen HM. Cancer secondary to chemotherapy. In: Witmer CM, Snyder RR, Jollow DJ, et al., eds. Biologic reactive intermediates IV: molecular and cellular effects and their impact on human health. New York: Plenum Press; 1991:619-25.
4. Linet MS, Cartwright RA. The leukemias. In: Schottenfeld D, Fraumeni FR Jr, eds. Cancer epidemiology and prevention. New York: Oxford University Press; 1996:841-92.
5. Mueller NE. Hodgkin's disease. In: Schottenfeld D, Fraumeni FR Jr, eds. Cancer epidemiology and prevention. New York: Oxford University Press; 1996:893-919.
6. Scherr PA, Mueller NE. Non-Hodgkin's lymphomas. In: Schottenfeld D, Fraumeni FR Jr, eds. Cancer epidemiology and prevention. New York: Oxford University Press; 1996: 920-45.
7. Hayes R, Songnian Y, Dosemeci M, et al. Benzene and lymphohematopoietic malignancies in humans. Am J Ind Med 2001; 40:117-26.
8. Fagioli F. Distinct cytogenetic and clinicopathologic features in acute myeloid leukemia after occupational exposure to pesticides and organic solvents. Cancer 1992; 70:77-85.
9. Dann EJ, Rowe JM. Biology and therapy of secondary leukemias. Best Pract Res Clin Haematol 2001; 14:119-37.
10. Crane MM, Keating MJ, Trujillo JM, et al. Environmental exposures in cytogenetically defined subsets of acute nonlymphocytic leukemia [published erratum appears in JAMA 1990; 263:662]. JAMA 1989; 262:634-9.
11. Rodella S, Ciccone G. Cytogenetics and occupational exposures in acute nonlymphocytic leukemia and myelodysplastic syndrome. Scand J Work Environ Health 1993; 19:369-74.
12. West RR. Cytogenetic abnormalities in the myelodysplastic syndromes and occupational or environmental exposure. Blood 2000; 95:2093-7.
13. Matanoski GM, Stockwell HG, Diamond EL, et al. A cohort mortality study of painters and allied tradesmen. Scand J Work Environ Health 1986; 12:16-21.
14. Tates AD. Biologic effect monitoring in industrial workers following incidental exposure to high concentrations of ethylene oxide. Mutat Res 1995; 329:63-77.
15. Theriault GP, Goldberg M, Miller AB, et al. Cancer risks associated with occupational exposure to magnetic fields among electric utility workers in Ontario and Quebec, Canada, and France: 1970-1989 [published erratum appears in Am J Epidemiol 1994; 139:1053]. Am J Epidemiol 1994; 139:550-72.
16. Dellarco VL, Generoso WM, Sega GA, et al. Review of the mutagenicity of ethylene oxide. Environ Mol Mutagen 1990; 16:85-103.
17. Zhang L. The nature of chromosomal aberrations detected in humans exposed to benzene. Crit Rev Toxicol 2002; 32: 1-42.
18. Blair A, Zheng T, Linos A, et al. Occupation and leukemia: a population-based case-study in Iowa and Minnesota. Am J Ind Med 2000; 40:3-14.
19. Willman CL. Molecular evaluation of acute myeloid leukemias. Semin Hematol 1999; 36:390-400.
20. Crane MM, Strom SS, Halabi S, et al. Correlation between selected environmental exposures and karyotype in acute myelocytic leukemia. Cancer Epidemiol Biomarkers Prev 1996; 5:639-44.
21. Perera FP. Molecular epidemiology: on the path to prevention? J Natl Cancer Inst 2000; 92:602-12.
22. Colt JS, Blair S. Parental occupational exposures and risk of childhood cancer. Envrion Health Perspect 1998; 106(Suppl):909-25.
23. Freedman DM, Stewart P, Kleinerman RA, et al. Household solvent exposures and childhood acute lymphoblastic leukemia. Am J Public Health 2001; 91:564-7.
24. Mayer J, Warburton D, Jeffrey AM, et al. Biologic markers in ethylene oxide-exposed workers and controls. Mutat Res 1991; 248:163-76.
25. Jaffe ES, Raffeld M, Medeiros LJ, et al. An overview of the classifications of non-Hodgkin's lymphomas: an integration of morphological and phenotypical concepts. Cancer Res 1992; 52(Suppl):5447s-5452s.
26. Hartge P, Devesa SS. Quantification of the impact of known risk factors on time trends in non-Hodgkin's lymphoma incidence. Cancer Res 1992; 52(Suppl): 5566s-5569s.
27. Ferreira OC Jr, Planelles V, Rosenblatt JD. Human T-cell leukemia viruses: epidemiology, biology and pathogenesis. Blood Rev 1997; 111:91-104.
28. Blattner WA. Human retroviruses: their role in cancer. Proc Assoc Am Physicians 1999; 111:563-72.
29. Beral V, Newton R. Overview of the epidemiology of immunodeficiency-associated cancers. J Natl Cancer Inst Monogr 1998; 23:1-6.
30. Baris D, Zahm SH. Epidemiology of lymphomas. Curr Opin Oncol 2000; 12:383-94.
31. Morales Suarez-Varela MM, Llopis Gonzalez A, Marquina Vila A, et al. Mycosis fungoides: review of epidemiological observations. Dermatology 2000; 201:21-8.
32. Davis DL, Hoel D, Fox J, et al. International trends in cancer mortality in France, West Germany, Italy, Japan, England, Wales, and the USA. Lancet 1990; 336:474-81.
33. Aguiar RC. Therapy-related chronic myeloid leukemia: an epidemiological, clinical and pathogenetic appraisal [published erratum appears in Leuk Lymphoma 1998; 30:665]. Leuk Lymphoma 1998; 29:17-26.
34. McDevitt JJ, Lees PS, McDiarmid MA. Exposure of hospital pharmacists and nurses to antineoplastic agents. J Occup Med 1993; 35:57-60.

35. McMichael AJ. Carcinogenicity of benzene, toluene and xylene: epidemiological and experimental evidence. IARC Sci Pub 1988; 85:3-18.

36. McMichael AJ, Spirtas R, Gamble JF, et al. Mortality among rubber workers: relationship to specific jobs. J Occup Med 1976; 18:178-85.

37. McMichael AJ, Spirtas R, Kupper LL. An epidemiologic study of mortality within a cohort of rubber workers. J Occup Med 1974; 16:458-64.

38. Finch SC, Linet MS. Chronic leukemia. Baillière's Clin Haematol 1992; 5:27-56.

39. Chase A, Huntly BJ, Cross NC. Cytogenetics of chronic myeloid leukemia. Best Pract Res Clin Haematol 2001; 14: 553-71.

40. Faderl S, Kantarjian HM, Talpaz M, et al. New treatment approaches for chronic myelogenous leukemia. Semin Oncol 2000; 27:578-86.

41. Tondel M, Persson B, Cartensen J. Myelofibrosis and benzene exposure. Occup Med (Lond) 1995; 45:51-2.

42. Bench AJ, Cross NC, Huntly BJ, et al. Myeloproliferative disorders. Best Pract Res Clin Haematol 2001; 14:531-51.

43. Cardis E, Gilbert ES, Carpenter L, et al. Combined analysis of cancer mortality among nuclear industry workers in Canada, the United Kingdom and the United States of America. Lyons, France: International Agency for Research on Cancer; 1995.

44. National Research Council. Health effects of exposure to low levels of ionizing radiation – Beir V. National Research Council, Committee on the Biologic Effects of Ionizing Radiations, Board on Radiation Effects Research, and Commission on Life Sciences. Washington DC: National Academy Press; 1990.

45. Linos A, Gray JE, Orvis AL, et al. Low-dose radiation and leukemia. N Engl J Med 1980; 302:1101-5.

46. Stewart A, Pennybacker W, Barber R. Adult leukemia and diagnostic x-rays. BMJ 1962; 2:882-90.

47. Gibson R, Graham S, Lillienfeld A, et al. Irradiation in the epidemiology of leukemia among adults. J Natl Cancer Inst 1972; 48:301-11.

48. Lyman GH, Lyman CH, Johnson W. Association of leukemia with radium groun dwater contamination. JAMA 1985; 254:621-6.

49. Collman GW, Loomis DP, Sandler DP. Childhood cancer mortality and radon concentration in drinking water in North Carolina. Br J Cancer 1991; 63:626-9.

50. Fuortes L. Leukemia incidence and radioactivity in drinking water in 59 Iowa towns. Am J Public Health 1990; 80:1261-2.

51. Laurier D, Valenty M, Tirmarche M. Radon exposure and the risk of leukemia: a review of epidemiological studies. Health Phys 2001; 81:272-88.

52. Gardner MJ, Snee MP, Hall AJ, et al. Results of case-control study of leukaemia and lymphoma among young people near a Sellafield nuclear plant in West Cumbria. BMJ 1990; 300:423-9.

53. Kinlen L. Evidence for an infective cause of childhood leukemia: comparison of a Scottish new town with nuclear reprocessing sites in Britain. Lancet 1988; ii:1323-7.

54. Kinlen LJ, Dickson M, Stiller CA. Childhood leukaemia and non-Hodgkin's lymphoma near large rurual construction sites, with a comparison with Sellafield nuclear site. BMJ 1995; 310:763-8.

55. Kinlen L. Infection, childhood leukaemia and the Seascale cluster. Radiol Protect Bull 2000; 226:9-18.

56. Greaves MF. Speculations on the cause of childhood acute lymphoblastic leukemia. Leukemia 1988; 2:120-5.

57. Greaves MF, Alexander FE. An infectious etiology for common acute lymphoblastic leukemia in childhood? Leukemia 1993; 7:349-60.

58. Greaves MF. Childhood leukemia. BMJ 2002; 324:283-7.

59. Aksoy M, Erdem S, Dincol G. Types of leukaemia in a chronic benzene poisoning: a study in thiry-four patients. Acta Haematol 1976; 55:65-72.

60. Aksoy M. Different types of malignancies due to occupational exposure to benzene: a review of recent observations in Turkey. Environ Res 1980; 23:181-90.

61. Vigliani EC, Forni A. Benzene and leukemia. Environ Res 1976; 11:122-7.

62. Infante PF, Rinsky RA, Wagoner JK, et al. Leukaemia in benzene workers. Lancet 1977; 2:76-8.

63. Rinsky R, Smith A, Hornung R, et al. Benzene and leukemia – an epidemiologic risk assessment. N Engl J Med 1987; 316:1044-50.

64. Hotz P. Biologic monitoring of vehicle mechanics and other workers exposed to low concentrations of benzene. Int Arch Occup Environ Health 1997; 70:29-40.

65. Zahm SH. Pesticides and childhood cancer. Environ Health Perspect 1998; 106(Suppl):893-908.

66. Daniels JL. Pesticides and childhood cancers. Environ Health Perspect 1997; 105:1068-77.

67. Blair A, Zahm SH. Agricultural exposures and cancer. Environ Health Perspect 1995; 103(Suppl):205-8.

68. Court Brown WM, Doll R. Mortality from cancer and other causes after radiotherapy for ankylosing spondylitis. BMJ 1965; 2:1327-32.

69. Sessink PJ, Bos RP. Drugs hazardous to healthcare workers. Evaluation of methods of monitoring occupational exposure to cytostatic drugs. Drug Safety 1999; 20:347-59.

70. McCunney RJ. Hodgkin's disease, work and the environment. J Occup Environ Med 1999; 41:36-46.

71. Savitz DA, Loomis DP. Magnetic field exposure in relation to leukemia and brain cancer mortality among electric utility workers [published erratum appears in Am J Epidemiol 1996; 144:205] . Am J Epidemiol 1995; 141:123-34.

72. Floderus B, Persson T, Stenlund C, et al. Occupational exposure to electromagnetic fields in relation to leukemkia and brain tumors: a case-control study in Sweden. Cancer Causes Control 1993; 4:465-76.

73. National Research Council. Possible health effects of exposure to residential electric and magnetic fields. Committee on the possible effects of electromagnetic fields on biologic systems. Washington DC: National Academy Press; 1997:1-356.

74. Portier C, Wolfe M. NIEHS Working Group. Assessment of health effects from exposure to power-line frequency electric and magnetic fields. NIH Publication No. 98. Research Triangle Park, North Carolina: NIEHS, NIH, USDHHS, PHS; 1998:1-508.

75. Wartenberg D, Dietrich F, Goldberg R, et al. A meta-analysis of studies of childhood cancer and residential exposure to magnetic fields. A report to the National Institute of Environmental Health Sciences. 2002.

76. Wartenberg D. Residential EMF exposure and childhood leukemia: meta-analysis and population attributable risk. Bioelectricmagnetics 2001; Suppl 5:S86-S104.

77. Ahlbom A, Day N, Feychting M, et al. A pooled analysis of magnetic fields and childhood leukemia. Br J Cancer 2000; 83:692-8.

78. Greenland S, Sheppard AR, Kaune WT, et al. A pooled analysis of magnetic fields, wire codes and childhood leukemia. Epidemiology 2000; 11:624-34.

79. Becker N, Berger J, Bolm-Audorff U. Asbestos exposure and malignant lymphomas – a review of the epidemiological literature. Int Arch Occup Environ Health 2001; 74:459-69.

80. McMichael AJ, Spirtas R, Kupper LL, et al. Solvent exposure and leukemia among rubber workers: an epidemiologic study. J Occup Med 1975; 17:234-9.

81. Acquavella JF, Leonard RC. A review of the epidemiology of 1,3-butadiene and chloroprene. Chem Biol Interact 2001; 135-136:43-52.

82. Lemen RA, Meinhardt TJ, Crandall MS, et al. Environmental epidemiologic investigations in the styrene-butadiene rubber production industry. Environ Health Perspect 1990; 86:103-6.

83. March HC. Leukemia in radiologists. Radiology 1944; 43:275-8.

84. Lynge E, Antitila A, Hemminki K. Organic solvents and cancer. Cancer Causes Control 1997; 8:406-19.

85. Steenland K, Stayner L, Greife A, et al. Mortality among workers exposed to ethylene oxide. N Engl J Med 1991; 324:1402-7.

86. Ries LAG, Eisner MP, Kosary CL, et al., eds. SEER Cancer Statistics Review, 1973-1998. Bethesda, Maryland: National Cancer Institute; 2001.

87. Beebe GW, Kato H, Land CE. Studies of mortality of A-bomb survivors. VI. Mortality and radiation dose. Radiat Res 1978; 75:138-201.

88. Caldwell GG, Kelley D, Zack M, et al. Mortality and cancer frequency among military nuclear test (Smoky) participants, 1957 through 1979. JAMA 1983; 250:620-4.

89. Stern FB, Waxweiler RA, Beaumont JJ, et al. A case-control study of leukemia at a naval nuclear shipyard. Am J Epidemiol 1986; 123:980-92.

90. Stevens W, Thomas DC, Lyon JL, et al. Leukemia in Utah and radioactive fallout from the Nevada test site. JAMA 1990; 264:585-91.

91. Archer VE. Association of nuclear fallout with leukemia in the United States. Arch Environ Health 1987; 42:263-71.

92. O'Brien TR, Decoufle P, Rhodes PH. Leukemia and ground water contamination [letter to the editor]. JAMA 1987; 257:317.

93. Cohen BL. Radon exposure in homes and cancer [letter to the editor]. Lancet 1991; 337:790-1.

94. Aksoy O, Dincol K, Erdem S, et al. Details of blood changes in 32 patients with pancytopenia associated with long-term exposure to benzene. Br J Ind Med 1972; 29:56-64.

95. Rinsky RA, Smith AB, Young RJ. Leukemia in benzene workers. Am J Ind Med 1981; 2:217-45.

96. Goldstein B. Is exposure to benzene a cause of human multiple myeloma? Ann N Y Acad Sci 1990; 609:225-30.

97. Goldstein BD. Clinical hematotoxicity of benzene. In: Benzene: occupational and environmental hazards – scientific update. Princeton, New Jersey: Princeton Scientific; 1989:55-67.

98. Vianna NJ. Lymphomas and occupational benzene exposure. Lancet 1979; i:1394-5.

30.3 **Bladder Cancer**

Avima M Ruder, Tania Carreón, Elizabeth M Ward, Paul A Schulte, William Halperin

It is well documented that the etiology of bladder cancer involves environmental risk factors. Occupational risks may account for 21–27% of bladder cancers among men in the United States,[1,2] an estimated 40,000 cases in 2001,[3] and 11% among the estimated 15,000 cases in women in 2001.[3,4]

Occupational exposure to aromatic amines has been known to cause bladder cancer since Rehn identified the first few cases in workers in the new organic chemical industry in 1895.[5] Since that time, numerous occupations and specific substances have been associated with an increased risk of bladder cancer (Tables 30.3.1 and 30.3.2). Beyond the certainties that specific aromatic amines have been demonstrated to be human occupational bladder carcinogens and that a broad range of occupations are at risk of bladder cancer, a well-informed approach to the prevention and management of bladder cancer depends on appreciating various controversies involved in its primary and secondary prevention and treatment. The reader is referred to a report of a national conference held in 1989[6] to delineate these issues. Many of these controversies, such as the relevance to human bladder cancer of findings from animal studies, the line between benign and malignant tumors, the appropriate screening regimen for workers exposed to bladder carcinogens, and whether early detection is worthwhile, remain relevant more than a decade later.

In addition to incidence and survival differences by social class, race, and gender,[7] new developments in understanding inherited risk factors, such as acetylator status and intermediate biomarkers, influence understanding of etiology, prevention and management.

ETIOLOGY
Epidemiology

Bladder cancer is the eighth most common neoplasm worldwide. An estimated 261,000 new cases of bladder cancer occur each year, with four-fifths of the cases occurring in men.[8] Incidence rates of bladder cancer vary about 10-fold, with higher rates in Western Europe and North America, and lower rates in Eastern Europe and several Asian countries.[9]

Cigarette smoking accounts for 47% of bladder cancer among men and 37% among women; smokers have twice the risk of non-smokers.[3] The contributions of coffee drinking and alcohol consumption to bladder cancer are equivocal. The World Health Organization estimates that bladder cancer cases can be subdivided into two broad categories based on etiology. (1) Those caused by tobacco and industrial carcinogens are predominantly transitional cell carcinomas and are common in industrialized countries. (2) Those due to bilharzia, human papilloma virus, and schistosomiasis infection[10,11] are more likely to be squamous cell carcinomas and are found chiefly in subtropical

and tropical countries. Thus, both types are, in principle, preventable.[12]

Bladder cancer is historically the neoplastic disease most strongly linked to occupational exposure to chemicals. Several occupations have been suspected to increase the risk of bladder cancer, but strong associations only exist for dye workers, aromatic amine manufacturing workers, leather workers, rubber workers, painters, truck drivers, and aluminum workers.[13] Table 30.3.1 presents the epidemiologic studies of occupational associations. Occupational exposures to chemicals such as arylamines, polycyclic aromatic hydrocarbons and other industry-related agents may explain some of the risk associated with these occupations.[14] Some of the relative risks for exposed workers are substantially higher than the two-fold increased risk for smokers. Table 30.3.2 includes specific chemicals or processes classified by IARC as carcinogenic to the human or canine bladder, combined with data on working populations potentially at risk. Over 200 chemicals have been confirmed as rodent bladder carcinogens; however, rodent bioassays do not appear to be a good model for human bladder cancer[15] (see 'Animal studies' section below).

A relationship between bladder cancer and exposure to chemical dyes was first established in 1895.[5] In the late 1930s, oral administration of the industrial arylamine 2-naphthylamine was shown to induce bladder cancer in dogs.[16] In 1954, Case et al. reported a 20-fold excess of bladder cancer in arylamine-exposed individuals, compared to the general population of England and Wales.[17] Since then, the most investigated bladder carcinogens have been 2-naphthylamine, benzidine, and 4-aminobiphenyl. Several studies have reported increased risks of bladder cancer in workers exposed to 2-naphthylamine and 4-aminobiphenyl, and have been reviewed elsewhere.[18]

One newly recognized factor that may have an occupational component is fluid intake. In a study of about 50,000 men, it was observed that drinking more fluids was associated with a significantly decreased rate of bladder cancer.[19] These results are consistent with the urogenous contact hypothesis, which proposed that the level of DNA adducts to 4-aminobiphenyl (a carcinogenic amine) could be decreased by increased fluid intake.[20,20a] Occupations that have exposure to carcinogens and limit the workers' ability to drink liquids could be at risk.

There is no known distinctive histologic feature for occupational bladder cancer. However, in some heavily exposed cohorts, cases regularly occur at ages 15 years younger than the median age at diagnosis of the general population,[17,21] in which the rate of bladder cancer increases substantially with age. Usually, the interval from first exposure to onset of symptoms is decades long; however, occupational cases have occurred surprisingly early after exposure, which substantiates the argument that cases with only a few years of latency may be occupationally induced. It has been estimated that the latency for chemically induced bladder cancer ranges from 4 to 45 years.[21,22]

Occupation /Industry	Study site, type, population	Increased morbidity relative risk	Increased mortality relative risk (95% CI)	Controlled for (95% CI)	Reference
Aluminum smelterers (10 yrs)	Canada, NCC, men	3.9 (1.6–9.6)*		smoking	Armstrong et al., 1986[58]
Armed services	Canada, CC, men	1.8 (1.2–2.7)			Howe et al., 1980[59]
Auto workers (>10 yrs)	US, CC, African–American men	4.7 (1.7–10.7)		age, smoking	Silverman et al., 1989[1]
Butchers	Sweden, CC, men	1.3 (1.0–1.6)			Malker et al., 1987[60]
Carpenters	US, CC, men	11.1 (3.3–37.0)		current smokers	Schumacher et al., 1989[61]
Carpenters	US, CC, white men	1.4 (1.1–1.8)		smoking	Silverman et al., 1989[2]
Chemical mfg. workers	UK, CC, men	2.2 (1.7–3.0)			Boyko et al., 1985[62]
Chemical mfg. workers	US, C, white men	2.6 (1.1–6.4)*		age	Schulte et al, 1985[63]
	US, C, African–American men	5.0 (2.2–11.3)*		age	
Chemical workers†	Sweden, CC, men	1.3 (1.1–1.5)			Malker et al., 1987[60]
Chemical workers	US, CC, white women	2.1 (0.9–5.1)*		smoking	Silverman et al., 1990[4]
Clerical workers	UK, CC, men	1.5 (1.1–1.9)			Cartwright, 1982[64]
Clerical workers	China, CR, men	1.3 (1.0–1.7)			Zheng et al., 1992[65]
Clerical workers (>10 yrs)	US, CC, African–American men	2.9 (1.2–6.2)		age, smoking	Silverman et al., 1989[1]
Construction workers	US, CC, white men	1.6 (1.1–2.5)*		smoking	Silverman et al., 1989[2]
Construction workers	US, C, Latino men		PMR 1.6 (0.9–2.8)		Schultz & Loomis, 2000[66]
Crafts workers	China, CR, women	1.2 (1.0–1.4)			Zheng et al., 1992[65]
Dental technicians	Sweden, CC, men	2.5 (1.3–4.3)			Malker et al., 1987[60]
Drivers	Argentina, CC, men	5.3 (2.3–12.2)			Iscovich et al., 1987[67]
Drivers	Denmark, CC	1.6 (1.1–2.3)*		sex, age, smoking	Jensen et al., 1987[68]
Drivers†	US, CC, white men	1.2 (1.1–1.4)*		smoking	Silverman et al., 1989[1,2]
Drivers, railroad	Germany, CC, men	3.0 (1.2–8.8)			Claude et al., 1988[69]
Drivers, taxi	US, CC, white men	6.3 (1.6–29.3)*		age, smoking	Silverman et al., 1986[87]
Drivers, truck	US, CC, white men	2.1 (1.4–4.4)*		age, smoking	Silverman et al., 1983[88]
Drivers, truck	Germany, CC, men	1.8 (1.1–2.8)*			Claude et al., 1988[69]
Drivers, truck	US, CC, white men	1.5 (1.1–2.0)		age, smoking	Silverman et al., 1986[87]
Drivers, truck	UK, CC, men		PMR 2.0 (P<0.05)		Baxter & McDowall, 1986[70]
Dry cleaners	US, CC, African–American men	2.8 (1.1–7.4)			Silverman et al., 1989[1]
Dry cleaners	US, C, African–American men		5.1 (1.4–13.1)	age	Ruder et al., 2001[71]
Dye mfg. workers	China, C, men	11.1 (3.6–25.9) 31.5 (20.4–46.4)	17.5 (7.5–34.5)	non-smokers smokers age	Bi et al, 1992[72]
Dye mfg. workers	UK, CC, men	3.5 (2.2–5.3)			Cartwright, 1982[64]
Dye mfg. workers	UK, CC, men	2.6 (1.8–3.7)		age, smoking	Boyko et al., 1985[62]
Dye mfg. workers	US, C, white men		5.2 (1.4–13.2)	age, exposure (azo dyes only)	Sathiakumar & Delzell, 2000[73]
Dyers, printers, textile ind.	US, CC, white men	4.4 (1.2–16.8)		smoking	Silverman et al., 1989[2]
Dye workers†	Canada, CC, men	4.1 (2.9–5.5)		latency ≥ 8 yrs	Risch et al., 1988[74]
Dye workers	Russia, C, men	3.9 (2.7–6.0)	2.8 (1.9–3.9)	age	Bulbulyan et al., 1995[75]
Dye workers	Russia, C, women	8.6 (4.6–80.0)	3.1 (1.5–5.7)	age	Bulbulyan et al., 1995[75]
Fabricators, assemblers, hand workers	US, C, African–American men		PMR 1.6 (0.9–2.9)		Schultz & Loomis, 2000[66]
Fabricators, etc.	US, Latino men		PMR 2.8 (1.0–7.9)		
Farm workers (field crops, vegetables)	Europe, CC, women	1.8 (1.0–3.1) *		age, smoking	't Mannetje et al., 1999[85]
Farm workers (nurseries)	Canada, CC, men	5.5 (1.2–51.1)			Howe et al., 1980[59]
Food counter workers	US, white men	2.6 (1.4–5.1)		age, smoking	Schoenberg et al., 1984[76]
Food counter workers	US, CC, white men	1.4 (0.9–2.1)*		smoking	Silverman et al., 1989[2]
Guards	Canada, CC, men	4.0 (1.3–16.4)			Howe et al., 1980[59]
Guards	Germany, CC, men	3.5 (1.2–9.9)*			Claude et al., 1988[69]
Janitors and cleaners	US, CC, white men	3.5 (1.6–7.7)		age, alcohol, smoking	Brownson et al., 1987[77]
Janitors	Germany, CC, men	3.5 (1.2–9.9)*			Claude et al., 1988[69]
Laborers in mfg. ind.	US, CC, white men	12.3 *			Silverman et al., 1989[2]
Laborers in metal ind.	US, African–American women		PMR 4.2 (1.1–16.8)		Schulz & Loomis, 2000[66]
Leatherworkers	US, CC, men	6.3 (3.1–11.3)*			Decoufle, 1979[78]
Leatherworkers	US, CC, women	4.4 (1.2–12.1)			Decoufle, 1979[78]
Lumber jacks	US, CC, white men	1.3 (1.0–1.5)*		smoking	Silverman et al., 1989[2]
Machine operators, tenders	US, C, Latino men		PMR 1.7 (1.0–3.1)		Schultz & Loomis, 2000[66]
Machinists	Sweden, CC, men	1.2 (1.1–1.3)			Malker et al., 1987[60]

Table 30.3.1 Occupations associated with increased risk of bladder cancer

Occupation /Industry	Study site, type, population	Increased morbidity relative risk	Increased mortality relative risk (95% CI)	Controlled for (95% CI)	Reference
Machinists, metal	Canada, CC, men	2.7 (1.1–7.6)			Howe et al., 1980[59]
Machinists†	US, CC, white men	1.3 (1.0–1.7)		smoking	Silverman et al., 1989[2]
Mail sorting clerks	Europe, CC, women	4.4 (1.0–19.5)		age, smoking	't Mannetje et al., 1999[85]
Mfg. workers	China, CR, women	1.2 (1.0–1.5)			Zheng et al., 1992[65]
Mfg. checkers, examiners, and inspectors	US, CC, white men	1.4 (1.1–1.8)*		smoking	Silverman et al., 1989[2]
Mfg. checkers	US, CC, white women	1.5 (1.0–2.3)		smoking	Silverman et al., 1990[4]
Mechanics	US, CC, white men	3.5 (1.4–9.1)		age, alcohol, smoking	Brownson et al., 1987[77]
Mechanics	Spain, CC, men	1.8 (1.2–2.7)		smoking, other jobs	Gonzalez et al., 1989[89]
Mechanics†	US, CC, white men	1.2 (1.0–1.4)		smoking	Silverman et al., 1989[2]
Mechanics, auto	US, CC, white men	10.2 (2.1–68.6)		smoking	Silverman et al., 1989[2]
Mechanics & repairers	US, C, Latino men		PMR 1.6 (0.7–3.7)		Schultz & Loomis, 2000[66]
Metal workers†	US, CC, white men	1.2 (1.0–1.4)		smoking	Silverman et al., 1989[2]
Metal workers	China, CR, men	1.4 (1.0–2.0)			Zheng et al., 1992[65]
Metal workers	Europe, CC, women	1.9 (1.1–3.6)*		age, smoking	't Mannetje et al., 1999[85]
Metal workers	US, women	1.4 (1.0–1.9)		smoking	Silverman et al., 1990[4]
Mining machine ops	US, CC, white men	2.9 (1.1–7.5)		age, alcohol, smoking	Brownson et al., 1987[77]
Mining workers	Germany, CC, men	2.0 (1.2–3.3)*			Claude et al., 1988[69]
Painters	Switzerland, C, men	1.7 (1.0–2.7)	2.1 (1.0–3.9)		Guberan et al., 1988[79]
Painters	Denmark, CC	2.5 (1.1–5.7)*		sex, age, smoking	Jensen et al., 1987[68]
Painters, artistic	US, CC, C, men	2.5 (1.1–5.7)*	PMR 3.5 (2.1–5.7)	smoking (incidence)	Miller et al., 1986[80]
Painters	US, CC, white men	1.5 (1.2–2.0)*		smoking	Silverman et al., 1989[2]
Painters	US, C, white men	1.2 (1.1–1.4)*		age	Steenland & Palu, 2000[81]
Paper pulp workers†	Sweden, CC, men	1.1 (1.0–1.3)			Malker et al., 1987[60]
Pesticide mfg. workers	Europe, C, men	35 (14–66)		smoking	Popp et al., 1992[82]
Petroleum processors†	US, CC, white men	2.4 (1.1–5.5)		smoking	Silverman et al., 1989[2]
Printers	Sweden, CC, men	1.2 (1.0–1.3)			Malker et al., 1987[60]
Printers	UK, CC, men	3.1 (1.4–6.8)			Cartwright, 1982[64]
Printers	US, CC, white men	2.1 (1.0–4.3)		smoking	Silverman et al., 1989[2]
Print machine operators	US, CC, white men	3.1 (1.1–8.9)		age, alcohol, smoking	Brownson et al., 1987[77]
Produce graders, packers	US, CC, white men	3.2 (1.1–9.3)		smoking, educ.	Silverman et al., 1989[2]
Precision prod. workers	US, C, African–American women		PMR 1.8 (1.0–3.3)		Schultz & Loomis, 2000[66]
Professional specialists	US, C, African–American men		PMR 1.4 (1.0–1.9)		Schultz & Loomis, 2000[66]
Rubber & plastics workers	China, CR, men	2.1 (1.2–3.4)			Zheng et al., 1992[65]
Rubber additive workers†	US, C	3.6 (1.9–6.3)			Ward et al., 1991[90]
Rubber processing workers	US, CC, white women	4.5 (1.1–21.9)		smoking	Silverman et al., 1990[4]
Salespeople	US, C, Asian men		PMR 2.1 (0.8–5.6)		Schultz & Loomis, 2000[66]
Salespeople, service, construction industries	US, CC, white men	2.2 (1.2–4.1)*		smoking	Silverman et al., 1989[2]
Salespeople	US, CC, white women	2.5 (1.0–6.0)*		smoking	Silverman et al., 1990[4]
Salespeople	Europe, CC, women	2.6 (1.0–6.9) 4.8 (1.2–18.7) (≥ 10 yrs)		age, smoking	't Mannetje et al., 1999[85]
Services, personal	US, Asian women		PMR 5.3 (1.6–16.8)		Schulz & Loomis, 2000[66]
Switchboard ops (> 10 yrs)	Europe, CC, women	8.1 (2.1–32.0)		age, smoking	't Mannetje et al., 1999[85]
Tailors	Germany, CC, men	2.7 (1.1–6.6)			Claude et al., 1988[69]
Tailors	Canada, CC, men	3.9 (1.3–14.2)		latency≥ 8 yrs	Risch et al., 1988[74]
Tailors, dressmakers	Europe, CC, women	1.4 (1.0–2.1)		smoking	't Mannetje et al., 1999
Technicians	US, C, African–American women		PMR 1.8 (0.8–3.8)		Schultz & Loomis, 2000[66]

Table 30.3.1 (Cont'd) Occupations associated with increased risk of bladder cancer

Occupation /Industry	Study site, type, population	Increased morbidity relative risk	Increased mortality relative risk (95% CI)	Controlled for (95% CI)	Reference
Telephone & telegraph ops	US, CC, white men	1.9 (0.9–4.0)*		smoking	Silverman et al., 1989[2]
Textile workers	Spain, CC, women	6.4 (1.3–30.0)		smoking, other jobs	Gonzalez et al., 1989[89]
Textile workers	Spain, CC, men	1.9 (1.1–3.1)		smoking, other jobs	Gonzalez et al., 1989[89]
Textile workers	Denmark, CC	1.7 (1.1–2.4)		sex, age, smoking	Jensen et al.. 1987[68]
Textile workers†	Italy, CC, women	1.9 (0.9–4.2)			Maffi & Vineis, 1986[86]
Tobacco processors	Europe, CC, women	3.1 (1.1–9.3)		age, smoking	't Mannetje et al., 1999[85]
Turners (lathe operators)	UK, CC, men	1.5 (1.2–1.8)			Cartwright, 1982[64]
Turners (lathe operators)	Germany, CC, men	2.3 (1.0–5.6)*			Claude et al., 1988[69]
Upholsterers	Germany, CC, men	2.7 (1.1–6.6)			Claude et al., 1988[69]
Weavers	Germany, CC, men	2.7 (1.1–6.6)			Claude et al., 1988[69]
Weavers	Spain, CC, men	3.5 (1.3–9.3)		smoking, other jobs	Gonzalez et al., 1989[89]
Weavers	Spain, CC, women	21.2 (1.5–298)		smoking, other jobs	Gonzalez et al., 1989[89]
Weavers	US, CC, white men	3.5 (1.3–9.3)		smoking	Silverman et al., 1989[2]
Welders	Canada, CC, men	2.8 (1.1–8.8)			Howe et al., 1980[59]
Welders, oxyacetylene	Italy, C, men		3.7 (1.2–8.6)	age	Merlo et al., 1989[83]

Only occupations explicitly mentioned in a study are included. Study types: CC (case-control), C (cohort), NCC (nested case-control), CR (linkage of case registry and census data)
* Dose–response demonstrated
† Higher risks were found for some subcategories of workers

Table 30.3.1 (Cont'd) Occupations associated with increased risk of bladder cancer

Based on mortality data from England and Wales, it was estimated that bladder cancer due to occupational exposures was responsible for half of the rate difference between high and low social classes because these exposures are concentrated in blue-collar jobs.[23] However, no evidence was provided associating the blue-collar jobs with exposure to bladder carcinogens.

Metabolic polymorphisms and bladder cancer

Interindividual variation is common for many metabolic enzymes. In some cases, the variability has been attributed to inherited polymorphisms.[24] Phenotypic and genotypic tests have shown that variation in xenobiotic metabolizing enzymes is associated with cancer risk and may have an influence on human susceptibility to genotoxic agents.

A limited number of studies of bladder cancer genetic susceptibility in populations exposed occupationally to arylamines has been published.[25–29] The results of a meta-analysis of all studies of acetylation status and bladder cancer in the general population suggest that certain groups with the NAT2 slow-acetylation phenotype are at greater risk of bladder cancer.[30] Additional studies are needed to establish if individuals could be at higher risk of bladder cancer given the presence of certain alleles that make them more susceptible. In the workplace, various metabolic polymorphisms could be acting in combination with occupational toxicants to produce risk. For occupational bladder cancer, polymorphic genotypes in the *NAT* (N-acetyltransferase) and *GST* (glutathione S-transferase) families of genes have been explored. Their joint effect, together with the effect of other genotypes, has not yet

been investigated. Moreover, the metabolic differences between monoarylamines and diarylamines, such as benzidine, warrant careful attention to the specific compounds to which each worker is exposed.

Animal models

Use of animal models to predict human bladder carcinogens has been problematic. Rats and mice are not susceptible to bladder cancer by most aromatic amines, including some highly potent occupational carcinogens. For aromatic amines, the Syrian hamster and dog were found to be better predictors for human bladder cancer than mice or rats, but this may not necessarily be the case for other chemical classes.[15] There has been considerable debate about the relevance to human bladder cancer of bladder tumors associated with urinary calculi in mice or rats or calcium phosphate-containing precipitates in rats. The International Agency for Research on Cancer (IARC), which has a formal program for identification of carcinogenic hazards to humans, has issued a consensus report on this subject.[31] Based on this consensus report, the IARC monograph program has recently classified saccharin in Group 3 (not classifiable as to carcinogenicity in humans) because the mechanism through which it is thought to cause bladder cancer in rats, formation of a calcium phosphate-containing precipitate, is not relevant to humans.[32]

Numerous classes of genotoxic chemicals have been identified as bladder carcinogens in rodents and some of these have been identified in humans, most notably, aromatic amines, nitrosamines, and cyclophosphamide. In contrast, non-genetoxic chemicals appear to be highly specific with regard to species strain, diet, agent, dose, and mechanism.

Compound name [variant name]	CAS#	IARC group	Source(s)	Potentially exposed occupations, numbers*
Aluminum (production)	7429–90–5†	1	Boffetta	al production workers
Arsenic & arsenic compounds	7440–38–2	1	Wilbourn	arsenical pesticide manufacturing workers; pesticide users
Auramine dye manufacturing	492–80–8†	1	Boffetta	dye mfg. workers
Benzidine	92–87–5	1	Boffetta	1,554 (NOES)
Benzidine-based dyes		2A	IARC 29;	28,442 (NOES)
Direct Black 38 [2,7-Naphthalenedisulfonic acid, 4-amino-3- {[4'-((2,4-diaminophenyl)azo) (1,1'-biphenyl)-4-yl]azo}-5-hydroxy-6-(phenylazo)-disodium salt]	1937–37–7		IARC Supp 7	dye manufacturing workers; dye-using workers – 44,500 (BLS)
Direct Blue 6 [2,7-Naphthalenedisulfonic acid, 3,3'-[(1,1'-biphenyl)- ((4,4'-diylbis(azo))bis(5-amino-4-hydroxy)-, tetrasodium salt]	2602–46–2			
Benzidine, 3,3'-dichloro-	91–94–1	2A	Wilbourn	
4-Biphenylamine [4-Aminobiphenyl]	92–67–1	1	Boffetta; Wilbourn	
Chemotherapy agents				
Chlornaphazine [(N,N-Bis(2-chloro-ethyl)-2-naphthylamine)]	494–03–1	1	Wilbourn	pharmaceutical mfg. workers, oncology nurses, pharmacists
Cyclophosphamide [2H-1,3,2-Oxazaphosphorine, 2-(bis(2-chloroethyl)amino)tetrahydro, 2-oxide]	50–18–0	1		27,171 (NOES)
Coal-tar pitches	65996–93–2	1	Wilbourn; Boffetta	roofers – 142,600 (BLS)
Coal tars	65996–89–6	1	Wilbourn; IARC Supp 7	roofers – 142,600 (BLS)
Diesel engine exhaust	various	2A	Wilbourn	truck drivers – 2,500,000+ (BLS)
p-Dimethylaminoazobenzene [Brilliant yellow]	60–11–7	2B	Wilbourn	dye-using workers – 44,500 (BLS)
Magenta dye manufacture	632–99–5†	1	Boffetta	dye mfg. workers
4,4'-Methylene bis (2-chloroaniline) [MOCA]	101–14–4	2A	Wilbourn	
Mineral oils, untreated and mildly treated	various	1	Wilbourn	metal machinists – 1 million+ (BLS)
2-Naphthylamine	91–59–8	1	Boffetta	275 (NOES)
Phenacetin [p-Acetophenetidide]	62–44–2	2A	Wilbourn	17,658 (NOES) pharmaceutical mfg.
Analgesic mixtures containing phenacetin	various	1	Wilbourn	workers, oncology nurses, pharmacists
Rubber industry (certain occupations)	various†	1	Boffetta	rubber additives workers
Tobacco smoke		1	Wilbourn	‡
p-Chloro-o-toluidine	95–69–2	2A	IARC, 2000; Wilbourn	
o-Toluidine [o-Aminoazotoluene]	97–56–3	2A	IARC, 2000; Wilbourn	rubber additives workers & dye workers

An RTECS search for substances associated with bladder tumors produced the original list, adapted from Ruder et al., 1990.[84] IARC classifications are adapted from Wilbourn et al. 1999[15] and Boffetta et al 1997.[23] Updates through Monograph 84 by the authors of this chapter. IARC ratings: 1, definite human bladder carcinogen; 2A, probable human bladder carcinogen. Compounds rated by Wilbourn et al.[15] as canine bladder carcinogens are included, but not those rated as exclusively rodent bladder carcinogens.

* Estimated numbers are from two sources: 1. (NOES) Chemical-specific numbers of workers potentially exposed are from the 1981–1983 National Occupational Exposure Survey. Note that all these workers would be reaching > 20 years latency about 2001–3; 2. (BLS) Estimates of numbers of workers in occupational categories are from the Bureau of Labor Statistics 1999 National Occupational Employment and Wage Estimates (http://stats.bls.gov/oes). These data do not consider turnover among employees, which would lead to a greater number of persons exposed than is suggested by estimates from specific points in time.
† These manufacturing processes involve exposure to a number of chemicals.
‡ No study to date has linked passive smoking to bladder cancer; several have found no association.

Table 30.3.2 Known and suspected human bladder carcinogens and estimated numbers of potentially exposed US workers

Use of molecular and genetic mechanism information may be helpful in identifying possible mechanisms involved for these non-genotoxic chemicals and, therefore, can be important for a rational evaluation of human risk.

CLINICAL ASPECTS
Pathology

Transitional cell carcinomas (TCC) are graded by the World Health Organization histologically by the degree of abnormality of the tissues[33] and staged by the American Joint Committee on Cancer – Union Internationale Contre

le Cancer by the extent to which they have spread.[34] One problem in the pathology of bladder tumors is the somewhat ambiguous line between the benign and the malignant, distinguishing between a papilloma, a papillary tumor with delicate fibrovascular stroma covered by a layer of epithelial cells indistinguishable from normal bladder mucosa, and a papillary carcinoma. This distinction should be viewed as a region where borders shift between pathologists, between institutions, and given the circumstances, even successive biopsies of the patient.

Some so-called benign papillomas display effects of inflammation and reactive or regenerative conditions so that they are classified by some pathologists as anaplastic, although most of them do not behave as malignant tumors. To make the situation more complicated, some papillary tumors do become aggressive. Robinson and Hall[33] summarized the results of several studies: about 2–5% of 'benign' papillomas progress to carcinoma. The use of biochemical, molecular and genetic characteristics of cells is beginning to provide pathologists with a way to reduce these uncertainties. Strong associations of various markers with progression, invasiveness, and metastatic potential may provide a way to distinguish between pathologic subtypes of bladder cancer in the future.[35]

Therapy

Strategies for diagnosis and therapy of occupational bladder cancer do not differ from those for bladder cancer resulting from non-occupational etiologies. A comprehensive guide to current treatment options by stage and grade has been assembled by the National Cancer Institute.[36] Treatment strategies do not appear to differ by histological type. Occupational bladder cancer does have a public health component: putative bladder carcinogens and high-risk populations that need to be followed with screening have been identified when exceptional cases of bladder cancer (i.e., in young non-smokers) were diagnosed.

Survival

The survival of patients with bladder cancer depends on the grade of anaplasia of the tumor and the stage of tumor invasion at time of diagnosis. SEER 1992–1997 5-year survival rates range from 94.5% for localized disease in white males to 0% for distant disease in African-American males. At each stage, women fare more poorly than men (except African-American women with distant disease) and African-Americans more poorly than whites. From 1974 to 1997 overall survival has improved from 48% to 65% in African-Americans and from 74% to 82% in whites. During the same period, incidence increased slightly overall from 14.6 to 16.7/100,000, in men from 25.6 to 29.0, and in women from 6.3 to 7.4.[37]

Survival also appears to depend on social class and race, which, of course, are somewhat correlated. A review of five studies on bladder cancer survival found about a 20% discrepancy overall between higher and lower income patients.[38] African-Americans are less likely than whites to develop bladder cancer; however, once diagnosed, African-Americans experience poorer survival: 64% 5-year survival vs. 82% for whites.[3]

PREVENTION
Techniques for early detection

Cytoscopy is effective in identifying visible tumors in the bladder. A cytoscope is a slender tube with a lens and a light that is inserted through the urethra, allowing the physician to visually inspect the urethra and bladder. Cytoscopy is invasive and not employed for asymptomatic individuals.[39]

Urine cytology is the accepted technique for detection of bladder cancer in asymptomatic individuals. Urine cytology microscopically identifies the presence of abnormal, malignant cells, which are shed into the urine of patients with bladder cancer.[39] Cytologic screening for bladder cancer has a sensitivity of about 70% and a specificity of 90–95%, depending on the grade and stage of the tumor,[40] which is comparable to screening tests for cervical cancer, breast cancer, and colon cancer.[41] Bladder cytology is effective in detecting preclinical stages of aggressive tumors and is substantially less effective in detecting low-grade tumors. There is widespread agreement that superficial well-differentiated papillary tumors rarely can be diagnosed definitively from voided urine cytology. In summary, cytology may be used to detect aggressive tumors, but these tumors may be advanced by the time they are discovered by this method. Cytology is less effective for low-grade tumors, which, although they are less aggressive, it would be desirable to find.[42]

The greatest determinant of the sensitivity of urine cytology is the level of cytopathologist expertise. Ancillary techniques have been tested to improve the sensitivity of urine cytology. Of the large variety of methods, the most promising techniques appear to be DNA flow cytometry and image analysis for the detection of nuclear aneuploidy. Other sensitive methods include immunocytochemistry to detect the presence of antigens that are commonly expressed in neoplastic urothelium but not in the normal urothelium, such as the Lewis X antigen, and immunohistochemical analysis for the detection of p53 overexpression.[43]

Hematuria screening, by urinalysis or by dipstick – a positive reaction for blood on urine-reagent-strip testing of asymptomatic people[44] – may be a more effective method than cytology for detecting low-grade early stage bladder tumors. The dilemmas with testing for hematuria are: (1) although almost all bladder tumors eventually cause hematuria, an infrequent examination may not be adequately sensitive, and (2) hematuria due to bladder cancer may be intermittent.[45] Although more frequent examinations increase the sensitivity of the test for bladder cancer, this method decreases the specificity of the test because it will detect other, non-malignant conditions causing hematuria, including cystitis, kidney disease, and urinary calculi.[3] The debate then focuses on the predictive value of a positive test result for hematuria or the probability that a positive test result will reflect bladder cancer rather than another problem. It has been suggested that 5–10% of patients with hematuria have bladder cancer and 10–20% have some other serious urinary tract disease. As a condition becomes more prevalent in a population, the predictive value of a positive test increases. Exposure of an individual to an occupational carcinogen, as well as the individual's age and other risk factors for bladder cancer, should ensure a higher underlying prevalence of bladder cancer and thus increase the predictive value of a screen for hematuria.[45] The American Urological

Association recommends that asymptomatic microhematuria be evaluated only when associated with a risk (such as occupational exposure to carcinogens) of disease.[46]

Tests of genetic factors are now being developed or assessed for evaluation of risk factors for bladder cancer. In addition to variations in metabolic phenotypes such as *N*-acetyltransferase, there are other genetic factors and acquired factors, such as recessive alleles for oncogenes, mutated tumor suppressor genes, and growth factors, that may place individuals at increased risk for bladder cancer independent of occupational exposure.[47] These genetic factors could add to any occupational risks for bladder cancer or multiply those risks. It is likely that the rapid pace of research will result in the identification of new predictive or prognostic markers in the near future.

A number of new techniques are being tested for use in bladder cancer screening. Most markers appear to have an advantage over urine cytology in terms of sensitivity, especially for detecting low-grade superficial tumors. However, most markers tend to be less specific than cytology, yielding more false-positive results. This scenario is more common in patients with concurrent bladder inflammation or other benign bladder conditions. A summary of the sensitivity, specificity and limitations of these methods is presented in Table 30.3.3.

The nuclear matrix protein (NMP) 22 test detects and measures urinary levels of a particular NMP called NuMA (nuclear mitotic apparatus). The NMP22 assay appears to be useful only to monitor, with high accuracy, for recurrence in patients with a past history of bladder cancer.[48]

The bladder tumor antigen (BTA) test detects the presence of a bladder tumor antigen in the urine of patients with bladder cancer. The BTA stat and the BTA trak assays are qualitative and quantitative assays, respectively. Both detect a human complement factor H-related protein in the urine, and both accurately identify two-thirds of patients with bladder cancer. Both are limited because of the high number of false-positive reactions compared to urine cytology in low-grade bladder tumors.[39]

The fibrin and fibrinogen degradation products (FDP) test is positive in two-thirds of patients with bladder cancer. The FDP test detects the degradation product of an extravascular fibrin clot produced by tumors. It is more sensitive than urine cytology and has a high specificity.[49]

Telomerase is an essential enzyme for cellular immortality and tumorigenesis. The telomeric repeat amplification protocol assay for telomerase in exfoliated cells can be used as a tumor marker. However, the low stability of telomerase in urine affects test sensitivity.[50] Inflammatory cells and stem cells have telomerase activity, and may be the source of false-positive tests.

Hyaluronic acid is a glycosaminoglycan that promotes tumor metastasis. High levels are detectable in the urine of patients with bladder cancer. Patients with high-grade TCC have elevated urinary hyaluronidase activity. A combination of both tests (HA-HAase test) yields a higher sensitivity than the sensitivity of individual tests,[51] but it has no better sensitivity than urine cytology for detecting low-grade lesions.

Recently, detection of survivin in urine has been suggested as a predictive molecular marker of bladder cancer. Survivin is an enzyme inhibitor of apoptosis that is selectively overexpressed in human cancers, but undetectable in most normal adult tissues. In a patient series, the sensitivity of the urine survivin test for new or recurrent bladder cancer was 100%, and the specificity was 90–100%, depending on the population tested.[52]

Test batteries

Combining tests can increase their sensitivity and specificity.[41] Series testing is used to increase specificity and reduce the number of false-positive results. Parallel testing is used to increase sensitivity and reduce the number of false-negative results. A new US/European research consortium wants to create a simple, cost-effective, non-invasive diagnostic test to replace cytoscopy and cytology, initiating multicenter trials to find which of seven molecular markers, alone or in combination, is the most accurate detector of bladder cancer.[53]

Screening programs

There are two reasons for screening a population exposed to a known or suspect bladder carcinogen. First, individu-

Test	Sensitivity	Specificity	Limitations
Urine cytology	17–70%	90–95%	Poor criteria to identify low-grade TCC*
BTA test	29–40%	68–91%	Low detection of grade I TCC. Poorer predictive value than urine cytology
BTA stat test	67–87%	40–70%	High false positive with gross hematuria, prostate cancer, BCG
BTA trak test	72%	43–48%	High false positive with UTI, stones, instrumentation
NMP22	48–80%	64–80%	High false positive with gross hematuria
FDP test	40–68%	80–96%	High false positive with gross hematuria
Telomerase	70–86%	60–90%	False negatives with gross hematuria, false positives with inflammation, complicated assay not widely available
HA-HAase test	90–92%	80–84%	No detection of grade I TCC

Modified from Brown, 2000[43]
* Abbreviations: BCG = bacillus Calmette-Guérin, BTA = bladder tumor antigen, FDP = fibrin/fibrinogen degradation products, HA-HAase = hyaluronic acid/hyaluronidase, NMP = nuclear matrix protein, TCC = transitional cell carcinoma, UTI = urinary tract infection

Table 30.3.3 Sensitivity and specificity of non-invasive bladder tumor markers

als may be screened so that their tumors can be detected early when they are more readily treated, resulting in less morbidity and higher survival rates. This type of screening is for the personal benefit of the individuals. The second rationale for screening is to detect disease in a population at the earliest time possible in order to ensure that more primary methods of disease prevention, such as engineering controls and use of personal protective devices, are effectively incorporated to prevent exposure.[54] The two motivations should be kept in mind in appreciating a consensus view that was reached at the 1989 conference on screening for bladder cancer in high-risk groups. For populations exposed to known carcinogens at high levels, cytologic examination and testing for hematuria was recommended at 6-month intervals. The rationale for including hematuria was to ensure the acceptability of the screening program by ensuring that low-grade tumors would be detected that otherwise may be missed by cytology.

For low-exposure groups, as may be found in patients suffering from conditions as a result of environmental exposures, cytology was recommended 2 years after the first exposure, then every 5 years thereafter. For a suspect carcinogen, at high-exposure levels, cytology was recommended every 6 months, as well as measurement of hematuria to detect low-grade tumors. The argument for detecting low-grade tumors, even though there may be limited personal benefit for the individual because most such tumors are less aggressive, was to provide information that exposure had not been adequately controlled. The panel was not enthusiastic about any recommendations for a suspect carcinogen at low levels of exposure.[55]

When weighing the benefits of a strategy of early detection, be it for the personal benefit of the worker or for the benefit of the workforce, it is necessary to consider the extent to which false-positive findings will be involved. A screening modality that leads to a disproportionate number of unnecessary follow-up and diagnostic procedures may not be cost effective or personally desirable. Moreover, the lengthening of the lead time, although possibly providing an extended opportunity for therapeutic intervention, also could provide a longer period of anxiety and distress for the worker.[54]

In contrast to the recommendations of the bladder cancer conference consensus panel, the US Preventive Services Task Force concluded that there was insufficient evidence that hematuria and cytology screening improved the prognosis for those found to have cancer, even within high-risk groups.[56] If the efficacy of hematuria and cytology screening is not established, then in monitoring high-risk populations, cystoscopy should be reserved as a diagnostic test in individuals who had positive results on cytology and hematuria. However, it should be remembered that in at least one high-risk group, the MBOCA cohort, bladder cancer was diagnosed in two individuals who had had negative hematuria by dipstick and cytology screening.[57] Perhaps the non-invasive screening batteries now under development will end this dilemma.

SUMMARY

Despite substitution and process changes to prevent or reduce worker exposure, a substantial number of workers continue to be exposed to bladder carcinogens. Much larger numbers have been exposed to bladder carcinogens in the past. Some of these workers may still be at risk for bladder cancer. Improved screening options for high-risk groups, as well as better treatment options, should continue to improve survival and quality of life for these individuals.

References

1. Silverman DT, Levin LI, Hoover RN. Occupational risks of bladder cancer in the United States: II. Non-white men. J Natl Cancer Inst 1989; 81:1480–3.
2. Silverman DT, Levin LI, Hoover RN, Hartge P. Occupational risks of bladder cancer in the United States: I. White men. J Natl Cancer Inst 1989; 81:1472–9.
3. American Cancer Society. Cancer facts and figures 2001. Atlanta: ACS, 2001.
4. Silverman DT, Levin LI, Hoover RN. Occupational risks of bladder cancer among white women in the United States. Am J Epidemiol 1990; 132:453–61.
5. Rehn L. Blasengeschwülste bei fuchsin-arbeitern [Urinary bladder tumors in dye workers]. Arch Klin Chir 1895; 50:588–600.
6. Schulte P, Halperin W, Ward E, Ruder A. Bladder cancer screening in high risk groups. J Occup Med 1990; 32:787–945.
7. Hartge P, Harvey ED, Linehan WM, et al. Unexplained excess risk of bladder cancer in men. J Natl Cancer Inst 1990; 82: 1636–40.
8. Parkin DM, Pisani P, Ferlay J. Global cancer statistics. CA Cancer J Clin 1999; 49:33–64.
9. Silverman DT, Hartge P, Morrison AS, Devesa SS. Epidemiology of bladder cancer. Hematol Oncol Clin North Am 1992; 6:1–30.
10. EL Mawla MD, EL Bolkainy MN, Khaled HM. Bladder cancer in Africa: update. Sem Oncol 2001; 28:174–8.
11. Lopez-Beltran A, Escudero AL. Human papillomavirus and bladder cancer. Biomed Pharmacother 1997; 51:252–7.
12. Koroltchouk V, Stanley K, Sthernsward J, Mott K. Bladder cancer: approaches to prevention and control. Bull WHO 1987; 65:513–20.
13. Silverman DT, Morrison AS, Devesa SS. Bladder cancer. In: Cancer epidemiology and prevention, 2nd edn. New York: Oxford University Press 1996;1156–79.
14. Zhang Z-F, Steineck G. Epidemiology and etiology of bladder cancer. In: Raghavan D, Scher HI, Leibel SA, Lang PH, eds. Principles and practice of genitourinary oncology. Philadelphia: Lippincott-Raven, 1997;215–22.
15. Wilbourn JD, Partensky C, Rise JM. Agents that induce epithelial neoplasms of the urinary bladder, renal cortex and thyroid follicular lining in experimental animals and humans: summary of data from IARC Monographs volumes 1–69. In: Capen CC, Dybing E, Rice JM, Wilbourn JD, eds. Species differences in thyroid, kidney and urinary bladder carcinogenesis. IARC Scientific Publications No. 147. Lyon: IARC, 1999;191–209.
16. Hueper WC, Wiley FH, Wolfe HD. Experimental production of bladder tumors in dogs by administration of beta-naphthylamine. J Industr Hyg Toxicol 1938; 20:46–84.
17. Case RAM, Hosker ME, MacDonald DB, Pearson JT. Tumors of the urinary bladder in workmen engaged in the manufacture and use of certain dyestuff intermediaries in the British chemical industry. Br J Ind Med 1954; 11:75–104.
18. Vineis P, Pirastu R. Aromatic amines and cancer. Cancer Causes Control 1997; 8:346–55.

19. Michaud DS, Spiegelman D, Clinton SK, et al. Fluid intake and the risk of bladder cancer in men. N Engl J Med 1999; 340:1390–7.

20. Oyasu R, Hupp ML. The etiology of cancer of the bladder. Surg Gynecol Obstet 1974; 138:97–108.

20a. Melicow MM. Tumors of the bladder: a multifaceted problem. J Urol 1974; 112: 467–78.

21. Schulte PA, Ringen K, Hemstreet GP, Ward E. Occupational cancer of the urinary tract. Occup Med 1987; 2:85–107.

22. Wallace OMA. Occupational urothelial cancer. Br J Urol 1988; 61:175–82.

23. Boffetta P, Kogevinas M, Westerholm P, Saracci R. Exposure to occupational carcinogens and social class differences in cancer occurrence. IARC Sci Publ 1997; 138:331–41.

24. Hayes RB. Genetic susceptibility and occupational cancer. Med Lav 1995; 86: 206–13.

25. Cartwright RA, Glashan RW, Rogers HJ, et al. Role of N-acetyltransferase phenotype in bladder cancer. Lancet 1982; ii(8303):842–5.

26. Hanke J, Krajewska B. Acetylation phenotypes and bladder cancer. J Occup Med 1990; 32: 917–18.

27. Hayes RB, Bi W, Rothman N, et al. N-Acetylation phenotype and genotype and risk of bladder cancer in benzidine-exposed workers. Carcinogenesis 1993; 14:675–8.

28. Rothman N, Hayes RB, Zenser TV, et al. The glutathione S-transferase M1 (GSTM1) null genotype and benzidine-associated bladder cancer, urine mutagenicity, and exfoliated urothelial cell DNA adducts. Cancer Epidemiol Biomark Prevent 1996; 5:979–81.

29. Shinka T, Ogura H, Morita T, Nishikawa T, Fujinaga T, Ohkama T. Relationship between glutathione S-transferase M1 deficiency and urothelial cancer in dye workers exposed to aromatic amines. J Urol 1998; 159:380–3.

30. Marcus PM, Vineis P, Rothman N. NAT2 slow acetylation and bladder cancer risk: a meta-analysis of 22 case-control studies conducted in the general population. Pharmacogenetics 2000; 10:115–22.

31. Capen CC, Dybing E, Rice JM, Wilbourn JD, and Workshop Participants. Consensus report. In: Capen CC, Dybing E, Rice JM, Wilbourn JD, eds. Species differences in thyroid, kidney and urinary bladder carcinogenesis. IARC Scientific Publications No. 147. Lyon: IARC, 1999;1–14.

32. International Agency for Research on Cancer. Saccharin and its salts. Lyon: IARC, 2003. http://wwwcie.iarc.fr/htdocs/monographs/vol73/73-19.html

33. Robinson MC, Hall RR. Histopathology of urothelial cancer: consensus or controversy? In: Hall RR, ed. Clinical management of bladder cancer. New York: Oxford University Press, 1999;25–65.

34. Droller MJ. Clinical presentation, investigation, and staging of bladder cancer. In: Raghavan D, Scher HI, Leibel SA, Lang PH, eds. Principles and practice of genitourinary oncology. Philadelphia: Lippincott-Raven 1997;249–59.

35. Fradet Y, Cordon-Cardo C. Tumor markers in the management of bladder cancer. In: Raghavan D, Scher HI, Leibel SA, Lang PH, eds. Principles and practice of genitourinary oncology. Philadelphia: Lippincott-Raven 1997;231–8.

36. National Cancer Institute. PDQ website, December 15, 2003. http://www.nci.nih.gov/cancerinfo/pdq/cancerdatabase.

37. Ries LAG, Eisner MP, Kosary CL, et al., eds. SEER Cancer Statistics Review, 1973–1998. Bethesda, MD: National Cancer Institute, 2001.

38. Kogevinas M, Porta M. Socioeconomic differences in cancer survival: a review of the evidence. IARC Sci Publ 1997; 138:177–206.

39. Pirtskalaishvili G, Konety BR, Getzenberg RH. Update on urine-based markers for bladder cancer. Postgrad Med J 1999; 106:85–94.

40. Hemstreet GP, Bonner RB, Hurst RE, Rao JY. Cytology of bladder cancer. In: Vogelzang NJ, Scardino PT, Shipley WV, Coffey DS, eds. Comprehensive textbook of genitourinary oncology. Philadelphia: Lippincott Williams & Wilkins, 2000;322–32.

41. Hulka B. Principles of bladder cancer screening in an intervention trial. J Occup Med 1990; 32:812–6.

42. Farrow G. Urine cytology in the detection of bladder cancer: a critical approach. J Occup Med 1990; 32:817–21.

43. Brown FM. Urine cytology: is it still the gold standard for screening? Urol Clin North Am 2000; 27:25–37.

44. Hall RR. 1999 The diagnosis of bladder cancer. In: Hall RR, ed. Clinical management of bladder cancer. New York: Oxford University Press 1999;1–20.

45. Messing E, Vaillancourt A. Hematuria screening for bladder cancer. J Occup Med 1990; 32:838–46.

46. Grossfeld GD, Wolf JS, Litwan MS, et al. Asymptomatic microscopic hematuria in adults: summary of the AUA best practice policy recommendations. Am Fam Phys 2001; 63:114–54.

47. Koenig F, Jung K, Schnorr D, Loening SA. Urinary markers of malignancy. Clin Chim Acta 2000; 297:191–205.

48. Soloway MS, Briggman JV, Carpinito GA, et al. Use of a new tumor marker, urinary NMP22, in the detection of occult or rapidly recurring transitional cell carcinoma of the urinary tract following surgical treatment. J Urol 1996; 156:363–7.

49. Schmetter BS, Habicht KK, Lamm DL, et al. A multicenter trial evaluation of the fibrin/fibrinogen degradation products test for detection and monitoring of bladder cancer. J Urol 1997; 158:801–5.

50. Lokeshwar VB, Soloway MS. Current bladder tumor tests: does their projected utility fulfill clinical necessity? J Urol 2001; 165:1067–77.

51. Lokeshwar VB, Block NL. HA-HAase urine test. A sensitive and specific method for detecting bladder cancer and evaluating its grade. Urol Clin North Am 2000; 27:53–61.

52. Smith SD, Wheeler MA, Plescia J, Colberg JW, Weiss RM, Altieri DC. Urine detection of survivin and diagnosis of bladder cancer. J Am Med Assoc 2001; 285:324–8.

53. Agres T. Finding a better way to identify bladder cancer. The Scientist 2001; 15 (June 25): 21.

54. Halperin WE, Ratcliffe J, Frazier TM, Wilson L, Becker SP, Schulte PA. Medical screening in the workplace: proposed principles. J Occup Med 1986; 28:547–52.

55. Halperin W, Cartwright RA, Farrow GM, et al. Where do we go from here? J Occup Med 1990; 32: 936–45.

56. United States Preventive Services Task Force. Guide to Clinical Preventive Services, 2nd edn, 1996. December 15, 2003. http://www.ahcpr.gov/clinic/cpsix.htm

57. Ward E, Halperin W, Thun M, et al. Screening workers exposed to 4,4′-methylenebis(2-chloroaniline) for bladder cancer by cystoscopy. J Occup Med 1990; 32:865–68.

58. Armstrong BG, Tremblay CG, Cyr D, Theriault GP. Estimating the relationship between exposure to tar volatiles and the incidence of bladder cancer in aluminium smelter workers. Scand J Work Environ Health 1986; 12:483–93.

59. Howe GR, Burch JD, Miller AB, et al. Tobacco use, occupation, coffee, various nutrients and bladder cancer. J Natl Cancer Inst 1980; 64:701–3.

60. Malker HSR, McLaughlin JK, Silverman DT, et al. Occupational risks for bladder cancer among men in Sweden. Cancer Res 1987; 47:6763–6.

61. Schumacher MC, Slattery ML. Occupation and bladder cancer in Utah. Am J Ind Med 1989; 16:89–102.

62. Boyko RW, Cartwright RA, Glashan RW. Bladder cancer in dye manufacturing workers. J Occup Med 1985; 27:799–803.

63. Schulte PA, Ringen K, Hemstreet GP, et al. Risk assessment of a cohort exposed to aromatic amines. Initial results. J Occup Med 1985; 27:115–21.

64. Cartwright R. Occupational bladder cancer and cigarette smoking in West Yorkshire. Scand J Work Environ Health 1982; 8:79–82.

65. Zheng W, McLaughlin JK, Gao YT, Silverman DT, Gao RN, Blot WJ. Bladder cancer and occupation in Shanghai, 1980–1984. Am J Ind Med 1992; 21:877–85.

66. Schulz M, Loomis D. Occupational bladder cancer mortality among racial and ethnic minorities in 21 states. Am J Ind Med 2000; 38:90–8.

67. Isovich J, Castellrito R, Esteve J, et al. Tobacco smoking, occupational exposure and bladder cancer in Argentina. Int J Cancer 1987; 49:734–40.

68. Jensen OM, Wahrendorf J, Knudsen JB, et al. The Copenhagen case-referent study on bladder cancer. Risks among drivers, painters and certain other occupations. Scand J Work Environ Health 1987; 13:129–34.

69. Claude JC, Prenzal-Beyme RR, Kunze E. Occupation and risk of cancer of the lower urinary tract among men. A case-control study. Int J Cancer 1988; 41:371–9.

70. Baxter PJ, McDowall ME. Occupation and cancer in London. An investigation into nasal and bladder cancer using the Cancer Atlas. Br J Ind Med 1986; 43:44–9.

71. Ruder AM, Ward EM, Brown DP. Mortality in dry cleaning workers: an update. Am J Ind Med 2001; 39:121–32.

72. Bi W, Hayes RB, Feng P, et al. Mortality and incidence of bladder cancer in benzidine-exposed workers in China. Am J Ind Med 1992; 21:481–9.

73. Sathiakumar N, Delzell E. An updated mortality study of workers at a dye and resin manufacturing plant. J Occup Environ Med 2000; 42:762–71.

74. Risch HA, Burch JD, Miller AB, et al. Occupational factors and the incidence of cancer of the bladder in Canada. Br J Ind Med 1988; 45:361–7.

75. Bulbulyan MA, Figgs LW, Zahm SH, et al. Cancer incidence and mortality among beta-naphthylamine and benzidine dye workers in Moscow. Int J Epidemiol 1995; 24:266–75.

76. Schoenberg JB, Stemhagen A, Mogielnicki AP, Altman R, Abe T, Mason TJ. Case-control study of bladder cancer in New Jersey. I Occupational exposure in white males. J Nat Cancer Inst 1984; 72:973–81.

77. Brownson RC, Chang JC, Davis JR. Occupation, smoking and alcohol in the epidemiology of bladder cancer. Am J Public Health 1987; 77:1298–300.

78. Decoufle P. Cancer risks associated with employment in the leather and leather products industry. Arch Environ Health 1979; 34:33–7.

79. Guberan E, Usel M, Raymond L, et al. Disability, mortality and incidence of cancer among Geneva painters and electricians: a historical prospective study. Br J Ind Med 1988; 46:16–23.

80. Miller BA, Silverman DT, Hoover RN, Blair A. Cancer risk among artistic painters. Am J Ind Med 1986; 9:281–7.

81. Steenland K, Palu S. Cohort mortality study of 57,000 painters and other union members: a 15 year update. Occup Environ Med 1999; 56:315–21.

82. Popp W, Schmieding W, Speck M, Vahrenholz C, Norpoth K. Incidence of bladder cancer in a cohort of workers exposed to 4-chloro-o-toluidine while synthesizing chlordimeform. Br J Ind Med 1992; 49:529–31.

83. Merlo F, Costantini M, Doria M. Cause specific mortality among workers exposed to welding fumes and gases: a historical prospective study. Sangyo I Daigaku Zasshi 1989; 11 (Suppl):302–15.

84. Ruder A, Fine L, Sundin D. National estimates of occupational exposure to animal bladder tumorigens. J Occup Med 1990; 32:797–805.

85. 't Mannetje A, Kogeninas M. Chang-Claude J, et al. Occupation and bladder cancer in European women. Cancer Causes Control 1999; 10:209–17.

86. Maffi L, Vineis P. Occupation and bladder cancer in females. Med Lav 1986; 77:511–4.

87. Silverman DT, Hoover RN, Mason TJ, Swanson GM. Motor exhaust-related occupations and bladder cancer. Cancer Res 1986; 46:2113–6.

88. Silverman DT, Hoover RN, Albert S, Graff KM. Occupation and cancer of the lower urinary tract in Detroit. J Natl Cancer Inst 1983; 70:237–45.

89. Gonzalez CA, Lopez-Abente G, Errezola M, et al. Occupation and bladder cancer in Spain: a multi-centre case-control study. Int J Epidemiol 1989; 18: 569–77.

90. Ward E, Carpenter, A, Markowitz S, Roberts D, Halperin W. Excess number of bladder cancers in workers exposed to ortho-toluidine and aniline. J Natl Cancer Inst 1991; 83:501–6.

30.4 **Renal Cancer**
Stuart L Shalat, Sandra N Mohr

Renal cancer is relatively rare, accounting for only 3% of all cancers diagnosed in the US. It is the 10th leading cause of cancer in men and the 14th in women. Perhaps because it has received less attention than other, more common tumors, the etiology of renal cancer, with respect to both general and occupationally related causes, is still not well understood. However, approximately one-third to one-half of all cases of renal cell carcinoma occur in patients with von Hippel–Lindau disease.[1] Other risk factors associated with renal cell carcinoma include smoking, obesity, history of kidney stones, and long-term use of phenacetin.[2]

Examination of risk of renal cancer in the workplace has included a variety of exposures, including metals (arsenic, cadmium, lead, and uranium), polyaromatic hydrocarbons (PAHs), organic solvents (including chlorinated compounds), asbestos, and other factors. Therefore, although renal cancer may be rare, the exposures that may confer increased risk to workers are not.

In the US in 1996, there were approximately 30,600 incident cases of renal cancer with approximately 12,000 deaths.[3] The disease is more common in men than women. Black men and women are at greater risk for the disease than whites. In 1997, age-adjusted incidence rates in the US were 12.2/100,000 in white males, 15.9/100,000 in black men, 6.4/100,000 in white women, and 7.9/100,000 in black women (SEER, 2000). The incidence rates for renal cancer peak in the sixth and seventh decades of life. Epidemiologic data from the National Cancer Institute's Surveillance Epidemiology and End Results (SEER) pro-gram followed from 1973 to 1997 suggest that the incidence of cancer in the kidney is rising. There has been an increase of 1.7% per year for men and 2.2% for women. This increase, however, also may be due to improvements in diagnostic records. Only 41% of male cases and 46% of female cases were localized at the time of diagnosis. The 5-year survival rate for renal cancer has shown slight improvement from approximately 50% in the early 1970s (all gender and race groups) to approximately 61% for cases diagnosed in the early 1990s.

CLINICAL ASPECTS

There are no distinguishing characteristics with regard to occupational etiology in the diagnosis and clinical course of renal cell carcinoma. Approximately 60% of cases present with hematuria, either gross or microscopic. The classic triad of flank pain, palpable abdominal mass, and hematuria is found in only 10% of patients. Most of the other presenting symptoms are systemic, including fever, weight loss, anemia, hypertension, and erythrocytosis. At the time of diagnosis, 30% of individuals have extensive metastatic disease. Renal tumors usually are detected by intravenous pyelography with tomography, or by ultrasound, followed up by a computed tomography (CT) scan. The CT scan is considered comparable to renal arteriography for the staging and characterization of the disease.

Classification

Renal cell carcinoma, also known as renal adenocarcinoma or hypernephroma, accounts for 90% of tumors in the kidney. The cancer arises from cells of the proximal convoluted tubule and its associated connective tissue. The Mainz classification is now widely utilized for renal cancer, as a result of several cytogenetic studies.[4] In this system, there are three histologically distinct forms of renal cell carcinoma:
- clear cell type (cholesterol-filled cells);
- chromophilic (eosinophilic or basophil-staining); and
- chromophobic.

Renal pelvic cancers involve the collecting systems of the kidney, and account for less than 10% of all renal neoplasms. These include collecting duct carcinoma and renal oncocytoma. The cancers usually are morphologically identical to transitional cell carcinomas seen in the bladder, and are associated with them in roughly 50% of cases.

Wilms' tumor, or nephroblastoma, is the third most common form of childhood cancer and represents about 5% of all kidney cancers. These tumors contain a variety of cell types, all derived from the mesoderm. The epithelial cell types may present as immature tubules or glomeruli.

Therapy

As discussed above, the annual number of new diagnoses of renal cell carcinoma is increasing. For patients with localized primary tumors, surgical resection remains the mainstay of therapy. Since renal cell carcinoma is characterized by a lack of early warning signs, a majority of patients present with metastatic disease. Several reviews of available treatment regimens have concluded that renal cell carcinoma is resistant to chemotherapy.[5–7] The result is that patients with distant metastatic disease (Stage IV) have a 5-year survival of less than 10%.[8] Recent studies have suggested possible improved survival for advanced renal cell carcinoma from interferon and/or interleukin (IL)-2 therapy, and, more recently, allogenic stem-cell transplantation; however, far more research is required and new agents and treatment programs need to be considered.[5,9]

GENERAL EPIDEMIOLOGY

Several epidemiologic studies have attempted to identify risk factors for renal cell carcinoma, which are shown in Table 30.4.1. These risk factors have been evaluated mostly through the use of case–control studies. Because of the high case-fatality rate occurring 1 year after diagnosis, the majority of these studies have had a fairly low response rate of 60% to 73%. In order to prevent a high percentage of non-response, some investigations have used proxy interviews

Established	Suspected	Reported*
Cigarette smoking	Obesity	Meat consumption
Phenacetin analgesics	Hypertension and/or antihypertensive medications	Kidney infections/stones
Hereditary disorders	Northeastern European ancestry	Acetaminophen analgesics
von Hippel–Lindau disease	Long-term hemodialysis	
* Causal association requires further research		

Table 30.4.1 Non-occupational risk factors for renal cell carcinoma

to substitute for deceased patients. This strategy, however, raises the problem of differential recall bias between proxy and direct patient interviews. These issues need to be taken into account when interpreting case–control studies of renal cancer.

Cigarette smoking has been consistently associated with renal cancer across several epidemiologic studies. In a population-based case–control study of 495 cases and 697 controls, McLaughlin and coworkers found an odds ratio for smoking of 1.6 for men, and 1.9 for women.[10] There was also a positive dose–response relationship in both sexes for years of tobacco use. Several other studies also found significant odds ratios for smoking in the 1.5–2.0 range. A large study from Australia recently confirmed the positive association for smoking, and estimated an attributable risk for renal cell cancer of 30% for men and 24% for women.[11]

Obesity has also been suggested as a risk factor for renal cell carcinoma. In a study by Yu and colleagues which assessed the effect of obesity, as measured by Quetelet's index 10 years before the onset of cancer, significant increases in odds ratios for both men and women were observed.[12] Maclure and Hankinson found that obesity was a predisposing factor for renal cell carcinoma among women in a case–control study of renal cell cancer.[13] A nested case–control study (cases, $n = 37$; controls, $n = 148$) of refinery and petrochemical workers used body mass index (BMI) and found a statistically significant increase in risk of kidney cancer.[14]

A positive association of premorbid hypertension and the risk of renal cell cancer has been demonstrated, but it remains unclear whether the effect is due to an increase in blood pressure or use of antihypertensive drugs. McCredie and Stewart found that both beta-blocker use and hypertension for more than 2 years were independently associated with renal cell cancer, but the use of diuretics was not.[15] In contrast, Yu and colleagues found that hypertension was not significantly associated with renal cell cancer after controlling for diuretic use in women.[12] Several prospective studies have also investigated the relationship of hypertension, antihypertensive medications, and renal cell cancer, but only one of these demonstrated an effect due to antihypertensive medication independent of high blood pressure.[16] In the same occupational study of refinery and petrochemical workers as previously mentioned, high blood pressure resulted in a large increase in risk, even when BMI was taken into account (OR = 4.5; 95% CI, 0.8–26).[14]

Phenacetin-containing analgesics have been consistently related to renal cell carcinoma in several epidemiologic studies. Acetaminophen has not yet been investigated as extensively. While Sandler and colleagues demonstrated an association of acetaminophen with chronic kidney disease, the risk of renal cancer associated with this analgesic is not currently known.[17]

Hereditary forms of renal cell cancer have also been identified. These cancers tend to occur earlier and are more likely to be bilateral and multifocal. It has been hypothesized that tumor development in individuals with these cancers may be associated with an alteration of a tumor suppressor gene at the short arm of chromosome 3.

Other risk factors that have been found to be associated with renal cell carcinoma include meat consumption, northeastern European ancestry, and prior kidney stones and infections. Coffee consumption has not been identified as a risk factor. Long-term users of renal dialysis, and those who develop acquired cystic kidney disease, have also been shown to have elevated numbers of renal cell cancer in several recent studies. These latter risk factors suggest that prior injury may predispose an individual to the development of renal cancer.

TOXICOLOGIC STUDIES

Many known carcinogens – for example, asbestos and lead – have been found to cause renal cancer in animals. Animal studies in mice also have shown a clear dose–response relationship between unleaded petrol vapor and renal cell cancer, suggesting a carcinogenic role for gasoline. Several organic compounds have been shown to induce renal cancer in animals, including vinylidene chloride, dichloroacetylene, nitrosamines, PAHs, aromatic amines, coumarins, and various dyes.

A toxicologic study by Walker and associates identified a gene that predisposes rats to develop renal cancer after exposure to a chemical carcinogen.[18] Those rats that carried a single mutation on chromosome 4 had a 70-fold increased risk of developing renal cortical tumors compared with wild rats. These results suggest the involvement of tumor suppressor genes in the development of this cancer; a mutation in one allele predisposes susceptibility to the development of cancer if a spontaneous mutation by an environmental carcinogen occurs in another allele. This study provides valuable insight into the mechanisms of carcinogenesis in kidney cancer. Some studies have examined the role of glutathione S-transferase (GST) and variations in some of the GST genes in the etiology of renal cell carcinoma. A population-based case–control study found that those with GSTT1 null gene were almost five times as likely to develop renal cell carcinoma.[19]

OCCUPATIONAL STUDIES

Epidemiologic research on the role of occupational factors in the development of renal cancer has been conducted through both large occupational cohort studies of cancer mortality and case–control studies. The former have the advantage of relatively specific information on exposure, while usually containing minimal information on potential confounders (i.e., smoking, BMI), while the latter usually are able to address the confounders but are often limited by imprecise information on occupational exposures. In addition, these studies pos-sess other weaknesses, such as difficulty in assessing exposures, recall bias, and lack of statistical power due to the relative rarity of the cancer.

While earlier large occupational cohort mortality studies were suggestive of increased cancer risk, recent studies have specifically addressed this issue. Since these studies have often not distinguished between different types of renal cancer, the following section only discusses occupational factors in relation to renal cell carcinoma. Table 30.4.2 shows the major exposures and occupations that have been examined in relation to renal cell carcinoma to date.

Hydrocarbons

Polyaromatic hydrocarbons

Little direct work has been conducted over the last decade to expand our knowledge on the role of PAHs in renal cell carcinoma. The combustion of organic materials, such as coke or coal, has been associated with renal cancer in several studies. Redmond and coworkers studied men who were employed between 1950 and 1955 at one of 10 coke plants.[20] After adjusting for potential confounders, they observed a relative risk of 7.5 for renal cell cancers among coke oven workers. Those workers were presumed to be exposed to byproducts of coke and coal combustion.

Coal tar pitch and petroleum coke combustion volatiles also appeared to be involved in the high rate of renal cancer mortality seen in Rockette and Arena's study of workers from 14 aluminum reduction plants.[21] Those individuals who worked in an area where carbon anodes were prebaked were exposed to volatile agents containing PAHs and showed an increased standardized mortality ratio (SMR) for renal cell carcinoma. In a case–control study in Canada, the authors found an increased risk of 1.7 for exposure to burning coal, after controlling for smoking.[22] Exposure to coal tar pitch also was found to be significantly associated with increased risk for renal cell cancer.

Petroleum-based hydrocarbons

Since the International Agency for Research on Cancer (IARC) conducted its last comprehensive review of epidemiologic studies of oil refinery workers in 1989, and classified the workplace environment as containing probable human carcinogens, a number of new studies, updates of cohorts, and meta-analyses have been published.[14,23–27] Petroleum products such as gasoline, chemicals found in distilled fuel oils or oil mist, and PAHs have been suggested as the possible carcinogens. Gasoline, in particular, has been suspected because of its high aromatic content.

Recently, two papers examined both active and terminated workers and retired workers separately.[23,28] These studies have observed a small increased risk for kidney cancer. In the active and current workers this reached statistical significance, with the point estimates for the SMRs virtually identical (active and terminated workers, SMR = 144; retirees, SMR = 140). A recent case–control

Occupations	Chemicals	Probable	Possible
Aluminum pot-room workers	PAHs	X	
Carbon electrode bakers	PAHs	X	
Coke oven workers	PAHs	X	
Dry cleaners	Perchloroethylene		X
Electric utility transformer repairmen	Organic solvents, PCBs		X
Ferrosilicon and silicon metal workers	Metal fume, organic solvents		X
Formaldehyde production	Formaldehyde		X
Foundry workers	Asbestos, metal fume, PAHs	X	
Gas station attendants	Gasoline	X	
Insulators	Asbestos	X	
Lead battery manufacturing	Lead		X
Lead smelter workers	Lead, arsenic		X
Newspaper pressmen	Lead, organic solvents	X	
Petrochemical and oil refinery workers	PAHs, gasoline, aliphatic hydrocarbons	X	
Phenol production	Phenol		X
Rocket-test stand workers	Hydrazine, TCE		X
Sheet metal workers	TCE		X
Uranium processing workers	Uranium, TCE		X
Welders	Asbestos, cadmium, organic solvents		X

PAHs, polyaromatic hydrocarbons; PCBs, polychlorinated biphenyls; TCE, trichloroethylene

Table 30.4.2 Occupational risk factors for renal cell carcinoma

study of kidney cancer in Canada found odds ratios of 3.9 (95% CI, 1.6–9.8) and 3.6 (95% CI, 1.4–8.8) in workers with an exposure to jet fuel or aviation gasoline.[29] Although further investigation is still clearly needed in this area, the available research does suggest that exposure to petroleum products in oil refineries, as well as in distribution, is likely to increase risk of renal cancer.

Organic solvents

A number of case–control studies have also found a positive association between hydrocarbons and renal cell carcinoma. McLaughlin and colleagues demonstrated a statistically significant increased relative risk of 2.6 for workers with 20 years or greater on the job.[10] In a case–control study of 210 cases of renal cell carcinoma, Kadamani and colleagues similarly found increased risk for moderate hydrocarbon exposure, with an odds ratio of 3.5 with high cumulative solvent exposure.[30] A greater than 3.4-fold risk was also associated with exposure to mixed non-chlorinated solvents in a large Finnish study of 672 cases of renal cell cancer. Whether other specific organic materials are renal carcinogens in human populations continues to be an area of active investigation. A review of the question of the potential role of trichloroethylene and perchloroethylene in renal cell cancer failed to reach any definitive conclusions.[31] The authors evaluated seven cohort studies and six case–control studies. Only three of the cohort studies and two of the case–control studies observed an excess, and in only one cohort study was the result statistically significant. It was concluded that future studies need to have large populations and quantitative exposure estimates to further characterize dose-related risk.

Other studies have been conducted with regard to the potential role of gene interaction (GST) in workers exposed to trichloroethylene.[32] Elevated odds ratios were observed for both those with GSTM1+ (OR = 2.7; 95% CI, 1.2–6.3) and those with GSTT1+ (OR = 4.2; 95% CI, 1.2–14.9). A more general review of this subject, that examined both the mechanistic issues as well as the occupational epidemiologic data, concluded that the issue was far from settled conclusively.[33]

With respect to other specific organic solvents, a cluster of renal cancer cases was observed in a group of workers employed in the repair and refurbishment of electrical transformers.[34] The exposures included organic solvent systems used in epoxy coatings for transformers, as well as polychlorinated biphenyls (PCBs), with which the transformers were filled. The authors suggested that the solvents may have acted as initiators, with the PCBs potentially acting as promoters.

A study of mortality in 8854 workers exposed to acrylamide observed only small increases in risk of kidney cancer (SMR 1.1; 95% CI, 0.7–1.6).[35] The study also failed to observe a dose response; however, this is not surprising with only 22 cases of kidney cancer in the cohort. Perhaps more importantly, when workers with mean intensity of exposure >0.02 mg/m^3 were considered (n = 5), the SMR increased to 1.7; although not statistically significant, this is suggestive of a possible causal linkage.

Metals

Cadmium

Cadmium, a potential animal carcinogen and a nephrotoxin, has also been associated with an increased risk of renal cancer. A case–control study by Kolonel identified 64 renal cancer cases in white males admitted to one hospital and 269 controls.[36] A relative risk of 2.5 was found for workers exposed occupationally to cadmium. In addition, a synergistic effect was demonstrated between smoking and cadmium exposure, with a relative risk of 4.4. A 1991 study in Finland of 338 cases of renal cell carcinoma also found a suggestion of elevated risks in individuals exposed to cadmium.[37] While studies are suggestive of an association of cadmium and renal cancer, further research is required to characterize this risk.

Lead

A mortality study in a cohort of lead smelter workers has been reported by Selevan and coworkers.[38] The exposure to lead in the smelting process was considered to be heavy, averaging over twice the consensus standard established in 1965 for air-borne lead exposure of 200 µg/m^3. An SMR of 301 (98 to 703), associated with five deaths, was found for kidney cancer in this study. In addition, a significant SMR of 392 for chronic kidney disease was found for exposure lasting more than 20 years. Results for both chronic renal disease and renal carcinoma have been variable in subsequent studies. A recent review and meta-analysis by Steenland and Boffetta of eight studies of lead smelter and battery workers – 40 total cases of renal carcinoma – found little evidence of lead as a risk factor for kidney cancer, observing a relative overall risk of 1.01 (95% CI, 0.7–1.4), with only two of the eight studies demonstrating a risk greater than 1.[39] The existing evidence for lead as a renal carcinogen thus remains inconclusive.

Steel, aluminum, ferrosilicon and silicon metal

Studies at steel and aluminum reduction plants have shown elevated rates of renal cancer in some workers. In addition, a recent study of ferrosilicon and silicon metal facilities in Norway observed a small excess of cancer of the kidney and ureter in both furnace (standardized incidence ratio [SIR] = 1.3; 95% CI, 0.66–2.38) and non-furnace (SIR = 1.7; 95% CI, 1.03–2.55) workers.[40] As discussed earlier, however, these risks are thought to be due to PAHs generated in processing, as well as organic solvents used in cleaning the metals; the role of these metals remains unclear.

Asbestos

A large number of studies have been carried out to examine the mortality of workers exposed to asbestos. While they have primarily focused on lung cancer, a number of studies have observed increased risk of kidney cancer as well. Selikoff's study of 17,800 insulators found 18 deaths due to renal cancer when 8.1 were expected, yielding an SMR of 222, which was statistically siginificant.[41] These results were supported by two other long-term cohort studies of use of asbestos products in Italian factory and shipyard workers. A recent meta-analysis of 37 cohort studies was carried out at the IARC.[42] As is often the case with cohort studies, the actual number of kidney cancer deaths was limited ($n = 169$). The pooled SMR for these studies was 1.1 (95% CI, 0.9–1.6).

The positive epidemiologic studies are supported by several toxicologic experiments of asbestos exposure. It is clear that it is possible for asbestos fibers to reach the kidney, presumably through the blood or lymphatic system. Autopsy studies of individuals have found asbestos bodies in the kidney. Amphibole fibers have also been demonstrated in urine. In conclusion, while there is evidence for a causal association between asbestos exposure and renal cancer, the magnitude of the risk is likely to be relatively small compared with that for lung cancer.

Uranium

There have been two studies that have observed an increased risk of renal cell carcinoma in workers processing uranium.[43,44] While the former study observed a dose–response association with radiation exposure in general, studies of ionizing radiation have not noted similar increases in risk.[45–49] In addition to ionizing radiation, other chemical exposures related to the processing may be confounders. Interestingly, in a study of 2514 workers at a uranium processing plant, in addition to renal cell carcinoma, the authors also observed increased mortality for chronic nephritis (OR = 1.9; 95% CI, 0.8–3.8).[43]

Other associated occupations

Several other occupations have been suggested to be associated with renal cell carcinoma, including ferrochromium workers, rocket-engine test-stand personnel, newspaper web pressmen, printers, and white-collar workers. The excess in kidney cancer (5 versus 1.6 expected) seen in one study of newspaper web pressmen is notable, given the substantial exposure to organic solvents as well as lead in this industry. A study of workers involved in rocket-engine testing found an association between exposure to hydrazine-based fuels and increased relative risk of death from bladder and kidney cancer (RR = 1.8; 95% CI, 0.6–5.1).[50] The authors indicate that there was significant exposure to trichloroethylene in the same procedures that utilized the hydrazine. The increased risk in white-collar workers, such as physicians, found in several studies, is thought to be related to increased levels of other risk factors associated with renal cell carcinoma, including obesity, meat and fat consumption, analgesic use, as well as increased diagnostic surveillance.

WILMS' TUMOR

The general epidemiology of Wilms' tumor has only recently been understood. There appears to be both a genetic and non-genetic form of this cancer. The genetic cases are more likely to be bilateral and show nephroblastomatosis on pathologic examination. The genetic form is not familial in nature but reflects mutations in the germ cells before conception.

A case–control study of 88 Wilms' tumor patients identified both maternal and paternal risk factors for Wilms' tumor.[51] The increase was highest in those whose fathers held jobs as machinists and welders during preconception (OR = 5.3; $P = 0.006$). Maternal use of hair dyes in the preconception period revealed a statistically significant odds ratio of 3.6. Other gestational risk factors included hypertension during pregnancy, tea drinking, and vaginal infection. Older maternal age was associated with the genetic form of Wilms' tumor. In a study carried out in England of paternal exposures and childhood cancer, the only statistically significant finding was for exposure to pesticides (proportional mortality ratio [PMR] = 1.6; 95% CI, 1.2–2.2).[52] A review was carried out of 48 published epidemiologic studies regarding childhood cancer and parental occupation.[53] Of the 48 studies, only five addressed the issue of Wilms' tumor, the previously cited Bunin et al. study[51] among them. One study attributed the increased risk to parental exposure to lead, the others to various occupations, including manufacturing of wood and furniture, iron and metal structures, and electrical contracting.[54] Another study found associations between maternal exposure to PAHs and Wilms' tumor.[51] The overall status of parental exposure and Wilms' tumor, certainly suggestive of an association, warrants further investigation.

References

1. Christenson PJ, Craig JP, Bibro MC, et al. Cysts containing renal cell carcinoma in von Hippel-Lindau diseases. J Urol 1982; 128:798-800.
2. McCredie M, Ford JM, Stewart JH. Risk factors for cancer of the renal parenchyma. Int J Cancer 1988; 42:13-16.
3. Sokoloff MH, deKernion JB, Figlin RA, et al. Current management of renal cell carcinoma. CA Cancer J Clin 1996; 46:284-302.
4. Diaz JI, Mora LB, Hakam A. The Mainz classification of renal cell tumors. Cancer Control 1999; 6:571-9.
5. Motzer RJ, Russo P. Systemic therapy for renal cell carcinoma. J Urol 2000; 163:408-17.
6. Motzer RJ, Vogelgang NJ. Chemotherapy for renal cell carcinoma. In: Raghaven D, Scher HI, Leibel SA, et al., eds. Principles and practice of genitourinary oncology. Philadelphia: Lippincott-Raven; 1991:885.
7. Yagoda A, Abi-Rached B, Petrylak D. Chemotherapy for advanced renal-cell carcinoma: 1983-1993. Semin Oncol 1995; 22:42-60.
8. Motzer RJ, Bander NH, Nanus DM. Renal-cell carcinoma. N Engl J Med 1996; 335:865-75.
9. Childs R, Chernoff A, Contentin N, et al. Regression of metastatic renal-cell carcinoma after nonmyeloblative allogenic peripheral-blood stem-cell transplantation. N Engl J Med 2000; 343:750-8.
10. McLaughlin JK, Mandel JS, Blot WJ, et al. A population-based case-control study of renal cell carcinoma. J Natl Cancer Inst 1984; 72:275-84.
11. McCredie M, Stewart JH. Risk factors for kidney cancer in New South Wales. I. Cigarette smoking. Eur J Cancer 1992; 28A:2050-4.

12. Yu MC, Mack TM, Hanisch R, Cicioni C, Henderson BE. Cigarette smoking, obesity, diuretic use and coffee consumption as risk factors for renal cell carcinoma. J Natl Cancer Inst 1986; 77:351-6.

13. Maclure M, Hankinson S. Analysis of selection bias in a case-control study of renal adenocarcinoma. Epidemiology 1990; 6:441-7.

14. Gamble JF, Pearlman ED, Nicolich MJ. A nested case-control study of kidney cancer among refinery/petrochemical workers. Environ Health Perspect 1996; 104:642-50.

15. McCredie M, Stewart JH. Risk factors for kidney cancer in New South Wales, Australia. II. Urologic disease, hypertension, obesity, and hormonal factors. Cancer Causes Control 1992; 3:323-31.

16. Grove JS, Nomure A, Stemmermann GN. The association for blood pressure with cancer incidence in a prospective study. Am J Epidemiol 1991; 134:942-7.

17. Sandler DP, Smith JC, Weinberg CR, et al. Analgesics use and chronic renal disease. N Engl J Med 1989; 320:1238-43.

18. Walker C, Goldsworthy TL, Wolf DC, Everitt J. Predisposition to renal cell carcinoma due to alteration of a cancer susceptibility gene. Science 1992; 255:1693-5.

19. Sweeney C, Farrow DC, Schwartz SM, et al. Glutathione S-transferase M1, T1, and P1 polymorphisms as risk factors for renal cell carcinoma: a case-control study. Cancer Epidemiol Biomarkers Prev 2000; 9:449-54.

20. Redmond CK, Ciocco A, Lloyd JW, Rush HW. Long-term mortality study of steelworkers. VI – Mortality from malignant neoplasms among coke oven workers. J Occup Med 1972; 14:621-9.

21. Rockette HE, Arena VC. Mortality studies of aluminum reduction plant workers; potroom and carbon departments. J Occup Med 1983; 25:549-57.

22. Sharpe CR, Rochon JE, Adam JM, Suissa S. Case-control study of hydrocarbon exposures in patients with renal cell carcinoma. Can Med Assoc J 1989; 140:1309-18.

23. Lewis RJ, Gamble JF, Jorgensen G. Mortality among three refinery/petrochemical plant cohorts. I. 1970 to 1982 active/terminated workers. J Occup Environ Med 2000; 42:721-9.

24. Lynge E, Andersen A, Nilsson R, et al. Risk of cancer and exposure to gasoline vapors. Am J Epidemiol 1997; 145:449-58.

25. Poole C, Dreyer NA, Satterfield MH, et al. Kidney cancer and hydrocarbon exposures among petroleum refinery workers. Environ Health Perspect 1993; 101(Suppl 6):53-62.

26. Rushton L. A 39-year follow-up of the U.K. oil refinery and distribution center studies: results for kidney cancer and leukemia. Environ Health Perspect 1993; 101(Suppl 6):77-84.

27. Wong O, Raabe G. A critical review of cancer epidemiology in the petroleum industry, with a meta-analysis of a combined databse of more than 350,000 workers. Regul Toxicol Pharmacol 2000; 32:78-98.

28. Gamble JF, Lewis EJ, Jorgensen G. Mortality among three refinery/petrochemical plant cohorts. II. Retirees. J Occup Environ Med 2000; 42:730-6.

29. Parent ME, Hua Y, Siemiatycki J. Occupational risk factors for renal cell carcinoma in Montreal. Am J Ind Med 2000; 38:609-18.

30. Kadamani S, Asal NR, Nelson RY. Occupational hydrocarbon exposure and risk of renal cell carcinoma. Am J Ind Med 1989; 15:131-41.

31. McLaughlin JK, Blot WJ. A critical review of epidemiology studies of trichloroethylene and perchloroethylene and risk of renal-cell cancer. Int Arch Occup Environ Health 1997; 70:222-31.

32. Bruning T, Lammert M, Kempkes M, et al. Influence of polymorphisms of GSTM1 and GSTT1 for risk of renal cell cancer in workers with long-term high occupational exposure to trichloroethene. Arch Toxicol 1997; 71:596-9.

33. Lash LH, Parker JC, Scott CS. Modes of action of trichloroethylene for kidney tumorigenesis. Environ Health Perspect 2000; 108:225-40.

34. Shalat SL, True LD, Fleming LE, Pace P. Kidney cancer in utility workers exposed to polychlorinated biphenyls (PCB's). Br J Ind Med 1989; 46:823-4.

35. Marsh GM, Lucas LJ, Yuok AO, Schall LC. Mortality patterns among workers exposed to acrylamide: 1994 follow up. Occup Environ Med 1999; 56:181-90.

36. Kolonel LN. Association of cadmium with renal cancer. Cancer 1976; 37:1782-7.

37. Partanen T, Heikkila P, Hernberg S, et al. Renal cell cancer and occupational exposure to chemical agents. Scand J Work Environ Health 1991; 17:231-9.

38. Selevan SSG, Landrigan PJ, Stern FB, Jones JH. Mortality of lead smelter workers. Am J Epidemiol 1985; 122:673-83.

39. Steenland K, Boffetta P. Lead and cancer in humans: where are we now? Am J Ind Med 2000; 38:295-9.

40. Hobbesland A, Kjuus H, Thelle DS. Study of cancer incidence among 8530 male workers in eight Norwegian plants producing ferrosilicon and silicon metal. Occup Environ Med 1999; 56:625-31.

41. Selikoff IJ, Hommond EC, Seidman HA. Mortality experience of insulation workers in the United States and Canada, 1948-1976. Ann N Y Acad Med 1979; 330:91-116.

42. Sali D, Boffetta P. Kidney cancer and occupational exposure to asbestos: a meta-analysis of occupational cohort studies. Cancer Causes Control 2000; 11:37-47.

43. Dupree-Ellis E, Watkins J, Ingle JN, Phillips J. External radiation exposure and mortality in a cohort of uranium processing workers. Am J Epidemiol 2000; 152:91-5.

44. Fraser P, Carpenter L, Maconochie N, et al. Cancer mortality and morbidity in employees in three United Kingdom Atomic Energy Authority 1946-86. Br J Cancer 1993; 67:615-24.

45. Beral V, Fraser P, Carpenter L, et al. Mortality of employees of the atomic weapons establishment, 1951-82. BMJ 1988; 297:757-70.

46. Cardis E, Gilbert ES, Carpenter L, et al. Effects of low doses and low dose rates of external ionizing radiation: cancer mortality among nuclear industry workers in three countries. Radiat Res 1995; 142:117-32.

47. Carpenter L, Higgins C, Douglas A, et al. Combined analysis of morality in three United Kingdom nuclear industry workforces, 1946-1988. Radiat Res 1994; 138:224-38.

48. Omar RZ, Barber JA, Smith PG. Cancer mortality and morbidity among plutonium workers at the Sellafield plant of British Nuclear Fuels. Br J Cancer 1999; 79:1288-301.

49. Ritz B. Cancer mortality among workers exposed to chemicals during uranium processing. J Occup Environ Med 1999; 41:556-66.

50. Ritz B, Morgenstern H, Froines J, Moncau J. Chemical exposures of rocket-engine test-stand personnel and cancer mortality in a cohort of aerospace workers. J Occup Environ Med 1999; 41:903-10.

51. Bunin GR, Mass CC, Kramer S, Meadows AT. Parental occupation and Wilms' tumor: results of a case-control study. Cancer Res 1989; 49:725-9.

52. Fear NT, Roman E, Reeves G, Pannett B. Childhood cancer and paternal employment in agriculture: the role of pesticides. Br J Cancer 1998; 77:825-9.

53. Colt JS, Blair A. Parental occupational exposures and risk of childhood cancer. Environ Health Perspect 1998; 106(Suppl 3):909-25.

54. Olshan AF, Breslow NE, Daling JR, et al. Wilms' tumor and parental occupation. Cancer Res 1990; 50:3212-17.

30.5 **Cancer of the Liver and Gastrointestinal Tract**
Howard Frumkin, Patricia Blackwell

The gastrointestinal tract, considered as a whole, is the most common site of cancer incidence worldwide.[1] It is also the most common cause of cancer mortality worldwide, and in the US ranks second to cancer of the pulmonary system in this regard.[2,3] This chapter considers occupational and environmental contributions to cancers at several sites: the esophagus, the stomach, the colon and rectum, the liver, the gallbladder, and the pancreas. These cancers are summarized in Table 30.5.1.

The cancers discussed in this chapter share several common features. Most are adenocarcinomas, with the exception of esophageal cancer, in which both squamous cell cancer and adenocarcinoma are common. Most of these cancers exhibit strikingly variable incidence rates in geographic comparisons and migrant studies, suggesting substantial contributions from environmental factors. Diet, infectious agents, and alcohol and tobacco use generally have been implicated more than chemical or other workplace exposures. Most gastrointestinal cancers do not cause symptoms until they are relatively far advanced, resulting in poor prognoses. The primary treatment is surgical. Unfortunately, with the important exception of colorectal cancer, effective means of early detection are not available.

SPECIFIC DISORDERS
Esophageal cancer

Etiology

An interesting feature of the epidemiology of esophageal cancer is its tremendous geographic variation, ranging over 500-fold from nation to nation and within nations. The highest rates occur in a belt from the Caspian littoral in Turkey and northern Iran, through the southern republics of Kazakhstan, Uzbekistan, and Turkmenistan, to northern and eastern China, as well as in parts of southern and eastern Africa, India, and Sri Lanka. Rates are much lower in most of Europe and North America. In the US, the incidence is higher in blacks than in whites, and is higher in males than in females. Throughout the world, esophageal cancer rates are higher in lower socioeconomic classes.[4]

This geographic and class variability strongly suggests environmental determinants, and many have been identified. Alcohol consumption and tobacco use are recognized as important causes, especially in developed nations and in Africa. In parts of China with a high incidence of esophageal cancer, domestic fowl also exhibit a high incidence of pharyngoesophageal tumors, suggesting a common environmental cause, perhaps nitrosamine contamination of water, fungal agents, or both. In India, the chewing of betel nuts is associated with esophageal cancer. The use of hot drinks also may be a risk factor. Dietary factors[5] may play a role; some populations with a high incidence of esophageal cancer eat high-grain diets low in vegetables, fruits, and animal products. Fumonisin B(1), a mycotoxin produced by *Fusarium verticillioides* that contaminates maize and other grains, especially in Africa, has been linked to esophageal cancer risk. Radiation is carcinogenic to the esophagus, and pre-existing conditions such as achalasia, lye injury, and Plummer–Vinson syndrome also are risk factors for esophageal cancer. Human papilloma virus is a suspected cause of esophageal squamous cell carcinoma, although results across studies have been inconsistent.[6]

Beginning in the early 1980s, a rising incidence of adenocarcinoma of the esophagus was noted, particularly in white males.[7] While squamous cell carcinoma remains the predominant histologic type for esophageal cancer worldwide, in some centers adenocarcinoma has come to predominate. Most cases of adenocarcinoma of the esophagus occur in individuals with Barrett's esophagus (intestinalized mucosa lining the lower esophagus[8]), related to gastroesophageal reflux. Of possible etiological factors investigated, obesity[9] is the best established.

Relatively few occupational exposures have been clearly associated with esophageal cancer.[10] Table 30.5.2 shows industries, exposures, and occupations for which such observations have been made. However, few firm conclusions can be drawn at present with regard to the observations in Table 30.5.2 for several reasons: most of the observations are unique and have not been corroborated; opposing evidence exists in some cases; and confounders such as smoking, alcohol use, and social class often were not adequately controlled. Interestingly, several studies have shown that farmers have a lower-than-expected rate of esophageal cancer; the significance of this observation is unclear.

There is relatively more information on asbestos exposure as a cause of esophageal cancer, but the evidence is equivocal.[11] Similarly, considerable evidence is available on the rubber industry, but this, too, is equivocal. Because worker exposures often vary within the same facility, exposure misclassification may have obscured a true association in some studies. Straif and collaborators[12] reported increased rates of esophageal cancer in rubber workers exposed to nitrosamines.

Other notable observations include an association between esophageal cancer and two exposures, sulfuric acid and carbon black, in the large case–control study database at Institut Armand-Frappier in Quebec,[13] an elevation of esophageal cancer among workers with potential exposure to silica dust and chemical solvents or detergents in data from the National Center for Health Statistics,[14] and an association between cutting oils and cancer of several gastrointestinal sites, including the esophagus, in several studies.[15]

Diagnosis, treatment, and prognosis
The diagnosis and treatment of esophageal cancer in the workplace do not differ from those of esophageal cancer in

Origin	Approximate US incidence (/100,000)	Major cell type	Five-year survival (%)
Esophagus	3.9	Squamous/adenocarcinoma	14.8
Stomach	6.7	Adenocarcinoma	22.6
Colon–rectum	43.9	Adenocarcinoma	62.0
Liver	4.3	Adenocarcinoma, angiosarcoma	5.5
Gallbladder	1–2	Adenocarcinoma	<10
Pancreas	8.8	Adenocarcinoma	4.6

Table 30.5.1 Cancers of the gastrointestinal tract

Industries and exposures	Occupations
Aluminum reduction plant	Brickmakers and brickmasons
Asbestos	Brewery workers
Automobile repair/body shops	Chimney sweeps
Benzidine	Diagnostic X-ray workers
Biogenic silica (sugar-cane workers)	Dry-cleaning workers
Bitumen	Dye workers
Carbon black	Firefighters
Cutting oils, mists	Janitors and cleaners
Hazardous waste sites	Laborers
Inorganic silica	Painters
Meatpacking	Plutonium workers
Metal working	Police officers
Mineral spirits	Restaurant workers
Nitrosamines	Roofers
Pesticides	Rubber workers
Petroleum products in potable water	Shoemakers
Phenol	Stonemasons
Polycyclic aromatic hydrocarbons	Textile workers
Printing	Wood and forestry workers
Pulp and paper	
Silica dust	
Styrene-butadiene polymerization	
Sulfuric acid	
Synthetic abrasives manufacturing	
Toluene	

Table 30.5.2 Industries, exposures, and occupations in which high rates of esophageal cancer have been reported

the general population, and these topics are beyond the scope of this text.

Opportunities for screening and early detection in the workplace

Screening for esophageal cancer has been attempted in high-incidence areas, using esophageal cytology specimens obtained with brush or abrasive balloon,[16] and in some studies using endoscopy with biopsy. Balloon cytology is more suitable to workplace screening because it is far more rapid and less invasive than endoscopy. However, the Chinese program was conducted as part of a study of the prevalence of epithelial dysplasia, and it did not yield full data on test sensitivity and specificity, opportunities for early treatment, outcomes, or screening costs. Moreover, no occupational groups have been identified with a risk of esophageal cancer even approaching that of northern China. Therefore, workplace screening cannot be recommended based on currently available data.

Gastric cancer

Etiology

Gastric cancer incidence varies substantially from region to region; among nations that collect data, gastric cancer mortality is highest in the Russian Federation, Kazakhstan, Chile, and Japan, and lowest in the US, Canada, New Zealand, and Australia. Migrant studies, especially of Japanese living in the US, have also revealed dramatic decreases in incidence over one or two generations. These observations strongly implicate environmental factors in the etiology of stomach cancer.

Whatever the environmental factors, they are likely to be associated with poverty, because many studies have shown a strong association between low socioeconomic status and gastric cancer incidence. Dietary factors are likely to be important. One dietary risk factor is nitrates and related compounds, which are found in dried, smoked, salted, and pickled foods, cured meats, green vegetables, and, sometimes, drinking water. Nitrates are converted to nitrites by oral bacteria and then to nitrosamines by combining with dietary secondary amines. On the other hand, many studies have found the consumption of fresh fruits and vegetables to be protective. Radiation can cause gastric cancer, whereas the evidence implicating cigarette smoking and alcohol consumption is less consistent. Other risk factors include blood group A, pernicious anemia, and, possibly, gastric ulcer disease. Cancer of the gastric cardia is thought to be similar to esophageal adenocarcinoma in etiology.

Several benign disorders of the stomach are considered premalignant; examples include chronic atrophic gastritis, *Helicobacter pylori* infection, intestinal metaplasia, and gastric dysplasia. When such a condition is associated with an occupational exposure, then the exposure may be considered a risk factor for gastric cancer. For example, methyl methacrylate exposure causes chronic gastritis, and, therefore, it has been considered a risk factor for gastric cancer in Russia.

In individual studies, a wide variety of occupational factors has been reported to be associated with gastric cancer[10,17,18] (Table 30.5.3). Again, many of these observations cannot support firm conclusions because they are for the most part uncorroborated, and there is opposing evidence in some cases. Most occupational studies have not controlled for social class, a potentially important confounder because both occupational status and the disease are class related.

Industries and exposures	Occupations
Acetylene production	Aluminum reduction workers
Air pollution (petrochemical	Brickmakers
plants)	Carpenters
Asbestos	Ceramic workers
Pulp and paper manufacturing	Chemical workers
Auto body/repair shops	Chemists
Azo dyes	Concrete workers
Styrene-butadiene polymerization	Divers
Coal dust	Dockers and freight handlers
Electronics manufacturing	Farmers
Ethylene oxide	Firefighters
Rubber manufacturing	Fishermen
Fertilizer manufacturing	Forestry workers
Gasoline (leaded)	Granite workers
Glass manufacturing	Hematite miners
Gold mining	Jewelry workers
Halogenated hydrocarbons	Machinists and metal
Hazardous waste sites	workers
Hydraulic fluids	Painters
Kerosene	Plumbers
Lead	Plutonium workers
Metal dust	Radium-dial painters
Magnesium production	Railroad workers
Silica	Shoemakers
Nickel/chromium plating	Steel foundry workers
Pesticides	Stonemasons
Petroleum refining and	Tin miners
petrochemicals	Tool and dye workers
Rock wool manufacturing	Truck drivers
Phenoxy herbicides	
Sulfuric acid	
Synthetic abrasives manufacturing	
Wood dust/furniture making	
Wood fuel use	

Table 30.5.3 Industries, exposures, and occupations in which high rates of gastric cancer have been reported

An interesting and frequent observation is the association of dusty work with gastric cancer risk. Data are available for coal dust, silica, and asbestos. *Coal dust* has emerged as a risk factor for gastric cancer in many studies.[19,20] The mechanism of gastric cancer induction by coal dust is unknown. Constituents such as polyaromatic hydrocarbons (PAHs) and metals may act as carcinogens, or nitrosation of coal dust constituents may create the active carcinogens. The risk of gastric cancer may be confined to coal miners with no or mild pneumoconiosis, perhaps because more severe pneumoconiosis entails defects in respiratory clearance that exposes the gastrointestinal tract.[19] Dusty trades[21,22] such as cement and quarry work, granite work, and other kinds of mining, many of which entail *silica* exposure, carry an elevated risk of gastric cancer. Finally, *asbestos* exposure has been associated with gastric cancer in numerous studies,[23–25] although not all studies confirm this association. The best estimate is that lifelong exposure to high levels of asbestos carries a relative risk of approximately 1.3.

Several other exposures deserve special mention. Workers exposed to *wood dust and its derivatives*, such as furniture makers and paper workers,[26] have been extensively studied and show a consistent increase in gastric cancer risk. *Farmers* also have higher rates in most studies.[27] Lead exposure has been associated with gastric

cancer, but results have been inconsistent across studies.[28] *Metalworking and related activities*[29] have been associated with an increased risk of gastric cancer in several studies. Although cutting oils have been implicated, other exposures such as solvents, abrasives, metals, and nitrosamine contaminants may play a role as well. Studies of workers in the *rubber industry*[30] have shown consistent elevations of gastric cancer.

Diagnosis, treatment, and prognosis
The diagnosis and treatment of gastric cancer in the occupational setting are identical to those occurring in the general population, and they are beyond the scope of this text. Prognosis is affected by the stage at diagnosis. Five-year survival ranges from 78% in AJCC stage IA disease to 7% for stage IV cases.[31]

Opportunities for screening and early detection in the workplace
Several techniques have been considered for gastric cancer screening. Large-scale gastric cancer screening has been conducted in Japan since the 1960s, using image-intensified photofluorography at fixed locations and in mobile vans. Reports of high sensitivity and specificity, earlier average stage at diagnosis, and improved survival[32] have appeared. However, even in the high-risk Japanese population, the positive predictive value of the test is probably less than 2%. In China and the former Soviet Union, screening programs have attempted to identify high-risk individuals based on symptoms, history, or both, followed by referral for gastroscopy. The efficacy and cost–benefit features of these programs have not been reported. Other screening methods that have been attempted elsewhere, generally in endemic areas of Asia, include an occult blood detector that is swallowed and extracted from the stomach after a few minutes and tests for monoclonal antibodies. Widely available tests for *H. pylori* may provide a cost-effective screening test to target individuals for antibiotic treatment or gastroscopy. The ratio of pepsinogen type I (PGI) to pepsinogen II (PGII) decreases in proportion to the extent of gastric atrophy, and is a potentially useful test for selecting individuals for cancer screening. However, because no screening method has been sufficiently characterized or subjected to randomized trials, and because no occupational groups in the US are known to have such a markedly elevated risk of gastric cancer, workplace screening for this tumor cannot be recommended at present.

Colorectal cancer

Etiology
Like other gastrointestinal cancers, colorectal cancer has a highly variable incidence across different populations and in migrant studies. Diet is known to play a major etiologic role.[33] High-fat diets confer increased risk, probably mediated by the production of endogenous bile acids. High fiber intake, and perhaps a high intake of calcium, folate, or yellow–green vegetables are associated with decreased

risk. Several studies have shown non-steroidal anti-inflammatory agents to lower the risk of colon cancer. Lichtenstein et al.,[34] in a twin study, calculated that 35% of colon cancer risk could be attributed to genetic factors. Several hereditary syndromes, such as familial polyposis, are associated with a substantial increase in the risk for colon cancer. Other risk factors for colorectal cancer include inflammatory bowel disease, ureterosigmoidostomy, *Streptococcus bovis* bacteremia, and, perhaps, cholecystectomy. Most colonic cancers arise from polyps, and the presence of polyps may be an independent risk factor.

Colon cancer rates vary by subsite of origin, and the incidence of cancer at different subsites varies by age, gender, race, and geographical region.[35] Recent evidence suggests that colorectal cancers arising at different sites within the colon may represent genetically distinct diseases. Consistent with this theory, several investigators have found that work-related elevations in colorectal cancer tend to be site specific. Advances in molecular biology and epidemiology may clarify this finding in coming years.

The level of physical activity is a risk factor for colorectal cancer, and may be work related. Numerous studies have demonstrated that sedentary employment is associated with an increased risk of colon cancer, whereas high levels of physical activity seem to be protective. Interestingly, the protective effect seems most striking in the proximal colon, whereas results are less consistent with regard to rectal cancer.

Beyond this observation regarding physical activity, few workplace exposures have been consistently linked with cancer of the lower gastrointestinal tract.[9] One exception is *asbestos*.[36] Frumkin and Berlin, in a meta-analysis,[23] calculated that substantial asbestos exposure confers a relative risk of about 1.6 for colorectal cancer, consistent with the value seen in the largest ongoing cohort study of asbestos workers. Smaller cohorts and studies of less intensely exposed workers have yielded less clear results. While evidence suggests that asbestos is a colorectal carcinogen, there remains some disagreement on this point.

Studies of the *rubber industry* have revealed a slightly elevated risk of colorectal cancer, although the risk is well below the relative risk for gastric cancer among rubber workers. Studies of *printers* and *pressmen* have shown a fairly consistent increase in colorectal cancer, as have studies of *automotive pattern and model makers*. *Wood dust* exposure in furniture makers has also been associated with colon cancer.[37] Other reports of exposed groups with increased colorectal cancer rates are shown in Table 30.5.4.

Diagnosis, treatment, and prognosis

The diagnosis and treatment of colorectal cancer are well described in standard texts and are not covered here. The prognosis depends upon how advanced the tumor is. Superficial tumors that do not cross the submucosa (stage A) have a 5-year survival better than 90%. Stage B tumors that infiltrate the muscularis or penetrate the bowel wall but do not involve lymph nodes have a 70% to 85% 5-year survival. Tumors that involve lymph nodes (stage C)

Industries and exposures	Occupations
Abrasives manufacturing	Accountants and auditors
Arsenic	Artists
Asbestos	Brewery workers
Automobile engine and parts manufacturing	Chemical workers
	Chemists
Bearing manufacturing	Designers and draftsmen
Bitumen	Dockworkers
Chlorination byproducts	Farmers (small intestine)
Clothing manufacturing (small intestine)	Firefighters
	Forest and soil conservationists
Coke byproducts	Fur dressers and dyers
Communications	Janitors and housekeepers
Copper smelting	(small intestine)
Crude oil	Lawyers and judges
Diesel exhaust	Leather workers
Dry cleaning (small intestine)	Machinists
Dyes	Millwrights
Electronics manufacturing	Pattern and model makers
Food manufacturing	Plutonium workers
Formaldehyde	Police officers
Fuel oil	Printers and pressmen
Gasoline exhaust	Radium-dial painters
Glass manufacturing	Salesmen and sales clerks
Grain dust	Tailors and furriers
Grinding wheel dust	Textile workers
Hazardous waste sites	Veterinarians
Meatpacking	Waiters
Metal dust	White-collar workers
Metal-working fluids	Woodworkers, furniture makers
Methyl methacrylate, ethyl acrylate	
Optical manufacturing	
Paint and coating manufacturing	
Pesticides	
Petroleum products trade	
Petroleum refinery	
Polypropylene manufacturing	
Rubber manufacturing	
Solvents	
Stress	
Synthetic fiber dust	

Table 30.5.4 Industries, exposures, and occupations in which high rates of colorectal cancer have been reported

have a 35% to 65% 5-year survival rate, and those with distant metastases have less than a 5% 5-year survival. Carcinoembryonic antigen (CEA), which is elaborated by colorectal and other tumors, may have a role in monitoring patients postoperatively for tumor recurrence.

Opportunities for screening and early detection in the workplace

For persons at average risk for colorectal cancer, the US Preventive Services Task Force[38] recommends home fecal occult blood testing annually, or periodic flexible sigmoidoscopy, or a combination of these approaches. While the Preventive Services Task Force does not specify the frequency of sigmoidoscopy, other groups[39,40] recommend 5-year intervals. According to Preventive Services Task Force recommendations, colonoscopy may be substituted for flexible sigmoidoscopy. Again, the test interval is not specified, but other groups[39,40] recommend every 10 years.

Double-contrast barium enema is considered a less effective option, and digital rectal examination has not been shown to be of use. Although flexible sigmoidoscopy may miss some proximal lesions, the increased expense and complication rate of colonoscopy render it a less cost-effective screening option. Insufficient data exist at present to evaluate the effectiveness of newer technologies, such as virtual colonoscopy or stool screening for DNA abnormalities.

Some workplace screening programs for colorectal cancer have been implemented, not because of any presumed job-related increase in risk, but because such screening was considered generally advisable and the workplace was a convenient screening site. Certainly, the workplace may be a suitable venue for cancer screening and other health interventions that are generally beneficial.

In specific industrial settings believed to confer increased risk – most notably among pattern makers, asbestos workers, and polypropylene manufacturing workers – screening programs have been implemented. These programs have generally achieved participation rates of 50% or less. Non-participants identified various reasons for their reluctance, including inconvenience, embarrassment, anxiety, a belief that the procedure was unnecessary, and a belief that they were at low risk, factors generally similar to those cited by non-participants in screening programs in the general population. Moreover, there is no evidence that colorectal cancer screening in any specific occupational group (beyond that recommended for the general public) results in decreased morbidity and mortality. Firm recommendations on workplace screening must await further data on the general utility of colorectal cancer screening and on specific risks of various occupational exposures.

Liver cancer: hepatocellular carcinoma

Etiology

Liver cancer is one of the most common cancers in Africa and Asia, although it is relatively uncommon in Western countries. The usual cell type is hepatocellular carcinoma (or hepatoma). Liver cancer is two to three times more common in men than in women, probably reflecting greater male exposure to the causative agents and perhaps hormonal factors as well. Three risk factors account for most hepatocellular carcinoma worldwide:

- hepatitis B or C[41] virus;
- alcohol; and
- aflatoxin.

Recent advances in molecular epidemiology have permitted investigation of possible interactions among these risk factors.[42] About 75% of cases occur in patients with cirrhosis. Hepatitis D virus is considered to contribute little if any risk of hepatocellular carcinoma.

Agents that induce liver cancer may do so by acting as initiators or promoters. Few occupations, industries, or environmental agents have been consistently associated with elevations of hepatoma incidence.[10,43] Steenland and Palu[44] reported an increase in liver cancer among painters.

Industries and exposures	Occupations
Abrasives manufacturing	Accountants
Aflatoxin-contaminated dust (oil mills, livestock feed processing)	Bartenders
	Brewery workers
Arsenic	Business executives
Arts, theater and recreation	Chemical plant maintenance
Asbestos	workers
Auto repair shops	Chimney sweeps
Automobile engine and parts manufacturing (machining/ assembly plant)	Construction workers
	Diagnostic X-ray workers
	Farmers
Benzene	Fishermen
Chemical industry	Grain millers
Diesel exhaust	Insulation workers
Dry cleaning	Insurance agents
Dye, paint and oil stores	Jewelry workers
Flower shops	Metal workers
Formaldehyde	Painters
Gasoline service stations	Physicians
Shoe manufacturing	Plumbers and pipefitters
Highway construction	Police officers
Incinerators, solid waste	Pressmen
Metal product manufacturing	Rubber workers
Nickel and chromium plating	Salesmen (travelling and door-to-door)
Nickel alloy production	Service workers
Paper and graphics industry	Slaughterhouse workers
Pesticides	Waiters
Polychlorinated biphenyls	Woodworkers
Restaurant and hotel industry	
Retail foods	
Rubber manufacturing	
Solvents	
Wool manufacturing	

Table 30.5.5 Industries, exposures, and occupations in which high rates of liver cancer have been reported

Cirrhosis was also increased within this group, but it was felt that alcohol consumption only partially accounted for the increased cancer incidence. Workers in nuclear weapons production plants have been reported to experience an increased incidence of liver cancer.[45] Although increases in liver cancer have been seen in some studies of rubber workers and asbestos workers, these findings are not consistent across most studies. A recent study of women workers found little evidence of occupational liver cancer increases.[46] Other observed elevations of liver cancer, mostly isolated, appear in Table 30.5.5.

Some occupational groups are heavily exposed to agents that are known to cause liver cancer but that are not normally considered occupational carcinogens. Thus, brewery workers show an increased risk of liver cancer, probably related to increased alcohol consumption. Similarly, healthcare workers and prostitutes may be exposed to hepatitis B virus, and grain handlers and other food preparation workers may be exposed to aflatoxin. Premalignant conditions also should be considered. Solvent-exposed workers have been shown to develop hepatic necrosis and potentially fibrosis, at least after massive accidental exposure; in such uncommon cases, occupational liver cancer must be considered a possibility, even if no risk has yet been demonstrated for the solvent, per se.

Diagnosis, treatment, and prognosis

Useful diagnostic measures include radionuclide scans, ultrasound examinations, and computed tomography (CT) and magnetic resonance imaging (MRI) scans, but the most informative non-invasive test is angiography. Both hepatomas and hemangiosarcomas are hypervascular, as distinguished from hepatic metastases. Tissue diagnosis is made following biopsy, either with a percutaneous needle or at surgery. The only definitive treatment is surgical excision, but this is often precluded by an underlying illness such as cirrhosis and by the extent of the disease. The prognosis is poor, with median survival well under 1 year.

Opportunities for prevention, screening and early detection in the workplace

The hepatitis B vaccine represents an important opportunity for primary prevention of hepatitis B in healthcare workers at risk for occupational exposure to the virus. In these workers, both standard medical practice and Occupational Safety and Health Administration (OSHA) requirements[47] dictate that the vaccine should be routinely offered. In addition, serologic testing of workers with documented exposure to body fluids infected with hepatitis A or B may identify individuals requiring follow-up.

Early detection of hepatoma has been attempted in high-risk populations in China, Taiwan, South Africa, Italy, Alaska, and elsewhere. In most cases, screening has been targeted at chronic carriers of hepatitis B antigen and patients with cirrhosis, groups with substantially elevated risk. Two tests have received the most attention: alpha-fetoprotein and high-resolution ultrasonography. Alpha-fetoprotein alone is less than 50% sensitive in detecting small hepatomas. Even in the setting of large tumors, the sensitivity is only 85% to 90%. The specificity is well under 50% in some studies, because alpha-fetoprotein may increase in hepatitis and for other unknown reasons. These values can be varied considerably by redefining the upper normal limit of the test. Ultrasound alone is about 90% sensitive and 70% specific. The most successful programs have used both tests sequentially, following up abnormal alpha-fetoprotein values with ultrasonographic examination. Most studies have been unable to demonstrate any improvement in resectability or survival following screening. Therefore, routine screening for liver cancer in occupational groups, most of which have much lower risk than populations of cirrhotics and hepatitis carriers, cannot be recommended at this time.

Liver cancer: hemangiosarcoma

Etiology

A second form of liver cancer, hepatic hemangiosarcoma, is much rarer than hepatocellular carcinoma and is much more closely identified with occupational causes.[48] The world literature includes several hundred cases to date. Non-occupational causes include *thorotrast* (thorium dioxide), an alpha-emitter that was used as a radiographic

contrast agent from about 1930 to 1955, and *steroid medications* (both anabolic steroids and estrogen preparations). There are two major occupational and environmental causes: *vinyl chloride* and *arsenic*. An Egyptian report[49] suggests that organophosphate and organochlorine pesticides may be associated with hepatic angiosarcoma, but because the patients described also were exposed to arsenicals, the other pesticides could not be clearly implicated.

Arsenic exposure (see Chapter 39.2) has occurred following the use of Fowler's solution for medical purposes; following contamination of drinking water in Mexico, Taiwan, Chile, China, Argentina, and elsewhere; and following occupational exposure in agriculture, smelting, and wine making. Many studies of arsenic-exposed populations have described elevations of rates of liver cancer, mostly hemangiosarcoma but also including hepatomas.

Vinyl chloride exposure (see Chapter 41) was first associated with hemangiosarcoma when an alert clinician noted a cluster of cases in a polyvinyl chloride plant in Louisville in 1974.[50] Since then, numerous studies have confirmed an increased risk of hemangiosarcoma and of hepatoma in exposed workers and in animals. Recent evidence suggests a role for specific k-ras-2 and p53 mutations.[51,52] Following deep reductions in occupational exposure to vinyl chloride in the US and Europe in the 1970s, hemangiosarcoma and hepatoma related to this substance have declined dramatically.

Diagnosis, treatment, and prognosis

Angiosarcoma is associated with non-specific symptoms such as anorexia, malaise, nausea, weight loss, and right upper quadrant pain. Physical examination usually reveals hepatomegaly by the time of presentation, and often reveals fever, jaundice, ascites, splenomegaly, and a liver bruit as well. Laboratory studies reveal abnormal liver function tests and often normochromic, normocytic anemia. Liver scan or ultrasound shows single or multiple filling defects, CT scan shows mixed-attenuation tumor mass, and hepatic angiography shows a hypervascular lesion.

Needle biopsy is risky because of the vascularity of the tumor, so open liver biopsy often is necessary to reach a diagnosis. Angiosarcoma arises from the endothelial or Kupffer cells that line the hepatic sinusoids, and it has a variable microscopic appearance (Fig. 30.5.1). In areas of the liver that are minimally involved, dilated sinusoids are lined by hypertrophied endothelial cells with atypical hyperchromatic nuclei. As the tumor advances, the sinusoids dilate and fill with malignant endothelial cells. Eventually, hepatocytes may be entirely replaced by massed tumor cells with extensive vascular channels. The malignant cells may have an epithelioid appearance similar to poorly differentiated carcinoma or a spindled appearance similar to fibrosarcoma, making microscopic diagnosis difficult.

Hepatic angiosarcoma can progress to hemorrhage, disseminated intravascular coagulation, or renal failure, and is rapidly fatal. Chemotherapy and radiotherapy have

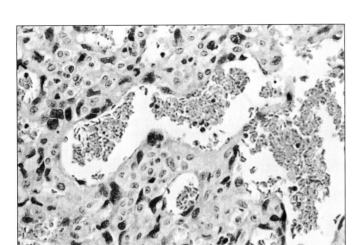

Figure 30.5.1: Histology of angiosarcoma of the liver. Solid cellular masses are separated by blood spaces. The tumor cells are elongated with pleomorphic, hyperchromatic nuclei and ill-defined cytoplasm (hematoxylin–eosin stain, ×250). (Courtesy of Dr Swan Thung.)

not been found to be helpful, and the role of local tumor resection and liver transplantation has not been defined.

Opportunities for screening and early detection in the workplace

Early detection of hemangiosarcoma has been attempted in vinyl chloride workers, but there is no evidence that outcomes are altered by such an effort. Primary prevention through containment of exposure rather than secondary prevention has proved feasible and extremely effective in the US; consequently, it is the preferred approach.

Gallbladder and biliary tract cancer

Cancer of the gallbladder and biliary tract is extremely rare in the US, and it is not generally considered occupational or environmental in origin. Cholangiocarcinoma has been induced experimentally in animals by feeding 3-methyl-4-dimethyl-aminoazobenzene.[53] Isolated observations[54] appear in Table 30.5.6, which cites reports of increased risk among forestry workers, rubber workers, automotive workers, textile workers, chemical workers, and shoemakers. Other industries in which some increase in risk has been observed include metal fabricating, aircraft, wood finishing, petroleum refining, and paper mills. Because workers in forestry, wood finishing, and paper mills have been

Industries and exposures	Occupations
Aircraft manufacturing	Automotive workers
Heavy metals	Chemical workers
Metal fabricating	Forestry workers
Paper mills	Shoemakers
Petroleum refining	Textile workers
Rubber manufacturing	
Wood finishing	

Table 30.5.6 Industries, exposures, and occupations in which high rates of biliary tract cancer have been reported

mentioned in this regard, it is interesting to speculate that a wood product may be specifically carcinogenic to the biliary tract. Shukla et al.[55] studied the relationship of biliary heavy metal concentrations and gallbladder cancer in an area of India with high drinking water concentrations of heavy metals. Thirty-eight patients with gallbladder cancer were found to have significantly elevated biliary levels of cadmium, chromium, and lead, compared with a control group of 58 patients presenting with benign cholelithiasis. This difference was particularly marked for biliary lead, with cases having a mean lead level of 58.38 mg/l, as compared with 3.99 mg/l for controls ($P<0.001$).

Pancreatic cancer

Etiology

Cancer of the pancreas varies among populations relatively less than other gastrointestinal cancers, ranging from a high incidence of 20.8 per 100,000 per year among black men in central Louisiana[56] to a low incidence of 1.4 per 100,000 per year among women in Mauritius. Most populations have an incidence of between 5 and 10 per 100,000 per year. Because it is almost invariably fatal, pancreatic cancer is the fourth leading cause of cancer mortality in the US.

Pancreatic cancer is clinically associated with diabetes, pancreatitis, and gallbladder disease, although the nature of these associations is unclear. Both demographic (advancing age, black race, male gender, Jewish religion) and dietary (carbohydrates, cholesterol, meat, salt, dehydrated food, preservatives, refined sugar, nitrosamines) factors have been associated with an increased risk of pancreatic cancer.[57] A protective effect has been reported for dietary fiber, vitamin C, fruits and vegetables, pressure cooking, and microwave cooking. Cigarette smoking increases the risk of pancreatic cancer several-fold.

Few occupational exposures have been clearly and consistently associated with pancreatic cancer.[10,58,59] Garabrant[60] reported a relative risk of 5 for *chemical workers* exposed to dichlorodiphenyltrichloroethane (DDT) and its metabolites. Several studies of *chemists* have shown an increased risk, all with relative risk less than 2. Workers in *petroleum refineries*, the *chemical industry*, and the *rubber industry* also have demonstrated an increased risk of pancreatic cancer, although results have been inconsistent in both settings. Finally, several studies of *mechanics* have suggested an increased risk of pancreatic cancer. Although each of these findings suggests a risk for chemical exposures, specific etiologic agents have not been identified. Other isolated occupational associations with pancreatic cancer are shown in Table 30.5.7.

Diagnosis, treatment, and prognosis

The diagnosis of pancreatic cancer is well described in standard texts and is not covered here. The only definitive treatment is surgical resection, either pancreaticoduo-denectomy (the Whipple procedure) or total pancreatec-

Industries and exposures	Occupations
Acetylene production	Automobile assembly workers
Aluminum reduction plants	Chemists
Aromatic amines	Corn wet-milling workers
Asbestos	Engineers
Chemical industry	Food, drink and tobacco
Chromates	workers
Coke byproducts	Furniture workers
Cotton dust	Jewelry workers
Dichlorodiphenyl trichlorethane	Mechanics
(DDT) and metabolites	Metal workers
Diesel exhaust	Photoengravers, lithographers
Dry cleaning	Pressmen
Dyestuffs	Radiologists
Electrical equipment	Truck and bus drivers
manufacturing	White-collar workers
Electronics manufacturing	
Farm implement and diesel	
equipment manufacturing	
Flour mills	
Ionizing radiation	
Leather tannery	
Methylene chloride	
Nickel and nickel compounds	
Paints, thinners, and varnishes	
Paper, printing and publishing	
Pesticides	
Petroleum refineries	
Rubber manufacturing	
Textile industry	
Wood and pulp mills	

Table 30.5.7 Industries, exposures, and occupations in which high rates of pancreatic cancer have been reported

tomy, but these are rarely possible because of tumor spread by the time of diagnosis. The prognosis is poor, with a median survival of less than 6 months.

Opportunities for screening and early detection in the workplace

No screening tests have proved useful in the early detection of pancreatic cancer.

References

1. Parkin, MD, Pisani P, Ferlay J. Global cancer statistics. CA Cancer J Clin 1999; 49:33-64.
2. Greenlee RT, Murray T, Bolden S, Wingo PA. Cancer statistics, 2000. CA Cancer J Clin 2000; 50:7-33.
3. Ries LAG, Eisner MP, Kosary CL, et al., eds. SEER Cancer Statistics Review, 1973-1997. Bethesda: National Cancer Institute; 2000.
4. Gammon MD, Schoenberg JB, Ahsan H, et al. Tobacco, alcohol and socioeconomic status and adenocarcinomas of the esophagus and gastric cardia. J Natl Cancer Inst 1997; 89:1277-84.
5. Kabat GC, Ng SKC, Wynder EL. Tobacco, alcohol intake, and diet in relation to adenocarcinoma of the esophagus and gastric cardia. Cancer Causes Control 1993; 4:123-32.
6. Talamini G, Capelli P, Zamboni G, et al. Alcohol, smoking and papillomavirus infection as risk factors for esophageal squamous-cell papilloma and esophageal squamous-cell carcinoma in Italy. Int J Cancer 2000; 86:874-8.
7. Devesa SS, Blot WJ, Fraumeni JF Jr. Changing patterns in the incidence of esophageal and gastric carcinoma in the United States. Cancer 1998; 83:2049-53.
8. Riddell RH. Early detection of neoplasia of the esophagus and gastroesophageal junction. Am J Gastroenterol 1996; 91:853-63.
9. Lagergren J, Bergstrom R, Nyren O. Association between body mass and adenocarcinoma of the esophagus and gastric cardia. Ann Intern Med 1999; 130:883-90.
10. Ward EM, Burnett CA, Ruder A, Davis-King K. Industries and cancer. Cancer Causes Control 1997; 8:356-70.
11. Kang SK, Burnett CA, Freund E, Walker J, Lalich N Sestito J. Gastrointestinal cancer mortality of workers in occupations with high asbestos exposures. Am J Ind Med 1997; 31:713-18.
12. Straif K, Weiland SK, Bungers M, et al. Exposure to high concentrations of nitrosamines and cancer mortality among a cohort of rubber workers. Occup Environ Med 2000; 57:180-7.
13. Parent M, Siemiatycki J, Fritschi L. Workplace exposures and esophageal cancer. Occup Environ Med 2000; 57:325-34.
14. Cucino C, Sonnenberg A. Occupational mortality from squamous cell carcinoma of the esophagus in the United States during 1991-1996. Dig Dis Sci 2002; 47:568-72.
15. Tolbert P. Oils and cancer. Cancer Causes Control 1997; 8:386-405.
16. Roth MJ, Liu SF, Dawsey SM, et al. Cytologic detection of esophageal squamous cell carcinoma and precursor lesions using balloon and sponge samplers in asymptomatic adults in Linxian, China. Cancer 1997; 80:2047-59.
17. Cocco P, Ward MH, Buiatti E. Occupational risk factors for gastric cancer: an overview. Epidemiol Rev 1996; 18:218-34.
18. Cocco P, Ward MH, Dosemeci M. Occupational risk factors for cancer of the gastric cardia. Analysis of death certificates from 24 US states. J Occup Environ Med 1998; 40:855-61.
19. Swaen GMH, Meijers JMM, Slangen JJM. Risk of gastric cancer in pneumoconiotic coal miners and the effect of respiratory impairment. Occup Environ Med 1995; 52:606-10.
20. Frumkin H. Cancer of the liver and gastrointestinal tract. In: Rosenstock L, Cullen MR, eds. Textbook of clinical occupational and environmental medicine, 1st edn. Philadelphia: WB Saunders; 1994:576-84.
21. Xu ZY, Brown LM, Pan GW, et al. Cancer risks among iron and steel workers in Anshan, China, Part II: Case-control studies of lung and stomach cancer. Am J Ind Med 1996; 30:7-15.
22. Simpson J, Roman E, Law G, Pannett B. Women's occupation and cancer: preliminary analysis of cancer registrations in England and Wales, 1971-1990. Am J Ind Med 1999; 36:172-85.
23. Frumkin H, Berlin J. Asbestos exposure and gastrointestinal malignancy: review and meta-analysis. Am J Ind Med 1988; 14:79-85.
24. Tsai SP, Waddell LC Jr, Gilstrap EL, Ransdell JD, Ross CE. Mortality among maintenance employees potentially exposed to asbestos in a refinery and petrochemical plant. Am J Ind Med 1996; 29:89-98.
25. Pang ZC, Zhang Z, Wang Y, Zhang H. Mortality from a Chinese asbestos plant: overall cancer mortality. Am J Ind Med 1997; 32:442-4.
26. Torén K, Persson B, Wingren G. Health effects of working in pulp and paper mills: malignant diseases. Am J Ind Med 1996; 29:123-30.
27. Blair A, Zahm SH. Agricultural exposures and cancer. Environ Health Perspect 1995; 103(Suppl 8):205-8.
28. Steenland K, Boffetta P. Lead and cancer in humans: where are we now? Am J Ind Med 2000; 38:295-9.
29. Calvert GM, Ward E, Schnorr TM, Fine LJ. Cancer risks among workers exposed to metalworking fluids: a systematic review. Am J Ind Med 1998; 33:282-92.
30. Straif K, Keil U, Taeger D, et al. Exposure to nitrosamines, carbon black, asbestos and talc and mortality from stomach, lung and laryngeal cancer in a cohort of rubber workers. Am J Epidemiol 2000; 152:297-306.

31. Stewart AK, Bland KI, McGinnis LS Jr, Morrow M, Eyre HJ. Clinical highlights from the National Cancer Data Base, 2000. CA Cancer J Clin 2000; 50:171-83.

32. Yoshida S, Saito D. Gastric premalignancy and cancer screening in high risk patients. Am J Gastroenterol 1996; 91:839-43.

33. Tomeo CA, Colditz GA, Willett WC, et al. Harvard Report on Cancer Prevention. Volume 3: prevention of colon cancer in the United States. Cancer Causes Control 1999; 10:167-80.

34. Lichtenstein P, Holm NV, Verkasalo PK, et al. Environmental and heritable factors in the causation of cancer. N Engl J Med 2000; 343:78-85.

35. Devesa SS, Chow WH. Variation in colorectal cancer incidence in the United States by subsite of origin. Cancer 1993; 71:3819-26.

36. Germani D, Belli S, Bruno C, et al. Cohort mortality study of women compensated for asbestosis in Italy. Am J Ind Med 1999; 36:129-34.

37. Innos K, Rahu M, Rahu K, Lang I, Leon D. Wood dust exposure and cancer incidence: a retrospective cohort study of furniture workers in Estonia. Am J Ind Med 2000; 37:501-11.

38. Preventive Services Task Force. Guide to Clinical Preventive Services: Report of the U.S. Preventive Services Task Force, 2nd edn. Baltimore: Williams & Wilkins; 1996.

39. Winawer SJ, Fletcher RH, Miller L, et al. Colorectal cancer screening: clinical guidelines and rationale. Gastroenterology 1997; 112:594-642.

40. Smith RA, Mettlin CJ, Davis KJ, Eyre H. American Cancer Society guidelines for the early detection of cancer. CA Cancer J Clin 2000; 50:34-49.

41. Tzonou A, Trichopoulos D, Kaklamani E, Zavitsanos X, Koumantaki Y, Hsieh CC. Epidemiologic assessment of interactions of hepatitis-C virus with seromarkers of hepatitis-B and -D viruses, cirrhosis and tobacco smoking in hepatocellular carcinoma. Int J Cancer 1991; 49:377-80.

42. Stern MC, Umbach DM, Yu MC, London SJ, Zhang ZQ, Taylor JA. Hepatitis B, aflatoxin B(1), and p53 codon 249 mutation in hepatocellular carcinomas from Guangxi, People's Republic of China, and a meta-analysis of existing studies. Cancer Epidemiol Biomarkers Prev 2001; 10:617-25.

43. Døssing M, Petersen KT, Vyberg M, Olsen JH. Liver cancer among employees in Denmark. Am J Ind Med 1997; 32:248-54.

44. Steenland K, Palu S. Cohort mortality study of 57 000 painters and other union members: a 15 year update. Occup Environ Med 1999; 56:315-21.

45. Gilbert ES, Koshurnikova NA, Sokolnikov M, et al. Liver cancers in Mayak workers. Radiat Res 2000; 154:246-52.

46. Heinemann K, Willich SN, Heinemann LA, DoMinh T, Mohner M, Heuchert GE. Occupational exposure and liver cancer in women: results of the Multicentre International Liver Tumour Study (MILTS). Occup Med (Oxford) 2000; 50:422-9.

47. Occupational Safety and Health Administration, United States Department of Labor. OSHA Regulations (Standards – 29 CFR) Bloodborne Pathogens – 1910.1030. 56 FR 64004, Dec. 06, 1991, as amended at 57 FR 12717, April 13, 1992; 57 FR 29206, July 1, 1992; 61 FR 5507, Feb. 13, 1996.

48. [No authors listed]. Epidemiological notes and reports. Angiosarcoma of the liver among polyvinyl chloride workers – Kentucky. 1974. Morbid Mortal Wkly Rep 1997; 46:97-101.

49. el Zayadi A, Khalil A, el Samny N, Hamza MR, Selim O. Hepatic angiosarcoma among Egyptian farmers exposed to pesticides. Hepatogastroenterology 1986; 33:148-50.

50. Creech JL Jr, Johnson MN. Angiosarcoma of the liver in the manufacture of polyvinyl chloride. J Occup Med 1974; 46:150-1.

51. Kielhorn J, Melber C, Wahnschaffe U, Aitio A, Mangelsdorf I. Vinyl chloride: still a cause for concern. Environ Health Perspect 2000; 108:579-88.

52. Weihrauch M, Benicke M, Lehnert G, Wittekind C, Wrbitzky R, Tannapfel A. Frequent k-ras-2 mutations and p16(INK4A)methylation in hepatocellular carcinomas in workers exposed to vinyl chloride. Br J Cancer 2001; 84:982-9.

53. Reddy KP, Buschmann RJ, Chomet B. Cholangiocarcinomas induced by feeding 3'-methyl-4-dimethylaminoazobenzene to rats. Histopathology and ultrastructure. Am J Pathol 1977; 87:189-204.

54. Malker HS, McLaughlin JK, Malker BL, et al. Biliary tract cancer and occupation in Sweden. Br J Ind Med 1986; 43:257-62.

55. Shukla VK, Prakash A, Tripathi BD, Reddy DCS, Singh S. Biliary heavy metal concentrations in carcinoma of the gallbladder: case-control study. BMJ 1998; 317:1288-9.

56. Weiderpass E, Partanen T, Kaaks R, et al. Occurrence, trends and environmental etiology of pancreatic cancer. Scand J Work Environ Health 1998; 24:165-74.

57. Lillimoe KD, Yeo CJ Cameron JL. Pancreatic cancer: state-of-the-art care. CA Cancer J Clin 2000; 50:241-68.

58. Alguacil J, Porta M, Benavides FG, et al. Occupation and pancreatic cancer in Spain: a case-control study based on job titles. PANKRAS II Study Group. Int J Epidemiol 2000; 29:1004-13.

59. Ojajärvi IA, Partanen TJ, Ahlbom A, et al. Occupational exposures and pancreatic cancer: a meta-analysis. Occup Environ Med 2000; 57:316-24.

60. Garabrant DH, Held J, Langholz B, Peters JM, Mack TM. DDT and related compounds and risk of pancreatic cancer. J Natl Cancer Inst 1992; 84:764-71.

30.6 Thyroid Neoplasia
Thomas E Hamilton

Thyroid cancer continues to be one of the most uncommon forms of carcinoma, although the prevalence has been increasing, with now over 15,000 cases and 1200 deaths annually in the US.[1] However, this information is misleading in terms of the impact of the condition on clinical practice. Thyroid carcinoma usually presents as a thyroid nodule, one of the most common clinical problems that physicians and healthcare professionals encounter. The prevalence of palpable thyroid nodules is as high as 4%–7% in the general population, thus making the evaluation of thyroid cancer common and important to understand.

In addition, during the last two decades, there has been increasing public interest and concern about the potential hazards of environmental exposures, particularly from radioactive iodine, stemming from nuclear accidents or nuclear weapons development. This concern was heightened in 1986 after the accident at the Chernobyl nuclear power facility, which released approximately 1.8×10^{18} becquerels (48 million curies) of radioactive iodine into the atmosphere. During that same year, the US Department of Energy revealed that large amounts of radioactive iodine (subsequently estimated to be 2.74×10^{16} becquerels [740,000 curies]) had been released into the atmosphere from the Hanford Nuclear Site in Washington State during plutonium production in the 1940s and 1950s.

CLINICAL EVALUATION
History

The evaluation of a thyroid nodule of environmental origin does not differ from that of a nodule found in general practice. Although most people presenting with thyroid nodules are asymptomatic, a complete history pertaining to the thyroid gland should be gathered, including time of onset, recent change in nodule size, and symptoms related to compression of vital structures in the neck, such as dysphagia and hoarseness.

Patients should be asked about past exposures to ionizing radiation, especially those that occurred 10 to 40 years prior to presentation. The most common risk to the thyroid gland involves prior head and neck treatment with external beam radiation therapy for disorders of childhood. These radiation exposures resulted from treatment of presumed enlargement of the thymus gland, facial acne, tonsillar enlargement, fungal infections of the scalp, and various infections of the cervical lymph nodes such as tuberculosis.[2] These treatments should be distinguished from diagnostic X-ray studies of the head and neck, which constitute little or no clinical risk for adults. Prior history of radiation treatment for non-thyroid malignancies such as for Hodgkin's lymphoma should also be obtained, since such exposures can also confer an increased risk of thyroid neoplasia.

Medications that may exert an indirect effect on the induction of thyroid neoplasms via the action of thyroid-stimulating hormone (TSH) include lithium and amiodarone. A family history of thyroid neoplasms should be obtained, and, if positive, specific inquiry for medullary histology should be made. Ethnic background and past residential history are important in determining the likelihood of dietary iodine that may promote the induction of thyroid neoplasia via TSH stimulation of the thyroid gland.

There is very little information about the effects of occupational, environmental, and medical exposures on thyroid cancer induction other than ionizing radiation. Although the evidence linking the risk of thyroid carcinoma to environmental radioiodine exposure has been mixed, a residential history should be obtained with emphasis on residence locations or military service around atmospheric nuclear test sites (e.g., Nevada Test Site, Marshall Islands), locations near nuclear weapons production facilities, or childhood residence near the Chernobyl reactor accident.

Physical examination

The thyroid gland is one of the more challenging areas of the body to examine and several important features deserve mention. The most important aspect of the examination is to have the patient swallow water. A full swallow enables the thyroid examiner to inspect the thyroid gland and to palpate the body of the gland more completely as it moves under the examiner's fingers, allowing the size, shape, and consistency of the gland to be noted. If discrete nodules are present, they should be described in detail and the size of each nodule recorded. A complete evaluation for thyroid abnormalities also should include listening for hoarseness; carefully examining the cervical lymph glands, eyes, skin, and hair; examining the deep tendon reflexes; and observing for the presence of tremor.

Laboratory examination

Routine thyroid function testing is generally normal in persons presenting with either a benign thyroid nodule or thyroid carcinoma. However, because 5% to 10% of thyroid nodules may function autonomously, measurement of TSH is indicated. Although thyroglobulin levels are important in detecting recurrent carcinoma after surgery and radioiodine therapy, this measurement is not sufficiently specific to warrant its use as an initial screening test. Use of fine needle aspiration for histologic assessment of suspect nodules is discussed in evaluation and treatment, below.

CLASSIFICATION

A general classification of malignant thyroid neoplasms is listed in Table 30.6.1. This classification belies the com-

Type	Prevalence (%)	Radiation association
Papillary adenocarcinoma	80–85	Yes
Follicular carcinoma	10–15	Yes
Medullary carcinoma	2–10	No
Undifferentiated (anaplastic) carcinoma	<5	Uncertain
Lymphoma	<1	No

Table 30.6.1 Pathologic classification of thyroid carcinoma

plexity of differentiating between benign and malignant lesions as well as among the subtypes within these categories. In addition, the international distribution of papillary and follicular histology is highly dependent on iodine sufficiency. Because the majority of thyroid carcinomas are papillary or follicular in histology and the association of nearly all environmental or occupational exposures is with papillary, the focus of the subsequent sections is on papillary and follicular carcinomas.

Papillary and follicular carcinomas

Etiology and epidemiology

Papillary and follicular carcinomas are both the most common thyroid cancers and also the ones most notably associated with occupational or environmental exposures, particularly ionizing radiation. These carcinomas comprise nearly 90% of all thyroid cancers.

Non-occupational factors

Age and sex are the two most important non-occupational risk factors for thyroid neoplasms. The prevalence of solitary thyroid nodules (both benign and malignant) is reported to be 2% to 4% in the US, with this number increasing to 7% to 8% in the seventh and eighth decades of life.[3] The common occurrence in women has been a consistent finding, with a female-to-male ratio of at least 3:1 in most studies. There is no clear evidence that ethnic background is an important risk factor for thyroid neoplasia, although individuals of Jewish descent have been shown to have a higher risk of radiation-induced thyroid neoplasms.

Although data exist to suggest that familial factors may be involved in the pathogenesis of thyroid carcinoma,

this issue is far from settled. It remains uncertain whether the presence of a papillary or follicular thyroid neoplasm in a person with a family history of thyroid carcinoma is any more frequent than in age- and sex-matched members of the general population without a family history of thyroid neoplasm. There does appear to be an increased risk of papillary thyroid cancer in persons with colonic adenocarcinoma.

MEDICAL RADIATION EXPOSURES
External gamma or photon radiation

The most thoroughly studied etiologic agent of thyroid cancer is ionizing radiation. The evidence that most strongly supports ionizing radiation as a cause of thyroid cancer has arisen from historic cases in which children were treated with external gamma radiation for benign diseases of the head and neck (Table 30.6.2). The first such case, reported in 1907, involved a young boy whose pre-sumed enlarged thymus gland was thought to be the cause of respiratory distress; he responded after treatment with external X-irradiation. Over the next several decades, ex-ternal beam radiation therapy was given for tonsillar enlargement, fungal infections of the scalp, facial acne, and cervical adenitis from tuberculosis. During the 1950s, several retrospective analyses indicated that adults with a history of childhood radiation exposure had a high prevalence of thyroid cancer.[4–6] Since these initial reports, multiple cohort studies have clearly established that childhood exposure to external gamma radiation is a risk factor not only for papillary and follicular thyroid carcinoma but also for benign nodules of the thyroid.[7–9] The magnitude of the risk has been estimated to be linearly dose dependent, with an excess relative risk per gray of 7.7 and highest for those exposed at young ages.[10]

Although most of these therapeutic regimens were abandoned by the late 1960s, the risk is still present because the latency for developing radiation-induced thyroid neoplasms has been shown to be 40 years or longer.

Therapeutic radioactive iodine

Much less information is available regarding the induction of thyroid carcinoma from medical uses of radioactive

Agent	Source	Mean thyroid dose estimate (Gy)	Effect	Reference
External gamma or photon radiation	Head and neck radiation treatments	0.09–1.36 (range)	Linear dose–response[*]	10
Diagnostic I-131	Diagnostic thyroid scans	1.1	No clear excess risk[†]	17
Therapeutic I-131	Patients with hyperthyroidism	na[¶]	No clear excess risk[‡]	12,13,15

* Pooled analysis of seven studies
† See text: excess risk documented but thought to be due to underlying condition
‡ See text: excess risk documented; however, it is uncertain whether it is related to I-131 exposure
¶ Doses not available; thyroid dose was generally targeted to be 60–100 Gy

Table 30.6.2 Risk of thyroid neoplasia from medical radiation exposures

iodine as compared with gamma or photon radiation. Large therapeutic doses of radioactive iodine have been used to treat Graves' hyperthyroidism. A large multicenter cooperative study in the 1970s assessed the long-term carcinogenic effects on the thyroid of iodine-131 (I-131) treatment in over 20,000 persons with Graves' disease and found no increase in thyroid cancer when compared with individuals who were treated with thyroidectomy (Table 30.6.2).[11] More recently, Ron and colleagues extended the follow-up of that cohort until 1990.[12] The mean age at radioiodine treatment was 46 years and the mean length of follow-up was 21.2 years. Although no excess risk was found in total cancer deaths, an increase in thyroid cancer was detected in patients treated with I-131 (standardized mortality ratio [SMR], 3.94; 95% confidence interval [CI], 2.52–5.86). However, the absolute risk was quite low, with few thyroid cancer deaths, and the increase was most pronounced in patients with toxic nodular goiter. Limitations of the study included treatment based on the medical condition, multiple statistical comparisons, and lack of individual dosimetry. The authors concluded that the increase in thyroid cancer deaths might reflect an association with thyrotoxicosis rather than I-131 treatment.

In a Swedish mortality study, which has also been extended, cancer mortality was evaluated in 10,552 hyperthyroid patients who were treated with I-131 between 1950 and 1975. Patients were matched with Swedish registry data and were followed for a mean of 15 years. The targeted thyroid dose was between 60 and 100 Gy. Ninety-five percent of the patients were older than 40 at the time of exposure. No increased risk of thyroid cancer was detected for persons followed for more than 10 years, with an SMR of 0.66 (95% CI, 0.08–2.37).[13,14]

The most recent investigation of the risk of thyroid cancer following radioiodine treatment of hyperthyroidism involved a population-based cohort of 7400 patients treated with I-131 between 1950 and 1991.[15] All cancer diagnoses and deaths from this cohort were compared with registry data for England and Wales. Overall cancer incidence and mortality were decreased; however, thyroid cancer incidence and mortality were increased (standardized incidence ratio [SIR], 3.25; 95% CI, 1.69–6.25: SMR, 2.78; 95% CI, 1.16–6.67). As in the study by Ron et al., there were small numbers of both thyroid cancer cases and deaths. The authors could not distinguish between thyrotoxicosis or radioiodine as the cause of the increased thyroid cancer incidence and mortality.

Diagnostic radioactive iodine

Although not in use now, I-131 was used previously at low doses for diagnostic thyroid scans to evaluate nodules or hyperthyroidism. Swedish investigators followed over 35,000 persons who had had diagnostic I-131 scans for a mean follow-up period of 20 years.[16] The average thyroid dose was 0.5 Gy. No significant increase in thyroid carcinoma was detected in this group when compared with expected rates for the general population. This cohort study has subsequently been extended through a follow-up period of 40 years.[17] The results of the extended follow-up differed in that an increase in thyroid cancer incidence was detected (SIR, 1.35; 95% CI, 1.05–1.71). However, the excess cases were apparent only among patients referred for suspicion of a thyroid tumor; no increased risk was found among those referred for other reasons. In addition, risk was not related to thyroid radiation dose, time since exposure, or age at exposure. The authors concluded that the excess appeared related to the underlying thyroid condition rather than radiation exposure. It should be noted that 93% of the cohort were over age 20 years when I-131 was administered. Thus, while this study shows little, if any, detectable risk of thyroid cancer in adults after exposure to low dose I-131, it likely cannot be used to assess the risk of similar doses to infants or children.

ENVIRONMENTAL EXPOSURES

As with medical exposures, the most common environmental agent thought to cause thyroid neoplasms is ionizing radiation. However, in contrast to studies of persons exposed to medical radiation, studies of environmental radiation exposure have been more difficult, primarily because of the difficulty in determining who was exposed and estimating individual thyroid radiation doses. The following sections characterize studies of populations exposed to environmental radiation and are summarized in Table 30.6.3.

Agent	Source	Mean thyroid dose (Gy) (range)	Effect	Reference
External gamma radiation	Japanese atomic bomb survivors	0.27 (0.01–3.99)	Linear dose–response*	10,19
Nuclear fallout (mixed radioiodines and external gamma)	Utah; weapons test fallout	0.17 (0–4.6)	ERR 0.7%/mGy†	29–32,34
	Chernobyl accident	0.15–1.0	Dramatic increase in children‡	
	Marshall Islands; weapons test fallout	2.8–21¶	Dose–response for total thyroid nodules**	20,24–26
Iodine-131	Hanford nuclear reservation; plutonium production	0.186 (0–2.8)	No effect detected	35

* Thyroid cancer only
† Excess relative risk for benign neoplasms and cancer combined
‡ Risk estimates not yet available; doses highly dependent on multiple factors, including region of residence
¶ Mean population estimated doses: 2.8 Gy for Utrik islanders, 21 Gy for Rongelap islanders
** No individual dosimetry available; strong linear dose–response using distance from test site as proxy for dose

Table 30.6.3 Risk of thyroid neoplasia from environmental ionizing radiation exposures

Natural background radiation

Although information is limited about the risk of thyroid cancer from variations in background radiation exposure, one study from China assessed thyroid nodularity in a region of high background radiation and compared it to a region with low background radiation exposure.[18] In 2000 elderly women, there was no difference in thyroid nodularity in women from high (14 cGy) and low (5 cGy) radiation areas.

External gamma or photon radiation

Persons exposed to atmospheric nuclear fallout from nuclear weapons testing or from nuclear attack such as in Hiroshima and Nagasaki may also be at increased risk for developing benign or malignant thyroid neoplasms. The increased risk of thyroid carcinoma from external gamma-radiation exposure among the Japanese survivors is well documented.[10,19] This exposure, resulting from an air burst of an atomic bomb, produced external whole-body penetrating photon radiation nearly instantaneously. A linear dose–response relationship was shown, with an increased relative risk for thyroid cancer. An age-related effect was also demonstrated, with those exposed before the age of 15 having the greatest risk and those exposed after age 15 having little or no increased risk of thyroid cancer.[10]

Radioactive iodine

The most widespread population exposures to radioactive iodine have occurred in the following locations:

- the Marshall Islands, where nuclear weapons were tested;
- the state of Utah and areas surrounding the Nevada test site, from US nuclear weapons testing;
- eastern Europe near the Chernobyl accident; and
- the United States Pacific Northwest, where nuclear weapons were produced at the Hanford test site.

Numerous other populations have been directly exposed (as opposed to indirect exposure from worldwide fallout) to weapons test fallout, such as at Semipalatinsk in the Kazakhstan area in the former Soviet Union, the Mayak nuclear power station, and the aboriginal population in Australia.

Marshall Islands

The Marshall Islanders represent one of the most intensively studied populations exposed to weapons test fallout. In contrast to the external gamma radiation from the atomic bomb attacks on Japan, the Marshall Islanders were exposed to particulate fallout radiation. Of at least 66 atomic tests detonated in the Marshall Islands between 1946 and 1958, the BRAVO thermonuclear test on March 1, 1954, produced the largest single radiation exposure to the Marshallese people. Extensive evaluation of this population by Brookhaven National Laboratory has shown an increase in benign and malignant thyroid nodules in persons living on the northern atolls of Rongelap and

Utrik.[20] Thyroid doses have been estimated to be primarily from a mixture of the short-lived radioiodines and, to a lesser extent, I-131 and external gamma radiation.[21,22]

Although the Brookhaven studies had maintained that fallout exposure from the BRAVO test affected only the Rongelap and Utrik atolls, additional dosimetry studies have suggested a much wider area of fallout exposure.[23,24] In addition, a retrospective cohort study of over 7000 Marshall Islanders showed that the prevalence of palpable thyroid nodularity (>/= 1.0 cm) decreased linearly with increasing distance from the Bikini test site.[25] These results were highly statistically significant and strongly suggested that fallout radiation affected a much wider region of northern and central atolls, including those used by Brookhaven as a control population.

Takahashi and colleagues recently attempted to independently assess the prevalence of thyroid nodularity in the Marshall Islanders and compare their results with those of the above 1987 study.[26] They reported a much higher prevalence of thyroid nodules in the population but only a borderline significant relationship between prevalence of thyroid nodules and distance to the Bikini test site. However, the authors' first result can be partially explained by the inclusion of ultrasound abnormalities in addition to palpable nodules in their criteria of thyroid nodules. Also, the very small numbers of persons screened from each atoll in the Marshall Islands produced unstable point prevalence figures and can explain the failure to find a relationship between thyroid nodule prevalence and distance from the Bikini test site.

Dose reconstruction for Marshall Islanders exposed to nuclear fallout is difficult. Because adequate individual dosimetry information was either not obtained or not available during the actual exposures in the 1950s, it is unlikely that future dose reconstruction efforts will be successful in further elucidating the risk of radiation-induced thyroid cancer in this population.

Nevada test site

Over 100 atmospheric nuclear tests were detonated at the Nevada test site between the years 1951 and 1958. Although recent reports have suggested that persons throughout the US might have been exposed to small amounts of radiation from radioiodine during the 1950s, the persons with some of the highest exposures were from southwestern Utah. Early studies of thyroid disease in Utah schoolchildren appeared to show no difference in thyroid disease outcomes compared to children from unexposed areas.[27] However, extension of this cohort study showed an excess of thyroid neoplasms which was associated with exposure to radioiodine from the Nevada test site.[28]

In that study, a relative risk of 3.4 for the period prevalence of thyroid neoplasms during 1965–1986 was observed for persons exposed to >400 mGy. A statistically significant excess relative risk of 0.7% per mGy was observed for total neoplasms, which included both benign follicular adenomas and thyroid cancers. Although positive dose–response trends were noted for total nodules or thyroid carcinoma, these were not statistically significant. The mean dose in the Utah exposed children was 170 mGy. Although the dose was reported to be primarily from I-131, the contribution of external radiation or short-lived radioiodines is uncertain.

Chernobyl

The 1986 accident at the Chernobyl power station near Kiev in the Ukraine is the most recent event that involved environmental exposure to radioiodine. Beginning in 1992, reports began to show increased rates of thyroid cancer in children who were exposed to radiation from the Chernobyl accident.[29,30] A marked increase in childhood thyroid cancer has since been documented in areas surrounding the Chernobyl reactor, especially in Belarus and Ukraine.[31–33] Pacini et al. have evaluated thyroid cancer registries in Belarus since 1986 and compared them with presumably unexposed cases from registries from France and Italy.[32] Of 472 cases of thyroid cancer from the six regions in Belarus, 52% were from the most exposed region of Gomel; the numbers of cases of thyroid carcinoma throughout Belarus roughly correlated to the degree of radioactive contamination. In addition, the cases from Belarus were younger, more aggressive at initial presentation, and more likely papillary in histology than the thyroid cancer cases from France and Italy. Similar increased rates of thyroid cancer occurring at young ages at exposure have been reported in the Ukraine.[34]

To date, there is limited individual thyroid dosimetry and therefore little published information assessing a dose–response relationship between Chernobyl radiation exposure and thyroid cancer. The type of radiation exposure presumably is largely due to I-131, although external radiation as well as short-lived radioiodines also contributed to the dose.

Hanford nuclear reservation

A second large population from the United States Pacific Northwest was exposed to atmospheric radioiodine during the 1940s and 1950s from the Hanford nuclear site. This information, released in 1986 by the US Department of Energy, resulted in the funding of two studies: the Hanford Environmental Dose Reconstruction project and the Hanford Thyroid Disease Study (HTDS), designed to determine whether or not thyroid disease, including thyroid neoplasia, was increased among individuals exposed to environmental I-131 from Hanford.

Results from the HTDS have found no evidence of an increase in thyroid neoplasia as a result of Hanford radiation exposure.[35] This study was based on the results of comprehensive thyroid evaluations in 3441 persons who were aged 0–7 years at the time of the radiation exposures, including duplicate thyroid physical examinations, thyroid ultrasound scans, and thyroid function testing. In addition, individual thyroid radiation doses were estimated for each person. In contrast to most of the above exposures involving mixtures of I-131, other short-lived radioiodines, and external gamma radiation, the Hanford exposures were primarily I-131 alone. No increase was found for either benign or malignant thyroid neoplasms in relation to radiation dose from radioiodine exposure. Factors that might have contributed to lack of a radiation effect include low thyroid doses, and chronic rather than acute exposures to radioactive iodine.

OCCUPATIONAL EXPOSURES

The risk of thyroid cancer in occupations involving ionizing radiation has not been well studied because the mortality rate is low and, therefore, is not detected in occupational mortality studies. One incidence study showed that thyroid cancer incidence in 27,000 medical diagnostic X-ray workers in China was significantly increased when compared with 25,000 physicians who did not use X-rays.[36] Although previous studies have not shown occupational exposures to diagnostic X-rays to be a risk factor for thyroid cancer, the patterns of risk associated with age, calendar time of employment, and duration of employment suggested that the excess thyroid cancer in this study might be caused by occupational exposure to X-rays. Although an increased risk of thyroid cancer has most commonly been the result of acute high doses of gamma radiation, this study suggests that chronic low doses of X-ray exposure may also confer excess risk.

More recently, several studies have assessed the risk of thyroid cancer in workers exposed to ionizing radiation. Fraser and colleagues analyzed a cohort of 39,718 atomic energy employees in the UK based on deaths from 1946 to 1986; they found no increase in thyroid cancer prevalence or mortality.[37] A second study of 95,217 radiation workers in the UK did show an increased SMR for thyroid cancer; however, there was no evidence for a trend with external radiation dose.[38] In a study of Danish employees in two radiotherapy departments, Andersson et al. found no increase in thyroid cancer among 4151 workers compared to the general population.[39] Antonelli and colleagues evaluated thyroid nodularity in 50 medical workers from a Pisa hospital who worked in high radiation exposure units and compared them to unexposed male workers. They found an elevated relative risk for thyroid nodularity in the exposed group and concluded that occupational exposure to radiation might be a risk factor for thyroid nodules. These results are somewhat limited by lack of individual dosimetry, small numbers of exposed workers, and diagnostic criteria for thyroid nodules which rely primarily on ultrasound abnormalities. No thyroid cancer was found in either the exposed or control group.[40]

The risk of thyroid cancer from radiation exposures from the Chernobyl accident in workers at the nuclear power station as well as those involved in clean-up has also been studied. Inskip and colleagues screened 2400 Estonian clean-up workers using ultrasound and needle biopsy of thyroid nodules.[41] They found no increase in thyroid disease that could be correlated with radiation dose.

Even less is known about occupational risks of thyroid cancer other than ionizing radiation, again because of the low incidence and mortality rate of the disease. In a study from Sweden, a record linkage between the Swedish Cancer Registry and census data reported an increased incidence of thyroid cancer in men working in petroleum refineries.[42] The association was found only in occupations working with crude oils and not in those involving volatile petroleum products. Whether this represents a real association from a hypothesis-generating study remains unclear.

A more recent case–control study (1272 cases, 2666 controls) from Canada explored the etiology of thyroid cancer and occupational exposures.[43] An adjusted odds ratio of 2.54 (95% CI, 1.11–5.83) was found for wood processing, pulp, and papermaking workers, who have multiple chemical exposures, including hydrocarbons. The authors concluded that additional studies with better exposure characterization would be warranted.

EVALUATION AND TREATMENT

The evaluation (and usually the treatment) of suspected environmentally or occupationally related thyroid neoplasms is not different from that of those which occur sporadically. The advent of fine-needle aspiration (FNA) has significantly changed the approach and evaluation of a thyroid nodule over the last 20 years, and now it is usually the initial diagnostic test following a TSH determination. There is controversy about the ability of thyroid ultrasound to predict histology, and the sensitivity and specificity of this modality are not adequate to reliably distinguish malignant from benign neoplasms.[44,45] Therefore, thyroid ultrasonography, as well as thyroid nuclear scans, are adjuncts to an experienced physical examination and FNA of nodules.

The treatment of thyroid carcinoma includes thyroidectomy and usually radioiodine ablation. The indication for radioiodine ablation is not influenced by whether the carcinoma is caused by an environmental or occupational exposure. Regardless of the extent of the initial thyroidectomy or whether radioiodine ablation and therapy is employed, the administration of thyroid hormone is indicated on a lifelong basis for thyroid hormone replacement and for TSH suppression, which decreases recurrence rates. The dose of thyroid hormone should be high enough to suppress TSH but to avoid clinical symptoms of hyperthyroidism.

External beam radiotherapy usually is reserved for palliative treatment of progressive or widely metastatic disease, for persons with focal bone metastases, and for those patients whose disease is inoperable. Clinical decisions in these cases must be made in consultation with the endocrinologist and radiation oncologist.

Chemotherapy (except radiosensitizers in conjunction with I-131 or X-ray therapy) has generally not been used in well-differentiated papillary or follicular carcinoma, primarily because most patients do well with the therapeutic regimens discussed earlier. Although chemotherapeutic regimens have been tried in widely metastatic disease, it is unclear whether they add any benefit beyond external beam radiotherapy.

Benign thyroid nodules

Any discussion regarding the management of thyroid carcinoma is incomplete without reviewing the management of benign thyroid lesions, because ruling out carcinoma confirms a benign lesion, which may occur in 2% to 4% of the general population. Two important issues are the management of benign nodules, and whether occupational or environmental causation changes the management.

The management of benign nodules can be difficult because of the possibility of false-negative FNA results and the question of whether TSH suppression with thyroid hormone is effective in causing regression of nodules. It can be difficult to decide whether a nodule is truly benign because FNA cytology cannot reliably distinguish follicular carcinoma from follicular adenoma. Because studies have shown that 10%–20% of follicular neoplasms diagnosed by FNA cytology are malignant, most authorities recommend thyroidectomy in persons with such cytology. The beneficial effect of TSH suppression on benign nodules is questionable both because of unproven effectiveness and also because of potential symptoms and long-term adverse effects of TSH suppression. Typically, benign thyroid nodules can be managed by periodic examinations to ensure that the nodule is not enlarging or causing compression symptoms. In persons with enlarging nodules or compression symptoms, thyroidectomy should be considered.

Evaluation of thyroid nodules in radiation-exposed patients

Does a history of prior head and neck radiation exposure change the management (or evaluation) of a thyroid nodule? Such a history has in the past compelled many clinicians to recommend thyroidectomy regardless of cytology or in lieu of biopsy. It is clear that a prior history of head and neck radiation exposure from X-rays increases the risk that a person will develop thyroid nodularity (both benign and malignant neoplasms). However, it is less clear whether such nodules are more likely to be malignant than are sporadic thyroid nodules. In addition, with the possible exception of carcinomas developing in children from the exposure at Chernobyl, there is no convincing evidence that radiation-induced thyroid carcinomas are more aggressive than those arising spontaneously. In fact, the majority of radiation-induced cancers have been of papillary histology, which has the best prognosis. Although persons with a benign nodule who have a history of radiation exposure should have careful and experienced lifelong yearly examinations of the thyroid, these nodules can generally be evaluated and managed in the same manner as the spontaneous nodule found in a person without prior radiation exposure.

Prognosis

The prognosis of well-differentiated thyroid carcinoma, in general, is good, and the long-term survival is in excess of 90%–95% of patients. Three prognostic factors have proved to be predictors of poor outcome: age at diagnosis, local tumor invasion, and distant metastases. The age range when prognosis worsens is probably between 40 to 50 years and less than 20 years. Except for poorly differentiated tumors, minor differences in tumor grade do not appear significant. To date, there is no strong evidence that the prognosis of papillary and follicular carcinomas that are caused primarily by ionizing radiation is different from the prognosis of sporadic carcinomas.

Screening of radiation-exposed populations

Persons having a history of environmental or occupational radiation exposures (including medical exposures) should be considered for routine thyroid surveillance. The question of who should have routine screening is complex because the documentation of increased risk has not been shown for all types of radiation exposures and depends on multiple factors, including age at exposure, thyroid dose, and perhaps whether the exposure was acute or protracted. Clearly, those individuals with a history of prior head and neck X-ray treatments for benign childhood conditions, as well as those with prior external gamma or photon exposures (including persons given radiation therapy for non-thyroid primary malignancies), should be screened. In addition, persons having documented exposures from nuclear weapons attack (e.g., Hiroshima or Nagasaki) or who received high doses from nuclear weapons testing (Marshall Islands, Nevada test site) should be screened.

Recommendations for screening after exposures to I-131 are much less clear. There is no convincing evidence that the medical use of I-131 in the treatment of hyperthyroidism or the diagnostic doses of I-131 formerly used in thyroid scans have caused an increased risk of thyroid neoplasms.

The largest screening programs have included the Marshall Islanders, who have been screened every 1 to 2 years with careful palpation of the thyroid gland and thyroid function testing. Screening programs in the US Midwest were performed in persons having a prior history of head and neck radiation treatments in childhood. Although these programs have increased the detection rate of thyroid nodules, it is not clear that detecting the nodules earlier has improved morbidity or mortality rates. Nonetheless, it seems prudent to screen on an annual basis persons who have been exposed to external gamma radiation, especially given the long latency of thyroid neoplasms.

The question of how exposed individuals should be screened is controversial, and screening is performed differently throughout the world. Certainly, a careful and experienced thyroid physical examination is important to detect clinically significant thyroid neoplasms (as well as thyroid function tests to detect hypothyroidism). The question of whether adjunctive diagnostic tests, such as thyroid ultrasound and thyroid nuclear scans, should be used is less clear. Ultrasound of the thyroid gland is definitely a more sensitive technique compared with physical examination. This increased sensitivity may increase the number of clinically palpable nodules that might be missed without ultrasound; however, a large number of non-palpable ultrasound-detected abnormalities will also be detected. The number of such ultrasound-detected abnormalities in the general population is estimated to be at least 5% to 10%, and in some studies, as high as 40% to 50%.[46,47] The biologic significance of these small non-palpable ultrasound findings is unclear, but such lesions are unlikely to represent important clinical neoplasms.

A recent study followed the natural history of thyroid ultrasound abnormalities identified 5 years earlier from random screening of an adult population in Finland.[48] In the original survey, 69 of 253 persons (27%) had ultrasound abnormalities. At follow-up, 35% of the nodules had grown, 24% of the nodules had diminished or disappeared, and 12% of persons screened had new nodules. Biopsies were performed in 10 of 12 persons with growing lesions, and in five of seven persons with new lesions. All biopsied lesions were benign. No malignancies were detected at follow-up. The authors con-cluded that thyroid ultrasound abnormalities occurring in a random adult population are unlikely to be clinically important. Because most clinically significant thyroid nodules are palpable and because false-positive ultrasound findings may lead to increased medical intervention, including thyroid surgery, the use of thyroid ultrasound as a screening test is generally not warranted at the present time.

Although thyroid nuclear scans may be useful as an adjunct to the physical examination, this test also is unwarranted as a screening diagnostic test. Although malignant neoplasms usually do not take up the tracer isotope, the finding of a cold nodule on a thyroid scan does not distinguish between a benign and a malignant lesion. In fact, more than 80% to 90% of such lesions found on thyroid nuclear scanning are benign.

The question of how long to screen exposed individuals is uncertain. However, because studies have shown the latency of thyroid neoplasia to be at least 40 years,[10] screening should be conducted annually on an indefinite basis.

In summary, persons with a clear history of external gamma or photon radiation to the head and neck should have lifelong screening for thyroid neoplasms. This should be conducted on an annual basis and include careful thyroid physical examination by an experienced thyroid examiner. Although thyroid ultrasound can improve sensitivity over thyroid palpation, it should be used only in this context and not as a general screening tool because of the high rate of ultrasound-detected abnormalities that have unclear clinical significance.

Persons who have a history of I-131 exposure need not have routine screening if this exposure was from a diagnostic thyroid scan. Persons with prior radioiodine therapy for Graves' disease will likely be followed for that problem. Persons who have a history of environmental exposure to I-131, especially if the exposure was during childhood, may benefit from screening. It would be reasonable for individuals who have a concern about such exposure to have a careful thyroid evaluation.

UNCOMMON THYROID CARCINOMAS

Of the uncommon types of thyroid carcinoma listed in Table 30.6.1, the most frequent is medullary thyroid carcinoma, which occurs in 2% to 10% of all cases. Medullary thyroid carcinoma has not been found to result from exposure to ionizing radiation or other occupational or environmental exposures.

The small- and large-cell anaplastic thyroid carcinomas are considered undifferentiated or poorly differentiated carcinomas and are highly lethal. One of their unusual features is that they may occur by transformation from well-differentiated papillary or follicular carcinomas. Although the factors involved in this transformation are not known, there has been some suggestion, although unconfirmed, that ionizing radiation might be a factor. This lesion has a very poor prognosis, with a survival time of usually 3 to 6 months.

Lymphomas of the thyroid gland are rare (less than 1% of all thyroid malignancies) and usually occur beyond the sixth or seventh decade of life. A strong association with autoimmune thyroiditis (Hashimoto's thyroiditis) has been found with thyroid lymphoma. The basis for this association is currently unknown. Again, no association has been found between lymphomas of the thyroid and ionizing radiation or other environmental or occupational exposures.

The clinical evaluation, treatment, and prognosis of these malignancies are beyond the scope of this text.

References

1. Figge J. Epidemiology of thyroid cancer. In: Wartofsky L, ed. Thyroid cancer. A comprehensive guide to clinical management. Totowa, New Jersey: Humana Press; 2000:77.
2. Schneider AB. Radiation-induced thyroid tumors. Endocrinol Metab Clin North Am 1990; 19:637-48.
3. Wang C, Crapo L. The epidemiology of thyroid disease and implications for screening. Endocrinol Metab Clin North Am 1997; 26:189-218.
4. Clark DE. Association of irradiation with cancer of the thyroid in children and adolescents. JAMA 1955; 159:1007-9.
5. Duffy F. Cancer of the thyroid in children: a report of 28 cases. J Clin Endocrinol Metab 1950; 10:1296-308.
6. Simpson CL, Hemplemann LH, Fuler LM. Neoplasia in children treated with x-rays in infancy for thymic enlargement. Radiology 1955; 64:840-5.
7. Ron, E, Modan B. Thyroid cancer and other neoplasms following childhood scalp irradiation. In: Boice JD, Fraumeni JF Jr, eds. Radiation carcinogenesis: epidemiology and biologic significance. New York: Raven Press; 1984:139.
8. Schneider AB, Recant W, Pinsky SM, et al. Radiation-induced thyroid carcinoma. Ann Intern Med 1986; 105:405-12.
9. Shore RE, Hildreth N, Dvoretsky P, et al. Benign thyroid adenomas among persons X-irradiated in infancy for enlarged thymus glands. Radiat Res 1993; 134:217-23.
10. Ron E, Lubin JH, Shore RE, et al. Thyroid cancer after exposure to external radiation: a pooled analysis of seven studies. Radiat Res 1995; 141:259-77.
11. Dobyns BM, Sheline GE, Workman JB, et al. Malignant and benign neoplasms of the thyroid in patients treated for hyperthyroidism: a report of the Cooperative Thyrotoxicosis Therapy Follow-up Study. J Clin Endocrinol Metab 1974; 38:976-98.
12. Ron E, Doody MM, Becker DV, et al. Cancer mortality following treatment for adult hyperthyroidism. Cooperative Thyrotoxicosis Therapy Follow-up Study Group. JAMA 1998; 280:347-55.
13. Holm LE, Dahlqvist I, Israelsson A, et al. Malignant thyroid tumors after iodine-131 therapy: a retrospective study. N Engl J Med 1980; 303:188-91.
14. Hall P, Berg G, Bjelkengren G, et al. Cancer mortality after iodine-131 therapy for hyperthyroidism. Int J Cancer 1992; 50:886-90.
15. Franklyn JA, Maisonneuve P, Sheppard M, et al. Cancer incidence and mortality after radioiodine treatment for hyperthyroidism: a population-based cohort study. Lancet 1999; 353:2111-15.
16. Holm LE, Wiklund KE, Lundell GE, et al. Thyroid cancer after diagnostic doses of iodine-131: a retrospective cohort study. J Natl Cancer Inst 1988; 80:1132-8.
17. Hall P, Mattsson A, Boice JD Jr. Thyroid cancer after diagnostic administration of iodine-131. Radiat Res 1996; 145:86-92.
18. Wang ZY, Boice JD Jr, Wei LX, et al. Thyroid nodularity and chromosome aberrations among women in areas of high background radiation in China. J Natl Cancer Inst 1990; 82:478-85.
19. Thompson DE, Mabuchi K, Ron E, et al. Cancer incidence in atomic bomb survivors. Part II: Solid tumors. Radiat Res 1994; 137:S17-S67.
20. Conard RA. Late radiation effects in Marshall Islanders exposed to fallout 28 years ago. In: Boice JD Jr, Fraumeni JR, eds. Radiation carcinogenesis: epidemiology and biologic significance. New York: Raven Press; 1984:57.
21. James RA. Estimate of radiation dose to thyroids of the Rongelap children following the BRAVO Event (Publication 12-273). Livermore, University of California Radiation Laboratory: US Department of Energy; 1964.
22. Lessard E, Miltenberger R, Conard R, et al. Thyroid absorbed dose for people at Rongelap, Utrik, and Sifo on March 1, 1954. (Publication BNL 51-882). Upton, New York, Brookhaven National Laboratory: US Department of Energy; 1985.
23. Harley JH, Hallden NA, Ong LD. Summary of gummed film results, 1959. 15th edn. New York: US Atomic Energy Commission, New York Operations Office, Health and Safety Laboratory; 1960; HASL-93, UC 41, Health and Safety, TID-4500.
24. Simon SL, Graham, JC. Findings of the first comprehensive radiological monitoring program of the Republic of the Marshall Islands. Health Physics 1997; 73:66-87.
25. Hamilton TE, van Belle G, LoGerfo JP. Thyroid neoplasia in Marshall Islanders exposed to nuclear fallout. JAMA 1987; 258:629-36.
26. Takahashi T, Trott KR, Fujimori K, et al. An investigation into the prevalence of thyroid disease on Kwajalein Atoll, Marshall Islands. Health Physics 1997; 73:199-213.
27. Rallison ML, Dobyns BM, Keating FR, et al. Thyroid nodularity in children. JAMA 1975; 233:1069-72.
28. Kerber RA, Till JE, Simon SL, et al. A cohort study of thyroid disease in relation to fallout from nuclear weapons testing. JAMA 1993; 270:2076-82.
29. Baverstock KF. Thyroid cancer in children in Belarus after Chernobyl. World Health Stat Q 1993; 46:204-8.
30. Kazakov VS, Demidchik EP, Astakhova LN. Thyroid cancer after Chernobyl [letter]. Nature 1992; 359:21.
31. Likhtarev AI, Sobolev BG, Kairo IA, et al. Thyroid cancer in the Ukraine. Nature 1995; 375:365.

32. Pacini F, Vorontsova T, Demidchik EP, et al. Post-Chernobyl thyroid carcinoma in Belarus children and adolescents: comparison with naturally occurring thyroid carcinoma in Italy and France. J Clin Endocrinol Metab 1997; 82:3563-9.

33. Tronko N, Bogdanova T, Kommisarenko I, et al. Thyroid cancer in children and adolescents in Ukraine after the Chernobyl accident (1986-1995). In: Karaoglou A, Sobolev BG, Kairo IA, et al., eds. The radiological consequences of the Chernobyl accident. ERU 16544 EN. Luxembourg: European Commission; 1996:683-90.

34. Sobolev B, Heidenreich WF, Kairo I, et al. Thyroid cancer incidence in the Ukraine after the Chernobyl accident: comparison with spontaneous incidences. Radiat Environ Biophys 1997; 36:195-9.

35. Hamilton, TE, Davis S, Kopecky KJ. The risk of thyroid neoplasia after exposure to iodine-131 from the Hanford Nuclear Site: implications for populations exposed to atmospheric radiation releases from nuclear accidents and nuclear testing. J Endocrinol Invest 1999; 22(6 Suppl):Abstr. 247.

36. Wang J, Inskip PD, Boice JD, et al. Cancer incidence among medical diagnostic x-ray workers in China, 1950 to 1985. Int J Cancer 1990; 45:889-95.

37. Fraser P, Carpenter L, Maconochie N, et al. Cancer mortality and morbidity in employees of the United Kingdom Atomic Energy Authority, 1946-86. Br J Cancer 1993; 67:615-24.

38. Kendall GM, Muirhead CR, MacGibbon BH, et al. Mortality and occupational exposure to radiation: first analysis of the National Registry for Radiation Workers. BMJ 1992; 304:220-5.

39. Andersson M, Engholm G, Ennow K, et al. Cancer risk among staff at two radiotherapy departments in Denmark. Br J Radiol 1991; 64:455-60.

40. Antonelli A, Silvano G, Bianchi F, et al. Risk of thyroid nodules in subjects occupationally exposed to radiation: a cross sectional study. Occup Environ Med 1995; 52:500-4.

41. Inskip PD, Hartshorne MF, Tekkel M, et al. Thyroid nodularity and cancer among Chernobyl clean-up workers from Estonia. Radiat Res 1997; 147:225.

42. Carstensen JM, Wingre G, Hatschek T, et al. Occupational risks of thyroid cancer: data from the Swedish Cancer-Environment Register, 1961-1979. Am J Ind Med 1990; 18:535-40.

43. Fincham SM, Ugnat AM, Hill GB, et al. Is occupation a risk factor for thyroid cancer? J Occup Environ Med 2000; 42:318-22.

44. Hegedus L, Karstrup S. Ultrasonography in the evaluation of cold thyroid nodules. Eur J Endocrinol 1998; 138:30-1.

45. Takashima S, Fukuda H, Nomura N, et al. Thyroid nodules: re-evaluation with ultrasound. J Clin Ultrasound 1995; 23:179-84.

46. Ezzat S, Sarti DA, Cain DR. Thyroid incidentalomas. Prevalence by palpation and ultrasonography. Arch Intern Med 1994; 154:1838-40.

47. Tan GH, Gharib H. Thyroid incidentalomas: management approaches to nonpalpable nodules discovered incidentally on thyroid imaging. Ann Intern Med 1997; 126:226-31.

48. Brander AE, Viikinkoski VP, Nickels JI, et al. Importance of thyroid abnormalities detected at US screening: a 5-year follow-up. Radiology 2000; 215:801-6.

30.7 Cancer of the Reproductive Organs
Lora E Fleming

INTRODUCTION

Although an area of increasing scientific interest, there is relatively little information on the role of occupational and environmental exposures in reproductive cancers. In particular, these exposures have not been closely studied in women because women traditionally were not believed to be at risk for major chemical or physical occupational or environmental exposures. For men, the lack of study has been, in part, because the incidence of testicular cancer peaks at a young age and that of prostate cancer peaks at an advanced age – patients that constitute populations predominantly outside the workforce.

Although all of the reproductive cancers have been found to have familial predispositions suggestive of genetic risk factors, recent work by Verkasalo et al[1] has shown the importance of environmental (and occupational) exposures in the development of cancers over a purely genetic predisposition. Verkasalo et al[1] used the Finnish Cancer Registry, Twin Cohort Study and Central Population Register to evaluate cancer risk among monozygotic versus dizygotic twins. Based on genetic modeling, inherited genetic risk factors accounted for 18% (95%CI = 4–32%) of cancer risk while unique environmental factors accounted for 75% (95% CI = 65–85%). In particular, the risk from unique environmental factors for prostate cancer was 58% (95% CI = 33–89%), and for breast/ovarian cancer 77% (95% CI = 52–96%). This chapter reviews the current knowledge of the contribution of occupational and environmental factors to the risk for reproductive cancers, summarized in Table 30.7.1.

In general, reproductive cancers due to workplace exposures present with the same signs and symptoms as the same type of cancer would in the general population (i.e., with a bleeding, growing mass; irregular menses; and localized pain), and they are diagnosed the same way. Differing age distributions from those found for the same cancer type in the general population may be a clue to an occupational or environmental exposure etiology. In addition, as far as we know, workplace reproductive cancers should be treated therapeutically in the same way, and should have a similar prognosis as these same cancers in the general population.

A unique aspect of reproductive cancers in the workplace is the possibility of primary and secondary prevention. Primary prevention can be practiced in those workplaces in which known or suspect reproductive carcinogens are used. This type of prevention can be accomplished by industrial hygiene and engineering, as well as by education of the workforce, to prevent exposure to potential carcinogens.

For those workers who appear to be at high risk for a particular reproductive cancer, or even for workers in general, the workplace also provides an unique venue for screening and education of at-risk workers where appropriate programs exist.[2,3] For example, both the testicular and breast self-examinations may be taught to all workers whether or not they are exposed to suspect reproductive carcinogens.

Endocrine disrupters

Before beginning a review of specific reproductive cancers, a brief discussion is necessary of recent research concerning chemicals that can act as endocrine disrupters and their possible role in the etiology of reproductive cancers, both occupationally and environmentally. A more detailed discussion of this topic is provided in Chapters 45 and 27.1.

It has been demonstrated that various natural and synthetic exogenous substances, such as the previously widely used organochlorine pesticide DDT, can bind and functionally interact with endogenous receptors. An environmental endocrine disrupter is an exogenous agent that interferes with the synthesis, secretion, transport, binding, action, or elimination of natural hormones in the body that are responsible for the maintenance of homeostasis, reproduction, development, and/or behavior.[4,5] Recent in-vitro and in-vivo studies have demonstrated that some exogenous substances can have estrogenic (xenoestrogens) and antiandrogenic effects.[4,5]

In the case of the organochlorine pesticide, DDT, the first interpretation of an estrogen-like action of DDT was noted in 1950, when the inhibition of testicular growth and secondary sexual characteristics of cockerels was reported.[6] Furthermore, it was subsequently demonstrated that both DDT and its metabolites were estrogen receptor agonists[7–9] and androgen receptor antagonists.[10] Numerous in-vitro testing procedures indicate that DDT is not a mutagen.[6] There is evidence, however, that DDT can act as a promoter of carcinogenesis. Specifically o,p'-DDT can support the growth of an estrogen-responsive tumor[6] in a specific and dose-dependent manner, and at a rate similar to estradiol[7].

The chronic effects of these chemicals are of particular concern. These compounds are highly persistent in the environment and have been found in animals[11] and in tree bark in the most remote locations worldwide.[12] The more volatile compounds have been found to globally redistribute to colder, higher latitudes by a distillation effect.[12] These compounds can have a half-life of the order of several years, and are resistant to the natural degradation pathways.[11] Their highly lipophilic properties and environmental persistence

Female	Male
Breast cancer	Testicular cancer
Ovarian cancer	Prostatic cancer
Uterine/endometrial cancer	Male breast cancer
Trophoblastic disease (choriocarcinoma & hydaditiform mole)	

Table 30.7.1 Cancers of the reproductive organs

result in their bioconcentration in the food chain.[11] Concern about chronic effects in humans, including cancer, is reasonable considering the ubiquity of exposure to these agents.

Initial evidence supported a possible role for endocrine disrupters such as DDT in the etiology of breast cancer.[13] However, as discussed below, more recent evidence not only does not uphold this association, but rather may focus future attention on the possible role of these endocrine disrupters in the male reproductive cancers.

CANCERS OF THE REPRODUCTIVE ORGANS IN THE FEMALE
Female breast cancer

Breast cancer is predominantly a disease of women. It will develop in at least 1 out of 11 women in the United States during their lifetimes. Each year in the United States, it accounts for over 30% of newly diagnosed cancers among women, with over 100,000 new cases and over 33,000 deaths. Throughout the world, it is very rare in girls before they reach menarche and until age 30, with a significant increase in incidence among postmenopausal women. Factors such as a high-fat diet and obesity appear to play an important role in breast cancer in postmenopausal women, whereas genetic (especially a history of premenopausal and/or bilateral breast cancer in a close female relative) and endocrine factors appear to be important for breast cancer in premenopausal women. Identification of BRCA gene mutations and associated breast cancer risk underscores the importance of genetic factors. Increased rates of breast cancer are found in industrialized countries, in urban areas, and in higher socioeconomic classes. Early first pregnancy and lactation appear to be protective factors.[14,15]

Ramazzini[16] noted in 1713 that certain groups of women (e.g., nuns) have a greater susceptibility to breast cancer; this susceptibility is probably related to lack of parity. In large epidemiologic studies of occupation and cancer, jobs with higher education were associated with increased breast and decreased cervical cancer rates;[17] this finding may have been confounded by socioeconomic class.[18] For example, King et al[19] found increased risk for breast cancer for teachers (proportionate mortality rate (PMR) 1.68) and registered nurses (PMR 1.20) in British Columbia from 1950 to 1984. Rix et al[20] found an increased risk among 1.4 million Danish working women since 1970, particularly among women professionals (lawyers, medical doctors, dentists, physiotherapists, and nurses), as did Morton[21] using the National Cancer Institute Surveillance, Epidemiology and End Results (SEER) program in the US, and Pollan[22] among Swedish working women. Coogan et al,[23] using a population-based case-control study in the US, found an increased risk only for administrative support occupations; Gunnarsdottir[24] found an increased risk of breast cancer for Icelandic nurses. Threlfall and associates[25] have suggested that this association with socioeconomic class and higher education may be due to low parity and older age at first birth, which are both risk factors associated with these types of jobs. Other reported occupational and environmental causes for female breast cancer are summarized in Table 30.7.2.[26]

Cantor et al[27] used mortality records from 24 states from 1984 to 1989 in a case control analysis of breast cancer risk, using a job matrix after adjusting for socioeconomic class. They found an increased risk of breast cancer with probable occupational exposure to styrene, several organic solvents (methylene chloride, carbon tetrachloride, formaldehyde), several metals/metal oxides, and acid mists. Petralia et al[28] found an association between the risk of estrogen receptor-positive breast cancers and occupational exposure to benzene. Aschengrau et al,[29] in a case-control study, found an insignificant increase in breast cancer among women with drinking water contaminated by tetrachloroethylene from the lining of drinking water pipes.

Ionizing radiation exposure is an established risk factor for breast cancer. This has been shown in a number of different exposure cohorts, including women who received repeated fluoroscopy for pulmonary tuberculosis, women receiving radiation treatments for mastitis, and survivors of the atomic bomb blasts in Hiroshima and Nagasaki, where marked increases in breast cancer were seen in women exposed to 10 rads or more (with peak at 100 rads and latencies typically of more than 10 years from exposure).[30,31] All of these cohorts demonstrated evidence of a linear

Possible causes/contributing factors	Occupation/group	References
Exposures		
External ionizing radiation	Survivors of Hiroshima and Nagasaki; flight attendants	30, 31, 35, 37, 41
Radium	Radium-dial painters	32, 33, 34
Permanent hair dyes, hair dyes	Cosmetologists	22, 63, 64, 65
Anti-rust oil (N-phenyl-1-naphthalene)	Factory workers	67
Various exposures	Ethylene oxide, styrene, several organic solvents, several metals/metal oxides, and acid mists	27, 28, 68
Occupations/industries		
Lamp manufacturing (methylene chloride, trichloroethylene, resin)	Factory workers (coiling and wiredrawing area)	66
Various occupations	Nuns, employers, managers, clericals, nurses, teachers, sales clerks, professionals (lawyers, medical doctors, dentists and physiotherapists), skilled tobacco workers, book binders, meat wrappers and cutters, secretaries and typists, radio and telegraph operators, pharmaceutical workers	

Table 30.7.2 Breast cancer: occupational and environmental causes

dose–response relationship between radiation exposure and risk of breast cancer. There also appears to be a significantly increased risk in women irradiated during adolescence; this finding is postulated to be due to increased sensitivity of stem cells in the developing and adolescent breast to ionizing radiation exposure.

There is a controversial relationship between radium dial painting and increased breast cancer.[32,33] In a cohort of women radium dial painters in the United States who were exposed before 1930,[34] breast cancer risk was increased with a highly significant dose–response relationship at high radium intake, but there was no indication of an association with duration of employment or any suggestion of the importance of age at first exposure (e.g., <20 years of age). Other factors in this controversy concern whether or not the increased risk of breast cancer is due to external exposure to ionizing radiation in the workplace or to the radium absorbed by work practices such as 'tipping' (placing the brushes in the mouth).

Whether or not women exposed to low-level ionizing radiation (such as occupational exposure to radiation for technicians or nurses) are at increased risk for breast cancer is not known. For example, Pukkala et al[35] found a statistically increased risk of breast cancer incidence (standardized incidence ratio (SIR) = 1.87; 95% CI 1.15–2.23) among Finnish flight attendants, but Boice et al[36] did not find a significant risk among certified women radiologic technologists in the US.[37] In a death certificate study, Loomis et al[38] found an increased risk of breast cancer mortality (odds ratio (OR) = 1.38; 95% CI = 1.04–1.82) among female electrical workers in the US. In particular, significant increased risks were reported for electrical engineers (OR = 1.73), electrical technicians (OR = 1.28), and telephone installers, repairers, and line workers (OR = 2.17).

With respect to non-ionizing radiation, Tynes et al[39] found an increased risk of breast cancer among Norwegian female radio and telegraph operators. Feychting et al[40] performed a case-control study of male and female breast cancer risk and residential magnetic field exposure. Female breast cancer risk was particularly increased for women diagnosed at <50 years of age with estrogen-positive tumors, however, with wide confidence limits (relative risk (RR) = 7.4; 95% CI = 1.0–178.1). However, this suggests at least a theoretical possibility of increased breast cancer risk associated with non-ionizing radiation, and has raised concern regarding low-level radiation for women who have undergone repeated mammographic examinations.[41]

Brainard et al[42] evaluated the hypothesis that breast cancer risk may be associated with a decrease in melatonin production secondary to increased exposure to artificial light at night and electromagnetic fields (EMFs). The authors concluded that there is no strong evidence of such an association, though they cautioned that even a small risk would have a substantial public health impact.

Male and female breast cancer incidences were both increased among employees in a Danish pharmaceutical plant where sex hormones, antibiotics, insulin and enzymes were produced.[43] Breast cancer incidence among female employees was significantly elevated (SIR = 1.5), particularly for the subgroup that started work at aged 30–39 for at least 1–9 years (SIR = 2.8).

As discussed above, early age at first pregnancy and breast feeding have long been observed to be protective factors in the development of breast cancer. While this is likely due to hormonal influences, this may have an impact on the body burden of fat-soluble environmental toxicants. Repeated breast feeding, as well as pregnancy itself, leads to a mobilization of a woman's fat stores, including any lipophilic substances such as the organochlorines, leading to a decrease in stored levels (and an increase in their breast-feeding infants).[44] This suggests that breast-feeding may be an important 'detoxification mechanism' for organochlorines and possibly explains in part the decreased risk of breast cancer associated with lactation.[13,44–46] In addition, various authors have proposed that pregnancy itself may protect against breast cancer due to the excretion of lipophilic organochlorines by the mother through the fetal fat and vernix caseosa.[46,47]

Several small studies have evaluated organochlorine levels in breast cancer tissue with variable results.[48–51] Westin and Richter,[45] among others, have argued that changing breast cancer trends over time in Israel may be related to changes in pesticide contamination in breast milk and other sources of milk, and the banning of organochlorine use in Israel. Wolff et al[13,52] showed a strong statistical association between DDE levels and breast cancer in a nested case-control study of women in New York City, even when controlling for a variety of other variables. However, the actual mean levels of DDE were quite low (11.0 ± 9.1 ng/mL cases vs 7.7 ± 6.8 ng/mL controls), presumably because women in New York City have had relatively little exposure to DDT and other organochlorines, even historically; similarly low levels were found in the nested case-control study of Kreiger et al.[53] Thus, the possible association found between DDE levels (and other similar organochlorine compounds with possible estrogenic action) and breast cancer needs to be investigated in populations with historically high organochlorine use. Wesseling et al[54] found significantly increased rates of breast cancer incidence in allegedly high pesticide use areas compared to low pesticide use areas in Costa Rica; no increased risk was found among women in North Vietnam, where there had been extensive use of DDT for malaria control.[55] To date women potentially exposed occupationally to organochlorines have in general not been found to have increased risks of breast cancer.[56–62]

A variety of studies have examined the possible relationship between breast cancer and exposure to permanent hair dyes.[63,64] Occupational exposure to hair dyes has also been examined. Among others, Pollan[22] and Teta et al[65] found significantly increased risk of cancers of the breast among cosmetologists, while other studies have found no increase among cosmetologists, hairdressers, manicurists, and beauticians. An increased frequency of the regular use of permanent hair dyes was found among those with breast cancer as opposed to controls in two studies. Of interest, in the past certain hair dyes (permanent and semi-permanent) were strongly mutagenic in the Ames test. A significant excess of chromosomal damage (mainly chromosomal breaks) has been reported in women with dyed hair, although this has not been found in those with occupational exposures (except when the hairdressers dyed their own hair) or in men with dyed hair.

A follow-up study of a cluster of tumors in women workers in a lamp manufacturing plant found increases in ovarian, uterine, and breast cancer in the coiling and wire drawing area of the plant, without identifying a definite exposure.[66] Women workers exposed to anti-rust oil, in particular N-phenyl-1-naphthalamine or its nitroso derivatives, were observed to have an increased rate of cancer, including uterine, ovarian, and breast cancers.[67] Breast cancer incidence was increased in a cohort of workers in an ethylene oxide plant, although there was no increase associated with cumulative exposure.[68] Pulp and paper industry workers in Spain had an insignificantly increased of breast cancer mortality.[69]

Prevention and early detection are best served by following the recommendations and schedules of the American Cancer Society for breast self-examination and mammography. Workplace screening may be an effective and under-utilized setting for breast cancer screening.[2] Particular attention should be paid to women with environmental or occupational exposure to ionizing radiation in terms of primary and secondary prevention.

Ovarian cancer

The lifetime risk of ovarian cancer among white women is 1–2% (less among African-American and Hispanic women), and the risk increases sharply with age. There are several different cell types (including germ cell, stromal and epithelial tumors), with different types predominating in different geographic populations. A variety of risk factors have been identified. In animals, oocyte loss is a prerequisite for tumor production, as well as gonadotropin stimulation. Low fertility is a risk factor, although there appears to be some protection with the use of birth control pills. There may be increased risk in humans and animals after the use of diethylstilbestrol (DES). There is a strong familial risk of ovarian cancer.[15,70]

In a review of occupation and mortality from reproductive cancers among women from 24 US states from 1884 to 1993,[71] ovarian cancer mortality risk was increased for certain professional groups, including managers, teachers, librarians, office workers, financial workers, and religious workers. Technical writers had the highest risk with a mortality odds ratio of 6.1. Among other occupations, waitresses, dental assistants, electricians and bus drivers had excess risk. Among African-American women, financial managers, elementary school teachers, librarians, designers, health technicians, administrative support occupations, child care workers and machine operators had the highest risk, with the occupation of financial managers demonstrating the greatest risk of mortality (MOR = 20.9). Industries with the highest risk included printing, publishing, soap and cosmetic manufacturing, machinery manufacturing, utilities, retail trade, finance, healthcare, legal services, education, professional services, and government. Rix et al[20] found an increased risk of ovarian cancer among 1.4 million working Danish women since 1970 among clerks. In a proportionate mortality study, King et al[19] found an increased risk for ovarian cancer for teachers (PMR 1.48) and registered nurses (PMR 1.56) in British Columbia from 1950 to 1984 (Table 30.7.3).

Shen et al,[70] reviewing the experience in European countries, observed an increased risk for ovarian cancer among hairdressers, beauticians and women employed in the printing industry, but concluded that the data were insufficient to conclude an occupational association. The authors judged that only exposure to talc had sufficient evidence for a modest to moderate increased risk. Vasama-Neuvonen et al[72] used the Finnish cancer registry to evaluate risk by occupational exposure of ovarian cancer using a job-exposure matrix. Occupational exposures to aromatic hydrocarbon solvents, man-made vitreous fibers, high levels of asbestos, diesel and gasoline engine exhausts were associated with insignificant increases in cancer risk; hairdressers and women in the printing industry were also at increased risk.

Exposure to ionizing radiation appears to be a risk factor for ovarian cancer (Table 30.7.3). Studies by Doll and Smith[73] of women who underwent radiation for ostensibly benign pelvic conditions showed a small increased risk for

Possible causes/contributing factors	Occupation/group	References
Exposures		
Ionizing radiation	Women survivors of atom bomb blast	74
Asbestos and talc	Gas mask assemblers, asbestos workers	72, 75, 76, 77, 78
Talc	Cosmetologists, hairdressers, pulp and paper workers	65, 70, 72, 79, 80, 81, 82, 83, 84
Occupations/industries		
Lamp manufacturing (methylene chloride, trichloroethylene, resin)	Factory workers (coiling and wire)	66
Various professions	Managers, teachers, librarians, office workers, financial workers, religious workers, waitresses, dental assistants, electricians, bus drivers, nurses, clerks, aerospace workers	19, 20, 70, 71, 85
Various industries	Printing, publishing, soap and cosmetic manufacturing, machinery manufacturing, utilities, retail trade, finance, health care, legal services, education, professional services, and government	71

Table 30.7.3 Ovarian cancer: occupational and environmental causes

developing ovarian carcinoma. This increased risk also was seen in a case-control study[74] of the atomic bomb survivors (6 versus 3.3 expected) in Hiroshima, but the risk did not appear in Nagasaki. The latter finding was possibly due to increased neutron exposure in Hiroshima.

Asbestos and talc exposures, both occupationally and environmentally, have been related to an increased risk of ovarian cancer; in the past, talc has been contaminated with asbestos. Women who worked as gas mask assemblers and with other asbestos products during World War II had an increased risk of ovarian cancer. This risk appears to be associated most strongly with crocidolite exposure. Asbestos can reach the ovary, and high fiber counts have been seen in women with para-occupational exposure to asbestos.[75-78]

An increased risk for ovarian cancer was reported in a study of female cosmetologists and hairdressers in British Columbia, a study of cosmetologists in Connecticut, and reviews of national cancer registries in Europe for cancer risk among hairdressers.[65,79-81] A NIOSH[82] retrospective survey of cancer in relation to occupations also found an increased relative risk for hairdressers and cosmetologists for ovarian cancer. In the case of cosmetologists, talc has been a hypothesized etiology. Langseth[83] found a significantly increased risk of ovarian cancer incidence (SIR = 1.5; 95% CI = 1.07–2.09) among Norwegian pulp and paper workers with possible exposure to talc and paper dust; Bulbulyan et al[84] also found an increased risk of ovarian cancer mortality (standardized mortality ration (SMR) = 2.9; 95% CI = 1.50–5.00) among women in the Russian printing industry with possible talc exposure. Of interest, talc particles have been found more frequently in ovarian tumors than in normal ovarian tissue. Several areas of controversy still exist. First, talc, including cosmetic talc, was contaminated with asbestiform fibrous particles in the past (including exposures in the 1970s); non-fibrous talc does not cause cancer in experimental animals. Furthermore, it is possible that the ovarian cancers actually represent undiagnosed mesotheliomas of the peritoneum.

A follow-up study[66] of a cluster of various tumors in women workers in a lamp manufacturing plant found increases in ovarian cancer in the coiling and wire drawing area. The etiologic agents are unknown; occupational exposures included methylene chloride, trichloroethylene, and various resins. Morgan et al[85] found an insignificant increased risk of ovarian cancer relative risk among aerospace workers with increased trichloroethylene exposure using job exposure matrix.

Wesseling et al[54] found significantly increased rates of ovarian cancer incidence in reported high pesticide use areas compared to low pesticide use areas in Costa Rica. However, other studies of pesticide-exposed working populations have not found an increased risk of ovarian cancer.[59-61,86]

Endometrial/uterine (corpus) cancer

The risk factors for uterine cancer resemble those of breast cancer except for the peak age incidence. The age-adjusted incidence for uterine cancer is approximately 30 per 100,000 women. However, the age-specific incidence peaks around 55–60 years, and the amount of uterine cancer is apparently increasing worldwide, although mortality has decreased substantially. There is an increased incidence of uterine cancer among higher socioeconomic classes, and in industrialized countries. Obesity (or increased estrogen production from non-ovarian sources) and endogenous estrogen are known risk factors for uterine cancer. There also is an increased risk with nulliparity. Uterine cancer originating from the endometrium (adenocarcinoma) is much more common than that originating from the myometrium (sarcoma); uterine sarcoma is very rare, although it is increased among African-American women in the United States.[15]

In a review of occupation and mortality from reproductive cancers among women from 24 US states from 1884 to 1993,[71] highest risk of endometrial cancer were seen among teachers in special education (MOR = 3.7), with increased risk also observed in public relations specialists (MOR 2.8) and religious workers (MOR = 2.7). Among African-American women, librarians, clergy and hand packers had the highest risks. By industry, endometrial mortality was highest in fishing and trapping (MOR = 4.8) and optometry (MOR = 4.8); manufacture of paper, metal products; education, and public administration. Rix et al[20] found an increased risk of uterine cancer among 1.4 million working Danish women since 1970 among traveling saleswomen, furriers, hairdressers, nurses and clerks. Dalager et al[87] reported that US military nurses who served in Vietnam had increased risk of uterine cancer mortality compared to other US military nurses. King et al[19] found an increased risk for ovarian cancer for teachers (PMR 1.56) in British Columbia from 1950 to 1984 (Table 30.7.4).

As discussed above with breast cancer, exposure to lipophilic organochlorines with estrogenic action theoretically may be associated with an increased risk of uterine cancer. As in the case of ovarian cancer, Wesseling et al[54] found significantly increased rates of uterine cancer incidence in high pesticide use areas in Costa Rica. However, to date women potentially exposed occupationally to organochlorines have not been found to have increased risks of uterine cancer.[57-60,88]

Possible causes/ contributing factors	Occupation/group	References
Occupations/industries		
Various professions	Teachers in special education, public relations specialists, religious workers, nurses, traveling saleswomen, furriers, hairdressers, clerks	19, 20, 21, 87
Various industries	Fishing and trapping; employment in optometry; manufacture of paper, metal products; education; and public administration	71

Table 30.7.4 Uterine cancer: occupational and environmental causes

Several studies of occupation and cancer have revealed a number of job categories with statistically increased risk for uterine cancer.[89] A NIOSH[82] retrospective survey of cancer in relation to occupation found an increased relative risk for hairdressers and cosmetologists for uterine body cancer, although this was not seen in other studies. A cohort study of cosmetologists[65] in Connecticut also observed a significant increased risk for cancer of the uterus.

In a large Swedish cohort study from 1971 to 1984, Floderus et al[90] analyzed jobs for possible occupational exposure to magnetic fields using a job matrix. An association was noted for uterine cancer among women workers with those jobs judged to have more definite occupational electromagnetic field exposures.

Prevention and early detection are best served by following the recommendations and schedules of the American Cancer Society for uterine biopsy. Particular attention should be paid to women with environmental or occupational exposure to estrogens in terms of primary and secondary prevention, although no increase in uterine cancer has been noted in workers such as farmers and pesticide applicators possibly exposed to estrogen analogues.

Cervical cancer

The peak in incidence for cervical cancer is around age 30, with a reported age-specific incidence of approximately 110 cases per 100,000 women. Cervical cancer is very rare in women who are not sexually active (e.g., nuns). The most important risk factors are increased and early sexual behavior, i.e., young age at first intercourse and high number of sexual partners. There is a more modest risk associated with exposure to sex hormones (prolonged use of combined oral contraceptives, injectable progesterones) and lower socioeconomic class. Worldwide, there has been a decrease in incidence, especially in developed nations, which is believed to be due to improved standards of living, as well as increased routine screening through the Pap smear. Cigarette smoking may be a risk factor, however smoking is also associated with lower socioeconomic class, a major confounder. Squamous cell cancer accounts for 85–90% of invasive cancers of the cervix, whereas 5–8% are adenocarcinomas (non-clear cell). Clear cell adenocarcinoma is seen almost exclusively in association with maternal DES exposure. Finally, several viruses have been studied for their possible oncogenic role in cervical cancer, including papilloma and herpes (especially HSV-2). The data strongly indicate that papilloma virus is the major risk factor for cervical cancer.[15,91]

A controversy has developed concerning the role of occupation (especially husband's occupation) and cervical cancer. Several researchers have noted that occupation (of the woman or spouse) is too closely associated with socioeconomic class to draw environmental inferences. However, widely different rates have been reported for cervical carcinoma of women classified by their spouse's occupation within the same socioeconomic class. Spouses of men with jobs involving exposures to dust, metals, chemicals, tar, and machine oil appear to have higher rates of cancer,

possibly due to indirect para-occupational genital exposures via the husband, but socioeconomic status continues to be a significant confounder.[92]

In a review of occupation and mortality from reproductive cancers among women from 24 US states from 1884 to 1993,[71] the highest risks were seen for cervical cancer among actors and directors (MOR = 4.1), typesetters and compositors (MOR = 3.3), and artists and performers (MOR = 3.1). Cervical cancer mortality risk was increased for certain service occupations: maids, cleaners, waitresses, and nursing aides. Increased risk among manufacturing occupations was observed for molding machine operators, printers and textile machine operators. Similar results in a proportionate mortality study were found by Alterman et al[93] using mortality data from the National Occupational Mortality Surveillance System from 1985 to 1990 for 27 states, and by Rix et al[20] among 1.4 million Danish working. Cellulose triacetate fiber workers exposed to methylene chloride with 20 or more years of employment were at increased risk of mortality (SMR = 8.02.; $P < 0.01$) from cervical cancer[94] (Table 30.7.5).

Florida women pesticide applicators and farmers[59,60] had an increased risk of cervical cancer incidence (SIR = 3.69; 95% CI = 1.84–6.61), without increased mortality. Sala et al[71] and Alterman et al[93] observed that among African-American women, farmers had a significantly increased risk for cervical cancer mortality (MOR = 1.7; 95% CI = 1.2–2.4). Other studies have also observed increased cervical cancer risk among farmers,[95,96] although not in all studies.[61,97]

A study of nurses found an increased risk of cervical cancer as well as other lower genital tract cancers with hair dye use; this risk persisted despite adjustment for smoking.[89] Increases in cancer of the cervix uteri and of the genitals (unspecified) were reported in a case-control study of female laundry and dry cleaning workers even after adjusting for socioeconomic class. Cervical cancer was increased (SIR = 1.71; 95% CI = 1.3–2.3) among waitresses in Norway,[98] particularly in the subcohort working in restaurants with liquor licenses. Of note, waitresses have been at particularly high risk for both passive and active smoking exposure.

Prevention and early detection are best served by following the recommendations and schedules of the American

Possible causes/ contributing factors	Occupation/group	References
Occupations/industries		
Various professions	Actors and directors, typesetters and compositors, artists and performers, maids, cleaners, waitresses, nursing aides, farmers	20, 54, 59, 60, 71, 93, 95, 96, 98, 99
Various industries	Molding machine operating, printers and textile machine operating	20, 71, 93, 94

Table 30.7.5 Cervical cancer: occupational and environmental causes

Cancer Society for PAP smear. Of note, a study by Savitz et al[99] comparing the risk of invasive carcinoma versus carcinoma in situ identified maids, cleaners and cooks as a group at particularly increased risk for invasive cervical cancer.

Miscellaneous: choriocarcinoma and hydatidiform mole

Choriocarcinoma, which arises from the trophoblastic epithelium of the placenta, usually is seen after hydatidiform mole, but can occur after a normal pregnancy (either aborted or progressing to term). Choriocarcinoma is very rare; in the US the incidence has been estimated at 1.4/million population. The risk of choriocarcinoma is about 1000 times greater after a pregnancy with hydatidiform mole than after normal pregnancy (choriocarcinoma is seen in 3% of hydatidiform moles). There also are increased risks associated with increasing maternal age, increasing parity, lower socioeconomic status, and exposure to exogenous sex hormones.[15,100]

An increased incidence of hydatidiform mole and choriocarcinoma has been reported among Southeast Asians (1 in 200 deliveries versus 1 in 2000 in Europe and the United States). Ha et al[101] examined the increased risk for gestational trophoblastic disease (hydatidiform mole and choriocarcinoma) in Vietnam since the spraying of the dioxin-contaminated Agent Orange as a case-control study. Adjusted odds ratio was increased among agricultural workers breeding pigs (OR = 5.7; 95% CI = 1.27–27.6) as well as increased meat intake, but no difference was noted for residence history with Agent Orange exposure or agricultural use of pesticides.

In a Japanese study,[102] cosmetic salespersons and beauticians were reported at increased risk for hydatidiform mole. It has been hypothesized that the increased risk of cancer may be related to exposure to a red pigment commonly used in Japan as a cosmetic. The same study also reported significantly increased risks of hydatidiform mole for textile dyers, printers, chemical workers, and fishermen.

CANCERS OF THE REPRODUCTIVE ORGANS IN THE MALE
Testicular cancer

Testicular cancer accounts for less than 1% (0.2% lifetime risk for US white males) of all male cancer deaths; nevertheless, it is the most commonly diagnosed malignancy in men aged 20–34 years with a 50% increase noted in the age-adjusted incidence between 1973 and 1990. The young age of onset tends to cast doubt on an occupational etiology, unless para-occupational factors such as indirect para-occupational exposures from parents are the cause. However, the incidence of testicular cancer has been rising over the last 50 years in industrialized countries (England, the United States, Japan, and Denmark), without an obvious connection to increased screening. There appears to be an increased risk with upper socioeconomic class (up to 2.5 times). Race still appears to be an important risk factor; it is generally rare among black populations. Other risk factors include higher socioeconomic class, testicular trauma, mumps, testicular atrophy, the solvent dimethylformamide, and radiation exposure.[15,103–105]

In several large epidemiologic studies examining occupation, an increased risk for testicular cancer has been found among a variety of disparate occupational groups (Table 30.7.6).[106,107] Paternal occupational exposure to metal or the food and beverage industry may be related to an increased risk of testicular cancer in Ontario.[108] In particular, non-seminoma tumors were associated with male parents who were miners, food and beverage processors, utilities employees, and other service workers, while seminomas were associated with male parents who were leather industry employees.[108]

Possible causes/contributing factors	Occupation/group	References
Exposures		
Dimethylformamide (DMF)	Navy aviation mechanics, leather tanners, US Navy personnel, British Navy airmen	135, 136, 137, 138, 139, 142, 145
Chromates, metal protective primers (zinc chromate, solvents)	Painters in Geneva	141, 145
Agricultural chemicals	Farmers, pesticide applicators, agricultural workers	59, 105, 131
Ionizing radiation	Employees of the United Kingdom Atomic Energy Authority	105, 109, 110
Tetrachloroethane	Workers in World War II (impregnation of clothing)	15
Carpets and textiles	Carpet and textile workers	151
Asbestos	Asbestos workers	147, 148
Extremes of temperature	Numerous occupations	112
Ferrosilicon	Furnace workers	113
Vinyl chloride	Plastics industry workers	149
Occupations/industries		
Professions	Podiatrists	152
Industrial exposures	Mill workers, oilfield natural gas workers, electrical, forestry, food manufacture, and preparation, printing workers, fishermen, and draughtsmen, metal workers	106, 107, 114, 129, 130

Table 30.7.6 Testicular cancer: occupational and environmental causes

A variety of other occupational and environmental exposures have been associated with an increased risk of testicular cancer. An increase in cancer of the testis was seen among 39,546 employees of the United Kingdom Atomic Energy Authority between 1946 and 1979.[109] Stenlund and Floderus[110] found a significantly increased risk for testicular cancer with occupational electromagnetic field exposure in a Swedish case control. Floderus et al,[111] in a large Swedish cohort study from 1971 to 1984, analyzed jobs for possible occupational exposure to magnetic fields using a job exposure matrix. An association was noted for testicular cancer among young male workers judged to have more definite occupational electromagnetic field exposures, although the authors noted that occupational heat exposure might also be an important factor. In a separate case control study[110] an increased risk, predominantly for non-seminoma tumors was noted with increased electromagnetic field occupational exposure.

In controlled studies, occupational exposure to temperature extremes was associated with increased risks of testicular cancer incidence.[112] Hobbesland et al[113] studied cancer incidence in 8 ferrosilicon and silicon metal plants in Norway. Testicular cancer incidence (SIR = 2.30) was elevated among the furnace workers. Metal workers had a significantly increased risk of testicular cancer (OR = 2.05; 95% CI = 1.17–3.58) in Germany.[114]

Although controversial, an increased risk of testicular cancer has been associated with exposure in utero to estrogens (such as DES) in animals and possibly in humans.[103,115–117] Of note, cryptorchidism, the only established risk factor for testicular cancer, is associated with in utero estrogen exposure. Cryptorchidism appears to also have an increasing incidence, especially in the more developed nations, paralleling the increase noted in testicular cancer incidence.[115,118]

Recent reports have raised the question of an overall worldwide significant decrease in human sperm counts, possibly related to the use of certain pesticides and their estrogen effects.[115,119–125] The latter issue has been given further credence by the historical link between profound male infertility and occupational exposure to the pesticide dibromochloropropane (DBCP). The pesticide dibromochloropropane (DBCP) causes sterility in human males exposed occupationally. It also is very toxic to the testis in animals (causing atrophy and degeneration), and it is carcinogenic (although not to the testis) in a variety of animal species. However, so far, DBCP has not been demonstrated to be carcinogenic to the testis (or other organs) in humans.[126,127] More recently, some of the organochlorines have been shown in animal models to be powerful antiandrogens.[115] These chemicals and their derivatives are environmentally persistent, and extremely lipophilic, leading to lifetime body burdens. Therefore, this is an area of great research interest.[128]

Several studies have found increased risks for testicular cancer among agricultural workers.[129] These include a case control study[130] of 347 people with histologically confirmed germ cell tumors of the testis, that demonstrated a significant odds ratio of 6.27, and a large case-control study (2434 cases) in England and Wales, that observed increased testicular cancer rates (OR > 3) among farmers. Fleming et al[59,60] performed a retrospective cohort study of 33,658 pesticide applicators licensed in Florida. Testicular cancer incidence was significantly elevated compared with the general population (SIR = 2.49; 1.58–3.74). In a cohort study in Sweden[56,131] an elevated, but non-statistically significant increase for testicular cancer was found among both agricultural workers and pesticide applicators. Mills[132] found a significant correlation (r = 0.41) for testicular cancer incidence in Hispanic males with atrazine occupational pesticide exposure. In a case-control study of testicular cancer, Hardell et al[133] found that embryonal testicular cancer, but not seminoma, was associated with reported history of farming (OR = 3.1; 95% CI 1.03–9.1) and exposure to farm animals (OR = 3.3; 95% CI 1.00–10.9); Kirstensen et al[134] found increased risk of seminoma associated with parental exposure to specific fertilizer regimens on farms. However, several other studies among agricultural workers do not support this finding.[54,56]

Occupational exposure to the bipolar solvent dimethylformamide (DMF) has been implicated as a suspect risk factor for testicular cancer in a variety of studies. This association was first seen in a cluster and subsequent retrospective cohort among navy aviation mechanics who used DMF and other solvents.[135] Boice et al[136] found significantly increased risk of testicular cancer associated with exposure to mixed solvents among aircraft manufacturing workers; Ryder[137] found significant increases in testicular cancer risk in a case-control study of the UK Royal Navy, particularly among Fleet Air Arm (OR = 1.90; 95% CI = 1.04–3.48), air engineers (OR = 2.32; 95% CI = 1.20–4.48), and aircraft handling (OR = 7.31; 95% CI = 1.81–29.53). Another cluster of testicular cancer was identified among leather tanners in a follow-up case-control study;[138,139] increased risk for development of seminoma was also found in male parents who had been involved in leather tanning.[140]

Increased testicular cancer was observed in two retrospective cohort studies: one among US Navy personnel with exposure to chromate-based paints and solvents (including possible DMF exposure),[141] and another study of painters in Geneva who were exposed to metal protective primers containing zinc chromate and a variety of solvents.[142] DMF is neither a known animal carcinogen nor mutagen, but it can cause testicular damage in animals. In a study conducted by a DMF manufacturer,[143,144] of 2530 potentially exposed employees, no increase in testicular cancer was observed. This has led Ducatman and others to hypothesize that DMF (a highly polar solvent) may act to increase tissue absorption of direct carcinogens such as chromates, cadmium, and other heavy metal pigments.[145,146]

Mesothelioma of the tunica vaginalis from the head of the epididymis (i.e., primary malignant testicular mesothelioma) has been reported in asbestos workers with 20 years of regular exposure and a latency period of greater than 20 years from first exposure;[147,148] no asbestos fibers were identified in the tumors.

Hardell et al[149] observed an increased risk of testicular cancer with self-reported polyvinyl chloride exposure; the odds ratio was 6.6 (95% CI = 1.4–32) with the majority seminomas. Cancer of the genital organs was moderately increased among men exposed to tetrachloroethane exposure during World War II in the impregnation of clothing for protection against mustard gas.[150] Testicular cancer was noted to be increased in a study of cancer mortality among Northern Georgia carpet and textile workers.[151] There have been two separate clusters reported of testicular carcinoma among podiatrists, with no obvious etiology.[152]

In certain working populations, such as those exposed to DMF, teaching testicular self-examination and testicular cancer screening may be warranted, given the markedly increased survival rate with early detection and treatment of this disease and its peak occurrence among working-aged men.

Prostate cancer

Prostate cancer is common, and is responsible for at least 27.5% of cancer cases among males and 13% of cancer deaths in the US. The highest rates are reported in industrialized Western countries. In 1981 in the United States, 70,000 men were newly diagnosed and 22,700 men died of prostate cancer. As a subgroup, African-American men in the United States have the highest incidence and mortality in the world. Because this incidence is not seen among African black men, some other risk factor such as dietary influences (e.g., fat intake) and occupational and environmental exposures may be involved. Prostate cancer is very rare in men younger than 50 years of age, and it is chiefly seen in older men. There appears to be an association with sexual behavior, in that the risk increases with an increase in the number of sexual partners and a history of repeated venereal infections. Ninety-five per cent of prostate cancers are adenocarcinomas.[15,153]

Hanchette and Schwartz[154] performed an ecological study of the geographic distribution of prostate cancer mortality within the US. Data on prostate cancer mortality for white men in 3073 counties in the continental US were compared to UV radiation levels at the county level and as a geographic trend. The authors demonstrated a significant north–south trend in mortality; higher mortality was demonstrated in the north and with lower levels of UV radiation. These results have been interpreted as providing possible support for a role of vitamin D as an antitumor agent in prostate cancer.

Farmers, teachers, welders, metal workers, mechanics, plasterers, textile workers, transport workers, fire fighters, nitrate workers, and rubber workers exposed to heavy metal oxides have all been reported to be at an increased risk of prostate cancer (Table 30.7.7). Cadmium is one of the few chemicals predominant in occupational exposures clearly associated with prostate cancer.[103,155–163]

An increased risk in cancer of the prostate has been reported among employees of the United Kingdom Atomic Energy Authority between 1946 and 1979; of interest, those with radiation monitoring showed a significant dose–response relationship.[109,164] At both Hanford and Oak Ridge National Laboratory, there were increases in prostate cancer without a dose–response relationship. Increases in cancer of the prostate have not been seen in other populations exposed to high doses of ionizing radiation, such as the atomic bomb survivors.[165,166] Increased risk of prostate cancer mortality was found among workers exposed specifically to kerosene during uranium processing.[167]

Prostate cancer has been suspected among workers exposed to cadmium, although this association is still somewhat controversial.[168] Potts[169] first reported on 74 men exposed for over 10 years to cadmium as battery workers, with three out of eight deaths due to prostate cancer. There are several small positive cohort studies. Holden[170] reported one case among 42 workers with 2–40 years of exposure to cadmium oxide occurring more than 20 years after first exposure; Kipling and Waterhouse[171] retrospectively studied 248 workers with at least 1 year of cadmium exposure and observed four deaths (0.58 predicted). A retrospective study by Lemen[172] of 292 workers with at least 2 years of exposure

Possible causes/contributing factors	Occupation/group	References
Exposures		
Cadmium	Battery workers, other workers, nickel-cadmium battery workers	169, 170, 171, 172, 173, 174, 175
Ionizing radiation	Employees of the United Kingdom Atomic Energy Authority; Employees at Hanford and Oak Ridge National Laboratory	109, 148, 164, 165
Agricultural chemicals	Horticultural workers, dairy farmers, farmers, pesticide applicators, golf course superintendents	59, 60, 158, 162, 188, 194, 204, 207, 221, 222
Rubber tire/batch preparation	Rubber tire workers, production workers	205, 206, 207, 208, 209, 210
DMF, acrylonitrile,	Acrylonitrile workers, textile workers	200, 201
Acetic acid, acetic anhydride	Production workers	203
Ferrosilicon, ferrochromium	Production workers, non furnace workers	113, 177, 178, 202
Organic chemicals	Swedish chemists	199
Androgens	Butchers, meat cutters, abattoir workers	195, 196, 197, 198
Occupations/industries		
Industrial/occupational activities (no obvious exposures)	Mechanics, blacksmiths, compositors, typesetters, ship fitters, plumbers, clergy, newspaper printing and publishing workers, coke oven workers, firefighters, pulp and paper, metal workers	69, 82, 159, 160, 161, 162, 163, 179, 180, 207

Table 30.7.7 Prostate cancer: occupational and environmental causes

in a cadmium smelter observed four deaths (versus 1.88 expected). In a meta-analysis, available data from the most recent follow-up of causes of death among cadmium workers in six different cohorts identified 28 cases among 522 nickel-cadmium battery workers (SMR = 162); a possible additional role of nickel was suggested. Two case control studies[173,174] of prostate cancer have found the relative risk to be about 1.7 for work in the cadmium trades.

In animals, there is definite evidence of carcinogenicity with cadmium exposure.[175] It also is hypothesized that prostate cancer may be related to crucial zinc-calcium interactions in the prostate. Of note, there has been no further evidence of an association between occupational exposure to nickel-cadmium batteries (cadmium oxide) and cancer of the prostate in longitudinal follow-up of a cohort, with four cases reported by Kipling,[171] nor in the United States cadmium production workers. However, this finding may be related to more recent lower occupational exposures.[176]

A number of studies have observed an association between working with metals and prostate cancer.[177,178] A review of studies of metal workers and repairmen by van der Gulden[163] found a slight but consistent excess of prostate cancer. An increased incidence of prostate cancer was found in a retrospective study of male workers producing ferrosilicon and ferrochromium; in another study of ferrochromium workers, a similar increase was observed. Hobbesland et al[113] studied prostate cancer incidence in eight ferrosilicon and silicon metal plants in Norway; prostate cancer incidence was increased among the blue-collar non-furnace workers. Costantino et al[179] reported that coke oven workers have an increased risk of prostate cancer as much as 4.45 times greater than non-coke oven workers, even as their risk of respiratory cancer is decreasing. Firefighters in Washington State were found to have an increased risk of prostate cancer incidence (SIR = 1.45; 95% CI 1.1–1.7) compared to the general population.[180]

Farmers and agricultural workers are the occupational groups most studied for prostate cancer risk. Compared with other occupational groups, farmers are reported to have a lower risk of cancer from all causes combined and most of the major types of cancer.[181–184] The observations that farmers have an elevated risk of prostate cancer, and are exposed to greater than average amounts of UV radiation, are at odds with the suggested protective effect of UV radiation, and thus vitamin D, on prostate cancer.[154] It is possible, however, that some environmental factor associated with farming and prostate cancer may be responsible and identifiable. For example, increased nitrate levels in drinking water in Spain were associated with an increased risk of prostate cancer mortality.[185]

A number of studies have examined the issue of increased prostate cancer among farmers and pesticide applicators.[162,186,187] One study[156] suggested that 38% of the excess prostate cancer mortality among African-Americans could be due to farming-related occupations. Mills[132] found a significant correlations for prostate cancer incidence and black males with atrazine (r = 0.67) and captan (r = 0.49) occupational pesticide exposure. In a case-control study of Checkoway et al,[188] farming was the most common occu-

pation among the prostate cancer patients (75% cases vs 38% controls). This association persisted even when adjusted for education, age, race and county of residence. Another case-control study of farming and prostate cancer risk in Iowa[189] observed an increased risk (RR = 1.7; 95% CI = 1.0–2.7%) of prostate cancer among farmers after adjustment for age, smoking, alcohol, and diet, compared to cancer-free controls selected from the cohort. The relationship was strengthened (RR = 2.0; 95% CI = 1.1–3.6) when localized well-differentiated tumors were excluded. Adjusting for family history only slightly attenuated the association. Iowa cancer mortality data has demonstrated that the risk of prostate cancer in farmers may have increased from 1971 to 1986.[189]

A number of literature reviews and meta-analyses of farming and cancer risk, including prostate cancer risk, have been performed with variable results.[54,157,181,190–193] Internationally, prostate cancer risk for farmers has been found to be consistently but only slightly elevated, with some variation across countries. Some of the variation is believed to be associated with differing types and amounts of pesticide and other farming exposures.

Two recent studies of pesticide applicators found positive associations between this occupational category and prostate cancer.[59,60,158] Dich and Wiklund[158] studied the cohort of 20,025 Swedish pesticide applicators. The total standardized incidence ratio (SIR) for prostate cancer was significantly but only mildly elevated at 1.13 (95% CI = 1.02–1.24). Fleming et al[59,60] performed a retrospective cohort study of 33,658 pesticide applicators licensed in Florida. Prostate cancer mortality [SMR = 2.38 (95% CI = 1.83–3.04)] and prostate cancer incidence [SIR = 1.92 (1.73–2.14)] were both significantly elevated. An investigation of golf course superintendents found a significantly increased risk of prostate cancer mortality (PMR = 2.93; 95% CI = 187–460).[194]

There is an ongoing controversy as to whether an increase in cancer of the prostate noted among butchers and meat cutters in the United Kingdom could be due to occupational exposure to androgens.[195,196] However, the levels of androgen exposure are believed to be insignificant, and increased prostatic cancer was not noted in a large cohort study of abattoir workers in the United States.[197,198]

An increase in prostate cancer was found among 857 Swedish chemists.[199] Chen and associates[200,201] noted an increase in prostate cancer in production workers exposed to DMF and acrylonitrile; this risk was not observed in workers who were exposed to only DMF. Of interest, an unexpected increase was seen previously in a cohort of acrylonitrile workers.[202] Whorton et al[203] observed a significant increase in prostate cancer mortality (SMR = 3.30; 95% CI = 1.21–7.19) among workers in a chemical plant making acetic acid and acetic anhydride for the synthesis of cellulose triacetate fibers. Textile workers have been noted to have an increased risk of prostate cancer in large epidemiologic surveys. However, in a case-control study in South Carolina, no relationship except among African-American males was found between working in the textile industry and prostate cancer.[204]

In the past, studies of rubber workers have shown an increase in the rates of cancer of the prostate, although no specific carcinogens were causally identified.[205-209] A recent meta-analysis by Stewart et al[210] concluded that occupational exposure to rubber and tire manufacture did not result in an increased risk of prostate cancer.

Although controversial, workplace sponsored prostate cancer screening can be instituted based on the length of employment and possible occupational risk factors of employees.[3]

Male breast cancer

Male breast cancer is rare, and studies have been very limited. Female to male incidence ratios vary from 70:1 to 130:1 around the world. It is known that males with altered estrogen, orchitis or orchiectomy, gynecomastia, and Klinefelter's syndrome are at greatest risk of developing breast cancer; there are also reports of familial clusters and an association with higher reported weight during adolescence. The strongest risk factors appear to be higher socioeconomic class, estrogen and radiation.[15,211]

A Swedish Cancer Environment Registry study[212] found increased incidences of male breast cancer in several occupations. The highest risk was found among men employed in making soap and perfume and among newspaper printers. Other increased rates were seen among a variety of occupations. In a large US national mortality study, Cocco et al[213] observed a significantly increased risk for employment in blast furnaces, steel works and rolling mills (OR = 3.4; 95% CI = 1.1–10.1) as well as motor vehicles manufacture (OR = 3.1; 95% CI = 1.2–8.2). Occupational exposures to electromagnetic fields, PAHs, herbicides and pesticides, and organic solvents were not associated with an increased risk.

Male and female breast cancer incidences were both increased among employees in a Danish pharmaceutical plant where sex hormones, antibiotics, insulin and enzymes were produced.[43] There were three male breast cancer cases with 0.4 expected. Hansen[214] also found an increased risk for male breast cancer incidence among workers potentially exposed to gasoline vapors and combustion products. The odds ratio for men potentially exposed more than 3 months ranged from 2.5 (95% CI = 1.3–4.5), to 5.4 (95% CI = 2.4–11.9) for men with first employment potential exposure before age 40.

Robinson et al[215] found a significantly increased risk of male breast cancer (PMR = 4.69; 95% CI = 128–720) among white male carpenters. This risk was associated with last employment in wood machining trades. Forastiere et al[216] found an increased risk of male breast cancer mortality (SMR = 14.36) based on only two cases.

An increase in male breast cancer has been observed in men with a variety of occupational exposures to electromagnetic fields in both the United States and Norway.[217] Demers and coworkers[218] reported the highest risk among electricians, telephone linemen, and electric power workers in a population-based case-control study. Rosenbaum et al[219] performed a case-control study using the New York State Tumor Registry between 1979 and 1988, with 71 male breast cancer cases. No increased risk was found for electromagnetic field exposure, although an increased risk was associated with occupational heat exposure. Stenlund and Floderus[110] did not find an increased risk for male breast cancer with occupational electromagnetic field exposure in a Swedish case-control study. Feychting et al[220] performed a case-control study of male and female breast cancer risk and residential magnetic field exposure with a non-statistically significant increased relative risk of 2.1 (95% CI = 0.3–14.1) for male breast cancer incidence.

References

1. Verkasalo PK, Kaprio J, Koskenvuo M, Pukkala E. Genetic predisposition, environment and cancer incidence: a nationwide twin study in Finland, 1976–1995. Int J Cancer 1999; 83:743–9.
2. Caplan LS, Coughlin SS. Worksite breast cancer screening programs: a review. AAOHN J 1998; 46:443–53.
3. Myers R, Vernon SW, Carpenter AV, et al. Employee response to a company sponsored program of colorectal and prostate cancer screening. Cancer Detect Prev 1997; 2:380–9.
4. Cheek AO, Vonier PM, Oberdoster E, Burow BC, McLachlan JA. Environmental signaling: a biologic context for endocrine disruption. Environ Health Perspect 1998; 106:5–8.
5. Crisp TM. Environmental endocrine disruption: an effects assessment and analysis. Environ Health Perspect 1998; 106:11–55.
6. Smith AG. Chlorinated hydrocarbon insecticides. In: Haynes W, Laws E, eds. Handbook of pesticide toxicology. San Diego: Academic Press Inc., 1991; 743–81.
7. Robinson AK, Sirbasku DA, Stancel GM. DDT supports the growth of an estrogen- responsive tumor. Toxicol Lett 1985; 27:109–13.
8. Robinson AK, Stancel GM. The estrogenic activity of DDT: correlation of estrogenic effect with nuclear level of estrogen receptor. Life Sci 1982; 31:2479–84.
9. Bustos SC, Diaz F, Tchernitchin AN. P,p'-DDT is an estrogenic compound. Bull Environ Contam Toxicol 1988; 41:496–501.
10. Kelce WR, Stone CR, Laws SC, Gray LE, Kemppainen JA, Wilson EM. Persistent DDT metabolite p,p'-DDE is a potent androgen receptor antagonist. Nature 1995; 375:581–5.
11. Cooper K. Effects of pesticides on wildlife. In: Hayes W, Laws E, eds. Handbook of pesticide toxicology. San Diego: Academic Press, 1991;463–96.
12. Simonich S, Hites R. Global distribution of persistent organochlorine compounds. Science 1995; 269:1851–4.
13. Wolff MS, Toniolo PG, Lee EW, Rivera M, Dubin N. Blood levels of organochlorine residues and risk of breast cancer. J Natl Cancer Inst 1993; 85:648–52.
14. Wolff MS, Collman GW, Barrett JC, Huff J. Breast cancer and environmental risk factors: epidemiologic and experimental findings. Ann Rev Pharm Tox 1996; 36:573–96.
15. Schottenfeld D, Fraumeni JF, eds. Cancer epidemiology and prevention. New York: Oxford University Press, 1996.
16. Ramazzini B. Diseases of workers. The Latin text of 1713. Wright WC, trans. New York: Hafner, 1964.
17. Milham S. Occupational mortality in Washington State 1950–1979. NIOSH Publication #83-116. Washington, DC: US Dept of Health and Human Services, 1983.
18. van Loon AJM, Burg J, Goldbohm RA, van den Brandt PA. Differences in cancer incidence and mortality among socioeconomic groups. Scand J Soc Med 1995; 2:110–20.
19. King AS, Threlfall WJ, Band PR, Gallagher RP. Mortality among female registered nurses and school teachers in British Columbia. Am J Ind Med 1994; 26;125–32.

20. Rix BA, Skov T, Lynge E. Socioeconomic group, occupation and incidence of breast and genital cancer among women in Denmark. Eur J Pub Health 1997; 7:177–81.

21. Morton WE. Major differences in breast cancer risks among occupations. J Occup Environ Med 1995; 37:328–35.

22. Pollan M, Gustavsson P. High risk occupations for breast cancer in the Swedish female working populations. Am J Pub Health 1999; 89:875–81.

23. Coogan PF, Clapp RW, Newcomb PA, et al. Variation in female breast cancer risk by occupation. Am J Ind Med 1996; 30:430–7.

24. Gunnarsdottir H, Rafnsson V. Cancer incidence among Icelandic nurses. J Occup Environ Med 1995; 37:307–12.

25. Threlfall WI, Gallagher RP, Spinelli JJ, Band PR. Reproductive variables as possible confounders in occupational studies of breast and ovarian cancer in females. J Occup Med 1985; 27:448–50.

26. Goldberg MS, Labreche F. Occupational risk factors for female breast cancer: a review. Occup Environ Med 1996; 53:145–56.

27. Cantor KP, Stewart PA, Brinton LA, Dosemeci M. Occupational exposures and female breast cancer mortality in the United States. J Occup Environ Med 1995; 37:336–48.

28. Petralia SA, Vena JE, Feudenheim JL, et al. Risk of premenopausal breast cancer in association with occupational exposure to polycyclic aromatic hydrocarbons and benzene. Scand J Work Environ Health 1999; 25:215–21.

29. Aschengrau A, Paulu C, Ozonoff D. Tetrachloroethylene contaminated drinking water and the risk of breast cancer. Environ Health Persp 1998; Supp14:947–53.

30. McGregor DH, Land CE, Choi K, et al. Breast cancer incidence among atomic bomb survivors, Hiroshima and Nagasaki, 1950–1969. J Natl Cancer Inst 1977; 59:799–811.

31. Land CE. Studies of cancer and radiation dose among atomic bomb survivors: the example of breast cancer. JAMA 1995; 274:402–7.

32. Bayerstock KF. UK luminizers survey misrepresented. J Occup Med 1985; 27:613.

33. Stebbings IH, Lucas HF, Stehney AF. Mortality from cancers of major sites in female radium dial workers. Am J Ind Med 1984; 5:4335–59.

34. Adams EE, Braes AM. Breast cancer in female radium dial workers first employed before 1930. J Occup Med 1980; 22:583–7.

35. Pukkala E, Auvinen A, Wahlberg G. Incidence of cancer among Finnish airline cabin attendants, 1967–1992. Br Med J 1995; 311:649–52.

36. Boice ID, Mandel JS, Doody MM. Breast cancer among radiologic technologists. JAMA 1995; 274:394–401.

37. Doody MM, Mandel JS, Boice JD. Employment practices and breast cancer among radiologic technologists. J Occup Environ Med 1995; 37:321–7.

38. Loomis DP, Savitz DA, Ananth CV. Breast cancer mortality among female electrical workers in the United States. J Natl Cancer Inst 1994; 86:921–5.

39. Tynes T, Hanevik M, Andersen A, Vistnes AI, Haldorsen T. Incidence of breast cancer in Norwegian female radio operators. Cancer Causes Control 1996; 7:197–204.

40. Feychting M, Forssen U, Rutqvist LE, Ahlbom A. Magnetic fields and breast cancer in Swedish adults residing near high voltage power lines. Epidemiology 1998; 9:392–7.

41. Land CE. Radiation and breast cancer risk. Prog Clin Biol Res 1997; 396:115–24.

42. Brainard GC, Kavet R, Kheifets LI. The relationship between electromagnetic field and light exposures to melatonin and breast cancer risk: a review of the relevant literature. J Pineal Res 1999; 26:65–100.

43. Hansen J, Olsen JH, Larsen AI. Cancer morbidity among employees in a Danish pharmaceutical plant. Int J Epidemiol 1994; 23:891–8.

44. Hayes WJ, Laws ER. Handbook of pesticide toxicology. San Diego: Academic Press Inc, 1991.

45. Westin JB, Richter E. The Israeli breast cancer anomaly. Ann NY Acad Sci 1990; 609:269–79.

46. Dewailly E, Ayotte P, Brisson J. Protective effect of breast feeding on breast cancer and body burden of carcinogenic organochlorines [Letter]. J Natl Cancer Inst 1994; 86:1255.

47. Levine RS, Dolin P. Pregnancy and breast cancer: a possible explanation for the negative association. Med Hypoth 1992; 38:276–83.

48. Wasserman M, Nogueira DP, Tomatis L, et al. Organochlorine compounds in neoplastic and adjacent apparently normal breast tissue. Bull Environ Contam Toxicol 1976; 15:478–84.

49. Unger M, Klaer H, Blichert-Toft M, Olsen J, Clausen J. Organochlorine compounds in human breast fat from deceased with and without breast cancer and in biopsy material from newly diagnosed patients undergoing breast surgery. Environ Res 1984; 34:24–8.

50. Falck F, Ricci A, Wolff MS, Godbold J, Deckers P. Pesticides and polychlorinated biphenyl residues in human breast lipids and their relationship to breast cancer. Arch Environ Health 1992; 47:143–6.

51. Zheng T, Holford TR, Mayne TR, et al. DDE and DDT in breast adipose tissue and risk of female breast cancer. Am J Epidemiol 1999; 150:453–8.

52. Wolff MS, Dubin N, Toniolo PG. Response [Letter]. J Natl Cancer Inst 1993; 85:1873–5.

53. Kreiger N, Wolff MS, Hiatt RA, Rivera M, Vogelman J, Orentreich N. Breast cancer and serum organochlorines: a prospective study among white, black and Asian women. J Natl Cancer Inst 1994; 86:589–99.

54. Wesseling C, Antich D, Hogstedt C, Rodriguez AC, Ahlbom A. Geographical differences of cancer incidence in Costa Rica in relation to environmental and occupational pesticide exposure. Int J Epidemiol 1999; 28:365–74.

55. Schecter A, Toniolo P, Dai LC, et al. Blood levels of DDT and breast cancer risk among women living in the north of Vietnam. Arch Env Contam Tox 1997; 33:453–6.

56. Dich J, Zahm SJ, Hanberg A, Adami H-O. Pesticides and cancer. Cancer Causes Control 1997; 8:420–43.

57. Adami H-O, Lipworth L, Titus-Emstoff L, et al. Organochlorine compounds and estrogen-related cancers in women. Cancer Causes Control 1995; 6:551–66.

58. Ahlborg UG, Lipworth L, Titus-Enstoff L, et al. Organochlorine compounds in relation to breast cancer, endometrial cancer, and endometriosis: an assessment of the biologic and epidemiologic evidence. Crit Rev Toxicol 1995; 25:463–531.

59. Fleming LE, Bean JA, Rudolph M, Hamilton K. Cancer incidence in Florida pesticide applicators. J Occup Environ Med 1999; 41:279–88.

60. Fleming LE, Bean JA, Rudolph M, Hamilton K. Mortality in Florida pesticide applicators. J Occup Environ Med 1999; 56:14–21.

61. Wiklund K, Dich J. Cancer risks among female farmers in Sweden. Cancer Causes Control 1994; 5:449–57.

62. Davidson NE. Environmental estrogens and breast cancer risk. Curr Opin Oncol 1998; 10:475–8.

63. Clemmesen J. Epidemiological studies into the possible carcinogenicity of hair dyes. Mutat Res 1981; 87:65–79.

64. Nasca PC, Lawrence CE, Greenwald P, et al. Relationship of hair dye use, benign breast disease and breast cancer. J Natl Cancer Inst 1980; 64:23–8.

65. Teta MI, Walrath J, Meigs JW, Flannery IT. Cancer incidence among cosmetologists. J Natl Cancer Inst 1984; 72:1051–7.

66. Shannon HS, Haines T, Bemholz C, et al. Cancer morbidity in lamp manufacturing workers. Am J Ind Med 1988; 14:281–90.

67. Jarvholm B, Lavenius B. A cohort study on cancer among workers exposed to an anti-rust oil. Scand J Work Environ Health 1981; 7:179–84.

68. Norman SA, Berlin JA, Soper KA, Middendorf BF, Stolley PD. Cancer incidence in a group of workers potentially exposed to ethylene oxide. Int J Epidemiol 1995; 24:276–84.

69. Sala-Serra M, Sunyer J, Kogevinas M, McFarlane D, Anto JM. Cohort study on cancer mortality among workers in pulp and paper industry in Catalonia, Spain. Am J Ind Med 1996; 30:87–92.

70. Shen N, Weiderpass E, Anttila A, et al. Epidemiology of occupational and environmental risk factors related to ovarian cancer. Scand J Work Environ Health 1998; 24:175–82.

71. Sala M, Dosemeci M, Zahm SR. A death certificate based study of occupation and mortality from reproductive cancers among women in 24 US states. J Occup Environ Med 1998; 40:632–9.

72. Vasama-Neuvonen K, Pukkala E, Paakkulainen H, et al. Ovarian cancer and occupational exposures in Finland. Am J Ind Med 1999; 36;83–9.

73. Doll R, Smith PG. The long-term effects of X-irradiation in patients treated for metropathia haemorrhagica. Br J Radiol 1968; 41:362–8.

74. Beebe GW, Kato H, Land CE. Mortality experience of atomic bomb burvivors, 1950–1974. Life Span Study, Report 8. Radiation Effects Research Foundation TRI-77, 1977.

75. Heller DS, Gordon RE, WesthoffC, Gerber S. Asbestos exposure and ovarian fiber burden. Am J Ind Med 1996; 29:435–9.

76. Acheson ED, Gardner MI. Pippard EC, Grime LP. Mortality of two groups of women who manufactured gas masks from chrysotile and crocidolite asbestos: a 40-year follow-up. Br J Ind Med 1982; 39:344–8

77. Newhouse ML, Berry G, Wagner JC, Turok ME. A study of the mortality of female asbestos workers. Br J Ind Med 1972; 29:134–41.

78. Wignall BK, Fox AJ. Mortality of female gas mask assemblers. Br J Ind Med 1982; 39:34–8.

79. Walrath J. Cancer incidence among cosmetologists. A dissertation presented to the faculty of the Graduate School of Yale University, 1977.

80. Spinelli JJ, Gallagher RP, Band PR, Threlfall WI. Multiple myeloma, leukemia and cancer of the ovary in cosmetologists and hairdressers. Am J Ind Med 1984; 6:97–102.

81. Boffeta PK, Andersen A, Lynge E, Barlow L, Pukkula E. Employment as hairdresser and risk of ovarian cancer and non-Hodgkins lymphomas among women. J Occup Med 1994; 36:61–5.

82. National Institute for Occupational Safety and Health. A retrospective survey of cancer in relation to occupation. PHS Publication #77 178. Washington, DC: US Government Printing Office, 1977.

83. Langseth H, Andersen A. Cancer incidence among women in the Norwegian pulp and paper industry. Am J Ind Med 1999; 36:108–13.

84. Bulbulyan MA, Ilychova SA, Zahm SH, Astashevsky SV, Zaridze DG. Cancer mortality among women in the Russian printing industry. Am J Ind Med 1999; 36:166–71.

85. Morgan RW, Kelsh MA, Zhao K, Heringer S. Mortality of aerospace workers exposed to trichloroethylene. Epidemiology 1998; 9:424–31.

86. Dich J, Zahm SI, Hanberg A, Adami H-O. Pesticides and cancer. Cancer Causes Control 1997; 8:420–43.

87. Dalager NA, Kang HK, Thomas TL. Cancer mortality patterns among women who served in the military: the Vietnam experience. J Occu Environ Med 1995; 37:298–305.

88. Dich J, Zahm SI, Hanberg A, Adami H-O. Pesticides and cancer. Cancer Causes Control 1997; 8:420–43.

89. Hennekens C, Speizer FE, Rosner B, et al. Use of permanent hair dyes and cancer among registered nurses. Lancet 1979; i:1390–3.

90. Floderus B, Stenlund C, Persson T. Occupational magnetic field exposure and site specific cancer incidence: a Swedish cohort study. Cancer Causes Control 1999; 10:323–32.

91. Bosch FX, Munoz N, de San Jose S. Risk factors for cervical cancer in Colombia and Spain. Int J Cancer 1009; 52:750–8.

92. Zakelj MP, Fraser P, Hazel L Cervical cancer and husband's occupation. Lancet 1984; i:510.

93. Alterman T, Burnett C, Peipins L, Lalich N, Halperin W. Occupational and cervical cancer: an opportunity for prevention. J Womens Health 1997; 6:649–57.

94. Gibbs GW, Amsel J, Soden K. A cohort mortality study of cellulose triacetate fiber workers exposed to methylene chloride. J Occu Environ Med 1996; 38:693–7.

95. Wesseling C, Ahlbom A, Antich D, et al. Cancer in banana plantation workers in Costa Rica. Int J Epidemiol 1996; 25:1125–31.

96. Blair A, Dosemeci M, Heineman EF. Cancer and other causes of death among male and female farmers from 23 states. Am J Ind Med 1993; 23:729–42.

97. Dich J, Zahm SI, Hanberg A, Adami H-O. Pesticides and cancer. Cancer Causes Control 1997; 8:420–43.

98. Kjaerheim K, Andersen A. Cancer incidence among waitresses in Norway. Cancer Causes Control 1994; 5:31–7.

99. Savitz DA, Andrews KW, Brinton LA. Occupation and cervical cancer. J Occu Environ Med 1995; 37:357–61.

100. Palmer JR. Advances in the epidemiology of gestational trophoblastic disease. J Reprod Med 1994; 39:155–62.

101. Ha MC, Cordier S, Bard D, et al. Agent Orange and the risk of gestational trophoblastic disease in Vietnam. Arch Environ Health 1996; 51:368–74.

102. Yuasa S. Association between hydatidiform mole and occupational groups of Japanese women. Jikeikai Med 1979; 26;153–7.

103. Boyle P, Zaridze DG. Risk factors for prostate and testicular cancer. Eur J Cancer 1993; 29A:1048–55.

104. Swerdlow AJ, Douglas AJ, Huttly SR, Smith PG. Cancer of the testis, socioeconomic status and occupation. Br J Ind Med 1991; 48:670–4.

105. Newell GR, Mills PK, Johnson DE. Epidemiologic comparison of cancer of the testis and Hodgkin's disease among young males. Cancer 1984; 54:1117–23.

106. McDowall ME, Balarajan R. Testicular cancer mortality in England and Wales 1971–1980: variations by occupation. J Epidemiol Commun Health 1986; 40:26–9.

107. Milham S. Neoplasia in the wood and pulp industry. Ann NY Acad Sci 1976; 271:294–300.

108. Knight JA, Marrett LD. Parental occupational exposure and the risk of testicular cancer in Ontario. JOEM 1997; 39:333–8.

109. Beral V, Inskip H, Fraser P, et al. Mortality of employees of the United Kingdom Atomic Energy Authority, 1946–1979. Br Med J 1985; 291:44.

110. Stenlund C, Floderus B. Occupational exposure to magnetic fields in relation to male breast cancer and testicular cancer: a Swedish case-control study. Cancer Causes Control 1997; 8:184–91.

111. Floderus B, Stenlund C, Persson T. Occupational magnetic field exposure and site specific cancer incidence: a Swedish cohort study. Cancer Causes Control 1999; 10:323–32.

112. Zhang ZF, Vena JE, Zielezny M, et al. Occupational exposure to extreme temperature and risk of testicular cancer. Arch Environ Health 1995; 50:13–18.

113. Hobbesland A, Kjuus H, Thelle DS. Study of cancer incidence among 8530 male workers in 8 Norwegian plants producing ferrosilicon and silicon metals. Occup Environ Med 1999; 56:625–31.

114. Rhomberg W, Schmoll HJ, Schneider B. High frequency of metal workers among patients with seminomatous tumors of the testis: a case-control study. Am J Ind Med 1995; 28:79–87.

115. Toppari J, Larsen JC, Christiansen P, et al. Male reproductive health and environmental xenoestrogens. Environ Health Perspect 1996; 104(supp14):741–823.

116. Towbly R. Assault on the male. Environ Health Perspect 1995; 103:802–5.

117. Yager JD, Liehr JG. Molecular mechanisms of estrogen carcinogenesis. Ann Rev Pharm Toxicol 1996; 36:203–32.

118. Santti R, Newbold RR, Makela S, Pylkkanen L, McLachlan JA. Developmental estrogenization and prostatic neoplasia. Prostate 1994; 24:67–78.

119. Carlsen E, Giwercman A, Keiding N, Skakkebaek NE. Evidence for decreasing quality of semen during past 50 years. Br J Med 1992; 305:609–13.

120. Wright L. Silent sperm. New Yorker, January 15, 1996.

121. Schettler T, Solomon G, Bums P, Valenti M. Generations at risk: how environmental toxins may affect reproductive health in Massachusetts. Cambridge: Greater Boston Physicians for Social Responsibility, 1996.

122. Strohmer H, Bo1dizsar A, Plockinger B, Geldner-Busztin M, Feichtinger W. Agricultural work and male infertility. Am J Ind Med 1993; 24:587–92.

123. Skakkebaek NE, Rajpert de Meyts E, Jorgensen N, et al. Germ cell cancer and disorders of spermatogenesis: an environmental connection? APMIS 1998; 106:3–11.

124. Jensen TK, Toppari J, Keiding N, Skakkebaek NE. Do environmental estrogens contribute to the decline in male reproductive health? Clin Chem 1995; 41:1896–901.

125. Giwercman A, Bonde JP. Declining male fertility and environmental factors. Endocrin Metab Clin North Am 1998; 27:807–30.

126. Whorton MD: Health effects of dibromochloropropane. In: Rom WN, ed. Environmental and occupational medicine, 2nd edn. Boston: Little, Brown, 1992; 903–10.

127. Moses M, Johnson ES, Anger WK, et al. Environmental equity and pesticide exposure. Tox Ind Health 1993; 9:913–59.

128. Fleming LE, Herzstein JA. Emerging issues in pesticide health studies. Occup Med State Art Rev 1997; 12:387–97.

129. Mills PK, Newel GR, Johnson DE. Testicular cancer associated with employment in agriculture and oil and natural gas extraction. Lancet 1984; i:207–10.

130. Swerdlow A J, Skeet RG. Occupational associations of testicular cancer in South East England. Br J Ind Med 1988; 45:225–30.

131. Wiklund K, Dich J, Hol L-E. Testicular cancer among agricultural workers and licensed pesticide applicators in Sweden. Scand J Work Environ Health 1986; 12:630–31.

132. Mills PK. Correlation analysis of pesticide use data and cancer incidence rates in California counties. Arch Env Health 1998; 53:410–13.

133. Hardell L, Nasman A, Ohlson CG, Fredrikson M. Case-control study on risk factors for testicular cancer. Int J Oncol 1998; 13:1299–303.

134. Kirstensen P, Andersen A, Irgens LM, Bye AS, Vagstad N. Testicular cancer and parental use of fertilizers in agriculture. Cancer Epiemiol Biomarker Prev 1996; 5:3–9.

135. Ducatman AM, Conwill DE, Crawl C. Germ cell tumors of the testicle among aircraft repairmen. J Urol 1986; 136:834–6.

136. Boice JD, Marano DE, Fryzek JP, Sadler CI, McLaughlin JK. Mortality among aircraft manufacturing workers. Occup Environ Med 1999; 56:581–97.

137. Ryder SI, Crawford PI, Pethybridge RJ. Testicular cancer an occupational disease? A case-control study of Royal Naval personnel. Naval Med Serv 1997; 83:130–46.

138. Frumin E, Brathwaite M, Towne W, et al. Testicular cancer in leather workers – Fulton County, New York. MMWR 1989; 38:105–14.

139. Levine SM, Baker DB, Landrigan PI, et al. Testicular cancer in leather tanners exposed to dimethylformamide. Lancet 1987; ii:1153.

140. Knight JA, Marrett LD, Weir HK. Occupation and risk of germ cell testicular cancers by histologic type in Ontario. J Occu Environ Med 1996; 38:884–90.

141. Guberan E, Use IM, Raymond L, et al. Disability, mortality, and incidence of cancer among Geneva painters and electricians: a historical prospective study. Br J Ind Med 1989; 46:16–23.

142. Garland FC, Gorham ED, Garland CF, Ducatman AM. Testicular cancer in US Navy personnel. Am J Epidemiol 1988; 127:411–14.

143. Chen JL, Fayerweather WE, Pell S. Cancer incidence of workers exposed to dimethylformamide and/or acrylonitrile. J Occup Med 1988; 30:813–8.

144. Chen JL, Kennedy GL. Dimethylformamide and testicular cancer. Lancet 1988; i:55.

145. Ducatman AM, Crawl JR, Conwill DE. Cancer clusters, causation and common sense. Chemtech 1988; 18:204–10.

146. Ducatman AM. Dimethylformamide, metal dyes, and testicular cancer. Lancet 1989; i:911.

147. Karunaharan T. Malignant mesothelioma of the tunica vaginalis in an asbestos worker. J Roy Coll Surg Edin 1986; 31:253–4.

148. Huncharek M, Klassen M, Christiani D. Mesothelioma of the tunica vaginalis testis with possible occupational asbestos exposure. Br J Urol 1995; 75:679–80.

149. Hardell L, Ohlson C-G, Fredrikson M. Occupational exposure to polyvinyl chloride as a risk factor for testicular cancer evaluated in a case-control study. Int J Cancer 1997; 73:828–30.

150. Norman JE, Robinette CD, Franmeni JF. The mortality experience of army World War II chemical processing companies. J Occup Med 1981; 23:818–22.

151. O'Brien TR, Decoufle P. Cancer mortality among Northern Georgia carpet and textile workers. Am J Ind Med 1988; 14:15–24.

152. Brahim F, Levine B, Lemer A. Testicular carcinoma in podiatrists. Curr Pod Med 1988; 37:17–18.

153. Ekman P, Pan Y, Li C, Dich J. Environmental and genetic factors: a possible link with prostatic cancer. Br J Urol 1997; 79(Supp12):35–41.

154. Hanchette C, Schwartz G. Geographic patterns of prostate cancer mortality. Cancer 1992; 70:2861–8.

155. Carter B, Carter H, Isaacs J. Epidemiologic evidence regarding predisposing factors to prostate cancer. Prostate 1990; 16:187–97.

156. Dosemeci M, Hoover RN, Blair A, et al. Farming and prostate cancer among African-Americans in the southeastern United States. J Natl Cancer Inst 1994; 86:1718–9.

157. van der Gulden J, Kolk J, Verbeek A. Work environment and prostate cancer. Prostate 1995; 27:250–7.

158. Dich J, Wiklund K. Prostate cancer in pesticide applicators in Swedish agriculture. Prostate 1998; 34:100–12.

159. Band PR, Le ZD, Fang R, Threlfall WJ, Gallagher RP. Identification of occupational cancer risks in British Columbia. J Occu Environ Med 1999; 41:233–47.

160. Golden AL, Markowitz SB, Landrigan PI. The risk of cancer in firefighters. Occup Med 1995; 10:803–20.

161. Krstev S, Baris D, Stewart P, et al. Risk for prostatic cancer by occupation and industry: a 24 state death certificate study. Am J Ind Med 1998; 34:413–20.

162. Krstev S, Baris D, Stewart P, et al. Occupational risk factors and prostate cancers in US blacks and whites. Am J Ind Med 1998; 34:421–30.

163. van der Gulden JWJ. Metal workers and repairmen at risk for prostate cancer: a review. Prostate 1997; 30:107–16.

164. Friedman L. Commentary on case-control study of prostatic cancer in employees of the United Kingdom Atomic Energy Authority. ONS Nursing Scan Onc 1994; 3:14.

165. Checkoway H, Matthew RM, Wolf SH, et al. Mortality among workers at the Oak Ridge National Laboratory. In: Proceedings of the 16th Midyear Topical Meeting of the Health Physics Society, 1983; 90–104.

166. Gilbert ES, Marks S. An analysis of the mortality of workers in a nuclear facility. Radiat Res 1979; 79:122–48.

167. Ritz B. Cancer mortality among workers exposed to chemicals during uranium processing. J Occu Environ Med 1999; 41:556–66.

168. Waalkes MPH, Rehm S. Cadmium and prostate cancer. J Tox Env Health 1994; 43:251–69.

169. Potts CL. Cadmium proteinuria – the health of battery workers exposed to cadmium oxide dust. Ann Occup Hyg 1967; 8:55–61.

170. Holden H. Further mortality studies in workers exposed to cadmium. In: Occupational exposure to cadmium. London: Cadmium Association, 1980; 23–4.

171. Kipling MD, Waterhouse JAH. Cadmium and prostatic carcinoma. Lancet 1967; i:730–1.

172. Lemen RA, Lee JS, Wagoner JK, et al. Cancer mortality among cadmium production workers. Ann NY Acad Sci 1976; 271:273–9.

173. Kolonel L, Winkelstein W. Cadmium and prostate cancer. Lancet 1977; ii:566–7.

174. Ross RK, McCurtis JW, Henderson BE, et al. Descriptive epidemiology of testicular and prostatic cancer in Los Angeles. Br J Cancer 1979; 39:284–92.

175. Piscator M. Role of cadmium in carcinogenesis with special reference to cancer of the prostate. Environ Health Perspect 1981; 40:107–20.

176. Thun MJ, Schnorr TM, Smith AB, et al. Mortality among a cohort of US cadmium production workers – an update. J Natl Cancer Inst 1985; 74:325–33.

177. Axelsson G, Rylander R, Schmidt A. Mortality and tumor incidence among ferrochromium workers. Br J Ind Med 1980; 37:121–7.

178. Langard S, Anderson A, Gylseth B. Incidence of cancer among ferrochromium and ferrosilicon workers. Br J Ind Med 1980; 37:114–20.

179. Costantino JP, Redmond CK, Bearden A. Occupationally related cancer risk among coke oven workers: 30 years of follow up. J Occu Environ Med 1995; 37:597–604.

180. Demers PA, Checkoway H, Vaughn TL, Weiss NS, Heyer NJ, Rosenstock L. Cancer incidence among firefighters in Seattle and Tacoma, Washington, US. Cancer Causes Control 1994; 5:129–35.

181. van der Gulden JWJ, Vogelzang PFJ. Farmers at risk for prostate cancer. Br J Urol 1996; 77:6–14.

182. Council on Scientific Affairs. Cancer risk of pesticides in agricultural workers. JAMA 1988; 260:959–66.

183. Maroni M, Fait A. Health effects in man from long term exposure to pesticides. Toxicology 1993; 78:1–180.

184. Dich J, Zahm SI, Hanberg A, Adami H-O. Pesticides and cancer. Cancer Causes Control 1997; 8:420–43.

185. Morales Suarez Varela MM, Llopis Gonzalez A, Tejerizo Perez ML. Impact of nitrates in drinking water on cancer mortality in Valencia, Spain. Eur J Epidemiol 1995; 11:15–21.

186. Alberghini V, Luberto F, Gobba F, Morelli C, Gori E, Tomesani N. Mortality among male farmers licensed to use pesticides. Med Lav 1991; 82:18–24.

187. Aronson KJ, Siemiatycki J, Dewar R, Gerin M. Occupational risk factors for prostate cancer: results from a case-control study in Montreal, Quebec, Canada. Am J Epidemiol 1996; 143:363–73.

188. Checkoway H, DiFerdinando G, Hulka BS, Mickey DD. Medical, life-style and occupational risk factors for prostate cancer. Prostate 1987; 10:79–88.

189. Parker AS, Cerhan J, Putnam S, Cantor K, Lynch C. A cohort study of farming and risk of prostate cancer in Iowa. Epidemiology 1999; 10:452–55.

190. Keller-Byrne JE, Khuder SA, Schaub EA. Meta-analysis of prostate cancer and farming. Am J Ind Med 1997; 31:580–6.

191. Acquavella J, Olsen G. Cancer among farmers: a meta-analysis. Ann Epidemiol 1998; 8:64–74.

192. Acquavella JF. Farming and prostate cancer. Epidemiology 1999; 10:452–4.

193. Cantor K, Silberman W. Mortality among aerial pesticide applicators and flight instructors: follow-up from 1965–1988. Am J Ind Med 1999; 36:239–47.

194. Kross BC, Burmeister LF, Ogilvie LK, Fuortes LJ, Fu CM. Proportionate mortality study of golf course superintendents. Am J Ind Med 1996; 29:501–6.

195. Heitzman RJ. Butchers and prostate cancer. Lancet 1987; i:453.

196. Lloyd MM, Lyster WR, Lloyd OL. Birth sex ratios and prostatic cancer in butchers. Lancet 1987; i:561.

197. James WH. Prostatic cancer, butchers and androgens. Lancet 1987; i:216–7.

198. Johnson ES. Prostate cancer and androgens. Lancet 1987; i:814.

199. Olin RG. The hazards of a chemical laboratory environment. A study of the mortality of two cohorts. Am Ind Hyg Assoc J 1978; 39:557–62.

200. Chen JL, Fayerweather WE, Pell S. Cancer incidence of workers exposed to dimethylformamide and/or acrylonitrile. J Occup Med 1988; 30:813–8.

201. Chen JL, Kennedy GL. Dimethylformamide and testicular cancer. Lancet 1988; i:55.

202. O'Berg MT, Chen JL, Burke CA, et al. Epidemiologic study of workers exposed to actylonitrile: an update. J Occup Med 1985; 27:835–40.

203. Whorton MD, Amsel J, Mandel J. Cohort mortality study of prostate cancer among chemical workers. Am J Ind Med 1998; 33:293–6.

204. Hoar SK, Blair A. Death certificate case-control study of cancers of the prostate and colon and employment in the textile industry. Arch Environ Health 1984; 39:280–3.

205. Goldsmith DF, Smith AH, McMichael A. A case-control study of prostate cancer within a cohort of rubber and tire workers. J Occup Med 1980; 22:533–41.

206. McMichael AJ, Andelkovic DA, Tyroler HA. Cancer mortality among rubber workers: an epidemiologic study. Ann NY Acad Sci 1976; 271:125–37.

207. Williams RR, Stegens NL, Goldsmith JR. Associations of cancer site and type with occupation and industry from the Third National Cancer Survey Interview. J Natl Cancer Inst 1977; 59:1147–85.

208. Bernadinelli L, De Marco R, Tinelii C. Cancer mortality in an Italian rubber factory. Br J Ind Med 1987; 44:187–91.

209. Straif K, Weiland SK, Werner B, Chambless L, Mundt KA, Keil U. Workplace risk factors for cancer in the German rubber industry. Occup Environ Med 1998; 55:325–32.

210. Stewart RE, Dennis LK, Dawson DV, Resnick MI. A meta-analysis of risk estimates for prostate cancer related to tire and rubber manufacturing operations. J Occu Environ Med 1999; 41:1079–84.

211. Mabuchi K, Bross DS, Kessler H. Risk factors for male breast cancer. J Natl Cancer Inst 1985; 74:371–5.

212. McLaughlin JK, Malker HRS, Blot WJ, et al. Occupational risks for male breast cancer in Sweden. Br J Ind Med 1988; 45:275–6.

213. Cocco P, Figgs L, Dosemeci M, Hayes R, Linet MS, Hsing AW. Case-control study of occupational exposures and male breast cancer. Occup Environ Med 1998; 55:599–604.

214. Hansen I. Elevated risk for male breast cancer after occupational exposure to gasoline and vehicular combustion products. Am J Ind Med 2000; 37:349–52.

215. Robinson CE, Petersen M, Sieber WK, Palu S, Halperin WE. Mortality of Carpenters' Union members in the US construction or wood products industries, 1987–1990. Am J Ind Med 1996; 30:674–94.

216. Forastiere F, Perucci CA, di Pietro A, et al. Mortality among urban policemen in Rome. Am J Ind Med 1994; 26:785–98.

217. Tynes T, Andersen A. Electromagnetic fields and male breast cancer [Letter]. Lancet 1990; ii:1596.

218. Demers P A, Thomas DB, Rosenblatt KA, et al. Occupational exposure to electromagnetic fields and breast cancer in men. Am J Epidemiol 1991; 134:340–7.

219. Rosenbaum PF, Vena JE, Zielezny MA, Michalek AM. Occupational exposures associated with male breast cancer. Am J Epidemiol 1994; 139:30–6.

220. Feychting M, Forssen U, Rutqvist LE, Ahlbom A. Magnetic fields and breast cancer in Swedish adults residing near high voltage power lines. Epidemiology 1998; 9:392–7.

221. Pearce NE, Sheppard RA, Fraser J. Case-control study of occupation and cancer of the prostate in New Zealand. J Epidemiol Commun Health 1987; 41:130–2.

222. Cerhan JR, Cantor KP, Williamson K, Lynch CF, Torner JC, Burmeister LF. Cancer mortality among Iowa farmers: recent results, time trends, and lifestyle factors (US). Cancer Causes Control 1998; 9:311–9.

30.8 **Brain Neoplasms**
Paul A Demers

In this chapter the classification, occurrence, and suspected occupational and environmental causes of intracranial neoplasms are discussed. Although even a benign tumor occurring in the enclosed space within the skull may eventually prove fatal if untreated, this chapter is concerned primarily with malignant brain tumors. Malignant tumors identified in epidemiologic studies and case series have often been found to be gliomas of the astrocytic series and, in particular, glioblastoma multiforme. However, most studies have not had the ability to differentiate between brain tumors of different histologies so that common non-malignant neoplasms, such as meningiomas, also are discussed. Extracranial nervous system tumors are not considered in this chapter because they are both extremely rare and have, in general, not been associated with occupational or environmental agents. Although the brain is a frequent site of metastasis, most commonly from the lung or breast, tumors whose origin is outside the brain also are not considered in this chapter.

CLASSIFICATION

Nervous system tumors are primarily classified according to the presumed cell type of origin. Table 30.8.1 presents the most common brain tumor histologic types. Gliomas are the most common malignant brain tumor. The majority of gliomas belong to the astrocytic series, of which grades 1 and 2 are referred to as astrocytoma, whereas grades 3 and 4 are referred to as malignant astrocytoma or glioblastoma multiforme. Lymphomas also may arise within the brain and are sometimes referred to as microgliomas. Meningiomas are the second most common brain tumor (after gliomas) and the most common non-malignant tumor. Nerve sheath tumors, also referred to as neuromas, are usually benign.

DESCRIPTIVE EPIDEMIOLOGY

The age-adjusted incidence rate for brain neoplasms in the United States is 7.0 per 100,000 people for men and 5.0 for women.[1] The corresponding mortality rates are 5.1 and 3.5, respectively. Although the incidence varies somewhat by country, Western Europe and Canada have rates similar to that of the United States, while Japan and some Asian countries have lower rates.[2] In the United States, the risk of brain cancer is higher among whites than blacks, Asians, and other racial groups.[1] In the US all women and African-American men appear to have lower rates of gliomas and higher risk of meningioma than white men.[3] The reason for the gender and racial differences is not known. A higher risk of brain tumors among men relative to women also has been observed in a number of other countries.[2]

Among adults, brain cancer incidence peaks between the ages of 65 and 75.[1] Brain cancer is the second most common malignancy in children (after leukemia). Approximately a fifth of both incident and fatal childhood cancers arise in the brain, and some histologic types occur almost exclusively in children. For example, medulloblastomas (primitive neuroectodermal tumors) account for almost a quarter of brain tumors among children but less than 2% of brain tumors among adults.

Five-year survival from brain cancer has improved in recent years and is approximately 30% for all malignant brain and central nervous system neoplasms in the US.[1] Survival is primarily determined by the histology of the tumor and the age at diagnosis rather than stage at diagnosis. Only 2% of persons diagnosed with glioblastoma multiforme survive 5 years, with younger individuals having a better prognosis.[3] Brain neoplasms may metastasize to other sites within the brain but rarely metastasize outside the central nervous system. However, the brain is a relatively common target of metastasis from other sites, such as the lung and breast.

The etiology of brain neoplasms is poorly understood. Although some genetic factors are suspected, only a small percentage of brain tumors are currently believed to be due to inherited factors. Head injuries, exposure to x-rays, and viruses are suspected of causing brain tumors, whereas intracranial lymphomas have been associated with immunosuppression.[3] Brain cancer rates have been rising in many industrialized countries in recent decades.[4] The increase has been observed primarily among individuals over 65 and has occurred in both males and females. It is unclear whether the increasing rates are due to changes in diagnostic practices or reporting procedures alone, or whether the true incidence is rising.

ENVIRONMENTAL AND OCCUPATIONAL CAUSES

The higher incidence of brain neoplasms observed in men relative to women, as well as the positive results of animal studies of chemical agents, have raised the suspicion that environmental exposures, possibly of occupational origin, may increase the risk of brain cancer. Based on the results of experimental studies using rodents, many occupational and environmental exposures are suspected of increasing the risk of brain neoplasms. In addition, epidemiologic studies have identified a wide range of occupations and industries with a higher risk for brain neoplasms than the general population, often without implicating any specific exposures. However, the results of many of these studies have been inconsistent and there are no occupational or environmental exposures widely accepted as causing brain neoplasms.

EXPERIMENTAL STUDIES OF ANIMALS

Animal experimentation with carcinogens has not always been useful in predicting the target organ for carcinogenesis in humans. However, in the case of brain neoplasms atten-

| Gliomas |
| Glioblastoma multiforme |
| Astrocytoma |
| Primitive neuroectodermal tumors |
| Oligodendroglioma |
| Ependymoma |
| Pineal tumors |
| Lymphoma |
| Meningeal tumors |
| Meningiomas |
| Meningeal sarcomas |
| Nerve sheath tumors |
| Acoustic neuromas |
| Pituitary tumors |

Table 30.8.1 Histologic classification of common primary brain tumors

| Vinyl chloride |
| Acrylinotrile |
| N-nitroso compounds |
| Inorganic lead |
| Diethyl and dimethyl sulfate |
| Ethylene oxide |
| 2-methylaziridine (propyleneimine) |
| 1,3-propane sultone |
| 7,12-dimethylbenz[a]anthrazene |

Table 30.8.2 Agents found to produce brain tumors in animals after systemic exposure

| Chemicals |
| Vinyl chloride |
| Formaldehyde |
| Solvents |
| Inorganic lead |
| Physical agents |
| Ionizing radiation |
| Electromagnetic fields |
| Occupations |
| Agricultural workers |
| Firefighters |
| Industries |
| Petroleum refining |
| Petrochemical production |
| Synthetic rubber production |
| Nuclear fuels and weapons fabrication |

Table 30.8.3 Chemicals, physical agents, occupations, and industries suspected of increasing the risk of brain cancer

tion has focused on animal studies in the hope of identifying the agent or agents responsible for the excess risks observed among workers exposed to multiple chemicals, such as in the petrochemical and rubber industries. The basis for such anticipation is that humans share common mechanisms with other mammals for excluding many foreign substances from the central nervous system. A large number of agents that can produce brain neoplasms under experimental conditions have been identified. These belong to a wide variety of families and include nitrosoureas, triazenes, hydrazines, and various polycyclic aromatic hydrocarbons.[5] In addition, there is evidence that lead acetate and subacetate may cause gliomas in rats. Although early experiments used direct implantation of chemicals into the intracranial space, later studies used systemic administration, which may be more relevant for assessing occupational or environmental risks. Agents that have produced brain tumors in animals after inhalation, ingestion, or exposure through the placenta are listed in Table 30.8.2.

Generally, there is insufficient epidemiologic evidence to either support or refute an association between these chemicals and brain cancer in humans. However, we have learned from animal experiments that the tissues of the central nervous system are susceptible to chemical carcinogens and that, despite the protection afforded by the blood–brain barrier, chemical agents that have been introduced via inhalation and ingestion have been able to produce intracranial tumors.

EPIDEMIOLOGIC STUDIES

Despite the availability of data from a large number of epidemiologic studies, the relationship between brain neoplasms and occupational and environmental exposures has not been clearly defined. There are a number of reasons why this is true. First, because of the rarity of brain cancer, most studies of occupational groups have lacked the statistical power to detect excesses, whereas those with a sufficient number of cases, such as case control or very large cohort studies, have typically lacked relevant exposure information. Second, many studies have historically relied on death certificates, which often lack the histologic type and also may not specify whether the brain tumor was malignant or benign. There is evidence that brain

cancers of different histologic types have different risk factors and, thus, the combination of all histologies could obscure existing associations. Last, some studies have found the incidence of brain cancer to be positively associated with higher socioeconomic status.[3] Whether this association is due to the fact that these individuals have a greater likelihood of diagnosis or autopsy or whether the actual risk of disease is different is not known, but socioeconomic status may be a potential confounding factor in some studies. Table 30.8.3 lists chemicals, physical agents, occupations, and industries reported to be associated with an increased risk of brain cancer in humans. However, in all cases there are conflicting studies, making it difficult to draw conclusions regarding causal relationships.

AGENTS AND OCCUPATIONS ASSOCIATED WITH NEOPLASMS
Vinyl chloride

In 1976, Maltoni reported on a relationship between inhalation of vinyl chloride and brain tumors in rats.[6] Around the same time, epidemiologic studies found an excess risk of brain cancer in exposed workers.[7,8] In general, the relative risks observed in these studies ranged from 1.5 to 2.5.[9] Among the few studies that have collected histologic information, a large proportion of the brain tumors were found to be glioblastoma multiforme. It is important to note that not all investigators have found an association. For example, a large collaborative study conducted by the International Agency for Research on Cancer did not find a strong association between brain neoplasms and exposure to vinyl chloride, and an update of one of the original cohorts observed only a small excess that was not associated with exposure.[10,11]

Formaldehyde

High rates of brain neoplasms have been seen in professional occupations potentially exposed to formaldehyde, such as embalmers, pathologists, morticians, and anatomists.[12] However, most studies of industrially exposed workers have not found an elevated risk.[12,13] Socioeconomic status has been suggested as a possible confounder, although one analysis that compared anatomists to psychiatrists, an occupational group with similar social and economic status, still found an elevated risk among anatomists.[14]

Inorganic lead

Several epidemiologic studies have observed an association between the risk of brain cancer and occupational exposure to lead. Antilla and colleagues found an excess risk of glioma among a large cohort of Finnish workers biologically monitored for blood lead.[15] An excess associated with both elevated blood lead and duration of lead exposure was observed. Cocco and colleagues found an association between brain cancer and intensity of lead exposure in a death certificate study using a job exposure matrix.[16] However, excesses have not been observed in most other studies of workers in lead exposed industries.[17] The studies which have observed an association have been given greater attention because the central nervous system is the target organ for other toxic effects of lead and because some lead salts have been found to be carcinogenic to animals.[5]

Organic solvents

Thomas and Waxweiler have suggested that organic solvents be considered as possible brain carcinogens because they are exposures that are held in common by several of the occupational groups identified as being at higher risk.[18] Heineman and colleagues observed an association between the risk of astrocytic brain cancers and exposure to methylene chloride, carbon tetrachloride, tetrachloroethylene, and trichloroethylene assessed through a job exposure matrix.[19] Rodvall and colleagues observed an excess risk associated with exposure to solvents, degreasers, and cleaning agents in a Swedish case-control study of gliomas.[20] Some studies of childhood cancer have observed an association between brain cancer and paternal exposure to paints.[21] However, evidence for an association between hydrocarbon exposure and childhood cancers appears to be less consistent.

Ionizing radiation

Exposure to ionizing radiation frequently has been reported to increase the risk of brain neoplasms. Studies of individuals who received scalp irradiation or full-mouth dental x-ray studies as children have found a higher risk of brain tumors.[3] Airline pilots, who are exposed to cosmic radiation during high altitude flights, have also been observed to be at an increased risk of brain cancer.[22] High rates of brain neoplasms also have been observed among workers at plants producing nuclear fuels or weapons in some studies.[23] Histology was reported for two of these studies, and gliomas were the predominant type observed. It is important to note that no association with radiation exposure was found in the nuclear industry studies, and it is unclear whether radioactive materials or some other exposure common to the plants is responsible.

Electromagnetic fields

A potential association between occupational exposure to electromagnetic fields (EMF) and brain neoplasms was first reported by Milham, who found a high rate in men whose usual occupation (from death certificate) involved potential exposure to EMF.[24] An association between employment in these occupations, which include electricians, utility workers, communications workers, welders, and electrical or electronic equipment repairers, technicians, and engineers, has been observed in a number of subsequent studies.[3] More recent studies have attempted to assess quantitative exposure to magnetic fields. The results of these studies have been mixed and the potential for confounding due to chemical or other exposures remains a limitation.[25] A recent meta-analysis of five studies which had used quantitative estimates of magnetic field exposure to estimate dose–response found evidence consistent with a small overall increase in relative risk.[25] Some studies have observed an increased risk of brain cancer among the children of men employed in operations with potential EMF exposure but a recent Swedish study which attempted to assess exposure quantitatively did not find an association.[21,26]

Agricultural work

Farmers and other agricultural workers are at lower risk than the general population for most types of cancer (other than possibly multiple myeloma and lymphomas), but a number of studies have found them to be at higher risk for brain neoplasms.[27] For example, Musicco and colleagues found an excess of gliomas among farmers in Northern Italy.[28] The excess was limited to those who had worked in the 1960s or later, leading the authors to speculate that it might be due to the introduction of pesticides, fertilizers, and herbicides around the same time. Excesses also have been seen in other studies among farmers or farm workers, and potential excesses also have been observed among other agricultural occupations such as pesticide applicators and agricultural extension agents.[27,29] Agricultural workers are potentially exposed to a variety of exposures including fertilizers, fuels, vehicle exhausts, organic dusts, and zoonotic bacteria and viruses, as well as insecticides, fungicides, and herbicides.[30] Some case control studies and a number of large state or national studies have found excess risks in various subpopulations of agricultural workers, but a consistent pattern has yet to emerge.[3,29] Several studies have also observed an association between paternal exposure to pesticides or employment in agricultural occupations prior to birth and the risk of childhood brain cancer.[31]

Firefighting

Smoke is a complex mixture of combustion products. Although the exact composition may vary significantly from fire to fire, smoke commonly contains a number of carcinogens such as polycyclic aromatic hydrocarbons, benzene, formaldehyde, and others.[32] Several studies have observed a two-fold excess of brain tumors among firefighters.[18,33–35] Several have not observed an association.[5,26] In addition, the relationship with duration of employment and other indicators of exposure in the positive studies has been weak, but given the variability in smoke exposure between fires these may only be poor surrogates for smoke exposure. The only study that examined the risk by number of fires fought observed a pattern that was compatible with a dose–response, but there were too few cases to draw firm conclusions.[18]

Rubber industry

Rubber manufacturing was one of the first industries to come under suspicion for an excess of brain cancer based on evidence that Ohio workers producing tires had a higher risk of brain neoplasms.[36] Although early studies implicated the tire curing and building processes, few studies have examined the risk among subpopulations defined on the basis of potential exposure. Most ensuing investigations have not found an excess of brain neoplasms among rubber workers, possibly indicating that exposure may have changed over time.[37] However, a case-control study of Shanghai women observed a five-fold excess among rubber workers and a five-fold excess was also observed among male rubber workers from Moscow.[38,39]

Petrochemical industry

Suspicions that petrochemical workers are at higher risk for brain neoplasms were raised in 1978 when a large cluster of cases was reported among former employees of a petrochemical company in Texas.[40] Following the discovery, a series of studies were initiated in order to determine whether or not an excess risk truly existed. In general, the results of the initial studies sponsored by government agencies and the Oil, Chemical, and Atomic Workers Union were consistent with a two-fold excess, and the histologies of the majority of tumors reported were either astrocytoma or glioblastoma multiforme.[41] However, studies sponsored by the industry at the same time generally found no excess risk. Much of this disparity may have been due to differences in study design (proportionate mortality versus cohort studies) and populations studied (all workers versus workers most likely to be exposed). More recent cohort studies have continued to yield mixed results and to suffer from the same limitations.[42] Several case control

studies have also observed an association between employment in the industry and brain neoplasms, but no association with any specific chemical exposure has been found.[43,44]

Parental exposure and childhood cancer

Numerous epidemiologic studies have examined the relationship between parental occupation and childhood brain cancer. Although no firm causal relationships have been established, suggestive associations have been observed with paternal exposure to paints, hydrocarbons, ionizing radiation, electromagnetic fields, and pesticides[21,31,45] The degree to which a father's exposure may influence an offspring's cancer risk is unclear, and few studies have examined maternal occupational exposures. Experimental studies have found animals that were exposed to carcinogens transplacentally or at young age to be particularly susceptible to brain neoplasms. However, it is unclear whether these studies are relevant to adult or childhood cancer in humans because of the long induction times observed in animal experiments.

CLINICAL EVALUATION

The diagnosis, clinical course, treatment, and prognosis of brain tumors associated with occupational or environmental exposures are no different from their non-occupational counterparts. Patients initially may present with a variety of symptoms including headache, seizures, personality changes, vomiting, loss of sensory functions, hemiparesis, hemiplegia, or ataxia depending on the tumor type and location.[46] Tumors are detected after the onset of symptoms using computed tomographic (CT) scanning or magnetic resonance imaging (MRI). Treatment may require surgery, radiotherapy, or chemotherapy, or some combination of these methods depending on the histology or location of the tumor.

Screening for brain neoplasms cannot be recommended at this time. It would be very difficult to identify a group of individuals who are clearly at higher risk given the ambiguity of much of the epidemiologic evidence, and unfortunately, there are no appropriate screening tests available. The utility of advanced diagnostic techniques, such as MRI, for improving or prolonging the life of asymptomatic patients when used for screening has yet to be proved, and the financial costs would be substantial.

References

1. Reis LAG, Kosary CL, Hankey BK, et al. Cancer statistics review 1973–1996. Bethesda: National Cancer Institute, 1999.
2. Parkin DM, Muir CS, Whelan SL, et al. Cancer incidence in five continents, Volume VI. IARC Scientific Publication No. 120. Lyon: International Agency for Research on Cancer, 1992.
3. Preston-Martin S, Mack WJ. Neoplasms of the nervous system. In: Schottenfeld D, Fraumeni JF, eds. Cancer epidemiology and prevention, 2nd edn. Philadelphia, WB Saunders, 1996.

4. Davis DL, Ahlbom A, Hoel D, Percy C. Is brain cancer mortality increasing in industrialized countries? Am J Ind Med 1991; 19:421–31.

5. National Toxicology Program. Ninth annual report on carcinogens. Research Triangle Park, NC: US Department of Health and Human Services, Public Health Service, 2000.

6. Maltoni C. Predictive value of carcinogenesis bioassays. Ann NY Acad Sci 1976; 271:431–43.

7. Doll R. Effects of exposure to vinyl chloride. Scand J Work Environ Health 1988; 14:61–78.

8. Waxweiler RJ, Stringer W, Wagoner JK, et al. Neoplastic risk among workers exposed to vinyl chloride. Ann NY Acad Sci 1976; 271:40–8.

9. Beaumont JJ, Breslow NE. Power considerations in epidemiologic studies of vinyl chloride workers. Am J Epidemiol 1981; 114:725–34.

10. Simonato L, L'Abbe KA, Anderson A, et al. A collaborative study of cancer incidence and mortality among vinyl chloride workers. Scand J Work Environ Health 1991; 17:159–69.

11. Wu W, Steenland K, Brown D, et al. Cohort and case-control of workers exposed to vinyl chloride: an update. J Occup Med 1989; 31:518–23.

12. IARC Working Group. Wood dust and formaldehyde. IARC monographs on the evaluation of the carcinogenic risk of chemicals to humans, vol 62. Lyon: International Agency for Research on Cancer, 1995.

13. Blair A, Stewart P, O'Berg M, et al. Mortality among industrial workers exposed to formaldehyde. J Natl Cancer Inst 1986; 6:1071–84.

14. Stroup NE, Blair A, Erikson GE. Brain cancer and other causes of death in anatomists. J Natl Cancer Inst 1986; 77:1217–24.

15. Anttila A, Heikkila P, Nykyri E, et al. Risk of nervous system cancer among workers exposed to lead. J Occup Environ Med 1996; 38:131–6.

16. Cocco P, Dosemeci M, Heineman EF. Brain cancer and occupational exposure to lead. J Occup Environ Med 1998; 40:937–42.

17. Steenland K, Boffetta P. Lead and cancer in humans: where are we now? Am J Ind Med 2000; 38:295–9.

18. Tornling G, Gustavsson P, Hogstedt C. Mortality and cancer incidence in Stockholm fire fighters. Am J Ind Med 1994; 25:219–28.

19. Heineman EF, Cocco P, Gomez MR, et al. Occupational exposure to chlorinated aliphatic hydrocarbons and risk of astrocytic brain cancer. Am J Ind Med 1994; 26:155–69.

20. Rodvall Y, Ahlbom A, Spannare B, Nise G. Glioma and occupational exposure in Sweden, a case-control study. Occup Environ Med 1996; 53:526–37.

21. Colt JS, Blair A. Parental occupational exposures and risk of childhood cancer. Environ Health Perspect 1998; 106(Suppl 3):909–25.

22. Ballard T, Lagorio S, De Angelis G, et al. Cancer incidence and mortality among flight personnel: a meta-analysis. Aviation Space Environ Med 2000; 71:216–24.

23. Alexander V. Brain tumor risk among United States nuclear workers. Occup Med 1991; 6:695–714.

24. Milham S. Mortality in workers exposed to electromagnetic fields. Environ Health Perspect 1985; 62:297–300.

25. Kheifets LI, Afifi AA, Buffler PA, et al. Occupational electric and magnetic field exposure and brain cancer: a meta-analysis. J Occup Environ Med 1995; 37:1327–41.

26. Feychting M, Floderus B, Ahlbom A. Parental occupational exposure to magnetic fields and childhood cancer (Sweden). Cancer Causes Controls 2000; 11:151–6.

27. Blair A, Malker H, Cantor KP, et al. Cancer among farmers, a review. Scand J Work Environ Health 1985; 11:397–407.

28. Musicco M, Sant M, Molinari S, et al. A case-control study of brain gliomas and occupational exposure to chemical carcinogens: the risk to farmers. Am J Epidemiol 1988; 128:778–5.

29. IARC Working Group. Occupational exposures in insecticide application and some pesticides. IARC monographs on the evaluation of the carcinogenic risk of chemicals to humans, vol 53. Lyon: International Agency for Research on Cancer, 1991.

30. Sanderson WT, Talaska G, Zaebst D, et al. Pesticide prioritization for a brain cancer case-control study. Environ Res 1997; 74:133–44.

31. Daniels JL, Olshan AF, Savitz DA. Pesticides and childhood cancers. Environ Health Perspect 1997; 105:1068–77.

32. Lees PSJ. Combustion products and other firefighter exposures. Occup Med State Art Rev 1995; 10: 691–707.

33. Aronson KJ, Tomlinson GA, Smith L. Mortality among fire fighters in metropolitan Toronto. Am J Ind Med 1994; 26:89–101.

34. Demers PA, Heyer NJ, Rosenstock L. Mortality among firefighters from three Northwest US cities. Br J Ind Med 1992; 49:664–70.

35. Vena JE, Fiedler RC. Mortality in a municipal workers cohort: IV. fire fighters. Am J Ind Med 1987; 11:671–84.

36. Monson RR, Fine LJ. Cancer mortality and morbidity among rubber workers. J Natl Cancer Inst 1978; 61:1047–53.

37. Thomas TL, Waxweiler RJ. Brain tumors and occupational risk factors: a review. Scand J Work Environ Health 1986; 12:1–15.

38. Heineman EF, Gao YT, Dosemeci M, et al. Occupational risk factors for brain tumors among women in Shanghai, China. J Occup Environ Med 1995; 37:288–93.

39. Solionova LG, Smulevich VB. Mortality and cancer incidence in a cohort of rubber workers in Moscow. Scand J Work Environ Health 1993; 19:96–101.

40. Waxweiler RJ, Alexander V, Leffingwell SS, et al. Mortality from brain tumors and other causes in a cohort of petrochemical workers. J Natl Cancer Inst 1983; 70:75–81.

41. Savitz DA, Moure R. Cancer risk among oil refinery workers, a review of epidemiologic studies. J Occup Med 1984; 26:662–70.

42. Cooper SP, Labarthe D, Downs T, et al. Cancer mortality among petroleum refinery and chemical manufacturing workers in Texas. J Environ Path Toxicol Oncol 1997; 16:1–14.

43. Demers PA, Vaughan TL, Schommer RR. Occupation, socioeconomic status, and brain tumor mortality: a death certificate-based case-control study. J Occup Med 1991; 33:1001–8.

44. Thomas TL, Stewart PA, Stemhagen A, et al. Risk of astrocytic brain tumors associated with occupational chemical exposures. A case-referent study. Scand J Work Environ Health 1987; 13:417–23.

45. Cordier S, Lefeuvre B, Filippini G, et al. Parental occupation, occupational exposure to solvents and polycyclic aromatic hydrocarbons and risk of childhood brain tumors (Italy, France, Spain). Cancer Causes Control 1997; 8:688–97.

46. Cairncross JG. Tumors of the central nervous system. In: Kelley WN, ed. Textbook of internal medicine. Philadelphia: JB Lippincott Company, 1992.

30.9 **Skin Cancers**
David E Cohen, Shirley Bassiri, Brian G Forrester, James Nethercott

INTRODUCTION

The skin is the largest organ of the body and a critical interface with the environment. During activities of routine daily living, work, and recreation, the integument is subjected to a legion of chemical and physical assaults that are typically neutralized through metabolic and homeostatic mechanisms. When these systems are overwhelmed, cutaneous and systemic disease may result. When evaluating occupational and environmental dermatoses, a variety of inflammatory, neoplastic, and infectious diseases may be encountered. Irritant and allergic contact dermatitis are the most common occupational dermatoses, and benign and malignant neoplasms may be associated with a variety of exposure patterns. Malignancies of the skin represent the most common human cancers.

The major divisions of the skin are the epidermis (comprising the outermost layer), the dermis (composed of collagen, elastin, and appendageal structures), and the subcutis (principally composed of fat). Cutaneous neoplasms may be encountered in all layers of the skin but the epidermis is the most common site.

The epidermis is subdivided into four histologically defined sections that represent the differentiation pathways of a mature skin surface: basal, spinous, granular, and cornified layers. The basal layer, or stratum germinativum, abuts the dermis and is composed principally of epidermal progenitor cells. These cells divide constantly to replenish those lost on the surface and consequently maintain epidermal integrity. One daughter of this mitotic activity will move upward toward the surface as it undergoes morphologic and biochemical changes in a process called terminal differentiation. These cells from the mitotic layer first move into the stratum spinosum, where they begin to differentiate, developing more extensive intracellular filaments and pronounced intercellular attachments at desmosomal junctions with adjacent cells.

With further upward movement toward the surface, the cells reach the granular layer, where they begin to accumulate keratohyalin granules in their interstices. Membrane-coating granules attach to the outer cellular membrane and can secrete substances into the intercellular space. This process begins to isolate the cells from one another. Finally, the cells reach the outer layer of the epidermis. The cells in the granular layer metamorphose from living nucleated cells to become dead cells filled with filaments and keratohyalin with only a faint outline left of residual intracellular organelles such as the nucleus. This outer layer of cells, the stratum corneum, forms the principal barrier to the loss of fluids and electrolytes from the body, and is the major barrier to percutaneous absorption of environmental agents and adverse effects from physical trauma and ultraviolet (UV) light.

The vast majority of the cells in the epidermis are keratinocytes in the various stages of differentiation outlined earlier. In addition, melanocytes or pigment cells are resident in the normal epidermis. The cells reside along the basement membrane, sharing the basal layer with the dividing keratinocytes. They have dendrites that contact and transfer melanin to keratinocytes in the epidermis above them. Melanin, the main pigment in skin, is produced in two forms: eumelanin, a brown pigment, and pheomelanin, a red-yellow pigment, that is produced in a specialized organelle called a melanosome. The melanin is formed via a series of enzymatic steps that begins with the conversion of tyrosine to dopaquinone. As the melanin is produced, it accumulates within the melanosome until the structure is mature. The melanosome is then transferred from the melanocyte dendritic tip to a keratinocyte via an incompletely characterized mechanism that may involve membrane fusion. Each melanocyte has a population of keratinocytes that it serves and to which it transfers melanin.

Melanosomes are larger in black skinned people compared to Caucasians, and the amount of melanin and melanosome is greater in black skin. Facultative increases in pigmentation are accomplished by increases in melanin and melanosome production typically after stimulation with UV light or local inflammation or hormone fluctuations (e.g., sun tanning, post-inflammatory hyperpigmentation). Physiologically, melanin is an effective ultraviolet light chromophore, protecting the epidermal and underlying dermal cells from UV radiation. Melanin confers this protection by absorbing photons of UV light and dissipating the energy absorbed through the melanin polymer structure so that damage to cellular structures and DNA is avoided. The melanocyte may undergo transformation, forming a variety of benign and malignant neoplasms ranging from benign nevi to malignant melanoma.

In addition to melanocytes and keratinocytes, the epidermis contains immunocompetent cells called Langerhans' cells. These cells are distinctive in that they stain selectively with gold salts and contain distinctive intracellular granules demonstrable by transmission electron microscopy called Birbeck's granules. They function as antigen-processing cells and transmit signals to lymphocytes, allowing the development of immune responses to antigens that they encounter. Langerhans' cells also produce lymphokines, which will activate other immunologically active cells (e.g., T cells, natural killer cells). The Langerhans' cells are susceptible to malignant transformation, which results in the T-cell lymphoma of the skin known as mycosis fungoides.

Finally, there is another cell found in the epidermis, known as the Merkel cell, whose function is unknown. Rarely, tumors of the skin arise from this enigmatic cell.

PATHOPHYSIOLOGY

Subcellular and cellular events are necessary prerequisites in the transformation of a normal skin cell to a malignant cell. Such a transformed cell ignores internal and environmental messages, becoming a malignant cell that grows to become a collection of cells with no defined borders or lifespan. This process in the pathogenesis of cancers such as squamous cell carcinoma (SCC), basal cell carcinoma (BCC) and malignant melanoma (MM) is referred to as carcinogenesis and is thought to involve multiple steps of assault to the cell and damage to cellular deoxyribonucleic acid (DNA).

Ultraviolet (UV) radiation plays a pivotal role in the initiation of skin damage and photocarcinogenesis. The basic mechanism of phototoxicity lies in DNA damage resulting in a mutation-like genetic change. It may involve mutation of tumor suppressor genes, oncogenes, and genes directly involved in control of the stability of the genome, such as the mismatch repair (MR) genes. The UV radiation forms dimers in DNA between adjacent pyrimidine residues. Damaged cells normally will respond to injury either by arresting cell growth to repair the damaged DNA or by inducing apoptosis (programmed cell death). The failure of these processes results in a proliferation of abnormal cells bearing genomic mutations. Consequent to the DNA alteration, this change is irreversible and persists throughout the subsequent life of the altered daughter cells. Three to seven mutations at different loci are estimated to be required for the transformation of a normal cell to a cancerous one. Besides UV radiation, polycyclic aromatic hydrocarbons (PAHs) are also well-known mutating agents.

Alterations in the expression of various tumor suppressor genes and oncogenes have been reported in skin carcinogenesis. The *P53* tumor suppressor gene, which is frequently mutated in human cancers, appears to be an early target in the development of UV radiation-associated skin cancers, and plays an important role in the development of BCC. Various studies have reported that 40–90% of BCCs show at least focal immunopositivity for *P53*. It is thought that UVR can result in mutations of *P53*, which stabilize the protein and are therefore detected by increased immunoreactivity. It is not known whether BCCs arising largely as a consequence of exposure to agents other than UVR that share the same disruption of *P53* function and, in particular, the same spectrum of mutations. In cutaneous melanoma, UVB has been shown to increase collagenase IV activity and angiogenesis, thereby promoting tumor aggressiveness, and *P53* involvement has been linked to melanocyte malignant transformation.

The instability of microsatellites (short repetitive DNA sequences) is a common event in the carcinogenic process, resulting in mutation in genes responsible for the mismatch repair process. Such mutated genes contribute to the control of cellular proliferation by regulating growth control genes, the prototype of which is the hMSH2 gene. This gene, situated on chromosome 2p21-22, has also been implicated in the pathogenesis of UV-associated skin cancers.[1]

NON-MELANOMA SKIN CANCER
Premalignant skin lesions

Actinic, or solar, keratoses (AKs) most commonly have the appearance of warts (Fig. 30.9.1), but are occasionally flat.

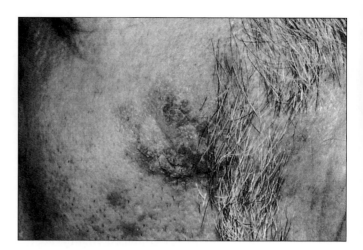

Figure 30.9.1: Actinic or solar keratosis.

These lesions develop on the sun-exposed skin and are usually evident on the face, hands, and non-hair-bearing scalp. Occasionally, they are exophytic and grow to form an excrescence or cutaneous horn. A variant of this occurs on the vermilion border of the lip as a focal area of thickening or erosion and is referred to as actinic cheilitis. It has been estimated that up to 20% of those persons with multiple AKs eventually develop one or more SCCs. Although the risk of metastases from SCCs evolving out of AKs on the skin is small (i.e., 0.5%), the risk is 11% in instances from actinic cheilitis.

While AKs are benign lesions, some have argued that they may be thought of as evolving lesions of squamous cell carcinoma in situ in which the altered keratinocytes remain restricted to the epidermis. The differentiation between SCC and AK may be very difficult, illustrating the continuum between these two entities; however, there is no dermal invasion in AK. There is evidence of actinic damage to the dermal tissue in AK, such as solar elastotic degeneration. The presence of degeneration of the elastin in the dermis allows one to conclude that there has been significant sun damage.

Common clinical forms of non-melanoma skin cancer

The most frequently occurring skin cancers known to be of environmental and occupational origin are the non-melanoma skin cancers (NMSC) that are derived from keratinocytes.[2] These include basal cell carcinoma and squamous cell carcinoma.

Basal cell carcinoma

BCC is a common tumor thought to be derived from an adult progenitor epithelial cell (either an altered basal cell in the epidermis or precursor cell from cutaneous adnexal structures) or, rarely, an aberrant primary germ cell in the case of the basal cell nevus syndrome (BCNS). There is experimental evidence derived from transplantation of BCCs that they need connective tissue stroma to be successfully transplanted.

BCCs can be relatively slow growing. For instance, it has been shown by using ³H-thymidine uptake by BCC tumors harvested from nude mice that there are large areas of quiescence or very slow growth in the tumor cell mass, with growth occurring mainly at the tumor nodule periphery. In addition, approximately 5% of BCCs demonstrate areas of spontaneous regression, although this process is almost always incomplete. The presence of amyloid in such tumors also suggests cell death is occurring, accounting for the slow progression of growth. The presence of Councilman's bodies in such tumors also suggests a significant role for cell degeneration in limiting tumor growth.

Metastasis of BCC is rare, with reported incidences of 0.0028–0.4%.[3] Of BCCs that metastasize, 70–86% occur in the head and neck region. Lesions in the ear and scalp region have been cited as the most likely to metastasize. Larger, more invasive tumors have a greater tendency to metastasize. Tumors smaller than 1 cm rarely metastasize. A history of radiation therapy may also be a risk factor for metastasis. The risk of metastases is greater in men than in women (2:1), and affected persons tend to be younger than other patients presenting with BCCs. However, there are no absolute prerequisites for metastasis.

Clinical variants of BCC correspond closely to their histologic subtypes. Although as many as 26 different categories of tumor have been described based on histologic appearance, they are often subdivided into four major variants: nodulocystic, adenoid, morpheaform, and superficial.

Nodulocystic BCC (Fig. 30.9.2) is the most common form and accounts for approximately 70% of all cases. It characteristically presents as a dome-shaped papule with superficial telangiectasia, raised, rolled margins and a 'pearly' translucent border. There are frequently signs of actinic damage on surrounding skin. It also may appear as an erosive, pimple-like or pigmented lesion. The pigmented sub-variant is not uncommon, particularly in skin of color, and may be clinically suggestive of malignant melanoma. Histologically, nodulocystic BCC is characterized by cellular clusters with peripheral palisading, whereby a parallel alignment of peripheral tumor cell nuclei occurs at right angles to nuclei of cells at the center of the nodule. Connective tissue stromal retraction at the periphery of the tumor is usually apparent. The tumor cells are uniform in size, polygonal in shape, and have scanty cytoplasm and variable mitotic activity. Typically, separation of the tumor cells from the stroma leaves gaps, related to a paucity of desmosomal junctions joining tumor cells to the underlying stroma as well as gaps in the basement membrane.

Adenoid BCC occurs in approximately 20% of cases and displays a gland-like growth pattern in tumor cell clusters. In contrast to true glandular tumors of the skin, adenoid BCC retains the typical peripheral nuclear palisading seen in nodulocystic BCC. Clinically, both adenoid and nodular BCCs have a similar appearance.

Approximately 5% of all BCCs are termed *morpheaform*, or sclerotic, BCCs because of intense connective tissue stromal proliferation characterizing the tumor's architecture. Clinically, it presents the greatest diagnostic challenge, as it may be difficult to detect. They either exhibit an irregular, scar-like appearance or present as a firm, yellowish, plaque-like lesion. The margins of the tumor are often difficult to determine clinically. Histologically, stromal retraction and peripheral palisading are not readily apparent. Unlike other BCCs, this type produces a cytokine that stimulates the synthesis of glycosaminoglycan by surrounding fibroblasts. The marked fibrotic response makes treatment more challenging by protecting the tumor cells so that total excision or Moh's chemosurgery is often required to eradicate the lesion.

The fourth type, the *superficial* BCC, presents as an erythematous faintly scaly patch with a subtle 'rolled' edge often only seen when the lesion is stretched manually on clinical examination. It may be mistaken for a benign dermatosis such as nummular eczema, dermatophytosis or psoriasis. It is the least common of the four main subtypes and has been associated with exposure to arsenic. Individuals with superficial BCC due to arsenic exposure usually also have arsenical keratoses, which have a distinctive histologic appearance due to the presence of vacuolated keratinocytes in the proliferating epidermal cells, as discussed in further detail later in the chapter. Superficial BCCs are more likely to be pigmented and, in a high percentage of cases, are multifocal and show a downward, bud-like growth of tumor nodules from the basal epidermis.

Variants of basal cell carcinoma Basal cell nevus syndrome and linear unilateral basal cell nevus with comedones are distinctly different from common BCCs in their appearance, natural history, and etiology. Although they may be of some importance in elucidating the underlying pathogenic mechanisms in BCC, they are not environmentally caused per se. BCNS may predispose an individual to an increased risk for the development of BCCs with x-ray exposure.[4]

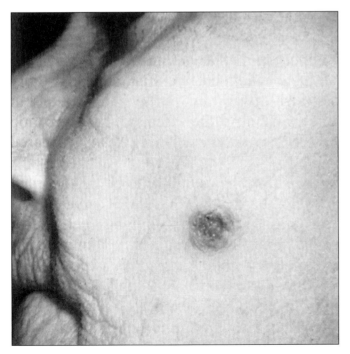

Figure 30.9.2: Nodulocystic basal cell carcinoma.

Squamous cell carcinoma

SCCs have the capacity to metastasize locally and to distant sites. Although the capacity for metastasis in SCC is greater than that of BCC, it is less than that of many cancers. It is estimated that only 0.5% of all SCCs derived from solar keratoses metastasize. For SCCs developing on skin that is not exposed to the sun the risk is 2–3% with a fatal outcome in 75% of cases. For SCCs of the lower lip (Fig. 30.9.3), the risk is even greater, with 16% metastasizing and half the patients succumbing to the disease.

The histologic variants of SCC include the conventional, adenoid, spindle-pleomorphic, small cell, clear cell, and verrucous forms. Only the two main subtypes, the conventional and adenoid forms, are discussed. Conventional SCCs display a connecting growth pattern of cords and nests of polygonal-shaped cells with enlarged nuclei and amphophilic cytoplasm. They are usually categorized by Borders' grades of differentiation as well differentiated, moderately differentiated, and poorly differentiated. Well-differentiated SCC tumor cells often are arranged in a concentric pattern enclosing keratin pearls, which are masses of enucleate keratin. Moderately differentiated SCCs are more deeply invasive, have greater mitotic activity, and have less propensity for keratin pearl formation. Poorly differentiated SCCs have little, if any, keratin formation and often are noted to have infiltrated the subcutis at the time of diagnosis. Adenoid SCC is a variant that exhibits a combination of glandular and squamous differentiation, and often is associated with AKs. The principal differentiating feature is the lack of invasion of epidermal cells into the reticular dermis in the AK.

Variants of squamous cell carcinoma   *Bowen's disease* is exhibited as a single lesion on sun-exposed or unexposed skin. It is a slow growing, erythematous patch that is often mistaken clinically for a superficial BCC. The histology is that of an AK but without evidence of solar degeneration in the dermis if the lesion is not in a sun-exposed area. The risk of metastases is higher than for SCCs associated with AKs, with percentages varying from 3% to 11% in reported series. Arsenic exposure is known to be associated with the

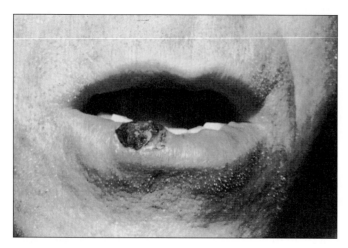

Figure 30.9.3: Squamous cell carcinoma of the lip.

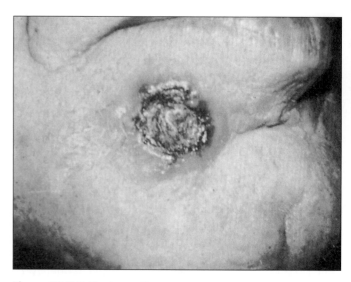

Figure 30.9.4: Keratoacanthoma.

development of BD lesions on skin that is not exposed to the sun.

Keratoacanthoma (KA), or self-healing squamous cell carcinoma, may occur as a solitary event or, rarely, affected individuals may develop multiple KAs. The lesion has a crater-like appearance, with the central portion filled with keratinous debris (Fig. 30.9.4).

In the more common solitary KAs, the lesions occur in older persons at a sun-exposed site. They erupt suddenly and grow rapidly for 4–6 weeks, following which they involute spontaneously to leave a depressed scar. It may take up to a year for complete resolution to occur. Larger lesions may cause severe disfigurement and fail to involute. Differentiation from an SCC may be difficult or impossible and occasionally, such lesions have metastasized. In the latter instances, it is suggested that the KAs were, in fact, SCCs.

Epidemiology of non-melanoma skin cancer

NMSC is the most common malignancy in the United States, accounting for one-third of all diagnosed cases of cancer. The American Cancer Society estimated that there are 1.3 million cases of NMSC diagnosed in the United States alone each year, with nearly 75% presenting as BCCs. The incidences of both SCC and BCC have been rising at an alarming rate.[5] Between 1980 and 1994, incidence rates of SSC rose by 235–350%, and those of BCC increased by 80%.

Basal cell carcinoma is the most common skin cancer in the United States, with an estimated 900,000 cases per year. It represents 75% of all cutaneous neoplasms and outnumbers squamous cell carcinoma by 3.3–4.5 to 1. It has also become the most commonly diagnosed malignancy in the world, with the highest annual incidence in Australia. The incidence of BCC is higher in men than in women and increases with age, usually occurring between the ages of 40 and 60 years. However, there has been a

Host factors	
Fair skin	
Blue eyes, blond or red hair	
Skin sensitivity to sun	
Older age	
Immunosuppression	
Photochemotherapy (PUVA)	
Occupational and environmental factors	**Typical exposure settings**
UV radiation	Outdoor workers: construction workers, roofers, agricultural workers, telephone-repair workers, highway workers, sailors, fishermen
Ionizing radiation	Radiation workers: uranium miners, radium workers, nuclear energy workers Medical uses: x-ray technicians, therapeutic radiation
Skin trauma	Construction workers, machinists, agricultural workers
Arsenic	Pesticide, herbicide workers, copper smelter workers Contaminated food, water, medicinals, treated wood
Polycyclic aromatic hydrocarbons (PAH)	Coal tar workers, petroleum workers, chimney sweeps, foundry workers, diesel engine workers

Table 30.9.1 Risk factors for non-melanoma skin cancer

rise in the number of cases among younger patients. Approximately 80% of BCCs occur in the head and neck. The nose is the most common site of occurrence, followed by the cheeks and forehead.

Risk factors for NMSC are listed in Table 30.9.1. Numerous studies have documented a particular phenotype that appears to be associated with NMSC. Important constitutional risk factors include fair skin, blue eyes, blond or red hair, childhood freckling, skin sensitivity to the sun, and an inability to tan. Darkly pigmented skin appears to be more resistant to the effects of UV radiation because of the protection of epidermal cells by the increased level of melanin.

Exposure to UV radiation also is known to be an important risk factor in the development of NMSC. NMSC occurs most frequently on areas most exposed to sunlight, such as the head, neck, arms, and hands. In Australia, where immigrants of Celtic origin experience near year-round sun exposure, the highest rates of NMSC in the world are found.[6] SCC appears to be more strongly related to sun exposure than BCC, because 20–30% of all BCCs are found on the relatively unexposed areas of the body, such as the trunk and eyelid. SCCs have been found to be more common with frequent or long-term sun exposure and southern geographic locations, where exposure to UV radiation is more intense.

Ultraviolet light and non-melanoma skin cancer

The association between sun exposure and skin cancer was first commented on over 100 years ago. UV radiation is further discussed in Chapter 33.2. Numerous epidemiologic and experimental studies have presented overwhelming evidence that UV radiation is the primary risk factor for NMSC.[7] This factor has important implications for the prevention of occupationally related skin cancer, because numerous occupations involve chronic, almost continuous exposure to sunlight.

The association between increasing age and the risk of NMSC is well known and is probably related to cumulative UV radiation dose. BCC has been found to be ten times more prevalent in elderly patients with severe actinic skin damage than in individuals of the same age without marked actinic damage. A history of sustaining multiple painful sunburns has been found to be associated with an increased risk of NMSCs and AKs. The carcinogenic effect of natural sunlight is possibly related primarily to ultraviolet B (UVB) in the 290–320 nm band.[8] This is the component of the UV spectrum that produces normal sunburn.

There is also experimental evidence for UV causation of NMSC. Although keratinocytes are more resistant to the effects of UV radiation than Langerhans' cells, they have been found to have a shortened lifespan and to show evidence of cellular damage after UV exposure. Nude mice irradiated with UVB radiation inevitably develop SCCs, but wavelengths above this range do not induce malignant skin tumors in mice.

UV radiation in the 320–400 nm band, known as UVA, also has been implicated in photocarcinogenesis.[9] UVA radiation can cause erythema of the skin but at dose levels 800–1000 times higher than the dose of UVB required. However, since UVA is much more prevalent in the solar spectrum than UVB, it may be responsible for as much as 15% of the erythema dose received at noon on a sunny day.

UV radiation in the 200–290 nm band, known as UVC, also is associated with skin carcinogenesis, but UVC is not causally related to skin cancer associated with sun exposure because it is completely absorbed by the stratospheric ozone layer. As the ozone layer is being depleted, rising incidences of NMSC have been observed. Industrial sources of UV, such as germicidal lamps and welding arcs, also emit UV below 290 nm. Workers exposed to UVC should be considered to have a potential carcinogenic exposure, and appropriate precautions to limit sun exposure should be taken.

The different topographic distribution of NMSC in men and women may be due to clothing styles and differences in occupational sunlight exposure. Skin cancers of all types occur more frequently on the ears of men and on the legs of women. These findings fit exposure patterns predicted from traditional hair and dress styles. The incidence rate for SCC in men is 3–4 times higher than in women, possibly related to greater outdoor occupational and recreational UV radiation exposure.

The relationship between UV radiation and SCC is more clear-cut than that for UV and BCC. In a study of Maryland fishermen, in whom exposure assessment was determined through a combination of a detailed occupational history with laboratory and field measurements, SCC prevalence was strongly correlated with UV exposure but BCC prevalence was consistent with a dose saturation effect, with a plateau at higher exposures.[10] About 33% of BCCs are found on relatively unexposed areas of the body. This suggests that different etiologic mechanisms may be operative in BCC and SCC.

The main bases on which UV radiation derived from sun exposure has been linked to the development of NMSC are as follows.

1. The preferential tendency for NMSC to occur on sun-exposed areas of the skin.
2. The increase in the incidence rate of NMSC as one examines populations closer to the equator, where there is greater exposure to UV radiation.
3. The higher incidence of NMSC in people with extensive outdoor exposures.
4. The predisposition of individuals with fair complexions, who sunburn easily, to develop NMSC.
5. The increased risk of NMSC in patients with a heritable disorder of defective repair of UV-induced DNA damage.

In recent years, increased solar irradiation as a consequence of stratospheric ozone depletion is thought to be partially responsible for the rising incidence rates of NMSC and has raised concern that the incidence of skin cancer will increase at even greater rates in the future.[11] A 50% drop in the ozone concentration overlying the Antarctic region has been observed. It has been estimated that every 1% decline in ozone concentration could result in a 2–6% increase in skin cancer. However, it is not likely that the sharp increase in skin cancer incidence observed in the past two decades is entirely due to ozone depletion. It is most likely that the increase is the result of changing behavioral patterns associated with increasing personal sun exposure.

Awareness of these behavioral patterns and the association with skin cancer has led to increasing use of sunscreens to protect against the harmful effect of solar UV radiation. The epidemiologic data suggest that sun protection will have the greatest impact if achieved as early as possible in life and that it will probably have an impact later in life, especially in those who had high childhood exposure to solar radiation. It is important that in implementing sun protection an increase in intermittency of exposure also be avoided.

The age at which exposure to the harmful effects of solar UV radiation occurs also may be an important factor in the pathogenesis of NMSC. In a study of solar keratotic lesions in Australians, it was found that British-born persons over the age of 40 who had migrated to Australia after age 20 had significantly fewer lesions than native-born Australians. This implies that a reduction in childhood and adolescent sun exposure may substantially reduce the incidence of solar keratoses and, by implication, SCC in adulthood.

Other physical agents in the environment associated with NMSC

Physical agents other than UV radiation have been associated with the development of NMSC, and include psoralen combined with UV therapy (PUVA), Grenz ray treatment, and ionizing radiation (Table 30.9.1).

Whether or not long-term PUVA therapy is associated with the development of NMSC has been debated for several years.[12] The immunologic effects of PUVA include depletion of Langerhans' cells, cutaneous anergy, and tolerance to skin grafting in laboratory animals. Thus, PUVA therapy could conceivably lead to an increased risk of skin cancer. High-dose PUVA therapy appears to increase the risk of developing NMSC, especially for SCC. In patients treated with more than 260 individual PUVA sessions, Stern and Lange[13] showed an 11-fold increase in squamous cell carcinomas compared with patients who had received fewer than 160 sessions. Of greater concern is the recent demonstration of an increase in malignant melanoma many years after the onset of PUVA treatments in patients who had received more than 250 treatments. Therefore, it seems prudent to limit exposure to PUVA to low doses if prolonged treatment is necessary and to provide medical surveillance for NMSC in patients who have received high doses in the past.

Grenz rays, also known as ultra soft x-rays or Bucky rays, have been used in the treatment of benign skin disease for more than 60 years. Grenz rays, given in usual therapeutic doses, appear to be associated with NMSC only rarely but may cause NMSC if given in high doses for prolonged periods.[14] Work-related SCC on the finger has been described in a dermatologist who was notoriously careless about exposing his hand directly to the Grenz ray when he treated patients.

Treatment with prolonged administration of low-dose ionizing radiation is associated with subsequent NMSC, particularly BCC.[15] Higher dose rate exposures appear to result in SCC, whereas lower dose exposures predominantly result in BCC. The latency period between first exposure to therapeutic ionizing radiation and the appearance of NMSC is presumed to be at least 20 years. In several studies, elevated risks in relation to therapeutic ionizing radiation were found to be confined to the site of radiation exposure and have ranged from an odds ratio of 3.30 to 5.7 for BCC to an odds ratio of 2.94 to 4.8 for SCC.

The first reported case of skin cancer due to x-ray exposure appeared in 1902. An x-ray technician who had exposed his hands directly to the x-ray beam for 4 years for demonstration purposes developed an invasive SCC of the dorsum of his hand, with regional lymph node metastases. The use of x-rays in the treatment of tinea capitis, facial acne, hypertrichosis, hemangioma, lupus vulgaris (cutaneous tuberculosis), toxic goiters, and eczema has been associated with the development of skin cancer. In a study of 2200 children receiving x-ray therapy for tinea capitis during the 1940s and 1950s, a relative risk of 6.1 was found for the development of NMSC compared with non-irradiated controls. In the 25% of the study population that had black skin, no cases of skin cancer occurred. Studies such as this suggest that UV exposure may interact with ionizing radiation exposure in the development of NMSC in susceptible individuals.

Chronic dermatitis following the application of ionizing radiation (e.g., chronic radiodermatitis) has been found to be associated with NMSC, possibly as a result of chronic epithelial regeneration, as well as due to direct damage to the DNA of the epidermal keratinocyte. Skin type is a factor in one's propensity to develop NMSC following ionizing radiation exposure. The SCC risk following irradiation may be highest in persons with a sun-sensitive phenotype.

Ionizing radiation as a result of exposure to radioactive materials has also been associated with skin cancer. Skin cancers have been reported to develop in areas of chronic radiodermatitis occurring in radium workers who had been exposed to radium for 10 years or more. For instance, the incidence of BCCs in Czechoslovakian uranium miners exposed to radium was shown to have increased, most markedly in miners with more than 10 years of exposure. This increase has been attributed to external α-particle radiation to the basal layer of the epidermis. Radioactive gold jewelry also has been documented to cause NMSC. In the early 1980s, the state of New York conducted a voluntary screening program for radioactive jewelry and found 200 contaminated items out of 160,000 pieces of jewelry screened, indicating the risk of such exposure is small.

Repeated high doses of diagnostic x-ray exposures, such as in multiple fluoroscopic examinations to evaluate artificial pneumothorax therapy for tuberculosis in the 1940s and 1950s, have also been associated with the development of NMSC in the skin where the radiation was delivered. BCCs developing in sites of such radiation exposure may be more invasive than other types of BCC.

Injury and the development of NMSC

The description of a malignant skin cancer developing at a site of previous trauma was first reported in 1828. It has been found that SCCs associated with burn scars, draining sinuses, and radiodermatitis have much higher rates of metastasis than other forms of SCC, with distant spread occurring in 20–30% of all such lesions. In a review of 1774 BCCs requiring Moh's micrographic surgery, 7.3% of the cancer subjects reported a history of trauma at the site previously. The trauma-associated lesions were larger, required more Moh's surgery stages to excise, and were more deceptive clinically than other BCC lesions. NMSC has been found to occur in old unstable scars of tattoos, lupus vulgaris (cutaneous tuberculosis), chronic leg ulcers, hair transplant sites, varicella scars, vaccination scars, and colostomy sites.

Using a combination of criteria from various authors, the following useful list has been formulated by Stoll and Crissey[16] as criteria to aid in the diagnosis of trauma-related skin cancer.
1. The skin must previously have been normal.
2. Adequate and authenticated trauma must have occurred, preferably confirmed and documented by medical personnel.
3. A positive diagnosis of a non-metastatic carcinoma must be made, and the tumor must be histologically consistent with the tissue of that site.
4. The carcinoma must originate from the exact point of injury.
5. A reasonable time interval (e.g., several years) between the trauma and the first appearance of the carcinoma must have elapsed.
6. There must be continuity of physical signs from the trauma event to the appearance of the carcinoma.

Chemical agents associated with the development of skin cancer

Percivall Pott first described the association of chemical exposure with the development of skin cancer in 1775, in his classic description of SCC of the scrotum associated with exposure to soot in chimney sweeps. Since then, a number of chemicals, compounds or industrial settings have been associated with an increased risk of skin cancer (Table 30.9.1). Arsenic, whether present in well water, medicinals, pesticides or industrial processes, is a well-documented cause of SCC and BCC, also discussed in Chapter 39.2. Substances containing polycyclic aromatic hydrocarbons (PAHs) such as coal tar pitch, mineral oil, and anthracene, also have been implicated in NMSC formation (see also Chapter 44). Other chemicals that have been suggested as potential skin carcinogens include PCBs, vinyl chloride, and other metals, but data are limited.[17–19]

An association between the smoking of tobacco and SCC has been recently observed, with an estimated relative risk of 2.0 of developing SCC among smokers after adjustment for age, sex, and sun exposure.[20] No significant association was found between smoking and other forms of skin cancer. Proposed mechanisms include tobacco smoke acting as a skin carcinogen inducing specific mutations in the *P53* gene or due to the loss of immune surveillance since tobacco smoke has been shown to suppress immunologic functions, and immunosuppressed patients (described below) have an increased risk of squamous cell carcinoma.

Arsenic

The acute lethal effects of arsenic have been known since the Middle Ages. The carcinogenic effect of long-term exposure to arsenic was not described until 1809, when Lambe linked drinking arsenic-contaminated water with malignant disease. Paris described cancer of the scrotum in workers exposed to arsenical fumes from copper smelting in 1822. The first description of arsenic-induced skin cancer and its relationship to hyperkeratosis in patients exposed to medicinal arsenic was by Hutchinson in 1887. Arsenic is unique in that skin tumors may be produced by ingestion, injection or inhalation in humans, as compared with the necessity for skin contact in most other cutaneous carcinogens. Only inorganic arsenic has been associated with cancer.

Epidemiologic evidence has shown strong associations between arsenic and cancers of the lung, skin, liver, kidney, and urinary bladder in humans.[21,22] However, until recently studies have been unable to show arsenic compounds as carcinogens in animal models, hindering mechanistic studies. While arsenic compounds are not mutagenic alone in standard bacterial and mammalian test systems, they have been shown to increase the mutagenicity of other DNA-damaging agents, including UV radiation in animal models.[23] Arsenite (inorganic trivalent arsenic), the likely environmental carcinogen, is thought to act as an enhancing agent (co-carcinogen) with a genotoxic partner such as UV radiation by inhibiting DNA repair and disrupting *P53* function. A recent study found that SCCs occurring in mice given both UV radiation and arsenite were much larger and more invasive than in mice given UV radiation alone. No tumors appeared in mice given arsenite alone.[24]

Arsenic may also cause the induction of gene amplification, the arrest of cells in mitosis, the replacement of phosphorus in the DNA chain, and the expression of heme oxygenase and *c-fos*. Other theories of carcinogenic modes include arsenic-induced chromosome abnormalities,[25] DNA damage due to oxidative stress from arsenic metabolites, and alterations in growth factors such as transforming growth factor-α (TNF-α), granulocyte macrophage-colony stimulating factor (GM-CSF), and interleukin-6, which then lead to cell proliferation and promotion of carcinogenesis.[26]

The major clinical manifestations of chronic arsenic poisoning are hyperpigmentation, hyperkeratosis, and NMSC, regardless of the source of exposure. Hyperpigmentation is the most frequently observed clinical skin response to chronic arsenic toxicity. The lesions are dark brown, and usually are present at sites of normally increased pigmentation, such as the axilla, groin or areola. Arsenic-induced hyperkeratosis, known as arsenical keratoses, usually occur on the palms and soles, and are exhibited as small, multiple, non-tender, indurated elevations, usually 0.4–1 cm in diameter. The nodules may coalesce into plaques or form large verrucous-appearing growths. Skin tumors associated with arsenic exposure include SCC, BCC, and Bowen's disease. Arsenic-induced tumors usually are multiple and often occur at sites not directly exposed to UV. Arsenic-induced SCC and BCC do not differ histologically from SCC and BCC arising from other exposures, although they appear to be clinically more aggressive.[27]

The use of inorganic arsenic in insecticides, herbicides, and fungicides has led to occupational, environmental, and dietary exposures. Although the commercial use and production of arsenic-containing substances have declined over the past few decades, it still remains an occupational hazard with the United States Bureau of Labor Statistics reporting 28 cases of occupational disease associated with arsenic from 1994 to 1995. In earlier decades, tobacco contained substantial amounts of arsenic, up to 40 mg/kg, as a result of the use of arsenical pesticides in agriculture. The inhalation of tobacco smoke from tobacco grown in the United States during the 1950s may have resulted in the intake of more than 100 micrograms of arsenic daily. Arsenic in well water also has been found to be associated with skin cancer. In a prevalence study of skin cancer in an area of Taiwan where arsenic-contaminated artesian wells had been in use for over 45 years, the authors found a positive dose–response relationship.[28] In the study population, the youngest skin cancer patient was age 24, the youngest with hyperpigmentation was age 3, and the youngest with hyperkeratosis was age 4. Examination of a nearby control population did not reveal any melanosis, hyperkeratosis or skin cancer.

The association between arsenic exposure and skin cancer in a worker with arsenic exposure is considered strongly suspicious if the following criteria are met.

1. The simultaneous occurrence of arsenical hyperkeratosis and hyperpigmentation, which occurs at lower doses than arsenic-associated skin cancer.
2. The occurrence of multiple skin cancers, often in areas not exposed to the sun.
3. The development of such skin cancer at a relatively young age.

Polycyclic aromatic hydrocarbons (PAHs)

Workers are exposed to PAHs from inhalation as well as skin contact. PAHs are the major concern in exposures found in coal gasification, aluminum production, iron and steel foundries, coke production, and occupations involved with diesel engine exhaust, carbon black, and coal tar. Complex mixtures containing some PAHs have been implicated as causes of skin cancer[29] and compose a large group of chemical carcinogens found in the workplace. These chemical complex mixtures include coal tar pitch, mineral oil, anthracene, chimney soot, shale oil, creosote, asphalt, crude paraffin waxes, cotton-mule spinning oil, and others.

PAHs have also been associated with lung, skin, breast, and bladder cancer.[30] PAH-induced carcinogenesis involves a number of steps including: (1) the enzymatic activation of the PAH into metabolites; (2) the covalent binding of the PAH metabolites to DNA; and (3) the induction of mutations that serve to initiate the transformation process as a result of PAH-DNA adducts. PAH can covalently bind to DNA, RNA, and proteins, but it is the amount of covalent interaction between PAH and DNA that correlates with carcinogenicity.[31]

The relationship of PAHs and SCC of the scrotum is well known. The development of SCC of the scrotum has been related to the presence of numerous pilosebaceous follicles on the scrotal skin. It is theorized that the lipid-soluble carcinogenic chemicals concentrate in sebum. Despite long-established knowledge of this association, scrotal tumors continue to occur in exposed workers.

Exposure of the skin to coal tar and other PAH-containing products can cause erythema and an acute burning sensation at the site of contact. Exposure to sunlight intensifies the burning sensation because these agents induce phototoxic contact dermatitis. Long-term contact has been implicated in chronic skin changes, including irregular areas of atrophy, patchy hyperpigmentation and hypopigmentation, wart-like papillomas (known in certain trades as tar warts), BCCs, and keratoacanthoma. The inhalation of volatilized PAHs may be associated with the development of skin cancer, but the importance of this route is uncertain because skin contact also generally occurs. Despite the laboratory modeling of cutaneous carcinogenesis of coal tar, decades long use of this therapeutic agent alone and with ultraviolet light (Geokerman therapy) have not demonstrated a clear increase in the incidence of skin cancer in treated individuals.[13,32]

Immunologic considerations in the development of NMSC

The interaction of the host's immune surveillance mechanism with tumor cells appears to be important in the development of NMSC. It is known that cell-mediated immune response declines with age, especially after age 50, leading to speculation that this decline may foster the development of skin cancer. Patients with primary immunodeficiency states have a much higher incidence of cutaneous malignancies than do normal individuals.[33,34] The high prevalence of skin cancer in immunosuppressed organ transplant recipients also implies a role for the immune system. One study found that the risk of developing BCC in renal transplant patients was 3.4 times greater than that of the general population, whereas for SCC it was 36 times greater. Risks of 1.4 times and 18 times normal for BCC and SCC, respectively, in immunosuppressed subjects have also been reported.

Immunosuppression induced by oral glucocorticoids in the absence of organ transplantation has also been associated with an increased risk of NMSC, and SCC in particular.[35] In patients infected with HIV, the incidence of epithelial neoplasms is markedly increased especially in oral, cervical, and anorectal sites.[36] BCCs have been reported on unexposed sites in HIV-seropositive patients, as has metastatic BCC, probably as a consequence of immunocompromise.

Langerhans' cells present in the epidermis play pivotal roles in the immune surveillance of the skin, with important functions in contact hypersensitivity reactions and foreign antigen presentation. UV radiation has been shown to deplete the epidermis of this important cell, with resultant decreases in delayed hypersensitivity reactions to dinitrofluorobenzene, a contact-sensitizing agent. Evidence also exists that epidermal Langerhans' cells in patients with BCC are abnormal, including altered Langerhans' cell morphology and disruption of the usually uniform Langerhans' cell network.

UV radiation also has been shown to decrease the total number of circulating T cells, as well as decrease the T-helper/T-suppressor cell ratio, and increase the number of T-suppressor cells. These studies suggest that exposure to UV radiation may alter T cell function, hampering immune rejection of malignantly transformed keratinocytes.

Further support for the importance of the immune surveillance system in the control of NMSC comes from the effectiveness of immunomodulators such as interferon and imiquimod in the treatment of BCC. In a clinical trial of 194 patients with BCC, the use of α-2-interferon resulted in a complete regression of 89% of patients treated with interferon.[37] The mechanism by which IFN-α produces regression of BCC relates to a considerable increase in the number of CD4+ T cells infiltrating the dermis and surrounding the BCC. The CD4+ cytotoxic T cells are capable of inducing apoptosis in their target cells via CD95 receptor–CD95 ligand interaction. In IFN-α-treated patients BCC cells express not only CD95 ligand but also CD95 receptor. Upon intralesional IFN-α treatment BCCs commit suicide by concomitant expression of both CD95 receptor and CD95 ligand.[38] More recently, the immune response modifier imiquimod has been demonstrated to induce cytokines including interferon-α and shown to be efficacious in the topical treatment of superficial BCC in clinical trials.[39]

Other host factors that may relate to the development of NMSC

It is known that patients who lack skin pigment (albinos) develop skin cancer at an early age. In the rare skin disease xeroderma pigmentosum (XP) there is a hereditary defect in the ability to repair damage to DNA induced by UV exposure. Patients with XP develop AKs, SCCs, BCCs, and malignant melanomas (MMs) early in life and succumb from metastatic disease, often in their second or third decade. The risk of developing skin cancer in XP patients is 2000 times greater than the general population, and heterozygotes also are at greater risk.[40] Differences in the ability to repair UV-induced DNA damage have been associated with the development of BCC in women.

MALIGNANT MELANOMA (MM)
Non-malignant skin lesions

Dysplastic nevus syndrome

Large and irregular shaped nevi were first described in 1978 in a family with a high incidence of MM. Such lesions are now known to occur without a familial association while still carrying an increased risk for the development of MM.

Lentigo maligna

This lesion, also known as the melanotic freckle of Hutchinson, occurs on the exposed surfaces of the elderly and usually is found on the face. It is an in situ MM. It is indolent and slowly evolves over many years to become a large brown patch with uneven coloration. It is estimated that 30–50% of such lesions eventually metamorphose into invasive MM.

Clinical types of malignant melanoma

MM tumors are derived from the epidermal melanocyte. Its common morphologic variants are superficial spreading melanoma (SSM), lentigo maligna melanoma (LMM), nodular melanoma (NM), and acral or mucosal lentiginous melanoma. Although these histologic types do not correlate with survival as was suggested by early studies, the classification remains useful as a way to characterize the several morphologic variants of MM that may be seen clinically. These conditions are briefly discussed in turn.

SSM is the most common type of MM and comprises 70% of the cases in the United States. The lesions are usually 1–2 cm in diameter when discovered and classically involve the trunk and extremities, usually proximal to the ankles and wrist. The tumor usually has a radial growth phase of 1–7 years prior to initiating a vertical growth pattern that results in the formation of nodules. The melanotic tumor cells appear uniformly malignant, with large nuclei and prominent nucleoli. The tumor cells are evident along the basal layer of the epidermis as well as being scattered through the upper epidermal strata. Clinically, one sees a patch of altered pigmentation with areas of recession of the pigment and areas of inflammation (Fig. 30.9.5). Regional node involvement or hepatic metastases may be evident if there is a nodule present due to vertical growth. In the absence of a nodular pattern of growth, there may be no extension of the tumor beyond the primary site.

NM represents approximately 15% of all cases of MM. It develops as an invasive nodule without lateral spread. The nodules may be dark gray or pink in color and usually arise more rapidly than other forms of melanoma. They may develop on any mucosal or cutaneous surface but usually are seen on the trunk. On examination, the patient has a black nodule, usually with an area of erythema around it. The history of the lesion may be as short as a few weeks and regional lymph node involvement or hepatic metastases are frequently evident.

LMM is the least common type of MM. Such tumors are seen in elderly patients with a history of sun exposure and occur almost exclusively on the face and neck. They arise out of persistent areas of hyperpigmentation known as lentigo maligna and appear as a brown patch with variegate pigmentation. Once these cells alter their growth pattern and invade the dermis, the lesion changes from an indolent lesion to one with the potential to metastasize.

Acral lentiginous melanoma and mucosal lentiginous melanoma occur more commonly in darker skinned patients. The acral variant usually occurs on the palms, soles, and subungual areas, with the mucosal surfaces being involved in mucosal lentiginous melanoma, as the name implies. The two subtypes are very similar histologically to LMM, although clinically acral and mucosal lentiginous melanomas tend to behave much more aggressively.

The prognosis in MM is highly dependent on the depth of penetration, which can be assessed by measuring the thickness of the lesion from the granular layer, or the ulcer base, to the lowest extent of the tumor cells. The most recent American Joint Committee on Cancer[41] guidelines classify melanoma into a TNM staging system whereby importance is placed on tumor thickness, the presence of histologic ulceration, the number of involved lymph nodes, and the presence of an elevated serum lactic dehydrogenase level.

Epidemiology of malignant melanoma

Similar to NMSC, the incidence of cutaneous MM has been rising rapidly.[42] The American Cancer Society estimated that there would be 53,600 new cases of MM in the United States in 2002 with 7400 deaths. MM accounts for nearly 4% of skin neoplasms but represents close to 80% of skin cancer mortality. From 1973 to 1994, the incidence of MM rose 120%, faster than most other cancers in the United States. MM now accounts for between 1% and 2% of all cancer deaths in the United States. The current lifetime risk for Americans of experiencing melanoma is approximately 1 in 75. Unfortunately, cancer registries have not been as effective in the collection of data related to MM as for other cancers because often the lesions are excised in doctors' offices and may not be captured for incidence statistics. It is unclear to what extent improvement in the collection of such data may account for the observed changes in incidence.

Ultraviolet light exposure and malignant melanoma

There is an inverse relationship between latitude of residence and MM incidence, and individuals with light complexion, blue eyes, and blond or red hair appear to be at greater risk for MM, similar to NMSC.[43] However, the relationship of MM to sunlight exposure is more complex than that of NMSC.[44] With the exception of LMM, which is associated with cumulative sun exposure and appears primarily on the face and sun-exposed areas, long-term continuous exposure to sunlight does not appear to be a risk factor for MM. MM risk is more closely related to intermittent intense rather than total UV exposure.[45] MM is more common in professional workers of relatively high socioeconomic status than blue collar and outdoor workers,[46–48] and in those with intermittent, intense UV exposure and sunburn in childhood. In fact, outdoor work has been found to be protective against the development of MM,[49] particularly in males who started work outside at a young age and continued for at least 10 years. The mechanism by which continuous sun exposure may be protective is unknown.

A number of studies support recreational and intermittent sunlight exposure as a risk factor for the development of MM. In Queensland, Australia, the occurrence of multiple sunburns has been used as a surrogate for acute high-dose UV radiation exposure, with an estimated relative risk of 2.4 for those categorized as having experienced six or more sunburns and a relative risk of 1.5 for those having had two to five sunburns in their lives. Another case-control study found that the MM incidence rate was

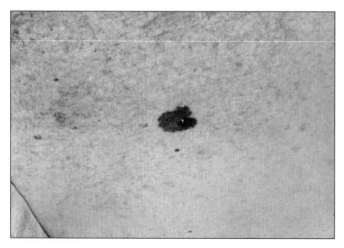

Figure 30.9.5: Superficial spreading malignant melanoma.

associated with frequent sunbathing between the ages of 15 and 24 and with exposure of the trunk while working outdoors.[50] Support for the intermittent exposure hypothesis also has come from studies of sunlamps and tanning booths. Increased risk for developing MM has been found to be associated with the use of artificial tanning devices. A case-control study found a 2.9-fold increase in MM risk in those who use UV lamps or sun beds; this risk increased as the duration of use increased.[51]

In addition to the manner in which one is exposed to UV radiation (e.g., intermittent or continuous), the age at which the UV exposure occurs is also an important factor. Among British immigrants to Australia, immigrants arriving before age 10 appear to have a risk of developing MM similar to that of native-born Australians. Immigrants arriving after the age of 15 were at one-quarter the risk. Other studies also have found an increased risk for MM with intense UV radiation exposure at an early age, with little risk occurring after the age of 30, and no risk associated with occupational exposure.[52] These studies lend support to the idea of a critical time period of exposure being necessary for the development of MM. Possible explanations that have been advanced for the association of UV exposure in childhood and adolescence with the risk of MM are as follows.

1. Melanocytes may be more sensitive to the sun in childhood.
2. More severe blistering sunburns in the teenage years occur due to adolescent behavior patterns.
3. Passing through critical stages of a multistep pathway for carcinogenesis early in life increases the chance of later completing the remaining stages of carcinogenesis.

Host and genetic factors also play a role in the interaction of UV radiation exposure and the development of MM. After UV exposure subjects whose population of melanocytes is relatively small experience greater increases in the size of their melanocyte population in both exposed and unexposed skin when compared with subjects with larger pre-exposure melanocyte populations. Therefore, individuals with low melanocyte density (e.g., redheads) may constitute a high-risk group for development of MM due to the fact that their melanocyte must enter a higher mitotic rate following UV radiation exposure than more pigmented individuals.[53]

Another host risk factor for MM is the propensity to freckle and develop nevi. It has been shown that the propensity to freckle is significantly higher in patients with MM than in controls. Increased numbers of melanocytic nevi have been associated with MM. The relative risk of developing MM has been found to be 30 in subjects with many nevi on the body. Increased risk of MM is seen in those with multiple, large or dysplastic nevi, a family history of MM, and dysplastic nevus syndrome.[54,55]

Suspected and reported chemical causes of malignant melanoma

Although light is an important factor in the development of MM, MM cannot be accounted for totally by UV radiation exposure. In keeping with this concept, it is notable that MM is ubiquitous in the vertebrate animal kingdom, from fish to higher forms of life in which UV radiation exposure often is limited due to the marked photoprotection offered by hair. The occurrence of acral lentiginous MM on the palms and soles of dark skinned individuals also argues against UV radiation as the sole causative factor.

Polychlorinated biphenyls (PCBs), which were previously used as insulating fluids in electrical transformers, capacitors, and switches, have been associated with melanoma. An epidemiologic study conducted among 138,905 men, mostly electrical power company workers, with long-term occupational exposure to polychlorinated biphenyls (PCBs) between 1950 and 1986 suggested that mortality from malignant melanoma increased with PCB exposure.[56] Rate ratios for melanoma relative to unexposed men ranged from 1.23 to 1.93 depending on the length of exposure. However, the preponderance of the epidemiologic studies suggests that PCB exposure and related congeners are only reliably associated with certain non-cancerous skin changes, acneiform eruptions, and eye irritation, and not with MM.[57–60]

Cutaneous MM has been associated with possible exposures in pulp and paper,[61] airline,[62] printing,[63] pharmaceutical,[64] telecommunications,[65] and petrochemical industries.[66] Although there is some limited experimental evidence to suspect chemical causes,[67] the human information is far too sparse to draw conclusions at this time. Consequently, the current theories on the pathogenesis of malignant melanoma have not been linked to chemical exposures except for psoralens in combination with UVA radiation (PUVA).[68]

MYCOSIS FUNGOIDES

First described by Alibert in 1806, mycosis fungoides (MF) is now known to be a chronic T-cell lymphoma (CTCL) of the skin that may involve the blood, resulting in a mononuclear cell leukemia called Sezary syndrome. Incidence rates for CTCL vary considerably from 0.13 to 0.9 per 100,000 people per year. It is somewhat more common in men and tends to develop in the middle years of life. Although usually presenting as slowly growing flat lesions that slowly increase in number, it may start as an erythroderma or sudden fulminant disease with rapidly enlarging ulcerating tumors. It has been linked with an association with various industrial exposures[69] and multiple cases of MF have been reported in immune-suppressed patients with a history of organ transplantation or human immunodeficiency virus infection.[70] The role of long-standing topical antigen exposure with chronic allergic contact dermatitis and subsequent development of this malignant T-cell tumor is intriguing but remains an unlikely etiologic scenario.

PREVENTION OF OCCUPATIONAL SKIN CANCER
Personal protective equipment

Protective clothing is most useful as a barrier to UV radiation exposure. If this does not produce heat stress or interfere with tasks at work, workers are more likely to comply. Hats with brims and sunglasses are also helpful. When clothing is not practical, topical sunscreen formulations can be used. It has been estimated that the use of sunscreens in childhood and adolescence could result in as much as a 78% reduction in the incidence of NMSC in adults.

Sunscreens should be used daily on individuals habitually exposed to the sun, by people with fair skin who freckle and sunburn easily, and by those who are hypersensitive to the sun. They fall into two broad categories of absorbing and reflecting agents. The absorbing agents contain chromophores that absorb photons of UV light and prevent its entry into the epidermis, thus preventing UV-induced injury. Early chemical sunscreen agents were frequently associated with allergic contact and photo-allergic contact sensitivity reactions and often discolored clothing. The common ingredients in current formulations are para-aminobenzoic acid (PABA) esters, cinnamates, and benzophenone and avobenzone. These products provide protection in the UVA and UVB spectrum and have the advantage of invisibility on the skin and thus they are cosmetically acceptable to most individuals.

Reflecting agents include substances like zinc oxide and titanium dioxide. Such agents provide excellent protection from UV, but are not invisible. Such products have enjoyed considerable use in high-altitude work. On the label of such products sold in the United States, a sun-protective factor (SPF) number is found. This number is the ratio between the time needed to produce a sunburn response in a normal person with the product divided by the time needed to do so without it. Greater photoprotection is provided at higher SPF numbers. A dry T-shirt alone only provides protection equal to a sunscreen with an SPF of 8. Once wet, its level of sun protection drops down to SPF 4.

Ionizing radiation can be effectively attenuated by the use of shielding devices such as gloves, aprons, and lead containers.

Protection from skin contamination with PAHs and other possible environmental causes of skin cancer can be accomplished by the use of appropriate gloves, gauntlets, uniforms, and aprons. Impervious materials should be used for these items since devices made of latex and vinyl may allow for the penetration of solvents. Frequent changes in the protective devices will give the best protection. Engineering alterations are preferred for situations where personal protection is necessary continuously.

Engineering controls

Enclosures can be constructed to limit exposure to UV radiation. Simple devices such as an awning over the work area of a fishing boat can significantly reduce UV radiation exposure. This equally applies to ionizing radiation sources.

In an experimental study of skin tumor induction in mice, lubricating oils that had been treated with a new form of severe hydro treatment to remove PAHs, did not induce skin tumors. Control groups of mice treated with unrefined crude oil and benzo[a]pyrene developed a significant number of skin tumors. Analysis of the hydro-treated

lubricating oil found a substantial decrease in the PAH concentration.[71] This shows that new severe hydro-treated lubricating oils have been converted from carcinogenic to less carcinogenic materials.

Medical surveillance

The surveillance program for workers with exposure that could lead to the development of skin cancer should involve a cutaneous examination. The procedure must be carried out in a well-lit room by staff experienced in such examinations. Early diagnosis in the case of MM may be life saving.[72] In the case of SCC, Bowen's disease, and actinic cheilitis, early intervention may significantly alter the outcome and prevent death of the worker. In the case of AKs, BCCs, and SCCs developing on sun-exposed skin, early intervention should reduce scarring and disfigurement. While surveillance programs are important in monitoring the efficacy of hygiene practices, regular annual integumentary examinations for individuals with exposure to UV light through occupation or recreation is advisable.

The implementation of preplacement and periodic examinations leads to the consideration that certain workers may be at greater risk of developing skin cancer. Some of these risk factors are evident on cutaneous examination. For instance, workers with fair skin, blue eyes, and red or blonde hair who freckle are more susceptible. Should such a worker choose to enter a job where there are higher levels of exposure to UV radiation and/or photo-sensitizers, he or she should be advised of the risk and careful skin self-examination and use of protective practices for work and recreational activities. It is likely that in the future, biomarkers of an increase in susceptibility to skin cancer may be available. Recent work suggests that women with BCC have a reduced ability to repair altered DNA in their peripheral white blood cells. These markers may offer additional ways to target workers who may be at increased risk and ensure that all steps are being taken to prevent the development of skin cancer, but should not be used to exclude workers from jobs with exposure to skin carcinogens.

References

1. Staibano S, Lo Muzio L, Pannone G, et al. P53 and hMSH2 expression in basal cell carcinomas and malignant melanomas from photoexposed areas of head and neck region. Int J Oncol 2001; 19:551–9.
2. Emmett EA. Occupational skin cancers. State Art Rev Occup Med 1987; 2:165–77.
3. Snow SN, Sahl W, Lo JS, et al. Metastatic basal cell carcinoma: report of five cases. Cancer 1994; 73:328–35.
4. Howell J. Nevoid basal cell carcinoma syndrome. Profile of genetic and environmental factors in oncogenesis. J Am Acad Dermatol 1984; 11:98–104.
5. Glass AG, Hoover RN. The emerging epidemic of melanoma and squamous cell skin cancer. JAMA 1989; 262:2097–100.
6. Marks R, Jolley D, Dorevitch AP, et al. The incidence of non-melanocytic skin cancers in an Australian population: results of a five-year prospective study. Med J Aust 1989; 150:475–8.
7. Diffey BL. Analysis of the risk of skin cancer from sunlight and solaria in subjects living in northern Europe. Photodermatology 1987; 4:118–26.

8. Stierner U, Rosdahl I, Augustsson A, et al. UVB irradiation induces melanocyte increase in both exposed and shielded human skin. J Invest Dermatol 1989; 92:561–4.

9. Staberg B, Wulf HC, Klemp P, et al. The carcinogenic effect of UVA irradiation. J Invest Dermatol 1983; 81:517–9.

10. Strickland PT, Vitasa BC, West SK, et al. Quantitative carcinogenesis in man: solar ultraviolet B dose dependence of skin cancer in Maryland watermen. J Natl Cancer Inst 1989; 81:1910–3.

11. Rundel RD, Nachtwey DS. Projections of increased non-melanoma skin cancer incidence due to ozone depletion. Photochem Photobiol 1983; 38:577–91.

12. Tanew A, Honigsmann H, Ortal B, et al. Nonmelanoma skin tumors in long-term photochemotherapy treatment of psoriasis. J Am Acad Dermatol 1986; 15:960–5.

13. Stern RS, Lange R. Non-melanoma skin cancer in patients treated with PUVA five to ten years after first treatment. J Invest Dermatol 1988; 91:120–4.

14. Frentz G. Grenz ray-induced nonmelanoma skin cancer. J Am Acad Dermatol 1989; 21:475–8.

15. Lichter MD, Karagas MR, Mott LA, Spencer SK, Stukel TA, Greenberg ER. Therapeutic ionizing radiation and the incidence of basal cell carcinoma and squamous cell carcinoma. The New Hampshire Skin Cancer Study Group. Arch Dermatol 2000; 136:1007–11

16. Stoll HL, Crissey JT. Epithelioma from single trauma. In: Helm F, ed. Cancer dermatology. Philadelphia: Lea & Febiger, 1979;25–30.

17. Gallagher RP, Bajdik CD, Fincham S, et al. Chemical exposures, medical history, and risk of squamous and basal cell carcinoma of the skin. Cancer Epidemiol Biomarkers Prev 1996; 5:419–24.

18. James RC, Busch H, Tamburro CH, et al. Polychlorinated biphenyl exposure and human disease. J Occup Med 1993; 35:136–48.

19. Langard S, Rosenberg J, Andersen A, Heldaas SS. Incidence of cancer among workers exposed to vinyl chloride in polyvinyl chloride manufacture. Occup Environ Med 2000; 57:65–8.

20. De Hertog SA, Wensveen CA, Bastiaens MT, et al. Leiden Skin Cancer Study. Relation between smoking and skin cancer. J Clin Oncol 2001; 19:231–8.

21. Pershagen G. The carcinogenicity of arsenic. Environ Health Perspect 1981; 40:93–100.

22. Tseng WP. Effects and dose–response relationship of skin cancer and blackfoot disease with arsenic. Environ Health Perspect 1977; 19:109–19.

23. Kitchin KT. Recent advances in arsenic carcinogenesis: modes of action, animal model systems, and methylated arsenic metabolites. Toxicol Appl Pharmacol 2001; 172:249–61.

24. Rossman TG, Uddin AN, Burns FJ, Bosland MC. Arsenite is a cocarcinogen with solar ultraviolet radiation for mouse skin: an animal model for arsenic carcinogenesis. Toxicol Appl Pharmacol 2001; 176:64–71.

25. Nordenson I, Beckman G, Beckman L, et al. Occupational and environmental risks in and around a smelter in northern Sweden. II. Chromosomal alterations in workers exposed to arsenic. Hereditas 1978; 88:47.

26. Petres J, Baron D, Hagedorn M. Effects of arsenic cell metabolism and cell proliferation: cytogenic and biochemical studies. Environ Health Perspect 1977; 19:223.

27. Shannon RE, Strayer DS. Arsenic-induced skin toxicity. Hum Toxicol 1989; 8:99–104.

28. Tseng WP, Chu HM, How SW, et al. Prevalence of skin cancer in an endemic area of chronic arsenicism in Taiwan. J Natl Cancer Inst 1968; 40:453–63.

29. Partanen T, Boffetta P. Cancer risk in asphalt workers and roofers: review and meta-analysis of epidemiologic studies. Am J Ind Med 1994; 26:721–40.

30. Boffetta P, Jourenkova N, Gustavsson P. Cancer risk from occupational and environmental exposure to polycyclic aromatic hydrocarbons. Cancer Causes Control 1997; 8:444–72.

31. Marston CP, Pereira C, Ferguson J, et al. Effect of a complex environmental mixture from coal tar containing polycyclic aromatic hydrocarbons (PAH) on the tumor initiation, PAH-DNA binding and metabolic activation of carcinogenic PAH in mouse epidermis. Carcinogenesis 2001; 22:1077–86.

32. Pion IA, Koenig KL, Lim HW. Is dermatologic usage of coal tar carcinogenic? A review of the literature. Dermatol Surg 1995; 21:227–31.

33. Kripke M. Immunology and photocarcinogenesis. J Am Acad Dermatol 1986; 14:149–55.

34. Gatti RA, Good RA. Occurrence of malignancy in immunodeficiency states. Cancer 1971; 28:84–9.

35. Karagas MR, Cushing GL Jr, Greenberg ER, Mott LA, Spencer SK, Nierenberg DW. Non-melanoma skin cancers and glucocorticoid therapy. Br J Cancer 2001; 85:683–6.

36. Aftergut K, Cockerell CJ. Update on the cutaneous manifestations of HIV infection. Clinical and pathologic features. Dermatol Clin 1999; 17:445–71.

37. Cornell RC, Greenway HT, Tucker SB, et al. Intralesional interferon therapy for basal cell carcinoma. J Am Acad Dermatol 1990; 23:694–700.

38. Buechner SA, Wernli M, Harr T, Hahn S, Itin P, Erb P. Regression of basal cell carcinoma by intralesional interferon-alpha treatment is mediated by CD95 (Apo-1/Fas)-CD95 ligand-induced suicide. J Clin Invest 1997; 100:2691–6.

39. Marks R, Gebauer K, Shumack S, et al. The Australasian Multicentre Trial Group. Imiquimod 5% cream in the treatment of superficial basal cell carcinoma: results of a multicenter 6-week dose–response trial. J Am Acad Dermatol 2001; 44:807–13.

40. Kraemer H, Lee M, Scotto J. DNA repair protects against cutaneous and internal neoplasia: evidence from xeroderma pigmentosum. Carcinogenesis 1984; 5:511–7.

41. Balch CM, Buzaid AC, Soong S-J, et al. Final version of the American Joint Committee on Cancer staging system for cutaneous melanoma. J Clin Oncol 2001; 19:3635–48.

42. Hall HI, Miller DR, Rogers JD, Bewerse B. Update on the incidence and mortality from melanoma in the United States. J Am Acad Dermatol 1999; 40:35–42.

43. Evans RD, Kopf AW, Lew RA, et al. Risk factors for the development of malignant melanoma. I: Review of case control studies. J Dermatol Surg Oncol 1988; 14:393–408.

44. Koh HK, Kligler BE, Lew RA. Sunlight and cutaneous malignant melanoma: Evidence for and against causation. Photochem Photobiol 1990; 51:765–79.

45. Armstrong BK. Kricker A. The epidemiology of UV induced skin cancer. J Photochem Photobiol B Biol 2001; 63:8–18.

46. Gallagher RP, Elwood JM, Threlfall WJ, et al. Socioeconomic status, sunlight exposure, and risk of malignant melanoma: the western Canada melanoma study. J Natl Cancer Inst 1987; 79:647–52.

47. Kirkpatrick CS, Lee JAH, White F. Melanoma risk by age and socioeconomic status. Int J Cancer 1990; 46:1–4.

48. Vagero D, Swerdlow AJ, Beral V, et al. Occupation and malignant melanoma: a study based on cancer registration data in England and Wales and in Sweden. Br J Ind Med 1990; 47:317–24.

49. Garland FC, White MR, Garland CF, et al. Occupational sunlight exposure and melanoma in the US Navy. Arch Environ Health 1990; 45:261–7.

50. Armstrong BK. Epidemiology of malignant melanoma: intermittent or total accumulated exposure to the sun. J Dermatol Surg Oncol 1988; 14:835–49.

51. Walter SD, Marrett LD, From L, et al. The association of cutaneous malignant melanoma with the use of sunbeds and sunlamps. Am J Epidemiol 1990; 131:232–43.

52. Weinstock MA, Colditz GA, Willett WC, et al. Nonfamilial cutaneous melanoma incidence in women associated with sun exposure before 20 years of age. Paediatrics 1989; 84:199–204.

53. Bell CMJ, Jenkinson CM, Murrells TJ, et al. Aetiologic factors in cutaneous malignant melanomas seen at a UK skin clinic. J Epidemiol Commun Health 1987; 41:306–11.

54. Holman CJ, Armstrong BK. Pigmentary traits, ethnic origin, benign naevi, and family history as risk factors for cutaneous malignant melanoma. J Natl Cancer Inst 1984; 72:257–66.

55. Holly EA, Kelly JW, Shpall SN, et al. Number of melanocytic nevi as a major risk factor for malignant melanoma. J Am Acad Dermatol 1987; 17:459–68.

56. Loomis D, Browning SR, Schenck AP, Gregory E, Savitz DA. Cancer mortality among electric utility workers exposed to polychlorinated biphenyls. Occup Environ Med 1997; 54:720–8.

57. Bertazzi PA, Riboldi L, Pesatori A, et al. Cancer mortality of capacitor manufacturing workers. Am J Ind Med 1987; 11:165–76.

58. Brown D. Mortality of workers exposed to polychlorinated biphenyls: an update. Arch Environ Health 1987; 42:333–9.

59. Gustavsson P, Hogstedt C, Rappe C. Short-term mortality and cancer incidence in capacitor manufacturing workers exposed to polychlorinated biphenyls (PCBs). Am J Ind Med 1986; 10:341–4.

60. Robinson CF, Petersen M, Palu S. Mortality patterns among electrical workers employed in the US construction industry, 1982–1987. Am J Ind Med 1999; 36:630–7.

61. Band PR, Le ND, Fang R, et al. Cohort cancer incidence among pulp and paper mill workers in British Columbia. Scand J Work Environ Health 2001; 27:113–9.

62. Nicholas JS, Butler GC, Lackland DT, Tessier GS, Mohr LC Jr, Hoel DG. Health among commercial airline pilots. Aviat Space Environ Med 2001; 72:821–6.

63. Dubrow R. Malignant melanoma in the printing industry. Am J Ind Med 1986; 10:119–26.

64. Thomas TL, Decoufle P. Mortality among workers employed in the pharmaceutical industry. A preliminary investigation. J Occup Med 1979; 21:619–23.

65. Deguire L, Theriault G, Iturra H, et al. Increased incidence of malignant melanoma of the skin in workers in a telecommunications industry. Br J Ind Med 1988; 45:824–8.

66. Wright WE, Peters JM, Mack TM. Organic chemicals and malignant melanoma. Am J Ind Med 1983; 4:577–81.

67. Pawlowski A, Lea PJ. Nevi and melanoma induced by chemical carcinogens in laboratory animals: similarities and differences with human lesions. J Cutan Pathol 1983; 10:81–110.

68. Stern RS, Nichols KT, Vakeva LH. Malignant melanoma in patients treated for psoriasis with methoxsalen (psoralen) and ultraviolet A radiation (PUVA). The PUVA Follow-Up Study. N Engl J Med 1997; 336:1041–5.

69. Morales Suarez-Varela MM, Llopis Gonzalez A, Marquina Vila A, Bell J. Mycosis fungoides: review of epidemiological observations. Dermatology 2000; 201:21–8.

70. Nahass GT, Kraffert CA. Cutaneous T-cell lymphoma associated with the acquired immunodeficiency syndrome. Arch Dermatol 1991; 127:1020–2.

71. McKee RH, Daughtrey WC, Freeman JJ, et al. The dermal carcinogenic potential of unrefined and hydrotreated lubricating oils. J Appl Toxicol 1989; 9:265–70.

72. Koh H, Lew R, Prout M. Screening for melanoma/skin cancer: theoretic and practical considerations. J Am Acad Dermatol 1989; 20:159–72.

Chapter 31
Occupational Injuries

Bruce H Alexander, Frederick P Rivara

BACKGROUND

Injuries are a leading cause of work-related morbidity and mortality among persons in the labor force, and are responsible for substantial financial loss and decreased productivity. The US Department of Labor estimated that from 1997 to 2001 an average of 6036 fatal work-related injuries occurred annually in the US, with 5915 being reported in 2001.[1] These numbers exclude losses due to the terrorist attacks of September 11, 2001, which accounted for an additional 2886 work-related fatalities. In the same time period, 4.9 million non-fatal injuries were reported by the Bureau of Labor Statistics.[2] The long-term and economic burden of work-related injuries is substantial. The National Safety Council (NSC) estimates that 3.9 million disabling occupational injuries occurred in the United States in 2001.[3] The total estimated costs for these injuries were $132.1 billion, which included $24.6 billion in medical costs alone.[3] Work-related injuries also result in enormous losses in worker productivity. Injuries sustained in 2001 caused an estimated 85 million lost workdays, and another 45 million lost workdays were attributed to injuries from previous years. The cumulative economic effect of these lost workdays totaled $69.2 billion in lost wages and productivity. On an individual basis, approximately $970 of every worker's annual productivity is absorbed by the costs of occupational injury. The true number and costs of work-related injuries are unknown, and the NSC estimates are subject to debate. However, there is little debate on the importance of work-related injuries and the need to improve injury prevention measures.

THE SCIENCE OF INJURY CONTROL

Over the last three decades, the field of injury control has developed a solid scientific basis by which a substantial reduction in the morbidity and mortality from trauma can be expected. Injuries are viewed as preventable problems, not as 'accidents' that occur without pattern, predictability or reason. Viewing injuries as 'accidents' fosters a sense of fatalism, in which a certain number of deaths and permanently disabling injuries are believed to be inevitable.

One of the basic premises of this approach to trauma is conceptually separating the injury (i.e., the trauma to the individual) from the events leading to the injury. A motor vehicle collision is separate from the injuries that may or may not occur in the collision; the injuries are not an inevitable outcome of such an event. Even if the collision cannot be prevented, the chance of injury may be substantially decreased through the use of seat restraints and vehicle design to protect the occupants. Likewise, a slip from a roof does not need to lead to a fall and injury, if the person is restrained with a safety harness.

Once injuries occur, the outcome (recovery, temporary or permanent disability, or death) is also influenced by the availability of adequate pre-hospital care at the scene, rapid transport to an appropriately equipped trauma center, and the provision of rehabilitation care to return the individual back to his or her level of functioning before the injury. The emphasis is on injury control, a more comprehensive concept than the more traditional approach, which encompasses only injury prevention. The paradigm of injury control incorporates etiologic research, interventions, and outcomes (Fig. 31.1).[4] Etiologic research explores not only the causes of injury and the factors that reduce the frequency and severity of injury, but also how the body responds to energy transfer during an injury event and the healing process. The intervention phase of injury control focuses on modifying risk factors to prevent an injury from occurring and ameliorating the negative effects of injury events and any injuries that occur. The final aspect of injury control is to change the outcomes of hazardous situations by reducing the rate and severity of injury, decreasing the costs of injury and their impact on productivity, improving trauma care, and the overall quality of life of injured workers.

A useful tool for examining injury problems and determining potential avenues for intervention is the matrix developed by Haddon (Table 31.1).[5] This takes the classic epidemiologic paradigm of agent, host, and environment and applies it to the pre-event, event, and post-event factors associated with the occurrence of injury. The matrix also separates the physical environment from the sociocultural environment of laws, expectations, and norms that affect injuries and prevention strategies.

A large body of research conducted over the last two decades has established that injury prevention strategies are likely to be most successful if they operate automatically, without needing repeated behavioral change on the part of the individual.[6] Thus, modification of the environment or of the product and vehicle to reduce the hazards associated with their use are likely to have the greatest impact on injuries. Examples of these successes are airbags, anti-lock brakes, interstate highways, rollover protection devices on tractors, and bulletproof partitions in taxicabs. Legislation and regulation have also proved to be effective

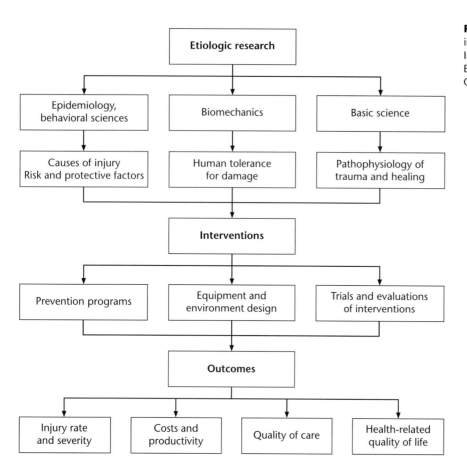

Figure 31.1: Conceptual model for occupational injury control. (Adapted from: Rivara FP. Introduction: the scientific basis for injury control. Epidemiol Rev 2003; 25:20–3 by permission of Oxford University Press.)

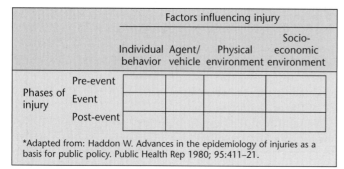

*Adapted from: Haddon W. Advances in the epidemiology of injuries as a basis for public policy. Public Health Rep 1980; 95:411–21.

Table 31.1 Haddon matrix*

adjuncts to decreasing the toll from injury. Mandatory seat belt use and motorcycle helmet laws have resulted in a substantial reduction of fatalities on the nation's highways. Gun control laws may help to curb the epidemic of homicides that occur both at home and at work.

The effectiveness of educational programs to change behavior is difficult to establish. Training workers in the proper use of equipment is a key safety measure in many industries. The fact that injuries are often associated with unsafe behavior attests to the difficulties inherent in this approach. Since its inception in 1971, OSHA has required engineering changes and workplace controls as the primary means of reducing hazards in the workplace.

The severity of an injury will vary depending on the mechanism and the underlying causal force. When evaluating the effectiveness of control programs or prioritizing prevention efforts, an understanding of the severity of injuries is necessary. Several algorithms for scoring the severity of injuries have been developed, although they have traditionally been directed toward predicting the survival and functional outcome of victims of very severe injuries. Some essential injury severity scoring systems include: the Abbreviated Injury Score (AIS), developed by the Association for the Advancement of Automotive Medicine,[7] that is primarily based on the diagnostic classification and location of injury, and the Injury Severity Score (ISS),[8,9] which is directly calculated from the most severe AIS scores of each body region and was developed as a method to characterize multiple injuries. Limitations of these scoring systems have led to the proposal of potential alternatives, including the New Injury Severity Score (NISS)[10] and the Anatomic Profile Score (APS),[11] that are intended to more accurately describe severity due to multiple injuries. More complex injury severity rating systems, which include physiologic parameters, have been specifically developed for evaluating patients in trauma centers.[12–14]

The above scoring systems, and several other proposed algorithms, are directed at the most severe injuries and often require substantial clinical information. A majority of the work-related injury burden may result in a range of

Indicators

- *Death*
- *Permanent total disability*: loss of functions necessary for work or routine life skills.
- *Permanent partial disability*: limits work or normal activities.
- *Time-loss injuries*: injuries that meet a minimum amount of time away from work, allowing the injured worker to collect worker compensation wage replacement. The criteria vary by state.
- *Return to work*: return to work or return to normal tasks. This may be influenced by the occupation and usual job tasks.
- *Re-assignment of work tasks/Restriction of work activities*: injury requires change in normal work duties. May or may not accompany reduction of income.

Care received

- *Hospitalization*: most severe injuries receiving medical treatment. Duration of hospitalization, procedures, and cost may correlate with severity. Usually only available through worker compensation insurance records.
- *Emergency room*: urgent care needed.
- *Physician office*: professional medical care needed. May or may not be urgent.
- *First aid*: these injuries are not generally reportable unless they result in a restriction or re-assignment of work activities.

Table 31.2 Potential indicators of severity for work-related injuries based on administrative data. Adapted from Haddon W. Advances in the epidemiology of injuries as a basis for public policy. Public Health Reports 1980; 95:411–421, by permission of Oxford University Press

permanent or temporary disability and medical care, but the relative severity of most of these injuries is not distinguishable using the existing scoring systems. Moreover, most of the available data for studying occupational injuries reside in administrative or surveillance databases, which may not contain the information necessary to calculate these injury severity scores. Alternative methods of evaluating injury severity for occupational injuries are based on the outcome of the injury and the immediate care received (Table 31.2). The most severe injuries are fatal, followed by those injuries resulting in either total or partial permanent disability. The level of medical treatment required, ranging from first aid to hospitalization, and other administrative variables, including time lost from work and re-assignment of usual tasks, can be used to classify injuries by severity. These methods, however, are not well validated and may be a function of occupation as well as the nature of the injury. An injured foot may not interfere with the work of a typist, but would prevent a construction worker from numerous activities.

SOURCES OF DATA FOR WORK-RELATED INJURIES

Data sources that characterize the injury problem and prioritize prevention measures are a fundamental element of injury prevention programs. Characterizing an injury problem and evaluating prevention efforts require effective means for injury surveillance. Data resources available for general injury surveillance and research include vital records, hospital discharge data, surveillance of emergency rooms, and trauma registries.[15,16] The extent to which these traditional sources of injury data can capture work-related injuries is quite variable. Several sources of data on occupational injuries in the United States are available; however, each source uses different methods of collecting information. The usefulness of these data requires an understanding of how the data are collected and their attendant limitations. The sources presented below represent the types of data routinely collected in the United States, but are by no means the only sources of data on occupational injuries.

Fatal work-related injuries

In 2002 an estimated four fatal work-related injuries occurred in the United States for every 100,000 persons employed. Historically, the number of work-related fatalities has been difficult to determine. In the United States, the Bureau of Labor Statistics and the National Institutes of Occupational Safety and Health (NIOSH) previously had systems that used different methods. The BLS primarily used employer reporting, while the NIOSH National Traumatic Occupational Fatality (NTOF) database relied solely on death certificate information collected by the National Center for Health Statistics. Other sources of information on fatal injuries, including OSHA reports, medical examiners, and workers' compensation claims, collected detailed information about fatal injury events, but did not capture most injuries. The available surveillance data were also used by other organizations, specifically the National Safety Council (NSC), to derive estimates of work-related fatalities.

The different approaches to fatality surveillance yielded markedly variable results and the lack of consistency represented a significant limitation. A review by Stout and Bell of the various reporting methods concluded that death certificates had the highest capture rate but only identified, on average, 81% of occupational fatalities, followed by medical examiner records (61%), workers' compensation claim data (57%), and lastly, OSHA records that identified only 32% of occupational fatalities.[17] A problem common to all systems was identifying the work-relatedness of a fatal injury. For example, identifying work-related fatalities from death certificates relies on the recorder to check the designated 'injury at work' box, a fact that is not always apparent to healthcare professionals treating the injury, or coroners and medical examiners. Incidents that happen on an employer's premises while the individual is conducting their job-related tasks are fairly readily identified. However, when the person is self-employed or the location of the incident is not at the work site (e.g., a fatal motor vehicle crash for a person in sales), the ability of most single systems to capture such incidents is limited. Consequently, a segment of the work-related fatalities is under-reported and it is unlikely these are distributed evenly by industry, occupation or cause.

Recognizing the limitations of existing systems, the BLS created the Census of Fatal Occupational Injuries (CFOI) in 1992.[2] This system uses multiple sources of information to identify cases of fatal work-related injuries, including death certificates, workers' compensation claims, newspapers, and investigations by OSHA or other state agencies. Each state is contracted to collect available data within the state and provide the BLS with the information. As with any surveillance system, the CFOI will not capture all fatal work-related injuries; however, the use of multiple data sources improves the probability of capture and will likely provide more information on the characteristics of the injured worker and cause of the injury.

Surveillance systems like CFOI are designed to enumerate cases, but are limited in their ability to identify contributing causes to the fatality. These depend on investigations of fatal injury incidents conducted by federal and state regulatory agencies. While these incident investigations are conducted too infrequently to qualify as classic surveillance systems, they provide a wealth of qualitative information on specific injury events and are examples of sentinel surveillance tools that can identify immediate problems. OSHA has developed the Integrated Management Information System (IMIS) based on OSHA inspection records. OSHA is responsible for workplace safety and health inspections in the 29 states and territories that do not have a state occupational health and safety plan. The other 23 states and two territories with state plans submit inspection reports to OSHA for the IMIS.

Other than routine inspections, a large number of OSHA inspections are performed in response to fatalities, which are required to be reported to OSHA within 48 hours of occurrence. OSHA does not investigate all fatalities but focuses on those that appear to be related to workplace safety. Inspections also are conducted in response to worker complaints and as a follow-up of citations from routine inspections. NIOSH has implemented the state-based Fatality Assessment and Control Evaluation Program[18] that conducts detailed investigations of specific types of fatal work-related injury incidents. Collection of these specific data can alert employers and workers to particular problems. NIOSH publishes a series of requests for assistance in preventing work-related injury and illness that is directed at identified problem areas,[19] for example trench cave-ins, falls through skylights, and work-related homicides.

Sources of injury morbidity data

In contrast to fatal injury events that represent the most severe work-related injuries, non-fatal work-related injuries may range from a minor injury that results only in a brief alteration of usual duties to one that results in permanent disability. Though less severe, non-fatal injuries occur over 1000 times more frequently than fatal injuries. The actual number of non-fatal work-related injuries is difficult to determine. In addition to the problems of designating work-relatedness, the mechanisms for surveillance may vary from state to state, with different definitions and rules for reporting. However, several sources of data are available to characterize the extent of the problem. Some of these data sources are amenable to etiologic research, while others are primarily useful as surveillance tools.

In the United States, national data are primarily available from the Bureau of Labor Statistics (BLS). The BLS compiles data on business and labor activities in the United States, including information on occupational injuries and illnesses occurring in the labor force. The primary source of data is the annual Survey of Occupational Injuries and Illnesses that is based on employer reports from approximately 180,000 private industry establishments. Additional information on mining and transportation activities is provided by the Department of Labor's Mine Safety and Health Administration (MSHA) and the Department of Transportation respectively. Selected establishments submit summarized data from the OSHA 200 forms to the BLS, indicating the number of occupational injuries and illnesses that occurred each year. Employers are required to report all injuries that are fatal and injuries that require medical care beyond first aid, result in loss of consciousness, lost work days or restriction of work, or transfer to another position. The average number of workers and total hours worked that year are collected, enabling rates to be calculated. Each establishment is classified by Standardized Industrial Code (SIC) according to its major enterprise. Annual survey data can be used to estimate the total number and rates of morbidity, mortality, and lost work-days due to occupational injury for each industry. Although this procedure identifies high-risk industries, the data lack information concerning the cause and type of the injury and specific high-risk groups identified by job classification or demographic characteristics.

At the state level, worker compensation claims data provide a reasonable estimate of the burden of non-fatal work-related injuries. The worker compensation insurance laws are state specific, with each state having a mechanism to characterize injury burden, therefore the data are not necessarily comparable between states. Most states require the reporting of fatal injuries and compensable injuries that result in time-loss, generally involving 3 days lost. In some states, such as Washington, the state is the sole-source provider of worker compensation insurance; thus all establishments that do not self-insure or are not covered by a federal program have claims processed by the state. In a majority of states the worker compensation insurance is issued by a third party insurer; thus collecting more than summary statistics is problematic. Nevertheless, worker compensation insurance claims can be a useful tool in monitoring non-fatal work-related injuries and identifying priority problem areas to target.

Other data sources

Several other sources of injury data that are not specific for occupational injuries are available and can be useful in identifying work-related injuries. The National Electronic Injury Surveillance System (NEISS), co-ordinated by the Consumer Product Safety Commission, surveys a sample of hospital emergency rooms throughout the country.[20] The NCHS collects fatality data, from which information on occupational fatalities can be extrapolated. The NCHS also collects injury morbidity data through the National Health Interview survey. The NSC does not collect original data on occupational injuries; however, it compiles data from other sources listed above and provides estimates of the occurrence and cost of occupational injuries.

CHARACTERISTICS OF OCCUPATIONAL INJURIES

Understanding the general distribution of occupational injuries by type of industry, occupation, and characteristics of the worker is necessary for establishing any injury prevention and control activities. These characteristics comprise the first layer of factors influencing the injury event, using the Haddon approach to injury control, and are distinct with increasing severity of injury.

Occupational fatalities

While the completeness of fatality surveillance data can be debated, the CFOI data effectively summarize the major factors related to fatal work-related injuries. In 2002 there were 5524 identified fatalities in the United States. The industry-wide rate was four fatalities for every 100,000 employed persons; however, this varied markedly by industry, occupation, and other characteristics. The highest rates were seen in the agriculture, mining, construction, and transportation industries (Table 31.3). The rates for agriculture and mining were more than five times the industry-wide average. Similar patterns have been identified by occupation type where construction laborers, farm occupations, and truck drivers had the highest rates of fatalities.

The most frequent types of fatal injury incidents were transportation related, falls, and homicides. Fully 43% (2381) of the 2002 fatalities were transportation-related incidents, of which 1372 occurred on highways. Accordingly, truck driving was an occupation with one of the highest fatal injury rates (25/100,000). Fatal fall injuries were predominantly falls from one level to another level, and 77% of the homicides were related to

firearms. Men account for 92% of the occupational fatalities with an annual rate that is 10-fold that of women (6.9 vs 0.69 per 100,000 persons employed); however, homicides account for 31% of fatalities in women, but only 9% in men (Fig. 31.2). The rates of occupational fatalities are similar for younger age groups, but begin to dramatically increase after age 65 (Fig. 31.3). Whether this increase is due to a higher rate of more severe injuries in this age group or a greater case-fatality rate associated with the elderly is not clear. In most traumatic injuries the elderly do have a substantially higher case-fatality rate than younger individuals.

	n	%	Rate*
Industrial division			
Construction	1121	20.3	12.2
Transportation	910	16.5	11.3
Agriculture	789	14.3	22.7
Services	680	12.3	1.7
Manufacturing	563	10.2	3.1
Government	554	10.0	2.7
Retail trade	487	8.8	2.1
Wholesale trade	205	3.7	4
Mining	121	2.2	23.5
Finance	87	1.6	1
Selected occupations			
Truck drivers	808	14.6	25.0
Farm occupations	519	9.4	28.0
Sales occupations	347	6.3	2.1
Construction laborers	302	5.5	27.7
Other laborers	181	3.3	14.2
Groundskeepers	146	2.6	15.0
Police and detectives	140	2.5	11.6
Electricians	116	2.1	13.5
Carpenters	108	2.0	6.9
Pilots and navigators	90	1.6	69.8
Total	5524	100	4.0

*Fatalities per 100,000 persons employed.

Table 31.3. Number and rate of fatal occupational injuries in the United States in 2002 as reported by the Bureau of Labor Statistics Census of Fatal Occupational Injuries

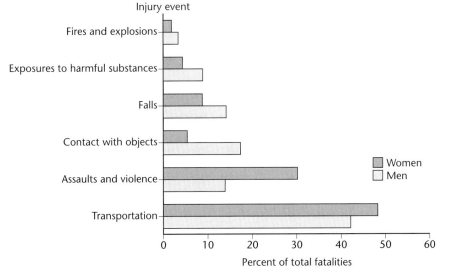

Figure 31.2: Gender distribution of fatal occupational injuries in the United States, 2002. (From the Bureau of Labor Statistics Census of Fatal Occupational Injuries.)

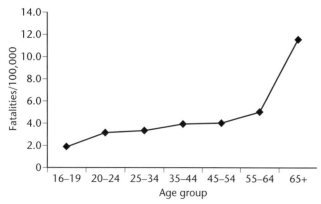

Figure 31.3: Rate of fatal occupational injuries by age group in the United States, 2002. (From the Bureau of Labor Statistics Census of Fatal Occupational Injuries.)

Identifying the industries and occupations with the highest occupational fatality rates provides some direction for injury prevention programs; however, it is necessary to identify the specific mechanism of injury to prevent further fatalities. The mechanism of injury will vary within an industry and occupational group. Among motor vehicle operators, highway fatalities account for 69% of fatal occupational injuries in truck drivers, while homicides account for only 2% of the fatalities. By contrast, 59% of fatalities among taxicab drivers are due to violence, whereas 37% of the deaths are roadway related. A clear difference between taxicab drivers and truck drivers is the degree to which they interact with the public. Similar differences are observed in the construction trades where the rate of fatal injuries among construction laborers is four times higher than for carpenters (27.7 vs 6.9/100,000); however, carpenters are much more likely to die from falls. These differences reflect the types of hazards inherent in the specific job activities.

Non-fatal occupational injuries

Unlike fatalities, non-fatal injuries lack a clear definition; in addition to determining the actual work-relatedness of an injury, it is important to understand which injuries are reportable. The BLS definition of a traumatic injury is an instantaneous event resulting in medical treatment beyond first aid or loss of consciousness, lost workdays, restriction of work or being transferred to another job. According to the BLS Annual Survey, the construction industry has the highest reported rates of injury, followed by agriculture (including forestry and fishing), manufacturing, and mining.[2] This ranking is essentially the same for the rate of lost workdays, a surrogate measure of severity. Mining, however, which had the fifth highest rate of injury, had the greatest number of lost workdays. Comparing the rankings of fatal and non-fatal injuries along with lost workdays identifies the high-risk industrial groups. Mining, transportation, construction, agriculture, and manufacturing are high-risk industries compared with services, retail and wholesale trade, and finance and real estate, which have relatively low injury rates.

The hazards identified in surveillance of fatal and non-fatal injuries will vary, even when the non-fatal injuries are severe. A comparison of fatal injuries and severe non-fatal injuries in Washington State revealed different patterns. For instance, roofers are at high risk of fatal fall injuries, based on national data, but burns are a significant cause of non-fatal injury. Similarly, in orchard workers fatalities were primarily due to motor-vehicle incidents, but the majority of hospitalized injuries were due to falls.[21]

TRENDS IN INJURY RATES

Rates of occupational injuries have not been stable over time, and trends vary by industry and occupation. The incidence of disabling injuries in manufacturing industries in the United States declined from the 1920s until approximately 1958, after which it appeared to rise. The incidence of injuries in the construction industry decreased from the 1940s until the mid-1950s; from approximately 1975, there has been a marked upward trend. Similar trends have been seen for injuries in wholesale and retail trade.[22] Conversely, the rate of fatal injuries in the mining industry dropped drastically over the last century as regulatory measures improved the safety records of mines.[23]

A general downward trend has been observed for both fatal and non-fatal injuries in the last two decades; however, the rates vary by industry and mechanism of injury. Fatality data indicate that the rate of motor vehicle-related deaths dropped in the transportation industry, but there was little improvement in the public administration, construction, and agriculture sectors. Within these long-term trends, there is cyclic fluctuation that has been observed to be associated with changes in the strength of the economy. For example, a 10% increase in the rate of new hires is associated with a 10.4% increase in injury rates, providing evidence that new workers have higher injury rates than their more experienced counterparts. Increases in productivity, measured as output per hour, are also associated with increases in injury rates.[24] The extent to which this increase is due to laxity in enforcement of safety practices in order to meet increased demand is uncertain.

Changes in occupational injury rates can serve as a measure of the effectiveness of prevention programs as well as pointing to areas in need of more effective interventions. However, the value of such data depends heavily on their quality and validity, as described earlier.

OCCUPATIONAL INJURY TYPES AND SETTINGS

Occupational injuries are characterized largely by the type of occupation or the type of injury. In either case there will be considerable heterogeneity within subsets of the population under study. In this section the characteristics of intentional injuries and agriculture-related injuries will be presented to demonstrate the scope of issues associated with specific injuries and their respective control interventioning.

Assaults and homicides

The classic perceptions of work-related injuries and fatalities evoke images of catastrophic events related to machinery, falls or explosions. The role of intentional injury in the workplace has been somewhat overlooked as a significant cause of morbidity and mortality. Homicide ranks as one of the leading causes of fatal occupational injury in the United States, accounting for the deaths of an estimated 609 workers in 2002 or 11% of all work-related fatalities.[1] While the rate of work-related homicide is two to three times greater for men than women, homicides are the leading cause of work-related death in women, accounting for approximately one-third of occupational deaths. Homicide is the second leading cause of death for workers aged 25–44, behind highway-related deaths, yet the rate of work-related homicide increases in workers over age 55. The majority of the homicides are committed by firearms. Assault-related injuries and fatalities are, to a large degree, specific to occupation. Surveillance data from 2002 indicate that 50–80% of the work-related fatalities in the technical, sales, and administrative support jobs are homicides.

A variety of surveillance systems have identified occupations at higher risk of homicide and assault; a common theme is the close interaction between the worker and the general public, often in isolation, including taxicab drivers, gas station and convenience store clerks, liquor store clerks, police officers, and security guards.[25,26] The occurrence of these fatal events is often associated with another crime, primarily robbery, and often in establishments with a prior history of such events.[27,28] In 1982 Baker and colleagues called for uniform standards to protect workers from homicides in the workplace;[29] however, none have been enacted to date. Possible prevention strategies include making cash registers visible from the street; the use of a drop safe at night for bills larger than $5; bulletproof barriers between driver and passenger in taxis; enclosed cashier booths in gasoline stations; protective vests for law enforcement personnel. Other strategies include the provision of training programs in conflict resolution and non-violent response; these have been implemented in some retail settings.

Non-fatal work-related assault is also a significant morbidity concern. As with homicides, the non-fatal work-related injuries occur disproportionately in occupations that have routine contact with the general public. The risks are higher for healthcare workers, social service workers, public transportation workers, and safety and corrections personnel.[27,30–33] Sexual assault in the workplace constitutes an important proportion of rape cases, but has received little attention in the occupational health and safety literature. The National Crime Victimization Survey has been used to characterize the victims of work-related physical assaults and robbery,[34] while occupational information is not collected by the FBI, nor reported in Uniform Crime Reports.

Violence and assault within the healthcare occupations have been evaluated for potential risk factors. Certain jobs that involve contact with high-risk patients, particularly patients with mental health conditions, are at highest risk.[35–37] Low staff-to-patient ratios may increase risk. The administrative recognition of risk as an inherent problem related to the job activities provides an opportunity to target intervention, including assault prevention training or presence of security guards. The success of interventions in workplace violence, however, has not been well documented, with several studies proving inconclusive.[38,39]

Agricultural injuries

Agriculture is one of the most dangerous industries in the United States. The annual death rate is 22.7 deaths per 100,000 workers compared with 4.0 deaths per 100,000 for the general private sector workforce.[1] Over the course of a typical 40–50-year career, farmers accrue a substantial lifetime risk of occupationally related mortality. Data on agricultural injuries include injuries to individuals involved with agricultural production, agricultural services, forestry, and fishing. Specifically, for agricultural crop production, livestock production and agricultural services, the rates of fatal injuries in 2002 were approximately 37.0, 12.5, and 13.8 per 100,000 workers, respectively.[1] The mortality for farmers 65 years of age and older appears to be two to three times that of younger workers.

Although agricultural machinery including tractors accounts for around 20% of minor farm injuries, they are responsible for more than half of all severe injuries that result in permanent disability, and about 40% or more of the fatalities. In contrast, injuries from animals are very rarely fatal but account for a sizeable proportion of mild injuries. Tractor-related injuries are the most common type of fatal agricultural trauma, accounting for 30–50% of all fatal injuries on the farm. Approximately one-half to three-fourths of these fatal incidents involve tractor rollovers. In the NTOF database, 69% of agricultural machinery deaths involve tractors, of which 52% were rollovers.[40,41]

One way to prevent these deaths is by using roll bars or crush-proof cabs, commonly referred to as rollover protection structures (ROPS), which were developed as early as 1959. In 1976, OSHA imposed standards requiring ROPS on all tractors used by employees, but this standard does not apply to the many tractor operators who are self-employed or farm family members. Furthermore, special legislation limited OSHA to inspect only farms employing more than 10 non-family members, effectively eliminating 89% of farms in the United States. A population-based study of tractor-related injuries in Minnesota indicated that only 42% of tractors were equipped with a ROPS,[42] which is representative of use in the US generally.[43] In contrast, mandatory standards for ROPS have been markedly effective in nearly eliminating tractor fatalities in Sweden. Since 1959, all new tractors in Sweden have had to be equipped with ROPS and since 1983 all workers, including employers and family members, had to be protected with ROPS on tractors.[44] A comparison of the number of fatalities, normalized to the number of tractors, suggests a 24-fold greater risk of tractor rollover fatalities in the US compared to Sweden.[43]

Other important sources of injury related to agricultural machinery include power take-off (PTO) devices and augers.[45] PTOs are rapidly rotating shafts on the tractor to power other machinery and account for 10–15% of fatal injuries and an even higher percentage of severe, disabling, but non-fatal traumatic injury. The injuries consist of fractures, severe soft tissue trauma, dislocations, nerve injuries and amputations. Although shielding is provided by the manufacturer, the shielding is often removed to make access to the PTO devices easier. Typically, a worker in proximity to an unshielded PTO shaft has an article of clothing pulled into the machine. As with ROPS, OSHA shielding regulations for PTOs apply only to inspected farms, thus most family farms and those with fewer than 11 employees are not covered.

As with ROPS, reliance on voluntary compliance by manufacturers and farmers appears to be ineffective. Grain augers are a source of serious and potentially devastating injuries. Invented by Archimedes to move water up a hill, modern augers and screw conveyors are widely used to transport wood, grain, meat, and other materials on the farm. The screw rotation of augers is 800 to 900 RPM with a pitch of 1:1. An auger with a 6-inch diameter moves material up the tube at 400 feet per minute or 7 feet per second. A finger that is caught in a tube will thus ascend a number of feet before the individual has time to react. The most common injuries are amputations, usually of fingers. Many of the injuries are at multiple levels because the spiral blades strike the limb several times as it is drawn up the tube. One half of those injured suffer significant permanent impairment.

The distribution of both fatal and non-fatal injuries is largely determined by the type of agriculture. In the Midwest, farm animals have been associated with up to 40% of the non-fatal farm-related injuries.[46] The risk of a farm animal-related injury is obviously related to the amount of contact an individual has with the animals, but is also influenced by the type of work done. For example, injuries among dairy cattle handlers will be affected by the amount of time doing specific tasks such as milking and hoof trimming.[47] Among California migrant workers, the tasks associated with injury included manual harvest, operating machinery, and cannery work.[48]

CHILDREN

Children make up a significant portion of the agricultural workforce and hence are exposed at an early age and often tragically to its hazards. Children may work for their parents; many more work alongside their migrant families as seasonal laborers. Like adults, children suffer injuries when engaged in agricultural work and the injuries are often severe. Children employed in agriculture production in California had elevated risks for death by machinery (OR = 81), animals (OR = 10), electricity (OR = 5), and non-traffic motor vehicles (OR = 3).[49] Minors under the age of 15 employed on farms in Washington State were over-represented in the number of claims filed by all minors;[50] furthermore, 26% of claims filed by minors employed in

agriculture were for serious injuries, compared with 16% for all other occupations. The rates of injury are higher for older adolescents, with males age 15–17 having the highest rates of injury.[51] While children employed in agriculture are clearly at substantial risk of injury, the extent of this problem has not been well characterized.

Estimates vary on the number of fatal injuries that occur among children and adolescents on farms each year, but range from 100 to approximately 300 children, with another 23,000 non-fatal injuries. Farm machinery accounts for one-third of deaths and nearly one-half of deaths of children under the age of 10 years. Firearms account for one in 10 deaths of children on farms, whereas farm animals are responsible for less than 2% of farm deaths among children, despite the relatively frequent exposure to this hazard.

There are very different attitudes and legislation for child farm labor compared with other employment of children in the workplace. Under the Fair Labor Standards Act, children as young as 12 and 13 years of age may be employed on any farm with the consent of their parents. These federal regulations are in marked contrast to those applying to non-agricultural occupations. For most other occupations, the basic minimum age is 16 years. Adolescents are especially prohibited from employment in manufacturing industries, which have a lower rate of fatalities than agriculture.

SUMMARY

In summary, occupational injuries are a complex problem requiring an array of preventive strategies. The first steps necessary for attacking the problem are (1) a change in orientation to one that views these injuries as events that are intrinsically preventable and (2) the use of a scientific approach to development of interventions. An important requirement for the success of this approach will be the development of adequate data systems in order to better understand the magnitude of the problem among specific populations, industries, and jobs at risk.

References

1. United States Department of Labor Bureau of Labor Statistics. National Census of Fatal Occupational Injuries in 2002. Washington, DC: Bureau of Labor Statistics, 2003.
2. United States Department of Labor Bureau of Labor Statistics. Workplace injuries and illnesses in 2001. Washington, DC: Bureau of Labor Statistics, 2002.
3. National Safety Council. Injury facts. Itasca, IL: National Safety Council, 2002.
4. Rivara FP. Introduction: the scientific basis for injury control. Epidemiol Rev 2003; 25:20–3.
5. Haddon W. Advances in the epidemiology of injuries as a basis for public policy. Public Health Rep 1980; 95:411–21.
6. Bonnie RJ, Fulco CE, Liverman CT, eds. Committee on Injury Prevention and Control, Institute of Medicine. Reducing the burden in injury: advancing prevention and treatment. Washington, DC: National Academy Press, 1999.
7. Association for the Advancement of Automotive Medicine Committee on Injury Scaling. The Abbreviated Injury Scale – 1990. Des Plains, IL: Association for the Advancement of Automotive Medicine, 1990.

8. Baker SP, O'Neill B, Haddon W, Long WB. The severity score: a method for describing patients with multiple injuries and evaluating emergency care. J Trauma 1974; 14:187–96.

9. Baker SP, O'Neill B. The injury severity score: an update. J Trauma 1976; 16:882–5.

10. Osler T, Baker SP, Long W. A modification to the Injury Severity Score that both improves accuracy and simplifies scoring. J Trauma 1997; 43:922–6.

11. Copes WS, Champion HR, Sacco WJ, et al. Progress in characterizing anatomic injury. J Trauma 1990; 3:1200–7.

12. Champion HR, Copes WS, Sacco WJ, et al. Improved predictions from A Severity Characterization of Trauma (ASCOT) over Trauma and Injury Severity Score (TRISS): results of an independent evaluation. J Trauma 1996; 40:40–49.

13. Champion HR, Copes WS, Sacco WJ. The major trauma outcome study: establishing norms for trauma care. J Trauma 1994; 36:499–503.

14. Champion HR, Sacco WJ, Copes WS, Gann DS, Gennarelli TA, Flanagan ME. A revision of the trauma score. J Trauma 1989; 29:623–9.

15. Horan JM, Mallonee S. Injury surveillance. Epidemiol Rev 2003; 25:24–42.

16. Pollack ES, Keimig DG, eds. Counting injuries and illnesses in the workplace: proposals for a better system. Washington, DC: National Academy Press, 1987.

17. Stout N, Bell C. Effectiveness of source documents for identifying fatal occupational injuries: a synthesis of studies. Am J Public Health 1991; 81:725–8.

18. NIOSH. Fatality Assessment and Control Evaluation (FACE) Program, 2003. Atlanta, GA: National Institute for Occupational Safety and Health, 2003.

19. NIOSH. NIOSH alerts on traumatic occupational injury topics. Atlanta, GA: National Institute for Occupational Safety and Health, 2003.

20. US Consumer Product Safety Commission. National Electronic Injury Surveillance System. Bethesda, MD: US Consumer Product Safety Commission, 2003.

21. Alexander BH, Franklin GM, Fulton-Kehoe D. Comparison of fatal and severe nonfatal traumatic work-related injuries in Washington state. Am J Ind Med 1999; 36:317–25.

22. Robinson JC. The rising long term trend in occupational injury rates. Am J Public Health 1988; 78:276–81.

23. Stout NA, Linn HI. Occupational injury prevention research: progress and priorities. Injury Prev 2002; 8(Suppl 4):IV9–14.

24. Robinson JC, Schor GM. Business-cycle influences on work-related disability in construction manufacturing. Milbank Quart 1989; 67:92–113.

25. Kraus JF, Blander B, McArthur DL. Incidence, risk factors and prevention strategies for work-related assault injuries: a review of what is known, what needs to be known, and countermeasures for intervention. Annu Rev Public Health 1995; 16:355–79.

26. Peek-Asa C, Erickson R, Kraus JF. Traumatic occupational fatalities in the retail industry, United States 1992–1996. Am J Ind Med 1999; 35:186–91.

27. Erickson RJ. Retail employees as a group at risk for violence. Occup Med 1996; 11:269–76.

28. Schaffer KB, Casteel C, Kraus JF. A case-site/control-site study of workplace violent injury. J Occup Environ Med 2002; 44:1018–26.

29. Baker SP, Samkoff S, Fisher RS, Van Buren CB. Fatal occupational injuries. JAMA 1982; 248:692–7.

30. Kraus JF, McArthur DL. Epidemiology of violent injury in the workplace. Occup Med 1996; 11:201–17.

31. Nelson NA, Kaufman JD. Fatal and nonfatal injuries related to violence in Washington workplaces, 1992. Am J Ind Med 1996; 30:438–46.

32. Peek-Asa C, Howard J, Vargas L, Kraus JF. Incidence of non-fatal workplace assault injuries determined from employer's reports in California. J Occup Environ Med 1997; 39:44-50.

33. McGovern P, Kochevar L, Lohman W, et al. The cost of work-related physical assaults in Minnesota. Health Serv Res 2000; 35:663–86.

34. Klein PJ, Gerberich SG, Gibson RW, et al. Risk factors for work-related violent victimization. Epidemiology 1997; 8:408–13.

35. Lee SS, Gerberich SG, Waller LA, Anderson A, McGovern P. Work-related assault injuries among nurses. Epidemiology 1999; 10:685–91.

36. Bensley L, Nelson N, Kaufman J, Silverstein B, Kalat J, Shields JW. Injuries due to assaults on psychiatric hospital employees in Washington State. Am J Ind Med 1997; 31:92–9.

37. Simonowitz JA. Healthcare workers and workplace violence. Occup Med 1996; 11:277–91.

38. Runyan CW, Zakocs RC, Zwerling C. Administrative and behavioral interventions for workplace violence prevention. Am J Prev Med 2000; 18:116–27.

39. Casteel C, Peek-Asa C. Effectiveness of crime prevention through environmental design (CPTED) in reducing robberies. Am J Prev Med 2000; 18:99–115.

40. Myers JR, Hard DL. Work-related fatalities in the agricultural production and services sectors, 1980–1989. Am J Ind Med 1995; 27:51–63.

41. Myers JR. National surveillance of occupational fatalities in agriculture. Am J Ind Med 1990; 18:163–8.

42. Lee TY, Gerberich SG, Gibson RW, Carr WP, Shutske J, Renier CM. A population-based study of tractor-related injuries: Regional Rural Injury Study-I (RRIS-I). J Occup Environ Med 1996; 38:782–93.

43. Reynolds SJ, Groves W. Effectiveness of roll-over protective structures in reducing farm tractor fatalities. Am J Prev Med 2000; 18:63–9.

44. Springfeldt B, Thorsen J, Lee BC. Sweden's thirty-year experience with tractor rollovers. J Agric Health Safety 1998; 4:173–80.

45. Gerberich SG, Gibson RW, French LR, et al. Machinery-related injuries: regional rural injury study – I (RRIS – I). Accident Analysis Prev 1998; 30:793–804.

46. Gerberich SG, Gibson RW, French LR, et al. Injuries among children and youth in farm households: regional rural injury study – I. Injury Prev 2001; 7:117–22.

47. Boyle D, Gerberich SG, Gibson RW, et al. Injury from dairy cattle activities. Epidemiology 1997; 8:37–41.

48. McCurdy SA, Samuels SJ, Carroll DJ, Beaumont JJ, Morrin LA. Agricultural injury in California migrant Hispanic farm workers. Am J Ind Med 2003; 44:225–35.

49. Schenker MB, Lopez R, Wintemute G. Farm-related fatalities among children in California, 1980–1989. Am J Public Health 1995; 85:89–92.

50. Heyer NJ, Franklin GM. Work-related traumatic brain injury in Washington State, 1988–1990. Am J Public Health 1994; 84:1106–9.

51. Rivara FP. Fatal and non-fatal farm injuries to children and adolescents in the United States, 1990–3. Injury Prev 1997; 3:190–4.

Section 4

Hazards in the Workplace and the Environment

Chapter 32
Mechanical Stressors

Thomas J Armstrong

INTRODUCTION

When work contributes significantly as a cause of musculoskeletal disorders (MSDs) or aggravates MSDs, regardless of their cause, the MSD is considered a work-related musculoskeletal disorder (WMSD). This chapter is intended to provide background to help healthcare providers assess work factors that may cause or aggravate MSDs. In particular it focuses on mechanical stressors, because there is significant literature supporting their contribution to WMSDs and to provide guidance for their assessment. It also focuses primarily on the upper limb, although many of the concepts are applicable to the back and other parts of the body. This chapter is not intended to make healthcare providers expert ergonomists or job analysts. Its goal is to help occupational physicians with: (1) walk-through inspections of worksites and (2) the clinical assessment of individual workers. In either case, the physician is likely to have limited time and resources. An understanding of these factors will enable the physician to work more closely with their working patients, managers, engineers, ergonomists, and occupational and physical therapists.

Mechanical stresses result from transfer of force between muscles and external work objects, e.g., equipment controls, parts and materials, and movements of the body to reach, grasp and move work objects. Within certain limits the body adapts to mechanical stress, and some stress is desirable to sustain physical fitness; however, there are limitations for adaptation. These limits may be influenced by chronic diseases, previous injuries, and other personal factors. As a result, susceptibility to MSDs varies from person to person and the 'dose–response' relationship between mechanical stresses and musculoskeletal disorders is modeled probabilistically. There is an established and growing body of literature that describes the relationship between work activities, mechanical stress, and musculoskeletal disorders. This literature provides guidance for the assessment of physical job demands and their contribution to WMSDs. The literature on WMSDs has been thoroughly reviewed by the Occuptional Safety and Health administration for development of a standard[1-3] that was subsequently withdrawn by the Congress for political reasons. Proposed standards have also been withdrawn in the state of Washington. The strong scientific basis for work-related musculoskeletal disorders has also been reviewed in two separate reports by the National Academy of Sciences in 1999[4] and 2001.[5]

WORK ACTIVITIES AND MECHANICAL STRESSORS

Figure 32.1 illustrates the relationship between job/task, the environment, and the internal loads on tendons, muscles and adjacent structures. It draws on models put forward by Armstrong et al[6] and the NRC[5] and NRC & IOM.[4] Job task demands specify quantity of work and performance expectations. To achieve this goal the worker must perform: (1) mental actions to obtain and process information and (2) physical actions to hold and use work objects (parts, materials, and controls). The physical actions involve the activation of muscles and the production of forces in the musculoskeletal system to produce the desired effects. Aside from accomplishing the desired work task, these actions are associated with physiologic and mechanical responses.

Physiologic responses start with the release of ions to initiate contraction of muscles; they also include consumption of metabolic substrates and production of metabolites. Depletion of substrates, accumulation of metabolites, and ionic imbalance are all associated with transient fatigue response that is manifest by loss of strength, loss of motor control and discomfort. Localized muscle fatigue is a transient response that typically develops and recovers in periods of minutes or hours.[7] Recovery begins with the cessation of work and, depending on its severity may require seconds to hours. As a practical matter, workers should not be experiencing effects of fatigue from one day to the next. Longer-term effects include tissue damage due to ischemia and free radical production. Tissue damage stimulates repair and adaptation of damaged tissue, which requires several weeks, assuming that the muscle is not re-injured.

Biomechanical responses include tissue stress and strain. Mechanical stress refers to force divided by the area over which is it distributed, and strain is the resulting deformation of the material divided by the unstressed dimensions of the material. Stress may also be used in broad reference to factors that disturb an individual's physical or mental state, and strain as a broad reference to the resulting disturbances. Tissue loads include the transmission of tensile forces from the muscles via tendons, and enable the body to maintain a mechanical equilibrium with the reaction forces associated with holding, using, and manipulating work objects. When the muscles pull on the tendons, tensile forces are produced in the direction of the long axis

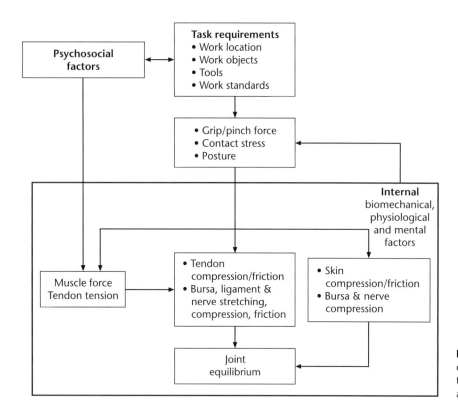

Figure 32.1: A conceptual model illustrating how external loads impose internal loads on the muscles, tendons, and nerves that may in turn cause or aggravate MSDs.

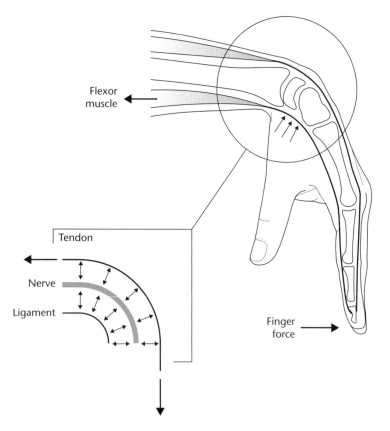

Figure 32.2: The wrist flexion or Phalen's test is widely used for diagnosis of carpal tunnel syndrome. Flexion of the wrist causes the finger flexor tendons to compress the median nerve against the flexor retinaculum.[8] The test may be accelerated by pinching at the same time, which produces tension on the finger flexor tendons and additional pressure on the nerve.[9]

of the tendon and cause it to stretch. Compression forces are produced between the tendons and adjacent anatomical surfaces that intrude into the space between the point of a tendon's origin and its insertion, which occur when joints are flexed or extended.

This concept is exploited in the Phalen's wrist flexion test[8] (Fig. 32.2) in which flexion of the wrist causes the median nerve to be compressed against the flexor retinaculum. Numbness and tingling in the areas innervated by the median nerve is a positive sign of carpal tunnel syndrome.

Smith et al[9] proposed that the test could be improved if patients forcibly pinched at the same time they flexed their wrist, because of increased tension on the finger flexor tendons and pressure on the median nerve. In addition to its diagnostic value, the Phalen's test demonstrates how certain postures of the body impose secondary loads on tendons and nerves and can contribute to WMSDs. Flexion or extension of a joint also causes the shape of the tissues around the joint structure to change and can produce increased fluid pressure. These pressure changes have been measured around the median nerve in the wrist, and shown to be sufficient to interfere with microcirculation.

Tissues demonstrate viscoelastic properties; that is, they undergo both elastic and viscous deformations. Elastic deformations are essentially instantaneous with the application of force. Similarly, recovery is also instantaneous with the removal of the load. Viscous deformation continues to increase after the load is applied. Similarly, recovery requires some period of time following removal of the force. As a result, tendons may continue to stretch if there is insufficient recovery time between successive exertions. Touch and proprioception involve tissue deformation, but tissue deformation also produces pain. As with muscle fatigue, muscle deformation and associated pain will recover with the cessation of work. Elkus and Basmajian[10] refer to intramuscular fatigue as the performance changes that occur as a result of changes inside the muscle, and extramuscular fatigue that occurs as a result of changes outside muscles.

Although tissue deformations are unlikely to result in acute tissue failure, e.g., tendon rupture, they may be sufficient to interfere with circulation and other physiologic functions. They may be sufficient to create micro tissue damage. In the short term, micro damage affects tissue and capillary permeability. This can lead to swelling following the cessation of work, and explains why many persons experience nocturnal numbness in their hands. Micro damage also stimulates degradation, repair, and adaptation of damaged tissues. This is a likely explanation for non-specific synovitis that results in proliferation of connective tissue and is commonly found inside the carpal tunnel. Thickening of the synovial membranes inside the carpal tunnel is a likely explanation of increased inter-carpal canal pressures in carpal tunnel patients[8,11] and secondary carpal tunnel syndrome.

It can be seen that there are multiple primary and secondary mechanisms of musculoskeletal disorders, but that they share a common link to the patterns of exertions. Figure 32.3 depicts a general response function to varying exertion intensities and frequency. Figure 32.3a depicts a case where there is sufficient time in between exertions for complete recovery. Figure 32.3b depicts a case in which the response is increased either as a result of a primary factor like loading of the muscle tendon unit, or as a result of co-factors (e.g., posture or vibration). In this case the recovery time is insufficient, so that the response is increased with each successive exertion. Additional recovery time is required to arrest the growing response. Figure 32.3c depicts a case where there is adequate recovery time, but an irregular work element results in an extreme response that is then aggravated with each successive response, shown in Figure 32.3d.

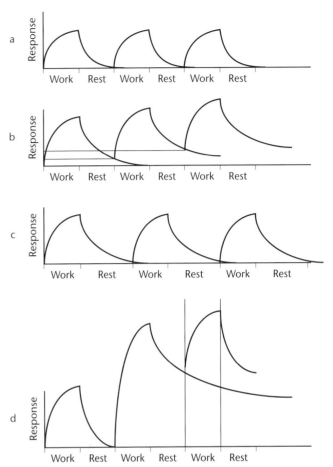

Figure 32.3: Four scenarios for repetitive work. In Case (a), the recovery periods are sufficient for complete recovery of biomechanical and physiologic disturbances that occur during the work periods. The work exposures to mechanical stresses have been increased in Case (b), such that the recovery periods are insufficient and the disturbances are cumulative. In Case (c), the recovery periods have been increased to compensate for the increased work levels in Case (b). In Case (d), the recovery periods are generally adequate until the worker is exposed to unusually high stresses as a result of an irregular work activity. Subsequent actions continue to aggravate the initial disturbance so that the worker is unable to achieve full recovery.

As shown in Figure 32.1, task demands are a primary determinant of the physical stressors that are placed on the worker's body and ultimately on the expression of symptoms. The load may be influenced by psychologic and sociologic factors.[4,5,12] Some of these other factors are not explicitly part of the work requirements, but pertain to the workplace (e.g., manager and coworker). Other factors do not pertain to the job at all, but influence how the worker responds to mechanical stressors, e.g., family concerns, personal attitudes and beliefs, or coping and cognitive skills. These factors may be broadly referred to as psychosocial factors. There is a growing body of literature regarding psychosocial factors, but there is not yet broad consensus on how to evaluate and manage these factors. Management of psychosocial factors is complicated by the personal nature of many of the issues, which may be considered confidential.

The concept of biologic and mechanical response to physical exertion provides the foundation for an expo-

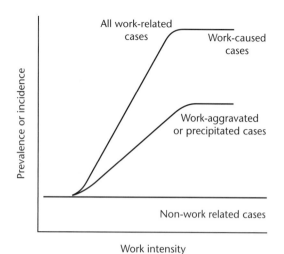

Figure 32.4: General dose–response curve for musculoskeletal disorders and exposure to various physical stressors. Some cases occur irrespective of work exposures. Other cases are due to aggravation of existing conditions and still others are primarily due to work exposures.

sure–response relationship. There is a growing body of epidemiological data that shows increased risk of MSDs with increasing intensity of handwork. Although there is not yet agreement on the best way to measure exposure or risk of MSDs, this is an important concept for those concerned with treatment. Figure 32.4 shows a general exposure–response relationship. Available literature demonstrates that: (1) there is a background risk of MSDs, even at the lowest level of exposure, and (2) the risk increases with increasing exposure. There is disagreement about the location of the inflection point where the risk of WMSDs begins to increase with increasing exposure. Part of the confusion can be attributed to different exposure and outcome metrics among investigators. It may be necessary for the healthcare providers and employers to aim for exposure levels that are below those that will cause an MSD in the absence of predisposing personal conditions.

A practitioner may elect to intervene with the onset of symptoms and in the absence of objective findings. Knowledge that the worker is experiencing persistent pain, and is exposed to a physical demanding job, will generally be more important to a practitioner than physiologic parameters such as intercarpal canal pressure, particularly since such physiologic data are not readily available. This approach is reflected in the current OSHA reporting regulations. Although there is a 'temporary' moratorium on the reporting of musculoskeletal disorders, the rules provide general guidelines for assessing the 'work-relatedness' of worker injuries and illnesses.

According to OSHA[13] section 1904.5a: 'Work-relatedness is presumed for injuries and illnesses resulting from events or exposures occurring in the work environment. . .' The regulations include specific exemptions such as: it is clear the condition resulted from activities to exposures outside of the workplace, the worker was participating in a 'voluntary' company fitness program or it was due to motor vehicle accidents while commuting to work, to communicable diseases unrelated to work or to mental illness. Section 1904.5(b)(5)

states: 'An injury or illness is a pre-existing condition if it resulted solely from a non-work-related event or exposure that occurred outside the work environment'. Section 1904.5(b) describes the meaning of significantly aggravated:

- One or more days away from work, or days of restricted work, or days of job transfer that otherwise would not have occurred but for the occupational event or exposure.
- Medical treatment in a case where no medical treatment was needed for the injury or illness before the workplace event or exposure, or a change in medical treatment was necessitated by the workplace event or exposure.

There is a high burden of proof on the employer and healthcare provider to show that a case is not work related. If there is a question about the contribution of work, Section 1904.5b says: 'You must evaluate the employee's work duties and environment to decide whether or not one or more events or exposures in the work environment either caused or contributed to the resulting condition or significantly aggravated a pre-existing condition'.

OSHA not withstanding, many employers will want information about jobs performed by injured workers so that they can investigate factors that might affect other workers or, that would pose a barrier to employment by affected workers.

JOB ANALYSIS

As a practical matter, the time that a healthcare provider has to assess a worker's exposure to mechanical stressors may be limited. This makes it important that the provider understand what a job analysis entails to effectively review the detailed analysis of others, to understand job factors that produce mechanical stress and to prescribe meaningful work restrictions.

It is important that the job analysis be systematic so that all possible stresses are identified. Several structured approaches have been proposed for assessing mechanical stressors. Selected systems are summarized in Table 32.1 along with the factors they include. These systems provide structured approaches for the analysis of jobs; however, systems developed in one setting are not necessarily applicable to others. For example, Keyserling et al[14] describe a checklist developed for automotive manufacturing. The checklist used cycle time of less than 30 seconds as the threshold for high repetition work. Although a 30-second threshold works well for some types of manufacturing work, it does not work well for others, e.g., keyboard data entry. In some cases, healthcare providers may find that all of the information required to apply a given analysis system is not available, and that the action limit or threshold cannot be fully assessed. Finally, even though a threshold may protect most workers, it is likely that some fraction will be affected, and that a healthcare provider will be asked to manage that fraction.

An alternative to the structured systems listed in Table 32.1 is an open-ended structured approach in which each factor is considered, in so far as necessary or possible.[15] The open-ended analyses require the user to recognize risk factors and exercise judgment about their severity and importance. They provide the user with the flexibility to increase the breadth and depth of the analysis as necessary

	Body parts	Repetition	Duty cycle	Dynamics	Work duration	Force	Posture	Contact stress	Low temp	Vibration
UAW-GM RFC Checklist developed & tested for automobile manufacturing	Upper limb & back	RFC I: Low >30s; Hi <30s RFCII: Low, Medium High[19]	Included in repetition	Included in repetition	No	Selected factors yes/no	Wrist, elbow, shoulder	Selected factors yes/no	Selected factors yes/no	Yes; three categories
RULA generic work, tested on office work[41]	Upper limb and torso	Yes; static >1 minute or repeated >4 times/min add one point to score	No	Static/dynamic	No	Loads <2kg, 2-10kg (intermittent or static/repeated), >10kg	Wrist, lower arm, upper arm, neck, trunk variable categories	No	No	No
REBA generic, no test data[42]	Whole body	Activity score increased if static >1 min, repeated, >4 times/min or very large movements	No	No	No	Load/force <5kg, 5-10kg, >10kg, shock	Wrist, lower arm, upper arm, neck, trunk, leg variable categories	No	No	No
Strain index, generic, tested on pork, poultry and light manufacturing[24]	Hand, wrist, forearm	Efforts/min <4, 4-8, 9-14, 15-20, ≥20	<10, 10-29, 30-49, 50-79, >80%	Very slow, slow, fair, fast, very fast	<1, 1-2, 2-4, 4-8, ≥8 hr/day	Light, somewhat hard, hard, very hard, near maximal	Hand/wrist five categories	No	No	No
ACGIH TLV for Monotask Hand Work Generic[18]	Upper limb	None to maximum, continuous scale	Included in repetition	Included in repetition	Applies to 4 or more hours per day	None to maximum, continuous scale	Defers to expert judgment	Defers to expert judgment	Defers to expert judgment	Separate guideline
Washington State generic office & mnfc[22]	Upper limb, trunk	Specified motions >4hr/day; intense keying >2hr/day	No	No	Yes, >2hr/day, >4hr/day	Exertion of fixed force holding unsupported objects of specified weights	Shoulder, neck, back, knees, various categories; hand/wrist posture combined with force metrics	Pounding with base of hand >1/min & >2hr/day	No	12 m/s² > 2.5 hr/day
Open ended[15] Generic	Upper limb & backs	Includes all factors to extent desired by analyst								
OCRA[17] generic, mnfc examples	Upper limbs	Ex/min (continuous scale)	% (continuous scale)	No	1, 2, 3-5, 6-8 hr	0-10 continuous	Shoulder, elbow, wrist, hand various categories	Yes	No	No
OWAS, whole body posture assessment, generic[43,44]	Whole body	No	% time spent in posture	No	No	No	Back, upper limb, lower limb various categories	No	No	No
Wrist Velocity[36] generic, test on mnfc wkers	Hand, wrist, forearm	Angular velocity & acceleration of wrist (continuous scale)	No	Angular velocity & acceleration of wrist (continuous scale)	No	No	Angular position of wrist (continuous scale)	No	No	No
Snook et al[45] generic, lab test only	Wrist flexions or extension/min	No	No	No	No	Finger force	No	No	No	No

Table 32.1 Summary of selected job analysis systems for assessing upper limb physical stressors

for a given situation. The open-ended analysis can be supplemented as needed with some of the standardized procedures listed in Table 32.1. The following section presents a generic open-ended approach. The job analysis is divided into two steps: (1) documentation and (2) assessment of mechanical stressors:

Documentation

The first step of the job analysis is documentation. The documentation is descriptive information about the job,[6,15-17] which is an aid to understanding what the worker does and determining his or her exposure to physical stressors. For example, repetitiveness may be related to a work standard that specifies a certain number of parts be assembled in a given amount of time, or that a certain amount of data be entered into a computer in a given amount of time. Posture stresses may result from the location of a work object or the shape of a tool. An understanding of what the worker does – even at a minimal level – will help the healthcare provider work more effectively with management to identify the causes of MSDs and to facilitate return to work. The following is a general outline of the necessary documentation information.

Table 32.2 provides a listing of the basic information that should be considered for documentation. How the documentation is performed will depend on the level of concern and available resources. Some organizations maintain a library of job information. Examples include job descriptions used by personnel for hiring and placement, work methods and standards data used by management for work allocation and production planning, and job safety analyses used by safety managers to identify unsafe work conditions. Often these data are not available in a form that healthcare providers can use.

Few healthcare providers have the luxury of visiting the worksite to observe or videotape jobs, to make direct measurements, or to interview workers and supervisors. They are most likely to perform the analysis when they see the worker/patient in their clinic, which may be offsite. As a result it may be necessary for someone to review the available documentation, observe and/or videotape the job, and to interview supervisors and workers. In the absence of this support, healthcare providers often have to obtain the needed information from workers at the same time they are evaluating or treating them. Table 32.3 provides a list of questions for obtaining descriptive job information from worker. These questions are intended as starting points. Additional questions may be required to achieve the desired level of detail. It will be helpful if the healthcare provider visits the worksites on a regular basis so that they have a background perspective for interpreting the worker's comments. Healthcare providers should understand that workplaces are highly dynamic, and work activities may vary from day to day or even hour to hour depending on the production demands, absenteeism and worker turnover.

The time required for completing documentation increases with job complexity. Complexity refers to the number of steps required to complete a job activity and how

1. Objective/purpose
The reasons the job is performed. These can be stated as simply as possible in list form.

2. Tasks
Groups or cycles of work elements that have a common objective. Tasks need not be performed in the same sequence, and one task may interrupt another. All jobs are composed of at least one task.

3. Production standards
The quantity of work that must be completed in a given amount of time. Standards may be stated as the number of parts per hour, the time per part, the line speed, or a work duration.

4. Work objects
Objects, such as parts and materials, on which work is performed. Work objects have attributes of size, shape, weight, hardness/softness, surface friction, location, orientation and temperature.

5. Tools and equipment
Objects or devices held or manipulated with the hands to do something to the work object, such as, insert fasteners, trim parts, or control. Tools and equipment have many of the same properties as work objects. Additionally they may require force to engage, activate or resist (reaction forces).

6. Workstation
The equipment that is used to hold or support work objects, equipment, or the worker, such as, the benches, chairs, and assembly lines. Workstations have important location, size and shape attributes.

7. Methods
A step-by-step description of the elements required to perform the task, such as, get part, inspect part, insert part, and drive screw. Steps can be listed for the right and left hand, but one list is sufficient if both hands do the same steps.

8. Environment
Where the work is performed and its physical characteristics, such as, inside, outside, and air temperature.

Table 32.2 Factors to include in job documentation. The level of detail may be adjusted according to the user's needs and resources

1. Does your job have an official name? Does it have a nickname (how do you refer to your job)?
2. In your own words, what is the purpose of your job?
3. How much are you expected to produce in a given minute, hour or shift – give averages and ranges?
4. Do you repeat the same work 'tasks' (e.g., get and assemble parts) over and over in the same way or do you perform different tasks (e.g., perform various maintenance, construction or office tasks as needed) in different ways from one time to the next? Please list the 'tasks' that you do. Indicate if they occur in the same or random order. Indicate approximately how many times per day and how long each is performed.
5. For each task list the things that you use: machines, hand tools, parts, and personal protective equipment (e.g., gloves). Also indicate if and how you interact with coworkers and clients.
6. Where is each task performed? Is it hot, cold or just right? Do your hands ever get cold?

* Detail may be added or removed depending on the needs and available resources

Table 32.3 Suggested questions for interview regarding work documentation* (can be modified as needed)

much those steps vary from one time to the next. At one extreme are simple mono-task jobs in which a few steps are completed in the same way in a few seconds, time after time. Examples of these jobs include transcription on a computer or feeding a machine in a production manufacturing setting. At the other extreme are complex multitask jobs with high inter-task and inter-cycle variability. Examples of complex jobs might include maintenance jobs in which the workers must diagnose and fix equipment, or software under a variety of conditions, or utility workers who rotate from job to job. Even short cycle time mono-task jobs may require significant time to ascertain all of the material, process and worker variations. Long cycle time jobs, multi-task jobs and jobs with irregular schedules may require considerably more time. While it often is not possible to do a rigorous analysis, it is important that the analyst recognize the uncertainties associated with their assessment.

Some employers videotape jobs and send them with the patient to the healthcare provider. Videotapes can be very helpful if the healthcare provider has time to review them; however, videotapes can be misleading. Video recordings are only a sample of what the worker does in a much larger work shift, with potential variation from day to day. For example, a brief interruption in the supply of parts may leave the worker briefly idle and create the impression that there is a lot of recovery time built into the job. Similarly, an irregular part may require extra attention and make it look like the worker has to hurry to keep up with the process. Unless the person making the videotape understands the job and takes care to record sequences that are representative, the recording may provide an incorrect impression. Video recordings are a two-dimensional representation of a three-dimensional system. As a result, there will inevitably be distortions and it may not be clear if the worker is reaching towards or away from the camera. It may be necessary to record multiple views to see all of the hand actions.

The job documentation provides a framework for considering what the worker does and lays a foundation for assessing the physical stressors. Even if a thorough documentation is not possible, knowledge of these issues will help the healthcare provider with their assessment of physical stressors and interact with workers and supervisors to more effectively manage cases. Careful documentation provides a framework for assessing mechanical stressors.

Assessment of mechanical stressors

Physical stressors are identified and quantified from:
1. Interviews of workers and supervisors
2. Observations (direct or using videotape)
3. Computations based on job specific attributes, and
4. Instrumentation.

This chapter focuses primarily on interviews and observations because they are most readily available to healthcare providers. Computations are only introduced to help the healthcare provider understand the basis for the observational methods.

Repeated and static exertions (hand activity level)

Repeated and sustained exertions refer to the time qualities of the exertions of the hand or other body parts. An exer-

tion can be defined as an event during which the physiologic or biomechanical demand is placed on the musculoskeletal system at rate greater than at which recovery occurs. Exertions are depicted in Figure 32.3 as increasing response, and recovery is depicted as decreasing response. The rate of response and recovery will be related to force, posture, contact, vibration and other work factors, as well as personal factors. An exertion often corresponds to a work element or step, such as getting the screw, putting it on the bit, and driving the screw, but one work element and exertion may run into the next without intervening recovery periods. The result may be fewer but longer discrete exertions with reduced recovery time. Important time qualities include exertion frequency, exertion time, and recovery time. As a practical matter, few jobs entail repetition of a single exertion all day, such as shown in Figure 32.3, although some keyboard data entry, transcription, certain food processing, and packing jobs may approximate this. Most jobs entail one or more sequences of exertions. Exertion frequencies, durations and duty cycles are reported as average values and/or as ranges (minimum and maximum).

The ACGIH[18] refers to repetition as hand activity level (HAL) and spells out the steps for calculating HAL for a detailed methods analysis. It also provides a scale for rating HAL from zero to ten, based on observations of the job or a video recording of the job, including six verbal anchor points based on work by Latko et al[19,20] (see Table 32.4a). The ACGIH also includes a recommended exposure limit for various combinations of repetition and force.

Ebersole and Armstrong[21] examined a procedure for applying the Latko scale in which two trained analysts

---

(a) Verbal anchor points used to rate repeated and sustained exertions of the hand*

0	Hands idle most of the time, no regular exertion
2	Consistent, conspicuous long pauses; or very slow motions
4	Slow steady motion/exertion, frequent brief pauses
6	Steady motion/ exertion; infrequent pauses
8	Rapid steady motion/ exertion; infrequent pauses
10	Rapid steady motion/ continuous exertion, difficulty keeping up

(b) The UAW-GM Risk Factor Checklist†

Low:	Hands/wrists pause to wait for equipment and/or parts
Medium:	Hands/wrists are in steady motion/pace. Infrequent opportunity for pauses
High:	Hands/wrists are in constant motion to keep up. No opportunity for pauses.

(c) The State of Washington Workplace Ergonomic Standard‡
The 'caution zone' is for an exposure to the following activity, occurring for more than one day per week and one week per year.
1. Repeating the same motion with the neck, shoulders, elbows, wrists, or hands (excluding keying activities) with little or no variation every few seconds more than 2 hours total per day
2. Performing intensive keying more than 4 hours total per day

* Hand activity level from 0 to 10.[18,19]
† Keyserling et al 1993[14] has been modified to include three ranges of repetition based on Latko et al.[19]
‡ Includes a checklist for assessing repetition.[22]

Table 32.4 Repeated and static exertions (hand activity level)

observed and rated jobs in real time, and after discussion re-rated the jobs by consensus. Six raters working in random combinations of two rated a total of 410 automobile assembly jobs. Ninety-one percent of the HAL ratings were within one point on a 0–10 scale.

The UAW-GM Risk Factor Checklist initially characterized repetition as low (work cycle time greater than 30 seconds) and high (work cycle time less than 30 seconds).[15] This checklist has subsequently been modified to include three levels of repetition: low, medium and high (see Table 32.4b). Medium and high risk are interpreted as having 'potential risk to some workers', further analysis is required for high exposures.

The State of Washington Workplace Ergonomic Standard includes a checklist for assessing job risk of musculoskeletal injuries.[22] The criteria for assessing repetition are included in Table 32.4c. Their criteria 'Repeating the same motion with the . . . wrists, or hands (excluding keying activities) with little or no variation every few seconds more than 2 hours total per day' could correspond to the middle and upper parts of the Latko[19] and ACGIH scales.[18] 'Performing intensive keying more than 4 hours total per day' corresponds to the upper limit of Latko and ACGIH scales.

Worker self-assessments. Table 32.5 includes a list for questions that can be asked of the worker to assess their perception of physical stressors. Question 1 pertains to repetition and asks the worker if they can work at his or her own pace. It also addresses if the worker has trouble keeping up and would indicate if the worker is near the upper end of the ACGIH Hand Activity Scale.[18] It may be

instructive to compare worker self-assessments of repetitions with those of a third party. Significant differences may indicate where the workers capacity is excessively challenged by the job demands.

Forceful exertion

Forces are exerted to hold or move the body or to hold or move work objects. Force is an important determinant of stresses on muscles, tendons and adjacent connective and nerve tissues. Force also is an important factor in muscle metabolic rates (Fig. 32.1). Tissue loads and metabolic rates may be influenced by posture. Recovery occurs when the hands are able to relax. The lowest force and greatest recovery occurs when workers are able to sit with their hands on their lap. A more likely scenario is sitting or standing waiting for a machine to cycle or respond; if the forearms are not supported, muscle activity to support the shoulder girdle may prevent recovery in the neck–shoulder region of the body. The mechanical relationship between external and internal loads is affected by the position of the body. As a result, greater muscle and tendon loads are required to work in some positions. For example, grip strength is typically four or five times greater than pinch strength. Force is also affected by work pace. Rapid or sudden motions will impose inertial loads and require higher muscle forces than for slow steady motions.

Force can be expressed on an absolute scale of newtons (kilograms or pounds). It also can be expressed on a relative scale of 0 to 10, where 10 corresponds to the greatest effort possible or 100%.

Using a relative scale of 0–10 makes it easier to compare the magnitude of force with other factors. If repetition is rated as 8 and force as 2, this would mean that it is a highly repetitive, but low force job. Physicians might focus more on the possible contribution of repetition than force to patient's MSD, and an engineer would focus more on steps to reduce repetition than force.

A relative force value can be calculated as the required force divided by the strength of an individual or population percentile and multiplying by ten:

Relative force (0–10) = Absolute force / Strength *10

A 0–10 scale was adopted by ACGIH so that it corresponded to the Hand Activity Level scale. Because strength varies from group to group, the relative force required for a given job will vary as well. For example, if a tool requires 350N of grip force to cycle, then the required force would be 10 for an average female, but only 5 for an average male. As a practical matter, the relative force will probably be one or two points greater for persons with high strength compared with low strength, because most people exert more than the minimum required force unless they are near their maximum.

A list of factors affecting hand force is included in Table 32.6. To understand the relationship between work requirements and force requirements, two examples are considered (Fig. 32.5a). In the first example, the worker is holding an object such as a toolbox or a suitcase. Flexing the fingers

---

1. Is there adequate time for your hands to rest between work cycles, between tasks or during breaks, or do you have to use your hands continuously to keep up? (note: your hands may be resting while you are performing tasks such as reading documents, walking to parts, etc.)
2. Are you able to repeatedly exert the force required to get, put, or assemble parts, or to hold and use tools throughout the work shift without excessive fatigue? What, if any, parts of your job seem to require excessive force? How frequently do they occur?
3. Does your job require you to assume any unusual or uncomfortable postures? As appropriate demonstrate extreme: a. wrist flexion and extension, b. wrist deviation, c. forearm rotation, d. elbow flexion, e. reaching overhead, f. reaching forward, g. reaching side to side, h. reaching back, i. neck rotation, j. neck flexion/extension, k. bending, l. twisting and m. squatting. What work activities require these postures? How frequently?
4. Do you strike, press, or rest your body against any hard or sharp objects (e.g., pound parts together, rest wrists on sharp edge of desk or keyboard, lean on elbow? Where? Frequency?
5. Does anything you hold or touch vibrate or shake? What? Where? Frequency?
6. Do your hands get cold? Where? Frequency?

* For greater quantification, workers can also be asked to rate their exposures on a scale of 0 to 10 and to indicate exposure duration and frequency. Assessments may be performed for each task and the overall job depending on job complexity, needs and resources.

Table 32.5 Suggested questions for interview regarding exposure to physical stressors*

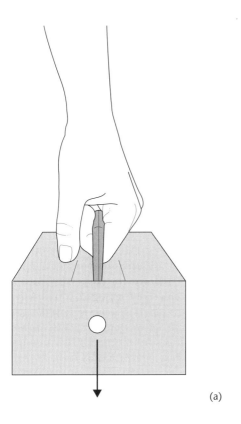

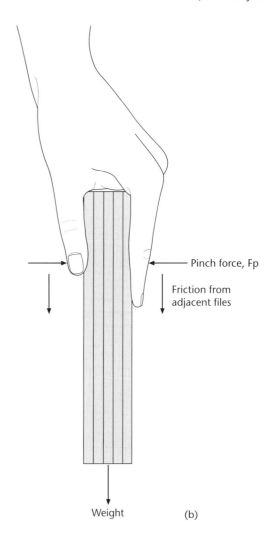

Pinch force, Fp

Friction from
adjacent files

Weight (b)

Figure 32.5: (a) Holding a tool box requires the worker to flex his fingers against the weight of the tool box. The force requirements of holding the tool box will be equal to the gravity and inertial forces on the tool box. (b) To pull the files from the file drawer the worker must pinch the file hard enough to overcome the weight, friction and inertial forces on the file.

Weight of work object or tool
Center of gravity versus center of grip
Friction between hand and work object/tool
Size/shape of work object/tool
Glove fit/stiffness/friction
Force to activate controls for machines/tools
Force required to join parts and engage tools
Reaction forces of tools as they start and stop
Mechanical assists that are used to support and transfer materials and tools
Tool maintenance
Quality control

Table 32.6 Factors affecting hand force

against the handle supports the object. The force exerted by the fingers on the work object must be exactly equal to force exerted on the toolbox by gravity. In this case the force requirements to hold the toolbox will be equal to its weight. The relative workload required to hold the toolbox can be calculated by dividing the task force requirements by the strength of the worker.

$$\text{Finger force} = \text{Weight of work object}$$

The force required to pick up the toolbox will be greater than the force required to hold it because of the inertial

forces. As workers approach their maximum strength they will generally slow down. Thus a strong worker may end up exerting as much force as a weak worker because they lift the object more quickly.

The second example shown in Figure 32.5b involves pulling and holding a file. In this case the fingers must press against the sides of the file to produce enough friction to overcome the force of gravity and frictional forces from adjacent files. A mathematical expression that describes the relationship between the force exerted by the hand, the weight of an object, and the slipperiness or coefficient of friction of the skin can be written:

$$\text{Finger force} \geq \text{File Weight} / 2 \text{ x Friction Coefficient}$$

This equation is written as an inequality because the worker can exert more than the minimum required force to hold the file. Friction is related to the object's material properties and moistness of the skin. Coefficients of friction for porous materials, such as paper and leather, are sensitive to moisture and range from 0.25 to 0.4 for dry skin and 0.4 to 0.7 for moist skin.[23] Coefficients of friction for non-porous materials such as aluminum, vinyl, and sandpaper are insensitive to moisture and range from 0.4 to 0.6.

The simplest case corresponds to holding the file at a stationary location in which the friction forces from adjacent files and inertial forces are zero. The required pinch force can therefore be expressed simply as:

Finger force = File Weight / 2 x Friction Coefficient

As an example, if a file folder weighs 15N and the coefficient of friction for moist skin and paper is 0.5, the minimum pinch force required to overcome gravity is calculated as 15N; if the coefficient of friction is 0.25 for dry skin, the pinch force is 30N. The required pinch force to hold the folder if the skin is moist is approximately equal to the weight of the folder. Handling of paper folders results in the drying of the skin and decreasing the coefficient of friction. Thus, the required pinch force for the dry skin is nearly twice the weight of the file.

Other factors affecting force include the balance of the work object in the hand, the use mechanical assistance, glove fit, stiffness and friction, part quality, and fit and tool maintenance (Table 32.6). Many of these factors are addressed in the UAW-GM Risk Factor Checklist.[14] Other systems such as the Strain Index,[24] the ACGIH,[18] and the State of Washington[22] leave it up to the user's professional judgment or the use of other methods.

The relative force can be calculated by dividing the force required by the strength of the hand in the position required to grip the work object. The file is held in pinch posture, so the pinch strength data from Table 32.7 are used to estimate strength. Approximately 99% of the males and 94% of the females with moist skin would be able to hold the folder and have a relative force less than 10. Only 89% of the males and 48% of the females with dry skin would be able to hold the folder and have a relative force less than 10. The relative force would range from 3 to 5 for average males and females with moist skin, and from 6 to 10 for average males and females with dry skin. Relative forces above 10 are not possible, which means persons with pinch strength less than that of a 5th percentile female would not be able to perform the task. Jobs that require 'pinching an unsupported object(s) weighing 2 or more pounds per hand, or pinching with a force of 4 or more pounds per hand, more than 2 hours total per day (comparable to pinching half a ream of paper) or 'gripping 10 or more pounds' would be designated by the State of Washington criteria as a caution zone job.[22]

This simple example shows how hand force is related to weight and friction. Hand force is related to weight and friction of the work object for other postures in addition to pinch. The relationship between finger force and muscle force varies significantly from one hand posture to another (Fig. 32.1). Generally, the lowest muscle forces for a given external load are found when the fingers can be closed around the object, such as holding a hammer or a suitcase. It can be seen from Table 32.7 that the hand is roughly 10 times stronger in power grip than in pinch. The finger flexor muscles have to work harder in pinch than in power grip to produce equivalent external forces.

It is possible to exert more than the required force. The pulps of the fingers are richly endowed with nerve endings, which provide feedback to the central nervous system when the object is slipping. The system does not provide perfect control, and the amount of force exerted will vary from person to person. As a practical matter, submaximal exertions will be greater than the minimum required. Armstrong et al[25] reported that subjects apply an average of three times the required force for keyboard jobs, at the low end of the scale. Westling and Johansson[26] refer to this excess force as a safety margin. Frederick and Armstrong[27] showed that the safety margin decreases with force as task strength requirements approach the maximum strength of the subject. Thus while strong subjects in theory do not have to exert as much force for a given task as weaker subjects, in practice stronger subjects tend to exert proportionally more effort than weaker subjects. As a result the relative workload difference between strong and weak subjects may vary from predicted. It has been suggested that the amount of force may be affected by psychological stressors, and provides a mechanism by which psychosocial stresses contribute to musculoskeletal disorders.[28] The sensitivity of the fingers and ability to control force may be altered by factors such as low temperatures and vibration, which alter the sensitivity of the fingers.

It should be apparent that the force required to perform a job typically varies from one work element to the next. It is possible to have a high maximum peak force while having a very low average force. The average force can be calculated as the sum of the average force times the time for each element, divided by the sum of the times. This is the same procedure that is used to calculate time-weighted averages for evaluating chemical TLVs. There is a debate about acceptable levels of average force. Physical endurance goes down precipitously when the average force increases above 15–20% (1.5–2.0 on a relative scale of 0–10), but workers may also experience adverse effects, such as acute and chronic muscle pain, as a result of prolonged and sustained exertions at lower levels. Some investigators argue that complete relaxation is necessary for a muscle to recover and avoid adverse effects of fatigue (see Bystrom and Fransson-Hall[7] and NRC[4,5] for a summary of this literature).

Posture	Population	5%tile	Male Average	95%tile	5%tile	Female Average	95%tile
Power grip[46]	Steel mill applicants	383.7	503 (72.5)	622.3	237.3	311 (44.8)	384.7
Power grip[47]	US Adults	333.8	487 (92.5)	639.2	186.4	308 (73.9)	429.6
Power grip[48]	Office workers	327.8	452 (75.5)	576.2		Not reported	
Pulp 3 pinch[49]	US Adults	23.5	48 (15.3)	73.8	15.0	30 (9.4)	45.9

* Values may vary greatly from one population to another. See text for discussion.

Table 32.7 Average, fifth percentile and ninety-fifth percentile grip and pinch strength data for adult males and females*

Observational methods do not have enough precision and accuracy to reliably rate absolute force levels between 1 and 2 on a scale of 0–10. However, it is often possible to determine which of two or more workers is exerting the most force within the low force range.[29]

The UAW-GM Risk Factor Checklist and the State of Washington ergonomic standard checklist use weights in pinch and grip postures as criteria for forceful exertions.

Worker self-assessments. In Table 32.5, force is assessed by asking the worker if they perceive their job as fatiguing. While this is basically a yes/no question, it does take into consideration other factors, e.g., repetition and posture. Also, workers will add qualifications, e.g., 'on days when we run a specific part'. The modified Borg[31] scale is widely used to obtain worker assessments on a scale from 0 to 10, which correspond to the relative force ratings described above. Workers are shown the scale and simply asked to rate the effort required to perform their job using the verbal anchor points shown in Table 32.8. By dividing the Borg score by 10 and multiplying by the worker's strength, the absolute force can be estimated. As a practical matter, we have found that a simple 10 cm horizontal line with 0 at one end and 10 at the other works as well as the Borg scale. Workers may be asked to rate the overall job or they may be asked to rate specific tasks or work elements, e.g., the insertion of a connector or use of a hand tool, etc.[30] In some cases it is instructive to obtain independent ratings from multiple workers. The Strain Index (Table 32.1) specifies five levels of force achieved on the Borg scale.[24]

Mechanical stresses from localized contact

A localized mechanical stress is defined as a force distributed over some part of the body. For example, resting an arm on the edge of a workstation causes the weight of the arm to be distributed over the area of contact between the arm and armrest; or gripping a tool causes the force required to activate the tool to be distributed between the handle of the tool and the hand. Localized mechanical stresses can be quantified by dividing the contact force by the area of contact. For example, if an armrest, 2 cm × 5 cm, is in complete contact with the fleshy area of the forearm and if the forearm is resting on the armrest with a force of 20 N, the average contact stress is 20 kPa. As a second example, consider an arm resting against the edge

of a work surface holding a keyboard. In this case, the area of contact is 2 cm × 0.5 cm, again assuming a resting weight of 20 N, the contact stress is calculated as 200 kPa. (For comparison a 75 kg person with a 10 × 10 cm heel would produce about 75 kPa pressure if they were to step on your foot with their full weight.) These are average stress concentrations. When the load is distributed over large fleshy areas by a soft surface, these are reasonable approximations of the actual contact stresses. When the forces are exerted against bony areas of the body, such as the elbow or on hard surfaces, then the force is not uniformly distributed and there will be areas of much higher and much lower stress.

The level of insult and discomfort increases with the magnitude of contact stress. Some parts of the body are more tolerant to contact stresses than others. For example, a contact force may be tolerated longer if it is distributed in the thenar eminences than over the median nerve at the wrist and palm. Nerve response to even brief percussion over the median nerve is brisk, explaining its use as a diagnostic test (Tinel's sign, Fig. 32.6). The steps for analyzing contact force are as follows.

Contact stresses can be rated on a scale of 0–10, as was described for repetition and force. One of the difficulties with rating contact stress is that the upper limit (i.e., scale designation of '10') is not always clearly defined. Also, some parts of the body are more tolerant to contact stresses

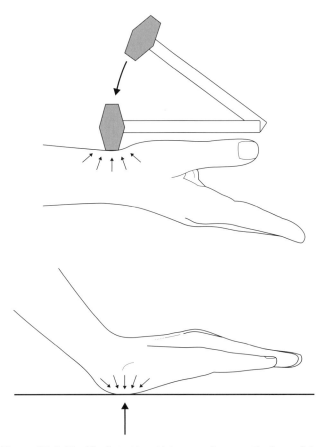

Figure 32.6: The Tinel's test in which percussion over the base of the palm demonstrates how contact stress at certain locations on the surface of the body can produce stress on underlying tissues.

0	Nothing at all
0.5	Very, very easy
1	Very easy
2	Easy
3	Moderately hard
4	Somewhat hard
5	Hard
6	
7	Very hard
8	
9	
10	Very, very hard

Table 32.8 Ten-point Borg scale for worker assessment of task force requirements

than others.[32] Even though a 10-point scale is used, it may be only possible to discriminate between high and low values or low, medium and high values.

Jobs that involve high contact stresses from pounding or exertions of connectors may still have low average values because the duration of the exertions is short as compared to the overall work cycle. High average values are sometimes observed where a worker rests his hand or forearms on hard or sharp surfaces.

The UAW-GM Risk Factor Checklist uses yes/no questions about contact with the fingers, palm, elbow and armpits with hard or sharp objects to identify contact stress hazards.[14] The Washington State workplace ergonomic standard criteria for a 'caution zone job' is: '(9) Using the hand (heel/base of palm) or knee as a hammer more than 10 times per hour more than 2 hours total per day'.[22]

Worker self assessments. In Table 32.5, contact stress is assessed by asking the worker if they strike, press or rest their body against any hard or sharp objects. The worker's hands often provide evidence of repeated contact via calluses, which can be observed in the clinic. In work settings, tape and packing materials on work equipment and on the worker's hands often provide evidence of contact stresses. Workers' bodies often show evidence of impact in the form of abrasions and calluses at specific locations contact with equipment (Fig. 32.7).

Posture stresses

All postures are stressful if they are maintained long enough. For example, lying in bed or sitting in an easy chair eventually becomes uncomfortable. Conversely, conspicuously stressful postures, such as stretching the arms above the head, may feel good for a brief period. Thus the question becomes: what makes one posture more stressful than another? First, some postures require more

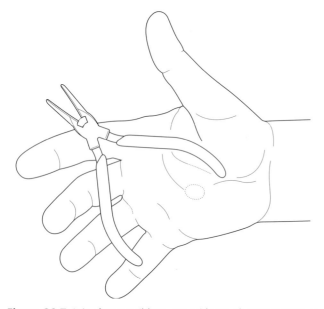

Figure 32.7: It is often possible to see evidence of contact stress on the surface of the body. For example, use of needle nose pliers can produce a major callus near the base of the palm.

effort than others. For example, the body must work harder to produce the same force with an outstretched arm or with a pinch grip than with the arms close to the body or with the hand in a power grip posture. Second, some postures result in greater internal stresses than others. The most common sites of these stresses are in tendons, nerves and blood vessels around joints. For example, exertion of the hand with a flexed wrist causes the flexor tendons to press against the median nerve (see Fig. 32.2). Precipitation of numbness and tingling in the median dermatome of the hand by this maneuver is considered a sign of carpal tunnel syndrome (Phalen's test).

Similarly, extreme extension of the wrist causes increased carpal canal pressure and stretching of the median nerve. Ulnar deviation of the wrist causes the extrinsic abductor and extensor tendons of the thumb to be stretched around the radial styloid process. Discomfort produced by forced deviation of the wrist with the fingers wrapped around the thumb is regarded as a positive sign of de Quervain's disease (Finkelstein's test). Stressful upper limb postures for repeated or sustained exertions include elevation of the elbows, reaching behind the torso, extreme elbow flexion, extreme forearm rotation, wrist deviation, flexion or hyperextension, and pinching. Joint angles can be measured in degrees and both peak and average values should be considered. Video methods have been proposed for assessing posture at fixed time intervals.[33,34]

Corlett et al[35] proposed a graphical scheme for rating each major joint based on its degree of rotation. Armstrong et al[33] proposed an ordinal scheme for rating postures in which each major joint of the upper limb was divided into three or more zones. The Strain Index uses a system in which wrist posture is divided into five zones: very good (neutral), good, fair, bad and very bad (maximum deviation).[24] The UAW-GM risk factor checklist specifies acceptable ranges of postures for each joint. Postures that exceed those ranges are given a star if it occurs less than one-third of the time or a star if it occurs more than one-third of the time. Postures or joint positions can be rated from 0 to 10 where 0 is neutral and 10 is maximum deviation – as was described for repetition, force and contact stress. In most cases it is possible to achieve an extreme joint position in two or more directions. For example, the wrist can be flexed or extended or deviated in a radial or ulnar direction. The elbow can be flexed and the forearm can be rotated. The shoulder can be flexed or extended, it can be abducted or adducted, or it can be rotated. Rating can be performed for the most extreme position of a given joint or each degree of motion can be rated individually. Posture ratings should include both peak and average values.

Instrumental methods are generally beyond the scope of this discussion; however, the proliferation of commercially available equipment increases the likelihood that it will be encountered by an occupational health physician. Goniometers that can be attached externally to joints and connected to data loggers are commercially available. As was shown in the introduction to this chapter, there are important reasons why wrist postures and movements may contribute to specific MSDs. Indeed, Marras and

Schonmarklin[36] have presented evidence that wrist velocity and acceleration measurements are associated with risk of cumulative trauma disorders. While these results are promising, further studies are needed to examine the relationship between joint postures and specific disorders before this equipment is widely used. Also, goniometers only measure posture and movement; they do not measure other factors such as force and contact stress. Presently this equipment is best used to answer narrowly defined questions about posture and as a research tool.

Worker self-assessments. In Table 32.5, posture stress is assessed by asking the worker if their job requires them to assume any unusual or uncomfortable postures. It is suggested that the physician demonstrate wrist flexion/extension and radial/ulnar deviation, extreme forearm rotation, extreme elbow flexion, extreme reaching, extreme neck motion, and, if appropriate, bending. Pictures can be used for greater standardization. The worker should then be asked where and how frequently the extreme postures are encountered. Workers also can be asked to rate posture comfort or discomfort for the overall job or specific tasks.[30]

Low temperature

Strength, dexterity, and sensitivity are profoundly affected by skin temperatures below 18 degrees C. Most people have experienced the effect of cold fingers when working outside on a cold day. People normally exert just enough or slightly more force than is required to keep objects from slipping out of their hand, but cooling the skin results in reduced sensory function and excess force. Sources of cold exposure include ambient air, work materials, and the exhaust air from tools.

Worker self-assessments. In Table 32.5 the worker is asked if his or her hands get cold. If the answer is 'yes', subsequent questions would focus on the frequency and duration as well as the cause, e.g., is it due to low ambient temperatures or due to localized cooling from handling cold materials?

Vibration

Hand–arm vibration (HAV) has been shown to be associated with a number of soft tissue disorders of the upper limb, secondary Raynaud's phenomenon being the most notable.[37] It is important to remember that HAV occurs in combination with other mechanical stressors. Workers undergo vibration exposure by holding something that vibrates. Thus, vibration exposure inevitably occurs in combination with repeated or sustained exertions. Additionally, these exertions may involve high forces, localized mechanical stresses, posture stresses, and exposure to low temperatures.

Although quantitative vibration measurements require specialized instrumentation and trained technicians, it is possible to estimate the intensity of exposure from information about the job and the tools. There are several important considerations in estimating the intensity of HAV from tools. The first consideration is the action of the tool. Tool action can be classified as rotary, in which the tool turns something, such as a threaded fastener or a grinder wheel, or as reciprocating, in which the tool moves something back and forth, such as a manual hammer, powered chipping hammer, or a rivet gun. Free running (not in contact with another object) industrial quality rotary tools that are well maintained should not exceed physiologic vibration limits; however, this may not be true for reciprocating tools. Some tools encompass both rotary and reciprocating parts. Examples include tools with internal combustion engines, such as lawn mowers and chain saws. Although these tools turn, they have reciprocating components such as pistons that may produce high vibration levels. Controls for machines and vehicles are another source of vibration exposure that should be considered. The State of Washington workplace ergonomics standard specifies maximum exposure duration limits for specified types of tools.[22] For example, the limit for impact wrenches, chain saws and percussive tools is 30 minutes per day, while the limit for grinders and sanders is 2 hours per day.

Worker self-assessments. In Table 32.5 the worker is asked if anything he or she holds or touches vibrates or shakes. Subsequent questions would investigate how frequently and how long if the worker answers affirmatively.

PLANT VISIT/WALK-THROUGH

Many physicians find that walk-through inspections of workplaces provide important background information for evaluating workers they see in clinic. They also afford an excellent opportunity to learn about the attitudes of workers and employers. Table 32.9a includes a list of useful background information. Information about what the plant does, processes, equipment, materials and numbers of workers provides an overview of the operations and potential exposures. Often this information can be obtained in advance, and can be used to plan the visit. Table 32.9b is intended for collection of data about physical stress exposures for individual jobs and tasks at the time of the visit. It is important to recognize that exposures may change from job to job, hour to hour, day to day and season to season, and that the walk-through only

Company name
Contact information
Location
Department/work area (list)
For each department/work area:
Description of service or product
List of production and service areas
Description of:
Products/services
Tools/equipment
Materials
General layout
Estimate of number of workers on each shift
Daily or seasonal variations
Source of information
Last update

Table 32.9a General worksite information that may be collected in advance of plant walk-through

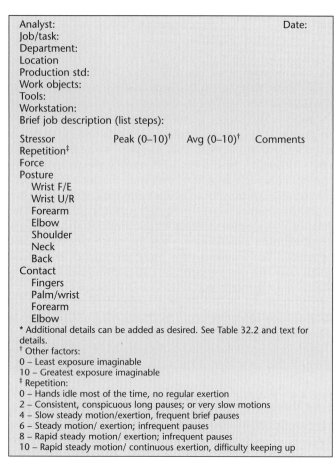

Analyst:			Date:
Job/task:			
Department:			
Location			
Production std:			
Work objects:			
Tools:			
Workstation:			
Brief job description (list steps):			

Stressor	Peak (0–10)[†]	Avg (0–10)[†]	Comments
Repetition[‡]			
Force			
Posture			
Wrist F/E			
Wrist U/R			
Forearm			
Elbow			
Shoulder			
Neck			
Back			
Contact			
Fingers			
Palm/wrist			
Forearm			
Elbow			

* Additional details can be added as desired. See Table 32.2 and text for details.
[†] Other factors:
0 – Least exposure imaginable
10 – Greatest exposure imaginable
[‡] Repetition:
0 – Hands idle most of the time, no regular exertion
2 – Consistent, conspicuous long pauses; or very slow motions
4 – Slow steady motion/exertion, frequent brief pauses
6 – Steady motion/ exertion; infrequent pauses
8 – Rapid steady motion/ exertion; infrequent pauses
10 – Rapid steady motion/ continuous exertion, difficulty keeping up

Table 32.9b Simple data collection forms for walk-through job surveys*

provides a sampling of some of the jobs at one point in time and may not be representative of the entire operation over the entire year or even the entire day. This can also be seen in a grocery store between the middle of the day and in the early evening or days immediately preceding holidays versus after holidays. Table 32.9a specifically asks for information on daily and seasonal variations. The walk-through should be designed to provide an overview, while allowing additional time to examine jobs with high exposures. Medical visit logs and OSHA records sometimes can be used to identify problem areas, but may be subject to statistical limitations due to small numbers, or variations in reporting.

An important source of information is from people at the plant – both workers and managers. It is helpful if both a management and worker representative accompany the physician on the walk-through. This is reinforced by a personal experience by the author during a walk-through inspection of a pork processing plant with a labor and a management representative. The management representative stated that he did not understand why people were having problems, because he himself had worked on the line for a number of years. The labor representative countered that they were previously running only 350 animals an hour through the plant, and now they were running 600. Also, the presence of the labor and management

representatives is usually reassuring to both workers and supervisors. A plant walk-through also provides an opportunity to involve others, e.g., other healthcare providers, engineers, and ergonomists who may be called upon to provide addition job information, develop job accommodations and treat patients.

Table 32.9b is intended for assessing exposures on individual jobs or job tasks, providing structure for the survey; it is not a definitive survey tool. The healthcare provider may want to request a detailed analysis using one or more of the tools listed in Table 32.1 as the need arises.

The walk-through survey should be documented in writing. It is likely that the healthcare provider will see workers from many plants and a written record will enable them to refresh their memory when they see a patient from that site. The written record also can be shared with the employer. This will help the healthcare provider and the employer reach a common understanding about the exposures. It also will give the employer feedback about exposures at that site so they can determine the feasibility of interventions.

The following examples illustrate how plant walk-through data can be used to supplement worker assessments in the clinic.

Office seating

By visiting an office worksite, the healthcare provider discovers to what degree jobs are clerical and involve keyboard and mouse work, filing, phoning, copying and meetings. It also might be discovered that some of the jobs entail repetitive handling of heavy files, while others involve prolonged interaction with the computer to compose documents with both text and graphical components. It may be determined that workers are using some new and some old furniture with varying degrees of adjustability. By inquiring about a patient's job title, job responsibilities and work equipment, the healthcare provider may be able to quickly assess the worker's exposure to mechanical stressors. Further discussion could focus on details unique to the case at hand. The following scenario illustrates the use of this job information.

A male worker from the office with persistent forearm, neck and shoulder pain visits a healthcare provider in his off-site clinic. It is quickly determined that the worker is an accounts manager who uses the computer and mouse to prepare financial reports and propose budgets. It is learned that the patient has a healthy lifestyle, with no evidence of chronic diseases, traumatic injuries, or excess recreation that might explain his symptoms. Finally it is learned that the worker had a recent deadline that required intense use of the computer and mouse and that he was working extended shifts and skipping breaks. It is also determined that the worker is 1.9 m tall (approximately 95th percentile), does not have an adjustable work surface for his keyboard, mouse, and monitor, and that his chair was difficult to adjust. By demonstrating the job, it appears that the worker has been spending 75% of his work shift, up to 12 hours a day, facing a computer monitor (non-adjustable) with his neck flexed to highly flexed and his hands on the keyboard or mouse. The remaining time is spent handling documents and on the phone (often held between the neck and shoulder). A work restriction in this case might specify how much time the worker is permitted to key each day, and frequency of breaks. It might specify the use of a headset or speakerphone. An evaluation of the workstation to investigate modifications and to make sure the worker understands how to adjust the workstation and chair should also be initiated. Restrictions should be specified for a fixed period time, at which point the worker and restrictions would be reassessed.

Kitchen appliance manufacturer

A second example involves a manufacturer of small kitchen appliances. It is learned that the jobs include: 200 general utility workers who may be assigned to any job on the assembly line, 10 materials handlers who operate fork lifts and load and unload stock, 20 maintenance workers who set up and service equipment, six custodial workers who perform housekeeping activities, and 30 administrative/clerical workers who work in the office. From discussions with production supervisors and observations of the assembly line, it is determined that the assembly jobs have a 1-minute cycle time. The workers do not appear to be rushing, but there are no definable rest periods. Using Table 32.4 it is estimated that the repetition varies from 4 to 7 on the scale of 10.

Most of the parts handled by assemblers are small, with weights below 1 pound. While the overall force requirements are low, some jobs require nearly all of the worker's strength to install harnesses and join electrical connectors. The small size of the connectors forces assemblers to use their finger tips in awkward locations. It is also observed that about one-third of the workers use small in-line and pistol-shaped power tools. Tool use varied from one fastener per cycle to six per cycle. While most of the workers do not appear to have any trouble holding and controlling tools, many appear to jerk their wrist as the tool starts and stops. Using the methods described above, peak forces for assemblers were rated from 2 to 10 on a scale of 10. Average forces are generally below 2 on a 10 scale, but some jobs are of concern because the force never reaches zero, enabling the hands to rest. These cases occur where workers hold tools in their hand continuously – even while performing non-tool related work elements. As a result, these workers may never fully recover during work cycles (see Fig. 32.3).

Contact stress on the hand – particularly on the finger-tips – results from grasping and handling of parts and tools. In some cases workers were observed joining parts by pressing and pounding on parts with the base of their palms. It was estimated peak finger and palm contact stresses are in the upper third of a 10-point scale (7–9 for some jobs), although the averages are all in the lower third of the scale 1–3.

Postures are observed to vary widely from one workstation to the next, as workers obtain and install parts and use tools. Some notable examples include shoulder stresses associated with overhead reaching to get suspended tools, reaching for parts in tote pans, and installing parts in the moving assemblies. Some involve wrist flexion and deviation, and extreme forearm rotation to grasp and position parts and tools. Peak shoulder, forearm, and wrist postures are 7–9 on the 10-point scales as described above for repetition, force and contact stress. For most workers the average values are below 3, but for some workers the average shoulder stress is above 5. These workers were sitting down and had to keep their elbows up to reach their work.

The only source of vibration exposure is the power tools. It was observed that only about one-third of the workers use power tools. The most fasteners installed with a tool are six, which require less than 6 seconds of the 1-minute cycle time. Air-powered screw drivers generally have low vibration unless they use slip clutches to regulate torque.[38] The major stress associated with the hand tools is posture and force.

The assembly area is at room temperature. The only exposure to low temperature is from occasional batches of parts that are brought in from an unheated warehouse in the cold season.

Similar information would be compiled for other jobs at this worksite, e.g., materials handling, maintenance, custodial activities. These jobs will be much harder to characterize because they involve multiple and often irregular work tasks. Multiple visits or assistance from ergonomists or industrial hygienists may be required to get information about all jobs. Medical visit records and OSHA logs may be used to determine which jobs have a history of injuries and to set priorities for evaluation.

One of the first work questions for a patient with MSD symptoms from this plant would pertain to which area of the plant or which job he or she was employed in and for how long. How far back the exposures are traced would depend on the history and duration of symptoms. If the symptoms are new, it may be necessary to go back only a few months. If they are longstanding, it may be necessary to go back several years. Workplace rotations are becoming more and more common, which can increase the time required to get a full work history. At the same time, work rotations may provide an opportunity to compare jobs to see if there is anything about one position relative to another that makes symptoms worse.

For example, it may be that the worker's hand symptoms are worse when performing assembly jobs that require power tools. From the plant visit, the physician knows that hand tools are only used for a small part of any one work cycle, and that the tools do not weigh much or require high torque levels. By asking the worker to demonstrate how the tools are held and how they are used, it is learned that they are held in the hand continuously, even while other assembly operations are being performed, and that worker has to reach over the assembly and point the tool back towards himself to drive two screws. By watching the worker simulate this in the clinic, it is determined that the job requires elevation of the shoulder (7 on a scale of

10), inward rotation of the forearm (8 on a scale of 10) and extreme wrist flexion (9 on a scale of 10).

Rather than restrict the worker from the use of all power tools, the restriction is crafted to emphasize avoidance of continuous holding of tools or exertions that require flexion of the wrist or extreme forearm rotation. Further qualifications could be added depending on the severity of the case. The restrictions could be decreased over time. For example, the first week could specify that the worker should not perform any job that provides less than 20 seconds recovery time for each minute and no wrist flexion or forearm rotation more than two-thirds of their range of motion. It might still say 'no continuous holding of tools'. The following week might reduce the recovery time to 10 seconds, no wrist flexion, and no extreme forearm rotation, and still forbid continuous holding of tools. The physician would have to either instruct the employee on how to interpret wrist flexion and forearm rotation or meet with appropriate plant representatives. In many cases plants will designate someone to coordinate work restrictions between management, engineers, and healthcare providers.

These two scenarios illustrate the assessment of work exposures in both plant walk-through and clinical settings. Quality job information is essential for assessing the contribution of work to MSDs and for developing effective work restrictions. It is assumed that the work assessment also considers and prescribes for non-work factors, e.g., existing medical conditions and outside activities that can also cause MSDs. Even in cases where an MSD is due to non-work related factors, work exposures still need to be considered to avoid aggravating those conditions and facilitating return to work.

ANALYSIS OF JOBS FROM THE CLINIC

In the absence of first-hand information or summary information from the plant, the healthcare provider will have to rely on his or her interview of the worker. The information included in Tables 32.2 and 32.3 should serve as general guidelines. The healthcare provider will have to explore details as dictated by the needs of the worker and permitted by time.

Recognizing the limitations inherent in a clinical assessment of a job, many physicians will issue very conservative work restrictions, e.g., no hand tools, no gripping greater than 10 pounds, nor repetitive work. These may pose a challenge for the plant to accommodate. Physicians who issue such restrictions may want to add some qualifying language to indicate that the restriction was issued in the absence of a formal job analysis and that such an analysis should be performed to clarify the work restriction. Depending on the time or the service arrangement with the employer, the physician might want to arrange to visit the plant or for a trained job analyst to visit the plant and provide more detailed job analysis.

Worker assessments are sometimes criticized for not being objective. Studies by Homan and Armstrong[39] found that workers in office settings tended to over-estimate their use of keyboards and mice by as much as 200% when compared with second party observations and electronic surveillance. The discrepancy between self-reports and external observations can be attributed to a difference in perspective and the analyst's failure to consider the worker's perspective. Most of the people were next to the computer and in some cases looking at the monitor. From their perspective they were using the keyboard. If the question is how much time they are using the keyboard, they should be asked that directly. They also should be asked what other activities they perform and how much time they devote to those tasks. Discrepancies can then be noted and discussed. It is important that the person asking the questions be perceived as neutral, and not express approval or disapproval.[40]

CAUSALITY

As mentioned above, present and proposed OSHA regulations presume that injuries are work related and place a high burden on employers to prove otherwise. Healthcare providers frequently are called upon to decide if specific MSD cases are related to a specific job or, in some cases, a specific activity or tool. Determining causality goes beyond the scope of this chapter; however, information about exposure to mechanical stressors is an important consideration in determining causality. Most musculoskeletal disorders can be caused by one or more factors. The available data may be insufficient to assign exact probabilities to any one or combination of factors with a high degree of certainty; however, the data may effectively address 'more probable than not' criteria for causation. It is possible to determine if and how much a given worker was exposed to a mechanical stressor or group of stressors. This information must be weighed against knowledge of other physical and mental factors that may affect a worker's risk. This issue is likely to remain within the realm of expert medical opinion and be subject to much controversy over workers' compensation claims for the foreseeable future. This controversy must not dissuade healthcare providers from assessing mechanical stressors and treating both the cause and the consequences of musculoskeletal disorders.

SUMMARY

Musculoskeletal disorders may be caused or aggravated by certain types of work activities. Recognized risk factors include: repetitive or prolonged force, contact stresses, postures, vibration, and low temperatures. The healthcare provider should consider, along with health and personal information, information about the workers' exposure to mechanical stresses. In most cases, healthcare providers do not have time to visit the worksite each time a worker with symptoms reports to them. Thus they often have to obtain information about the job from the worker. It is helpful if the healthcare provider conducts regular walk-through inspections of workplaces so that they have a background for interviewing the worker and interpreting their responses. It is helpful if the healthcare provider understands how work contributes to musculoskeletal disorders, and uses a structured approach in obtaining and interpreting clinical and workplace data.

References

1. Occupational Safety and Health Administration. Occupational safety and health standards: ergonomics program final rule. Fed Reg 2000; 65(220):68261–870.
2. Keyserling WM. Workplace risk factors and occupational musculoskeletal disorders. Part 1: A review of biomechanical and psychophysical research on risk factors associated with low-back pain. AIHAJ 2000; 61:39–50.
3. Keyserling WM. Workplace risk factors and occupational musculoskeletal disorders. Part 2: A review of biomechanical and psychophysical research on risk factors associated with upper extremity disorders. AIHAJ 2000; 61:231–43.
4. National Research Council and the Institute of Medicine. Musculoskeletal disorders and the workplace: low back and upper extremities. Washington, DC: National Academy Press, 2001.
5. National Research Council Committee on Human Factors. Work-related musculoskeletal disorders report, workshop summary, and workshop papers. Washington, DC: National Academy Press, 1999.
6. Armstrong TJ, Buckle P, Fine LJ, et al. A conceptual model for work-related neck and upper-limb musculoskeletal disorders. Scand J Work Environ Health 1993; 19:73–84.
7. Bystrom S, Fransson-Hall C. Acceptability of intermittent handgrip contractions based on physiologic response. Hum Factors 1994; 36:158–71.
8. Phalen GS. The carpal-tunnel syndrome. Clinical evaluation of 598 hands. Clin Orthop 1972; 83:29–40.
9. Smith EM, Sonstegard DA, Anderson WH Jr. Carpal tunnel syndrome: contribution of flexor tendons. Arch Phys Med Rehabil 1977; 58:379–85.
10. Elkus R, Basmajian JV. Endurance in hanging by the hands. Why do people hanging by their hands let go? Am J Phys Med 1973; 52:124–7.
11. Armstrong TJ, Castelli WA, Evans FG, et al. Some histological changes in carpal tunnel contents and their biomechanical implications. J Occup Med 1984; 26:197–201.
12. Feuerstein M. Biobehavioral mechanisms of work-related upper extremity disorders: a new agenda for research and practice. Am J Ind Med 2002; 41:293–7.
13. Occupational Safety and Health Administration. Regulations (Standards – 29 CFR) Determination of work-relatedness – 1904.5. Cincinatti: OSHA, 2002.
14. Keyserling WM, Stetson DS, Silverstein BA, et al. A checklist for evaluating ergonomic risk factors associated with upper extremity cumulative trauma disorders. Ergonomics 1993; 36:807–31.
15. Keyserling WM, Armstrong T, et al. Ergonomic job analysis: a structured approach for identifying risk factors associated with overexertion injuries and disorders. Appl Occup Environ Hyg 1991; 6:353–63.
16. Barnes RM. Motion and time study: design and measurement of work. New York: Wiley, 1980;407.
17. Colombini D. An observational method for classifying exposure to repetitive movements of the upper limbs. Ergonomics 1998; 41:1261–89.
18. ACGIH. Hand activity level. 2002 threshold limit values for chemical substances and physical agents and biologic exposure limits. Cincinnati: American Conference of Governmental Industrial Hygienists, 2002;109–19.
19. Latko WA, Armstrong TJ, Foulke JA, et al. Development and evaluation of an observational method for assessing repetition in hand tasks. Am Ind Hyg Assoc J 1997; 58: 278–85.
20. Latko WA, Armstrong TJ, Franzblau A, et al. Cross-sectional study of the relationship between repetitive work and the prevalence of upper limb musculoskeletal disorders. Am J Ind Med 1999; 36:248–59.
21. Ebersole M, Armstrong TJ. Inter-rater reliability for hand activity level (HAL) and force metrics. Baltimore: Human Factors and Ergonomics Society, 2002.
22. Washington State. WAC 296-62-051 Ergonomics. 2002. http://www.lni.wa.gov/wisha/ergo/
23. Buchholz B, Frederick LJ, Armstrong TJ. An investigation of human palmar skin friction and the effects of materials, pinch force and moisture. Ergonomics 1988; 31:317–25.
24. Moore JS, Garg A. The strain index: a proposed method to analyze jobs for risk of distal upper extremity disorders. Am Ind Hyg Assoc J 1995; 56:443–58.
25. Armstrong TJ, Foulke JA, Martin BJ, et al. Investigation of applied forces in alphanumeric keyboard work. Am Ind Hyg Assoc J 1994; 55:30–5.
26. Westling G, Johansson RS. Factors influencing the force control during precision grip. Exp Brain Res 1984; 53:277–84.
27. Frederick LJ, Armstrong TJ. Effect of friction and load on pinch force in a hand transfer task. Ergonomics 1995; 38:2447–54.
28. Bongers PM, de Winter CR, Kompier MA, et al. Psychosocial factors at work and musculoskeletal disease. Scand J Work Environ Health 1993; 19: 297–312.
29. Pascarelli EF, Kella JJ. Soft-tissue injuries related to use of the computer keyboard. A clinical study of 53 severely injured persons. J Occup Med 1993; 35:522–32.
30. Armstrong T, Punnett L, et al. Subjective worker assessments of hand tools used in automobile assembly. Am Ind Hyg Assoc J 1989; 50:639.
31. Borg GA. Psychophysical bases of perceived exertion. Med Sci Sports Exerc 1982; 14:377–81.
32. Fransson-Hall C, Kilbom A. Sensitivity of the hand to surface pressure. Appl Ergon 1993; 24:181–9.
33. Armstrong TJ, Foulke JA, Joseph BS, et al. Investigation of cumulative trauma disorders in a poultry processing plant. Am Ind Hyg Assoc J 1982; 43:103–16.
34. Fransson-Hall C, Gloria R, et al. A portable ergonomic obser-vation method (PEO) for computerized on-line recording of postures and manual handling. Appl Ergon 1995; 26:93–100.
35. Corlett E, Madeley S, et al. Posture targeting: a technique for recording working postures. Ergonomics 1979; 22:357–66.
36. Marras WS, Schoenmarklin RW. Wrist motions in industry. Ergonomics 1993; 36:341–51.
37. ACGIH. Hand-arm (segmental) vibration. 2002 threshold limit values for chemical substances and physical agents and biologic exposure indices. Cincinnati: ACGIH Worldwide, 2002;120–3.
38. Radwin RG, Armstrong TJ. Assessment of hand vibration exposure on an assembly line. Am Ind Hyg Assoc J 1985; 46:211–9.
39. Homan, MM, Armstrong T. Evaluation of three methodologies for assessing work activity during computer use. Am Ind Hyg Assoc J 2003; 64:48–55.
40. McCormick E. Task analysis. Handbook of industrial engineering. New York: John Wiley, 1982;2.4.4–2.4.6.
41. McAtamney L, Corlett E. RULA: a survey method for the investigation of work-related upper limb disorders. Appl Ergon 1993; 24:91–9.
42. Hignett S, McAtamney L. Rapid entire body assessment (REBA). Appl Ergon 2000; 31:201–5.
43. Karhu O, Kansi P, et al. Correcting working postures in industry: a practical method for analysis. Appl Ergon 1977; 8:199–201.
44. Karhu O, Harkonen R, et al. Observing working postures in industry: examples of OWAS application. Appl Ergon 1981; 12:13–17.
45. Snook SH, Vaillancourt DR, Ciriello VM, et al. Psychophysical studies of repetitive wrist flexion and extension. Ergonomics 1995; 38:1488–507.

46. Schmidt RT, Toews JV. Grip strength as measured by the Jamar dynamometer. Arch Phys Med Rehab 1970; 51:321–7.

47. Imrhan, SN, Loo CH. Trends in finger pinch strength in children, adults, and the elderly. Hum Factors 1989; 31:689–701.

48. Josty IC, Tyler MP, et al. Grip and pinch strength variations in different types of workers. Br J Hand Surg 1997; 22:266–9.

49. Dempsey PG, Ayoub MM. The influence of gender, grasp type, pinch width and wrist position on sustained pinch strength. Int J Ind Ergon 1996; 17:259–73.

Chapter 33
Radiation

33.1 Ionizing Radiation

H Gregg Claycamp, Niel Wald

EXPOSURE SETTINGS

Ionizing radiation is composed of electromagnetic energy or high-energy subatomic particles that have sufficient energy to break atomic bonds in absorbing materials, including biologic tissues. The high-energy electromagnetic radiation includes x-rays and gamma rays, while the particulate radiations include electrons, protons, neutrons, alpha particles or other subatomic particles. Everyone is exposed to ionizing radiation from natural sources, with additional exposure from technology-enhanced or artificial sources. The principal natural sources of ionizing radiation are: (1) cosmic rays, which originate in outer space, (2) terrestrial radiations, which emanate from radium, thorium, uranium, and other radioactive elements in the earth's crust, and (3) internal radiations, which are emitted by potassium-40, carbon-14, and other radioactive isotopes ('radionuclides') normally contained within living tissues. The principal artificially derived sources of radiation exposures include x-ray machines, particle accelerators, nuclear reactor or accelerator produced radionuclides and numerous lesser sources.

The average dose received annually worldwide from natural sources of ionizing radiation amounts to about 80% of the total average annual dose (Table 33.1.1). Typically more than one-half of the naturally derived radiation dose is from indoor radon (primarily ^{222}Rn) and its radioactive progeny occurring in the home. Medically derived radiation exposures, amounting to about 20% of the average annual dose, fall primarily on the elderly and the ill. Occupational exposures from ionizing radiation contribute little to the worldwide population average annual dose (Table 33.1.1); however, to occupationally exposed individuals, the average annual dose on a worldwide basis approaches 1 mSv per year. Other groups in the population who receive greater than average doses are those who reside at high elevation (e.g., Denver, Colorado), where cosmic rays may be twice as intense, or those residing in areas where the earth's content of uranium and/or radium is comparatively high. Cigarette smokers can also receive up to 200 mSv per year to the lung from the polonium-210 that is present naturally in tobacco products. Finally, sources of small doses to the population include natural radioactive minerals in building materials, phosphate fertilizers and crushed rock, radiation-emitting components of television sets, smoke detectors, and other consumer products.

Ionizing radiation is a hazard that can be encountered in many different occupations (Table 33.1.2). Workers in both radiation and non-radiation occupations that use radiation-emitting devices or materials have widely variable exposures depending on their work assignments and working conditions (Fig. 33.1.1). The average yearly dose equivalent of whole-body radiation received occupationally by monitored workers in the United States who do not work at nuclear reactors is less than 1 mSv (Table 33.1.3) – similar to the dose received from natural background irradiation. Most workers in Table 33.1.3 receive doses that are less than or near the lower detection limits of personnel dosimeters, and relatively few workers (<1%) reach the maximum permissible dose limit of 50 mSv in any given year. It is also important to note that the average annual doses to radiation workers have declined steadily over several decades, primarily as a result of effective radiation protection programs.

Exposure to ionizing radiation in the ambient and occupational environments differs not only in amount, but oftentimes by the type of ionizing radiation. Much ambient and medical exposure is from external sources of ionizing radiation in the form of x-rays or gamma rays. These radiations are from the very high frequency end of the electromagnetic energy spectrum, beginning near ultraviolet light energies (about 0.0001 joule) to several joules of energy per gamma ray. X- and gamma rays are highly penetrating forms of ionizing radiation that can easily impart energy to any part of the body not effectively shielded from them. Typically, lead or other high-density materials are used to shield workers from high-intensity sources of x- or gamma rays. Radionuclides in the environment or the work place might emit gamma rays but might also give off radioactive particles such as alpha particles, beta particles or, rarely, neutrons. These particles have different properties from x-rays and gamma rays in terms of their ability to penetrate tissue and with respect to the biologically effective dose (discussed below). For example, high-energy beta particles can readily penetrate millimeters of soft tissues in the body whereas alpha particles are poorly penetrating and can be effectively blocked by the dead layers of the epidermis. Thus, alpha-emitting radionuclides can cause hazardous exposures only when they are deposited internally.

Each radioactive element or radionuclide has its own unique pattern of radioactive decay with a characteristic half-life (the time over which one-half of a given compound's radiation will be released) and decay scheme – the types and energy of the emitted ionizing radiation. What is most relevant medically is that the types of radiation released for each radionuclide are known and, therefore, the theoretical total absorbed dose can be modeled

Source	Average annual effective dose equivalent (mSv)	Percent of total
Natural		
Cosmic radiation and cosmogenic radionuclides	0.31	11
Terrestrial external	0.46	16
Terrestrial internal (excluding radon)	0.23	8
Internal radon-222 and its decay products	1.28	44
Total natural	2.28	79
Medical radiation		
Diagnostic medical radiation	0.3	10
Therapeutic medical radiation	0.3	10
Industrial		
Radionuclides in medical, educational and industrial applications	<0.001	0.0003
Nuclear fuel cycle	0.03	0.0103
Occupational	0.001†	0.0003
Total artificial	0.632	21
Total	2.91	

* Compiled from data in UNSCEAR 1993.[19]
† The occupational figure is averaged over the entire population. Occupational doses approach 1 mSv per year on a worldwide basis.

Table 33.1.1 Average annual dose equivalent from various sources of ionizing radiation*

Aircraft pilots and crews	Petroleum refinery workers
Cathode ray tube makers	Physicians
Dental assistants	Pipeline oil flow testers
Electron microscope makers	Pipeline welders
Electron microscopists	Radiographers
Electrostatic eliminator operators	Plasma torch operators
Fire alarm makers	Radar tube makers
Gas mantle makers	Radiologists
High-voltage vacuum tube makers	Radium laboratory workers
	Television tube makers
High-voltage vacuum tube users	Thickness gauge operators
Industrial fluoroscope operators	Thorium-aluminum alloy workers
Industrial radiographers	
Inspectors using, and workers located near, sealed gamma ray sources	Thorium-magnesium alloy workers
	Thorium ore producers
Klystron tube operators	Underground metal miners
Luminous dial painters	Uranium mill workers
Nuclear submarine workers	X-ray aides
Nuclear reactor workers and operators	X-ray diffraction operators
	X-ray technicians
Oil well loggers	X-ray tube makers
Ore assayers	

* Modified from Kahn K, Ryan K, Sabo A, et al. Ionizing radiation. In: Levy BS, Wegman DH, eds. Occupational health. Boston: Little, Brown, 1983;189–206.

Table 33.1.2 Workers who may be exposed to ionizing radiation*

Types of work	Numbers of exposed workers annually	Average dose equivalent per year (mSv)
Nuclear fuel production	13,870	0.42
All defense activities	115,000	0.6
Nuclear reactors	186,000	2.18
Industrial uses (monitored workers)	274,000	0.55
Medical applications	734,000	0.42

* Data from UNSCEAR 1993.[19]

Table 33.1.3 Estimated numbers of monitored US workers exposed to ionizing radiation, with their estimated annual doses*

clide. Thus, radioactive isotopes of iodine will be taken up in the thyroid; heavy metals like radium or radioactive strontium will be stored in bones; and radioactive sodium will follow stable sodium through tissues. The characteristics of some common radionuclides to which humans are exposed are summarized in Table 33.1.4.

DOSE ASSESSMENT

The international unit of absorbed dose from ionizing radiation is the *gray* (Gy), which equals 1 joule of absorbed energy per kilogram of absorbing medium, e.g., tissue. Formerly, 'radiation absorbed dose' or the *rad* was used for this measure (and still is by the US Nuclear Regulatory Commission): the conversion is 1 Gy = 100 rad. Different types of ionizing radiation elicit different amounts of tissue injury for a given amount of dose. The relative biologic effectiveness (RBE) is a term that designates the ratio of doses from standard gamma or x-rays to that of a test radiation for a given level of effect, under a given biologic endpoint. RBE varies for different biologic endpoints (e.g., lethality, mutation, erythema, etc) and as a function of dose, making the measure impractical for use in health protection programs. Thus, a physical quantity representing the rate of energy transfer per unit path length of tissue – linear energy transfer or 'LET' – is used as a surrogate measure of the RBE (radiation weighting factors for various radiation types provided in Table 33.1.5).

The LET of the radiation is used to weight the radiation dose by the relative biologic effectiveness, creating a unit of *dose equivalent*. For many years, the unit 'radiation equivalent man' or *rem* was used to indicate the dose equivalent. More recently, the sievert (Sv) was adopted internationally as the official unit of dose equivalent. Since the radiation weighting factor is dimensionless, the base units of Sv remain in joules per kilogram (1 Sv = 1 J/kg). The conversion between Sv and rem also remains as 1 Sv = 100 rem. A Sv of equivalent dose is defined as the dose in Gy multiplied by the LET weighting, or Q-factor, for the type of radiation (Table 33.1.5). Thus, 1 Gy of alpha particles delivers an effective dose of 20 Sv to exposed tissue because the LET for alpha particles is 20-fold that for x-rays. For low-LET radiation, such as gamma rays or beta particles, the absorbed dose in Gy equals the biologically effective dose in Sv.

for a given exposure scenario. This is particularly true for external exposures from x-rays, gamma rays, and some particles; however, the absorbed dose from radionuclides deposited internally depends on the chemical properties of the element and/or the chemical to which the radionuclide is bound. The target organ(s), retention and elimination for radionuclide will be completely governed by the chemical – not radiological – properties of the radionu-

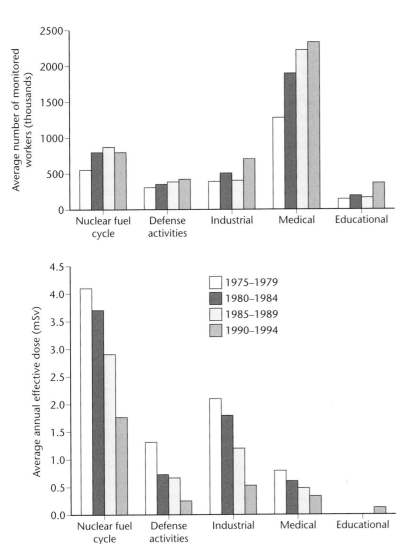

Figure 33.1.1: Numbers of monitored radiation workers and average annual effective dose in the US radiation industry. Adapted from UNSCEAR.[14]

Radionuclide	Half-life	Typical source of exposure	Emission(s)	Target organ
Tritium (^{3}H)	12.3 yr	Biomedical research, nuclear weapons, power plants	Beta	Body water
Strontium (^{90}Sr)	27 yr	Nuclear fallout	Beta	Bone
Technetium(^{99}Tc)	6 hr	Medical diagnosis	Beta, gamma	Not stored
Iodine (^{131}I)	8 day	Medical diagnosis and therapy	Beta, gamma	Thyroid
Cesium (^{137}Cs)	30 yr	Radiation sources	Gamma	Bone
Radon (^{222}Rn)	3.8 day	Indoor environment; mines	Alpha	Lung
Uranium (^{238}U)	4.5 billion yr	Weapons production	Alpha, beta	Lung, Kidney
Plutonium (^{239}Pu)	20,000 yr	Weapons production, reactors	Alpha	Lung

Table 33.1.4 Characteristics of commonly encountered radionuclides

Ionizing radiation may also be measured in other ways important for health effects assessment. The former unit representing the *quantity* of radioactive material is the curie (Ci), which was originally defined as the number of radioactive transitions ('radioactive decays') per second in 1 gram of pure radium-226. This quantity is 3.7×10^{10} transitions per second. The new SI unit of radioactivity is the becquerel (Bq), which is defined simply as 1 transition per second. Thus, 1 Ci = 3.7×10^{10} Bq. Users of radioisotopes or radionuclides purchase them by the curie or becquerel; or, in the case of *radiolabeled* chemicals used as tracers in biomedical research, the typical units are Ci or Bq per millimole or per gram of the labeled chemical. In the atmosphere or in drinking water, the concentration of radionuclide is typically expressed in picocuries (pCi) per liter or becquerels (Bq) per cubic meter.

A special case for units of air-borne radioactivity is encountered in uranium and certain other types of mining environments. The direct assessment of air-borne radon radioactivity is complicated by the fact that the products of the radioactive transition of radon are also radioactive. In order to account for the complex equilibrium among these air-borne radionuclides, a unit of measure was defined based on the total amount of energy emitted by

Type of radiation and energy range	Radiation weighting factor (w_r)
Photons (x-rays, gamma rays) of all energies	1
Electrons (beta particles)	1
Neutrons by energy:	
< 10 keV	5
10–100 keV	10
>100 keV to 2 MeV	20
2–20 MeV	10
>20 MeV	5
Protons, other than recoil protons, energy > 2 MeV	5
Alpha particles, fission fragments, heavy nuclei	20

*From: The International Commission on Radiological Protection (ICRP). Recommendations of the International Commission on Radiological Protection. ICRP Publication 60. Ann ICRP 1991; 21:1–3.

Table 33.1.5 Radiation weighting factors for various linear energy transfers*

Tissue or organ	Tissue weighting factor (w_T)
Gonads	0.20
Bone marrow (red)	0.12
Colon	0.12
Lung	0.12
Stomach	0.12
Bladder	0.05
Breast	0.05
Liver	0.05
Esophagus	0.05
Thyroid	0.01
Skin	0.01
Bone surface	0.01
Remainder	0.05

* From: The International Commission on Radiological Protection (ICRP). Recommendations of the International Commission on Radiological Protection. ICRP Publication 60. Ann ICRP 1991; 21:1–3.

Table 33.1.6 Tissue weighting factors for radiation protection*

the mixture of radionuclides. This unit is the working level (WL), or 1.3×10^5 MeV per liter of air. When radon and its progeny radionuclides are in equilibrium, the WL is equivalent to about 100 pCi/L. The working level month (WLM) is a measure of the cumulative occupational exposure defined as an exposure of 1 WL in the atmosphere for 170 hours – a 'working month'.

The various tissues and organs of the body may receive different radiation doses, depending on the circumstances of exposure. The risk of injury to a specific tissue depends on the dose to that tissue. It is therefore important to know the distribution of the radiation dose. The *effective dose* is the sum of the dose equivalents to the individual organs of the body, weighted by factors that represent the relative risk that injury in these tissues contributes to detriment for the entire individual (Table 33.1.6). The weighting factor is derived from the risk of cancer in the specific tissue, the probability of death from cancer in that tissue, the relative loss of life expectancy and the age-weighted risks of cancer in specific tissues.[1] In the case of the gonads, the detriment includes the risks to offspring (i.e., genetic effects) from radiation doses in the exposed individual. The apportionment of risk by the tissue-specific factors enables a risk

weighting of a radiation dose in cases in which the external exposure is non-uniform. According to this system of risk-weighted dosimetry, a dose selectively delivered to the lung ultimately involves 12 times more detriment (risk) than does a radiation dose delivered to the thyroid, for example (Table 33.1.6).

Evaluation of the radiation dose

Radiation doses to individuals can be evaluated using instruments to measure the radiation emitted by sources and/or by calculations estimating the intensity of radiation exposure and the resulting dose. Dose estimates in radiation protection programs provide valuable assurance that occupational risks are understood and managed appropriately. In radiation oncology, knowledge of doses to both the tumor and to normal tissue is essential for effective radiation therapy. Dosimetry in diagnostic radiology and nuclear medicine is necessary for quality assurance in imaging and to ensure that an unnecessary radiation dose to the patient is avoided. Finally, an evaluation of radiation doses in accidents provides a basis for prognosis, treatment, and patient management.

In protection programs, personnel monitoring with film badges, thermoluminescent dosimeters or digital pocket dosimeters is frequently used to assess exposures from external sources. Regular monitoring of radiation-exposed workers is usually required if it is possible that the individual might receive one-tenth of an annual occupational dose limit during normal workplace procedures. Personnel monitoring is typically supplemental to measurements of radiation sources using instruments such as ionization chambers. If the results from personnel monitoring or direct reading instruments are not available, mathematical modeling of the radiation fields may be used to provide an estimate of dose. The duration of the exposure, the relative positions of the source with respect to the exposed individual, and the presence of any shielding materials are important factors in completing the calculation. In radiation accidents, accurate descriptions of these variables are invaluable steps toward providing reliable dose estimates.

It is important to distinguish between situations in which an individual is exposed only to the radiation from an external source and those in which the individual is exposed to radioactive materials as the result of a release of such material into the environment, resulting in deposition on or in the body. An evaluation of the dose resulting from external exposure requires knowledge of the intensity of the radiation and the damage that the various types of radiation can cause. In general, particles can penetrate tissue far less readily than x-rays or gamma rays so they can cause effects only on tissues near which they are deposited or stored in the body. For this reason, they are termed internal emitters. The different types of radiation also differ by their relative ability to impart energy or injury to tissue (e.g., Table 33.1.5).

In accident cases in which the patient was exposed to external sources of gamma rays, x-rays, beta particles or alpha particles, patient management does not present radiation safety problems because the patient is not made radioactive by these exposures. However, in accidents in which radioactive materials are deposited on or in the body, or are generated within the body by external exposures from neutron sources, radiation exposure to the patient continues as long as these materials are present. Special handling may be needed because the material may be transferred to others or contaminate the environment An evaluation of surface contamination may be made using a portable Geiger counter or scintillation probe that could detect the radiation from this material on skin or other surfaces. Alternatively, a wipe test may be made by wiping the surface with paper or cotton and analyzing the sample with a suitable detector.

An evaluation of the dose caused by internal exposure is based on calculations using knowledge of the type of material present, its quantity, its distribution in the body, and the change in quantity and distribution as a function of time. These factors may be determined directly using radiation detectors placed external to the body; by sampling body fluids, tissues or excreta and analyzing these in suitable bioassay instruments; or by dose modeling. The physical and biochemical characteristics of the material, use of dosimetry, or other radiation detectors determine the appropriate method. A whole-body counter is a shielded scintillation detector system used to evaluate the quantity of radioactive material in the body when radiation from that material can be detected outside the body. The gamma camera is employed in nuclear medicine to determine the distribution of radiopharmaceuticals administered for diagnostic purposes. These instruments may be applied to the evaluation of accidents in appropriate cases. Bioassay techniques require the careful preparation of samples and analysis with specialized laboratory instruments such as the well or liquid scintillation counter. The evaluation of radiation dose is a specialized task that may be performed by health or medical physicists, addressing both radiation dose and associated risks.

MANAGEMENT AND PREVENTION

The prevention of radiation injury is the primary goal of radiation protection programs. To this end, all unnecessary exposures to radiation should be minimized and permissible occupational exposure must be kept as low as reasonably achievable (ALARA). The operating limits on the doses of radiation that may be delivered to members of the public and to radiation workers are not expected to prevent all mutagenic, carcinogenic and teratogenic effects (because thresholds for these effects *may* not exist) but they should keep the risks of these effects within acceptable bounds. The minimization of unnecessary radiation exposures requires careful design of the workplace, equipment, and work procedures; thorough training and supervision of workers; and implementation of an appropriate radiation protection program, including systematic oversight and monitoring by health physicists. The radiation protection

program also should include plans for coping with radiation accidents, including a delineation of the lines of authority for managing such accidents, a knowledge of the local medical facilities that are capable of evaluating and treating radiation accident victims, and arrangements for handling and transporting radioactive victims.

CLINICAL EFFECTS
Types and subcellular mechanisms of radiation Injury

Ionizing radiation, in contrast to non-ionizing radiation, is capable of depositing enough localized energy in living cells to disrupt the atoms and molecules on which it impinges, producing ions and free radicals in the process, thus giving rise to the biochemical changes that may lead to injury. The distance between successive atomic collisions along the path of an impinging radiation depends on the energy, mass and electrostatic charge of the radiation. In the case of the alpha particle, the collisions typically occur so close together that the particle gives up all of its energy while traversing only a few cells. Thus, if emitted externally, alpha particles pose little risk of injury, even to the skin. In the case of x-rays or gamma rays, on the other hand, the collisions typically occur so far apart from one another that the radiation may penetrate through the entire body.

The molecular changes produced by a given dose of radiation and, in turn, the probability of cellular injury depend on the microscopic distribution of the energy that is deposited in the cell. In general, the relative biologic effectiveness of radiation increases with the ion density – or LET (linear energy transfer) – of the radiation. Hence, a given amount of energy deposited in the cell by alpha particles is more likely to cause injury than the same amount of energy deposited by x-rays. Because of the differences in potency, doses of different types of radiation are customarily normalized by LET-dependent weighing factors (Table 33.1.5) when they are evaluated for purposes of risk assessment or radiation protection.

Although a large enough dose of radiation, in principle, can alter any molecular constituent of the cell, DNA is the most critical biologic target because of the limited redundancy of the genetic information it contains, i.e., damage to a single gene, if unrepaired, may kill or profoundly alter the affected cell. A dose of radiation large enough to kill the average dividing cell (approximately 2 Sv) causes hundreds of lesions in its DNA. Most such lesions are repairable, however, with the result that the ultimate fate of a given lesion depends on the outcome of DNA repair processes as well as on the initial lesion itself. An irreparable lesion in DNA is more likely to be produced by densely ionizing radiation (e.g., a proton or an alpha particle) than by sparsely ionizing radiation (e.g., an x-ray or a gamma ray). Unrepaired or misrepaired damage to DNA, manifested in the form of mutations, has been well documented in many types of cells. At a given genetic locus, the frequency of mutations characteristically increases linearly with radiation dose approximating 10^{-5} to 10^{-6} per Sv.

Radiation-induced damage may also involve chromosome breakage, thereby giving rise to changes in chromosomal structure and number. The combined frequency of translocations, dicentrics, rings, and other chromosomal aberrations increases linearly with the dose in the range below 1 Sv, approximating 0.1 per cell per Sv in human lymphocytes irradiated in vitro. The frequency of such aberrations has also been observed to increase with the dose in the lymphocytes of atomic bomb survivors, radiation workers and persons residing in areas of elevated natural background radiation. The dose–response relationship for such changes has been characterized well enough so that the aberration frequency can serve as a useful early biologic dosimeter in radiation accident victims.

Damage to genes, chromosomes and other vital organelles may be lethal to the affected cells, especially dividing cells, which are particularly radiosensitive as a class. The survival of dividing cells, measured in terms of proliferative capacity, tends to decrease exponentially with increasing dose: 1–2 Gy generally suffice to reduce the surviving fraction by about 50%. Although the killing of individual cells is a stochastic process, too few cells are killed by a dose below 0.5 Gy to cause clinically detectable changes in most tissues and organs, except those of the embryo. Thus, there are substantial thresholds for the acute effects of radiation, which vary from organ to organ as noted subsequently.

Acute radiation injury

Tissues in which the cells proliferate rapidly are generally the first to exhibit injury. Mitotic inhibition and cytologic abnormalities may be detectable immediately after intensive irradiation in such tissues, in contrast to fibrosis, other degenerative changes and neoplasia, which may not appear until months, years, or decades later. Because of homoeostatic mechanisms, including the repair of DNA damage and compensatory proliferation of surviving stem cells, tissues generally suffer less injury from a given dose if the radiation is accumulated gradually over a period of days or weeks than if it is absorbed in a single brief exposure. The injury from a given dose is also generally less severe if only a fraction of a tissue is exposed than if all the cells in the tissue are exposed. A brief summary of the effects of radiation on key organs and on the whole body follows but more detailed information is available in specialized texts, such as the publication by Mettler and Upton.[2]

Skin

Erythema may occur within minutes or hours after exposure, depending on the radiation dose, energy, and the size of the area irradiated. The threshold for erythema in a 10 cm^2 field varies from 6 to 8 Sv of gamma rays or x-rays delivered in a brief exposure, to more than 30 Sv delivered in daily exposures over a period of weeks. After rapid exposure to a dose of 6 Sv or more, the erythema typically appears within hours, lasts a few hours, and is then followed 2–4 weeks later by one or more waves of deeper and more prolonged erythema and epilation. A dose as large as 10–20 Sv delivered acutely may cause transepithelial injury with moist desquamation and possibly necrosis of the skin within 2–4 weeks.

Bone marrow and lymphoid tissue

A dose of 2–3 Sv delivered rapidly to the whole body will kill enough mature lymphocytes as well as their precursors to produce severe lymphopenia, reaching a minimum within 48 hours. There will also be enough precursor hemopoietic cell damage to cause severe depression of the granulocyte and platelet counts within 3–5 weeks. A dose above 3–5 Sv without medical treatment is likely to result in fatal infection and/or hemorrhage during that vulnerable period (Table 33.1.7), with almost immediate aplasia of lymphoid tissues, lymphopenia and depression of the immune response.

Gastrointestinal tract

Stem cells of the intestinal mucosa are killed in sufficient numbers by an acute dose of 10 Sv to produce ulceration of the overlying epithelium. If a large enough area of the mucosa is affected, the injury may result in a fatal, dysentery-like syndrome within 1–2 weeks (Table 33.1.7).

Gonads

Acute exposure of both testes to a dose as low as 0.15 Sv will kill enough spermatogonia to depress the sperm count for months, beginning about 6 weeks after exposure. A dose of more than 2 Sv will cause more prolonged and possibly permanent sterility. Acute exposure of both ovaries to a dose of 1.5–2.0 Sv will, similarly, cause temporary sterility, and a dose of 2.0–3.0 Sv can cause permanent sterility, depending on the age of the woman at the time of exposure.

Lens of the eye

Irradiation of the lens can cause the formation of lenticular opacities within a matter of months. The threshold for a vision-impairing cataract is estimated to vary from 2–3 Sv absorbed by the lens in a single brief exposure to 5.5–14 Sv absorbed over a period of months.

Respiratory tract

The respiratory tract can withstand considerable localized radiation injury, such as may result from intensive irradiation of a small part of the lung. When all or most of both lungs are heavily irradiated, however, a fatal pneumonitis can result within 1–6 months. The lethal dose for 50% of a theoretical population for this reaction is about 8–10 Gy for gamma rays delivered in a single brief exposure. Those who survive the acute inflammatory phase of the reaction may succumb later to pulmonary fibrosis or cor pulmonale. The pathogenesis of the lesion involves a complex series of reactions apparently resulting from damage to alveolar cells and pulmonary vasculature.

This pulmonary pattern has been recognized in patients treated with radiation therapy, as well as occupational exposures, including firemen who dealt with the Chernobyl reactor fire and radiation workers involved in more recent industrial accidents in Israel and Japan in

Acute dose equiv (Sv)	Incidence (%)	Latency hours	Syndrome or organ involved	Characteristic symptoms	Critical period after exposure	Therapy	Prognosis	Lethality (%)	If injury is fatal	
									Death within	Cause of death
1–2	0–50	>3	Bone marrow	Mild leukopenia and thrombopenia	2–6 weeks	Symptomatic	Excellent	0–10	Months	Infections and/or hemorrhage
2–5	50–90	1–2	Bone marrow syndrome	Thrombopenia, leukopenia, hemorrhage, infections, epilation	2–6 weeks	Transfusions of leukocytes and platelets, supportive care (isolation, antibiotics, fluids), cytokines, stem cell transplantation	Uncertain depending on success of therapy	0–90	Weeks	Infections and/or hemorrhage
5–10	100	0.5–1	Bone marrow syndrome	Thrombopenia, leukopenia, hemorrhage, infections, epilation	2–6 weeks	Cytokines, stem cell transplantation, transfusions of leukocytes and platelets. Supportive care (isolation, antibiotics, fluids)	Uncertain depending on success of therapy	0–90	Weeks	Infections and/or hemorrhage
10–15	100	0.5	Intestinal syndrome	Diarrhea, fever, electrolytic imbalance	3–14 days	Palliative	Very poor	90–100	2 weeks	Enterocolitis, shock
>50	100	<1	Neurologic syndrome	Cramps, fever, ataxia, lethargy, impaired vision, coma	1–48 hours	Symptomatic	Hopeless	100	1–4 hours	Cerebral edema

Table 33.1.7 Features of the acute radiation syndrome

whom the hematologic damage was effectively treated. It includes respiratory failure associated with interstitial edema and pneumonitis. This has appeared within 1–3 months after radiation therapy of 8–9 Gy to the chest and within 3–30 days in seven Chernobyl-injured workers.

Total body radiation injury

Intensive irradiation of the whole body or a major part of it may cause sufficient simultaneous damage to several key organ systems, such as the hematopoietic system, the gastrointestinal tract, nervous and cardiovascular systems, to produce the collection of signs and symptoms known as the acute radiation syndrome. This syndrome is characterized by a succession of manifestations that can be grouped temporally into a prodromal stage, a latent period, a stage of manifest illness, and, finally, for survivors, recovery. The duration and severity of the associated phenomena are strongly related to the magnitude of the evoking exposure. With increasing dose, the syndrome may be dominated clinically by the consequences of malfunctioning of a particular system; hence, the acute radiation syndrome has been subdivided into the hematologic, gastrointestinal, neurovascular and pulmonary forms. The overall pattern of the acute radiation syndrome is summarized in Table 33.1.7.

Regardless of which form of the syndrome ultimately dominates the clinical course, the early or prodromal symptoms characteristically include anorexia, nausea, and vomiting (and diarrhea at higher dose levels), occurring within a few hours after irradiation. These are primarily transient neurogenic phenomena, which are then followed by a symptom-free interval of dose-related duration, until the onset of manifest illness (Table 33.1.7). The ensuing clinical phenomena fall into three or four general patterns.

The hematologic form, reflecting bone marrow suppression, with deficit in the production of hematologic cell lines, is triggered by about 1 Gy or more. This form is characterized by infections, particularly including oropharyngitis, mucositis, enteritis, pneumonitis, and septicemia between the third to fifth postexposure week. Infections include opportunistic bacteria, viruses and fungi. Also prominent are the external and internal hemorrhagic manifestations associated with thrombocytopenia, including petechiae, purpura, epistaxis, hematemesis, melena, hematuria and internal bleeding.

Somewhat higher levels of exposure of about 10 Gy or more can lead to gastrointestinal sequelae related to the insufficiency of cell production necessary to maintain the integrity of the gastroenteric mucosal lining. Beginning by the end of the first postexposure week, signs of malnutrition, dehydration, electrolyte disturbances, and gastrointestinal infec-tion and bleeding become increasingly prominent.

Still higher levels of radiation exposure, exceeding about 20 Gy, can elicit a neurovascular response after a short latent period including ataxia, somnolence, coma alternating with hyperexcitability, and convulsions accompanied by hypotension, hypothermia, and death within hours to 1 or 2 days.

Clinical evaluation strategy

The signs and symptoms of radiation injury are nonspecific; the clinical evaluation of an irradiated person requires integration and synthesis of pertinent information from the individual's exposure record, medical history, physical examination and laboratory data. In managing a radiation accident victim, even if the patient was heavily irradiated or contaminated, an evaluation of burns, smoke inhalation, mechanical trauma or other forms of injury should be performed. Contaminated clothing should be removed promptly, isolated in a plastic bag, and labeled to denote radioactivity; the victim should be isolated; and the contaminated area sealed off as soon as possible. The management of the radiation injuries themselves (Table 33.1.7) will vary depending on their severity and the particular organs that are affected.

Because the nature and severity of any injury that may result from exposure to radiation depend on the size and anatomic distribution of the dose, assessment of the dose is a useful adjunct to the clinical evaluation of an exposed person. Present maximum permissible exposure limits for radiation workers are sufficiently restrictive to prevent detectable impairment of organ function under normal conditions of occupational exposure. However, if a sizable proportion of the entire body is more heavily irradiated, a rapid assessment of the extent of anticipated injury will greatly facilitate subsequent clinical management.

Physical dosimetry can be helpful, but processing of dosimeters and careful reconstruction of the exposure events usually requires significant time. Fortunately, there are a number of biologic dosimeters that can help to provide early information about the extent of injury for which to prepare. Much can be learned by a careful history, physical examination and sequential complete blood counts, including differential analysis, platelet and reticulocyte counts. If feasible, peripheral blood cytogenetic examinations should be performed. The early prognostic information to be gained by clinical observations and blood counts alone is summarized in Table 33.1.9. A listing of useful early procedures, with the time of appearance of some key findings, and the minimum exposure that evokes them, is provided in Table 33.1.8. This simplified approach can be helpful when assessing large groups of people, as well as with individual patients.

Procedure	Finding	Approximate time of onset	Minimum exposure required
History	Nausea, vomiting	Within 48 hours	1.5 Gy
Physical examination	Erythema	Within 48 hours to days	3.0 Gy
Blood count and differential	Hair loss	Within 2 weeks	3.0 Gy
Chromosomal analysis	Lymphocytes < 1000/mm³	Within 24–48 hours	1.0 Gy
	Dicentrics, rings, and/or fragments	Within hours	0.10 Gy

Table 33.1.8 Radiation injury evaluation procedures and their results in relation to time and magnitude of radiation exposure

Evaluation procedures
1. Observe and record time of onset of clinical signs and symptoms
2. Perform daily blood count

Findings	Potential outcome
Nausea, vomiting, diarrhea within minutes. Ataxia, disorientation, shock, coma in minutes to hours	Neurovascular syndrome
Nausea and/or vomiting and some blood count derangement in 2 days	Minor hematologic syndrome
Marked leukocyte and lymphocyte count derangement in 3 days	Major hematologic syndrome
Diarrhea within 4 days and marked platelet derangement within 6 to 9 days	Gastrointestinal syndrome

Table 33.1.9 Preliminary evaluation of acute radiation injury following overexposure

Treatment considerations

The management of acute radiation injury has evolved on an empirical basis largely from experience with populations exposed to atomic weapons and radiation therapy, as well as accidental exposure to a variety of occupational sources. Such treatment can be divided into supportive and intensive care, reviewed in a consensus symposium in mid-1989, the proceedings of which have been published.[3] Supportive care includes provision of a pathogen-free environment; early administration of antibiotics for prophylactic treatment of the upper respiratory and the gastrointestinal tracts; utilization of intravenous nutrients, fluids and blood components; and active therapy of any overt infections that develop.

A more intensive form of therapy that has been used in the treatment of the hematologic form of acute radiation injury has been bone marrow or stem cell transplantation from umbilical cord blood, peripheral blood, and fetal tissue. This therapy was originally developed in the 1960s with support from the US Atomic Energy Commission to improve understanding and treatment of radiation injury, but quickly entered broader clinical use to treat leukemias, other neoplastic disorders and some genetic disorders. Various protocols for stem cell administration have now been employed in 30,000–40,000 patients worldwide, and this population is currently increasing by 10–20% per year.[4,5] In this form of antileukemic therapy, a conditioning regimen of total body irradiation of about 10–12 Gy in one brief exposure or 15 Gy divided over 3–7 days is generally given, preceded by preconditioning with antineoplastic therapy, and followed by transfusion of bone marrow or stem cells.

In a literature review of relevant case series published from 1981 to 1987, with sufficient pertinent data over a 60-day follow-up period, seriously ill patients had a postirradiation 60-day survival rate of 85–90%. Bone marrow transplantation was first used to treat radiation injury 3–4 weeks after accidental radiation overexposure following a reactor accident in Vinca, Yugoslavia, in 1958 without clear evidence of a positive effect on outcome.[6,7] The first successful such use of bone marrow transplantation followed the Pittsburgh accelerator accident in 1965 in which one of the three industrial accelerator workers involved had a mean

whole-body exposure of about 6 Gy and much higher extremity doses that eventually led to quadruple amputations. In a transplantation from an identical twin, hematologic recovery began about 10 days after the transplantation, which was performed on the ninth postexposure day.[8]

Thirteen of the approximately 200 patients with acute radiation syndrome treated in Moscow and Kiev after the Chernobyl reactor accident received bone marrow transplants, and six were given fetal liver cells. Two of the former and none of the latter survived. Both survivors rejected the transplant by 36 days postexposure, although transient engraftment may have aided survival. It must be emphasized that all these patients had whole-body exposures above 6 Gy, with thermal and radiation burns exceeding 50% of the skin surface, as well as other trauma complicating recovery.

The poor results of hematopoietic stem cell transplantation at Chernobyl must be weighed against those obtained in poor-risk medical patients undergoing radiation therapy and in industrial accidents. The method probably warrants consideration in radiation accident patients with life-threatening exposures in the range of 8–12 Gy or higher, with an individual risk–benefit judgment required a case-by-case basis.

The clinical use of hematopoietic growth factors is another recent therapeutic development that may obviate the problems of finding appropriate bone marrow donors and ensuring that the overall benefits of transplantation outweigh risks. The identification of various hematologic growth factors began in the 1960s, with recombinant gene technology leading to availability of myeloid (GCSF, interleukin-3, PIXY321), myeloid/macrophage (GM-CSF), myeloid/lymphoid (SCF), macrophage/monocyte (M-CSF), lymphoid (interleukin-2), erythroid (erythropoietin or EPO) and megakaryocytic (MGDF/TPO) growth factors. In general, these factors enhance the survival, proliferation and differentiation of the committed progenitor cells of the various cell lines.

The potential value of these factors for radiation accident patients with hematologic injury is apparent, despite uncertainties associated with any new therapy. The first scientific report of the use of granulocyte-macrophage colony-stimulating factor was in eight patients exposed to cesium-137 contamination in a 1987 incident in Goiania, of whom four survived.[9]

The same factor was used to treat three patients in an industrial sterilization unit accident in San Salvador in 1989. All recovered from the hematologic effects, although one died 8.5 months later from radiation pneumonitis and other complications.[10] A third accident involved a radiation worker in Israel in 1990, who received a bone marrow transplant and interleukin-3 following massive exposure that proved fatal within 36 days.[11] Other accident patients, including a worker at an irradiation facility in Belarus in 1991[12] and two workers in Tokaimura, Japan, 1999, survived the hematologic impairment period only to succumb later to the respiratory injury. Successful management of pulmonary injury remains an unmet challenge in treating acute whole-body high-dose radiation overexposure.

The gastrointestinal form of acute radiation syndrome has not been treated successfully in either victims of Chernobyl or earlier accidents. It should be noted, however, that many patients with hematologic diseases who undergo stem cell transplants have survived after exposures to 10–15 Gy, an exposure level that would be expected to produce some gastrointestinal damage without such aggressive therapy. Similar results in animal studies suggest that additional use of leukocyte growth factors may enhance the survival of accident victims exposed to such levels of ionizing radiation. The neurovascular and, as noted above, the pulmonary manifestations of high-dose total-body radiation exposure remain therapeutic challenges.

Local injury

External radiation sources can produce localized tissue injury. Such injuries constitute the most frequent form of occupational overexposure, usually involving the hands. Correct diagnosis depends on an accurate history and observation of transient waves of erythema after exposures of about 3–6 Sv. These may be followed by bullae formation in the 'wet' form of radiodermatitis associated with exposures of about 10–20 Sv, occurring within 1–3 weeks depending on dose. Treatment is supportive, but tissue grafting may become necessary for healing. Over the longer term, a reactive obliterative endarteritis may compromise regional blood supply, necessitating amputation of the necrotic tissue.

Radionuclide contamination

Accidental radionuclide contamination may involve the external surfaces of the body and internal deposition by inhalation, ingestion, or through traumatic injuries. Following (or during) any necessary emergency treatment of life-threatening injuries, prompt action including decontamination, is desirable to avoid incorporation of surface activity, to enhance decorporation of any actual intake, and to minimize psychological sequelae. A clinical challenge is the large number of variables that must be considered in dealing with such exposures, including the physicochemical and metabolic characteristics of the radioactive compound involved, routes of entry, and sites of deposition. NCRP Report number 65 is a practical monograph providing guidance in the management of these clinical problems.[13] Isolation measures and use of personal protective equipment by healthcare providers and emergency responders may be required.

External surface contamination can be treated by applying the least irritating agents first, such as soap and water. Insufficient results may require increasingly strong measures, such as abrasive soap, detergents, oxidizing agents, complexing agents, or chelating agents. Cleansing efforts should be terminated when all significant radioactivity or unbound activity has been removed, or when there is evidence of hyperemia or abrasion of the skin that might enhance transcutaneous movement of radioactivity.

For radionuclide inhalation, naso-oropharyngeal irrigation is indicated. After inhaled material is deposited in the lungs, there is no simple effective agent to use. For a major deposition of a highly hazardous, long-lived isotope, bronchopulmonary lavage has been used, but this requires general anesthesia and management by an experienced pulmonologist.

In cases of radionuclide ingestion, which may be associated with inhalation, naso-oropharyngeal lavage is also indicated. Unless performed immediately, emesis or gastric lavage are not likely to be useful. Purgatives will accelerate the transit time of material through the gastrointestinal tract, reducing the mucosal contact time and absorption.

For contaminated lacerations, thorough irrigation and surrounding skin decontamination are necessary steps before any effort at closure. The use and extent of surgical debridement and possibly of excision of contamination, must be individualized based on clinical judgment. After these initial measures have been taken, evaluation of the amount of residual internal radioactivity, its medical significance, and the rate of spontaneous decorporation will determine the need for further treatment. This assessment may involve bioassays of excreta and whole-body radioactivity measurements. If necessary, there exist several approaches to decorporation, including dilution, blocking, mobilization and chelation. Appropriate agents for various important radionuclides are provided in Table 33.1.10.

Combined injury

Importantly, the existence of one type of radiation injury does not preclude the concurrent presence of another, nor does radiation injury prevent the simultaneous occurrence

Method	Isotope	Agent
Dilution	^{3}H	Water
	^{32}P	Phosphorus (Neutra-Phos)
Blocking	^{137}Cs	Ferric ferrocyanide (Prussian blue)
	^{131}I, ^{99m}Tc	KI (Lugol's solution)
	^{89}Sr, ^{85}Sr	Aluminum phosphate (Phosphogel)
		Aluminum hydroxide (Amphojel)
		Sodium alginate (Gaviscon)
Mobilization	^{86}Rb	Chlorthalidone (Hygroton)
Chelation	^{252}Cf, ^{242}Cm, ^{241}Am,	Diethylenetriaminepentaacetic acid
	^{239}Pu, ^{144}Ce, rare earths,	
	^{143}Pm, ^{140}La, ^{90}Y, ^{65}Zn, ^{46}Sc	Disodium acetate (Versenet Na), penicillamine
	^{210}Pb	(Cyrimine)
	^{203}Hg, ^{60}Co	Penicillamine

Table 33.1.10 Methods for elimination of some important internally emitting radionuclides

of other trauma. This can result in combined injury, the severity of which may exceed those of the individual component parts. This has been seen in catastrophic situations, such as the atomic bombings of Hiroshima and Nagasaki, Japan, and the explosion and fire at the Chernobyl nuclear power station near Kiev, Ukraine. There are significant differences in clinical management, such as the timing of surgical intervention and the choice of pharmaceuticals under these circumstances. The combined effects of low-dose, chronic intermittent radiation exposure and exposure to other agents is an area receiving increasing recent attention, as they are more representative of the majority of the workers exposed to radiation. A discussion of these issues is included by Mettler and Upton,[2] and in more detail in the United Nations 2000 report.[17]

Psychologic stress

Common to most accident incidents, regardless of the extent of actual radiation injury and/or radionuclide contamination, is anxiety and fear in the people who perceive themselves involved. Historic incidents, such as the Hiroshima and Nagasaki atomic bombings, the nuclear weapons tests at Bikini and Nevada, and accidents at Three Mile Island and Chernobyl, and all their repercussions have received extensive media coverage. It is therefore necessary to anticipate concern on the part of patients, relatives, and those who perceive themselves as possibly affected. Helpful measures include prompt dissemination of honest factual information and provision of evidence that the situation is understood, and that a practical plan for clinical management is in place and can be implemented as needed. Appropriate prior education of individuals potentially encountering radiation is important in preventing panic.[19]

Mass radiation terrorism or accident casualties

There are three broad areas to consider in preparing to address the potential problems associated with terrorist activities involving radiation exposure on a large scale. One requisite is an understanding of the potential radiation sources such as radiation dispersal devices (RDD) and the consequent health effects, including the psychosocial ones, and their care. Another is knowledge concerning incident command and control procedures at federal, state and local levels, as well as the crucial aspects of communication and information flow to the public. These include cleanup recommendations and guidance on dose limitations for the impacted public as well as for the responders. A third requisite is familiarity with emergency planning, response resources and personnel training for radiation events.

For those for whom radiation has only been familiar as a research subject or tool in industry, or as a clinical or experimental therapeutic modality, the reality is that the likelihood of being called upon to assist in the event of an accidental or deliberate radiation incident is increasing. The National Council on Radiation Protection and Measurement (NCRP) has published NCRP Report number 65, a patient-oriented monograph on the *Management of Persons Accidentally Contaminated with Radionuclides*[13] and NCRP report number 138, *Management of Terrorist Events*

Involving Radioactive Material,[14] which cover the basic public health information with which to anticipate, prepare for, recognize and deal with a deliberate public assault involving radionuclides. The information and resource listings in these reports make it useful for every 'responder' and medical organization to have reference copies at each site where such information might be needed on an emergency basis. Other guides are also available.[15,16]

Chronic effects

Effects on cancer incidence

Radiation workers were among the first to demonstrate the carcinogenic effects of irradiation. Historic examples include: (1) carcinomas of the skin in pioneer radiologists and x-ray workers, (2) leukemias in early radiologists, (3) osteogenic sarcomas and carcinomas of the cranial sinuses in early radium watch dial painters, and (4) lung cancers in pitchblende and other underground hard-rock miners. Although the risks of such cancers in radiation workers are drastically reduced as a result of modern radiation protection standards, the extent to which radiation workers might be at risk for cancer remains a concern. Radiation thus continues to be among the most thoroughly investigated of occupational carcinogens.

The neoplasms induced by irradiation characteristically take years or decades to develop, and they are indistinguishable from neoplasms induced by other environmental, occupational or lifestyle causes. Moreover, the induction of radiation-related cancers has been detectable only after relatively large radiation doses (>0.5 Gy) and has varied with the type of neoplasm as well as age and gender of the exposed individual. The dose–incidence data for most neoplasms are consistent with a multistage, linear non-threshold relationship. Overall, the extent to which the risk of cancer might be increased by low-level radiation exposures cannot be estimated except by extrapolation from dose–response relationships based on highly exposed populations, extrapolating to low radiation doses.

Among various dose–incidence models for estimating the risks of low-level radiation [R(d)], the one that has been judged to fit the currently available data best is a multiplicative model of the form:

$$R(d) = R_0 [1 + F(d)g(b)]$$

where R_0 denotes the age-specific background risk of death from a specific type of cancer, d is the radiation dose, $F(d)$ is a function of dose that is linear for cancers other than leukemia and linear-quadratic for leukemia (i.e., $f(d) = a_1 d$ or $f(d) = a_2 d + a_3 d^2$), and $g(b)$ is a risk function dependent on other parameters, such as gender, age at exposure, and time after exposure.

Epidemiologic data from atomic bomb survivors and other irradiated populations have been used to estimate lifetime incidence and mortality risks for various cancers (Fig. 33.1.2).[17] The risk projections derived from these data provide a range of estimates for the lifetime risk from cancer

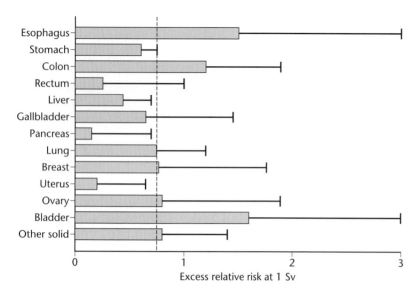

Esophagus
Stomach
Colon
Rectum
Liver
Gallbladder
Pancreas
Lung
Breast
Uterus
Ovary
Bladder
Other solid

0   1   2   3
Excess relative risk at 1 Sv

Figure 33.1.2: Excess relative risk of mortality (and 90% CI) from specific solid cancers in atomic bomb survivors. An excess relative risk = 1 is a 100% increase in risk or a doubling of the background mortality for the tumor type. The data shown are standardized for females exposed at age 30 years. The dashed line is the excess risk for all cancers combined. Data from UNSCEAR.[14]

mortality (Table 33.1.11). The result of radiation risk analysis summarized in Table 33.1.11 demonstrates that the risk of exposure-induced death (REID) from solid cancers, after exposure to an acute whole-body dose of 1 Sv, is about 6.5–9.9% (combined male and female population). The range of estimates here is generated by the type of risk projection model and whether the risk is calculated as a multiple of the normal cancer risk (relative risk, or RR) or an absolute increase above the normal cancer risk (absolute risk or AR). The corresponding REID for leukemia is about 1.19% after a dose of 1 Sv. The estimates of REID after acute doses of 0.1 Sv – twice the annual occupational dose limit in the US – are 0.7–1.1% for solid cancers and 0.06% for leukemia (Table 33.1.11).

Much of the difference between the upper and lower estimates in the estimated ranges results from uncertainty regarding longer latencies of 40 years or greater following irradiation. Although the risk of leukemia in irradiated populations has been observed to reach a peak and then decrease within 25 years following exposure, latencies for other cancer types may remain elevated. To determine the extent to which the risk of cancer in persons irradiated during childhood may be elevated relative to the general population will require further follow-up of atomic bomb survivors and other exposed populations.

In addition to the uncertainty about the length of time that cancer risk remains elevated following irradiation, other sources of uncertainty that complicate assessment of the risks of low-level irradiation include: (1) uncertainty about the shape of the relevant dose–incidence relationship, (2) uncertainty about the extent to which the carcinogenic effects of a given dose may be affected by variations in the distribution of the radiation time and space, (3) uncertainty about the degree to which the risk of a given cancer may vary with age at irradiation, sex, smoking habits, diet and other factors, and (4) uncertainty about the accuracy of the dose measurements, diagnoses, and other data on which the estimates are based. Because of these uncertainties, the existing risk estimates must be interpreted with caution.

Projection model	Risk model	Male	Female	Both
Solid cancer mortality (dose of 1 Sv)				
Age at exposure	RR*	8.5	16.4	12.5
	AR	8.5	11.5	9.9
Attained age	RR	6.2	12.4	9.3
	AR	5.4	7.6	6.5
Leukemia mortality (dose of 1 Sv)				
Age- and time-varying	AR	1.13	1.25	1.19
Solid cancer mortality (dose of 0.1 Sv)				
Age at exposure	RR	0.9	1.9	1.4
	AR	0.9	1.3	1.1
Attained age	RR	0.7	1.4	1.0
	AR	0.6	0.8	0.7
Leukemia mortality (dose of 0.1 Sv)				
Age- and time-varying	AR	0.06	0.06	0.06

* RR: risk relative to unexposed cancer risk; AR: absolute risk
Data from UNSCEAR 2000.[14]

Table 33.1.11 Estimates of lifetime risk of exposure-induced death (REID, in percent) following an acute whole-body exposure to a population of all ages

Caution must also be exercised in extrapolating from the estimates tabulated Table 33.1.11 to predict the risk of cancer following the accumulation of a given dose over a period of weeks, months, or years. For instance, the carcinogenic effects of low-LET radiation in laboratory animals are reduced by a factor of 2–10 if the exposure is sufficiently prolonged to allow recovery through homeostatic processess.[18] Because comparable human data on the comparative carcinogenicity of protracted low-LET irradiation are lacking, it is not possible to specify the extent to which the projections tabulated (Table 33.1.11) may overestimate the doses accumulated over longer periods; however, it is conceivable that they may overestimate risk by a factor of two or greater.

Epidemiologic studies of underground uranium, iron, zinc, lead, and fluorspar miners, who were exposed to elevated concentrations of radon, have convincingly demonstrated excess lung cancer from exposures to the high LET radiations emitted from radon (^{222}Rn) and its radioactive progeny.[19] The observation that indoor radon contributes more than 50% of the annual effective dose equivalent received by the population from all radiation sources, together with the dose–risk relationships derived from the miner studies, indicate that indoor radon exposures may account for up to 10% of all lung cancers. Indoor radon may thus represent the most significant risk factor for lung cancers in the non-smoking population. The National Research Council's Committee on the Health Effects of Exposure to Radon (BEIR VI) recently estimated the attributable risk for lung cancer death from domestic exposure to radon (using 1985–89 mortality rates) to be as great as 27% in never-smokers, and 14% in ever-smokers. Using the BEIR VI risk models, the absolute number of radon-related lung cancer deaths in the US in 1995 would be 15,400 or 21,800, depending on the risk model used for estimation. Among these deaths, an estimated 2100 or 2900 would have occurred among never-smokers.

While the risk of lung cancer from domestic radon exposures cannot be directly validated from existing residential studies, the exposure–response relationships are consistent with occupational miner data, when the latter are restricted to exposures under 50 WLM. However, a large-scale study of county-based lung cancer mortality and average indoor radon concentration resulted in an exposure–response relationship that differs markedly from the BEIR VI exposure–risk models.[20] Given current epidemiologic methodologies, it is unlikely that differences among risk assessment models can be resolved. Some of the uncertainties that affect the estimates of low-dose lung cancer risks from indoor radon include those listed in Table 33.1.12. While significant uncertainties regarding dose–response relationship remain, most risk assessments of lung cancer in residential settings have generally supported the issuance of guidelines limiting residential radon exposure.

The average dose of radiation received by members of the United States population from natural sources other than radon approximates 1 mSv (100 mrem) per year, which is estimated to account for less than 3% of all cancers in the population. Epidemiologic studies to determine the extent to which the rates of cancer may actually vary with natural background radiation have been inconclusive. In certain studies, the rates of cancer have been found to vary inversely with natural background radiation levels, a relationship interpreted by some observers as evidence of beneficial (or hormetic) effect of low-level irradiation;[21] however, the relationship has not persisted after controlling for the effects of altitude and other confounding variables. Although the risk associated with low levels exposure to natural background radiation is uncertain, the studies to date generally support the risk estimates tabulated in Table 33.1.11.

In reference to occupationally exposed populations, a significant excess of leukemia has been found in only one of 17 recent studies of radiation workers, without a significantly positive dose–response relationship in nine studies assessing radiation dose. These findings suggest that the average risk of leukemia in today's radiation workers is no larger than predicted from extrapolation models discussed above. Notably, risk for multiple myeloma has been observed to be elevated in several occupationally exposed cohorts, including workers at the Hanford nuclear facility (Washington State); the disease has not increased in frequency in the majority of cohorts investigated.

Increased cancer rates have been reported in some cohorts of radiation workers. The mortality rate from lung cancer, for example, was reported to increase with cumulative occupational exposure in workers at Oak Ridge National Laboratory. However, the increase was not significant in non-monthly workers, nor were there any deaths from lung cancer in male monthly workers whose accumulated doses exceeded 40 mSv. In the group as a whole, moreover, the lung cancer mortality rate was less than two-thirds of that would have been expected from national rates. Hence, the findings must be interpreted with caution. Excesses of other forms of cancer also have been reported occasionally in various occupationally exposed cohorts; however, because of methodologic problems and other sources of uncertainty that arise in studies involving low-level exposures, the findings are of equivocal public health significance.

In the vicinity of Sellafield, Dounreay, and other nuclear installations in the United Kingdom, the occurrence of clusters of childhood leukemia has suggested the possibility of radiation release; however, the releases are estimated to have increased total radiation dose by less than 2% above background. In contrast, large-scale studies of cancer in populations having very high natural radiation backgrounds (i.e., several times usual background) have not revealed significant increases in cancers. Also noteworthy is the fact that mortality rates for childhood leukemia in United States counties containing nuclear installations have revealed no significant excess.

The aftermath of Chernobyl

Although there have been significant health consequences of the Chernobyl reactor accident in 1986, uncertainties regarding chronic cancer risk remain, due to problems in

1. Uncertainty arising from the model relating lung cancer risk to exposure:
   a. Uncertainties in parameter estimates in the underground miner data
   b. Uncertainties in application of the lung cancer exposure–response model and in its application to residential exposure to the general US population.
2. Uncertainty arising from difference in radon progeny dosimetry in mines and in homes.
3. Uncertainty arising from estimating the exposure distributions for the US population exposure distribution model.
4. Uncertainty in the demographic data used to calculate lifetime risk.

Table 33.1.12 General sources of uncertainty in estimates of lifetime risk of lung cancer mortality resulting from exposure to radon in homes

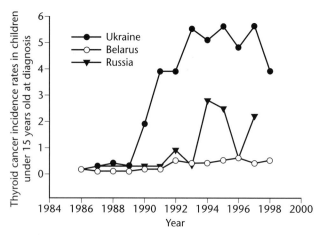

Figure 33.1.3: Thyroid cancer incidence among populations exposed to the Chernobyl accident. The data are for thyroid cancer diagnosed in children under 15 years old at the time of diagnosis. Adapted from UNSCEAR.[14]

assessing individual doses, cancer reporting methods, baseline disease rates, and short latency since the accident. In spite of these limitations, it is apparent that an increase in thyroid cancer exists in children exposed to radioactive iodine (principally ^{131}I) released during the accident[17] (Fig. 33.1.3). The observations of thyroid cancer are consistent with the fact that the thyroid in children is known to be one of the most radiosensitive tissues in the body.[21]

While leukemia is usually considered to be a sentinel disease in irradiated populations, and can occur with a latency period of less than 2–3 years, no increased risk of leukemia related to radiation exposure has been validated among residents living near Chernobyl or among clean-up workers. Some reports attempted to attribute findings of leukemia in these groups to radiation exposures from the accident; however, these were flawed by use of national health registries using different reporting methods. A finding of no increased leukemia risk was reported in a 1997 case-control design.[23]

Solid tumors other than thyroid cancers have not yet been reported in populations exposed from the Chernobyl accident; however, the longer latencies required for solid tumors has not allowed an accurate assessment of risk to date.

Effects on the growth and development of the embryo

During critical stages of organogenesis, exposure to as little as 0.25 Sv has been observed to cause malformations in many animal models. In humans, a dose-dependent increase in the prevalence of mental retardation and decreases in intelligence quotient scores and scholastic performance were observed among atomic bomb survivors of Hiroshima and Nagasaki who were between the eighth and fifteenth weeks of prenatal development at the time of exposure.

Heritable abnormalities

Heritable effects of radiation have yet to be demonstrated conclusively in human germ cells, despite a search for such

effects among the children of the atomic bomb survivors. On the basis of the data from mouse models, the dose required to double the frequency of heritable mutations in germ cells is estimated to exceed 1 Sv. It is inferred that less than 1% of all genetically determined diseases is attributable to natural background irradiation.

References

1. International Commission on Radiological Protection. Recommendations of the International Commission on Radiological Protection. ICRP Publication 60. Ann ICRP 1991; 21:1–3.
2. Mettler FA Jr, Upton AC. Medical effects of ionizing radiation, 2nd edn. Philadelphia: WB Saunders, 1995;214–306.
3. Wald N. The acute radiation syndromes and their medical management. In: Mossman K, Mills WA, eds. The biologic basis of radiation protection practice. Baltimore: Williams & Wilkins, 1992;184–201.
4. Thomas ED, Blume KG, Forman SJ. Hematopoietic cell transplantation, 2nd edn. Malden: Blackwell Science, 1999.
5. Ball ED, Lister J, Law P. Hematopoietic stem cell therapy. New York: Churchill Livingstone, 2000.
6. Jablon S, Hrubec Z, Boice J. Cancer in populations living near nuclear facilities. A survey of mortality nationwide and incidence in two states. JAMA 1991; 265:1403–8.
7. Mathe G, Jammet H, Pendic B, et al. Transfusions et greffes de moelle osseuse homologue chez des humains irradies a haute dose accidentellment. Rev Etudes Clin Biol 1959; V:226–38.
8. Gilberti MY, Wald N. The Pittsburgh radiation accident: 23 year follow-up of clinical and psychological aspects. In: Ricks RC, Berger M, O'Hara F, eds. The medical basis for radiation accident preparedness III: psychological perspectives. New York: Elsevier, 1991;199–206.
9. International Atomic Energy Agency. The radiological accident in Goiania. Vienna: IAEA, 1988.
10. International Atomic Energy Agency. The radiological accident in San Salvador. Vienna: IAEA, 1990.
11. International Atomic Energy Agency. The radiological accident in Soreq. Vienna: IAEA, 1993.
12. International Atomic Energy Agency. The radiological accident at the irradiation facility in Nesvizh. Vienna: IAEA, 1996.
13. National Council on Radiation Protection and Measurement (NRCP). Management of persons accidentally contaminated with radionuclides. Report No. 65. Bethesda: NRCP, 1980.
14. National Council on Radiation Protection and Measurement (NCRP). Management of terrorist events involving radioactive material. Bethesda: NRCP, 2001.
15. Armed Forces Radiobiology Research Institute. Medical management of radiological casualties handbook, 2nd edition. Bethesda: AFRRI, 2003. http://www.afrri.usuhs.mil.
16. Smith JM, Spano MA. Interim guidelines for hospital response to mass casualties from a radiological incident. Atlanta: Division of Environmental Hazards and Health Effects, National Center for Environmental Health, CDC/HHS, 2003.
17. United Nations Scientific Committee on the Effects of Atomic Radiation. Sources and effects of ionizing radiation. UNSCEAR 2000 Report to the General Assembly With Annexes. New York: United Nations, 2000.
18. National Academy of Sciences, National Research Council, Advisory Committee on the Biologic Effects of Ionizing Radiation. The effects on populations of exposure to low levels of ionizing radiation (BEIR V). Washington, DC: National Academy Press, 1990.
19. National Academy of Sciences, National Research Council, Advisory Committee on the Biologic Effects of Ionizing Radiation. Health effects of exposure to radon (BEIR VI). Washington, DC: National Academy Press, 1999.

20. Cohen BL. Test of the linear-no threshold theory of radiation carcinogenesis for inhaled radon decay products. Health Phys 1995; 68:157–74.
21. Calabrese EJ, Baldwin LA. Radiation hormesis: its historical foundations as a biologic hypothesis. Hum Exp Toxicol 2000; 19:41–75.
22. United Nations Scientific Committee on the Effects of Atomic Radiation. Sources and effects of ionizing radiation. UNSCEAR 1993 Report to the General Assembly With Annexes. New York: United Nations, 1993.
23. Ivanov VK, Tsyb AF, Konogorov AP, et al. Case-control analysis of leukemia among Chernobyl accident emergency workers residing in the Federation, 1986–1993. J Radiol Protect 1997; 17:137–57.

33.2 **Non-Ionizing Radiation**

Christopher J Martin, Alan M Ducatman

INTRODUCTION

Non-ionizing radiation is a general term for the various frequencies of the electromagnetic spectrum that lack the energy to ionize the molecules in living cells. The continuum of non-ionizing radiation is conventionally subdivided into bands expressed as frequency for radiofrequency radiation and wavelength for optical radiations (ultraviolet, visible, infrared and lasers, Figure 33.2.1). Table 33.2.1 gives the frequency ranges and acronyms associated with radiofrequency bands. Part of the ultraviolet (UV) spectrum overlaps into the domain of ionizing radiation, but will be discussed here for comprehensiveness. Radiant heat is technically part of the non-ionizing spectrum, but is dealt with separately in Chapter 34.

Non-ionizing radiation is not a new concept – the adverse effects of infrared (IR) radiation on the eye were first recognized in 1786. However, concerns about the potential hazards of lower frequencies of non-ionizing radiation have led to intense study in recent years. The ubiquitous nature of these exposures means that research efforts, differences in interpretation of epidemiological data, policy initiatives, and societal concerns regarding non-ionizing radiation are assured for the next decade. Society also faces a major disease epidemic and vast economic cost related to UV radiation effects.

In addition to a review of the known and suspected health effects associated with each band of non-ionizing radiation, three specific sources will be discussed: cellular telephones, video display terminals (VDTs), and lasers. Table 33.2.2 summarizes the known or suspected health effects associated with each form of non-ionizing radiation discussed in this section.

SUB-EXTREMELY LOW FREQUENCY (SELF) AND EXTREMELY LOW FREQUENCY (ELF)

Exposures

The generation, transport, and use of electricity are associated invariably with ELF and SELF fields. However, it is technically confusing to refer to long-wavelength SELF and ELF fields as radiation. When the wavelength is very long, exposed subjects will be enveloped within one wavelength of the source. The physical characteristics of such confined fields dictate that the relative energy effects will be trivial compared with radiation of shorter wavelengths. For alternating current (AC) what the exposed subject experiences is an induction field, in which charges from the nearby electromagnetic source induce currents and charges on and within the exposed body. In contrast, direct current (DC) induces little secondary current in the body and only if the body moves within the field. Remembering this technical

difference will help the reader understand the confusion between the very low imparted energies and the real, possibly important, physiologic responses of cells to induction fields.

Electric and magnetic field components are necessarily generated together – so-called electromagnetic fields (EMF). The strength of the magnetic field increases with the flow of electric current, while both fields decrease rapidly with distance from the source. However, while electric fields are easily shielded or distorted by intervening objects, magnetic fields are not. Because of this phenomenon, accurate measurement of exposure to electric fields is, for practical purposes, almost impossible. Accordingly, the magnetic field has been implicated in relation to health outcomes. The logic of this is clear, yet there is no reason to rule out the electric field as causing health effects.

Magnetic fields are measured in units of milliGauss (mG) in the United States or microTesla (μT) in most other countries, with 1 μT equal to 10 mG. There are both natural and anthropogenic sources of EMF. The earth's magnetic field ranges from a low of about 250 mG (25 μT) at the equator to a high of 650 mG (65 μT) at either pole. Since the earth's EMF consists of DC only, far less secondary current is induced in comparison with anthropogenic (AC) sources.

A prominent source of exposure in and outside of the workplace is the power line. Types of power lines include powerful transmission lines (69 to 765 kV), distribution primaries (5 to 35 kV), and distribution secondaries (110 to 220 V). Residential magnetic field exposures from household electrical wiring typically vary between 0.6 and 2.5 mG (0.06 to 0.25 μT).[1] Magnetic fields are also generated by the use of any electrically powered device, including home appliances (Table 33.2.3). When in close proximity, these sources may provide greater exposures than that of the largest nearby power lines.

Health effects

Health physicists have been complacent historically in regard to low frequencies of non-ionizing radiation. This type of energy is orders of magnitude less than natural background ionizing radiation, and naturally occurring electromagnetic fields (such as the earth's static magnetic field) are several orders of magnitude more intense than those induced by power lines.

However, in 1979, considerable concern arose following the publication of a now famous case-control study of childhood cancer by Wertheimer and Leeper.[2] These investigators reported statistically significant excesses of leukemia, brain cancer and total cancer associated with residential EMF exposure. A surrogate measure of exposure ('wire codes', a summary index of wire type, configuration and distance from the residence) was substituted for field exposure measurements. Many subsequent studies using this or more refined exposure metrics have now revisited the question of electromagnetic field exposures and childhood

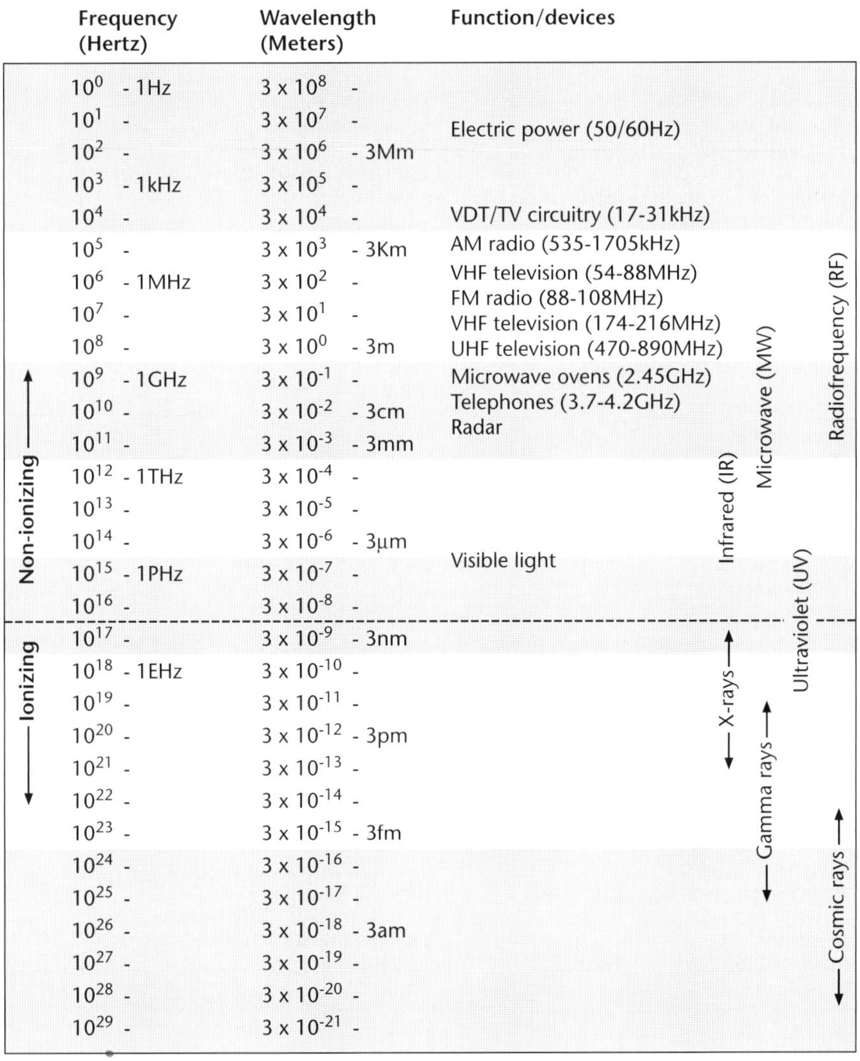
Frequency (Hertz)
Wavelength (Meters)
Function/devices
10^0 - 1Hz | 3 x 10^8 -
10^1 - | 3 x 10^7 -
10^2 - | 3 x 10^6 - 3Mm
10^3 - 1kHz | 3 x 10^5 -
10^4 - | 3 x 10^4 -
10^5 - | 3 x 10^3 - 3Km
10^6 - 1MHz | 3 x 10^2 -
10^7 - | 3 x 10^1 -
10^8 - | 3 x 10^0 - 3m
10^9 - 1GHz | 3 x 10^-1 -
10^10 - | 3 x 10^-2 - 3cm
10^11 - | 3 x 10^-3 - 3mm
10^12 - 1THz | 3 x 10^-4 -
10^13 - | 3 x 10^-5 -
10^14 - | 3 x 10^-6 - 3μm
10^15 - 1PHz | 3 x 10^-7 -
10^16 - | 3 x 10^-8 -
10^17 - | 3 x 10^-9 - 3nm
10^18 - 1EHz | 3 x 10^-10 -
10^19 - | 3 x 10^-11 -
10^20 - | 3 x 10^-12 - 3pm
10^21 - | 3 x 10^-13 -
10^22 - | 3 x 10^-14 -
10^23 - | 3 x 10^-15 - 3fm
10^24 - | 3 x 10^-16 -
10^25 - | 3 x 10^-17 -
10^26 - | 3 x 10^-18 - 3am
10^27 - | 3 x 10^-19 -
10^28 - | 3 x 10^-20 -
10^29 - | 3 x 10^-21 -
Electric power (50/60Hz)
VDT/TV circuitry (17-31kHz)
AM radio (535-1705kHz)
VHF television (54-88MHz)
FM radio (88-108MHz)
VHF television (174-216MHz)
UHF television (470-890MHz)
Microwave ovens (2.45GHz)
Telephones (3.7-4.2GHz)
Radar
Visible light
Non-ionizing
Ionizing
Radiofrequency (RF)
Microwave (MW)
Infrared (IR)
Ultraviolet (UV)
X-rays
Gamma rays
Cosmic rays

Figure 33.2.1: The electromagnetic spectrum, including non-ionizing (above) and ionizing radiation spectra. Radiations are expressed both by frequency (Hertz), increasing and wavelength (meters), decreasing, as energy levels increase from top to bottom.

Frequency range	Acronym*
0–30 Hz	SELF
30–300 Hz	ELF
0.3–3 kHz	VOICE F
0–30 kHz	VLF
30–300 kHz	LF
0.3–3 MHz	MF
3–30 MHz	HF
30–300 MHz	VHF
0.3–3 GHz	UHF
3–30 GHz	SHF
30–300 GHz	EHF
0.3–3 THz	SEHF

* E, extremely; F, frequency; H, high; L, low; M, medium; S, super/sub; U, ultra; V, very.

Table 33.2.1 Frequency bands of the electromagnetic spectrum

cancer. None has duplicated the original strongly positive results of the original study. A nested case-control study combining data from five occupational cohorts in three countries estimated a relative risk of 1.12 (95% confidence interval 0.98–1.28) for brain cancer, and 1.09 (95% confidence interval 0.98–1.21) for leukemia for each year of exposure of 100 mG (10 μT).[3]

Studies of workers with high field exposures have not been fully consistent, but do generate viable additional hypotheses for liver, breast, kidney, pituitary gland, and melanoma as cancer outcomes potentially associated with EMF exposures.

The International Agency for Research on Cancer (IARC) reviewed the data on the carcinogenicity of ELF radiation.[4] This review noted that the most consistent finding from pooled analyses was an approximately two-fold increase in childhood leukemia from residential power line exposure where magnetic field strengths exceeded 4 mG (0.4 μT). While this finding was felt not to be due to chance, it may have been affected by selection bias. No consistent evidence was found between ELF radiation and other childhood tumors or adult cancers at any site. Overall, ELF radiation was classified by IARC as 'possibly carcinogenic to humans' (Group 2B), based on the childhood leukemia association.

EMF exposure has also been associated with increased risk for a variety of non-cancer outcomes including neurodegenerative and psychiatric diseases. Studies have reported an elevation for amyotrophic lateral sclerosis most consistently,[5] although Alzheimer's disease, Parkinson's disease, and depression have also been implicated.[6] Elevations in cardio-

Name	Frequency or wavelength	Potential sources	Known or (suspected) health concerns
Extremely low	30–300 Hz	Power lines Video display terminals Mobile phones Electric appliances Natural sources	(leukemia, brain, breast cancer) (neurodegenerative disease) (cardiovascular disease) (depression) (adverse reproductive outcomes)
Radiofrequency/Microwave	3 kHz–300 GHz	Telecommunication equipment Cellular phones Radar RF heaters/sealers Medical equipment Radio Television	Thermal damage Cataracts (hypertension) (hypogonadism) (non-thermal effects – headache, malaise) (testicular cancer)
Infrared	760 nm–1 mm	Hot objects (molten glass, metals)	Eye damage – cataracts, choroidal damage and retinal burns Burns
Visible	400–760 nm	Sun and artificial light	Eye strain Injuries

Ultraviolet	100–400 nm	Sun
		Welding
		Lasers
		UV lamps (tanning, laboratory, germicidal)
			Seasonal affective disorder
			Skin
			  Acute:
			    Sun burn
			    Phototoxicity
			    Photosensitivity
			  Chronic:
			    Cancer
			    Solar elastosis
			    Solar lentigines
			    Telangiectasia
			Eye
			  Acute:
			    Keratoconjunctivitis
			  Chronic:
			    Cortical cataracts
			    Spheroidal degeneration
			    Pingueculae and pterygia
			    (macular degeneration)

Laser	200 nm–10 μm	Laser pointer Biomedical laser Industrial processes (welding, cutting, drilling) Military use (range finders) Fiberoptic communication	Retinal burns Skin/tissue burns (Infection, toxic/mutagenic gases)

Table 33.2.2 Overview of known and suspected health effects of non-ionizing radiation

Source	Median magnetic field in milliGauss at 6 inches
Refrigerator	2
Coffee maker	7
Washing machine	20
Dishwasher	20
Electric blanket	21.8*
Microwave oven	200
Vacuum cleaner	300
Can opener	600

* Average at 2 inches
Modified from *EMF in your environment* (EPA 1992) and information courtesy of the Center for Devices and Radiological Health, US Food and Drug Administration.

Table 33.2.3 Strength of EMF exposures from common household appliances

vascular mortality[6] and adverse reproductive outcomes (birth defects[8] and miscarriages[9]) have also been observed.

In summary, a number of studies using increasingly sophisticated exposure metrics have now accumulated, indicating either no association or the possibility of a modest association between EMF and brain cancer or leukemia. More recent endpoints of other cancer types, non-neoplastic disease, and adverse reproductive outcomes are less well studied. The inability to assign exposure status accurately has been a pervasive problem in the epidemiology of EMF. A further constraint is the rarity of most of the outcomes under study, which has limited the ability of even large studies to achieve sufficient sample size. Some have argued that little is to be gained through further studies on brain cancer and leukemia; what is now required is a breakthrough on the biologic understanding of the effects of EMF which can inform future epidemiological investigations.[10] In view of the expanding list of potential outcomes, the relevance of any new line of research to policy making or public concern should be borne in mind.[11]

Recommendations and prevention

As noted, the strength of EMF falls off sharply with distance from source, and electrical (but not magnetic) fields are easily shielded. Although electrical devices must usually be turned on to generate magnetic fields, electrical fields are maintained unless units are also unplugged.

A general strategy of 'prudent avoidance' has been advocated as a measure to deal with the possible hazard of ELF radiation. This refers to simple, minimally disruptive, low-cost measures to reduce exposures even in the absence of clear evidence of risk. Examples of prudent avoidance include routing high-powered lines away from schools, unplugging electric blankets before going to bed, and standing away from electrical appliances during operation. Several countries have adopted prudent avoidance as a regulatory policy for EMF.

However, given the complex, ubiquitous nature of EMF exposures, the utility of such policies is unknown and perhaps unknowable. More detailed guidance on limiting exposures has been provided by the International Commission on Non-Ionizing Radiation Protection (ICNIRP).[12]

VIDEO DISPLAY TERMINALS (VDTS)

VDTs are potentially associated with relatively high electromagnetic field exposure levels, therefore many of the hazards discussed previously apply to this source. A specific concern regarding a possible reproductive hazard from VDT exposure arose when clusters of adverse reproductive outcomes were reported in frequent users in the 1970s and 1980s. However, several extensive studies subsequently failed to find an association, leading NIOSH to conclude in 1998 that VDTs do not represent a reproductive risk.[13]

An additional concern, most prominent in Nordic countries, is skin rashes (so called 'screen dermatitis') and other symptoms ('sensitivity to electricity') in VDT users. Double blind studies, in which such individuals are unaware of when the electromagnetic field has been turned on or off, have failed to consistently reproduce such symptoms.[14]

Visual fatigue is common among computer users, especially when poor screen resolution and room lighting decrease the legibility of the electronically displayed information. There is little doubt of the existence of focusing or accommodation fatigue following prolonged computer use.

The ergonomic aspects of VDT work are important, but they are unrelated to electromagnetic fields and are discussed elsewhere (Chapter 15).

RADIOFREQUENCY (RF) RADIATION, INCLUDING MICROWAVES
Exposure measurements

These bands are generally defined to include the frequencies from about 3 kilohertz to 300 gigahertz, corresponding to wavelengths of 1 mm to 3 km in air. The intensity of RF fields includes both an electric and magnetic component. At distances of several wavelengths from the source (the so-called 'far field'), the two are related and intensity is described by the power density in units of milliwatts per square centimeter (mW/cm²). Near field measurements must include separate electric and magnetic field measurements in units of volts per meter (V/m) and amperes per meter (A/m) respectively.

The amount of energy absorbed from RF radiation also varies with the frequency of the source and the dimensions of the exposed body. Because of this, an additional quantity, the specific absorption rate (SAR) in units of watts per kilogram (W/kg) has been used more recently.

A variety of telecommunications devices operate within these frequencies (Fig. 33.2.1 and Table 33.2.1). Much of the concern about RF radiation has focused on microwave exposures produced by radar, telecommunication devices, diathermy machines and microwave ovens. One extensively studied source of RF radiation is cellular phones, which is dealt with in a separate section.

Health effects

A major difference between RF and ELF exposures is that RF exposures, especially RF exposures in the microwave band, may have thermal effects. Unlike other forms of heat stress, the degree, rate, and distribution of heating are less predictable. It is well recognized that heating of deep tissue by RF radiation can occur without skin heating, thereby creating a risk of serious thermal damage without the normal warning signs.

Case reports of overexposure to microwave radiation are limited and usually involve military radar sources. Outcomes have included erythema and a heating sensation acutely followed by hypertension and psychiatric symptoms lasting several months, the latter attributed by some authors to post-traumatic stress disorder.[15] Hypogonadism in a man has also been described.[16] Although the belief and warning literature remain widespread, current microwave ovens no longer pose a risk of interference with cardiac pacemakers.

Microwave-induced cataracts have been produced in experimental animals and reported, rarely, in humans. The experimental cataractogenesis is of two types. Rapid and complete lens opacification occurs after overwhelming exposures, while low-intensity microwaves may cause small, apparently reversible lenticular opacities after a latent period of several weeks. The posterior subcapsular cortex of the lens is most commonly involved when the transmitting source is not applied directly to the eye. While human studies are extremely limited, the present consensus is that very high intensity (greater than 1.5 kW/m²) exposures are required to produce detectable eye damage.

A case series of six men exposed to high levels of RF radiation in the very high frequency (VHF) range of 100 MHz through work on transmission mast antennas describes a variety of non-specific, multisystemic symptoms (headache, diarrhea, malaise) without objective abnormalities.[17]

Additional non-thermal effects of RF radiation have been demonstrated in animal studies and include behavioral alterations, changes in immune cells, and adverse reproductive outcomes.

In response to specific concerns about a link between testicular cancer and traffic radar devices used by police, the US National Institute for Occupational Safety and Health (NIOSH) published a review of this literature in 1995.[18] This report indicated that present day exposures appeared to be low in this setting, and that no assessment could be made regarding the chronic, non-thermal effects from this source in view of the extremely limited number of scientific studies since the mid-1980s. A recent cohort study of 40,581 Korean War veterans with potentially high exposure to radar found no evidence of increases for brain cancer, testicular cancer, or overall mortality.[19]

Prevention and recommendations

Shielding, warning signs and personal protective devices should be used for any source of high-intensity RF exposure that can cause acute thermal effects. Electrical injury associated with powerful RF sources should be considered in all engineering designs. Specific recommendations for the safe use of traffic radar devices have been provided by NIOSH.

Exposure limits have varied widely, due to disagreement on the need to protect against non-thermal effects. An OSHA standard of 10 mW/cm² is designed to protect against thermal effects only, while the American Conference of Governmental Industrial Hygienists (ACGIH) recommendation based on a whole body SAR < 0.4 W/kg is more stringent.

CELLULAR TELEPHONES

Use of cellular telephones has increased dramatically in the US and worldwide in the last decade. At the beginning of 2001, there were an estimated 108 million phone subscribers in the US alone, with about 46,000 new subscriptions per day. Cell phone use is higher in other parts of the world, such as Scandinavia. The cell phone used at the beginning and through the last decade was analogue. Voice messages are transmitted by varying either the amplitude or frequency of the radiowave. A progressive shift to digital cell phones is underway today. Digital messages are transmitted as rapidly pulsed digits. Thus, the technology studied to date is not identical to the technology that will be used by increasing numbers of people in the future.

Exposure

Cellular telephones and cell phone base stations transmit and receive RF signals in the microwave range, between 800 and 2000 MHz, with specific emphasis on 824–894 MHz for the phone unit. As noted in the section on RF and microwaves, this wavelength is capable of causing cellular heating by inducing electrical currents and by increasing molecular movement. Cell phone power outputs are typically so small (around 0.25 w) that the small changes in tissue heat that they might induce are much less than

occurs with normal bodily functions. In contrast to the subtle hypotheses concerning induced heating fields or currents and possible chronic CNS outcomes, acute hazards of cell phones are easy to visualize. Operators of moving vehicles are deprived of the use of one hand while keying or holding a cell phone and may experience 'exposure distraction', especially while keying and talking.

Health hazards

Three well-performed studies have now evaluated the relationship between cell phone use and cancer, with an emphasis on brain cancer, salivary gland cancer, and leukemia. One of these studies, using a nationwide retrospective cohort based on subscriber data linked to a national cancer registry, is quite large.[20] These investigations do not support the hypothesis of an association between cell phone use and cancer outcomes. These findings are reassuring, and indicate that the average user of the analog technology will not experience significantly increased cancer risk during a relatively short latency period. Longer term studies are in progress; these should address issues of peak exposures, longer latencies and, over time, new technologies. Anecdotal reports of headaches are common in cell phone users. No adequate epidemiologic data address this question.

In contrast to the initial reassuring news about cell phones and cancer, cell phone use during motor vehicle operation should be assumed to create hazards for drivers, passengers, and those nearby. Preliminary data show a marked increase in accident rates among cell phone users. 'Hands-free' phones were not protective. Driving left of center and striking fixed objects are among excess outcomes in preliminary data. It is possible that this hazard will also improve with better technology (hands-free phones with voice-activated dialing). Additional well-funded studies of chronic health hazards are underway, but the data concerning the outcome of merely talking are not encouraging, and have already come under regulatory scrutiny in areas.

Cell phones do interfere with cardiopulmonary monitoring devices and other equipment in the hospital setting. Mayo Clinic researchers deemed the interference important enough to potentially interfere with the interpretation of data or cause the equipment to malfunction in 7.4% of 526 tests.[21] Digital and analogue phones produced different kinds of interference. Most alarming was interference with mechanical operations of a ventilator. They conclude that malfunctions and interference are less likely if the phone is kept at least 60 inches from sensitive equipment. Banning the use of cell phones in patients' rooms or procedure areas is suggested to be an adequate precaution.[20]

Prevention and recommendations

While waiting for the definitive follow-up of already reassuring data about cell phones and cancer, those concerned with exposure can minimize it by: not using cell phones or minimizing use; obtaining a cell phone with relatively lower power or that directs RF away from the user. Some manufacturers provide these RF data. Consultants for the World Health Organization have cited the precautionary principle in recommending prudent minimization of cell phone use, and have emphasized minimization of use by children. These recommendations are not based on data, but on gaps in data relating to plausible latency, study follow-up time, and evolving technology.

In contrast, acute hazards from cell phone use next to patient care equipment and in moving vehicles are assumed to be real, a reality supported by disconcerting preliminary data. Cell phone use, including 'dialing' operations and even hands-free communication, should be regulated until studies document that safer technologies address both attention and control. Designed studies of distracted attention with present technology and epidemiologic evaluation of health outcomes (accidents, injuries) will be appropriate, and logically more important than the studies concerning hypothesized chronic hazards.

INFRARED (IR) RADIATION
Exposures

All objects with temperature above absolute zero emit IR radiation. IR-A extends from 760 nm to 1.4 µm and borders on visible light. IR-B extends from 1.4 to 3.0 µm. IR-C has the longest wavelength and is furthest from visible light (3.0 µm to 1 mm). IR-A is also referred to as 'near IR' and IR-C as 'far IR'. IR-A is sometimes perceptible to the eye as a dull, red glow. IR-B and IR-C are invisible. Sources of significant IR include the sun, furnaces, molten glass, welding arcs, IR heaters and dryers. A variety of lasers also emit IR; lasers are discussed in a separate section.

Health effects

Biologic systems exposed to IR experience a corresponding rise in the temperature of the absorbing tissue. IR is absorbed by tissue water and, therefore, is non-penetrating; energy transfer is directly to the outer surfaces. Normal skin has good warning properties (pain) for thermal injury caused by IR (see Chapter 34). Unfortunately, the eyelid and eye do not have adequate thermal warning properties.

Critical to an understanding of the effects of IR radiation is an appreciation that with decreasing wavelength, the bands become more energetic but also less penetrating. Therefore, the physiologic effects of IR-C are confined to heating of superficial tissues. However, excessive ocular exposure to IR-A may lead to damage to the lens (cataracts), choroid and retina. IR-B can damage the cornea, conjunctiva and aqueous humor. The focusing ability of the eye may concentrate IR-A energy onto a localized point on the retinal pigment epithelium, leading to burns. Retinal burns may vary in severity from discrete peripheral lesions, which do not affect the visual field, to local or even global hemorrhage, leading to blindness.

Historically, chronic IR-A exposure was associated with posterior cortex cataract formation, as in glass and furnace workers or others who handle molten materials at temperatures greater than 1500 degrees C. When prevalent, this condition appeared to require intense, unprotected exposure for several years. With mechanization of glass manufacture and use of protective goggles, this condition has become rare.

Recommendations and prevention

Permissible exposures to IR-C relate to heating and vary with ambient temperature. There are no legal exposure limits for IR-A or IR-B (except in the case of laser use). The ACGIH provides a recommended threshold limit value intended to be protective for near-infrared effects on the eye, which varies depending upon the spectral characteristics and position of the worker.

Protective eyewear for workers with significant IR exposures should include appropriate infrared filters.

VISIBLE LIGHT
Exposure

The human eye detects light in the narrow band between 760 nm (red end) and 400 nm (violet end), with peak sensitivity at 555 nm. Light perception is partly a photochemical process. Light is measured in units of footcandles or SI units of lux, with 1 lux = 0.093 footcandles. Consideration should also be given to the quality of visible light, including the amount of glare, contrast, brightness and color.

Health effects

Inadequate amounts or poor quality of lighting have obvious effects of reduced worker performance and increased injury rates. Lighting has also been found to contribute to complaints which may initially be ascribed to air quality in the indoor environment. Although animal studies have shown that chronic exposure to excessively bright light may lead to premature degeneration of the cones responsible for color vision, there is no evidence that normal amounts of visible light exhaust human photochemical processes or produce chronic eye damage. Excessive luminance in the visual field (glare) may overcome the adaptive abilities of the pupil and retina. Glare reduces visual perception and causes visual fatigue. Severe glare can cause reversible iritis and blepharospasm.

Many individuals use bright artificial light therapeutically for the prevention of depression in seasonal affective disorder (SAD). Possible mechanisms include effects of light upon melatonin, serotonin, and cortisol regulation. Numerous clinically designed but obviously non-blinded studies have addressed this belief. Most show a positive outcome for light intensities up to 10,000 lux (workplace light is typically 200–400 lux), without adverse effects.[22]

An interesting controversy relating indoor lighting to human health is the question of full-spectrum light, which, by including wavelengths in the ultraviolet (UV) range, more closely replicates the spectrum of natural daylight. Advocates of full-spectrum light believe that the absence of the full-spectrum emissions from traditional indoor fluorescent lighting represents a source of physical and psychologic harm. They point out that full-spectrum light is natural and used in the treatment of seasonal affective disorder. Their suggestion is that UV frequencies should also be emitted from fluorescent lighting, but the preventive value of this recommendation is uncertain.

A role for excessive exposure to light at night, possibly acting in conjunction with electromagnetic fields, in the development of breast cancer has also been proposed (see section on SELF and ELF).

Recommendations and prevention

The most important consideration for this spectrum is to ensure that an appropriate amount and suitable quality of lighting is present in the workplace. For activities such as reading and writing, a work surface should have a minimum of 215 lux (20 footcandles) of appropriate quality light. The investigation of buildings with concerns about air quality should also include an assessment of indoor lighting. A useful summary with references on lighting is provided by the Environmental Protection Agency.[23]

In the absence of data, occupational physicians should not make full-spectrum light a workplace recommendation.

ULTRAVIOLET (UV) RADIATION
Exposures

Ultraviolet (UV) radiation extends in a narrow band between 400 to 100 nm. The UV band is subdivided into UV-A (400–315 nm), UV-B (315–280 nm), and UV-C (280–100 nm). As with all forms of radiant energy, with decreasing wavelength, the bands become more energetic but less penetrating. Therefore, UV-A is the least energetic but penetrates deepest into skin. UV-C is the most energetic and potentially damaging but is unable to penetrate the superficial layers of non-viable epidermis. UV-B is intermediate between the two.

The most important source of UV radiation is the sun. Although UV-C is the most energetic band and capable of greatest tissue damage, it lacks the ability to penetrate the earth's stratosphere. Therefore, the UV bands of environmental concern are UV-A and UV-B. All three bands may be produced by artificial sources of UV radiation, which are listed in Table 33.2.4.

Health effects

The harmful effects of UV light are caused largely by UV-B, although UV-A is a more common exposure and has been more recently recognized to have important health effects. UV-C is so readily absorbed by air and superficial skin cells that, in the rare event of exposure, it is unlikely to cause even residual erythema. Because of generally poor penetration properties, UV radiation effects are confined to the

Ultraviolet lamps
germicidal (air, water sterilization)
tanning beds
curing of resins (dental bonds, circuit boards), coatings, and inks
medical (PUVA)
photochemical processes (agricultural chemical, pharmaceutical production)
graphic arts
laboratory (spectrophotometers)
Electric arcs
welding
furnaces
UV lasers

Table 33.2.4 Artificial sources of UV radiation

skin and eyes and, depending on the degree of exposure, may be either acute or chronic in nature.

The main cause of both sunburn (solar erythema) and melanogenesis is UV-B. Sunburn usually appears 1–6 hours following exposure and fades after 3 days. Severe sunburn may cause blistering and destruction of the skin surface, with a risk of secondary infection. Human skin is partially protected from this hazard by melanin pigment production and thickening of the stratum corneum through keratinization in response to sunlight. Dark-skinned people are better protected than are light-skinned people. Although there is some immediate darkening of the skin in normally tanned individuals, the tanning process consists primarily of melanogenesis, which begins shortly after exposure and becomes visible within about 3 days.

UV-A is a less potent cause of sunburn. However, solar UV-A penetrates to the earth's surface to a greater extent than UV-B and effects from the two are additive. UV-A is also the cause of phototoxic and photosensitivity reactions (discussed in Chapter 29.2) and contributes to skin cancer and photoaging.

Sun exposure causes a constellation of chronic morphologic changes in the skin (see also Chapter 29.2). These consist of increased keratinization (solar keratosis), changes in underlying connective tissue (solar elastosis), vascular changes (telangiectasia), and pigment alterations (solar lentigines). Outdoor activities, ranging from agricultural work to outdoor construction, are associated with these changes. Similar to acute sun damage, dark-skinned individuals are relatively protected from these chronic outcomes.

The most important UV outcome is skin cancer (see also Chapter 30.10). Recent increases in all three major types of skin cancer have been linked to UV radiation exposure, most clearly to UV-B but with limited evidence implicating UV-A as well. Basal cell carcinoma is more strongly associated with peak exposure episodes (sunburn) while squamous cell carcinoma is very strongly associated with cumulative exposure. The relationship of melanoma to sun exposure is complex and involves a combination of both acute and cumulative exposure, with the strongest single exposure factor being a history of sunburn. Recent epidemiological data indicate that melanoma mortality is now declining in some parts of the world, concordant with preventive efforts in these regions.[24] A completely preventable cause of adverse effects stems from the use of UV tanning devices for cosmetic purposes. Corneal and retinal injuries, first- and second-degree skin burns and increased risk of melanoma have all been reported from this source.

The acute effects on the eye from UV radiation include photokeratoconjunctivitis (see also Chapter 20.1). Since human eyesight perceives UV poorly, acute damage may occur before the individual is aware of exposure. Keratitis and conjunctivitis are dramatic, but they are usually self-limited and heal within several days. Potential sources of this exposure include electric arc welding ('welder's flash'), germicidal UV lamps, and intense environmental sun exposure in colder climates ('snow blindness') or on water. Chronic ocular outcomes of UV exposure are a major concern. Exposures in the middle of the UV-B spectrum induce cataract formation most effectively, with a clear dose–response relationship.[25] Cortical cataracts are most prevalent in geographic areas where solar radiation is high and in outdoor workers.[26] In contrast, the incidence of nuclear cataracts appears to be unaffected by UV exposure.

Pinguecula and pterygium are localized areas of benign conjunctival thickening associated with prolonged UV exposure. Pingueculae are found adjacent to the limbus, more frequently on the nasal side. When the lesion crosses onto the cornea it is called a pterygium. Although both may be a cosmetic concern, symptoms only arise when a pterygium obstructs vision or causes astigmatism. Spheroidal degeneration (also known as climatic droplet keratopathy) is a form of corneal degeneration characterized by the presence of fine yellowish drops underneath the conjunctival or corneal epithelium which is usually asymptomatic. In addition to geographic associations with areas of increased UV exposure, spheroidal degeneration, pingueculae and pterygia have all been reported at higher frequency among outdoor workers[27] and in welders.[28]

Concern has also arisen about a possible relationship between long-term exposure to ultraviolet radiation and heightened risk of age-related macular degeneration, but limited studies to date have presented conflicting results.

Prevention and recommendations

Efforts should be made to reduce both UV-A and UV-B exposure. Recreational exposures that may lead to repetitive cycles of sun burning should be particularly avoided. Light-skinned, blue-eyed, freckled individuals are at greatest risk. Increased appreciation for outdoor recreation, increased residence time in sunbelt areas, and loss of ozone in the earth's atmosphere are likely to accentuate the risk and need for preventive interventions.

Exposure to natural UV radiation can be reduced by avoiding the midday sun (10am to 2pm). The National Weather Service and the Environmental Protection Agency have developed a daily UV Index for many US cities which estimates the risk of overexposure ranging from 0 (minimal) to 10+ (very high). Residents are advised to take special care when the index is 5 or higher.

Skin exposure can be reduced by wearing a wide-brimmed hat and long-sleeve clothing. Sunscreens represent the least desirable level of protection. In addition to compliance concerns, the protective effect of sunscreens for longer wavelengths of UV-A and chronic photodamage is unclear.[29]

Ocular exposure can be reduced through protective eyewear which blocks both UV-A and B. Although many companies now offer 'UV absorbing' contact lenses, there are limited studies that indicate reduced efficacy relative to comparable approved sunglasses – the latter should still be worn.[30] Arc welders' photokeratoconjunctivitis can be prevented with appropriate face shields.

LASERS
Exposures

A laser (Light Amplification by Stimulated Emission of Radiation) is a device emitting intense monochromatic radiation, continuously or in pulses. The wavelength of lasers overlaps that of the IR, visible and UV spectra. The hazard arises from the high intensity of the laser beam. IR lasers include the neodymium:yttrium, aluminum garnet and carbon dioxide lasers. Visible light lasers include dye, helium–neon, and krypton lasers. UV lasers include excimer lasers. These excited dimers of argon–fluoride or xenon–chloride are used for tissue excision purposes. Laser classification according to the recently revised American National Standards Institute (ANSI) and associated hazards are described in Table 33.2.5.[31]

Health effects

The most consistent hazard of lasers is related to non-beam effects such as electrocution or ignition of surrounding flammable materials by these powerful devices. There is also a significant acute hazard to the eye, skin, and deeper tissues from exposure to the beam depending on the wavelength, intensity, and duration of exposure of the laser.

Class of laser	Potential danger
I	Essentially harmless
II	Essentially harmless (do not stare at the laser)
*IIIa and IIIb	Hazardous
	Direct viewing is very dangerous
	Specular reflections are also dangerous
	Skin exposure is harmful
*IV	Extremely hazardous
	Direct viewing must not occur
	Specular reflections extremely dangerous
	Diffuse reflections extremely dangerous
	Skin exposure extremely hazardous
	Fire hazard

Note: When class III and IV lasers are fully embedded into an enclosed system that has full safety interlocks, the system may be classified as a class I system.
* Protection is required.

Table 33.2.5 ANSI laser classification

Laser injury is determined primarily by beam power (Table 33.2.5). The eye is the organ most vulnerable to acute damage, partly because the cornea and lens focus visible and near IR laser energy to small areas on the retina. At the point of focus, radiant exposure can be increased by more than five orders of magnitude. Both direct and reflected beams may cause eye damage. Pupil size, focusing ability, and myopia or aphakia may also influence the amount of retinal damage. Direct laser injury may cause partial or complete loss of small or large visual fields, depending on the extent and position of damage in the retina.

A great deal of concern has arisen recently over the increasingly widespread use of laser pointers, which may be deliberately directed to the eyes in an effort to distract or 'dazzle' the victim. Although permanent retinal damage has rarely been reported from laser pointers (most of which are class II or IIIa), this requires uninterrupted eye contact in excess of 10 seconds, making inadvertent injuries unlikely.[32]

Until recently, the indirect hazards of medical laser use have been less recognized. Laser surgery or any other tissue use of class IV lasers will inevitably generate smoke. In addition to being malodorous, there is evidence that this plume contains viable infectious agents (both viruses[33] and bacteria[34]) toxic gases (benzene, hydrogen cyanide, and formaldehyde),[35] and is mutagenic.[36] Medical use of UV lasers has also been calculated to increase UV exposure by the equivalent of 1 day of sunbathing.[37]

Prevention and recommendations

Detailed information on the safe operation of lasers can be found in ANSI Z136.1, 2000 Guidelines for the Safe Use of Lasers. Several important points of relevance to the occupational health provider are discussed below.

Ideally, lasers should be enclosed during use. Unfortunately, this is often impossible in research uses. Laser-using facilities must also be carefully designed to prevent reflections. They should be well lit so that the pupils are not dilated.

The eyes and skin are best kept out of the beam by interlock devices, which turn off the laser electronically or provide physical barriers between the operators or bystanders and the beam during operations. Not all research or medical laser activities are amenable to interlock protection. Laser surgery is a prime example. In such circumstances, personal protective devices are then used. Eye shielding must be selected in accordance with the wavelength of the laser used and should include side shielding. Absorptive filters are generally preferred over reflective types because absorptive filters are reliable regardless of the incident angle of the beam. A problem with optical density markings on laser-protective eye wear has been uncertainty with the reliability of the manufacturers' markings concerning transmittance. Independent checks are not truly achievable with available equipment so it is important to identify reliable suppliers.

Another problem with eye protection is that complete protection from visible beams blinds the user, interfering

with safety and efforts at beam alignment. In our experience, this tempts scientists to remove their eye protection to align the beam. For this reason, we recommend eye shields that are largely, but not absolutely, protective for open visible beam alignment operations. Under these circumstances, scientists will be afforded the eye protection necessary while their ability to view hazards and align the beam is adequately maintained. Laser users ought to assume that any ruby or neodymium laser capable of causing material surface ablations is also above the safe limits for viewing diffuse reflections. Laser retinal injuries continue to occur, despite the well-known safety precautions.

Specialty applications may present particular hazards. The optical hazards of beam splitters and the wavelength consequences of doubling crystals are understood by users but are not translated into safety practice. Installation and repair of fiber-optic communication systems is potentially hazardous; visualization of tightly packed energized cables or optically aided visualization of individual fibers may cause injury. Laser-equipped weapons present potentially uncontrolled hazards, which may be encountered in warfare, training simulations, or war games. Laser welding applications are often open-beam configurations with class IV lasers. There is usually significant diffuse reflection within 2 m of the target, whose direction becomes difficult to predict because of the use of process-shielding gases. Barriers, eye wear, and gloves are mandated for open laser welding.

Skin protection is also important for the operation of non-interlocked class IV lasers. The American Medical Association Council on Scientific Affairs makes specific recommendations for skin protection against carbon dioxide laser burns in surgical fields, using wet towels and sponges.[38] Carbon dioxide–nitrogen lasers emit invisible UV energy, so burns may potentially be severe before the hazard is appreciated. Barrier protection is required. Recommendations to control smoke from medical lasers have been described by NIOSH.[35]

Occupational physicians are asked frequently about medical surveillance for users of class IIIb and IV lasers. There are clear, acute hazards associated with laser use, but the existence of a chronic hazard amenable to medical surveillance is uncertain. Epidemiologic studies addressing chronic effects of laser exposure are not currently available, and new lasers and uses for lasers are introduced continually; so the absence of future chronic hazards should not be assumed. In particular, efforts should be made to reduce UV scattering in laboratories, to protect skin and eyes, and to follow workers who may receive substantial UV exposures.

For established programs experiencing no difficulties, it makes sense to obtain preplacement evaluations, evaluations at the time of suspected laser incidents, and termination evaluations.. Evaluations include ocular history, visual acuity, macular function (Amsler grid or similar pattern), contrast sensitivity (Arden sine wave or similar pattern), and fundoscopic evaluation with careful documentation of abnormalities.

Acknowledgment

The authors would like to thank Dr Gilles Thériault of McGill University for his review of a draft of this chapter.

References

1. Kaune WT, Stevens RG, Callahan NJ, Severson RK, Thomas DB. Residential magnetic and electric fields. Bioelectromagnetics 1987; 8:315–35.
2. Wertheimer N, Leeper E. Electrical wiring configurations and childhood cancer. Am J Epidemiol 1979; 109:273–84.
3. Kheifets LI, Gilbert ES, Sussman SS, et al. Comparative analyses of the studies of magnetic fields and cancer in electric utility workers: studies from France, Canada, and the United States. Occup Environ Med 1999; 56:567–74.
4. International Agency for Research on Cancer. Non-ionizing radiation, Part 1: Static and extremely low-frequency electric and magnetic fields (19–26 June 2001). Vol. 80. Lyon: IARC, 2001.
5. Li C-Y, Sung F-C. Association between occupational exposure to power frequency electromagnetic fields and amyotrophic lateral sclerosis: a review. Am J Ind Med 2003; 43:212–20.
6. Ahlbom A. Neurodegenerative diseases, suicide and depressive symptoms in relation to EMF. Bioelectromagnetics 2001; S132–43.
7. Savitz DA, Liao D, Sastre A, Kleckner RC, Kavet R. Magnetic field exposure and cardiovascular disease mortality among electric utility workers. Am J Epidemiol 1999; 149:135–42
8. Blaasaas KG, Tynes T, Lie RT. Residence near power lines and risk of birth defects. Epidemiology 2003; 14:95–8.
9. Li D-K, Odouli R, Wi S, et al. A population-based prospective cohort study of personal exposure to magnetic fields during pregnancy and the risk of miscarriage. Epidemiology 2002; 13:9–20.
10. Savitz DA. Invited commentary: electromagnetic fields and cancer in railway workers. Am J Epidemiol 2001; 153:836–8.
11. Savitz DA. Health effects of electric and magnetic fields: are we done yet? Epidemiology 2003: 14:15–17.
12. International Commission on Non-Ionizing Radiation Protection. Guidelines for limiting exposure to time-varying electric, magnetic, and electromagnetic fields (up to 300 GHz). Health Phys 1998; 74:494–522.
13. National Institute of Occupational Safety and Health. Video display terminals, 3rd edn. Publication Number 99-135. Cincinatti: NIOSH, 1999.
14. Lonne-Rahm S, Andersson B, Melin L, Schultzberg M, Arnetz B, Berg M. Provocation with stress and electricity of patients with 'sensitivity to electricity'. J Occup Environ Med 2000; 42:512–6.
15. Forman SA. Sublethal exposure to microwave radar. JAMA 1998; 259:3129.
16. Rosenthal DS, Beering SC. Hypogonadism after microwave radiation. JAMA 1968; 205:105–7.
17. Schilling CJ. Effects of exposure to very high frequency radiofrequency radiation on six antenna engineers in two separate incidents. Occup Med 2000; 50:49–56.
18. National Institute for Occupational Safety and Health. Occupational exposure of police officers to microwave radiation from traffic radar devices. Publication Number PB95-261350. Cincinatti: NIOSH, 1995.
19. Groves FD, Page WP, Gridley G, et al. Cancer in Korean War navy technicians: mortality survey after 40 years. Am J Epidemiol 2002; 155:810–18.
20. Johansen C, Boice JD, McLaughlin JK, Olson JH. Cellular telephones and cancer – a nationwide cohort study in Denmark. J Natl Cancer Inst 2001; 93:203–7.
21. Tri JL, Hayes DL, Smith TT, Severson RP. Cellular phone interference with external cardiopulmonary monitoring devices. Mayo Clin Proc 2001; 76:11–15.
22. Gaster B. Light therapy for seasonal affective disorder. Alternative Medicine Alert 2001; April:40–43.
23. United States Environmental Protection Agency. Lighting fundamentals. EPA 430-B-95-007; 1997.
24. Severi G, Giles GG, Robertson C, Boyle P, Autier P. Mortality from cutaneous melanoma: evidence for contrasting trends between populations. Br J Cancer 2000; 82:1887–91.
25. West S. Ocular ultraviolet B exposure and lens opacities: a review. J Epidemiol 1999; 9(6 Suppl):S97–101.
26. Risk factors for age-related cortical, nuclear, and posterior subcapsular cataracts. The Italian-American Cataract Study Group. Am J Epidemiol 1991; 133:541–3.
27. Taylor HR, West SK, Rosenthal FS, Munoz B, Newland HS, Emmett EA. Corneal changes associated with chronic UV irradiation. Arch Ophthalmol 1989; 107:1481–4.
28. Norn M, Franck C. Long-term changes in the outer part of the eye in welders. Prevalence of spheroid degeneration, pinguecula, pterygium, and corneal cicatrices. Acta Ophthalmol 1991; 69:382–6.
29. Gasparro FP. Sunscreens, skin photobiology, and skin cancer: the need for UVA protection and evaluation of efficacy. Environ Health Perspect 2000; 108(Suppl 1):71–8.
30. Anstey A, Taylor D, Chalmers I, Ansari E. Ultraviolet radiation-blocking characteristics of contact lenses: relevance to eye protection for psoralen-sensitised patients. Photodermatol Photoimmunol Photomed 1999; 15:193–7.
31. American National Standards Institute. American National Standard for the safe use of lasers, ANSI Z136.1. New York: National Standards Institute, 2000.
32. Yolton RL, Citek K, Schmeisser E, Reichow AW, Griffith T. Laser pointers: toys, nuisances, or significant eye hazards? J Am Optom Assoc 1999; 70:285–9.
33. Garden JM, O'Banion MK, Sheinitz LS, et al. Papillomavirus in the vapor of carbon dioxide laser-treated verrucae. JAMA 1988; 259:1199–202.
34. Capizzi PJ, Clay RP, Battey MJ. Microbiologic activity in laser resurfacing plume and debris. Lasers Surg Med 1998; 23:172–4.
35. NIOSH Hazard Controls. Control of smoke from laser/electric surgical procedures. HC11. Publication No. 96-128. Cincinatti: NIOSH, 1999.
36. Plappert UG, Stocker B, Helbig R, Fliedner TM, Seidel HJ. Laser pyrolysis products –genotoxic, clastogenic and mutagenic effects of the particulate aerosol fractions. Mutat Res 1999; 441:29–41.
37. Sterenborg HJ, de Gruijl FR, Kelfkens G, van der Leun JC. Evaluation of skin cancer risk resulting from long term occupational exposure to radiation from ultraviolet lasers in the range from 190 to 400 nm. Photochem Photobiol 1991; 54:775–80.
38. American Medical Association, Council on Scientific Affairs. Lasers in medicine and surgery. JAMA 1986; 256:900–7.

Chapter 34
Thermal Stressors

Oyebode A Taiwo, Mark R Cullen

Thermal stress on workers represents perhaps the oldest recognized occupational hazard. Thermal stresses, and their consequent health effects, are created by exposure to extreme ambient temperatures, high humidity, physical activity, and the use of specialized clothing and gear. Although these problems have been alleviated to a large extent in developed countries by modern climate control, problems related to thermal stress remain widespread among industrial workers everywhere. Indeed, new problems in thermal stress have been created by advancing technologies, even as old ones have disappeared. Although reliable data on the incidence and prevalence of the major sequelae are not available from most parts of the world, compensation files and hospital admissions records document that disorders related to heat and cold exposure continue to be reported.

Thermal stresses are also important outside the workplace, particularly in vulnerable populations, such as infants and elderly and homeless persons. So great is the problem in these groups that it is generally viewed as beyond the scope of environmental medicine and will not be addressed in this text. Similarly, thermal burns, which are extremely important in both occupational and non-occupational settings, have been extensively reviewed in existing surgical texts and are also beyond the scope of this book. Accordingly, this chapter will focus on exposures to heat and cold in the occupational setting, the major clinical problems that these stresses create, and current strategies for their prevention and treatment.

HEAT STRESS
Exposure settings

Occupational heat stress or heat load is the combination of external factors of heat on the worker. This includes environmental conditions (temperature, humidity, heat index), work demands (nature of job, duration), and clothing requirements. The resulting heat strain is the immediate physiologic response of the body to heat stress. This includes an increase in body temperature, heart rate, and sweating.[1]

The potential for a work environment to produce heat stress sufficient to interfere with function depends on three largely independent factors:
- the amount of heat generated by the worker over time;
- the external heat load; and
- the capacity for effective heat removal.

The amount of heat generated by the worker is related to the intensity and type of work performed. For example, heavy physical work generates a larger amount of heat than medium, light or sedentary work. The external heat load is a function of the ambient temperature plus the radiant temperature. The latter occurs from sources such as heating elements, fires, or sunlight and provides an additional load. The capacity for heat removal can be determined by environmental evaluation. Low humidity and high air movement against the skin strongly favor heat removal. Clothing covering the skin, especially if it is impermeable to water, will impede heat removal. Protective clothing has become increasingly important in some occupations, such as hazardous waste removal, to block exposures to chemicals, or biotechnology work, to protect work products.[2,3]

The assessment of potential heat stress requires simultaneous knowledge of six factors:
- ambient temperature;
- radiant temperature;
- relative humidity;
- air velocity;
- physical activity level; and
- clothing cover and permeability.

Air temperature, radiant temperature, humidity, and air velocity can be measured by separate devices or collectively measured with a single device, i.e., the wet bulb globe thermometer. Various indices, including the corrected effective temperature and the wet bulb globe thermometer index, calculate the thermal stress on workers better than temperature alone.[4] However, given the quantitative importance of the work intensity itself as the major source of heat stress, excess reliance on these environmental measures may be misleading. Therefore it is essential to evaluate all sources of heat gain as well as the potential for heat loss to assess adequately the overall risk for incurring heat-related disorders.[5]

A four-stage strategy for evaluation and prevention of risk due to work in thermal environments has been proposed.[6] In the first stage, a screening tool is used to detect the majority of the risk factors related to safety, health, and well-being of the employees and workplace. The conclusion would be to determine if there is a need for further investigation. The second stage consists of close observation of the climatic and working conditions over the entire year to identify particular circumstances, specific tasks, and unusual working conditions where problems might exist and to determine solutions to eliminate the problems. The third stage, analysis, usually conducted by occupational hygienists, is carried out where a heat-stress problem remains after stage 2; therefore it will deal with specific conditions and usually involves measurement. The objective is to find technical solutions and, where exposure is unavoidable, to define organizational solutions and short-term protection measures. At the end of this stage, most of the conditions should be under control. If an unacceptable risk of heat stress remains, further assistance of an expert will be required for studying these unusual circumstances, using specific investigational techniques such as plane radiant thermometry, clothing permeation, or oxygen consumption measures. Not all four stages need be performed; the procedure stops when adequate solutions have been implemented.

Physiology

Body temperature represents a balance between heat production and heat loss. The maintenance of body function requires that the temperature of vital internal organs be at or near 37°C. Body heat is primarily produced by continuous metabolic activity. A resting adult produces about 75 kcal of heat per hour as a byproduct of the basal metabolism. Physical activity adds heat to the body at a greater rate than does a hot environment. Work activities can range from 80 to 700 kcal/hour (Table 34.1). Heat is also gained from the environment, either through radiation from the sun, the heated ground, reflected radiation from the sky or radiant sources such as furnaces.

Heat loss occurs through four mechanisms: conduction, convection, radiation, and evaporation. Conduction is the heat exchange between two surfaces in direct contact. It is generally the least important mechanism of heat loss since behavioral thermoregulation generally intervenes. Convection is the heat transferred from a surface to a gas or fluid, usually air or water molecules circulating in the body. As the air in the immediate contact of the skin is warmed, heated molecules move away and cooler ones replace them and, in turn, are warmed up and the process continues. Radiation is the transfer of heat between the body and its surroundings by electromagnetic waves. The magnitude of heat loss or gain by radiation depends on the temperature difference between the skin and the surrounding environment, and the body surface area. Evaporation

is the conversion of a liquid to the gaseous phase. Evaporation of water takes place from the lungs and skin.

The body will attempt to unload the excess heat gained, to maintain a normal body temperature. The body's primary defense against overheating is sweating. Each liter of sweat that completely evaporates from the skin removes 600 kcal from the body. Although a healthy adult can produce up to 1.5 liters of sweat per hour, the ability of this sweat to carry heat from the body depends on its ability to be evaporated. Thus, sweat loss by dripping, absorption onto clothing, and climactic conditions (such as high humidity and slow air movement) impedes heat loss. Only small amounts of heat are lost by radiation or by direct convective transfer to air.

Heat is distributed throughout the body by convection in the blood stream. Thermal sensors in the brain respond to the increased blood temperature and relay signals to a central integrative area in the hypothalamus, which, in turn, directs thermoregulatory effectors to conserve or unload the excess heat gained. Heat loss responses induce increased rates of blood flow to the skin and sweating. These responses promote an increase in the rate of heat transfer from the body core to the environment. The increased heat transfer from the core to the skin occurs as a result of increased convection in the elevated skin blood flow, and the increased transfer from the skin to the environment is achieved partly by the increased radiation and convection and, primarily, by the evaporation of sweat. When the rate of heat dissipation becomes equal to the rate of heat production, the body temperature becomes stable.

The absolute rise in body temperature in any heat gain condition is a function of the speed of the heat dissipation response. A relatively fast response will result in less heat being stored in the body and, thus, in a smaller rise in deep-body temperature on reaching a steady state. A rise in body core temperature of more than 2°C to 2.5°C will be accompanied by side effects that reduce both performance and the ability to prolong activity. These effects are primarily the result of a progressive redistribution of blood flow and, hence, of blood volume toward the skin. A reduction in central circulating blood volume acts to reduce the filling pressure of the heart. If compensatory reflexes are not activated, the ability of the heart to maintain an adequate blood flow will diminish, resulting in a fall in arterial blood pressure and blood flow to the brain. As blood flow to the brain is reduced, the effect will be a feeling of light-headedness or dizziness, disorientation, and, eventually, a loss of consciousness. The physiologic compensatory responses to a fall in the heart's filling pressure include an increased heart rate and constriction of non-essential vascular beds, including those of the skin. The latter reflex serves to shift blood to the body's core, thereby helping maintain central blood volume and, thus, flow to the brain and contracting muscles. A relatively fast thermoregulatory mechanism, resulting in relatively lower body heat storage, provides a greater margin of safety and time before compensatory responses need to be invoked.[7]

With the occurrence of heat stress and a subsequent loss of body water by sweating, substantial changes may occur

Activity	Rate (kcal/hr)
Bicycling	360–600
Climbing stairs	360–720
Construction tasks	300–600
Domestic work	75–300
Driving	120–180
Heavy labor/factory work	210–400
Light assembly/inspection	90–160
Machine operator/manual trade	120–240
Office work (sitting)	75–120
Resting (sitting or lying)	60–90
Standing (inactive)	90–120
Swimming	300–880
Walking on a flat surface (3–5 km/hr)	300–400

Table 34.1 Rate of heat generation for common occupational activities

in the composition of body fluid. Sodium and potassium are both lost in sweat, at concentrations that rise as sweating is prolonged. The decline in renal blood flow accompanying heat stress stimulates the renin–aldosterone axis to conserve sodium, but this may exacerbate potassium losses. Antidiuretic hormone release is stimulated because of the decrease in central blood volume. The plasma osmolality increases because of excess water loss and inadequate sodium delivery to the distal nephrons accompanying the reduced renal blood flow.

Although these changes are physiologically stressful, adverse health effects will occur only if the heat stress exceeds the individual's heat tolerance capacity. In otherwise healthy individuals, factors predisposing the worker to hyperthermia include salt and/or water depletion, fever, infection, and obesity.[8] Workers with underlying diseases, even if controlled clinically and not routinely disabling, may be at particularly high risk. Common risk factors include cardiovascular disease, alcoholism, diabetes mellitus, and hyperthyroidism.[9–11] In addition to these factors, any disorder of sweat production, including miliaria or a prior episode of heat stroke, cystic fibrosis, scleroderma, healed burns, or dermatitis may be a serious problem (Table 34.2).[12] Among the more prevalent risk factors in the workforce is the use of therapeutic or recreational drugs. Agents that have proven or suspected effects are listed in Table 34.3, but any agent that may interfere with

autonomic function, vascular tone, motor activity, or cardiovascular responses should be considered likely to lower the threshold at which thermoregulation fails and the core temperature begins to rise.[13,14]

After the body's core temperature starts to rise, pathologic responses ensue. Acutely, hyperthermia may contribute to the development of hepatic necrosis and pancreatitis. Fibrinolysis and activation of platelet activity may lead to disseminated intravascular coagulation (DIC). Skeletal and myocardial muscle is disrupted, leading to rhabdomyolysis and myocardial necrosis. Renal function, already compromised by low renal blood flow, may be more severely disrupted by the outpouring of myoglobin and uric acid from this cascade. Ultimately, the central nervous system is affected by the heat, DIC, and metabolic disturbances.[15,16]

Heat acclimatization

Many of the physiologic alterations induced by heat stress are attenuated by the process of heat acclimatization. To become heat acclimated, an individual must undergo gradually increased exposures to both heat stress and exercise stress. Furthermore, these must occur on a regular basis over a period of about 2 weeks to be maximized. Although some changes may occur from heat stress alone without physical activity, such as during very hot times of the year, only regular and repeated exposures to heat and activity induce acclimatization sufficient to alter heat tolerance substantially.[17,18] Heat acclimatization is characterized by the following.

1. *Enhanced cardiovascular fitness*. This includes increased maximal oxygen uptake in the muscles, increased plasma volume, increased cardiac stroke volume and contractility, and reduced heart rate for a given cardiac output.[19]
2. *Altered sweat*. The sweating onset for a given thermal load occurs sooner, and the maximum sweating rate is increased. Furthermore, the sodium concentration of sweat is markedly decreased, thereby acting to conserve the body's sodium store.[20,21]
3. *Enhanced renal function*. The glomerular filtration rate may increase up to 20% over baseline, largely as a result of cardiovascular changes.[19,21]

The net effect of these changes is such that acclimated workers have a markedly enhanced tolerance for heat stress. This fact forms the basis for an administrative control over heat-related disturbances; the gradual introduction of new or non-acclimated workers to jobs with high thermal stress.

Classification of disorders resulting from thermal stress

ACUTE DISORDERS OF SYSTEMIC HEAT STRESS

Heat syncope
Heat edema
Heat tetany

Normal persons	Predisposing diseases
Salt and/or water depletion	Cardiovascular disease
Infection	Diabetes mellitus
Fever	Malnutrition
Lack of acclimatization	Acute or chronic alcoholism
Obesity	Electrolyte disturbances
Drugs (Table 34.3)	Hyperthyroidism
Advanced age	Impaired sweat production
	Miliaria
	Sweat gland injury after prior heat stroke
	Cystic fibrosis
	Scleroderma
	Healed thermal burns

Modified from Knochel JP. Heat stroke and related heat stress disorders. Dis Mon 1989; 35:301-77.

Table 34.2 Risks predisposing to exhaustion and heat stroke

Alpha and beta (sympathetic) blocking agents
Anticholinergics
Antidepressants
Antihistamines
Calcium channel blockers
Cocaine
Diuretics
Dopaminergics
Ethanol
Lithium
Neuroleptics
Sympathomimetics

Table 34.3 Drugs that may enhance risk for heat stress-induced disorders

Heat cramps
Heat exhaustion
   Predominant water depletion
   Predominant salt depletion
Exertional heat stroke

SUBACUTE EFFECTS OF HEAT STRESS
Infertility
Teratogenesis

SKIN DISORDERS CAUSED BY HEAT STRESS
(see Chapter 29.2)
Erythema ab igne
Miliaria

MAJOR DISORDERS CAUSED BY HEAT STRESS

Although the major heat-related disorders can be separated from each other on clinical grounds, there is considerable overlap; therefore, they should be considered as a series of syndromes along a single spectrum.

Heat syncope

Clinical pattern
Heat syncope is a relatively benign disorder that occurs primarily in the unacclimated worker as a result of vasodilatation and diminished venous return during the early adaptation to heat stress. It is indistinguishable clinically from syncope caused by postural hypotension of any cause. There may be postural symptoms preceding an actual syncopal event. Workers with low blood volumes related to diuretic use or those receiving pharmacologic agents that impede autonomic function are at highest risk.[22,23]

Evaluation
Individuals who experience postural dizziness or frank syncope after unaccustomed exertion in the heat are readily diagnosed; sinus tachycardia and mild postural hypotension should be evident, along with sweating. The body temperature is generally normal, unless a febrile illness has predisposed the patient to this event. Cardiac and central nervous system causes of syncope can generally be excluded by the history and physical examination. Vasovagal episodes are distinguished because of their presentation with bradycardia rather than tachycardia.

Treatment
The most important steps in management are placing the patient in a recumbent position to maximize blood flow to the brain and administering salt and water. This rarely requires an intravenous line because the patients are usually stable and able to drink sitting up long enough to replenish lost fluids and electrolytes. Further testing or prolonged observation is generally unnecessary.

Course and prognosis
Patients generally recover quickly and completely after fluid administration. There are no further steps necessary other than recognition that heat stress is excessive, at least for the particular affected person, and must be modified before a return to work, generally on a subsequent day.

Heat edema

Clinical pattern
Heat edema represents a second clinical response to the physiologic adaptation of unacclimated workers to heat stress. Generally within 1 to 2 days after first exposure, new-onset dependent edema may occur (or an increase in pre-existing peripheral edema). This is probably caused by relative oliguria and hyperaldosteronism, although other hormonal factors such as insulin and growth factor may be involved.[23]

Evaluation
This diagnosis should be made by the history and physical examination with attention to excluding coincident cardiovascular events. Further diagnostic testing is not indicated unless the edema persists for more than a few days.

Treatment
Because body fluid expansion is part of the acclimatization process, steps to interfere with this, such as diuretics or salt restriction, are strongly contraindicated. Patients with predisposing risks for edema or complications, such as congestive heart failure, should be excluded from further exposures to heat stress; others may carry on.

Course and prognosis
The disorder is self-limiting and will disappear as the glomerular filtration rate and cardiac output rise during the acclimatization process. There are no sequelae or evidence that individuals who experience this problem are at particular risk for other heat-related health problems.

Heat tetany

Clinical pattern
Heat tetany is a third benign disorder, generally occurring in the unacclimated individual early after heat stress. The cause is central hyperventilation, leading to systemic alkalemia. Symptoms such as perioral paresthesia and signs of frank tetany generally resolve when the patient is removed to a cooler area, usually before medical attention can be obtained.[23]

Evaluation
The diagnosis should be considered based on the history. In an individual without underlying health problems, the major differential diagnosis is with hyperventilation syndrome or panic disorder. Although the manifestations

and laboratory findings of hypocarbia and high partial pressure of oxygen are identical, heat tetany should be distinguished from these other causes because of the stigma associated with them, the different treatment modalities, the likelihood of recurrence, and the proper assignment of cause. Rarely, determination of serum calcium and arterial blood gases may be necessary to exclude more serious disorders.

Treatment

Removal from the heat stress is all that is required. In general, affected workers should have their heat loads modified to prevent recurrences prior to full acclimatization.

Course and prognosis

This disorder is completely benign and has no implication other than that mentioned in regard to a modification of the heat load.

Heat cramps

Clinical pattern

Heat cramps are characterized by brief, intermittent, and often excruciating cramping pain in the muscles that have been subjected to excessive work. The most common muscle groups affected are the muscles of the extremities. The cramps typically occur late in a workday or after the muscles have cooled, e.g., in the shower. In severe cases, there may be muscle necrosis with leakage of creatinine and muscle enzymes, although frank myoglobinuria with renal involvement has not been described in this setting. The basis for heat cramps is hyponatremia. Acclimated workers are at far greater risk because of the adaptation that allows them to sweat far greater volumes than in the control state.[24] Although adaptation to heat reduces the concentration of sodium in the sweat, the marked increase in sweat volume results in far greater total sodium losses than would otherwise be possible. The replacement of water losses without replacement of salt losses creates the condition in which heat cramps occur.[22,23]

Diagnosis

Similar to other heat-related disturbances, the pattern of the illness in the typical setting is usually diagnostic. The body temperature is usually normal and the individual sweats normally or there is excessive sweating. Heat cramps must be distinguished from the more common cramps that occur during strenuous work. Common cramps generally last longer but will resolve completely with rest and massage; they are unrelated to systemic fluid and electrolyte imbalances. A determination of serum electrolyte levels will distinguish the two conditions. It is also important to distinguish simple heat cramps from the more life-threatening syndrome of heat exhaustion (see later), in which cramps may also occur. As a matter of definition, if cramps occur together with constitutional symptoms (such as fatigue, weakness, headache, gastrointestinal

upset, or mental status changes), the diagnosis of heat exhaustion is appropriate.

Treatment

The key to treatment is the correction of hyponatremia by the administration of fluids containing adequate concentrations of sodium. This can almost always be done orally in cases of simple heat cramps. Rest alone is not sufficient because the condition often occurs in the resting state after a work shift. If continued heat stress is present, as in very hot climates, the control of heat cramps is easier if the patient is removed to a cooler area where sweating will slow or stop.

Course and prognosis

Heat cramps, although benign in and of themselves, are a premonitory sign of decompensation caused by heat stress. Unlike syncope, tetany, and edema, the condition is not self-limited and will resolve only after sodium losses are replaced. More importantly, continued work under conditions of heat stress without replacement may lead to heat exhaustion, with a possibility of heat stroke supervening unexpectedly at any time.

Heat exhaustion: predominant salt-depletion type

Clinical pattern

When water replacement of sweat is adequate but salt replacement is not, heat exhaustion of the salt-depletion type, with or without cramps, may occur. Unlike simple heat cramps, this syndrome typically occurs during periods of heat stress and is more common in unacclimatized individuals, although all workers are at risk.[23] The predominant symptoms are nausea, vomiting, dizziness, weakness, and anxiety; alterations of mental status are often seen, although they are not profound early. Thirst is generally minimal or absent because plasma volume and intracellular volume are generally well preserved at the expense of the interstitial spaces, which lack oncotic forces. Clinically, the patients appear clammy and pale. Normal skin elasticity may be lost as a result of depletion of the interstitial fluid. The body temperature is normal or may be low unless heat stroke supervenes. The urine volume may also be normal. In the unacclimated worker, cardiovascular strain may be evidenced by hypotension and tachycardia. Similar to heat cramps, hyponatremia is uniformly present in this condition.

Diagnosis

As in other heat-related disorders, the history and signs described should be sufficient to make the correct diagnosis. The presence of cramps suggests hyponatremia. The biggest differential consideration is coincident viral syndrome, which this disorder might mimic. A demonstration of low serum sodium levels and response to salt replacement should serve to differentiate these two.

Treatment

Because this disorder typically begins during conditions of heat stress, removal to a cool place is essential to slow the ongoing salt losses. The specific treatment is replacement of sodium, usually with additional water because the total body water may also be somewhat low. Fluids of normal tonicity should be administered orally or intravenously until the symptoms have cleared, the pulse has normalized, and the urine flow is high and contains adequate (i.e., > 10 mEq/l) sodium. In the rare individual whose serum sodium has fallen to very low levels (i.e., < 120 mEq/l), replacement should be paced to avoid a too rapid correction with its inherent risk of central pontine myelinolysis.[25,26] An important consideration is avoidance of aspirin use or any non-steroidal anti-inflammatory drugs for this disorder, because of anecdotal reports of paradoxical hyperthermic responses to these agents in this setting.

Course and prognosis

Treated individuals should recover completely. Obviously, patients would not be returned to heat stress until total correction has occurred and the conditions that led to this extremely serious outcome have been investigated and corrected.

Heat exhaustion: predominant water-depletion type

Clinical pattern

This severe disorder of heat stress is heralded by changes in mental status, starting as anxiety and weakness, but frequently advancing to confusion, agitation, and delirium. Patients usually complain of thirst but may be incoherent. Signs include evidence of dehydration, oliguria, and hyperthermia; hyperventilation and tetany also may occur.

The underlying disturbance is failure to replace water losses related to sweating, with subsequent volume loss and hypernatremia. Because thirst itself is not impaired until late in the course of the illness, the setting of heat exhaustion of this type is typically one in which access to water is restricted, as in construction, farming, military work, and mining.[23] However, thirst is the least sensitive of the body's sensory systems and should not be relied on to signal the body water deficit adequately, especially in older workers.

Diagnosis

Although recognition of this disturbance is crucial and often life saving, it should present few problems diagnostically unless the history of heat stress is unavailable because of the patient's mental status. In the setting of delirium or coma without a history, the diagnosis should be evident from the signs of total body volume depletion and hyperthermia, combined with hypernatremia. Ruling out coincident sepsis may be difficult if the history is not available; stress leukocytosis and hypocapnia do not distinguish between the two. Similarly, in a diabetic subject, serum glucose levels may rise rapidly and raise consideration

of non-ketotic hyperosmolar coma. In either case, neither consideration of infection and search for a source nor concern about underlying metabolic disturbance should distract the clinician from the recognition that the manifestations of heat exhaustion of this type may occur from heat stress alone.

Treatment

Unlike all the preceding disorders, heat exhaustion of the water-depletion type is a medical emergency because heat stroke, with cardiovascular collapse and rapid rise of body core temperature, may supervene at any moment. Therefore, victims should be emergently transported to a hospital rather than attempting oral fluid replacement on site.

The mainstay of treatment is the administration of water, with or without sodium. If hypotension is evident, half-normal or even normal saline should be given. After the blood pressure is stable, hypotonic solutions, such as 5% dextrose in water, should be given, with the goal to correct the serum sodium level at a rate of 1 to 2 mEq/l/hour. There is a serious risk of cerebral edema from a too rapid correction.

Course and prognosis

Although full recovery is the rule, improvement in mental status may be delayed for several days, well after the fluid and electrolyte disturbances have corrected. Needless to say, the worker's return to heat stress after the hospital discharge must be done cautiously and only after full appreciation of the circumstances that led to the event.

Heat stroke

Clinical pattern

The hallmark of heat stroke is the ultimate failure of heat-dissipating mechanisms to compensate for heat stress, with a rapid rise in the core body temperature to more than 40°C and often much higher. Profound dysfunction of central nervous system activities occurs, with depression of the level of consciousness, often preceded by delirious or even psychotic behavior. Circulatory collapse with hypotension is frequent. The signs on the physical examination may be variable, depending on the setting and severity of the episode. In exertional heat stroke, unlike the classic picture of this disease in the elderly patient, sweating and other compensatory mechanisms may still be active when the patient is first seen, so skin may or may not be hot and dry.[27] Despite peripheral evidence of volume depletion, pulmonary edema may be present as a result of myocardial involvement. Focal neurologic signs may be present because of direct central nervous system involvement or secondary to seizures, which typically occur during the early cooling phase, although often before the patient arrives at the hospital. The laboratory findings are striking. Muscle enzymes are invariably elevated, with often spectacular creatine phosphokinase (CPK) levels. The serum potassium concentration is usually low, but it

Feature	Classic	Exertional
Age group	Very young, very old	Working age
Health status	Chronic illness common	Usually healthy
History of recent febrile illness	Unusual	Common
Drug use	Autonomic antagonists, diuretics, neuroleptics	Amphetamines, cocaine
Sweating	Usually absent	Often present
Respiratory alkalosis	Dominant	Mild
Lactic acidosis	Absent or mild	Often marked
Acute renal failure	<5% of patients	30% of patients
Rhabdomyolysis	Seldom severe	Severe
Hyperuricemia	Modest	Severe
Creatine phosphokinase/aldolase	Mildly elevated	Markedly elevated
Hypocalcemia	Uncommon	Common
Disseminated intravascular coagulation	Mild	Marked
Hypoglycemia	Uncommon	Common

Modified from Knochel JP. Heat stroke and related heat stress disorders. Dis Mon 1989; 35:301-77.

Table 34.4 Comparison of classic and exertional heat stroke

may be elevated if muscle and other cell necroses are advanced and renal failure has begun. Serum uric acid and phosphate levels are often elevated because of tissue damage, and hepatic enzyme concentrations are also frequently elevated. Generally, the serum creatinine level is high because of muscle cell lysis and renal failure. At the same time, evidence of DIC is usually evident, with thrombocytopenia and abnormal clotting parameters. Blood gas measurements may demonstrate respiratory alkalosis, but lactic acidosis is usually the dominant acid–base disorder. If the liver is extensively involved, serum glucose levels may be low. The urine, if there is any, typically shows myoglobin and pigmented casts.[15,28] The differences between heat stroke seen in the occupational setting and the classic disease of infants and elderly persons are summarized in Table 34.4.

Diagnosis

The only diagnostic issues are early recognition and appropriate and expectant classification of the involved organ systems. Before total decompensation, patients still sweating may not appear hyperthermic. Therefore, when heat stroke is considered, the rectal temperature must be obtained immediately. After hyperthermia is demonstrated, two important drug-related conditions with differing mechanisms and treatments must be ruled out. The first is malignant hyperthermia, which results from administration of anesthetic agents in susceptible subjects.[29] This can usually be excluded because of the setting and the presence in that disorder of profound muscle rigidity. The malignant neuroleptic syndrome, caused by haloperidol, phenothiazines, and lithium, also is characterized by profound muscle rigidity and striking extrapyramidal movement abnormalities.[30] An important differentiating characteristic of each of these drug-induced conditions is the continued rise in core temperature until treated; core temperature begins to fall in heat stroke after the patient is removed from the thermal stress.

Treatment

The management of this life-threatening disorder should be undertaken by a team experienced in intensive care medicine. Because of the complexities of the neurologic, cardiovascular, renal, metabolic, and hematologic disturbances, the details of such care are beyond the scope of this text. The basic steps in early intervention are summarized here.

1. As with any other life-threatening condition, airway support, effective ventilation, and circulatory support must be ensured. After intravenous access has been established, baseline studies should be obtained. The next most crucial step is rapid body cooling. This is most easily accomplished by spraying the naked patient with cool mist while using fans to enhance airflow over the body. This method reduces temperature by 0.06°C to 0.16°C per minute. The common practice of placing icepacks on the body surface is not effective and may be counterproductive because icepacks can increase peripheral vasoconstriction and may induce shivering.[31] Lavaging the stomach with iced saline solution has also been found to be no more effective than the evaporation procedure.[32] Rapid cooling should be continued until the core temperature is below 39°C. The control of seizures, which often occur during cooling, may be accomplished with diazepam. Shivering, which also generates heat, can be controlled by the use of phenothiazines.

2. Cardiovascular adequacy must be maintained. Although the intravascular volume may initially be low, fluids should be given cautiously because of the intense vasoconstriction that will occur with cooling. The possibility of pulmonary edema from a volume overload must be considered, given the likelihood of myocardial damage from the heat stroke. Monitoring of central pressures, with a Swan-Ganz catheter, can assist with this aspect of management.

3. Acid–base and electrolyte disturbances must be corrected. If the serum potassium level is depressed, careful repletion is essential. Renal output and function must be carefully watched to avoid rapid hyperkalemia. Disturbances in plasma tonicity should be corrected by the choice of fluid administered. If the blood glucose level is low, high dextrose-containing

solutions must be given that are consistent with the demands of serum osmolarity correction.

4. Renal function must be optimized. Because of the invariable insult to the nephrons from myoglobinemia, extreme hyperuricemia, hypokalemia, dehydration, and impaired cardiac output, acute renal failure is likely. The most important step is maximizing the renal blood flow by maintaining the cardiac output and blood volume and by cooling, which will reshunt the blood back to the visceral organs. Beyond these measures, ensuring the patient's survival and minimizing the sequelae will depend on attention to the specific organ complications of the disease. Treatment of DIC, renal failure, myocardial infarction, hepatic insufficiency, and neurologic manifestations is no different in this setting than in catastrophic illnesses of other origins, such as overwhelming sepsis.

Course and prognosis

The course of the acute illness will depend on the extent of involvement of the vital organs and their response to treatment. Many patients will require prolonged stays in intensive care units. Despite this, with ideal care, as many as 95% of all patients will survive the episode, although they may be left with residual damage to one or more of the involved organs. Among those who recover fully, it is important to recognize that the sweat glands are often affected by an episode of heat stroke and may not recover normal function for many weeks, if ever. For this reason, patients who recover from heat stroke should be excluded from heat exposure for at least 4 weeks. Subsequent return should be carefully monitored to determine whether the patient's tolerance for heat has been diminished permanently. Needless to say, the circumstances of exposure must be rectified.

Reproductive effects of heat stress

There is a growing body of literature reporting that routine heat stress is associated with decrements in sperm production. A quantitative study of populations examined during cool seasons and again in the summer has shown drops in the baseline sperm counts of 20% or more during warmer weather.[33] That this has an impact on actual reproductive success is suggested by the seasonal differences in birth rates in temperate climates, with the lowest rates occurring in the spring and the highest in the fall.[34] This effect appears to be of sufficient magnitude to merit consideration in the workup of male infertility. Similarly, confounding by heat exposure must be taken into account in studies of the reproductive impact of other environmental agents (see Chapter 27.2). There is also growing speculation that thermal stress to the developing fetus may be teratogenic in humans. Experimental data in animals suggest a significant potential for retardation of central nervous system development after even brief periods of intense heat exposure early in gestation. It has been hypothesized, but not proved, that working women in the first and early second trimester may be at risk. These data have not been confirmed in well-controlled human studies.[35,36]

PREVENTION OF HEAT STRESS DISORDERS

The prevention of disorders resulting from heat stress involves a combination of environmental and administrative controls. The use of personal protective equipment has no direct protective role for this hazard but is discussed because of its importance as a contributory risk factor that can be modified.

Environmental control

When possible, direct control of temperature, humidity, air velocity, and radiant sources should be used where strenuous, heat-generating activities will occur. In some settings, this can be effectively combined with other engineering tools, e.g., the delivery of large quantities of fresh air to underground miners cools the air and replaces stale air. When temperature itself cannot be controlled, the potential value of manipulating the other variables should not be underestimated, e.g., the use of rapid air circulation and dehumidification or shielding of sources, such as furnaces, in metals refining or processing operations.

Personal protective equipment

It has been already noted that devices used to control other hazards may promote heat stress. Uniforms and protective clothing may be maladaptive in this regard.[2] Conversely, there are few devices to enhance heat removal. The goal, therefore, is to minimize the impact of clothing and gear. When possible, direct exposure of the skin surface to the ambient environment will enhance sweat evaporation and heat removal. The only negative consideration is exposure of the skin to radiant sources such as the sun. When the skin must be covered, the goal is to maximize the air movement through the clothing (pumping action) to support evaporation of further sweat. Impermeable garments, although advantageous for workers exposed to chemical or biologic hazards, block evaporation completely. Newer materials are now being marketed that effectively support breathing of the clothing while preventing permeation of liquids from the outside in.[37] Whether these will prove effective compromises between competing hazards remains to be determined in field studies.

Administrative controls

Given that climatic controls are often unfeasible, especially for outside work, administrative controls must form a preventive program. There are four mainstays: acclimatization, work scheduling, fluid and salt supplementation, and surveillance.

As noted above, the human body undergoes quantitatively large adaptations to heat stress over a period of about 2 weeks with regular exposure. Taking due precautions, workers exposed to uncontrolled heat stress must go through acclimatization, a graded program for 2 weeks before work as usual may commence safely. During this time, the loads must be sufficient to cause some cardiovascular stress, e.g., tachycardia, but not severe enough to induce even the minor disorders described above. Symptoms such as syncope or tetany should flag the need to slow the process and evaluate the adequacy of other administrative controls. Workers who are absent from work for more than 1 week, either on vacation or as a result of illness, need to be reacclimatized before resuming regular work. This is particularly true in the case of illness, which itself may predispose to heat exhaustion or stroke.

Work scheduling is a time-honored way to minimize the risk from heat-induced illness. Depending on the nature of the load, providing rest intervals sufficient to allow removal of any burden that has resulted in the elevation of temperature and to allow an opportunity to replace the salt and water losses is an invaluable control technique. Most cases of major heat disorder have occurred during stresses in which rest was not incorporated into the work schedule.

Replacement of salt and water losses is crucial. Workers must have access to water at all times. Where losses will exceed more than 1 to 2 liters during a work shift, salt must also be provided, either in tablet form or in salt-containing beverages/electrolyte drinks. However, to prevent heat exhaustion and hypernatremia, it is imperative that salt supplements never be given in the absence of free access to salt-free drinking water. Electrolyte drinks are more effective because they are formulated to optimize the provision of energy, water, and essential electrolytes, particularly sodium, and are more palatable than salt tablets.[38,39]

Finally, an active surveillance program of heat-exposed workers is vital. All must be examined before the onset of acclimatization to evaluate their underlying risks for heat-related illness. The decision to allow a worker to proceed should be based on a careful evaluation of data. Table 34.2 lists the conditions that may predispose the worker to the life-threatening effects of heat stress. Although the choice is generally straightforward for individuals with serious conditions, such as cardiovascular disease or complications of diabetes, it is more difficult for the young hypertensive worker receiving medication or the moderately obese worker. In such cases, it may be advisable to proceed under close medical scrutiny or elect a job change; sometimes, a simple change in medical management may lower the risk, such as elimination of diuretics. Pregnant women should probably not participate in jobs that require acclimatization. Non-pregnant women, in general, appear to have a lower risk for developing hyperthermia than do their male counterparts.[34]

Beyond initial screening and modification of medical or work regimens as indicated, continued surveillance is highly advisable. Periodic questionnaires and examinations may provide further clues that existing controls are inadequate or that particular individuals may be more sensitive than average to thermal stresses.

COLD STRESS
Exposure settings

Because the normal physiologic state at comfortable ambient temperatures involves positive heat production with its obligatory removal, only excessive, uncompensated heat losses contribute to cold stress. The most prevalent mechanism is by excess convective transfer of heat from the skin into the air or water. Radiative losses are smaller, and losses caused by evaporation of sweat cease to be a problem because cold itself inhibits sweating. Work activities themselves are protective because they generate heat; sedentary activities favor a net heat loss.

Two aspects of cold stress must be considered: systemic and local. Systemic cold stress occurs when heat loss exceeds heat production (as during outdoor activities in cold climates), refrigeration work (as in food processing), and body immersion (as in diving). Although these exposures have been associated with potentially important clinical sequelae, there is not, in general, much potential for uncontrolled progression to frank hypothermia in workers.

Local exposures to cold, usually involving the extremities, are far more common. These occur frequently in outdoor workers who cannot perform their tasks wearing gloves, such as in the maritime industries, in military activities, and in any setting of systemic cold exposure in which an extremity is unprotected. Because the local effects may be somewhat delayed, prolonged exposures are commonplace. It is important to recognize that local exposures need not be to freezing or subfreezing temperatures to be deleterious to local tissues; prolonged exposure at temperatures as high as 10°C may induce acute and chronic effects.

Physiology

The responses to cold stress can also be divided into systemic and local. When the total heat loss from the body begins to exceed the heat production, cardiovascular, neuroendocrine, and metabolic adaptations occur. The most striking of these is enhanced sympathetic and adrenergic discharge, with a marked increase in skin vascular resistance and a relative shunting of blood centrally. This simultaneously reduces heat losses from the body and protects the internal organs from cooling. The net effect on systemic vascular resistance and cardiac output is variable in the healthy individual. However, in the individual with pre-existing vascular lability, such as essential hypertension, there is evidence of exaggerated pressor responses. Similarly, adrenergic stimulation is believed to enhance platelet aggregation, at least in those with an underlying predisposition. Cold exposure is often accompanied by enhanced spontaneous muscle activity to generate additional heat (shivering). Interestingly, although people chronically exposed to cold appear to be better adapted in that they may comfortably wear fewer clothes and shiver less to a given stimulus, there is not a well-delineated cold adaptation comparable to the acclimatization induced by heat.[40]

The local responses to cold are more complex and clinically important. With the decrease in local temperature, peripheral vascular resistance increases as a result of local and systemic factors. This occurs spasmodically, with cyclic decreases in the skin temperature interspersed with transient increases. Accompanying this response, there is endothelial leakage and stasis of the blood flow, leading to local tissue injury. With severe or prolonged temperature decreases, vascular necrosis and thrombosis occur. Exposures to temperatures below freezing also have a direct effect on non-vascular tissues. Ice crystals form, leading to high intracellular osmolality. This causes direct mechanical trauma on the cells, especially axons and melanocytes, leading to depigmentation and axonopathies that persist long after the soft tissue and skin changes have healed.[41-43]

Classification of disorders resulting from cold stress

SYSTEMIC EFFECTS OF COLD

Hypothermia
Essential hypertension
Thromboembolic disease
Menstrual disorders

LOCAL EFFECTS OF COLD (see Chapter 29.2)

Chilblains
Immersion foot
Frostbite

COLD-PRECIPITATED DISORDERS
(see Chapter 29.2)

Raynaud's phenomenon
Cold urticaria

MAJOR DISORDERS ASSOCIATED WITH COLD STRESS
Hypothermia

Clinical pattern

Hypothermia is defined as core body temperature less than 35°C. Primary hypothermia occurs when normal heat conservation mechanisms cannot overcome low environmental temperature. Secondary hypothermia occurs when heat conservation mechanisms are disturbed by underlying disease. Such states may interfere with hypothalamic temperature regulation, shivering, redistribution of blood, and ability to leave the environment. Hypothermia is most likely to occur in infants (whose large body surface area predisposes them to rapid heat loss) and the elderly (who may have impaired ability to sense decreasing tempera-

ture, to limit heat loss by peripheral vasoconstriction, or to shiver). Drugs that alter the sensorium (e.g., alcohol) or other drugs that act on the central nervous system (e.g., barbiturates, phenothiazines) may inhibit the body's response to cold and thus increase susceptibility to cold. Risk of hypothermia is increased by hypothyroidism, hypopituitarism, hypoadrenalism, diabetes, sepsis, and head injury.[44] Decreased core temperature establishes the diagnosis and severity of hypothermia and determines appropriate treatment.

In mild hypothermia, defined as core temperature ranging from 32°C to 35°C, patients are pale, cool, and have maximally vasoconstricted blood flow to the skin. Patients may shiver uncontrollably, and have varying degrees of mental status change. These patients have tachycardia, tachypnea, and cold diuresis induced by increased cardiac output and, as a result, increased renal perfusion.

In moderate hypothermia, core temperature ranges from 28°C to 32°C. Symptoms are more severe, and may include impaired mental status, muscle rigidity with absent reflexes, and dilated pupils. The shivering reflex is lost, and the blood pressure, heart rate, and respiratory rate decrease. Cardiac arrhythmia is common, and electrocardiography may show the pathognomonic J-point elevation or Osborne wave.[45] At this point, with no ability to generate heat, the patient cools to the ambient temperature and dies if warming is not accomplished.

Severe hypothermia (core temperature less than 28°C) causes the patient to appear dead. Blood pressure is not recordable, respiratory rate is extremely slow, the patient is in a coma, pupils are dilated and fixed, and reflexes are absent. Atrial arrhythmia may be present, and ventricular fibrillation may easily be induced, even by moving the patient slightly. This type of arrhythmia resists pharmacologic or electrical cardioversion without core rewarming; however, magnesium sulfate, quinidine, or bretylium tosylate may be helpful in these cases.[46,47]

Treatment

The goal of initial treatment for hypothermia is prevention of further heat loss. Basic life support should be initiated, ensuring adequate airway and circulation. Cardiopulmonary resuscitation is indicated in patients who have a non-perfusing cardiac arrhythmia. Severe peripheral vasoconstriction in hypothermic patients typically makes pulses difficult to palpate, therefore pulse should be examined for a full minute to help avoid inappropriate chest compression. Oxygen and intravenous fluids should be warmed before being given to a hypothermic patient.[48] Passive rewarming, such as moving the patient to a warm shelter, removing wet clothes, and application of a dry blanket, should be attempted initially in all hypothermic patients and may suffice for mildly hypothermic patients who are otherwise healthy. Active external rewarming techniques can supplement passive rewarming and include application of exogenous heat sources (heating blankets, heating lamps, hot packs). More invasive techniques for core rewarming may include peritoneal dialysis or hemodialysis.[49-51]

Essential hypertension

There has been experimental evidence that the risk for and progression of essential hypertension correlates with vascular reactivity to cold, usually measured by the cold pressor test, in which arterial blood pressure is measured before and after a systemic cold stimulus.[52] Moreover, among people with essential hypertension, slightly elevated blood pressure has been observed during winter months.[53,54]

The question is raised, therefore, whether actual exposure to chronic cold stress may either cause elevated blood pressure or enhance progression in hypertensive patients to more serious levels of blood pressure elevation. At present, it is premature to extend this speculation into clinical decision making, other than to consider a modification of the work environment for those with hypertension.

Thromboembolic disease

Two important lines of evidence raise concern that cold exposure may enhance the risk for thromboembolic disease, particularly coronary artery disease and cerebrovascular accident. First, it has been well established that the risk for these disorders in different regions of the world follows a temperature gradient that other risk factors cannot explain alone. Second, cold exposure has been shown to enhance acutely the levels of factors that induce platelet aggregation, such as thromboglobulin and platelet factor IV, probably as a consequence of adrenergic stimulation.[55] Although these two independent observations are insufficient to identify causality between cold exposure and the risk for major diseases, they suggest that further exploration of these associations is warranted. It may be prudent to exclude subjects with active vascular disease, e.g., poorly controlled angina or congestive heart failure, from chronic cold exposure.

Menstrual disorders

Anecdotal evidence suggests that dysmenorrhea is more prevalent in cold climates and during colder seasons. To date, no other menstrual or other reproductive system effects have been ascribed to cold exposure.

PREVENTION OF DISORDERS CAUSED BY COLD STRESS

In general, climatic control is impossible in situations in which cold stresses occur, e.g., out of doors or in refrigeration work where cold is essential. The keys to control, therefore, are a modification of work to minimize the exposure opportunity, education to recognize early symptoms of local injury, and the use of protective equipment. Medical surveillance plays a minimal role, i.e., it is limited to the examination of workers who undertake cold exposure occupations to identify those few who might be at special risk. Continued monitoring for the ill effects of cold, other than for the purpose of scientific enquiry, is probably not warranted.

Dedication

Ethan Nadel, who co-authored this chapter in the first edition, died before the preparation of this revision, which still bears his stamp.

References

1. Havenith G, Luttikholt VG, Vrijkotte TG. The relative influence of body characteristics on humid heat stress response. Eur J Appl Physiol Occup Physiol 1995; 70:270-9.
2. Bernard TE. Heat stress and protective clothing: an emerging approach from the United States. Ann Occup Hyg 1999; 43:321-7.
3. Crockford GW. Protective clothing and heat stress: introduction. Ann Occup Hyg 1999; 43:287-8.
4. Brief RS, Confer RG. Comparison of heat stress indices. Am Ind Hyg Assoc J 1972; 32:11-16.
5. American Conference of Governmental Industrial Hygienists. Heat stress and strain. Documentation of the threshold limit values for physical agents. Volume 1. Cincinnati: ACGIH; 2001.
6. Malchaire J, Gebhardt H, Piette A. Strategy for evaluation and prevention of risk due to work in thermal environments. Ann Occup Hyg 1999; 43:367-76.
7. Rowell LB. Cardiovascular aspects of human thermoregulation. Circ Res 1983; 52:367-79.
8. Chung NK, Pin CH. Obesity and the occurrence of heat disorders. Mil Med 1996; 161:739-42.
9. Andersen I, Jensen PL, Junker P, et al. The effects of moderate heat stress on patients with ischemic heart disease. Scand J Work Environ Health 1976; 2:256-68.
10. Desruelle AV, Boisvert P, Candas V. Alcohol and its variable effect on human thermoregulatory response to exercise in a warm environment. Eur J Appl Physiol Occup Physiol 1996; 74:572-4.
11. Shirreffs SM, Maughan RJ. Restoration of fluid balance after exercise-induced dehydration: effects of alcohol consumption. J Appl Physiol 1997; 83:1152-8.
12. Dixit SN, Bushara KO, Brooks BR. Epidemic heat stroke in a midwest community: risk factors, neurological complications and sequelae. Wis Med J 1997; 96:39-41.
13. Epstein Y, Albukrek D, Kalmovitc B, et al. Heat intolerance induced by antidepressants. Ann N Y Acad Sci 1997; 813:553-8.
14. Vassallo SU, Delaney KA. Pharmacologic effects on thermoregulation: mechanisms of drug-related heatstroke. J Toxicol Clin Toxicol 1989; 27:199-224.
15. Ellis FP. Heat illness. II. Pathogenesis. Trans R Soc Trop Med Hyg 1976; 70:412-18.
16. Lumlertgul D, Chuaychoo B, Thitiarchakul S, Srimahachota S, Sangchun K, Keoplung M. Heat stroke-induced multiple organ failure. Ren Fail 1992; 14:77-80.
17. Ellis FP. Heat illness. III. Acclimatization. Trans R Soc Trop Med Hyg 1976; 70:419-25.
18. Shvartz E, Shapiro Y, Magazanik A, et al. Heat acclimatization, physical fitness, and responses to exercise in temperate and hot environments. J Appl Physiol 1977; 43:678-83.
19. Wyndham CH, Rogers GG, Senay LC, Mitchell D. Acclimatization in a hot, humid environment: cardiovascular adjustments. J Appl Physiol 1976; 40:779-85.
20. Mitchell D, Senay LC, Wyndham CH. Acclimatization in a hot, humid environment: energy exchange, body temperature, and sweating. J Appl Physiol 1976; 40:768-78.
21. Senay LC, Mitchell D, Wyndham CH. Acclimatization in a hot, humid environment: body fluid adjustments. J Appl Physiol 1976; 40:786-96.
22. Dinman BD, Horvath SM. Heat disorders in industry. A reevaluation of diagnostic criteria. J Occup Med 1984; 26:489-95.
23. Khosla R, Guntupalli KK. Heat-related illnesses. Crit Care Clin 1999; 15:251-63.
24. Scott J. Heat-related illnesses. When are they a true emergency? Postgrad Med 1989; 85:154-6.

25. Lampl C, Yazdi K. Central pontine myelinolysis. Eur Neurol 2002; 47:3-10.

26. Oya S, Tsutsumi K, Ueki K, Kirino T. Reinduction of hyponatremia to treat central pontine myelinolysis. Neurology 2001; 57:1931-2.

27. Lee-Chiong TL Jr, Stitt JT. Heatstroke and other heat-related illnesses. The maladies of summer. Postgrad Med 1995; 98:26-8, 31-3, 36.

28. Tham MK, Cheng J, Fock KM. Heat stroke: a clinical review of 27 cases. Singapore Med J 1989; 30:137-40.

29. Wappler F. Malignant hyperthermia. Eur J Anaesthesiol 2001; 18:632-52.

30. Adnet P, Lestavel P, Krivosic-Horber R. Neuroleptic malignant syndrome. Br J Anaesth 2000; 85:129-35.

31. Kielblock AJ, Van Rensburg JP, Franz RM. Body cooling as a method for reducing hyperthermia: an evaluation of techniques. S Afr Med J 1986; 69:378-80.

32. White JD, Riccobene E, Nucci R, Johnson C, Butterfield AB, Kamath R. Evaporation versus iced gastric lavage treatment of heatstroke: comparative efficacy in a canine model. Crit Care Med 1987; 15:748-50.

33. Levine RJ, Mathew RM, Chenault CB, et al. Differences in the quality of semen in outdoor workers during summer and winter. N Engl J Med 1990; 323:12-16.

34. Kenney WL. A review of comparative responses of men and women to heat stress. Environ Res 1985; 37:1-11.

35. Edwards MJ, Shiota K, Smith MS, Walsh DA, Hyperthermia and birth defects. Reprod Toxicol 1995; 9:411-25.

36. Milunsky A, Ulcickas M, Rothman KJ, et al. Maternal heat exposure and neural tube defects. JAMA 1992; 268:882-5.

37. Burnbarger S. Reducing the hazards of high heat. A new fabric technology is put to the test and comes a winner. Occup Health Saf 2000; 69:44-6, 48, 50.

38. Burke LM, Read RS. Dietary supplements in sports. Sports Med 1993; 15:43-65.

39. Maughan RJ, Goodburn R, Griffin J, et al. Fluid replacement in sport and exercise – a consensus statement. Br J Sports Med 1993; 27:34-5.

40. Wittmers LE Jr. Pathophysiology of cold exposure. Minn Med 2001; 84:30-6.

41. Hamlet MP. Prevention and treatment of cold injury. Int J Circumpolar Health 2000; 59:108-13.

42. Murphy JV, Banwell PE, Roberts AH, McGrouther DA. Frostbite: pathogenesis and treatment. J Trauma 2000; 48:171-8.

43. Reamy BV. Frostbite: review and current concepts. J Am Board Fam Pract 1998; 11:34-40.

44. Hirvonen J. Some aspects on death in the cold and concomitant frostbites. Int J Circumpolar Health 2000; 59:131-6.

45. Cheng D. The EKG of hypothermia. J Emerg Med 2002; 22:87-91.

46. Kanzenbach TL, Dexter WW. Cold injuries. Protecting your patients from the dangers of hypothermia and frostbite. Postgrad Med 1999; 105:72-8.

47. Sallis R, Chassay CM. Recognizing and treating common cold-induced injury in outdoor sports. Med Sci Sports Exerc 1999; 31:1367-73.

48. Giesbrecht GG. Emergency treatment of hypothermia. Emerg Med (Fremantle) 2001; 13:9-16.

49. Owda A, Osama S. Hemodialysis in management of hypothermia. Am J Kidney Dis 2001; 38:E8.

50. Spooner K, Hassani A. Extracorporeal rewarming in a severely hypothermic patient using venovenous haemofiltration in the accident and emergency department. J Accid Emerg Med 2000; 17:422-4.

51. Tveita T. Rewarming from hypothermia. Newer aspects on the pathophysiology of rewarming shock. Int J Circumpolar Health 2000; 59:260-6.

52. Lafleche AB, Pannier BM, Laloux B, Safar ME. Arterial response during cold pressor test in borderline hypertension. Am J Physiol 1998; 275(2 Pt 2):H409-15.

53. Donaldson GC, Robinson D, Allaway SL. An analysis of arterial disease mortality and BUPA health screening data in men, in relation to outdoor temperature. Clin Sci (Lond) 1997; 92:261-8.

54. Winnicki M, Canali C, Accurso V, Dorigatti F, Giovinazzo P, Palatini P. Relation of 24-hour ambulatory blood pressure and short-term blood pressure variability to seasonal changes in environmental temperature in stage I hypertensive subjects. Results of the Harvest Trial. Clin Exp Hypertens 1996; 18:995-1012.

55. Sessler DI. Complications and treatment of mild hypothermia. Anesthesiology 2001; 95:531-43.

Chapter 35
Noise

Derek E Dunn, Peter M Rabinowitz

Noise is one of the most prevalent workplace hazards. Hearing loss caused by noise is also one of the oldest known occupational diseases. Ramazzini identified noise-induced hearing loss in the 1700s at a time when the noise was almost exclusively from the hammers of carpenters, blacksmiths, or other smiths. The general mechanization of industry, farming, and transportation not only has increased the occupational range that exposes workers to noise but also, for the first time, has introduced significant exposures to uninterrupted or continuous noise.

While most research into the adverse effects of noise has focused on damage to the auditory system (see also Chapter 20.2), some studies have also examined the non-auditory effects of noise on the cardiovascular and other organ systems. Noise in settings other than the workplace, such as homes near an airport, is also a rising environmental concern. Because these exposures, however, are not usually as intense as those in the occupational setting, this chapter will primarily focus on the hazardous effects of excessive noise exposure in the workplace.

OCCUPATIONAL NOISE EXPOSURE SETTINGS

Today, the majority of workers exposed to noise levels potentially damaging to their hearing are employed in manufacturing. The Occupational Safety and Health Administration (OSHA) estimates that in the United States alone, more than 8 million manufacturing workers are occupationally exposed to noise greater than 80 dBA (decibels measured using a sound level meter's 'A' weighted scale). These workers do not include the more than 3 million employed in agriculture, mining, construction, transportation, or the Federal government. The number of workers in the American manufacturing sector who have hearing loss from occupational noise is estimated to be more than 1 million; one half of these workers have moderate to severe hearing impairment. One worker in four exposed to 90 dBA of noise during a working lifetime will have hearing loss attributable to occupational noise exposure. Surveys of machinery noise indicate that more than 50% emit noise levels between 90 and 100 decibels (dB), and approximately 50% of the industrial work environments have noise levels between 85 and 95 dB. Fewer than 6% of the machines surveyed by the National Institute for Occupational Safety and Health (NIOSH) produce noise levels below 85 dB.

Despite the prominence of noise in manufacturing, significant numbers of people in other occupations (e.g., construction, agriculture, mining, transportation, and the armed forces) are also exposed to hazardous noise. Data reveal that 50% of construction workers and 57% of carpenters employed for over 20 years have hearing impairment at age 50. By age 50, 90% of coal miners have a hearing loss. Table 35.1 lists some of the occupations for which hazardous noise exists. Table 35.2 lists the average and range of noise levels for selected industries. Table 35.3 identifies some of the common noisy tools.

NON-OCCUPATIONAL EXPOSURES

Outside the workplace, individuals may be exposed to a wide range of noise sources capable of causing damage. Approximately 60 million Americans own firearms[1] and many use them without adequate hearing protection. Other non-occupational sources of noise include chain saws, power tools, amplified music, and recreational vehicles, such as snowmobiles. While community noise sources, such as airport and traffic noise, may not be of sufficient intensity to damage hearing, those noises may increase the risk of non-auditory effects, e.g., sleep disturbances, cardiovascular changes, and psychological changes.

SOUND AND NOISE
Basic properties of sound

The mammalian auditory system is sensitive to sound pressure waves, which are rapid fluctuations in the ambient air pressure. Something must create a disturbance in the ambient air pressure to generate the sound pressure waves. The source of the disturbance is usually a vibrating object or a sudden expansion of gases, such as occurs in an explosion. The basic traits of the sound pressure waves that allow us to distinguish one sound from another are amplitude (loudness), frequency (pitch), and temporal pattern. Amplitude and frequency may vary independently of one another. For example, a pure tone has one frequency (i.e., the number of times per second that the changes in the ambient air pressure occur), but may vary in intensity or loudness.

Definition of noise

Noise (sometimes referred to as unwanted sound) is composed of many pure tone frequencies that interact

Industry group	Employment levels (thousands)	Percent exposed
Fishing and forestry	82	6.1
Mining	82	13.0
Construction	2535	7.9
Manufacture (total)	15,241	23.0
Ordnance	33	42.1
Food	1402	29.7
Tobacco	80	19.2
Textiles	232	25.3
Apparel	918	14.4
Lumber and wood	161	40.4
Furniture	295	26.8
Paper	571	36.8
Printing	1239	12.2
Chemical	996	7.0
Petroleum	195	31.4
Rubber and plastic	534	32.7
Leather	155	12.6
Stone, clay and glass	700	23.1
Primary metals	1347	37.0
Fabricated metals	1350	37.0
Machines, non-electric	1539	18.6
Electrical machines	1501	7.6
Transportation equipment	1224	29.7
Instruments	386	7.1
Miscellaneous	384	21.0
Transportation	3311	5.6
Trade	9283	2.2
Finance	1946	0.4
Services	5803	1.6

Based on data from NIOSH. National Occupational Hazard Survey. Washington, DC: Department of Health, Education, and Welfare, Public Health Service, Center for Disease Control, National Institute for Occupational Safety and Health, DHEW (NIOSH) Publications No. 74-127, May 1974, pp. 177–213; and DHEW (NIOSH) Publications No. 78-114, July 1977.

Table 35.1 Numbers and percentages of workers in the United States exposed to noise levels 85 dBA or greater by industry group and by industry within the manufacturing group

Industry	Average noise level (dB)*	Range of noise (dB)
Food	87	72–95
Textiles	88	82–104
Apparel	78	77–82
Lumber	85	73–105
Paper, printing, publishing	89	70–102
Chemical	95	73–106
Leather	92	73–115
Stone, clay, glass	90	68–112
Metals	95	73–115
Fabricated metal	89	68–108
Machinery	88	80–113
Aircraft	87	78–94

*Note: These levels are for the general work area; noise levels near the machines were higher. Maximum noise levels at the sound source exceeded 110 dB for lumber and chemicals. Source noise levels exceeded 120 dB for metals, machinery, and aircraft.

Table 35.2 Work area noise levels for industry

Tools	Minimum and peak octave band noise levels (75–9600 Hz)
Riveting/chipping	75–125
Saws	70–100
Planers	70–109
Steam and air tools	70–105
Tumblers	77–95
Grinders	70–105
Welding	68–103
Lathes	65–100
Drills/milling	73–95
Furnaces	70–100
Mixers	55–98

Table 35.3 Range of sound pressure for typical tools

referred to as continuous or steady-state noise. If the same noise has significant drops in intensity or ceases, it is classified as interrupted noise. Impact or impulse noise is characterized by a sudden rise in its intensity, followed by a quick decay in intensity. The relative hazard to hearing from exposure to continuous, interrupted, impact, or impulse noise depends on the combination of the intensity, duration, and frequency making up the noise.

The human ear is capable of responding to sound pressures that span an enormous intensity range. In the frequencies near 1000 hertz (Hz) (where hearing is most sensitive), the ratio of the intensity of a painfully loud sound to the intensity of a barely audible sound is 10^{15} to 1. Ratios such as 1,000,000,000,000,000:1 are too cumbersome to handle in routine calculations, but the logarithm of the ratio (e.g., the log of 10^{15} = 15) yields units that are more manageable. The 15 logarithmic units that span the range of human auditory sensitivity are called Bels in honor of Alexander Graham Bell, an early investigator of auditory communication. Because it is necessary to make sound pressure measurements with more precision than is possible using the Bel, the Bel is divided into 10 units called decibels. A decibel is the common unit for measuring sound pressure level (SPL) and reflects the log of the ratio between the measured SPL and a reference SPL. The formula for calculating a decibel level is as follows:

$$dB = 20 \log p1/p0$$

where p1 is the measured SPL, and p0 is the reference SPL. The lowest sound pressure level that can be detected by the average young adult is 0.0002 dynes/cm^2, and this value is used as the reference SPL, p0. Consequently, SPL is a measure of decibels above 0.0002 dynes/cm^2. Table 35.4 shows typical levels of common sounds and noises.

Measurement of noise

Noise is directional and is affected by objects and people in its path. Sound levels vary with distance from the source and are affected by many other factors. Care must be taken to obtain accurate measurements, and numerous noise measurement instruments are available for a range of noise environments and tasks.

The basic instrument used for the measurement of SPL is the sound-level meter. Sound-level meters are made to be held in the hand while readings are taken. Most of these

with one another to yield a sound with a complex mixture of loudness and pitch. A noise with a given frequency composition that is more or less constant in intensity is

Sound level (dB)		
	130	Airplane motor
	120	Pneumatic chipper
		Loud rock music, sandblasting
	110	
	100	Subway train passing
OSHA 8 hr. PEL	90	
OSHA hearing conservation action level	85	Truck passing
	80	
	70	Residential vacuum cleaner
	60	Normal conversation
	50	Car at 50 feet
	40	Quiet office
	30	
	20	Whispers, rustling leaves
	10	
	0	Human hearing threshold

Table 35.4 The approximate measured level in dB of common noises and sounds. Values of the United States Occupational Safety and Health Administration (OSHA) permissible exposure limit (PEL) and action level are noted for comparison

meters are equipped with at least two weighting systems. The A scale is designed to approximate the sensitivity of the human ear, giving less weight to the lower frequencies of the hearing range. The C scale is almost linear in its weighting, counting all frequencies in the range as nearly equal. The A scale is specified by OSHA in its hearing conservation standard for the workplace and is more commonly used for measurements taken to evaluate noise exposure. Measurements made with sound-level meters are reported in dBA or dBC (C-weighted decibels).

For workplace noise evaluations, OSHA specifies that an instrument meeting the accuracy requirements of a type 2 sound-level meter, as specified by the American National Standards Institute (ANSI), must be used in the slow-response mode. The slow-response mode integrates SPL over a longer period than does the fast-response mode. These instruments, even if equipped with a fast response, are not appropriate for measuring impulse or impact noise (brief, loud bursts of noise, such as those created by a drop forge or a stamping machine).

While the overall dose of noise to workers is of concern, the type 2 sound-level meter measures the SPL at a given moment only. Therefore, the noise dosimeter has been developed to integrate SPL over longer periods. Dosimeters are typically worn by workers for an entire shift. The instrument is small and clipped to a belt or placed in a pocket, and the microphone is clipped to the shoulder to measure almost ear-level noise.

The dosimeter provides an approximation of the total noise dose over time, such as during a work shift. In situations where workers do not spend an entire shift in constant noise of the same quality and loudness, OSHA recommends a dosimeter that calculates a percent of allowable dose on an 8-hour time-weighted average (TWA). The underlying assumption regarding noise dose is that the effect of noise on the target organ (ear) is a function of the noise intensity and its duration. Thus, 100% corresponds to 8 hours spent at levels of 90 dBA or 4 hours

spent at 95 dBA; 50% corresponds to 85 dBA for an 8-hour shift and is the action level triggering the OSHA hearing conservation standard. The assumptions incorporated by these conversions are a 5-dBA doubling rate (although sound energy actually doubles every 3 dBA) and the inclusion of all continuous, intermittent, and impulsive sound levels from 80 to 130 dBA. These assumptions, while convenient for regulatory compliance, may not accurately reflect the way sound causes morphological or physiologic changes in the auditory system.

Combined sound-level meters and dosimeters are sold with built-in computers that calculate and store data. Many will store peak exposures, allow the option of selecting a different noise threshold or doubling the rate, calculate the percent dose, indicate the equivalent time-weighted exposure, or have other options, such as printing out a minute-by-minute history of the entire sampling period.

Octave-band analyzers, networks that separately characterize the noise by its component frequency bands, can be added to some sound-level meters, allowing for a more detailed characterization of the noise composition. This capability is most helpful in designing controls for noise because different frequencies are controlled or attenuated most effectively by different approaches or materials.

CLINICAL EFFECTS OF NOISE EXPOSURE
Noise-induced hearing loss (see also Chapter 20.2)

Noise damages the sensory hair cells in the auditory end organ (cochlea). Once significantly damaged, the auditory sensory cells cannot repair themselves nor can medical procedures restore normal function. The sensory hair cells are responsible for initiating the neural impulses that carry information to the brain regarding the sounds in our environment. The human cochlea has one row of inner hair cells and three rows of outer hair cells. The outer rows of hair cells run the length of the cochlea and have sometimes been viewed as the site of sensitivity for very low-intensity sounds near our hearing threshold. The hair cells responding to the higher frequency sounds are located nearer the basal end of the cochlea, and those most sensitive to lower frequency sounds are found toward the apical end of the cochlea.

Some exposures to noise or other ototraumatic agents lack sufficient intensity or duration to result in permanent damage to the auditory system. At these subtraumatic doses, the auditory system exhibits a temporary shift in hearing sensitivity that returns to normal with time away from the hazardous exposure. However, when the ototraumatic exposure results in the destruction of auditory hair cells, the loss of hearing is permanent. After the sensory hair cells that respond to a given frequency are destroyed, we no longer hear the sounds at that frequency.

Hair cell damage from noise usually affects the rows of outer hair cells before damaging the inner hair cells. The hair cells sensitive to high frequencies in the basal turn of the cochlea are more susceptible to noise-induced damage than are hair cells in the apical end of the cochlea. As a consequence of the difference in relative susceptibility of hair cells to trauma from noise exposure, the early stage of noise-induced hearing loss usually is characterized by decreased ability to hear very soft high-frequency sounds.

Noise-induced hearing loss usually occurs gradually, unless there is exposure to extremely intense sound. In the early stages of hearing loss, changes in sensitivity resulting from noise exposure may be detectable only by audiometric testing. Without a hearing test to identify the beginning of a loss in auditory sensitivity, the subtle destruction of the auditory sensory cells progresses with continued exposure to noise until the resulting hearing loss begins to impair the person's ability to communicate or hear necessary sounds.

Hearing loss due to combined exposures to noise and other factors

It is clear that some workplace chemicals are damaging to the auditory system and can cause or aggravate work-related hearing loss. These include chemicals having neurotoxic potential, such as organic solvents and heavy metals. Other suspect factors include heat and hand-arm vibration. The scope of this chapter does not permit an overview of this subject matter. However, references on ototoxic chemicals are included in the Further Reading.

NON-AUDITORY EFFECTS OF NOISE EXPOSURE

Excessive exposure to noise is also thought to be an environmental stressor, independent of the problems of hearing loss. Accordingly, most of the research on the non-auditory effects of noise has focused on physiologic functions that may be influenced by the stress induced by noise exposure. The suspected mechanism for stress is heightened activity of the sympathetic nervous system, resulting in increased levels of 'stress' hormones, such as cortisol and catecholamines. These stress-induced physiologic functions include behavioral, reproductive, sleep, and cardiovascular responses.

Psychological effects of noise

Annoyance, irritability, and performance decrement have been associated with noisy work environments. Annoyance is reported more often in response to higher intensity sound levels and longer exposure times. Irritability increases when the noise is unpredictable and uncontrollable.

Loud noise in the workplace has been associated with increased accidents and lower productivity rates. However, the results of laboratory studies have failed to define clearly the effect of noise on task performance. In fact, some levels of background noise have been shown to improve task performance. Noise may also play a role in exacerbating symptoms related to indoor air quality (see

Chapter 50). Increased rates of non-specific symptoms, such as fatigue among building inhabitants, have been associated with increased background noise levels.[2]

Reproductive effects

The literature concerning the effects of occupational noise exposure on human pregnancy is sparse. Studies in rodents, however, have shown that excessive noise exposure is related to decreased fetal weight and increased litter resorption. These effects occur simultaneously with increases in plasma and uterine catecholamine levels, resulting in vasoconstriction. The reduced blood flow to the uterus can, therefore, cause these adverse reproductive effects. However, experimental studies in large mammals have not demonstrated an effect of noise exposure on the pregnancy outcome.

Clinical studies of noise measurements in utero have shown an average noise attenuation of 10–15 dB at frequencies near 4–5 kilohertz (kHz). Low-frequency sounds (0.125 kHz) have been shown to be enhanced in utero by an average of 3.7 dB. Given the low attenuation, it is plausible that there are direct effects of noise exposure to the fetus.

A cross-sectional Canadian study of auditory damage after perinatal noise exposure investigated the hearing of children aged 4–10 years. Based on maternal noise exposure during pregnancy, a three-fold increased risk was found for high-frequency hearing loss in children whose mothers were exposed to noise of 85–95 dB. There was also a significant increase of hearing loss specifically from low-frequency noise exposure. The study also found an interactive effect with other contributors to hearing loss, including jaundice or incubation at birth. Other factors that may have led to hearing loss after infancy were not controlled for in this study.

However, no clear evidence exists for an effect of noise on most reproductive outcomes. Given the noise levels found in utero, the most plausible adverse effect is auditory damage in children. More studies are needed to confirm this.

Sleep disturbance due to noise

The effect of environmental noise on sleep, while not studied extensively, is a common concern expressed by the public. Some estimates indicate that as much as a third of the urban population rates sleep disturbance as the most annoying effect of noise. Intermittent noise is more likely to decrease the duration of deep sleep while continuous noise may actually increase the percentage of time in deep sleep. Despite these effects on sleep patterns, research has not conclusively shown that sleep disturbance resulting from noise causes chronic health effects.

Cardiovascular effects of noise exposure

As early as the 1970s occupational noise exposure was associated with increased blood pressure, but nearly 30 years later the role of noise exposure on blood pressure and/or hypertension remains unclear.[3] In laboratory animals, brief noise exposure produces an acute elevation of blood pressure and a chronic elevation from long-term noise exposure.[4,5] Experimental studies in humans have also shown short-term increases in diastolic pressure in subjects exposed to noise between 90 and 100 decibels.[6] A possibility exists that long-term increases in blood pressure due to noise could lead to chronically elevated blood pressure. The suspected mechanism is increased activity of the sympathetic nervous system and increased levels of hormones, such as cortisol.[6,7]

Given that exposure to high noise levels is common, any relation between noise and increased blood pressure has potentially large public health significance. Studies suggest an increase in blood pressure of approximately 2 millimeter mercury (mmHg) is due to noise exposure above 85 dBA. It is estimated that a 2 mmHg reduction in diastolic blood pressure would result in a 17% decrease in the prevalence of hypertension, a 6% reduction in the risk of coronary disease, and a 15% reduction in risk of stroke.[8] Although not conclusive, studies have found positive relationships between noise (or hearing loss) and hypertension. The more relevant studies are reviewed briefly below:

Tarter et al. studied 150 white men and 119 black men in the United States who had been exposed to noise at or above 85 dBA for at least 5 years. Hearing impairment and years worked were both significantly related to blood pressure and the prevalence of hypertension among black workers (32%), but not white workers (22%).[6]

Green et al. studied 162 noise-exposed male workers in Israel. Average diastolic blood pressure (DBP) and systolic blood pressure (SBP) were significantly higher among the high-noise exposed versus (vs) the low-noise exposed. No differences were seen for older workers.[9]

Hirai et al. conducted a study of noise and blood pressure among 868 male Japanese workers. Current blood pressure measurements were compared with measurements from 10 years earlier. There were no noise-associated differences in current blood pressure, blood pressure over time, or current hearing impairment and hypertension.[4]

Zhao et al. evaluated 1101 Chinese female textile workers. Current noise level, family history of hypertension, and a high-salt diet were significant predictors of hypertension, while years worked had no effect.[10]

Tomei et al. investigated 75 high-noise exposed and 225 low-noise exposed Italian workers. The high-noise exposed group had significantly increased hypertension (20% vs 8%). Hypertension was also significantly increased in those with hearing loss. The most marked increase in hypertension occurred in those with longer high-noise exposures.

Lang et al. studied 1844 male French workers, of whom 346 were exposed to noise at or above 85 dBA. Mean blood pressure was no higher in the high-noise group. However, it was significantly higher for workers with more than 25 years employment.[11]

Figaro et al. examined 8078 Italian workers exposed above 80 dB and 733 workers exposed below 80 dB.

Significantly higher blood pressures were found in the high-exposed group, especially for those aged 50–60. The high-exposure group had a significantly greater prevalence of hypertension, especially in older workers.[12]

Hessel and Sluis-Cremer studied 2197 South Africa miners for noise and blood pressure over a 30-year period. These authors found no differences in blood pressure related to noise either cross-sectionally or longitudinally.[13]

Kristal-Boneh et al. conducted a cross-sectional study of 3105 Israeli noise-exposed workers. No effect of noise level was found on blood pressure. However, heart rate increased during the workday for those with high-noise exposures, but not for those with low-noise exposures.[14]

Sokas et al. used records to study 2135 men in a variety of companies with high-noise levels in the Middle East. Approximately one-third of these workers had some degree of hearing loss. Hearing loss predicted an increase in resting blood pressure predominantly in the younger-aged group and within certain ethnic groups.[15]

Talbott et al. investigated 329 males in a high-noise exposure plant and 314 males in a low-exposure plant. Cumulative noise exposure was a significant predictor of blood pressure at the high-exposure plant, but not at the low-exposure plant.

Melamed and Bruhis studied 35 industrial workers exposed to noise levels above 85 dBA and measured their urinary cortisol. Cortisol, a stress hormone, usually peaks in the morning and then declines during the day. The workers wearing hearing protection experienced decreasing cortisol levels during the day as expected. Those not wearing hearing protection experienced cortisol levels at the end of the day that were similar to pre-work morning measurements and significantly higher than expected.[7]

The literature suggests an effect of noise on hypertension, but the studies are not conclusive. Two studies found effects only in those with long exposures (presumably older workers), while two found effects predominantly in younger workers. One study found effects only in blacks, but not whites.

Vibroacoustic disease

Recent studies have examined the effects of long-term exposure to large pressure amplitude and low frequency (LPALF) noise (noise ≥ 90 dB TWA, ≤ 500 Hz).[16] Such exposures may occur in certain aviation and aerospace settings. A number of extra-auditory effects have been reported, including neurological and cardiovascular degenerative changes. The number of individuals studied to date remains small, and a clear cause-and-effect relationship remains to be established.

PREVENTION OF NOISE EXPOSURE IN THE WORKPLACE

Attempts by industry to reduce noise exposure in the workplace usually focus on reducing the risk of noise-induced hearing loss. Efforts to prevent occupational noise-induced hearing loss are essential when one considers the numbers of workers exposed to occupational job-related noise and the proportion who suffer hearing loss as a consequence.

Regulations for hearing conservation in the workplace

The Occupational Safety and Health (OSH) Act requires that workers be protected from excessive noise exposure. The original 1971 standard laid the foundation for a control strategy that was updated and detailed in 1983. Although obviously this standard applies only to American workers covered by OSHA, the basic principles apply to all settings in which noise exposure threatens health.

1971 OSHA noise standard

The 1971 OSHA noise standard requires that workers not be exposed to noise in excess of 90 dBA, TWA for 8 hours. Higher dBA levels are permitted (not to exceed 115 dBA), but each increase of 5 dBA reduces the permitted exposure time by 50%, e.g., 95 dBA for 4 hours or 100 dBA for 2 hours. This relationship between noise level and exposure time is referred to as the 5-dB doubling rate. Table 35.5 gives an expanded list of allowable noise exposures. Exposure to impulse or impact noise is limited to a peak pressure of 140 dB. The 1971 standard requires that a hearing conservation program be instituted whenever noise exposures exceed the allowable noise exposure; however, it does not specify the required components of an effective hearing conservation program.

1983 Hearing Conservation Amendment

In 1983, OSHA amended the 1971 noise standard. The 1983 amendment includes details of the components of an effective hearing conservation program and requires that a program be initiated when worker noise exposures exceed 85 dBA, TWA. The OSHA-mandated hearing conservation program includes monitoring noise exposure, periodic hearing testing of noise-exposed workers, applying noise abatement and/or administrative controls, providing hearing protectors to employees, offering an employee education program, and keeping records.

Monitoring

The company is required to identify workers whose noise exposure exceeds the limits defined in the 1971 noise standard. Workers have the right to observe, or have a representative observe, the noise assessment procedures. Assessment of the noise exposure may be accomplished by using a variety of instruments, e.g., basic sound-level meters, noise dosimeters, integrative sound-level meters, and graphic level recorders. It is possible for people with simple devices and limited training in noise measurement to determine whether the occupational noise environment requires that workers be included in a hearing conservation program. However, it is appropriate to consult a professional who has extensive experience in noise measurement to obtain a precise description of the work area noise map and to determine the effectiveness of noise control or the administrative changes on the workers' noise exposures.

Periodic audiometry

Under the standard, hearing testing must be provided annually at no cost to workers exposed to 85 dBA, TWA or more. Specific procedures are mandated for daily, yearly, and biannual audiometer calibration. Audiometry must be provided by a qualified tester (audiologist, physician, or technician) or supervised by an audiologist, physician, or otolaryngologist. Initial audiograms serve as a baseline reference against which subsequent audiograms are compared. An average shift of 10 dB at 2000, 3000, and 4000 Hz is referred to as a standard threshold shift (STS). If STS is determined to have occurred, the worker must be notified in writing of the STS, retrained in hearing protector use, and refitted with hearing protectors.

Noise control

OSHA requires that 'feasible' engineering or administrative controls be implemented to reduce noise exposures that exceed the permissible exposure limits (PELs). Only if such controls do not reduce noise sufficiently can hearing protection be considered. The methods of preventing workers from suffering hearing loss as a result of exposure to loud noise in the workplace are the following, in order of preference.

1. Noise reduction by engineering controls that decrease the noise emitted to the work environment from sources.
2. Administrative or work practice controls that involve limiting the amount of time each worker spends in a noisy environment so that the overall exposure meets the noise standard.
3. Hearing protection wherein the worker wears an earmuff or plug, attenuating the noise at the ear to a permissible level below the standard.

Engineering controls are vastly preferred because they address the elimination of a hazard, making all the complex programs required to track and limit the damage completely unnecessary. Engineering controls reduce the noise in the environment by a change in the process or its machinery, such as damping a vibrating part, replacing noisy metal gears by quieter plastic ones, muffling an air discharge, or myriad other options. When the noise cannot be eliminated or reduced at the source, enclosures

Duration per day (hours)	Sound level dBA slow response
8	90
6	92
4	95
3	97
2	100
1.5	102
1	105
0.5	110
0.25 or less	115

Table 35.5 Permissible noise exposures

of noise-attenuating material can be constructed to reduce the amount of noise escaping into the environment, thus reducing the number of noise-exposed workers to those who must be close to the source. Noise-absorbing surface coatings or baffles can reduce overall noise levels by reducing reverberation. This is generally only effective when used in conjunction with a method of source reduction.

The effectiveness of noise controls is dependent on the source (type) of the noise and its frequency. Noise reduction is often a complex and difficult task, but much has been learned. Effective controls for more processes are constantly being developed.

Administrative controls are not favored because they are based on the unproved assumption that the effects of noise are linear with respect to time and consistent over frequencies, as weighted in decibels on the A scale. Furthermore, careful limitation of the amount of time each worker spends in noisy areas is extremely cumbersome to enforce. Maintenance workers, for example, are sent where they are needed when they are needed. To restrict an electrician from entering a noisy area to fix a needed production machine because he or she has already received his or her noise quota is difficult.

Hearing protectors

Hearing protection is not an optimal solution. Major drawbacks to hearing protectors are that they must be worn to be effective and that they must fit properly. Many people find hearing protectors uncomfortable and annoying and resist wearing them. To encourage acceptance, a variety of types of hearing protectors should be provided, allowing workers to choose those that are most comfortable. Training is necessary to ensure that hearing protectors are worn correctly. Hearing protection is more effective at attenuating higher frequency noise. Some are designed to be particularly effective against certain frequencies. If an individual already has a high frequency hearing loss, a 'flat attenuation' hearing protector may be more appropriate. The two types of common hearing protection are:

1. Earmuffs that cover the external ear. They also must sit firmly against the head, leaving no opening for the noise to pass through.
2. Ear plugs that fit into the external ear canal. Disposable plugs are made of foam or batting. Premolded plastics in all shapes, colors, and sizes are available, as are custom-molded plugs. They must be correctly inserted.

When hearing protection is required by OSHA, it must be sufficient to reduce noise levels to or below the TWA of 85 dB. The acceptability of a given ear plug or earmuff may be determined using the noise reduction rating (NRR) that is provided with every type of hearing protector. The noise dose, as measured by a dosimeter with a C scale, is converted to a TWA in decibels. The NRR is then subtracted from the dose in decibels, and the result must be less than 85 dB to be acceptable. If no C-weighting scale is available and an A-weighting network dosimeter is used, a factor of 7 dB must be subtracted from the NRR before it is subtracted from the exposure. For example, if the 8-hour TWA exposure measured on the A scale is 105 dBA and the NRR is 29, the effective attenuation is 29 dB minus 7 dB = 22 dB. The level of protection is then 105 minus 22 = 83 dB, which is acceptable to OSHA. This 'de-rating' of the NRR is employed because the NRR has been found to correlate poorly with the actual attenuation obtained by workers on the job.

Education and record keeping

All employees mandated to be in the hearing conservation program are required to receive education annually concerning the effects of noise on hearing, information regarding the purpose of audiometric testing, and correct personal hearing protection use.

The standard also requires records to be kept of noise assessments (2 years) and audiometric tests (for the period of employment). These records are to be made available upon request to the employee or his/her representative. The records are to be transferred to, and maintained by, new owners, should the company be sold.

CONCLUSION

Since noise-induced hearing loss is a cumulative process, strategies to prevent occupational hearing loss must also take into account non-occupational noise exposures. Education to inform individuals about hazards of exposures to noise from firearms, amplified music, and recreational machinery, including chain saws and snowmobiles, is important. Individuals should wear hearing protection when unable to avoid such noise sources. For other sources of non-occupational noise, such as aircraft and traffic noise, community noise ordinances may provide guidelines about necessary exposure limits, especially during sleeping hours.

Dedication

Dr Derek Dunn died while this chapter was in press. During his long and productive tenure at NIOSH, he was a major force in advocating research and prevention of noise induced hearing loss and was a mentor and friend to many. His passing, in mid-career, was a major loss to the field.

References

1. Dobie R. Prevention of noise-induced hearing loss. Arch Otolaryngol Head Neck Surg 1995; 121:385–91.
2. Niven RM, Fletcher AM, Pickering CA, et al. Building sickness syndrome in healthy and unhealthy buildings: an epidemiological and environmental assessment with cluster analysis. Occup Environ Med 2000; 57:627–34.
3. Talbott E, Findlay RC, Kuller L, et al. Noise-induced hearing loss: a possible marker for high blood pressure in older noise-exposed populations. J Occup Med 1990; 32:690–7.
4. Hirai A, Takata M, Mikawa M, et al. Prolonged exposure to industrial noise causes hearing loss but not high blood pressure: a study of 2124 factory laborers in Japan. J Hypertension 1999; 9:1069–73.
5. Peterson EA, Augenstein JS, Tanis DC, et al. Noise raises blood pressure without impairing auditory sensitivity. Science 1981; 211:1450–1.
6. Tarter SK, Robins TG. Chronic noise exposure, high frequency hearing loss, and hypertension among automotive assembly workers. J Occup Med 1990; 32:685–9.

7. Melamed S, Bruhis S. The effects of chronic industrial noise exposure on urinary cortisol, fatigue, and irritability. J Occup Med 1996; 38:252–6.

8. Cook N, Cohen J, Hebert P, Taylor J. Implications of small reductions in diastolic blood pressure for primary prevention. Arch Intern Med 1995; 10:701–9.

9. Green M, Schwartz K, Harari G, Najenson T. Industrial noise exposure, ambulatory blood pressure, and heart rate. J Occup Med 1991; 33:879–83.

10. Zhao Y, Zhang S, Selvin S, Spear R. A dose–response relation for noise-induced hypertension. Br J Ind Med 1991; 48:179–84.

11. Lang T, Fouriaud C, Jacquinet-Salord M. Length of occupational noise exposure and blood pressure. Arch Occup Environ Health 1992; 63:369–72.

12. Figaro R, Zoppi A, Vanasia A, Marasi G, Villa G. Occupational noise exposure and blood pressure. J Hypertension 1994; 12:475–9.

13. Hessel P, Sluis-Cremer G. Occupational noise exposure and blood pressure: longitudinal and cross-sectional observations in a group of underground miners. Arch Environ Health 1994; 29:128–34.

14. Kristal-Boneh E, Melamed S, Harari G, Green M. Acute and chronic effects of noise exposure on blood pressure and heart rate among industrial employees: the Cordis study. Arch Environ Health 1995; 50: 298–304.

15. Sokas R, Moussa M, Gomes J, et al. Noise-induced hearing loss, nationality and blood pressure. Am J Ind Med 1995; 28:281–8.

16. Castelo Branco NAA, Rodriguez E. The vibroacoustic disease – an emerging pathology. Aviat Space Environ Med 1999; 70(3 suppl):A1–6.

Further reading

Abel SM. The non-auditory effects of noise and annoyance: an overview of the research. J Otolaryngol 1990; 1(suppl):2–12.

Andren L, Hansson L, Eggerstein R, et al. Circulatory effects of noise. Acta Med Scand 1983; 213:31–5.

Babisch W, Ising H, Gallacher JE, Sweetnam PM, Elwood PC. Traffic noise and cardiovascular risk: the Caerphilly and Speedwell studies, third phase – 10-year follow up. Arch Environ Health 1999; 54:210–6.

Barregard L, Axelsson. Is there an ototraumatic interaction between noise and solvents? Scand Audiol 1984; 13:151–5.

Berger EH, Royster LH, Thomas WG. Presumed noise-induced permanent threshold shift resulting from exposure to an A-weighted Leq of 89 dB. J Acoust Soc Am 1978; 64:192–7.

Clark WW, Bohl CD, Davidson LS, et al. Evaluation of a hearing conservation program at a large industrial company. J Acoust Soc Am 1987; 82(suppl 1):S113(A).

Cohen A. Industrial noise and medical, absence and accident record data on exposed workers. In: Proceedings of the International Congress on "Noise as a Public Health Problem," Dubrovnik, Yugoslavia, 1973; 441–5.

Cohen A. The influence of a company hearing conservation program on extra-auditory problems in workers. J Safety Res 1976; 8:146–62.

Cook RO, Nawrot PS, Hamm CW. Effects of high-frequency noise on prenatal development and maternal plasma and uterine catecholamine concentrations in the CD-1 mouse. Toxicol Appl Pharmacol 1982; 66:338–48.

Dunn DE. Noise damage to cells of the organ of Corti. Semin Hear 1988; 9:267–78.

Dunn DE. Making a commitment to effective hearing conservation. Appl Ind Hyg 1988; 3:F16–18.

Dunn DE, Morata TC. Current opinion: industrial noise and hearing conservation. Otolaryngol Head Neck Surg 1997; 5:330–3.

Earshen JJ. Sound measurement: instrumentation and noise descriptors. In: Berger EH, Ward WD, Morrill JC, et al, eds.

Noise and hearing conservation manual. Akron, OH: American Industrial Hygiene Association, 1986.

Eggertsen R, Svensson A, Magnusson M, et al. Hemodynamic effects of loud noise before and after central sympathetic nervous stimulation. Acta Med Scand 1987; 221:159–64.

Fechter LD. A mechanistic basis for interactions between noise and chemical exposure. Arch Complex Environ Studies 1989; 1:23–8.

Federal Register. 36 Fed. Reg. 10518. Occupational Safety and Health Administration: Occupational noise exposure standard. Chapter XVII, part 1910, subpart G, 1910.95, 1971.

Federal Register. 48 Fed. Reg. 9738-9785. Occupational Safety and Health Administration: Occupational noise exposure: hearing conservation amendment, final rule, 1983.

Fouriaud C, Jacquinert-Salord MC, Degoulet P, et al. Influence of socioprofessional conditions on blood pressure levels and hypertension control. Am J Epidemiol 1984; 120:72–86.

Franks J, Davis R, Kreig E. Analysis of a hearing conservation program data base: factors other than workplace noise. Ear Hear 1989; 10:273–80.

Garcia AM, Carcia A. Occupational noise as a cardiovascular risk factor. Schrift Ver Wass Bod Luft 1993; 88:212–22.

Gamallo A, Alario P, Gonzalezabad G, et al. Acute noise stress, ACTH administration, and blood pressure alteration. Physiol Behav 1992; 51:1201–5.

Hartikainen-Sorri AL, Kirkinen P, Sori M, et al. No effect of experimental noise exposure on human pregnancy. Obstet Gynecol 1991; 77:611–5.

Hartikainen-Sorri AL, Sorri M, Tuimala R, et al. Occupational noise exposure during pregnancy: a case-control study. Int Arch Occup Environ Health 1988; 60:279–83.

Hempstock TI, Hill E. The attenuations of some hearing protectors as used in the workplace. Ann Occup Hyg 1990; 34:453–70.

Johanning E, Wilder DG, Landrigan PJ, et al. Whole body vibration exposure in subway cars and review of adverse health effects. J Occup Med 1991; 33:605–12.

Johnson BL, ed. Prevention of neurotoxic illness in working populations. New York, NY: John Wiley and Sons, 1987;140–61.

Kjjellberg A. Subjective, behavioral, and psychophysiological effects of noise. Scand J Work Environ Health 1990; 16(suppl 1):29–38.

Knipschild P, Meijer H, Salle H. Aircraft noise and birth weight. Int Arch Occup Environ Health 1983; 48:131–6.

Kristensen TS. Cardiovascular diseases and the work environment. Scand J Work Environ Health 1989; 15:165–279.

Kurppa K, Rantala K, Nurminen T, et al. Noise exposure during pregnancy and selected structural malformations in infants. Scand J Work Environ Health 1989; 15:111–6.

Lalande NM, Hetu R, Lambert J. Is occupational noise exposure during pregnancy a risk factor of damage to the auditory system of the fetus? Am J Ind Med 1986; 10:427–35.

Lim DJ, Dunn DE. Anatomic correlates of noise-induced hearing loss. Otolaryngol Clin North Am 1976; 12:493–513.

Melamed S, Harari G, Green MS. Type A behavior, tension, and ambulatory cardiovascular reactivity in workers exposed to noise stress. Psychosom Med 1993; 55:185–92.

Meyer RM, Aldrich TE, Easterly CE. Effects of noise and electromagnetic fields on reproductive outcomes. Environ Health Perspect 1989; 81:193–200.

Morata TC. Study of the effects of simultaneous exposure to noise and carbon disulfide on workers' hearing. Scand Audiol 1989; 18:53–8.

Morata TC, Dunn DE, Kretchmer LW, Lemasters GK, Keith RW. Effects of occupational exposure to organic solvents and noise on hearing. Scand J Work Environ Health 1993; 19:245–54.

Morata TC, Dunn DE, Sieber WK. Occupational exposure to noise and ototoxic organic solvents. Arch Environ Health 1994; 49:359–65.

Morata TC, Franks JR, Dunn DE. Unmet needs in occupational hearing conservation. Lancet 1994; 344(8920):479.

Morata TC, Nylen PR, Johnson A-C, Dunn DE. Auditory and vestibular functions after single or combined exposure to toluene: a review. Arch Toxicol 1995; 69:413–43.

Morata TC, Dunn DE, eds. Occupational hearing loss, occupational medicine. In: State of the art reviews, vol. 10. Philadelphia, PA: Hanley and Belfus, Inc, 1995.

Morata TC, Engle T, Durao A, et al. Hearing loss from combined exposures among petroleum refinery workers. Scand Audiol 1997; 26:141–9.

Morata TC, Fiorini AC, Fischer FM, et al. Toluene-induced hearing loss among rotogravure printing workers. Scand J Work Environ Health 1997; 23:294–303.

Morata TC. An epidemiological study of the effects of exposure to noise and organic solvents on workers' hearing and balance [Dissertation]. Cincinnati, OH: University of Cincinnati, 1990.

Morata TC, Dunn DE, Sieber KW. American workers exposed to noise and potentially ototoxic chemicals: a review. Sitges, Spain: Abstracts of Association, 1989.

National Hearing Conservation Association. Bang bang, you're deaf. Hearing Conservation News 1988; 6(3):1B3.

NIOSH. Criteria for a recommended standard: occupational exposure to noise. Publication No. 73-1101. Cincinnati, OH: U.S. Department of Health, Education, and Welfare, Health Services and Mental Health Administration, National Institute for Occupational Safety and Health, DHEW (NIOSH), 1972

NIOSH. National occupational hazard survey. Publication No. 74-127. Washington, DC: Department of Health, Education and Welfare, Health Services and Mental Health Administration, National Institute for Occupational Safety and Health, DHEW (NIOSH), 1974;177–213.

NIOSH. National occupational hazard survey. Publication No. 78-114. Washington, DC: Department of Health, Education and Welfare, Health Services and Mental Health Administration, National Institute for Occupational Safety and Health, DHEW (NIOSH), 1977.

NIOSH. Proposed national strategies for the prevention of leading work-related diseases and injuries (part 2: noise-induced hearing loss). Cincinnati, OH: US Department of Health and Human Services, Public Health Service, Centers for Disease Control, National Institute for Occupational Safety and Health, DHHS, 1988;51–63.

NIOSH. Criteria for a recommended standard: occupational noise exposure. Publication No. 98-126.Cincinnati, OH: US Department of Health and Human Services, Public Health Service, Centers for Disease Control and Prevention, National Institute for Occupational Safety and Health, DHHS (NIOSH), 1998.

Nurminen T, Kurppa K. Occupational noise exposure and course of pregnancy. Scand J Work Environ Health 1989; 15:117–24.

Occupational Safety and Health Act of 1970. 29 United States Code. Public Law 91-596. 91st Congress, S. 2193. December 29, 1970.

OSHA. Occupational Safety and Health Administration: final regulatory analysis of the hearing conservation amendment. Report No. 723-860/752 1B3. Washington, DC: Government Printing Office, 1981.

Richards DS, Frentzen B, Gerhardt KJ, et al. Sound levels in the human uterus. Obstet Gynecol 1992; 80:186–90.

Royster JD, Royster LH. Hearing conservation programs, practical guidelines for success. Chelsea, MI: Lewis Publishers, 1990; 7–22.

Royster LH, Royster JD. Education and motivation. In: Berger EH, Morrill LH, Royster LH, eds. Noise and hearing conservation manual. Akron, OH: American Industrial Hygiene Association, 1986; 383–416.

Sataloff RT, Sataloff RT J. Occupational hearing loss. New York, NY: Marcel Dekker, 1987; 623–36.

Stewart AP. The comprehensive hearing conservation program. In: Lipscomb DM, ed. Hearing conservation in industry, schools and the military. Boston, MA: Little, Brown, 1988; 203–30.

Talbot E, Gibson L, Burks A, Engberg R, McHugh K. Evidence for a dose–response relationship between occupational noise and blood pressure. Arch Environ Health 1999; 54:71–8.

Talbot E, Hlemkamp J, Matthews K, et al. Occupational noise exposure, noise-induced hearing loss, and the epidemiology of high blood pressure. Am J Epidemiol 1985; 121:501–14.

Tomei F, Fantini S, Tomao E, Baccolo TP, Rosati MV. Hypertension and chronic exposure to noise. Arch Environ Health 2000; 55:319–25.

Tomei F, Tomao E, Papaleo B, Baccolo T, Alfi P. Study of some cardiovascular parameters after chronic exposure to noise. Int J Cardiol 1991; 33:393–400.

Verbeek JHAM, van Dijk FJH, de Vries FF. Non-auditory effects of noise in industry. Int Arch Occup Environ Health 1987; 59:51-54.

Weiss B. Neurotoxic risks in the workplace. Appl Occup Environ Hyg 1990; 5:577–84.

Welch BL, Welch AS. Physiologic effects of noise. New York, NY: Plenum Press, 1970.

Westman JC, Walters JR. Noise and stress: a comprehensive approach. Environ Health Perspect 1981; 41:291–309.

Wu TN, Chiang HC, Huang JT, Chang PY. Comparison of blood pressure in deaf-mute children and children with normal hearing: association between noise and blood pressure. Int Arch Occup Environ Health 1993; 65:119–123.

Wu TN, Ko YC, Chang PY. Study of noise exposure and high blood pressure in shipyard workers. Am J Ind Med 1987; 12:431–8.

Yiming Z, Shuzheng Z, Selvin S, et al. A dose–response relation for noise induced hypertension. Br J Ind Med 1991; 48:179–84.

Ylikowski ME. Self-reported elevated blood pressure in army officers with hearing loss and gunfire noise-exposure. Milit Med 1995; 160:388–90.

Chapter 36
Baromedicine

Louis F James, Gabrielle Morris, David A Youngblood

INTRODUCTION

Continuing technologic advance has led mankind commercially, academically and recreationally into previously prohibited environments. Ambient barometric and hydrostatic pressure changes have a profound influence on physiology and therefore human performance and health. Baromedicine is still emerging as a discrete discipline. It is a conglomerate of related elements of engineering science, hyperbaric medicine, undersea diving medicine, aviation medicine, space medicine, high altitude medicine, and all of their underlying basic sciences. These disciplines share common concerns stemming from the effects on humans and their activities of significant departures from the ambient pressures experienced between sea level and modest elevations. The body of information it contains has grown rapidly in recent years.

While this co-operative effort has been essential, it has produced some unfortunate difficulties, such as a dozen more or less equivalent units of pressure encountered in the literature, a result of parochial traditions in the contributing disciplines. The subject encompasses some important clinical entities and a few less so. Since Paul Bert's seminal work of 1878,[1] no monograph on the subject has been forthcoming, although the body of information is sufficient to warrant it, and human progress continues to advance on an exponential scale as we continue to press the pressure frontier which is so fraught with risk.

HISTORY

This chapter is intended as an overview, and the more serious reader is directed to the sources listed at the end for more exhaustive treatments of specific aspects of baromedicine . Humans have undoubtedly experienced the effects of large barometric pressure variations since they developed sufficient awareness and ventured up mountains and into and under the sea, but scant early reference to problems encountered exists. In the late 16th century, Spanish travelers in the Peruvian Andes first clearly reported the phenomenon of mountain sickness.[2] True appreciation, however, began only with the 17th and 18th century formulations of the basic laws of classical physics, leading to understanding of the atmosphere, and consequently, ambient pressure. The inquisitive mind of Robert Boyle in 1670 observed and reported on a moving bubble in the unblinking eye of a snake he had placed in a vacuum chamber, but did not elaborate on the finding.[3] The development of underwater diving apparatus for salvage and construction, and the caisson for bridge and tunnel building in the 19th century exposed large numbers of individuals to increased ambient pressure, with the emergence of decompression sickness, first known as caisson worker's disease, which became well recognized with high attack rates resulting in frequent disability and death. Simultaneously, hydrogen and hot air balloons were invented and, with the extreme altitudes attained, resulted in profound hypoxia and death, even with the experience of simulated altitude training in a pressure chamber and supplemental oxygen aboard.[1]

Paul Bert, in France, trained in engineering, law and medicine, became interested in pressure physiology, and systematically investigated it. In 1878, after 8 years of intense work, he published his definitive and seminal work, La Pression Barometrique, Recherches de Physiologie Experimentale (Barometric Pressure, Researches in Experimental Physiology)[1], and in so doing became the unquestioned founder of the field of pressure medicine and physiology. The work is a monograph of 1178 richly illustrated pages containing an exhaustive literature review that completely summarized all known and theoretical information on the subject, as well as detailed descriptions of 670 ingenious and meticulously executed original experiments, encompassing the entire pressure spectrum. His discussions were superbly reasoned and his conclusions so sound and comprehensive that they remain scarcely challenged to the present. The work stands today not only as a monumental scientific achievement, but also as an exemplary model of scientific investigation, and there has been no serious attempt to comprehensively update it.

In the intervening century or more since Bert, major strides have been made expanding on his work. Work exposures to depth and decompression rates were adjusted to reduce the incidence of decompression disorders. Workers had long reported amelioration of decompression symptoms upon returning to work under pressure. Although as early as 1854 Pol and Watelle,[4] in France, recommended repressurization as therapy for decompression sickness, there is no record of it being employed until 1889 when Moir constructed and proved the effectiveness of a treatment chamber.[5] By 1909 this had been confirmed and reports by Keays[6,7] had made the use of treatment chambers routine. J. S. Haldane, in 1907, working on commission by the British Royal Navy, published the first theoretically based and successful decompression procedures for diving. His work has formed the basis for all modern refinements.

In the 1920s, aviation medicine was born of necessity and formalized in the 1940s, with the natural extension to space in the following decades. The unanticipated frequency of decompression sickness in aviators flying high-altitude military missions over Europe in the 1940s led eventually to the design of pressurized cabins in commercial and military aviation. The pressure-related discipline of undersea medicine, somewhat younger, was formally established in the 1960s. Although the advantages of 100% oxygen breathing had been known since Bert, it was only then that it was incorporated into decompression sickness treatment protocols, drastically reducing long treatment times and improving outcomes.[8] Today, the new field of hyperbaric medicine, primarily concerned with the therapeutic effects of tissue oxygen tensions elevated by pressure delivery, has been established.[9] Altitude (terrestrial) medicine is also coming of age, with increased understanding of low pressure environments.

Even today, however, with a sophisticated understanding of pathophysiology and stringent safety measures, work protocols and on-site treatment facilities in most industrial and military diving operations, decompression illness regularly occurs, resulting in serious permanent sequelae. In recreational diving, with its large number of exposures and where fitness, training and operational safety standards cannot possibly meet those of industry and the military, such mishaps are far more frequent. The hazards of extreme ambient pressure environments will continue to pose a serious challenge far into the future.

PHYSICS

An appreciation of the direct and indirect effects of pressure on human physiology requires a basic understanding of gas physics, including Boyle's, Dalton's, and Henry's laws. Below is a brief description of these. More in-depth treatments of this topic are available in texts devoted to physics.

Boyle's law

Robert Boyle, physicist and chemist of the late 1600s, described the inverse mathematical relationship between gas pressure and volume. Holding temperature and amount constant, as pressure is increased the volume of a gas decreases. Conversely, as pressure is decreased the volume of a gas increases (Table 36.1). A useful form of Boyle's mathematical formula is: $P_1V_1 = P_2V_2$, where P is pressure and V is volume (subscripts denote beginning and ending values respectively).

Dalton's law of partial pressures

Dalton explained the relationship between total gas pressure and the partial pressures of the individual component gases of the mixture, all of which add up to equal the total pressure. Gases in the atmosphere (air), include nitrogen (N_2), oxygen (O_2), helium (He), hydrogen (H_2), carbon dioxide (CO_2), argon (Ar), carbon monoxide (CO), and other trace gases. The partial pressure of each is denoted by the capital letter 'P' in front of the gas symbol. For example PO_2 is the symbol for the partial pressure of oxygen. Partial pressures change relative to depth or altitude. The percent or fraction of a gas in a mixture is denoted by the capital letter 'F' in front of the gas symbol. For example FO_2 is the symbol for the fraction or percentage of oxygen in the gas mixture. The sum of all fractions or percentages must always equal one, or 100%, respectively. The fraction of a gas does not change with depth or altitude. The partial pressure of a gas (Pg) is equal to the total pressure (P) times the fraction or percentage of the gas (Fg):

$$P \times Fg = Pg.$$

Although various mixes of gases are used in commercial diving, the gas mix most commonly used by divers is air, composed almost entirely of nitrogen ($FN_2 \cong 0.79$ or 79%), and oxygen ($FO_2 \cong 0.21$ or 21%) (Fig. 36.1). At the surface, where the total pressure is 1 atmosphere absolute (1 ATA), the partial pressures of oxygen and nitrogen are calculated as follows (for these examples, the pressure unit ATA is used, however other pressure units may be used):

oxygen: $P \times FO_2 = PO_2$; 1.00 ATA × 0.21 = 0.21 ATA
nitrogen: $P \times FN_2 = PN_2$; 1.00 ATA × 0.79 = 0.79 ATA

At a depth of 33.08 FSW, or 2 ATA, the partial pressures of oxygen and nitrogen are calculated as follows:

oxygen: $P \times FO_2 = PO_2$; 2.00 ATA × 0.21 = 0.42 ATA
nitrogen: $P \times FN_2 = PN_2$; 2.00 ATA × 0.79 = 1.58 ATA

Determination of partial pressures for gases in mixtures other than air is easily accomplished by applying the partial pressure formula (Table 36.2).

ATA (atmospheres absolute)	Depth (FSW/MSW) or altitude (feet/meters)	Relative volume	Relative bubble diameter (%)
0.5	18,000 feet / 5486 meters	2	126%
0.7	10,000 feet / 3048 meters	1.4	112%
1	0	1	100%
2	33.08 FSW / 10.03 MSW	1/2	79%
3	66.16 FSW / 20.26 MSW	1/3	69%
4	99.24 FSW / 30.39 MSW	1/4	63%
5	132.32 FSW / 40.52 MSW	1/5	58%

Table 36.1 Pressure and volume at altitude and depth. FSW, feet of seawater; MSW, meters of seawater.

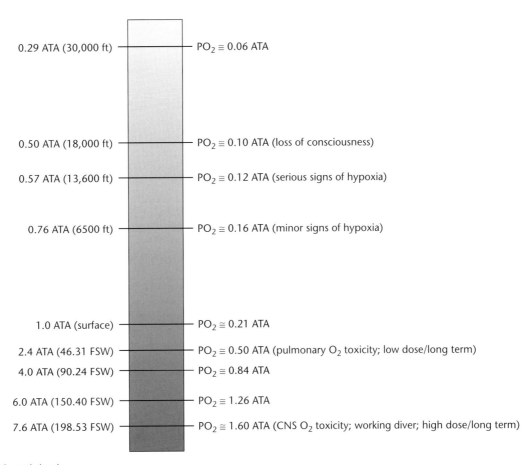

Figure 36.1: PO_2 at altitude and depth

Total pressure ATA (atmospheres absolute)	Depth (FSW/MSW) or altitude (feet/meters)	FO_2 / PO_2 (air)	FN_2 / PN_2 (air)
0.19	40,000 feet / 12,192 m	0.21 / 0.04	0.79 / 0.15
0.3	30,000 feet / 9144 m	0.21 / 0.06	0.79 / 0.24
0.5	18,000 feet / 5486 m	0.21 / 0.11	0.79 / 0.40
0.7	10,000 feet / 3048 m	0.21 / 0.15	0.79 / 0.55
1	0	0.21 / 0.21	0.79 / 0.79
2	33.08 FSW / 10.03 MSW	0.21 / 0.42	0.79 / 1.58
3	66.16 FSW / 20.26 MSW	0.21 / 0.63	0.79 / 2.37
4	99.24 FSW / 30.39 MSW	0.21 / 0.84	0.79 / 3.16
5	132.32 FSW / 40.52 MSW	0.21 / 1.05	0.79 / 3.95

Table 36.2 Partial pressures of oxygen and nitrogen at altitude and depth. FSW, feet of seawater; MSW, meters of seawater.

Henry's law

Henry's law states that the amount of a gas that dissolves in, or is given off from, a liquid is proportional to the partial pressure of that gas at the liquid's surface. This forms the basis of our understanding of decompression theory and decompression sickness. As an air-breathing diver descends, the ambient pressure increases and the PN_2 in the diver's lung increases according to Dalton's law of partial pressures. This creates a N_2 gradient between the diver's lungs and blood. Per Henry's law, under these conditions N_2 dissolves into the blood. From the blood, N_2 dissolves into other body tissues at varying rates depending on the N_2 solubilities of different tissues (called

compartments). If the diver remains at a particular depth and pressure, eventually N_2 equilibrium will be reached, and the diver becomes 'saturated'. There will be no further gain or loss of N_2 as long as the diver remains at 'saturation' (stable depth and pressure). Most dives do not achieve saturation, as this takes many hours.

At the conclusion of the dive, the diver begins to ascend and ambient pressure decreases. As ambient pressure decreases so does the PN_2 in the diver's lungs, thus creating a N_2 gradient, now in the opposite direction. In response to this gradient, N_2 moves out of the diver's blood. A slow ascent, perhaps with periodic stops (called decompression stops), may allow N_2 to pass from the blood into the lungs without significant clinical bubble formation.

However, a more rapid ascent may allow N_2 bubbles to form in the blood or tissues causing a pathologic condition known as decompression sickness (DCS), or 'the bends'. Dive tables were developed in an effort to provide the diver with guidelines regarding depth, dive time, ascent rate, and decompression stops, which generally aid in the prevention of DCS; however, they do not guarantee against its occurrence. The amount of gas that will dissolve in a liquid or tissue (C), is equal to the solubility constant (k) for the particular liquid or tissue, multiplied by the partial pressure of the gas (Pg, measured in ATA) at the liquid's surface:

$$C = k \times Pg$$

All gases behave in this manner. However, metabolized gases such as O_2 generally do not cause DCS.

FITNESS TO DIVE

Human physiology is affected by changes in pressure. Some effects may be pathologic, potentially causing disease, injury, or even death. Additionally, some medical conditions that may be well managed or relative annoyances on dry land may be life threatening in the underwater environment. Evaluation of fitness to dive is therefore an important component of the occupational medicine physician's role in support of patients who are considering or are already engaged in this activity.

Diving is generally a shared activity, and the interdependency between team divers may place all at risk should one become incapacitated. Unlike recreational diving, which is for the most part an optional activity (i.e., does not have to be done if one is not feeling well or if environmental conditions are not favorable), occupational diving usually demands participation at the convenience of the employer or the needs at hand. Additionally, unlike recreational diving, occupational divers may be called upon to dive in relatively unfriendly conditions. This is particularly true for public safety divers who may dive during conditions in which someone has become lost or injured, or has died.

Approach

In general, any condition that may predispose a potential diver to altered or loss of consciousness, interfere with the ability of gas to expand or contract (per Boyle's law), or cause erratic or irresponsible behavior may be disqualifying. Additionally, SCUBA diving, like any potentially strenuous physical activity, requires a level of general physical fitness appropriate for safe participation.

Age

Minimum age
Though children are not likely to present for occupational diving fitness evaluation, the practitioner may be asked to evaluate a child for participation in recreational dive training or academic dive activities (summer camps, school programs, etc). Very little data exist regarding how children are affected by hyperbaric exposure and decompression relative to adults. Potential areas of concern include the relatively high prevalence of asthma in children when compared to adults. Additionally, the effects of 'silent' bubbles on bony epiphyses are unknown. It is not known if children are at an inherently greater or lesser risk for decompression illness, or if they experience decompression illness differently than adults. Behavioral issues exist as well. Addition-ally, the child must possess the capacity to understand and appreciate the risks of diving. It is vital that all divers possess the physical, emotional, and intellectual ability to learn unique skills, become proficient at them, and then judge their appropriate use. Further study is needed in order to address the questions of risk, injury, and long-term sequelae.

Advanced age
By and large, existing diving fitness guidelines focus on medical and physical criteria rather than upper age limit. People who meet the medical and physical criteria are generally deemed fit to dive, regardless of advanced chronological age.

Cardiac

Generally speaking, any organic heart disease may be cause for rejection unless it is considered by a cardiologist to be hemodynamically unimportant. Cardiovascular disqualifiers include ischemic heart disease, all types of cardiomyopathies, hemodynamically significant valvular disease, cyanotic heart disease, and any rhythm disturbance that might cause in-water incapacity.

Murmurs
Innocent murmurs are common in children, and decline in adolescence. The older the subject, the less likely that the murmur is innocent. Therefore, any murmur heard should be presumed 'guilty until proven otherwise'.

Cardiomegaly
Cardiomegaly should be evaluated prior to clearance to dive. The very fit may have large ventricular volumes and therefore 'innocent' cardiomegaly. The physician is cautioned against making this assumption, and an assessment should be done.

Valvular disease
Significant stenosis of valves is generally disqualifying for diving. Patients with valvular stenosis may have difficulty increasing their cardiac output in response to exercise stress. Mitral stenosis is associated with an increased risk for atrial fibrillation and the development of systemic emboli and strokes. Additionally, the physician must consider the likelihood of further deterioration of the valve over time. Immersion causes high central blood volume which, when coupled with mitral stenosis, may lead to increased risk for

pulmonary edema. Aortic stenosis may lead to angina, syncope, and heart failure. Mitral valve prolapse is common and usually not a disqualifying condition, if asymptomatic. The issue of diving after valve replacement is best addressed by a cardiologist. Considerations include post-replacement medications (anticoagulants), associated problems (chamber enlargement, risk for emboli or arrhythmia), chest surgery vs percutaneous pulmonary valvotomy. These cases need to be considered on their own merits.

Hypertension

High blood pressure is associated with multiple conditions including stroke, coronary artery disease, infarcts, angina, aortic aneurysm, peripheral vascular disease, and other end-organ disease. These conditions may cause sudden incapacity, which may be devastating in the underwater environment. The risk for these events increases as hypertension becomes worse or is left uncontrolled. Additionally, some antihypertensive medications such as betablockers may reduce exercise capacity. The National Oceanic and Atmospheric Administration (NOAA) Diving Program 'cut-off' resting blood pressure is 145/90 mmHg on repeated examination.[10]

Ischemic heart disease

Patients with symptomatic ischemic heart disease are predisposed to significant problems including angina, sudden death, and arrhythmias. These may cause sudden incapacity. Any evidence of coronary insufficiency or myocardial ischemia is disqualifying. Grafts do not usually result in complete revascularization and about 20% are occluded after about one year. Risk of reocclusion of a single vessel 'opened' by angioplasty is highest during the first 3 months after the procedure. Therefore after successful surgery, patients may be fit to dive after a period of observation.

Arrhythmias

Arrhythmias other than sinus arrhythmia and ventricular extrasystoles should be evaluated by a cardiologist. Other EKG findings of concern include, but are not limited to, pathological Q waves, ST segment elevation and depression, and should be evaluated as well.

Shunts

There is some evidence, though not conclusive, suggesting an association of intercardiac shunts, such as patent foramen ovale, which may allow bubbles to enter the arterial circulation leading to increased risk for decompression illness, particularly arterial gas embolism (AGE).[11]

Pulmonary

Asthma

Several theoretical concerns exist regarding asthma and diving, including the potential effects of airway obstruction. Traditional concern regards air trapping and the risk of embolization on ascent. There may be some evidence that asthmatics are over-represented in the statistics from the Divers Alert Network (DAN) data on diving fatalities.[12] However, the data do not clearly support that the cause of the deaths was directly asthma related. It may be that asthmatics are at higher risk for decompression illness. Additional study is needed in this area. Also at issue is whether or not an individual with asthma has adequate exercise tolerance to safely participate in strenuous underwater diving activities. In addition to strenuous exercise, underwater diving typically involves breathing cold, dry air, and the potential for water aspiration, which may trigger an asthmatic episode.

Some diving medicine physicians utilize challenge testing in an attempt to simulate some of the stresses to which divers are exposed. At a minimum, divers with a history of asthma should undergo exercise challenge and spirometry. Those who have significant exercise-induced bronchoconstriction are at increased risk for exercise intolerance and therefore should not dive. Methacholine challenge testing is not as helpful in the determination of diving fitness.

Chest x-rays

Until recently chest films were a routine part of the initial diving fitness evaluation, and at regular intervals thereafter, often annually. While initial evaluation may reveal previously undetected pulmonary or cardiac abnormalities, subsequent radiographs have not been shown to be of significant value. More recent guidelines suggest initial radiography, and thereafter chest radiography should not be carried out as routine, but rather at the discretion of the examining diving physician.[13]

ENT

Ears

The diver must be able to equalize middle ear pressures on demand. This is usually accomplished by a gentle Valsalva maneuver, forcing air through the Eustachian tube into the middle ear. This ability can be confirmed during physical exam by direct otoscopic observation of TM movement with Valsalva maneuver. Both TMs should appear healthy and move crisply with this maneuver.

Perforations not completely healed and closed are disqualifying, and should be evaluated by an otolaryngologist. Likewise, an otolaryngologist's opinion should be sought for potential divers who have undergone surgical tympanic membrane repair or other significant otic procedures. Due to the potential for hearing loss due to barotrauma or DCS, audiometric evaluation is necessary for baseline and periodic assessment.

Acute otitis media is a temporary disqualifier. Once resolved with no indication of residual Eustachian tube dysfunction, the diver may resume diving. Chronic otitis media may be disqualifying, and should be evaluated by an otolaryngologist. Acute mild external otitis is not an absolute disqualifier, though treatment is generally more effective if water exposure is curtailed. Treatment regimes include antibiotic eardrops, combination antibiotic-topical steroid drops, and topical acidifying preparations including Domoboro's solution, acetic acid drops, and boric acid powder. Divers with recurrent external otitis should be evaluated further, including culture and appropriate antibiotic treatment. Many occupational divers use preparations including Domoboro's solution or boric acid powder in an effort to prevent external otitis. During periods of daily immersion, boric acid powder may be gently puffed into the external ear canal once a day using an ear syringe.

Nose and sinus

In order to allow for pressure equalization, sinus openings must be patent. Polyps or other blockages may lead to inability to equalize with changing pressure. Temporary blockage may occur during upper respiratory tract infections or allergic rhinitis. These conditions are usually only temporarily disqualifying. Chronic or structural blockage should be evaluated by an otolaryngologist familiar with diving medicine. Chronic or seasonal allergic rhinitis are often treated with the long acting 'non-sedating' antihistamines. With adequate control of symptoms, and the ability to crisply autoinflate the middle ears, these conditions are generally not disqualifying. In contrast, treatment with shorter-acting medications such as some over-the-counter cold remedies may relieve symptoms temporarily, even allowing for adequate autoinflation. However there exists a real risk that the medication effects may 'wear off' at depth, allowing blockage, potentially leading to air trapping on ascent and subsequent barotrauma. Therefore, the use of these medications is generally discouraged.

Oropharynx

The diver must be able to hold a regulator mouthpiece securely with adequate bite and lip seal. Dental appliances (dentures, orthodontic devices, etc) must not interfere with this. Teeth in poor repair may contain spaces that may trap air leading to tooth discomfort and barotrauma with changing air pressure.

Ophthalmology

Visual acuity and correction

The nature of the particular task the diver is expected to perform may dictate visual acuity criteria, but at minimum the diver must be able to read his or her gauges underwater.

Diving after refractory correction procedures

Radial keratotomy (RK) involves the making of small corneal incisions in order to correct refractive deficiency. Theoretically, a decrease in the strength and integrity of the cornea may result with subsequent increased risk of eye injury due to blunt trauma or barotrauma such as severe mask squeeze. However, literature search revealed no reports of this actually occurring. Many diving medicine physicians recommend that a diver wait 3 months after an uncomplicated RK procedure before returning to diving. Lasik procedure involves laser-assisted reshaping of

the cornea and subsequent corneal flap replacement. In order to allow healing and absorption of any bubbles beneath the corneal flap, many diving medicine physicians recommend a 2-week wait after an uncomplicated Lasik procedure before return to diving.[14]

Corrective lenses

Some divers use masks with built-in prescription lenses. Use of contact lenses poses several concerns. In the event of a flooded or lost mask, contact lenses may be lost. Hard contact lenses may cause corneal irritation, believed due to gas bubbles that form between the cornea and the contact lens. There seem to be fewer problems associated with the use of soft contact lenses, and their use is generally accepted.[15]

Other ophthalmologic procedures

Uncomplicated cataract procedures, once fully healed, are generally not considered disqualifying for diving. Healing times vary depending on the cataract procedure, but by 3 months diving is generally permitted.

Diabetes

Insulin-dependent diabetes mellitus (IDDM) is, at this time, generally considered a disqualification for occupational diving. This is due to the potential for a hypoglycemic event and subsequent incapacitation under water. Studies are underway to better understand how diving affects the diver with IDDM, and to better understand the associated risks. It is likely there may be circumstances in which diving, and perhaps occupational diving, with IDDM is not considered disqualifying.[16]

Gastroenterologic

Acute conditions such as gastroenteritis are disqualifying until resolved. Chronic gastroenterologic conditions may or may not be disqualifying, and should be considered on a case by case basis. Divers with ostomies generally have little difficulty as long as intestinal gas is allowed to escape or expand unhindered. Of note, 'continent' ileostomy is a type that does not allow gas to readily escape, and is therefore disqualifying. Divers with hernias that may potentially trap gas should not dive until repaired and healed. Gastroesophageal reflux syndrome may be disqualifying if not well controlled.

STANDARDS AND GUIDELINES

Standards and guidelines involving commercial and scientific diving are too lengthy to list here, but are available through the Occupational Safety and Health Administration (OSHA),[17] US Coast Guard (USCG),[18] National Oceanic and Atmospheric Administration (NOAA),[10] and organizations such as the Association of Diving Contractors (ADC)[19] and the American Association of Underwater Scientists (AAUS).[20]

ALTITUDE: THE HYPOBARIC ENVIRONMENT

Barometric pressure decreases exponentially with increasing elevation such that the sea level value of 760 mmHg is halved to 380 mmHg at 18,000 feet and falls to a mere 0.6 mmHg at 50,000 feet, posing a serious challenge to human physiology. Recent rapid increases in commercial, military and recreational activities at high altitudes have focused increasing attention on them. Human compensatory physiologic mechanisms ordinarily allow for excursions of healthy individuals from sea level to elevations of approximately 8000 feet, at a modest rate, without significant noticeable detrimental effects. Beyond that, problems occur with increasing frequency and severity as the altitude or ascent rate increases. While some of the finer details of the pathogenesis of these problems remain unclear, the basic etiologies can be traced directly to the physical reduction in ambient pressure encountered on ascent and to its rate.

Foremost among the effects of reduced atmospheric pressure is a reduction of available oxygen in the inspired air, leading to tissue hypoxia, with its myriad implications and consequences. The direct effect of reduced pressure per se contributes to the risks as well. The sudden or rapid reduction of ambient pressure in the aviation and space operational environments may produce gas embolic phenomena and local mechanical tissue damage by the evolution of free bubbles from supersaturated dissolved gasses or by their introduction into the circulation from the rupture of overpressured pulmonary alveoli. Prolonged travel and activity at high terrestrial altitude results in the risk of developing a variety of subacute or chronic hypoxia-related conditions, some of which have proven debilitating and fatal. Ascending to altitude immediately following hyperbaric exposure, such as in underwater diving, is frequently associated with evolved gas disorders. The difference in the temporal characteristics of terrestrial and aviation activities results in different clinical pictures. The field of altitude medicine contains a vast body of information.

High-altitude illness (HAI)

The more serious reader's attention is directed to excellent exhaustive and scholarly treatments of this subject by Hackett[21] and Hutgren,[22] and especially to Deitz's internet website.[23] The mountaineering axiom, 'It is OK to get altitude illness. It is not OK to die from it'[23] attests not only to the intrepid spirit of these stalwart adventurers, but also to the general prevalence and wide range of severity encountered. The pathophysiology of all its variations is founded in subacute and chronic tissue hypoxia, with varying individual sensitivities of organ systems. The prominent feature is a cascade of events ending in intractable edema. The mechanisms are primarily normal compensatory responses that perform well enough at low altitudes and initially at higher ones, but over time eventually go awry and produce an intolerable physiologic state.

Vascular chemoreceptors mediate hyperventilation and increased cardiac output leading to hypocarbia with uncompensated alkalosis, resulting in increasing vascular and pulmonary alveolar permeability, extravasation, edema and pulmonary hypertension. The most sensitive organs are the lung and the brain.

A marked degree of individual susceptibility exists which approximates a normal Gaussian distribution and is consistent over time, making previous experience the only reliable predictor of future risk. A significant degree of acclimatization can occur in travelers from low altitudes, but it never matches the physiologic performance of indigenous populations, which is presumably due to genetic and/or perinatal adaptation. Three, more or less discrete, clinical pictures are most commonly seen, with differing implications. A handful of essentially benign conditions such as isolated peripheral edema, particularly in women, have been reported and the finer details of this constellation of disorders are still being clarified.

Acute mountain sickness (AMS)

This syndrome is characterized by malaise, fatigue, anorexia, dyspnea, chest wall ache, headache, nausea, vertigo, memory and sensory disturbances, disturbed sleep resulting from dreams and periodic (Cheyne-Stokes) breathing, and occurring usually within 24 hours of arrival at altitude. Some of these symptoms are present in virtually all high-altitude travelers, often without noticeable impairment but debilitating and incapacitating in some, increasingly with altitude and rate of ascent, and leading to attack rates of 70–80% and more. Findings include hyperventilation from increased tidal volume rather than tachypnea, chest rales, tachycardia and arrhythmia, peripheral edema, vomiting, pallor, cyanosis, retinal hemorrhages, ataxia and incoordination, and mental dullness. Some spontaneous improvement may be noted with time but progressive worsening may indicate the onset of one of the next two syndromes.

High-altitude pulmonary edema (HAPE)

To paraphrase the words of C. Gresham Bayne, the lung is the stupidest organ in the body since it knows only one way to react to insult and that is to fill with fluid.[24] Such is the case with persistent hypoxemic insult. The only practical difference between HAPE and any other pulmonary edema is etiology. Increased alveolar membrane permeability and pulmonary hypertension result in extravasation and accumulation of fluid in the alveoli, producing impaired gas exchange and deeper hypoxemia. The clinical picture is familiar and consists of fatigue, weakness, rales, dyspnea, tachypnea, tachycardia, cough, frothy sputum (sometimes blood-tinged), cyanosis, incapacitation, stupor, coma, and death. Systems to quantify severity have been developed, but respiratory rates over 30 and approaching 40 are ominous. Management is directed at the cause. This condition must be taken seriously since fatality rates can reach 12% and more, depending on circumstances.

High-altitude cerebral edema (HACE)

The central nervous system manifestations of severe HAI are often encountered without significant pulmonary features, indicating a variation in individual tissue sensitivity to hypoxemia. Edema of the cerebral tissues is the primary contributing factor in HACE, although in some instances simple anoxia may be responsible, and the term high-altitude encephalopathy (HAE) has been considered.

The onset of HACE can be insidious, beginning with mild headache and cognitive, affective, sensory, and motor disturbances with a variety of findings. HACE can progress at a variable rate to frank ataxia, paresis, confusion, dementia, coma and death. Papilledema and elevated cerebrospinal fluid pressures are common but not universal findings, and autopsies have demonstrated cerebral edema, often with hemorrhage. Prompt treatment of mild to moderate cases ordinarily results in eventual full recovery, but delayed treatment or severe cases carry a risk of residual neurologic deficit. The true nature of HACE is still being debated since it is much less frequently encountered than HAPE. Prudence dictates a high index of suspicion for and rapid response to this disorder.

Management of HAI

Prevention and treatment of HAI employ behavioral, pharmacological and pressure measures. Acclimatization by controlling ascent rates markedly reduces the incidence and severity of AMS, but is essentially ineffective in reducing the risk and morbidity of HAPE and HACE, once these complications have occurred. Slower ascent rates are more effective, but operational considerations may press for more rapid ones. Recommendations vary, but 1000–1500 feet per day seems to be a standard with decreasing rates at increasing altitudes. Day-long periods of rest are essential during acclimatization, and absolute bed rest is essential in the treatment of HAI, since physical exertion may drastically lower arterial oxygen tensions and exacerbate the problem. Routine use of oxygen during acclimatization and ascent effectively reduces the risk of AMS, but has little effect on the risk of developing HAPE or HACE. It is, however, essential in the treatment of all three. Oxygen should be applied at high flow rates or, better still, with a demand valve and a tightly sealing oronasal mask when used therapeutically. This equipment is cumbersome to transport, which somewhat limits its usefulness.

The traditional sulfonamide carbonic anhydrase inhibiting agent acetazolamide (Diamox) and, more recently, the corticosteroid dexamethasone (Decadron) have been consistently shown to be useful prophylactically and therapeutically for HAI, although adequate controlled studies are still lacking.[25] Both clearly reduce the risk of AMS and ameliorate the symptoms. Acetazolamide mitigates hypocarbia and alkalosis. Adverse effects are mild and tolerable, but its use is sharply limited to a week or less due to rapidly developing tachyphylaxis. Recommended regimens vary from 250 mg to 750 mg daily in divided doses. Dexamethasone ameliorates cerebral edema. At doses of 8–16 mg daily it seems equally effective, with an adverse effect of depression on abrupt secession, which may be successfully averted by tapering.

While no clear benefit of either drug has been demonstrated in treating HAPE or HACE, their use is generally recommended on the grounds that it will surely help some individuals, and is not likely to harm. Numerous trials of diuretics, e.g., furosemide, to combat edema and calcium channel blocking agents, e.g., nifedipine, to moderate cardiac output have failed to demonstrate effectiveness. The sine qua non for the successful treatment of HAI is repressurization. Immediate and rapid evacuation to lower altitude is mandatory but often logistically impossible, particularly with an uncooperative or moribund patient in remote irregular terrain, in potentially adverse weather conditions.

The recent introduction of reliable, simple and effective but sturdy lightweight and portable hyperbaric chambers has undoubtedly already proved lifesaving. Widespread use could conceivably all but eliminate fatalities from HAPE and HACE, were it not for the historical tendency of people to use such technology to extend the limits of the operational envelope, thereby maintaining risk levels. These devices permit on site repressurization with dramatic resolution of even severe symptoms, which enables or greatly facilitates the required eventual evacuation. Treatment times are reported as 2–4 hours for HAPE and 4–6 hours for HACE.[23] The pressure attainable within these chambers is limited by pressure relief valves dependent on the differential across the chamber wall, and is therefore dependent on ambient pressure at the altitude of use.

Altitude decompression illness and acute hypoxia

The operational characteristics of space and aerial flight present a milieu of more rapid and extreme pressure changes than terrestrial altitude activities, which leads to a different set of clinical syndromes. The effect of pressure in this altitude environment has, for many decades, been amply addressed, along with many other important factors, in the discipline of aerospace medicine. Excellent discussions are readily available in standard writings in this field.[26–29]

Decompression illness

This useful term includes decompression sickness (DCS) and air/gas embolism (AGE). Except for primary etiology, their pathophysiology is much the same, with clinical pictures often indistinguishable, except at times on the basis of history, and their management is virtually identical. More detailed treatment of the subject is found in this chapter under depth medicine.[30-32] DCS results from free gas evolved from tissues that become supersaturated, primarily with the relatively inert gas nitrogen on ascent to altitude. Bubbles can occur in the circulation or tissues. Most aviation DCS occurs in military and space activities, where exposures are more rigorous than in commercial aviation, but the popularity of diving, with air travel soon after, has produced cases.

Pain-only DCS (Type I) is most frequent, and is characterized by moderate to severe deep aching pain in the joints and bones, primarily of the appendicular skeleton – the shoulders and knees being common sites. It is presumably produced by local tissue bubbles or embolism from the circulation.

Central nervous system DCS (Type II) is less common but more serious. Spinal involvement predominates, as demonstrated by paresthesia, anesthesia, paresis and paralysis. Brain symptoms are much less common and can take a wide variety of forms including headache, vertigo, ataxia and behavioral changes. Bubbles have been demonstrated in animal and human CNS tissue and circulation. Pulmonary DCS (chokes) accounts for perhaps 10% of aviation DCS cases. It manifests as substernal distress, dyspnea, cough and apprehension. The mechanism is thought to be an overwhelming of the pulmonary circulation by bubbles, leading, again, to pulmonary edema. Other factors, such as hypoxic alveolar gas, probably account for the difference in occurrence rates seen in aviation and diving.

Arterial gas embolism (AGE) is the term used to describe an embolism of gas introduced directly into the circulation from ruptured alveoli. This can be caused by the barotrauma resulting from reduced ambient pressure over trapped gas; risk factors include underlying pulmonary pathology (e.g., asthma and obstructive lung disease), and breathing patterns coupled with rapid ascent or pressure loss. Manifestations are often cerebral and devastating, such as collapse, coma and death, but are also frequently milder, simulating those of Type II DCS such that clinical distinction is sometimes not possible. Skin manifestations of DCI such as rash and subcutaneous emphysema are usually of little significance except to raise the suspicion of more serious accompanying conditions.

Management of DCI

Prevention is accomplished by a variety of effective procedural and mechanical means. The axiom 'Anything will eventually fail, whether man or machine', however, prevails and DCI is an ongoing problem. Breathing 100% oxygen for a period of time prior to exposure removes some dissolved nitrogen from the body and reduces the risk of developing symptoms. Oxygen delivery systems that variably meter percentages and even supply positive pressure depending on altitude are in use and are effective, as are mechanically pressured vessels such as cabins and space suits, all of which provide adequate alveolar partial pressures of oxygen within operational limits. The mainstay of treatment consists of 100% inspired oxygen delivered by mask and, in more severe cases, in a pressurized vessel. Treatment protocols used by the United States Air Force are representative.[30] Pain that resolves spontaneously on return to ground level is treated minimally, while the more severe and persistent symptoms require modified United States Navy chamber Tables 5 and 6, involving about 2.25 hours and 5 hours respectively in a hyperbaric chamber.

Acute hypoxia

The brain and heart are the most critically sensitive organs to sudden oxygen deprivation. Complete exclusion of oxygen from inspired gas at sea level leads to loss of consciousness in minutes and cessation of cardiac activity shortly after, as arterial and tissue oxygen tensions drop precipitously, and death is not far behind. Moreover, exposure to reduced ambient pressure at altitude results in the rapid exit of tissue oxygen through the lungs, accelerating tissue hypoxia markedly. Breathing ambient air suddenly at an atmospheric pressure of 25,000 feet, results in a time of useful consciousness that varies between 3 and 5 minutes, and at 40,000 feet is measured in short seconds. Most commercial flights operate between 30,000 and 40,000 feet and manned military and research operations extend far higher.

Barotrauma

Gas trapped in body cavities, such as dental defects, the middle ear and sinuses, by Eustachian dysfunction or sinusitis, often results in pain, sometimes with transudation, on descent. Except for discomfort, these conditions are seldom of consequence. Sympathomimetic amine decongestants, topically or systemically, are useful in prevention and treatment.

DEPTH MEDICINE
Barotrauma

The undersea and hyperbaric environments are harsh in comparison to others; a mere 33-foot descent beneath the sea is a greater pressure change than 30,000 feet of altitude. Because of these rapid pressure changes, barotrauma becomes the most common occupational hazard of the hyperbaric environment. Barotrauma can occur on ascent or descent where gas-containing cavities fail to equalize with ambient pressure. It ranges from the mild skin 'squeeze' of a dry suit to the catastrophic bursting of a lung.

Ear barotrauma may be confined to the external ear canal if wax, earplugs, or a hood blocks the external meatus. It is usually mild and easily prevented. Middle ear barotrauma of descent is much more common. It is caused by the failure to equalize the middle ear cavity through the Eustachian tube, and if descent continues without equalization, pain becomes intense until relieved by rupture of the eardrum. Unless a dry diving helmet is worn the ruptured eardrum can flood the middle ear with water, causing sudden vertigo.

Vertigo sometimes occurs during descent, when Eustachian tube function is delayed in one ear, but vertigo is more common with middle ear barotrauma of ascent as the unequal expansion of gas within the middle ear stimulates the vestibular end-organ of the inner ear. A 'blocked' ear during ascent can dangerously impede a return to the surface. Occasionally a facial nerve may be affected, causing unilateral facial weakness. It is important to distinguish this condition from a potentially serious case of decompression sickness. Inner ear barotraumas may be a serious consequence of any of the other types of otic barotrauma just described. Since the inner ear is not accessible to viewing with an otoscope, the symptoms are the key to a presumptive diagnosis: tinnitus, ataxia, vomiting, and vertigo are all associated with inner ear barotraumas, and the diagnosis is confirmed by serial audiometry and electronystagmography.

Inner ear barotraumas may be due to a fistula of the round window with leakage of perilymph from the inner ear into the middle ear, or due to hemorrhage; hence it is important to immediately take the following precautions.

1. Avoid straining, nose blowing, Valsalva maneuver, or any physical exertion that could increase cerebrospinal fluid pressure; avoid diving or flying.
2. Strict bed rest with the head elevated for several days. Diazepam will help control vertigo.
3. Monitor otological changes: if hearing does not improve in 24 hours, if it deteriorates, or incapacitating vertigo is present, consider operative intervention with middle ear exploration and grafting the round and oval windows.

Sinus barotrauma is most often over the frontal sinus during descent, but can occur during ascent, particularly after long dives breathing a dry compressed gas, which causes drying of the sinus mucosa, or if sinus polyps are present. In rare instances, rupture of the sinuses can cause pneumocephalus. The trigeminal nerve may also be affected by sinus barotraumas and cause numbness in the face and upper lip, as well as pain in the upper teeth. Again, it is important to recognize this complex as being associated with sinus barotraumas and not decompression sickness.

Dental barotraumas may be the result of carious teeth or gas spaces in deteriorating fillings. A particularly common form of dental barotraumas of ascent occurs in saturation diving when helium slowly diffuses beneath fillings during weeks at depth then expands during the relatively rapid decompression, causing pain as the saturation complex nears the surface and oftentimes 'popping' the filling out in the process.

'Squeeze' is the common term for the barotrauma caused by relatively rigid appurtenances in contact with a diver, such as masks, suits, or 'hard hat' helmets. Problems usually occur in relatively shallow depths since that is where the greatest changes in relative volume occurs; the most common cause is an uncontrolled descent such as falling off an underwater stage slung under a ship for maintenance work by a diver, but simply leaping over the side without an attentive tender also occurs. At depth, the problem is often due to a failure of the non-return valve. The consequences can be catastrophic.

Pulmonary barotrauma

Pulmonary barotrauma of ascent or 'burst lung' is life threatening. It is more common in sport divers than commercial divers, but it can occur anywhere that free ascent occurs, including breath-hold divers and swimmers who descend to a relatively shallow depth and 'share' a breath of air from a friend's regulator; or in aviators training in underwater escape devices, if they breathe from an emergency gas supply and fail to exhale during ascent. Survivors trapped in submerged automobiles or boats are at risk as they breathe in a bubble of trapped – and compressed – air and may not know to exhale during an escape ascent.

Pulmonary barotraumas may present as pulmonary tissue damage, pneumothorax, mediastinal emphysema, or cerebral arterial gas embolism – separately or in any combination. Mediastinal emphysema may be deceptively mild in its presentation with voice changes, retrosternal discomfort, dysphagia, and subcutaneous emphysema of the neck and supraclavicular area. Older texts often dismissed mediastinal emphysema as trivial and requiring nothing more than breathing 100% oxygen for a few hours. This author strongly disagrees with this dismissal, since the same pathophysiology is present as cerebral gas embolism. In the field, we take the stance that mediastinal emphysema may herald much more serious involvement and deserves aggressive treatment. Since this often means recompression, be wary of the presence of a pneumothorax, since it may become a tension pneumothorax on ascent. Be prepared to relieve the tension pneumothorax with a suitable needle/catheter attached to a Heimlich valve.

Cerebral arterial gas embolism is the most ominous complication of pulmonary barotrauma, as gas from the ruptured lung enters the pulmonary veins and the systemic circulation with a predilection for the cerebral and coronary vessels, with devastating effects. These patients may show transient improvement, but it is unlikely to be sustained. Do not be lulled into any delay in seeking definitive treatment.

Treatment of pulmonary barotraumas should be prompt and predicted upon a worst-case presentation, i.e., the presence of cerebral arterial gas embolism despite more benign presentations. Since many of these cases will be divers with an unknown amount of inert gas in their tissues, deep recompressions should be avoided. For example, a compression chamber application of 165 FSW could constitute an unrecognized repetitive dive and complicate matters by causing decompression sickness during 'ascent' to the oxygen breathing depth of 60 FSW. A USN Table 6[33] is an excellent compromise under these circumstances. It is important to treat promptly based upon signs, symptoms and suspicion; one must be prepared to provide circulatory and respiratory support in the recompression chamber. Diagnostic studies may be performed later to confirm diagnosis.

Pulmonary barotrauma of descent, 'lung squeeze', is uncommon but can occur in breath-hold diving, failure of a non-return valve in surface supplied diving, or simply descending at a rapid rate with an inadequate gas supply or volume. Recompression is not warranted; 100% oxygen should be provided by mask en route to a definitive care facility.

Inert gas narcosis

Inert gas narcosis is a clinical syndrome caused by increased partial pressure of inert gas, and is characterized by impaired mental status, which for some resembles alcohol intoxication. One of the most memorable descriptions of inert gas narcosis is Jacques Cousteau's accounting of 'rapture of the deep', in which he described his own experiences with nitrogen narcosis (the form of inert gas narcosis experienced by divers breathing air). Depth of onset varies with the individual. For many, narcotic effects become apparent at about 100 FSW, and impairment increases with depth. Signs and symptoms include loss of judgment and skill, a false feeling of wellbeing, lack of concern for job or safety, inappropriate laughter, euphoria, and inability to correctly recall events during narcosis.[34] Severe narcosis may result in bizarre behavior, hallucinations, or loss of consciousness. Treatment consists of controlled ascent to a shallower depth, sometimes only a few feet, where the effects rapidly reverse. Commercial divers who must maintain greater depths may avoid or minimize inert gas narcosis by breathing gas mixtures containing helium, which does not tend to cause narcosis, in the place of nitrogen.

CNS oxygen toxicity

CNS oxygen toxicity can occur in divers at depths where the PO_2 equals about 1.6 ATA, or about 250 FSW for the diver breathing air. Susceptibility is largely dependent on activity, and people at rest can usually tolerate a PO_2 of about 2.0 ATA without experiencing symptoms of CNS oxygen toxicity.[33,34] Time at depth is also an important factor (roughly 5–50 minutes) but there is much variation. The acronym VENTID may help in remembering the associated signs and symptoms: Visual disturbances including tunnel vision; Ear ringing; Nausea; Tingling, twitching or muscle spasms, especially face and lips; Irritability, restlessness, euphoria, anxiety; Dizziness, dyspnea. These signs and symptoms must not be ignored, as they may be closely followed by convulsion, which, while not life threatening in and of itself, but may result in drowning. Convulsion may also occur without warning.

Decompression sickness

Decompression sickness is the presence of gas bubbles in blood or tissues following their release from solution. In the purest sense, the mere presence of these bubbles constitutes disease even if they are subclinical and asymptomatic, inasmuch as their presence is abnormal and may result in impairment to the microcirculation. As these bubbles grow, they may distort and damage tissue directly.

Attempts at classification are confusing and imprecise: their utility is limited to the selection of treatment tables by laymen and the generation of statistics retrospectively. Type I describes 'simple' or 'pain only' decompression sickness, and Type II or 'serious' decompression sickness, which includes symptoms other than pain or skin involvement involving neurological, cardiovascular, respiratory, or gastrointestinal symptoms. Since so-called 'Type I DCS' often evolves to Type II – or may merely reflect an inadequate examination; a more useful classification is to simply describe the organs affected.

To add further confusion to the classification issue we now have Type III DCS, based on the serious decompression sickness which evolves when gaseous microemboli from pulmonary barotraumas 'seed' the circulation in the presence of an inert gas load from a dive, often with a catastrophic outcome.

The presence of signs or symptoms within 6 hours following a dive should be presumed to be decompression sickness until proven otherwise. Never 'rule out' decompression sickness based on reports that the dive was within the no-decompression limits or that an appropriate table was followed. A subclinical or 'silent' pulmonary microembolism can seed the circulation with microemboli, which will grow in the presence of even modest amounts of tissue supersaturation, sometimes with disastrous consequences.

Presentations of DCS

The most overlooked presentations are fatigue and personality changes. The latter are best determined by questioning friends or family members. Musculoskeletal symptoms are common, often poorly localized, progressing to a dull ache but waxing and waning in intensity. Neurological presentations are varied and may be focal or diffuse; many are thought to be the result of arterialization of venous gas emboli as pulmonary artery pressures increase and right-to-left shunts occur, particularly if a patent foramen ovale is present. Neuropsychologic testing and SPECT scanning may identify cognitive impairment in the aftermath of acute treatment. Low-pressure hyperbaric oxygen therapy may be useful in these brain-injured divers and therapeutic response can be tracked by SPECT scanning. Spinal cord damage, occurring most often in the white matter involving the mid-thoracic, upper lumbar, and lower cervical levels, has also responded to serial low-pressure hyperbaric therapy.

Cerebellar inner ear lesions may be difficult to differentiate acutely if they present as 'staggers' but the vertigo of inner ear DCS is more commonly associated with deep mixed-gas dives. Violent vertigo with nystagmus is sudden in onset, usually while still under pressure in a diving bell or chamber, and is often associated with a shift in the composition of breathing gases. Prompt recompression and oxygen-rich treatment gas can avoid permanent disability, but care must be taken to differentiate inner ear DCS from inner ear barotraumas since rapid compression of the latter could exacerbate the injury. Diazepam is useful in controlling the vertigo and vomiting in cases of inner ear DCS or barotraumas.

Pulmonary DCS, 'the chokes', is an ominous presentation with cough and pain on deep inspiration. A classic finding, little used among today's health-conscious divers, is 'Behnke's sign' – a severe cough triggered by inhaling cigarette smoke. It is important to note that 'the chokes' represents a bubble overload of the pulmonary circulation, since the asymptomatic trapping of bubbles in the pulmonary circulation probably occurs on most non-saturation dives.

Decompression sickness is no longer common among commercial divers with well-tested decompression tables and recompression chambers readily available. Catastrophic cases do occur with equipment failure or 'blow up' (rapid ascent), and the incidence can approach epidemic level among indigenous diver-fisherman in remote areas of the world. Do not be lulled into a false sense of security by seemingly trivial signs or symptoms. DCS can progress rapidly, and the end-point can be death.

Management of diving accidents

Practitioners of occupational medicine should participate in advance planning for the management of diving and other hyperbaric accidents such as underwater construction, or offshore petroleum exploration, and tunnel projects. Since the physician is unlikely to be on site, it is important to establish a program with the employer to provide medical personnel with hyperbaric training in addition to conventional competence in advanced cardiac and trauma life support. These diving and hyperbaric medical technicians communicate with the supervising physician, offer immediate care, provide a working diagnosis, stabilize, and accompany the patient to the definitive care facility. Accompanying the patient is essential since the hyperbaric exposure may be overlooked in an injured diver or tunnel worker arriving at a busy emergency department and delayed recognition could be disastrous.

Pressure, oxygen, and time are the key elements of recompression therapy. There are no substitutes; emergency transportation to the nearest recompression chamber is mandatory. Even if apparent recovery occurs en route, transportation to the chamber must continue, since recurrences can be serious. By the same token, one should be reluctant to leave the sanctuary of an offshore chamber for an uncertain shore-side hospital destination until certain that any diving injuries have been thoroughly stabilized.

Most cases of barotraumas and decompression sickness in commercial diving operations occur in a decompression chamber or at a site where a chamber is available. As a consequence, definitive treatment – pressure, oxygen, and time – is possible. When a recompression chamber is not on site, first efforts should be toward obtaining telephone consultation, communication with the nearest suitable recompression chamber, and arranging appropriate transportation. On-scene immediate care in the absence of a chamber should be continued until reaching a recompression facility.

1. Provide 100% oxygen by demand valve and a double-seal mask. Do not be concerned about oxygen toxicity. Most previously healthy divers will tolerate this regimen for up to 24 hours with only brief interruptions for food, liquids, etc.
2. Establish intravenous access and maintain adequate intravascular volume, tissue perfusion, and the elimination of inert gas. Normal saline and lactated Ringer's solution are acceptable. Provide fruit juices and balanced electrolyte beverages to maintain urine output at 1–2 mL/kg/hr.
3. If spinal cord decompression sickness is present, an indwelling urinary catheter may be required.
4. Avoid steroids and/or aspirin. Their use is unproven and could be deleterious in certain situations. Consider

diazepam for the control of vertigo and vomiting in inner ear DCS.

Communication and transportation

Depending upon location and circumstances, the consulting hyperbaric physician may be able to direct emergency care and transportation to a chamber or hospital, but in some cases the physician must go to the accident site or chamber. These hyperbaric emergency physicians must be trained and physically fit for prolonged hyperbaric exposure in a chamber in order to provide medical care during decompression. During the trip to the site, on-scene personnel should arrange to communicate with a second shore-based physician to ensure continuity of care.

Emergency evacuation of hyperbaric casualties should be preplanned. If close enough to a recompression chamber, surface transportation may be faster than waiting for an aircraft. If aircraft are unpressurized, the flight should be planned at an altitude of 1000 feet – or less if practicable. When possible, aircraft should be utilized which can maintain sea-level pressure throughout the flight. As a compromise, lightweight portable recompression chambers may be utilized to maintain a minimum of sea-level pressure in unpressurized aircraft.

Coordination is the key to a successful hyperbaric casualty evacuation. The coordinating facility must track every aspect: failure to coordinate has caused casualties to arrive unannounced at a hyperbaric facility shut down for maintenance or where an operating crew has not been notified. Physicians unfamiliar with hyperbaric injuries have innocently delayed recompression while diligently seeking a more familiar diagnosis. The hyperbaric physician and hyperbaric technician accompanying the patient must cut through well-intentioned but misguided delay in order to obtain specific recompression therapy in cases of decompression sickness and arterial gas embolism.

References

1. Bert P. La pression barometrique, recherches di physiologie experimentale. Paris: G. Massonet cie., 1878. (English translation, Hitchcock MA, Hitchcock FA. Barometric pressure, researches in experimental physiology. Columbus, Ohio: College Book Co., 1943. Reprinted by Undersea Medical Society, 1978.)
2. de Acosta J. Historia natural y moral de las indias: en que se trata de cosas notables del cielo, de los elementos, metales, plantas, y animales. Seville, 1590
3. Boyle R. New pneumatical observations about respiration. Phil Trans R Soc 1670; 5:2035–56.
4. Pol B, Watelle TJJ. Memoire sur les effects de la compression de l'air applique au creusement des puits a hoville. Ann d'Hyg Pub Med Legate Paris 1854; Ser2(1):147–54.
5. Hill L. Caisson sickness and the physiology of work in compressed air. London: Edward Arnold, 1912.
6. Keays FL. Compressed air illness with a report of 3692 cases. Researches from the Department of Medicine, Cornell University Medical College 1909; 2:1–55.
7. Keays FL. Compressed air illness. American Labor Legislation Review 1912; 2:192–205.
8. Goodman MW, Workman RD. Minimal recompression, oxygen-breathing approach to treatment of decompression

sickness in divers and aviators. US Navy Experimental Diving Unit Research Report 5-65, 1965.

9. Kindwall EP, Whelan HT. Hyperbaric medicine practice, 2nd edn. Flagstaff, AZ: Best Publishing Company, 1999.

10. National Oceanic and Atmospheric Administration Diving Program, Training and Certification, Medical Criteria, Standards. January 2002. http://www.ndc.noaa.gov/tc_medical_standards.html

11. Wilmhurst P, Davidson C, O'Connell G, Byrne C. Role of cardiorespiratory abnormalities, smoking and dive characteristics in the manifestations of neurological decompression illness. Clin Sci 1994; 86:297–303.

12. Van R, Ugoccioni D, eds. DAN's report on decompression illness: diving fatalities and project dive exploration. Durham, NC: Divers Alert Network, 2001.

13. Elliott DH, ed. Medical assessment of fitness to dive. Ewell, England: Biomedical Seminars, 1995.

14. Butler FK. High-pressure ophthalmology. Alert Diver 1998; May/June.

15. Brown MS, Siegel IM. Cornea-contact lens interaction in the aquatic environment. CLAO J 1997; 23:237–42.

16. Dear GL. Diabetes and diving. Alert Diver 1997; Jan/Feb.

17. Occupational Safety and Health Administration (OSHA). Title 29 CFR Part 1910 Subpart T and Title 29 CFR Part 1926 Subpart Y. January 2002. http://www.osha-slc.gov/

18. US Coast Guard. Diving Regulations, Title 46 CFR Part 197 Subpart B, January 2002. http://www.access.gpo.gov/nara/cfr/waisidx_98/46cfr197_98.html

19. Association of Dive Contractors. Consensus standards. Houston, TX: Association of Dive Contractors, 2000.

20. The American Academy of Underwater Sciences. Standards for scientific diving. Nahant, MA: American Academy of Underwater Sciences, 2001.

21. Hackett PH, Roach RC. High altitude illness. In: Auerbach PS, ed. Wilderness medicine: the management of wilderness and environmental emergencies, 4th edn. St. Louis: Mosby, 2001.

22. Hultgren HN. High altitude medicine. Stanford: Hultgren Publications, 1997.

23. Deitz TE. The high altitude medicine guide. Hood River, 2000. www.high-altitude-medicine.com

24. Bayne CG. Personal communication.

25. Dumont L, Mardirosoff C, Tramer MR. Efficacy and harm of pharmacological prevention of acute mountain sickness: quantitative systematic review. BMJ 2000; 321:267–72.

26. Heimbach RD, Sheffield PJ. Decompression sickness and pulmonary overpressure accidents. In: Dehart RL, ed. Fundamentals of aerospace medicine, 2nd edn. Philadelphia: Lippincott Williams and Wilkins, 1996.

27. DeHart RL. The atmosphere. In: DeHart RL, ed. Fundamentals of aerospace medicine, 2nd edn. Philadelphia: Lippincot Williams and Wilkins, 1996.

28. Sheffield PJ, Heimbach RD. Respiratory physiology. In: DeHart RL, ed. Fundamentals of aerospace medicine, 2nd edn. Philadelphia: Lippincot Williams and Wilkins, 1996.

29. Sheffield PJ, Stork RL. Protection in the pressure enviornment. In: DeHart RL, ed. Fundamentals of aerospace medicine, 2nd edn. Philadelphia: Lippincot Williams and Wilkins, 1996.

30. Kimbrell PN. Treatment of altitude decompression sickness. In: Moon RE, Sheffield PJ, eds. Treatment of decompression illness. Kensington: Undersea and Hyperbaric Medicine Society, 1996;43.

31. Pilmanis AA. Altitude decompression sickness. In: Moon RE, Sheffield PJ, eds. Treatment of decompression illness. Kensington: Undersea and Hyperbaric Medicine Society, 1996;28.

32. Powell MR. Decompression in space: manifestations and treatment. In: Moon RE, Sheffield PJ, eds. Treatment of decompression illness. Kensington: Undersea and Hyperbaric Medicine Society, 1996;53.

33. Rutkowski D. Recompression chamber life support manual, 4th edn. Key Largo, FL: Hyperbarics International Inc., 1995.

34. Joiner JT, ed. NOAA diving manual: diving for science and technology, 4th edn. Flagstaff, AZ: Best Publishing Company, 2001.

Chapter 37
Biologic Factors

37.1 Animal Exposures

James A Merchant, Peter S Thorne, Stephen J Reynolds

Exposures to animals are an important cause of respiratory disease in the workplace.[1,2] There are three types of occupational settings that have provided research information on a wide range of exposures arising from animals and their housing environments: epidemiologic data on respiratory symptoms and functional changes, clinical presentation, and prevention strategies. These categories of exposures include (1) concentrated animal feeding operations (CAFOs) for swine and poultry, (2) dairy farming, and (3) exposure to laboratory animals at work and to pets at home.

The US population at risk in agriculture is large, including an estimated 12 million farmers, farm family members who participate in farming, and other agricultural workers, including migrant workers. Of this number, approximately 750,000 persons are exposed in livestock confinement and an estimated 500,000 persons are exposed in dairy farming. Hundreds of thousands work as laboratory animal handlers, technicians, and investigators. The respiratory diseases that arise from animal exposures in these populations include allergic and irritant rhinitis, acute and chronic bronchitis, asthma, allergic alveolitis, bronchiolitis, and toxic pneumonitis. This chapter does not address other occupational diseases arising from exposure to animals, which include occupational dermatoses and zoonotic diseases (see Chapters 29.1, 29.2, and 37.2), nor does it address the significant risk of injury that livestock, dairy farmers, and animal handlers face through their exposure to animals.

OCCUPATIONAL AND ENVIRONMENTAL EXPOSURES
The livestock environment

Technologic improvements in animal husbandry, including the use of enclosed and controlled environments, have substantially increased the efficiency of livestock production, especially for swine and poultry, over the last 30 years. Because of the intensive nature of these farming practices, workers are exposed to high concentrations of air-borne dusts and gases.[3] Enclosed livestock facilities typically consist of simple one-story, pole barns with windows or curtained walls and fans for ventilation. Temperature, feed quality, and other factors are monitored and adjusted by the farmer to facilitate efficient animal growth. Capacity may range from several hundred animals per building, in some swine facilities, to more than 50,000 chickens in some poultry facilities. In the case of both swine and chickens, manure is collected in pits or lagoons,

located either under or adjacent to the building. Manure in turkey facilities typically accumulates directly on bedding material, consisting of wood chips, sunflower hulls or peat, and may not be cleaned out for several years. Workers may spend up to 40 hours per week inside these facilities. Tasks include supplying, checking and cleaning feed and watering systems, culling dead or ill animals, inoculating, collecting blood samples, cleaning manure systems and pumping out manure pits, tilling bedding (turkey facilities), mixing and applying antimicrobials and insecticides, and moving animals out of these confinement facilities for shipment.[4]

Environmental agents measured in swine and poultry barns include a complex mixture of organic dusts, microorganisms, and irritant gases.[5] Dusts have been found to contain plant material (bedding and feed); animal-derived particles (skin cells, hair, feathers, droppings, urine); bacteria and fungi; microbial toxins (endotoxins); feed additives including antibiotics and other antimicrobials; pesticides; and ammonia, hydrogen sulfide, methane, nitrogen oxides, and odoriferous vapors from microbial action in manure.[6] Air sampling studies have found total dust concentrations typically range from about 4 to 40 mg/m^3, with respirable dust levels much lower, ranging from 0.5 to 5.0 mg/m^3. Daily time-weighted average concentrations often exceed the current Occupational Safety and Health Administration (OSHA) permissible exposure limit (PEL) of 15 mg/m^3 for total nuisance particulates and 5 mg/m^3 for respirable dusts.[7] Endotoxins, lipopolysaccharide portions of the cell wall of gram-negative bacteria, have been measured at levels ranging from 1 to 3000 ng/m^3, again often well in excess of a proposed guideline of 9 ng/m^3.

Air-borne concentrations of culturable bacteria have been found to range from 10^4 to 10^7 colony-forming units per cubic meter of air (CFU/m^3), and although total viable fungal concentrations usually have been low (less than 500 CFU/m^3), isolated findings of much higher concentrations (exceeding 50,000 CFU/m^3) have been reported. Hydrogen sulfide, a potent respiratory irritant and toxin, which has the odor of rotten eggs, is produced by anaerobic bacterial activity in manure pits. Hydrogen sulfide levels typically remain far below 10 parts per million (ppm), but agitation of liquid manure pits, which is often necessary for pumping, may release short-term concentrations high enough to kill workers and animals (700 to 2000 ppm). Ammonia, a highly reactive and alkaline irritant gas produced from microbial degradation of urea and uric acid, has been found at concentrations higher than 100 ppm in some poultry operations, far in excess of the current OSHA PEL of 25 ppm averaged over an 8-hour time period, and may exceed the short-term (15-minute) exposure limit (STEL) of 35 ppm.[8,9] Ammonia levels tend to be much lower in confined swine operations, typically closer to 5 to 10 ppm. Air-borne concentrations of dusts and gases are highest during activities such as tilling bedding, pumping out manure pits, and during animal handling. Seasonal effects are also evident, with air-borne concentrations of these agents being much higher during the winter, when buildings are closed.

The dairy environment

The dairy barn environment consists of numerous air-borne substances arising from a diversity of operations that occur in the course of daily dairy farming. Each of the principal tasks – feeding, milking, manure handling, distribution of bedding, silage handling, and tillage – is associated with its own spectrum of potentially hazardous agents. Dairy farming has recently experienced considerable consolidation with fewer but larger operations and increasing automation. Exposures encountered by dairy farmers are characterized by continuous exposure to moderately high bioaerosols punctuated by very high short-term dust exposures.[10] Mixing and distribution of feed may generate dusts that are heavily laden with bacteria, fungi, microbial toxins, and feed additives, such as vitamins, minerals, and medications. Bedding, chopping, and pitch-forking of hay may produce levels of air-borne fungi and thermophilic bacteria as high as 10^{10} organisms/m^3, accompanied by grain mite and pollen exposures.[11]

Other sources of bedding, such as sawdust or shredded newspaper, may also introduce high bioaerosol levels. Silo loading is associated with potentially lethal exposures to nitrogen oxides, whereas silo unloading can lead to extremely high exposure to micro-organisms and their toxins, potentially leading to organic dust toxic syndrome (ODTS) or farmer's lung disease (FLD, an allergic alveolitis).[12] Manure handling is associated with exposures to endotoxin dust and bacteria, as well as urine proteins, ammonia, and hydrogen sulfide. Air-borne dust concentrations in milking parlors are lower than in stanchions, but may constitute higher breathing zone concentrations of antigenic cattle epithelium. Many dairy farmers do not have parlors and milk their cows in the barn, often while they feed. Infrequent, but high exposure tasks include silo or grain bin clean-out and silo uncapping when total dust exposures often exceed 150 mg/m^3. Approximately once daily, lime (CaCO$_3$) is spread to control micro-organisms in a process that produces high short-term exposure. This material may contain fibrogenic crystalline minerals, including asbestos.

Air-borne total dust levels during routine operations typically fall in the range of 0.2–4 mg/m^3 in winter, when barn ventilation is reduced to conserve heat, and are somewhat lower in summer. Respirable dust levels account for a highly variable proportion of this dust, depending on the tasks performed during the sampling period, but generally represent less than 30% of the total dust. When bedding is dropped from a loft, chopped or pitch-forked, total dust

concentrations increase by an order of magnitude. Bioaerosol sampling in a sample of 25 Wisconsin dairy barns found culturable mesophilic bacteria at a geometric mean concentration of 1.8×10^6 CFU/m^3, thermophilic bacteria at 3×10^3 CFU/m^3, and fungi at 6×10^4 CFU/m^3. In the United States, the air-borne fungi typically include common environmental molds such as *Aspergillus*, *Penicillium*, *Fusarium*, *Mucor*, *Cladosporium*, and *Alternaria*, in addition to several yeast genera. Assessment of total micro-organisms, both culturable and non-culturable, has shown that up to 90% of the air-borne micro-organisms may be non-culturable. The largest study of levels of air-borne endotoxin in dairy barns reported a geometric mean inhalable endotoxin concentration of 74 ng/m^3, with substantial variability (range of 4–3480 ng/m^3). Mycotoxins present in air-borne conidia (mold spores) have rarely led to measurable concentrations in air samples, although we have detected deoxynivalenol (vomitoxin) and fumonisin B1 at 1–5 micrograms/m^3.

A number of studies have tested the serum of dairy farmers and found elevated levels of immunoglobulin reactivity to fungi, thermophilic bacteria, and storage mite antigens.[13] Recent studies have identified storage and predator mites in dairy barn dust samples including *Lepidoglyphus destructor*, *Acarus siro*, *Tyrophagus putrescetiae*, *Caloglyphus berlesei*, *Chortoglyphus arcuatus*, *Glycyphagus ornatus*, and *Euroglyphus maynei*. In addition, specific radioallergosorbent test (RAST) inhibition assays have identified air-borne levels of *L. destructor* reactivity as high as 12 micrograms/m^3.

Exposures to excessive levels of gases and vapors also occur in dairy farming. During silo filling, nitrogen oxides are formed through enzymatic degradation of plant nitrates, producing NO, NO$_2$, and N$_2$O$_4$. Exposure to nitrogen dioxide is of particular concern and, from hours to several days after filling the silo, it often exceeds the PEL of 3 ppm and may be as high as 2000 ppm. Ammonia concentrations in the vapor phase in dairy barns often exceed the PEL of 25 ppm, with additional exposure from ammonia adsorbed to dry aerosols. In addition to these exposures, dairy farmers, like other farmers, are frequently exposed to gas or diesel engine exhaust, pesticide aerosols, welding fumes, and a host of other occupational aerosols and vapors that may be produced in the many tasks involved in farming.

The laboratory animal environment

Animals raised for meat production account for 99.7% of the total use of animals in the United States. The other 0.3% (some 15 million animals) are used in research and toxicologic testing. Of these laboratory animals, 97% are birds, reptiles, amphibians, and rodents. The most commonly used mammals are mice, rats, hamsters, guinea pigs, and rabbits. Other species in common use include gerbils, opossums, ferrets, cats, dogs, sheep, swine, and non-human primates. Non-mammalian species commonly handled by laboratory animal workers include pigeons and other birds, reptiles and amphibians, and cockroaches.

Aeroallergens are associated with all of the above-named species. These immunogenic bioaerosols arise from urine proteins, salivary proteins, epithelial cells, fecal proteins (especially avian) or sebaceous secretions. In addition to these allergens, laboratory animal workers come in contact with microbial bioaerosols, endotoxins, and antimicrobials and other chemicals used in cleaning operations. Concentrations of dust from feed or bedding materials also can be significantly elevated. Certain tasks, such as cage washing, often have been identified as producing high levels of immunogenic dust.[14] During cage cleaning, the soiled bedding material (commonly shredded paper, wood shavings, or ground corn cob) is dumped into a waste receptacle so that danders, urine proteins, micro-organisms, and fecal material become air-borne. Although total dust exposures are higher when fresh bedding is placed in cages, exposures to these dusts are less immunogenic and, therefore, less likely to lead to respiratory symptoms.

For animal handlers, cross-shift total personal dust concentrations typically range from 0.1 to 1.5 mg/m³, whereas respirable levels range from below detection to 0.2 mg/m³.

Concentrations of rat urine aeroallergens have been measured in rat facilities at about 1 μg/m³, with 70% of the aerosol being respirable. Laboratory animal technicians, who most commonly develop allergies to rodent species, frequently cite performance of animal surgery or euthanizing animals as processes that exacerbate their symptoms. Animal bites are common and are one likely route of sensitization to animal proteins.

CLINICAL EFFECTS

Adverse health effects that may arise from these several animal exposures include bronchitis, asthma, bronchiolitis, allergic alveolitis, chemical pneumonitis, pulmonary edema, and organic dust toxic syndrome (ODTS) (Table 37.1.1). The epidemiology and clinical presentation are only briefly reviewed in this chapter as more detailed accounts on upper airway disorders (Chapter 20.3), asthma (Chapter 19.2), irritant bronchitis (Chapter 19.4), hypersensitivity pneumonitis (Chapter 19.6), and acute inhalational injury (Chapter 19.5) are found elsewhere in this text. Although the prevalence and distribution of respiratory diseases vary between these three types of exposures, they all share a common characteristic of exposure to the bioactive constituents of organic dust, the primary cause of airway inflammation.

Health effects arising from livestock exposures

The most common respiratory manifestation of airway inflammation from exposure in animal confinement facilities is bronchitis. Chronic cough has been found in 45–75% of workers and chronic phlegm has been found in 35–50% of workers in studies of Iowa swine confinement workers, which is consistently higher than that for non-swine confinement farmers (35% and 15%, respectively).[7,15,16] Symptoms of chest tightness (20%) and breathlessness (10%) also are more common among confinement workers than among non-confinement farmers (5% and 2%, respectively).[17] The pattern of symptoms is similar among poultry farmers, but the prevalence is typically lower.[18]

A study of 303 Canadian poultry farmers found a significant difference in symptoms among workers in caged chicken rearing barns compared to those in barns with floor raised birds.[19] Symptoms reported for caged system and floor system workers were: cough (35% and 25%), phlegm (30% and 25%), wheeze (10% and 5%), and shortness of breath (25% and 20%). These symptoms are all found to be higher among workers who smoke cigarettes, which is less common among farmers than blue collar workers. It has been shown that swine confinement farmers are more likely than other farmers to have significant cross-shift decrements in expiratory flow rates, and airway hyper-responsiveness and clinical asthma are not uncommon in this working population.[20,21] Cross-sectional studies of swine confinement workers have demonstrated evidence of more chronic airways obstruction compared with other farmers, and prospective evaluation has found that cross-shift decline in FEV_1 was a significant determinant of progressive loss of lung function over time.[22,23]

While there is evidence that removal of affected workers from exposure influences the results of these studies, cross-shift declines in FEV_1 have been found to be a significant predictor of annual decline in FEV_1.[24–26] The vast majority of farmers with bronchitis are able to continue to work in livestock confinement operations; however, those with airway hyper-responsiveness or asthma are rarely able to continue this type of work.[27] If asthmatic farmers are unable to hire workers to run their confinement operations, they may be forced to close down their livestock facilities, usually at a considerable cost, and are often unable to continue farming.

Two toxic exposures have been observed among CAFO workers. ODTS has been found in about 10% of Iowa swine confinement farmers.[15] This syndrome is most common among new workers or following an especially high exposure

Occupation	Exposure	Respiratory conditions
Swine farmers Poultry farmers	Organic dust Animal particles Bacteria and fungi Microbial toxins Feed additives Pesticides Irritant gases	Chronic bronchitis Asthma Bronchiolitis Toxic pneumonitis Rhinitis Organic dust toxic syndrome
Dairy farmers	Organic dust Feed additives Thermophilic bacteria and fungi Microbial toxins Storage mites Pesticides Irritant gases	Chronic bronchitis Asthma Allergic alveolitis (farmer's lung) Bronchiolitis Toxic pneumonitis (silo filler's lung) Rhinitis
Laboratory animal handlers, technicians, and investigators	Organic dusts Animal proteins Bacteria and fungi Microbial toxins Biocides and cleaning chemicals	Organic dust toxic syndrome Rhinitis Asthma Allergic alveolitis (rare) Chronic bronchitis

Table 37.1.1 Exposures and respiratory conditions among workers exposed to animals

in a confinement facility.[28] It also is reported among these farmers when they clean out grain bins, which often results in high exposure to moldy grain. Symptoms, which begin 4–12 hours after exposure, include cough, fever, myalgia, fatigue, and occasionally, dyspnea. This flu-like illness rarely requires hospitalization. A second toxic exposure that has been reported on numerous occasions is toxic pneumonitis, often with acute respiratory distress syndrome (ARDS), most commonly associated with agitation or pumping of liquid manure out of a pit. High concentrations of hydrogen sulfide gas exposure may result in respiratory distress, followed by ARDS and often death. Farmers who have survived such an episode describe hearing all of their animals hitting the floor at the same time (none survive) and having to run from the building to avoid this lethal exposure. Farmers who recover from ARDS are typically left with bronchiolitis obliterans, airway hyper-responsiveness, and severe pulmonary impairment.

Several recent studies have found that growing up on a farm, especially if exposed to farm animals in early life, decreases the risk of allergic disease, including atopic asthma. While not all studies have found this to be consistently the case, some studies suggest that endotoxins may be conveying a protective effect through modulation of the immune response, resulting in lower rates of atopy and allergic diseases including allergic rhinitis, airway hyper-responsiveness, and asthma. However, as asthma is a multifactorial disease, numerous risk factors must be assessed, including the livestock environment. Such assessments are often lacking or incomplete in published papers on this topic. When children work in CAFOs they will experience the same types of exposure as other farm workers, and thereby experience an increased risk to asthma despite any modulation of the immune response.

Clinical effects arising from dairy farming exposures

As with swine and poultry livestock farmers, the most common clinical finding is that of chronic bronchitis arising from exposure to organic dusts and other irritants in the dairy environment. However, the inter-relationship between symptoms and exposures is complex. A series of studies of Wisconsin dairy farmers have found that those with antibodies to organisms (*Saccharopolyspora rectivirgula*, *Thermoactinomyces vulgaris*, *Saccharomonospora viridis*, *Aspergillus fumigatis*, *T. candidis*, and *T. sacchari*) thought to cause farmer's lung disease (FLD) had a significantly higher prevalence of chronic cough and phlegm, a finding that might be explained by larger dairy herds and their higher microbial exposures.

Serologic assessments of Wisconsin dairy farmers by immunoassay have found that a positive serology to one or more of these organisms occured in as many as 75% of individuals in of one large population-based cohort. Acute respiratory symptoms, including cough, fever, chills or dyspnea, occurring 4–12 hours after exposure to moldy hay or silage, were found in 17% of these dairy farmers, most of whom were seropositive. There is some evidence that those with

acute respiratory symptoms with dairy barn exposure are more likely to be sensitized to storage mites. However, many of these episodes occurred with silo unloading or chopping of bedding with very high exposures, and are most likely to represent ODTS rather than the acute phase of FLD.[12] Because these symptoms are relatively common among dairy farmers, and because the frequency of a positive FLD serology is so high, it is difficult to distinguish between an acute episode of FLD and ODTS. Bronchoalveolar lavage in a nested-case-control study of this population showed little evidence of a lymphocytic response (evidence of FLD) among antibody-positive farmers with acute respiratory symptoms. This finding is consistent with the finding of a low prevalence of 4.2 cases per 1000 of clinically confirmed cases of chronic FLD in the original study of this large cohort. Serology status was not associated with diminished lung function in this population. Apart from the well-documented finding that dairy farmers with confirmed FLD have progressively diminished lung function with continued exposure, dairy farmers have been found to have surprisingly well-preserved lung function, even after years of exposure.

The other significant lung disease that is occasionally observed among dairy farmers is toxic pneumonitis, and occasionally ARDS, from inhalation of oxides of nitrogen in a recently filled silo (silo filler's lung). Although this exposure, which is now widely recognized among dairy farmers, occasionally results in fatal ARDS, it more commonly causes toxic pneumonitis, which may result in residual airway hyper-responsiveness and asthma. Both ODTS and silo filler's lung occur following filling the silo. ODTS typically occurs with removal of the moldy silage on top of the plastic cap placed over the fermented silage, and is characterized by a febrile illness, with numerous constitutional symptoms occurring 4–12 hours after exposure. Silo filler's lung usually occurs hours to several days following filling of the silo. Exposure most commonly occurs when the farmer enters a partially filled silo and is exposed to the brownish, highly irritating nitrogen oxide gases. The onset of symptoms of cough and breathlessness may be delayed for several hours and is dependent on the extent of exposure, but the febrile and constitutional symptoms typical of ODTS do not develop. Immediate, often intensive, medical treatment is necessary for silo filler's lung but is rarely needed for ODTS.

Clinical health effects resulting from exposure to laboratory animals

A number of cross-sectional epidemiologic studies of allergies to laboratory animals have shown a prevalence of allergy (allergic rhinitis, asthma, skin wheal formation or urticaria) to laboratory animals ranging from 15% to 33%.[29–31] The prevalence of asthma in these studies has ranged from 1% to 12%. Authors frequently noted that asthmatics and others sensitized to laboratory animals often were transferred because of their sensitization or removed themselves from this occupational exposure.[32] Allergic alveolitis is rare but has been reported from exposure to rat urine. Workers exposed to laboratory animals have been found to be significantly more likely to have work-related symptoms of coughing, wheezing, and chest tightness than controls who have not been exposed to animals. Exposed workers also have been found to have airway hyper-responsiveness more often, and to have positive skin tests to a number of common laboratory animals including rats, mice, guinea pigs, hamsters, and gerbils.[33] Symptoms of laboratory animal allergy often are associated with a history of atopy.

Exposure assessments strongly suggest that the incidence of laboratory animal allergy is dose related.[34,35] Recent studies using RAST-inhibition assays for animal antigens now provide a quantitative approach for assessment of dose–response relationships and a methodology to monitor strategies aimed at reducing these immunogenic exposures. Workers with laboratory animal allergy are frequently found to be sensitized to several animal species. Previous sensitization to animals as pets, most commonly to cats, becomes evident among new employees exposed within the first days on the job. Workers who are atopic are much more likely to become sensitized, especially at low levels of exposure. Among workers not previously sensitized, the latent period until sensitization may begin in weeks and is usually less than 1 year. There is now evidence that environmental control of these immunogenic exposures delays or prevents sensitization in some laboratory workers.[36] There is further evidence that endotoxin exposure is a determinant of respiratory symptoms among laboratory workers not sensitized to mice, thereby extending the need also to control this exposure.[37]

MANAGEMENT AND PREVENTION

Epidemiologic studies of workers exposed to animals provide the keys to management and prevention of these respiratory diseases. There is evidence of a dose–response relationship between exposure and respiratory effects in all three of these occupational settings. It also is clear that early recognition of asthma, toxic pneumonitis, and allergic alveolitis (although very uncommon) is critically important to treatment and management of workers with these conditions.[38] Finally, use of dust control, appropriate work practices, and personal protective equipment to reduce or eliminate exposures is important in all three of these occupational settings.

Management of affected individuals

The most common respiratory conditions arising from these exposures are chronic bronchitis and ODTS, both of which are manifestations of airway inflammation. Management of individuals with these conditions necessarily and primarily involves reduction of their exposure to organic dusts and other irritants and, if the individual is a smoker, smoking cessation. Because control of exposures in agricultural settings is difficult, management of the farmer with chronic bronchitis usually involves careful and continuing use of appropriate respiratory protection. Negative pressure respirators or powered air-purifying respirators often are useful and are especially important in settings that involve very heavy exposures. The worker must be instructed in the maintenance, repair, and replacement of filters and the respirator. Although most workers are able to continue to work with the help of respiratory protection, those with significant airway obstruction, asthma, frequent expectoration, and those who find wearing a respirator unacceptable may require transfer to less dusty environments. In the case of farming, this approach may prove difficult or impossible.

Each of these occupational settings may result in occupational asthma. As with other forms of occupational asthma, it is important that the worker be separated from exposures that will exacerbate and worsen the worker's asthma. For this reason, farmers and laboratory workers exposed to animal environments that are thought to cause asthma must be counseled, very seriously, about the risks of continued occupational exposure. With farmers, it may be possible for them to delegate enough of the high exposure tasks that they can continue farming with respiratory protection and appropriate medical management. Some workers with laboratory animal allergy may be able to continue work with the use of appropriate personal protective clothing and an efficient respirator. However, if the asthma continues, these workers will need to be removed from animal exposures. This may require a costly career change for some farmers, for full-time animal handlers and for investigators who work directly with laboratory animals.

Management of toxic pneumonitis and ARDS requires the physician always to be alert to these rare respiratory disorders among farmers. Intensive care may be necessary and early intervention with steroids is important, a treatment that must often continue for several weeks following presentation. Medical management with steroids, leukotriene inhibitors and bronchodilators for asthma, a frequent sequela of toxic pneumonitis, often is necessary. With successful treatment, lung function may improve over a period of several months to 2 years. Workers with mild cases of toxic pneumonitis often make a full recovery, but more severe cases and those who had ARDS are typically left with significant, irreversible impairment.

Prevention

Prevention of respiratory disease among those exposed to animals requires a variety of approaches. Because some agricultural exposures are life threatening or may cause acute toxic injury, it is critically important that farmers understand and recognize the exposure risks in certain agricultural settings. All farmers with manure pits must be made aware of the very significant risk of potentially fatal exposures to hydrogen sulfide gas with agitation and pumping of liquid manure. Under no circumstance should a farmer ever enter a pit. If a pit must be entered, an air-supplied respirator with a full face piece must be used. This may entail working with the local fire department or hazardous materials unit. Farmers should work in pairs when pumping pits, remove their animals from the building over the pit, and ventilate the pit and building during pumping. Similarly, dairy farmers must be made aware of the potentially fatal exposure to oxides of nitrogen they may face if they enter a recently filled silo. This practice should be avoided, if at all possible. Dairy farmers should work in pairs in loading and unloading silos, use safety harnesses, and employ effective respiratory protection if entering the silo is necessary. An air-supplied respirator should be used if a silo filled with nitrogen oxide gas must be entered, and an efficient negative pressure or powered air-purifying respirator should be used during silo uncapping.

At the present time, there are no specific dust standards for exposures in these work settings. There are US OSHA standards for control of hydrogen sulfide and ammonia, but enforcement of standards in farming is virtually nonexistent. Because there is evidence of dose–response relationships between some of these exposures and some measures of respiratory disease, efforts should always be made to reduce exposures, which often can be high.[7] Occupational exposure limits for total dust (2.8 mg/m^3) and ammonia (7.5 ppm) have been recommended by researchers for livestock confinement buildings. Engineering controls such as the use of more efficient ventilation systems, canola oil sprinkling systems in animal confinement facilities, and improved manure management practices, often can significantly reduce exposures to organic dust and irritant gases and vapors.[39–41] Improved work practices that include use of appropriate personal protective equipment, more frequent cleaning of animal quarters, and routine use of negative pressure respirators or powered air-purifying respirators in dusty areas, can help reduce exposure to these several agents.[42]

Industrial hygiene controls are being instituted more frequently in an attempt to control exposure to animal allergens among laboratory animal workers. These controls include use of negative-pressure or powered air-purifying respirators for high-risk tasks, increased general exhaust in animal care facilities, carefully balanced ventilation systems that direct airflow from clean areas to dirty areas, performance of animal surgery and necropsy in laminar flow or fume hoods, and use of specialized cage-dumping stations that are equipped with high-efficiency particulate air filters and operate under negative pressure.[43] All of these measures can reduce aeroallergen exposures significantly. Under some conditions of positive pressure, certain caging systems designed to maintain experimental animals in a pathogen-free environment increase the aeroallergen levels in the animal suite and result in higher exposures to workers. Such caging systems should be fitted for direct exhaust or should be located in a room with higher air exchange rates.

References

1. Dosman JA, Cockcroft DW, eds. Principles of health and safety in agriculture. Boca Raton, FL: CRC Press, 1989.
2. Merchant JA. Agricultural respiratory disease. Semin Respir Med 1986; 7:211–24.
3. Popendorf W. Health effects of organic dusts in the farm environment. Report on agents. Am J Ind Med 1986; 10:251–9.
4. Duchaine C, Grimard Y, Cormier Y. Influence of building maintenance, environmental factors, and seasons on air-borne contaminants of swine confinement buildings. J Sci Occup Environ Health Safety 2000; 61:56–63.
5. Reynolds SJ, Parker D, Vesley D, et al. Occupational exposure to organic dusts and gases in the turkey growing industry. Appl Occup Environ Hyg 1994; 9:493–502.
6. Douwes J, Thorne PS, Pearce N, Heederik D. Bioaerosol health effects and exposure assessment: progress and prospects. Ann Occup Hyg 2003; 47:187–200.
7. Donham KJ, Reynolds SJ, Whitten P, et al. Respiratory dysfunction in swine production facility workers: dose–response relationships of environmental exposures and pulmonary function. Am J Ind Med 1995; 27:405–18.
8. Donham KJ, Cumro D, Reynolds SJ. Synergistic effects of dust and ammonia on the occupational health effects of poultry production workers. J Agromed 2002; 8:57–76.
9. Jones W, Morring K, Olenchock SA, et al. Environmental study of poultry confinement buildings. Am Ind Hyg Assoc J 1984; 45:760–6.
10. Kullman GJ, Thorne PS, Waldron PF, et al. Organic dust exposures from work in diary barns. Am Ind Hyg Assoc J 1998; 59:403–13.
11. Lange JL, Thorne PS, Kullman GJ. Determinants of viable bioaerosol concentrations in dairy barns. Ann Agric Environ Med 1997; 4:187–94.
12. May JJ, Pratt DS, Stallones L, et al. A study of dust generated during silo opening and its physiologic effects on workers. In: Dosman JA, Cockcroft D, eds. Principles of health and safety in agriculture. Boca Raton, FL: CRC Press, 1989;76–9.
13. Campbell AR, Swanson MC, Fernandez-Caldas E, et al. Aeroallergens in dairy barns near Cooperstown, NY, and Rochester, MN. Am Rev Respir Dis 1989; 140:317–20.
14. Eggleston PA, Newill C, Ansari A, et al. Task-related variation in air-borne concentrations of laboratory animal allergens: studies with Rat n 1. J Allergy Clin Immunol 1989; 84:347–52.
15. Merchant JA, Donham KJ. Health risks from animal confinement units. In: Dosman JA, Cockcroft D, eds. Principles of health and safety in agriculture. Boca Raton, FL: CRC Press, 1989;58–63.
16. Zejda JE, Hurst TS, Rhodes CS, et al. Respiratory health of swine producers. Focus on young workers. Chest 1993; 103:702–9.
17. Choudat D, Goehen M, Korobaeff M, et al. Respiratory symptoms and bronchial reactivity among pig and dairy farmers. Scand J Work Environ Health 1994; 20:48–54.
18. Reynolds SJ, Parker D, Vesley D, et al. Cross-sectional epidemiological study of respiratory disease in turkey farmers. Am J Ind Med 1993; 24:713–22.
19. Kirychuk SP, Senthilselvan A, Dosman JA, et al. Respiratory symptoms and lung function in poultry confinement workers in Western Canada. Can Respir J 2003; 10:375–80.
20. Radon K, Garz S, Schottky A, et al. Lung function and work-related exposure in pig farmers with respiratory symptoms. J Occup Environ Med 2000; 42:814–20.
21. Smid T, Heederik D, Houba R, Quanjer PH. Dust- and endotoxin-related acute lung function changes and work-related symptoms in workers in the animal feed industry. Am J Ind Med 1994; 25:877–88.
22. Kirychuk S, Senthilselvan A, Dosman JA, et al. Predictors of longitudinal changes in pulmonary function among swine confinement workers. Can Respir J 1998; 5:472–8.
23. Vogelzang PF, van der Gulden JW, Folgering H, et al. Endotoxin exposure as a major determinant of lung function decline in pig farmers. Am J Respir Crit Care Med 1998; 157:15–18.
24. Reynolds SJ, Donham KJ, Whitten P, et al. Longitudinal evaluation of dose–response relationships for environmental exposures and pulmonary function in swine production workers. Am J Ind Med 1996; 29:33–40.
25. Schwartz DA, Donham KJ, Olenchock SA, et al. Determinants of longitudinal changes in spirometric function among swine

confinement operators and farmers. Am J Respir Crit Care Med 1995; 151:47–53.

26. Senthilselvan A, Dosman JA, Kirychuk SP, et al. Accelerated lung function decline in swine confinement workers. Chest 1997; 111:1733–41.

27. Vogelzang PF, van der Gulden JW, Folgering H, et al. Longitudinal changes in bronchial responsiveness associated with swine confinement dust exposure. Chest 2000; 117:1488–95.

28. Vogelzang PF, van der Gulden JW, Folgering H, van Schayck CP. Organic dust toxic syndrome in swine confinement farming. Am J Ind Med 1999; 35:332–4.

29. Bryant DH, Boscato LM, Mboloi PN, Stuart MC. Allergy to laboratory animals among animal handlers. Med J Aust 1995; 163:415–8.

30. Bush RK. Mechanism and epidemiology of laboratory animal allergy. ILAR J 2001; 42:4–11.

31. Kibby T, Powell G, Cromer J. Allergy to laboratory animals: a prospective and cross-sectional study. J Occup Med 1989; 31:842–6.

32. Fuortes LJ, Weih L, Pomrehn P, et al. Prospective epidemiologic evaluation of laboratory animal allergy among university employees. Am J Ind Med 1997; 32:665–9.

33. Hollander A, Doekes G, Heederik D. Cat and dog allergy and total IgE as risk factors of laboratory animal allergy. J Allergy Clin Immunol 1996; 98(3):545–54.

34. Heederik D, Venables KM, Malmberg P, et al. Exposure–response relationships for work-related sensitization in workers exposed to rat urinary allergens: results from a pooled study. J Allergy Clin Immunol 1999; 103:678–84.

35. Hollander A, Heederik D, Doekes G. Respiratory allergy to rats: exposure–response relationships in laboratory animal workers. Am J Respir Crit Care Med 1997; 155:562–7.

36. Heederik D, Thorne PS, Doekes G. Health based occupational exposure limits for high molecular weight sensitizers: how long is the road we must travel? Ann Occup Hyg 2002; 46:439–46.

37. Pacheco KA, McCammon C, Liu AH, et al. Air-borne endotoxin predicts symptoms in non-mouse-sensitized technicians and research scientists exposed to laboratory mice. Am J Respir Crit Care Med 2003; 167:983–90.

38. Kruize H, Post W, Heederik D, et al. Respiratory allergy in laboratory animal workers: a retrospective cohort study using pre-employment screening data. Occup Environ Med 1997; 54:830–5.

39. Kirychuk S, Donham K, Reynolds S, et al. Oil/water sprinkling intervention in a swine building. International Symposium on Dust Control in Animal Production Facilities Congress Proceedings. Aarhus, Denmark: Scandinavian Congress Center, 1999;335–42.

40. Nonnenmann MW, Rautiainen RH, Donham KJ, et al. Vegetable oil sprinkling as a dust reduction method in a swine confinement. International Symposium on Dust Control in Animal Production Facilities Congress Proceedings. Aarhus, Denmark: Scandinavian Congress Center, 1999;271–278.

41. Senthilselvan A, Zhang Y, Dosman JA, et al. Positive human health effects of dust suppression with canola oil in swine barns. Am J Respir Crit Care Med 1997; 156:410–7.

42. Taivainen AI, Tukiainen HO, Terho EO, Husman KR. Powered dust respirator helmets in the prevention of occupational asthma among farmers. Scand J Work Environ Health 1998; 24:503–7.

43. Ziemann B, Corn M, Ansari AA, Eggleston PA. The effectiveness of the Duo-Flo Bioclean unit for controlling airborne antigen levels. Am Ind Hyg Assoc J 1992; 53:138–45.

37.2 **Plant and Vegetable Exposures**

James A Merchant

Exposure to plant dusts, or vegetable dusts, as they are commonly called, and their products represents perhaps the earliest and still the most prevalent form of occupational and environmental exposure to respiratory hazards. These exposures vary in their nature, their concentration, their health effects, and their relative risk. In the United States, where agriculture now involves less than 2% of the population, those with significant occupational and environmental exposure to these hazards still number in the millions. In developing countries, 50–70% of the population may be engaged in agriculture. Most of what we know about respiratory conditions arises from occupational studies, but community exposures to plant dusts have been documented to cause environmental asthma. Allergic rhinitis and asthma, both of which arise from occupational vegetable dust exposures, also result from exposure to grass and tree pollens, ragweed, and other common aeroallergens, and are common in the general population, but may be considered occupational hazards among those sensitive individuals whose jobs expose them to aerosols of these plants. Similarly, many plant exposures may result in a wide range of dermatologic conditions. These conditions are addressed in Chapter 29.

OCCUPATIONAL AND ENVIRONMENTAL EXPOSURES

A classification of occupational and environmental respiratory exposures to plant materials, commonly exposed occupations, and reported health effects is found in Table 37.2.1. Although this classification is not exhaustive, it does provide a useful summary of the variety and exposure settings of plant materials.

Exposure settings

There is a common pattern to occupational and environmental exposures to plant products. The largest population at risk is that engaged in agriculture. Plant exposures typically begin with harvesting of agricultural products. Harvesting of plants may result in significant respiratory exposures, including those transporting grain products for storage or to terminals for further transport for processing. Agricultural harvesting is typically a family affair, involving wives, children, and elderly, often retired farmers. Seasonal migrant farm workers and other seasonal workers also are exposed. Although all of these agricultural subgroups have some respiratory exposure, they have a far greater risk of traumatic injury (see Chapter 31).

Storage of plant products on the farm may result in still other respiratory exposures. Commodity prices often dictate whether the farmer will sell his or her crop, or store it on the farm or in the local elevator. Storage on the farm may result in very significant exposures to spoiled grain, especially when grain bins are cleaned out, or to moldy silage when a silo is uncapped. Another important silo exposure arising from fermentation of silage are oxides of nitrogen. Vegetable dust exposure also occurs with grinding of grain for feeding of livestock and in handling processed grain in the form of animal feed. Antibiotics, often added to feed as growth promotants, and other antimicrobials add further potential respiratory hazards. Those who work in grain elevators typically face a very substantial exposure to grain dust. Grain handlers also are frequently exposed to respiratory irritant and neurotoxic fumigants, including carbon disulfide and methyl bromide, which often are used to suppress pest infestation of grain.

A second population at risk is community residents living in proximity to grain-handling facilities. Studies of epidemic asthma in New Orleans suggested that grain dust was the cause, and soybean dust was documented to cause epidemic community asthma in Barcelona arising from unloading and processing of soybeans. The extent to which transportation, storage, and processing of plant materials may contribute to community asthma is still poorly understood and is a priority for environmental health research.

The third major population at risk of exposure to plant products is the processors. Although grain and wood products are not subject to processing in the agricultural setting, plants yielding vegetable fibers typically are. The ginning of cotton to remove cottonseed results in the initial occupational exposure to cotton dust. Similarly, the retting of flax, especially traditional water retting, and the initial step in processing grain may also result in very substantial exposures. These agricultural operations remove vegetable material arising from the leaf and stem of plants, but they also result in entrainment of vegetable dust in the vegetable fiber or grain. As a result, the initial processes used in textile processing and grain milling may result in high exposures to these vegetable dusts. As textile, grain, and wood products move down the processing line, substantially greater numbers of workers are potentially at risk.

The fourth category of those exposed to these products is the end-users, including certain occupational groups and some consumers who may be environmentally exposed. Although these occupational groups, and especially the environmentally exposed consumers, have not been extensively studied, asthma is well documented among those using flour for baking and those using certain wood products for furniture making and woodworking. As a result, exposure to vegetable dusts remains an important source of occupational and environmental respiratory disease, including allergic rhinitis, asthma, bronchitis, airway obstruction, and rarely, hypersensitivity pneumonitis.

Environmental measurement

Assessment of environmental exposures to plant products involves both characterization of the constituents and

Dust types	Occupations	Respiratory conditions
Vegetable fibers		
Cotton	Ginners, textile	Byssinosis
Flax	workers, bedding	Acute febrile
Soft hemp	and upholstery	syndromes
Sisal	workers, and	Non-specific
Jute	rope and twine	airway obstruction
Hard hemps	makers	Chronic bronchitis
Sunn (Indian hemp)		Rhinitis
Henequen		
Mauritius hemp		
Manila		
St. Helena hemp		
Kapok		
Grain dusts		
Corn	Farm workers,	Occupational
Rye	grain handlers,	asthma
Spring wheat	millers, bakers,	Hypersensitivity
Durum wheat	food processors	pneumonitis
Barley		Acute febrile
Oats		syndromes
Rice		Non-specific
Soy bean		airway obstruction
Castor bean		Chronic bronchitis
		Rhinitis
Wood dusts		
Western red cedar	Sawmill workers,	Occupational
California redwood	carpentry,	asthma
Cedar of Lebanon	cabinet making,	Hypersensitivity
Cocabolla	furniture making,	pneumonitis
Iroko	wood processing	Non-specific
Oak		airway obstruction
Mahogany		Chronic bronchitis
Abiruana		Rhinitis
African maple		
Tanganyika aningre		
Central American		
walnut		
Kejaat		
African zebra wood		
Other plants		
Coffee	Cutters, packers,	Occupational
Black tea	blenders,	asthma
Herbal teas	processors	Non-specific
Tobacco		airway obstruction
Gum acacia	Printers and gum	Chronic bronchitis
Gum tragacanth	manufacturers	Rhinitis

Adapted from World Health Organization Study Group. Recommended health-based occupational exposure limits for selected vegetable dusts. Report Series 684. Geneva: World Health Organization, 1983.

Table 37.2.1 Respiratory conditions among workers exposed to vegetable dusts

quantitation of the exposure. Exposures to vegetable dusts are complex. With harvesting of plant products, some inorganic soil particles are retained, and become a part of the occupational or environmental exposure. Although the occupational aerosol arises predominantly from the plant itself, it is commonly contaminated with microorganisms, most commonly gram-negative bacteria and their endotoxins, as well as fungi and their glucans and other mycotoxins. Other contaminants include insects, such as grain weevils and storage mites; hairs, feathers, and excreta of rodents and birds; and residual antimicrobials and agricultural chemicals, including fertilizers, pesticides,

herbicides, fungicides, and fumigants. Vegetable dusts also may contain constituents of weeds that contaminate the plant crop; these may be irritants or sensitizers in themselves.

The sampling strategy adopted for assessment of these exposures depends on the aim of the survey.[1] The most common approach has been measurement of total dust using a personnel sampling device with an open-faced filter. Work in the agricultural setting and in storage of plant products often results in massive exposures to the vegetable dust and its contaminants. For instance, exposures to total dust in farming and grain handing typically range from 2 to 3 mg/m^3 to well over 100 mg/m^3 in some instances. Exposure concentrations in the processing of plant products typically range from 0.5 mg/m^3 to greater than 10 mg/m^3. In some settings, such as the cotton textile industry, studies have demonstrated that total dust measurements often contained highly variable fractions of respirable dust and, therefore, have not been considered reliable indicators of risk. The vertical elutriator was developed and used as an area sampler to measure inhalable dust (15 micrograms in aerodynamic diameter), the biologically active fraction that penetrates the large and small airways. This sampling device has proved to provide reliable measurements of vegetable dust in the manufacturing setting, but it is not suitable for agricultural or general environmental assessment of these exposures in which use of total dust samplers is still preferred.

Research studies have developed a variety of sampling techniques to capture, quantify, and speciate bacteria and fungi contaminating vegetable dusts. Sampling filters have been found to be satisfactory sampling media for assessment of endotoxin and certain mycotoxins. Entomologic assessment of insects and mites that commonly contaminate these exposures is now giving way to the use of immunochemical testing, which is both more sensitive and quantitative. Endotoxins have been found to be important biologically active ingredients of plant exposures and, in the case of cotton dust, have been shown to be related in a linear dose–response fashion to decline in lung function across a work shift. Storage mites increasingly are being found to be important contaminants of plant products and to be responsible for some of the allergic rhinitis and asthma among those persons exposed.

CLINICAL EFFECTS

The various health effects that arise from exposure to vegetable dusts are summarized in Table 37.2.1. They will be only briefly discussed here because more detailed accounts on upper airway disorders (Chapter 20.3), asthma (Chapter 19.2), byssinosis and other cotton-related lung diseases (Chapter 19.3), irritant bronchitis (Chapter 19.4), and hypersensitivity pneumonitis (Chapter 19.6) are found elsewhere in the text. Although these health effects vary somewhat depending on the specific plant exposure, the nature of the contamination of the plant material, and the concentration of the exposure, occupational and environmental exposures to plant products cause both acute and chronic conditions or diseases.[2] Ramazzini[3] first made this observation in 1705:

'. . . for there flies out of this matter a foul mischievous powder, that entering the lungs by the mouth and throat, causes continual coughs and gradually makes way for an asthma. . . . But in the long run if they find their affliction grows upon them they must look out for another trade; for 'tis a sordid profit that's accompanied with the destruction of health'.

Acute health effects

Acute health effects, especially from high exposures to respirable plant products, are common.[4,5] Acute health effects may be divided into those characterized by symptomatic responses and those that may be characterized predominantly by functional responses. Although those who are symptomatic often have a measurable functional response, there is considerable variability between those who present with functional abnormalities and those who present with symptoms. Acute health effects characterized by symptoms include both irritant and allergic rhinitis, irritant and allergic asthma, and febrile and constitutional symptoms typical of organic toxic dust syndrome (OTDS). Functional abnormalities include decline in expiratory flow rates over a work shift and/or work week and heightened airway responsiveness following an occupational exposure as short as 1 week.

Acute upper airway symptoms

Occupational exposure to certain vegetable dusts results in inflammation and drying of the nasal mucosa. This problem commonly leads to a diminished sense of smell, to a chronic irritant rhinitis, and occasionally to chronic sinusitis and recurrent epistaxis. Some of the exposures listed in Table 37.2.1 result in a specific IgE response and allergic rhinitis among some exposed individuals. Nasal lavage of exposed workers typically demonstrates an inflammatory response.

Acute lower airway symptoms

Nearly all workers with high exposures to vegetable dusts exhibit a dry cough, and many develop chest tightness. Both of these symptomatic responses are dose related, are more frequent among smokers, and occur more commonly after an absence from work. Textile workers, who usually do not work weekends, commonly exhibit these symptoms at the beginning of the work week; for instance, Monday cough and chest tightness are the clinical hallmarks of byssinosis.[6–10] With further exposure during the work week, the worker appears to develop a tolerance to the dust, and experiences diminished or no cough or chest tightness on Tuesday or later in the week. With further exposure and lung impairment, chest tightness may occur each day of the work week. New workers or visitors to these work sites, who have a history of asthma, may develop severe asthma after a single significant exposure to vegetable dust, even if the individual has not experienced asthma for several years. Workers who develop asthma almost always remove themselves from these jobs or are identified by medical surveillance programs and moved to jobs that reduce the risk of exposure.

Acute febrile syndromes

Two febrile syndromes have been described among workers exposed to vegetable dusts. It is likely that they differ only in the concentration and circumstance of exposure and share a common etiology: exposure to mycotoxins and endotoxins from gram-negative organisms that are indigenous to vegetable dust. Among workers regularly exposed to high concentrations of vegetable dust for the first time, or after a prolonged absence from exposure, an acute febrile response is often observed for the first several days of employment. This febrile illness, sometimes called mill fever or grain fever, is accompanied by constitutional symptoms of myalgias and fatigue. With further exposure, the worker is said to become 'seasoned' and these symptoms typically disappear.

Among workers exposed to plant products that are heavily contaminated with micro-organisms, such as moldy grain, moldy hay or spotted cotton – especially in poorly ventilated areas such as grain bins, silos or box cars – a severe febrile illness may ensue. With high exposures, workers experience very high rates of a flu-like illness consisting of fever, chills, myalgias, arthralgias, fatigue, cough, and occasionally, shortness of breath. These symptoms predictably begin 6–8 hours after exposure and often continue for many days, but rarely require hospitalization and respiratory assistance. It is common for the affected worker to complain of fatigue for several days or weeks following this illness. This syndrome is now recognized as organic dust toxic syndrome or ODTS. The much rarer, acute phase of farmer's lung disease (FLD, an allergic alveolitis) may also arise from exposure to fungi, thermophilic bacteria, or both. However, FLD differs from ODTS in that it may occur from lower exposures, does not occur in clusters, is progressive with continuing exposure, and may lead to a chronic granulomatous lung disease.

Acute functional responses

Workers exposed to vegetable dusts have been observed to have modest declines, usually 5–10%, in expiratory flow rates over a work shift.[11] Of all o f these measures, FEV_1 has been found to be the least variable and, hence, the most reliable indicator of this response. As a result, cross-shift change in FEV_1 has become a commonly used test for medical surveillance and epidemiologic studies (Fig. 37.2.1).[12] As with acute lower respiratory symptoms, a decline in FEV_1 is related to concentration of inhalable dust and endotoxin in a linear dose–response fashion.[13,14] Although smoking has not been consistently found to have an effect on this measure, it does appear to enhance this response at higher levels of exposure. It has been observed that the FEV_1 and the forced vital capacity (FVC) often are proportionally reduced, with an increase in residual volume (RV) indicative of air trapping. While lower respiratory symptoms of chest tightness and declines in expiratory flow rates are common among exposed workers,

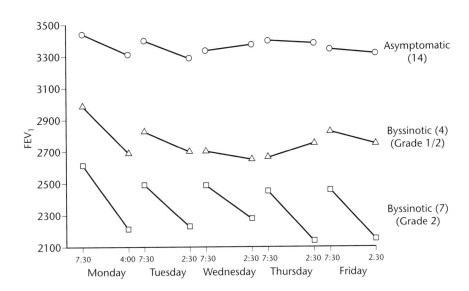

Figure 37.2.1: The pattern of functional response to cotton dust during work week among different types of responders. (With permission from Merchant JA, Halprin GM, Hudson AR, et al. Evaluation before and after exposure – the pattern of physiological response to cotton dust. Ann NY Acad Sci 1974; 221:38–43 © 1974 New York Academy of Sciences, USA.)

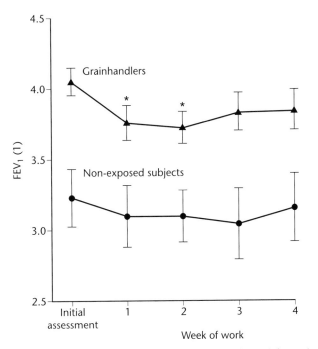

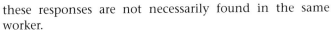

Figure 37.2.2: Forced expired volume in one second (FEV_1) for grain handlers (triangles) and non-exposed subjects (circles) at initial assessment and at end of each week of work. Mean ± SEM * $p<0.05$ compared with initial assessment. (From James AL, Zimmerman MJ, Ee H, et al. Exposure to grain dust and changes in lung function. Br J Ind Med 1990; 47:466–72.)

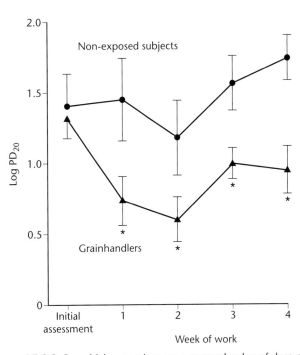

Figure 37.2.3: Bronchial responsiveness, expressed as log of dose of methacholine provoking a 20% fall in baseline FEV_1 (log PD_{20}) for grain handlers (triangles) and non-exposed subjects (circles) at initial assessment and at end of each week of work. Mean ± SEM * $p<0.05$ compared with initial assessment. (From James AL, Zimmerman MJ, Ee H, et al. Exposure to grain dust and changes in lung function. Br J Ind Med 1990; 47:466–72.)

these responses are not necessarily found in the same worker.

Recent studies have demonstrated that although symptoms and the decline in FEV_1 observed following these exposures usually resolve within a day or two, (Fig. 37.2.2) airway hyper-responsiveness commonly persists (Fig. 37.2.3).[15] Prospective studies of respiratory symptoms and lung function suggest that those with acute respiratory symptoms are at greater risk of the development of chronic airway obstruction from chronic exposure to vegetable dusts.[16]

Chronic health effects

With prolonged exposures to vegetable dust, as commonly occurs in the cotton textile industry and among grain handlers, some workers will develop chronic bronchitis and irreversible airway obstruction.[17,18] While not as easily demonstrated as are acute health effects, these chronic effects also are dose related.

Data from the cotton textile industry indicate that even low doses of cotton dust (below the OSHA standard of

0.2 mg/m^3) may not be fully protective, especially if the worker continues to smoke.[14,19] Although chronic bronchitis frequently occurs within the first few years of employment, significant airway obstruction usually is not observed until after 10 years of employment. With prolonged occupational exposure to moderate or high concentrations of these vegetable dusts, some workers may develop severe and disabling chronic airway obstruction. Cigarette smoking has been found to be an important additive risk factor to both chronic bronchitis and chronic airway obstruction among these workers. Although removal of workers with acute responses from these exposures makes prospective evaluation of this question more difficult, those with the acute responses of chest tightness and significant cross-shift declines in FEV$_1$ do appear to have accelerated annual declines in FEV$_1$. This observation adds to the importance of recognition of acute responses to vegetable dusts for both clinical and preventive applications. Thus with improved dust control in the cotton textile industry, which resulted from a standard based on acute dose–response data, the proportion of workers with chronic airway diseases has significantly declined.

MANAGEMENT AND PREVENTION

Epidemiologic studies of workers exposed to vegetable dusts have provided very good guidance for clinical management. Many of the tests employed in epidemiologic studies have been applied to medical surveillance programs for exposed workers. Similarly, some of the environmental measurement techniques, notably the use of the vertical elutriator in the cotton textile industry, have been adopted for environmental monitoring of some of these workplaces. Because both acute and chronic health effects are dose related, dust control is the foundation for all other elements of management and prevention. With increasing confidence that acute health effects are predictors of chronic health effects for these exposures, dose–response studies of acute respiratory symptoms and changes in lung function are gaining greater importance as indicators of appropriate permissible limits (PELs).

Management of affected individuals

Management of workers affected by these exposures is extremely important. Medical surveillance methods mandated by the United States OSHA Cotton Dust Standard still provide useful guidance. Exposed workers should have annual medical evaluations during which respiratory symptoms, smoking status, and FEV$_1$ before and after a Monday work shift should be documented. Those with acute respiratory symptoms or significant and replicable declines in FEV$_1$ (>5%) should be transferred to a low dust exposure area and monitored at least semiannually. Workers with significant airway obstruction (FEV$_1$ less than 2 standard deviations [SDs] of predicted) should similarly be transferred to low-exposure areas. Those workers who exhibit rapid declines in lung function or moderate to

severe airway obstruction (<60% of predicted for race, sex, age, and height) should be referred for a full pulmonary evaluation to determine their eligibility or need for reassignment to a job involving no exposure to vegetable dust and/or workers' compensation.

Workers who develop clinical asthma from their exposure to vegetable dust must be evaluated very carefully. Some with asthma may be transferred to low-dust areas, which may result in asthma control. Respiratory protective devices may be useful with mild asthma. If such a move appears to be successful, these individuals must be followed closely (at least every 3 to 6 months) to assess respiratory symptoms and lung function. With worsening asthma or a progressive decline in lung function – even at a low level of exposure – it is then very important to transfer the worker to a work area that is free of vegetable dust and other respiratory irritants. For some, asthma may be so severe that continued work is not possible, even in an area that is free of respiratory irritants. In these cases, the only recourse may be to assist the worker in seeking workers' compensation.

Prevention

Prevention of acute and chronic health effects arising from exposure to vegetable dusts and assessment of risk depends on assessment and control of dust levels. Dose–response studies of several vegetable dusts, including cotton and mixed grains, have resulted in recommended PELs for each of these exposures. In the United States cotton textile industry, in which assessment of dose has depended on use of the vertical elutriator, OSHA has set a PEL of 0.2 mg/m^3 for exposure to cotton dust in preparation and yarn processing areas, and a PEL of 0.75 mg/m^3 for slashing and weaving areas where biologically inactive, but inhalable, material is added to the process.[14] Over the decades that have followed regulation of cotton dust, considerable progress has been made by the cotton textile industry through the use of new technology, exhaust ventilation, and improved work practices. Based on dose–response studies of grain handlers, which have depended on measurement of total dust, the American Conference of Governmental Industrial Hygienists (ACGIH) has recommended a Threshold Limit Value (TLV) of 4 mg/m^3 for mixed grain dust. Based on the documented adverse health effects, these dose–response relationships, and the risk of grain dust explosions, concentrations of grain dust have been reduced over time (Fig. 37.2.4).

Routine medical surveillance of workers with these exposures is also necessary. The medical surveillance plan implemented through the US OSHA Cotton Dust Standard has proven to be both practical and effective in management of workers with adverse health effects. As dust is controlled, the numbers of workers with adverse health effects decrease, and these medical surveillance programs become more easily managed. Other aspects of prevention include attention to work practices to reduce exposure, appropriate use of personal protective equipment, notification of workers regarding the risks of these and other hazardous exposures, and appropriate record keeping of both medical and

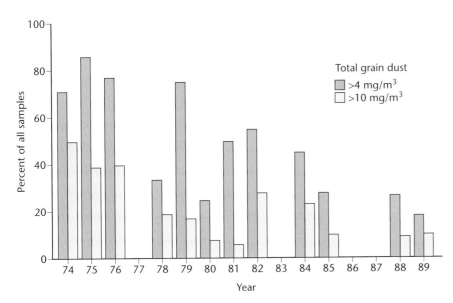

Figure 37.2.4: Proportion of personal dust samples (total grain dust) measuring greater than 4 mg/m^3 (dark bars) or greater than 10 mg/m^3 (pale bars) for Vancouver terminal grain elevators 1974–1989; total number of samples overall = 781 (100). (With permission from Chan-Yeung M, Emerson DA, Kennedy SM. State of the art – the impact of grain dust on respiratory health. Am Rev Respir Dis 1992; 145:476–87. Official Journal of the American Thoracic Society © American Lung Association.)

environmental data. In settings where dust control is not possible, as often occurs in farming, the appropriate use of respirators can diminish exposure. Finally, prospective epidemiologic studies of these vegetable dust exposures and their respiratory disease outcomes will refine our understanding of the natural history of health effects arising from these exposures, improve techniques to measure biologically relevant dose, and yield more innovative dust control and prevention methods.

References

1. Fishwick D, Allan LJ, Wright A, Curran AD. Assessment of exposure to organic dust in a hemp processing plant. Ann Occup Hyg 2001; 45:577–83.
2. Chan-Yeung M, Enarson DA, Kennedy SM. State of art – the impact of grain dust on respiratory health. Am Rev Respir Dis 1992; 145:476–87.
3. Ramazzini B. Diseases of workers, 1713. Translation by George Rosen. New York: Hafner Publishing Company, 1964.
4. Anto JM, Sunyer J, Rodriguez-Roisin R, et al. Community outbreaks of asthma associated with inhalation of soybean dust. N Engl J Med 1989; 320:1097–102.
5. Chan-Yeung M, Lam S. State of art – occupational asthma. Am Rev Respir Dis 1986; 133:686–703.
6. Christiani DC, Wegman DH, Eisen EA, et al. Cotton dust and gram-negative bacterial endotoxin correlations in two cotton textile mills. Am J Ind Med 1993; 23:333–42.
7. Deetz DC, Jagielo PJ, Quinn TJ, et al. The kinetics of grain dust-induced inflammation of the lower respiratory tract. Am J Respir Crit Care Med 1997 155:254–9.
8. Monso E, Magarolas R, Badorrey I, et al. Occupational asthma in greenhouse flower and ornamental plant growers. Am J Respir Crit Care Med 2002; 165:959–60.
9. Obata H, Dittrick M, Chan H, Chan-Yeung M. Occupational asthma due to exposure to African cherry (Makore) wood dust. Intern Med 2000; 39:947–9.
10. Smith TA, Lumley KPS. Work-related asthma in a population exposed to grain, flour and other ingredient dusts. Occup Med 1996; 46:37–40.
11. James AL, Zimmerman MJ, Ee H, et al. Exposure to grain dust and changes in lung function. Br J Ind Med 1990; 47:466–72.
12. Merchant JA, Halprin GM, Hudson AR, et al. Evaluation before and after exposure – the pattern of physiologic response to cotton dust. Ann NY Acad Sci 1974; 221:38–43.
13. Castellan RM, Olenchock SA, Kinsley KB, Hankinson JL. Inhaled endotoxin and decreased spirometric values. N Engl J Med 1987; 317:605–10.
14. Merchant JA, Lumsden JC, Kilburn KH, et al. Dose–response studies in cotton textile workers. J Occup Med 1973; 15:222–30.
15. Kline, J, Jagielo PJ, Watt JL, Schwartz DA. Bronchial hyper-reactivity is associated with enhanced grain dust-induced airflow obstruction. J Appl Physiol 2000; 89:1172–8.
16. Glindmeyer HW, Lenfante JJ, Jones RN, et al. Exposure-related declines in the lung function of cotton textile workers. Am Rev Respir Dis 1991; 144:675–83.
17. Huy T, De Schipper K, Chan-Yeung M, Kennedy SM. Grain dust and lung function – dose–response relationship. Am Rev Respir Dis 1991; 144:1314–21.
18. Tanaka H, Saikai T, Sugawara H, et al. Workplace-related chronic cough on a mushroom farm. Chest 2002; 122:1080–5.
19. World Health Organization Study Group. Recommended health-based occupational exposure limits for selected vegetable dusts. Technical Report Series 684. Geneva: World Health Organization, 1983.

Chapter 38
Psychologic Stressors and Work Organization

James W Grosch, Steven L Sauter

Job stress is an everyday reality for many workers and a growing concern in the field of occupational safety and health. This is especially true in light of recent changes in the workplace (e.g., increasing work hours; non-standard employment practices) and increasing evidence that stress has serious implications for worker health. Although job stress is still a subject of some uncertainty to many occupational safety and health professionals, research over the past four decades has taught us much about the sources, effects, and prevention of stress in the workplace.

This chapter begins with a brief historical perspective on job stress and then presents an overview of current knowledge organized around three fundamental questions.
- What is job stress?
- How is job stress related to occupational safety and health?
- How can the adverse effects of job stress be reduced or prevented?

JOB STRESS: HISTORICAL PERSPECTIVE AND OVERVIEW

The field of occupational stress coalesced in the 1960s, arising amidst growing concerns over worker alienation, job dissatisfaction, and mental health problems, concerns which originated during the Industrial Revolution, with the implementation of mass production technologies and the re-design of jobs. Mass production methods and the introduction of scientific management principles at the end of the 19th century resulted in the simplification and fragmentation of jobs into highly repetitive and routine tasks, and the treatment of workers as commodities motivated purely by economic rewards.

The well-known Western Electric Hawthorne studies[1] and other studies beginning in the 1920s, however, drew attention to the fact that social and psychologic factors that had been given little attention served as important motivators for workers. The Hawthorne investigators realized that the increased attention, feedback, and freedom from supervisory control given to workers in the context of studies on the effects of lighting and other physical environmental factors had an important independent effect on productivity. These landmark observations paved the way for what would later become the human relations movement and efforts to 'humanize' the workplace. They also set the stage for a new field of research on the effects of social and psychologic aspects of work on the satisfaction, health, and mental health of workers.

In 1935, Robert Hoppock surveyed the entire population of New Hope, Pennsylvania, and discovered substantial occupational differences in satisfaction, with unskilled manual laborers exhibiting the least satisfaction and professional and managerial workers exhibiting the most satisfaction.[2] In studies of automotive workers in the 1940s, Walker and Guest found that the rigid pacing and fragmentation of work in the automotive assembly line led to high levels of stress and discontent among workers.[3] Ciulla reported annual turnover of 100–250% in automobile assembly work in the early decades of the 20th century.[4] Observations similar to Walker and Guest's findings were reported in other industrial settings by Kornhauser in his seminal book *Mental health of the industrial worker*.[5]

Before long, theories and models of occupational stress began to emerge in both the US and Europe. Research in Sweden by Bertil Gardel, Lennart Levi and their colleagues at the Karolinska Institute identified the lack of control and limited opportunities for learning and social interaction characteristic of industrial work as important risk factors for stress and illness among workers.[6] Notably, these factors occupy a central place in the present day 'demand-control' model of job stress popularized by the work of Robert Karasek.[7,8] Robert Kahn drew attention to work roles (role conflict and ambiguity) as risk factors for job stress in the early 1960s[9] and, together with colleagues at the University of Michigan Institute for Social Research, pioneered epidemiologic studies and theoretical developments in job stress in the US. Particularly notable in this regard was the highly influential study of job stress and health that investigated the impact of nearly two dozen facets of job demands in 23 occupations on somatic complaints and psychophysiologic outcomes.[10]

Job stress research subsequently flourished in the US and Europe. Beehr[11] observed that prior to 1972 not a single entry could be found under the heading 'occupational stress' in the index of 'Psychological Abstracts', but the number of abstracts then grew exponentially. In the US, much of this growing momentum could be attributed to leading figures such as Alan McLean of the Center for Occupational Mental Health, Cornell University, who worked with industry, labor, and government organizations to host major conferences on stress at work in the 1960s and 1970s.[12] The US Department of Health,

Education and Welfare also played a key role. In 1965, a task force appointed by the Surgeon General expressed concern that 'millions of American workers, as a direct result of their occupations, are exposed to health damage . . . increasingly from psychological stress' and appealed for greater attention in the occupational health field to this problem.[13] In 1971 a task force was convened by Elliot Richardson (then Secretary of the Department of Health, Education and Welfare) and in 1974 issued the highly acclaimed report *Work in America*[14] that concluded that workers and society are bearing serious medical costs that have their genesis in preventable workplace stressors. In this same period, Congress passed the Occupational Safety and Health Act that gave broad recognition to behavioral factors and stress as etiologic agents for occupational disease and injury, and charged NIOSH with the responsibility for investigating these factors.[15]

Today there exists widespread appreciation of the threat that stress poses to the health of workers and organizations. In the US, nearly half the states legitimize 'mental injury' from stressful working conditions as a compensable condition under workers' compensation,[16] and these types of claims grew dramatically throughout the 1980s until legislative reforms reduced their numbers. Northwestern National Life Insurance (now Reliastar) reported that stress-related disability claims comprised 13% of all disability claims processed in 1990 – up from 6% in 1980.[17]

Most recently, concerns have been expressed that the rapid restructuring of jobs and the workforce evidenced in the tumultuous 1990s and continuing today may further heighten the risk of stress among workers.[18] Data from the Families and Work Institute, for example, show a marked increase from 1977 to 2001 in the percentage of workers who report that they work very hard (70–88%) and never have enough time to get things done on the job (40–60%). During roughly this same period, prime-age working couples increased their annual work time by nearly 700 hours.[19] Although available information fails to confirm an increase in reported job stress in the last decade, the prevalence of reported job stress during this period remains high. US representative data obtained from the General Social Survey show that the percentage of workers who reported their jobs to be 'often' or 'always' stressful was 39% in 1989 and 36% in 1998.[20] These figures are in reasonable agreement with other recent data suggesting that stressful working conditions are very prevalent. For example, in the 1991 Northwestern National Life study, 40% of workers reported their jobs to be 'very' or 'extremely' stressful. In 1997, the Families and Work Institute reported that 26% of workers said they were 'often' or 'very often' burned out or stressed by their jobs, and 36% felt 'often' or 'very often' used up at the end of the day.[21]

These high levels of reported stress take on special significance in the presence of recent data on the economic and health burden of stress in the American workforce. Data from the Bureau of Labor Statistics Survey of Occupational Injuries and Illnesses show that lost-time cases due to job stress are among the most serious in terms of the length of the disability period. In 1997, the median absence period

was 23 days, more than four times the median for all other injuries and illness.[22] Adding to these data is sobering information on increased healthcare utilization among workers reporting high levels of stress in the workplace. In a 1998 study of 4600 employees, healthcare costs were 46% greater for workers reporting high levels of stress compared to workers reporting low levels of stress. The increment rose to nearly 150% for workers reporting high levels of both stress and depression.[23]

Together with improved recognition of the scope and organizational costs of stress in the workplace, research has led to a better scientific understanding of the stress process – risk factors, mechanisms, safety and health effects, and of interventions to prevent stress at work. In following sections of this chapter current knowledge on these topics is summarized, beginning with an overview of different conceptual approaches to stress and the stress process.

WHAT IS JOB STRESS?

As concern about job stress has grown, the different ways in which stress is defined and conceptualized have expanded.[24–26] These approaches, in emphasizing different elements of the stress experience, provide a sense of how our understanding of job stress has evolved over the past few decades.

Job stress as a response

Perhaps the most obvious approach is to focus on how the body responds to a threatening situation. In this case, stress is viewed as a dependent variable and conceptualized in terms of changes that an individual experiences in physiologic, emotional, and behavioral functioning. Walter Cannon, an early investigator of the physiologic aspects of emotion, described the 'flight or fight response' that typically occurs when a organism perceives a threat. Although this response can be adaptive in some situations, Cannon argued that it can also be harmful, particularly when it involves the repeated activation of the sympathetic nervous system and the endocrine system.[27]

Hans Selye extended this physiologic perspective and introduced a triphasic model, called the general adaptation syndrome, to describe an individual's response to a stressful situation.[28] In the alarm phase, the body reacts with an increase in adrenal activity, as well as cardiovascular and respiratory functioning. During the resistance stage, the individual either takes action to overcome the external threat or learns to adjust to it. Finally, if continued wear and tear on the body takes place, exhaustion occurs involving a depletion of physiologic resources and an increased likelihood of illness or disease. Underlying this model is Selye's definition of stress as a 'non-specific response of the body to any demand made upon it'.[28] Although we now know that there can be subtle differences in how the body reacts to different types of external threats,[29] Selye's model provides a useful first step in understanding how repeated stress can result in disorders, such as cardiovascular disease, musculoskeletal problems, hypertension, and immune-related deficiencies.

Job stress as a stimulus

An alternative perspective is to view stress as being 'out there' or part of the external environment. This approach has its roots in engineering and the focus on understanding what happens when an outside force or demand is applied to an object. In this case, stress is an independent variable that produces harm when an individual's tolerance level is exceeded. Symonds[30] summarized this view when he stated that 'stress is that which happens to the man, not that which happens in him; it is a set of causes not a set of symptoms'. Much of the impetus for this perspective comes from early industrialization when the primary concern regarding worker health centered on the physical work environment (e.g., heat, noise, social density) that could be measured objectively. This view has contributed to the cataloging of different sources of job stress and a desire to develop objective measures that do not necessarily depend on individual perception.

Current models of job stress

Defining job stress solely in terms of either a response or a stimulus has inherent limitations. Both of these approaches are static, overly simplistic, and reflect only one component of the stress experience. They largely ignore individual differences that can moderate the impact of stressful conditions, as well as perceptual and cognitive processes that may ultimately determine how a worker interprets and responds to a stressful situation. Most contemporary theorists agree that job stress is best thought of as an interaction between a person and his or her work environment. In other words, job stress does not lie solely in the individual or in the situation, but rather, in the degree of 'fit' between the two.[31,32] Job stress terminology has also come to reflect an interactionist perspective, with 'stressor' referring to adverse events in the work environment and 'strain' referring to the physiologic and emotional responses to those events.

Despite a general consensus on job stress as an interaction, contemporary theories of job stress vary with regard to the features in the person or work environment they emphasize. These theories can be viewed as falling onto a continuum that ranges from a *clinical perspective*, which emphasizes primarily individual-level processes, to a *public health perspective*, which emphasizes job and organizational-level factors. To some degree, this continuum still reflects the response and stimulus biases of earlier approaches, but it also provides a much richer view of the range of factors that need to be considered in understanding the causes and consequences of job stress.

Clinical perspective

Clinical models of job stress acknowledge the importance of the individual in the stress process, and factors such as coping and stress management tend to play an important

role in prevention strategies. One area receiving a great deal of attention is the appraisal process, or how an individual evaluates the environment, the threats it may pose, and ways of coping with those threats. Lazarus[33,34] argued that appraisal is a fundamental element of the job stress experience and proposed two different types: primary appraisal in which an individual initially determines whether or not a situation presents a risk (stressful or not), and secondary appraisal in which an individual determines the availability of different coping options for dealing with the stress.

Appraisal is conceptualized as a dynamic, or transactional, process that develops over time through an ongoing relationship between an individual and the work environment. Lazarus's theory also focuses on identifying different types of coping strategies.[35] For example, workers may adopt a coping strategy that is problem focused and involves an attempt to alter the situation by changing either one's behavior or some aspect of the environment. Alternatively, workers may choose an emotion-focused strategy that involves an attempt to regulate or manage the strain experienced from a particular event. This basic dichotomy has inspired other experts on stress to develop more elaborate taxonomies of coping strategies that can be found in the literature (e.g., Pearlin et al[36]). Most authors emphasize that there is no single best coping strategy, and effectiveness must be evaluated in light of individual characteristics and the specific work context.

The emphasis on appraisal and coping advocated by Lazarus can be found in a number of theories on job stress, usually referred to as 'transactional' models of job stress. Cox and Mackay,[37] for example, proposed that stress occurs when there is an imbalance between the perception of environmental demands and a worker's ability to cope with those demands. The impact of this imbalance is determined through a five-stage sequence that includes: cognitive appraisal of work demands, a judgment of one's ability to cope with the demands, awareness of changes in wellbeing, evaluation of the effectiveness of coping strategies and, finally, stress that affects future perceptions of work demands and selection of coping strategies. Consistent with Lazarus's view, the emphasis rests with understanding how workers perceive, interpret, and individually react to their environment.

A more current approach to job stress focusing on the individual is advocated by Siegrist,[38] who goes further than Lazarus in targeting specific features of the work environment. Siegrist proposed that chronic strain results from a perceived imbalance between the efforts required of an individual and the rewards he or she receives for that effort. In other words, strain occurs when there is a combination of high effort and low reward at work. Siegrist defined effort as consisting of both extrinsic (e.g., work demands and pressure) and intrinsic (e.g., coping pattern) dimensions. Rewards were measured by combining the financial, self-esteem, and status outcomes a worker receives from a job. According to the model, an imbalance between effort and rewards (i.e., high effort/low reward condition) produces 'a state of emotional distress with special propensity to autonomic arousal and associated strain reactions'. Initial findings indicate a significant link between perceptions of effort/reward imbalance and cardiovascular risk factors, such as hypertension and altered lipoproteins. Although additional research is needed to further evaluate the assumptions of the Siegrist model and its applicability to other health outcomes, this approach highlights the importance of an aspect of the workplace – namely, the perceived fairness of costs and benefits experienced by employees – that is seldom emphasized in other theories of job stress.

Public health perspective

Public health models of job stress differ from clinical models in that they tend to place more emphasis on the work experience itself as a risk factor for job stress, and work reorganization as the primary strategy for preventing stress at work. Two factors in this tradition that have long been associated with heightened levels of strain are excessive work demands and lack of control over one's work environment. A widely recognized model incorporating both of these dimensions was proposed by Karasek[7] and is referred to as the demands–control model.

Figure 38.1 presents this model in terms of four different combinations of control (also referred to as 'decision latitude') and demands (high versus low). A key prediction of the model is that demands and control interact so that workers falling into quadrant IV (high demands, low control) experience the highest levels of job strain and an increase in the risk of illness (e.g., cardiovascular disease). However, workers in quadrant III, with active jobs, who experience high demands *and* high control, are at less risk of strain. In other words, a high degree of control offsets the harmful effects of high work demands. The other two quadrants are also seen as producing reduced strain, although workers in quadrant I may report problems associated with monotony or boredom. Unlike the Siegrist or Lazarus models, the demands–control perspective does not place much emphasis on individual differences or worker attempts to cope with the strain they experience. Karasek's model has been widely tested and has received a moderate level of support, although empirical evidence for an inter-

active effect (in contrast to an additive effect) between control and demands is generally weak and inconsistent. In addition, the model has recently been expanded to include the dimension of social support, which is seen as a factor that can reduce the harmful effects of a job that has high demands and low control.

Many other organizational-level factors have been implicated with regard to worker strain. For example, Robert Kahn and his colleagues emphasized the importance of *role demands* that workers face.[9] These demands include stressors such as *role ambiguity* (i.e., lack of clarity about work expectations) and *role conflict* (i.e., incompatible work demands) and have been linked to a variety of adverse health outcomes.[26] *Job insecurity* has also received a great deal of attention, particularly as organizations downsize their workforces and increasingly rely on temporary, or contingent, workers. Much of this research focuses on unemployment (actual or anticipated) and its association with outcomes such as poor health, depression, and suicide.[39] Specific work practices such as *shift work* and *long working hours* have also been studied with regard to their potential negative impact on workers.

In order to include a broad range of variables in a single framework, researchers have developed process models that draw on variables from a variety of theories and empirical studies.[40–42] Figure 38.2 illustrates the NIOSH job stress model developed by Hurrell and Murphy.[42] This model views stress as an interaction between working conditions, or stressors, and individual worker characteristics that results in acute strain reactions which, if continued over time, lead to illness and injury. Job stressors include those already described (e.g., control, role demands), as well as variables taken from other theoretical perspectives.

An important feature of the NIOSH model is the identification of factors that can moderate or buffer the health impact of job stressors. For example, personality can play an important role in how an individual reacts to a stressful environment. Two personality constructs receiving increasing attention in recent years are the Type A behavior pattern and self-efficacy. Type A individuals are characterized by high levels of competitiveness, achievement striving, time urgency, and aggressiveness. Individuals displaying this pattern, and particularly those with high levels of hostility, may be more prone to develop cardiovascular heart disease.[43] In contrast, individuals with high self-efficacy are confident in their abilities and believe they are capable of successfully completing a given task. Research indicates that this quality may help individuals remain resilient in the face of stressful working conditions.[44] Despite these moderators, the emphasis of the NIOSH model rests with organizational and job-based stressors, which are viewed as having the most significant and direct impact on the acute reactions and illnesses ultimately experienced by workers.

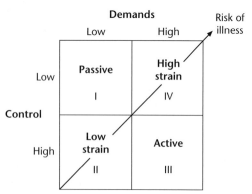

Figure 38.1: The demand and control model of job strain. (Adapted from Karasek R, Theorell T. Healthy work: stress productivity and the reconstruction of working life. New York: Wiley & Sons, 1990).

Conclusions

Of all the theories reviewed thus far, none has met with universal acceptance. Indeed, a number of methodologic

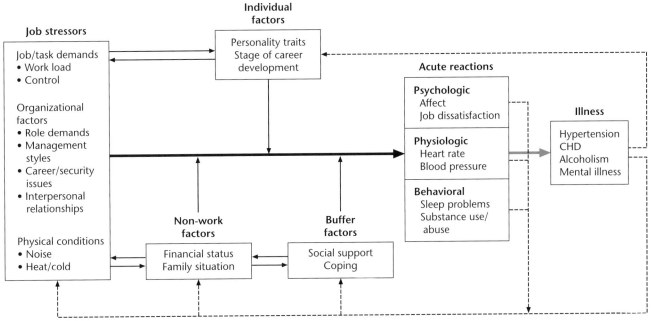

Figure 38.2: A process model of job stress and health. (From Hurrell JJ, Murphy LR. Psychological job stress. In: Rom WN, ed. Environmental and occupational medicine, 3rd edn. Boston: Little, Brown and Company, 1998).

challenges remain if our understanding of job stress is to progress in the future. These include the further development of improved measures for assessing risk factors for stress at work (e.g., assessments by coworkers, managers, objective measures) and greater reliance on prospective studies that follow workers over time. However, current theories of job stress provide different focal points that are useful in diagnosing and treating stress-related problems. Whether we adopt a clinical or public health perspective, job stress needs to be viewed as a complex interactive process involving both the workplace and the individual that, if left unchecked, can have serious consequences for a worker's health and safety.

HOW IS JOB STRESS RELATED TO OCCUPATIONAL SAFETY AND HEALTH?
Potential pathways linking job stress and health outcomes

Before discussing specific outcomes associated with job stress, the different pathways through which stress may affect safety and health should be addressed. Figure 38.3 presents a model based on the work of Cohen and Rodriguez,[45] who focused on understanding the link between psychologic and physical disorders. The model is intended to be heuristic in nature and makes no attempt to include all possible variables or pathways affecting the development of a particular health disorder (e.g., individual differences and cultural variables are omitted). However, the four pathways identified in the model provide a useful conceptualization of how stress can result in health

disorders that has implications for both treatment and prevention.

Biologic pathways

Changes in physiologic functioning represent the most direct pathway between stress and health and have been studied in both human and animal subjects. These changes can be categorized as either non-specific (occurring with most affective states) or specific (occurring with some affective states more than others). Two non-specific changes involve the activation of the sympathetic-adrenal-medullary (SAM) system and the hypothalamic-pituitary-adrenocortical (HPA) axis. SAM activation involves sympathetic arousal and release of adrenaline and noradrenaline from the adrenal medulla, two catecholamines that stimulate organ systems throughout the body, leading to a heightened state of physiologic activation (e.g., increased heart rate, blood pressure, skin conductivity, and respiration). HPA activation, on the other hand, is characterized by the release of three main hormones. Initially, corticotropin-releasing hormone is secreted by the hypothalamus, causing the pituitary gland to release adrenocorticotropic hormone. This stimulates the adrenal cortex which, in turn, releases corticosteroids. One of the most important corticosteroids is cortisol, which works to increase the level of fatty acids and glucose in the blood stream. Research suggests that excessive activation of SAM and HPA contributes to a variety of disorders, including coronary heart disease, essential hypertension, increased susceptibility to infectious disease, atherosclerosis, and chronic inflammatory responses, such as rheumatoid arthritis.[46]

Physiologic changes can also show specificity with regard to the nature of the external threat. For example, research

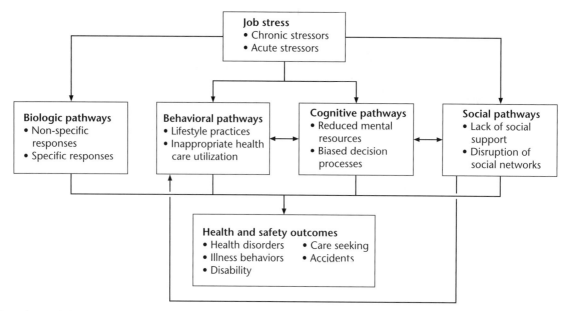

Figure 38.3: Pathways linking job stress to health and safety outcomes (based on a model developed by Cohen S, Rodriguez MS. Pathways linking affective disturbances and physical disorders. Health Psychol 1995; 14:374–80).

suggests that anxiety-producing situations are associated with increased levels of adrenaline, whereas increased levels of noradrenaline are associated with aggression-producing situations.[29] Similarly, in terms of specific job stressors, Frankenhaeuser[47] has proposed that the body's response is different for work that is demanding versus work in which there is a lack of control. In the former case, adrenaline levels are thought to increase; in the latter case cortisol levels are also raised because the worker is more likely to feel distress or unhappiness.

Behavioral pathways

Stressful situations and events can also lead to behaviors that make an individual more vulnerable to health problems. These behaviors can be viewed as maladaptive coping strategies that may provide some relief in the short term, but hold serious health consequences over the long term. The list of behaviors linked to job stress includes smoking,[48] alcohol consumption, lack of exercise, poor diet,[49] being overweight,[50] non-medical drug use,[51] and poor sleeping habits.[52] In addition, stress at work may influence whether or not an individual seeks out appropriate healthcare services for a problem, and the degree to which workers are willing and able to follow safety practices at work that should reduce the risk of accident or injury.

Cognitive pathways

Job stress can also influence how an individual thinks about or appraises a given situation at work. This appraisal process includes specific beliefs that develop about the harm or threat posed by an event, its causes and controllability. In terms of health perception, research suggests that stress can lead to different biases in how a worker interprets various physical symptoms and decides at what point it is appropriate to seek diagnosis or treatment.[53] Also,

cognitive responses to stress can result in mental fatigue and a reduced ability to attend to other tasks. As a result, there may be less time and energy to focus on other demands, leading to arousal, reduced performance, and other symptoms of strain.

Social pathways

The value of social support from family, friends, and coworkers has long been studied by stress researchers. Although social support is often included in job stress models as a moderator variable (see Fig. 38.2), it can also be viewed as an outcome variable that is itself influenced by job stress. For example, stress can reduce an individual's ability to maintain or build social networks that provide the necessary resources for coping with difficult situations.[54] When social networks are disrupted, an individual may have less incentive to follow good health practices and may be less likely to seek care for a given health problem.

An important feature of Figure 38.3 is that the four pathways described above interact, so that, for example, a change in social functioning might produce a change in cognition and behavior which, in turn, increases susceptibility to a physical illness over time. This model highlights the complexity of the stress process and the fact that job stressors have a variety of avenues through which they can influence a worker's health and safety. The actual pathways a job stressor activates are undoubtedly influenced by many factors at both the individual and organizational level.

Safety and health outcomes affected by job stress

In addition to identifying pathways, a good deal of research has focused on identifying the potential outcomes associated with job stress. A brief overview of this research is provided below and is divided into three broad categories: physical health, mental health, and organizational-level outcomes.

Physical health outcomes

Cardiovascular heart disease (CHD) Much of the research on CHD focuses on the two job stressors identified in the Karasek model (see Fig. 38.1): work demands and job control. For example, in a large prospective cohort study of British civil servants, low job control, both self-reported and externally assessed, was associated with an increased risk of new coronary heart disease. This risk remained after adjustment for lifestyle and personality factors, suggesting that the job control–heart disease association is independent of personal characteristics.[55] Numerous other studies have examined the importance of job control and job demands with regard to a broad range of CHD outcomes, including high blood pressure, angina, myocardial infarction, elevated concentrations of fibrinogen, and subclinical carotid atherosclerosis. Overall, the findings suggest that a significant role is played by both of these job stressors, although there are notable exceptions (e.g., Hlatky et al[56]) and methodologic issues exist regarding how demands and control should be defined and measured.[57] Research on other job stressors has found increased CHD risk for specific work practices, such as shift work and overtime work, as well as for more general psychosocial factors, such as reduced job complexity and social support, and job insecurity.[58]

Musculoskeletal disorders Some of the most common job stressors that have been studied with regard to musculoskeletal disorders include mentally demanding work, monotony, reduced coworker and supervisor support, time pressure, reduced job control and reduced opportunities for rest breaks. Overall, evidence suggests that these types of stressors are associated with work-related low back pain and, less consistently, with work-related upper extremity disorders.[59] These findings are impressive given the range of different research methodologies that have been employed. However, more remains to be learned regarding the biologic pathways through which job stress produces musculoskeletal problems, and the degree to which job stressors and physical demands interact.[60]

Immune deficiency disorders Numerous studies suggest that the physiologic changes associated with stress (e.g., release of cortisol) can have a serious impact on the immune system. Laboratory research has established that psychologic stress can produce changes in the level of antibodies in the blood and the level of many white blood cells.[61] Exposure to even brief periods of stress may influence levels of natural killer cells and lymphocytes. Changes in immune functioning, however, are very complex and seem to depend not only on the type of stressor, but also on what type of coping strategy the individual is using to deal with the situation. Health problems that have been linked to stress-induced immune suppres-

sion include asthma, rheumatoid arthritis, a wide range of infectious diseases, and recovery from illnesses such as pneumonia and the flu.[46] Although one might expect that immune suppression would be linked to increased risk for cancer, there is little direct evidence to support this association.[62]

Gastrointestinal problems A good deal of research has focused on the relationship between stress and the development of ulcers caused by factors such as pepsinogen levels or inadequate secretion of bicarbonate and mucus. In a review of this literature, Suls concluded that, although humans exposed to acute stress in the context of severe physical trauma are prone to ulcers, the evidence for an association with psychologic job and life stressors is weak.[63] Evidence that job (or life) stress causes elevated levels of pepsinogen and acid secretion, or that ulcer patients experience more work stressors is inconsistent. Additional research has recently focused on irritable bowel syndrome (IBS) and non-ulcer dyspepsia (NUD). Again, evidence for a link with job stress is weak. Although IBS and NUD patients tend to report greater anxiety levels, it is not clear whether this is a precursor or a consequence of gastrointestinal ailments.

Mental health outcomes

Emotional distress and depression There is a substantial body of research examining the link between job stress and different indices of emotional distress, including depression, anxiety, and fatigue. Some of these studies are conducted at the occupational level and report that certain occupations (e.g., machine operators, painters, kitchen workers) experience higher levels of depressive symptoms than other occupations.[64] Attempts to identify workplace factors that underlie these differences have focused on a wide variety of job stressors, including control/autonomy, time pressure, job security, work demands, role conflict and ambiguity, and perceptions of fairness. In a review of this literature, Jex and Beehr[65] concluded that measures of emotional distress (or affect) are one of the strongest correlates of job stress. Additional longitudinal research is needed, however, to more carefully examine the causal nature of this relationship.

Burnout Job burnout can be considered a special case of emotional strain and is characterized by feelings of cynicism, exhaustion, and inefficacy.[66] Burnout has been studied principally with regard to human service professionals (e.g., teachers, nurses, social workers) who develop strong emotional relationships with clients or coworkers as part of their work. The causes of job burnout vary somewhat with the occupational group being studied, but include many of the stressors reviewed earlier in this chapter. Particular attention has been given to the importance of role conflict, lack of autonomy, and the absence of social support.[24]

Suicide Much of the research on risk factors for suicide has focused on the role of specific life events, including those that occur in the workplace. In several studies, changes at work that affect job security, such as losing a job, are associated with an increased risk of suicide or attempted suicide.[39,67] Since suicide is a rare event, most of this research has relied on the retrospective analysis of large archival datasets. As a result, it is difficult to rule out the role of other factors, such as prior mental health status or social support, which might also increase suicide risk. In any event, the link between suicide and work events (e.g., layoff, demotion) appears to be at least as strong as that between suicide and non-work events (e.g., illness of a spouse, death of a close friend).[68]

Organizational-level outcomes

Job dissatisfaction, absenteeism, and turnover Probably the most widely cited organizational-level response to job stress is job dissatisfaction. Although research indicates that these two variables are strongly correlated, this finding may also reflect a certain degree of conceptual overlap in terms of what each variable is attempting to measure. Job stress has also been consistently associated with employee withdrawal behavior, in the form of increased absenteeism, turnover, and willingness to retire early.[26]

Job performance A recent review reports that the link between job stress and job performance varies greatly across studies and, on average, does not appear to be particularly strong.[69] One reason for this conclusion is that job performance is a multidimensional concept, with not all dimensions showing the same relationship with stress. Evidence suggests that performance dimensions containing either an emotional or a social component are more likely to be associated with stress. Examples include counterproductive behaviors at work (e.g., stealing), organizational citizenship behaviors (e.g., helping coworkers), and workplace aggression. Interestingly, these are aspects of a worker's behavior that are only rarely covered in traditional performance reviews, suggesting that organizations need to adopt a broader perspective of what constitutes good job performance.

Accidents As with job performance, the relationship between job stress and accidents is complex. An important model linking job stress to an increased risk of workplace accidents has been developed by Murphy et al.[70] The first stage of this model focuses on acute, short-term reactions experienced by workers under stress (e.g., anxiety, fatigue, low motivation). These reactions, in turn, lead to decreased worker capacity (e.g., slower reaction time, inattention, impaired reasoning) and a greater likelihood of engaging in unsafe work practices (e.g., improper equipment operation, risky behavior). Unsafe work practices increase the probability of near misses and accidents, two events that can also function as a source of stress, thus reactivating the cycle. Although each step of the model has empirical support, more research is needed to further identify workplace factors that moderate the relationship between job stress and accidents. Recently, one factor receiving attention is safety climate, which refers to the shared perceptions of workers about the level of safety in their organization. Research suggests that certain job stressors (e.g., excessive work demands) lead to a poor safety climate and an increase in accidents.[71]

Healthcare expenditures Research suggests that workers who report being troubled by stress are also more likely to have higher healthcare expenditures.[23] Whether this finding is because stressed individuals experience more health problems requiring treatment, or are more inclined to seek medical attention for the conditions they do experience (or both) is in need of further study. In this research, stress is often measured as a global response (e.g., Are you concerned about stress at work?). As a result, more information about the actual features of the workplace that produce this response and the need for increased healthcare services is needed. Additional evidence for a link with healthcare expenditures comes from intervention research that shows a beneficial impact of health promotion programs (which include a focus on stress reduction) on healthcare utilization.[72]

HOW CAN THE ADVERSE EFFECTS OF JOB STRESS BE REDUCED OR PREVENTED?

Although this chapter focuses on job stress and the adverse effects of prolonged physiologic arousal, it has long been acknowledged that some degree of arousal and activation is necessary in order to reach optimum levels of performance.[32] But when job stress becomes too intense or persistent over time, many serious health consequences can result. A major challenge facing organizations is to develop strategies for reducing or preventing job stress before it impacts health and safety. As with job stressors, job stress interventions can be viewed as falling along a clinical–public health continuum, in which the focus gradually shifts from the worker to the organization.

Types of interventions to reduce job stress

Clinical perspective

Sometimes referred to as 'stress management training', the clinical approach focuses on making individuals more resilient to the demands of the work environment, often by modifying how a worker responds to a given stressor. Because this strategy does not eliminate the stressor, it is categorized as involving either *secondary prevention* (i.e., reducing the effects of the stressor) or *tertiary prevention* (i.e., providing treatment).[73] In either case, this approach represents a form of 'damage control' in which the outcomes, rather than the sources, of job strain are addressed. Intervention techniques based on this approach are derived principally from clinical and counseling psychology. As a result, these techniques tend to be fairly generic and applicable to wide variety of situations, not just those in the workplace.[74]

Examples of clinical intervention techniques include:

- Progressive muscle relaxation training
- Cognitive-behavioral skills training (e.g., modifying the appraisal process, time management)
- Biofeedback training
- Meditation
- Employee assistance programs (EAPs) (e.g., counseling services)
- Health promotion or 'wellness' programs (e.g., exercise programs, health education).

For all of these interventions, the principal goal is the same: to help workers modify their appraisal of stressful situations and/or deal more effectively with the symptoms of stress. These interventions typically involve sessions that last for an hour or more and are offered on a regular (e.g., weekly) basis. They can range from a few days of training or treatment to many weeks. Stress management training is also commonly offered in the context of EAPs and health promotion programs, and the organization usually makes a commitment to provide appropriate facilities and personnel, unless the services are offered off site.

A recent review of the research literature on clinical-based interventions found moderately strong evidence that these techniques help reduce stress related symptoms and somatic complaints, at least in the short term.[75] Less convincing evidence, however, exists for an improvement in job or organizational-relevant outcomes, such as absenteeism and job satisfaction. Given that clinical interventions do not involve an actual modification of the work environment, this finding should not be too surprising.

Murphy[75] concluded that the question of which intervention technique works best depends on the specific outcome under consideration. For example, biofeedback seems to have its strongest impact on physiologic outcomes (e.g., blood pressure), whereas cognitive-behavioral skills training shows better results for psychologic outcomes (e.g., anxiety). In addition, the most positive findings across various health outcomes were obtained with a combination of two or more techniques. The pairing of progressive muscle relaxation with cognitive-behavioral skills training was the most frequently reported combination. Finally, there is some evidence that clinical interventions can reduce healthcare costs, although additional studies are needed to further examine this potential benefit.

Public health perspective

The public health approach focuses on either eliminating or modifying sources of stress in the work environment. This strategy can be described as *primary prevention*, in that the goal is to change some aspect of the organization or job itself. At least in theory, primary prevention would seem preferable to the clinical approach since it targets factors earlier in the stress process.

Elkin and Rosch[76] summarize a wide range of public health interventions, including those that:

- Redesign the task
- Establish flexible work schedules
- Increase employee participation in decision making
- Change or redefine job roles
- Provide social support and feedback
- Restructure work units and lines of authority
- Establish fair human resource policies.

These interventions focus on changing some of the most commonly experienced workplace stressors, such as lack of control, excessive workload, job insecurity, role conflict, or poor interpersonal interactions. To implement them generally requires more resources and a greater long-term commitment from an organization than clinical interventions, since they usually cannot be introduced without affecting an organization's overall culture. Although these interventions target common job stressors, they are also adopted for non-stress reasons, such as a desire to improve organizational effectiveness or increase worker productivity.

Research on the effectiveness of public health interventions lags behind that on clinical interventions, largely because attempts to systematically change organizational factors are far less common.[74] The preference for clinical interventions reflects a number of factors, including a concern for the costs and risks associated with organizational change, and the view held by some managers that job stress is an individual problem rather than an organizational one. Research studies that do exist on public health interventions often have methodologic flaws (e.g., lack of appropriate control groups), making determination of causal relationships difficult. Although there is some evidence that techniques such as increasing worker participation in decision making can reduce strain, two recent reviews found that organizational interventions have not been clearly shown to substantially affect symptoms like distress or anxiety.[77,78] This conclusion may partly reflect the difficulty of applying rigorous research designs to actual work settings, or to a mismatch between the type of intervention studied and the methods used to evaluate its effectiveness.[18] More research is clearly needed before we know which public health interventions hold the most promise for reducing job strain.

Guidelines for interventions to reduce job stress

One issue that is clear from current research is that no single intervention should be seen as a panacea. By their nature, interventions, whether focused on the worker or the organization, are complex processes that sometimes produce unintended effects. As a result, how an intervention is implemented is probably as important as the type of intervention that is chosen.[79] A few simple guidelines for implementing job stress interventions include the following.

1. Follow a careful planning process

An intervention is more likely to succeed if it is the result of a thorough analysis of job stressors and strains. Cooper et al[24] recommend conducting a *stress audit* that involves collecting detailed information via self-report questionnaires (e.g., occupational stress inventory), interviews, observations, archival data, and even diaries kept by workers. The goal is to identify both individual and organizational factors that function as stressors and assess their impact on levels of strain experienced by workers. The next step involves selecting *targeted interventions* that are specific to the stressors that have been identified. This may require choosing between a clinical or public health strategy (i.e., primary, secondary, or tertiary prevention); however, in many cases it may be desirable to combine elements from both approaches. Finally, it is important to conduct a *focused evaluation* of the intervention, choosing criteria that examine a variety of specific outcomes, and not just a global improvement in wellbeing.

2. Involve workers in the design and evaluation of the intervention

A critical factor in an intervention's success is that workers need to accept the program and feel that it adequately addresses their needs and concerns. All too often, interventions are implemented by consultants or managers without adequate worker input. Involving workers takes advantage of their knowledge of the workplace and focuses attention on the process through which an intervention is selected and implemented. It is worker perception of this process that often determines the long-term viability of a program.

3. Obtain support for the intervention from all layers of the organization

A related factor is the need to build commitment for an intervention from all levels of an organization, including management, unions, and employees. If an intervention is implemented in isolation, without buy-in from all groups, it is likely to be perceived as a token gesture. Organization-wide support communicates that job stress is a serious issue that all sides are willing to take responsibility for addressing.

4. Base intervention on a conceptual model

An intervention is likely to fail if it focuses only on symptoms and does not adequately address the underlying problem(s) affecting workers. A conceptual model provides a useful framework for capturing the complexity of the stress process, and identifying the short- and long-term consequences of stress, potential moderating variables, and the nature of the relationship between stressors and strains. A number of conceptual models for stress interventions are currently available (such as those described earlier in this chapter), but these models remain underutilized by practitioners.[74]

Additional guidance for organizations on implementing and evaluating job stress interventions can be found in several sources, including *Stress at work*,[80] *Tackling work-related stress*,[81] and *Research on work-related stress*.[25]

CONCLUSIONS

As organizations and work practices continue to evolve, job stress and its effects on workers will inevitably remain a concern. Although more needs to be learned about the relationship between job stressors and strains, sufficient evidence exists to conclude that job stress can adversely impact occupational safety and health and that a variety of interventions are available for reducing or preventing job stress. After four decades of research, we have also gained an increased appreciation of the complexity of the stress process itself and the variety of ways in which worker safety and health can be affected. On a broader level, an understanding of job stress is crucial to the goal of creating 'healthy organizations'[82] in which worker safety and wellbeing go hand in hand with an organization's concern for productivity and profit.

References

1. Roethlisberger FJ, Dickson WJ. Management and the worker. Cambridge, MA: Harvard University Press, 1939.
2. Hoppock R. Job satisfaction. New York: Harper and Brothers, 1935.
3. Walker CR, Guest RH. Man on the assembly line. Boston: Harvard University. Press, 1952.
4. Ciulla JB. The working life. New York: Three Rivers Press, 2000.
5. Kornhauser A. Mental health of the industrial worker. New York: Wiley & Sons, 1965.
6. Levi L, ed. Society, stress, and disease: vol. 1. The psychosocial environment and psychosomatic diseases. Proceedings of an international interdisciplinary symposium held in Stockholm, April 1970. New York: Oxford University Press, 1971.
7. Karasek RA. Job demands, decision latitude, and mental strain: implications for job redesign. Admin Sci Quart 1979; 24:285–307.
8. Karasek R, Theorell T. Healthy work: stress productivity and the reconstruction of working life. New York: Wiley & Sons, 1990.
9. Kahn RL, Wolfe DM, Quinn RP, Snoek JD, Rosenthal RA. Organizational stress: studies in role conflict and ambiguity. New York: Wiley & Sons, 1964.
10. Caplan RD, Cobb S, French JRP, van Harrison R, Pinneau SR. Job demands and worker health. DHEW (NIOSH) Publication No. 75-160. Washington DC: US Government Printing Office, 1975.
11. Beehr TA. The themes of social-psychological stress in work organizations: from roles to goals. In: Riley AW, Zaccaro SJ, eds. Occupational stress and organizational effectiveness. New York: Praeger, 1987; 71–102.
12. McLean A. The reduction of occupational stress: an overview. In: McLean A, Black G, Colligan M, eds. Reducing occupational stress: proceedings of a conference held in White Plains New York, May, 1977. DHEW (NIOSH) Publication No. 78-140. Washington DC: US Government Printing Office, 1978;1–7.
13. US Department of Health, Education, and Welfare. Protecting the health of eighty million Americans: a national goal for occupational health. Washington DC: US Government Printing Office, 1966.
14. Work in America. A report of a special task force to the Secretary of Health Education and Welfare. Cambridge, MA: MIT Press, 1974.
15. Cohen A, Margolis B. Initial psychological research related to the Occupational Safety and Health Act of 1970. Am Psychol 1973; 28:600–6.
16. Elisburg D. Workplace stress: legal developments, economic pressures, and violence. In: Burton JF, ed. 1995 Workers' compensation yearbook. Horsham, PA: LRP Publications, 1995; I-217–I-222.

17. Northwestern National Life Insurance Company. Employee burnout: America's newest epidemic. Minneapolis, MN: Northwestern National Life Insurance Company, 1991.

18. Sauter SL, Brightwell WS, Colligan MJ, et al. The changing organization of work and the safety and health of working people. DHHS (NIOSH) Publication No. 2002-116. Cincinnati, OH: National Institute for Occupational Safety and Health, 2002. Available at: http://www.cdc.gov/niosh/02-116pd.html

19. Bluestone B, Rose S. Public policy brief no. 39: the unmeasured labor force – the growth in work hours. Blithewook, Annandale-on-Hudson, NY: The Jerome Levy Economics Institute of Bard College, Bard Publications Office, 1998.

20. General Social Survey 1972–2000 Cumulative Codebook. http://www.icpsr.umich.edu/GSS/. Date accessed: June 6, 2002.

21. Bond JT, Galinsky E, Swanberg JE. The 1997 national study of the changing workforce. New York: Families and Work Institute, 1998.

22. Webster T, Bergman B. Occupational stress: counts and rates. Compensation and Working Conditions Online 1999; 4:1–4. http://www.bls.gov/opub/cwc/1999/Fall/brief4.htm

23. Goetzel RZ, Anderson DR, Whitmer RW, Ozminkowski RJ, Dunn, RL, Wasserman J. The relationship between modifiable health risks and healthcare expenditure: an analysis of the multi-employer HERO health risk and cost database. J Occup Environ Med 1998; 40:843–54.

24. Cooper CL, Dewe PJ, O'Driscoll MP. Organizational stress. Thousand Oaks, CA: Sage, 2001.

25. Cox T, Griffiths A, Rial-González E. Research on work-related stress. Luxembourg: European Agency for Safety and Health at Work, 2000.

26. Kahn RL, Byosiere P. Stress in organizations. In: Dunnette MD, Hough L, eds. Handbook of industrial and organizational psychology, vol. 3, 2nd edn. Palo Alto, CA: Consulting Psychologists Press, Inc, 1992; 571–650.

27. Cannon WB. The wisdom of the body. New York: Norton, 1931.

28. Selye H. Stress in health and disease. Oxford, UK: Butterworths, 1976.

29. Cox T. Stress, 2nd edn. New York: Macmillan, 1985.

30. Symonds CP. Use and abuse of the term flying stress. In: Air Ministry, Psychological disorders in flying personnel of the Royal Air Force, investigated during the war, 1939–1945. London: HMSO, 1947.

31. French JRP, Caplan RD, van Harrison R. The mechanisms of job stress and strain. Chichester, NY: Wiley & Sons, 1982

32. McGrath JE. Stress and behavior in organizations. In: Dunnette MD, ed. Handbook of industrial and organizational psychology. Chicago, IL: Rand McNally, 1976;1351–95.

33. Lazarus RS. Psychological stress and the coping process. New York: McGraw-Hill, 1966.

34. Lazarus RS. Psychological stress in the workplace. J Soc Behav Personality 1991; 6:1–13.

35. Folkman S, Lazarus RS. An analysis of coping in a middle aged community sample. J Health Soc Behav 1980; 21:219–39.

36. Pearlin L, Lieberman ML, Menaghan E, Mullan JT. The stress process. J Health Soc Behav 1981; 19:2–21.

37. Cox T, Mackay CJ. A transactional approach to occupational stress. In: Corlett EN, Richardson J, eds. Stress, work design, and productivity. Chichester, NY: Wiley & Sons, 1981.

38. Siegrist J. Adverse health effects of high-effort/low-reward conditions. J Occup Health Psychol 1996; 1:27–41.

39. Kasl SV, Rodriguez E, Lasch KE. The impact of unemployment on health and well-being. In: Dohrenwend B, ed. Adversity, stress, and psychopathology. New York: Oxford University Press, 1998;111–31.

40. Beehr TA, Newman JE. Job stress, employee health, and organizational effectiveness: a facet analysis, model, and literature review. Personnel Psychol 1978; 31:665–99.

41. Cooper CL, Marshall J. Occupational sources of stress: a review of the literature relating to coronary heart disease and mental ill health. J Occup Psychol 1976; 49:11–28.

42. Hurrell JJ, Murphy LR. Psychological job stress. In: Rom WN, ed. Environmental and occupational medicine, 3rd edn. Boston: Little, Brown and Company, 1998;905–14.

43. Rosenman RH. Relationships of the type A behavior pattern with coronary heart disease. In: Goldberger L, Breznitz S, eds. Handbook of stress: theoretical and clinical aspects. New York: The Free Press, 1993;449–76.

44. Schaubroeck J, Merritt D. Divergent effects of job control on coping with work stressors: the key role of self-efficacy. Acad Manage J 1997; 40:738–54.

45. Cohen S, Rodriguez MS. Pathways linking affective disturbances and physical disorders. Health Psychol 1995; 14:374–80.

46. Hendrix WH. Physiologic effects of stress in the workplace. In: Jones JW, Steffy BD, Bray BW, eds. Applying psychology in business. Lexington, MA: Lexington Books, 1991;722–32.

47. Frankenhaeuser M. The psychobiology of workload, stress, and health: comparison between the sexes. Ann Behav Med 1991; 13:197–204.

48. Jonsson D, Rosengren A, Dotevall A, Lappas G, Wilhelmsen L. Job control, job demands and social support at work in relation to cardiovascular risk factors in MONICA 1995, Goteborg. J Cardiovasc Risk 1999; 6:379–85.

49. Lindquist TL, Beilin LJ, Knuiman MW. Influence of lifestyle, coping, and job stress on blood pressure in men and women. Hypertension 1997; 29:1–7.

50. Niedhammer I, Goldberg M, Leclerc A, David S, Bugel I, Landre MF. Psychosocial work environment and cardiovascular risk factors in an occupational cohort in France. J Epidemiol Commun Health 1998; 52:93–100.

51. Storr CL, Trnkoff AM, Anthony JC. Job strain and non-medical drug use. Drug Alcohol Depend 1999; 55:45–51.

52. Kageyama T, Nishikido N, Kobayashi T, Kurokawa Y, Kaneko T, Kabuto M. Self-reported sleep quality, job stress, and daytime autonomic activities assessed in terms of short-term heart rate variability among male white-collar workers. Ind Health 1998; 36:263–72.

53. Pennebaker JW. The psychology of physical symptoms. New York: Springer-Verlag, 1982.

54. Cohen S. Psychosocial models of social support in the etiology of physical disease. Health Psychol 1988; 7:269–97.

55. Bosma H, Stansfeld SA, Marmot MG. Job control, personal characteristics, and heart disease. J Occup Health Psychol 1998; 3:402–9.

56. Hlatky MA, Lam LC, Lee KL, et al. Job strain and the prevalence and outcome of coronary artery disease. Circulation 1995; 93:327–33.

57. Schnall PL, Landsbergis PA, Baker D. Job strain and cardiovascular disease. Annu Rev Public Health 1994;15:381–411.

58. Schnall PL, Landsbergis P, Baker D, eds. The workplace and cardiovascular disease. Occup Med State Art Rev 2000; 15 (1). Philadelphia, Hanley and Belfus.

59. National Research Council. Musculoskeletal disorders and the workplace: low back and upper extremities. Washington DC: National Academy Press, 2001.

60. Sauter SL, Swanson NG. An ecological model of musculoskeletal disorders in office work. In: Moon S, Sauter S, eds. Beyond biomechanics: psychosocial aspects of musculoskeletal disorders in office work. London: Taylor and Francis, 1996;3–21.

61. Ursin H. Immunological reactions. In: Stellman JM, ed. Encyclopaedia of occupational health and safety, vol. II, 4th edn. Geneva: International Labour Office, 1998;34.57–34.59.

62. Fox BH. Cancer. In: Stellman JM, ed. Encyclopaedia of occupational health and safety, vol. II, 4th edn. Geneva: International Labour Office, 1998;34.60–34.61.

63. Suls J. Gastrointestinal problems. In: Stellman JM, ed. Encyclopaedia of occupational health and safety, vol. II, 4th edn. Geneva: International Labour Office, 1998;34.59–34.60.

64. Grosch JW, Murphy LR. Occupational differences in depression and global health: results from a national sample of US workers. J Occup Environ Med 1998; 40:153–64.

65. Jex SM, Beehr TA. Emerging theoretical and methodological issues in the study of work-related stress. In: Rowland K, Ferris G, eds. Research in personnel and human resources management, vol. 9. Greenwich, CT: JAP Press, 1991;311–65.

66. Maslach C, Schaufeli WB, Leiter MP. Job burnout. Annu Rev Psychol 2001; 52:397–422.

67. Platt S, Pavis S, Akram G. Changing labour market conditions and health: a systematic literature review (1993–1998). Dublin, Ireland: European Foundation for the Improvement of Living and Working Conditions, 1999.

68. Grosch JW. Job transitions associated with suicide: results from the National Mortality Followback Survey. Unpublished manuscript, 2000.

69. Jex SM. Stress and job performance. Thousand Oaks, CA: Sage Publications, 1998.

70. Murphy LR, DuBois D, Hurrell JJ Jr. Accident reduction through stress management. J Business Psychol 1986: 1:5–18.

71. Murphy LR, Gershon RM, DeJoy D. Stress and occupational exposure to HIV/AIDS. In: Cooper CL, ed. Handbook of stress medicine. Boca Raton, FL: CRC Press, 1996;176–90.

72. Ozminkowski RJ, Ling D, Goetzel RZ, et al. Long-term impact of Johnson and Johnson's health and wellness program on healthcare utilization and expenditures. J Occup Environ Med 2002; 44:21–9.

73. Cooper CL, Cartwright S. An intervention strategy for workplace stress. J Psychosom Res 1997; 43:7–16.

74. Ganster DC, Murphy LR. Workplace interventions to prevent stress-related illness: lessons from research and practice. In: Cooper CL, Locke EA, eds. Industrial and organizational psychology: linking theory with practice. Malden, MA: Blackwell Publishers, 2000;34–51.

75. Murphy LR. Stress management in work settings: a critical review of the health effects. Am J Health Prom 1996; 11:112–35.

76. Elkin A, Rosch P. Promoting mental health at the workplace: the prevention side of stress management. Occup Med State Art Rev 1990; 5:739–54.

77. Briner RB, Reynolds S. The costs, benefits, and limitations of organizational level stress interventions. J Organiz Behav 1999; 20:647–64.

78. Parkes KR, Sparkes TJ. Organizational interventions to reduce work stress: are they effective? A review of the literature. Contract Research Report No. 193/198. Oxford, UK: University of Oxford, Health and Safety Executive, 1998.

79. Murphy LR. Occupational stress management: current status and future directions. In: Cooper CL, Rousseau D, eds. Trends in organizational behavior, vol. 2. New York: Wiley & Sons, 1995; 1–14.

80. NIOSH. Stress at work. DHHS (NIOSH) Publication No.2002-107. Cincinnati, OH: National Institute for Occupational Safety and Health, 1999. Available at: http://www.cdc.gov/niosh/99-101pd.html

81. Health and Safety Executive. Tackling work-related stress. Norwich, UK: HMSO, 2001.

82. Jaffe DT. The healthy company: research paradigms for personal and organizational health. In: Sauter SL, Murphy LR, eds. Organizational risk factors for job stress. Washington, DC: American Psychological Association, 1995.

Chapter 39
Metals and Related Compounds

39.1 Aluminum
Oyebode A Taiwo

EXPOSURE SETTINGS

Aluminum is the most abundant metal that occurs naturally in soil and constitutes about 8% of the earth's surface. It is not found in its metallic state, but in combination with other elements and compounds, including oxygen, fluorine, and silica. Bauxite, the principal source of aluminum, consists of a mixture of minerals formed by the weathering of aluminum-bearing rocks and occurs primarily in tropical and subtropical areas. Commercial bauxite deposits exist currently in Australia, South America and the West Indies. These deposits are extracted by open-cast mining. Aluminum production from extracted bauxite involves three main steps: (1) refining of bauxite to yield alumina, (2) electrolytic reduction of alumina to yield aluminum, and (3) aluminum casting into ingots.

Bauxite refining to yield aluminum oxide or alumina uses the Bayer process, whereby bauxite is digested under high temperature and pressure in a strong solution of caustic soda (sodium hydroxide). The resulting hydrate is crystallized and calcined to alumina in a kiln. Alumina is then reduced to aluminum by the Hall-Héroult process during which alumina is dissolved in molten cryolite (sodium aluminum fluoride) contained in a large carbon or graphite lined steel container known as a pot. An electric current flows between a carbon anode made of petroleum coke and pitch and a cathode formed by the lining of the pot. Molten aluminum is deposited at the bottom of the pot during this process and is siphoned off for use in casting ingots.

There are two main types of aluminum smelting technology – Söderburg and Pre-bake. The Söderburg technology uses anodes baked in the pot itself, while the Pre-bake technology uses anodes that are pre-baked in a separate facility. During reduction the pot emits fumes that contain hydrofluoric acid, sulfur dioxide, carbon, alumina and fluoride dusts. Polyaromatic hydrocarbons (PAHs) are also emitted, with higher PAH emissions found in Söderburg pots compared to Pre-bake pots. The aluminum produced is cast into ingots for subsequent manufacturing use.

Aluminum and its alloys enjoy widespread use in the construction, automotive, and aircraft industries. The electrical industry also makes use of aluminum for overhead distributions and power lines, electrical conductors, and insulated cables and wires. Aluminum is a common constituent of jewelry and cooking utensils and is also used extensively in packaging, including food containers, aluminum foil and beverage cans. Aluminum powder is used in paints, protective coatings and pyrotechnics production. Aluminum compounds are also used as: aluminum chloride in rubber and wood preservative manufacturing; aluminum borate in glass and ceramic production; aluminum chlorhydrate as an ingredient in deodorants; aluminum isopropoxide in soap and paint production; and aluminum trioxide as an absorbent and abrasive. In addition to its presence in many manufactured products, aluminum is universally present in variable and often trace amounts in food and water.

CLINICAL EFFECTS
Acute

There is little evidence to suggest that aluminum exposure by any route, i.e. inhalation, dermal, or gastrointestinal, is associated with any significant acute health effects.

Chronic

The occupational respiratory disorders associated with chronic exposure to aluminum dust and fumes include potroom asthma, chronic bronchitis, pulmonary fibrosis, and granulomatous lung disease. Potroom asthma, a syndrome characterized by both immediate and late asthmatic response, is associated with work in aluminum production. The annual incidence has been estimated to be approximately 2%, with prevalence as high as 10% in long-term workers. The specific mechanism is not known; however, fluorides and other respiratory irritants encountered in this environment have been suggested as the cause (see Chapter 19.2).[1,2] Non-specific airway response to dust characterized by cough and mucous production has also been described in workers in aluminum production; cross-sectional studies of these workers have shown decrement in lung function over many years.[3]

Aluminosis or Shaver's disease – a rare progressive pneumoconiosis of historic interest, characterized by upper lung predominance, peripheral emphysema, and frequent pneumothoraces – has been attributed to chronic aluminum exposure. Recent evidence suggests that exposure to aluminum oxide may also induce pulmonary fibrosis. However, exposure to a mixture of other dusts at low levels (free silica and asbestos) may explain this pathology (see Chapter 19.11).[4]

There are case reports in workers exposed to aluminum dust presenting with alveolitis and granulomas similar to those found in sarcoidosis and chronic beryllium disease.[5-7] This disease is characterized by a T lymphocytic alveolitis principally composed of CD4+ (helper) lymphocytes, but differing from sarcoid by the identification of aluminum within the granulomas. Blastic transformation of the patient's peripheral blood lymphocytes in the presence of aluminum compounds has also been reported.[8] These findings suggest that this pathologic picture may represent an early stage of aluminum-induced fibrosis. The existence of aluminum-induced lung disease remains controversial, in part because of its extensive use and the rarity of the lung disease attributed to this metal, making the significance of isolated case reports unclear.

The aluminum reduction process has been associated with excess lung and bladder cancer incidence. This increased cancer risk is related to the polyaromatic hydrocarbons used and generated in the reduction process.[9,10] This is covered more extensively in Chapters 44, 30.1 (lungs) and 30.3 (bladder).

Aluminum has been implicated as a potential toxic agent in the etiology of various neurologic disorders. Its neurotoxicity has been studied most extensively in dialysis patients who have developed dialysis encephalopathy, the clinical presentation of which includes speech impairment, dementia, apraxia, myoclonus, asterixis and focal seizure. These patients also develop a related microcytic anemia, as well as a severe form of osteomalacia that is resistant to calcium and vitamin D therapy.[11] Autopsy findings in these patients have shown elevated levels of aluminum in brain, liver and bone. The source of aluminum exposure has been traced to the water used to prepare the dialysate and orally administered aluminum phosphate binders.[12] Dialysis encephalopathy is largely preventable by elimination of aluminum from the dialysate; however, a few cases still occur from contamination of the dialysis fluid and consumption of aluminum-containing drugs.

There has been considerable interest in the potential role of aluminum in causing Alzheimer's disease. Identifying potential genetic and environmental risk factors for Alzheimer's disease is an active area of research. Some studies have reported high concentrations of aluminum in the brains of patients with Alzheimer's disease, while others have not.[13-16] A number of epidemiologic studies have reported a positive association between the prevalence of Alzheimer's disease and aluminum levels in drinking water, while other studies have not.[17] The amount of ingested aluminum from drinking water is very small in relation to other dietary sources; therefore, a direct toxic effect is unlikely.

'Potroom palsy', a progressive neurologic disorder characterized by incoordination, poor memory, impairment in abstract reasoning and depression, has been described in aluminum potroom workers.[18] Studies of other potroom workers have reported subclinical tremors, impaired visuo-spatial organization and a slight decline in psychomotor tempo.[19] Exposure to toxins in the potroom of the aluminum plant is the suspected cause of these neurologic symptoms; however, the exact causative agents are not known. Other studies have shown no difference in neurological function between potroom workers and comparison workers.[20,21] In conclusion, aluminum remains a plausible, but as yet unproven, cause of neurologic disease, based on limited but intriguing experimental, pathologic, and epidemiologic evidence.

DIAGNOSIS, EVALUATION AND TREATMENT

Biologic monitoring of exposure to aluminum usually is limited to quantification of parent compounds in blood and urine. Similar sensitive methods for detecting levels at low doses (parts per billion) also are available for other body tissues, but these are usually reserved for experimental purposes. Mean levels of aluminum in plasma or serum in those without occupational exposure have been reported to be less than 10 µg/L. Levels in workers exposed to aluminum have been found to be considerably higher (two or more times), with the highest levels of blood aluminum found in those undergoing dialysis (100–200 µg/L).[22] Urine levels also are consistently higher in exposed groups and likely reflect a longer period of recent exposure than do those from blood, although studies have been inconsistent in this regard.[23] More important, there is no evidence that measured plasma or urine aluminum levels are an adequate reflection of either respiratory or neurologic toxicity.

Based on current evidence, asymptomatic workers exposed to aluminum fumes or dusts should undergo periodic evaluation of respiratory symptoms and spirometry testing. The development of respiratory symptoms or presence of abnormal lung function should prompt further evaluation including chest radiographs. Workers with unexplained neurologic symptoms should also have a full neurologic evaluation, including consideration of neuropsychologic testing.

The primary approach to prevention is the institution of engineering control measures to reduce respirable levels of aluminum in the workplace. Treatment measures are limited to removal of workers with early respiratory or neurologic disease from further exposure.

Acknowledgment

This chapter is an update of Chapter 30.1; Aluminum, by Linda Rosenstock which was published in the 1st edition.

References

1. Abramson MJ, Wlodarczyk JH, Saunders NA, et al. Does aluminum smelting cause lung disease? Am Rev Respir Dis 1989; 139:1042–57.
2. O'Donnell TV. Asthma and respiratory problems – a review. Sci Total Environ 1995; 163:137–45.
3. Townsend MC, Enterline PE, Sussman NB et al, Pulmonary function in relation to total dust exposure at a bauxite refinery and alumina-based chemical products plant. Am Rev Respir Dis 1985; 132:1174–80.
4. Jederlinic PJ, Abraham JL, Churg A et al. Pulmonary fibrosis in aluminum oxide workers. Investigation of nine workers, with pathologic examination and microanalysis in three of them. Am Rev Respir Dis 1990; 142:1179–84.
5. Brancaleone P, Weynand B, De Vuyst P, et al. Lung granulomatosis in a dental technician. Am J Ind Med 1998; 34:628–31.

6. Chen WJ, Monnat RJ, Chen M, et al. Aluminum-induced pulmonary granulomatosis. Hum Pathol 1978; 9:705–11.

7. Musk AW, Greville H, Tribe AE. Pulmonary disease from occupational exposure to an artificial aluminium silicate used for cat litter. Br J Ind Med 1980; 37:367–72.

8. De Vuyst P, Dumortier P, Schandene L, et al. Sarcoid-like lung granulomatosis induced by aluminum dusts. Am Rev Respir Dis 1987; 135:493–7.

9. Armstrong B, Tremblay C, Baris D, et al. Lung cancer mortality and polynuclear aromatic hydrocarbons: a case-cohort study of aluminum production workers in Arvida, Quebec, Canada. Am J Epidemiol 1994; 139:250–62.

10. Tremblay C, Armstrong B, Theriault G, et al. Estimation of risk of developing bladder cancer among workers exposed to coal tar pitch volatiles in the primary aluminum industry. Am J Ind Med 1995; 27:335–48.

11. Visser WJ, Van de Vyver FL. Aluminium-induced osteomalacia in severe chronic renal failure (SCRF). Clin Nephrol 1985; 24(Suppl 1):S30–6.

12. Alfrey AC. Dialysis encephalopathy. Clin Nephrol 1985; 24(Suppl 1):S15–19.

13. Doll R. Review: Alzheimer's disease and environmental aluminum. Age Ageing 1993; 22:138–53.

14. Forbes WF, Hill GB. Is exposure to aluminum a risk factor for the development of Alzheimer disease? – Yes. AICH Neurol 1998; 55:740–1.

15. Munoz DG. Is exposure to aluminum a risk factor for the development of Alzheimer disease? – No. AICH Neurol 1998; 55:737–9.

16. Yokel RA. The toxicology of aluminum in the brain: a review. Neurotoxicology 2000; 21:813–28.

17. Flaten TP. Aluminium as a risk factor in Alzheimer's disease, with emphasis on drinking water. Brain Res Bull 2001; 55:187–96.

18. White DM, Longstreth WT, Rosenstock L, et al. Neurologic syndrome in 25 workers from an aluminum smelting plant. Arch Intern Med 1992; 152:1443–8. [Erratum appears in Arch Intern Med 1993; 153:2796.]

19. Bast-Pettersen R, Drablos PA, Goffeng LO, et al. Neuropsychological deficit among elderly workers in aluminum production. Am J Ind Med 1994; 25:649–62.

20. Dick RB, Krieg EF, Sim MA, et al. Evaluation of tremor in aluminum production workers, Neurotoxicol Teratol 1997; 19:447–53.

21. Letzel S, Lang CJ, Schaller KH, et al. Longitudinal study of neurotoxicity with occupational exposure to aluminum dust. Neurology 2000; 54:997–1000.

22. McCarthy JT, Milliner DS, Kurtz SB, et al. Interpretation of serum aluminum values in dialysis patients. Am J Clin Pathol 1986; 86:629–36.

23. Lauwerys RHP. Aluminum. In: Lauwerys RR, Hoet P, eds. Industrial chemical exposure: guidelines for biologic monitoring, 2nd edn. Boca Raton: Lewis, 1993;15–19.

39.2 **Arsenic**
Alfred Franzblau

EXPOSURE SETTINGS

Almost all arsenic for human use is obtained in the form of arsenic trioxide (As_2O_3), a byproduct of smelting of ores of copper, lead, or zinc. Worldwide production is 75,000 to 100,000 tons per year.[1] Arsenical compounds are encountered in a broad spectrum of industrial settings, including smelting, manufacture of glassware, specialty industrial chemicals, creation of alloys of lead and copper, and semiconductors, but 80% is used in agricultural applications such as pesticide manufacturing and application, wood preservatives, and feed additives for cattle. The first widely used manufactured pesticide was copper acetoarsenite (in the mid-19th century). NIOSH estimates that approximately 900,000 workers have potential occupational exposure to arsenic each day.

In the occupational setting inorganic arsenic compounds, such as arsenic trioxide, are usually absorbed via inhalation of air-borne dust. Arsine (AsH_3), a gas at room temperature and pressure, deserves special mention because of its unique acute toxicity. The organic arsenicals, e.g. pesticides, have greater potential for transcutaneous absorption.

Ingestion usually is only a significant route of exposure outside the workplace, particularly ingestion of ground water contaminated with inorganic arsenical compounds, usually from natural sources. Ingestion of arsenic-contaminated water has attracted increased attention in recent years because of concern related to potential health effects, and the large numbers of people exposed, especially in countries such as Bangladesh, India, Pakistan, and China. Ingestion of foods that naturally contain arsenic, particularly fish, shellfish, or seaweed, is also a major source of arsenic exposure, although the species of arsenic usually present in these sources are relatively non-toxic (e.g., arsenobetaine). Environmental exposure to arsenic has been documented to occur via inhalation of air-borne arsenic-containing dust among residents living downwind from large industrial sources of arsenic emissions, such as arsenic smelters.[2]

Arsenical compounds occupy an interesting historical position because of their frequent use as medicines and poisons. Arsenicals were used to treat syphilis (e.g., arsphenamine) in the first half of the 20th century, and Fowler's solution (1% potassium arsenite) was used for psoriasis and asthma until the 1960s. Arsenic trioxide is nearly tasteless, has the appearance of sugar, and is lethal in small doses, and so for centuries was a preferred homicidal and suicidal agent.[1] Lewisite, a vesicant war gas, was first used in World War I. Table 39.2.1 summarizes the different arsenical species, their chemical formula, and usual source of exposure.

CLINICAL EFFECTS
Acute

Acute arsenic intoxication usually occurs via ingestion of arsenic, specifically arsenic trioxide, with homicidal or suicidal intent, although there have been reports of unusual cases resulting from occupational or environmental exposure.[3] The minimal lethal dose is 100–200 mg of As_2O_3. Arsenic pentoxide (As_2O_5) is approximately half as toxic as the trivalent form, although the clinical syndrome produced is identical (much of the pentavalent arsenic is converted to the trivalent form in vivo). The onset of symptoms can vary from minutes to hours, depending on whether the arsenic is in solution, and recent food consumption. Inorganic arsenic compounds are acute gastrointestinal irritants, leading to nausea, vomiting (possibly with blood), and abdominal cramps. Electrocardiographic abnormalities reflecting myocardial toxicity consist of broadening of the QRS complex, flattening of T-waves, and ST segment depression. Patients may develop severe central nervous system toxicity manifested by encephalopathy. Death is usually the result of circulatory collapse due to fluid and electrolyte loss.

If the patient survives the immediate acute effects, the person is at risk of developing numerous delayed systemic toxic effects. Painful peripheral neuropathy, appearing one or two weeks after an acute ingestion, is initially sensory with a stocking–glove distribution, but can progress to include sensory and motor deficits. Following cessation of exposure the neuropathy usually worsens for a number of weeks and then stabilizes. Subsequent improvement is slow, and recovery may never be complete. Severe cases have been confused with Guillain–Barré syndrome.[4]

Reversible bone marrow suppression, with leukopenia and granulocytopenia, anemia, increased relative eosinophil count, and megaloblastic changes in the marrow can occur. Cutaneous effects vary from nothing to slight erythema to exfoliative erythroderma. Mees lines (sharply demarcated transverse white lines in the nails) usually appear 2–3 weeks following an acute exposure. Mild to moderate elevation of liver enzymes can occur.

Arsine (AsH_3) is a colorless gas with a slight garlic odor. Following acute exposure, there is an asymptomatic period lasting up to 24 hours; the duration of latency is inversely proportional to the degree of exposure. Initially, patients describe headache, lightheadedness, weakness, nausea, and vomiting. The classic triad consists of abdominal pain, hematuria, and jaundice due to arsine-induced intravascular hemolysis. The liver may be enlarged on examination. The usual cause of death is acute renal failure resulting from precipitation of free hemoglobin in renal tubules. If the patient survives the acute event, peripheral neuropathy, Mees lines and other sequelae may appear as noted above.

Chronic

Chronic arsenic exposure, usually related to inorganic arsenic such as arsenic trioxide, induces a multi-organ system disease, with primary non-malignant effects on the skin, nervous system, and vasculature. A number of stud-

Name	Chemical formula	Usual source of exposure	Urinary metabolite
Arsenic trioxide	As_2O_3 or As_4O_6	Smelting/industrial sources/naturally occurring in drinking water	As_2O_3 Monomethylarsonate Dimethylarsinate
Arsenic pentoxide	As_2O_5 or As_4O_{10}	Smelting/industrial sources/naturally occurring in drinking water	As_2O_3 and As_2O_5 Monomethylarsonate Dimethylarsinate
Arsine	AsH_3	Industrial applications/semiconductor manufacture/accidental formation	Monomethylarsonate Dimethylarsinate
Monomethylarsonate	$CH_3AsO(OH)_2$	Metabolic product of inorganic arsenic exposure	Mostly excreted unchanged as monomethylarsonate and some dimethylarsinate
Dimethylarsinate	$(CH_3)_2AsO(OH)$	Metabolic product of inorganic arsenic exposure	Mostly excreted unchanged as dimethylarsinate
Arsenobetaine	$(CH_3)_3AsCH_2COOH$	Common arsenical species found in certain sea foods	Mostly excreted unchanged as arsenobetaine
Gallium arsenide	GaAs	Used in semiconductor manufacture	Not water soluble and poorly absorbed; mostly excreted in feces
Lewisite	$ClCH=CH-AsCl_2$	War gas (vesicant)	–

Valence states:
+V Arsenates
+III Arsenites
0 metallic arsenic

Table 39.2.1 Common arsenic species, usual sources of exposure and urinary metabolites

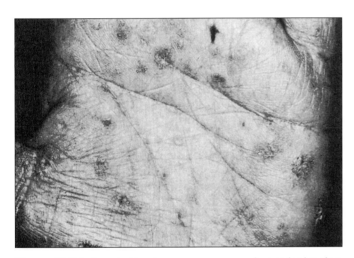

Figure 39.2.1: Arsenical keratoses, common on palms and soles after oral ingestion of arsenicals. These lesions are premalignant, but skin cancers also occur in patients without keratoses or hyperpigmentation. (Reprinted with permission from Braverman I. Skin signs of systemic disease. Philadelphia: WB Saunders, 1971.)

ies have shown an increased risk for diabetes with chronic, high exposures.[5] Non-malignant cutaneous effects include follicular and eczematous dermatitis due to a direct irritant effect, Mees lines, hyperpigmentation or melanosis (interspersed with small areas of depigmentation), and arsenical keratoses usually on the palms and soles from systemic absorption (Fig. 39.2.1).[6]

Clinical and pathologic findings of the peripheral nerves are similar to changes observed following acute exposure (i.e., an axonopathy), but slower and more insidious in onset.

Peripheral vascular disease may appear initially as Raynaud's phenomenon, and progress to acrocyanosis and frank gangrene, so-called 'blackfoot disease' which has been described in Silesia, Taiwan, and, most recently, Bangladesh.[7,8] More recent studies have linked chronic, high-level arsenic exposure to hypertension, increased mortality from heart disease, and cerebrovascular disease,[9–12] although the mechanisms are not well understood. An increased risk of myocardial infarction has been detected among arsenic smelter workers.

Additional non-malignant chronic toxic effects can include megaloblastic bone marrow suppression; liver enlargement, elevated serum liver enzymes, and possibly cirrhosis; and possible central nervous system effects including impaired cognition and personality changes.

Skin and lung cancer are the most well-established malignant effects of chronic arsenic exposure. Basal cell carcinomas, squamous cell carcinomas, and Bowen's disease have been reported with a positive dose–response relationship at high levels of exposure in drinking water,[6,13] as well as with occupational exposures. A characteristic feature of arsenic-associated cutaneous malignancies is their origin, which is frequently multicentric and on areas of the body typically not associated with UV exposure-related skin cancers. There is no known relationship between arsenic exposure and melanoma.

Increased risk of lung cancer has been well documented among arsenic-exposed workers, including arsenic smelter workers and workers involved with arsenical pesticides,[14,15] further discussed in Chapter 30.2. Studies of non-occupationally exposed cohorts, primarily persons exposed via arsenic in drinking water, have reported increased rates of cancer at multiple sites, primarily bladder, kidney, lung, liver, and hemopoietic malignancies.[12,16–19]

Some authors have suggested that the potential cancer risks to the general population from arsenic in drinking water, even at levels at or below the current EPA arsenic maximum contaminant level (MCL) of 50 micrograms/liter, may be substantial – in the same range as environmental tobacco smoke and radon in homes.[20] The Safe Water Drinking Act Amendments of 1996 mandated that the EPA must promulgate a new regulation for arsenic in drinking water in the future. Any new regulation, such as 10 micrograms/liter (the concentration for arsenic in drinking water recommended by the World Health Organization), or lower, will be costly. A major challenge is that risk estimates at low levels of exposure are based almost entirely on extrapolation of results from studies conducted outside the United States among persons exposed to arsenic levels in water that were much greater than the current MCL of 50 micrograms/liter, typically greater than 150 micrograms/liter, and as high as 2000 micrograms/liter.

DIAGNOSIS, EVALUATION, AND TREATMENT

There are no significant long-term mobilizable stores of arsenic in the body, and the half-life of arsenic in urine following low to moderate exposure is approximately one day; higher exposures result in some prolongation of half-life. Thus, biologic monitoring of chronic arsenic exposure is difficult even just a few weeks after cessation of exposure. Biologic monitoring of urine is useful for documenting current overexposure to arsenic compounds. The best approach is to collect a 24-hour urine specimen, although a spot urine sample can be useful. The total volume should be noted, and measurement of arsenic, creatinine, and specific gravity (the latter two allow correction for renal function and hydration, respectively) should be performed.

Ideally, the specimen should be obtained following two or three days abstention from known arsenic-containing food items, such as shellfish or seaweed. A 'normal' urinary arsenic concentration is less than 100 micrograms/liter, and the concentration will usually be less than 30 micrograms/liter in the absence of significant consumption of the arsenic-containing foods noted above. Assay techniques that can distinguish toxic arsenic species from those derived from ingestion of seafood exist, but are usually more expensive.

Because of the availability of sulfhydryl groups in keratin, absorbed arsenic tends to bind to hair and nails. The slow growth of these structures makes them useful as integrated measures of exposure to arsenic during the preceding months (normal: less than 1 microgram arsenic/gram). However, these tissues can be contaminated by external exposure, and so should be handled carefully and the results interpreted with some caution. Because of rapid clearance, the concentration of arsenic in blood is difficult to interpret and therefore is not a useful index of exposure.

Chelation with dimercaprol (British Anti-lewisite, or BAL), D-penicillamine, or dimercaptosuccinic acid (DMSA) can promote the excretion of absorbed arsenic in the setting of acute intoxication. Although chelation serves to accelerate the alleviation of acute symptoms, there is little evidence that such therapy has any impact on the chronic consequences of acute arsenic poisoning (e.g., peripheral

neuropathy or encephalopathy[21]). Following ingestion, attention should be directed toward gastrointestinal lavage and fluid and electrolyte replacement. There is no clear role for chelation in treatment of persons with chronic arsenic exposure. Early maintenance of high urine flow will reduce the risk of acute renal failure in persons with arsine exposure.

PREVENTION

Industrial arsenic exposure is prevented by appropriate engineering controls. Biologic monitoring of urine arsenic can assess the adequacy of such controls. Persons with a history of occupational exposure to arsenic smelter dust are required by OSHA to obtain regular chest radiographs, although the efficacy of such screening has not been demonstrated. Persons with arsenic exposure that has resulted in chronic non-malignant cutaneous changes (e.g., hyperkeratoses, hyperpigmentation) should have regular skin examinations to detect early malignant changes, and are at increased risk of skin and possibly various internal cancers. In the general environment most absorption of toxic arsenic species results from ingestion of contaminated drinking water; therefore testing of water supplies will detect exposure.

References

1. Tchounwou PB, Wilson B, Ishaque A. Important considerations in the development of public health advisories for arsenic and arsenic-containing compounds in drinking water. Rev Environ Health 1999; 14:211–29.
2. Milham S, Strong T. Human arsenic exposure in relation to a copper smelter. Environ Res 1974; 7:176–82.
3. Franzblau A, Lilis R. Acute arsenic intoxication from environmental arsenic exposure. Arch Environ Health 1989; 44:385–90.
4. Donofrio PD, Wilbourn AJ, Albers JW, Rogers L, Salanga V, Greenberg HS. Acute arsenic intoxication presenting as a Guillain-Barre-like syndrome. Muscle Nerve 1987; 10:114–20.
5. Rahman M, Tondel M, Ahmad SA, Axelson O. Diabetes mellitus associated with arsenic exposure in Bangladesh. Am J Epidemiol 1998; 148:198–203.
6. Schwartz RA. Arsenic and the skin. Int J Derm 1997; 36:241–50.
7. Engel RR, Hopenhayn-Rich C, Receveur O, Smith AH. Vascular effects of chronic arsenic exposure: a review. Epidemiol Rev 1994; 16:184–209.
8. Subramanian K, Kosnett M. Human exposures to arsenic from consumption of well water in West Bengal, India. Int J Occup Environ Health 1998; 4:217–30.
9. Chen CJ, Wu MM, Lee SS, Wang JD, Cheng SH, Wu HY. Atherogenicity and carcinogenicity of high-arsenic artesian well water. Arteriosclerosis 1988; 8:452–60.
10. Chiou HY, Huang WI, Su CL, Chang SF, Hsu YH, Chen CJ. Dose–response relationship between prevalence of cerebrovascular disease and ingested inorganic arsenic. Stroke 1997; 28:1717–23.
11. Hsueh YM, Wu WL, Huang YL, Chiou HY, Tseng CH, Chen CJ. Low serum carotene level and increased risk of ischemic heart disease related to long-term arsenic exposure. Atherosclerosis 1998; 141:249–57.
12. Tsai SM, Want TN, Ko YC. Mortality for certain diseases in areas with high levels of arsenic in drinking water. Arch Environ Health 1999; 54:186–93.

13. Tseng WP, Chu HM, How SW, Fong JM, Lin CS, Yeh S. Prevalence of skin cancer in an endemic area of chronic arsenicism in Taiwan. J Nat Cancer Inst 1968; 40:453–63.

14. Enterline PE, Henderson VL, Marsh GM. Exposure to arsenic and respiratory cancer: a reanalysis. Am J Epidemiol 1987; 125:929–38.

15. Jarup L, Pershagen G, Wall S. Cumulative arsenic exposure and lung cancer in smelter workers: a dose–response study. Am J Ind Med 1989; 15:31–41.

16. Cuzick J, Sasieni P, Evans S. Ingested arsenic, keratoses, and bladder cancer. Am J Epidemiol 1992; 136:417–21.

17. Hopenhayn-Rich C, Biggs ML, Fuchs A, et al. Bladder cancer mortality associated with arsenic in drinking water in Argentina. Epidemiology 1996; 7:117–24.

18. Smith AH, Goycolea M, Haque R, Biggs ML. Marked increase in bladder and lung cancer mortality in a region of Northern Chile due to arsenic in drinking water. Am J Epidemiol 1998; 147:660–9.

19. Tsuda T, Babazono A, Yamamoto E, et al. Ingested arsenic and internal cancer: a historical cohort study followed for 33 years. Am J Epidemiol 1995; 141:198–209.

20. Steinmaus C, Moore L, Hopenhayn-Rich C, Biggs ML, Smith AH. Arsenic in drinking water and bladder cancer. Cancer Invest 2000; 18:174–82.

21. Heyman A, Pfeiffer JB, Willett RW, Taylor HM. Peripheral neuropathy caused by arsenical intoxication: a study of 41 cases with observations on the effects of BAL (2,3, Dimercapto-Propanol). N Engl J Med 1956; 254:401–9.

39.3 **Beryllium and Cobalt**
Kathleen Kreiss

BERYLLIUM
Exposure settings

Beryllium is a lightweight metal that is transparent to x-rays and has neutron-moderating properties that make it an integral part of nuclear applications in weapons, energy, and research. It lends unique properties of high strength to metals to which it is alloyed, chiefly beryllium copper, with a beryllium content of 2–4%. Beryllium oxide is an insoluble salt with high heat conductivity, which leads to its use in specialty ceramics and in chip manufacture for semiconductors. Soluble beryllium salts are intermediates in beryllium refining and alloy manufacture. Historically, beryllium phosphors were used in fluorescent light manufacture. Their use was discontinued in 1949 because of the recognition of chronic beryllium disease in that industry.

Beryllium exposure occurs in nuclear industries, metal reclamation, beryllium ceramics manufacture, and beryllium extraction. In addition, metal workers and users of alloys, such as dental laboratory technicians, may be exposed to beryllium. In alloys, the beryllium content may be unknown or unrecognized as a hazard.

Since beryllium was recognized as a lung hazard in Europe in the 1930s, beryllium exposure–response relationships have been puzzling. Beryllium disease is an immunologic, cell-mediated hypersensitivity reaction, and most beryllium-exposed workers never develop lung disease. The few (5–15%) workers who develop beryllium disease usually have a disease latency of years,[1] that makes reconstruction of prior exposures difficult. However, beryllium disease has occurred in persons with only very limited exposure to beryllium, sometimes for very brief periods.[2] Within beryllium-using industries, cases of beryllium disease have occurred among secretaries, security guards, and even persons working in plants previously using beryllium containing materials without ongoing production.[1,3-5] Among beryllium disease cases, no relationship exists between tissue burden of beryllium and severity of disease.

In addition to bystander cases within industry, environmental cases of beryllium disease historically occurred among residents living close to exhaust stacks of beryllium extraction plants and among those with household exposure to dust-laden work clothes of beryllium workers.[1,6] Modeling of beryllium concentrations from stack effluents estimated environmental exposures to be three orders of magnitude less than in the plant, but the prevalence of beryllium disease in the plant and environments were similar. More recently, substantial lowering of air concentrations below the 2 µg/m³ permissible exposure limit did not decrease incidence of beryllium sensitization in new employees compared to employees previously exposed to higher air concentrations also below the exposure limit.[2] The failure to protect new employees by lowering air concentrations raises concern that skin exposure may affect sensitization risk.

These environmental, household, and industrial bystander cases signify the difficulty in ascertaining whether a biologically significant beryllium exposure has occurred in the workplace or in a patient with granulomatous or interstitial lung disease. All patients with sarcoidosis should be evaluated for the possibility of previous occupational or environmental beryllium exposure.[7] Within beryllium-using industries, surveillance for beryllium disease is appropriate for the populations with passive, intermittent, or inadvertent beryllium exposure, as well as for the traditional beryllium worker. Since beryllium metal and oxide particulate is biologically persistent, persons leaving the beryllium industry remain at risk for beryllium sensitization and disease the rest of their lives.

Although quantitative exposure–response relations are puzzling, cross-sectional studies of beryllium workers nearly always document process-related risk.[2-5,8] High-risk processes do not always have the highest beryllium mass concentrations in air.[8] This observation suggests that exposure characteristics apart from air-borne mass are more pertinent risk predictors.

Measurement

The current OSHA permissible exposure limit for beryllium of 2 µg/m³ time-weighted average was derived in 1949 by analogy to another toxic metal, lead, in rough proportion to the relative atomic weights of the two metals. The short-term (30 minute) exposure limit is 25 µg/m³, and some Department of Energy nuclear facilities had a housekeeping standard of 25 µg/ft² for surface contamination. The time-weighted average exposure historically recommended by NIOSH is 0.5 µg/m³. Recent workplace surveillance documents beryllium disease with average exposures well below these standards and sensitization within a few months of employment at exposures near the detection limit of methods used for workplace air sampling.[2] Most studies using qualitative or quantitative estimates of historical exposures have not demonstrated that cumulative exposure or exposure duration is a risk factor for disease,[3-5,8] but average or peak exposure may be important, particularly in plants with uniform size distributions across processes.[2,4,9]

Total beryllium concentration in air does not predict hazard, and alternative exposure metrics such as submicrometer particle number concentration appear promising[10,11] as risk factors for beryllium disease. Indices of skin contamination and integrity are currently under evaluation as predictors of sensitization risk. Among the sensitized, latency is important for disease expression,[2,3] but it is not yet clear whether the exposure requirements for beryllium disease differ from those for sensitization.[9]

Clinical effects

High levels of exposure to beryllium salts were thought to result in acute toxic pneumonitis in the 1940s, which was frequently self-limited, but sometimes progressed to irreversible chronic beryllium disease. Contact dermatitis affected a large percentage of workers early in the development of the extraction industry in the United States. The pathophysiology of acute beryllium disease remains unclear, and cases have not been reported in several decades. Its disappearance has been attributed to control of industrial exposures after the standard was developed.

The chronic granulomatous lung disease recognized today occurs among persons who develop lymphocyte reactivity to beryllium. Prevalence rates of sensitization in cross-sectional workforce screening are commonly about 10% if blood samples are split between two laboratories.[2,4,8,12] Among the sensitized, disease rates at the time of initial clinical evaluation vary between about 40% and 100%, with additional disease cases developing over years of follow-up. Sensitized workers with short latencies since first beryllium exposure are less likely to have beryllium disease.[2] Whether all beryllium-sensitized persons develop lung disease with follow-up is still unknown. Beryllium metal, alloy, and salts are implicated in the risk of sensitization and chronic beryllium disease (see also Chapter 19.7). Beryllium-contaminated wounds may require surgical excision of a granulomatous tissue response.

Beryllium-exposed cohorts and beryllium disease cases have a small excess risk for lung cancer,[13,14] and the International Agency for Research on Cancer has designated beryllium and beryllium compounds as human carcinogens. Quantitative exposure–lung cancer relationships are evident for average and maximum beryllium exposures and for cumulative exposure when historical exposure estimates are lagged 10 and 20 years.[15]

Clinical evaluation

Beryllium-exposed workers who develop cough, exertional dyspnea, or interstitial abnormalities on chest x-ray study need clinical evaluation for chronic beryllium disease (see also Chapter 19.7). In the setting of interstitial lung disease, the diagnosis can be made if cell-mediated immunity to beryllium is demonstrated by an abnormal lymphocyte proliferation test to beryllium salts (BeLPT) in either a blood sample or bronchoalveolar lavage sample. Blood samples sometimes are normal in cases of pathologically confirmed beryllium disease, and lavage samples are sometimes normal in smokers with excess lavage macrophages, which interfere with the lymphocyte response. Prior coordination with the laboratory performing the lymphocyte proliferation test is critical because cells must be cultured within 24 hours. Pathologic confirmation of granulomatous lung disease or lymphocytic alveolitis may be necessary in cases in which interstitial lung disease is not otherwise demonstrable by chest x-ray study or physiologic testing. The pathologic diagnosis usually can be made on transbronchial biopsy and bronchoalveolar lavage.

Asymptomatic beryllium-sensitized workers identified in workplace screening with the BeLPT typically undergo clinical evaluation with bronchoalveolar lavage and transbronchial lung biopsy. Those with beryllium disease re-

quire careful follow-up to ascertain when treatment should begin. Those with only sensitization require follow-up for development of disease. The natural history of beryllium sensitization and disease is under active study in relation to exposure and genetic characteristics.

Prevention

Primary prevention of beryllium sensitization among new employees has proven refractory to lowering beryllium air concentrations, apart from some modest effect in specific processes such as machining, in which sensitization rate has been decreased following enclosure and local exhaust.[2] The regulatory limit of 2 $\mu g/m^3$ does not protect against sensitization. In the absence of a quantitative basis for risk assessment, employers must consider a combination of engineering controls at the exposure source, scrupulous surface cleaning to lower potential skin contamination and resuspension, and personal protective equipment to reduce respiratory and dermatologic exposures to as low as reasonably achievable. Prevention of lung disease depends on prevention of sensitization and a beryllium lung burden.

Screening workforces for beryllium sensitization with the blood beryllium lymphocyte proliferation test is the cornerstone of prevention. Exposure surveillance does not assure a safe workplace. To date, no workforce of at least 100 employees screened with the beryllium lymphocyte proliferation test has been reported to be free of sensitization cases. To prioritize prevention needs, blood screening data should be linked with work and task history to document whether specific processes confer increased risk of beryllium sensitization and disease. Since past beryllium and process experience results in persistent risk, employers should consider sensitization in new employees as sentinels for inadequate current prevention efforts. In the beryllium industry, screening without surveillance analyses of risk factors results in missed opportunities to guide prevention efforts.

In the past, workplace surveillance for chronic beryllium disease has included a review of respiratory symptoms, a chest examination, spirometry, chest radiograph, and sometimes diffusing capacity. These tests are all insensitive in comparison to the blood lymphocyte proliferation test, which identifies persons with subclinical beryllium disease as well as those persons at high risk of developing beryllium disease because they have become sensitized. The traditional tests are best reserved for symptomatic workers who sometimes lack a blood lymphocyte proliferation response; in these instances, objective abnormalities on chest radiograph or longitudinal decreases/abnormalities in pulmonary physiology can support referral for bronchoscopic biopsy and lavage to establish a diagnosis of beryllium disease.

Screening of beryllium-exposed workers for cell-mediated hypersensitivity with BeLPT has a role in both primary and secondary prevention. Primary prevention requires seeing each sensitization case as a call for prevention based on linking screening information with exposures and task-based risks in surveillance. For secondary prevention, beryllium-sensitized workers without lung granulomas should probably be restricted from further beryllium exposure and followed carefully for the development of beryllium disease. Similarly, beryllium-sensitized workers with subclinical lung granulomas should be removed from exposure and followed to determine the need for treatment with corticosteroids.

No established role for biologic monitoring exists other than the BeLPT. Specifically, urine beryllium determinations have not proved useful or well correlated with exposure or risk of disease. Indeed, tissue and body fluid levels often are below detection limits in persons with beryllium disease.

Genetic characteristics are associated with beryllium disease risk[16-18] and are under intense investigation. Although the crude marker of HLA-DP^{glu69} confers a 5–10-fold risk of disease in some cohorts, the 30–40% prevalence of this set of alleles in worker populations results in poor positive predictive value. As many as a quarter of beryllium disease cases in population-based case series lack one of these alleles, limiting negative predictive value as well. Until allele-specific risk information becomes available, genetic analyses may not be of most value in confidential genetic counseling of prospective employees. It is not yet clear whether genetically susceptible beryllium workers can decrease their historically incurred risk by lowering or ceasing beryllium exposure. Counterbalancing the considerable ethical and discrimination issues surrounding genetic analyses of workers in a non-research setting is the prospect that longitudinal studies can define exposure–response relations for the substantial proportion of beryllium workers with enhanced susceptibility. Scientists also hope that genetic mechanistic information may open up more specific therapies for primary and secondary prevention of beryllium disease.

COBALT
Exposure settings

Cobalt is a hard magnetic metal that is used in alloys for permanent magnets, tool steels requiring high strength, and diverse metals in the electrical, automobile, and aircraft industries. Cobalt is used as the binder in cemented tungsten carbide, also known as hard metal, which is employed in wear-resistant tools, drill tips, and abrasives. Cobalt compounds are used as pigments; dryers for lacquers, paints, inks, and enamels; catalysts in polyester resin systems; animal feed additives; and foam stabilizers. Cobalt is found commonly in the glass, ceramic, photographic, printing, dental laboratory, and electroplating industries.

The industries in which cobalt-related respiratory disease occurs include tungsten carbide manufacturing and tool grinding, diamond polishing, porcelain painting, and cobalt extraction. Cobalt-related dermatitis is described in most of these industries, ceramics manufacturing, use of and manufacturing of printers, manufacturing of animal feed, and in European cement workers.

Measurement

The current US permissible exposure limit for cobalt is 50 µg/m^3, and the American Conference of Governmental Industrial Hygienists has proposed a limit of 20 µg/m^3. Whether these exposure limits protect the hypersensitive individual is unknown. Also unknown is the precise dose and route of exposure that results in hypersensitivity. Chronic airflow limitation effects occur with cobalt exposures well below the proposed standard.[19,20] No exposure standards exist in the United States for cobalt compounds.

Clinical effects

The occupational chest illnesses associated with cobalt exposure include giant cell pneumonitis, interstitial fibrosis, asthma, impaired ventilatory function, and non-inflammatory cardiomyopathy. Exposure–response relationships for cobalt are puzzling. In part, this may be because different cobalt-associated diseases may have different exposure–response relationships. Giant cell pneumonitis (see Chapter 19.7) occurs with hard metal exposure and in diamond polishing in which cobalt is used as a bonding agent for microdiamonds; however, this hard metal disease (cobalt lung in diamond polishers) does not seem to occur with cobalt exposure in the absence of particulate.[21] Asthma and giant cell pneumonitis are likely caused by specific immunological mechanisms, which occur at low prevalence and with variable latency. The characteristics of the sensitizing dose resulting in these diseases are largely unexplored. Cobalt-contaminated coolants used in the wet grinding of hard metal have been associated with a higher risk of hard metal disease, chest symptoms, and pulmonary function decrements despite very low cobalt levels, possibly because ionized cobalt aerosols are more biologically effective.[19,22] Ionized cobalt aerosols may not be associated with higher risk for cobalt asthma.[23] Non-specific pulmonary function decrements appear to be exposure related.[24]

A 1940 report of hard metal disease documented a 30% prevalence of radiologic abnormalities in hard metal workers. Such high prevalences are no longer found in cross-sectional studies in the United States or Japan, where prevalences of cobalt-related lung disease (asthma and/or interstitial disease) of 0.6–7% have been found. Diamond polishers who have been exposed to cobalt alone have prevalences of occupational lung disease (both asthma and fibrosis) of almost 1%.[20]

Cobalt dermatitis sometimes is accompanied by cell-mediated immunity, which can be documented with cobalt-specific lymphocyte proliferation tests. No consistent correlation exists between skin sensitization, demonstrated by patch testing, or cobalt dermatitis and cobalt-related lung disease. Cobalt was historically used to stimulate erythropoiesis in the treatment of anemia and may cause mild marrow stimulation after occupational or environmental exposure. Cardiomyopathy resulting from cobalt exposure, outside of several outbreaks in drinkers of beer to which cobalt had been added, has very rarely been reported.[25]

Some evidence exists that cobalt is a human carcinogen for lung cancer. The International Agency for Research on Cancer classified cobalt and its compounds as possible human carcinogens in 1991. Since that time, both positive and negative findings have been reported.[26-28]

Clinical evaluation

Bronchoalveolar lavage has shown diverse cellular abnormalities among cases of hard metal disease, including abnormalities in asymptomatic exposed workers suggestive of subclinical alveolar effects.[29] The diagnosis of cobalt lung/hard metal disease is confirmed by the demonstration of characteristic multinucleated giant cells in bronchoalveolar lavage fluid or lung biopsy. Interstitial fibrosis in cobalt workers has a non-specific pathology. No specific immunologic tests are known to be associated with cobalt lung disease, although this is an area of investigation. Cobalt-associated asthma has been demonstrated by specific inhalation challenge and, infrequently, by cobalt-specific antibody. Cobalt dermatologic sensitivity can be confirmed by patch testing and, in some cases, by cobalt-specific lymphocyte transformation tests using blood samples. The demonstration of cobalt cardiomyopathy in beer drinkers was epidemiologic and relied on examination of tissue levels in fatal or heart transplanted cases; clear clinical criteria for attribution of cardiomyopathy to cobalt do not exist.

Prevention

Engineering controls to lower cobalt exposures appear to have lowered historical prevalences of cobalt-related interstitial fibrosis, and epidemiologic evidence exists that abnormalities found on x-ray study are more prevalent among persons with high average exposures. However, cases exist following short and low exposures, consistent with an immunologic mechanism. The risk of cobalt asthma may be related to the exposure level, as reflected in attack rates by process group in hard metal workers, even when mean cobalt measurements were below the previous standard of 100 $\mu g/ m^3$.

No specific screening tests exist to identify those at risk of cobalt-related respiratory disease before exposure, although hard metal disease has been statistically associated with genetic alleles for the HLA-DPβ1 chain sharing a glutamic acid at position 69.[30] For workers developing cobalt-related asthma, giant cell pneumonitis, or less specific interstitial fibrosis, removal from cobalt exposure is mandatory. The natural history of cobalt-related lung disease is variable, with some cases of asthma or interstitial disease improving with cessation of exposure, and a substantial minority progressing despite exposure cessation and treatment.[31,32] Hard metal disease has recurred in a unilateral transplanted lung despite no further exposure nor documented spillage from the native affected lung,[33] suggestive of an autoimmune mechanism.

Cobalt dermatitis is a hypersensitivity reaction, and prudence dictates minimization of skin contact in the unsensitized individual and avoidance in those persons responding to cobalt in patch tests or lymphocyte transformation tests. Cobalt particulate has been shown to penetrate skin, as reflected in cobalt urinary excretion.[34]

Surveillance for cobalt asthma and interstitial lung diseases should include a review of respiratory symptoms, spirometry, diffusing capacity, and chest radiographs. In symptomatic workers, cross-shift spirometry, peak flow measurements, and tests of specific or non-specific bronchial reactivity may be helpful in establishing the relation of asthma to exposure and removal from exposure. Pulmonary function testing, including diffusing capacity, and radiographs are often insensitive indicators of interstitial disease,[35,36] and normal results should not affect the threshold for diagnostic evaluation in cobalt-exposed workers with dyspnea on exertion or persistent cough (see Chapter 19.7).

Biologic monitoring for cobalt exposure using blood or urine samples has been performed in studies of cobalt exposure. Urine excretion of inhaled cobalt has multiphase kinetics that does not allow easy correlation between end-shift urinary and ambient air levels, particularly for insoluble forms of cobalt. For soluble cobalt compounds, measurement of urine or blood cobalt at the end of the work week may be useful in assessing recent exposure.[34,37]

References

1. Eisenbud M, Lisson J. Epidemiologic aspects of beryllium induced non-malignant lung disease: a 30-year update. J Occup Med 1983; 25:196–202.
2. Henneberger PK, Cumro D, Deubner D, Kent M, McCawley M, Kreiss K. Beryllium sensitization and disease among long-term and short-term workers in a beryllium ceramics plant. Int Arch Occup Environ Health 2001; 74:167–76.
3. Kreiss K, Wasserman S, Mroz MM, Newman LS. Beryllium disease screening in the ceramics industry: blood lymphocyte test performance and exposure disease relations. J Occup Med 1993; 35:267–74.
4. Kreiss K, Mroz MM, Newman LS, Martyny J, Zhen B. Machining risk of beryllium disease and sensitization with median exposures below 2 ug/m^3. Am J Ind Med 1996; 30:16–25.
5. Kreiss K, Mroz MM, Zhen B, Martyny JW, Newman LS. Epidemiology of beryllium sensitization and disease in nuclear workers. Am Rev Respir Dis 1993; 148:985–91.
6. Eisenbud M. Origins of the standards for control of beryllium disease (1947–1949). Environ Res 1982; 27:79–88.
7. Newman LS, Kreiss K. Non-occupational beryllium disease masquerading as sarcoidosis: identification by blood lymphocyte proliferative response to beryllium. Am Rev Respir Dis 1992; 145:1212–4.
8. Kreiss K, Mroz MM, Zhen B, Wiedemann H, Barna B. Risks of beryllium disease related to work processes at a metal, alloy, and oxide production plant. Occup Environ Med 1997; 54 605–12.
9. Viet SM, Troma-Krajewski J, Rogers J. Chronic beryllium disease and beryllium sensitization at Rocky Flats: a case-control study. AIHAJ 2000; 61:244–54.
10. Kent MS, Robins TG, Madl AK. Is total mass or mass of alveolar-deposited air-borne particles of beryllium a better predictor of the prevalence of disease? A preliminary study of a beryllium processing facility. Appl Occup Environ Hyg 2001; 16:539–58.
11. McCawley M, Kent M, Berakis M. Ultrafine beryllium number concentration as a possible metric for chronic beryllium disease. Appl Occup Environ Hyg 2001; 16:631–8.

12. Kreiss K, Newman LS, Mroz MM, Campbell PA. Screening blood test identifies subclinical beryllium disease. J Occup Med 1989; 31:603–8.

13. Steenland K, Ward E. Lung cancer incidence among patients with beryllium disease: a cohort mortality study. J Natl Cancer Inst 1991; 83:1380–5.

14. Ward E, Okun A, Ruder A, Fingerhut M, Steenland K. A mortality study of workers at seven beryllium processing plants. Am J Ind Med 1992; 22:885–904.

15. Sanderson W, Ward E, Steenland K, Petersen M. Lung cancer case-control study of beryllium workers. Am J Ind Med 2001; 39:133–44.

16. Richeldi L, Sorrentino R, Saltini C. HLA-DPB1 Glutamate 69: a genetic marker of beryllium disease. Science 1993; 262:242–4.

17. Richeldi L, Kreiss K, Mroz M, et al. Interaction of genetic and exposure factors in the prevalence of berylliosis. Am J Ind Med 1997; 32:337–40.

18. Wang Z, White PS, Petrovic M, et al. Differential susceptibilities to chronic beryllium disease contributed by different Glu69 HLA DPB1 and DPA1 alleles. J Immunol 1999; 163:1647 53.

19. Kennedy SM, Chan-Yeung M, Marion S, Lea J, Teschke K. Maintenance of stellite and tungsten carbide saw tips: respiratory health and exposure-response evaluations. Occup Environ Med 1995; 52:185–91.

20. Nemery B, Casier P, Roosels D, et al. Survey of cobalt exposure and respiratory health in diamond polishers. Am Rev Respir Dis 1992; 145:610–6.

21. Lison D, Lauwerys R, Demedts M, Nemery B. Experimental research into the pathogenesis of cobalt/hard metal lung disease. Eur Respir J 1996; 9:1024–8.

22. Sjogren I, Hillerdal G, Andersson A, Zetterstrom O. Hard metal lung disease: importance of cobalt in coolants. Thorax 1980; 35:653–9.

23. Kusaka Y, Iki M, Kumagai S, Goto S. Epidemiological study of hard metal asthma. Occup Environ Med 1996; 53:188–93.

24. Kusaka Y, Iki M, Kumagai S, Goto S. Decreased ventilatory function in hard metal workers. Occup Environ Med 1996; 53:194–9.

25. Jarvis JQ, Hammond E, Meier R, Robinson C. Cobalt cardiomyopathy. A report of two cases from mineral assay laboratories and a review of the literature. J Occup Med 1992; 34:620–6.

26. Moulin JJ, Wild P, Romazini S, et al. Lung cancer risk in hard-metal workers. Am J Epidemiol 1998; 148:241–8.

27. Tüchsen F, Jensen MV, Villadsen E, Lynge E. Incidence of lung cancer among cobalt-exposed women. Scand J Work Environ Health 1996; 22:444–50.

28. Wild P. Lung cancer mortality in a site producing hard metals. Occup Environ Med 2000; 57:568–73.

29. Forni A. Bronchoalveolar lavage in the diagnosis of hard metal disease. Science Total Environ 1994; 150:69–76.

30. Potolicchio I, Mosconi G, Forni A, Nemery B, Seghizzi P, Sorrentino R. Susceptibility to hard metal lung disease is strongly associated with the presence of glutamate 69 in HLA-DPβ chain. Eur J Immunol 1997; 27:2741–3.

31. Pisati G, Zedda S. Outcome of occupational asthma due to cobalt hypersensitivity. Science Total Environ 1994; 150:167–71.

32. Zanelli R, Barbic F, Migliori M, Michetti G. Uncommon evolution of fibrosing alveolitis in a hard metal grinder exposed to cobalt dusts. Science Total Environ 1994; 150:225–9.

33. Frost AE, Keller CA, Brown RW, et al. Giant cell interstitial pneumonitis. Disease recurrence in the transplanted lung. Am Rev Respir Dis 1993; 148:1401–4.

34. Linnainmaa M, Kiilunen M. Urinary cobalt as a measure of exposure in the wet sharpening of hard metal and stellite blades. Int Arch Occup Environ Health 1997; 69:193–200.

35. Suardi R, Belotti L, Ferrari MT, et al. Health survey of workers occupationally exposed to cobalt. Science Total Environ 1994; 150:197–200.

36. Ruokonen EL. Linnainmaa M, Seuri M, Juhakoski P, Soderstrom KO. A fatal case of hard-metal disease. Scand J Work Environ Health 1996; 22:62–5.

37. Lison D, Buchet J-P, Swennen B, Molders J, Lauwerys R. Biologic monitoring of workers exposed to cobalt metal, salt, oxides, and hard metal dust. Occup Environ Med 1994; 51:447–50.

39.4 **Cadmium**
Alfred Franzblau

EXPOSURE SETTINGS

Cadmium was first isolated in 1817, and it has no known nutritional function in man. No ore is mined specifically for its cadmium content. Cadmium (Cd) is derived as a byproduct from smelting of other metals, primarily zinc, with some derived from ores of copper and lead.[1] In recent years recycling of cadmium from nickel-cadmium batteries has become more significant. Usage patterns of cadmium have changed in the last two decades, with increased use in batteries and reduction in other uses. Currently, the largest application of cadmium is in nickel-cadmium batteries (70% in the United States). Other major uses include stabilizers in polyvinyl chloride plastics, such as cadmium stearate (17%); plating and coatings on ferrous and non-ferrous metals (8%); specialized alloys, particularly copper; some specialized electrical devices; and pigments (e.g., cadmium sulfide, cadmium sulfoselenide).[1] Occupational exposure has been documented in each of these processes.

An important application, particularly from the perspective of occupational exposure, is cadmium in silver solder and in welding electrodes, although most solder no longer contains cadmium. Cadmium has a low boiling point (765°C), so welding on cadmium-plated materials, or use of cadmium-containing solder or welding electrodes, creates cadmium fume and the potential for acute pulmonary toxicity. The EPA has banned cadmium-related fungicides from many uses.

Cigarettes normally contain 1–2 micrograms Cd per cigarette, due to naturally occurring Cd in tobacco leaves, of which approximately 5–10% can be absorbed.[2] Hence, smokers have greater exposure and higher body burden of cadmium compared with non-smokers, and cadmium biomarkers are correlated with the number of cigarettes smoked per day.[3] The cadmium content of each cigarette may be increased up to 20 micrograms in a contaminated work setting. Increased ingestion of cadmium can also result from contamination of food in the work environment.

Skin absorption of cadmium is negligible, and gastrointestinal absorption is usually about 5% of the ingested amount. The latter can be increased to 20% with iron deficiency or low calcium intake. Pulmonary absorption, which is the main route of occupational exposure, can be up to 50%, depending on particle size and solubility. For most people who are non-smokers and who do not have occupational exposure, the primary route of absorption is via ingestion, estimated to be about 30 micrograms/day.[1] Certain grains will selectively concentrate cadmium present in soil or water.[4] Thus, environmental contamination with cadmium can result in substantial human over-exposure due to ingestion of contaminated foods.[5,6] At least one major episode of clinical cadmium-related toxicity has been traced to this route of exposure (itai-itai disease in Japan[5]).

CLINICAL EFFECTS
Acute

Inhalation exposure to cadmium fumes, usually associated with welding or silver soldering, can result in a syndrome that can be confused with metal fume fever (MFF). It may be possible to identify cadmium as a possible etiologic factor since cadmium fumes have a characteristic yellowish color, while zinc fumes are white. Clinical effects can be delayed up to 24 hours. Symptoms include shortness of breath, fever, weakness, and respiratory insufficiency. With mild exposure, these effects may resolve within a few days, similar to MFF. Following more intense exposure, patients will not improve after one or two days, and may develop acute chemical pneumonitis and pulmonary edema, with typical findings on physical examination and laboratory test results (rales, hypoxia, elevated leukocyte count, patchy infiltrates on chest radiographs, impaired gas transfer). If death from respiratory insufficiency does not occur, recovery can be prolonged, and permanent (restrictive) pulmonary dysfunction may result.[7]

Cadmium salts are direct irritants to the gastrointestinal mucosa. Ingestion of large quantities causes nausea, vomiting, abdominal cramps, diarrhea, and shock from fluid loss. Symptoms develop within minutes of ingestion.

Chronic

The kidneys are the critical target organs among persons with chronic cadmium exposure. Other reported effects include pulmonary emphysema; slight anemia; liver dysfunction; disruption of calcium, phosphate and vitamin D metabolism with consequent osteoporosis, osteomalacia and formation of calcium renal stones; anosmia and possible ulceration of the nasal septum; yellowing of teeth. Increased risk of lung and prostate cancer have been suggested but not proved.

Absorbed cadmium is initially transported in the blood, primarily within red blood cells, to other tissues. The major repositories are kidney, liver, and muscle; these three tissue depots can account for up to 70% of the body burden. Cadmium stimulates the production of a low molecular weight binding protein, metallothionein, which binds the metal in tissue, plasma, and within red blood cells. Cadmium released from tissue, in the form of cadmium-metallothionein complex, is filtered at the renal glomerulus, and the complex is efficiently reabsorbed in the proximal renal tubules. Reabsorbed cadmium accumulates in proximal renal tubular cells. If the cadmium within renal tubular cells exceeds a certain threshold (approximately 100–300 micrograms Cd/gram wet weight of renal tissue), the cells are damaged, and function is impaired. The clinical result is decreased capacity of proximal tubular reabsorption, initially with loss of 'tubular' proteins in urine. The latter include β-2 microglobulin, retinol binding proteins, and N-acetyl-β-glucosaminidase (NAG). In addition, there is marked increase in urinary excretion of cadmium due to loss of cadmium that had been sequestered within renal tubular cells that were damaged.

With more pronounced damage to renal tubules, the proteinuria is increased, and there is also loss of other components of glomerular filtrate, such as calcium, phosphate, amino acids, other acids, and glucose. 1-Hydroxylation of 25-hydroxy-vitamin D_3 may be impaired, since this occurs within tubular cells. Eventually, glomerular function can become compromised, resulting in albuminuria, decreased glomerular filtration rate, and elevated serum creatinine. Once initiated, these processes may not be reversible (depending on severity), and, in fact, may progress even following cessation of exposure, although cadmium-induced proteinuria rarely exceeds 2 grams per day.[8]

Increased incidence of calcium-containing renal calculi has been documented to occur among occupationally exposed groups, particularly among those with longer, more intense exposure (hence greater body burden) and renal dysfunction.[9] Overt bone disease, i.e., osteomalacia, osteoporosis and pseudo-fractures, related to hypercalciuria, hyperphosphaturia, and decreased 1-hydroxylation of 25-hydroxy-vitamin D_3 has also been recorded, although these tend to occur in conjunction with decreased dietary intake of calcium and hormonal effects such as post-menopausal status. The latter was the case in Toyama Prefecture, Japan, where people consumed rice grown in fields that had been irrigated with cadmium-contaminated industrial effluent. The major clinical presentation, proteinuria with osteomalacia and bone pain, occurred primarily among postmenopausal women and was termed 'itai-itai' (ouch-ouch) disease. More recently, lower-level environmental (as opposed to industrial) exposures to cadmium have been associated with increased risk of bone fractures,[10] and increased excretion of NAG, β-2 microglobulin, and retinol binding proteins.[11]

Inhalation of cadmium fumes appears to contribute to the development of emphysema, chronic bronchitis, and COPD among exposed workers, independent of cigarette smoking.[12] A history of acute, cadmium-induced chemical pneumonitis is not required, and this effect appears to be dose related.

The anemia observed in association with cadmium exposure has been a mild, reversible depression of hemoglobin. The mechanism is not entirely clear, but there is evidence suggesting that cadmium interferes with iron absorption, and may have a slight hemolytic effect.

The liver is one of the major sites of cadmium deposition. Liver dysfunction is uncommon, but can manifest as slight elevation of hepatic enzymes in serum.

Epidemiologic cohort studies have identified an elevated risk of death from lung cancer and prostate cancer among workers with long-term cadmium exposure,[13–16] although it has been difficult to control for confounding by concurrent occupational exposures to other lung carcinogens.

DIAGNOSIS, EVALUATION, AND TREATMENT

When evaluating persons with acute inhalation exposure to metal fumes, inquiry must be made concerning the possible presence of cadmium. Lack of awareness may be compounded by cadmium being present as only a trace component. The initial clinical picture can be confused with the benign condition, metal fume fever. Measurement of blood cadmium levels is considered a reasonable marker for recent cadmium exposure. However, with acute respiratory exposure blood cadmium may not be elevated and such test results might be delayed long after therapy may need to be initiated. Urinary cadmium levels, discussed below, can help assess cadmium body burden, but are not a good indicator of acute exposure. Therapy is primarily supportive. Chelation is risky since cadmium mobilized from pulmonary and other tissues is likely to be deposited in the kidneys, and thus precipitate or accelerate the development of renal dysfunction. Cadmium-induced chemical pneumonitis should be suspected in a welder who appears much more ill than would be typical in metal fume fever, or who fails to recover from apparent metal fume fever in the normal course.

Since the kidneys are the primary target organ with chronic cadmium exposure, and renal manifestations of cadmium toxicity are not reversible, the goal is to monitor workers to prevent the development of kidney dysfunction. The critical parameter for predicting toxicity is body burden or, more precisely, the renal burden of cadmium. Research methods for direct, in-vivo assessment of kidney burden of cadmium exist (e.g., neutron activation analysis), but are not practical clinical tools. The practical alternatives involve measurement of a variety of biologic parameters that reflect renal burden of cadmium or early nephrotoxicity.

On initiation of chronic exposure, cadmium levels in whole blood increase several-fold during the first few months, and then plateau. With cessation of exposure, cadmium in whole blood decreases following a two-compartment model, with an initial rapid clearance phase ($t_{1/2}$ of approximately 100 days), followed by a much slower phase ($t_{1/2}$ of about 10 years).[17] Thus, measurement of cadmium in whole blood during ongoing exposure mostly reflects exposure during preceding months. However, increased blood cadmium can occur with relatively low body burden (e.g., after only a few months of exposure), and moderate cadmium levels in blood may be detected after prolonged absence of exposure, despite near critical body burden. In non-occupationally exposed persons, whole blood cadmium is usually well below 1 microgram Cd/100 ml whole blood, smokers have slightly higher levels than non-smokers.

Cadmium is excreted primarily via the urine. Among persons without occupational exposure, urine cadmium levels are generally below 2 micrograms Cd/g urinary creatinine. Smokers may have slightly higher levels than non-smokers. During ongoing exposure, and prior to saturation of cadmium-binding sites within the kidneys, most filtered cadmium is reabsorbed in the proximal tubules, and so there may be only slight elevation of urinary cadmium. Urinary cadmium at this stage roughly reflects body burden. When binding sites within the kidney become saturated, urinary cadmium increases, and reflects 'overflow' of that which cannot be reabsorbed. At the onset of renal dysfunction, urinary cadmium increases dramatically, reflecting loss of cadmium that had been sequestered in proximal tubular cells. Even if exposure were to cease at this point, urinary cadmium would remain markedly elevated as more cadmium is lost from the kidney, and cadmium continues to be redistributed to the kidneys from non-renal tissue stores. The probability of renal dysfunction is increased when urinary cadmium exceeds 10–20 micrograms Cd/g urinary creatinine.[8,17] Persons with cadmium-induced renal dysfunction generally have urine levels above this threshold.

The earliest sign of renal dysfunction is increased excretion of low molecular weight proteins that would normally be reabsorbed in the proximal tubule. Classically, this has been detected by measuring β-2 microglobulin in urine (normal: less than 200 micrograms/g urinary creatinine). Measurement of retinol binding protein or NAG are alternative choices; retinol binding protein has the advantage that it is more stable in urine in the range of physiologic pH, but is not routinely available.

In persons with suspected renal dysfunction, a thorough evaluation should include measurement of serum electrolytes, BUN and creatinine, cadmium in blood and urine, full characterization of proteinuria, determination of whether renal calculi are present, a thorough screening for alternative or contributory factors to renal disease, and search for non-renal effects of cadmium exposure (e.g., pulmonary function tests, anosmia, liver dysfunction, yellowing of teeth). Renal histology is that of tubulo-interstitial nephritis, as opposed to glomerular disease, and tissue cadmium content is elevated. Possible metabolic bone disease is prevented or treated with calcium and vitamin D supplementation. As suggested above, chelation therapy is probably risky since cadmium mobilized from non-renal body stores would tend to add to the kidney burden, and is not recommended. Also, removal of cadmium from renal sites would not help since kidney dysfunction is believed to be irreversible.

PREVENTION

Biologic monitoring of exposed workers, including urinary and blood cadmium, and urinary β-2 microglobulin, is recommended. The OSHA Cadmium Standard mandates reassessment of the worker's exposure and further medical evaluation at certain action levels (such as urine Cd > 3 micrograms/g creatinine or blood Cd > 5 micrograms/l), and removal from exposure at higher biologic monitoring levels (urine Cd > 7 micrograms/g creatinine, blood Cd > 10 micrograms/l). Chest x-ray and pulmonary function testing are also recommended for cadmium-exposed workers.

If possible, other materials should be substituted for cadmium. When this is not an option, exposures should be reduced through engineering controls, improved work practices, protective clothing, good housekeeping, and other standard approaches. Workers should be educated about cadmium, so that they can take appropriate steps when exposed to cadmium-containing materials.

References

1. Agency for Toxic Substances and Disease Registry (ATSDR). Toxicological profile for cadmium. Atlanta, GA: US Department of Health & Human Services, Public Health Service, Agency for Toxic Substances and Disease Registry, 1999.
2. Shaham J, Meltzer A, Ashkenazi R, Ribak J. Biologic monitoring of exposure to cadmium, a human carcinogen, as a result of active and passive smoking. J Occup Environ Med 1996; 38:1220–8.
3. dell'Omo M, Muzi G, Piccinini R, et al. Blood cadmium concentrations in the general population in Umbria, Central Italy. Sci Total Environ 1999; 226:57–64.
4. Cabrera C, Ortega E, Lorenzo M-L, Lopez M. Cadmium contamination of vegetable crops, farmlands, and irrigation waters. Rev Envir Contam Toxicol 1998; 154:55–81.
5. Nogawa K, Kido T. Biologic monitoring of cadmium exposure in itai-itai disease epidemiology. Int Arch Occup Environ Health 1993; 65:S43–S46.
6. Nordberg GF, Jin T, Kong Q, et al. Biologic monitoring of cadmium exposure and renal effects in a population group residing in a polluted area in China. Sci Total Environ 1997; 199:111–4.
7. Townshend RH. A case of acute cadmium pneumonitis: lung function tests during a four-year follow-up. Br J Ind Med 1968; 25:68–71.
8. Roels HA, van Assche FJ, Oversteyns M, de Groof M, Lauwerys RR, Lison D. Reversibility of microproteinuria in cadmium workers with incipient tubular dysfunction after reduction of exposure. Am J Ind Med 1997; 31:645–52.
9. Järup L, Elinder CG. Incidence of renal stones among cadmium exposed battery workers. Br J Ind Med 1993; 50:598–602.
10. Staessen JA, Roels HA, Emelianov D, et al. Environmental exposure to cadmium, forearm bone density, and risk of fractures: prospective population study. Lancet 1999; 353:1140–4.
11. Buchet JP, Lauwerys R, Roels H, et al. Renal effects of cadmium body burden of the general population. Lancet 1990; 336:699–702.
12. Davison AG, Fayers PM, Taylor AJ, et al. Cadmium fume inhalation and emphysema. Lancet 1988; 1(8587):663–7.
13. Armstrong BG, Kazantzis G. Prostatic cancer and chronic respiratory and renal disease in British cadmium workers: a case control study. Br J Ind Med 1985; 42:540–5.
14. Elinder CG, Kjellstrom T, Hogstedt C, Andersson K, Spang G. Cancer mortality of cadmium workers. Br J Ind Med 1985; 42:651–5.
15. Sorahan T. Mortality from lung cancer among a cohort of nickel cadmium battery workers: 1946–84. Br J Ind Med 1987; 44:803–9.
16. Thun MJ, Schnorr TM, Smith AB, Halperin WE. Mortality among a cohort of US cadmium production workers – an update. J Natl Cancer Inst 1985; 71:325–33.
17. McDiarmid MA, Freeman CS, Grossman EA, Martonik J. Follow-up of biologic monitoring results in cadmium workers removed from exposure. Am J Ind Med 1997; 32:261–7.

39.5 Chromium
Alfred Franzblau, David H Garabrant

EXPOSURE SETTINGS

Metallic chromium was first isolated in 1797, and by the second decade of the 19th century chromium compounds had become important in industrial processes (e.g., potassium dichromate used as a mordant in textile dyeing). Following on soon after the discovery of their industrial utility were early descriptions of toxic effects of exposure to chromium compounds. Chromium and its compounds are widely used in industry.

The toxic effects of chromium are related primarily to exposure to the hexavalent [chromium(VI)] compounds, which are called chromates. Chrome alloys such as stainless steel [zero valence, chromium(0)] and trivalent chromium [chromium(III)] compounds have important and widespread industrial applications, but these compounds are generally less toxic than the hexavalent forms. NIOSH has estimated that over 305,000 workers in the United States are potentially exposed to chromium compounds, of which 196,000 are exposed to hexavalent chromium compounds.

In the occupational setting, exposure occurs by inhalation or skin contact with chromium-containing mist, dust, or fumes, or via direct contact with aqueous chromium solutions (e.g., in tannery workers). Ingestion of chromium salts or solutions can cause significant toxicity or death due to gastrointestinal irritation and renal failure, but this is not an important route of exposure in the industrial setting.

Chromium is derived from chromite ores (e.g., iron dichromate, $FeOCr_2O_3$), and exposure can occur among workers employed in the various roasting processes involved in the processing of ore and production of common commercially useful compounds (e.g., sodium or potassium chromate and dichromate, ammonium dichromate, and chromium oxide). Significant exposure also occurs during stainless steel production, stainless steel welding, and among users of chromium compounds. Chrome electroplating operations provide an opportunity for exposure to mist of plating bath solutions, which usually contain chromium trioxide (CrO_3), a potent irritant. Important exposure to chromium compounds also occurs in leather tanning (basic trivalent chromic sulfate, $Cr_2[SO_4]_3$, plus hexavalent forms), production and use of chromium-based paint pigments (yellow pigments based on lead chromate and zinc chromate), metallurgic operations (grinding or welding chrome alloy materials), use of cement (many cements contain trace amounts of various soluble hexavalent chromium compounds), textile dyeing (chromic oxide [Cr_2O_3] and chromic sulfate), manufacture of refractory products, and glassmaking (chromic oxide). Chrome compounds have produced toxicity among workers in a variety of smaller industries, including lithography, wood preserving, match production, paper pulp manufacture, and crayon making.[1]

Total chromium exposures in US air are typically below 0.01 micrograms/m^3 in rural areas and 0.01–0.03 micrograms/m^3 in urban areas. Occasionally, levels above 0.5 micrograms/m^3 have been measured. The proportion of total chromium comprising chromium(VI) varies but is often 20–30%. In the US, occupational permissible exposure limits are 1000 micrograms/m^3 for chromium metal and insoluble salts, 500 micrograms/m^3 for chromium(III) compounds, and 100 micrograms/m^3 for chromic acid and chromates [carcinogenic chromium(VI) compounds]. Thus, ambient environmental exposures are typically at least two orders of magnitude below occupational exposures.[2]

CLINICAL EFFECTS

Chromium(III) and chromium(VI) arc the oxidation states of chromium most commonly encountered by humans. Water-soluble chromium(III) compounds are not well absorbed into the body and enter cells poorly. Water-soluble chromium(VI) compounds (such as CrO_4^{2-}) are far more toxic because they are actively transported into cells in place of other structurally similar anions, such as phosphate (PO_4^{2-}). Inside the cell, chromium(VI) is reduced via reactive intermediates ultimately to chromium(III), which binds tightly to cellular ligands and is largely responsible for toxicity. Chromium(III) is an essential nutrient for humans and is involved in the metabolism of glucose. Average daily consumption of Cr(III) is 60 micrograms/day from food, with intake of 50–200 micrograms/day recommended.

Soluble hexavalent chromium compounds tend to be strong oxidizing agents. They also penetrate skin and mucous membranes more effectively than trivalent forms. These properties may explain, in part, the potent irritant properties of soluble hexavalent chromium compounds.

Cutaneous exposure to mist, dust, or chromium solutions can result in simple skin irritation. The classic cutaneous chromium lesion is the chrome ulcer, or chrome hole. This lesion was first described in 1827 and may be a relatively painless, although deep, punched-out wound that can penetrate into underlying tissue layers including cartilage, but usually not bone. Secondary bacterial infections are common. On removal of the affected individual from exposure, healing may require months and leave a residual scar. These lesions occur at sites of greatest exposure, such as over bony prominences of the hands and forearms, although they have been described on the lower extremities when work practices have been particularly poor. They also tend to occur at sites of skin trauma, such as incidental nicks or cuts. They are not related to chrome sensitization.[3]

The mucous membranes also suffer irritant consequences, including erythema of the throat, conjunctival irritation, nasal itching and soreness, edema of the uvula, coryza, epistaxis, ulceration of the nasal mucosa, and nasal septal perforation. With very high exposures, a high prevalence of nasal septal perforations may occur (greater than 50% in some settings) with rapid onset, in some cases less than 1 week, following initiation of employment. Because the damaged cartilage is not the most anterior portion, there may not be any apparent external deformity of the nose. Sinusitis and nasal polyps also have been noted among exposed workers, and rare cases of perforation of the tympanic membranes have been described.

Inhalation of chromium mist, dust, or fumes can produce acute bronchoconstriction, probably through a direct irritant mechanism. Chronic bronchitis and persistent abnormalities in pulmonary function have not been described following cessation of exposure. Allergic asthma due to chromium is uncommon, with fewer than two dozen cases documented in the published literature. Immediate, late, and dual bronchoconstrictive responses may occur. The immunologic mechanisms that have been reported for asthma include chromium-specific IgE (in one case of an immediate reaction) and a cell-mediated response (in one case of a delayed reaction).[4]

In addition to their direct irritant effects, chrome compounds (usually dichromates or hexavalent forms) also are potent cutaneous sensitizers.[5] Chromium allergic contact dermatitis is the most common occupational dermatosis among male patients. Exposure can be occult owing to the ubiquitous nature of chromium. Eczematous skin lesions usually are found in areas of greatest exposure, such as the hands and arms. Sensitization to chromium tends to persist for years, even after cessation of exposure, based on persistence of positive patch tests among workers who have been sensitized[6] (see also Chapter 29.1).

A number of hexavalent chromium compounds are established human carcinogens, including calcium chromate, chromium trioxide, lead chromate, strontium chromate, and zinc chromate.[7] Epidemiologic studies have documented increased rates of respiratory cancer (lung and nasal, primarily) among workers in the chromate production industry and the chromate pigment industry[8] (see Chapter 30.2). Of interest, studies of stainless steel welders and in the ferrochromium alloy industry have given inconclusive results regarding cancer risks, even though exposure to chromium(VI) is appreciable in these settings.[9] There is scant evidence that metallic chromium and chromium(III) compounds are carcinogenic in humans or animals and these materials are currently *not classifiable as to their carcinogenicity to humans* (IARC Group 3).[1] Lung cancers associated with exposure to hexavalent chromium compounds have prolonged latencies (delay from onset of exposure), generally lasting more than 20 years. There is no unique or predominant histology. Although some studies have indicated excesses of other cancers (such as gastrointestinal cancers) in the bichromate producing industry and the chromate pigment industry, these results are inconsistent. Chromium(VI) compounds generally are not regarded as causing cancers outside the respiratory tract.

Mild impairment of proximal renal tubular function, manifested by an increased excretion of β-2 microglobulin and retinol binding protein, has been documented among active chrome platers. There is no apparent effect on glomerular function, as reflected in the excretion of albumin. Tubular dysfunction appears to be reversible on cessation of exposure. Acute tubular necrosis with renal failure has been observed in rare cases following massive dermal absorption of chromium (e.g., falling into a vat of hot chromic acid). These observations of low molecular weight proteinuria and acute tubular necrosis raise the possibility that long-term exposure to chromates may be a risk factor for persistent renal injury.

DIAGNOSIS, EVALUATION, AND TREATMENT

The pharmacokinetics of chromium in humans are complex. Absorbed hexavalent chromium is mainly excreted in the urine. With ongoing exposure, the half-life in urine ranges from 15 to 41 hours. Detailed kinetic studies suggest a three-compartment model for chromates, with half-lives of about 7 hours, 15–30 days, and 3–5 years. Therefore, measurement of chromium in urine can be used to document recent exposure to chromates, although the concentration of chromium in urine is not correlated with toxicity.[10,11] The correlation between chromium(III) exposure and urine chromium levels is poor and urine monitoring is not felt to be useful for these exposures. In non-occupationally exposed populations urinary chromium is usually less than 5 micrograms/g of creatinine.[2] Because of a lack of adequate data, blood, hair, and nail levels of chromium are not interpretable at present and should not be relied upon in assessing exposure.[12]

If not prevented, chrome ulcers should be identified early and workers with such lesions should be removed from exposure until complete healing has occurred. Treatment of other acute cutaneous and mucous membrane effects of chromium exposure also requires reduction of exposure. Patch testing can be used to distinguish between irritant dermatitis and allergic contact dermatitis. Topical steroid preparations may be beneficial in treatment of both entities. Because sensitization tends to be long lasting, affected workers may experience adverse social and economic consequences because of the need to find alternative employment.

The clinical approach to and prognosis of patients with lung cancer who have had occupational exposure to chromium compounds are the same as for other patients with lung cancer. There is evidence that the chromium content of pulmonary tissue from chromium-exposed workers with lung cancer is higher than among persons without lung cancer matched for smoking history, and also is higher than those with lung cancer but without any history of occupational chromium exposure. However, the diagnostic value of such measurements in an individual case is unclear. The histologic appearance and cell types of respiratory cancers related to carcinogenic chromium(VI) exposure do not have any defining characteristics.

PREVENTION

If alternative materials are not available, then engineering controls that minimize or eliminate chromium exposure must be applied. In addition, prevention of chrome ulcers and other irritant effects of chromium compounds depends on the education of workers concerning the importance of industrial cleanliness and the use of personal protective equipment. Such measures should be supplemented with regular examinations of the skin and nose to detect early signs of irritant effects.

Assessment of pulmonary function and chest radiographs is recommended in workers with inhalational chromium exposure.

In some processes, substitution of trivalent chromium for hexavalent chromium, as in electroplating baths, can be beneficial in reducing the incidence of sensitization. Chromium sensitization among cement workers can be prevented by adding ferrous sulfate ($FeSO_4$) immediately before mixing, when most skin contact occurs. The quality of the cement is not impaired, but the hexavalent chromium present in the cement is reduced and precipitated as chromium sulfate, an insoluble trivalent species. This procedure is already in practice in Scandinavia.

References

1. IARC. Chromium, nickel, and welding. Lyon, France: International Agency for Research on Cancer, 1990;49–256.
2. ATSDR. Toxicological profile for chromium. Washington, DC: US Department of Health and Human Services, 2000;1–419.
3. Burrows D. The dichromate problem. Int J Dermatol 1984; 23:215–20.
4. Bernstein IL, Nemery B, Brooks S. Metals. In: Bernstein IL, Chan-Yeung M, Malo J-L, Bernstein DI, eds. Asthma in the workplace, 2nd edn. New York: Marcel Dekker, 1999;501–21.
5. Fregert S. Chromium valencies and cement dermatitis. Br J Dermatol 1981; 105:7–9.
6. Peltonen L, Fraki J. Prevalence of dichromate sensitivity. Contact Derm 1983; 9:190–4.
7. National Toxicology Program. Ninth report on carcinogens. Research Triangle Park, NC: National Institute for Environmental Health Sciences, US Dept of Health and Human Services, 2000.
8. Langard S, Vigander T. Occurrence of lung cancer in workers producing chromium pigments. Br J Ind Med 1983; 40:71–4.
9. Moulin JJ, Wild P, Haguenoer JM, Faucon D, DeGaudemaris R, Mur JM. A mortality study among mild steel and stainless steel welders. Br J Ind Med 1995; 50:234–43.
10. Welinder H, Littorin M, Gullberg B, Skerfving S. Elimination of chromium in urine after stainless steel welding. Scand J Work Environ Health 1983; 9:397–403.
11. Lindberg E, Vesterberg O. Urinary excretion of chromium in chromeplaters after discontinued exposure. Am J Ind Med 1989; 16:485–92.
12. Lauwerys RR, Hoet P. Industrial chemical exposure. Guidelines for biologic monitoring, 2nd edn. Boca Raton, FL: Lewis Publishers, 1993;55–70

39.6 Nickel
Alfred Franzblau, David H Garabrant

EXPOSURE

First isolated in 1751, nickel is abundant in the earth's crust (ranking 24th), and has multiple industrial applications. Current major industrial uses include stainless steel making, other alloys and superalloys, electroplating, plus lesser amounts used in cast iron, chemicals, batteries, ceramics and as industrial catalysts.[1] It is also a nutritionally important element, although a specific deficiency state has not yet been defined in man.

Most occupational nickel exposure occurs via inhalation of fume or dust, or skin contact with salts, alloys, or solutions. Diet is an important source of nickel exposure and is believed to be 100–800 micrograms/day (although less than 5% is typically absorbed), and contributes 80–94% of the total body burden of nickel among non-exposed populations.[2]

NIOSH has estimated that 250,000 persons in the United States have occupational exposure to inorganic nickel, and OSHA has estimated that 709,000 workers are possibly exposed to nickel and its compounds. Most exposed workers are involved in refining, smelting, machining, casting, welding, battery making, or grinding steel or other nickel alloys. Exposure to nickel salts is important in nickel plating operations. Release of air-borne nickel dusts from nickel refining and smelting operations has resulted in documented exposure to persons living downwind from such plants. Because of widespread use of nickel alloys in jewelry and other common consumer products, cutaneous exposure of the general population is prevalent. A small but significant problem is hypersensitivity of patients 'exposed' to implanted nickel-alloy bioprostheses; implanted prosthetic devices may employ alloys containing up to 35% nickel.

A small number of workers have potential exposure to nickel carbonyl (Ni[CO]$_4$). Formed by passing carbon monoxide over nickel-containing materials, it is a volatile, colorless liquid that boils at 43 degrees C. Sometimes described as 'musty', the gas lacks any strong or penetrating odor. This compound presents a considerable hazard in refining of nickel using the Mond process, gas plating, and also in synthesis of acrylates for paints and plastics. Exposure is usually via inhalation of the gas, although transcutaneous absorption of liquid presumably could be significant.

ABSORPTION, EXCRETION, AND BIOLOGIC MONITORING

Absorption of nickel compounds is related to their solubility, with nickel carbonyl being highly soluble, most nickel salts being soluble, and nickel oxides and sulfides being relatively insoluble. Gastrointestinal absorption of soluble nickel compounds is rapid, but only about 1–5% is absorbed. Absorption of metallic nickel and insoluble nickel compounds from the gastrointestinal tract is very small.

Absorption and clearance of inhaled insoluble nickel compounds (for example, nickel compounds in welding fumes) from the lungs is slow, occurring over months. Dermal absorption of nickel and nickel compounds is minimal.[3]

Absorbed nickel is rapidly excreted in the urine, with a half-life of 20–60 hours. Nickel concentrations in plasma and urine reflect recent exposure to soluble nickel compounds and therefore can be used to monitor such exposures. In contrast, concentrations of nickel in plasma and urine do not reflect exposures to insoluble nickel compounds, thus limiting the utility of biologic monitoring for most industrial nickel exposures. Among non-exposed populations, mean nickel concentrations in serum/plasma are in the range 0.14–0.63 micrograms/l, in blood < 0.05–3.8 micrograms/l, and in urine 0.9–3.2 micrograms/l and 1.5–1.6 micrograms/g creatinine.[4] The use of hair and fingernail samples as indices of internal exposure is not reliable and has not been demonstrated to have any clinical utility.[5]

CLINICAL EFFECTS
Acute

Nickel carbonyl is the most acutely toxic nickel compound. Acute exposure to nickel carbonyl results in a two-phase illness that is dominated by pulmonary involvement. The first phase has almost immediate onset, and consists of multiple non-specific systemic complaints (fever, chills, nausea, lightheadedness, headache, dyspnea, and chest pain). These are easily confused with the 'flu' or acute bronchitis, and may resolve after a few hours. The second phase develops after 12–36 hours, but can be delayed up to five days. Acute chemical pneumonitis dominates the clinical picture, with cough, dyspnea, tachycardia, and cyanosis. Encephalopathy, due to cerebral edema and possibly hemorrhage, can also occur. Death may result from respiratory failure. Recovery from acute nickel carbonyl exposure can be prolonged because of slowly resolving pneumonitis.

Additional acute responses resulting from exposure to nickel compounds include irritation of mucous membranes, contact dermatitis, and/or asthma in sensitized individuals. Allergic dermatitis can result from exposure to either nickel salts, such as nickel sulfate among nickel platers, or metallic nickel or nickel alloys (see Chapter 29.1). The latter is exemplified by cutaneous reactions to jewelry, buttons, and other clothing items that contain nickel. Up to 15% of women in the general population, who have no history of occupational nickel exposure, are sensitized to nickel, based on patch testing.[6] Dentists may also have a high prevalence (16%) of nickel sensitization.[7] Industrial 'nickel itch' can present in a number of ways, including: itching or burning papular erythema in interdigital areas with spread to exposed areas on the upper extremities; or papular or papulovesicular dermatitis with some lichenification, similar to atopic dermatitis or neurodermatitis. Eruptions distant from the site of metal contact have also been described.

Asthmatic reactions to nickel compounds, usually salts such as nickel sulfate, are unusual, but well documented.[8] Reactions can involve immediate, delayed, and dual bronchospastic responses.

Chronic

Increased incidence of cancer of the lungs and nasal cavities has been documented among nickel refinery workers in numerous epidemiologic studies from different geographic locations (see Chapter 30.2).[9] Other malignancies in humans are not established to be causally associated with exposure to nickel and its compounds. The precise agent(s) responsible for nickel carcinogenesis in man is uncertain, but insoluble dusts (nickel subsulfide – Ni_3S_2; nickel oxides – NiO and Ni_2O_3), soluble dusts (nickel sulfate, nitrate, or chloride - $NiSO_4$, $NiNO_3$, $NiCl_2$), nickel carbonyl, nickel pellets/dust, nickel acetate, nickel hydroxide, and nickel fluoride have been documented to be carcinogenic in various animal models.

The International Agency for Research on Cancer (IARC) classifies nickel compounds as carcinogenic to humans (Group 1), based on evidence of carcinogenicity of nickel sulfate and the combination of nickel sulfides and oxides encountered in the nickel refining industry. Metallic nickel and nickel alloys have also been evaluated, with inadequate evidence for carcinogenicity in humans for both metallic nickel and nickel alloys, but sufficient evidence in animals for metallic nickel and limited evidence in animals for nickel alloys and nickel carbonyl. Thus, metallic nickel is classified as possibly carcinogenic to humans (Group 2B).[9] The US National Toxicology Program (NTP) classifies nickel and certain nickel compounds (nickel acetate, nickel carbonate, nickel carbonyl, nickel hydroxide, nickelocene, nickel oxide, and nickel subsulfide) as reasonably anticipated to be human carcinogens.[10] It should be noted that this classification is different from the designation given by NTP to agents that are known to be carcinogenic to humans. Overall, it appears that insoluble nickel compounds (oxides and sulfides) are carcinogenic, while the carcinogenicity of soluble nickel compounds by inhalation cannot be determined because of conflicting data.[11]

IARC has conducted a separate evaluation of the carcinogenicity of surgical implants and other foreign bodies, many of which contain nickel alloys. Implanted foreign bodies of metallic nickel and certain nickel alloys are classified as possibly carcinogenic to humans (Group 2B), while orthopedic implants of complex composition and dental materials are not classifiable as to their carcinogenicity (Group 3).[12]

As with most occupational malignancies, nickel-related tumors resemble those of non-occupational origin, but there are some features of nickel-related lung cancers and nasal cancers that are noteworthy. The sites of tumor occurrence appear related to airflow patterns and particle deposition in the nose and tracheobronchial tree.

Premalignant metaplastic changes in the nasal mucosa and nasal cancers typically originate at the anterior tips of the middle turbinates and spread along the lateral nasal walls and sinuses. The histology of sinus cancers among nickel workers is predominantly squamous cell. Nickel-related lung cancers tend to arise in the larger bronchi, and there may be a slight disproportionate increase in squamous cell histology.[13]

Despite numerous studies showing an increased risk of malignancy among nickel refinery workers, an increased risk of cancer among end-users of nickel compounds or products has not been documented unambiguously. Nevertheless, it is prudent to consider nickel dusts as potential human carcinogens, and to employ appropriate control measures.

Repeated or chronic exposure to nickel carbonyl may induce pulmonary fibrosis, even in the absence of a history of acute intoxication and ARDS.

Exposure to nickel aerosols (e.g., nickel sulfate – $NiSO_4$) has been associated with chronic rhinitis, sinusitis, perforation of the nasal septum, and anosmia. These effects are irritant reactions, and not immunologically mediated. Workers in electrolytic nickel refineries and those employed in nickel plating operations are at greatest risk.

Nickel alloys are frequently employed in various internally implanted medical devices, including orthopedic prostheses, cardiac pacemaker electrodes, replacement cardiac valves, and metal sutures. Such devices can induce cutaneous allergic reactions, including urticaria, eczematous changes, and pemphigoid lesions.

DIAGNOSIS, EVALUATION, AND TREATMENT

Nickel carbonyl is the only nickel compound that has caused acute inhalation poisoning. Nickel carbonyl poisoning must be suspected on the basis of the history because prevention of acute poisoning, including pneumonitis, and a favorable outcome depend on early diagnosis and treatment. Sodium diethyldithiocarbamate (dithiocarb, DDC) is an investigational drug that has been an effective antidote for nickel carbonyl poisoning in animal studies when administered parenterally soon after exposure. Although it has been used in several hundred patients, there are no adequately controlled studies to establish its clinical effectiveness in the treatment of human poisoning by nickel carbonyl.[14] An adult oral dose of 35–45 mg DDC/kg in divided doses in the first 24 hours, then 400 mg every 8 hours until the urine nickel concentrations are near normal and the patient is symptom free has been recommended.[15] Critically ill patients may be treated parenterally with 12.5 mg sodium DDC/kg. Patients with more than 100 micrograms Ni/liter of urine in the first 8 hours postexposure, or in whom severe nickel carbonyl exposure is suspected, are candidates for treatment. Poisoning cases in which there is more than minor irritation of the upper respiratory tract should also undergo evaluation for acute chemical pneumonitis and carbon monoxide exposure.[3]

Because of chemical similarity to disulfiram, patients treated with dithiocarb must avoid alcohol so as not to experience an 'Antabuse' reaction. Studies provide no support for use of other common metal chelating agents, such as BAL, penicillamine, or EDTA. Otherwise, the therapy of acute nickel carbonyl exposure is supportive.

Patch testing with nickel sulfate can be used to distinguish irritant from allergic contact dermatitis due to nickel. Allergic reactions to nickel compounds generally mandate removal from exposure since even limited exposure of sensitized individuals will induce a response (i.e., asthma or contact allergic dermatitis). Enhanced in vitro lymphocyte proliferation using nickel acetate in lymphocytes obtained from sensitized individuals has been reported, but this test is an investigational tool and not widely available. Immediate response to skin prick testing may also be used to identify sensitized individuals. Routine screening of asymptomatic workers with patch tests to identify nickel sensitivity is not indicated. Cutaneous nickel hypersensitivity persists for years after cessation of exposure and ongoing dermatitis may persist because of contact with jewelry, buckles, and other apparel.

Treatment of nickel hypersensitivity among persons with implanted prostheses may require removal and replacement with non-nickel containing devices.

PREVENTION

Nickel and/or nickel compounds are carcinogens, therefore exposure to air-borne dust and fumes must be minimized. Nickel refinery workers should have regular medical examinations that include inspection of the nasal mucosa and chest radiography. Because of severe acute toxic potential, nickel carbonyl must be contained in enclosed systems to prevent human contact. Minimization of cutaneous exposure should reduce the likelihood of development of cutaneous sensitization or irritant effects.

References

1. ATSDR. Toxicological profile for nickel (update). Washington, DC: US Department of Health and Human Services, 1997;1–262.
2. Von Berg R. Toxicology update: nickel and some nickel compounds. J Appl Toxicol 1997; 17:425–31.
3. Barceloux DG. Nickel. Clin Toxicol 1999; 37:239–58.
4. Herber RFM. Review of trace element concentrations in biologic specimens according to the TRACY protocol. Int Arch Occup Environ Health 1999; 72:279–83.
5. Lauwerys RR, Hoet P. Industrial chemical exposure. Guidelines for biologic monitoring, 2nd edn. Boca Raton, FL: Lewis Publishers, 1993;55–70
6. Menne T, Borgan O, Green A. Nickel allergy and hand dermatitis in a stratified sample of the Danish female population: an epidemiological study including a statistic appendix. Acta Dermatovener 1982; 62:35–41.
7. Wallenhammar L-M, Ortengren U, Andreasson H, et al. Contact allergy and hand eczema in Swedish dentists. Contact Derm 2000; 43:192–9.
8. Malo JL, Cartier A, Doepner M, Nieboer E. Occupational asthma caused by nickel sulfate. J Allergy Clin Immunol 1982; 69:55–9.
9. IARC. Nickel and nickel compounds. Lyon, France: International Agency for Research on Cancer, 1990;257–445.
10. National Toxicology Program. Ninth report on carcinogens. Research Triangle Park, NC: National Institute for Environmental Health Sciences, US Department of Health and Human Services, 2000.
11. Haber LT, Erdreicht L, Diamond GL, Maier AM, Ratney R. Hazard identification and dose response of inhaled nickel-soluble salts. Regul Toxicol Pharmacol 2000; 31:210–30.
12. IARC. Surgical implants and other foreign bodies. Lyon, France: International Agency for Research on Cancer, 1999;1–256.
13. Sunderman FW, Morgan LG, Andersen AA, Ashley DL. Histopathology of sinonasal and lung cancers in nickel refinery workers. Ann Clin Lab Sci 1989; 19:44–50.
14. Bradberry SM, Vale JA. Therapeutic review: do diethyldithiocarbamate and disulfiram have a role in acute nickel carbonyl poisoning? J Toxicol Clin Toxicol 1999; 37:259–64.
15. Sunderman FW. Use of sodium diethyldithiocarbamate in the treatment of nickel carbonyl poisoning. Ann Clin Lab Sci 1990; 20:12–21.

39.7 **Fluorine and Related Compounds**
Stephanie Carter, Noah S Seixas

SOURCES OF EXPOSURE

Fluorine is a fairly ubiquitous element, forming 0.03% of the earth's crust, predominantly as the mineral fluorspar (calcium fluoride), as cryolite (sodium aluminum fluoride), and in phosphate rock.[1] Fluorine is the most electronegative of elements and is a powerful oxidizer, being able to form ionic or covalent fluoride compounds with all elements except helium, neon, and argon.[2] Fluorine gas (F^2) is a pale yellow gas used as a rocket fuel and in chemical processing to produce uranium hexafluoride, fluorocarbons, and other organic and inorganic fluoride compounds. Hydrogen fluoride (anhydrous, or in water as hydrofluoric acid), produced by the addition of sulfuric acid to calcium fluoride, is used as a catalyst in petroleum refining (alkylation), in etching glass, and metal cleaning in the electronics and semiconductor industries.

Simple salts of fluoride (including sodium, calcium, copper, stannous, and zinc fluorides) find a wide range of uses in steel making, pesticides, drinking water and toothpaste additives, in electroplating, lumber treatment, glass, enamel, ceramics manufacture, and as lubricants and fluxing agents for welding. Other fluoride compounds have specialized uses in industry: cryolite as a flux in aluminum reduction smelters; magnesium fluosilicate in concrete and waterproofing applications; polychlorofluorocarbons (e.g., Freon and Halon) as aerosol propellants and fire suppressors; and fluoropolymers (e.g., Teflon, Tedlar) have numerous specialized applications.

An estimated 183,000 US workers may be occupationally exposed to fluoride,[3] while elevated community exposures may occur near aluminum smelters or phosphate fertilizer facilities, and during volcanic eruptions. Lower levels of exposure through toothpaste ingestion, fluoridated water supplies, and diet are almost ubiquitous in industrialized nations.[4]

ACUTE HEALTH EFFECTS

Both fluorine and hydrogen fluoride (HF) gas are severe irritants to the eyes, mucous membranes, and respiratory tract (see Chapters 19.5 and 29.1). Upon contact with skin or mucous membranes, HF quickly dissociates to form hydrofluoric acid. Chemical burns of the skin can also occur from contact with F_2 or HF. In the US, at least 1000 cases of exposure to liquid hydrofluoric acid and/or hydrogen fluoride occur each year.[5] Fluorine concentrations between 100 and 200 ppm result in burns, which appear similar to a thermal burn, and heal relatively quickly. Skin contact with hydrofluoric acid produces deep burns, possibly contacting bone, which can be exceedingly slow to heal. Prompt medical treatment through water irrigation and neutralization is required to limit the severity of these burns. If the concentration and degree of exposure are sufficient, the fluoride ions can remove enough calcium and/or magnesium to induce cardiac arrhythmias, damage the liver and kidney,

and cause neuromuscular hyperirritability.[5] Contact with hydrofluoric acid at concentrations greater than 50% produces immediate burning pain. At lower acid concentrations (especially below 20%), the symptoms may be unnoticed or delayed, thus delaying prompt treatment and allowing deep burns and systemic effects.[6]

Polymer fume fever is a flu-like acute response to the pyrolysis products of fluoropolymers, mold-release agents, and potentially other fluorocarbons (see Chapter 19.5). Symptoms of polymer fume fever include initial irritation followed 3–6 hours later by fever, chills, and general myalgia.[7] The pyrolysis products thought to be responsible for the effects vary depending on the amount of oxygen available and the pyrolysis temperature. Of most importance is carbonyl fluoride, which converts to hydrogen fluoride upon contact with moisture in the respiratory tract. Smokers are at increased risk of polymer fume fever due to smoking fluoropolymer-contaminated cigarettes. Chemical pneumonitis and adult respiratory distress syndrome (ARDS) have also been reported after inhalation exposure from HF-containing consumer products.[8]

CHRONIC HEALTH EFFECTS

The most well-known effect of chronic exposure to fluoride is bony fluorosis, an increased bone density or, in severe cases, skeletal deformities and spinal rigidity. The occurrence of fluorosis was first described in an occupationally exposed cohort in 1932 in which 30 of 78 cryolite-exposed workers had radiologic findings ranging from increased bone density to hyperosteoses.[9] Skeletal changes and possibly associated musculoskeletal complaints have continued to be observed among relatively highly exposed working populations. Kaltreider et al[10] reported a high prevalence of fluorosis among aluminum smelter workers with more than 10 years of exposure to fluoride levels of 2.4–6.0 mg/m^3. A follow-up of a small group ($n = 56$) of these workers 7–8 years later showed no further increase in bone density.[11] Possible and definite fluorosis was observed in 14% and 6.2%, respectively, of 2258 aluminum workers with relatively long exposure histories.[12] One study of aluminum workers suggests that musculoskeletal symptoms and increased rates of fracture may occur even in the absence of radiologic evidence of fluorosis.[13]

Fluorosis occurs as a result of the selective affinity of fluoride for bone and formation of fluorapatite. Despite the increased bone density associated with fluoride exposure, the possible benefits of fluoride in the treatment of osteoporosis are uncertain, with some studies indicating a higher risk of bone fracture, and animal studies indicating lower bone strength associated with fluoride exposure. The benefits of small amounts of fluoride in the prevention of dental caries have been well demonstrated. However, higher fluoride exposures during tooth formation in early childhood results in striation and mottling of teeth, while still higher levels may result in more severe dental discoloration and pitting, with decreased tooth strength and an increase in cavities.[4]

Occupational asthma has frequently been observed among aluminum potroom workers exposed to fluorides.[14] No specific causative agent has been identified in relation to asthma in this setting, though fluorides have been suspected. Current hypotheses are focusing on an irritant-induced mechanism with exposures to sulfur dioxide and HF as the primary suspected agents.

Other than bony fluorosis, there is no clear evidence of chronic systemic health effects of fluoride exposures. Gastrointestinal symptoms have been observed among groups with accidental high exposures or oral ingestion of fluoride compounds, probably due to irritation or erosion of the gastric mucosa.[4] Several epidemiologic studies have considered the effect of various fluoride compound exposures on cancer mortality in occupational and community cohorts. Each of these studies, however, has had important potential confounding exposures that may have explained any increased cancer rates observed. For instance, elevated cancer rates among aluminum smelter or fluoride workers[15,16] are more likely associated with carcinogens in coal tar pitch volatiles than fluoride exposures. The International Agency for Research on Cancer (IARC) has reviewed the available literature on fluoride exposure through drinking water, and concluded that there was no evidence of carcinogenicity from epidemiologic studies and insufficient evidence from animal studies.[17]

PREVENTION

Prevention of acute effects of fluorine or HF exposure is accomplished by preventing exposures, including short-term peak levels, from exceeding established guidelines (Table 39.7.1). The odor threshold for both HF and F_2 is approximately 0.1–0.2 ppm, exhibiting reasonable warning properties. In large part, the exposure limits are based on the prevention of irritation of the eyes and upper respiratory tract, although fluorosis is also prevented at these concentrations.[1]

The ACGIH[1] and OSHA PEL[18] for fluorine differ substantially (1 ppm and 0.1 ppm, respectively). This difference is based largely on the importance placed by OSHA on animal studies. ACGIH relied more heavily on more recent workplace studies that suggested that exposures above 0.1 ppm did not result in significant health effects or irritation.

Hydrogen fluoride exposure limits are based on HF as a primary irritant of the eyes, skin, and respiratory tract. ACGIH recommends a more conservative ceiling limit (3 ppm) to prevent skin reddening and burning of the eyes and nose seen in human studies. The OSHA PEL and NIOSH REL designate both TWA and STEL limits based mainly on prevention of more severe respiratory irritation and fluorosis.

Emergency response planning guidelines developed by the American Industrial Hygiene Association (AIHA) for HF and F_2 indicate levels of exposure below which nearly all individuals can be exposed for 1 hour without experiencing mild or transient health effects, developing health effects that may impair ability to protect themselves, or experiencing life-threatening health effects. For HF, these limits are 2, 10, and 50 ppm, respectively; for F_2, the limits are 0.5, 5, and 20 ppm.[19]

Irritation is reported at fluoride particulate concentrations of 5–10 mg/m^3. Changes in bone density appear to be prevented by maintaining exposures less than 2.6 mg/m^3 (ACGIH). All major US exposure-setting organizations concur with the 2.5 mg/m^3 limit for particulate fluoride including major international organizations. However, the German Maximum Allowable Concentration (MAK) includes a short-term level of 12.5 mg/m^3 averaged over a period of 30 minutes.

Because respiratory protection is commonly used in areas of high fluoride particulate, biologic monitoring may be used to evaluate the body burden at a particular point in time. Table 39.7.2 provides a summary of the suggested biologic monitoring levels for fluoride. Urinary levels are corrected for concentration by adjustment either with creatinine concentration or specific gravity. Creatinine adjustment requires that the creatinine concentration be within specified limits. ACGIH recommends monitoring fluoride in urine and assuring that levels are maintained below 3 mg fluoride per gram creatinine for spot samples taken prior to a work shift, or 10 mg/g Cr at the end of the work shift. Background levels of fluoride in urine, related to food and water intake, rarely rise above 2 mg/l, with most below 1 mg/l.

Air-purifying respiratory protection should utilize acid gas cartridges. For exposures lower than the exposure

Exposure guideline source	Fluoride (mg/m^3)	Hydrogen fluoride (ppm)	Fluorine (ppm)
ACGIH – TLV	2.5[TWA]	3[C]	1[TWA], 2[STEL]
NIOSH – REL	2.5[TWA]	3[TWA], 6[STEL]	0.1[TWA]
NIOSH – IDLH	500	30	25
OSHA – PEL	2.5[TWA]	3[TWA], 6[STEL]	0.1[TWA]

TWA: Time weighted average, over 8 hours.
STEL: Short term exposure limit, over 15 minutes.
C: Ceiling, concentration not to be exceeded.
REL: Recommended exposure limit.
IDLH: Immediately dangerous to life or health.

Table 39.7.1 Occupational exposure guidelines

Reference	Units	Pre-shift	Post-shift	Screening creat. (mg/l) or SG adjustment (g/ml)
(ACGIH 1996)[1]	(mg F/g creatinine)	3	10	Cr.: 300–3000
(DFG 1998)[22]	(mg F/g creatinine)	4	7	Cr.: 500–2500
(NIOSH 1975)[23]	(mg F/L)	4	7	SG: 1.024 g/ml

Table 39.7.2 Recommended biologic exposure indices for fluorides

Contact location	Water irrigation	Neutralization
Eyes	15 minutes	1% calcium gluconate
Skin	5 minutes	2.5% calcium gluconate or 0.13% iced benzalkonium chloride
Lung	NA	2.5% calcium gluconate by nebulizer

From: Segal E. First aid for a unique acid: HF. Chemical Health Safety 1998; Sept/Oct: 25–8.

Table 39.7.3 Guidelines for HF burn treatment[5]

limits specially impregnated filters may also afford some protection. Use of full-face respirators has the advantage of providing protection from splashes and reducing eye irritation. Work areas where there is a potential for large gas releases of HF or F_2 should have fixed-point gas alarms or other exposure indicators, and firewater deluge systems to minimize cloud formation. Additional information on management systems for safe operations and maintenance of HF operations, including methods to identify surface contamination and leaks, is available.[20]

EVALUATION AND TREATMENT

Immediate medical treatment is necessary for skin or significant inhalation exposure to hydrofluoric acid/hydrogen fluoride, with focus on irrigation with water followed by neutralization gels or solutions[6] (see Chapters 19.5, 29.1, and 20.1). Brief treatment guidelines are given in Table 39.7.3.

Further assessment should include electrolyte levels (Ca, Mg, K), ECG if potential for cardiac arrhythmia is present, and chest x-rays for significant inhalation exposure or liquid contact with face/neck. HF can penetrate the fingernails without exhibiting external evidence, requiring advanced treatment through removal of the nails or calcium gluconate by IV. For further information on emergency treatment of HF burns, see Wilkes 2001.[21]

Workers chronically exposed to fluorides such as aluminum potroom workers who develop respiratory symptoms should undergo pulmonary evaluation for possible asthma, including spirometry and peak flow measurements (see Chapter 19.2). Evaluation and treatment are similar for other workers with non-sensitizing irritant induced asthma (see Chapter 19.2). Bony fluorosis should be considered in workers with prolonged higher exposures who develop musculoskeletal complaints (see Chapter 23.5). X-ray findings include sclerosis and exostoses. There is no specific treatment of fluorosis beyond removal from further exposure.

References

1. ACGIH. Fluorides. Documentation for the Threshold Limit Values and Biologic Exposure Indices for chemical substances in the work environment. Cincinnati, OH: American Conference of Governmental Industrial Hygienists, 1996;657–9.
2. Hawley G, Lewis R. Hawley's condensed chemical dictionary. New York: Van Nostrand Reinhold, 1993.
3. NIOSH. National occupational exposure survey (1980–1983). Cincinnati, OH: US Department of Health and Human Services, National Institute for Occupational Safety and Health, 1989.
4. ATSDR. Draft toxicological profile for fluorine, hydrogen fluoride, and fluorides. Atlanta, GA: Agency for Toxic Substances and Disease Registry, US Department of Health and Human Services, 2001;308.
5. Segal E. First aid for a unique acid: HF. Chemical Health Safety 1998; Sept/Oct:25–8.
6. Bertolini JC. Hydrofluoric acid: a review of toxicity. J Emerg Med 1992; 10:163–8.
7. Shusterman D. Polymer fume fever and other fluorocarbon pyrolysis-related syndromes. Occup Med 1993; 8:519–31.
8. Bennion J, Franzblau A. Chemical pneumonitis following household exposure to hydrofluoric acid. Am J Ind Med 1997; 31:474–8.
9. Moller F, Gudjonsson S. Massive fluorosis of bones and ligaments. Acta Radiol 1932; 13:269–94.
10. Kaltreider N, Elder M, Cralley LV, Colwell MO. Health survey of aluminum workers with special reference to fluoride exposure. J Occup Med 1972; 14:531–41.
11. Dinman B, Elder M, Bonney TB, Bovard PG, Colwell MO. A 15-year retrospective study of fluoride excretion and bony radiopacity among aluminum smelter workers – Part 4. J Occup Med 1976; 18:21–3.
12. Czerwinski E, Nowak J, Dabrowska D, Skolarczyk A, Kita B, Ksiezyk M. Bone and joint pathology in fluoride-exposed workers. Arch Environ Health 1988; 43:340–3.
13. Carnow B, Conibear S. Industrial fluorosis. Fluoride 1981; 14:172–81.
14. Abramson M, Wlodarczyk J, Saunders NA, Hensley MJ. Does aluminum smelting cause lung disease? Am Rev Respir Dis 1989; 139:1042–57.
15. Grandjean P, Olsen JH, Jensen OM, Juel K. Cancer incidence and mortality in workers exposed to fluoride. J Natl Cancer Inst 1992; 84:1903–9.
16. Ronneberg A, Langmark F. Epidemiologic evidence of cancer in aluminum reduction plant workers. Am J Ind Med 1992; 22:573–90.
17. IARC. Inorganic fluorides used in drinking-water and dental preparations. Lyon: International Agency for Research on Cancer, World Health Organization, 1982.
18. OSHA. Code of Federal Regulations. Air Contaminants. Washington, DC: Occupational Safety and Health Administration, 1985;29.
19. AIHA. Emergency response planning guidelines. Fairfax, VA: American Industrial Hygiene Association, 1999.
20. API. Safe operation of hydrofluoric acid alkylation units. Washington, DC: American Petroleum Institute, 1999;48.
21. Wilkes G. Hydrofluoric acid burns. eMedicine 2001; May 7, 2(5). http://www.emedicine.com/emerg/topic804.htm
22. DFG. List of maximum allowable concentrations (MAKs) and biologic tolerance values (BATs) for 1998. Munich, Germany: Commission for the Investigation of Health Hazards of Chemical Compounds in the Work Area, 1998.
23. NIOSH. Criteria for a recommended standard: occupational exposure to inorganic fluorides. Washington, DC: US Department of Health, Education and Welfare, Public Health Service, National Institute for Occupational Safety and Health, 1975;191.

39.8 **Lead**
Jacqueline M Moline, Philip J Landrigan

Lead is an ancient metal. Because of its malleability and low melting point, humans have used lead since prehistoric times to make statues, jewelry, water pipes, and drinking vessels.[1] The salts of lead have long been valued for their brilliant colors. The quantity of lead used since 1940 surpasses the total used in all previous centuries. This heavy recent use reflects industrial applications as well as the use of lead as a fuel additive. In the mid-1970s, nearly 200,000 tons of lead were consumed annually in gasoline in the United States.[2] Virtually all of this lead was emitted into the environment from vehicles in a finely particulate form and caused widespread contamination of air, dust, soil, drinking water and food crops. In the United States and in many western European countries, the use of leaded gasoline has decreased sharply since 1976, and population mean blood lead levels have decreased by 90% as a result.[3] Leaded gasoline continues, however, to be used widely in Eastern European and developing nations.[4]

OCCUPATIONAL LEAD EXPOSURE

A wide variety of industrial populations are at risk of occupational exposure to lead (Table 39.8.1). In the United States more than 3 million workers are estimated by NIOSH to be potentially exposed to lead in their work. Occupational exposure to lead is regulated in the United States by the OSHA lead standard, first promulgated in 1978. This standard sets limits on air-borne lead exposure as well as on permissible levels of lead in blood. It has been successful in reducing the most serious industrial exposures to lead. However, this standard is enforced inadequately and occupational exposure to lead remains widespread in the United States. Workers at highest risk are those in smaller industries such as secondary lead smelters and automobile radiator repair shops.

A major industrial group that previously had been exempted from the protection of the United States lead standard were construction workers. Major outbreaks of lead poisoning were observed among workers who cut lead-painted steel structures such as bridges with oxyacetylene torches and among renovation workers who remove lead paint from older homes. The heating and burning of lead paint by these workers can create a highly respirable fume consisting of air-borne lead particles less than 1 μm in diameter; inhalation of lead fumes can produce acute lead poisoning within days or even hours. In 1993, the OSHA lead standard was extended to cover the construction and demolition trades. A sharp decline in their exposures to lead and their blood lead levels resulted.[5,6]

Occupational exposure to organic lead, principally tetraethyl lead (TEL), can occur in the manufacture of this compound for use as a fuel additive as well as in the cleaning of tanks and pipes that have contained TEL. Typically, in TEL manufacturing, exposures to organic and inorganic lead occur simultaneously.

Measurement of occupational exposure

Assessment of occupational exposure to inorganic lead requires measurement of lead levels in both air and blood. Air lead levels are measured by standard industrial hygiene techniques. The determination of lead in air provides direct information on sources and levels of exposure, information that is essential for controlling exposures to lead in the workplace. The OSHA standard (1993) for the permissible exposure level of lead in workplace air is 50 micrograms/m³, expressed as an 8-hour time-weighted average.[7] As is discussed below, this standard can no longer be considered adequately protective of workers' health, because lead toxicity has been observed in workers whose lead exposures do not exceed the current OSHA standard, and because fetal lead poisoning can occur in the offspring of female lead workers well below this level.[8]

Measurement of the blood lead level complements determination of lead levels in air. The finding of an elevated blood lead level identifies those workers who may have had uniquely high exposures that are not detected by air monitoring. For those workers in the United States covered by the OSHA lead standard, anyone found to have a blood lead level of 50 micrograms/dl or above must be removed from the high-exposure job (termed 'medical removal protection'). A worker is not allowed to return to a high-exposure job until the blood lead level has fallen to below 40 micrograms/dl. To prevent workers with elevated lead levels from being economically penalized during medical removal protection, the OSHA standard requires that these workers must continue to receive their full rate of pay (pay rate retention) while they are working in the less hazardous job.

ENVIRONMENTAL LEAD EXPOSURE

In the general population, children are the group most heavily exposed and most susceptible to the toxic effects of lead. The mean blood lead level of children in the United States is about 3 micrograms/dl.[9] A decline of 90% in blood lead levels occurred among American children from 1976 to 1997 as a consequence of removal of lead from gasoline. In contrast, lead use in gasoline as well as in industry remains widespread in nations undergoing transition to industrialization; environmental contamination and blood lead levels of workers and residents of communities near polluting industries in these countries have been reported to be dangerously elevated.[4]

According to the Centers for Disease Control and Prevention (CDC), blood lead levels of 10 micrograms/dl and higher in children indicate excessive exposure.[10] Blood lead levels of 10 mg/dl and above are associated with subclinical lead toxicity in children. More recently, consideration has been given to further decreasing the blood lead standard for children in light of recent data showing subclinical toxic-

Battery makers
Brass workers
Bronzers
Cable makers/splicers
Chemical operators
Demolition workers
Firing range personnel
Foundrymen
Glass makers/polishers
Gunstock/barrel makers
Jewelers
Lead burners
Painters
Pigment makers
Pipe cutters
Pottery workers
Printers (lino/electrotype)
Ship burners
Solderers
Stained glass makers
Tetraethyl lead manufacturers
Welders

Table 39.8.1 Major occupations associated with risk of inorganic lead poisoning

ity at blood levels below 10 mg/dl.[10a,10b] The CDC estimates that over 400,000 children in the United States have blood lead levels above 10mg/dl. The proportion of children with elevated blood lead levels is particularly high among minority inner-city populations, and among such children, the CDC estimates that as many as 35% of preschool children still have elevated blood lead levels.[9]

Lead-based paint is the major concentrated, high-dose source of lead for American children. Most cases of acute, symptomatic pediatric lead poisoning are caused by ingestion of dust derived from lead-based paint. Although new applications of interior lead-based paint are banned, an estimated 27.1 million housing units in the United States built before 1950 still contain lead-based paint. Since 1979, the maximum allowable concentration of lead in domestic paint has been regulated by the United States Consumer Product Agency at 0.06 parts per million.

Air, dust, soil, drinking water, cosmetics, dietary and herbal supplements, and soiled parental work clothing are additional potential sources of exposure to lead for children and for all members of the population. Children, because of their normal oral exploratory behavior, are at high risk of ingesting lead from dust and soil.[11,12] In 2001 the US Environmental Protection Agency (EPA) developed standards for lead in dust and soil, which were now consistent with existing US Department of Housing and Urban Development guidance levels for home dust levels. This was critical, since Lanphear et al found that a strong relationship between interior dust level landing and children's blood lead levels exists below the levels in the prior guidelines of 100 micrograms/ft^2 for floors, 500 micrograms/ft^2 for interior window sills, and 800 micrograms/ft^2 for window troughs.[13] The new dust standard is 40 micrograms/ft^2 for floors and 250 micrograms/ft^{2}on window sills; soil levels must be below 400 parts per million (ppm) in play areas and 1200 ppm average for bare soil in the rest of the yard. Current lead in drinking water is due principally to the widespread use of lead solder to join pipe in water

service lines. Acidic drinking water can leach lead from solder and also from lead pipes.

An analysis of sources of lead poisoning in urban children found that in infants younger than 1 year of age the principal sources were household renovation with lead paint removal (40%), ingestion of lead paint chips (20%), preparation of infant formula with lead-contaminated drinking water (18%), exposure to lead-contaminated parental work clothing (2%), congenital poisoning (2%), and sources unknown (18%). By contrast, the same study found that sources of lead poisoning for older children (18 through 30 months) were home renovations (4%), paint chip ingestion (87%), and sources unknown (9%).[14]

Cases of lead poisoning through ingestion of contaminated herbal supplements or infant formula prepared in lead-contaminated vessels have been documented.[15] The habit of sniffing leaded gasoline is an important source of lead poisoning for children in certain rural populations.[16]

Measurement of environmental exposure

Determination of lead levels in blood is the principal means of assessing the lead exposure of children. This assay should be conducted in a laboratory that has been licensed by the CDC or by comparable authorities and that participates satisfactorily in quality control and quality assurance programs. Hand-held portable blood lead instruments have been developed for use in the field. They complete the analysis in 2–3 minutes, appear highly reliable, and have been approved for use since 1997.[9]

Assessment of lead exposure in the general environment requires analysis by standard chemical and physical techniques. Lead levels in paint may be determined by portable, hand-held x-ray fluorescence (XRF) detectors. Determination of lead levels in air is undertaken under the requirements of the EPA's air lead standard; the community air lead standard in the United States is 1.5 micrograms/m^3 of air, computed as a quarterly average. Lead in drinking water is most reliably determined in a first-draw morning sample, when water has had an opportunity to sit in contact overnight with any lead in pipes or in solder. The current EPA safe drinking water standard for lead in drinking water is 0.15 mg/l (15 parts per billion). Lead concentrations in dust and soil are determined by standard chemical techniques.

CLINICAL EFFECTS IN ADULTS
Acute inorganic lead toxicity

Intense occupational exposure to lead over a brief period of time can cause a syndrome of acute lead poisoning.[17] Characteristics of this syndrome are abdominal colic, constipation, fatigue, hemolytic anemia, peripheral neuropathy, and in some cases, alteration of central nervous system function. A gingival lead line is occasionally seen. In profound cases, full-blown acute encephalopathy with coma, convulsions, and papilledema may occur; in milder cases, only fatigue, headache or personality changes may be evident as manifestations of the neurologic toxicity of lead. Mild liver involvement, limited to modest elevations in serum glutamic-oxaloacetic transaminase (SGOT), and musculoskeletal pains and arthritic symptoms are common. Basophilic stippling may be seen in the red blood cells. Usually, these finding occur when the blood lead level is very high, 70 micrograms/dl or more.[18,19]

Chronic inorganic lead toxicity

Chronic inorganic lead intoxication is an insidious illness that is highly prevalent among persons chronically overexposed to lead. Symptoms include arthralgias, myalgias, headache, weakness, depression, loss of libido, impotence, and vague gastrointestinal difficulties. The classic abdominal colic of acute lead poisoning is usually absent. Anemia may occur, accompanied in some cases by an increased reticulocyte count. Thyroid and adrenal function often are depressed. Hypertension may be present. Sperm counts can be depressed in men and fertility reduced in women. Measurement of renal function may reveal impairment of glomerular clearance; decreased tubular urate clearance resulting in hyperuricemia is common. Late effects of inorganic lead intoxication include chronic renal failure, gout, chronic encephalopathy, and hypertension.[19,20]

The definition of chronic lead intoxication has, in recent years, been expanded by the recognition that lead can cause toxic injury at levels of exposure that only a decade ago were thought to be safe. The term *subclinical toxicity* denotes this concept that relatively low-dose exposure to lead may cause harmful effects to health in the absence of symptoms and signs that are evident on the standard clinical examination. The underlying premise is that there exists a spectrum of toxicity in which clinically apparent effects have their asymptomatic subclinical counterparts, which are detected through special testing.[21,22]

The effects of lead on organ system function

Hematologic toxicity

Anemia is a classic clinical manifestation of acute lead toxicity (see also Chapter 21).[17] The severity and prevalence of lead-induced anemia are correlated directly with the blood lead level in both adults and children.[23] It is important to note that the presence of anemia is not required for a diagnosis of lead poisoning; at lower levels of excessive lead exposure the hemoglobin concentration is most often within the normal range. Most patients with chronic and late-effects of lead poisoning also have normal blood hemoglobin levels.

Lead-induced anemia is the result of multiple mechanisms: impairment of heme biosynthesis, acceleration of red blood cell destruction, and an inhibition of erythropoietin production in the kidney.

Lead-induced inhibition of heme biosynthesis is due first to inhibition of the cytoplasmic enzyme, δ-aminole-

vulinic acid dehydratase (ALA-D). This effect is dose related. It is noted initially at blood lead levels of 10–20 micrograms/dl and is virtually complete at levels of 70–90 micrograms/dl. The mitochondrial enzyme ferrochelatase is the next most sensitive enzyme in the heme biosynthetic pathway inhibited by lead. Ferrochelatase catalyzes the transfer of iron from ferritin into protoporphyrin to form heme. Inhibition of ferrochelatase causes increased excretion of coproporphyrin in the urine and accumulation of protoporphyrin (a zinc-requiring enzyme, also called zinc protoporphyrin [ZPP]) in the erythrocytes.[24,25]

Lead-induced acceleration of red blood cell destruction leading to hemolysis reflects toxicity to the red blood cell membranes and results probably from the inhibition of lead by the enzymes 5′-nucleotidase and ATPase. Erythropoietin, a glycoprotein hormone principally secreted by the proximal renal tubule, regulates red blood production. Chronic exposure to lead appears to inhibit secretion of erythropoietin, and may also act directly on erythrocyte progenitor cells in the bone marrow.[26]

Neurologic toxicity

Neurologic toxicity of lead in adults In the peripheral nervous system, the myelin sheaths surrounding the motor axons are the principal target of lead (see also Chapter 28). Lead-induced pathologic changes in these fibers include segmental demyelination and axonal degeneration. Extensor muscle palsy with wrist drop or ankle drop hasbeen recognized as the classic clinical manifestation of the peripheral motor neurologic toxicity of lead since the time of Hippocrates. Unlike other toxic neuropathies, this motor neuropathy may show left–right asymmetry. Mild to moderate sensory dysfunction also may be evident in lead neuropathy, and in such cases the clinical picture is one of mixed motor–sensory neuropathy, often with asymmetric features.

Recent studies of peripheral neurologic function in persons exposed to lead have used electrophysiologic probes to determine whether exposures insufficient to produce clinically evident signs and symptoms can cause covert abnormalities.[27] With the development of increasingly sensitive test methodologies, these studies have been able to detect peripheral neurologic toxicity at progressively lower blood lead levels. For example, Seppalainen et al, in a prospective study of new entrants to the lead industry, reported slowing of motor conduction velocity in the ulnar nerve at blood lead levels as low as 30–40 micrograms/dl.[28] In the central nervous system, high-dose acute exposure to lead causes encephalopathy characterized clinically by obtundation, coma, and convulsions. Among persons who recover from acute lead encephalopathy, a high proportion are left with significant neuropsychologic deficits, including reduced intelligence, shortened attention span, and instability of mood.[23]

The question of whether lead causes asymptomatic impairment in central neurologic function in adults at doses insufficient to produce clinical encephalopathy has been the subject of extensive research. Early investigations of this issue have shown a correlation between lead exposure and diminished neuropsychologic performance in a group of asymptomatic adult workers, all of whom had blood lead levels below 70 micrograms/dl.[29] The functions most severely impaired were those dependent on visual intelligence and visual-motor co-ordination. An increased prevalence of fatigue and short-term memory loss was observed in lead smelter workers that increased as blood lead levels rose. Other studies also found evidence of depressed mood and other central neurologic deficits in lead workers with blood lead levels in the range 40–70 micrograms/dl.[23] Stewart et al reported that past exposure to lead, assessed by elevated bone lead content, was associated with persistent decrements in neurobehavioral test results in a group of organolead workers.[30] Additional studies are required to confirm this finding, to elucidate toxic mechanisms, and to ascertain whether or not toxic effects occur at lower blood lead levels. A further implication of the finding that lead may cause insidious injury to the central nervous system is the possibility that some as yet unknown proportion of cases of presenile dementia, motorneuron disease (amyotrophic lateral sclerosi [ALS]),[30a] and other chronic neurologic and psychiatric conditions in adults may be the result of chronic exposure to lead. Such exposure may result in an accelerated attrition of neurons that becomes clinically evident with age.[30] These possible associations are currently the focus of research efforts.

Pediatric neurologic toxicity of lead   Lead is now recognized to cause subclinical neurologic toxicity in children at much lower levels of exposure than in adults (see also Chapter 28). The earliest suggestion of this toxicity came from studies by Byers and Lord in the 1940s of the survivors of acute lead poisoning. These early investigations demonstrated the presence of permanent neuropsychologic sequelae, including learning disabilities and shortening of attention span as well as highly aggressive behavior in children who had recovered from acute lead encephalopathy.[31]

The existence of subclinical lead neuropathy in asymptomatic children was then confirmed in a series of cross-sectional neuroepidemiologic studies undertaken by Needleman and colleagues in the mid-1970s.[32] These landmark investigations found an association between asymptomatic increased exposure to lead and decreased intelligence. Children with elevated body lead burdens, corresponding to blood lead levels of 25–55 micrograms/dl, were found to have mean verbal IQ scores 4.5 points lower than similar children with lower lead burdens. This deficit remained evident when results were adjusted for parental education, childhood illness, socioeconomic status, and other biologic and social variables. Subsequent long-term follow-up studies have shown that these deficits in IQ are associated with learning difficulties, reading problems, an increased rate of failure to graduate from secondary school and an increase in violent behavior. Needleman has noted that a 4.5 point downward shift in mean IQ produces a 50% reduction in the number of gifted children (IQ above 120) in a population, and a 50% increase in the number of retarded children (IQ below 80).[32,33]

The data from these cross-sectional studies have been further corroborated by data from a series of prospective epidemiologic studies of newborn children, followed from birth through the first several years of life. Each of these studies found that cord blood lead levels at birth as low as 15–20 micrograms/dl were associated with decrements in childhood intelligence.[34–37] Lead poisoning has also been associated with decreased hearing. An inverse relationship between blood lead levels and height has also been noted. Most recently, an analysis of data from the US National Health and Nutrition Evaluation Survey (NHANES) suggests that a negative association between lead and neurobehavioral function is evident in children at blood lead levels as low as 5–10 micrograms/dl.[38]

In recognition of the extreme sensitivity of the developing nervous system to low levels of lcad, the CDC has periodically revised the definition of childhood lead poisoning. Currently, the CDC considers a blood lead level of 10 micrograms/dl or higher as evidence of excess lead burden.[10] (The previous definition of lead toxicity, prior to 1992, was a blood lead level of 25 micrograms/dl or above.) Children with blood lead levels of 10 micrograms/dl or above must be provided medical follow-up and environmental monitoring, as is described in the section on clinical management. The therapeutic goal is to identify and reduce the child's environmental exposures to lead, so as to reduce the threat of subclinical neurotoxicity and to prevent re-exposure. In the near future, CDC may further reduce the blood lead standard for children.[10a,10b]

Renal toxicity

The cells lining the proximal tubules of the nephron appear to be the tissue in the kidney that is most highly sensitive to lead (see also Chapter 25).[20] In children with acute, high-dose lead poisoning, injury to these cells occasionally results in the development of acute Fanconi syndrome, in which glucose, amino acids, and phosphates are spilled in the urine in large quantities. This syndrome typically is reversible, and it is not known whether or not it predisposes the individual to long-term sequelae. Fanconi syndrome is not commonly seen in adults exposed to lead.

At blood lead levels below 25 micrograms/dl, lead inhibits the metabolic activation (hydroxylation) of vitamin D, a transformation that takes place in the cells lining the proximal tubules.[39] Also in these cells, at blood lead levels of 40–80 micrograms/dl, lead induces the formation of dense intranuclear inclusion bodies consisting of a lead protein complex.[20] These inclusion bodies persist for approximately 1 year. Hyperuremic gout, apparently resulting from increased reabsorption of uric acid by the tubular cells, is a third metabolic consequence of lead-induced renal impairment.

Chronic nephropathy, which may progress to kidney failure, is the classic late manifestation of chronic lead toxicity in the kidneys. It appears to result from long-term, relatively high-dose exposure to lead, but dose–response relationships have not been well defined. Individuals with chronic low-level lead exposure have abnormal urinary excretion of n-acetyl glucosaminidase (NAG) compared to controls, suggesting renal tubular dysfunction may occur after chronic low-level lead exposure. Population-based studies, such as the Normative Aging Study, also demonstrated a deleterious effect of lead in kidney function when body burdens of lead were assessed.[40–42]

The evolution of lead nephropathy usually is silent. The central event appears to be the progressive destruction of tubular cells and their replacement by fibrosis. Clinically obvious manifestations of impairment, such as elevations in BUN and serum creatinine, do not ordinarily become evident until 50–70% of the nephrons have been destroyed. Pathologically, chronic lead nephropathy is characterized by interstitial fibrosis with atrophy and dilation of the tubules and relative sparing of the glomeruli; intranuclear inclusions are infrequent, and the kidneys are small and shrunken. The pathologic picture may be indistinguishable from changes of chronic hypertension, which usually coexists (see later).[20]

Excess mortality from renal disease has been observed in several epidemiologic studies of lead workers. In each of these investigations, a two- to threefold increase has been noted in deaths from chronic nephritis, and in one of the investigations a positive association was observed between duration of employment in a lead smelter and mortality from chronic nephritis.[43,44]

Lead and hypertension

Hypertension has long been associated with lead toxicity, in both animal and epidemiologic studies. Early in the last century, long-term, high-dose exposure to lead was reported to be associated with an increased incidence of hypertension and cerebrovascular disease.[17] With the reduction in lead exposure that has occurred in most industries, these overt associations are now noted less commonly. Also, these exposures may have occurred many years prior to the development of hypertension, making this causal association less obvious.

However, population studies have investigated the effect of blood lead, even relatively low blood lead levels, on hypertension. An analysis of the NHANES II survey data revealed that lead was a significant contributor to hypertension in the US population.[45] Hypertension has also been associated with elevated bone lead levels.[45a] In addition, Schwartz et al found left ventricular hypertrophy was correlated with blood lead levels, demonstrating that lead was not merely raising blood pressure but also contributing to end-organ damage.[46] An analysis of the data from the Normative Aging Study also found an association between body burdens of lead and hypertension.[41]

Different mechanisms for lead-induced hypertension and renal failure have been proposed, including an increased responsiveness to α-2 adrenoreceptor stimulation after lead ingestion, and alterations in cAMP-dependent availability of calcium for contractile processes in vascular and cardiac myocells. Other potential mechanisms of action include increases in endothelin-3 concentration, decreases in endothelium-derived relaxing factor, and alterations in renin activity.[47,48]

From the perspective of disease prevention, it is most important to prevent hypertension in lead workers. Elevations in blood pressure, even at low levels, are associated with significantly increased rates of mortality from heart disease and stroke. A biomedical surveillance program of workers exposed to lead, therefore, should incorporate as a specific aim the prevention of elevated blood pressure. Periodic determination of blood pressure should be a routine component of the biomedical monitoring of workers exposed to lead.

Reproductive toxicity of lead

Male lead workers, especially those newly exposed to lead, can have evidence of decreased fertility (see also Chapter 27.2). Decreased sperm counts, abnormal sperm morphology, and decreased sperm motility have been noted in several studies when lead levels were above 40 micrograms/dl.[18,49] Animal studies indicate that blood lead concentrations greater than 30–40 micrograms/dl are associated with impairment of spermatogenesis and reduced concentrations of androgens. Changes in endocrine profiles have been noted in men with lead levels over 60 micrograms/dl. Men currently employed in lead trades may have reduced fertility, as measured by increased time to conception in their wives.[50] The effects of lead on male reproductive function at lower levels are more uncertain.

In women, lead at high doses can also be toxic to reproductive function (see also Chapter 27.2). Clinical reports, most of them from the first half of the 20th century, describe an increased incidence in spontaneous abortion among female lead workers as well as in the wives of male lead workers.[51] Low-level maternal lead exposure may increase the risk of spontaneous abortion.[52]

A difficult problem in the prevention and clinical management of the reproductive toxicity of lead is the finding that lead may cause neurologic damage to the fetus at blood levels as low as 5–10 micrograms/dl, substantially below the current OSHA standard for blood levels of lead in workers. Lead passes virtually unimpeded across the placental barrier, and the neurologic impairment that it produces in the fetus appears to be irreversible.[34,35] This problem is further compounded by the fact that under the metabolic stress of pregnancy, lead may be mobilized from bony stores of the mother to enter her blood and thus the blood of the fetus.[52a] Thus, if a woman who has previously had chronic lead exposure or who has suffered lead poisoning becomes pregnant, there may be mobilization of skeletal lead with resultant fetal exposure.

It is not known whether or not exposure of the father to lead before conception results in fetal injury.

The prevention of fetal lead encephalopathy requires that blood lead levels of prospective mothers be kept below 10 micrograms/dl, not only during pregnancy but also in the years preceding conception.[21] If this principle is followed, exposure of the fetus to currently absorbed lead, as well as to lead released from previously accumulated bony stores, should be prevented. If a woman who has previously had elevated blood lead levels wishes to become pregnant, it may be reasonable to recommend either an x-ray fluorescence examination of bone to determine the body burden of lead or to perform a chelation mobilization challenge test prior to conception (see below). If extensive bony lead stores are demonstrated by either of these tests, delay in conception may be indicated. In women with a history of exposure to lead, blood lead levels should be monitored frequently throughout pregnancy.

Carcinogenicity

Lead has been found to produce renal cancers in experimental studies in mice, rats, and hamsters. Positive dose–response relationships were observed between lead dose and tumor incidence. Also, brain tumors have been noted in rats exposed to lead.[4] Lead is currently considered by the International Agency for Research on Cancer (IARC) to be a probable human carcinogen (group 2A) based on 'Sufficient' animal data and 'limited' human data.[53]

Experimentally, lead exposure inhibits DNA repair and appears to interact with zinc binding sites on human protamine, an important DNA-associated protein, and lead may also cause changes in the conformational structure of P53, a tumor suppressor gene. These findings suggest that rather than altering DNA directly, lead may increase the carcinogenicity of other mutagens.

Epidemiologic studies of lead workers have shown excess kidney cancer in 5 of 6 published cohort mortality studies. Also 4 of these 6 studies have shown excess numbers of tumors of the brain and central nervous system.[54,55]

Most of the epidemiologic studies on the carcinogenicity of lead do not present adequate data in dose–response relationships. At present, there have been insufficient reported cases in humans to enable a definite conclusion to be reached as to whether or not lead causes human cancer.

Organic lead

One organic compound of lead, TEL, was widely used in the United States as an antiknock agent in gasoline and is still used extensively in developing nations. While overall exposure to TEL has declined significantly, individuals who work as producers, blenders, and persons who clean and maintain tanks are at risk of poisoning by TEL. It is a volatile liquid which, unlike inorganic lead, is absorbed readily through the skin.

Exposure to TEL produces a syndrome that is different from inorganic lead poisoning. TEL poisoning is limited largely to acute or subacute central nervous system signs and symptoms. Early symptoms of insomnia and anorexia are followed by muscle irritability. Agitated encephalopathy resembling delirium tremens occurs in cases of severe poisoning. Increased deep tendon reflexes and cerebellar signs (tremors and ataxia) are characteristic in severe cases.[56]

CLINICAL EVALUATION
Clinical evaluation strategy for adults

The diagnosis of inorganic lead intoxication in adults requires (1) demonstration of excess lead absorption, (2)

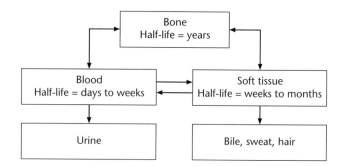

Figure 39.8.1: The three-compartment model for distribution of lead in the body. Estimates of half-life are given for each compartment. In the steady state almost all lead is stored in bone, so only very small amounts are excretable by other compartments. (From: Rabinowitz MB, Wetherill GW, Kobble JD. Kinetic analysis of lead metabolism in healthy humans. J Clin Invest 1977; 58:260–70.)

documentation of impairment in an organ system consistent with the effects of lead, and (3) exclusion of other causes of impairment. An assessment of increased lead absorption requires an understanding of the distribution and kinetics of lead. Lead is not distributed homogeneously in the human body. Instead, it is dispersed among several physiologically distinct compartments that differ from one another in their size and in the bioavailability of their lead (Fig. 39.8.1).[57]

Lead in blood comprises approximately 1% of the body lead burden; most of the lead in blood is red cell bound. The half-life of lead in blood is about 36 days. Elevation of the level of lead in blood provides the single best indicator of recent, acutely increased lead absorption. Thus, the blood lead level provides good information on lead absorption in persons with relatively brief exposure, such as construction workers or new entrants to the lead industry. The blood lead level rises rapidly within hours after an acute exposure episode and remains elevated for several weeks.

Normal adult blood lead levels in the United States are below 10 micrograms/dl. Clinical symptoms generally appear at blood lead levels of 30–40 micrograms/dl and become more frequent and severe as levels rise further.[23] Under the OSHA lead standard, as was noted earlier, workers with blood lead levels above 50 micrograms/dl must be immediately removed from lead exposure, and they cannot return to work with lead until their levels have fallen below 40 micrograms/dl.

Ninety to ninety-nine percent of absorbed lead is contained within the calcified tissue of skeleton and teeth in adults. In children, the portion is approximately 70%. There is evidence that the half-life of lead in bone is different for cortical and trabecular bone sites, but both half-lives are in the range of 15–25 years.[57]

In persons with long-term exposure to lead and substantially elevated bony lead stores, the blood level correlates poorly with current exposure. Under these conditions, the blood lead level appears principally to reflect release of stored lead from deep tissue compartments, principally the skeleton, and the influence on the blood lead level on release of lead from those compartments is proportional to the amount of stored lead. For this reason, the blood lead level is of only limited value in assessing dose–response relationships for the long-term consequences of lead exposure such as renal disease, hypertension, and chronic neurologic impairment. Also, the storage and later release of large amounts of lead in bone account for the long persistence of elevated blood lead levels in older retired lead workers who have ceased exposure to lead.

K-shell x-ray fluorescence (XRF) analysis is now a well-established technique for accurate, non-invasive and relatively rapid assessment of chronic lead exposure. It directly measures levels of lead in bone.[58,59] The radiation dose delivered is de minimus (approximately 1/500th of the average dental x-ray effective dose for a tibia lead measurement of an adult, and approximately 1/20th for a 1-year old).[58]

Zinc protoporphyrin (ZPP) or free erythrocyte protoporphyrin (FEP) levels reflect the toxic effect of lead on the erythrocytic enzyme ferrochelatase. FEP levels begin to rise in adults when blood lead levels exceed 30–40 micrograms/dl. Once elevated, FEP levels tend to stay above background for several months, which is substantially longer than acutely elevated blood lead levels.

A combination of normal FEP value and high blood lead level indicates very recent exposure that has not yet had opportunity to poison heme metabolism. The long persistence of elevations in ZPP creates a problem in the use of this test as a screening tool for lead exposure in occupationally exposed adults. Because the ZPP level remains elevated long after the blood lead level has fallen, this test does not discriminate between recent and past exposure. Therefore, it is of only ancillary value in evaluating occupational lead exposure.

In the past, the gold standard for determination of total body lead burden was the measurement of urinary lead excretion after intramuscular injection of 1 g of calcium EDTA (given mixed with lidocaine). Several studies have now shown that chelatable lead in general, and EDTA-chelatable lead in particular, bear little relation to bone lead stores.[30,60] Bone lead measurements using the x-ray fluorescence technique[60a] have therefore become the de facto standard for assessing body lead burden, because they sample the overwhelmingly largest pool of lead in the body. Chelatable lead remains the clinical gold standard but may be better viewed as an indicator of soft tissue bioavailable lead burden.

No other standard clinical test or laboratory finding is either very sensitive or specific for lead poisoning. Clinically evident anemia occurs only in relatively far-advanced cases of lead poisoning; thus, the diagnosis of lead poisoning cannot await the appearance of anemia. Basophilic stippling in the red blood cells is seen in most patients with acute hemolysis and occasionally in patients with chronic hemolytic syndromes; it is not specific to lead poisoning. Lead lines on the gums are uncommon except in cases of severe poisoning and may be difficult to recognize in patients with poor dental hygiene.

Complete blood counts and routine blood chemistry determinations should be performed as baseline measurements in asymptomatic workers exposed to lead. Other baseline tests that may be of value include creatinine clearance, BUN, and uric acid. Blood pressure should be measured regularly. Blood lead levels should be obtained on a periodic basis in lead workers. If the whole blood lead level exceeds 40 micrograms/dl, these tests should be repeated monthly; blood lead levels over 50 micrograms/dl require immediate removal of workers from lead-exposure, and they may not return to work in a lead-exposed job until there have been two lead-levels below 40 micrograms/dl.

Measurement of the urine lead level is of little value in monitoring populations exposed to inorganic lead; the test is too highly variable to be reliable. Similarly, hair lead analysis is not considered reliable for monitoring purposes.[61]

Clinical evaluation strategy for children

Preschool children in the United States should be screened routinely for lead poisoning according to guidelines developed by the CDC and the American Academy of Pediatrics.[62,63] These guidelines replace universal screening for all children, and target screening to geographic areas with older housing stock, and to communities where a substantial proportion of 1 and 2 years olds have elevated blood lead levels. Determination of the blood lead level is the principal technique for assessing increased lead absorption in children. Recent evidence suggests this can be accomplished safely and accurately using a capillary tube sample obtained by needle-stick. In some areas, an alternative is measurement on a filter paper. Elevated levels must be confirmed on a venous sample and tested in an accredited laboratory.

Guidelines for the interpretation of blood lead levels in children were developed by the CDC. Because recent data suggest that adverse health effects may occur in children at blood lead levels as low as 5–10 micrograms/dl, the CDC guideline of 10 micrograms/dl may need to be revised.[10a,10b] Currently, the CDC guidelines define a level above 10 micrograms/dl as excessive.[10]

A multi-tier approach for the evaluation of childhood blood lead levels has been developed by CDC and is reproduced in Table 39.8.2; this table also indicates the follow-up activities appropriate for each level of exposure.[10]

Provocative or challenge chelation with EDTA can be used to determine whether a child with an initial blood lead level of 25–44 micrograms/dl will respond to chelation therapy with a brisk lead diuresis. A dose of 500 mg EDTA/m^2 is administered intravenously over 1 hour. Urine is then collected for 8 hours, and the test is considered positive if the ratio of lead excreted (in micrograms) to the amount of EDTA infused (in milligrams) is greater than 0.6.[64] This test is recommended for use only in centers where large numbers of lead-exposed children are routinely evaluated. Children whose blood lead levels are 45 micrograms/dl and above should not receive a provocative chelation test; instead, they should be referred immediately to a pediatric center for appropriate chelation therapy. The use of XRF to assess bone lead stores is beginning to replace challenge chelation as a tool for assessing body lead burden in children.[22]

BLL* (µg/dl)	Action
<10	Reassess or rescreen in 1 year. No additional action necessary unless exposure sources change.
10–14	Obtain confirmatory blood lead levels, provide family lead education. Provide follow-up testing, within 3 months Refer for social services, if necessary.
15–19	Provide family lead education. Provide follow-up testing, with confirmatory blood lead level within 1 week. Refer to social services, if necessary. If BLLs persist (i.e., 2 venous BLLs in this range at least 3 months apart) or worsen, proceed according to actions for BLLs 20–44.
20–44	Provide co-ordination of care (case management). Confirm blood lead level within 1 week. Provide clinical management. Provide environmental investigation. Provide lead hazard control.
45–69	Within 48 hours, begin co-ordination of care (case management), including chelation with clinicians experienced in lead toxicity therapy. Environmental investigation, and lead hazard control.
70 or higher	Hospitalize child and begin medical treatment immediately. Begin co-ordination of care (case management), environmental investigation, and lead hazard control immediately.

* A diagnostic BLL is the first venous BLL obtained within 6 months of an elevated screening BLL.

Table 39.8.2 Interpretation of blood lead test results and follow-up activities: class of child based on blood lead concentration

Clinical evaluation strategy: organic lead

Organic lead (TEL) intoxication is difficult to diagnose without a history of exposure. Blood or urine lead levels and FEP levels are not predictably elevated in TEL poisoning; increased values are useful, but normal or borderline values may be seen in mild poisoning. Cerebrospinal fluid examination usually is normal.

MANAGEMENT
Management of lead poisoning in adults: acute intoxication

In all cases, the most important first step is the immediate removal from exposure to lead. Decisions to chelate should be based on several factors, including the blood lead level, current symptoms, and signs of lead-associated toxicity and duration of exposure. Chelation should be considered for blood levels greater than 80 micrograms/dl, especially when there are central or peripheral nervous system effects. For blood lead levels of 60–80 micrograms/dl, decisions regarding chelation should be made on a case-by-case basis, depending on clinical signs and symptoms. For individuals with blood lead levels less than 60 micrograms/dl, chelation is usually not required unless they have significant symptoms or unusual circumstances (such as a desire to conceive in a short time frame).

There are multiple chelating agents available. The best established agent is intravenous calcium EDTA. This treatment requires hospitalization, and should be surpervised by an experienced physician. The usual dose is 1 g of calcium EDTA (in 250 ml of 5% dextrose in water) infused slowly over 1–2 hours once or twice a day for 5 successive days. The patient should also receive intravenous hydration during the chelation. Daily determinations of kidney function, potassium levels and a urinalysis should be obtained; treatment should be discontinued if there is evidence of renal dysfunction or hematuria. Blood lead levels should be determined before treatment and after treatment ceases. It is common for a 'rebound' in blood lead levels to occur after chelation, and treatment of this rebound may require subsequent courses of chelation.

Oral chelation with DMSA (2,3 dimercaptosuccinic acid) has become widely used in adults as an alternative to intravenous EDTA, although the FDA approved DMSA only for children with lead levels over 45 micrograms/dl.[64,65] In adults, chelation with DMSA has been well tolerated and results in drops in blood lead levels similar to EDTA therapy. Dosages have varied, but treatment regimens of 10 mg/kg in three divided doses for 5 days have been used with success.[65a] Individuals with higher lead levels may require longer treatment; dosages of 10 mg/kg three times a day for 5 days followed by 10 mg/kg twice a day for 14 days (a total of 19 days) can be used. Hepatic and kidney function should be checked along with platelet counts. As with chelation with EDTA, a rebound in blood lead levels may occur, necessitating subsequent course of chelation. Oral chelation should never be used prophylactically during ongoing lead exposure as it enhances systemic absorption of lead.

Management of chronic lead intoxication

Patients with chronic manifestations of lead toxicity and high body burdens have been treated similarly to those with acute exposure, although the efficacy of treatment in such patients has not been proved. Studies are needed to confirm whether chelation therapy of adults with chronic lead intoxication results in amelioration of long-term effects such as gout, hypertension or renal insufficiency, as has been suggested.[42] The administration of chelating agents to persons with chronic lead intoxication must be approached with great care, because they often have impairment of renal function.

Chronic administration of oral chelation agents to workers who continue to be exposed to unacceptably high levels of lead in their work has been used by some unscrupulous employers as a means of reducing blood lead levels while not reducing levels of lead in air in the workplace. The practice is unethical and represents medical malpractice.[23] Moreover, the chronic administration of chelating agents may itself cause renal impairment or aggravate lead nephropathy, particularly in persons with continuing lead exposure.

Management of organic lead poisoning

The treatment for TEL poisoning is primarily support; chelation with calcium EDTA has been tried with variable efficacy. Sedation and careful observation are required in severe cases, often for prolonged periods.

Management of pediatric lead poisoning

Lead poisoning in children should be managed according to the detailed guidelines issued in 1991 by the CDC.[10] This approach is summarized in Table 39.8.2. Heavy emphasis is placed at every level on screening children and preventing further exposure.

All children with blood lead levels of 45 micrograms/dl and above require therapeutic chelation plus immediate removal from all sources of exposure to lead. Symptomatic lead poisoning in a child constitutes a medical emergency, and the child should be hospitalized immediately in a pediatric referral center.

DMSA, a chelating agent licensed by the Food and Drug Administration in 1991, has become the therapeutic agent most widely used for the treatment of childhood lead poisoning. It is available in 100-mg capsules. The recommended initial daily dose is 10 mg/kg or 350 mg/m^2 every 8 hours for 5 days, followed by 10 mg/kg or 350 mg/m^2 every 12 hours for 14 days.[65] A course of treatment, therefore, lasts 19 days. If additional courses of treatment are needed, a minimum of 2 weeks of rest between courses is recommended, unless blood lead levels indicate the need for immediate retreatment. In extreme cases of lead poisoning, intravenous CaNa$_2$EDTA is recommended.

When EDTA is used alone, it may aggravate symptoms in patients with very high blood levels. Therefore, EDTA always should be used in conjunction with BAL when the blood lead level is greater than 70 micrograms/dl or when overt symptoms of clinical lead poisoning are present in children. In such cases, the first dose of BAL always should precede the first dose of EDTA by at least 4 hours. (BAL is not used in adults.)

Doses of BAL are administered by deep intramuscular injection. The initial dose is 75 mg/m^2 of body surface area. The total daily dose of BAL is 450 mg/m^2/day in divided doses of 75 mg/m^2 every 4 hours. Once the initial dose of BAL is given and an adequate urine flow is established, EDTA is given in a dose of 1500 mg/m^2/day. EDTA is given as a continuous intravenous infusion in dextrose and water or in a 0.9% saline solution.

It is important to use only CaNa$_2$EDTA in treating children with lead poisoning. Na$_2$EDTA (disodium edetate) should never be used for treating children with lead poisoning because it can induce tetany and possibly fatal hypocalcemia.

Clinical management of asymptomatic lead-poisoned children with blood lead levels high enough to require chelation is similar to the management of symptomatic children. If the blood lead level is between 45 and 69 micrograms/dl, chelation treatment should be limited to DMSA only. If the level is 70 micrograms/dl or above, EDTA and BAL should be used, as described above. Patients who have received therapeutic courses of EDTA, with or without BAL, may use DMSA for subsequent treatment after an interval of 4 weeks.

Because lead can cause neurologic impairment at levels below 45 micrograms/dl, children with elevated lead levels between 22–44 micrograms/dl have been chelated in the past.[66] However, a recent multicenter study of chelation in children with lead levels in this range found no long-term improvement in cognitive function after chelation, and thus found no evidence to support the use of DMSA at levels below 45 micrograms/dl.[67]

It is most important that blood lead levels be rechecked frequently after treatment in all children who have been chelated. There is danger (1) of rebound blood lead levels subsequent to mobilization of lead from bony lead stores and (2) of re-exposure of a child to an unabated environmental source. Both of these possibilities should be strictly guarded against.

PREVENTION
Prevention of occupational lead poisoning

Air-borne exposure to both organic and inorganic lead in the workplace must be strictly limited by enclosure of hazardous processes, ventilation, and other engineering controls. At the present time, the OSHA lead standard mandates that occupational exposures to lead be held below 50 micrograms/m^3 of air, expressed as an 8-hour, time-weighted average. However, studies have shown clearly that toxic adverse effects can occur in lead workers at levels of exposure below this standard. An additional component of the current occupational lead standard is the existence of a biologic exposure limit regulating the permissible amount of lead in the blood. Recent research has demonstrated that clinical or subclinical toxic effects can occur at and below the current biologic exposure limit of 50 micrograms/dl of whole blood. A physician may remove a worker with a lower blood level if lead poisoning is diagnosed and restrict the worker from return to exposure until approved by the physician.

If the lead standard is reduced in the future, increasing reliance will need to be placed on the use of respirators in the workplace. In the hierarchy of industrial controls, process enclosure and ventilation take precedence over the use of respirators. However, respirators must be used when engineering approaches are not adequate to fully protect workers.

Prevention of childhood lead poisoning

The key to preventing childhood lead poisoning is prevention of exposure to lead.[62,68] The most urgent need in preventing children's environmental exposure to lead is to reduce exposure to lead-based paint. Whenever a child is found to have an elevated blood lead level, a vigorous search should be instituted for sources of all lead-based paint, as well as for other lead sources in the child's home and in other locations where the child may spend any significant part of the day. The child should not be allowed to return to a contaminated home or other contaminated environment until removal of lead-based paint has been completed. Moreover, no child and no pregnant woman should be allowed to be present in a home while abatement is occurring because of the high risk of their sustaining heavy lead exposure during abatement. In addition, special care must be taken for children undergoing chelation treatment, since they are at risk for further lead absorption if exposed to lead during treatment.

Control of lead in drinking water is most easily achieved by running the water for 3–5 minutes in the morning to flush the line before obtaining water for morning drinks or infant formula. System-wide alkalinization of drinking water systems will be required to prevent leaching of lead from pipes by acidic water.

Lead from interior house dust is best removed by first removing the lead-based paint that is the usual source of lead in dust. The contaminated dust is then removed by wet mopping.

Lead in soil is most effectively managed in most areas by leaving it in place and covering it with fresh topsoil and vegetation. In some cases, however, when contamination is intense and prospects for establishing plant cover are low, removal of topsoil may be required, followed by replacement with clean fill.

Prevention of lead poisoning in the community requires frequent screening of children for lead and community-wide surveys to identify lead hazards. Also, outreach and educational programs are necessary.

Screening of children for lead poisoning requires obtaining a brief history to ascertain a child's exposure to lead followed by measurement of blood lead level.

In 1991, the CDC recommended that all preschool children in the United States be screened for lead.[10] Subsequently, the CDC issued guidelines for state and local health authorities to enable them to decide on an appropriate lead screening policy, based on the housing stock and the prevalence of elevated lead levels in the community.[63] For communities with 27% or more of the housing stock built before 1950, or more than 12% of all 1–2 year olds with elevated lead levels, universal screening is recommended. For communities without a defined program for lead screening, universal screening is also advised. Priority groups for screening have been established, as shown in Table 39.8.3. Children in high-priority groups should be screened more frequently.

CONCLUSION

Ultimate control of lead poisoning in both adults and children will be achieved by eliminating all unnecessary uses of lead and by replacing lead with safer substitute materials whenever possible. It may be anticipated in the years ahead that the use of lead as an industrial material will diminish in developed countries; use in developing countries seems likely to continue for the foreseeable future.

– Children living in or regularly visiting a house or childcare facility built before 1950
– Children living in poverty
– Children with siblings or playmates who have or had lead poisoning
– Children of parents with occupational or environmental lead exposure
– Children with developmental delays whose oral behaviors put them at risk
– Immigrant children, including adoptees
– Children who may be exposed to lead-containing folk remedies

Table 39.8.3 Priority groups for screening of young children

References

1. Ramazzini B. De morbis artificum diatribe (translated by W C Wright). Chicago, IL: University of Chicago Press, 1713.
2. National Academy of Sciences. Lead: air borne lead in perspective. Washington, DC: National Academy Press, 1972.
3. Brody DJ, Pirkle JI, Kramer RA, et al. Blood lead levels in the US population: phase I of the third National Health and Nutrition Examination Survey (NHANES III, 1988 to 1991). JAMA 1994; 272:277–83.
4. Landrigran PJ, Boffetta P, Apostoli P. The reproductive toxicity and carcinogenicity of lead: a critical review. Am J Ind Med 2000; 38:231–43.
5. Levin SM, Goldberg M. Clinical evaluation and management of lead-exposed construction workers. Am J Ind Med 2000; 37:23–43.
6. Vork KL, Hammond SK, Sparer J, et al. Prevention of lead poisoning in construction workers: a new public health approach. Am J Ind Med 2001; 39:243–53.
7. US Department of Labor, Occupational Safety and Health Administration. 29 CFR Part 1926: Lead Exposure in Construction; Interim Final Rule. Fed Reg 1993; 58(No. 84): May 4.
8. Landrigan PJ, Silbergeld E, Froines JR, et al. Lead in the modern workplace (editorial). Am J Public Health 1990; 80:907–8.
9. Centers for Disease Control and Prevention. Update: blood lead levels – United States, 1991–1994. MMWR 1997; 46:141–6.
10. Centers for Disease Control. Preventing lead poisoning in young children. Atlanta, GA: Centers for Disease Control, 1991.
10a. Lanphear BP, Dietrich K, Auinger P, et al. Cognitive deficits associated with blood lead concentrations <10 microg/dL in US children and adolescents. Public Health Rep 2000; 115(6):521-9.
10b. Canfield RL, Henderson CR Jr, Cory-Slechta DA, et al. Intellectual impairment in children with blood lead concentrations below 10 microg per deciliter. N Engl J Med 2003; 348(16):1517-26.
11. Lanphear BP, Hornung R. Eberly S. Patterns of environmental lead exposure during early childhood. Proceedings of the IARC Gargnano Conference O.3, 1999.
12. Lanphear BP, Burgoon DA, Rust SW, et al. Environmental exposures to lead and urban children's blood lead levels. Environ Res 1998; 76:120–30.
13. Lanphear BP, Matte TD, Rogers J, et al. The contribution of lead-contaminated house dust and residential soil to children's blood lead levels. Environ Res 1998; 79:51–68.
14. Shannon MW, Graef JW. Lead intoxication in infancy. Pediatrics 1992; 89:87–90.
15. Markowitz SB, Nunez CM, Klitzman S, et al. Lead poisoning due to hai ge fen: the porphyrin content of individual erythrocytes. JAMA 1994; 271:932–4.
16. Fortenberry JD. Gasoline sniffing. Am J Med 1985; 79:740–44.
17. Legge Sir T. Industrial maladies. Oxford: Oxford University Press, 1934.

18. Cullen MR, Kayne RD, Robins JM. Endocrine and reproductive dysfunction in men associated with occupational inorganic lead intoxication. Arch Environ Health 1984; 39:431–40.

19. Cullen MR, Robins JM, Eskanazi B. Adult inorganic lead intoxication. Presentation of 31 new cases and review of recent advances in the literature. Medicine 1982; 62:2321–47.

20. Goyer RA, Rhyne B. Pathological effects of lead. Int Rev Exper Pathol 1973; 12:10–77.

21. Landrigan PJ. Toxicity of lead at low dose. Br J Ind Med 1989; 46:593–6.

22. Todd AC, Wetmur JG, Moline JM, et al. Unraveling the chronic toxicity of lead: an essential priority for environmental health. Environ Health Perspect 1996; 104(Suppl 1):141–6.

23. Baker EL Jr, Landrigan PJ, Barbour AG, et al. Occupational lead poisoning in the United States: clinical and biochemical findings related to blood lead levels. Br J Ind Med 1979; 36:314–22.

24. ATSDR. Toxicological Profile for Lead. PT 92-12. Atlanta, GA: Agency for Toxic Substances and Disease Registry, 1993.

25. Mushak P, Davis JM, Crocetti AF, Grant LD. Prenatal and postnatal effects of low level lead exposure: integrated summary of a report to the US Congress on childhood lead poisoning. Environ Res 1989; 50:11–36.

26. Osterode W, Barnas U, Geissler K. Dose dependent reduction of erythroid progenitor cells and inappropriate erythropoietin response in exposure to lead: new aspects of anaemia induced by lead. Occup Environ Med 1999; 56:106–9.

27. Tassler PL, Schwartz BS, Coresh J, et al. Associations of tibia lead, DMSA-chelatable lead, and blood lead with measures of peripheral nervous system function in former organolead manufacturing workers. Am J Ind Med 2001; 39:254–61.

28. Seppalainen AM, Hernberg S, Vesanto R, Kock B. Early neurotoxic effects of lead exposure: a prospective study. Neurotoxicology 1983; 4:181–92.

29. Hanninen H, Hernberg S, Manterer P, et al. Psychological performance of subjects with low exposure to lead. J Occup Med 1979; 20:683–9.

30. Stewart WF, Schwartz BS, Simon D, et al. Neurobehavioral function and tibial and chelatable lead levels in 543 former organolead workers. Neurology 1999; 52:1610–7.

30a. Kamel F, Umbach DM, Munsat TL, et al. Lead exposure and amyotrophic lateral sclerosis. Epidemiology 2002; 13(3):311–9.

31. Byers RK, Lord EE. Late effects of lead poisoning on mental development. Am J Dis Child 1943; 66:471–83.

32. Needleman HL, Gunnar C, Leviton A, et al. Deficits on psychologic and classroom performance of children with elevated dentine lead levels. N Engl J Med 1979; 300:689–95.

33. Campbell TF, Needleman HL, Riess JA. Bone lead levels and language processing performance. Dev Neuropsychol 2000; 18:171–86.

34. Bellinger D, Leviton A, Waternaux C, et al. Longitudinal analyses of prenatal and postnatal lead exposure and early cognitive development. N Engl J Med 1987; 316:1037–43.

35. Dietrich KN, Succop PA, Berger O, et al. Lead exposure and cognitive development of urban preschool children: the Cincinnati lead study cohort at age 4 years. Neurotoxicol Teratol 1991; 13:203–11.

36. McMichael AJ, Baghurst PA, Wigg NR, et al. Port Pirie cohort study: environmental exposure to lead and children's abilities at the age of four years. N Engl J Med 1988; 319:468–75.

37. Wasserman GA, Liu X, Lolacono NJ et al. Lead exposure and intelligence in 7-year-old children: the Yugoslavia prospective study. Environ Health Perspect 1997; 105:956–62.

38. Lanphear BP, Dietrich K, Auinger P, Cox C. Cognitive deficits associated with blood lead concentrations <10 micrograms/dL in US children and adults. Public Health Rep 2000; 115:521–9.

39. Rosen JF, Chesney RW, Hamstra A, et al. Reduction in 1,25-dihydroxyvitamin D in children with increased lead absorption. N Engl J Med 1980; 302:1128–31.

40. Hu H, Aro A, Payton M, et al. The relationship of bone and blood lead to hypertension: the normative aging study. JAMA 1996; 275:1171–6.

41. Kim R, Rotnitzky A, Sparrow D, et al. A longitudinal study of low-level lead exposure and impairment of renal function: the normative aging study. JAMA 1996; 275:1177–85.

42. Lin JL, Ho HH, Yu CC. Chelation therapy for patients with elevated body lead burden and progressive renal insufficiency: a randomized, controlled trial. Ann Intern Med 1999; 130:7–13.

43. Henderson DA. The etiology of chronic nephritis in Queensland. Med J Aust 1958; 1:377–86.

44. Morgan JM, Hartley MW, Miller RE. Nephropathy in chronic lead poisoning. Arch Int Med 1966; 118:17–29.

45. Pirkle JL, Schwartz J, Landis R, Harlan WR. The relationship between blood lead levels and blood pressure and its cardiovascular risk implications. Am J Epidemiol 1985; 121:246–58.

45a. Glenn BS, Stewart WF, Links JM, et al. The longitudinal association of lead with blood pressure. Epidemiology 2003; 14(1):30–6.

46. Schwartz J. Lead, blood pressure and cardiovascular disease in men. Arch Environ Health 1995; 50:31–7.

47. Victery W. Evidence for effects of chronic lead exposure on blood pressure in experimental animals: an overview. Environ Health Perspect 1988; 78:72–6.

48. Victery W, Vander AJ, Shulak AM. Lead, hypertension and the rennin-angiotensin system in rats. J Lab Clin Med 1982; 99:354–62.

49. Lancranjan I, Popescu HI, Gavenscu O, et al. Reproductive ability of workmen occupationally exposed to lead. Arch Environ Health 1975; 30:396–401.

50a. Sallmen, Lindbohm M-L, Anttila A, et al. Time to pregnancy among the wives of men occupationally exposed to lead. Epidemiology 2000; 11:141–7.

51. Selevan SG, Hornung R, Kissling GE, et al. Reproductive outcomes in wives of lead exposed workers. DHHS Pub. No. PB8:5-220879. Cincinnati, OH: National Institute for Occupational Safety and Health, 1984;1–42.

52. Lindbohm M-L, Sallmen M, Anttila A, et al. Paternal occupational lead exposure and spontaneous abortion. Scand J Work Environ Health 1991; 17:95–103.

52a. Gomaa A, Hu H, Bellinger D, et al. Maternal bone lead as an independent risk factor for fetal neurotoxicity: a prospective study. Pediatrics 2002; 110:110–118.

53. International Agency for Research on Cancer. Lead and lead compounds. Lyon, France: IARC, 2004.

54. Fu H, Boffetta P. Cancer and occupational exposure to inorganic lead compounds: a meta-analysis of published data. Occup Environ Med 1995; 52:73–81.

55. Steenland K, Boffetta P. Lead and cancer in humans: where are we now? Am J Ind Med 2000; 38:295–9.

56. Chang LW. The neurotoxicity and pathology of organomercury, organolead and organotin. J Toxicol Sci 1990; 15(Suppl 4):125–51.

57. Rabinowitz MB, Wetherill GW, Kobble JD. Kinetic analysis of lead metabolism in healthy humans. J Clin Invest 1977; 58:260–70.

58. Landrigan PJ, Todd AC. Direct measurement of lead in bone: a promising biomarker (editorial). JAMA 1994; 271:239–40.

59. Todd AC, McNeil FE, Fowler BA. In vivo x-ray fluorescence of lead in bone. Environ Res 1992; 59:326–35.

60. Lee BK, Schwartz BS, Stewart W, et al. Provocative chelation with DMSA and EDTA: evidence for differential access to lead storage sites. Occup Environ Med 1995; 52:13–19.

60a. Todd AC, Chettle DR. Calculating the uncertainty in lead concentration for in vivo bone lead x-ray fluorescence. Phys Med Biol 2003; 48(13):2033–9.

61. Steindel SJ, Howanitz PJ. The uncertainty of hair analysis for trace metals. JAMA 2001; 285:83–5.

62. American Academy of Pediatrics. Committee on Environmental Health. Screening for elevated blood lead levels. Pediatrics 1998; 101:1072–78.

63. Centers for Disease Control and Prevention. Screening young children for lead poisoning: guidance for state and local public health officials. Atlanta, GA: Centers for Disease Control and Prevention, 1997.

64. Markowitz M. Lead poisoning: a disease for the next millennium. Curr Probl Pediatr 2000; 30:62–70.

65. Graziano JH. Role of 2,3-aminocaptosuccinic acid in the treatment of heavy metal poisoning. Med Toxicol 1986; 1:155–62.

65a. Markowitz SB, Nunez CM, Klitzman S, et al. Lead poisoning due to hai ge fen. The porphyrin content of individual erythrocytes. JAMA 1995; 273(1):24–5.

66. O'Connor ME, Rich D. Children with moderately elevated lead levels: is chelation with DMSA helpful? Clin Pediatr 1999; 38:325–31.

67. Rogan WJ, Dietrich KN, Ware JH, et al. The effect of chelation therapy with succimer on neuropsychological development in children exposed to lead. N Engl J Med 2001; 344:1421–6.

68. Etzel RA, Balk SJ, eds. Handbook of pediatric environmental health. Elk Grove Village, IL: American Academy of Pediatrics, Committee on Environmental Health, 1999.

39.9 **Mercury**

Alfred Franzblau, Mary Carol Fromes

EXPOSURE

According to NIOSH, over 150,000 people in the United States have potential occupational exposure to mercury or its compounds, including elemental mercury, inorganic mercury salts, and organic mercurials.[1] The largest fraction of this group is employed in jobs that entail low-level chronic or intermittent exposure to elemental mercury, such as chemical and science technicians, nurses and dental technicians, and machine operators. Those workplaces that have greatest potential for clinically significant mercury exposure are more directly involved with industrial production and use of elemental mercury, such as chloralkali plants, cinnabar mining and processing, and manufacture and use of instrumentation containing elemental mercury.

The absorption and toxicity of mercury are largely a function of the form of mercury and route of exposure. The term 'organic mercury' may be confusing in this context, since it includes short-chain alkyl compounds and also long-chain alkyl and non-alkyl organic compounds (e.g., phenyl mercury). The latter tend to be rapidly metabolized in vivo, with splitting of mercury from the organic moiety, and thus have toxic profiles similar to elemental mercury or the inorganic salts. In short-chain alkyl mercury compounds (e.g., methyl mercury salts and dimethyl mercury), mercury remains covalently bound to carbon for a prolonged period in vivo, which in part explains the different pharmacokinetics and toxic profile of the short-chain alkyl mercury compounds.[2]

Elemental mercury is a liquid at room temperature with a substantial vapor pressure. Most occupational mercury exposure results from inhalation of elemental mercury vapor; pulmonary retention is more than 80%. Dermal absorption/exposure can also be significant, particularly for organic mercury compounds. Ingestion of mercury compounds is not a major route of exposure in the work setting, in part because gastrointestinal absorption of elemental mercury is poor (approximately 0.10%).

Gastrointestinal absorption is the major route of mercury exposure among the general population, and is implicated in a number of tragic toxic episodes (e.g., Minimata, Japan (see Chapter 53). The distinguishing feature is that mercury species associated with exposure in the general population are primarily short-chain alkyl mercury compounds (organic mercury or methyl mercury) derived from food, particularly large fish such as tuna and swordfish. Inorganic mercury discharged from industrial sources is metabolized to short-chain alkyl compounds by microorganisms, which are consumed by higher organisms. The alkyl mercury compounds have a prolonged half-time in animal tissues, and become concentrated in the food chain. More than 95% of ingested alkyl mercury is absorbed in humans. The average daily absorbed dose of mercury among persons without occupational exposure is estimated to be 10–20 micrograms, largely from mercury in the food chain.[1]

Some forms of mercury exposure which were previously important are now only of historical significance. Mercury and mercury compounds were used widely as medicinal agents. In the Middle Ages mercurial compounds were employed in treatment of syphilitic sores; until just after World War II, mercury compounds were an important constituent of teething powders given to infants; and mercurial diuretics were the mainstay of diuretic therapy until displaced by furosemide and ethacrynic acid in the 1960s.[3] The classic description of 'mad hatters' resulted from exposure to mercuric nitrate used as a carrotting agent in preparation of animal skins for production of hats. Mercury compounds employed in the production of hats were replaced with less toxic agents during the late 19th and early 20th centuries. Certain organic mercury compounds once were used widely as fungicidal agents in paints (e.g., phenylmercuric acetate and phenylmercuric proprionate). This use stopped in the United States in the early 1990s.[1]

Mercury exposure related to dental amalgam deserves special mention. Such exposure must be divided into two distinct categories: mercury exposure of dentists and dental technicians (a form of occupational exposure mentioned previously), and exposure of patients who have tooth fillings consisting of mercury amalgam. Dental amalgam, which has been in use for approximately 150 years, typically consists of (by weight) 50% mercury, 35% silver, 9% tin, 6% copper, and a trace amount of zinc.[1] A single filling (involving the multi-surface grinding portion of a molar) contains between 750 and 1000 milligrams of elemental mercury. Millions of mercury amalgam tooth fillings are put in place each year in the United States.

Occupational exposure of dental personnel to mercury has been well documented. In surveys conducted between 1975 and 1983, average urinary mercury among dentists in the United States was 14.2 micrograms per liter, well above the mean of the general population.[4] Following an educational campaign on mercury hygiene sponsored by the American Dental Association, similar surveys in 1985 and 1986 documented that mean mercury levels in urine among dentists had dropped to 5.8 and 6.7 micrograms per liter, respectively.[5] In 1995, the mean level had fallen to 4.94 micrograms per liter.[6]

Characterization of mercury exposure to patients with amalgam tooth fillings has been somewhat confused. In the early 1970s, technologic advances made it possible to measure mercury in intraoral air, leading to a flurry of publications that applied this technique. It was documented that in patients with amalgam tooth fillings, various routine activities (e.g., tooth brushing, chewing gum, and professional manipulations such as cleaning or polishing) resulted in marked transient elevations of intraoral mercury concentrations. Unfortunately, many of the assumptions and modeling procedures employed initially to estimate an overall absorbed dose of mercury related to amalgam fillings were flawed. More recent measurements and analyses have shown that among subjects with multiple amalgam tooth surfaces (13–48 surfaces), the average daily absorbed dose of mercury is 1.7 micrograms (range: 0.4–4.4 micrograms), which is small in comparison to the usual daily dose of non-occupationally exposed persons (10–20 micrograms per day).[7] The influence of such 'internal exposure' on urinary mercury concentration (a more universal standard of inorganic mercury exposure) was correlated with the number of amalgam tooth surfaces, but was small[8] when compared with the major source of environmental mercury, dietary intake.

CLINICAL EFFECTS
Acute

Acute high-level exposure to elemental mercury vapor primarily affects the respiratory system. Clinical effects include metal fume fever, bronchial irritation, and acute chemical pneumonitis. Within hours of exposure (which need last only a few minutes), subjects begin to experience dyspnea, chest pains, cough, chills, weakness, and possibly hemoptysis. These can be accompanied by lightheadedness, nausea, and vomiting. Tachypnea and rales may be noted, and laboratory studies can demonstrate leukocytosis, hypoxemia, diffuse infiltrates on chest radiographs, and impaired diffusion capacity. Respiratory failure and death can occur. Gingivitis and mercurial stomatitis can develop in the weeks following recovery from the acute event. Patients may have residual restrictive impairment of pulmonary function and reduced diffusing capacity.[9]

Some mercury compounds are direct cutaneous irritants. However, it is likely that the frequency of true hypersensitivity to mercury compounds has been overestimated in the past due to use of mercuric chloride ($HgCl_2$) as a patch test reagent at concentrations which were frankly corrosive. Elemental mercury is only rarely a cause of allergic contact dermatitis. Documented cases of allergic dermatitis usually result from sustained exposure to organic mercurial compounds. Fewer than 50 cases of mercury hypersensitivity (e.g., stomatitis and/or dermatitis) related to dental amalgam are reported in the literature published in the 20th century. It adds some perspective to recall that dental amalgam contains other metals which are potential sensitizers (e.g., copper), and that other metals commonly used in dental appliances (e.g., gold, nickel, cobalt, and chromium) are well-documented sensitizers.

Ingestion of mercuric chloride ($HgCl_2$, corrosive sublimate) may be lethal, making it a common method of suicide in the past. Clinical manifestations include direct gastrointestinal irritation with fluid loss and shock, as well as acute renal failure. The latter results from accumulation of mercury in proximal renal tubules with consequent acute tubular necrosis.[3]

Chronic

Classic mercurialism usually results from exposure to elemental mercury vapor or inorganic salts, and the primary target organs are the nervous system, oral cavity, and kidneys. The neurologic expressions include: fine intention tremor of the extremities, tongue and lips; psychologic disturbances consisting of nervousness, irritability, and pathologic shyness (erethism); mental confusion; and peripheral polyneuropathy (sensorimotor axonopathy) affecting the lower extremities more than the upper. Oral cavity disorders can include gingivitis, stomatitis, salivary gland swelling, and excessive salivation. Unless severe, the clinical manifestations tend to abate following cessation of exposure. Only minor neurologic abnormalities were documented in a recent study of chloralkali workers examined an average of six years after their exposure to mercury ended.[10] Remote (in time) occupational mercury exposure appears to interact with normal aging processes (i.e., natural neuronal attrition) so as to unmask prior exposure-related subclinical effects, particularly peripheral polyneuropathy and tremor, among workers with high past exposures.[11]

Absorbed inorganic mercury is preferentially concentrated in the renal proximal tubules, but tubular dysfunction is unusual in the occupational setting. Glomerular disease with nephrosis is the most common, though infrequent, manifestation of renal dysfunction among occupationally exposed individuals. Interestingly, pathologic findings include interstitial and/or glomerular immune-complex nephritis, suggesting that mercury-related glomerular disease may have an immunologic mechanism. Proteinuria usually abates following removal from exposure.[3]

Short-chain alkyl mercury compounds (organic mercury) are a potential exposure hazard in the general environment in addition to the work setting, and have distinct pharmacokinetic and toxic profiles. With chronic exposure the clinical manifestations usually have a gradual onset. Following a single, massive exposure, there is usually a latency of several weeks before the appearance of clinical abnormalities. The spectrum of effects is similar regardless of the time course of exposure, and the primary target is the nervous system.[12]

The clinical effects of short-chain alkyl mercury compounds are distinct from classic mercurialism; salivation, stomatitis, and erethism do not occur. The effects include: neurasthenia (weakness, fatigue, headache, poor recall and concentration, emotional instability, and intellectual deterioration in severe cases); numbness and tingling in fingers, toes, mouth, lips, and tongue; global ataxia involving impairment of speech, swallowing, gait, writing, and truncal movements; spasticity and intention tremor; impairment of hearing; concentric constriction of visual fields; and possible seizures. If exposure occurs prenatally, the clinical expression may be cerebral palsy in the newborn or a less severe presentation, such as psychomotor retardation. There appears to be increased susceptibility to, and preferential concentration of, alkyl mercury in the fetus, since mothers of affected infants may have lower tissue levels, and not demonstrate clinical effects.[12]

A rare form of inorganic mercury poisoning which has been described only in children is acrodynia. The mechanism of acrodynia is poorly understood, but is best described as an uncharacterized form of 'hypersensitivity' to mercury. The syndrome usually begins weeks or months after onset of exposure to mercury. It consists of: severe pain and cramps in the extremities; muscle weakness in the pectoral and pelvic regions; nerve dysfunction in the lower extremities; characteristic cutaneous manifestations (pink or red macular rash on the hands and/or feet, with desquamation); pruritus; irritability and mood swings; intermittent low-grade fevers; abdominal cramps; photophobia; increased perspiration; hypertension; hypotonia; and tachycardia. The diagnosis is confirmed by documentation of elevated urine mercury in a 24-hour specimen, but the concentration is frequently below the usual range associated with typical, chronic mercury poisoning.

Allegations of mercury exposure being associated with various immunologically mediated diseases (e.g., multiple sclerosis related to mercury dental amalgam) are without foundation.

DIAGNOSIS, EVALUATION, AND TREATMENT

Acute inhalational exposure to a high concentration of elemental mercury vapor (greater than 1–3 mg/m^3 for a few hours) is a life-threatening medical emergency. With development of acute pneumonitis, subjects require aggressive supportive respiratory care. Chelation with penicillamine, dimercaprol, or dimercaptosuccinic acid (DMSA) can help to accelerate the urinary excretion of mercury following acute high exposure. Although it is necessary to rely on the history and clinical picture to make the initial diagnosis and begin therapy, measurement of mercury in 24-hour urine specimens (frequently in the thousands of micrograms per liter of urine) confirms exposure.

Acute ingestion of mercuric chloride, usually with suicidal intent, is also a medical emergency. Chelation can mobilize mercury from tissue, specifically the kidneys. Hemodialysis, possibly with cysteine infusion, can remove mercury from the body.[1]

The early clinical manifestations of chronic mercury poisoning are non-specific, and therefore confirmatory laboratory tests, specifically biologic monitoring, are important. Appropriate biologic monitoring techniques are predicated on the pharmacokinetics of different mercury compounds. Elemental mercury, inorganic mercury salts, and organic (non-short-chain alkyl) compounds of mercury are rapidly cleared from blood and metabolized in vivo to the mercuric form (Hg^{++}), primarily excreted via the urine. The half-life of the total body burden is about 30–60 days, although there is great variability among the different organs (e.g., retention in brain tissue may be of the order of years).[1] Short-chain alkyl mercury compounds are not metabolized quickly, and are more evenly distributed to all body tissues due to their lipid solubility. Ninety percent of short-chain alkyl mercury in blood is bound within red blood cells. Excretion of alkyl compounds is primarily via feces due to excretion in bile. There is efficient enterohepatic circulation, and the half-time in the body is about 70 days.[13]

In light of the preceding observations, recent or chronic ongoing exposure to elemental mercury, mercuric salts, and non-short-chain alkyl compounds is assessed best via measurement of mercury in urine, preferably 24-hour specimens. Measurement of mercury in blood can also be used for this purpose during the first few days following cessation of exposure. However, dietary habits can confound the interpretation of blood measurements since short-chain alkyl compounds found in certain foods also appear in blood, but not in urine. Clinical abnormalities of classic mercurialism are usually not found among chronically exposed workers with urine levels maintained below 300 micrograms Hg/l,[1] and the World Health Organization endorses 50 micrograms Hg/g of creatinine as an appropriate biologic threshold value for persons exposed to inorganic and elemental mercury. Persons without occupational exposure to mercury usually have urine levels below 5 micrograms Hg/g creatinine. The correlation of urine or blood levels of mercury with toxicity is poor.

Measurement of mercury in whole blood or hair appears to reflect body burden of the short-chain alkyl compounds (predominantly methyl mercury). For reasons outlined previously, urinary levels are not useful in assessing exposure to short-chain alkyl mercury compounds. Levels in blood or hair that exceed 20 micrograms Hg/100 ml or 50 micrograms Hg/g, respectively, may be associated with early toxicity. WHO endorses a threshold value of 10 micrograms Hg/100 ml in blood. The validity of hair analysis for trace elements has been questioned. Analysis of hair from one individual by multiple commercial laboratories may yield significantly different results.[14]

With documentation of exposure and findings consistent with chronic (classic) mercury poisoning, the primary therapeutic maneuver is removal from exposure. In most cases, the natural elimination of mercury coincides with gradual clinical improvement of neurologic, oral cavity, and renal abnormalities. Although chelation may accelerate urinary excretion of mercury, such aggressive therapy may result in worsening of patients' clinical conditions, since mobilization of mercury from body stores may increase toxicity in the kidney and cause greater deposition in the brain. Penicillamine may present less of a hazard in this regard, and may also be more effective in ameliorating the nervous system effects of mercury.[13] Because of the potential for renal damage due to mercury, assessment of tubular and glomerular proteinuria should be considered.

Removal from exposure is also the primary therapeutic approach for persons exposed to short-chain alkyl mercury compounds, commonly a reduction in fish consumption or other potential dietary sources. Chelation is not effective in accelerating the excretion of organic mercury or improving clinical outcome. However, there is promise in approaches directed at interrupting enterohepatic circulation of alkyl mercury compounds excreted in bile, such as ingestion of non-absorbable mercury-binding substances (e.g., polythiol resins).[13]

PREVENTION

Process substitution, appropriate engineering controls, good industrial hygiene and housekeeping practices, worker education, and, when necessary, use of personal protective equipment should reduce or prevent occupational exposure to mercury. Workers with potential exposure to elemental, inorganic, or non-short-chain alkyl mercury compounds should be monitored via measurement of mercury in 24-hour urine specimens. Periodic assessment of mercury in whole blood should be used to monitor workers with exposure to short-chain alkyl mercury compounds. Pregnant women, or women intending to become pregnant in the near future, should limit their intake of foods known to contain elevated levels of mercury (e.g., swordfish, tuna, etc.).[1] Hypersensitivity reactions to mercury in dental amalgam are exceedingly rare and usually self-limited; removal of amalgam tooth fillings for this reason is almost never justified.

References

1. Agency for Toxic Substances and Disease Registry. Toxicological profile for mercury. Atlanta, GA: Agency for Toxic Substances and Disease Registry, US Department of Health and Human Services, Public Health Service, 1999.
2. Clarkson TW. Recent advances in the toxicology of mercury with emphasis on the alkylmercurials. CRC Crit Rev Toxicol 1972; 1:203–34.
3. Wedeen RP. Occupational renal disease. Am J Kidney Dis 1984; 3:241–57.
4. Naleway C, Sakaguchi R, Mitchell E, Muller T, Ayer WA, Hefferren JJ. Urinary mercury levels in US dentists, 1975–1983: review of Health Assessment Program. J Am Dent Assoc 1985; 111:37–42.
5. Naleway C, Chou H-N, Muller T, Dabney J, Roxe D, Siddiqui F. On-site screening for urinary Hg concentrations and correlation with glomerular and renal tubular function. J Public Health Dent 1991; 51:12–17.
6. Martin MD, Naleway C, Chou H-N. Factors contributing to mercury exposure in dentists. J Am Dent Assoc 1995; 126:1502–11.
7. Berglund A. Estimation by a 24-hour study of the daily dose of intra-oral mercury vapor inhaled after release from dental amalgam. J Dent Res 1990; 69:1646–51.
8. Olstad ML, Holland RI, Pettersen AH. Effect of placement of amalgam restorations on urinary mercury concentration. J Dent Res 1990; 69:1607–9.
9. Lilis R, Miller A, Lerman Y. Acute mercury poisoning with severe chronic pulmonary manifestations. Chest 1985; 88:306 9.
10. Frumkin H, Letz R, Williams PL, et al. Health effects of long-term mercury exposure among chloralkali plant workers. Am J Ind Med 2001; 39:1–18.
11. Albers JW, Kallenbach LR, Fine LJ, et al and the Mercury Workers Study Group. Neurological abnormalities associated with remote occupational elemental mercury exposure. Ann Neurol 1988; 24:651–9.
12. Bakir F, Damluji SF, Amin-Zaki L, et al. Methylmercury poisoning in Iraq. Science 1973; 181:230–41.
13. Joselow MM, Louria DB, Browder AA. Mercurialism: environmental and occupational aspects. Ann Intern Med 1972; 76:119–30.
14. Seidel S, Kreutzer R, Smith D, McNeel S, Gilliss D. Assessment of commercial laboratories performing hair mineral analysis. JAMA 2001; 285:67–72.

39.10 Copper, Manganese, Thallium, Vanadium, Zinc

Alfred Franzblau, Mary Carol Fromes

COPPER

Exposure

Copper was one of the earliest metals utilized by man. The word was derived from the Greek for Cyprus ('Kyprios'), which was known for its rich deposits of this reddish-brown metal. Romans referred to the metal as 'aes cyprium' (ore of Cyprus) and later as 'cuprum'. The English word evolved from this latter term.[1]

The toxicity of copper is dependent on its chemical form and mode of exposure. Copper salts tend to be more toxic than metallic copper, although the latter is more widespread in industrial settings. Copper is also an essential trace metal, and humans have evolved homeostatic mechanisms for control of copper balance. Derangements of these mechanisms, as occurs rarely in certain dietary circumstances or inherited diseases, leads to severe illness (Indian childhood cirrhosis, Menkes' syndrome, or Wilson's disease), but these will not be discussed further.[2]

Copper is extremely malleable, and possesses high thermal and electrical conductivity. Industrial exposure to copper occurs primarily via inhalation of fume in the setting of welding on copper-containing metal objects, or formation of copper alloys (e.g., bronze or brass). Grinding or polishing of copper-coated materials can release very fine metallic copper dust that is respirable. Copper sulfate is used widely as a fungicide and algaecide. Skin contact with copper salts or metal dust can result in cutaneous reactions, but these are rare. Copper salts, particularly the sulfate, are most toxic when ingested. Copper can leach out of copper-containing beverage containers or pipes when the pH is acidic, and result in clinically significant soluble copper exposure.[2]

Clinical effects

The most prominent consequence of industrial copper exposure is metal fume fever (MFF) resulting from inhalation of copper fume while welding or brazing (see Chapter 19.5). Finely divided metallic copper dust may cause the same condition. The clinical syndrome is identical to MFF caused by other metal fumes (e.g., zinc, nickel, etc.). Symptoms consist of delayed onset (up to 24 hours) of fever, chills, headache, nausea, vomiting, myalgia, malaise, shortness of breath, non-productive cough, and sometimes a metallic taste. These symptoms usually abate within 24–48 hours, and resolve without specific therapy in a few days.[3] Transient infiltrates may be noted on chest radiographs.

However, the association of copper inhalation with MFF has recently been called into question.[4] A critical review of published reports on this topic has revealed only a small number of original case reports, and that copper exposures were not always measured properly in these studies. This has led to speculation that the workers described as having MFF related to copper may actually have inhaled fumes or dusts contaminated with other metals known to be associated with this syndrome.

Air-borne copper sulfate exposure is associated with mucous membrane irritation, rhinitis, and cough. Cutaneous sensitization to copper or copper salts is probably rare.[1]

An uncommon occupational pulmonary problem associated with copper exposure is 'vineyard sprayer's lung,' which has only been described among agricultural workers in Portugal. It is related to inhalation of 'Bordeaux mixture', a 1–2.5% solution of copper sulfate neutralized by hydrated lime. Bordeaux mixture is applied manually to combat mildew on grape vines. Typically, patients can present with restrictive lung disease after many years of exposure. Chest radiographs can reveal diffuse reticulonodular or miliary changes. Pathologic findings of interstitial lung fibrosis, granulomas, and pigmentation with copper deposition have been reported. Granulomas may also be found in other organs, such as the liver, indicating that this entity can mimic sarcoidosis. There is suggestive evidence that there may be an increased incidence of lung cancer among patients with this disorder, but no population-based or cohort studies have been performed.[5]

Although first described in the 17th century among coppersmiths, green hair (due to exogenous deposition of copper) among copper workers has all but disappeared. Occasional reports of green hair continue to appear, but are usually related to showering or swimming in water with a high copper content.[6] When the copper content of water exceeds 5 mg/l, a mild blue-green tint may be visible.[2] In these circumstances the metal is leached from copper pipes by acidic water, or is derived from copper salts used as algaecides in swimming pools. Discoloration from copper is a sign of external exposure and not systemic toxicity.[6]

Systemic toxicity of copper or its salts is seen almost exclusively in association with ingestion. Copper sulfate solution is inexpensive, so at one time ingesting it was a preferred method of suicide in some regions of India. Multiple system effects may be seen among victims. Copper is a direct irritant of the gastrointestinal mucosa, causing nausea, vomiting, and burning in the epigastrium. A metallic taste is frequently noted after ingestion.[7] Once copper is absorbed, it is deposited in the liver, where accumulation can lead to centrilobular necrosis. If enough copper is absorbed, the patient is at risk of massive hemolytic anemia, with subsequent development of acute renal failure and attendant complications. Copper leached from copper-containing water pipes or beverage containers can also produce gastrointestinal irritation.[2]

Diagnosis, evaluation, treatment, and prevention

Clinically, the most useful approach for assessing occupational exposure to copper is to obtain a good history and documentation of the industrial process. Indices for biologic monitoring for copper are not well established, although there are a few reports in which blood concentration or urinary excretion of copper have been employed. The primary difficulties are that there are wide normal ranges for copper levels in blood and urine, and these can vary substantially due to intercurrent medical illnesses.[3]

Following removal from exposure, therapy for copper-related illness is usually supportive. Chelation therapy is only employed in the setting of Wilson's disease, which causes copper to accumulate in the liver and other organs. Zinc acetate has also been used to treat Wilson's disease because zinc induces production of intestinal metallothionein, which binds copper and prevents its movement into the blood by forming complexes with the metal in intestinal cells.[2] Metal fume fever is self-limited and generally has no long-term consequences. Engineering controls, worker education, and personal protective equipment are the primary measures to prevent copper-related illness in the occupational setting.

MANGANESE
Exposure

Manganese is an essential trace element with a typical intake of 1–5 mg/day. Under normal circumstances manganese can be identified in small quantities in most human tissues. It is the second most abundant heavy metal in the earth's crust (0.1%), after iron. Although there are thousands of facilities in the United States that manufacture, process, or produce manganese, almost no manganese ore has been mined in the US since the late 1970s. Manganese ore is imported from Australia, Brazil, Mexico, Morocco, and South Africa.[8] Industrially, it is used primarily in production of steel (85–90% of all tonnage). Other significant applications include dry-cell batteries, matches, fireworks, chemicals, glass, ceramics, paints, inks, dyes, animal feed supplements, antiknock compounds, welding rods, drugs, fungicides, fertilizers, as an intravenous contrast agent (i.e., mangafodipir) for magnetic resonance imaging (MRI), purification of water, and as a preservative of rubber and wood products.[8]

Industrial (inorganic) manganese exposure typically occurs via inhalation of dust or fume. Cutaneous and gastrointestinal absorption are negligible (except in the setting of iron deficiency), which, in part, explains why almost all reported cases of chronic manganism have occurred in an occupational setting rather than in relation to environmental contamination. Manganese-associated illness has been described primarily among workers in dusty operations associated with mining, transportation, crushing, and sieving of manganese-bearing ore.[9] Historical

dust levels of 250 mg Mn/m^3, and higher, have been reported with these processes. Cases of disease have also been reported among industrial end-users of manganese, such as workers employed in smelters producing ferromanganese alloys, foundry men, ceramics workers, welders using manganese-coated welding rods, and those who perform burning or grinding of ferromanganese alloy steel.[10,11] Cutaneous absorption of (organic) manganese can be significant among agricultural workers who spray manganese-containing fungicides, such as Maneb (manganese ethylenebisdithiocarbamate) or Mancozeb (zinc manganese ethylenebisdithiocarbamate).[12] Patients on total parenteral nutrition and/or with severe liver dysfunction can demonstrate increased manganese in blood and characteristic changes on brain MRI, and may have signs consistent with manganese toxicity.[13–16]

Considerable controversy has developed over the potential for human exposure and adverse health effects related to use of methylcyclopentadienyl manganese tricarbonyl (MMT) as an octane booster in gasoline.[17] The concern is that widespread use of MMT in gasoline with consequent dispersion of manganese salts via tailpipe emissions could parallel the environmental impact related to decades of use of tetraethyl lead in automotive fuel. However, recent data and environmental models suggest that the contribution of MMT in gasoline to air-borne respirable manganese particulate, and the absorbed daily dose of manganese, is low in relation to existing background levels.[18] Nevertheless, further research is needed to better characterize the potential for adverse health effects, particularly among more susceptible subpopulations.[19]

Clinical effects

Acute

Manganese salts can act as minor irritants to skin, eyes, and mucous membranes. Inhalation of fume of manganese oxide can cause metal fume fever (see Chapter 19.5). Potassium permanganate ($KMnO_4$) is corrosive to tissue due to its potent oxidizing capability.

Pulmonary function deficits, bronchitis, asthma, and/or an increased incidence of pneumonia (but not pneumoconiosis) have been reported among manganese-exposed workers, and also persons living in the vicinity of manganese-emitting plants (e.g., smelters). Some of these reports are from the early to middle part of the 20th century, prior to the availability of antibiotics, and the clinical and epidemiologic descriptions are limited.[20] In some cases, 'manganese pneumonia' has been noted to be resistant to antibiotic therapy, and there is some animal evidence to suggest that manganese exposure may increase susceptibility to bacterial infections. Manganese may directly cause inflammation of pulmonary tissue, and may also serve to increase susceptibility to bacterial infection. However, in an epidemiologic study of non-malignant respiratory disease mortality among ferroalloy plant workers, Hobbesland et al[21] did not find any consistent relationship between manganese exposure and pneumonia.

Nevertheless, manganese dusts and fumes may be possible aggravating factors in the development of the pulmonary effects noted above, but additional causes should not be overlooked if evaluating possible pulmonary disease among manganese-exposed industrial workers, or those living adjacent to manganese-emitting plants.

Chronic

The primary health concern related to manganese exposure is development of a neurologic syndrome, termed manganism, which was first described by Couper in 1837.[22] He reported on five men employed grinding manganese dioxide for the manufacture of bleach. Subsequently, hundreds of cases from a variety of industrial circumstances have appeared in the medical literature.

Clinical manifestations of manganism can occur after a variable length of time, depending upon intensity of exposure, individual susceptibility, and possibly the type of ore (a mixture of $Mn_2O_3/MnSiO_3$ may be more damaging than MnO_2, although data are limited). The mechanism by which manganese produces neurotoxicity has not been clearly established. Rare cases have developed after just one or two months of exposure, while others have become recognized only following more than 20 years of employment. The crude 'length of exposure' may be a misleading parameter, as illustrated by cases involving industrial workers with longstanding manganese exposure who develop manganism within months following breakdown of ventilation equipment and consequent increase in manganese exposure.[11]

More recently, neuropsychologic screening of exposed workers has uncovered subclinical or mild impairments that might otherwise not have come to clinical attention, and at levels of exposure that had been considered 'acceptable'.[23–27] Based in part on these findings, the American Conference of Governmental and Industrial Hygienists (ACGIH) lowered the 8-hour time-weighted average threshold limit value (TLV) from 5.0 mg Mn/m^3 to 0.2 mg Mn/m^3.[28]

The earliest effects of manganism are non-specific and usually subjective, such as anorexia, asthenia, apathy, somnolence, headaches, and reduction in spontaneous social interaction. Patients can appear depressed or excited. A minority may experience a brief period of aggressiveness, increased sexual activity, hallucinations, and at times pressured or incoherent speech. These manifestations of excitement are termed 'manganese psychosis'. Patients with both depressive and excitatory effects mistakenly have been referred to psychiatrists for evaluation.

With continued exposure speech can be affected, with loss of variation of pitch. Diction is slowed and inarticulate, often with stuttering. In advanced manganism, there can be almost complete muteness. The facies become fixed in expression ('masque manganique'), although it is possible to make voluntary facial movements. Episodes of inappropriate laughter or weeping can occur. Patients are noted to develop clumsiness, especially of the upper limbs. On examination, one finds an increase in reflexes, particularly in the lower extremities, and adiadochokinesia.

Patients in the advanced stages are notable for aggravation of the above signs and symptoms, the development of disturbances of gait (e.g., the 'cock walk'), and possibly resting tremor. Micrographia can be apparent on samples of writing.

Manganism appears to be a progressive condition even after cessation of exposure, particularly once it has advanced to clinically overt stages.[29] Long-term follow-up of manganese-exposed industrial workers with subclinical impairments is variable; the neurologic findings typically do not progress, but they may or may not improve after reduction or elimination of exposure.[30,31]

Although many similarities with idiopathic Parkinson's disease (PD) have been noted, important clinical and pathologic distinctions have been described more recently. Patients with manganism tend to have more psychiatric disturbances early in their history, less frequent resting tremor, more frequent dystonia, and are less likely to be responsive to PD drugs such as levodopa.[32,33] A distinguishing gait disturbance found among patients with manganism, but not those with PD, is the 'cock walk'.[32] In humans (and animal models) the pathologic lesions of manganism are more diffuse (i.e., in the pallidium, caudate nucleus, putamen, and possibly cortex) than among persons with idiopathic PD (i.e., primarily in pigmented areas such as the substantia nigra). Lewy bodies are usually present in the substantia nigra in patients with PD, but usually not among patients with manganism.[32] MRI scans of patients with manganism can demonstrate characteristic changes thought to represent the accumulation of manganese in brain tissue.[13–16,32] Patients with idiopathic PD usually have normal MRI scans. Fluorodopa positron emission tomography (PET) scanning is reported to be abnormal in PD, but normal in manganism.[34]

Diagnosis, evaluation, and treatment

Diagnosis of manganism requires a history of exposure, and typical findings on medical examination. As noted above, the early effects can be subtle and non-specific. Unfortunately, valid and accurate methods of biologic monitoring for assessing exposure to, or body burden of, manganese are not well established. Manganese is excreted primarily in bile and feces, and only a small percentage in urine.[8] The total body half-life varies from 15 to 35 days. In the blood, most manganese is bound within red blood cells. Individual manganese levels in blood and urine are not well correlated with recent or past exposure, and thus should not be relied upon as definitive evidence in assessing exposure. In contrast, group mean concentrations of manganese in blood or urine correlate with recent exposure in epidemiologic studies.[27] Challenge tests with EDTA to determine if the body burden is increased are not helpful. As noted above, MRI scans may show increased manganese uptake in the brain.[14,32] In spite of numerous reports of successful application of hair analyses, these are difficult to interpret for the usual reasons: there is no standard method for washing, and external contamination can be difficult to distinguish from internal deposition.

Treatment of manganism is primarily removal from exposure. Chelation has not been shown to have any consistent benefit. Treatment with drugs used for idiopathic PD, such as levodopa and 5-hydroxytryptophan, has been advocated in the past,[35,36] but less success has been noted more recently.[32] A small double-blind study of levodopa among patients with chronic manganism did not show any positive effects.[33]

Prevention

Engineering control of exposures is the mainstay of prevention of manganese-related occupational disease. Pre-employment and periodic medical examinations of exposed workers should include attention to personality changes and movement disorders in order to detect early manganism, when it will have the highest potential for reversal with removal from exposure. Most human health studies on MMT in gasoline have been based on healthy adult males, with a focus on neurotoxicity. Human data pertaining to possible reproductive, developmental or other effects, especially at low levels of exposure, are limited, and further studies are needed to address these issues.

THALLIUM
Exposure

Thallium was discovered in 1861, and within two years it was known to be highly toxic. Despite such knowledge, thallium compounds were employed as medicinal agents for almost 60 years. Uses during the late 19th and early 20th centuries included the treatment of syphilis, tuberculosis, and ringworm. It was also employed as a depilatory.[37] Numerous instances of iatrogenic toxicity were documented.[38]

In 1920, thallium compounds were first used as pesticides in Germany. Subsequently, ingestion of thallium-containing rodenticides, usually thallium sulfate, was a common cause of thallium poisoning, particularly among children. These compounds, and many other thallium formulations, have excellent transcutaneous, gastrointestinal, and pulmonary absorption. In 1972, thallium rodenticides were banned in the United States, with a consequent decrease in the incidence of such episodes. However, the problem of ingestion of thallium rodenticides continues elsewhere in the world.

Industrial exposures to thallium compounds can result in acute and chronic disease, but now are rare. Thallium is a byproduct of the combustion of flue dust, the smelting or refining of zinc and lead, and cadmium production, but it has not been produced in the United States since 1981. Thallium has limited industrial applications, with only small amounts currently utilized, of the order of a few thousand pounds per year in the United States. Thallium is a component of crystals employed in equipment for detection and signaling of long wavelength radiation and spectrometers, and photoelectric cells. Solutions of organic thallium salts are used to perform gravimetric separation of minerals. Thallium compounds are also used in certain low temperature thermometers, as an additive to cement, in pigments, and in other specialized products. Grinding or machining of thallium alloys has resulted in occupational exposure.[39]

Environmental exposure to thallium has been documented in a number of instances. Soil and water contain minute quantities of thallium. In the past, episodes of environmental exposure involved ingestion of foods, such as bread, in which grain had been treated excessively with thallium-containing pesticides. More recently, persons living in the vicinity of a cement plant in Germany that emitted thallium were reported to have excessive absorption and toxicity. Toxicokinetic analyses revealed that thallium absorption in this population was correlated with consumption of locally grown vegetables.[40]

Radioactive thallium isotopes (thallium-201) are used in nuclear medicine, but the quantities injected are small. Thallium toxicity has not been reported in this setting.

Clinical effects

Acute

Thallium has high acute toxicity. The minimum lethal dose for an adult is 1g or less. Neuropathy, gastrointestinal irritation, and hair loss form the classic triad of acute thallium intoxication. Gastrointestinal upset (abdominal pain, nausea, vomiting, diarrhea or constipation, and hemorrhagic gastritis) can occur within hours of ingestion of large doses. Peripheral neurologic changes, initially painful parasthesias, can appear within a few days, followed by motor neuropathy. Multiple levels of the nervous system can suffer injury, including cranial nerves (particularly the optic and vagus nerves), autonomic function, spinal cord, and areas of the cortex and basal ganglia. Convulsions have been described. Alopecia is delayed for two or three weeks, and can become total. Other organ systems can also be affected. Liver enzymes (ALT, AST, alkaline phosphatase) can become elevated, and centrilobular necrosis has been reported. Renal function may deteriorate due to tubular necrosis. In fatal cases, focal necrosis of skeletal and myocardial muscle has been documented at autopsy. The latter probably plays a role in refractory arrhythmias, although vagal neuropathy may also be responsible.[41] Thallium is teratogenic in a number of animal species.

Histopathologic studies of nerves following thallium poisoning disclose axonal degeneration.[41] As with many toxic axonopathies, recovery is slow, inversely related to severity of injury and duration of exposure, and may be incomplete.

Mees' lines can be seen two to three weeks following an acute ingestion. In some cases a blue line appears in the gingiva within two or three days.[42]

Chronic

Effects of chronic thallium exposure represent a subset of the acute effects noted previously, but with slower and more insidious onset. In this setting, gastrointestinal symptoms are less prominent or absent, and alopecia is the most classic finding. The pattern of hair loss is unusual in that it can be complete on the head, but axillary and facial hair (e.g., eyebrows) are spared. Sensorimotor peripheral neuropathy completes the clinical picture. Patients may also experience a variety of non-specific symptoms, such as disordered sleep, headache, fatigue, and emotional disturbances.[43]

Diagnosis, evaluation, and treatment

Aside from an accurate history, the best test for documenting thallium exposure is measurement of thallium in urine, preferably a 24-hour sample. The concentration of thallium in urine of unexposed persons is less than 1.5 micrograms per liter, or 1.0 microgram per gram of creatinine. Determination of blood concentration of thallium is not useful since the metal tends to be rapidly cleared and to reside intracellularly. In this respect ionic thallium tends to behave like potassium. Hair analyses are also unreliable for the usual reason: external deposition cannot be distinguished from internal incorporation of the metal. Thallium is excreted predominantly via the kidneys with a half-life in urine of approximately 30 days. Unfortunately, aside from documenting exposure, the thallium concentration in urine cannot be used to predict clinical effects or outcome.

Cessation of exposure and general supportive measures are the primary therapeutic modalities for acute intoxication. Most signs of toxicity resolve with cessation of exposure, but effects on the nervous system may be permanent. Attempts at specific treatment of acute thallium poisoning are aimed at displacing thallium from tissues and increasing excretion. Although there may be increased excretion of the metal, no therapeutic approach has demonstrated significant or unequivocal improvement in clinical outcome, and some approaches are associated with clinical deterioration, at least initially (e.g., potassium supplementation). Potassium supplements may displace thallium from its intracellular compartment and may also enhance the renal excretion of thallium by competing with it for resorption at the distal tubule. Potassium ferricyano-ferrate II, or Prussian Blue, is another potential therapy for thallium poisoning. This dye is given because thallium is concentrated in stomach acid and bile, and the alkaline pH of the small intestine allows the metal to be exchanged for potassium in Prussian Blue, which may facilitate fecal excretion of thallium and end its enterohepatic circulation. Chelation with a variety of agents is another possible approach. Peritoneal and hemodialysis are of limited usefulness because thallium is primarily an intracellular toxin.[42]

Prevention

Thallium is no longer applied as a medicinal agent, and its use as a rodenticide has been banned in most countries. Care must be exercised to prevent thallium from entering the human food chain, either from inadvertent human consumption of thallium-treated grain or vegetable products, or environmental contamination of farm areas with thallium, as occurred near the German cement plant noted above. Because of its extreme toxicity, workers with potential exposure should be educated about its effects, and industrial exposure prevented by appropriate work practices and engineering controls. Measurement of thallium in urine is helpful to assess whether occupational exposure has occurred.

VANADIUM
Exposure

Vanadium usually is recovered as a byproduct of mining of other metals, such as uranium, iron, copper, zinc, and lead. The largest fraction of vanadium use is for various alloys of iron, molybdenum, bronze, brass, and aluminum. Smaller amounts are employed in chemical processes as catalysts (ammonium vanadate and vanadium pentoxide), in ceramics, dyeing processes, inks, insecticides, photographic developer, color phosphors for television, and glass production. Most foods contain minute amounts of vanadium. Vanadium may be an essential trace element, although a deficiency state is not recognized.[44] It is known to have insulin-mimetic properties in humans and other mammals.

Inhalation of vanadium dust or fume, particularly the pentoxide, is the most common route of industrial exposure. Vanadium is poorly absorbed from the gastrointestinal tract or transcutaneously. It can cause a local irritant or hypersensitivity reaction when in contact with skin, mucous membranes, or upper respiratory tract. Industrial exposure (inhalation) can occur whenever there is release of vanadium dust or fume, such as mining, milling, and refining, although such exposures are usually minor.[45]

Shellfish have a relatively high content of vanadium, which explains why it is a trace constituent of crude oil and coal. The concentrations in crude petroleum vary considerably, from 0.1 ppm (certain domestic crudes) up to 1400 ppm (crude from western Venezuela).[46] Combustion results in deposition of vanadium in bottom ash (as high as 15.3%) and crusted deposits, or clinker, on the inside of boilers (up to 35%).[47] Numerous reports have documented vanadium dust and fume exposure (in the form of pentoxide) among workers involved in cleaning and refurbishing of oil- and coal-fired boilers.[48]

Clinical effects

The most significant pattern of illness observed among workers exposed to vanadium dust is that of irritation of the upper respiratory tract. Depending on the concentration in air, workers can begin to experience symptoms within hours of onset of exposure, including: cough; wheezing; irritation of the eyes, nose, and throat; hemorrhagic bronchitis; and, rarely, chemical pneumonitis. Pulmonary function tests have been variable among symptomatic subjects, but have included reductions in forced vital capacity (FVC), forced expiratory volume in one second (FEV_1), peak expiratory flow, and mean mid-expiratory flow (FEF_{25-75}). Symptoms and decrements in pulmonary function usually resolve within one or two weeks following cessation of exposure, although bronchial hyper-responsiveness may persist for several months.[49]

The potential for rapid onset of symptoms with a first exposure suggests that the mechanism is irritant and not immunologic, although some reports have noted an apparent increase in sensitivity on subsequent exposures, which would suggest the possibility of an immunologic response, as would high levels of IgE documented in some individuals with bronchial hyper-responsiveness following vanadium exposure.[49]

Vanadium skin rashes are usually of an irritant nature. However, positive patch tests have been noted in some cases. With particularly heavy exposure a green discoloration of the tongue has been described, which is due to oral deposition of inhaled vanadium dust, and is not a sign of systemic toxicity. There is no evidence to suggest that chronic pulmonary dysfunction or emphysema results from vanadium exposure. In addition, vanadium has not been implicated as a human carcinogen.

Diagnosis, evaluation, and treatment

There is no specific treatment for vanadium-induced illness. Symptomatic individuals should be removed from exposure, and therapy is supportive.

Biologic monitoring of vanadium in urine and blood are possible approaches to documenting recent exposure. The concentration of vanadium in whole blood is normally below 0.1 microgram per deciliter, and less than 1.0 microgram per gram of creatinine in urine. The half-life in urine is 20–40 hours following cessation of exposure. Although documentation of exposure is feasible, it has been difficult to correlate vanadium levels in air with urinary excretion.[50]

Prevention

Industrial operations that have the potential for creating vanadium dust or fumes should employ appropriate engineering controls, such as wet drilling in mining operations. Persons involved in cleaning or refurbishing of coal- or oil-fired furnaces, particularly boilermakers and others who might work inside the firebox, should use appropriate respiratory protection. The occurrence of a case of vanadium-related pulmonary disease mandates an investigation and implementation of control measures. At present there is insufficient evidence to justify routine biologic monitoring of workers potentially exposed to vanadium.

ZINC
Exposure

Zinc is ubiquitous in the environment. It is a trace component of many foods and an essential nutrient. It is also one of the oldest metals used by humans. Despite its long history of use, its most prevalent industrial toxicity, metal fume fever, was not described until the early part of the 19th century. Zinc exposure can occur in a variety of industries. However, it is the inhalation of freshly formed zinc oxide fume that is of primary concern. Such exposure occurs in processes where volatilization of zinc is possible (e.g., welding on galvanized materials, in brass foundries, etc.).[51]

Zinc vaporizes at 907 degrees C. The vapor reacts with ambient oxygen to form zinc oxide, which then precipitates to form a fume. Particle size is critical, and the freshly formed particles of zinc oxide are respirable, typically in the range of 0.2–1.0 microns. With passage of time, the small particles may flocculate, resulting in larger particles that deposit in upper airways when inhaled, thus making them less hazardous. Transcutaneous absorption of zinc oxide is insignificant, and oral toxicity is minimal.

Other salts of zinc, particularly zinc chloride, are irritating to skin and mucous membranes. Zinc chloride is used in smoke generators and in certain soldering fluxes, and can therefore become volatilized.[51]

Zinc-bearing ores usually contain at least trace amounts of arsenic, cadmium, and other potentially toxic metals. Processes that result in volatilization of zinc can therefore also cause exposure to these other metals. The toxicities of these other metals can be overlapping, as in the acute effects of cadmium on the lungs (i.e., metal fume fever and chemical pneumonitis), or distinct (e.g., release of arsenic and hydrogen with formation of arsine gas during the process of acid-stripping and galvanizing of steel products).

Clinical effects

Acute

Metal fume fever (MFF) has appeared under a variety of titles including brass founder's ague, brass chills, zinc fever or chills, spelter's shakes, glavo, metal shakes, brazier's disease, foundry fever, and 'the smothers'. Almost all cases have been reported in association with processes that include vaporization of zinc; a few have been reported in association with grinding, buffing, or sanding of zinc-coated surfaces. Tolerance may be a factor in the development of this condition, as reflected in the additional eponym 'Monday morning fever'; an absence from exposure may increase one's susceptibility. Seasonal variation, with increased incidence during winter, has been reported, although this probably reflects greater exposure resulting from reduced natural ventilation during colder months.

The clinical syndrome of MFF is well described. Usually within 2–10 hours following inhalational exposure to zinc oxide fume, workers begin to experience dryness and soreness in the throat with cough, followed by fever (sometimes over 103 degrees F), chills, malaise, hoarseness, chest tightness, and myalgias. There can also be profuse sweating, rigors, thirst, nausea, vomiting, and a metallic taste in the mouth. Findings are quite variable, depending on the severity of the episode. Rales and/or wheezes may be present during the acute phase. Laboratory test results are also variable, and can include: elevation of the white blood count (reported over 30,000/mm³ in some cases) with left shift; impairment of pulmonary function (decreased FVC, FEV_1, and diffusion capacity); scattered infiltrates on chest radiographs; and mild hypoxemia on blood gas analysis.[52]

There is evidence that MFF results when respirable particles of zinc oxide elicit an inflammatory response in the lungs. Bronchoalveolar lavage performed 20 hours after volunteers were exposed to zinc oxide fume or air demonstrated increased levels of polymorphonuclear leukocytes and inflammatory mediators (such as tumor necrosis factor-α and interleukin-8) in the lavage supernatant after exposure to zinc oxide compared to air.[53]

Zinc chloride is also a direct irritant of mucous membranes, and exposure can result in the usual constellation of clinical effects of the eyes, nose, and throat. Because of its marked hygroscopicity, zinc chloride can cause direct irritation to exposed skin. Inhalation of zinc chloride fume is a cause of occupational asthma.[54] Massive inhalational exposure has resulted in chemical burns of bronchial mucosa, chemical pneumonitis, and adult respiratory distress syndrome, which may occur weeks after exposure and may be fatal.[55]

Diagnosis, evaluation, and treatment

Diagnosis of MFF depends primarily on the symptoms, and the clinical and occupational histories. Zinc levels in blood and urine are not correlated with disease severity and therefore are not useful.[51] The differential diagnosis typically includes flu, acute bronchitis, bacterial pneumonia, or hypersensitivity pneumonitis. Distinction of MFF due to zinc oxide exposure from MFF related to exposure to other metals that can cause MFF is not possible clinically, although the presence of additional toxic effects related to other metals should be sought as these may require specific therapies. The syndrome usually resolves completely within 24–48 hours. Chronic consequences are not well documented. Treatment is supportive, including fluids, and use of antipyretics/analgesics.

Common 'folk remedies' for MFF employed by workers include drinking warm milk to treat the acute illness and to prevent illness. Drinking of peppermint oil derivatives has also been reported. These treatments have no documented value, but they are also not believed to be harmful.

Prevention

As with many conditions, the key to prevention is to avoid exposure. Employer and worker awareness of the presence of a potential hazard is critical. Engineering controls should be employed to prevent inhalation of zinc oxide fume or to reduce exposure to acceptable levels. These measures can be supplemented with personal respiratory protection where needed.

References

1. Cohen SR. A review of the health hazards from copper exposure. J Occup Med 1974; 16:621–4.
2. Barceloux DG. Copper. J Toxicol Clin Toxicol 1999; 37:217–30.
3. Armstrong CW, Moore LW Jr, Hackler RL, Miller GB Jr, Stroube RB. An outbreak of metal fume fever. Diagnostic use of urinary copper and zinc determinations. J Occup Med 1983; 25:886–8.
4. Borak J, Cohen, H, Hethmon TA. Copper exposure and metal fume fever: lack of evidence for a causal relationship. AIHAJ 2000; 61:832–6.
5. Villar TG. Vineyard sprayer's lung. Clinical aspects. Am Rev Respir Dis 1974; 110:545–55.
6. Lampe RM, Henderson AL, Hansen GH. Green hair. JAMA 1977; 237:2092.
7. Chuttani HK, Gupta PS, Gulati S, et al. Acute copper sulfate poisoning. Am J Med 1965; 39:849–54.
8. Agency for Toxic Substances and Disease Registry (ATSDR). Toxicological profile for manganese (update). Atlanta, GA: Agency for Toxic Substances and Disease Registry, US Department of Health and Human Services, Public Health Service, 2000.
9. Rodier J. Manganese poisoning in Moroccan miners. Br J Ind Med 1955; 12:21–35.
10. Emara AM, El-Ghawabi SH, Madkour OI. Chronic manganese poisoning in the dry battery industry. Br J Ind Med 1971; 28:78–82.
11. Wang JD, Huang CC, Hwang YH, Chiang JR, Lin JM, Chen JS. Manganese induced parkinsonism: an outbreak due to an unrepaired ventilation control system in a ferromanganese smelter. Br J Ind Med 1989; 46:856–9.
12. Ferraz HB, Bertolucci PH, Pereira JS, Lima JG, Andrade LA. Chronic exposure to the fungicide maneb may produce symptoms and signs of CNS manganese intoxication. Neurology 1988; 38:550–3.
13. Fell JM, Reynolds AP, Meadows N, et al. Manganese toxicity in children receiving long-term parenteral nutrition. Lancet 1996; 347(9010):1218–21.
14. Nagatomo S, Umehara F, Hanada K, et al. Manganese intoxication during total parenteral nutrition: report of two cases and review of the literature. J Neurol Sci 1999;162:102–5.
15. Ono J, Harada K, Kodaka R, et al. Manganese deposition in the brain during long-term total parenteral nutrition. Jpn J Parenteral Enteral Nutr 1995; 19:310–2.
16. Spahr L, Butterworth RF, Fontaine S, et al. Increased blood manganese in cirrhotic patients: relationship to pallidal magnetic resonance signal hyperintensity and neurological symptoms. Hepatology 1996; 24:1116–20.
17. Frumkin H, Solomon G. Manganese in the US gasoline supply. Am J Ind Med 1997; 31:107–15.
18. Lynam DR, Roos JW, Pfeifer GD, Fort BF, Pullin TG. Environmental effects and exposures to manganese from use of methycyclopentadienyl manganese tricarbonyl (MMT) in gasoline. Neurotoxicology 1999; 20:145–50.
19. Lyznicki JM, Karlan MS, Khan MK. Manganese in gasoline. Council on scientific affairs, American Medical Association. J Occup Environ Med 1999; 41:140–3.
20. Lloyd Davies TA. Manganese pneumonitis. Br J Ind Med 1946; 3:111–35.
21. Hobbesland A, Kjuus H, Thelle DS. Mortality from nonmalignant respiratory diseases among male workers in Norwegian ferroalloy plants. Scand J Work Environ Health 1997; 23:342–50.
22. Couper J. On the effects of black oxide of manganese when inhaled into the lungs. Br Ann Med Pharm 1837; 1:41–2.
23. Iregren A. Psychological test performance in foundry workers exposed to low levels of manganese. Neurotoxicol Teratol 1990; 12:673–5.
24. Lucchini R, Selis L, Folli D, et al. Neurobehavioral effects of manganese in workers from a ferroalloy plant after temporary cessation of exposure. Scand J Work Environ Health 1995; 21:143–9.

25. Mergler D, Huel G, Bowler R, et al. Nervous system dysfunction among workers with long-term exposure to manganese. Environ Res 1994; 64:151–80.

26. Roels H, Lauwerys R, Buchet JP, et al. Epidemiological survey among workers exposed to manganese: effects on lung, central nervous system and some biologic indices. Am J Ind Med 1987; 11:307–27.

27. Roels HA, Ghyselen P, Buchet JP, Ceulemans E, Lauwerys RR. Assessment of the permissible exposure level to manganese in workers exposed to manganese dioxide dust. Br J Ind Med 1992; 49:25–34.

28. American Conference of Governmental Industrial Hygienists. Documentation of threshold limit values, 6th edn. Cincinnati, OH: ACGIH, 1996.

29. Huang CC, Chu NS, Lu CS, Chen RS, Calne DB. Long-term progression in chronic manganism: ten years of follow-up. Neurology 1998; 50:698–700.

30. Crump KS, Rousseau P. Results from eleven years of neurological health surveillance at a manganese oxide and salt producing plant. Neurotoxicology 1999; 20:273–86.

31. Roels HA, Ortega Eslava MI, Ceulemans E, Robert A, Lison D. Prospective study on the reversibility of neurobehavioral effects in workers exposed to manganese dioxide. Neurotoxicology 1999; 20:255–71.

32. Calne DB, Chu NS, Huang CC, Lu CS, Olanow W. Manganism and idiopathic parkinsonism: similarities and differences. Neurology 1994; 44:1583–6.

33. Lu CS, Huang CC, Chu NS, Calne DB. Levodopa failure in chronic manganism. Neurology 1994; 44:1600–2.

34. Wolters EC, Huang CC, Clark C, et al. Positron emission tomography in manganese intoxication. Ann Neurol 1989; 26:647–51.

35. Barbeau A. Manganese and extrapyramidal disorders (a critical review and tribute to Dr George C. Cotzias). Neurotoxicology 1984; 5:13.

36. Mena I, Court J, Fuenzalida S, et al. Modification of chronic manganese poisoning treatment with L-DOPA or 5-OH tryptophane. N Engl J Med 1970; 282:5–10.

37. Bank WJ, Pleasure DE, Suzuki K, Nigro M, Katz R. Thallium poisoning. Arch Neurol 1972; 26:456–64.

38. Munch JC. Human thallotoxicosis. JAMA 1934; 102:1929–34.

39. Agency for Toxic Substances and Disease Registry. Toxicological profile for thallium. Atlanta, GA: Agency for Toxic Substances and Disease Registry, US Department of Health and Human Services, Public Health Service, 1992.

40. Dolgner R, Brockhaus A, Ewers U, Wiegand H, Majewski F, Soddemann H. Repeated surveillance of exposure to thallium in a population living in the vicinity of a cement plant emitting dust containing thallium. Int Arch Occup Environ Health 1983; 52:79–94.

41. Galvan-Arzate S, Santamaria A. Thallium toxicity. Toxicol Lett 1998; 99:1–13.

42. Innis R, Moses H. Thallium poisoning. Johns Hopkins Med J 1978; 142:27–31.

43. Richeson EM. Industrial thallium intoxication. Ind Med Surg 1958; 27:607–19.

44. Barceloux DG. Vanadium. J Toxicol Clin Toxicol 1999; 37:265–78.

45. Vintinner FJ, Vallenas R, Carlin CE, Weiss R, Macher C, Ochoa R. Study of the health of workers employed in mining and processing of vanadium ore. AMA Arch Ind Health 1955; 12:635–42.

46. US Dept of Health and Human Services. Toxicological profile for vanadium. Atlanta, GA: US Department of Health and Human Services, Public Health Service, 1992.

47. Lees REM. Changes in lung function after exposure to vanadium compounds in fuel oil ash. Br J Ind Med 1980; 37:253–6.

48. Levy BS, Hoffman L, Gottsegen S. Boilermakers' bronchitis. Respiratory tract irritation associated with vanadium pentoxide exposure during oil-to-coal conversion of a power plant. J Occup Med 1984; 26:567–70.

49. Irsigler GB, Visser PJ, Spangenberg PAL. Asthma and chemical bronchitis in vanadium plant workers. Am J Ind Med 1999; 35:366–74.

50. Kawai T, Seiji K, Wantanabe T, Nakatsuka H, Ikeda M. Urinary vanadium as a biologic indicator of exposure to vanadium. Int Arch Occup Environ Health 1989; 61:283–7.

51. Agency for Toxic Substances and Disease Registry. Toxicological profile for zinc (update). Atlanta, GA: Agency for Toxic Substances and Disease Registry, US Department of Health and Human Services, Public Health Service, 1994.

52. Gordon T, Fine JM. Metal fume fever. Occup Med 1993; 8:505–17.

53. Kuschner WG, D'Alessandro A, Wintermeyer SF, Wong H, Boushey HA, Blanc PD. Pulmonary responses to purified zinc oxide fume. J Invest Med 1995; 43:371–8.

54. Weir DC, Robertson AS, Jones S, Burge PS. Occupational asthma due to soft corrosive soldering fluxes containing zinc chloride and ammonium chloride. Thorax 1989; 44:220–3.

55. Hjortso E, Qvist J, Bud MI, et al. ARDS after accidental inhalation of zinc chloride smoke. Intensive Care Med 1988; 14:17–24.

Chapter 40
Organic Solvents and Related Compounds

Ingvar Lundberg, Christer Hogstedt, Carola Lidén, Gun Nise

Organic solvents constitute a chemically diverse group of liquids characterized by their ability to dissolve oils, fats, resins, rubber, and plastics. Organic chemistry emerged in the early 1800s, and expanded during the second half of that century, with the development of large-scale distillation of coal tar. It thus became possible to obtain specific hydrocarbon compounds such as the aromatic solvents, with a wide variety of applications in the chemical industry. Later, coal tar was largely substituted by petroleum as the raw material for production of these solvents, including aliphatic hydrocarbons, alcohols, and petroleum distillates such as naphtha or white spirit.

Chlorine is a byproduct in the alkali industry, and the commercial exploitation of this byproduct for the chlorination of the aliphatic hydrocarbons led to the introduction of the chlorinated solvents during the 1920s. Reports on the toxicity of these solvents to exposed workers appeared soon after their introduction on to the market.

CHEMICAL STRUCTURE, USE AND EXPOSURE

Solvents may be divided into a number of categories based on their chemical structures. These categories are described in Tables 40.1 and 40.2, together with some physicochemical properties and the main areas of use of common solvents.

The National Institute for Occupational Safety and Health estimated that 9.8 million workers were exposed to solvents in the United States in the first half of the 1970s. In the 1980s, around 400,000 workers in Denmark, or approximately 15% of the Danish labor force, were estimated to be occupationally exposed to solvents on a daily basis. In 1984 over 49 million tons of organic solvents were produced in the United States. Thus, exposure to organic solvents is common and constitutes one of the most important occupational chemical hazards. However, in the industrialized world the exposure level has decreased in many occupations during recent decades. In Sweden only about 6% of the workforce report solvent exposure during at least one-quarter of the work shift in the early 1990s. Table 40.3 lists several occupations that continue to involve significant solvent exposure.

ENVIRONMENTAL MEASUREMENTS

Measurements of solvent vapor concentrations are performed for different reasons, e.g., to compare workers' exposure with hygienic standards, to control the effect of different interventions, to evaluate the exposure levels associated with complaints, or to assess exposure in cross-sectional or retrospective studies.

The exposure measurements are performed in different ways, depending on the aim of the investigation. When a possible adverse effect from solvent exposure is studied, the concentration of the solvent itself or its metabolites in the target organ is of interest. This concentration depends not only on the air concentration, but also on the skin uptake, workload, and other factors. However, on most occasions, the solvent dose to the relevant tissue cannot be obtained, and only the air concentration in the breathing zone can be measured. The measurements have to be planned and performed in cooperation with an experienced industrial hygienist to ensure reliable and representative results. Use of biologic sampling, including measurement in blood and metabolites in urine, is available for some solvents (see Biologic monitoring).

Sampling methods

When the individual worker's exposure is measured, a portable sampling device is used. A small battery-operated membrane pump, which draws the air through a small glass tube packed with some adsorbent, is commonly used. Activated charcoal, a coconut-based carbon, is the most common adsorbent for solvent sampling. This adsorbent can be used for the collection of the most commonly used solvents. However, methanol and ethanol cannot be sampled on activated charcoal, as desorption may result in underestimation of the exposure.

Modified polystyrene polymers, including XAD, Tenax, Chromosorb, and Porapak, are adsorbents with a lower capacity. They are primarily used to sample high molecular weight non-volatile solvents. Most adsorption tubes consist of two separate sections, one for sampling and one for backup. If solvents are found in the backup section during analysis, the sample has been overloaded and will not give a reliable result.

Progress in vapor sampling has been achieved by the use of continuously collecting passive monitors. The exposed worker carries a small badge with an adsorbent. No sampling pump is needed because the sampling is controlled by diffusion. According to Fick's first law of diffusion, the mass uptake is a direct function of the badge sampling rate, the ambient concentration, and the sampling time. The manufacturers distribute lists of sampling rates for various solvents. The adsorbent used in the passive monitors is usually activated charcoal. The sampling area of most

Chemical class of hydrocarbon	Solvent	Boiling point at 101.3 kPa (°C)	Vapor pressure at 25°C (kPa)	Flash point (°C)	Water solubility (weight %)	Partition coefficients			Odor threshold (ppm)
						w/a	b/a	o/a	
Aliphatic	n-Hexane	156	16	<-20	<0.1	-	-	-	-
Aromatic	Benzene	80	10	-11	<0.1	3	8	490	-
	Toluene	111	2.9	4	<0.1	2	16	1470	0.03–3
	Xylenes	138–144	0.6–1.1	23–30	<0.1	2	42	4050	20–40
	Styrene	146	0.6	32	0.3	5	40	5000	0.05–25
Halogenated	Methylene chloride	40	45	none	2	7	9	150	50–80
	Chloroform	61	21	none	0.7	4	10	400	200
	Carbon tetrachloride	77	12	none	<0.1	0	2	360	25–50
	Trichloroethylene	87	8	none	0.1	1.5	9	700	20–100
	Tetrachloroethylene	121	1.9	none	<0.1	0	13	1900	50–70
	Methyl chloroform	74	13	none	<0.1	1	2	350	75–100
Esters	Ethylacetate	77	10	-4	9	-	-	-	50–200
Ketones	Acetone	56	25	-19	100	400	250	90	200–450
	Methyl ethyl ketone	80	9	-7	27	250	200	260	<25
	Methyl-n-butyl ketone	127	0.4	23	-	110	130	1640	-
	Methyl-iso-butyl ketone	117	0.7	14	2	80	90	930	<100
Alcohols	Methanol	64	13	11	100	-	-	-	400–2000
	Ethanol	78	6	12	100	-	-	-	350
	Iso-propanol	82	4	12	100	-	-	-	200
	n-Butanol	118	0.6	29	8	-	-	-	15–25
Glycol ethers	Ethylene glycol	197	<0.01	111	100	-	-	-	-
	2-Ethoxyethanol	135	0.5	40	100	-	-	-	-
	2-Ethoxyethyl acetate	156	0.2	49	23	-	-	-	-
Misc.	Carbon disulfide	46	40	-30	0.3	1	2	-	1
	Dimethylformamide	153	0.4	58	100	-	-	-	-
	Tetrahydrofuran	65	19	-14	100	-	-	-	-
	Limonene	178	0.3	45	0.5	2	42	5700	30
	Ethylene oxide	10	-	<-18	infinite	-	-	-	260
Petroleum distillates	Naphthas	27–221	-	-	-	-	-	-	-
	White spirit	150–200	<0.7	35–40	-	<0.1	-	-	variable

- Data not found or not applicable; w, water; a, air; b, blood; o, oil.
Data from: Fiserova-Bergerova V. Gases and their solubility: a review of fundamentals. In: Fiserova-Bergerova V, ed. Modeling of inhalation exposure to vapors: uptake, distribution, and elimination, Vol II. Boca Raton: CRC Press, 1983;3-28;[38] Sato A, Nakajima T. Partition coefficients of some aromatic hydrocarbons and ketones in water, blood and oil. Br J Ind Med 1979; 36:213-34;[39] Shmunes E. Solvents and plasticizers. In: Adams R, ed. Occupational skin disease. 2nd edn. Philadelphia: W.B. Saunders Company, 1990.[40]

Table 40.1 Physicochemical properties, partition coefficients and odor thresholds of commonly used solvents

Solvent (World production in metric tons 10^3 1996)	Main uses
n-Hexane	Component in gasoline and solvent in production of plastic and rubber, in printing of laminated products, in extraction of vegetable oil (use of the pure solvent has diminished because of toxicity).
Benzene (20,124)	In chemical syntheses (of nitrobenzenes, halogenated derivatives, aromatic amines, styrene, phenols and others). In unleaded gasoline for antiknock properties. Solvent for paints, inks, rubber, plastics (although uncommon in industrialized countries because of toxicity).
Toluene (7881)	In the production of benzene and toluene diisocyanate and solvent in paints, coatings, inks, adhesives, and in the leather and pharmaceutical industries. In gasoline to improve octane rating.
Xylenes (12,802)	Solvent in paints, lacquers, and varnishes; in rubber manufacturing; in plastics and leather industries; in the manufacture of insecticides and pharmaceuticals. In gasoline to improve octane rating.
Styrene (15,415)	Solvent in polyester resins, particularly in the manufacturing of glass Fiber-reinforced plastics.
Methylene chloride	Aerosol propellant, paint stripper, degreasing. Solvent for oils, fats, bitumen. Extraction at low temperatures, such as decaffeination of coffee. Manufacturing of photographic films.
Chloroform	Production of fluorocarbons (use limited because of toxicity).
Carbon tetrachloride	Production of fluorocarbons and solvent in rubber and chemical industries (use limited because of toxicity).
Trichloroethylene (113)	Vapor degreasing and cleaning of metallic and electronic parts.
Tetrachloroethylene	Dry cleaning and vapor degreasing.
Methyl chloroform	In vapor degreasing and cleaning of metallic parts and solvent in printing trades, in office machinery, in electrical industries, insecticides. Extractant for oils, fats, and resins. As an aerosol propellant.
Ethyl acetate	Solvent in paints, varnishes, lacquers, inks, and synthetic rubbers. Used in the manufacturing of photographic films, linoleum, plastic wood, artificial silk, and leather. In the cleaning of textiles.
Acetone (2104)	Solvent for resins, fats, lacquers, oils, cotton, cellulose acetate, acetylene. Employed in paint, varnish, lacquer, rubber, plastics, and chemical manufacturing industries.
Methyl ethyl ketone	Solvent in manufacturing of paints, varnishes, and lacquers; in the electronics industry; and in the manufacturing of synthetic resins.
Methyl-n-butyl ketone	In glues and cleaning fluids (current use is limited because of toxicity).
Methyl-isobutyl ketone	Solvent in paints, varnishes, and lacquers.
Methanol (13,438)	In production of formaldehyde. Used in shellac, lacquers, and other surface coatings. Used as a cleaner for surface coatings, metal, and resins. Solvent in rubber industry, for rotogravure inks, and duplicator fluids. Extractant in chemical processes. Intermediate in syntheses of methylated chemicals. Denaturant in ethanol.
Ethanol	Solvent in paints, varnishes, and lacquers and in the manufacture of plastics, drugs, plasticizers, and cosmetics. Used in chemical synthesis of acetaldehyde, ethyl ether, chloroethane, butadiene, and others.
Iso-propanol	Solvent for oils, gums, and resins. Deicing agent for liquid fuels, defogging, and antifreeze products. Used in the manufacture of many cleaning and degreasing agents, including packet products for antiseptic wiping. It is used in several chemical syntheses and as an extractant.
n-Butanol (3000)	Solvent in paints and lacquers and for synthetic and natural polymers. Used for extraction and dehydration
Butanols (2494)	in the pharmaceutical industry.
Ethylene glycol (5075)	Used as a deicer and as an antifreeze formulation in heating and cooling systems. As a solvent in lacquers, inks, adhesives, and resins.
2-Ethoxyethanol	Solvent in paints, lacquers, car painting, and silk screen printing.
2-Ethoxyethyl acetate	Solvent in paints, lacquers, car painting, and silk screen printing.
Carbon disulfide (205)	Used in the production of rayon fibers. Used in the manufacture of optical glass and in semiconductors.
Dimethylformamide (100)	Solvent for vinyl-based polymers in the manufacture of films, fibers, and coatings; for making polyurethane lacquers for clothing and accessories made of synthetic leather; and for fibers and films based on polyacrylonitrile.
Tetrahydrofuran	Solvent in glues, paints, varnishes, inks, and wetting and dispersing agents in textile processing.
Limonene	Degreasing operations.
Ethylene oxide (4830)	Intermediate in production of various chemicals, for example 1,2-ethane and glycol ethers. Antimicrobial sterilant.
Naphthas (143,757)	Solvents in paints, lacquers, varnishes, agrochemicals, industrial cleaning, and others.
White spirit (3495)	Solvent in paints, lacquers, varnishes, agrochemicals, and industrial cleaning.

Data from 1996 Industrial Commodity Statistics Yearbook, Productions Statistics (1987–1996). Department of Economic and Social Affairs, Statistics Division, United Nations, New York 1998

Table 40.2 Common solvents and their main uses

passive monitors is large compared with that of the tubes, explaining why the risk of contamination through splashing has to be considered. Furthermore, knowledge of the influence on each solvent's sampling rate from different solvents in a mixed exposure is still limited, and should be considered when mixed solvents are present.

Direct-reading instruments, usually portable, which continuously take samples from the air, may be used to follow changes in the solvent concentration during different work operations. The detectors in such portable instruments are often of an infrared or photoionization type. The solvent concentration might be recorded on a printer or collected into a data logger for later evaluation. The calibration of these instruments is important, and this procedure is rather complicated for many instruments. When a solvent mixture (like painter's naphtha) is measured, the instrument must be calibrated with the mixture used in the process, otherwise, there is a risk of under- or overestimating exposure. Some direct-reading instruments are also sensitive to changes in temperature and humidity.

The indicator tube, a glass tube filled with chemical material that changes color on contact with the sampled solvent, is the simplest direct-reading sampling device. The solvent air concentration is obtained by comparing the

Painting with solvent-based paints, particularly spray painting and painting large areas (mixed solvents)

Paint manufacturing, particularly manual cleaning of equipment with solvents (mixed solvents)

Production of glass fiber-reinforced polyester plastics, particularly lamination of large areas as in the production of boats (styrene)

Floor laying (mixed solvents)

Rotogravure printing and screen printing (toluene, mixed solvents)

Metal degreasing (commonly 1,1,1-trichloroethane)

Dry cleaning (commonly perchloroethylene)

Table 40.3 Occupations that may involve heavy solvent exposure

colors produced to a set of standard colors or by measuring the length of the stain produced. Grab samples with indicator tubes describe the conditions at the moment of sampling, and give a rough estimate of the exposure level. However, the results can be misleading due to the effects of variable factors, such as temperature and humidity, inexperience in interpreting the results, and lack of specificity of detection methods.

Sampling strategy

When measurements are performed to compare the solvent exposure level with hygienic standards, a personal sampling device should be used, e.g., a portable pump with adsorption tube or a passive monitor. Air from the worker's breathing zone is monitored during the whole shift, usually 8 hours. It is important that cleaning operations are included in the sampling time because such work often involves heavy exposures. The shift may be covered by only one sample, but it is advisable to divide it into at least two sampling periods. If there is a great variation in the exposure, several continuous samples during the shift will give more information about the conditions, which is valuable for determining intervention approaches.

The direct-reading instruments are often small enough to be used for personal monitoring. Such instruments are also suitable to investigate vapor leakage from different operations and the distribution of the solvents in the workplace from the emitting area. Furthermore, they give an immediate picture of the air concentration; alternatively, the adsorption tubes and the passive monitors have to be sent to a laboratory for analysis. However, used together with personal sampling devices, a good picture of both the time-weighted average exposure and the variation of the air level is obtained. Such information is of importance when efforts are made to lower the worker's exposure.

The distribution of solvent vapors might be visualized by sampling with a direct-reading instrument at several locations in the working area within a short period, so-called map sampling. Such a map is valuable during the discussion of the most suitable interventions. In addition, a direct-reading instrument together with a video camera provides educational information on the exposure levels associated with different working habits.[1]

Grab samples randomly monitored during the shift will depict the variation of the exposure level. The geometric mean of these samples will roughly illustrate the average exposure level during the shift. The larger the variation in exposure, the more grab samples are needed.

All measurements have to be well documented. The report should contain information on the reason for sampling, the sampling method, the sampling periods, and the production conditions. The reader of a measurement report needs such information to interpret the results correctly. When retrospective exposure assessment is performed for epidemiologic studies of health effects from long-term solvent exposure, well-documented measurement reports are of particular importance. A further discussion of sampling principles is provided on Chapter 4.2.

DECREASING EXPOSURE LEVELS IN INDUSTRY

The preventive measures taken against solvent-related health hazards are manifest in the lists of hygienic standards that are published in most industrialized countries. During the last 20 years there has been a substantial reduction of regulatory standard levels in most countries. In some countries, such as those in Scandinavia, the hygienic standard level reductions have been more pronounced than those of the American Conference of Governmental Industrial Hygienists (ACGIH).

Among the common solvents, the reduction of standard levels is substantial for methylene chloride. The finding that this solvent was metabolized to carbon monoxide caused a dramatic reduction between 1970 and 1980. The potential carcinogenicity of the compound, as shown in animal experiments, led to a further reduction (in 1990) to less than one-fifth of the 1970 standards. The low standard for benzene in most countries is related to its hematotoxicity and carcinogenicity. The reproductive effects of 2-methoxyethanol have led to a substantially decreased exposure limit. For most other solvents, the hygienic standards are commonly based on neurotoxic and irritant effects, and the differences between those of the Scandinavian countries and those of the ACGIH probably reflect different assessments of the importance of such effects.

It is likely that improved standards have resulted in a reduction in the number of heavily exposed workers in the industrial branches of larger operations. This is particularly true in the case of automation, which reduces the number of workers and moves the remaining workers away from the production process. The decrease of toluene exposure among rotogravure printers in Sweden is shown in Figure 40.1. However, in small and medium sized enterprises the exposure level may still be high or even increase due to lack of knowledge and resources.

REDUCING EXPOSURE BY DIMINISHING SOLVENT CONTENT IN PAINTS

In trades involving end-use of solvents (e.g., painters), the possibilities of reducing the exposure by closed systems

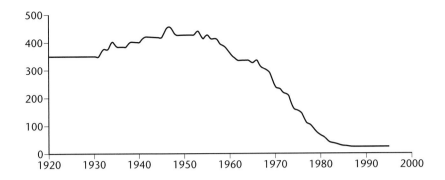

Figure 40.1: The decrease of the average toluene exposure level in rotogravure printing. During the period 1948–1985 five factories are included in the estimation (further development of data presented in Svensson et al[37]).

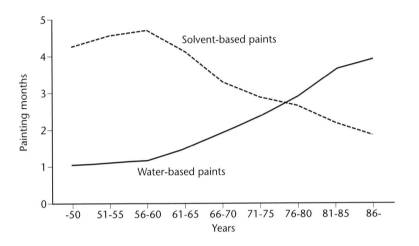

Figure 40.2: The time spent painting with solvent-based and water-based paints among Swedish house painters.

and exhaust ventilation are much smaller than in industry. In fact, among painters, efforts to reduce exposure to solvents have followed another route, namely, reducing the solvent content in paints by replacing the solvent-soluble binders with water-soluble alternatives. This tendency is obvious in all industrialized countries, although the pace of substitution may vary. The use of solvent-based paints and water-based paints among Swedish house painters can be seen in Figure 40.2. The replacement of solvent-based paints has continued and in 1995 as many as 97% of the paints used indoors were water based.

PHARMACOKINETICS
Uptake and distribution

Uptake through the lungs
During occupational exposure, solvents may be taken up through the lungs or through the skin; uptake through the gastrointestinal tract is negligible. Generally, the lungs provide the most important absorption route. The most important determinant of pulmonary uptake is the solubility of the solvent in the blood. Even for solvents that are readily absorbed through the lungs, the uptake cannot exceed approximately 80%, with the remainder exhaled because of dead-space ventilation. The uptake at rest for methylene chloride, trichloroethylene, toluene, xylene, and styrene is between 50% and 70% of the amount inhaled.

Physical activity is the major important modifying factor on the toxicokinetics of organic solvents. The amount of

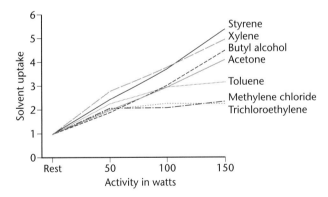

Figure 40.3 Solvent uptake at different workloads. (Data from Strand I. Effect of physical exercise on uptake, distribution, and elimination of vapors in man. In: Fiserova-Bergerova V, ed. Modeling of inhalation exposure to vapors: uptake, distribution, and elimination. Vol II. Boca Raton: CRC Press, 1983;107–30.)

solvent taken up per time unit increases during exercise. Figure 40.3 shows the uptake of some common solvents during rest and exercise. Male volunteers were exposed to different solvents during 30 minutes of rest followed by 30 minutes of exercise at 50 W (light work), 100 W (medium work load), and 150 W (heavy work), respectively. The solvents in the figure may be divided into two groups. Those in the first group, i.e., styrene, xylene, acetone, and butyl alcohol, are more soluble in the blood and tissues than the solvents in the second group, i.e., methylene chloride, trichloroethylene, and toluene. This is shown by the fact that, in the first group, there was a linear increase of solvent uptake with increasing workload that was caused by increasing ventilation. In the second group, the uptake increased at 50 W, but remained fairly constant when the workload was further increased, indicating that an equilibrium had been reached. Thus, it is important to determine the workload when considering the potential health effects of, particularly, the solvents in the first group.[2]

The amount of solvent taken up by a body tissue depends mainly on the solubility of the solvent in that tissue, but the blood flow through the tissue is also of importance. The change in adipose tissue blood flow during exercise increases uptake. Thus the toluene concentration in adipose tissue was ten times higher after light physical exercise compared to rest, although the respiratory uptake and the blood toluene only doubled.[3] The effects that most solvents have in common, i.e., on the nervous system and the skin, are to a large extent dependent on their lipophilicity. In experiments with human volunteers, the distribution of different organic solvents to the subcutaneous fat has been investigated. Obese subjects, compared with thin ones, retained more solvents. It was also observed that, on average, 5% of xylene, 8% of styrene, 9% of methylene chloride, and 17% of the total amount of toluene taken up by the body was retained in fat deposits. These figures are influenced not only by the fat solubility of the solvent, but also to a large extent by the degree of biotransformation of each solvent. The half-life of methylene chloride in fat tissue was around 8 hours, compared to 3–5 days for toluene, styrene and xylene.

In studies on occupationally exposed workers, it has been shown that the body fat accumulates a significant amount of some solvents, implying a residual continuous low-dose solvent exposure during work-free periods.

Uptake through the skin
Solvent compounds may be absorbed through the skin in considerable amounts, and may thus contribute to the total body burden. Skin absorption may occur in settings of single solvent compounds or to products containing solvent mixtures, such as cleansing and greasing agents, and in some cases to vapors.

The uptake of a solvent through the skin varies widely between different solvents. Factors of importance are water solubility, lipid solubility and volatility. Most readily absorbed are solvents that are easily soluble in water and in lipophilic compounds, i.e., having amphiphilic properties. Risk assessments of skin absorption of solvents have benefited from calculations of permeability coefficients, based on the logarithm of the partitioning coefficient between octanol and water (log $P_{o/w}$). Other factors influencing the rate of skin absorption of solvents are environmental factors such as humidity, temperature, air velocity, vehicle, occlusion and exposure time.

Skin exposures to glycolethers and dimethylformamide are hazardous as they contain a lipophilic and a hydrophilic portion. Skin absorption from vapors is also significant. The absorption of glycolethers is enhanced by

their relatively low volatility and high boiling point, which allows them to remain on the skin surface for long periods. For most common solvents, significant skin exposures are needed before the skin absorption reaches the level of lung uptake. For example, if both hands are kept in a xylene bath for 15 minutes, uptake will be equal to the respiratory uptake from air exposure to 100 ppm during the same period. This does not apply to dimethylformamide, for which the skin uptake may be substantially higher than the respiratory uptake during normal industrial working conditions.

Lists of hygienic standards often contain a special notation, skin, to mark whether a substance is efficiently absorbed through this route. The notations are, in general, based on limited data, and the absence of the notation should not be interpreted to mean that dermal exposure is negligible. The number of solvents with a skin notation has, in recent years, been much extended in the US and several European countries. Benzene, carbon disulfide, carbon tetrachloride, dimethylformamide, 2-ethoxyethanol, methanol, methylene chloride, methyl-n-butyl ketone, n-butanol, styrene, toluene and xylene are some of the solvents with a designation of significant skin absorption.

Biotransformation and elimination

Absorbed solvents are usually biotransformed to more water-soluble metabolites that may be excreted in the urine. The main site for metabolism is the liver. Up to 95% of the xylene and styrene absorbed, and up to 80% of the total amount of trichloroethylene and toluene absorbed, is biotransformed. However, some common solvents like methylchloroform and perchloroethylene are metabolized to a small extent and largely excreted unchanged by exhalation. Excretion of unchanged solvent by exhalation increases during physical activity. The exhalation of toluene, styrene and trichloroethylene were approximately doubled at light physical work compared with rest.[4]

Biotransformation has important implications in the evaluation of solvent toxicity and in the assessment of solvent exposure.[5] Solvents may be biotransformed into reactive metabolites that are more toxic than the mother compound. For example, the trichloromethyl radical obtained from carbon tetrachloride is responsible for the hepatotoxicity of this solvent. In fact, solvents that show acute, dose-related hepatotoxicity, such as chloroform and dimethylformamide, are often hepatotoxic through reactive metabolites. Similarly, the peripheral neurotoxicity of n-hexane and methyl-n-butyl ketone is caused by the metabolites of these solvents. Metabolites from other solvents, including the epoxides produced from trichloroethylene and styrene, may result in carcinogenic effects.

Non-toxic metabolites from other solvents may be used to estimate the dose of the solvent that has been absorbed (see section on biologic monitoring later in this chapter).

Biotransformation and individual susceptibility
The rates of oxidative metabolism vary substantially among different individuals, sometimes reflecting genetic poly-

morphisms, leading to potential differences in susceptibility to solvent effects. The metabolism of specific solvents may be altered through a variety of factors. Solvents have been shown to interact with each other; for example toluene and xylene seem to inhibit competitively the metabolic degradation of each other because they compete for the same enzymes for side-chain hydroxylation.[6] Toluene and xylene inhibit the biotransformation of benzene, thus protecting experimental animals from the hematotoxicity of benzene. Ingested ethyl alcohol inhibits the metabolic degradation of toluene and xylene, increasing blood levels and decreasing the rate of elimination from the blood of these solvents, thus enhancing central nervous system effects. Drugs (e.g., acetaminophen) and smoking may also decrease the elimination of toluene from the blood. Dietary factors may play a role, and a diet with a low carbohydrate intake probably enhances the metabolism of several solvents. Tobacco smoking enhances the metabolism of numerous organic solvents.

HEALTH EFFECTS

This section focuses on the effects common to all organic solvents or to large groups of solvents, namely, mucous membrane irritant effects, and effects on the skin and central nervous system. It also provides information on potential common effects involving other tissues. Specific effects on other tissues will be addressed in the following section.

We differentiate between short- and long-term exposures, denoting exposures of hours to days and months to years, respectively. We also distinguish among acute, subchronic, and chronic effects. Acute effects are readily reversible after the discontinuation of exposure. Subchronic effects are most often reversible within 6 months and always within 1 year. Chronic effects are not reversible, only partly reversible, or reversible after more than 1 year.

As a caveat, it should be noted that practically all studies on which our knowledge is based have been performed in developed countries. We cannot exclude the possibility that the effects may be different when undernourished workers with other diseases, particularly liver diseases, are exposed. All comments on safe levels for different solvents and various effects should be understood to have this limitation.

Irritant effects

Most solvents produce irritant effects on the mucous membranes of the eyes, nose, and throat. A burning sensation is induced from the stimulation of trigeminal afferent nerve endings of the eyes and nose; cough is produced from the stimulation of laryngeal nerve endings in the pharynx, hypopharynx, and laryngeal regions. However, all common solvents have weak irritant properties in comparison with intense irritants, such as toluene diisocyanate, acrolein or formaldehyde. The eyes are often sensitive. Heavy exposures are commonly associated with bronchitic symptoms of cough, as well as chest tightness, and a feeling of breathlessness. At very high exposures, a number of common solvents, such as toluene, xylene, and methylene chloride,

can induce pulmonary edema or chemical pneumonitis (see Chapter 19.6).

Different solvents have varying potentials to irritate mucous membranes. It is probable that irritation is mediated through an interaction between the solvent and receptor proteins located in the lipid bilayer of the cell membrane. Animal experiments and practical experience suggest that butanol, styrene, toluene, xylene and methyl ethyl ketone are irritating at comparatively low concentrations, while higher concentrations are needed for irritant effects from ethyl acetate, isopropanol, methanol, acetone, and ethanol.[7] The reason for the differences in potency between these solvents is unclear. It is a common experience that, when entering, for example, a paint factory, most visitors feel some irritation, particularly of the eyes. Mild irritant effects may occur at exposure levels below current hygienic standards; however, this irritation disappears within minutes. Adaptation to the irritant effects seems to occur for many solvents, but the mechanism behind this adaptation is not known.

Skin

Contact dermatitis represents 90% of occupational skin diseases (see Chapter 29.1). The most common localization of contact dermatitis is the hands. Hand eczema is most frequently an irritant contact dermatitis caused by skin irritation, but may on occasion represent allergic contact dermatitis resulting from a contact allergy. Dermal exposure to organic solvents has been estimated to be responsible for up to 20% of occupationally induced dermatitis.[8] The main effects of organic solvents on the skin are irritant, including contact dermatitis and acute burns. Dermal sensitization rarely occurs. Other effects are subjective irritation, whitening, contact urticaria, generalized dermatitis, and systemic toxicity due to percutaneous absorption. The skin may be exposed to organic solvents when cleaning the hands with solvents or cleaners containing solvents, by spills, lack of proper protective equipment, or poor hygienic practice, and lack of appropriate cleaning facilities at work.

Skin irritation

The mechanism and nature of skin-related solvent injuries differ.[9] Organic solvents have a defatting action on the skin. Repeated exposure may easily develop into an irritant contact dermatitis with dryness, erythema, edema, scaling and fissures. Prolonged exposure and occlusion may cause chemical burns. The irritation results in increased water loss and facilitated uptake of other substances.

Low-boiling-range (<250 degrees C) petroleum solvents have the greatest defatting action and potential to cause dermatitis. Aromatic solvents are more potent irritants than aliphatic solvents. Skin contact with perchloroethylene and several other halogenated solvents may cause erythema, blistering, burns, or exfoliation of the skin. This may occur if clothes have not been properly dried after dry cleaning with perchloroethylene or trichloroethylene.

Alcohols are claimed to be less irritating than the aldehydes or ketones. The potential to cause irritation decreases as the molecular size increases. The alcohols act as drying agents, resulting in xerosis and subsequent irritant contact dermatitis. Ketones are mild skin irritants. Esters are, in general, more potent skin irritants than the corresponding alcohols.

Carbon disulfide is one of the most irritating solvents. Dimethyl sulfoxide (DMSO) is used as an industrial solvent and also in veterinary medicine. DMSO is readily absorbed through the skin. Its systemic toxicity, however, is low but it may facilitate the percutaneous absorption of other substances.

Sensitization

Because organic solvents often cause irritant contact dermatitis, they may facilitate dermal sensitization to workplace allergens. Contact allergy to organic solvents themselves, however, is rare.[8]

Turpentine was previously a common solvent for paints, but its use has declined. It is still added to oil-based paints and varnishes and is used as an ingredient in other industrial and commercial products. Turpentine of Swedish and Finnish origin was previously a common cause of allergic contact dermatitis among painters. American, French, and Portuguese turpentines are less potent sensitizers. 2,3-Carene is regarded as the main allergen in turpentine. Turpentine contains several mono-terpenes, and their oxidation products are sensitizers.

d-Limonene, a citrus solvent, is an organic solvent increasingly used in metal cleaning, and it has many other uses. It is a major fragrance component and is used as a perfume ingredient in various products. Allergenic oxidation products are created with air exposure of d-limonene. The main allergens are limonene oxide, l-carvone and limonene hydroperoxides. In addition to allergic reactions, irritant effects can occur. The oxidation of d-limonene can be prevented by avoidance of air exposure and by the addition of antioxidant.[10] Case reports exist of contact allergy to the alcohols methanol, ethanol, ethylene, glycol and propylene glycol, and there are a few reports of contact allergy to styrene and dioxane. Contact urticaria has been caused by xylenes, alcohols, DMSO and, in single cases, by other solvents.

Protective equipment

Protective gloves should be used to prevent dermal exposure to organic solvents. Gloves are manufactured in different types, according to their use and thickness, by different methods, and from several polymeric materials, with variable resistance to chemicals. Commonly used latex gloves are permeable to a number of solvent compounds. When selecting protective gloves, permeation test data must be considered, as well as the risk of contamination and adverse effects related to gloves (e.g. allergy related to glove material).[11] Barrier creams are far less efficient than protective gloves in reducing percutaneous absorption of organic solvents.[12]

Diagnosis

Skin lesions caused by organic solvents do not have a specific clinical picture. The diagnosis is based on dermatologic examination and the history of dermatitis, exposure to organic solvents, other chemicals, and skin irritants. Hand eczema is the most common solvent-induced dermatologic lesion. Dermatitis on the face and other contact distributions are also caused by organic solvents, whether by aerosol or through hand contamination. Dermatitis on the neck and flexures may be caused by solvents in working clothes, including those that have dry cleaned and not properly dried. Hand eczema is often caused by a combination of several factors, such as exposure to solvents, water, detergents, other skin irritants, and contact allergens. Atopic dermatitis and hand eczema in atopic patients are often aggravated by exposure to organic solvents. Patch testing should be carried out in the case of persistent dermatitis. The contact allergens that often cause hand eczema in association with solvent exposure are rubber chemicals in protective gloves, preservatives in creams, soaps, paints, perfumes, nickel, chromate, and colophony. Contact allergy to oxidized d-limonene should also be considered.

Treatment and prognosis

Clinical management of dermatitis caused by organic solvents should emphasize the avoidance of dermal exposure to solvents and exposure to other skin irritants. Solvent-induced dermatitis should be treated similarly to other forms of dermatitis with topical corticosteroids and emollients. Systemic corticosteroids are indicated only in severe cases (see Chapter 29.1). Mild hand eczema may clear spontaneously. Hand eczema, however, often becomes chronic or recurrent, as a result of repeated exposure to skin irritants and contact allergens. Hand eczema in persons with atopic dermatitis often becomes more chronic than in others. Contact allergies are frequently persistent. In the case of contact allergy to a solvent (i.e., to d-limonene or turpentine), contact must be avoided in the future. Hand eczema caused by exposure to solvents may necessitate a change of job, especially in cases where exposure cannot be avoided.

Central nervous system

In the middle of the 19th century, the process of vulcanization of rubber was developed, and carbon disulfide was found to be a suitable solvent to use in the process. Soon after its introduction, the French physician August-Louis Delpech described severe neuropsychiatric effects among rubber workers, and was able to identify carbon disulfide as the causative agent. The exposure to carbon disulfide was extremely high in a large number of small workshops in Paris, and many workers became ill.

Delpech discerned two phases in the development of carbon disulfide poisoning. The first appeared rapidly, sometimes after only a few hours of exposure. It was characterized by an excitatory phase followed by collapse. The other phase developed much more slowly and was frequently chronic. It was associated with fluctuations in mood, insomnia, memory problems, loss of sensation in different parts of the body, and impotence. A few of the workers became clinically psychotic. The symptoms described by Delpech seem approximately to fit with modern concepts of the acute and chronic effects of solvents on the central nervous system[13] (see Chapter 28.1).

Acute effects

Short-term high-level exposures to organic solvents produce narcotic effects. In fact, several solvents (e.g., trichloroethylene and chloroform) have been used medically as general anesthetics. The narcotic effect of a solvent is directly related to its solubility in fat, and associated bioavailability in lipid-rich cerebral tissues. Acute symptoms include headache, dizziness, confusion, a feeling of inebriation, and, if the exposure continues, unconsciousness and death. Such symptoms have been common in several heavily exposed occupations. The acute symptoms are reversible after the discontinuation of exposure, but may increase sensitivity to future exposures.

A vast number of laboratory investigations have been carried out to elucidate the relationships between acute solvent exposures and neuropsychiatric symptoms and neurobehavioral test results. In general, these studies have confirmed that irritant and prenarcotic symptoms occur in a dose-related manner. It is apparent that current solvent hygienic standards in some countries are too high to protect workers completely from these acute central nervous system effects.

Subchronic and chronic effects

Most workers are exposed to mixtures of aromatic and aliphatic solvents, and the majority of these workers are exposed to solvents in paints and lacquers. The most important occupational groups include different kinds of painters (e.g., house painters and car painters) and paint manufacturing workers. The solvent mixtures often contain painter's naphtha (brush painting), xylene, or toluene (industrial painting) as main components.

Exposure to mixed solvents has for a long time been associated with long-lasting central nervous system symptoms and case reports have appeared throughout the previous century. The interest in these complaints grew in the 1970s and 1980s when Scandinavian investigators reported excesses of disability pensions caused by neuropsychiatric disorders in solvent-exposed occupational groups. At the same time, several cross-sectional studies, also from Scandinavian countries, reported excess neuropsychiatric symptoms and impaired neuropsychologic performance in house painters, car painters, and workers exposed to jet fuel. Studies from Switzerland, Holland, the USA and other countries have later verified similar excesses of disability pensions caused by neuropsychiatric conditions.

Several cross-sectional studies from different countries have reproduced the findings of excess neuropsychiatric symptoms and impaired neuropsychologic performance among workers with long-term exposure to solvents, but some studies have been unable to reproduce the findings. There are compelling reasons for the discrepancies in some cases. These include very low solvent exposures or exposure mainly to water-soluble solvents with a low potential to induce neurologic damage. In other cases, the reasons for the discrepancies remain unclear.

The studies cited show that long-term solvent exposure has been consistently associated with similar symptoms related to the central nervous system. Most of the early studies were performed in Scandinavian countries, and the existence of a clinical syndrome caused by solvents was first accepted in those countries. During the 1980s, the concept gained wider acceptance, and two international workshops with participation of most researchers in the field reached consensus on the potential association and refined the classification of neurobehavioral disorders caused by solvents.

Three studies[14-16] published between 1988 and 1999 were designed to minimize bias related to the healthy worker effect. In two,[14,15] painters were examined who had been union members for more than 10 years before the data collection started, and regardless of trade or activity at the time of examination. Symptoms compatible with functional or structural brain damage were observed in excess among painters compared with comparison groups. However, there were very mild effects on psychometric test scores when painters were compared as a group with referent groups. In both studies there was evidence of exposure–response relationships, such that painters with lower cumulative exposure often performed better, painters with intermediate exposure often equal to, and painters with higher exposure often worse than the comparison group. Mikkelsen et al[14] attribute this mainly to a less fortunate choice of the referent group, while Lundberg et al[15] suggest that it may be a selection effect among painters, resulting in lower exposure among painters with greater potential for upward social mobility.

In the study by Daniell et al[16] abnormal psychometric test scores were more common among previously exposed than previously non-exposed retired workers. Hence there is still some debate as to what extent long-term occupational solvent exposure may contribute to chronic effects on the central nervous system. Further research is needed to study whether there is a selection out of solvent-exposed work related to neuropsychologic performance, to clarify the association, to gain information on which types of solvent exposures are most likely to cause effects, on potentially toxic concentrations, and on the reversibility of the syndromes. However, there is currently sufficient support for the association of high long-term solvent exposure with long-lasting psycho-organic symptoms to consider this a clinical reality.

The central nervous system effects of specific solvents are discussed in the section on effects from specific agents. However, all solvents seem to elicit similar central nervous system symptoms.

Symptoms and signs

The symptoms described in case reports and cross-sectional studies of solvent-exposed workers include memory problems, concentration difficulties, affective changes (such as aggressiveness, irritability and depression), fatigue, vertigo, decreased libido, sleeping problems, and hyperautonomic symptoms (such as palpitations and increased sweating). The frequent headaches described among those with acute symptoms related to heavy exposures are also common after long-term exposure. The time of appearance of the symptoms and their severity is believed to depend on the previous exposure level. At least some years of exposure are typically required for the symptoms to become chronic, even in heavily exposed occupations.

Diagnosis of solvent-induced CNS effects

The diagnosis of solvent-induced neuropsychiatric dysfunction mainly rests on the clinical evaluation of the previously mentioned symptoms and exposure history. The development of the symptoms is often insidious. Initially, the symptoms may disappear over weekends and holidays, but over a period encompassing years they will become chronic. In the end, they will typically be perceived by the individual and their relatives as a fundamental change in mental status and personality.

Patients will complain about changes in their ability to work, to participate in social activities, to function sexually, and to manage relationships. They do not remember what to bring or where to go; they stop participating in organized activities and playing music or cards or doing other hobbies which they used to enjoy and in which they may have been skilful. They may be accompanied to the physician by a spouse because they have severe memory deficiencies and because they are afraid.

It is vital that the examining physician inquires about such functional changes, professionally and socially, to elucidate the cognitive and personality changes that have occurred, often over a period of years. The diagnosis of a solvent syndrome is clinical, and is based on a thorough exploration of the intellectual, memory, and affective changes, from the premorbid personality, that has caused the patient to seek medical advice.

Some of the symptoms, such as memory problems and concentration difficulties, may also be demonstrated as an impairment in the corresponding functions assessed in neuropsychologic tests. Such tests were originally developed to measure mild forms of brain damage, and have been widely used in the diagnosis of early stages of dementia. The neuropsychologic test batteries in common use measure several functions thought to be sensitive to neurotoxic exposures (non-hold tests) and some functions that are considered insensitive or less sensitive (hold tests). The latter type of tests are used to evaluate premorbid neurobehavioral function, assuming that the original level was the same in all functions. The assumption is based on dementia testing, but may be highly variable on an individual basis. There has been a fair correlation between the results in tests measuring different types of intellectual functioning. The use of different test batteries in epidemiologic studies has created some difficulties in the interpretation of results. Therefore, the World Health Organization has developed a test battery suitable for the detection of group differences in working populations, as well as development of entirely computerized test batteries.[17]

The demands put on a test battery for clinical purposes may be different than those on a battery used for assessing group differences. The test battery in clinical use should not only discriminate exposed and non-exposed individuals, but should also assess as many functions as possible to provide a profile of the abilities and deficits of a given individual. A basic requirement for tests used in clinical practice is the existence of reference data to enable the comparison with a healthy population without neurotoxic exposures of the same age, social class, and gender. The tests used in Scandinavian countries cover at least the verbal ability (hold tests), cognitive non-verbal functions (often unchanged by exposure), psychomotor function (non-hold test), perceptual speed (non-hold tests), and short-term memory (non-hold tests). A number of tests that are used in Scandinavia and the United States in the clinical evaluation of individuals with suspected solvent-induced neuropsychiatric disorders are listed in Table 40.4.

It is important that the tests are performed and interpreted by an appropriate trained neuropsychologist or psychologist. The evaluation of the premorbid functioning in relation to the present, within the different functions measured and between hold tests and non-hold tests, may be subtle and requires experience (see Chapter 28.1).

The ability of several other methods to predict the diagnosis of solvent-induced changes has been assessed in different studies; the results are in general discouraging. Although differences have been detected between exposed and non-exposed groups, and between persons with and without the diagnosis, this diverse group of tests, including electroencephalographic studies, computed tomographic scans, magnetic resonance tomography of the brain, liquor proteins, regional cerebral blood flow, and evoked potentials, have been difficult to interpret. The group differences are too small and the interindividual differences too large for these methods to be of value in an individual case.

The vertigo experienced by many long-term solvent-exposed workers is a feeling of unsteadiness and movement. Solvent-induced disturbances in the vestibulo-oculomotor system may often be the origin of such symptoms. Solvent-

Test types	Examples of tests
Hold tests	Verbal comprehension vocabulary (WAIS) Similarities (WAIS) Synonyms
Semi-hold tests	Cognitive non-verbal function. Block design (WAIS)
Non-hold tests	Picture completion (WAIS) Figure classification Psychomotor function simple reaction time (WHO) Santa Ana (WHO) Purdue peg board Pursuit aiming (WHO) Perceptual speed Digit symbol (WAIS, WHO) Trail making Short-term memory Benton visual retention (WHO) Digit span (WAIS WHO)

WAIS denotes that the test is included in the Wechsler Adult Intelligence Scale. WHO denotes that the test is included in the WHO neurobehavioral core test battery

Table 40.4 Psychometric tests

exposed workers, particularly those with toxic encephalopathy, have shown rather pronounced disturbances in vestibulo-oculomotor functioning. However, methods to measure vestibulo-oculomotor malfunction seem also to provide little help in the diagnosis of individuals.

Exposure evaluation

Exposure evaluation is crucial in the diagnosis of solvent-related central neurologic syndromes. Solvent exposure may occur in many occupations, but there are large quantitative and qualitative differences between the exposure conditions in different jobs, companies, and countries. Lipid-soluble solvents, such as the common aromatic, aliphatic, and chlorinated hydrocarbons, are much more likely to cause chronic central nervous system effects than are the more water-soluble solvents, such as the common alcohols, ketones and esters.

A thorough evaluation of lifetime solvent exposure is crucial in the assessment of a patient with possible solvent-induced changes. The evaluation should concern all exposed employment, as well as specific work hygiene conditions, and all hobby-related exposures (see Chapter 3). Jobs that are associated with high solvent exposures are listed in Table 40.3.

Even in heavily exposed jobs, the worker is usually solvent exposed during only part of the workday, and may not be exposed during some periods. Others have large amounts of overtime, or an additional job where they are heavily exposed. The exposure level is usually dependent on the size of the area from which the solvent may evaporate and the temperature. Solvent uptake is modified by the workload and respiratory rate, the use of respirators and gloves, and the availability of engineering and ventilation controls. To evaluate particularly heavy exposures, it is useful to ask about the occurrence and frequency of symptoms of acute intoxication, including light-headedness and feelings of inebriation. Many painters, floor layers, and paint manufacturing workers have fainted on their jobs because of intoxication. In some instances, the exposure evaluation may be challenging, and collaboration with a trained industrial hygienist may be warranted.

Syndromes associated with solvent exposure

The following is a classification of solvents syndromes, with some modifications, agreed on in two international meetings in 1985.[18]

1. Type I: Symptoms only. The patients have non-specific symptoms of fatigue, memory and concentration disturbances, affective changes, and sleeping problems. Psychometric tests show no impairment. The symptoms are most often reversible within 6 months and always within 1 year after discontinuation of exposure.

2. Type IIa: Personality or mood change. There is a marked and sustained alteration in personality with obvious affective changes such as increased depressivity or aggressivity, fatigue, diminished impulse control, and decreased motivation. Psychometric test results are usually normal. It is unclear to what degree these symptoms are reversible.

3. Type IIb: Impairment in intellectual function. There is difficulty in concentration, impairment in memory, and decreased learning capacity. There may also be minor neurologic signs. Psychometric test results are affected. After the discontinuation of exposure, this syndrome may remain stationary or improve. Progression should not be expected.

4. Type III: Dementia. This condition involves global deterioration in intellect and memory and is often accompanied by neurologic signs. Psychometric test results are severely affected. This syndrome is caused by repeated, severe overexposure and is not reversible after discontinuation of exposure. Non-occupational etiologies include glue sniffing.

It is assumed that progressively higher exposure levels are required to elicit the syndromes from types I to III, but the relative importance of peak exposures versus cumulative exposure, the importance of age when the exposure occurs, and other factors are not well characterized. However, the cumulative exposure, as summed up in exposure months, is often related to the severity of the changes and may be used in the clinical evaluation. Clinical experience indicates that heavier exposures may have a relatively greater influence on brain function than lower exposures.

In the authors' experience, the Type IIa syndrome is not well delineated from Type IIb. The patients usually have complaints concerning intellectual functions and personality and mood changes, but only some of the patients show changes in neuropsychologic test results. In Scandinavia, the Type IIb syndrome, which requires changes in neuropsychologic test findings, has been labeled a chronic toxic encephalopathy. To diagnose a type IIb syndrome, a significant impairment, compared with the appropriate reference values, in at least two functions (e.g., memory, perceptual speed and accuracy, and psychomotor performance) is required, together with smaller differences in verbal ability.

In Sweden there is consensus on some diagnostic requirements concerning a chronic toxic encephalopathy (Type IIb syndrome) elicited by solvents; these are (1) long and/or intense exposure to solvents (often of many years duration), (2) relevant symptoms as described above, and (3) consistent changes on neuropsychologic testing in settings where exposure data are available. Long and intense exposure may be assumed to have occurred if average 8-hour exposure over at least 10 years has corresponded to more than 250 mg/m^3 of painters' naphtha (or equivalent exposure to other lipopholic solvents). In Sweden, such exposures were common among painters until the mid 1970s.

Time course and prognosis

The symptoms and neuropsychologic impairment seem to progress as long as the solvent exposure continues. After discontinuation of solvent exposure, symptoms of psychological distress are often alleviated, although full recovery is seldom achieved. The impairment in neuropsychologic tests commonly remains stationary. Progress is not to be expected, either for symptoms or for neuropsychologic test results.[19]

Differential etiologies and differential diagnoses

The symptoms produced by long-term solvent exposure are common in everyday life. They may be elicited by a wide variety of psychologic and psychosocial factors and by different neurotoxic exposures. They may also occur without any immediately apparent reason. The time of occurrence is crucial in determining whether or not the symptoms are the result of solvent exposure. The chronic symptoms associated with solvent-induced CNS injury may develop with a concomitant feeling of change in the perception of oneself and the environment after a prolonged exposure to solvents for several years.

Symptoms and neuropsychologic impairment may occur as a consequence of excessive alcohol consumption. In settings of concurrent solvent hepatoxicity, the pattern of hepatic enzymes may be useful, AST/ALT ratio is atypically less than in alcohol-related hepatitis (see chapter 26.1). Moreover, alcoholism will usually be apparent if the patient is followed over some period. Depression may result in a clinical syndrome similar to solvent-induced encephalopathy; it may be differentiated from the solvent-induced syndrome by its rather sudden reversibility within a certain period. Depression associated with chronic encephalopathy is usually more severe, and less responsive to antidepressant therapy. Evidence of cognitive impairment disproportionate to that which occurs in depression is also helpful in diagnosing a solvent-induced effect.

It is reasonable to presume interactive effects. The presence of these conditions does not, by itself, exclude solvents as a contributing cause of the disorder. Previous meningitis or encephalitis and previous head trauma with loss of consciousness may also produce chronic encephalopathy. It is thus important that the patient interview covers such causes. Other differential diagnoses involve ischemic brain disease, brain tumors, and presenile and senile dementia. These causes may be identified by laboratory evaluations such as electroencephalography, computed tomographic scans, evoked potentials and magnetic resonance imaging (MRI). The time course of presenile and senile dementia is also different from that of solvent-induced encephalopathy, with a progressive and often rapid, deterioration of intellectual functions. If the diagnosis is uncertain, neurologists and psychiatrists with experience in psycho-organic syndromes and their differential diagnoses should be consulted.

Treatment

Cognitive therapy may be useful in selected individuals though results are often disappointing. Patients with chronic toxic encephalopathy offered a 10-week rehabilitation program involving intellectual training, with particular emphasis on memory and group discussions, experienced an initial significant improvement in symptoms and neuropsychologic test results measuring memory. While a continuing improvement in emotional symptoms was still present at 6 months, cognitive and somatic symptoms had returned to the original level. Only tests associated with verbal memory continued to show improvement. In a recent follow-up 7 years after the rehabilitation program, substantial improvement was found with respect to social functioning and stress-related symptoms among patients who had participated, as well as not participated, in the program. In neither of the groups was there any improvement in neuropsychologic tests. Thus this particular program did not show a sustainable effect.[19]

However, too little effort has been devoted to the treatment of chronic toxic encephalopathy. Although the identification of neurotoxic hazards implies that primary prevention is achievable, and thus is the most important aim of occupational health studies, it is important not to ignore the potential for rehabilitation for those with a chronic work-related disease. Methods obviously need to be developed to improve the rehabilitation of patients with central nervous dysfunction related to solvent exposure, and there is a need for further studies to evaluate the effect of rehabilitation programs. Early retirement should be the last option and should only be considered when work rehabilitation has failed, or in very severe cases.

Additional CNS effects

Solvent exposure may decrease olfactory function at exposure levels below current hygienic standards in industrialized countries. The specific site of the action is unknown, although it has been speculated that the olfactory neuron is the target. It has also been shown in experimental studies that aromatic solvents may induce hearing loss. It is unclear whether these findings have clinical relevance at current exposure levels in industry; however, interaction with noise-induced hearing loss is a concern. It also seems likely that solvent exposure may impair color vision. Various studies have suggested that solvent exposure may contribute to many other disorders such as multiple sclerosis, Parkinson's disease, Alzheimer's disease and epilepsy, but several studies have failed to confirm these results.

Some studies have suggested an excess of alcoholism diagnoses in solvent-exposed occupations, and studies of toluene-exposed printers and animal experiments indicate that solvent exposure may contribute to excess alcohol consumption, possibly through a desire either to avoid withdrawal from or to prolong the acute central nervous system effects of occupational solvent exposure.

Peripheral nervous system

Some studies performed on groups exposed to mixed solvents have indicated impaired peripheral nerve functioning, as evidenced by group differences in some electrophysiologic variables. Jet fuel may be particularly prone to induce a mild neuropathy. However, the effects of mixed solvents seem to be subclinical in the large majority of exposed workers, and some studies have been unable to demonstrate such an effect. The effects of n-hexane, methyl-n-butyl ketone, styrene, and toluene on the peripheral nervous system are discussed in the section on the effects of specific agents.

Liver

A number of halogenated solvents are classic hepatotoxins (see Chapter 26.1). The 1,1,2,2-tetrachloroethane used in the aeronautics industry during World War I caused employees to develop jaundice with subacute hepatic necrosis developing over a period of weeks. Carbon tetrachloride and chloroform will be discussed in the section on the effects of specific agents.

Several epidemiologic studies have been performed to determine the hepatotoxicity of long-term exposure to such solvents. Most of these studies are cross-sectional and use routine hepatic enzymes as the outcome. These studies have reported variable results with mixed solvent exposure; a number of studies have demonstrated elevations in serum bile acids. Some recent studies suggest that fatty liver disease, not reflected by liver enzymes, may occur as an effect of solvent exposure,[20,21] but further confirmation is needed. The interaction between common solvents and other agents that may render these solvents hepatotoxic has not been well characterized.

As a rule, hepatic effects from solvents are avoided if the hygienic standards are respected, and hepatic effects should not readily be anticipated if neuropsychiatric effects are absent. Among patients with raised hepatic enzymes, suspected to be caused by solvents, removal from exposure for a 2–4-week period may play a useful diagnostic and therapeutic role (see Chapter 26.1).

Kidney

For many decades, it has been known that certain solvents, particularly chlorinated compounds like carbon tetrachloride, as well as ethylene glycol, may induce renal failure in humans after acute exposures through a mechanism of acute tubular necrosis. Acute solvent intoxication from a number of common solvents has been associated with renal failure in case reports. Several cross-sectional studies have found increases in the excretion of glomerular or tubular proteins, erythrocytes, and enzymes in groups exposed to common solvents and solvent mixtures. In aggregate, these studies have not localized a unique anatomic lesion. In recent years, most of the interest concerning solvent nephrotoxicity has been devoted to the possible induction of glomerulonephritis (see Chapter 25) Case referent studies have demonstrated a significant association between solvent exposure and glomerulonephritis, while some epidemiologic studies have not demonstrated an association. A low power to detect small increases in the relative risk associated with this uncommon condition has likely contributed to this discrepancy.

In patients in whom occupational causes of proteinuria have been ruled out, it is important to interview them concerning their solvent exposure.

Circulatory system

Among those who abuse solvents for their inebriating properties, there has been an excess of sudden deaths during the intoxication. Experiments in dogs have shown that the likely reasons for these deaths are disturbances in the cardiac rhythm, which are mediated by norepinephrine. The solvents may make the myocardium more sensitive toward endogenous norepinephrine or increase the amount of norepinephrine reaching the heart by decreasing its uptake and degradation. The effects have been seen only at very high exposure levels, and should not be expected in occupational settings unless significant intoxication is present. Carbon disulfide and methylene chloride have effects related to the function of the heart. These are discussed in the section on the effects of specific agents.

Blood

Benzene is a bone marrow toxin that may cause pancytopenia (see the following section on effects of specific agents). Ethylene glycol ethers have also been implicated in hypoplastic syndromes (see Chapter 21). Several studies have indicated that exposures to mixed solvents may induce some lymphocytosis in exposed compared with non-exposed populations, possibly as an effect of irritative effects and associated inflammation. The clinical relevance of this has not been characterized.

Carcinogenicity and mutagenicity

Benzene is a potent leukemogen. Several studies have demonstrated an excess risk of lung cancer and cancer of the bladder among painters. Based on an evaluation of these studies, the International Agency for Research on Cancer has considered painting an occupation at increased risk of cancer. A number of studies have also shown increases of non-Hodgkin's lymphomas and myelomas in occupational groups exposed to mixed solvents, though this association has not been well characterized. The risk for carcinogenicity associated with styrene, methylene chloride, trichloroethylene, perchloroethylene, carbon tetrachloride, and chloroform is discussed in the section on the effects of specific agents.

Reproductive effects

General information on reproductive and developmental effects is found in Chapter 27.2. Glycol ethers with short alkyl groups, 2-methoxy- and 2-ethoxyethanol are teratogenic and testicular toxins at rather low doses in experimental animals. This observation has entailed a shift to glycol ethers with longer alkyl chains in general industrial use.

It seems well established that high exposure to solvent mixtures among pregnant women will increase the risk of spontaneous abortions. Among specific solvents, the best evidence is available for toluene. However, decreasing occupational exposures in recent decades have likely resulted in reduced risk for spontaneous abortions. A number of studies have suggested that maternal and paternal exposure to mixed solvents may increase the risk of congenital malformations. However, no specific type of defect or syndrome has repeatedly been associated with solvent exposure. The summary evidence on effects of organic solvent exposure on female and male fecundity is so far inconclusive. Thus, several studies have suggested that occupational organic solvent exposure during pregnancy may damage the fetus. Current hygienic standards are usually not based on the possibilities of reproductive effects, and it seems warranted to keep solvent exposure of pregnant women far below these standards.

Specific agents

This section will mainly address specific effects of individual solvent compounds. Irritant effects and effects on the skin will not be discussed, although the agents listed certainly share such effects with other solvents. Similarly, the solvents listed may elicit the same central nervous symptoms as described in previous sections in this chapter.

n-Hexane and Methyl-n-butyl ketone
During the 1960s and early 1970s, several outbreaks of polyneuropathy were described among shoe and leather workers in countries that used glues containing n-hexane. The workers developed glove and stocking symmetric sensory dysfunction in the hands and feet, with the feet normally being affected first. In more severe cases, motor function was also affected, manifested by proximal muscular weakness. The air concentrations of n-hexane in these cases were high, with average exposures above 100 ppm. Occupational groups with lower exposure, 20 ppm and above, have shown indications of a subclinical polyneuropathy manifested as mean value decrements zneurophysiologic test results, including nerve conduction velocities. Symptoms of polyneuropathy have also been described among workers exposed to methyl-n-butyl ketone. The cases show sensory impairment with loss of superficial pain, sensitivity to temperature change and diminished light touch and vibration in the toes. Methyl ethyl ketone is not thought to be toxic to peripheral nerves by itself, but may potentiate the effect of n-hexane and methyl-n-butyl.

Animal experiments have shown that the peripheral neurotoxicity of n-hexane and methyl-n-butyl ketone is caused by a common metabolite, 2,5-hexanedione. In fact, it has been shown that other diketones with the same distance between the ketone groups share this ability to damage peripheral nerves. These metabolites appear to cause a disturbance in the axonal transport in large myelinated fibers. Nerve biopsy specimens show axonal swelling followed by myelin retraction at the nodes of Ranvier, and masses of neurofilaments in the axons. Axonal degeneration starts distally.

If signs of polyneuropathy are present, the most important treatment is removal from exposure. After discontinuation of exposure, recovery occurs slowly, reflecting the regeneration of peripheral nerve axons. Residual permanent impairment has been noted in severely injured individuals. It has been possible to find substitutes for methyl-n-butyl ketone in almost all applications, and the use of this solvent should be limited.

Benzene
Heavy benzene exposures are known to induce pancytopenia (see Chapter 21). The first account of this association was published in 1897[22] and described four female workers who died from aplastic anemia after a few months of benzene exposure. Since then, a vast number of case reports have been published. It is unclear if the granulocytes, erythrocytes, or platelets are differentially susceptible to benzene. Pancytopenia is typically dose dependent and is unlikely to appear until the time-weighted average exposure levels have reached at least one order of magnitude above the current hygienic standards in industrialized countries.

Benzene is an established human carcinogen. The first case reports on the association between benzene exposure and leukemia were published in 1928. During the 1960s and 1970s, large series of cases of leukemias among benzene-exposed workers were published, and these reports later were confirmed by convincing epidemiologic and experimental evidence.

It was previously believed that benzene induced acute myelogenous leukemia only, but more recent studies have strongly indicated that other forms of leukemia and lymphomas may be caused by benzene exposure. Exposure–response calculations in recent studies have suggested that benzene may pose a significant cancer risk at low exposure levels. Exposure to 1 ppm of benzene, 8 hours per day, 5 days per week during 40 years was in one study estimated to increase the risk of leukemia by about 70%.[23] The US EPA currently estimates the lifetime risk of cancer associated with exposure to 1 ppm of benzene to range from 7.1×10^{-3} to 2.5×10^{-2}.[24] The time from first exposure until the diagnosis of the tumor is shorter, 10 years on average, for benzene-induced leukemias than for most other occupational cancers.

There are no well-validated screening tests for early diagnosis of benzene-induced hematopoietic malignancies. To monitor exposed populations, cytogenetic methods may be used. Benzene induces chromosomal aberrations in peripheral blood lymphocytes. A recent study has shown that a time-weighted average exposure of 0.3 ppm may induce an increased number of micronuclei in peripheral blood B-lymphocytes.

Benzene-induced tumors are not known to have distinct features. They are diagnosed and treated in the same way as are the same tumors induced by other causes. Restriction from further benzene exposure is essential in diagnosed cases.

Toluene
Toluene is used as a sniffing agent, and several case series have been published of symptoms and signs among long-term sniffers. Tremor, ataxia, and memory impairment are the most commonly encountered findings, but heart dysrhythmias (including death), decreased sense of smell, optic atrophy, hearing impairment, and peripheral neuropathy may also occur. In workers with long-term occupational exposure, there is an increase in neuropsychiatric symptoms.[25]

Styrene
Styrene may induce a mild neuropathy predominantly of a sensory type, as evidenced by sensory nerve conduction

velocities. The neuropathy may manifest itself as increased pain and tingling in the limbs, although the effects at time-weighted average air concentrations around 100 ppm and below are typically subclinical. The effects seem to be largely reversible over a period of 4 weeks. Styrene is suspected of being carcinogenic based on the fact that its metabolite, styrene oxide, is an established carcinogen. However, styrene oxide seems to be readily degraded in humans. Cytogenetic effects have been found in workers exposed to comparatively low levels of styrene, i.e., around 25 ppm. There are a few animal carcinogenicity studies with somewhat contradictory results. Epidemiologic studies carried out in the glass-reinforced plastics industry, in which styrene exposures are highest, have been inconclusive to date. The International Agency for Research on Cancer has concluded that styrene is possibly carcinogenic to humans (group 2B).[26]

Methylene chloride

Methylene chloride is metabolized to carbon monoxide. The hygienic standard for carbon monoxide has been set to avoid carboxyhemoglobin (COHb) levels above 5%, because such levels have been reported to increase ischemic symptoms among patients with angina pectoris. Exposures to 100 ppm of methylene chloride may produce COHb levels just above 5%. However, the biotransformation to COHb becomes saturated if the exposure exceeds 250 ppm, and COHb levels above 10% among non-smokers are unlikely to be the result of methylene chloride exposure. The epidemiologic studies performed thus far have found an incidence of heart disease in methylene chloride exposed workers that is comparable to the incidence in the control populations. Methylene chloride causes several types of tumors in experimental animals, and the evidence for carcinogenicity was considered sufficient by the International Agency for Research on Cancer. However, the few epidemiologic studies carried out so far have shown inconclusive results for classification as a Group 2B agent (possibly carcinogenic to humans).[27]

Carbon tetrachloride and chloroform

The use of carbon tetrachloride as a solvent has been accompanied by numerous case reports of hepatoxicity, including hepatic and renal necrosis. Chloroform is also, hepatotoxic although at higher doses. It has been shown that the hepatotoxicity of these solvents is caused by the metabolic activation with formation of reactive metabolites that attack macromolecules in the hepatocytes, as well as lipid peroxidation.

These solvents interact with agents capable of inducing the microsomal enzyme system of the liver. Accordingly, barbiturates and alcohol may potentiate the hepatotoxicity. There is also a convincing report of an interaction between occupational exposure to isopropyl alcohol in conjunction with carbon tetrachloride. Usually, the hepatic effects resolve after discontinuation of exposure, depending on the degree of injury.

After heavy short-term exposures, carbon tetrachloride may induce renal failure in humans as a result of acute tubular necrosis. Carbon tetrachloride causes hepatic cancer in animal experiments, and cases of hepatic cancer have also been described in exposed humans. It is possible that the carcinogenicity of carbon tetrachloride is associated with its potential to induce toxic hepatic damage. Chloroform causes hepatic and renal tumors in rodents. The acute solvent toxicity to these tissues might contribute to the carcinogenicity.

Trichloroethylene

In a classic study published in 1955, Grandjean and coworkers showed an increased prevalence of neuropsychiatric symptoms with increasing exposure among workers exposed to trichloroethylene in the mechanical engineering industry.[28] They also diagnosed a psycho-organic syndrome characterized by intellectual impairment with memory deficiencies and affective changes. A strong exposure–response relationship was observed with the prevalence of this syndrome increasing at higher exposure levels. The authors concluded that the prevalence of neuropsychiatric symptoms and signs was definitely increased at exposure levels above 40 ppm.

Trichloroethylene exposure at high concentrations may induce trigeminal neuropathy with facial numbness and weakness of the masticatory muscles. In fact, this observation led to the unsuccessful use of trichloroethylene as a remedy for trigeminal neuralgia. However, trigeminal neuropathy does not seem to occur at the exposure levels currently prevalent in industrialized countries.

There are a few case reports of serious hepatic injury after occupational exposure to trichloroethylene and methyl chloroform. Trichloroethylene can interfere with alcohol metabolism in the liver. Flushing of the face and neck and severe nausea are induced if alcohol is ingested in conjunction with high exposure to these solvents. Accordingly, the clinical picture mimics the effects of the drug disulfiram (Antabuse).

There is significant evidence of the carcinogenicity of trichloroethylene in experimental animals. In humans three highly relevant cohort studies have demonstrated an excess incidence of liver and biliary tract cancers as well as non-Hodgkin lymphomas. The IARC has concluded that trichloroethylene is group 2A (probable human carcinogen).[29]

Perchloroethylene

Women working in laundries and dry-cleaning jobs seem to have an increased risk of primary hepatic cancer. Exposure to chlorinated solvents, particularly perchloroethylene, is a likely cause. Several studies have also shown excesses of non-Hodgkin lymphomas, esophageal and cervical cancers among perchloroethylene-exposed workers. The IARC has classified perchloroethylene as probably carcinogenic to humans (group 2A) based on sufficient evidence in experimental animals and limited epidemiological evidence.[29]

Methanol

Methanol may damage the retina and induce blindness after ingestion of sufficient amounts. Occupational exposure, however, does not seem to induce ocular toxicity because the bioavailability by the inhalation route is not sufficient for this effect to occur.

Ethylene glycol

Ethylene glycol may induce acute tubular necrosis and renal failure in humans after ingestion. However, this effect has not been seen after occupational exposures because the low volatility of the compound precludes sufficiently high air exposures.

Carbon disulfide

Carbon disulfide has pronounced central nervous system effects. Psychoses are well-described among heavily exposed workers. Exposure to carbon disulfide may also contribute to the development of Parkinson's disease. Decreased libido and loss of potency have been repeatedly reported among exposed men.[30]

Exposure to carbon disulfide has been shown to increase the incidence of myocardial infarction in several studies (see Chapter 24). Carbon disulfide alters fat metabolism and increases arteriosclerosis. A successful preventive program directed toward carbon disulfide-induced coronary disease was instituted in a Finnish viscose rayon plant.[31] In the early 1970s, the carbon disulfide concentrations in the plant were lowered from 30 ppm and above to 10 ppm, and workers with coronary risk factors were removed from exposure. Because of these measures, the previously heavily elevated coronary mortality rate was reduced to levels in the general population by 1980, with an estimated 40 lives saved among a cohort of 343 men.

Dimethylformamide

There are several recent reports on the hepatotoxicity of dimethylformamide, which currently seems to be the most widely used of the hepatotoxic solvents. The hepatotoxicity of dimethylformamide depends on metabolic activation. This solvent is easily absorbed through the skin, which makes it particularly dangerous. Usually, the hepatic effects resolve after the discontinuation of exposure. Dimethylformamide may also interfere with alcohol metabolism in the liver. Severe nausea and flushing of the face and neck may occur if alcohol is ingested in conjunction with exposure to this solvent. Accordingly, the effect is similar to that of the drug disulfiram.

Tetrahydrofuran

Tetrahydrofuran is a common component of glues and may produce hepatic and renal damage at high concentrations.

Ethylene oxide

Ethylene oxide is a gas at room temperature and is a highly reactive agent. It irritates the respiratory tract and the skin, and may induce allergic contact dermatitis. High exposures greater than 500 ppm have induced peripheral neuropathy. Ethylene oxide is mutagenic in bacterial test systems and animal experiments. Cytogenetic studies in humans have shown dose-related chromosomal changes. Ethylene oxide is carcinogenic to experimental animals,

with leukemia and brain cancer being induced in a dose-related manner. In epidemiological studies, the most frequently reported association has been with lymphatic and hematopoietic cancer; stomach and breast cancer excesses have also been reported. The International Agency for Research on Cancer[26] considers ethylene oxide carcinogenic to humans, based on limited evidence in humans and sufficient evidence in experimental animals.

BIOLOGIC MONITORING

For some common solvents, the solvent itself or some metabolite may be measured in end-exhaled air, blood, or urine to monitor the amount of the solvent taken up by the body. Biologic monitoring has advantages compared with air-concentration measurements because it accounts not only for the respiratory uptake at rest, but also for the workload and uptake through the skin. Biologic monitoring may also be used to assess the function of personal protective equipment. However, the common use of biologic monitoring is still as an alternative to air-exposure measurements, and the following comments will mostly concern such practice.

Inhalation exposure and uptake may vary considerably from day to day as well as within shift, due to fluctuation of the solvent concentration in air. Concentrations in the biologic determinants (i.e., the solvent or its metabolite) change in a similar fashion. Therefore, determinants with short biologic half-life indicate current or very recent exposure, while determinants with long half-life indicate the integrated exposure over an extended time period. These conditions are important to remember when interpreting results of biologic monitoring.[32]

Table 40.5 lists the solvents for which the ACGIH has proposed or is considering biologic exposure indices (BEI), i.e., a biologic standard intended to measure approximately the same exposure level as the threshold limit values proposed by the ACGIH. However, the BEIs themselves are not shown because proposed standards vary by country and tend to shift substantially over time. To obtain currently acceptable limits, the reader may refer to the standards published by the health and safety authorities in each country.

It seems that urinary metabolites of trichlorethylene and styrene provide the most commonly used biologic indicators of solvent exposure. Usually, the combined urinary excretion of mandelic acid and phenylglyoxylic acid gives a better estimate of the preceding styrene exposure than any of these styrene metabolites separately. However, mandelic acid is often used alone and is an acceptable indicator of styrene exposure at low exposure levels. Measurements of styrene in the blood or exhaled air show large interindividual differences and should not be used to quantify the exposure.

Trichloroethanol and trichloroacetic acid are excreted in the urine after trichloroethylene exposure. Trichloroacetic acid has a long half-life, around 3 days, and will integrate the exposure over several days. Trichloroethanol has a much shorter half-life and may give a reasonable estimate

Solvent	Indicator	Comments
n-Hexane	2,5-Hexanedione in urine	Exposure quantitation at low exposures
Benzene	S-Phenylmercapturic acid in urine	Background level
	Muconic acid in urine	Background level
Toluene	Hippuric acid in urine	Non-specific, insensitive. Toluene exposures around 100 ppm needed to mirror exposure
	Toluene in blood	
	O-cresol in urine	Background level
Xylene methyl	Hippuric acid in urine	Exposure quantitation at low exposure
Styrene	Mandelic acid	Non-specific
		Exposure quantitation at low doses
	Phenylglyoxylic acid in urine	Exposure quantitation at low doses
	Styrene in blood	Indicator of exposure
Trichloroethylene	Trichloroethanol and trichloroacetic acid in urine	Non-specific, exposure quantitation at low doses
	Free trichloroethanol in blood	Non-specific indicator of exposure
	Trichloroethylene in blood and end-exhaled air	
Methyl ethyl ketone	Methyl ethyl ketone in urine	
Carbon disulfide	2-Thiothiazolidine-4-carboxylic acid in urine	
Dimethylformamide	N-methylformamide in urine	
	N-Acetyl-S-(N-methylcarbamoyl) cysteine in urine	Indicator of exposure
Methyl chloroform	Methyl chloroform in end-exhaled air	Large interindividual variation
	Total trichloroethanol and trichloroacetic acid in urine	Large interindividual variation, non-specific indicator of exposure
	Total trichloroethanol in blood	Non-specific
Perchloroethylene	Perchloroethylene in end-exhaled air	
	Perchloroethylene in venous blood	
	Trichloroacetic acid in urine	Large interindividual variation. Non-specific indicator of exposure
Acetone	Acetone in urine	Non-specific
Chlorobenzene	Total 4-chlorocatechol and total p-chlorophenol in urine	Non-specific
2-Ethoxyethanol and 2-ethoxyethyl acetate	2-Ethoxyacetic acid in urine	
Ethyl benzene	Mandelic acid in urine	Non-specific
Methanol	Methanol in urine	Non-specific, background level
Methyl isobutyl ketone	Methyl isobutyl ketone in urine	

Table 40.5 Biologic monitoring of solvents

of the exposure during a particular shift. The combined excretion of the metabolites has also been suggested to estimate the exposure.[33]

Hippuric acid is a toluene metabolite, but it is also a metabolite of benzoic acid. Thus, it is often present in the urine in significant amounts without any toluene exposure. Toluene exposures below 100 ppm could not be effectively quantified by hippuric acid excretion.[34] In the future, toluene in the venous blood may prove to be a successful method for biologic monitoring of toluene exposure.

Benzene exposure can be determined by analyzing phenylmercapturic acid in urine. The method is sensitive and can detect even low-level environmental exposures. Although exhaled air analysis, in general, is unreliable for exposure quantification, it seems that benzene levels in exhaled air currently are the best estimate of benzene exposure.

Methyl hippuric acids are specific metabolites of the corresponding xylene isomers. They give a reliable estimate of xylene exposure. However, because the xylenes are usually used in solvent mixtures, the practical use of this indicator has been limited.

MONITORING OF EXPOSED GROUPS

Most solvents share the ability to irritate mucous membranes and to affect the central nervous system and the skin. In general, the monitoring of exposed groups should focus on these effects. Skin problems are easily diagnosed, and the exposure conditions causing the damage are often apparent. However, subtle effects on the central nervous system are not easily diagnosed. These effects cause vague and non-specific symptoms that generally lack objective correlates. Thus, questionnaires have been developed to monitor the solvent effects on groups of exposed workers.

The Swedish Q16 questionnaire, reproduced in Figure 40.4, is a simple 'yes or no' instrument containing 16 questions. It was developed from clinical experience with long-term solvent-exposed workers. Understanding of the questions was checked between exposed workers, physicians, and psychologists. The questions were investigated for reliability through test–retest procedures and for validity by showing the anticipated dose–response relationships in exposed and non-exposed groups. The intercorrelations

Questionnaire 16 (Q16)

Question	Yes	No

1. Do you have a short memory?

2. Have your relatives told you that you have a short memory?

3. Do you often have to make notes about what you must remember?

4. Do you often have to go back and check things you have done such as turned off the stove, locked the door, etc?

5. Do you generally find it hard to get the meaning from reading newspapers and books?

6. Do you have problems concentrating?

7. Do you often feel irritated without any particular reason?

8. Do you often feel depressed without any particular reason?

9. Are you abnormally tired?

10. Are you less interested in sex than what you think is normal?

11. Do you have palpitations even when you don't exert yourself?

12. Do you sometimes feel an oppression in your chest?

13. Do you perspire without any particular reason?

14. Do you have a headache at least once a week?

15. Do you often have a painful tingling in some part of your body?

16. Do you have any problems with buttoning and unbuttoning?

Figure 40.4: The Swedish Q16 questionnaire, developed from clinical experience with long-term solvent-exposed workers.

between the replies to the different questions were also checked. The Q16 has been used in several languages but is validated only in the Swedish version. Recent reports have shown that the Q16 is efficient in encephalopathy.[35] A review of the experiences of the Q16 from its use in different countries is available.[36]

At present, the Q16 seems to be the best instrument available to monitor the solvent effects in groups exposed particularly to solvent mixtures. If an individual gives six or more yes replies, this should be considered an indication for an interview with a physician to elucidate the character and origin of the symptoms. If the symptoms have occurred after a period of heavy solvent exposure and there is no other obvious explanation, it may be reasonable to refer the patient to a occupational health department for further examination, including psychometric testing.

Apart from the effects on the central nervous system, it might be necessary to investigate the specific effects of some compounds. For example, carbon tetrachloride, chloroform, and dimethylformamide cause hepatic effects that may be monitored with conventional liver tests. These solvents are also nephrotoxic, and their nephrotox-icity could be monitored with tests assessing tubular and glomerular functions (see Chapter 25). A few hexacarbon solvents may damage peripheral nerves at high concentrations, and monitoring for this effect may be appropriate. In general, however, compliance with present hygienic standards in industrialized countries should protect the large majority of exposed workers from such specific effects.

References

1. Rosen G, Andersson I. Video filming and pollution measurement as a teaching aid in reducing exposure to air-borne pollutants. Ann Occup Hyg 1989; 1:137–44.
2. Astrand I. Effect of physical exercise on uptake, distribution, and elimination of vapors in man. In: Fiserova-Bergerova V, ed. Modeling of inhalation exposure to vapors: uptake, distribution, and elimination. Vol. II. Boca Raton: CRC Press, 1983;107–30.
3. Löf A, Johansson G. Toxicokinetics of organic solvents. A review of modifying factors. Crit Rev Toxicol 1998; 28:571–650.
4. Baelum J. Human solvent exposure. Factors influencing the pharmacokinetics and acute toxicity. Academic dissertation. Institute of Environmental and Occupational Medicine. Aarhus, Denmark: University of Aarhus, 1990.

5. Sato A, Nakajima T. Pharmacokinetics of organic solvent vapors in relation to their toxicity. Scand J Work Environ Health 1987; 13:81–93.

6. Riihimaki V, Hfuminen O. Xylenes. In: Snyder R, ed. Ethel Browning's toxicity and metabolism of industrial solvents, 2nd edn. Amsterdam: Elsevier, 1987.

7. Nelson KW, Ege JF Jr, Ross M, et al. Sensory response to certain industrial solvent vapors. J Ind Hyg Toxicol 1943; 25:282–5.

8. Boman A, Wahlberg JE. Organic solvents. In: Kanerva L, Elsner P, Wahlberg JE, Maibach HI, eds. Handbook of occupational dermatology. Berlin, Heidelberg: Springer Verlag, 2000;679–87.

9. Boman AS. Irritants – organic solvents. In: van der Valk PGM, Maibach HI, eds. The irritant contact dermatitis syndrome. Boca Raton: CRC Press, 1996;95–103.

10. Karlberg A-T, Magnusson K, Nilsson U. Influence of an anti-oxidant on the formation of allergenic compounds during auto-oxidation of d-limonene. Ann Occup Hyg 1994; 38:199–207.

11. Mellstrom GA, Boman A. Protective gloves. In: Kanerva L, Elsner P, Wahlberg JE, Maibach HI, eds. Handbook of occupational dermatology. Berlin, Heidelberg: Springer Verlag, 2000;417–25.

12. Wahlberg JE, Boman A. Prevention of contact dermatitis from solvents. Cuff Prob Dermatol 1996; 25:57–66.

13. O'Flynn RR, Waldron HA. Delpech and the origins of occupational psychiatry. Br J Ind Med 1990; 47:189–98.

14. Mikkelsen S, Joergensen M, Browne E, et al. Mixed solvent exposure and organic brain damage. Acta Neurol Scand 1988; 78(suppl):118.

15. Lundberg I, Michelsen H, Nise G, et al. Neuropsychiatric function among housepainters with previous long-term heavy exposure to organic solvents. Scand J Work Environ Health 1995; 21(suppl 1):1–44.

16. Daniell WE, Clavpoole KH, Checkoway H, et al. Neuropsychological function in retired workers with previous long-term occupational exposure to solvents. Occup Environ Med 1999; 56:93–105.

17. Anger WK, Sizemore OJ, Grossman SI, Glasser JA, Letz R, Bowler R. Human neurobehavioral research methods: impact of subject variables. Environ Res 1997; 73:18–41.

18. World Health Organization. Organic solvents and the central nervous system. Environmental Health 5. Copenhagen: WHO, 1985.

19. Åbjörnsson G, Palsson B, Bergendorf U, et al. Long-term follow-up of psychological distress, social functioning, and coping style in treated and untreated patients with solvent-induced chronic toxic encephalopathy. J Occup Environ Med 1998; 40:801–7

20. Brodkin C, Daniell W, Checkoway H, et al. Hepatic ultrasonic changes in workers exposed to perchloroethylene. Occup Environ Med 1995; 52:679–85.

21. Lundqvist G, Flodin U, Axelson O. A case-control study of fatty liver disease and organic solvent exposure. Am J Ind Med 1999; 35:132–6.

22. Santesson CG. Ueber chronische Vergiftungen mit Steinkohltheerbenzin; vier TodesfDlle. Arch Hyg 1897; 31:336–76.

23. Rinsky R, Smith A, Hornung R, et al. Benzene and leukemia. An epidemiologic risk assessment. N Engl J Med 1987; 316:1044–50.

24. Environmental Protection Agency. Carcinogenic effects of benzene: an update. Washington DC: US Environmental Protection Agency, 1998.

25. Antti-Poika M, Kalliokoski P, H Onninen O. Toluene. In: Snyder R, ed. Ethel Browning's toxicity and metabolism of industrial solvents, 2nd edn. Amsterdam: Elsevier, 1987.

26. International Agency for Research on Cancer. IARC Monographs on the Evaluation of Carcinogenic Risks to Humans. Volume 60. Some industrial chemicals. Lyon: IARC, 1994

27. International Agency for Research on Cancer. IARC Monographs on the Evaluation of Carcinogenic Risks to Humans. Volume 71. Lyon: IARC, 1999.

28. Grandjean E, Munchinger R, Turrian V, et al. Investigations into the effects of exposure to trichlorethylene in mechanical engineering. Br J Ind Med 1955; 12:131–42.

29. International Agency for Research on Cancer. IARC Monographs on the Evaluation of Carcinogenic Risks to Humans. Volume 63. Lyon: IARC, 1995.

30. Tas S, Lauwerys R, Lison D. Occupational hazards for the male reproductive system. Crit Rev Toxicol 1996; 26:261–307.

31. Nurminen M, Hernberg S. Effects of intervention on the cardiovascular mortality of workers exposed to carbon disulphide: a 15 year follow up. Br J Ind Med 1985; 42:32–5.

32. Droz PO. Biologic monitoring I: Sources of variability in human response to chemical exposure. Appl Ind Hyg 1989; 4:F-20–24.

33. Droz PO, Fernandez JG. Trichloroethylene exposure. Biologic monitoring by breath and urine analysis. Br J Ind Med 1978; 35:35–42.

34. Nise G. Urinary excretion of o-cresol and hippuric acid after toluene exposure in rotogravure printing. Int Arch Occup Environ Health 1992; 63:377–81.

35. Pauling T, Ogden I. Screening and neuropsychological assessment of spray painters at risk for organic solvent neurotoxicity. Int J Occup Environ Health 1996; 2:286–93.

36. Lundberg I, Hogberg M, Michelsen H, Nise G, Hogstedt C. Evaluation of the Q16 questionnaire on neurotoxic symptoms and a review of its use. Occup Environ Med 1997; 54: 343–50.

37. Svensson BG, Nise G, Englander V, Attewell R, Skerfving S, Maller T. Deaths and tumours among rotogravure printers exposed to toluene. Br J Ind Med 1990; 47:372–9.

38. Fiserova-Bergerova V. Gases and their solubility: a review of fundamentals. In: Fiserova-Bergerova V, ed. Modeling of inhalation exposure to vapors: uptake, distribution, and elimination. Vol. II. Boca Raton: CRC Press, 1983;3–28.

39. Sato A, Nakajima T. Partition coefficients of some aromatic hydrocarbons and ketones in water, blood and oil. Br J Ind Med 1979; 36:231–4.

40. Shmunes E. Solvents and plasticizers. In: Adams R, ed. Occupational skin disease, 2nd edn. Philadelphia: WB Saunders, 1990.

Chapter 41
Chemicals in the Plastics, Synthetic Textiles, and Rubber Industries

Steven Markowitz

PLASTICS INDUSTRY

Plastic materials are one of the fastest growing parts of the chemical industry in the United States. The industry produced 86 billion pounds of plastics in 2000 and experienced a 34% increase in production from 1967 to 2000. This industry employs 2% of the workforce in the United States and is geographically spread throughout the country in many thousands of plants that manufacture and process plastic resins and compounds. The plastics industry represents a $330 billion economic sector.

Much of this industry's growth has been facilitated by rapid changes in plastics technology, which in turn enable increasingly diverse uses of plastics materials. Although the bulk of plastics is used in packaging and consumer products, newer uses of plastics are being developed, especially in building and construction, in which more than 20% of all plastics is currently used. Plastic materials have significantly displaced glass and wood for many industrial and commercial purposes and are rapidly encroaching on the traditional domain of numerous metals.

The prominence of the plastics industry necessarily has important ramifications for occupational health, especially in terms of the size of the exposed population and the nature and range of potential exposures. In 2000, the plastics industry employed 2.4 million workers in approximately 21,000 establishments in the United States. The majority of these workplaces and their workers are involved in processing plastics and in the fabrication of products, with many fewer involved in transforming basic materials into plastic resins. This workforce is potentially exposed to thousands of chemical substances that are used in the production and modification of plastics. Like most chemical substances in the workplace, many of the chemicals used to make plastics have not been fully evaluated for toxicity. Hence, the clinician is faced with an increasingly daunting task of understanding the relationship between the health problems of workers and their complex and frequently unstudied occupational exposures.

It is necessary, therefore, to use a sound general approach in the evaluation of workers and others who may be exposed to chemical agents in the formation, processing, and combustion of plastics. Such an approach requires a basic understanding of the plastics industry, recognition of the opportunities for exposure to various toxins, knowledge of the well-documented serious hazards in the industry, and finally, an appreciation of the relative deficiency in the current scientific database on the potential health effects of plastics materials.

The production of finished plastic pieces has three principal components: (1) the synthesis of plastic polymers, (2) the mixing and compounding of additives to the resin material, and (3) the conversion of the compounded polymer into useful products (Fig. 41.1). These components are achieved in different and distinct processes, use largely different sets of materials, and usually occur at different worksites. Hence, although there may be some overlap in hazards that are related to these components of the plastics industry, sufficient differences exist to warrant recognition of the specific hazards that accompany each.

The manufacture of the plastic polymer is achieved by converting basic raw materials (which are simple organic chemicals, usually derived from petroleum fractions) from the monomeric state to the relatively pure polymer, which is called a resin. A monomer is a low molecular weight molecule with the capacity to combine covalently with itself to form a repeating chain, termed a polymer. The resultant high molecular weight polymer consists of a backbone with attached side groups of radicals. Polymers vary in the chemical nature of their backbone and side groups and, thereby, have different properties. Other factors, such as the distribution of molecular weight, degree of crystallinity, and extent of cross linking between polymer chains, also determine the physical properties and, therefore, potential utility of plastic polymers. Two or more different monomers can be reacted in different combinations, usually in the presence of a catalyst, such as an organometal compound, to form a copolymer.

The first phase of production of plastics, polymerization, is usually achieved in large-scale operations performed in closed systems (Fig. 41.1). The exposure may be to the raw materials, the chemical intermediates, the catalysts, or the polymer products. Significant exposure to plastic monomers is, for the most part, restricted to this phase of plastics manufacturing. Workers employed in this phase of the industry experience a variable degree of exposure, depending on the age and capitalization of the plant and the type of job performed by the worker. The resins produced in this industry are usually formulated into pellets, granules, or powders for shipment to plants that compound and process the resin.

Plastic resins are usually mixed or compounded with additives to acquire added desired qualities in the second phase of plastics manufacture (Fig. 41.1). Although the

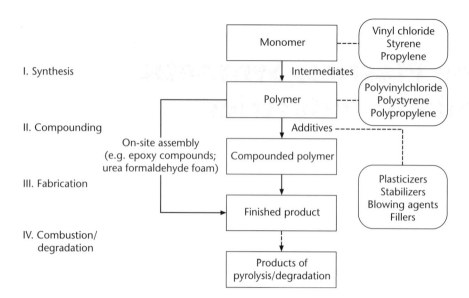

I. Synthesis

II. Compounding

III. Fabrication

IV. Combustion/
degradation

Figure 41.1: General paradigm for plastics production, fabrication into products, and degradation.

chief health concerns in this phase center on the potential hazards associated with the additives, exposure to the polymer and residual monomer leaching from the polymer should not be neglected. These additives include plasticizers to enhance flexibility, fillers to provide bulk, reinforcers to lend strength, blowing agents to act as a foaming mechanism, impact modifiers to improve strength and process ability, stabilizers to prevent thermal degradation and oxidation, antistatic agents to reduce friction and/or electrical charges, and others with self-explanatory functions, such as flame retardants, catalysts, lubricants, and colorants. By the tonnage used, the major additives are fillers, reinforcing fibers, and plasticizers, which account for more than 75% of the total volume of additives.

Additives are principally divided into two groups: (1) fillers and reinforced fibers, which are usually minerals and metals, and (2) chemical additives, which most often involve organic chemicals. The major fillers in order of the quantities used include calcium carbonates, kaolin and other silicates, carbon black, and wood flour. More than three-quarters of all fillers are used in polyvinyl chloride and unsaturated polyester products. Fiberglass is the chief reinforcement fiber used in plastics. Among the chemical additives, phthalates, including diethylhexyl phthalate and diisodecyl phthalate, represent the most important plasticizers used, with additional limited use of epoxy compounds and organic phosphates. The major colorant is titanium dioxide pigment, with a much lesser role played by cadmium, chromium, and iron oxide. Among the organic pigments, phthalocyanine blue and phthalocyanine green are the most important agents.

The major stabilizers include, in order of importance, barium-cadmium soaps, lead compounds, organotins, and calcium-zinc soaps. The additives significantly expand the range of potentially hazardous exposures of workers in the plastics industry.

In the third phase of plastics manufacture, the transformation of compounded resins into finished products requires the application of heat and/or pressure to the formulated materials, and subsequent shaping by molding, blowing, and other processes. Even in this final phase, workers in the plastics processing industry may be exposed to unreacted monomers, intermediates, or additives retained in the formulated resin materials. Overheating of resins may lead to the formation of combustion products that have not been fully characterized, but may be toxic. Finally, finishing processes, such as cutting and grinding of materials, may create polymer dust exposure; although this step of the plastics production industry has been traditionally considered the least hazardous.

Selected important plastics systems do not follow these orderly phases. The various components of finished epoxy resins and polyurethane foams (see subsequent sections) are often assembled and reacted at the site of use of the finished products. The potentially hazardous exposures presented by the agents involved may therefore not be restricted to a relatively circumscribed group of workers at centralized sites where conditions may be carefully controlled. Rather, the field use of these plastics may lead to uncontrolled occupational and environmental exposures to relatively large numbers of users who are unfamiliar with the attendant hazards.

Workers other than those directly employed in the plastics industry may have important exposures to plastics and related materials. Combustion products of plastics represent a major concern to fire fighters because residences and offices are increasingly filled with these products. Users of plastics products, such as food wrappers, are exposed to combustion products, such as hydrogen chloride and phosgene, and have developed respiratory disease as a result. The hazards inherent in the use of plastics materials are clearly not confined to the plastics industry workforce.

Table 41.1 lists the most important plastic polymers and synthetic textiles in the order of the volume currently produced in the United States. Plastics are broadly categorized as thermoplastics, which can be reprocessed, and thermosets, which are chemically altered with application of heat and, therefore, cannot be reheated without losing

Polyethylene
Polypropylene
Vinyl chloride/polyvinyl chloride
Fluoropolymers (Teflon)
Epoxy resins
Amino resins
Acrylics (including acrylamide)
Polyurethane
Plastic additives
Polyamides (nylon)
Polyesters
Rayon

Table 41.1 Major plastics and synthetic textiles

Organ/disease	Examples of agents
Skin	Epichlorohydrin
Contact dermatitis (allergic and irritant)	Formaldehyde
Vitiligo	Hydroquinone
Toxic epidermal necrolysis	Acrylonitrile
Scleroderma-like changes	Vinyl chloride
Lung	Ethyl acrylate
Irritation	Formaldehyde
	Epichlorohydrin
	Isocyanates
Asthma	Phthalic anhydride
	Isocyanates
	Trimellitic anhydride
	Epichlorhydrin
Hypersensitivity pneumonitis	Isocyanates
	Anhydrides (phthalic, trimellitic)
Pneumoconiosis	Phenolic resin dust
Polymer fume fever	Polyvinyl chloride
	Polytetrafluoroethylene
Bone	
Acro-osteolysis	Vinyl chloride
Liver	
Hepatitis	Vinyl chloride
Cirrhosis	Vinyl chloride
Nervous system	
Peripheral neuropathy	Methyl methacrylate
	Styrene
	Acrylamide
Encephalopathy	Vinyl chloride
	Styrene
Cancer	
Brain	Formaldehyde (suspected)
	Vinyl chloride (reported)
Leukemia	Formaldehyde (reported)
	Acrylonitrile (reported)
	Vinyl chloride (reported)
Lymphoma	Styrene (suspected)
Liver (hemangiosarcoma)	Vinyl chloride (known)

Table 41.2 Selected occupational diseases in the plastics and synthetic textiles industry

essential properties. Most of the polymers in Table 41.1 are thermoplastics, with the exception of the phenolics, polyurethanes, epoxies, urea, and melamine, which are thermosets.

Table 41.2 presents an overview of the spectrum of diseases that have been observed following exposure to one or more agents used in the plastics industry. Of principal concern have been the organs of direct contact, the skin and the respiratory system, including effects of irrita-

tion, allergy, and carcinogenicity. Additional details are presented by the specific agent in the following sections.

Polyethylene

Ethylene

Polyethylene is an important bulk plastic with high- and low-density forms. Low-density polyethylene is used principally in the manufacture of films, sheets, and layered packaging materials. High-density polyethylene is usually molded into containers, toys, and housewares.

In the polymerization phase, ethylene is the monomer used to produce polyethylene. Indeed, ethylene is the raw material used in the greatest volume in the plastics industry and ranks among the ten chemicals with the highest tonnage produced in United States. Ethylene is used in the formation of other monomers or intermediates, such as styrene, ethylene oxide, and vinyl chloride, which are used to make polystyrene, polyurethane, and polyvinyl chloride (PVC), respectively. Small amounts of ethylene are also used as a refrigerant and as a fruit-ripening agent. Ethylene is derived from the cracking of petroleum and, to a lesser extent, from the processing of natural gas. Ethylene production in the United States was 40 billion pounds in 1994.

Ethylene is highly combustible when exposed to heat or flame, and can react vigorously with oxidizing chemicals. It acts as a simple asphyxiant, posing a hazard by the displacement of oxygen from the breathing atmosphere. The anesthetic potential of ethylene has been exploited clinically; however, its tendency to produce hypoxia, its explosiveness, and its variable clinical utility have limited its use. The clinical experience with its use as an anesthetic agent has limited relevance to the occupational setting because the concentrations of ethylene used in anesthesia were much higher than those typically experienced in the workplace. A review by the International Agency for Research against Cancer (IARC) in 1987 identified no data on ethylene's carcinogenicity from human or animal studies.

The thermal degradation products of polyethylene include carbon monoxide, acrolein, and formaldehyde. Asthma has been reported among workers heating polyethylene film as part of food-wrapping activity; the film used reportedly contained no additives. However, this entity is much more often reported in food wrappers exposed to the pyrolytic products of PVC film.

Polypropylene

Propylene

Polypropylene is a bulk plastic characterized by relative strength, heat resistance, and durability. It is used principally in molded products and in fibrous form in carpeting and clothing. Polypropylene materials, such as pipes and moldings, are also increasingly welded in small workshops to produce custom items. Such use presents opportunities for exposure to polypropylene combustion products outside the more widely recognized exposures entailed in the manufacture of polypropylene.

The polymer is formed from propylene in the presence of a solvent (e.g., xylene or butyl alcohol) and an organometal catalyst (e.g., titanium trichloride). Propylene, like ethylene, is obtained through the cracking of petroleum hydrocarbons. Although it is mainly used as a monomer in the formation of polypropylene, it also serves as a fuel and as a raw material in the production of acrylonitrile, isopropyl alcohol, polyurethane, epoxy resins, and other plastics. It is second only to ethylene as a raw material in plastics manufacturing, with approximately 23 billion pounds produced and used in the United States in 1994, primarily to make 15.7 billion pounds of polypropylene. Like ethylene, propylene is highly flammable when mixed with air or oxygen. The liquid form of propylene can cause freezing burns of the skin or eyes. It is a simple asphyxiant, and it can produce progressive symptoms and signs of hypoxia with increased exposure.

While polypropylene manufacture has generally been regarded as a safe industrial process, epidemiologic studies have raised concern regarding an association with colorectal cancer. An epidemiologic study of workers in polypropylene manufacture demonstrated a 5.6-fold elevation in colorectal cancer incidence, occurring chiefly among workers less than 60 years of age and with a duration of employment of at least 20 years.[1] A subsequent company-sponsored colorectal polyp screening program found an increased prevalence of colorectal adenomatous polyps in the same workforce, especially among mechanical and process workers with a latency of at least 20 years.[2] A detailed case-control analysis indicated that the excess prevalence of polyps was limited to two processes within the plant, and was probably not due to confounding.[3] In the only other relevant study, from a synthetic textile plant, workers employed for more than five years in the polypropylene and cellulose triacetate extrusion unit showed a 5.5-fold excess in colon cancer incidence and mortality.[4]

Vinyl chloride, polyvinyl chloride, and related chemicals

Vinyl chloride

Vinyl Chloride

Vinyl chloride ranks among the top 20 chemicals in terms of the volume produced in the United States, with 13.8 billion pounds manufactured in 1994. It is principally produced by the thermal cracking of ethylene dichloride. Almost the entire production of vinyl chloride in the United States is devoted to the manufacture of PVC, which is used to make pipes, wire and cable coating, packaging material, housewares, and automotive parts. Small amounts of vinyl chloride are used to make mixed polymers, such as vinyl chloride-vinyl acetate, vinyl chloride-acrylonitrile, and vinyl chloride-vinylidine chloride.

Nervous system effects Vinyl chloride is an anesthetic at high levels of air-borne exposure in the range of 3000–10,000 ppm. Symptoms of central nervous system toxicity, including headache, lightheadedness, and dizziness, were commonly reported by workers in PVC polymerization plants until the 1970s; even loss of consciousness was not uncommon. After the carcinogenic effect of vinyl chloride was reported in 1974, the air-borne levels of exposure to vinyl chloride decreased dramatically, leading to the disappearance of notable central nervous system symptoms. Of interest is a study reporting a mild distal axonal neuropathy in the majority of vinyl chloride workers at a PVC polymerization plant in Italy.[5]

Skeletal and vascular effects Vinyl chloride causes acro-osteolysis, a unique syndrome consisting of resorption of bone from the terminal phalanges of the fingers and toes, Raynaud's syndrome, and scleroderma-like skin alterations. This syndrome was first reported in the late 1950s, and was documented in 3–6% of workers studied in the 1960s and the 1970s. Variable changes include cortical bone defects (termed transverse or half moon) in the distal phalanges of the fingers and toes, with subsequent complete resorption of bony tufts in severe cases. These bony abnormalities have a characteristic appearance on x-ray; the large bones are occasionally involved, with the appearance of cystic lesions and areas of increased radiolucency; there may also be alterations in the patella and sacroiliac joint. Bony lesions are usually painless.

Raynaud's syndrome in the hands and feet may be seen in a small percentage of exposed workers as part of the acro-osteolysis syndrome. More commonly, symptoms of numbness, tingling, and sensitivity to cold are reported, without the dramatic vascular changes characterized by Raynaud's syndrome. Some workers also have thickened and tense skin that is suggestive of scleroderma. The pathogenesis of this disorder is not known but may involve a primary effect of vinyl chloride on the arteries and arterioles of the extremities. Alternatively, immunologic alterations may be important in the pathogenesis of this disease, as suggested by the fact that cryoglobulins have been reported in a large percentage of acro-osteolysis cases.

Historically, acro-osteolysis occurred among workers with high levels of exposure to vinyl chloride, most often among workers who clean PVC reactor vessels with exposure to vinyl chloride in the thousands of parts per million; fewer cases have occurred following drastic reductions in exposure.

An interesting case of Raynaud's phenomenon and severe polymyositis in association with anti-Jo1 antibody was recently reported in a man with long-term vinyl chloride exposure.[6] Whether vinyl chloride initiates a myopathic process has not been otherwise investigated.

Hepatic effects Vinyl chloride causes non-malignant and malignant liver disease, including inflammation and a characteristic periportal fibrosis (see Chapter 26.1). The observed hepatotoxicity ranges from the asymptomatic presence of liver function abnormalities to hepatic fibrosis with accompanying portal hypertension, esophageal varices, and splenomegaly. Hepatic fibrosis may be present without abnormalities in liver function tests. The pathology of vinyl chloride-associated hepatotoxicity includes a characteristic pattern of hepatoportal sclerosis, capsular, and subcapsular fibrosis; and focal irregular dilatation of the sinusoids. Cross-sectional studies of workers in the mid-1970s found that 10–25% of vinyl chloride workers had liver function abnormalities, not all of which could be ascribed to the chemical. Excess hospitalization rates for liver cirrhosis were found among Taiwanese vinyl chloride workers.[7] A marked increase in cirrhosis-related mortality was observed in the combined European vinyl chloride industry study.[8]

Cancer Vinyl chloride-induced cancer was first demonstrated in animals in 1971. Three years later, hemangiosarcoma of the liver was observed in three vinyl chloride workers. The association of this rare tumor with vinyl chloride was further confirmed by the reporting of a total of 27 cases among vinyl chloride workers in the United States and Europe by 1975. Like arsenic and thorotrast, vinyl chloride is one of the few agents known to cause hemangiosarcoma of the liver. Most afflicted workers have had long-term vinyl chloride exposure, and the disease has developed following a 10–15-year latency period. As of 1999, there were approximately 200 reported cases of vinyl chloride-associated angiosarcoma of the liver, mostly from the US and Europe.[9]

Vinyl chloride has been associated with other cancers, although none have demonstrated the strength and consistency of the relationship between vinyl chloride and hemangiosarcoma of the liver. The largest study to date, involving 3191 deaths among 10,109 workers at 37 plants in the United States, was undertaken by Mundt and others on behalf of the Chemical Manufacturers Association (CMA).[10] Significant increases in cancer of the brain, connective tissue, and soft tissue were identified, especially among workers with 20 or more years of cumulative exposure to vinyl chloride. Smaller Swedish[11] and German studies have also found an increase in brain cancer risk among vinyl chloride workers, although a major British study[12] and the European cohort study as a whole[8] did not observe the same magnitude of risk. Wong and associates, who investigated the US cohort prior to Mundt, found an increase in the risk of cancer of the biliary tract and of hepatic tumors other than hemangiosarcoma;[13] this has recently been confirmed in a Taiwanese study.[14] An excess lung

cancer risk has been reported in some smaller studies, but has not been corroborated in larger studies. Increased cancer risk among vinyl chloride workers has also been observed for malignant melanoma, thyroid cancer, and lymphopoietic cancers.

Respiratory effects Vinyl chloride and PVC are associated with a variety of non-malignant respiratory diseases. In a large cross-sectional study reported in 1976, Lilis and others found that approximately 20% of workers at two PVC polymerization facilities had linear-reticular and, less frequently, nodular opacities on chest x-ray studies.[15] Subsequent cross-sectional studies of PVC manufacturing workers also showed small opacities on the chest radiographs, although at lesser rates.[16] Both obstructive and restrictive dysfunction has been observed. Notably, the study with the highest rate of pneumoconiotic opacities also demonstrated the highest rate of pulmonary function abnormalities.[17] The accumulated data suggest that there may be more than one disease process present in these studies, characterized by both pulmonary fibrosis and chronic obstructive pulmonary changes. Wong and coworkers found a significant excess in mortality from chronic obstructive pulmonary disease in vinyl chloride and PVC workers, providing further evidence that vinyl chloride and PVC, especially the latter, cause chronic airway obstruction of clinical significance.[13]

There have been additional case reports of granulomatous pulmonary reactions and desquamative interstitial pneumonitis in association with exposure to PVC dust. Of interest is a report of a PVC worker with dyspnea, irregular opacities on chest x-ray studies, and restrictive pulmonary dysfunction, who underwent a lung biopsy. The results showed pulmonary fibrosis and a granulomatous reaction. Similar pathologic findings have been produced in rats exposed to PVC dust.[18] In another case report, a group of investigators have documented a case of interstitial pneumonitis verified by histopathologic studies in a worker cleaning PVC from a reaction vessel.

The pyrolytic products of PVC film and associated adhesive labels can cause respiratory irritation and asthma, commonly known as meat wrappers' asthma. This was first noted in case reports in the early 1970s, and has been corroborated by cross-sectional epidemiologic studies of meat wrappers. In this work setting, PVC plastic wrap is cut with a hot knife, causing PVC degradation and production of hydrogen chloride and di(2-ethylhexyl) adipate. Pyrolysis of an accompanying price label adhesive, when present, may produce other allergenic agents, such as phthalic anhydride and dicyclo-hexylphthalate, with independent bronchospastic responses.

Vinylidine chloride

Vinylidine Chloride

Vinylidine chloride is used primarily in the formation of copolymers with vinyl chloride or acrylonitrile. It is produced from ethylene dichloride and vinyl chloride through successive chlorination and dechlorination reactions. The combustion products include hydrogen chloride. Vinylidine chloride is an irritant to the eyes, mucous membranes, and lungs. Exposure to high concentrations in the air causes narcosis. Chronic exposure to vinylidine chloride has been shown to cause fetal, hepatic, and renal damage in animals.

Vinylidine chloride causes neoplasms in animals, including renal adenocarcinomas.[19] It is mutagenic in short-term bacterial assays. The two epidemiologic studies completed to date showed no increase in cancer deaths among vinylidine chloride-exposed workers, but were limited by the occurrence of few deaths and a short latency.[19]

Ethylene dichloride

Ethylene Dichloride

Ethylene dichloride, or 1,2-dichloroethane, is a chemical intermediate in the production of vinyl chloride. It is additionally used in the manufacture of acrylic adhesives, rubber cement, leather and metal cleaners, and rubber goods. Approximately 18 billion pounds of this agent were used in the United States in 1993. Ethylene dichloride has an odor that is generally considered pleasant and may not be detectable at levels that are hazardous. Important combustion products include phosgene, hydrogen chloride, acetylene, and vinyl chloride, presenting an irritant and carcinogenic hazard.

Early Eastern European reports of morbidity associated with occupational exposure to ethylene dichloride in a variety of industries indicate that irritation of the mucous membranes, liver function abnormalities, and central nervous system symptoms can result from chronic exposure to this chemical. Ethylene dichloride has also been found in the breast milk of women occupationally exposed to the agent, necessitating an avoidance of exposure in women during breast feeding.

In a recent review (1999), IARC concluded that there is sufficient evidence of the carcinogenicity of ethylene dichloride in animals, and therefore it is a potential human carcinogen.[19] In general, epidemiologic studies suggest ethylene chloride may contribute to a significant elevation in mortality from lymphatic and hematopoietic cancer and, in one study, cancer of the stomach, although there were other coexisting exposures.[19]

The National Institute for Occupational Safety and Health (NIOSH) has recommended that workers exposed to ethylene dichloride receive an annual examination, including a medical and work history, assessing cardiovascular, pulmonary, neurologic, and liver function; the benefit of specific surveillance tests in this setting is unproven.

Fluoropolymers

Tetrafluoroethylene

Polytetrafluoroethylene (PTFE) is a polymer of tetrafluoroethylene with the commercial name Teflon. PTFE, when heated to 315–475 degrees C, produces polymer fume fever, an illness clinically similar to metal fume fever. First described 40 years ago, this syndrome is characterized by fever, chills, malaise, cough, and chest pain. Some individuals may also experience joint pains, nausea, and vomiting. Polymer fume fever is usually a self-limited illness that occurs within several hours following exposure to the pyrolytic products of PTFE, and resolves within a few days. Although most affected workers have only the described symptoms, there have been case reports of pulmonary edema occurring as part of the clinical picture of polymer fume fever. Complete resolution of the syndrome following an attack is typical, although long-term studies have not been performed. One case report found pathologic evidence of interstitial pulmonary fibrosis in a worker after repeated episodes of polymer fume fever.

Polymer fume fever has occurred in a variety of environments in which PTFE has been used, including generation of PTFE aerosol as a mold-release spray. PTFE-impregnated or contaminated material can also be a source of exposure.[20] The pyrolysis required for the syndrome to develop may occur as a result of the industrial process or as a result of the burning of contaminated cigarettes (e.g., smoking during work breaks). The exact pyrolytic products responsible for the syndrome have not been identified, but suspected agents include carbonyl fluoride, tetrafluoroethylene, hydrogen fluoride, and other fluorinated compounds.

Epoxy resins

Epoxide Ring

Epoxy resins are polymers containing an epoxide ring, which are formed through the reaction of uncured resin material with a curing agent. The uncured resin consists of epichlorohydrin, diluents, fillers, and pigments. The principal diluents are glycidyl ethers, especially the diglycidyl ether of bisphenol A, and various solvents. Important curing agents include acid anhydrides and aliphatic and aromatic amines. Epoxy resins differ from many other plastics in that they are cured at the site of use of the final product. Epoxy resins are used as adhesives, laminating materials, reinforcing agents, and surface coatings.

While most of the health effects of epoxy resins have now been associated with specific components of the resin, some health problems have been associated with epoxy resins per se. Lymphocytopenia was identified in a screening program of pattern and model makers, particularly automobile-manufacturing workers, who have myriad exposures. A history of epoxy resin and plastic dusts exposures provided the highest relative risks for low lymphocyte counts.[21] Shipyard workers using epoxy resin-based paints showed higher rates of cough, dyspnea, and cross worksheet declines in FEV_1 compared to unexposed shipyard painters.[22]

Epichlorohydrin

Epichlorohydrin

Epichlorohydrin is widely used in the manufacture of epoxy resins, pharmaceuticals, plasticizers, adhesives, and various elastomers. The current Occupational Safety and Health Administration (OSHA) Permissible Exposure Limit is 2 ppm as an 8-hour time-weighted average, although NIOSH has recommended that the exposure be at the lowest level possible.

Epichlorohydrin is a strong irritant and allergen, and principally affects the skin, mucous membranes, and respiratory tract. There is limited evidence of hepatotoxicity in humans. Animal studies have demonstrated both liver and kidney injury following exposure to epichlorohydrin.

Epichlorohydrin is an animal carcinogen. Elevated rates of chromosomal aberrations and sister chromatid exchanges have been documented in workers exposed to epichlorohydrin.[23] Several cohort mortality studies have been completed, including investigations at two major United States epichlorohydrin-producing facilities. An earlier finding of excess leukemia in a cohort mortality study was not confirmed in a recent update of the same cohort.[24,25] However, a nested case-control study of lung cancer in a different epichlorohydrin-exposed cohort demonstrated an excess risk of lung cancer associated with epichlorohydrin exposure.[26] A European study with a limited number of deaths, and low statistical power identified no increased risk of lung cancer. IARC classifies epichlorohydrin as a probable human carcinogen.[19]

Epichlorohydrin is a possible reproductive toxin. Oral administration of epichlorohydrin produces irreversible infertility in male rats, after a single high dose. In limited human studies to date, no alterations have been noted in sperm count and morphology or in the fertility status of workers exposed to epichlorohydrin.

Glycidyl ethers

Glycidyl ethers are principally used with epichlorohydrin to form epoxy resins. The diglycidyl ether of bisphenol A is the major agent used in this class; others include n-butyl

Glycidyl Ether

glycidyl ether and phenyl glycidyl ether. These agents are clearly responsible for some of the irritation and sensitization that have been observed among epoxy resin manufacturing workers; however, the relative disease-producing role of the glycidyl ethers as compared to epichlorohydrin and various amines may be difficult to determine. Newly introduced glycidyl ethers, such as ortho-cresyl glycidyl ether and diethylene glycol diglycidyl ether, also cause allergic contact dermatitis.[27]

Animal studies show that some glycidyl ethers may cause testicular atrophy in rodents, as well as a range of hematopoietic abnormalities, including atrophy of lymphoid tissue and bone marrow toxicity. Studies of these effects in humans have not been completed, but the repeated demonstration of these effects in animals has raised substantial concerns.

Diglycidyl resorcinol ether is a confirmed animal carcinogen, and there is limited evidence that the diglycidyl ether of bisphenol A is an animal carcinogen. The potential carcinogenicity of the glycidyl ethers in humans has not been well investigated.

Acid anhydrides

Acid Anhydride

This family of chemicals includes well-known agents, such as phthalic anhydride, trimellitic anhydride, and maleic anhydride, and other lesser known agents, such as tetra-chlorophthalic anhydride, hexahydrophthalic anhydride, and himic anhydride, all of which have been shown to cause human disease. Acid anhydrides have a variety of uses and are commonly employed agents in industry. As noted previously, acid anhydrides are used as curing or hardening agents for epoxy resins. They are also used in the production of plasticizers, polyester resins, and alkyd resins, the latter of which are important in the formulation of paints, varnishes, and reinforced plastics. Phthalic anhydride is the most commonly utilized agent, with a volume of nearly 1 billion pounds produced in the United States in 1994.

Clinical effects Acid anhydrides are severe direct irritants and have caused chemical burns of the skin, corneal ulceration, epistaxis, and hemoptysis. These severe irritant effects were more common in the 1940s and 1950s, when the exposure levels were considerably higher than they are at present.

Hypersensitivity to acid anhydrides may result in allergic rhinitis, conjunctivitis, urticaria, and asthma. Indeed, acid anhydrides are among the most well-documented agents capable of producing occupational asthma. Several dozen published reports have been cited as documenting acid anhydride-induced asthma, mostly caused by phthalic anhydride and, to a lesser extent, trimellitic and maleic anhydride.[28]

Inhalation challenge tests have documented acid anhydride-induced asthma. Nearly all patients that have been tested to date show a dual response to bronchoprovocation, including an initial fall of the forced expiratory volume in 1 second (FEV_1) within the first hour, and a second decline in FEV_1 several hours after exposure. Very low exposures to acid anhydrides in the bronchoprovocation protocol are often sufficient to induce the asthmatic response in sensitized individuals.

Almost all workers with acid anhydride-induced asthma have immunoglobulin E (IgE) antibody that is specifically reactive to an acid anhydride-protein conjugate, as demonstrated by RAST testing. Such specific IgE antibody can also be found, although uncommonly, in workers without asthma who are merely exposed to acid anhydride. More recently, an IgG antibody specific for acid anhydride was identified in exposed patients with asthma, but may not represent a specific marker of clinical hypersensitivity.

Most documented cases of acid anhydride-related asthma occur within the first few years of exposure. As in other causes of occupational asthma, the symptoms may improve after leaving the work environment, but bronchospasm sufficient to require medication has been demonstrated to persist following cessation of exposure.

Another syndrome associated with exposure to acid anhydrides is a condition described as 'trimellitic flu' (also known as 'late respiratory distress syndrome'), which has been shown to occur following exposure to trimellitic or phthalic anhydride. This syndrome includes myalgias, malaise, fever, and respiratory symptoms, which occur following a workshift. The chest x-ray studies in affected workers are usually normal, but may document the presence of extrinsic allergic alveolitis. Except for the prominence of respiratory symptoms, this syndrome is similar to polymer or metal fume fever. An immunologic origin for this syndrome is likely; however, a direct toxicity of the relevant acid anhydride has not been excluded.

Besides direct irritation, asthma, rhinitis, and late respiratory distress syndrome, trimellitic anhydride has been shown to cause, albeit rarely, pulmonary hemorrhage, also called pulmonary disease-anemia syndrome.[29] This syndrome is characterized by hemoptysis, pulmonary infiltrates, and hemolytic anemia. Lung biopsy results show non-specific alterations of acute lung injury. This syndrome, which has usually followed high exposure to trimellitic anhydride, may be severe and requires emergency medical attention. Whether this response represents hypersensitivity or direct toxicity is unknown.

The mortality of workers exposed to acid anhydrides has not been well investigated. A case-control study of lung cancer in a factory in Italy, that produced and used,

phthalic anhydride reported a significant increase in lung cancer after controling for cigarette smoking.[30] The extent to which phthalic anhydride may be responsible for the observed excess lung cancer risk is unclear. The limited animal studies performed to date have not confirmed that phthalic anhydride is a carcinogen.

Evaluation The clinical evaluation of symptomatic workers varies according to the clinical syndrome that is present. In cases of asthma, inhalation challenge testing is generally not necessary when the presence of asthma and the acid anhydride exposure are both documented. Measuring the level of acid anhydride-specific IgE antibody may be helpful. The diagnosis of the late respiratory distress syndrome may be delayed unless a high level of clinical suspicion is maintained. Any exposed worker with symptoms suggestive of a syndrome involving pulmonary hemorrhage requires immediate evaluation.

Biologic monitoring of a number of the phthalic anhydrides is possible, assessing metabolites in urine or serum.[31] Protein adducts have also been measured and show excellent correlation with urinary metabolites; and these have the advantage of providing a measure of cumulative exposure of several months rather than current exposure.[32]

Prevention Awareness by exposed workers and their physicians about the spectrum of health problems associated with the acid anhydrides is essential. Exposure should be restricted to as few workers as possible, and to the lowest achievable levels. There is some evidence that very low levels of phthalic anhydrides may not be associated with disease; a recent longitudinal study showed that a large number of workers exposed to a mean of < 2 micrograms/m^3 did not develop any evidence of respiratory disease during a three-year period.[33] Nonetheless, minimizing exposure is essential. Proper engineering controls, supplemented by personal protective equipment, are the mainstays of prevention. In general, early identification of individuals who demonstrate clinical hypersensitivity to acid anhydrides is prudent to reduce or eliminate the exposure.

Amino resins

Amino resins are produced by the combination of formaldehyde and an amine, principally melamine or urea. The primary products include urea-formaldehyde foam, adhesives, laminates, and various textile finishing materials designed to reduce creases. In addition to possible occupational exposures, this class of materials has posed potential environmental concerns to consumers using formaldehyde-based products.

Formaldehyde

Formaldehyde is a widely used raw material in the manufacture of plastic resins and other commercially important products. It has found broad industrial application because of its high reactivity, low cost, and colorless nature. One half of all formaldehyde production in the United States is

O
‖
H — C — H

Formaldehyde

used to make urea-formaldehyde and phenolic resins. The dominant uses of these formaldehyde-based resins are in the production of plywood, particle board, foam insulation, and a variety of molded plastic items. The remaining formaldehyde production is used to make melamine, pentaerythritol, hexamethylenetetramine, fertilizers, and other materials. Formaldehyde has an important use in the textile industry; it forms the basis of products that render textiles crease proof, flame resistant, and shrink proof. Formaldehyde has antiviral and antibacterial properties and has been used extensively in cosmetics, embalming fluids, and selected medicines. The United States produced approximately 7.6 billion pounds of aqueous formaldehyde in 1993.

Clinical effects   Formaldehyde has a pungent odor and is highly irritating to the skin, eyes, and lungs. Sensitivity to formaldehyde varies, and some irritant effects can be experienced at or below the current legal standard of 0.1 ppm PEL, established by OSHA. Exposure to this chemical may result in tolerance, although 1–2 hours following cessation of exposure, the characteristic odor and effect of formaldehyde once again become apparent. The severe effects on the lungs after high exposure may include chemical pneumonitis or pulmonary edema.

Formaldehyde has been known to cause skin sensitization since the early 1900s. It has been linked to asthma, although not commonly. Such formaldehyde-induced asthma may be related to its irritant properties; there is also evidence of an immunologic mechanism. A six-year follow-up study of workers who produced urea-formaldehyde observed that exposed workers experienced similar respiratory symptoms as an unexposed group, but exposed non-smokers suffered a mean decline in FEV_1 that was 50% higher than unexposed non-smokers; no similar exposure-related effect was seen among smokers.[34]

Formaldehyde causes dose-related, site-specific cancer in animals. Studies in the late 1970s and early 1980s demonstrated an unequivocal increase in squamous cell carcinoma in the nasal passages in rats; the evidence was sufficient for IARC to conclude that formaldehyde is an animal carcinogen. Formaldehyde is a potent mutagen and genotoxic agent, inducing mutations, elevated rates of lymphocyte sister chromatid exchanges, and chromosomal aberrations.

In 1995, IARC revised its designation of formaldehyde as a probable human carcinogen (group 2A).[35] Epidemiologic evidence favors a causal link between formaldehyde and nasopharyngeal and sinonasal cancer. Additional studies variably show excess rates of other types of cancer such as leukemia and cancer of the lung and brain; interpretation has been challenging, given confounding occupational exposures and heterogeneity of findings according to type of workers (e.g., professionals versus industrial workers).[36,37]

Evaluation and prevention   The evaluation of suspected work-related health problems among formaldehyde-exposed workers should center on the known irritant and allergic effects of this chemical on the skin, mucous membranes, and respiratory tract. With respect to medical surveillance, formaldehyde is one of the few agents for which OSHA has specific provisions. These provisions include a medical questionnaire, physical examination, and spirometry, that apply to all workers who are exposed to formaldehyde at or above the action level (OSHA PEL 0.75 ppm time-weighted average) or at or above the short-term exposure level (2 ppm for 15 minutes). Physicians should be aware that OSHA requires the employer to provide the examining physician with a copy of its formaldehyde standard, a description of the worker's job duties, relevant exposure monitoring data, information concerning personal protective equipment, and the results from previous medical examinations.[38]

Urea

O
‖
H — N — C — N — H
  | |
  H   H

Urea

Urea is used in combination with formaldehyde to produce resins and adhesives, and is also used in the production of melamine. Urea is among the top 20 most commonly produced agents in the United States, with most of its use devoted to the production of fertilizer and livestock feed. Urea has low toxicity in the occupational setting. Most of the human experience with urea exposure is related to the former medicinal use of urea as a diuretic agent.

Melamine

H — N — H
    |
    C
   ⫽ ⟍
  N   N
  | ‖
H—N—C   C—N—H
  | ⟍ ⫽ |
  H   N   H

Melamine

Melamine is an important chemical substance, which is usually mixed with formaldehyde to make amino resins for use in laminates, molding compounds, surface coatings, paper coatings, textile printing, and adhesives. Melamine and urea production combined was 3.2 billion pounds in the United States and Canada in 2000. Melamine can be hazardous when burned because its pyrolytic products include hydrogen cyanide.

Melamine has produced urinary calculi with associated epithelial hyperplasia and transitional cell carcinoma of the bladder in rats. The human toxicity of melamine is obscured by its usual mixture with formaldehyde and other agents with better documented toxicity. A review of animal studies by IARC in 1987 noted that there was insufficient evidence concerning the animal carcinogenicity of melamine.[39]

Acrylics

Methyl Acrylate

The acrylics are a group of plastics having in common the formation of polymers of acrylate esters. The principal acrylic monomers include methyl methacrylate, methyl acrylate, ethyl acrylate, and butyl acrylate. These are high-volume monomers. There are a large number of acrylate-based compounds, which may be used in combinations, thereby complicating characterization of occupational health effects.

These polymerized esters are best known as substitutes for glass under the trade names of Lucite (methyl acrylate) and Plexiglas (ethyl acrylate). They can be easily molded and have been widely used in the production of dentures and surgical prostheses. They are also widely used as surface coatings; as coatings for textiles, paper, and leather; and as a component of adhesives.

The acrylic monomers are variably irritating to the mucous membranes, skin, and respiratory tract, with ethyl acrylate having the highest irritant potency. The odor threshold of ethyl acrylate is below 1 ppm and, therefore, should serve as a warning prior to the development of irritant effects. Methyl methacrylate is known to be irritating at less than twice the permissible level established by OSHA. These monomers are also known to produce dermal sensitization. Recent studies of acrylic-induced contact dermatitis include a broad range of acrylates, and suggest that some of the more recently introduced acrylates may be potent sensitizers.[40] Asthma has been associated with acrylates in case reports for at least 20 years, but a recent epidemiologic study implicates acrylate-based materials, especially rapidly drying glues, as having some of the highest relative risks among occupational exposures known to cause asthma.

Methyl methacrylate has limited nervous system toxicity. Dental technicians who molded methyl methacrylate by hand experienced finger paresthesias. Sensory nerve conduction velocities of the digits were significantly slowed, possibly representing direct local toxicity to the nerves. A single case of a dental technician with long-term exposure to methyl methacrylate and generalized peripheral neuropathy has been reported.[41] Another cross-sectional study of workers exposed below the permissible exposure level set by OSHA reported a high prevalence of headaches, increased prevalence of pain in the extremities, loss of memory, fatigue, and sleep disturbances.

Ethyl acrylate is unique among the acrylic monomers as an established animal carcinogen. Epidemiologic studies of methyl methacrylate-exposed workers producing polymer in the United States and England have suggested an increased risk of colon cancer, but results are mixed and inconclusive.[42]

Hydroquinone

Hydroquinone

Hydroquinone is an important polymerization inhibitor for acrylic monomers and vinyl acetate, and is a raw material in the production of rubber antioxidants. Hydroquinone is also important as a photographic developer and reducer.

Hydroquinone is irritating to the skin, mucous membranes, and respiratory tract. Exposure to air-borne hydroquinone has been known to produce corneal ulcers. This chemical has also rarely been associated with the development of vitiligo. Oral ingestion of hydroquinone produced gastrointestinal irritation, as evidenced by nausea, vomiting, abdominal cramps, and diarrhea, in several dozen American sailors who inadvertently drank hydroquinone-contaminated water when the ship's water system was connected to automatic photodeveloping machines on the ship.[43]

In a French factory, workers chronically exposed to hydroquinone had reduced ventilatory capacity (FEV_1) and flow rates in comparison with the control group, suggesting that hydroquinone may produce airway obstruction. Elevated levels of IgG and IgE were also found in the hydroquinone-exposed group.[44]

Hydroquinone is an animal carcinogen, producing renal adenomas in rats.[45] Epidemiologic studies are negative to date, but have involved few people, limiting statistical power.[46] Hydroquinone is a metabolite of benzene and may be responsible, at least in part, for the leukemogenesis caused by benzene.[47] IARC currently rates hydroquinone as not classifiable with respect to human carcinogenicity.

Acrylamide

Acrylamide

Polyacrylamide, the polymeric form of acrylamide, is not generally considered a plastic material but is relevant, because the industrial production process is similar to that of the plastics. Polyacrylamide is principally used to bind and remove suspended solids from waste water, to increase water viscosity in oil recovery processes, to strengthen and retain fibers and pigments in paper making, and to coat surfaces. Minor uses include textile treatment, cosmetic preparations, gel chromatography, and electrophoresis.

The principal routes of exposure of acrylamide are through dermal contact and inhalation. Retention of the monomer in the polymer has been a concern, although improvements in the polymerization process have led to a decrease in monomer to less than 1% of the polymer resin.

Peripheral neuropathy is the dominant effect of acrylamide (see also Chapter 28.2). First described in 1953, the symptoms of the sensorimotor neuropathy include weakness, diminution of all sensory modalities, and evidence of sympathetic nervous system involvement, including excessive sweating and cold extremities. Distal changes in the nerves of the extremities precede proximal involvement. Limited central nervous system involvement may occur, as demonstrated by ataxia, vertigo, and alterations in mood, orientation, and memory. Desquamation of the skin of the palms and soles has accompanied the neurologic illness in exposed workers.

Acrylamide is a recognized animal carcinogen. In a mortality study of 8508 workers who manufactured acrylamide, an elevation in thyroid and lung cancer was found, though without apparent dose relation to acrylamide exposure.[48] A statistically significant excess of pancreatic cancer was also found among workers with higher acrylamide exposure, with some evidence of a dose–response relationship. Additional insight about the potential for acrylamide to cause human cancer awaits further follow-up of this cohort and additional studies. IARC considers acrylamide to be a probable human carcinogen.[49]

Hemoglobin adducts of acrylamide have been used as a biomarker of internal dose and have demonstrated a dose–response relation with peripheral nervous system symptoms.[50]

Polyurethane

The polyurethanes are mainly used to make rigid and flexible foams and surface coatings. They are formed through the reaction of isocyanates and di- or polyfunctional alcohols. Additional materials, such as amines and glycols, may be used in small amounts. Isocyanates are the most important occupational health hazard in polyurethane manufacture and application.

Isocyanates

$$R{-}N{=}C{=}O$$

Isocyanate

Isocyanates are an important family of low molecular weight chemicals; the most notable examples are toluene diisocyanate (TDI), methylenediphenyl diisocyanate (MDI), and hexamethylene diisocyanate (HDI). The industrial use of isocyanates exploits their high chemical reactivity, making them useful as cross-linking agents. The production of TDI alone was 875 million pounds in the United States in 1994.

Isocyanates are of particular interest in occupational medicine because of their capacity to cause respiratory disease at remarkably low levels of exposure. The current OSHA standard for exposure to TDI, for example, is 0.005 ppm (5 parts per billion), which is several orders of magnitude lower than the OSHA time-weighted averages for most industrial chemicals.

Diisocyanates, especially TDI and MDI, are principally used in the production of polyurethane foams, which may be rigid or flexible. MDI is more commonly used for rigid foam, whereas flexible foam is produced with TDI. Rigid foams are often generated at the site of use, principally as insulation material, and may present opportunities for uncontrolled exposures. Polyurethane foams are used in upholstery, insulation material, and packaging. Isocyanates are also used in the production of adhesives, rubbers, surface coatings, elastomers, and spray paints. Workers at risk for isocyanate-related disease include those who manufacture isocyanates, those who manufacture or apply polyurethane products (such as foam), and those who use polyurethane products (such as varnishes and spray paints).

Isocyanates vary in their capacity to produce disease. MDI has a vapor pressure several hundred times lower than that of TDI and HDI, and it is therefore much less volatile than the latter agents. If used under similar conditions, MDI produces lower ambient isocyanate levels than does TDI or HDI. Although HDI has the same vapor pressure as TDI, the former often exists as three molecules bound together, lowering its vapor pressure and decreasing its likelihood of significant air-borne isocyanate exposure to vapor. However, all isocyanate compounds present an exposure risk in aerosol form, during spraying or generation of mists.

Clinical effects Isocyanates cause significant respiratory disease in humans (Table 41.3). The respiratory toxicity of TDI was first documented in animal experiments in 1941, prior to the significant commercial use of isocyanates. Important commercial use of isocyanates occurred following the Second World War and did not begin in the United States until 1953. The first report of human respiratory toxicity of TDI was by French investigators in 1951. Many cases of isocyanate respiratory disease were reported soon thereafter, and by 1962 a review article of the published literature cited 222 cases of respiratory illness caused by TDI exposure.

Respiratory irritation results from isocyanate exposure, affecting both the upper and lower airways, with symptoms ranging from cough and mucus production to chemical pneumonitis and pulmonary edema, as occurred with methyl isocyanate exposure during the Bhopal incident in

Direct irritation of the respiratory tract
Asthma
Chronic obstructive pulmonary disease
Hypersensitivity pneumonitis
Pulmonary disease-anemia syndrome (hemorrhagic pneumonitis)

Table 41.3 Respiratory diseases associated with isocyanates

1984. Irritant symptoms resulting from isocyanate exposure occur in a dose-related fashion with many workers experiencing irritation of the nose and throat at or above 30–70 ppb of TDI, with significant lower respiratory tract irritation at higher levels of exposure. Notably, a ten-year follow-up of some of the victims of the Bhopal methyl isocyanate leak indicates a high prevalence of persistent respiratory symptoms and small airway dysfunction.[51]

In recent decades isocyanate-induced asthma has become the most common form of occupational asthma (see also Chapter 19.2).[52] This is the most common and best studied respiratory effect of the isocyanate group of compounds. Isocyanate-induced asthma occurs with variable latency following the initial exposure, although characteristically the asthma develops within two years of exposure. The asthma develops at air-borne isocyanate levels that are well below those producing the irritant symptoms previously described. Exposures below the current time-weighted average standard of 5 ppb for TDI have been shown to cause sensitization and asthma; this may be the result of higher transient peak exposure levels. After a worker has become sensitized to isocyanates, respiratory symptoms may appear at levels far below permissible limits. Once sensitized, asthma often becomes persistent, with non-specific bronchial hyper-reactivity. Although antiasthmatic therapy may control or prevent symptoms in affected individuals, a lethal attack of asthma may unexpectedly occur. There are several reports in the literature of deaths among young TDI- or MDI-sensitized workers receiving antiasthmatic therapy, following continued exposure to isocyanates at work. In addition, therapy may not alter the natural history of asthma, and continued exposure to isocyanates may lead to more severe and sustained reactions that may generalize to agents other than isocyanates.

After complete cessation of exposure, respiratory symptoms and bronchial hyperactivity may continue for years. In a long-term follow-up of 245 cases of isocyanate-induced asthma, Finnish investigators found that over 80% still had asthmatic symptoms ten years following initial diagnosis.[53]

Workers affected by isocyanate-induced asthma typically have bronchospastic symptoms several hours after the initial exposure, that is, at the end of the work day or a delayed response in the evening after work. On returning to work the following day, a similar temporal pattern recurs. Isocyanate inhalation challenge tests demonstrate a similar pattern of late physiologic response, as well as dual responses. Three important caveats exist about the use of the specific inhalation challenge tests. First, isocyanate inhalation challenge tests may be positive in affected workers, despite normal methacholine challenge tests. Second, the isocyanate inhalation challenge test may yield a false-negative result if testing is performed after a significant amount of time elapses since the last exposure to the offending agent. Third, availability of such testing is limited, and can only be performed at specialized medical centers with experience in specific inhalation challenge testing.

Population-based studies of TDI-exposed workers show that 5–20% of workers exposed to TDI may become sensitized to the chemical. There seems to be no relationship between a history of allergy or atopy and the development of isocyanate-induced asthma. The pathogenesis of isocyanate asthma has yet to be fully elucidated. Isocyanate-specific IgE antibodies have been demonstrated in some isocyanate-sensitive individuals by radioallergosorbent testing, but exposure to isocyanates in the absence of respiratory symptoms has also been associated with the development of such antibodies in workers. It appears that only a small proportion of isocyanate-sensitive individuals, i.e., approximately 20%, have these IgE antibodies. IgE antibodies are, thus, highly specific but not very sensitive indicators of isocyanate-induced asthma. Alternative, though not mutually exclusive, mechanisms for bronchospasm include pharmacologic effects on adrenergic receptors and direct inflammatory effects; the epidemiologic and clinical data strongly suggest an immunologic basis. The role of a cell-mediated response to isocyanates is currently under active investigation.

Longitudinal observation of occupational groups exposed to TDI has demonstrated that chronic airflow limitation may develop in individuals who are not specifically sensitized to it. An investigation of polyurethane foam manufacturing plant workers showed an excessive decline in FEV_1 during a two-year follow-up at exposure levels less than 1–9 ppb.[54] A prospective study of workers at a new TDI manufacturing factory showed an excessive decline in lung function only in non-smokers with the highest cumulative TDI exposure. Most TDI exposures in this study were below 5 ppb.[55] In an earlier British study of workers exposed to levels of TDI of 20–50 ppb or higher, no differences in respiratory symptoms or pulmonary function were observed between the study group and a control group of unexposed workers. Different study methods and settings may in part explain the variable findings in these studies.

Both TDI and MDI have been shown to cause hypersensitivity pneumonitis.[56] Although much less common than asthma, extrinsic allergic alveolitis may occur in at least 1% of isocyanate workers with symptoms. IgG antibodies against the offending isocyanates are usually found in the serum and bronchoalveolar lavage fluid. Isocyanates have also recently been reported to cause hemorrhagic pneumonitis.[57] A recent case report described dyspnea, hemoptysis, patchy pulmonary infiltrates, and high serum levels of isocyanate-specific IgE and IgG antibodies in a spray painter with exposure to multiple isocyanates. This may be the same syndrome as the pulmonary disease–anemia syndrome that has been reported among workers exposed to phthalic anhydride.

There has been recent interest in the risk of cancer associated with isocyanates. According to an IARC evaluation in 2000, animal experiments demonstrate sufficient evidence of carcinogenicity to designate TDI an animal carcinogen; there is limited evidence of carcinogenicity for MDI.[58] Epidemiologic studies are limited but show possible excess in non-Hodgkin's lymphoma, rectal cancer, and pancreatic cancer.[59]

Evaluation and prevention The diagnosis of isocyanate-induced asthma is based on a history of exposure to isocyanates and the presence of the characteristic temporal bronchospastic response. Inhalation challenge testing with isocyanate test material may be useful in confirming the causal relationship, particularly when methacholine challenge testing is negative or, in questionable cases, where it is necessary to demonstrate the specificity of bronchospasm to isocyanate exposure. After isocyanate-related asthma develops in a worker, it is essential that he or she be removed from any further isocyanate exposure.

Workers who are routinely exposed to isocyanates should be educated about the respiratory effects of such exposure and should undergo a biannual respiratory symptom review and spirometry. There is currently no rational basis for excluding atopic individuals from jobs involving potential exposure to isocyanates.

Plastics additives

Azodicarbonamide

Azodicarbonamide is a blowing agent for a variety of plastic and rubber polymers, including PVC, polyurethane, polyethylene, acrylonitrile-butadiene-styrene resins, and elastomers. It is widely used as an additive in the plastics industry, although not in a high volume relative to the polymers with which it is compounded. When heated, azodicarbonamide releases a large amount of gas, which produces the desired blowing effect.

This chemical has been known for the past 20 years to produce asthma. The asthma usually develops within the first year after onset of exposure. There is a characteristic late bronchospastic response, i.e., at the end of a work-shift or during the evening following exposure. Because there may be other allergenic agents in the work environment where this chemical is used, the diagnosis of azodicarbonamide-induced asthma is dependent on a clear temporal relationship between the exposure and related symptoms, as well as demonstration of bronchial hyper-reactivity on specific inhalation challenge test.[60] Cross-sectional studies of workers exposed to this chemical in both a manufacturing facility and plastic injection molding facility observed that as many as 20% of workers may have bronchospastic symptoms in association with azodicarbonamide exposure.[61] Allergic contact dermatitis has also been reported in a few exposed individuals.

Hexamethylenetetramine and other amines

Hexamethylenetetramine (hexamine) is an important amine used predominantly as a curing agent for urea-formaldehyde and phenolic resins. Hexamine is also used in the rubber industry to prevent vulcanized rubber from 'blocking', as well as an accelerator. Approximately 80 million pounds of this agent were produced in the United States in 1994. Hexamine hydrolyzes to ammonia and formaldehyde in an aqueous environment and has thus been used as a oral antibacterial agent (e.g., mandelamine).

Its pyrolytic products include nitrogen oxides, carbon monoxide, carbon dioxide, and formaldehyde.

It has been known for decades that hexamine is a skin and respiratory irritant. A recent cross-sectional study of workers at a hexamine production plant observed no relation between respiratory symptoms and pulmonary function abnormalities, though workers were well aware of irritant dermatitis caused by hexamine.[62] Oral hexamine use in clinical settings been noted to cause gastro-intestinal distress, bladder irritation, dermatitis, and urticaria.

A variety of other amines have been associated with the development of asthma, including dimethylethanolamine, ethylenediamine, piperazine, and dimethylaminopropylamine. Because numerous amines are used in curing plastic resins, including phenolic, epoxy, and polyurethane resins, it is reasonable to expect that these agents may contribute to the occupational asthma that occurs in resin production. The role of amines may be obscured by the presence of other allergenic agents, such as isocyanates and anhydrides. In a recent Swedish study, Belin and coworkers documented airway obstruction in workers in a polyurethane foam-producing plant in which the air-borne concentration of isocyanates was extremely low and the air-borne concentration of a catalytic amine, N-methylmorpholine, was 10,000 times higher than that of the isocyanates.[63] Even when the role of isocyanates and other well-recognized allergens cannot be excluded, it is worth considering the potential role of amines when respiratory symptoms are present in workers with these multiple exposures.

Diethylhexyl phthalate (DEHP)

DEHP and other phthalates are the major agents used as plasticizers, which impart flexibility to plastic compounds. These additives may represent a substantial amount, as much as 20–40% by weight, of plastics such as PVC. Other polymers in which these plasticizers are used include synthetic rubber and polystyrene. DEHP, also known as dioctyl phthalate, is an irritant of the skin and respiratory tract. Animal studies have shown evidence of testicular, renal, developmental, and pulmonary toxicity associated with DEHP exposure; similar toxicity in humans has not been well described.[64]

Of considerable interest is whether DEHP represents a human carcinogen. A review by IARC in 2000 concluded that DEHP was not classifiable as to carcinogenicity in humans.[57] There is sufficient evidence that DEHP causes cancer in animals, particularly liver tumors in mice and rats. Adequate human epidemiologic data are not available for the assessment of possible carcinogenic effects in humans. However, the carcinogenicity of DEHP in animals has generated concern, not only because of the potential occupational exposure to DEHP, but also as a result of the potential exposure to the general public through leaching of DEHP from plastic bags used to store blood and intravenous solutions. Biologic monitoring of DEHP metabolites in urine has been demonstrated to be a useful means of quantifying exposure.[65]

SYNTHETIC TEXTILES

Synthetic textiles are fibrous forms of plastics. The overall production process described in Figure 41.1 also applies to this subgroup of plastics. Indeed, many of the materials used in plastics production are also used in the manufacture of synthetic textiles. Examples include styrene and the anhydrides. Surprisingly few data are available specifically on the occupational health aspects of finished synthetic fibers.

Nylon

Nylon

Nylon is formed through one of two means: (1) by the condensation of an acid, such as adipic acid, and an amine, such as hexamethylenediamine, or (2) by the polymerization of a lactam, such as caprolactam. Adipic acid is the major organic acid used as a raw material in the production of nylon. A small amount of adipic acid is additionally used in the production of polyurethane resins, plasticizers, and synthetic lubricants. Caprolactam is almost exclusively used in the manufacture of nylon, i.e., polycaprolactam. Nylon fibers are used in textiles, tire cords, and related fabrics; nylon plastics are molded to form various consumer products, including housewares and appliances.

Adipic acid and caprolactam are irritating to the eyes, skin, and throat. There is additionally a convincing case report of a worker with moderately severe asthma after repeated exposure to adipic acid. The worker had an immediate bronchospastic reaction following inhalation of a low dose of adipic acid; the reaction was prevented by a prior administration of cromolyn sodium.

In a mortality study of nylon manufacturing workers, there was a statistically significant excess in mortality from bladder cancer, which occurred largely in workers after 20 years from first employment. Another type of nylon (nylon 11) using a different monomer, 11-aminoundecanoic acid, caused transitional cell carcinomas of the urinary tract in rats. No human data relating to exposure to nylon 11 or its monomer are yet available.

Polyester

Polyester

Polyesters are produced by the condensation of an acid anhydride, such as phthalic anhydride, and an alcohol, such as ethylene glycol. The polyester polymer can be subsequently mixed with other materials, such as styrene and hydroquinone. The hazards associated with these raw materials are described in other sections.

Polyester polymer has demonstrated mucous membrane and respiratory toxicity. Workers grinding buttons made of polyester resin commonly report irritation of the throat and eyes during exposure to polyester dust. These symptoms were corroborated by mild but statistically significant decrements in mid-expiratory flow rates during 8-hour work shifts. A later report by the same investigators observed reduced preshift mid-expiratory flow rates and an excess in cough, phlegm, and dyspnea in exposed workers compared with a control group.

A mortality study of workers manufacturing polyester resin reported an increased rate of lung cancer among production workers, although this elevation was not statistically significant. A significant excess was observed in maintenance workers; cigarette smoking did not appear to be the cause of the observed excess in lung cancer.[66]

Rayon

$$S=C=S$$

Carbon Disulfide

Viscose rayon, also known as artificial silk, is one of the earliest synthetic fibers, with production beginning in the early 1900s. Rayon is formed through the treatment of alkali cellulose with carbon disulfide. Carbon disulfide, a highly volatile solvent, causes most of the toxicity experienced by rayon manufacturing workers. The toxicity of carbon disulfide has been known for 150 years and has been the subject of many reports in the first half of the 20th century. Carbon disulfide causes prominent central nervous system effects, ranging from headaches, dizziness, and irritability in mild cases, to mania, hallucinations, delirium, suicidal ideations, and coma (carbon disulfide psychosis) in severe cases. The solvent also causes a sensorimotor peripheral neuropathy.[67] Carbon disulfide has been associated with an increased risk of coronary artery disease. Exposure to carbon disulfide has been more effectively controlled in recent years, preventing more severe neurologic illness so well documented in the first half of the 20th century (see also Chapter 28, neurology).

SYNTHETIC RUBBER INDUSTRY

The use of synthetic rubber far outweighs that of natural rubber, accounting for approximately 70% of all rubber production. Although the number of applications of synthetic rubbers has increased in recent years, overall growth has been modest, with a 30% increase in production during the two decades from 1967 to 1988. Of the rubber polymers, styrene-butadiene polymer is the most important, representing nearly 40% of the entire production of elastomers. Other rubber polymers in decreasing order of volume produced include polybutadiene, ethylenepropylene, butadiene-acrylonitrile (nitrile), and polychloroprene (neoprene).

Like the plastics industry, the synthetic rubber industry has distinguishing characteristics that are essential to the recognition of the occupational hazards of the industry. The synthetic rubber industry shares the basic paradigm of production common to the plastics industry, i.e., the production of a polymer, also known as an elastomer, which is further processed into a finished product. The processing of rubber polymers represents the major sector of the synthetic rubber industry, including tire manufacture, and is highly complex compared with most plastics-processing operations. The synthetic rubber industry uses hundreds, if not thousands, of chemical agents, many of them additives. Furthermore, the profile of agents used in the industry has changed significantly over time, necessitating caution in applying the results of studies of health effects in prior decades, especially those evaluating carcinogenic risks of the industry, for currently exposed workers.

Given the large number of agents used, formation of complex and sometimes uncharacterized chemical mixtures, and relative complexity of the manufacturing process in the rubber industry, many epidemiologic studies of the rubber industry characterize exposures by the department or step in the manufacturing process, rather than by the specific exposures of individual workers. When possible, the role of individual agents, such as styrene, benzene, and β-naphthylamine in producing disease has been identified. More commonly, diseases have been associated with working in a department, such as mixing or curing, or another step in the production process.

The production of finished rubber materials requires two separate manufacturing processes, namely: (1) the formation of raw polymer, and (2) the conversion of the polymer to the finished rubber product. The first step is similar to that of plastic polymer production, with large-scale operations using bulk materials in enclosed systems. Because the number of important monomers and their polymeric forms are relatively few, the scope of the occupational health problems intrinsic to polymer production is more limited, though not fully characterized. The transformation of the raw polymer to finished rubber goods may be simple, similar to the comparable processes in plastics production, or it may be highly complex, such as in the 40-step process required to make tires. Major steps in the complex production of tires and selected other rubber goods are shown in Table 41.4.

Each step may involve characteristic and identifiable exposure or exposures to unknown chemical intermediates or byproducts of chemical reactions occurring throughout the production process.

Production step	Potential exposures
1. **Mixing or compounding:** combining the raw polymer with additives	Elastomers Reinforcers (carbon black) Fillers (amorphous silica, clays) Vulcanizers (sulfur, selenium) Accelerators (thiurams, thiocarbamates) Retarders (salicylic acids) Activators (zinc oxide, stearic acid) Plasticizers (phthalates) Antioxidants (phenylenediamines) Extenders (mineral oils) Pigments (titanium, cadmium, organic dyes) Solvents Processing aids (aromatic mineral oils)
2. **Milling:** thorough blending and heating of assembled ingredients	Fumes of elastomers and/or additives Antitacking agents (kaolin, soaps)
3. **Extrusion and calendering:** shaping and cutting of rubber compound and application of rubber onto textile fabrics or steel cords	Solvents (naphtha, hexane, toluene) Adhesives Formaldehyde
4. **Assembly:** fabricating the desired piece	Solvents (haptene, methanol, naphtha) Mold-release agents (silicones, soaps) Tacking agents (phenolic resins)
5. **Curing or vulcanization:** applying heat and pressure to the piece in a mold, press, or autoclave to effect cross-linking reactions	Mold-release agents Lubricants (solvent based) Curing fumes (complex mixtures)
6. **Finishing:** trimming, grinding, cleaning, and painting to produce the final product	Solvents Rubber dust Inks and paints

Table 41.4 Steps in synthetic rubber production

Styrene

Styrene

Styrene is an essential monomer in several of the most important rubber polymers, and it is additionally used in plastics production. The production of styrene in the United States in 2000 was 10.8 billion pounds and is increasing steadily. More than one-half of all styrene production is used to make polystyrene, the third leading plastic polymer after PVC and polyethylene. Most of the remainder is co-polymerized with acrylonitrile and/or butadiene to form elastomers. A small but important use of styrene is as a cross-linking agent and diluent in unsaturated polyester resin application, particularly in the boat-building industry, where excessive styrene exposure has been well documented.

Styrene is an irritant to the mucous membranes and respiratory tract at air-borne levels of 100 mid-expiratory 200 ppm, two to four times OSHA's current permissible exposure level of 50 ppm. Acute exposures to 50 ppm styrene in experimental settings are documented to cause irritation.

The impact of styrene exposure on the lungs is not well understood. Several cross-sectional studies of exposed workers demonstrate elevated rates of respiratory symptoms including chest tightness and wheezing. These symptoms have not been accompanied by well-characterized changes in pulmonary function. This important topic deserves further study.

Styrene has demonstrated hepatotoxicity in animals and in humans.[68] In a large cross-sectional study of polystyrene workers, the elevated γ-glutamyl transpeptidase activity was associated with high styrene exposure. No other liver function tests showed a relationship to styrene exposure. A recent study of two groups of workers exposed to styrene below 50 ppm were found to have mild subclinical hepatic injury as evidence by increased levels of bilirubin, alkaline phosphatase, and hepatic transaminases in exposed workers compared with controls (see also Chapter 26.1).[69]

Styrene is toxic to the central and peripheral nervous systems.[70–72] Exposure to high levels of styrene causes light-headedness, headache, and altered balance (as evidenced by an abnormal Romberg's test). A high prevalence of abnormal electroencephalograms has been found among styrene-exposed workers in a number of studies. Studies of subclinical toxicity using neurobehavioral tests demonstrate abnormalities in psychomotor performance, visual memory, and vigilance. There is also limited evidence that styrene can affect verbal learning and logical memory, at or below 50 ppm. Neurologic symptoms and selected neurobehavioral deficits (visuomotor performance and perceptual speed) may persist for several years following cessation of exposure.[73] In the few neurophysiologic studies evaluating the effects of styrene on the peripheral nervous system, sensory nerve conduction deficits have been consistently found, including workers with styrene exposure below 50 ppm.

Exposure to styrene has been weakly associated with an increase in a variety of lymphatic and hematopoietic malignancies, including leukemia, lymphoma, and multiple myeloma, in numerous epidemiologic studies. Other studies have not confirmed these associations. Study groups have had varying degrees of exposure to potentially confounding carcinogens, such as benzene, acrylonitrile, and butadiene, obscuring the relationship between styrene exposure and cancer. There is only limited evidence that styrene is an animal carcinogen. However, styrene-7,8-oxide, a metabolite of styrene in humans, is a confirmed animal carcinogen. IARC has rated styrene as a possible carcinogen (Group 2B) since 1994, based on limited evidence in experimental animals and inadequate evidence in humans. IARC designates styrene-7,8-oxide as a probable human carcinogen (Group 2A).[49]

Acrylonitrile

Acrylonitrile

Acrylonitrile is used principally in the manufacture of rubber copolymers and acrylic fibers. Acrylonitrile is among the top 50 chemicals produced in the United States, with 2.5 billion pounds produced domestically in 1993. Acrylonitrile production has grown rapidly. Approximately one-quarter of the acrylonitrile is copolymerized with butadiene and/or styrene to form acrylonitrile-butadiene-styrene, styrene-acrylonitrile, and butadiene-acrylonitrile (nitrile) resins. These elastomers are three of the major synthetic rubbers currently manufactured.

Clinical effects
Acrylonitrile is a well-known irritant to the mucous membranes and skin. Toxic epidermal necrosis had been reported among patients who were exposed to a fumigant containing carbon tetrachloride and acrylonitrile. Acrylonitrile may be hepatotoxic, but the nature and extent of the toxicity are not clear.

Systemic acrylonitrile poisoning can cause headaches, fatigue, nausea, and light-headedness initially, but may cause severe asphyxia and death in some cases. Much of the acute toxicity of acrylonitrile likely results from the metabolism of acrylonitrile to form cyanide, which is further metabolized to thiocyanate. Treatment of acute acrylonitrile toxicity is similar to that of cyanide poisoning, i.e., with amyl nitrate and sodium thiosulfate, although therapeutic efficacy may be limited by the formation of cyano metabolites other than cyanide that are not amenable to these antidotes. The role of hydroxycobalamin to bind cyanide and its metabolites is being explored.

Acrylonitrile is a well-documented animal carcinogen. Numerous epidemiologic studies have been completed in the US and in Europe and do not show consistent elevations in cancer risk. The largest US study demonstrated an elevation in risk of lung cancer among acrylonitrile workers in the highest quintile of cumulative exposure.[74] IARC considers acrylonitrile to be a probable human carcinogen (Group 2A).[19]

Evaluation and prevention
Clinical evaluation of acrylonitrile-exposed workers should center on the dermatologic, respiratory, and central nervous system effects of the agent. Biologic monitoring may be conducted through measurement of urine acrylonitrile or thiocyanate levels. Facilities using acrylonitrile should have an easily accessible cyanide poisoning antidote kit. Proper training in the use of the kit should be conducted.

OSHA-mandated annual medical surveillance provisions include a complete work and medical history, physical examination, chest x-ray studies, and screening for occult stool blood. Liver function tests are also advisable.

1,3-Butadiene

1,3-Butadiene

1,3-Butadiene is used principally as a comonomer in the manufacture of polymers with acrylonitrile and styrene or as a monomer in the formation of polybutadiene. Less important uses are as an intermediate in the production of adiponitrile, polychloroprene, and captan. The US production of 1,3-butadiene was 3.1 billion pounds in 1993.

At high levels of exposure, 1,3-butadiene is an irritant and can produce central nervous system depression. Despite the volume of 1,3-butadiene produced in the United States, few cases of toxicity have been reported. Initial symptoms of acute toxicity include blurred vision, drowsiness, fatigue, headache, and nausea.

In 1996, OSHA lowered the permissible exposure level for 1,3-butadiene to 1 ppm as an 8-hour time-weighted average with a short-term limit of 5 ppm. In recognition of its carcinogenicity, NIOSH recommends that occupational exposure to 1,3-butadiene be at the lowest feasible concentration. The principal health concern about 1,3-butadiene is its carcinogenicity. In 1998, IARC reviewed available studies on 1,3-butadiene and designated it as a Group 2A carcinogen, with sufficient evidence in animals and limited human evidence of carcinogenicity. In animal assays, 1,3-butadiene causes tumors at multiple sites in multiple species, including lymphomas in mice. Epidemiologic studies link exposure to 1,3-butadiene to leukemia and lymphomas.[75]

Biomonitoring for 1,3-butadiene exposure can be achieved in research settings through the measurements of urinary metabolites [1,2-dihydroxy-4-(N-acetylcysteinyl)-butane and 1-hydroxy-2-(N-acetylcysteinyl)-butene] and hemoglobin adducts, the latter being most highly associated with measures of 1,3-butadiene exposure.[76]

HEALTH HAZARDS

As noted previously, exposures in rubber manufacturing are numerous, complex, and often not fully characterized. Hence, the occupational health problems associated with the manufacture of rubber goods, especially tire production, have been described and are best reviewed by the specific activity within the industry or by the whole industry rather than by exposure to individual agents.

Skin disease

Rubber additives are the principal agents responsible for the dermatitis observed among rubber workers and consumers who wear rubber articles. Allergic skin reactions have been associated most frequently with mercaptobenzothiazole, phenylenediamine derivatives, and thiuram accelerators. Irritant dermatitis has also been caused by a number of different agents.

Respiratory disease

Rubber manufacturing causes chronic lung disease. Increased rates of cough, phlegm production, dyspnea, and wheezing have been reported in the mixing, milling, and curing departments of tire factories. Pulmonary function testing of exposed groups has shown predominantly obstructive changes [reduction in FEV_1, and/or FVC_1 (forced vital capacity ratio)] measured prior to work shifts. Cross-shift declines in FEV_1 have also been documented for rubber workers exposed to adhesives containing hexamethylenetetramine and resorcinol.

Talc, which was commonly used as an antitacking agent, has caused frank talcosis in rubber workers, and has been associated with respiratory morbidity and airway obstruction, even in the absence of chest radiographic abnormalities. When crystalline silica with a high content of the crystalline moiety was used as a substitute for talc, silicosis resulted. Carbon black exposure may also produce a pneumoconiosis.

Cancer

The cancer experience of rubber manufacturing workers has been the subject of intense epidemiologic research during the last four decades. Although the complexity of the industry has led to considerable variability in the carcinogenic risks measured, certain conclusions are warranted. An excess risk of death from bladder cancer (standardized mortality ratios ranging from 200 to 500) was observed in earlier studies and is believed to be the result of antioxidants containing β-naphthylamine. More recent cohort and case control studies show lower levels of risk, i.e., less than twofold, or, frequently, no increase in risk. Interestingly, a sixfold increase in risk has recently been observed among workers using the aromatic amines, toluidine and aniline, to produce a rubber accelerator.[77]

Excesses of leukemia and, to a lesser extent, lymphoma are observed among rubber workers.[78] Workers in a variety of parts of the industry, especially calendering, curing, and tire building, experienced a two- to fourfold increase in leukemia compared with reference populations. Benzene may be an important etiologic agent given the widespread use of this solvent in the industry in past decades.

Other cancer sites reported to show increased risk among rubber workers are the lung and stomach (standardized mortality ratios ranging from 100 to 250). In addition, the rates of cancer of the prostate and colon have been elevated in several studies; the evidence in favor of an occupational etiology for these cancer sites is considered to be limited by IARC. Finally, one or more studies have noted increases in the rates of cancer of the brain, thyroid, and pancreas. A review of the studies pertaining to the relationship between employment in the rubber industry and cancer can be found in the IARC monograph on the rubber industry.[79]

References

1. Acquavella JF, Douglass TS, Phillips SC. Evaluation of excess colorectal cancer incidence among workers involved in the manufacture of polypropylene. J Occup Med 1988; 30:438–44.
2. Acquavella JF, Douglass TS, Vernon S, et al. Assessment of colorectal cancer screening outcomes among workers involved in polypropylene manufacture. J Occup Med 1989; 31:785–91.
3. Acquavella JF, Owen CV, Bird MG, et al. An adenomatous polyp case-control study to assess occupational risk factors following a workplace colorectal cancer cluster. Am J Epidemiol 1991; 133:357–67.
4. Goldberg MS, Thériault G. Retrospective cohort study of workers of a synthetic textiles plant in Quebec: II. Colorectal cancer mortality and incidence. Am J Ind Med 1994; 25:909–22.
5. Perticoni GF, Abbritti G, Cantisani TA, et al. Polyneuropathy in workers with long exposure to vinyl chloride: electrophysiologic study. Electromyogr Clin Neurophysiol 1986; 26:41–7.
6. Serratrice J, Granel B, Pache X, et al. A case of polymyositis with anti-histidy1-t-RNA synthetase (Jo-1) antibody syndrome following extensive vinyl chloride exposure. Clin Rheumatol 2001; 20:379–82.
7. Du C-L, Wang J-D. Increased morbidity odds ratio of primary liver cancer and cirrhosis of the liver among vinyl chloride monomer workers. Occup Environ Med 1998; 55:528–32.
8. Ward E, Boffetta P, Andersen A, et al. Update of the follow-up of mortality and cancer incidence among European workers employed in the vinyl chloride industry. Epidemiology 2001; 12:710–8.
9. Kielhorn J, Melber C, Wahnschaffe U, et al. Vinyl chloride: still a cause for concern. Environ Health Perspect 2000; 108:579–88.
10. Mundt KA, Dell LD, Austin RP, et al. Historical cohort study of 10,109 men in the North American vinyl chloride industry, 1942–72: update of cancer mortality of 31 December 1995. Occup Environ Med 2000; 57:774–81.
11. Hagmar L, Akesson B, Nielsen J, et al. Mortality and cancer morbidity in workers exposed to low levels of vinyl chloride monomer at a polyvinyl chloride processing plant. Am J Ind Med 1990; 17:553–65.
12. Jones RD, Smith DM, Thomas PG. A mortality study of vinyl chloride monomer workers employed in the United Kingdom in 1940–1974. Scand J Work Environ Health 1988; 14:153–60.
13. Wong O, Whorton MDZ, Foliart DE, et al. An industry-wide epidemiologic study of vinyl chloride workers, 1942–1982. Am J Ind Med 1991; 20:317–34.
14. Wong R-H, Chen PC, Du C-L, et al. An increased standardized mortality ratio for liver cancer among polyvinyl chloride workers in Taiwan. Occup Environ Med 20002; 59:405–9.
15. Lilis R, Anderson H, Miller A, et al. Pulmonary changes among vinyl chloride polymerization workers. Chest 1976; 69:299–305.
16. Mastrangelo G, Manno M, Marcer G, et al. Polyvinyl chloride pneumoconiosis: epidemiological study of exposed workers. J Occup Med 1979; 21:540–2.
17. Miller A, Teirstein AS, Chuang M, et al. Changes in pulmonary function in workers exposed to vinyl chloride and polyvinyl chloride. Ann NY Acad Sci 1975; 246:42–52.
18. Lilis R. Vinyl chloride and polyvinyl chloride exposure and occupational lung disease. Chest 1980; 78:826–8.
19. International Agency for Research Against Cancer. IARC summary and evaluation, volume 71. Lyon: IARC, 1999.
20. Albrecht WN, Bryant MS. Polymer-fume fever associated with smoking and use of a mold-release spray containing polytetrafluoroethylene. J Occup Med 1987; 29:817–9.
21. Demers PA, Schade WJ, Demers RY. Lymphocytopenia and occupational exposures among pattern and model makers. Scand J Work Environ Health 1994; 20:107–12.
22. Rempel D, Jones J, Atterbury M, et al. Respiratory effects of exposure of shipyard workers to epoxy paints. Br J Ind Med 1991; 48:783–7.
23. Dabney BJ. Cytogenetic findings on employees with potential exposure to epichlorohydrin. In: Sorsa M, Morppa H, eds. Monitoring of occupational genotoxicants. New York: Alan R. Liss, 1986;59–73.
24. Enterline PE, Henderson V, Marsh G. Mortality of workers potentially exposed to epichlorohydrin. Br J Ind Med 1990; 47:269–76.
25. Tsai SP, Gilstrap EL, Ross CE. Mortality study of employees with potential exposure to epichlorohydrin: a 10 year update. Occup Environ Med 1996; 53:299–304.
26. Barbone F, Delzell E, Austin H, et al. A case-control study of lung cancer at a dye and resin manufacturing plant. Am J Ind Med 1992; 22:835–49.
27. Angelini G, Rigano L, Fori C, et al. Occupational sensitization to epoxy resin and reactive diluents in marble workers. Contact Derm 1996; 35:11–16.
28. Venables KM. Low molecular weight chemicals, hypersensitivity, and direct toxicity: the acid anhydrides. Br J Ind Med 1989; 46:222–32.
29. Zeiss CR, Wolkonsky P, Chacon R, et al. Syndromes in workers exposed to trimellitic anhydride. Ann Intern Med 1983; 98:8–12.
30. Riboli E, Bai E, Berrino F, et al. Mortality from lung cancer in an acetylene and phthalic anhydride plant. Scand J Work Environ Health 1983; 9:455–62.
31. Lindh CH, Jönsson AG, Welinder H. Biologic monitoring of methylhexahydrophthalic anhydride by determination of methylhexahydrophthalic acid in urine and plasma from exposed workers. Int Arch Occup Environ Health 1997; 70:128–32.
32. Rosqvist S, Johannesson G, Lindh CH, et al. Total plasma protein adducts of allergenic hexahyrophthalic and methylhexahydrophthalic anhydrides as biomarkers of long-term exposure. Scand J Work Environ Health 2001; 27:133–9.
33. Grammer LC, Shaughnessy MA, Kenamore BD, et al. A clinical and immunologic study to assess risk of TMA-induced lung disease as related to exposure. J Occup Environ Med 1999; 41:1048–51.
34. Nunn AJ, Craigen, Darbyshire JH, et al. Six year follow up of lung function in men occupationally exposed to formaldehyde. Br J Ind Med 1990; 47:747–52.
35. International Agency for Research Against Cancer. IARC summary and evaluation, volume 62. Lyon: IARC, 1995.
36. Blair A, Stewart PA, Hoover RN. Mortality from lung cancer among workers employed in formaldehyde industries. Am J Ind Med 1990; 17:683–99.
37. Vaughan TL, Stewart PA, Teschke K, et al. Occupational exposure to formaldehyde and wood dust and nasopharyngeal carcinoma. Occup Environ Med 2000; 57:376–84.
38. United States Department of Labor. 29 CFR Parts 1910 and 1926. Occupational exposure to formaldehyde: final rule. Occupational Safety and Health Administration. Fed Reg 1987; 52:46291–312.
39. International Agency for Research on Cancer. IARC Summary and evaluation, supplement 7. Lyon: IARC, 1987.
40. Kanerva L, Estlander T, Jolanki R, et al. Occupational allergic contact dermatitis caused by exposure to acrylates during work with dental prostheses. Contact Derm 1993; 28:268–75.
41. Donaghy M, Rushworth G, Jacobs JM. Generalized peripheral neuropathy in a dental technician exposed to methyl methacrylate monomer. Neurology 1991; 41:1112–6.
42. Tomenson JA, Bonner SM, Edwards JC, et al. Study of two cohorts of workers exposed to methyl methacrylate in acrylic sheet production. Occup Environ Med 2000; 57:810–7.
43. Hooper RR, et al. Hydroquinone poisoning aboard a Navy ship. MMWR, 1978; 28:237–8.
44. Choudat D, Neukirch F, Brochard P, et al. Allergy and occupational exposure to hydroquinone and to methionine. Br J Ind Med 1988; 45:376–80.
45. Kari FW, Bucher J, Eustis SL, et al. Toxicity and carcinogenicity of hydroquinone in F344/N rats and B6C3F1 mice. Food Chem Toxicol 1992; 30:737–47.

46. Pifer JW, Hearne FT, Swanson FA, et al. Mortality study of employees engaged in the manufacture and use of hydroquinone. Int Arch Occup Environ Health 1995; 67:267–80.

47. Joseph P, Klein-Szanto AJP, Jaiswal AK. Hydroquinones cause specific mutations and lead to cellular transformation and in vivo tumorigenisis. Br J Cancer 1998; 78:312–20.

48. Marsh GM, Lucas LJ, Youk AO, et al. Mortality patterns among workers exposed to acrylamide: 1994 follow up. Occup Environ Med 1999; 56:181–90.

49. International Agency for Research Against Cancer. IARC summary and evaluation, volume 60. Lyon: IARC, 1994.

50. Hagmar L, Tornqvist M, Nordander C, et al. Health effects of occupational exposure to acrylamide using hemoglobin adducts as biomarkers of internal dose. Scand J Work Environ Health 2001; 27:219–26.

51. Cullinan P, Acquilla S, Dhara VR. Respiratory morbidity 10 years after the Union Carbide gas leak at Bhopal: a cross sectional survey. Br Med J 1997; 314–38.

52. Rosenman KD, Reilly MJ, Kalinowski DJ. A state-based surveillance system for work-related asthma. J Occup Environ Med 1997; 39:415–25

53. Piirila PL, Nordman H, Keskinen HM, et al. Long-term follow-up of hexamethylene diisocyanate-, diphenylmethane diisocyanate-, and toluene diisocyanate-induced Asthma. Am J Respir Crit Care Med 2000; 162:516–22.

54. Wegman DH, Peters JM, Pagnotto L, et al. Chronic pulmonary function loss from exposure to toluene diisocyanate. Br J Ind Med 1977; 34:196–200.

55. Deim JE, Jones RN, Hendrick DJ, et al. Five-year longitudinal study of workers employed in a new toluene diisocyanate manufacturing plant. Am Rev Respir Dis 1982; 126:420–8.

56. Baur X. Hypersensitivity pneumonitis (extrinsic allergic alveolitis) induced by isocyanates. J Allergy Clin Immunol 1995; 95:1004–10.

57. Patterson R, Nugent KM, Harris KE, et al. Immunologic hemorrhagic pneumonia caused by isocyanates. Am Rev Respir Dis 1990; 141:226–30.

58. International Agency for Research Against Cancer. IARC summary and evaluation, volume 77. Lyon: IARC, 2000.

59. Bolognesi C, Baur X, Marczynski B, et al. Carcinogenic risk of toluene diisocyanate and 4,4-methylenediphenyl diisocyanate: epidemiological and experimental evidence. Crit Rev Toxicol 2001; 31:737–72.

60. Normand JC, Grange F, Hernandez CD, et al. Occupational asthma after exposure to azodicarbonamide: report of four cases. Br J Ind Med 1989; 46:60–62.

61. Whitehead LW, Robins TG, Fine LJ, et al. Respiratory symptoms associated with the use of azodicarbonamide foaming agent in a plastics injection molding facility. Am J Ind Med 1987; 11:83–92.

62. Merget R, Topcu M, Friese K, et al. A cross-sectional study of workers in the chemical industry with occupational exposure to hexamethylenetetramine. Int Arch Occup Environ Health 1999; 72:533–8.

63. Belin L, Wass U, Audunsson G, et al. Amines: possible causative agents in the development of bronchial hyperreactivity in workers manufacturing polyurethanes from isocyanates. Br J Ind Med 1983; 40:251–7.

64. Tickner JA, Schettler T, Guidotti T, et al. Health risks posed by use of di-2-ethylhexyl phthalate (DEHP) in PVC medical devices: a critical review. Am J Ind Med 2001; 39:100–11.

65. Dirven HAAM, van den Broek PHH, Arends AMM, et al. Metabolites of the plasticizer di(2-ethylhexyl)phthalate in urine samples of workers in polyvinylchloride processing industries. Int Arch Occup Environ Health 1993; 64:549–54.

66. Hours M, Cardis E, Marciniak A, et al. Mortality of cohort in a polyamide-polyester factory in Lyon: a further follow up. Br J Ind Med 1989; 46:665–70.

67. Chu CC, Huang CC, Chen RS, et al. Polyneuropathy induced by carbon disulphide in viscose rayon workers. Occup Environ Med 1995; 52:404.

68. Harkonen H, Lehtniemi A, Aitio A. Styrene exposure and the liver. Scand J Work Environ Health 1984; 10:59–61.

69. Brodkin CA, Camp J, Moon J-D, et al. Serum hepatic biochemical activity in two populations of workers exposed to styrene. Occup Environ Med 2001; 58:95–102.

70. Muti A, Muzzucchi A, Rustichelli P, et al. Exposure-effect and exposure-response relationships between occupational exposure to styrene and neuropsychological functions. Am J Ind Med 1984; 5:275–86.

71. Cherry N, Gautrin D. Neurotoxic effects of styrene: further evidence. Br J Ind Med 1990; 47:29–37.

72. Murata K, Araki S, Yokoyama K. Assessment of the peripheral, central, and autonomic nervous system function in styrene workers. Am J Ind Med 1991; 20:775–84.

73. Viaene MK, Pauwels W, Veulemans H, et al. Neurobehavioural changes and persistence of complaints in workers exposed to styrene in a polyester boat building plant: influence of exposure characteristics and microsomal epoxide hydrolase phenotype. Occup Environ Med 2001; 58:103–12.

74. Blair A, Stewart PA, Zaebst DD, et al. Mortality of industrial workers exposed to acrylonitrile. Scand J Work Environ Health 1998; 24:25–41.

75. Rice JM, Boffetta P. 1,3-Butadiene, isoprene and chloroprene: reviews by the IARC monographs programme, outstanding issues, and research priorities. Epidemiology 2001; 135–136:11–26.

76. Albertini RJ, Sram RJ, Vacek PM, et al. Biomarkers for assessing occupational exposures to 1,3-butadiene. Chem Biol Interact 2001; June 1:135–136:429–53.

77. Ward E, Carpenter A, Markowitz S, et al. Excess number of bladder cancers in workers exposed to ortho-toluidine and aniline. J Natl Cancer Inst 1991; 83:7.

78. Markowitz S, Levin K. Continued epidemic of bladder cancer in workers exposed to ortho-toluidine in a chemical factory. Occup Environ Med 2004; in press.

79. International Agency for Research Against Cancer. Monographs on the evaluation of the carcinogenic risk of chemicals to humans: the rubber industry, vol. 28. Lyon: IARC, 1982.

Chapter 42
Organic Nitrogen Compounds

Joel D Kaufman, Chris Carlsten

Organic nitrogen compounds, such as amines, amides, nitrates and nitrochemicals, encompass a wide range of specific agents, with industrial applications usually related to their highly reactive chemical nature. This chemical reactivity also frequently affects biologic systems, and makes nitrogen compounds important hazards in the work environment. Some of these chemicals have figured prominently in the history of occupational health and, as a result, occupational exposures have been markedly reduced or eliminated. In many other cases, however, when an agent is not considered replaceable, or when the health effects are not sufficiently well recognized to force substitution of a less toxic chemical, exposure remains an important concern.

EXPOSURE SETTINGS

Forty years ago, the recognized occupational health effects of organic nitrogen compounds primarily concerned exposure to the benzidine dyes in the dye-making and textile industries, and to the nitrates in the manufacture of explosives. Although concern about these agents remains, the largest group of agents in this class today are chemical reagents used in a variety of advanced technologic applications, including resin systems and advanced composite materials. In addition, the health effects of some nitrogen-containing agents have been exploited for medicinal purposes, and many of these agents are encountered in the pharmaceutical industry. Other agents are created as intermediates in chemical manufacturing processes or are used routinely as laboratory reagents. The biotechnology industry and research community use many organic nitrogen compounds; achieving exposure controls in the laboratory represents a continuing challenge. Still other agents are primarily encountered as drugs of abuse (e.g., amyl nitrate) and will not be addressed here. A summary of organic nitrogen compounds, including applications and health effects, is provided in Table 42.1.

ENVIRONMENTAL MANAGEMENT

No guidelines apply to managing all of the wide-ranging hazards presented by this group of chemical agents. One general problem with these chemicals is that the skin represents a major route of exposure, often accounting for a large fraction of the systemic bioavailable dose. Occupational and environmental management strategies, therefore, cannot rely only on reducing the air-borne concentration of the contaminant, but must also provide barriers to skin exposure. The choice of gloves and other skin protection strategies must be tailored to the particular agent; glove materials that are impermeable to some agents may not provide an effective barrier to other organic nitrogen compounds.

CLINICAL EFFECTS

Organic nitrogen compounds vary tremendously in their toxic effects, but some general patterns exist and can be used to understand the nature of the occupational and environmental hazards. Major categories of effects appear repeatedly throughout this group, and a discussion of each of these follows. Table 42.1 indicates which of the common effects can be seen with individual agents and lists other important toxic effects.

Methemoglobinemia and hemolytic anemia

A variety of nitrogen-containing substances, including certain nitrates, nitrites, and aromatic amines, have the capacity to oxidize the heme moiety in the hemoglobin of erythrocytes, resulting in methemoglobin (MetHb), which is darkly pigmented and a poor carrier of oxygen. The agents that produce this effect are classified methemoglobin-formers. Methemoglobinemia can result in tissue hypoxia, with cyanosis and the potential for ischemic complications.

Occupational or environmental contact with MetHb-formers is common, but the agents differ in their ability to oxidize hemoglobin. In addition, the physiologic response to these agents is variable, although some of the differences are predictable. Individuals who are heterozygous for the traits that cause congenital methemoglobinemia (hemoglobin M disease or MetHb reductase deficiency) are at increased risk for complications with exposure, and those with glucose-6-phosphate dehydrogenase (G-6-PD) deficiency are much more likely to experience hemolytic anemia when exposed to these oxidizing agents.

Methemoglobinemia may develop following exposure to chemical agents (e.g., sodium nitrite in food processing or a variety of amine dyes), pharmaceutical agents (e.g., nitroglycerin [NTG], topical anesthetics, or dapsone), explosive materials (e.g., di- or trinitrotoluene, or nitrite-contaminated well water). A selected list of organic nitrogen MetHb-formers, primarily from occupational exposures, is included in Table 42.1.

Agent	Use	MetHb	Vas	Car*	Irr	Sens♦	Hep	Comments/Notes
Aliphatic Amines								
Alkyl monoamines								
methylamine	intermediate for dyes, pesticides	–	–	–	M/R/D	–	–	as with allylamine, may increase atherosclerosis in susceptible individuals (i.e. diabetics)
ethylamine	catalyst in epoxy resins, corrosion inhibitor	–	–	–	M/R/D	–	–	
Alkyl secondary amines								
diethyl amine, dimethylamine	corrosion inhibitor, solvent, chem. intermed. in chemicals	–	–	–	M/R/D	–	–	alkali with corrosive effects
ethylene imine (aziridine)	chem. ingred. in agricultural & textile chemicals, coatings	–	–	?	M/R/D/	D	?	temporary hazy blue vision (corneal effect) possible CNS, renal effects. Hepatotoxic in rats
propylene imine	chem. intermed. in laboratory; used in polymers, dyes, fuels	–	–	?	M/R/D	D	–	renal toxicity in animals
(methyl aziridine)	rubber, pharmaceut; flocculant in petroleum refining							
hexane diamine	corrosion inhibitor, chem. intermed. for resins; in dyes	–	–	–	M/R/D	–	–	
Alkyl polyamines								
diethylene triamine	curing agent/chem. intermed. in resins	–	–	–	M/D/R	D/R	–	corneal erosion
dimethylethylamine	catalyst in foundry sand cores and urethane foam mfg., chem. intermed.	–	–	–	M/D/R	–	–	anosmia
tetramethylene diamine (TEMED)	used in gel electrophoresis	–	–	–	M/D	D	–	
triethylamine	curing agent for polymers, urethane form, solvent emulsifiers, quaternary ammonium compounds, pesticides, dyes, water repellents	–	–	–	M/R/D	–	?	corneal effects
Amino Alcohols								
dimethanolamine	pharmaceuticals, amino resin stabilizer dyes, corrosion inhibitors, spray coatings	–	–	–	–	R	–	
ethanolamine	chem. intermed. for emulsifiers, detergents, pharmaceut. corrosion inhibitor, cosmetics, gas scrubbing agent	–	–	–	M/R	R	–	
triethanolamine	intermediate or ingredient in pharmaceuticals, cosmetics, solvents, soaps, emulsions	–	–	–	M/D	D	–	alkaline effects predominate, less irritating than others in class
phenylpropanolamine	pharmaceutical	see note	+	–	–	–	–	severe hypertension if taken in excess; methemoglobin via methyl nitrite, a reagent in production
Aromatic Nitros and Amines								
aminophenol	Dye: in fur, cosmetics, textiles, photo developer, chelating resin for waste water; chem. intermed. in pharmaceut.	+	–	–	–	D	–	
aminobiphenyl	manufacture of resins, rubber	–	–	†	–	–	–	bladder cancer
o-anisidine (methoxyaniline)	dyestuffs, chemical intermediate	+	–	?	D	D	–	animal carcinogen
aniline	dye, chem. intermed. rubber processing	+	–	?	M	–	–	'toxic oil syndrome'
benzidine	dye making, rubber hardener, chem. reagent	+	–	†	D	D	–	bladder cancer

Table 42.1 Toxicity of organic nitrogen compounds

Agent	Use	MetHb	Vas	Car*	Irr	Sens◆	Hep	Comments/Notes
chloroaniline	curing agent for polyurethane; intermed. in manufacture of dyes, solvents, pesticides	+	–	?	–	–	+	mutagen; renal toxin in rats
chlorodinitrobenzene	lab reagent, explosives, dyes	+	–	?	D	D	–	retrobulbar neuritis, peripheral neuropathy dermatitis: vesiculopapular or exfoliative
diaminodiphenyl sulfone (DDS or dapsone)	pharmaceutical (antibiotic); curing agent for composite and epoxy resin systems	+	–	–	–	–	+	hemolytic anemia
dichlorobenzidine	dyestuffs, curing agent in plastics, rubbers	–	–	*	D	–	–	animal carcinogen
diethylaniline	herbicide manufacture	+	–	?	–	–	–	
dimethoxybenzidine	dyestuff (blue)	–	–	?	–	–	–	
dimethylaminoazobenzene	dyestuffs, fat indicator (Sudan stain), analytic reagent	–	–	†	D	D	–	
dimethylaniline	chem. intermed. for dyes, vanillin, lab reagent, catalyst in resin systems	+	–	?	–	–	–	CNS depression
dinitrobenzene	chem. intermediate for man–made fibers, dyes, explosives; lab reagent	+	–	–	R	–	?	hemolytic anemia; ocular toxicity
dinitrophenol	wood preservative, pesticide, lab reagent, chem. intermed. in dyes, photo developers	–	–	–	M/D	+	+	uncouples oxidative phosphorylation with resulting chemical asphyxia, hepatic/renal failure
dinitrotoluene	explosives, dyes, chem. intermed. in isocyanate production	+	+	†	–	–	+	2,6 but not 2,4-isomer is animal carcinogen (see text) hemolytic anemia
3,3'-dichlorobenzidine	dye-making, curing agent in plastics, rubber, urethane	–	–	†	D/R	–	–	animal carcinogen
methylene dianiline	chemical mfg, curing agent for resins, urethanes and epoxies	–	–	†	M/D	D	+	cholestatic hepatitis, skin staining
4,4'-diaminodiphenyl-methane methylene bis-2-chloroaniline (MOCA or M-BOCA)	corrosion inhibitor, dyemaking curing agent for urethane, epoxy, and other resin systems	+	–	†	–	–	–	hematuria as acute effect
naphthylamine	chem. intermed. for dyes, rubber, pesticides	+	–	†	–	–	–	hemorrhagic cystitis as acute effect, 2-naphthylamine is human carcinogen while evidence for 1-naphthylamine not strong
nitroaniline	red/yellow, orange dyes; corrosion inhibitor, chem. intermed.	+	–	–	–	–	+	hemolytic anemia
nitrobenzene	chem. intermed. for pharmaceut. dyes, pesticides, Isocyanate, preservative/constituent of paints, polishes, scents, dyes, explosives	+	–	?	M/D	–	+	hemolytic anemia; animal carcinogen
4-nitrophenol	leather treatment; lab reagent, fungicide, biocide	+	–	–	M	–	–	possible renal toxin
nitrotoluene	dyestuffs, explosives, detergents	+	–	–	–	–	–	
phenylenediamine	cosmetics, dyestuffs, photog. chemicals, metal cutting oils, chem. agent in polymers, fibers	–	–	–	D/M	R/D	–	potent sensitizer with usual exposure; rhabdomyolysis/acute tubular necrosis, hemolytic anemia in poisoning
picric acid	explosive, fuel additive	–	–	–	D/M	D	+	acute renal failure; skin staining; poisoning may be similar to dinitrophenol
trinitrotoluene	explosive	+	–	–	M/D	–	+	skin staining; aplastic anemia; cataracts
toluidine	dyestuffs, exchange resins, rubber processing	+	–	†	M	–	–	hemorrhagic cystitis, ortho isomer is probably human carcinogen
2,4-toleunediamine	photographic developer, dyestuffs, intermed. for TDI	+	–	?	M/D	D	?	see text; skin staining; gastritis; animal carcinogen

Table 42.1 (Cont'd) Toxicity of organic nitrogen compounds

Agent	Use	MetHb	Vas	Car*	Irr	Sens◆	Hep	Comments/Notes
Aliphatic Nitro Chemicals								
nitromethane	chemical coatings, fuels, explosives, solvent	–	–	–	M/D/R	–	–	CNS effects – narcosis
nitroethane	solvent, propellant, chem. intermed.	–	–	†	R/M/D	–	+	
2-nitropropane	solvent in paint and other spray coatings, propellant, fuel additive, chem. intermed.	+	–	†	M	–	+	fulminant hepatic failure, CNS effects – intoxication, headache
tetranitromethane	fuel additive, lab reagent, explosive	+	–	?	M/R/D	–	+	very potent respiratory irritant, mild methemoglobiemia
chloropicrin (trichloronitromethane)	pesticide, rodenticide, soil fumigant	–	–	–	R/M/D	–	–	severe gastroenteritis if ingested, severe pneumonitis if inhaled, reports of cardiac necrosis
Aliphatic Nitrates								
cyclonite or RDX (trimethylene trinitramine)	explosive	–	–	–		–	–	epileptiform seizures w/o sequelae
ethylene glycol dinitrate	explosive, fuel	+	+	–	–	–	–	skin staining
nitroglycerin	pharmaceuticals, explosives	+	+	–	–	D	–	CNS effects – headache, chronic
propylene glycol dinitrate	explosive, fuel	+	+	–	R	–	–	metabolite (propylene glycol) is possible renal toxin
pentaerythritol tetranitrate (Penitrate)	pharmaceuticals, explosives	+	+	–	–	–	–	
Nitrites								
methyl nitrite, ethyl nitrite, butyl nitrite, amyl nitrite	pharmaceuticals, deodorants, fuel additives, chem. intermed.	+	+	?	–	–	–	see text for discussion of cancer risk
Miscellaneous								
acetamides	solvent, plasticizer, stabilizer	–	–	?	mild	–	–	animal carcinogen
acetonitrile	solvent in hydrocarbon extractions, nail removers, high pressure liquid chromatography (HPLC) reagent	–	–	–	M	–	–	metabolized to cyanide and formic acid, management should be as for cyanide
acrylamide	see text	–	–	†	D	D	–	neurotoxin – see text; alopecia areata
acrylonitrile	comonomer, used in rubber, plastics, coatings, adhesives, acrylic fiber, chem. intermediate, pesticides	–	–	†	R	D	+	headache, nausea CNS effects, partially metabolized to release cyanide
benzotriazole	anticorrosive chem. intermediate, lab reagent, plastics stabilizer	–	–	–	R/?	D	–	
1,1-dimethylhydrazine (UDMH)	rocket fuel, organic chemicals, chemical intermediate	–	–	?	M/R/D	–	+	CNS effects, animal carcinogen
1,2-diphenylhydrazine	anti-sludging agent, chemical intermediate, reagent flame retardant	–	–	†	–	–	–	limited information on general toxicity
hexamethylene tetramine (HMT or methenamine)	pharmaceuticals; curing agent for resins used in plastics and explosive manufacture	–	–	–	R	D/R	–	GI irritation; possible kidney toxicity
hydrazine (sulphate)	pharmaceuticals, organic chemicals, rocket fuel, lab reagent, soldering flux	–	–	†	R/D/M	D?	+	central, peripheral neurotoxin; liver toxin
melamine	laminate resins (frequent comonomer with formaldehyde)	–	–	see note	–	–	–	CNS effects; bladder cancer in rats secondary to melamine-induced stones
morpholine	solvent for resins; defoaming agent, emulsifier, corrosion inhibitor,	–	–	–	D/R/M	–	–	corneal edema, ulceration

Table 42.1 (Cont'd) Toxicity of organic nitrogen compounds

Agent	Use	MetHb	Vas	Car *	Irr	Sens◆	Hep	Comments/Notes
piperazine	chemical intermediate pharmaceuticals, insecticides, plastics	–	–	–	–	D/R	–	urticaria; anticholinergic and extrapyramidal symptoms
piperidine	pharmaceuticals, dyes, explosives, solvents, lab reagent, fuel additive, curing agent for resins	–	–	–	D/M/R	–	?	Possible CNS depression
pyridine	pharmaceuticals	–	–	–	R/D/M	–	+	renal toxic, CNS depression
pyrrolidine	chem. intermed.: pharmaceuticals, pesticides, rubber curing agent for epoxies	–	–	–	M/R	–	–	
quinoline	pharmaceuticals, paints, dyestuffs, lab reagent, corrosion inhibitor, fungistat	–	–	?	R/M	–	–	CNS depression

MetHb: Methemoglobinemia; Vas: Vasoactive; Car: Carcinogenicity; Irr: Irritant; Sens: Sensitization; Hep: Hepatotoxicity.
+ indicates a preponderance of evidence in support of the effect; – indicates a preponderance of evidence unsupportive of the effect; and ? indicates equivocal evidence
† For cancer, indicates this agent should be considered a probable or certain human carcinogen; ? this agent is an animal carcinogen or potent genotoxic agent, although sufficient human evidence is lacking. It should be considered a possible human carcinogen; – based on available information, carcinogenic activity is not suspected.
M, this agent is a mucous membrane (eye, nose, throat) irritant; R, this agent is a lower respiratory tract irritant associated with acute effects and the potential for delayed pulmonary edema; D, this agent is a skin irritant.
◆ R, this agent has been noted to sensitize the respiratory system and is associated with asthma; D, this agent has been noted to sensitize the skin and is associated with allergic contact dermatitis.

Table 42.1 **(Cont'd)** Toxicity of organic nitrogen compounds

Although many nitrogen-containing compounds cause methemoglobinemia in animal studies, the effect is not clinically significant in all cases. For some chemicals, such as nitromethane, the agent's heme-oxidizing potency is too weak to cause toxicity in most occupational or environmental settings. For other agents, such as propylene glycol dinitrate, other toxic effects (vasoactive effects, in this case) are present and require attention at lower exposure levels than MetHb formation.

MetHb levels have been proposed for biologic monitoring of exposure to nitrate chemicals. Currently, dose–effect relationships for this response are not sufficiently predictable to use these levels for ongoing monitoring, although there is great potential for development of methods for biologic monitoring in the future. In instances when a recent high level of exposure to a potent MetHb-former (such as aniline) is suspected, however, MetHb concentration can provide a useful confirmation.

Acute and chronic effects

Significant methemoglobinemia has effects typical of other causes of tissue hypoxia. The severity of clinical effects, which can range from no symptoms to coma, depends on the degree of poisoning, presence of concomitant anemia, hypoxemia (from lung or heart disease), or ischemic vascular disease. Typical early complaints include headache and fatigue. Findings of acrocyanosis, with bluish discoloration of the fingertips, toes, ears, and lips, often precede any symptoms. Methemoglobinemia has no specific chronic effects, aside from those associated with hypoxic injury.

Clinical evaluation

Cyanosis unresponsive to oxygen administration and 'chocolate brown' blood (when dried on filter paper) strongly suggest the diagnosis of methemoglobinemia; laboratory evidence of normal oxygen saturation and elevated MetHb concentration provides confirmation. The initial evaluation should identify a history of relevant exposure, as well as family or personal history of anemia or hemoglobinopathy. Laboratory studies should include hemoglobin determination, oxygen saturation level, and spectrophotometric measurement of MetHb. Recently, several commercial oximeters, including a bedside device, have been shown to be better than conventional photometric analysis in terms of reproducibility and accuracy of methemoglobin concentration measurements.[1] Further studies are necessary to determine whether the instruments perform equally well under diverse clinical circumstances; importantly, methylene blue administration will interfere with these measurements. The presence of Heinz bodies and evidence of hemolytic anemia on a peripheral blood smear indicate a more severe oxidant stress on red blood cells and raise the suspicion of an underlying G-6-PD deficiency.

Management

Unless symptomatic, methemoglobinemia should be treated simply by removing the offending exposure. When treatment is needed, methylene blue (MB) is administered intravenously (1 mg/kg). Recently, high-dose riboflavin has been shown in vitro to be effective in reducing nitric oxide-induced MetHb,[2] but it is not yet clear whether this is safe or effective in clinical practice. N-acetylcysteine, while reducing MetHb in vitro, failed to do so in a randomized, controlled trial of human volunteers.[3] In severe cases unresponsive to MB, if significant hemolysis is present, or if the patient has known G-6-PD deficiency (so that methylene blue is contraindicated because of its additional oxidant activity), exchange transfusion should be provided as initial therapy. In such cases automated red blood cell exchange may be superior to conventional exchange.[4]

Prevention

Reducing potential exposure to MetHb-formers is the cornerstone of prevention. Attention must be paid to inhalational, dermal, and oral routes of exposure. At present, the use of MetHb in biologic monitoring, while specific, may be inaccurate in assessing the potential exposure hazards. In environments in which exposure is suspected, the presence of elevated MetHb levels should trigger engineering modifications; however, normal spot MetHb levels are insufficient to determine that exposure levels are safe.

There is no question that certain individuals (e.g., those with G-6-PD or MetHb reductase deficiency and those with hemoglobin M disease) are at increased risk from the health effects of exposure to nitrogen compounds that oxidize heme. Current environmental control techniques can achieve exposure levels that protect even these sensitive workers. If such workers are identified in a worksite with potential MetHb-former exposure, they should be screened periodically with complete blood counts, MetHb level and peripheral blood smears to be certain that adverse effects are not occurring. Blood work every 6 weeks for the first 3 months, followed by blood work every 6 months, is an appropriate schedule for most sensitive individuals. The finding of significant methemoglobinemia or hemolysis, even if asymptomatic, warrants medical removal while the offending exposure is reduced.

Vasoactive effects and coronary artery disease

The activity of nitrate esters on the vascular system was first exploited when NTG was employed to reduce blood pressure in 1847. The related occupational hazard was first noted shortly after Nobel incorporated NTG into dynamite in the late 19th century; untoward vasodilatory effects were described in dynamite workers and their families. Since that time, the effects of NTG have been extensively used for pharmacologic purposes; NTG and other nitrates are major medications in treatment regimens for coronary artery disease. The potential for vasoactive nitrates to cause occupational hazards persists during the use and production of associated pharmacologic agents, explosives, related propellants, and chemical products.

Two clinical vascular syndromes of occupational nitrate toxicity are clearly described, characterized by acute vasodilation and withdrawal vasospasm. Some evidence also exists for a third syndrome, in which chronic occupational exposure to certain nitrates may increase the risk of atherosclerotic coronary artery disease. The vasoactive agents typically implicated are NTG, ethylene glycol dinitrate (nitroglycol or EGDN), and propylene glycol dinitrate (or Otto Fuel II torpedo propellant).

Acute effects

With acute exposure to nitrate vasoactive compounds, general vasodilation occurs. Symptoms include a severe and usually throbbing headache, flushing, palpitations, light-headedness, nausea, vomiting, and occasionally alcohol intolerance. Physical examination may demonstrate hypotension, tachycardia, and evidence of vasodilation. In heavily exposed individuals with pre-existing coronary artery disease, the generalized vasodilation combined with reflex tachycardia may reduce coronary artery perfusion pressure and precipitate angina.

Habituation occurs if exposure to the vasodilating nitrates continues over several days, and the exposed individual may no longer notice the acute effects. With continued exposure, the vascular system develops a dependence on nitrates. As a result, withdrawal from exposure can be accompanied by vasoconstriction, with resulting headache, angina, myocardial infarction, or in extreme cases sudden cardiac death. Worldwide, dozens of cases of sudden death, typically occurring on a Monday morning (after a weekend away from exposure), were reported among explosives workers in the 1950s. Angina and sudden Monday death were described in individuals in whom coronary artery disease could not be demonstrated either by arteriography or autopsy. Sporadic cases continue to occur.[5] The typical toxicokinetics of nitrates, with withdrawal effects occurring shortly after exposure ends, do not explain the timing of the angina and sudden death that occurs days after removal from exposure, and prior to re-exposure, in occupationally habituated individuals.

Chronic effects

Whether or not any of the above effects lead to significantly increased long-term cardiovascular risk in current or former workers is unclear. Earlier studies by Hogstedt and colleagues did not show such an association.[6] Two cohorts of Swedish dynamite workers (EGDN and NTG exposed) demonstrated an excess of chronic heart and cerebrovascular disease, most notably among those with greater than 1 year of exposure and 20 years of latency since their first exposure. Deaths occurred long after exposure ended. A subsequent study with larger populations did not detect an increase in long-term mortality, though it did find higher risk of acute mortality in those less than 45 years old.[7] In a recent small case-control study,[8] occupational history of exposure to dynamite was not significantly associated with greater risk of myocardial infarction (including events distant in time from original exposure). At this time it is prudent to consider chronic nitrate exposure a potential but unconfirmed risk factor for atherosclerotic cardiovascular disease.

Clinical evaluation

The approach to the individual with vasoactive nitrate exposure is guided by the clinical presentation. All possible information on the type and duration of likely exposure, and the timing of last contact, should be obtained. In the setting of acute exposure or withdrawal vasoconstriction, a history of vasodilatory symptoms and headache or angina should be elicited. Physical examination, including orthostatic blood pressure measurement, supplemented by 12-lead electrocardiography, will guide the management. With several of these agents (e.g., Otto Fuel II), yellow skin staining can confirm both the presence and at least one route of exposure. Because these agents also oxidize hemoglobin, the MetHb level should be measured.

Management

The treatment is directed by the clinical presentation. Removal from exposure is the first step, and if dermal exposure is suspected, the exposed skin should be carefully washed. If marked postural blood pressure changes are found, fluid resuscitation with intravenous normal saline is indicated. In the appropriate exposure withdrawal setting (8–72 hours since the last exposure), evidence of ischemia by history or electrocardiographic studies indicates vasoconstriction, which should be managed conventionally. Dermal, sublingual, or intravenous NTG should be considered acutely to treat the severe withdrawal symptoms of the nitrate-habituated worker; subsequent withdrawal can then be managed in a supervised medical setting. The management of the chronic vascular effects is no different from that related to any other cause.

Prevention

Before exposure levels were controlled, nitrate-habituated explosives workers recognized the symptoms of withdrawal and prevented them by inserting NTG into their hat bands to maintain vasodilation through the weekend. Concern surrounding nitrate-withdrawal deaths led to precautions that reduced exposure to nitrates in munitions production. Continued vigilance is required to keep exposures low as new agents and processes are introduced.

For many vasoactive organic nitrogen compounds, including EGDN, dermal exposure can be the major source of systemic absorption and bioavailability; therefore, isolated control of air concentrations is inadequate to control exposure. Given the capability of engineering controls, inhalation and dermal exposures should be kept at a level below the threshold of the vasoactive effect, which varies for each agent. If this goal is met, it should never be necessary for workers to use nitrates or other vasodilators to prevent withdrawal symptoms.

In developed countries, it has been customary to screen potential nitrate-exposed workers with some combination of physical examination and resting and exercise electrocardiographic studies, and to exclude individuals with abnormal results for workplace exposures. Although these tests may seem prudent, there is no good evidence that this type of screening is effective in reducing morbidity or mortality, and the false-positive rate for such tests is likely

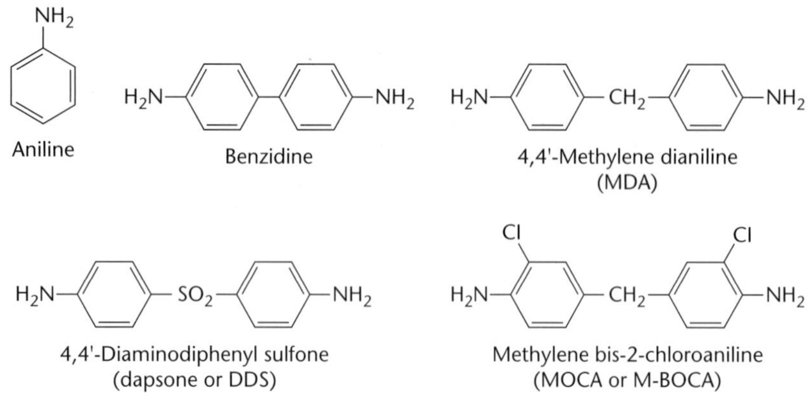

Figure 42.1: Aromatic amines in wide use, currently or in the past.

to be unacceptable in a working population. In addition, cases of sudden death have occurred in young, previously healthy individuals who have 'passed' these screening tests, indicating that the screening tests cannot effectively predict susceptible individuals. It is likely that the level of exposure, and not merely susceptibility, is most important in determining adverse effects. It remains judicious to limit occupational exposure to vasoactive organic nitrogen agents for individuals with a clinical history of coronary artery disease, cardiomyopathy, or life-threatening arrhythmias. In addition, exposed workers should be well informed about the toxicity of these agents, and regularly asked about the presence of headache, light-headedness, or other evidence of exposure; if symptoms are found, action should be taken to identify and reduce the exposure.

Biologic monitoring may have a role in the management of exposure to vasoactive organic nitrogen agents. Such methods are particularly attractive because of significant dermal absorption, that can be quantitated by determining the internal dose. Unfortunately, measuring the urine and serum levels of nitrates and their associated metabolites has not yet proven valid or practical for measurement of biologic exposure. For example, measurement of serum EGDN from the arm vein may represent the local concentration resulting from skin absorption and, hence, may overestimate systemic levels. Several new techniques, including gas chromatography-mass spectrometry and high-performance liquid chromatography, have been advanced to rival the traditional batch Griess assay for quantitative nitrate measurements. At this point, methodologic issues limit using these assays for routine monitoring. Methemoglobin levels, as noted above, remain non-specific and indicative only of gross exposure rather than a specific dose–effect relationship.

CARCINOGENESIS

Concern over the carcinogenicity of organic nitrogen agents stems from two lines of research regarding various chemical classes as follows: (1) several aromatic amines are demonstrated carcinogens by human epidemiologic and animal investigations, and (2) certain N-nitrosamines, which are potent animal carcinogens, may be encountered

directly or as a metabolite of an occupational or environmental exposure.

Aromatic amines

The structure for aromatic amines in wide use is shown in Figure 42.1. Benzidine and related aromatic amines (e.g., beta-naphthylamine, 4-aminobiphenyl, and related compounds listed in Table 42.1) were found in early epidemiologic studies to be the cause of excess bladder cancers in occupational cohorts. The relative risk of bladder cancer ranged from 8 to 87 among dyestuff, research, and rubber workers with significant exposures. These agents have subsequently been demonstrated to be potent animal carcinogens. Transitional cell cancer of the urinary bladder, renal pelvis, or ureter are the typical tumors seen in humans, primarily because of the urinary concentration of these genotoxic agents and their metabolites. Animal studies have also shown other bladder, liver, breast, and lung tumors related to carcinogenic aromatic amine exposure.

Although the use of these chemicals as dyestuffs has been curtailed, related chemicals that are probable human carcinogens are still used extensively in many industries. For example, agents such as methylene dianiline (MDA) and methylene bis-2-chloroaniline (M-BOCA) are curing agents in some contemporary resin systems. It can be expected that other carcinogenic aromatic amines, although less well studied, will find their way into advanced technologic processes. To illustrate, MDA and M-BOCA have been replaced in some applications by diethylene toluene diamine, an aromatic amine agent about which little toxicologic information is available.

N-Nitroso compounds and nitrate exposure

The general structure of nitroso chemicals and some examples are shown in Figure 42.2. Virtually all nitroso compounds have been found to be potent animal carcinogens, with malignant tumors occurring in many organs (respiratory tract, gastrointestinal tract, liver, kidney, bladder, and brain), relatively independent of the route of

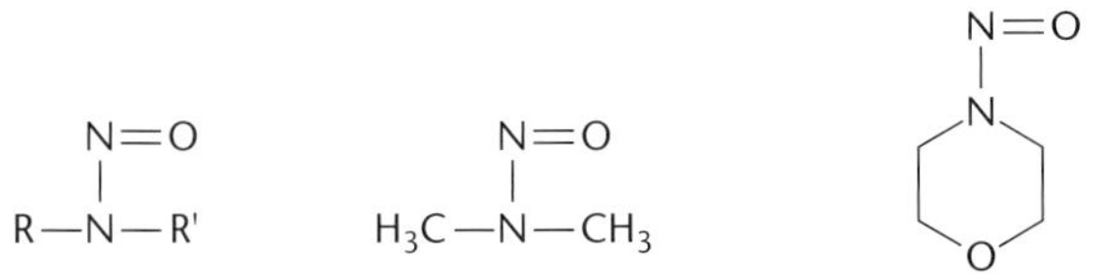

Nitrosamine (generic) — N,N-Dimethyl nitrosamine or n-Nitrosodimethylamine — N-Nitrosomorpholine

Figure 42.2: Structure of generic and representative nitrosamines.

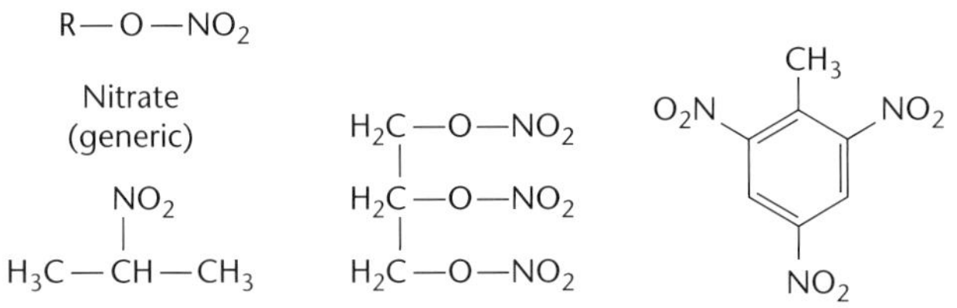

Nitrate (generic) — 2-Nitropropane — Nitroglycerin — 2,4,6-Trinitrotoluene

Figure 42.3: Generic nitrate structure and common nitro compounds.

administration. In rodent studies, symmetric dialkylnitrosamines (where the two R groups are the same, such as N-nitrosodimethylamine) tend to produce tumors in the liver, lung, kidney, or bladder; the esophagus is a more frequent target organ for tumors caused by asymmetric nitrosamines.

In occupational settings, exposure is primarily encountered in the form of a chemical reagent, reaction intermediate, or contaminant. Exposed groups have included rocket fuel production workers, pesticide formulators, rubber workers, tannery workers, and laboratory workers. The use of sodium nitrate as a corrosion inhibitor in lubrication systems can lead to the formation of N-nitroso compounds and volatile exposure. Contamination of ground-water sources can lead to environmental exposure by ingestion route.

Public health concern has arisen over the potential for in vivo nitrosamine formation as a result of exposure to ingested amines, nitrates, and nitrites. Exogenous nitrate (Fig. 42.3) can be reduced to nitrite by colonizing bacteria, and nitrite leads to the development of N-nitroso compounds in the digestive tract. This pathway has resulted in carcinogenesis in laboratory animals. In addition, there is evidence to support the notion that dietary nitrite and nitrate intake may explain some of the large geographic differences in gastric, esophageal, nasopharyngeal, and colorectal cancer rates. The nitrate concentrations of cured and smoked meats are among the highest found in foods. However, the relationship between gastric cancer and occupational, environmental, or dietary nitrate exposure remains unclear. Recent epidemiologic studies have not consistently supported a strong relationship between dietary nitrate intake and cancer.[9] However, as studies have focused on individual nitroso compounds and more specific dietary histories, this relationship may become better understood. One large recent study found that N-nitrodimethylamine specifically was associated with colorectal but not other cancers.[10] Another showed an association between nitrites/nitrosamines and nasopharyngeal cancer predominantly when the intake was high in early childhood.[11] It remains prudent to keep dietary nitrite exposure to a minimum.

Contamination of drinking water by nitrates is an issue of concern. The main source of nitrate is typically from fertilizer leaching into ground water,[12] though unusual sources, such as contamination from boiler fluid additives,[13] also occur. Since these situations can result in chronic exposure situations, often high enough to result in methemoglobinemia and possibly spontaneous abortions,[14] concern over chronic health effects is reasonable.

Prevention and management

Exposure to carcinogens must be prevented, and regulations generally are designed to eliminate or keep such exposures to a minimum. Rapid monitoring is not yet practical, although several new biochemical techniques designed for measuring nitric oxide radicals may be helpful in the future. Cancers related to organic nitrogen compounds are managed according to standard oncologic practice. If a cohort of workers is identified as being at elevated risk for a certain type of occupational cancer (such as workers exposed to a bladder carcinogenic aromatic amine), it is appropriate to implement a medical surveillance program.

HEPATOXICITY

Given the chemical reactivity of organic nitrogen compounds, it is not surprising that several agents in this group are potent hepatotoxins. A few of these chemicals will be discussed briefly here. Further details on the clinical presentation, evaluation, management, and prevention of hepatotoxicity are found in Chapter 26.1.

Trinitrotoluene

The structure of common nitro compounds such as trinitrotoluene is provided in Figure 42.3. An estimated 500 workers who were exposed to the explosive trinitrotoluene (TNT) in Great Britain during World War I developed severe clinical hepatitis manifested by jaundice and a mortality rate of 25%. The incidence of hepatic effects was estimated to be approximately 5% of exposed individuals. The usual pattern of hepatotoxicity was characterized by subacute or acute hepatic necrosis. The onset of clinically apparent disease may be delayed for up to 4 months following initial exposure, although biochemical markers, such as elevated aspartate aminotransferase, alanine aminotransferase, and bilirubin levels, and histologic abnormalities are typically present earlier. This chemical is reported to cause measurable methemoglobinemia without overt cyanosis at exposure levels lower than those associated with hepatitis. If hepatic necrosis occurs, it can persist for months following removal from exposure. If exposure ends prior to extensive liver damage, the prognosis for recovery is good. Aplastic anemia has also been reported with TNT exposure. Trinitrotoluene-exposed individuals should be monitored with liver function studies, methemoglobin levels, hematocrit, and white blood cell count.

2-Nitropropane

The animal hepatocarcinogen 2-nitropropane (2-NP) (Fig. 42.3), widely used as a solvent in spray coatings and epoxy resin systems, can cause fulminant hepatitis following brief, high-level exposure.[15] The pathophysiology likely involves free radical formation and rapid hepatocyte necrosis. After a single overexposure episode, there can be a deceptive period without overt clinical illness, followed by progressive hepatic failure over the course of days to weeks. The National Occupational Exposure Survey estimated that 185,000 American workers were exposed to 2-NP in 1980. Inadequate epidemiologic and laboratory knowledge exists regarding the toxicologic and pharmacokinetic properties of this chemical to determine a specific dose–effect relationship. As a result, although hepatotoxic effects are usually noted at exposure levels greater than 25 ppm, no safe level of exposure has been established. When substitution of this ingredient is not possible, exposed workers should be educated regarding its toxicity and provided with proper protection from inhalational and dermal exposure. Agents containing significant concentrations of 2-NP should not be used in confined space without well-engineered ventilation or supplied air respiratory protection. Neither biologic monitoring nor medical surveillance guidelines are currently available.

Methylene dianiline (MDA)

MDA (4, 4'-diaminodiphenylmethane) is used in the production of methylenediphenyl diisocyanate (MDI) and commonly encountered as a curing agent in reinforced plastics or 'advanced composites'. It is a hepatotoxin and a probable human bladder carcinogen. The hepatotoxic effects can be variable, but one clear pattern is cholestatic jaundice from bile duct injury,[16] which is otherwise unusual among occupational hepatotoxins. In many cases, pruritus is the dominant initial symptom, and the most prominent laboratory abnormalities may be elevations of the alkaline phosphatase and bilirubin levels, rather than the transaminase levels. Portal inflammation and bile stasis, without extensive parenchymal injury, characterize the histologic picture of the acute cholestatic injury. If exposure ends before fibrosis occurs, the prognosis for full recovery is thought to be good.

MDA is absorbed through the skin, with prominent dermal route of exposure; biologic monitoring should ideally supplement other exposure indices. Dermal pads or glove testing have not yet been standardized, and still do not quantify actual in-vivo exposure. Urine concentration can theoretically be used to more practically integrate recent dermal exposure. However, while development of a 'dermal occupational exposure limit' via urinary MDA excretion remains promising,[17,18] practical workplace applications have yet to be established. Excretion rates peak at 6–11 hours following dermal exposure (slower than

for inhalational exposure), so urine monitoring should ideally be conducted several hours after exposures. In practice, post-shift monitoring has been common. While some had previously recommended 70 µg MDA per gram of creatinine as a urinary action level to reduce exposure to MDA, this is likely not low enough to ensure compliance with the current (1992) Occupational Safety and Health Administration (OSHA) MDA standard. Under this standard, which recognizes the potential carcinogenicity of MDA, the air-borne permissible exposure limit is 10 parts per billion as a time-weighted average, and MDA biomonitoring is not required.

SENSITIZATION AND IRRITATION

Organic nitrogen compounds, especially amino compounds such as the polyamines, have the capacity to act as antigens or haptens, with resulting potent sensitizing properties. The syndromes of allergic contact dermatitis, allergic rhinitis or sinusitis, and asthma typically require removal from exposure. A history of atopy does not accurately predict who will be affected by these exposures. These compounds, which are frequently encountered as curing agents in epoxy resin or urethane foam systems, can also be potent skin and mucosal irritants, which makes diagnosis and management more challenging.

The primary toxic effect of many organic nitrogen compounds is irritation of the skin, mucous membranes, or respiratory tract. As a general rule, any of the agents that cause respiratory irritation can, at high exposure levels, also precipitate lower respiratory injury with toxic pneumonitis or pulmonary edema.

DERMATOLOGIC EFFECTS

The most common skin manifestations of the agents in this group are allergic and irritant contact dermatitis. However, skin staining is also caused by many nitrosylated compounds and is important not only as a dermatologic cosmetic problem, but also to verify dermal (and probably systemic) exposure to a potentially toxic agent. The skin staining can be yellow to orange, or occasionally black and tattoo-like. Agents that commonly stain the skin include nitric acid, trinitrotoluene, EGDN, MDA, and dinitrophenol. Skin staining sometimes appears only hours to days after the exposure, when the chemical is oxidized on the skin, or when the chemical is incorporated into the skin's protein.

NEUROLOGIC EFFECTS

Although neurotoxic properties are not prominent among the organic nitrogen compounds, two agents, acrylamide and dimethylaminopropionitrile (DMAPN), are important exceptions. They cause characteristic toxic peripheral neuropathies. In addition, retinotoxic effects of several aromatic amines have been described. 1,4-bis(4-aminophenoxy)-2-phenylbenzene (a component of some advanced composite materials) damaged photoreceptors in rats.[19]

Although the rat retina may regain partial function with time, and ocular damage from occupational exposure has not been clearly demonstrated in humans,[20] the retinotoxicity of this compound raises concern about related aromatic diamines. Methylene dianiline has been reported to have similar retinotoxicity in guinea pigs and in one documented human exposure.[21]

Acrylamide

Reactive acrylamide monomer is encountered as an intermediate in the manufacture of polyacrylamides, which are widely used in laboratory electrophoretic gels and other synthetic products. It is used in dam foundations and tunnels and as a flocculation agent to separate solids from aqueous solutions, which is useful in mining operations, in the disposal of industrial waste, and in the purification of water supplies, among other applications as a polymer in industry. Acrylamide causes a fairly typical toxic distal neuropathy, with mixed sensory and motor findings. Early findings can include numbness, paresthesias, or hyperesthesias of the lower legs or feet, as well as complaints of coldness or muscle weakness. Only the reactive monomer is toxic; polyacrylamides are regarded as non-toxic. Acrylamide is well absorbed by the dermal route.

In certain applications, N-methylolacrylamide – which is likely a less potent neurotoxin – has become a substitute for acrylamide. Isocyanate-containing resins have been proposed as substitutes as well, but this substitution cannot be justified on a health basis due to the respiratory hazard created.

An epidemiologic investigation in a polymerization factory found a dose–response relationship between the air-borne acrylamide concentration and symptoms of peripheral neuropathy, with effects seen at exposure levels near the current OSHA exposure limit of 0.3 mg/m^3. A lower level of 0.03 mg/m^3 was subsequently adopted but later rolled back under court order in 1992 as part of the PEL revisions. NIOSH and ACGIH continue to recommend 0.03 as a time-weighted average, and several states also enforce this level.

In subacute or chronic intoxication, central nervous system signs, such as ataxia, can occur; encephalopathy has been noticed in significant acute poisoning. The neurologic effects[22] frequently improve with removal from exposure. A syndrome with desquamation and sweating of the hands has been observed to accompany the peripheral neuropathy of acrylamide toxicity. In addition, fingertip dermatitis occurs following dermal exposure to acrylamide, and the presence of this finding indicates a level of exposure that is associated with neurotoxicity.

Hemoglobin adducts have been proposed as a proxy for exposure to acrylamide.[23] Hb adducts have been demonstrated to be present in acrylamide-exposed populations in which neurotoxic effects were documented.[24] While the presence of adducts is associated with exposure in epidemiologic studies, the usefulness in evaluating individual workers remains uncertain, and concern remains regarding confounding effects with concurrent smoking. Given

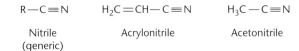

Figure 42.4: Nitriles. All contain the CN moiety, which may be released in vivo as cyanide ion.

acrylamide's status as a suspected carcinogen, exposures should be kept well below the levels associated with either dermatitis or neurotoxicity.

Dimethylaminopropionitrile (DMAPN)

Two clusters of neurogenic bladder dysfunction associated with DMAPN were reported in 1980,[25] with use of this agent as a catalyst in the manufacture of polyurethane foam. The pattern of neuropathy was unusual, in that it produced urinary symptoms, such as retention and hesitancy, more prominently than limb symptoms. The clinical syndrome also included sexual dysfunction, insomnia, and some muscle weakness and paresthesias. For unknown reasons, DMAPN appears to affect the sensory fibers of the sacral region selectively. Although the toxicologic mechanism for the neurotoxicity remains obscure, evidence exists that DMAPN exposure may result in in-vivo release of cyanide (as can all nitriles, see Fig. 42.4), and that it may inhibit certain glycolytic enzymes.[26] This agent has largely been eliminated from the workplace, although certain other aliphatic aminonitriles are suspected of sharing its neurotoxic risk.

References

1. Dotsch J, Demirakça S, Hahn D, et al. Accuracy of methemoglobin measurements: comparison of six different commercial devices and one manual method. Crit Care Med 1999; 27:1191–4.
2. Dotsch J, Demirakça S, Kratz M, et al. Comparison of methylene blue, riboflavin, and N-acetylcysteine for the reduction of nitric oxide-induced methemoglobinemia. Crit Care Med 2000; 28:958–61.
3. Tanen DA, LoVecchio F, Curry SC. Failure of intravenous N-acetylcysteine to reduce methemoglobin produced by sodium nitrite in human volunteers: a randomized controlled trial. Ann Emerg Med 2000; 35:369–73.
4. Golden PJ, Weinstein R. Treatment of high-risk, refractory acquired methemoglobinemia with automated red blood cell exchange. J Clin Apheresis 1998; 13:28–31.
5. RuDusky BM. Acute myocardial infarction secondary to coronary vasospasm during withdrawal from industrial nitroglycerin exposure – a case report. Angiology 2001; 52:143–4.
6. Hogstedt C, Axelson O. Mortality from cardio-cerebrovascular diseases among dynamite workers – an extended case-referent study. Ann Acad Med Singapore 1984; 13:399–403.
7. Stayner LT, Dannenberg AL, Thun M, et al. Cardiovascular mortality among munitions workers exposed to nitroglycerin and dinitrotoluene. Scand J Work Environ Health 1992; 18:34–43.
8. Gustavsson P, Plato N, Hallqvist J, et al. A population-based case-referent study of myocardial infarction and occupational exposure to motor exhaust, other combustion products, organic solvents, lead, and dynamite. Stockholm Heart Epidemiology Program (SHEEP) Study Group. Epidemiology 2001; 12:222–8.

9. Eichholzer M, Gutzwiller F. Dietary nitrates, nitrites, and N-nitroso compounds and cancer risk: a review of the epidemiologic evidence. Nutr Rev 1998; 56:90–105.

10. Knekt P, Jarvinen R, Dich J, et al. Risk of colorectal and other gastro-intestinal cancers after exposure to nitrate, nitrite and N-nitroso compounds: a follow-up study. Int J Cancer 1999; 80:852–6.

11. Ward MH, Pan WH, Cheng YJ, et al. Dietary exposure to nitrite and nitrosamines and risk of nasopharyngeal carcinoma in Taiwan. Int J Cancer 2000; 86:603–9.

12. Gelberg KH, Church L, Casey G, et al. Nitrate levels in drinking water in rural New York State. Environ Res 1999; 80:34–40.

13. Shih R. Methemoglobinemia attributable to nitrite contamination of potable water through boiler fluid additives – New Jersey, 1992 and 1996. MMWR 1997; 46:202–4.

14. Grant W. Spontaneous abortions possibly related to ingestion of nitrate-contaminated well water –LaGrange County, Indiana, 1991–1994. MMWR 1996; 45:569–72.

15. Harrison R, Letz G, Pasternak G. Fulminant hepatic failure after occupational exposure to 2-nitropropane. Ann Intern Med 1987; 107:466–8.

16. Kanz, MF, Wang A, Campbell GA. Infusion of bile from methylene dianiline-treated rats into the common bile duct injures biliary epithelial cells of recipient rates. Toxicol Lett 1995; 78:165–71.

17. Bos PM, Brouwer DH, Stevenson H, et al. Proposal for the assessment of quantitative dermal exposure limits in occupational environments: Part 1. Development of a concept to derive a quantitative dermal exposure limit. Occup Environ Med 1998; 55:795–804.

18. Brouwer DH, Hoogendoorn L, Bos PM, et al. Proposal for the assessment to quantitative dermal exposure limits in occupational environments: Part 2. Feasibility study for application in an exposure scenario for MDA by two different dermal exposure sampling methods. Occup Environ Med 1998; 55:805–11.

19. Lee KP, Valentine R. Pathogenesis and reversibility of retinopathy induced by 1,4-bis(4-aminophenoxy)-2-phylbenzene (2-phenyl-APB-144) in pigmented rats. Arch Toxicol 1991; 65:292–303.

20. Leong BK, Lund JE, Groehn JA, et al. Retinopathy from inhaling 4,4′-methylenedianiline aerosols. Fundam Appl Toxicol 1987; 9:645–58.

21. Roy, CW, McSorley PD, Syme IG. Methylene dianiline: a new toxic cause of visual failure with hepatitis. Hum Toxicol 1985; 4:61–6.

22. Myers J, Macun I. Acrylamide neuropathy in a South African factory: an epidemiologic investigation. Am J Ind Med 1991; 19:487–93.

23. Bergmark E. Hemoglobin adducts of acrylamide and acrylic workers, smokers and non-smokers. Chem Res Toxicol 1997; 10:78–84.

24. Hagmar L, Tornqvist M, Nordander C, et al. Health effects of occupational exposure to acrylamide using hemoglobin adducts as biomarkers of internal dose. Scand J Work Environ Health 2001; 27:219–26.

25. Keogh J, Petronk A, Wertheimer D. An epidemic of urinary retention caused by dimethylaminopropionitrile. JAMA 1980; 243:746–9.

26. Mumtaz MM, Farooqui MY, Ghanayem BI, et al. The urotoxic effects of N,N′-dimethylaminopropionitrile. 2. In vivo and in vitro metabolism. Toxicol Appl Pharmacol 1991; 110:61–9.

Chapter 43
Metal Working Fluids

Peter S Thorne, Nancy L Sprince

INTRODUCTION

Metal working fluids (MWF) are materials used in transforming cast metal forms into finished metal products or components with precise dimensions. The scores of parts in automotive engines and transmissions are familiar examples. Machining processes include cutting, boring, hobbing, tapping, grinding, lapping, and honing. Each process requires the use of MWF tailored to the specific properties of the metals. The MWF serve three primary functions: removal of heat from the machine tool and the product, lubrication at the contact point between the product and the tool or abrasive, and removal of swarf. Swarf is the debris generated from the metal and the abrasive in the cutting or grinding process. In addition, MWF are formulated to inhibit corrosion during and after machining of the products, and to extend the life of cutting, boring, or grinding tools.

Three classes of MWF are in widespread use. First are the straight oils that are solvent-refined petroleum oils or high oleic agricultural-based lubricants without added water. Soluble oil MWF and semi-synthetic MWF represent the second class and are water-based emulsions that typically contain 3–15% oils when in use. The third class is the synthetic MWF that have no added oil and are used where high lubricity is not needed. The soluble oil and synthetic MWF have been used extensively in the past two decades. The chemical and microbiologic characteristics of these classes of MWF are described below in greater detail.

Occupational exposure to MWF is widespread and common for workers engaged in the manufacture of automobiles and trucks, farm equipment, aircraft, heavy machinery, and military hardware. Estimates of the number of US workers exposed to MWF vary. In their most recent National Occupational Exposure Survey, the National Institute for Occupational Safety and Health (NIOSH)[1] estimated that a total of 400,000 workers were exposed full time to MWF and 830,000 were exposed part time.[2] The United Automobile, Aerospace and Agricultural Implement Workers Union (UAW) has estimated that one-third of their one million members are exposed to MWF. The nature of the exposures and the resulting health effects depend on the types of MWF in use, the metals being machined, the operations performed, ventilation systems employed, and the degree of exposure. Early health concerns, reflecting the widespread use of straight oils, included lipoid pneumonia, oil acne and folliculitis, and skin cancer attributable to polycyclic aromatic hydrocarbons in poorly refined straight oils. The introduction

and widespread use of the water-based MWF have shifted concerns to contact dermatitis, respiratory effects, and the potential carcinogenicity of these MWF, which contain a number of chemicals and contaminants including chemical irritants, biocides, and micro-organisms, discussed further below.

CHARACTERISTICS OF METAL WORKING FLUIDS

The properties of the multitudes of commercially available MWF are quite variable and are proprietary. MWF are generally supplied by vendor companies that are separate from the manufacturer that uses the fluids. The MWF market is highly competitive and detailed product specifications are closely guarded secrets. The emulsion and synthetic MWF are supplied by the vendors as 'neat' concentrates that are diluted about 20-fold with water prior to use. Once in use, further additions are made including biocides and fungicides, anti-foaming agents, emulsifiers, corrosion inhibitors, potassium hydroxide, and additional MWF concentrate. Thus MWF used ('in-use' MWF) may contain a number of contaminants and substances not present in the concentrated 'neat' MWF supplied by the vendor.

Straight oils contain no water and are composed of paraffinic and naphthenic mineral oils or bio-based oils. These oils may be made from highly refined base oils or mildly treated, minimally refined oils. Some products also contain animal or vegetable oils. Additives such as sulfurized active fats, non-active fats and base oils, sulfurized-phosphorized hydrocarbons, polychlorinated paraffins, fatty esters, and antirust agents are common. Due to their higher cost, waste disposal problems, and inferior heat removing properties, use of straight oils has decreased somewhat in favor of synthetic MWF and emulsions. However, they continue to be essential for fine polishing operations such as honing. Recent advances in plant genetics have contributed to the advancement of bio-based lubricants. Oxidative stability, or the tendency to polymerize at high temperature, has been a problem with vegetable oils. However, soybeans have now been genetically engineered to produce a highly stable oil that is 84% oleic acid. Bio-based MWF formulated with high oleic soybean oils perform as well as petroleum-based fluids for some applications and present fewer disposal problems, including disposal costs, which can be substantial.

Emulsions (soluble oils and semi-synthetic fluids) are frequently made from higher viscosity base stocks rather than straight cutting oils. Prior to use, these oils and special additives are diluted with water to provide an emulsified fluid with the cooling properties of water and the lubricating properties of oils. Surface-active emulsifying agents are added to facilitate the miscibility of the oil and the water phases. The emulsifying agents generally consist of sodium and amine soaps, such as sodium naphthenates, rosinates and sulfonates. Other additives include coupling agents such as alcohols, glycols, and glycol ethers, and corrosion inhibitors, amines, fatty oils and sulfurized fatty oils. In addition, biocides for control of micro-organisms and compounds that increase lubricity are added. The terms soluble and semi-synthetic oil are used interchangeably by some, while others distinguish them by the degree of emulsification of the oils they contain. Typical components of neat soluble oil MWF are water (20–60%), light and heavy hydro-treated naphthenic petroleum distillates (20–40%), soluble petroleum sulfonic acids (5–20%), tall oil fatty acids (1–10%), plus diethanolamines, chloroalkanes, iminoethanols, oxazolidines, diaminoalkanes, and a variety of biocides. The pH of these emulsions is normally maintained above 8.5.

Synthetic MWF are water-based alkaline solutions containing ethanolamines and acid salts along with borates or phosphates added as corrosion inhibitors. Surfactants and silicones are added to provide detergent and lubricating properties to the blend. The operating pH of these fluids is usually about 9.0. Biocides of a variety of types are usually added by the user to control microbial growth since these synthetic fluids provide a medium suitable to support bacteria, yeasts, and molds. Synthetic cutting fluids are preferred in high-speed production machining operations because of their superior heat removal and stability characteristics.

A number of constituents may be contained within in-use fluids that were not associated with the neat MWF. After some period of use any of the MWF can reach 0.5–5% contamination with tramp oil (hydraulic fluid or oil that leaks past the seals of machining tools). In plants with large machining operations the MWF are present in as much as 5 million liter quantities and travel from the point of use to large sumps (20,000–400,000 liters) via flumes located beneath the floor. Thus, anything spilled onto the floor may pass into the MWF. Since the coolants are rarely discarded these foreign materials can accumulate. In addition, microbial degradation and thermal cracking of the MWF constituents lead to the formation of new and complex chemicals not in the original formulation.

MWF exposures are regulated under the OSHA permissible exposure limit (PEL) for oil mist that applies to 'heavy mineral oil mist, paraffin oil mist, white mineral oil mist'. The current OSHA time-weighted average (TWA) PEL is 5 mg/m^3. PELs have been promulgated for relatively few of the other components found in MWF. In 1998, NIOSH published its Criteria for a Recommended Standard: Occupational Exposure to Metalworking Fluids.[3] In so doing it recommended that metal working fluid aerosol exposures be limited to 0.4 mg/m^3 (thoracic mass fraction)

based on a 10 hour per day, 40 hour per week TWA. Table 43.1 is a listing of many of the OSHA PELs, NIOSH recommended exposure limits (RELs), and ACGIH threshold limit values (TLVs) that pertain to environments where MWF are used. The ACGIH lists a TLV for 'oil mist, mineral' of 5 mg/m^3 for the TWA when sampling only the aerosol fraction and has issued a 2002 notice of intended change to 0.2 mg/m^3 TWA for the inhalable mass fraction (Table 43.1).

Exposure limits for other compounds potentially found in the machining environment are also provided in Table 43.1. Ammonia, sulfur dioxide, and hydrogen sulfide are vapors that may be present from microbial action on fluids. Ethanolamines, formaldehyde, glutaraldehyde, and chlorine may be in the formulation to inhibit microbial growth or may be released from biocides. Metals such as cadmium, chromium, and nickel may exist as suspended dust or as compounds in various oxidation states. Exposure limits for aluminum, iron, and zinc dust (not listed) are all above the 5 mg/m^3 limit for oil mist.

All classes of MWF can support the growth of micro-organisms, but those containing water (soluble oil, semi-synthetic, and synthetic MWF) are especially prone to gross contamination with aerobic bacteria, yeast, and molds. Control of microbial growth is achieved principally by maintaining pH above 8.8, large scale filtration of the in-use MWF, continuous circulation of the fluids through sumps and flumes, and the addition of biocides directly or as a component of the MWF concentrate. The most commonly used biocides include isothiazolones, formaldehyde-yielding biocides such as triazines, and phenolic biocides such as O-phenyl phenol. With these control measures, viable microbial concentrations in the bulk MWF up to 10^5/ml for bacteria and 10^3/ml for fungi are generally regarded as acceptable so long as the organisms present are not pathogens or allergens. Excursions to 10^6–10^7/ml should prompt actions such as large scale centrifugation and reprocessing of the fluid, and addition of more MWF concentrate or biocide. When viable microbial concentrations reach 10^8–10^9/ml the system is usually considered unrecoverable without major reprocessing, biocide addition, and addition of neat MWF, and often would be discarded.

There have been several studies in which investigators have identified the culturable organisms contained within freshly sampled, water-based MWF, summarized in Table 43.2. In general, the most commonly found genera of mesophilic bacteria are Pseudomonas and Acinetobacter. However, in certain systems the spectrum of biocide sensitivity may dictate which organisms predominate. We have sampled several large systems that contain triazine biocides in which the predominant mesophilic bacteria were *Micrococcus luteus*. With a different biocide, perhaps some other genus could compete more effectively. Repeated system treatments with isothiazolone biocides can select for more resistant organisms such as mycobacteria. These organisms may also be more likely to induce pulmonary diseases, most notably hypersensitivity pneumonitis (HP). Sometimes fungi can be the primary

Substance	CAS No.	OSHA PEL TWA	ST or C	NIOSH REL TWA	ST or C	ACGIH TLV* TWA	ST or C	Comment
Metalworking fluid aerosol	-	-	-	0.5 mg/m³ total 0.4 mg/m³ thor	-	-	-	-
Oil mist, mineral	[8012-95-1]	5 mg/m³	-	5 mg/m³	ST 10 mg/m³	0.2 mg/m³	ST 10 mg/m³	Poorly-mildly refined: suspected human carcinogen ACGIH NIC: 0.2 mg/m³ TWA inh
Oil mist, vegetable	[68956-68-3]	15 mg/m³ total 5 mg/m³ resp	-	10 mg/m³ total 5 mg/m³ resp	-	10 mg/m³	-	-
Ethanolamines tri-ethanolamine	[102-71-6]	-	-	-	-	5 mg/m³	-	
di-ethanolamine	[111-42-2]	-	-	3 ppm	-	2 mg/m³	-	
ethanolamine	[141-43-5]	3 ppm	-	3 ppm	ST 6 ppm	3 ppm	ST 6 ppm	
Ammonia	[7664-41-7]	50 ppm	-	25 ppm	ST 35 ppm	25 ppm	ST 35 ppm	
Chlorine	[7782-50-5]	-	C 1 ppm	-	C 0.5 ppm	0.5 ppm	ST 1 ppm	
Hydrogen sulfide	[7783-06-4]	-	C 20 ppm	-	C 10 ppm	10 ppm	15 ppm	ACGIH NIC: 1 ppm TWA
Sulfur dioxide	[7446-09-5]	5 ppm	-	2 ppm	5 ppm	2 ppm	5 ppm	
Formaldehyde	[50-00-0]	0.75 ppm	ST 2 ppm	0.016 ppm	C 0.1 ppm		C 0.3 ppm	Suspected human carcinogen, sensitizer Sensitizer
Glutaraldehyde	[111-30-8]	-	-	-	C 0.2 ppm	-	C 0.05 ppm	Suspected human carcinogen
Cadmium & cmpds total dust respirable dust	[7440-43-9]	0.005 mg/m³	-	Lowest feasible conc.	-	0.01 mg/m³ 0.002 mg/m³	-	
Chromium & inorganic cmpds	[7440-47-3]	-	-	-	-	-	-	Cr VI compounds are known human carcinogens
Cr metal Water-soluble Cr VI cmpds Insoluble Cr VI cmpds		1.0 mg/m³ 0.5 mg/m³ 0.1 mg/m³	-	0.5 mg/m³ 0.5 mg/m³ 0.001 mg/m³	-	0.5 mg/m³ 0.05 mg/m³ 0.01 mg/m³	-	
Nickel & cmpds elemental Ni soluble inorganic Ni cmpds insoluble inorganic Ni cmpds	[7440-02-0]	1 mg/m³	-	0.015 mg/m³	-	1.5 mg/m³inh 0.1 mg/m³inh 0.2 mg/m³inh	-	Insoluble inorganic compounds are known human carcinogens
Endotoxin	-	-	-	-	-	-	-	200 EU/m³ Dutch occupational health standard

*Threshold limit value (TLV) as published in 2004 by the American Conference of Governmental Industrial Hygienists. TWA = 8-hr time-weighted average concentration.
NIC = Listed under notice of intended change in 2002.
Total = total particulate mass
Thor = thoracic particulate mass
Inh = inhalable particulate mass
Resp = respirable particulate mass
C = ceiling limit
ST = short term exposure limit

Table 43.1 Recommended exposure limits for compounds potentially found in the metal working fluid environments

Gram-negative bacteria
Pseudomonas sp.
    P. putida
    P. fluorescens
    P. pseudoalcaligenes
    P. stutzeri
    P. aeruginosa
Xanthomonas maltophilia
Acinetobacter sp.
Enterobacter sp.
Serratia sp.
Citrobacter sp.
    C. diversus
    C. freundii
Escherichia coli
Proteus vulgaris
Morganella morganii
Klebsiella
    K. pneumoniae
    K. oxytoca
Shewanella putrefaciens
Yersinia pseudotuberculosis
Aeromonas hydrophilia
Ochrobactrum anthropi
Flavobacterium odoratum
Alcaligenes faecalis
Achromobacter sp.
Gram-positive bacteria
Bacillus sp.
    B. subtilis
    B. cereus
    B. pulvifaciens
    B. brevis
    B. pasteurii
    B. polymyxa
Micrococcus sp.
    M. luteus
    M. varians
Corynebacterium sp.
Aeromonas viridans
Rhodococcus sp.
Staphylococcus sp.
Streptococcus sp.
Mycobacteria
M. abscessus
M. chelonae
M. fortuitum
M. immunogens
Fungi
Candida sp.
Fusarium sp.
Geotrichum sp.
Stachybotrys sp.
Cephalosporium sp.

From Mattsby-Baltzer et al 1989,[72] Lonon et al 1999, Foxall-Van Aken et al 1986, Thorne et al 1996,[5] Zacharisen et al 1998.[75]

Table 43.2 Microorganisms commonly found in soluble oil, semi-synthetic and synthetic metal working fluids

contaminants. The predominant yeast is usually Candida, while Fusarium spp. are the most common molds.

EXPOSURE ASSESSMENTS

In the course of large machining operations MWF are sprayed onto the area where the tool contacts the product at flow rates in the range of 5–50 l/min. The tools, and in some cases the products, are spinning at high speeds as well as moving laterally. Thus, coarse droplets and fine aerosols may be dispersed widely. These aerosols are available for inhalation as well as dermal deposition. Geometric mean (GM) air-borne particulate concentrations of 0.16–1.24 mg/m^3 have been reported in published studies over the past 10 years (Table 43.3). NIOSH has reported a steady decrease in aerosol concentrations over the past three decades.[3]

In facilities where large volumes of MWF are used, much of the aerosol is respirable. Chan et al[4] studied the size characteristics of MWF aerosols in a transmission plant and found the gravimetric respirable aerosol fraction to range from 19% to 55%. Concentrations generally fluctuated between 0.5 and 2 mg/m^3 with both larger sizes (2–20 μm) and smaller sizes (0.1–1 μm) of aerosols. Thorne et al studied size distributions of MWF aerosols in a large engine plant using eight-stage cascade impactors positioned where machinists stood.[5] The calculated mean of the aerodynamic mass median diameters was 3.1 μm and the mean of the geometric standard deviations (GSD) was 3.0 μm. Woskie and coworkers reported similar, respirable MWF aerosols in a large machining facility with small single machine sumps,[6] a mean aerodynamic mass median diameter of 3.4 μm and a GSD of 3.0 μm.

Bioaerosol exposures have been assessed carefully in several studies (Table 43.3). While the most important source is generally the MWF themselves, other sources of bioaerosols coexist in these environments and are often overlooked. Biofilms may develop on machinery or in air handling systems and these may contribute to the bioaerosol load. Biofilms in ventilation systems, many of which recirculate air after coarse filtration, may act as an amplification site for the organisms arising from the MWF. During some periods of the year, bioaerosols (especially fungi) may be carried in significant concentrations in the make-up air from outside. The concentrations of air-borne culturable micro-organisms in machining facilities typically fall in the range of 10^2–10^3 CFU/m^3 (colony forming units/m^3) with levels from 10^4–10^6 CFU/m^3 viewed as excessive. It may happen that the levels of viable organisms are in the normal range but if one measures the total organisms (culturable and non-culturable) the values are one to three orders of magnitude higher. This may be the case if culture-based sampling methods are not selected properly to support the growth of the predominant organisms. It may also be the case after major biocide additions to a system that resulted in the sloughing of biofilms or the loss of viability of microbes in the MWF. There are no promulgated standards or recommended exposure limits for bioaerosols in the machining environment. Available methodology for bioaerosol sampling has been recently reviewed.[7]

Several studies have evaluated the role of air-borne endotoxins as a causative agent for acute respiratory health effects from MWF. Endotoxins arise from the cell wall of gram-negative bacteria and have been shown to induce cross-shift pulmonary function changes in occupationally exposed cotton workers, grain handlers, swine farmers, and potato processors.[8] Several studies in the metal working environment have assessed exposures to endotoxin (Table 43.3). Geometric mean values were generally below

	MWF type	Site note	N	GM	GSD	Reference
Particulate matter, mg/m³						
Personal inhalable	Soluble oil	Small sumps[a]	139	0.17	1.8	6
	Straight oil	Small sumps	74	0.19	1.8	6
Area total	Soluble oil	Old engine line[b]	12	1.24	2.1	5
	Soluble oil	New engine line	8	0.74	1.4	5
Personal total	Mixed	Job shops[c]	68	0.31	2.4	31
Total aerosol*	Soluble oil	Transmission plant[d]	–	0.33	0.04–1.44**	33
Personal total	Straight oil	Lathe work only[e]	23	0.16	1.8	76
Personal inhalable	Straight oil	Lathe work only	23	0.45	2.0	76
[e]Culturable micro-organisms, CFU/m³						
Bacteria	Soluble oil	Small sumps	67	184	3.3	6
	Straight oil	Small sumps	61	140	3.0	6
Mesophilic bacteria	Soluble oil	Old engine line	16	362	3.4	5
	Soluble oil	New engine line	16	186	2.2	5
	Soluble oil	Transmission plant	–	17,200	740–148,500**	33
Fungi	Soluble oil	Old engine line	16	31	5.7	5
	Soluble oil	New engine line	16	24	2.3	5
	Soluble oil	Transmission plant	–	1060	228–9420**	33
[f]Total organisms, microbes/m³						
Area total	Soluble oil	Old engine line	17	69,600	3.0	5
	Soluble oil	New engine line	17	36,700	2.1	5
	Soluble oil	Transmission plant	44	620,000	20,000–4,000,000**	33
Endotoxin, EU/m³						
Personal inhalable	Soluble oil	Small sumps	46	8.1	4.6	6
	Straight oil	Small sumps	25	6.2	4.7	6
	Soluble oil	Transmission plant	189	40.3	2.7–984**	33
Area total	Soluble oil	Old engine line	19	19.2	7.1	5
	Soluble oil	New engine line	12	14.3	4.9	5
	Soluble oil	Transmission plant	45	24.8	2.5–240**	33

[a]No central MWF sumps. Many machining operations were sampled in a large machining plant; 88% of the operations had single machine sumps with MWF volume less than 3750 liters.[6]
[b]A very large engine plant was sampled, including four areas on an old transfer line and four areas on a newly installed line with extensive controls. MWF were handled in large central sump systems 75,000–750,000 liters.[5].
[c]Apprentices in 13 small job shops working on single machine sumps with low MWF volumes. Soluble oil, synthetic and straight oil MWF were used.[31]
[d]A very large transmission plant was sampled including two areas serviced by three central MWF systems, two with soluble oil and one with semi-synthetic MWF.[33]
[e]Twenty-three workers doing the same operation (lathe work) in one facility wore a 37 mm total particulate sampler and an IOM inhalable particulate sampler.[76]
[e]Colony forming units (CFU)/m³.
[f]Total culturable + non-culturable bacteria and fungi.
*Measured using MiniRam which quantifies aerosol by light scattering.
**Range.

Table 43.3 Concentrations of airborne particulates measured in the machining environment

the 50 EU/m³ no-effect threshold suggested by the Dutch Expert Committee on Occupational Safety.[9] Our recent studies of bulk MWF have found endotoxin concentrations ranging from 160 to 20,000 EU/ml. If soluble oil MWF containing 90% water and endotoxin at 20,000 EU/ml is aerosolized to a water-free particulate mass concentration of 1 mg/m³, the air-borne endotoxin level would be about 200 EU/m³.

Endotoxin is an important causal agent of pulmonary inflammation in a host of occupational settings.[8] Because of the recognized presence of endotoxin at elevated concentrations in some machining environments, several studies have systematically evaluated endotoxin sampling methods. While a European occupational exposure guideline for endotoxin of 200 EU/m³ has been adopted,[10] no permissible exposure limits or recommended exposure limits have emerged in the United States. This may be due, in part, to a lack of rigorously harmonized sampling and analysis methods. In 1994, Thorne et al published methods for endotoxin assay in bulk metalworking fluids and in air samples.[5] Methods for assay of endotoxin in bulk MWF were evaluated by Brown et al[11] who found improved recovery of endotoxin from synthetic and semi-synthetic MWF using pyrogen-free

water with added Tween 20.[11] Without systematic evaluation, the American Society for Testing and Materials (ASTM) established a standard for estimation of air-borne endotoxin in machining environments. Subsequent systematic comparison by Thorne and coworkers[13] of this method with four alternatives demonstrated poorer performance of the ASTM method than the alternatives.

Exposure assessment of many other contaminants of the machining environment is well established. These include vapors such as formaldehyde and hydrogen sulfide as well as metals such as cadmium or chromium. Methods of air sampling for the toxicants listed in Table 43.1 are available from the NIOSH Manual of Analytical Methods.

HEALTH EFFECTS

Health effects associated with exposure to MWF are listed in Table 43.4 and discussed below.

Skin

Because many jobs in metal working require manual operations, the workers' hands and forearms receive direct

Skin
Oil folliculitis/oil acne
Oil keratoses
Pigment abnormalities
Irritant and allergic contact dermatitis
Skin cancer (including scrotal)
Respiratory tract
Occupational asthma
Hypersensitivity pneumonitis
Cross-shift reductions in FEV_1 (variable results among the studies)
Increased non-specific bronchial reactivity
Increased respiratory symptoms compared with unexposed
Cancer (substantial evidence)
Larynx
Bladder
Skin (scrotum)
Pancreas
Rectum

Table 43.4 Health effects associated with exposure to metalworking fluids

exposure to the MWF. In addition, aerosol deposition, splashing, wet clothing, and transfer from hands allow MWF to contact skin in other parts of the body. Skin trauma from small metal fragments increases the potential for percutaneous absorption of MWF constituents. Straight oils have been associated with oil folliculitis/oil acne, oil keratoses, pigment abnormalities, skin cancer, and some cases of contact dermatitis, while water-based fluids more often cause irritant and allergic contact dermatitis.

Oil folliculitis (oil acne) (see also Chapter 44), resulting from chemical irritation and plugging of the follicular opening, has been reported in workers exposed to straight oils. The lesions include perifollicular papules, pustules, and comedones. The areas affected initially are the backs of the hands, fingers, and forearms. The thighs and abdomen may also be affected because of contact with oily clothing. The folliculitis, which is seen shortly after initial exposure to straight oils, may last for months. Keratolytic agents, antibiotics and isotretinoin have been used for treatment. Prevention of recurrences depends on decreased exposure to oils, appropriate hand washing, and protective clothing. One study showed decreases in the prevalence of oil acne over time associated with: (1) changes in the tool-setting operation, (2) a change from acid-refined to solvent-refined oils, and (3) provision of free work clothes.[1]

The most common skin disease in workers exposed to water-based MWF is contact dermatitis (see also Chapter 29.1). In a study of newly hired machinists exposed to neat mineral oil MWF, the prevalence of contact dermatitis increased rapidly in the first three weeks of exposure and then remained constant at about 50%.[14] Several studies have shown that time spent in contact with wet fluids is a risk factor for contact dermatitis from MWF. Other risk factors noted in epidemiologic studies are cigarette smoking, semi-synthetic MWF exposure compared with soluble MWF exposure,[15] and increasing age.[16] Conflicting results have been published concerning atopy as a risk factor.[15,16] Prevalences vary widely among studies (6–67%), in part because of differences in the diagnostic criteria and variability in types and extent of exposure. The

rate of dermatitis is about two- to fourfold higher among workers exposed to MWF in studies comparing them with unexposed workers.[3] Among groups of exposed workers, a pattern of intermittent outbreaks of dermatitis superimposed on a background of endemic contact dermatitis has been described.

The combination of irritant and allergic dermatitis is frequent. Some studies have reported an allergic component in close to one-half of exposed workers with contact dermatitis. Alkalinity, irritating emulsifiers, and microtrauma from metal shavings are cited as the chief contributing factors for irritant contact dermatitis resulting from water-based MWF. Biocides in high concentrations, solvents used for degreasing, and strong detergents used for hand washing may contribute to skin irritation in those working with MWF.

Allergic contact dermatitis has been attributed to many components and additives of water-based MWF acting as sensitizers, including biocides, emulsifiers, corrosion inhibitors, pressure stabilizers, preservatives, antioxidants, and fragrances. Biocides have been cited as the most frequent causes, particularly among those who add the concentrated biocide solution to the in-use MWF. Common types of biocide associated with dermatitis include formaldehyde releasers and isothiazolinones. Sensitization to metals including chromium, nickel, and cobalt has been reported in metal workers with dermatitis. It is not clear whether the cause was dissolved metals in the cutting fluids or direct contact with the metals in current or past employment.

Contact dermatitis resulting from water-based MWF can present early on as a fine follicular eczema, followed later by a patchy, papular eczema on the backs of the hands and forearms. Although the clinical course is variable, many cases become chronic. One study of machine operators with soluble oil dermatitis reported high prevalence rates of chronic, non-healing dermatitis two years after the diagnosis, in those with and without ongoing MWF exposure. The prevalence rates of chronic, non-healing dermatitis were 78% and 70%, respectively.[17] There may be a better prognosis for a subgroup of exposed workers with contact dermatitis from MWF if they are removed from exposure before the dermatitis has lasted longer than three months.[18] Another study of machine operators examined at a dermatology clinic reported persistent dermatitis in 82% 1–5 years after evaluation. Discontinuing exposure did not improve the prognosis.[19]

Diagnosis

In general, the clinical pattern of oil folliculitis caused by straight oils is readily distinguished from the eczematous dermatitis resulting from water-based MWF. However, both irritant and allergic contact dermatitis may occur from exposure to some straight oils and their additives. Patch testing (see Chapter 29.1) may be useful in some cases, but is limited by both false-positive and false-negative results, as well as problems with clinical correlation due to the multifactorial etiology of contact dermatitis in workers exposed to MWF.

Treatment

Clinical treatment of individual workers with contact dermatitis from MWF does not differ from the general management of occupational contact dermatitis (see Chapter 29.1). Limiting or eliminating contact with MWF, use of non-irritating cleansers, application of emollient creams, and topical steroids are frequent recommendations.

Prevention

Measures for preventing occupational dermatitis caused by MWF are similar to those used to prevent other occupational dermatoses and include limiting exposure, protective gloves and clothing, worker education, and identification and removal of allergens. No studies have addressed the efficacy of plant-wide surveillance programs for the early detection of contact dermatitis. Nonetheless, surveillance coupled with strategies for decreasing or eliminating exposures in those affected may be useful in light of the high prevalence of contact dermatitis and the chronic nature of the dermatitis in many cases.

The prevention of oil folliculitis appears to be less of a problem than that for contact dermatitis. The prevalence is decreasing because of the increased use of water-based fluids, and the literature suggests easier treatment and prevention by routine measures of personal hygiene and protective clothing, including protective gloves, aprons, and footwear.

Respiratory tract

The reported respiratory effects of MWF in exposed workers include occupational asthma, hypersensitivity pneumonitis, cross-shift declines in FEV_1, and increases in non-specific bronchial reactivity. Respiratory symptoms, including cough and phlegm, have been reported in some studies without associated functional change. Lipid (lipoid) pneumonia has been reported historically in some workers exposed to MWF, but there is a paucity of recent reports. Legionnaire's disease due to contaminated MWF in an automotive plant has been reported.[20]

Hypersensitivity pneumonitis (see also Chapter 19.6)

Reports of clusters of cases of respiratory disease consistent with hypersensitivity pneumonitis (HP) occurring at several automotive industry plants began appearing in the mid-1990s[21] and were discussed at a 1996 NIOSH conference.[22] Several additional clusters of HP have more recently been reported in groups of workers exposed to MWF.[23–25] Most cases occurred at plants in which MWF aerosol exposures were maintained below 0.5 mg/m³.

Although the cause or causes of these clusters have not been definitely identified, aerosolized microbial contaminants from water-based MWF (including soluble, synthetic, and semi-synthetic MWF) are thought to be the most likely source. Recent attention has focused on unusual organisms found in water-based MWF, including fungi, gram-positive bacteria, and *Mycobacterium immunogenum*, a newly proposed non-tuberculous species closely related to *M. chelonae*. It has been suggested that use of biocides to control the more common gram-negative bacteria in MWF may lead to the emergence of unusual organisms responsible for HP. Although case definition varied across the studies, at least 44 biopsy-confirmed cases of HP have been reported from ten plants. Biopsies showed granulomatous inflammation consistent with HP. In several cases, clinical improvements or resolution have been reported after removal from exposure to MWF. Some studies have emphasized a close association between HP and asthma in workers exposed to MWF, the likelihood that some cases may be missed due to the non-specific presentation and the unfamiliarity of healthcare providers in recognizing and diagnosing HP (see Chapter 19.6).

Recommendations for medical surveillance and monitoring of workers exposed to MWF from the OSHA Scientific Advisory Committee on MWF[26] have emphasized that a single physician-diagnosed case of HP should be viewed as a sentinel event triggering active surveillance of exposed workers, in addition to review of MWF fluid management records and environmental assessment of microbial species in MWF present at the onset of disease. Recommended medical monitoring tools include baseline and periodic questionnaires addressing respiratory and systemic symptoms and pulmonary function testing. Further clinical evaluation would be indicated for workers with persistent respiratory or non-specific symptoms and/or abnormalities on baseline or periodic tests (discussed in Chapter 19.6). Routine use of chest radiographs and serologic tests for antibodies was not recommended for surveillance purposes.

Asthma (see also Chapter 19.2)

Data concerning the relationship between exposure to MWF and asthma come from several sources, including case reports of asthma reproduced by specific challenge testing and sentinel event surveillance data. In addition, cross-sectional studies have compared questionnaire-derived prevalences of asthma in exposed workers with unexposed controls. Taken together, the evidence is convincing for an association between MWF exposure and occupational asthma.

Case reports[27–29] have focused on individual workers who have been evaluated clinically after they presented with possible occupational asthma. In the largest case series,[28] 25 patients referred to an occupational respiratory clinic for possible occupational asthma were classified with definite or equivocal occupational asthma based on results of serial peak flow measurements. Of the 13 with definite occupational asthma, latency period ranged from immediate to 41 years. Nine had a history of workplace exposure only to soluble MWF, while one had only straight oil exposure and two had both soluble and straight MWF exposure. Six of the 13 underwent specific inhalation challenge testing with various MWF and constituents. Three of the six had positive challenge tests to unused soluble MWF, one reacted only to used soluble MWF, and two had inconclusive results. Another report[27] described two machinists with occupational asthma who had positive specific inhalation challenge responses to a component of used MWF, triethanolamine, with latencies of over ten years and eight years respectively. Specific inhalation challenge tests were positive to heated MWF containing triethanolamine but not triethanolamine-free MWF in one case and to cold pure triethanolamine in the other. Both patients had persistent asthma symptoms requiring medication six months after stopping workplace exposure.

Results from the Sentinel Event Notification System for Occupational Risk assessing work-related asthma in Michigan from 1988 to 1994 showed that MWF was the second leading cause of work-related asthma.[30] They reported 86 cases (identified from physicians, hospitals, and worker compensation claims) from 45 plants, 22 of which had air sampling for MWF. Exposure at only one plant exceeded the OSHA TWA of 5 mg/m³ for oil mist. About 20% of 755 fellow workers of the sentinel cases reported work-related asthma symptoms. The results also suggested that workers exposed to soluble, semi-synthetic, and synthetic MWF were more likely to report respiratory symptoms, including work-related asthma, than workers exposed to mineral oils alone.

Because of transfer of workers affected by asthma to new work environments, it is difficult to assess exposure–response relationships and relative risk for asthma among currently exposed workers. Several recent studies suggest that workers exposed to MWF have a 2–3-fold increased risk for asthma symptoms.[3] Increases in non-specific bronchial hyper-responsiveness have been reported in workers exposed to MWF in several studies, with positive associations between bronchial responsiveness and cumulative exposure to both soluble oil and synthetic MWF.[31,32]

Respiratory symptoms

A number of cross-sectional respiratory morbidity studies have compared respiratory symptoms between workers exposed to MWF and unexposed controls, recently reviewed by NIOSH.[3] All studies showed an increase in at least one respiratory symptom among the exposed. Symptoms with significantly elevated odds ratio in at least one study included cough, phlegm, chronic bronchitis, wheeze on most days, chest tightness, dyspnea, and acute eye, nose and throat irritation, with about a 2–7-fold increase in respiratory symptoms among the exposed. Two of these studies[33,34] reported exposure–response relationships between aerosol exposure and respiratory symptoms. One study reported a specific exposure–response relationship between respiratory symptoms and air-borne levels of culturable fungi and bacteria.[33] All types of MWF were associated with increases in respiratory symptoms, although two studies[33,34] suggested that synthetic or semi-synthetic MWF were associated with higher odds ratios than soluble MWF. Several studies reported cross-shift worsening of respiratory symptoms[30,33,35,36] and improvements off work.[34] Air-borne aerosol concentrations varied among the studies, although mean concentrations were all less than 3 mg/m³.

Chronic lung function effects

Several cross-sectional studies[32,33,35,37] have examined baseline FEV_1 and FVC in workers exposed to MWF compared with unexposed controls (see also Chapter 19.4.) They have found either no difference[32,33,37] or a slightly lower baseline FEV_1 and/or FVC among exposed workers.[35,38] Associations between current total culturable bacteria and baseline FEV_1;[33] current exposure to soluble oil MWF and baseline FEV_1;[35] and lifetime exposure to straight oils and baseline FVC[38] have been reported. Due to the healthy worker effect, such studies, as well as studies of acute effects (see below), may underestimate the respiratory effects of MWF exposure.

Acute lung function effects

Results of studies assessing acute cross-shift reductions in FEV_1 among workers exposed to MWF compared with unexposed workers have produced variable results. Two studies reported a higher prevalence of cross-shift FEV_1 decrement in exposed workers.[36,39] In one the highest risk was for those exposed to synthetic fluids and effects were observed at aerosol levels as low as 0.2 mg/m³. The other study[36] found, among exposed workers with lower baseline lung function, exposure–response relationships with thoracic particulate and viable plus non-viable bacteria. Two other studies reported no significant difference between exposed and unexposed workers.[33,35] One of these latter studies,[35] however, showed that higher exposures to MWF (above 0.15 mg/m³ in their study) were associated with more frequent declines in cross-shift FEV_1 when both exposed and control workers were combined.

Lipid (lipoid) pneumonia

Although reported historically, there have been few recent reports of lipoid pneumonia in MWF-exposed workers. Histopathologically confirmed lipoid pneumonia was reported in a subject exposed to a water-based coolant, a straight oil lubricant, and kerosene in a steel rolling tandem mill.[40] His chest radiograph was reportedly normal, and restriction was found on pulmonary function tests. Other case studies have reported interstitial changes in exposed workers.[41–43] However, no increase in respiratory morbidity was observed in two occupationally exposed groups.[44,45] However, no chest radiographs were performed in either study. The one major respiratory morbidity study that included both chest radiographic and pulmonary function evaluation in exposed workers compared with office workers showed no evidence of parenchymal abnormalities attributable to exposure.[46] The frequency, risk factors, and course of lipid (lipoid) pneumonia caused by MWF exposure are not well defined at this time.

Cancer

The presence of carcinogens in MWF has prompted numerous investigations of cancer in exposed workers.[13,47–58] Difficulties in evaluating these studies include variability in exposures and their classification, lack of exposure data in many, small numbers in some, and lack of information about confounding variables, such as cigarette smoking. NIOSH reviews of cancer mortality studies[3,60] have found substantial evidence for associations between MWF and cancers of the larynx, rectum, pancreas, skin/scrotum, and bladder, and more limited evidence for associations with stomach, lung, esophagus, prostate, colon, brain, and hematopoietic cancers.

With regard to the cancer sites linked with MWF by substantial evidence, the magnitude of risk, expressed as rate ratios, varied among the cancer sites. For laryngeal cancer, the rate ratios above 1.0 ranged from 1.05 to 2.5; for cancer of the rectum, 1.09 to 3.07; for cancer of the pancreas, 1.03 to 3.7; for skin/scrotal cancer, 1.06 to 10.5; for bladder cancer, 1.04 to 2.99.

For cancers of the skin/scrotum, larynx, and rectum, there is evidence to suggest a specific association with straight MWF exposure. For cancer of the pancreas, the evidence points to associations with synthetic fluids used for grinding and with straight MWF used for machining.

Metal working fluid exposures in these cancer mortality studies occurred prior to the mid-1970s. Because many changes have occurred in MWF since that time, it is not possible to extrapolate cancer risks from exposure after the mid-1970s from these earlier data. Temporal changes in carcinogenicity over time are likely, given the changes that have occurred in MWF over the last several decades. It has been suggested that changes in composition, reductions in polycyclic aromatic hydrocarbons and nitrosamine levels, and generally lower MWF exposure levels may reduce the carcinogenicity of MWF observed in future studies.

Medical surveillance and monitoring of exposed workers

NIOSH and the OSHA Metalworking Fluid Scientific Advisory Committee (SAC) have made recommendations for medical monitoring of workers exposed to MWF to enable early detection of respiratory and skin disorders caused by MWF. Both included recommendations for baseline and periodic examinations including standardized questionnaire (addressing symptoms and medical history), skin examination, and baseline spirometry. Both emphasized the need for monitoring workers in areas with known increased exposure to MWF and areas where sentinel cases of asthma, HP, or dermatitis have occurred. The OSHA SAC also made recommendations about medical removal, return to work, and medical removal protection of earnings, employment rights, and benefits. Medical surveillance in relation to cancer prevention among workers exposed to MWF has not been addressed.

Toxicology studies

Relatively few animal toxicology studies have been done to assess the acute and chronic effects of water-based MWF. Prior to 1990, several investigators studied oil mist inhalation representing automobile lubricating oil, cable oils, military foggers, food oils, and mineral oil.[61–66] Few histopathologic changes or alterations in pulmonary function were observed below 100 mg/m^3, and in several studies exposures exceeding 1000 mg/m^3 did not yield significant differences from control animals.

More recently, toxicology studies have investigated the health effects of water-based MWF in irritation, inflammation, mucous cell hyperplasia, and HP models in mice, rats, and guinea pigs. Such studies have confirmed that MWF exposure at levels comparable to those present in today's workplaces can cause lung inflammation, airway hyperresponsiveness and HP, and have begun to identify the most likely etiologic agents in MWF. One study[67] used a mouse pulmonary irritation model to study the responses arising from acute exposures to aerosolized metal working fluids. The straight oil they tested was less irritating, both as neat and in-use MWF, than the synthetic fluid or the oil emulsions. Pulmonary irritation was minimal for MWF at gravimetric concentrations less than about 50 mg/m^3. Three-hour exposures produced histopathologic changes (mild to moderate interstitial pneumonitis and bronchopneumonia) at the 24-hour time point in some mice, with little difference between new and in-use fluids.

Gordon[68] conducted inhalation studies in guinea pigs to assess the acute respiratory effects as indicated by measurement of specific airway conductance (sGaw). Aerosolized in-use soluble oil MWF samples yielded 3000 EU/m^3 endotoxin at 1 mg/m^3 aerosol concentration and 19,000 EU/m^3 endotoxin at 10 mg/m^3. The sGaw decreased 0%, 7%, and 40% upon exposure to 1, 10, and 100 mg/m^3, respectively, with greater responses upon inhalation of in-use MWF than unused MWF diluted similarly in terms of decrease in sGaw and several bronchoalveolar lavage assays. Gordon and Harkema[69] exposed rats to aerosols of used and unused MWF at 1 or 10 mg/m^3, 3 hr/day for three days and investigated production of mucosal substances in airway cells. Exposure to used MWF at 10 mg/m^3 (containing 8000 EU/m^3 endotoxin) produced mucous cell metaplasia in the nasal septum and mid-level airways. Metaplasia was also observed with unused MWF at this exposure level.

Thorne and coworkers have conducted studies of the pulmonary effects of inhaled MWF and their associated endotoxin and bioaerosols in animal models of acute lung inflammation and in subchronic models of HP. One such study[70] demonstrated that in-use soluble oil MWF contaminated with endotoxin and gram-negative bacteria (*Pseudomonas aeruginosa*) induced lung inflammation in a dose-dependent manner from 100 to 50,000 EU/m^3 of endotoxin activity, including marked neutrophilia and elevated pro-inflammatory cytokines, such as TNF-α and IL-6. The corresponding unused fluid produced responses no different from sham-exposed mice. Filter sterilization of the in-use fluid did not diminish the inflammatory potency of the MWF. Further studies in guinea pigs[5] demonstrated acute pulmonary function changes with exposures as low as 3 mg/m^3 for in-use MWF and 30 mg/m^3 for neat fluids. Experiments in which the appropriately diluted neat MWF was spiked with endotoxin supported the hypothesis that endotoxin may be the most important agent for pulmonary inflammatory responses to MWF.

HP represents a cell-mediated immunologic pulmonary disease displaying a Th$_1$ phenotype, associated with cytokines interferon-γ (IFN-γ), IL-2, and IL-12. Lung responses to in-use MWF samples have recently been evaluated using a murine model for HP.[71] These studies investigated the potential for MWF contaminated with Mycobacterium species to induce HP and characterized the physiologic and immunologic responses to these MWF exposures. Mice were exposed by nasal aspiration to live *Mycobacterium chelonae* bacteria (isolated from an in-use MWF sample), live *Saccharopolyspora rectivirgula* bacteria (positive control), saline (negative control), or endotoxin (inflammation control). Mice were exposed for three weeks, followed four days later by acute challenge with the MWF. The positive control agent for HP, *S. rectivirgula*, induced significantly more total cells, lymphocytes and monocytes in lung lavage; an increased CD4+/CD8+ ratio; elevated IL-12 levels; and marked pulmonary lymphocytosis on histologic exam when compared to saline-treated controls. Mice treated with mycobacteria alone or MWF containing this organism had significantly elevated lung weights, total lavage cells, neutrophils, and increased CD4+/CD8+ ratio as compared to saline controls. However, when *M. chelonae* was administered at twice the dose of *S. rectivirgula*, cellular and cytokine responses were still lower than those observed in the *S. rectivirgula*-treated mice. These data suggest that mycobacteria-contaminated MWF produce HP-like changes in the mouse but with lower potency, a distinct response profile and a more focal pathology than induced by *S. rectivirgula*.

SUMMARY

A substantial number of workers are exposed to MWF in a wide range of industries. Although the health effects associated with MWF exposures have been studied for some time, developing a clear understanding has been complicated by the fact that the fluids contain multiple and variable substances and contaminants, and have changed considerably in their formulation. Importantly, even MWF with a consistent neat formulation differ markedly over time and between systems when in use, both chemically and microbiologically. This has made difficult the process of identifying causative agents for suspected adverse health effects. In the past two decades there has been a transition from oil-based to water-based MWF. Coincident with this has been a shift in the major health concerns. Whereas previously oil folliculitis and skin cancer were the major dermatologic concerns, now irritant and allergic contact dermatitis are potential important problems. Earlier concerns about respiratory disease focused on lipid (lipoid) pneumonia and the possibility of lung cancer. Now there is concern for asthma, bronchitis and HP. Epidemiologic studies have identified varying results with regards to MWF exposures and cross-shift pulmonary function changes.

Animal toxicology studies have identified mechanisms of MWF-induced inflammation and HP. Adoption of appropriate medical monitoring and surveillance programs is an important consideration for workers exposed to MWF. Attempts to identify causative agents in MWF include these toxicology studies and exposure monitoring for chemical irritants, biocides, micro-organisms, microbial toxins, and

studies of the influence of changes in formulation on airborne levels. Improved design of new machining equipment with enhanced containment and local exhaust to reduce aerosol distribution, carefully directed nozzles, and elimination of high pressure air jets for fluid removal have served to reduce exposures in new or retooled production lines. An important policy area is setting exposure limits to prevent effects that have been observed among workers exposed below current standards. The research and control efforts mentioned above should help to reduce exposures and the health risks associated with MWF.

References

1. NIOSH. National Occupational Hazard Survey: volume III. Survey analysis and supplemental tables. DHEW (NIOSH) Pub no. 78–114. Cincinnati, OH: US Department of Health and Human Services, Public Health Service, Centers for Disease Control, National Institute for Occupational Safety and Health, Division of Surveillance, Hazard Evaluations and Field Studies, 1978;216–29.
2. NIOSH. National Occupational Health Survey (NOES), 1981–83. Unpublished dataset. Cincinnati, OH: US Department of Health and Human Services, Public Health Service, Centers for Disease Control, National Institute for Occupational Safety and Health, Division of Surveillance, Hazard Evaluations and Field Studies, 1983.
3. NIOSH. Criteria for a recommended standard: occupational exposure to metalworking fluids. Cincinnati, OH: US Department of Health and Human Services, Public Health Service, Centers for Disease Control, National Institute for Occupational Safety and Health, Division of Surveillance, Hazard Evaluations and Field Studies, 1998.
4. Chan TL, D'Arcy JB, Siak J. Size characteristics of machining fluid aerosols in an industrial metalworking environment. Appl Occup Environ Hyg 1990; 5:162–70.
5. Thorne PS, DeKoster JA, Subramanian P. Environmental assessment of aerosols, bioaerosols, and air-borne endotoxin in a machining plant. Am Ind Hyg Assoc J 1996; 57:1163–7.
6. Woskie SR, Virji MA, Kriebel D, et al. Exposure assessment for a field investigation of the acute respiratory effects of metalworking fluids. I. Summary of findings. Am Ind Hyg Assoc J 1996; 57:1154–62.
7. Heederik D, Thorne PS, Douwes J. Biologic agents – monitoring and evaluation of bioaerosol exposure. In: Perkins J, ed. Modern industrial hygiene, vol 2. Biologic aspects. Cincinnati, OH: American Conference of Governmental Industrial Hygienists, 2003. p. 293–327.
8. Thorne PS. Inhalation toxicology models of endotoxin and bioaerosol-induced inflammation. Toxicology 2000; 152:13–23.
9. Dutch Expert Committee on Occupational Standards. Endotoxins: health-based recommended exposure limit. A report of the Health Council of the Netherlands. Publ. No. 1998/03WGD. Rijswijk: Health Council of the Netherlands, 1998.
10. Douwes J, Thorne PS, Pearce N, Heederik D. Biologic agents – recognition. In: Perkins J, ed. Modern industrial hygiene, vol 2. Biologic aspects. Cincinnati, OH: American Conference of Governmental Industrial Hygienists, 2003. p. 219–292.
11. Brown ME, White EM, Feng, A. Effects of various treatments on the quantitative recovery of endotoxin from water-soluble metalworking fluids. Am Ind Hyg Assoc J 2000; 61: 517–20.
12. Thorne PS, Bartlett KH, Phipps J, Kulhankova K. Evaluation of five extraction protocols for quantification of endotoxin in metalworking fluid (MWF) aerosol. Ann Occup Hyg 2003; 47:31–6.
13. Järvholm B, Fast K, Lavenius B, et al. Exposure to cutting oils and its relation to skin tumours and premalignant skin lesions

on the hands and forearms. Scand J Work Environ Health 1985; 11:365–9.

14. Goh CL, Gan SL. The incidence of cutting fluid dermatitis among metalworkers in a metal fabrication factory: a prospective study. Contact Derm 1994; 31:111–5

15. Sprince NL, Palmer JA, Popendorf W, et al. Dermatitis among automobile production machine operators exposed to metal-working fluids. Am J Ind Med 1996; 30:421–9.

16. Berndt U, Hinnen U, Iliev D, Elsner P. Hand eczema in metalworker trainees – an analysis of risk factors. Contact Derm 2000; 43:327–32.

17. Pryce DW, Irvine D, English JSC, et al. Soluble oil dermatitis: a follow-up study. Contact Derm 1989; 21:28–35.

18. Menno T, Marbach H. Hand eczema, 2nd edn. Boca Raton, FL: CRC Press, 2000;235–49.

19. Shah M, Lewis FM, Gawkrodger DJ. Prognosis of occupational hand dermatitis in metalworkers. Contact Derm 1996; 34:27–30.

20. Herwaldt LA, Gorman GW, McGrath T, et al. A new Legionella species, Legionella feeleii species nova, causes Pontiac fever in an automobile plant. Ann Intern Med 1984; 100:333–8

21. Centers for Disease Control and Prevention. Biopsy-confirmed hypersensitivity pneumonitis automobile production workers exposed to metalworking fluids, Michigan, 1994–1995. MMWR 1996; 45(28):606–10. Available from: http://www.cdc.gov/mmwr/preview/mmwrhtml/00043265.htm.

22. Kreiss K, Cox-Ganser J. Metalworking fluid-associated hypersensitivity pneumonitis: a workshop summary. Am J Ind Med 1997; 32:423–32.

23. Fox J, Anderson H, Moen T, et al. Metal working fluid-associated hypersensitivity pneumonitis: an outbreak investigation and case-control study. Am J Ind Med 1999; 35:58–67.

24. Hodgson MJ, Bracker A, Yang C, et al. Hypersensitivity pneumonitis in a metal-working environment. Am J Ind Med 2001; 39:616–28.

25. Centers for Disease Control and Prevention. Respiratory illness in workers exposed to metalworking fluid contaminated with nontuberculous mycobacteria, Ohio 2001. MMWR 2002; 51(16):394–52. Available from: http://www.cdc.gov/mmwr/preview/mmwrhtm/mm5116a4.htm.

26. United States Department of Labor, Occupational Safety and Health Administration. Chapter 8: Deliberations related to best practice: medical monitoring and surveillance. Available from: http://www.osha.gov/SLTC/metalworkingfluids/mwf_finalreport_ch8.

27. Savonius B, Keskinen H, Tuppurainen M, Kanerva L. Occupational asthma caused by ethanolamines. Allergy 1994; 49:877–81.

28. Robertson AS, Weir DC, Burge PS. Occupational asthma due to oil mists. Thorax 1988; 43:200–5.

29. Hendy MS, Beattie BE, Burge PS. Occupational asthma due to an emulsified oil mist. Br J Ind Med 1985; 42:51–4.

30. Rosenman KD, Reilly MJ, Kalinowski D. Work-related asthma and respiratory symptoms among workers exposed to metal-working fluids. Am J Ind Med 1997; 32:325–31.

31. Kennedy SM, Chan-Yeung M, Teschke K, Karlen B. Change in airways responsiveness among apprentices exposed to metalworking fluids. Am J Respir Crit Care Med 1999; 159:87–93.

32. Massin N, Bohadana AB, Wild P, et al. Airway responsiveness, respiratory symptoms, and exposures to soluble oil mist in mechanical workers. Occup Environ Med 1996; 53:748–52.

33. Sprince NL, Thorne PS, Popendorf W, et al. Respiratory symptoms and lung function abnormalities among machine operators in automobile production. Am J Ind Med 1997; 31:403–13.

34. Greaves IA, Eisen EA, Smith TJ, et al. Respiratory health of automobile workers exposed to metal-working fluid aerosols: respiratory symptoms. Am J Ind Med 1997; 32:450–9.

35. Kriebel D, Sama SR, Woskie S, et al. A field investigation of the acute respiratory effects of metal working fluids. I. Effects of aerosol exposures. Am J Ind Med 1997; 31: 756–66.

36. Robins T, Seixas N, Franzblau A, et al. Acute respiratory effects on workers exposed to metalworking fluid aerosols in an automotive transmission plant. Am J Ind Med 1997; 31:510–24.

37. Ameille J, Wild P, Choudat D, et al. Respiratory symptoms, ventilatory impairment, and bronchial reactivity in oil mist-exposed automobile workers. Am J Ind Med 1995; 27:247–56.

38. Eisen EA, Smith TJ, Kriebel D, et al. Respiratory health of automobile workers and exposures to metal-working fluid aerosols: lung spirometry. Am J Ind Med 2001; 39:443–53.

39. Kennedy SM, Greaves IA, Kriebel D, et al. Acute pulmonary responses among automobile workers exposed to aerosols of machining fluids. Am J Ind Med 1989; 15:627–41.

40. Cullen MR, Balmes JR, Robins JM, et al. Lipoid pneumonia caused by oil mist exposure from a steel rolling tandem mill. Am J Ind Med 1981; 2:51–8.

41. Jones JG. An investigation into the effects of exposure to an oil mist on workers in a mill for the cold reduction of steel strip. Ann Occup Hyg 1961; 3:264–71.

42. Foe RB, Bigham RS. Lipid pneumonia following occupational exposure to oil spray. JAMA 1954; 155:33–4.

43. Proudfit JP, van Ordstrand HS, Miller CW. Chronic lipoid pneumonia following occupational exposure. Arch Ind Hyg 1950; 1:105–11.

44. Ely TS, Pedley SF, Hearne FT, et al. A study of mortality, symptoms, and respiratory function in humans occupationally exposed to oil mist. J Occup Med 1970; 12:253–61.

45. Goldstein DH, Benoit JN, Tyroler HA. An epidemiologic study of an oil mist exposure. Arch Environ Health 1970; 21:600–3.

46. Järvholm B, Bake B, Lavenius B, et al. Respiratory symptoms and lung function in oil mist-exposed workers. J Occup Med 1982; 24:473–9.

47. Acquavella JF, Leet TL. A cohort study among workers at a metal components manufacturing facility. J Occup Med 1991; 33:896–900.

48. Decoufle P. Further analysis of cancer mortality patterns among workers exposed to cutting oil mists. J Natl Cancer Inst 1978; 61:1025–30.

49. Eisen EA, Tolbert PE, Monson RR, et al. Mortality studies of machining fluid exposure in the automobile industry: I. A standardized mortality ratio analysis. Am J Ind Med 1992; 22:809–24.

50. Järvholm B, Lavenius B. Mortality and cancer morbidity in workers exposed to cutting fluids. Arch Environ Health 1987; 42:361–6.

51. Mallin K, Berkeley L, Young Q. A proportional mortality ratio study of workers in a construction equipment and diesel engine manufacturing plant. Am J Ind Med 1986; 10:127–41.

52. Park RM, Mirer FE. Mortality at an automotive stamping and assembly complex. Am J Ind Med 1996; 30:664–73.

53. Park RM, Wegman DH, Silverstein MA, et al. Causes of death among workers in a bearing manufacturing plant. Am J Ind Med 1988; 13:569–80.

54. Park R, Krebs J, Mirer F. Mortality at an automotive stamping and assembly complex. Am J Ind Med 1994; 26:449–63.

55. Rotimi C, Austin H, Delzell E, et al. Retrospective follow-up study of foundry and engine plant workers. Am J Ind Med 1993; 24:485–98.

56. Silverstein M, Park R, Marmor M, et al. Mortality among bearing plant workers exposed to metalworking fluids and abrasives. J Occup Med 1988; 30:706–14.

57. Tolbert PE, Eisen EA, Pothier LJ, et al. Mortality studies of machining fluid exposure in the automobile industry: II. Risks associated with specific fluid types. Scand J Work Environ Health 1992; 18:351–60.

58. Vena JE, Sultz HA, Fiedler RC, Barnes RE. Mortality of workers in an automobile engine and parts manufacturing complex. Br J Ind Med 1985; 42:85–93.

59. Kazerouni N, Thomas TL, Petralia SA, Hayes RB. Mortality among workers exposed to cutting oil mist: update of previous reports. Am J Ind Med 2000; 38:410–6.

60. Calvert GM, Ward E, Schnorr TM, Fine LJ. Cancer risks among workers exposed to metalworking fluids: a systematic review. Am J Ind Med 1998; 33: 282–92.

61. Costa DL, Amdur MO. Respiratory response of guinea pigs to oil mists. Am Ind Hyg Assoc J 1979; 40:673–9.

62. Lushbaugh CC, Green JW, Redemann CE. Effects of prolonged inhalation of oil fogs on experimental animals. Arch Ind Hyg 1950; 1:237–47.

63. Selgrade MK, Hatch GE, Grose EC, et al. Pulmonary effects due to short-term exposure to oil fog. J Toxicol Environ Health 1987; 21:173–85.

64. Shoshkes M, Banfield W, Rosenbaum SJ. Distribution, effect, and fate of oil aerosol particles retained in the lungs of mice. Arch Ind Hyg 1950; 1:20–35.

65. Skyberg K, Skaug V, Glyseth B, et al. Subacute inhalation toxicology of mineral oils, C_{15}–C_{20} alkylbenzenes, and polybutene in male rats. Environ Res 1990; 53:48–61.

66. Wagner WD, Wright PG, Stokinger HE. Inhalation toxicology of oil mists. I. Chronic effects of white mineral oil. Am Ind Hyg Assoc J 1964; 25:158–68.

67. Schaper M, Detwiler K. Evaluation of the acute respiratory effects of aerosolized machining fluids in mice. Fundam Appl Toxicol 1991; 16:309–19.

68. Gordon T. Acute respiratory effects of endotoxin-contaminated machining fluid aerosols in guinea pigs. Fundam Appl Toxicol 1992; 19:117–23.

69. Gordon T, Harkema JR. Mucous cell metaplasia in the airways of rats exposed to machining fluids. Fundam Appl Toxicol 1995; 28:274–82.

70. Thorne PS, DeKoster JA, Subramanian P. Pulmonary effects of machining fluids in guinea pigs and mice. Am Ind Hyg Assoc J 1996; 57:1168–1172.

71. Thorne PS, Lester B, Dodd A, O'Neill ME, Duchaine C. Responses to *Mycobacterium chelonae* from metal working fluids differ from *Saccharopolyspora rectivirgula* in a murine model of hypersensitivity pneumonitis. Toxicologist 2004; in press.

72. Mattsby-Baltzer I, Sandin M, Ahlström B, et al. Microbial growth and accumulation in industrial metal-working fluids. Appl Environ Microbiol 1989; 55:2681–89.

73. Lonon MK, Abanto M, Findlay RH. A pilot study for monitoring changes in the microbiological component of metalworking fluids as a function of time and use in the system. Am Ind Hyg Assoc J 1999; 60:480–85.

74. Foxall-Van Aken S, Brown Jr. JA, Young W, et al. Common components of industrial metal-working fluids as sources of carbon for bacterial growth. Appl Environ Microbiol 1986; 51:1165–69.

75. Zacharisen MC, Kadambi AR, Schlueter DP, et al. The spectrum of respiratory disease associated with exposure to metal working fluids. J Occup Environ Med 1998; 40:640–47.

76. Wilsey PW, Vincent JH, Bishop MJ, Brosseau LM, Greaves IA. Exposures to inhalable and 'total' oil mist aerosol by metal machining shop workers. Am Ind Hyg Assoc J 1996; 57:1149–53.

Chapter 44
Oils and Petroleum Derivatives

Oyebode A Taiwo, Ben Hur P Mobo Jr

Petroleum refining has evolved continuously in response to changing consumer demand for better and different products. Present-day refineries produce a variety of products that can be classified broadly as fuels, petrochemical feed stocks, solvents, process oils, and lubricants. Physically similar materials may also be derived from other organic minerals, such as coal, woods, and other vegetable matter. Because of their physical and chemical properties, these simple derivatives of naturally occurring substances have found an enormous number of uses in energy, construction, and primary metal manufacturing industries such as steel and aluminum.

This chapter provides an overview of information useful in the recognition and prevention of health effects related to exposures to petroleum-derived fuels and their combustion products, as well as petroleum derivatives such as semi-solid tars, pitch, coke, and asphalt.

PETROLEUM-DERIVED FUELS AND COMBUSTION PRODUCTS

Petroleum or crude oil is a naturally occurring liquid mixture containing thousands of different hydrocarbon molecules as well as sulfur, oxygen, nitrogen, and trace metals such as vanadium, iron, arsenic, and nickel. Petroleum, which literally means 'rock oil', is formed by the decay of organic matter such as marine organisms and vegetation. While the chemical and physical properties of crude oil vary widely from source to source, the petroleum-derived products are primarily influenced by the refining processes. The refining operation typically commences with desalting, a process that removes inorganic salts, water, and water-soluble compounds. Crude oils are then sent for distillation, which physically separates the oil into fractions based on range of boiling points. The resultant fractions undergo further processing depending on product specifications and economic factors. Some of the common petroleum-derived products are listed in Table 44.1.

Exposure setting

Given the ubiquity of petroleum production and use, as well as the complexity of refining processes, the potential for occupational exposure to physical and chemical agents in a petroleum operation is significant. In addition, environmental exposure may ensue following industrial spills, home accidents, and refueling procedures. Some of the chemicals present in refining operations are listed in Table 44.2. Their potential health effects are discussed in other chapters. The most important petroleum-derived products, gasoline and its constituents, and diesel and kerosene fuels, are discussed in this section.

Gasoline and gasoline constituents

Gasoline or petrol is a complex liquid mixture of saturated and unsaturated hydrocarbons used for internal engine combustion. It typically contains 62% paraffins (or alkanes), 7% olefins (or alkenes), 31% aromatics, and small amounts of alcohols, ethers, and additives.[1] In the past, additives included organolead compounds, which were phased out in the 1970s due to their adverse health effects. The health effects of these compounds are discussed in Chapters 39.7 and 40, respectively. These components were replaced with methyl tertiary butyl ether (MTBE), fuel ethanol, ethyl tertiary butyl ether, and tertiary amyl ether. Of these, the most prevalent additive is MBTE, which is present in 15% of today's gasoline formulations.

Human health effects of gasoline and its constituents

The main route of exposure to gasoline is inhalation of vapors. Symptoms of acute exposure include mucosal membrane irritation and central neurologic effects (headache, nausea, dizziness, blurred vision, and mental confusion).[2] Coma and death may ensue within minutes following a high-level exposure, with no evidence of respiratory distress.[3,4] Long-term effects of occupational exposure to gasoline include chronic headache, fatigue, memory loss, and psychomotor and visuomotor dysfunction. Chronic gasoline abuse through sniffing can also cause ataxia, tremors, and encephalopathic changes.[5]

A limited number of animal studies have shown a relationship between exposure to gasoline vapor and the development of cancer.[6–9] Human epidemiologic studies on lung cancer, kidney cancer, leukemia, and multiple myeloma have not shown statistically significant increases following chronic gasoline vapor exposure.[10,11] However, recent studies have reported a 3.5-fold increased risk of nasal cancer in service station workers[12] and an increased risk of male breast cancer among workers in trades with exposure to gasoline and combustion products.[13]

Fuel oils

Kerosene and diesel oil are among the most common petroleum-derived products, and are generally classified as

Products	Common uses	Number of carbon atoms	Boiling point range (°C)
Natural gas	Fuel, chemical	1–2	–164 to –88
Liquified gas	Fuel gas	3–4	–44 to +1
Petroleum ether	Solvents	4–5	20 to 60
Gasoline	Motor gasoline	5–10	32 to 210
Naphtha	Cleaning fluids	5–10	65 to 204
Fuel oil	Kerosene, aviation fuel	5–16	40 to 300
Gas oil	Diesel fuel, heating	9–16	204 to 371
Waxes	Sealant	≥20	204 to 400
Bottoms	Asphalts	≥20	≥499

Table 44.1 Common petroleum fractions

Arsenic
Benzene
Butadiene
Carbon monoxide
Chlorine
Chromium
Cobalt
Ethylene glycol
Formaldehyde
Heptane
Hexane
Hydrogen sulfide
Iron
Mercury
Methyl tertiary butyl ether
Nickel
Nitrogen oxides
Sulfur dioxide
Toluene
Vanadium
Welding fumes
Xylene

Table 44.2 Chemicals potentially present in refining operations

fuel oils. Kerosene, or fuel oil number 1, is heavier than gasoline and lighter than lubricant oils, and is commonly used as a heating fuel, cooking fuel, degreasing agent, and a solvent for asphalt coating. Diesel oil, or fuel oil number 2, is principally a blend of petroleum-derived compounds. Its grade varies with the alkane, alkene, cyclic alkane, and aromatic composition. Generally, kerosene and diesel oil have similar toxicologic profiles.

Human health effects of fuel oils

Fuel oils are less volatile than gasoline; therefore, dermal contact and ingestion are important routes of exposure. Inadvertent or intentional ingestion of fuel oils can lead to aspiration and may result in lipoid pneumonia, which is discussed later in this chapter.

Several skin conditions have been reported with exposure to diesel and kerosene, in both acute and chronic settings. These include irritant contact dermatitis due to the defatting effects of skin contact with fuel oil; allergic contact dermatitis, attributed to isothiazolines in diesel oil; and acne/folliculitis due to plugged skin follicles.[14–17] Dermal contact with fuel oil has also been associated with increased incidence of skin cancer in animal studies, though this is not established in human studies. The mech-

anism of action is presumably related to the effects of polycyclic aromatic hydrocarbons (PAHs) contained in fuel oil.

Health effects of fuel oils have been reviewed by the Agency for Toxic Substances and Disease Registry (ATSDR), and include respiratory, gastrointestinal, renal, hepatic, cardiovascular, and hematological effects.[18]

VEGETABLE OILS

Oils derived from vegetable materials are primarily used as food products and, to a lesser extent, as lubricants and dispersants. Vegetable oils are highly biodegradable, and generally free of toxicity. The main work-related health effects are due to dermal exposure leading to irritant and allergic dermatitis.[19–21] Two health effects are toxic oil syndrome (TOS), due to ingestion of contaminated vegetable oil, and lipoid pneumonia, caused by inhalation of oil mists (from vegetable, mineral, and fuel oils).

Toxic oil syndrome

TOS was first described in an epidemic that appeared in Spain in 1981. Nearly 20,000 people were affected and 457 died from this condition. TOS is attributed to the ingestion of rapeseed cooking oil adulterated with an aniline derivative,[22] although the syndrome has never been reproduced in animal studies. Withdrawal of the rapeseed oil from the market resulted in marked decline of new cases.

The clinical course of TOS is variable. During the first 2 months of disease, the presentation variably includes fever, cough, rash, dyspnea, myalgia, pulmonary edema, and eosinophilia. Few patients have complete remission after the acute phase. Over the subsequent months, most patients develop skin tenderness, severe myalgia, subcutaneous edema, abnormal liver function tests, and pulmonary hypertension. During the early chronic phase, from 4 to 24 months, disease manifestations include weight loss, joint contracture, polyneuropathy, scleroderma, and sicca syndrome. In the late chronic phase, the disease is characterized by muscle cramps, chronic musculoskeletal pain, Raynaud's phenomenon, and carpal tunnel syndrome.[23]

TOS has also been associated with other autoimmune diseases, particularly the eosinophilia–myalgia syndrome (EMS), due to ingestion of contaminated L-tryptophan products. An aniline derivative has been identified as a potential common contaminant in both syndromes.[24]

Lipoid pneumonia

Lipoid pneumonia is a lung disease characterized by alveolar lipid accumulation from either endogenous or exogenous sources. Endogenous lipoid pneumonia, also referred to as 'cholesterol' or 'golden' pneumonia, has been described in the setting of bronchiolitis obliterans, Wegener's granulomatosis, bronchial obstruction from tumor, tissue necrosis following radiotherapy and chemotherapy, fat emboli, pulmonary alveolar proteinosis, and lipid storage disease.[25]

In contrast, exogenous lipoid pneumonia is caused by aspiration or inhalation of fatty materials, including animal fats, mineral oil, vegetable oil, and fuels. It was first described in 1925 by Laughlen during autopsy of patients who had received mineral oil nose drops or oral laxatives. Exogenous lipoid pneumonia has since been reported in various occupational and non-occupational settings. Some of these cases are listed in Table 44.3. The most frequent occupational exposure has occurred in the setting of oil mist or spray inhalation by metal workers.[26]

Inhaled or aspirated mineral oils can enter the tracheobronchial tract without eliciting a cough reflex. Once deposited, they impair the mucociliary transport system. Lipids are rapidly taken up by alveolar macrophages, and the lipid–macrophage complex induces the release of inflammatory and fibrogenic mediators, which lead initially to inflammatory consolidation and later to fibrosis.

Risk factors associated with development of lipoid pneumonia include extremes of age, impaired swallowing and cough reflexes, mental status change, history of gastroesophageal reflux, neurologic or psychiatric illness, and prolonged recumbent position.[27,28]

The clinical manifestations of lipoid pneumonia vary. Many patients are asymptomatic while others present with non-specific symptoms like cough, dyspnea, chest pain, hemoptysis, fever, fatigue, and weight loss.[27] More than half of patients have normal physical findings. Others may have dullness to percussion, crackles, wheezing, and finger clubbing.[29]

Laboratory examinations may be normal, but elevated erythrocyte sedimentation rate and leukocytosis with neutrophilic predominance may occur. Pulmonary function tests may show a restrictive pattern; however, normal, mixed, and pure obstructive patterns have also been reported in a few cases.[27] Decreased diffusing capacity and exercise-induced hypoxemia have also been reported.[25]

The radiographic pattern of lipoid pneumonia is variable. Unilateral and bilateral ground glass opacities, as well as normal radiographic patterns, have been reported. Right and left lung fields are almost equally involved. Most cases involve multiple lobes, with some preponderance in the posterior and lower zones.[27] Alveolar consolidations, alveolar nodules, atelectasis, cavitary lesions, and small pleural effusion have also been reported (Fig. 44.1). Computed tomographic scan and magnetic resonance imaging may demonstrate presence of fat within the lung tissue (Fig. 44.2).

Bronchoalveolar lavage may show visible, if not stainable, oil droplets. Cytologic examination may demonstrate positive intracytoplasmic lipid staining of alveolar macrophages, which is fairly specific for lipoid pneumonia (Fig. 44.3). However, the test sensitivity has been variable, in part due to technique difficulty.

In summary, because of the non-specific clinical presentation of lipoid pneumonia, a thorough exposure history is

Offending substance	Exposure setting	Route of exposure
Oil mists	Machine shops	Inhalation
Vegetable and animal oil	Fire extinguisher tester	Inhalation
Kerosene	Fire eater	Inhalation
Petroleum-coated tobacco	Tobacco smoke	Inhalation
Hair spray	Hairspray use	Inhalation
Shellac	Spray	Inhalation
Mineral oil sprays	Metal turner, cashier, insect extermination	Inhalation
Petroleum jelly	High-altitude pilot	Aspiration
Diesel-contaminated water	Survivors of torpedoed ships during WW1 and WW2	Aspiration
Olive oil	Mouthwash use	Aspiration
Lip balm	Excessive use	Aspiration

Table 44.3 Exogenous lipoid pneumonia

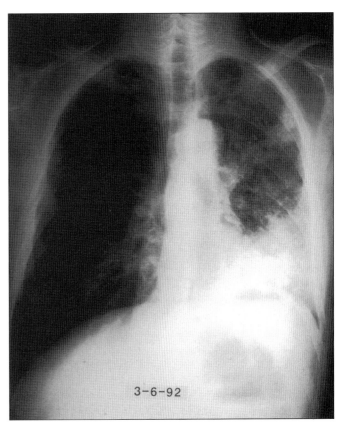

Figure 44.1: Exogenous lipoid pneumonia. The chest roentgenogram shows a dense consolidation in the left lung field with diffuse increased opacification in the remaining left lung. The right lung is inflated, but otherwise normal. (Reproduced with permission from Spickard and Hirschmann.[29])

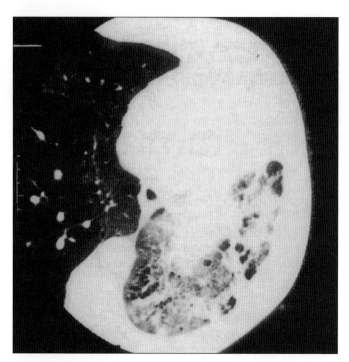

Figure 44.2: Exogenous lipoid pneumonia. High-resolution computed tomographic scan of the thorax demonstrates extensive airspace filled with fat in the left lung, with mild involvement of the right lung. Bronchiectasis is present in the left, and emphysema in the right lung. (Reproduced with permission from Spickard and Hirschmann.[29])

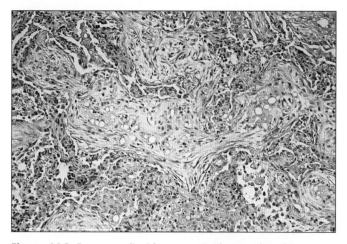

Figure 44.3: Exogenous lipoid pneumonia. The open lung biopsy specimen reveals numerous lipid-laden macrophages with prominent small vacuoles. In the center, intra-alveolar organization and fibrosis are present, the large vacant spaces representing accumulations of mineral oil (hematoxylin–eosin stain, ×80). (Reproduced with permission from Spickard and Hirschmann.[29])

essential. A high index of suspicion is warranted due to the fairly low sensitivity and specificity of available diagnostic studies. The cornerstone in the management of lipoid pneumonia is cessation of exposure, treatment of underlying infection, and provision of supportive care. Oral corticosteroids have been used with variable results. Prevention of exposure to aerosolized oil can be achieved through enclosure or automation of the process, and local exhaust ventilation.

PITCH, ASPHALT, COKE, TARS, AND RELATED MINERAL DERIVATIVES
Exposure settings

Pitch, asphalt, coke, and tars are chemically related dense semi-solid carbonaceous materials that are used widely in construction and in the production of metals such as steel and aluminum. These materials are derived from petroleum (pitch), coal (coke and tars), wood (tars), or naturally occurring asphalt.

Crude coal tar is a byproduct from the formation of coke from coal. The coal tar is then distilled to yield a number of chemical oils, coal tar pitch, and creosote. Coal tar pitch is primarily used as a binder for electrodes in the aluminum reduction process and as the adhesive in membrane roofs. Creosote is a wood preservative used in railroad ties, marine pilings, and telephone poles.

Asphalt, also known as bitumen outside North America, is the residue from the fractional distillation of crude petroleum. It also occurs as a natural deposit residue from the evaporation and oxidation of liquid petroleum. Asphalt is primarily used for paving roads, waterproofing and roofing, electrical insulation, sound insulation, and pipe coating.

All of these materials are composed of high molecular weight, aliphatic and aromatic hydrocarbons with trace amounts of sulfur or metals. Although physically similar, these materials are chemically diverse. The health effects are largely related to the content of PAHs.

PAHs are a group of chemicals formed during incomplete combustion of almost any fuel. They occur in association with domestic heating, vehicle exhaust, waste incinerators, certain industrial activities, as well as cigarette smoking. They are transported through the atmosphere in the vapor phase and absorbed on particulate matter. PAHs are distributed widely in the human environment at low concentrations. With higher levels in many industrial environments, significant exposure occurs in workplaces such as gas works and coke, aluminum, iron, and steel plants, where these materials are handled.

Exposure in workers is primarily by dermal or inhalation routes. At low temperature, these materials are minimally volatile; their physical characteristics make it difficult to generate respirable dusts, therefore the major exposure route is dermal. Skin absorption of PAHs contributes significantly to total body burden and can account for over 50% of total uptake.[30–33] Application of these agents is often performed at high temperature, especially in processes such as primary metal manufacture, like aluminum reduction, steel coking, or in coal gasification. Roofers, road workers, and manufacturers of construction materials also heat them as part of their regular work. This results in the generation of both vapors and fume volatiles (e.g., coal tar volatiles). These volatiles may contain high concentrations of respirable PAHs.

Human health effects

PAHs are carcinogens with both primary DNA-binding and cancer-promoting properties in various experimental models. The carcinogenic potential of individual chemicals varies by many orders of magnitude.[34,35] PAHs almost always occur in mixtures; therefore the carcinogenicity to humans cannot be linked to individual chemicals. Furthermore, because the proportions of specific PAHs are entirely different in each material, the overall carcinogenic potential of a given material cannot be inferred by measuring one or two other marker compounds, such as benzo[a]pyrene, as is often assumed.[36]

A strong association between chronic PAH exposure and lung cancer in coke and gas manufacturers[37,38] and lung and bladder cancer among workers in aluminum smelters[39–41] has been demonstrated in epidemiologic studies. Epidemiologic studies have also observed increased risk for laryngeal, renal cell, colorectal, and pancreatic cancers.[42–44]

Workers exposed to tars and related compounds are also at increased risk for skin cancers, primarily of the squamous type (see Chapter 30.10). Because construction workers may also have a high potential for exposure to ultraviolet light, synergistic effects may be important.[42,45] Heating of tars and related compounds also creates the potential for serious burns, because the hot materials will adhere to the skin and continue to transfer heat until cooled or removed surgically.

The evidence for human carcinogenicity of creosote and asphalt remains limited, owing to relatively few studies published to date, and to methodological limitations, such as insufficient sample size and latency effects. Asphalt fumes contain primarily long-chain hydrocarbons and a lower PAH concentration compared to coal tar fumes. While epidemiologic studies on the carcinogenicity of asphalt have raised concerns, further characterization of risk is required to allow definitive conclusions.[46–48]

Prevention

Primary measures to prevent inhalation and dermal contact by coal tar pitch volatiles and similar agents are essential, especially when they are heated. Monitoring for benzene-soluble material (BSM) that includes all the particulate coal tar pitch volatiles is recommended. Several studies on PAHs in ambient air have demonstrated that benzo[a]pyrene is found consistently in different mixtures and correlates well with total exposure; therefore it is also used as an indicator compound for the presence of PAHs in the workplace. However, it should not be assumed that PAH control has been achieved based on the air levels of benzo[a]pyrene or other easily measured marker compounds; rather, the total levels of particulate should be kept to the absolute minimum.

As an adjunct for prevention, urinary 1-hydroxypyrene (1-OHP) is a useful biologic marker for occupational exposure to PAHs in several work environments. This biomarker serves as an efficient complement to air-borne sampling, because of the significant dermal absorption of these compounds.[49] However, no direct relationship has been established between 1-OHP and cancer risk, therefore it is not a useful tool for quantitative risk assessment.[50,51] Other metabolites, such as thioethers, or more mechanistically important compounds, such as PAH–DNA adducts, have not proved to be easily measurable or amenable to quantifying exposures of interest.[52,53]

References

1. Caprino L, Togna GI. Potential health effects of gasoline and its constituents: a review of current literature (1990-1997) on toxicological data. Environ Health Perspect 1998; 106:115-25.
2. Reese E, Kimbrough RD. Acute toxicity of gasoline and some additives. Environ Health Perspect 1993; 101:115-31.
3. Ainsworth R. Petrol-vapour poisoning. BMJ 1960; 1:1547-8.
4. Yorukoglu D, Sen S, Saygin B. Sudden death from inhalation of petrol vapour. Anaesthesia 1999; 54:302.
5. Burbacher TM. Neurotoxic effects of gasoline and gasoline constituents. Environ Health Perspect 1993; 101:133-41.
6. Belpoggi F, Soffritti M, Maltoni C. Methyl-tertiary-butyl ether (MTBE) – a gasoline additive – causes testicular and lymphohaematopoietic cancers in rats. Toxicol Ind Health 1995; 11:119-49.
7. Mennear JH. Carcinogenicity studies on MTBE: critical review and interpretation. Risk Anal 1997; 17:673-81.
8. Short BG, Burnett VL, Swenberg JA. Elevated proliferation of proximal tubule cells and localization of accumulated alpha 2u-globulin in F344 rats during chronic exposure to unleaded gasoline or 2,2,4-trimethylpentane. Toxicol Appl Phamacol 1989; 101:414-31.
9. Standeven AM, Wolf DC, Goldsworthy TL. Interactive effects of unleaded gasoline and estrogen on liver tumor promotion in female B6C3F1 mice. Cancer Res 1994; 54:1198-204.
10. Rosamilia K, Wong O, Raabe GK. A case-control study of lung cancer among refinery workers. J Occup Environ Med 1999; 41:1091-103.
11. Wong O, Trent L, Harris F. Nested case-control study of leukaemia, multiple myeloma, and kidney cancer in a cohort of petroleum workers exposed to gasoline. Occup Environ Med 1999; 56:217-21.
12. Lynge E, Andersen A, Nilsson R, et al. Risk of cancer and exposure to gasoline vapors. Am J Epidemiol 1997; 145:449-58.
13. Hansen J. Elevated risk for male breast cancer after occupational exposure to gasoline and vehicular combustion products. Am J Ind Med 2000; 37:349-52.
14. Bruynzeel DP, Verburgh CA. Occupational dermatitis from isothiazolinones in diesel oil. Contact Dermatitis 1996; 34:64-5.
15. Das M, Misra MP. Acne and folliculitis due to diesel oil. Contact Dermatitis 1988; 18:120-1.
16. Fischer T, Bjarnason B. Sensitizing and irritant properties of 3 environmental classes of diesel oil and their indicator dyes. Contact Dermatitis 1996; 34:309-15.
17. Koschier FJ. Toxicity of middle distillates from dermal exposure. Drug Chem Toxicol 1999; 22:155-64.
18. Agency for Toxic Substances and Disease Registry (ATSDR). Toxicological profile for fuel oils. US DHHS Contract No. 205-93-0606. June 1995.
19. Aalto-Korte K. Allergic contact dermatitis from tertiary-butylhydroquinone (TBHQ) in a vegetable hydraulic oil. Contact Dermatitis 2000; 43:303.
20. Keane FM, Smith HR, White IR, et al. Occupational allergic contact dermatitis in two aromatherapists. Contact Dermatitis 2000; 43:49-51.

21. Sanchez-Perez J, Garcia-Diez A. Occupational allergic contact dermatitis from eugenol, oil of cinnamon and oil of cloves in a physiotherapist. Contact Dermatitis 1999; 41:346-7.

22. Kilbourne EM, Bernert JT Jr, Posada de la Paz M, et al. Chemical correlates of pathogenicity of oils related to the toxic oil syndrome epidemic in Spain. Am J Epidemiol 1988; 127:1210-27.

23. Alonso-Ruiz A, Calabozo M, Perez-Ruiz F, et al. Toxic oil syndrome. A long-term follow-up of a cohort of 332 patients. Medicine 1993; 72:285-95.

24. Bell SA. The toxic oil syndrome: an example of an exogenously induced autoimmune reaction. Toxic oil syndrome. Mol Biol Rep 1996; 23:261-3.

25. Pugath RD, Mark EJ. Case records of the Massachusetts General Hospital. Weekly clinicopathological exercises. Case 33-1999. A 57-year-old woman with a pulmonary mass. N Engl J Med 1999; 341:1379-85.

26. Cullen MR, Balmes JR, Robins JM, et al. Lipoid pneumonia caused by oil mist exposure from a steel rolling tandem mill. Am J Ind Med 1981; 2:51-8.

27. Gondouin A, Manzoni P, Ranfaing E, et al. Exogenous lipid pneumonia: a retrospective multicentre study of 44 cases in France. Eur Respir J 1996; 9:1463-9.

28. Rome L, Murali G, Lippmann M. Nonresolving pneumonia and mimics of pneumonia. Med Clin North Am 2001; 85:1511-30, xi.

29. Spickard A 3rd, Hirschmann JV. Exogenous lipoid pneumonia. Arch Intern Med 1994; 154:686-92.

30. Sanders CL. Percutaneous absorption of [7.10-14C]benzo[a]pyrene and [7,12-14C]dimethylbenz[a]anthracene in mice. Environ Res 1984; 33:353-60.

31. Vanrooij JG. Dermal exposure to polycyclic aromatic hydrocarbons among primary aluminium workers. Med Lav 1992; 83:519-29.

32. VanRooij JG. Absorption of polycyclic aromatic hydrocarbons through human skin: differences between anatomical sites and individuals. J Toxicol Environ Health 1993; 38:355-68.

33. VanRooij JG. Estimation of individual dermal and respiratory uptake of polycyclic aromatic hydrocarbons in 12 coke oven workers. Br J Ind Med 1993; 50:623-32.

34. Braga RS, Barone PM, Galvao DS. Identifying carcinogenic activity of methylated polycyclic aromatic hydrocarbons. J Mol Struct (Theochem) 1999; 464:257-66.

35. Jacob J. The significance of polycyclic aromatic hydrocarbons as environmental carcinogens. Pure Appl Chem 1996; 68:301-8.

36. Culp SJ, Gaylor DW, Sheldon WG, et al. A comparison of tumors induced by coal tar and benzo[a]pyrene in a 2-year bioassay. Carcinogenesis 1998; 19:117-24.

37. Constantino JP, Redmond CK, Bearden A. Occupationally related cancer risk among coke oven workers: 30 years of follow-up. J Occup Environ Med 1995; 37:597-604.

38. Redmond CK. Cancer mortality among coke oven workers. Environ Health Perspect 1983; 52:67-73.

39. Armstrong B, Tremblay C, Baris D, et al. Lung cancer mortality and polynuclear aromatic hydrocarbons: a case-cohort study of aluminum production workers in Arvida, Quebec, Canada. Am J Epidemiol 1994; 139:250-62.

40. Mastrangelo G, Fadda E, Marzia V. Polycyclic aromatic hydrocarbons and cancer in man. Environ Health Perspect 1996; 104:1166-70.

41. Tremblay C, Armstrong B, Theriault G, et al. Estimation of risk of developing bladder cancer among workers exposed to coal tar pitch volatiles in the primary aluminum industry. Am J Ind Med 1995; 27:335-48.

42. Boffetta P, Jourenkova N, Gustavsson P. Cancer risk from occupational and environmental exposure to polycyclic aromatic hydrocarbons. Cancer Causes Control 1997; 8:444-72.

43. Romundstad P, Haldorsen T, Andersen A. Cancer incidence and cause specific mortality among workers in two Norwegian aluminum reduction plants. Am J Ind Med 2000; 37:175-83.

44. Silverstein M, Maizlish N, Park R, et al. Mortality among workers exposed to coal tar pitch volatiles and welding emissions: an exercise in epidemiologic triage. Am J Public Health 1985; 75:1283-7.

45. Everall JD, Dowd PM. Influence of environmental factors excluding ultra violet radiation on the incidence of skin cancer. Bull Cancer 1978; 65:241-7.

46. Chiazze L Jr, Watkins DK, Amsel J. Asphalt and risk of cancer in man. Br J Ind Med 1991; 48:538-42.

47. Partanen T, Boffetta P. Cancer risk in asphalt workers and roofers: review and meta-analysis of epidemiologic studies. Am J Ind Med 1994; 26:721-40.

48. Partanen TJ, Boffetta P, Heikkila PR, et al. Cancer risk for European asphalt workers. Scand J Work Environ Health 1995; 21:252-8.

49. Levin JO, Rhen M, Sikstrom E. Occupational PAH exposure: urinary 1-hydroxypyrene levels of coke oven workers, aluminium smelter pot-room workers, road pavers, and occupationally non-exposed persons in Sweden. Sci Total Environ 1995; 163:169-77.

50. Ovrebo S, Real C, Haugen A, et al. Studies of biomarkers in aluminum workers occupationally exposed to polycyclic hydrocarbons. Cancer Detect Prev 1995; 19:258-67.

51. Strickland P, Kang D, Sithisarankul P. Polycyclic aromatic hydrocarbon metabolites in urine as biomarkers of exposure and effect. Environ Health Perspect 1996; 104:927-30.

52. Kriek E, Rojas M, Alexandrov K, et al. Polycyclic aromatic hydrocarbon-DNA adducts in humans: relevance as biomarkers for exposure and cancer risk. Mutat Res 1998; 400:215-31.

53. Kubiak R, Belowski J, Szczeklik J, et al. Biomarkers of carcinogenesis in humans exposed to polycyclic aromatic hydrocarbons. Mutat Res 1999; 445:175-80.

Chapter 45
Persistent Organic Pollutants

Jeffrey Derr, Peter Orris

'Persistent organic pollutants' (POPs), 'persistent toxic substances' (International Joint Commission), and 'persistent, bioaccumulative, and toxic pollutants' (US Environmental Protection Agency) are terms used to describe a group of organic carbon-based chemical compounds that possess a number of characteristics that distinguish them from most environmental pollutants. POPs are compounds that bioaccumulate, biomagnify, persist in the environment, and demonstrate a capacity for long-range geographic transport. While dominated by organochlorine compounds, POPs include a variety of chemical classes with the common property of biopersistence.

BIOACCUMULATION, BIOMAGNIFICATION, AND ENVIRONMENTAL PERSISTENCE

POPs have a prolonged half-life in the human body, and are extraordinarily slow to be metabolized and excreted. Due to their lipophilic properties, they tend to accumulate and concentrate in fatty compartments, including breast milk. The end result is that the concentration of the pollutant in the organism becomes far greater than in the surrounding environment, a process termed bioaccumulation.

Because organisms tend to accumulate concentrations of POPs in their tissues that are greater than the concentrations found in the food that they consume, tissue concentrations tend to be higher in organisms that are higher in the food chain. Through this process of biomagnification, large mammals, including humans, are often at the apex of these food chains and accumulate some of the highest levels of POPs in their fatty tissues. POPs enter the food chain through air-to-plant-to-animal and water/sediment-to-fish pathways. Most, though not all, human exposure to POPs occurs through food consumption. The usual processes that lead to environmental breakdown of pollutants include hydrolysis (breakdown by water), photodegradation (breakdown by light), and biodegradation (breakdown by micro-organisms). POPs are relatively resistant to most of these processes. For most POPs, hydrolysis does not play a major role. In general, photodegradation of POPs via photochemically generated free radicals is a more important mechanism than direct photolysis (direct breakdown by ultraviolet light). Photodegradation of POPs in water takes place at a rate approximately one-tenth that of air and is of minimal importance in the dark sediments of the lakes and oceans. Therefore, half-lives of POPs in aquatic sediments are prolonged, and POPs

bioaccumulate in organisms that feed in and around these sediments. Photodegradation in soil is limited to the top 1 mm of soil. Anaerobic biodegradation of POPs takes place in soil and aquatic environments, and its rate is dependent on a variety of factors, particularly temperature. For instance, the Baltic Sea half-life of dioxin, a classic POP, is 8 days in air, 167 days in water, and 37,500 days in soil and sediment.[1] These times are longer than would be expected in warmer environments. Prolonged half-lives in sediments and soil, where photodegradation is limited, demonstrate the importance of this mechanism in the breakdown of POPs.

LONG-RANGE TRANSPORT

Though a variety of global pathways have been identified, the relatively low volatility of POPs favors distribution to colder, higher latitudes through a process know as 'global distillation or fractionization'.[2] Oceans, fresh-water bodies, and land contain concentrations of POPs that are greater than that found in air. These reservoirs are in continuous equilibrium with the atmosphere. POPs enter and leave these reservoirs repeatedly as they move northward in a process described as the 'grasshopper effect'. Much of the re-deposition to the reservoirs following volatilization occurs via precipitation. More volatile compounds tend to migrate farther from their source than do less volatile ones; thus, less heavily chlorinated biphenyl compounds have greater transport due to higher volatility. Weather patterns dictate that most atmospheric transport to the Arctic occurs during the winter and spring. Similar patterns have been described for Antarctica. Deposition of contaminated river sediments into the Arctic seas provides a significant, but less important, mechanism of POP transport to Arctic regions. Because of this Arctic accumulation of POPs, populations indigenous to these regions are at risk for substantial exposure. This is especially true because their diets are heavily dependent on Arctic mammals in which POPs have already been heavily biomagnified.

Because of this dispersion process, reduction of POPs in the environment must be controlled on a global level. To this end, the United Nations Environmental Programme (UNEP) has identified 12 POPs in need of the most urgent attention.[3] Nine organochlorine pesticides are cited including aldrin, chlordane, DDT, dieldrin, endrin, heptachlor, hexachlorobenzene (HCB), mirex, and toxaphene. Polychlorinated dibenzodioxins (dioxins or PCDDs), polychlorinated dibenzofurans (furans or PCDFs), and polychlorinated biphenyls (PCBs) are also included.

Additional work is being done to develop a consensus process for defining additional chemicals as POPs that warrant elimination. UNEP initiated negotiations on an international binding agreement that will reduce or eliminate the release of the 12 currently identified POPs into the environment. Over 120 countries were involved in this negotiative process, culminating in a treaty adopted in May 2001.

DIOXINS, FURANS, AND PCBS

Dioxins, furans, and coplanar 'dioxin-like' PCBs are the POPs that have received the most attention regarding environmental and human toxicity. Although there are some differences between the groups of compounds, research over the last decade has revealed a common mechanism of action that has led them to be assessed together in terms of their environmental impact.

Structure

While many isomeric forms exist, certain dioxins, furans, and PCBs are considered 'dioxin-like' compounds with the potential for behaving like 2,3,7,8-tetrachlorodibenzo-p-dioxin (2,3,7,8-TCDD), the most toxic molecule in this group and the one most often referred to as 'dioxin'. Current research suggests that all dioxin-like compounds have similar mechanisms of action and cause similar environmental and health effects. Like all POPs, they are hydrophobic and resistant to biodegradation and metabolism; therefore, they are environmentally persistent and accumulate in the fatty tissues of animals and humans. 2,3,7,8-TCDD has a human half-life of slightly over 7 years, and researchers use this value for mixtures of dioxin-like compounds in pharmacokinetic modeling. Individual dioxin-like compounds have half-lives ranging from less than 1 year to 10 years.

Dioxins, furans, and PCBs each have slightly different ringed structures with chlorine substituted at various locations on the rings (Fig. 45.1). The specific location of the chlorine molecules determines whether or not the compound is considered dioxin-like. The range of possible substitutions results in 75 chlorinated dioxin compounds (PCDDs), 135 chlorinated furan compounds (PCDFs), and 209 PCBs. Each of these individual compounds is referred to as a congener. To have dioxin-like activity, dioxins and furans must be, at a minimum, substituted with chlorine at all four lateral positions. Therefore, only seven PCDDs and 10 PCDFs are considered to have dioxin-like activity. Because PCBs must have four or more lateral chlorines with no more than a single substitution in the ortho (inner) positions to have dioxin-like activity, only 12 of these compounds are classified as such. This PCB configuration results in a flat, or coplanar, molecule that resembles the planar PCDDs and PCDFs.

Brominated dioxin and furan congeners, as well as polybrominated biphenyl congeners used as flame retardants, are grouped exactly the same as their chlorinated counterparts with similar biochemical properties. There are also mixed chlorinated and brominated congeners. All of these compounds are felt to have some dioxin-like activity, though less is known regarding their biologic effects.

Mechanisms

In 1976, it was shown that dioxin binds with high affinity to the aryl hydrocarbon receptor (AhR), an intracellular cytosolic protein that serves as a nuclear transcription factor. Once dioxin binds AhR, the complex enters the cell nucleus, where it combines with the AhR nuclear translocator (Arnt). This complex then attaches to enhancer/promoter regions of DNA to induce transcription. While the precise natural mechanism of the AhR has not been characterized, it appears to interact with a variety of

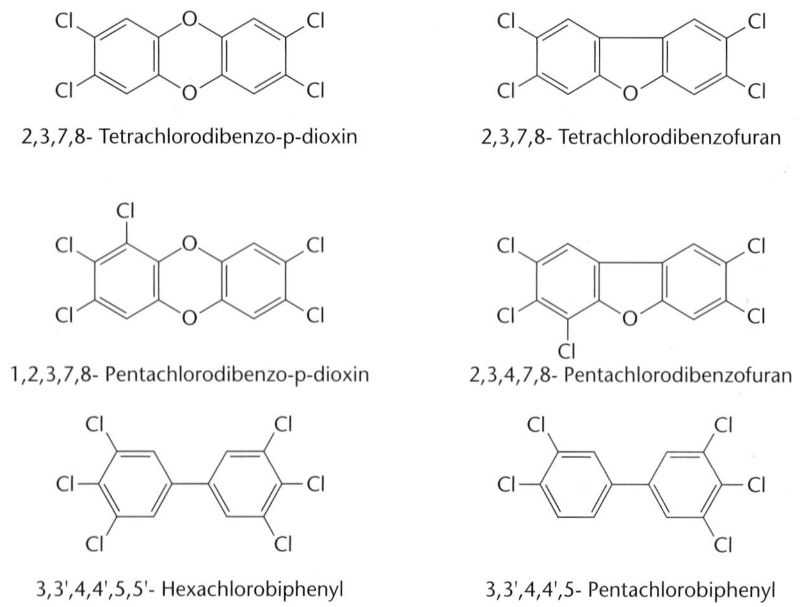

2,3,7,8- Tetrachlorodibenzo-p-dioxin

2,3,7,8- Tetrachlorodibenzofuran

1,2,3,7,8- Pentachlorodibenzo-p-dioxin

2,3,4,7,8- Pentachlorodibenzofuran

3,3',4,4',5,5'- Hexachlorobiphenyl

3,3',4,4',5- Pentachlorobiphenyl

Figure 45.1: Structure of some polychlorinated dioxins, furans and biphenyl compounds.

ligands to produce effects; thus, it is less specific than most hormone receptors. The receptor's presence across both vertebrate and invertebrate species, along with the tremendous degree of interspecies homology, suggests an important evolutionary function. The best-studied interaction is dioxin's association with the promoter region of the CYP1A1 gene, which results in induction of cytochrome P4501A1 enzyme activity. This enzyme facilitates metabolism and excretion of lipophilic substrates, such as polycyclic aromatic hydrocarbons (PAHs), by oxidizing them to more water-soluble derivatives. Thus, the AhR and the biochemical pathways it induces may have a natural role that involves detoxification of these and other environmental and dietary carcinogens.[4] However, prolonged activation of these pathways, and activation during developmentally critical periods, may be responsible for the adverse effects of dioxin-like chemicals.

While the AhR appears to be the dominant mechanism of action for dioxin-like compounds, it is worth noting that other modes of toxicity may be extant, especially for PCBs. In most PCB mixtures, dioxin-like PCBs comprise an extremely small fraction of the total, and health impacts from other congeners must be considered. For example, one animal study showed that carcinogenicity of Aroclor 1260 is not AhR dependent in rodents.[5]

The 'toxic equivalency factor' (TEF) concept

2,3,7,8-TCDD is the prototypical and most potent dioxin-like compound. The other congeners have a toxic potency that is less than that of 2,3,7,8-TCDD. Sources of dioxin often produce complex mixtures of the different congeners. Additionally, as dioxins persist and biomagnify, the congener make-up of the original environmental input changes due to different solubilities, volatilities, and rates of degradation/metabolism among the different congeners. Different ratios and types of dioxin-like compounds among different samples make comparisons of potency and adverse effects between cases very difficult. Therefore, the concept of toxic equivalency factors has been adopted. 2,3,7,8-TCDD has been assigned a TEF of 1.0, and the various other congeners have been assigned a TEF that is some fraction of 1.0 (Table 45.1). The total potency of any dioxin mixture can be determined by weighting the amount of each congener present in the mixture by its respective TEF. This gives a total amount (toxic equivalence, TEQ) of dioxin-like compounds in terms of 2,3,7,8-TCDD that is expressed in a variety of ways, including grams per year TEQ when referring to environmental inputs, or picograms per gram lipid TEQ when referring to serum levels.

The TEFs are derived both from in-vivo and in-vitro studies, and are felt to be conservative estimates that avoid underestimating risk of exposure to these compounds. Because of uncertainties in setting TEFs, they are to be considered 'an order of magnitude estimate' of potency, rather than a specific measure of toxicity. TEFs refer only to responses mediated via the AhR, and do not account for non-AhR-mediated effects. The most widely used TEF

Selected dioxin-like compounds	TEF
2,3,7,8-Tetrachlorodibenzo-p-dioxin (2,3,7,8-TCDD or 'dioxin')	1
2,3,7,8-Tetrachlordibenzofuran (2,3,7,8-TCDF)	0.1
1,2,3,7,8-Pentachlorodibenzo-p-dioxin (1,2,3,7,8-PeCDD)	0.5
2,3,4,7,8-Pentachlorodibenzofuran (2,3,4,7,8-PeCDF)	0.5
3,3',4,4',5,5'-Hexachlorobiphenyl (PCB 169)	0.01
3,3',4,4',5-Pentachlorobiphenyl (PCB 126)	0.1

Table 45.1 Toxic equivalency factors (TEFs) for selected polychlorinated dibenzodioxins, polychlorinated dibenzofurans, and polychlorinated biphenyls (PCBs)

system was developed by the World Health Organization (WHO) and was reviewed and updated by consensus conference in 1997.[6]

Critics of the TEF approach cite excessive uncertainty in TEF estimates and the possibility of non-additive interactions among the various congeners as major limitations.[7,8] Additionally, some studies show that natural AhR agonists (e.g., PAHs) found in dietary meat products and cigarette smoke result in much higher daily intake of TEQs and more readily elicit a biochemical response than TEQs derived from dioxin-like substances. This calls into question the relative significance of trace levels of dioxin-like TEQs compared to relatively high exposure to naturally occurring AhR agonists.[8] Even with these potential limitations, TEFs are used as a risk assessment tool to approximate relative potencies of mixtures of dioxin-like compounds and show good correlation with health effects in peer-reviewed studies.[7]

Sources

Dioxins and furans are not intentionally produced for human use; rather, they are byproducts of manufacturing and incineration processes involving chlorinated compounds. Because of its high reactivity, chlorine reacts rapidly with any organic matter it encounters. Though this is an extremely beneficial property for chemical synthetic processes, it also means many unintended byproducts are created as contaminants.[9] Thus, the production of pentachlorophenol (PCP; a pesticide previously used as a wood preservative), 2,4,5-trichloro-phenoxyacetic acid (a herbicide), polyvinyl chloride (PVC; a common plastic), and any other chlorinated organic material can result in byproducts containing dioxins. These waste products have been responsible for several instances of ambient environmental contamination and health concerns, as occurred at Love Canal and at Times Beach, Missouri.[10]

Other industrial waste sources include bleaching processes in the pulp and paper industry and dry-cleaning distillation residues. Point sources of combustion resulting in dioxin contaminants include municipal and hazardous waste incinerators, copper smelting, and sintering plants, while more diffuse sources include automobile exhaust and home heating emissions. Incineration of medical waste, which contains large amounts of organically bound chlorine in the form of PVC plastic, has also been identified as a major source.[11] Accidents such as PCB fires and building fires can be a significant source of dioxin exposure. Finally, natural events such as forest fires and volcanic eruptions result in some dioxin formation.

PCBs are chemically stable, relatively inflammable compounds with good insulating properties that were produced commercially in the US from 1929 through 1976. Because of their chemical characteristics, they were used as coolants and lubricants in electrical transformers and capacitors, as flame retardants, and as weatherproofers. They have also been mixed with pesticides to prolong their residual activity. Aroclor is the most commonly referred to trade name for PCBs, and the various formulations are assigned a number (e.g., Aroclor-1221 or Aroclor-1232) depending on the relative amount of the various PBC congeners. Dioxin-like PCB congeners are only found in trace amounts in commercial PCB preparations. However, because approximately 1.2 million tons of PCBs have been produced worldwide, these commercial preparations serve as the largest source of dioxin-like PCB congeners and contaminate the environment when PCB-containing equipment and materials are improperly disposed of. Like dioxins, PCBs are formed and emitted during combustion of chlorinated material.[12] Finally, when PCBs accidentally burn or are significantly heated during use, dioxins and furans are created that add to the toxicity of any pre-existing dioxin-like PCB congeners in the mixture.

Elimination of PCP and PCB production, substitution of chlorine-free bleaching agents in the paper industry, and use of smokestack emission controls have decreased dioxin input into the environment.[13] However, current environmental contaminants remain significant. The major environmental input sources are municipal waste incineration, copper smelting, medical waste incineration, coal combustion by utilities, sintering plants, industrial wood combustion, and sewage sludge incineration.

The 'endocrine disruption' hypothesis

Dioxin-like compounds and other organochlorines have been characterized as carcinogenic, developmental, endocrinologic, immunologic, and reproductive hazards. Multiple environmental observations of developmental and reproductive abnormalities in wildlife have been observed.[14] Although the less persistent toxicants dibromochloropropane and ethylene dibromide have also been put forth as the etiologic agents responsible for alligator population decline in an ecologic habitat,[15] the organochlorine pesticide DDT and other persistent pesticides are widely felt to be responsible. Following an accidental release of DDT into Lake Apopka, Florida, male juvenile alligators were shown to have diminished testosterone levels unresponsive to luteinizing hormone stimulation. Testes showed abnormal morphologic organization, and phalli were abnormally small. Normal sexual maturation did not occur, and reproductive capacity was diminished.[16]

Examples of endocrine abnormalities in wildlife have bolstered research on hormonally active agents in humans.

An endocrine disruptor has been defined by the Environmental Protection Agency (EPA) as an 'exogenous agent that interferes with the synthesis, secretion, transport, binding, action, or elimination of natural hormones in the body that are responsible for the maintenance of homeostasis, reproduction, development, and/or behavior'.[17] A further discussion of this topic is provided in Chapter 27.1. Exogenous chemicals have been identified that mimic estrogen compounds; act as anti-estrogens, anti-androgens, and anti-progesterone compounds; and interfere with thyroid hormone function. Human health concerns are related to potential disruption of sex steroid axes, including abnormal sexual differentiation, diminished reproductive capacity, and endometriosis and breast cancer in females. Diminished sperm production and testicular cancer may be a result in males. Alteration in thyroid function related to PCB exposure in the prenatal period appears to adversely affect neurologic development.[18,19] Additionally, as demonstrated by diethylstilbestrol (DES), compounds with estrogenic effects can result in transplacental effects after in-utero exposure. In the case of DES, clear-cell adenocarcinoma of the vagina, increased rates of cryptorchidism, and other reproductive abnormalities occurred in offspring of women administered DES during pregnancy.[20] Developmental exposure to endocrine disruptors is especially concerning because the absence of adult feedback mechanisms in the developing fetus may result in adverse effects at very low doses.[17] In fact, a reverse dose–response curve may be in effect, where effects that occur at low doses are not seen at higher doses due to receptor saturation.

Because exposure to most hormonally active agents occurs at very low concentrations, and may depend on exposure during certain critical periods of development, current risk assessment methodologies relying on high-dose studies and classic dose–response curves may not be sensitive enough to detect effects of endocrine disruptors. The Safe Drinking Water Act Amendments of 1996 and the Food Quality Protection Act of 1996 have mandated that the US EPA develop testing methodologies that determine whether chemical com-pounds have endocrine effects in humans. Because previous multi-generation reproductive studies that focused on fertility, fecundity, and growth of offspring have been found to be relatively insensitive for endocrine disturbance, and fail to provide insight into underlying mechanisms of biologic disruption, new test batteries examining more sensitive parameters, such as female estrous cyclicity and sperm quality, are being designed to screen potential environmental contaminants for endocrine-disrupting effects. These test batteries will use in-vitro and in-vivo animal assays to evaluate interactions with estrogen, testosterone, and thyroid hormone.[21] Accounting for the effect of complex mixtures of endocrine disruptors that are likely to occur in an exposed human population adds an additional level of complexity to the risk assessment process.

The 'endocrine disruption' hypothesis is consistent with the AhR mechanism of action for 2,3,7,8-TCDD. AhR agonists have been shown to disrupt thyroid homeostasis and induce teratogenicity. AhR-dependent effects of dioxin also include diminished testosterone levels, disruption of pituitary feedback, and anti-estrogenic activity.[4] Biochemical and animal assays, as well as environmental observations of wildlife, provide considerable evidence for endocrine disruption.[22,23] However, studies of human health effects that may result from endocrine disruption remain conflicting and equivocal. This is likely a function of the limitations of epidemiologic research in detecting health effects in populations that result from a complex series of biochemical events, in response to varied exposures involving potentially dozens of endocrine-disrupting chemicals. A further discussion of endocrine disruption can be found in a National Academy of Sciences publication that addresses the current state of knowledge on this topic.[24]

HEALTH EFFECTS OF DIOXIN-LIKE COMPOUNDS
High-dose exposures

Yusho and Yucheng[25]

In 1968, 1866 people in southern Japan developed a severe clinical illness known as 'Yusho syndrome'. Similarly, 2061 people developed a similar constellation of signs and symptoms in Taiwan in 1979 that were labeled as 'Yucheng syndrome'. In both instances, it was determined that the syndrome developed following consumption of rice bran cooking oil that was contaminated during the cooking process with PCBs and PCDFs from heat exchangers. 'Yusho' and 'Yucheng' each mean oil disease in Japanese and Chinese, respectively. Symptoms included loss of appetite, nausea, pruritus, distal paresthesias, joint pain, headache, and bronchitic pulmonary symptoms. Signs included eyelid swelling, Meibomian gland hypersecretion, conjunctival changes, visual disturbances, chloracne (see below), pigmentation changes in the skin and nails, and liver function biochemical abnormalities. Follow-up has indicated increased cancer mortality in poisoning victims. Significant excess mortality was seen for malignant neoplasms at all sites in males, with considerably increased mortality for cancer of the liver in both males and females (statistically significant only in males). Offspring exposed in utero were born with grayish dark-brown skin, had nail and eyelid changes, and exhibited growth retardation. Cognitive delay has also been observed in these children.[26]

Seveso

In 1976, thousands of people in the town of Seveso, Italy, were exposed to 2,3,7,8-TCDD that was released from a trichlorophenol production plant as a result of an accidental uncontrolled exothermic reaction. Immediately following the release, an excessive number of deaths were noted among animals, particularly poultry and rabbits. Chloracne (193 cases) was the most prominent acute manifestation among the exposed. Follow-up clinical studies revealed some evidence of neuropathy, immunologic changes, and a change in sex ratio, with an excess of female offspring in parents exposed to TCDD. Additional long-term follow-up identified excess cardiovascular and respiratory mortality, increased incidence of diabetes, and an elevated occurrence of gastrointestinal, lymphatic, and hematopoietic malignancies.[27]

Chloracne

Chloracne is a chronic, refractory dermatosis that is characterized by follicular hyperkeratosis (see Chapter 29.2). There is predominance of open over closed non-inflamed comedones. Milia develop and combine to form straw-colored cysts. In contradistinction to acne vulgaris, comedones and cysts concentrate over the malar crescent of the face, in the 'crow's foot' area lateral to the eyes, behind the ears, and in the axillae and scrotum. However, because the two conditions are often clinically and histologically indistinguishable, a history of exposure to dioxin-like compounds is frequently the only clue to the diagnosis of chloracne.[28] Chloracne results from exposure to a variety of halogenated organic compounds, and is a common feature of significant overexposure to dioxin-like compounds. Other symptoms consistent with exposure to the causative agent may be present concurrently with the skin condition. Chloracne occurs within 2 months of exposure and may persist for decades after exposure has ceased. As indicated in Table 45.2, the level of dioxin-like compounds required to develop chloracne is 30–60 times the background levels seen in the general population.[29] Neuberger et al. show that blood TCDD levels may remain elevated for many years in patients with chloracne.[30]

Low-dose exposures

As noted above, assessment of the chronic health effects of POPs presents a clinical challenge. The following health effects summary focuses on human data that is inconclusive in many cases and will require further investigation. Hopefully, improvements in our ability to detect endocrine disruption and its outcomes in animal models will provide knowledge that will facilitate more conclusive epidemiologic evaluations.

Breast cancer

Human data addressing the association between dioxin-like compounds and breast cancer are limited. An occupational cohort of women exposed to TCDD demonstrated an approximately twofold increased risk of breast cancer mortality, with a standardized mortality ratio (SMR) of 2.15 (95% confidence interval [CI] 0.98–4.09).[31,32] Seveso victims have shown a non-significant decrease in breast cancer risk. Nested case-control studies from 1994 and 1997 that examined the association between PCB levels and breast cancer found no significant relationship.[33,34] Additionally, a 1998 study from Denmark noted that PCBs were not associated with increased breast cancer risk.[35]

Other cancers

In a follow-up study of workers accidentally overexposed to 2,3,7,8-TCDD, there was no significant increase in overall

Exposure group	Years since exposure	Toxicant	Average levels (lipid basis)*	Range (lipid basis)*
9 Chlorphenoxy herbicide production workers with documented chloracne in 1972 and no further exposure[30]	18	2,3,7,8-TCDD	340 pg/g	98–659 pg/g
7 Chinese pentachlorophenol production workers with chloracne[29]	<1	Dioxins and furans	Not reported	1200–22,000 pg/g TEQ
9 Chinese pentachlorophenol production workers without chloracne[29]	<1	Dioxins and furans	Not reported	400–650 pg/g TEQ
228 members of German general population (1989)[58]	N/A	Dioxins and furans	43.74 pg/g TEQ	Not reported
69 members of German general population (1995)[58]	N/A	Dioxins and furans	24.06 pg/g TEQ	Not reported
50 young Japanese women 1993–1994[60]	N/A	Dioxins and furans	21.0 pg/g TEQ	9.1–37.0 pg/g TEQ
85 members of German general population[56]	N/A	Dioxins and furans	42 ppt TEQ	Not reported
100 members of the US general population[56]	N/A	Dioxins and furans	41 ppt TEQ	Not reported
5 blood bank samples from Kansas City, MO[57]	N/A	Dioxins and furans	23 ppt TEQ	Not reported
	N/A	PCBs	46 ppt TEQ	Not reported
	N/A	Dioxins, furans, and PCBs	69 ppt TEQ	Not reported

*ppt equals pg/g
PCBs, polychlorinated biphenyls; TCDD, tetrachlorodibenzodioxin; TEQ, toxic equivalence

Table 45.2 Body burdens of dioxin-like compounds in selected populations (blood lipid basis)

or cancer-related mortality. Subgroup analyses revealed that the most highly exposed workers (those with chloracne) had an elevated SMR for malignant neoplasms only after 20 years of follow-up (SMR, 201; 90% CI, 122–315). No single tumor type showed a significant increase, but colorectal cancer (SMR, 344; 90% CI, 94–888) and tumors of the trachea, bronchus and lung (SMR, 252; 90% CI, 99–350) showed the strongest trends towards significance.[36]

Another cohort study of workers with ongoing background exposure to TCDD showed a statistically significant increase in overall cancer mortality among the entire cohort, with an elevated risk of death from soft tissue sarcoma and respiratory cancers in the most highly exposed workers after 20 years of latency.[37] Workers in an herbicide plant contaminated with TCDD had an increase in overall cancer mortality, with increased death from cancers of the lung and hematopoietic system when compared to a similar non-exposed occupational referent group.[31] Some association between soft tissue sarcomas and TCDD and higher chlorinated dioxins has also been noted.[32,38]

In a 1997 case–control study, a dose–response relationship between serum PCB levels and non-Hodgkin's lymphoma was observed, with an odds ratio for the highest serum levels of 4.5 (95% CI, 1.7–12.0).[39] This was potentiated by seropositivity for Epstein–Barr virus (EBV), with an odds ratio of 22.3 (95% CI, 4.3–115.0) for elevated PCB levels with elevated EBV titers. The presence of elevated PCB levels in human populations has been proposed as an explanation for the worldwide increase in the incidence of this tumor in recent decades.[39] In 1997, the International Agency for Research on Cancer (IARC) characterized TCDD as a known human carcinogen (Group 1) based on the evidence in animals and human epidemiology.[40]

Developmental abnormalities

Studies assessing cognitive development in children prenatally exposed to PCBs due to maternal fish consumption have demonstrated decrements in gross motor function and visual recognition memory, as well as significant IQ decrements in more vulnerable children. Recent studies have confirmed these findings, suggesting particular sensitivity of the developing fetal brain.[18,19] No relationship has been found between cognitive developments and breast-feeding with PCB-contaminated milk.

Thyroid dysfunction

A significantly increased rate of primary hypothyroidism has been seen in a cohort of workers exposed to poly-brominated biphenyls (PBBs).[41] In another cohort, elevations in free thyroxine index were seen in workers with the highest body burdens of TCDD.[42] There has been some correlation between elevated neonatal thyroid-stimulating hormone (TSH) levels and PCB exposure, but studies are conflicting.[43,44] A further discussion of thyroid dysfunction is provided in Chapter 27.1.

Immune system dysfunction

Studies of adults occupationally exposed to PCDD/PCDFs have shown no consistent evidence of immune dysfunction, other than possible impairment of lymphocyte function with very high exposure.[45,46] However, the developing immune system is likely more sensitive. Animal studies suggest prenatal exposure to these compounds may cause long-lasting immunologic incompetence. Additionally, prenatal 2,3,7,8-TCDD exposures may interfere with normal development of self-tolerance and predispose to autoimmune disease.[47] Recent work has shown an increased risk of chickenpox and ear infections in young children with higher exposure to PCBs.[48]

Reproductive effects

As noted above, progeny of Seveso victims demonstrated a female-predominant altered sex ratio. Additional studies are underway to assess reproductive outcomes in this population.[49] Human studies have failed to demonstrate a consistent correlation between dioxin-like compounds and endometriosis.[49] However, an animal model for dioxin-induced endometriosis has demonstrated that endometrial changes may be promoted by interference with progesterone action.[50]

Although controversial, a recent meta-analysis confirmed that sperm density has been declining in Western countries.[51] It has been speculated that hormonally active com-pounds may be contributing to this phenomenon. A further discussion of reproductive effects is provided in Chapter 27.2.

Diabetes

A study of Vietnam veterans has shown increased prevalence of type II diabetes in personnel exposed to Agent Orange.[52] A potential mechanism includes estrogen-like effects, leading to hyperinsulinemia, with subsequent insulin resistance.[53]

Other effects

In adults potentially exposed to 2,3,7,8-TCDD, elevation of gamma-glutamyltransferase (GGT), with normal levels of other hepatic enzymes, has been observed. Studies have also shown possible increases in cardiovascular disease[54] and abnormal lipid metabolism. Oxidative stress mediated by the AhR may be a potential mechanism for these and other effects, but requires confirmation.

RISK ASSESSMENT CONSIDERATIONS FOR DIOXIN-LIKE COMPOUNDS

As discussed above, most human exposure to dioxin-like compounds occurs via dietary intake. By analyzing dioxin and furan concentrations in food and considering American consumption rates, average daily adult intake for these compounds has been estimated to be 0.3–3.0 pg/kg body weight (bw)/day TEQ.[55] Because dioxin-like PCBs were not included in this analysis, and may make up 35% of the total daily intake of dioxin-like compounds, the actual adult consumption rate may be 0.5–5.0 pg/kg bw/day TEQ. Diets rich in fish, meat, and dairy products may increase consumption several fold, depending on background contamination levels. On a body weight basis, intake of dioxin-like compounds is greater for young children. Because these chemicals are concentrated in breast milk, breastfed infants are at higher risk of exposure and may have consumption rates 12–18 times higher than adults during the first year of life.

Body burdens of dioxin-like compounds have been evaluated and are usually reported on a lipid basis due to their lipophilic characteristics. The lipid fraction of blood or whole milk is separated from the non-lipid components, and lipid basis calculations are reported as amount of dioxin per gram of lipid, rather than amount per gram of tissue. Parts per trillion (ppt) calculated on a lipid basis is equivalent to picograms per gram of lipid. Schecter et al. noted that the body burden of PCDDs/PCDFs in Germany and the US is approximately 40 ppt TEQ on a blood lipid basis (Table 45.2).[56] Blood bank samples from Kansas City

found the PCDD/PCDF body burden to be only 23 ppt TEQ but also showed that dioxin-like PCBs contributed 46 ppt TEQ, for a total of 69 ppt TEQ on a blood lipid basis.[57] PCDD/PCDF levels reported by Wittsiepe et al. show that body burdens present in the German general population are decreasing.[58] Levels found in Japan are consistent with other observations.[59,60]

Based on animal and epidemiologic data, several agencies have recommended exposure limits for dioxin-like compounds. In 1990, the WHO established a tolerable daily intake (TDI) for 2,3,7,8-TCDD of 10 pg/kg bw/day based on animal studies and kinetic modeling. In 1998, the WHO met again to evaluate new health effects evidence (particularly endocrine disruption) and incorporated the TEQ concept into the TDI. Based on the review, a daily intake of dioxin-like compounds of 1–4 pg/kg bw TEQ was recommended.[61] The IARC classified 2,3,7,8-TCDD as carcinogenic to humans (IARC Group 1) in 1997, but noted that other dioxin-like compounds were not classifiable as to their carcinogenicity in humans (IARC Group 3) due to limited experimental and epidemiologic evidence.[40] The National Institute for Occupational Safety and Health (NIOSH) recognizes 2,3,7,8-TCDD as a potential occupational carcinogen and recommends that exposure be limited to the lowest concentration feasible. Both NIOSH and the Occupational Safety and Health Administration (OSHA) have established exposure limits for air-borne concentrations of PCBs.

In 1994, the US EPA issued a dioxin draft reassessment stating that the unit cancer risk for dioxin-like compounds is 1.0×10^{-4} (pg/kg-d)$^{-1}$ TEQ. In its 2000 reassessment, through accumulation of new data on cancer outcomes in occupationally exposed cohorts,[31,36,37] the EPA has recommended a new value of 5.0×10^{-3} (pg/kg-d)$^{-1}$ that represents a 50-fold increase in its estimate of carcinogenic risk for dioxin-like compounds.[62,63] Using an analytic format applied by Schecter and Olson,[64] the risk from dioxin exposure in the US population can be estimated. If the new EPA unit cancer risk is used in this calculation, a risk level several orders of magnitude greater than the EPA's usual acceptable risk level for environmental exposures is obtained, suggesting that potentially thousands of cancer cases per year may be directly linked to dioxin exposure. Like all risk assessment processes, the evaluation of dioxin's carcinogenicity has sparked tremendous criticism and controversy in the scientific and industrial communities, and the proposed risk level has not been formally accepted by the EPA for practical application. Further research will be required to characterize the risk of dioxin and other POPs.

OTHER PERSISTENT ORGANIC POLLUTANTS

The remaining POPs currently targeted for elimination are organochlorine pesticides, which are discussed in detail in Chapter 48. Generally, these agents act as central nervous system stimulants following acute exposure.

Compound	General comments	Current use and exposures	Ecologic considerations	Chronic health effects (carcinogenicity per IARC)	Exposure limits
Aldrin and dieldrin	Both used as insecticides in soil; aldrin metabolized to dieldrin in living systems	Banned in most developed countries; aldrin used as termiticide in parts of SE Asia, Africa, and S America; misapplications for indoor termite control occur; dermal and inhalational exposures from occupational application and indoor environment of treated homes	Binds soil, causing prolonged soil half-life; readily volatilized and redistributed	Not classifiable regarding human carcinogenicity (IARC Group 3), but 1998 study from Denmark showed possible dose–response in humans for breast cancer;[35] neurologic changes include headache, dizziness, muscle twitches, abnormal EEGs, peripheral neuropathy, and psychologic illness; possible Parkinson's disease; may affect immune response; hepatotoxicity and renal toxicity in animals	Dieldrin:OSHA PEL 0.25 mg/m³ air NIOSH – lowest feasible
Chlordane	Insecticide used in fire ant control and other broad-spectrum agricultural applications	Production ended in 1976 in US, 1997 worldwide; used extensively to control termites, and air-borne exposure after indoor spraying may be most significant source of current exposure; stockpiles still in use in some countries	Residues found in soil up to 20 years after application; transport to Arctic readily occurs	Possible human carcinogen (IARC Group 2b); exposure following indoor application may increase rates of bronchitis, sinusitis, and migraines and may cause neurobehavioral changes; exposed workers have shown increased rates of cerebrovascular disease	OSHA PEL 0.5 mg/m³ air NIOSH REL 0.5 mg/m³ air US EPA 0.002 mg/L water
DDT (dichlorodiphenyl-trichloroethane)	Insecticide used in agriculture and to control the mosquito vectors of malaria; readily metabolized in living systems to DDE, a stable and equally toxic compound	WHO endorses phasing out worldwide use, but still promotes limited governmental programs to control malaria; use banned in many countries, but some indoor and agricultural spraying still occurs	Concentrates in sediments; still found in US soil and sediments 20 years after use discontinued; highly concentrated in Arctic food chain	Possible human carcinogen (IARC Group 2b) based on liver tumors in rodents; commonly studied in relation to breast cancer, with conflicting results; in 1993, a nested case–control study in New York found a significant dose–response relationship between serum DDE and breast cancer;[65] however, similar studies in 1994 and 1997 found no significant relationship;[33] there was no association noted between DDT levels and lymphoma;[39] case–control studies among farmers have shown no consistent correlation between DDT use and non-Hodgkin's lymphoma after adjustment for use of other pesticides;[66] many examples of estrogenic endocrine disruptive effects in wildlife; diffuse nervous system abnormalities	OSHA PEL 1 mg/m³ air NIOSH – lowest feasible
Endrin	Rodenticide; also an insecticide used on cotton, corn, and rice; related to aldrin and dieldrin, but more toxic; produces extremely toxic metabolites	Banned in most countries	Half-life in soil up to 12 years	Not classifiable as a human carcinogen (IARC Group 3); animal studies suggest that endrin may increase reactive oxygen species in the liver and brain and may lead to improper bone formation	
Heptachlor	Termiticide, insecticide used in agriculture and for fire ant control; found in chlordane preparations as an impurity; metabolized to heptachlor epoxide	Production ended in 1997, but use continues in many countries; exposure occurs via ingestion of treated foods contaminated with residues and via inhalation in the indoor environment of treated homes; most frequently detected organochlorine in US cattle	Long-range transport and atmospheric deposition via rainwater have been documented	Possible human carcinogen (IARC Group 2b) shown to inhibit breast epithelial cell communication; also may act as tumor promoter; occupational exposure may increase risk of bladder cancer; liver carcinomas in rats; increased risk of cerebrovascular disease in exposed workers	OSHA PEL 0.5 mg/m³ air NIOSH – lowest feasible US EPA 0.0004 mg/L water

Table 45.3 Characteristics of nine organochlorine pesticides targeted as persistent organic pollutants[3]

Compound	General comments	Current use and exposures	Ecologic considerations	Chronic health effects (carcinogenicity per IARC)	Exposure limits
Hexachlorobenzene (HCB)	Used as a fungicide for seed treatment; produced as byproduct during chlorinated chemical production and municipal incineration of waste similar to dioxins	Minimal ongoing production and direct use; acute high exposure due to human consumption of HCB-treated seeds in Turkey during the late 1950s resulted in a porphyria cutanea tarda-like syndrome, and breastfed children of exposed mothers developed the dramatic 'pembe yara' syndrome (aka 'pink sore', a low-grade cellulitis that quickly deteriorates into a limb- or life-threatening soft tissue infection)	Deposition and bioaccumulation in Arctic regions has been documented	Known animal and possible human carcinogen (IARC Group 2b): CNS, liver, and spleen damage shown in animals; low doses in animals have been shown to alter adrenal cortex function	
Mirex	Insecticide used for fire ant control in SE US; previous use as fire retardant in plastics, paints, and electrical equipment largely banned; breaks down to more toxic photomirex in presence of sunlight	Ongoing insecticide use in some countries; food primary source of intake, but food levels generally below recognized tolerances	Very stable and persistent; resists biodegradation; half-life of up to 10 years in sediment; deposition and bioaccumulation in Arctic regions have been documented	Minimal human data; possible human carcinogen (IARC Group 2b) based on animal studies; immune suppression in animals; endocrine disruption in animals well documented	
Toxaphene	Insecticide and ascaracide; used particularly on cotton crops	Most widely used insecticide in US by 1975; banned by the US EPA in 1982, stockpiles used through 1986; Argentina and Mexico continue to allow restricted use; very prominent residue on foods in 1980s, but current residue levels are generally below acceptable limits	One of most dominant freshwater organochlorine residues in US and Canada, with most transported via atmospheric deposition from C America and southern US; high Arctic concentrations	Limited human data; mutagenicity in mammalian cells and liver cancer in animals has resulted in classification as a possible human carcinogen (IARC Group 2b); has shown estrogenic and anti-estrogenic effects; may affect behavior and learning	Germany 0.1 mg/kg wet weight for fish US EPA 0.005 mg/L water

Table 45.3 (Cont'd) Characteristics of nine organochlorine pesticides targeted as persistent organic pollutants[3]

Headache, nausea and vomiting, dizziness, muscle weakness, ataxia, and seizures may occur. Coma, respiratory failure, and death may result from large overexposures. Some of the organochlorines may precipitate seizure at relatively low doses, even in the absence of other health effects. Though the evidence is stronger for some, many organochlorine pesticides are suspected of having hormonally active effects, raising concern over carcinogenic, developmental, endocrinologic, immunologic, and reproductive effects. Specific details for nine of the best-studied organochlorine compounds are shown in Table 45.3.

CLINICAL EVALUATION

In general, the appropriate clinical evaluation for patients concerned about exposures to PCBs, dioxins, and dibenzofurans focuses heavily on risk communication and avoidance of future exposures. History should emphasize sources of exposure, as well as health and reproductive function. Physical examination should be directed towards organ systems of concern, including skin, thyroid, lymphatic, breast, genitourinary, and hepatic systems. No special diagnostic tests or therapeutic regimen are recommended to avoid or prevent future health effects in most cases. While not specific, liver function tests, thyroid function, and complete blood count may be useful. Blood or lipid levels of these toxicants are occasionally helpful in etiologic assessment and as an aid to accurate risk communication. No therapeutic modality has been proven effective in reducing the half-life of these compounds in the human body. NIOSH provides excellent references for laboratory evaluation of persons exposed to PCBs, aldrin, dieldrin, chlordane, DDT, and endrin on their web page at www.cdc.gov/niosh/nmed/nmed0000.html. Local reference laboratories should be contacted for details regarding test specifications and interpretation, as well as specimen collection requirements.

References

1. Sinkkonen S, Paasivirta J. Degradation half-life times of PCDDs, PCDFs and PCBs for environmental fate modeling. Chemosphere 2000; 40:943-9.
2. Burkow IC, Kallenborn R. Sources and transport of persistent pollutants to the Arctic. Toxicol Lett 2000; 112-113:87-92.
3. Fisher BE. Most unwanted. Environ Health Perspect 1999; 107:A18-23.
4. Okono ST, Whitlock JP Jr. The aromatic hydrocarbon receptor, transcription, and endocrine aspects of dioxin action. Vitam Horm 2000; 59:241-64.
5. Safe SH. Polychlorinated biphenyls (PCBs): environmental impact, biochemical and toxic responses, and implication for risk assessment. Crit Rev Toxicol 1994; 24:87-149.
6. Van den Berg M, Birnbaum L, Bosveld AT, et al. Toxic equivalency factors (TEFs) for PCBs, PCDDs, PCDFs for humans and wildlife [see comments]. Environ Health Perspect 1998; 106:775-92.
7. Starr TB, Greenlee WF, Neal RA, Poland A, Sutter TR. The trouble with TEFs [letter; comment]. Environ Health Perspect 1999; 107:A492-3.
8. Safe S. Limitations of the toxic equivalency factor approach for risk assessment of TCDD and related compounds. Teratog Carcinog Mutagen 1997; 17:285-304.
9. Thornton J. Pandora's poison: chlorine, health, and a new environmental strategy. Cambridge, MA: MIT Press; 2000.
10. Tiernan TO, Taylor ML, Garrett JH, et al. Sources and fate of polychlorinated dibenzodioxins, dibenzofurans and related compounds in human environments. Environ Health Perspect 1985; 59:145-58.
11. Thornton J, McCally M, Orris P, Weinberg J. Hospitals and plastics. Dioxin prevention and medical waste incinerators [see comments]. Public Health Rep 1996; 111:299-313.
12. Alcock RE, Behnisch PA, Jones KC, Hagenmaier H. Dioxin-like PCBs in the environment-human exposure and the significance of sources. Chemosphere 1998; 37:1457-72.
13. Fiedler H. Sources of PCDD/PCDF and impact on the environment. Chemosphere 1996; 32:55-64.
14. Peterson RE, Theobald HM, Kimmel GL. Developmental and reproductive toxicity of dioxins and related compounds: cross-species comparisons. Crit Rev Toxicol 1993; 23:283-335.
15. Semenza JC, Tolbert PE, Rubin CH, Guillette LJ Jr, Jackson RJ. Reproductive toxins and alligator abnormalities at Lake Apopka, Florida. Environ Health Perspect 1997; 105:1030-2.
16. Guillette LJ Jr, Gross TS, Masson GR, Matter JM, Percival HF, Woodward AR. Developmental abnormalities of the gonad and abnormal sex hormone concentrations in juvenile alligators from contaminated and control lakes in Florida. Environ Health Perspect 1994; 102:680-8.
17. Crisp TM, Clegg ED, Cooper RL, et al. Environmental endocrine disruption: an effects assessment and analysis. Environ Health Perspect 1998; 106(Suppl 1):11-56.
18. Jacobson JL, Jacobson SW. Intellectual impairment in children exposed to polychlorinated biphenyls in utero. N Engl J Med 1996; 335:783-9.
19. Patandin S, Lanting CI, Mulder PG, Boersma ER, Sauer PJ, Weisglas-Kuperus N. Effects of environmental exposure to polychlorinated biphenyls and dioxins on cognitive abilities in Dutch children at 42 months of age. J Pediatr 1999; 134:33-41.
20. Giusti RM, Iwamoto K, Hatch EE. Diethylstilbestrol revisited: a review of the long-term health effects. Ann Intern Med 1995; 122:778-88.
21. Kavlock RJ. Overview of endocrine disruptor research activity in the United States. Chemosphere 1999; 39:1227-36.
22. Taylor MR, Harrison PT. Ecological effects of endocrine disruption: current evidence and research priorities. Chemosphere 1999; 39:1237-48.
23. Tyler CR, Jobling S, Sumpter JP. Endocrine disruption in wildlife: a critical review of the evidence. Crit Rev Toxicol 1998; 28:319-61.
24. National Research Council (U.S.) Committee on Hormonally Active Agents in the Environment. Hormonally active agents in the environment. Washington DC: National Academy Press; 1999.
25. Ikeda M. Comparison of clinical picture between Yusho/Yucheng cases and occupational PCB poisoning cases. Chemosphere 1996; 32:559-66.
26. Lai TJ, Guo YL, Yu ML, Ko HC, Hsu CC. Cognitive development in Yucheng children. Chemosphere 1994; 29:2405-11.
27. Bertazzi PA, Bernucci I, Brambilla G, Consonni D, Pesatori AC. The Seveso studies on early and long-term effects of dioxin exposure: a review. Environ Health Perspect 1998; 106(Suppl 2):625-33.
28. Orris P, Worobec S, Kahn G, Hryhorczuk D, Hessl S. Chloracne in firefighters [letter]. Lancet 1986; 1:210-1.
29. Coenraads PJ, Olie K, Tang NJ. Blood lipid concentrations of dioxins and dibenzofurans causing chloracne. Br J Dermatol 1999; 141:694-7.
30. Neuberger M, Landvoigt W, Derntl F. Blood levels of 2,3,7,8-tetrachlorodibenzo-p-dixoin in chemical workers after chloracne and in comparison groups. Int Arch Occup Environ Health 1991; 63:325-7.
31. Manz A, Berger J, Dwyer JH, Flesch-Janys D, Nagel S, Waltsgott H. Cancer mortality among workers in chemical plant contaminated with dioxin. Lancet 1991; 338:959-64.

32. Kogevinas M, Becher H, Benn T, et al. Cancer mortality in workers exposed to phenoxy herbicides, chlorophenols, and dioxins. An expanded and updated international cohort study. Am J Epidemiol 1997; 145:1061-75.

33. Krieger N, Wolff MS, Hiatt RA, Rivera M, Vogelman J, Orentreich N. Breast cancer and serum organochlorines: a prospective study among white, black and Asian women. J Natl Cancer Inst 1994; 86:589-99.

34. Hunter DJ, Hankinson SE, Laden F, et al. Plasma organochlorine levels and the risk of breast cancer. N Engl J Med 1997; 337:1253-8.

35. Hoyer AP, Grandjean P, Jorgensen T, Brock JW, Hartvig HB. Organochlorine exposure and risk of breast cancer. Lancet 1998; 352:1816-20.

36. Zober A, Messerer P, Huber P. Thirty-four-year mortality follow-up of BASF employees exposed to 2,3,7,8-TCDD after the 1953 accident. Int Arch Occup Environ Health 1990; 62:139-57.

37. Fingerhut MA, Halperin WE, Marlow DA, et al. Cancer mortality in workers exposed to 2,3,7,8-tetrachlorodibenzo-p-dioxin. N Engl J Med 1991; 324:212-18.

38. Saracci R, Kogevinas M, Bertazzi PA, et al. Cancer mortality in workers exposed to chlorophenoxy herbicides and chlorophenols. Lancet 1991; 338:1027-32.

39. Rothman N, Cantor KP, Blair A, et al. A nested case-control study of non-Hodgkin lymphoma and serum organochlorine residues. Lancet 1997; 350:240-4.

40. McGregor DB, Partensky C, Wilbourn J, Rice JM. An IARC evaluation of polychlorinated dibenzo-p-dioxins and polychlorinated dibenzofurans as risk factors in human carcinogenesis. Environ Health Perspect 1998; 106(Suppl 2):755-60.

41. Bahn AK, Mills JL, Snyder PJ, et al. Hypothyroidism in workers exposed to polybrominated biphenyls. N Engl J Med 1980; 302:31-3.

42. Calvert GM, Sweeney MH, Deddens J, Wall DK. Evaluation of diabetes mellitus, serum glucose, and thyroid function among United States workers exposed to 2,3,7,8-tetrachlorodibenzo-p-dioxin. Occup Environ Med 1999; 56:270-6.

43. Feeley MM. Workshop on perinatal exposure to dioxin-like compounds. III. Endocrine effects. Environ Health Perspect 1995; 103(Suppl 2):147-50.

44. Longnecker MP, Gladen BC, Patterson DG Jr, Rogan WJ. Polychlorinated biphenyl (PCB) exposure in relation to thyroid hormone levels in neonates. Epidemiology 2000; 11:249-54.

45. Jung D, Berg PA, Edler L, et al. Immunologic findings in workers formerly exposed to 2,3,7,8-tetrachlorodibenzo-p-dioxin and its congeners. Environ Health Perspect 1998; 106(Suppl 2):689-95.

46. Michalek JE, Ketchum NS, Check IJ. Serum dioxin and immunologic response in veterans of Operation Ranch Hand. Am J Epidemiol 1999; 149:1038-46.

47. Holladay SD. Prenatal immunotoxicant exposure and postnatal autoimmune disease. Environ Health Perspect 1999; 107(Suppl 5):687-91.

48. Kaiser J. Society of Toxicology meeting. Hazards of particles, PCBs focus of Philadelphia meeting [news]. Science 2000; 288:424-5.

49. Eskenazi B, Mocarelli P, Warner M, et al. Seveso Women's Health Study: a study of the effects of 2,3,7,8-tetrachlorodibenzo-p-dioxin on reproductive health. Chemosphere 2000; 40:1247-53.

50. Bruner-Tran KL, Rier SE, Eisenberg E, Osteen KG. The potential role of environmental toxins in the pathophysiology of endometriosis. Gynecol Obstet Invest 1999; 48(Suppl 1):45-56.

51. Swan SH, Elkin EP, Fenster L. The question of declining sperm density revisited: an analysis of 101 studies published 1934-1996. Environ Health Perspect 2000; 108:961-6.

52. Henriksen GL, Ketchum NS, Michalek JE, Swaby JA. Serum dioxin and diabetes mellitus in veterans of Operation Ranch Hand. Epidemiology 1997; 8:252-8.

53. Michalek JE, Akhtar FZ, Kiel JL. Serum dioxin, insulin, fasting glucose, and sex hormone-binding globulin in veterans of Operation Ranch Hand. J Clin Endocrinol Metab 1999; 84:1540-3.

54. Vena J, Boffetta P, Becher H, et al. Exposure to dioxin and nonneoplastic mortality in the expanded IARC international cohort study of phenoxy herbicide and chlorophenol production workers and sprayers. Environ Health Perspect 1998; 106(Suppl 2):645-53.

55. Schecter A, Startin J, Wright C, et al. Congener-specific levels of dioxin and dibenzofurans in U.S. food and estimated daily dioxin toxic equivalent intake. Environ Health Perspect 1994; 102:962-6.

56. Schecter A, Furst P, Furst C, et al. Chlorinated dioxins and dibenzofurans in human tissue from general populations: a selective review. Environ Health Perspect 1994; 102(Suppl 1):159-71.

57. Schecter A, Stanley J, Boggess K, et al. Polychlorinated biphenyl levels in the tissues of exposed and nonexposed humans. Environ Health Perspect 1994; 102(Suppl 1):149-58.

58. Wittsiepe J, Schrey P, Ewers U, Selenka F, Wilhelm M. Decrease of PCDD/F levels in human blood from Germany over the past ten years (1989-1998). Chemosphere 2000; 40:1103-9.

59. Iida T, Hirakawa H, Matsueda T, Nagayama J, Nagata T. Polychlorinated dibenzo-p-dioxins and related compounds: correlations of levels in human tissues and in blood. Chemosphere 1999; 38:2767-74.

60. Iida T, Hirakawa H, Matsueda T, Takenaka S, Nagayama J. Polychlorinated dibenzo-p-dioxins and related compounds: the blood levels of young Japanese women. Chemosphere 1999; 38:3497-502.

61. van Leeuwen FX, Feeley M, Schrenk D, Larsen JC, Farland W, Younes M. Dioxins: WHO's tolerable daily intake (TDI) revisited. Chemosphere 2000; 40:1095-101.

62. Kaiser J. Toxicology. Just how bad is dioxin? [news]. Science 2000; 288:1941-4.

63. Kaiser J. Dioxin draft sparks controversy [news]. Science 2000; 288:1313-4.

64. Schecter A, Olson JR. Cancer risk assessment using blood dioxin levels and daily dietary TEQ intake in general populations of industrial and non-industrial countries. Chemosphere 1997; 34:1569-77.

65. Wolff MS, Toniolo PG, Lee EW, Rivera M, Dubin N. Blood levels of organochlorine residues and risk of breast cancer. J Natl Cancer Inst 1993; 85:648-52.

66. Baris D, Zahm SH, Cantor KP, Blair A. Agricultural use of DDT and risk of non-Hodgkin's lymphoma: pooled analysis of three case-control studies in the United States. Occup Environ Med 1998; 55:522-7.

Chapter 46
Mineral Dusts: Asbestos, Silica, Coal, Manufactured Fibers

Gregory R Wagner, Frank J Hearl

INTRODUCTION

Mineral is the term traditionally applied to naturally occurring inorganic substances having definable and consistent physical properties and chemical composition. By conventional contemporary usage, mineral also refers to similar substances of organic origin, such as coal, as well as manufactured materials of mineral origin, such as ceramic fibers or slag wool. Dusts generated in the mining, milling, manufacture, and use of minerals have long been recognized as causes of serious lung diseases. This chapter provides an overview of information useful in the recognition and prevention of diseases related to mineral dust exposure. As with any agents causing chronic disease, hazard recognition and environmental surveillance and control are key to disease prevention and are thus a primary focus of this section.

ASBESTOS
Exposure settings

Asbestos is a generic name used in referring to a group of fibrous minerals that have exceptional resistance to degradation by heat, acids, bases, or solvents. Asbestos is defined in US regulations as the minerals chrysotile, crocidolite, amosite, tremolite asbestos, actinolite asbestos, and anthophyllite asbestos, although there are other hazardous fibrous minerals such as erionite, richterite, and winchite with similar characteristics.

Asbestos fibers can be classified based on their physical and chemical structures as serpentine (curved) or amphiboles (straight and needle-like). The most commonly used asbestos fiber is chrysotile asbestos, which now comprises over 95% of worldwide production, and is the only serpentine asbestos of importance. Amphibole asbestos, used more in the past, includes commercially used amosite (mined in South Africa) and crocidolite, and non-commercially used anthophyllite, tremolite, and actinolite, which can potentially contaminate other mineral ores or cause environmental rather than occupational asbestos-related disease. The relative potency of the different forms of asbestos in causing both malignant and non-malignant asbestos-related conditions has been a source of controversy, complicated in part by the fact that each form is rarely pure, but may contain small amounts of other fiber types; anyone who has worked with asbestos for many years likely was exposed to several fiber types. Chrysotile is generally considered less potent for mesothelioma induction than certain amphiboles, but still may be a cause. Crocidolite is considered the most potent fiber for mesothelioma.

The asbestos minerals are not combustible and have a high melting point and low thermal and electrical conductivity. These and other useful properties resulted in the development of thousands of commercial uses for asbestos. Asbestos has been in widespread use for more than a century. Before 1900, less than 10,000 metric tons per year were used in the US. The use of asbestos for products including clutch and brake linings, packing and gaskets, asbestos flooring, and thermal and electrical insulation, led to increased demand. By 1950, the annual US demand for asbestos grew to over 660,000 metric tons, and increased to over 801,000 metric tons by 1970.[1-3] Since the early 1970s, regulatory action and liability concerns have reduced or eliminated many uses in the US and elsewhere. Complete or partial asbestos bans are in place in at least 20 countries, and asbestos use will be banned throughout the European Union in 2005.

There are six classes of products in which the use of asbestos is currently banned by the US Environmental Protection Agency (EPA):

- corrugated paper;
- rollboard;
- commercial paper;
- specialty paper;
- flooring felt; and
- new uses of asbestos.

Since the 1970s, the US demand for asbestos products has dropped to the current levels of 14,600 metric tons in 2000.[4]

Recent total US production of asbestos fell from 9550 metric tons in 1996, to an estimated production of 5260 metric tons in 2000. Worldwide production and usage have been relatively stable, declining from 2.1 million metric tons in 1996 to 1.9 million metric tons in 2000. In 2000, the major continuing uses for asbestos were roofing products, gaskets, and friction products. Nevertheless, millions of tons of asbestos insulation remain installed, and removal and disposal create continuing exposure potential. In some situations, asbestos-bearing materials may be sealed with a coating to minimize release of inhalable fibers. This only defers the problem of exposure until major renovation or demolition is required. Today, most domestic exposure occurs in construction workers exposed to installed asbestos products or during asbestos abatement and removal activities. Exposure may also occur when asbestos is found as a contaminant in other commercially useful minerals, including, talc, clays, vermiculite, magnetite, marble, and metal ores.

The Occupational Safety and Health Administration (OSHA) estimated in its 1994 Asbestos Standard that about 700,000 US workers were potentially exposed to asbestos in general industry and shipyards.[5] Many more have been exposed in the past. Table 46.1 lists occupations where significant asbestos exposure has occurred and may continue to occur. Asbestos products have been so widely used that a complete list of potential exposure settings would include virtually all workplaces.

Acoustic product installers
Asbestos cement product makers and users
Asbestos grout makers and users
Asbestos millboard makers and users
Asbestos millers
Asbestos miners
Asbestos paper makers and users
Asbestos plaster makers and users
Asbestos insulators
Asbestos tile makers and installers
Asphalt mixers
Automobile repair workers
Boiler makers
Beer makers
Brake lining makers
Brake refabricators
Chemical workers
Clay workers
Construction workers
Demolition workers
Electric appliance workers
Electrical equipment workers
Electrical wire makers
Food processing workers
Gasket makers
Glass workers
Iron ore (taconite) miners and millers
Insulation workers
Loggers
Machinery makers
Maintenance and custodial workers
Nursery (agricultural) workers
Oil and gas extraction workers
Paint makers
Petroleum refinery workers
Primary metal industry workers
Plumbers and pipefitters
Railroad repair workers
Roofers
Rubber makers
Reinforced plastics makers
Shipyard workers
Stone workers
Talc miners and workers
Textile workers
Transportation equipment makers and repairers
Transportation workers
Vermiculite miners and workers

Table 46.1 Occupations with potential asbestos exposure

Environmental measurement

The techniques for environmental measurement of asbestos can be divided into two general categories. *Qualitative analysis* determines whether or not asbestos is present in a bulk material and estimates the relative amount and mineral type of asbestos present. Qualitative analysis can be done using polarized light microscopy, X-ray diffraction, or transmission electron microscopy. The results from qualitative analysis are usually given as percent asbestos on a projected area or a weight/weight basis. *Quantitative analysis* counts the number of fibers or structures present in a measured volume of air. Two principal techniques are generally used for quantitative analysis. Light microscopy with phase contrast enhancement is commonly used for the routine quantitative fiber measurements needed for comparison to occupational exposure limits. Transmission electron microscopy may be needed when thin fibers (<0.25 μm) are present. Fibers smaller than 0.25 μm are invisible using light microscopy techniques. When performing quantitative fiber analysis, the associated analytic capabilities of these microscopes limit the level of qualitative information (fiber-type identification) that can be gathered on individual fibers. Results from quantitative analysis are usually given as fibers per cubic centimeter or structures per cubic centimeter.[6,7]

Clinical effects

Specific asbestos-related diseases are discussed in detail in Chapters 19.8 and 30.2.

Acute effects
Aside from a non-specific mild respiratory and skin irritant effect, no clinically observable acute effects of asbestos exposure have been documented. Asbestos warts or corns have been described within weeks or months of initial skin exposure to asbestos fibers. These are small nodular lesions, sometimes on an inflammatory base, resulting from a granulomatous reaction to the presence of a foreign body.

Chronic effects
Non-malignant diseases such as pulmonary fibrosis, pleural fibrosis, benign pleural effusion, and chronic bronchitis, as well as a variety of malignancies, including cancers of the respiratory tract, malignant mesothelioma of the pleura or peritoneum, and gastrointestinal cancers, can result from occupational or environmental asbestos exposure. All are chronic conditions of insidious onset occurring after latencies of one or more decades. Each of the non-malignant or malignant effects of asbestos exposure may occur independently of the others. With the exceptions noted below, none is pathognomonic for asbestos dust exposure. Clinical manifestations are non-specific.

Pulmonary fibrosis may be recognized as a result of mandated surveillance of current asbestos workers or through diagnostic evaluation of symptoms of persistent cough and exertional dyspnea of insidious onset. The chest

X-ray demonstrates small irregular opacities at the lung bases. Alternatively, fibrosis may be noted on pathologic examination of lung tissue removed during evaluation of a suspicious or malignant lung lesion, even when the preoperative chest X-ray shows no interstitial changes.[8]

Pleural fibrosis, in the form of discrete plaques or diffuse thickening of the pleura, can occur independently of pulmonary fibrosis. One or more discrete pleural plaques may be recognized along the diaphragm or along the lateral chest walls. Bilateral plaques and plaques with visible calcification seen in individuals with a credible history of asbestos exposure and sufficient latency are presumed to have resulted from the asbestos exposure, although unilateral plaques may result from asbestos exposure, and non-calcified plaques occur more commonly than calcified ones. Pleural plaques undetected by conventional radiographs are often visualized using computed tomography (CT). Diffuse pleural fibrosis often involving blunting or obliteration of the costo-phrenic angle on chest X-ray is also seen as a result of asbestos exposure. This may be associated with significant pulmonary function abnormality, although mild pulmonary dysfunction can also be associated with the presence of pleural plaques.[9]

Benign pleural effusions, lasting weeks to months before spontaneous resolution, occur in asbestos-exposed workers, often within the first two decades following first exposure. These are sterile and without malignant cells. Associated symptoms may be minimal. There are suggestive data associating the eventual development of extensive diffuse pleural fibrosis with antecedent pleural effusions. Chronic bronchitis, persistent cough with phlegm, in general occurs more often in people working in dust than in those who do not, when compared to others with similar smoking habits. This observation has been confirmed in some cohorts of asbestos workers.

Restrictive physiology with a reduced carbon monoxide diffusion capacity, characteristic of diffuse interstitial fibrosis, is typically seen in patients with asbestosis. Inflammation and fibrosis of the respiratory bronchioles can also occur as a manifestation of asbestos exposure, even in the absence of asbestosis visible on chest X-ray. Mild pure airflow obstruction from asbestos exposure (demonstrable as an increased loss of FEV_1 in the absence of other adverse exposures such as cigarette smoke) has been found in some asbestos-exposed workers. Some have observed FEV_1 deficits in asbestos workers with pleural fibrosis. Others have documented progressive loss of FEV_1 in asbestos-exposed workers as they develop symptoms.[10] Higher degrees of lung function loss are associated with increasing pulmonary function deficits.[11]

Respiratory tract cancers are the most common cancers associated with occupational asbestos exposure. These are pathologically indistinguishable from other respiratory tract cancers. Cancers of the lung and larynx are seen more frequently in workers occupationally exposed to asbestos than in others with comparable smoking habits. Latency averages about 25 years from first asbestos exposure. Combined exposure to asbestos and cigarette smoke puts workers at extremely high risk for development of respiratory tract cancers. There is evidence that smoking cessation results in diminished lung cancer risk over time in individuals who have had prior asbestos exposure. Some have asserted that asbestos only causes lung cancer in workers who have already developed pulmonary fibrosis, although evidence for this is limited and increased risk of lung cancer with or without visible fibrosis is well documented in a number of occupational groups.[12] Since both the development of fibrosis and the development of lung cancer are dose-related phenomena, unambiguous resolution of this controversy is challenging.

Malignant mesothelioma of the pleura, peritoneum, or mediastinum in the presence of a credible history of asbestos exposure, occurring after a reasonable latency, are considered 'sentinel health events' presumptively resulting from exposure to the mineral fibers, most often asbestos. Mesothelial cells are thought to be transformed through direct interaction with asbestos fibers. Malignant mesothelioma has been reported with minimal exposure to asbestos; cohorts with high levels of exposure experience high rates of this cancer. Latency between first exposure and mesothelioma development is, on average, longer than that for bronchogenic cancer, averaging 30–35 years. The tumors grow rapidly and are virtually universally fatal, with no effective curative surgical or chemotherapeutic interventions found to date.

Cancers of the gastrointestinal tract, including cancer of the esophagus, stomach, pancreas, colon, and rectum, occur more frequently in most occupational cohorts heavily exposed to asbestos, although the risk is substantially less than for lung cancer.

Other cancers, including certain lymphomas and kidney cancer, have been observed more frequently in some, but not all, asbestos-exposed cohorts. Complex interrelationships between multiple adverse occupational exposures, including asbestos, may in part account for the diversity of malignancies associated with exposure.

Clinical evaluation and management

Clinical management of patients with a history of asbestos exposure requires a combination of medical screening, health counseling, appropriate and timely medical interventions, and emotional support based upon a realistic appraisal of the risks resulting from the exposure. If exposure is continuing, exposure control is critical, and health surveillance consistent with that mandated by the Occupational Safety and Health Administration (OSHA) is warranted. Given current restrictions on asbestos use, exposure has often ceased by the time healthcare is sought. Nevertheless, the biologic persistence of the fibers and the long latency between exposure and disease justify special attention to former asbestos-exposed workers. Also, individuals with asbestos-related diseases may be involved in litigation that may place certain responsibilities on the healthcare provider.

Medical screening involves the performance of tests directed toward the identification of significant diseases or conditions before the diseases become clinically apparent.

Effective treatments or interventions should be available which can improve the outcome of the disease. Screening for disease in an individual is a secondary prevention strategy, distinguishable from public health or workforce surveillance efforts that also involve medical testing. Also, tests done exclusively for screening purposes differ in intent from those performed for diagnostic purposes or to provide information useful in health counseling.[13]

Theoretically, any of the diseases for which asbestos-exposed individuals are at risk would be potential targets for screening in the course of routine medical care. However, most fail to justify the conduct of screening tests. For example, screening for malignant mesothelioma will not result in improved outcome until effective interventions are available. Respiratory tract cancer screening among high-risk groups, using periodic chest X-ray and sputum cytology, has failed to reduce significantly the number of cancer deaths in those screened compared to others receiving routine care. Newer approaches to lung cancer screening using low-dose spiral CT scanning are under evaluation and have demonstrated promising results in selected circumstances.[14]

No effective intervention has been identified to modify the course of pulmonary or pleural fibrosis resulting from asbestos exposures which are no longer continuing. However, the identification of one or more of these conditions combined with appropriate health counseling may help motivate patients to control or eliminate exposure to other pulmonary toxins, particularly tobacco smoke.

When exposure is continuing, however, the presence of abnormalities on chest X-ray justifies recommendations to increase the level of respiratory protection or eliminate the exposure altogether, since the development of fibrosis appears to be dose related and continuing exposure might cause more rapid deterioration. Thus, periodic chest X-rays are indicated for active asbestos workers. Also, when there is ongoing exposure, the ability to use respiratory protective equipment should be monitored closely by periodic examinations including pulmonary function testing.

Gastrointestinal cancer screening, using tests for occult blood in the stool and periodic sigmoidoscopy or colonoscopy, has been recommended by the US Preventive Services Task Force, the American Cancer Society, and others, as being effective in the general population. Given the increased risk of gastrointestinal cancer in asbestos-exposed individuals, this practice should be encouraged. No studies have yet shown benefit from either earlier initiation or more frequent performance of these screening procedures because of increased risk in this group.

Health counseling for patients currently or formerly exposed to asbestos must be directed toward control or elimination of exposure to all current pulmonary hazards, particularly asbestos dust and tobacco smoke. The importance of smoking cessation in asbestos-exposed patients, whether or not they have manifested any of the stigmata of asbestos-related diseases, cannot be overemphasized. The combination of asbestos exposure and tobacco smoke is far worse than either alone. During the decade following smoking cessation, lung cancer risk gradually drops but remains significantly elevated as a result of the asbestos exposure. No healthcare encounter with a current or former asbestos worker should omit inquiry into tobacco use and reinforcement of a smoking cessation message to all current tobacco users.

To date, evidence that dietary modification may diminish cancer risk is unconvincing; however, research into this important question continues. Studies of former asbestos workers with X-ray abnormalities have failed to provide evidence justifying recommendations of specific dietary supplements or other dietary modifications for these patients. Given the risk status of exposed individuals and the limited number of interventions available, prudent advice based on the best available current recommendations from the National Cancer Institute should be offered.

Medical interventions depend upon the diseases manifested by the patient and do not differ appreciably from those that should be offered others with comparable diseases with other etiologies. For example, asbestos-associated malignancies have not been shown to respond any better or worse to conventional surgical techniques or chemotherapy than cancers of unknown or other etiologies. The course of pulmonary fibrosis caused by asbestos exposure is generally slowly progressive to indolent and has not been shown to be affected by any particular intervention. Some have tried decortication procedures to relieve restriction caused by the rare cases of massive diffuse pleural thickening. Such treatments must depend upon the particular circumstances of the individual patient.

Medical therapies should be directed toward early identification and treatment of infection and relief of any element of bronchoconstriction. Evidence of hypoxemia should be sought and treated in severely impaired patients. Desaturation with exercise or during sleep should stimulate consideration of intermittent or continuous oxygen therapy.

Comprehensive educational and support programs directed toward patients with chronic respiratory impairment and their families have been of benefit to some. These programs often direct attention toward significant changes resulting from the disease, such as the need for environmental controls, the onset of sexual dysfunction, or the discouragement resulting from involvement in protracted and incomprehensible litigation. Voluntary organizations such as the American Lung Association may offer referral to pulmonary rehabilitation programs and patient support groups.

Litigation seeking redress for injury from asbestos and finances to purchase necessary healthcare is common in the US among people with asbestos-associated diseases. Physicians caring for these patients must be prepared to provide timely reports when requested by the patient or the patient's representative. Standard diagnostic criteria may be useful in preparation of such reports.[15] The fact that the patient is involved in litigation should not affect diagnostic or therapeutic decisions. Legal issues are considered in detail in Chapter 56.

Prevention

Control or elimination of exposure to asbestos-containing materials is the only absolutely effective strategy for prevention of asbestos-related diseases. Although substitute materials are being used in many current settings, the asbestos already in place will result in ongoing exposure to maintenance, mechanical, and construction workers for decades to come. Disease prevention in these workers will depend in great measure on recognition of the potential for exposure and strict compliance with health and safety regulations. Comprehensive regulations promulgated under the Occupational Safety and Health Act, intended to prevent asbestos-associated diseases, focus not only on exposure control but also on issues of training and surveillance.

Exposure limits

In the US, occupational exposure is limited to 0.1 fiber/cm^3 as a time-weighted average (TWA) over an 8-hour workday for general industry. There is a 1.0 fiber/cm^3 excursion limit averaged over a 30-minute sampling period. If exposure exceeds either the TWA or the excursion limit during the year, periodic exposure sampling, training, and surveillance are required.[16]

Monitoring

Initial personal sampling is required for all workers who may reasonably be expected to be exposed at or above the TWA and/or excursion exposure limits. Additional monitoring is required with a frequency such that the exposure of the worker is adequately described.

Regulated areas

Respiratory protection is required in areas where exposures exceed the TWA and/or excursion exposure limits. Hazard communications requirements, including the posting of warning signs and other restrictions on access, apply in any area with asbestos-containing materials or potentially asbestos-containing materials.

Control

Engineering and work practice controls are the preferred methods for maintaining exposure levels below the TWA and/or excursion exposure limits.

Respiratory protection

A strict program of respiratory protection using NIOSH-certified respirators, periodic fit testing, and training is mandated. The use of 'disposable' filtering facepiece respirators is not permitted. The employer must provide a tight-fitting positive-pressure respirator that provides adequate protection, instead of any negative-pressure respirator, if the employee chooses to use this type of respirator.

Training

All workers exposed above the TWA and/or excursion exposure limits must be trained initially and at least yearly thereafter. Items to include are:

- the health hazards of asbestos exposure;
- the relationship between asbestos and smoking in producing lung cancer;
- operations which could result in exposure;
- the importance of control procedures;
- proper use and limitations of respirators; and
- details of the medical surveillance program.

Medical surveillance

In the US employers must provide a medical surveillance program for all workers exposed above the TWA and/or excursion exposure limits, at no cost to the workers. A baseline pre-placement examination must include a medical and work history; a complete physical examination with emphasis on the respiratory, cardiovascular, and digestive tract systems; a standardized respiratory questionnaire; a full-sized PA chest radiograph; spirometry including FEV$_1$ and FVC; and any other tests deemed appropriate by the examining physician.

After the baseline examination, periodic examinations including an abbreviated questionnaire, periodic chest X-ray, and spirometry are mandated. The questionnaire is administered at baseline, then in an abbreviated form annually. Spirometry and a physical examination are performed at baseline, then annually. A chest radiograph must be offered:

- every 5 years for workers under 35 years and/or with less than 10 years since first asbestos exposure;
- every 2 years for workers aged 36–45 with over 10 years since first asbestos exposure; and
- every year for workers over age 45 with over 10 years since first exposure.

Medical examinations and testing are performed or conducted under the supervision of a licensed physician and at a 'reasonable time and place'. Chest X-ray interpretation is done according to the International Labour Office (ILO) classification system by a reader trained, tested, and certified by NIOSH (B reader), a board eligible or certified radiologist, or 'an experienced physician with known expertise in pneumoconioses'. The examining physician is responsible for making a determination as to whether the worker has any medical condition that would put him or her at increased risk of 'material health impairment'. There is mandatory worker and employer notification of the examining physician's opinion resulting from the overall assessment of the test results. Records of the interpretation of the examination along with supporting information must be kept by the employer for 30 years, whether or not the test results are abnormal.

There are no data reported which permit evaluation of the effectiveness of the current regulations for prevention of all asbestos-associated diseases. NIOSH has recommended that exposure to asbestos fibers be limited to 0.1 fibers/cm^3 time-weighted averaged over a 100-minute sampling time, based on the technical limits of fiber monitoring rather than on absolute health protection.

Although compliance with current exposure standards should substantially diminish the burden of asbestos-associated disease in the future, there are still many settings where significant asbestos exposure occurs before controls are put in place or where strict adherence to health protection programs is absent. When the possibility of asbestos exposure is determined after eliciting an occupational history, the healthcare provider should also inquire about the existence of a health protection program in the workplace.

SILICA

Exposure settings

Silicon is the second most common element in the earth's crust. The combination of silicon and oxygen, SiO_2, called silica, is found in amorphous or crystalline forms. Respirable crystalline silica causes silicosis. Heating can change amorphous silica into crystalline forms. The chief form of crystalline silica is α-quartz (hereafter simply 'quartz'). Quartz is a mineral found in most classes of rock, which is the principal source of exposure in many occupations (Table 46.2). Silica sand contains large amounts of quartz. Silica sand is used to produce glass, pottery, silica brick, mortar, and abrasives. Crystalline silica, as sand or aggregate, is added to cement to form concrete. Finely ground silica, also known as silica flour, is used in paints, porcelain, scouring soaps, and as wood filler. The clear rock crystal is of great value for electronic equipment. The colored varieties of crystalline silica are used as gems or ornamental materials.

Tridymite and cristobalite are chemically identical to quartz but differ in crystalline structure. These two minerals are used extensively as filtering and insulating media and as siliceous refractory materials for furnace linings and silica bricks. Flints contain crystalline silica and have been used for centuries because of their hardness and heat resistance.[17,18]

Description	Workers exposed
Masonry, plastering	13,800
Heavy construction	6300
Painting, paper hanging	3000
Iron and steel foundries	800
Metal services	400

Table 46.3 Estimation of workers exposed to at least 10 times the NIOSH REL for crystalline silica

In the US, occupational exposure to crystalline silica occurs in several large categories of industry. Using data from the National Occupational Exposure Survey (NOES) conducted from 1982 to 1983, and applying 1986 Bureau of the Census County Business Patterns, NIOSH estimated that 1.7 million workers are potentially exposed to one or more substances containing silica. Compliance data collected by OSHA inspectors indicate that within the exposed population, there are significant numbers of workers with continuing overexposures to crystalline silica. Table 46.3 lists the number of workers estimated to be exposed to at least 10 times the NIOSH recommended exposure limit (REL), which is approximately five times higher than the prevailing legal limit in the US, i.e., the permissible exposure limit or PEL.[19]

Occupational exposures to crystalline silica also occur throughout the mining industry. Over 300,000 coal, metal, and non-metal miners in stone or ground quarries are exposed to silica. Users of mined or quarried materials in activities such as road building, general construction, and railroad maintenance may be exposed to significant levels of quartz dust.

Environmental measurement

Silica often occurs in combination with other minerals whose composition may include silicon, aluminum, and varying amounts of magnesium, iron, calcium, and other elements. The term 'free silica' is sometimes used to describe SiO_2 that is not combined with other elements. Environmental measurement of silica involves two phases:
- collection of the sample using an appropriate sampling technique; and
- chemical analysis of the collected material.

Two types of samples are routinely collected: bulk dust and respirable dust. *Bulk samples* are collected to determine the average crystalline silica content of the dust in an environment. Once the average silica content is determined, an overall exposure limit for respirable dust can be computed in order to limit silica exposure. *Respirable dust samples* collect air-borne dust on a filter using a particle-size classifier such that the particle collection efficiency mimics the performance of the human respiratory system. It is possible to quantify individuals' exposure to low levels of silica using personal respirable dust samples.

Chemical analysis of both bulk dust and respirable dust samples may be done using X-ray diffraction (XRD) or infrared analysis (IR). A chemical technique involving acid digestion can also be used for bulk samples. The acid digestion technique was the basis for early (pre-1970) silica

Abrasive blasting
Abrasives
Boiler scaling
Cement production workers
Ceramics
Coal mining and milling
Fillers (paint, rubber, etc.)
Foundry work (ferrous and non-ferrous)
Glass manufacture
Insulation production and installation
Metal mining and milling
Micaceous earth excavation
Mining, quarrying and tunneling
Non-metallic mining and milling
Plastic manufacturing
Pottery making
Refractory materials
Road working
Rubber manufacturing
Scouring soap manufacturing
Tile and clay production
Tunneling
Vitreous enameling

Table 46.2 Selected occupations and industries involving exposure to free crystalline silica

analyses. Using phosphoric acid, the amorphous silica and silicate minerals from the bulk dust are digested, leaving the crystalline silica residue for quantification. The percent crystalline silica determined from the bulk analysis can be multiplied by air-borne respirable dust concentration to estimate worker exposure to air-borne crystalline silica. Using respirable dust personal samples, worker dust exposures are measured directly with subsequent crystalline silica analysis by IR or XRD on each individual respirable dust sample.[20]

Clinical effects

The health effects of silica exposure are discussed more fully in Chapters 19.1 and 30.2.

Acute effects

No acute effects of silica exposure have been documented.

Chronic effects

Silicosis is the pneumoconiosis resulting from fibrotic reactions to lung deposition of inhaled crystalline quartz dust. Disease latency and time course depend on the intensity and duration of dust inhalation. Particle size distribution and surface characteristics, as well as the crystalline structure of the quartz particle, may affect toxicity. A characteristic pathologic entity, the silica nodule, results from pulmonary response to inhaled and retained silica. These nodules may coalesce with resulting tissue destruction and disruption of the normal thoracic architecture. This is known as progressive massive fibrosis. Silicosis that occurs within a few years of the initiation of exposure is sometimes referred to as accelerated silicosis. Disease with a more indolent time course, often not identified for one or more decades from first exposure, is sometimes referred to as chronic silicosis. Accelerated and chronic silicosis most likely result from the same disease mechanisms, differing only in time course. A distinct condition, referred to as acute silicosis, may result from a different mechanism. It is a rapidly progressive disease which develops after inhalation of high concentrations of fine silica particles. Acute silicosis has pathologic characteristics similar to alveolar proteinosis.[21]

All forms of silicosis can progress in the absence of ongoing silica dust exposure, and people with occupational silica exposure may not manifest chest X-ray abnormalities until well after retirement. Although silicosis is irreversible, the likelihood of progressive impairment from accelerated or chronic silicosis is presumably diminished through early identification of disease and cessation of exposure. Once acute silicosis is present, interventions have not been shown to favorably influence disease outcome. Experimental therapies or interventions which are not widely available, such as bronchoalveolar lavage and lung transplantation, have been attempted for workers with acute silicosis and for some with total pulmonary incapacity due to progressive massive fibrosis.

Silicosis was listed as an underlying or contributing cause of death on 187 death certificates in the US in 1999.

Surveillance data suggest that death certificate records significantly underestimate the extent of the problem.

The risk of tuberculosis is greater in workers with silicosis than in the general population. Tuberculosis is probably more common in silica-exposed workers even without diagnosed silicosis. Tuberculosis can cause significant morbidity and mortality, particularly if unrecognized and untreated. While effective treatments are available, treatment failures and relapses are reported to occur more commonly in people with silicosis.

Emphysema, bronchitis, and airways obstruction appear to occur more commonly in silica-exposed workers than in the general population. The risk is most likely dose dependent. In general, these conditions cause significant morbidity and can cause premature mortality. Early intervention with control or cessation of adverse pulmonary exposures (including dust and tobacco smoke) may result in reversal of bronchitis symptoms and presumably diminish the rate of progression of airways obstruction.

Lung cancer as a result of silica exposure is the subject of ongoing scientific investigation. After intensive review, the International Agency for Research on Cancer (IARC) has stated that there is sufficient evidence to conclude that inhaled crystalline silica from occupational sources is a human carcinogen,[18] and NIOSH has recommended control of exposure based on the importance of reducing silicosis risk and the conclusion that crystalline silica should be considered a potential occupational carcinogen.[17] Some investigators suggest that silicosis rather than silica exposure is the key risk factor. In any event, as with lung cancer from asbestos exposure, there is no indication that silica dust-associated lung cancers differ from other lung cancers. No effective methods of early identification leading to successful intervention have been identified. Because both silica exposure and lung cancer are so common, even a small increase in relative risk of disease resulting from the exposure could result in a significant number of excess cases.

Clinical evaluation and management

A silica-exposed worker with chest symptoms should be evaluated in the normal fashion with a comprehensive history, focused physical examination, and a logical sequence of medical testing. Medical history should concentrate on adverse pulmonary exposures, including occupational exposure to dusts and fumes and tobacco use. A history of significant chest trauma, pulmonary infections, and cardiovascular disease is relevant. The extent to which current pulmonary problems interfere with normal levels of functioning should be documented. In general, a diagnosis of silicosis is made on the basis of an abnormal chest radiograph along with a credible history of silica exposure.

General clinical management issues for treatment of silicosis are no different than for other chronic pulmonary diseases. Elimination of adverse exposures, patient and family support and education, and interventions directed at optimization of the level of function and minimizing time lost to infection are appropriate. Because of the increased risk of mycobacterial infection in patients with silicosis, tuberculin skin testing and evaluation of risks and potential benefits of treatment should be pursued (see also Chapter 19.9).

Silicosis can progress in the absence of additional exposures, presumably through an iterative process of macrophage ingestion of retained silica particles followed by cell death (liberating inflammatory and fibrogenic mediators), and reingestion. In order to interrupt this process, some have suggested that bronchoalveolar lavage could diminish the body burden of silica. At this time, such therapies should be considered experimental and be performed only in the context of a clinical trial. Lung transplantation has also been attempted for far-advanced disease.

Prevention

Primary prevention

Although the effects of exposure to free silica have been known for many years, silicosis continues to prevail among workers in the dusty trades. The critical strategy for prevention of silicosis is prevention of exposure. The OSHA PEL for general industry is based on the measurement of respirable dust (including silica and non-silica components) and comparing that measurement to the following formula:

$$PEL = 10 \text{ mg/m}^3 / (\% \text{ quartz} + 2)$$

The effect of the formula is to limit respirable dust containing 100% quartz below 0.1 mg/m^3, and to limit respirable dust below 5.0 mg/m^3 for quartz-free dusts. The OSHA limit for the two other forms of crystalline silica, cristobalite and tridymite, is half the limit allowed for quartz.[22] Both NIOSH and the American Conference of Governmental Industrial Hygienists (ACGIH) recommend exposure limits of 0.05 mg/m^3 for all crystalline forms of silica.[23,24] Complicating the situation, OSHA uses a different and older standard for the construction industry, nominally requiring a count of the number of particles collected. Today, few laboratories are equipped or trained to do the microscopic particle counting that is required, consequently respirable mass measurements are sometimes used in conjunction with mass-to-count conversion factors to compare measurements to the exposure limits. The exposure limit for all forms of crystalline silica in the construction industry is determined from the following formula:

$$PEL = 250 \text{ mppcf} / (\% \text{ quartz} + 5)$$

where mppcf stands for million particles per cubic foot of air sampled.

The Mine Safety and Health Administration (MSHA) uses a crystalline silica standard equivalent to the OSHA standard for metal and non-metal mines. For underground coal mines, the respirable dust standard is 2.0 mg/m^3

for coal mine dust with less than 5% crystalline silica. When coal mine dust exceeds 5% quartz, the respirable dust standard (RDS) is calculated using the formula:

$$RDS = 10 \text{ mg/m}^3 / (\% \text{ quartz})$$

Silica dust is generated when silica-bearing soil, rock, or ore is drilled, blasted, cut, dug, or otherwise disturbed. There is no obvious way to determine if the material being processed contains silica other than to perform chemical analyses described earlier in this chapter. As a result, many exposures to crystalline silica go undetected simply because the exposure is not sampled and analyzed for silica. In mine settings, veins of silica may intertwine with veins of desirable ore. Crushed rock and gravel may have varying degrees of silica based on the specific location where the material originated. The best approach for protecting workers health is to sample and analyze the materials being mined or processed frequently.

Once the potential for exposure to silica is established, effective preventative measures are almost always available. These measures include substitution of materials and engineering controls. OSHA and MSHA have established legal standards for compliance, setting exposure limits at approximately 100 µg/m^3 described by the PEL and RDS formulae above; and a REL has been established by NIOSH at 50 µg/m^3. Any measure to control exposure should use these limits to determine the need for engineering controls and their adequacy. The selection of a specific control strategy that maintains exposures below these limits will be determined by the economic and technical feasibility of that particular strategy in each situation.

In abrasive blasting, where risk is high because of the generation of fine particles of 'freshly fractured' silica, it is often possible to replace the silica being used with a less toxic substitute. When using silica, even when the abrasive blaster operator is protected with an air-supplied respirator, blaster helpers and other process workers in the area may be exposed. There are alternative materials available that can be used as an abrasive agent in lieu of silica sand. Although those materials may also be hazardous, and the material liberated during blasting is often toxic, appropriate substitution combined with personal protective equipment can reduce the health risks for the blaster and other nearby workers.

The most common engineering control available in most settings is ventilation. In non-mining industries, ventilation is usually subdivided as blowing and exhausting ventilation and dilution ventilation. Particularly harmful dusts are often removed from the exhaust stream using bag-house filters to prevent general environmental contamination. Industrial applications where these controls have been successfully applied include, among others, foundries, ceramic industries, crushing, grinding, and screening.

In mining environments, the dust control problems are different. Drilling and grinding operations present high exposure potential at surface mines. Since these operations are typically open to the environment, ventilation is not a practical solution. There are two alternative strategies that can be applied: enclosure and dust suppression. The operator's cab in equipment used at surface mines can be enclosed and designed to deliver air-conditioned filtered air to the operator; however, other workers who are not machine operators may continue to be exposed. It may be possible to enclose the point of dust generation. Water injection, water spraying, and the use of wetting agents are means of dust suppression which have been used at both surface and underground mines.

At underground mines, dust control can be achieved through forced ventilation systems. Underground operations may also use high-pressure water sprays, water injection drilling, and other wetting methods to suppress the generation of dust at its source.

Finally, there are a number of ways to do most jobs. Redesigning task performance, utilizing engineering equipment to reduce dust exposure, or altering work practices can be effective. Educational efforts, labeling of quartz-containing materials, and posting of hazardous work sites can assist workers in recognizing the dangers of exposure to dust and the benefits to be gained by altering work practices to reduce exposure to the minimum achievable level.

Secondary prevention

Workplace-based medical screening of silica-exposed workers is generally recommended, using periodic questionnaires, chest X-rays, and lung function tests. The effectiveness of screening efforts has not yet been published. Chest radiographs may detect silicosis in some workers at a point when the disease is asymptomatic, but X-rays may be insensitive to other silica effects. In most exposure settings, a PA chest radiograph repeated every 3 years for asymptomatic workers should be sufficient. More frequent examinations should be conducted if an abnormality is demonstrated and exposure continues. Spirometry is another tool for screening and surveillance. Spirometry is inexpensive, acceptable, and readily available. Lung function testing should be performed using equipment and methods meeting American Thoracic Society-recommended standards (see Chapter 19.1). Spirometry can demonstrate restrictive or obstructive abnormalities, either of which may result from silica dust exposure. Once patients test below population-based 'normal' values, disease is generally well established. Using the patient's own baseline spirometry values for comparison may provide an earlier indication of the development of a problem. In this case, a drop of 15 percentage points from the baseline 'percent predicted' value for either FEV_1 or FVC (e.g., from 105% of predicted FEV_1 to 90% of predicted) should suggest the need for additional evaluation.

A number of state health departments require reporting of cases of silicosis as 'sentinel events'. Investigations of reported cases can identify new cases and lead to prevention of disease in workers not yet affected. Case identification and reporting are no substitute for primary disease prevention through exposure control; they are, however, critical components of an overall program of prevention requiring the cooperation of primary healthcare professionals.

Although silicosis is often thought to be a disease of primarily historical interest, current exposure conditions continue to produce significant disease and even death from silicosis. Exposure is so widespread that workers, employers, and healthcare providers must maintain a high index of suspicion that any work in a dusty trade may result in the development of this serious pulmonary disease.

COAL
Exposure settings

Coal is organic material that has been fossilized after millions of years of pressure and temperature extremes. Coal is used as a basic fuel for numerous industries requiring a source of heat; some coal is also used for residential heating. A relatively small amount of coal is used for production of gaseous and liquid fuels.

The primary occupations that are exposed to coal dust are those associated with the actual mining and processing of coal. Other workers may have significant exposures through coal handling operations. The method of mining has an effect on the dust concentration level in which a miner may work. Usually, coal miners who are employed at the working face (the area of the mine where the actual extraction of coal occurs) of underground mines have the highest coal mine dust exposures. In 2000, there were approximately 76,000 workers in the coal mining industry in the US.

Environmental measurement

Coal dust health standards

In the US, respirable dust levels in both underground and above-ground coal mines have been regulated since 1969. The current US exposure limit for respirable coal mine dust is 2.0 mg/m^3.[25] A lower limit is applicable if more than 5% of the dust is quartz. Exposures to coal mine dust in general industry occur primarily in the steam generation of electricity.

The basic sampling unit used in the US for measuring respirable dust consists of a battery-powered personal sampling pump which draws dust-laden air through a particle pre-separator (generally a cyclone) and onto a pre-weighed filter at a controlled flow rate for an 8-hour shift. The large particles are removed by the pre-separator, and the smaller respirable dust is collected on the filter. Because the exposure limit is for 'respirable coal mine dust', no special chemical analysis is needed; the filters are weighed and the measured mass collected is divided by the volume of air sampled, to calculate the worker's daily exposure.

Coal dust particle size distributions and regional effects

The current coal mine dust standard was intended to prevent deposition of fine particles in the non-ciliated alveolar air spaces. A study of particle size distributions in underground coal mines found that a substantial fraction of mine dust consists of larger particles capable of deposition in the upper airways. Chronic bronchitis is also prevalent in coal miners and may be related in part to the deposition of larger particles in the ciliated, conducting airways. Dust control techniques designed to obtain compliance with the respirable dust standard do not necessarily reduce the thoracic dust exposures.

Clinical effects

The health effects of coal mining are discussed further in Chapter 19.10.

Acute effects

A few studies have identified a relatively acute drop in FEV_1 among some, but not all, miners during the first months to years following first exposure to coal mine dust. The clinical and prognostic significance of this drop is unclear and is the subject of ongoing investigations.

Chronic effects

Coal workers' pneumoconiosis (CWP) is one of the lung diseases arising from inhalation and deposition of coal dust in the lungs and the reaction of the lungs to the dust. CWP is a chronic, irreversible disease of insidious onset, usually requiring 10 or more years of dust exposure before becoming apparent on routine chest radiographs. It is characterized by macular and nodular pigmented lesions in the lungs, which may be visible radiographically as small or large opacities. When only small opacities are present, the condition is called simple CWP or chronic CWP. Progressive massive fibrosis (PMF) or complicated CWP are terms used when radiographic shadows greater than 1 cm, attributable to coal dust exposure, are present. CWP, particularly in advanced stages or when PMF is present, has been associated with pulmonary incapacity and increased morbidity and mortality. The occurrence of CWP is dependent on the intensity and duration of coal mine dust exposure. CWP, in some instances, progresses after cessation of exposure, although this seems to be less common and the progression less aggressive than that resulting from retained silica dust.

CWP was listed as an underlying or contributing cause of death on over 1417 death certificates in the US in 1996. As exposure conditions have improved, the average age at death among men with CWP has increased and approximates the average age at death of all men in the US. Since chest X-ray abnormalities may be visible in the absence of clinical disease in some individuals, there may be a 'preclinical' stage during which CWP can be identified. Although reduction or elimination of exposure to coal mine dust in workers with chest X-rays showing category 1 abnormalities, by ILO criteria, would presumably result in decreased progression of disease and in fewer cases of PMF, statistical modeling based on large data sets in the UK and the US suggests that this benefit may not prove very great.

Dust control strategies in the US, initiated in the early 1970s, were directed at preventing miners from developing ILO category 2 CWP. Miners with category 1 CWP were offered work in jobs with a maximum dust exposure of $1 \, mg/m^3$. It was anticipated that this would result in the virtual elimination of PMF. This strategy has not been completely successful, in part because PMF can appear on a background of category 1 CWP or, rarely, category 0.

Chronic bronchitis, emphysema, and airways obstruction (accelerated loss of FEV_1) are more common in workers exposed to coal mine dust than in others with comparable tobacco use habits. All of these conditions appear to be dose related. Chronic bronchitis symptoms may be reversible if adverse exposures are controlled early. Presumably, the rate of loss of FEV_1 could be diminished through reduction or elimination of dust exposure, although the rate of loss that should trigger intervention and the optimal timing for intervention remain the subject of investigation. Chronic bronchitis, emphysema, airways obstruction, and CWP all result from exposure to coal mine dust and may occur in various combinations. The chest X-ray is not a reliable predictor of the likelihood of airways obstruction associated with dust exposure.[26] In general, diminished FEV_1 is associated with morbidity and premature mortality. Dust exposure unlikely to result in the development of CWP or PMF may still cause or contribute to clinically significant airways obstruction.[27]

Coal mine dust may contain varying proportions of crystalline quartz. CWP may be indistinguishable from silicosis on chest X-ray.

Excess risk of stomach cancer has been reported with coal mine dust exposure, although the level of increased risk is not great and the population prevalence of this condition is generally low (see Chapter 30.5).

Clinical evaluation and management

Miners with lung disease generally present for evaluation either of progressive dyspnea or an acute chest illness. Because a federal benefits program compensates miners with severe impairment, some miners present for consultation or evaluation of their qualification for these benefits. In other instances, the possibility of disease from coal mine dust exposure is an incidental finding in a routine health evaluation.

A clinical evaluation should include a comprehensive medical and occupational history, with a focus on the pulmonary and cardiovascular systems. Since miners with lung disease often become involved in benefits applications and significant weight is given to the assessment of the primary care physician, the history should be carefully taken and well documented. The onset and evolving course of symptoms such as dyspnea, cough, and sputum production should be described. Any changes in normal life activities should be explored in detail. For example, many miners describe the need to abandon hobbies such as hunting, or may report the modification of sexual activity as a result of increasing pulmonary impairment. Work decisions, such as a job transfer from a strenuous or dusty job to one that is less demanding physically, are significant. Since disease development is frequently insidious, it is often helpful to ask about the abilities of the patient in comparison with non-exposed contemporaries. Careful inquiry should also be made into adverse pulmonary exposures on and off the job, including tobacco use.

A comprehensive physical examination is appropriate, although findings are not specific. It is, however, often helpful to determine if other conditions associated with work exposures are present, such as noise-induced hearing loss or musculoskeletal disorders, which should be evaluated and treated.

Testing may include chest radiography, which should be interpreted by someone skilled in recognition of the pneumoconioses, preferably a certified B-reader. Spirometry should be performed using methods and equipment meeting American Thoracic Society recommendations. Other measures of lung function may be helpful in certain clinical settings but do not need to be performed routinely.

Care for miners with chronic lung disease should attempt to maximize their level of functioning and minimize life disruption. Ongoing dust exposure should be controlled to the extent possible, with transfer to a low-dust job recommended for working miners. Where other adverse exposures such as tobacco smoke can be identified, they should be eliminated. Bronchodilators provide symptomatic relief for some. Infections should be treated early and monitored carefully. Immunization against influenza and pneumococcal disease should be encouraged. Tuberculosis does not complicate CWP as it does silicosis.

In coal mining areas, the US Department of Labor has assisted in the development of clinic- or hospital-based respiratory disease treatment programs for miners and their families. Patient and family education can reinforce the therapeutic interventions of the primary care provider and provide emotional support.

Prevention

Primary prevention

The primary means of preventing dust-related illnesses is to limit the exposure of all workers through the use of engineering controls.[28] These include dilution ventilation and dust suppression. The MSHA prescribes minimum ventilation requirements for face operations, primarily to control the emission of methane from freshly fractured coal. The fresh air also reduces the dust concentration through mixing with the dust-laden air exhausting out of the return air tunnels. Dust suppression usually involves a system of water sprays near the cutting head of continuous mining machines or longwall shears. Dust exposures can also be reduced on an individual basis through the use of approved particulate air-purifying respirators. Respirator usage is usually voluntary and is not considered by MSHA to be an acceptable means for the operator to reduce exposures to respirable dust. However, many miners choose to wear respirators, particularly during the dust-producing mining operations. There is some evidence that use of respirators is associated with preservation of lung function.

Exposure limits in the US for coal mine dust are enforced by MSHA. Mine operators must take periodic dust samples during normal working conditions and send them to MSHA for weighing and analysis. The integrity of this program has been brought into question after MSHA's allegations of widespread tampering with dust sampling. The mandatory operator sampling program is supplemented by periodic inspections by MSHA personnel. Recent information suggests that the current dust exposure limit might not be fully protective, and NIOSH has recommended a lowering of the dust limit along with changes in the program of inspection and enforcement.[29]

Secondary prevention

Medical surveillance, directed toward the early identification of CWP through periodic radiographic examinations, is available for all underground coal miners in the US through the Coal Workers' X-ray Surveillance Program administered by NIOSH. Miners with CWP may exercise a right to work in a reduced dust environment of 1 mg/m^3 and have their exposures sampled more frequently. There is currently no screening or surveillance program directed toward the prevention of airways obstruction, which can cause significant morbidity among miners. Primary healthcare providers should consider performing periodic spirometry using techniques and equipment meeting the American Thoracic Society recommendations as a guide to care and education of patients exposed to coal mine dust. A drop of 15 percentage points or more from baseline 'percent predicted' values of FEV$_1$ should suggest the need for more intensive investigation and additional preventive interventions.

In the years following adoption of the current coal mine dust exposure regulations, an average of over 2000 former miners have continued to die each year in the US with CWP as an underlying or contributing cause of death. Thousands of others suffer from significant airways disease caused, at least in part, by their coal mine dust exposure. There must be continued attention to early disease identification and preventive intervention in order to supplement dust control efforts and prevent the continuing progression of these diseases.

MAN-MADE MINERAL FIBERS
Exposure settings

Man-made mineral fibers (MMMF), also called synthetic or man-made vitreous fibers, include a variety of manufactured materials with excellent insulating properties. Not true minerals, they are amorphous silicates manufactured into a fibrous form. MMMF are grouped according to their origin into glass fiber (from glass), ceramic fiber (from kaolin clay), and mineral wool (from rock or slag). Increasingly used as asbestos substitutes, they have thousands of applications in industrial and non-industrial settings. They are used for thermal and acoustic insulation and plastic reinforcement in everything from buildings, ships, and automobiles, to home appliances, industrial kilns, and furnaces.

Managers and administrators
Civil engineers
Mechanical engineers
Chemists (except biochemists)
Electrical and electronic technicians
Chemical and science technicians
Production coordinators
Warehouse clerks (receiving, recording, and issuing)
Janitors and cleaners
Supervisors (mechanics and repairers)
Engine mechanics (aircraft, bus, truck, and stationary)
Heavy equipment mechanics
Industrial machinery repairers
Mechanics (heating, air conditioning, and refrigeration)
Brick masons and stonemasons
Tile setters
Carpenters
Drywall installers
Painters (construction and maintenance)
Plasterers
Plumbers (pipe fitters and steam fitters)
Insulation workers
Roofers
Sheet metal duct installers
Structural metal workers
Boilermakers
Sheet metal workers
Plant and system operators
Machine operators (grinding, abrading, buffing/polishing)
Machine operators (metal, plastic, stone, and glass working)
Packing and filling machine operators
Slicing and cutting machine operators
Crushing and grinding operators
Oven operators (furnace and kiln)
Assemblers
Production manager (inspectors, checkers, and examiners)
Production testers, samplers, weighers, and helpers
Truck drivers (heavy and light)
Crane and tower operators
Industrial truck and tractor equipment operators
Material moving equipment operators
Construction laborers
Stock handlers and baggers
Vehicle washers and equipment cleaners
Hand packers and packagers

Table 46.4 Workers potentially exposed to man-made fibers

Exposure to MMMF occurs during production, fabrication, and application of materials. Over 500,000 US workers are potentially exposed to MMMF (Table 46.4), and that number is likely to increase.

Environmental measurement

The sampling protocol for MMMF is virtually identical to that for asbestos. The sample is collected on a filter for microscopic examination. The current literature indicates that in addition to biopersistence and durability, health effects relate to the length and diameter of the fibers; therefore, some size selectivity must be employed in either the sampling or analysis. The technique for asbestos sampling, as described earlier in this chapter, is the most common measurement technique.

Clinical effects

The health effects of MMMF are discussed in greater detail in Chapters 19.11 and 30.2.

Acute effects

Acute respiratory and skin irritation occur frequently among workers newly exposed to mineral fibers. Irritation has been reported most often in glass wool workers, but it can result from contact with other fibers. Although usually self-limited, these problems may cause workers to leave employment.

Chronic effects

Some studies have shown excess lung cancer risk in glass fiber and mineral wool production workers. Synthetic fibers vary widely in their physicochemical characteristics, and carcinogenic potential most likely relates to the biopersistence and solubility of inhaled fibers, with the most persistent and durable fibers – those most like asbestos – posing the greatest risk. IARC has recently reviewed the relevant scientific literature and concluded that the more biopersistent materials such as refractory ceramic fibers and some special-purpose glass wools are possible human carcinogens (IARC Group 2B). IARC has reclassified the more commonly used vitreous fiber glass wool and slag wool as not classifiable as to their carcinogenicity (IARC Group 3).[30] The US National Toxicology Program classifies ceramic fibers of respirable size as reasonably anticipated to be a human carcinogen.[31]

Epidemiologic investigations have suggested that exposure to mineral fibers may be associated with the development of low profusions of chest X-ray opacities consistent with a diagnosis of pneumoconiosis in some workers. In addition, refractory ceramic fiber production workers have been found to develop pleural plaques and pleural thickening which increases with increased latency.[32] These asbestos-like effects suggest the possibility that other asbestos-like health effects, particularly lung cancer, could result from refractory ceramic fibers. Mineral fiber exposure may also increase the risk of chronic bronchitis.

Clinical evaluation and management

When workers newly exposed to MMMF complain of intense pruritus with a minimum of visible dermatologic changes, the etiology is readily apparent. At times, fibers can be seen microscopically after cellophane tape is pressed against exposed skin. Workers presenting with skin irritation from mineral fiber exposure should be encouraged to minimize exposure through use of appropriate protective equipment and should be reassured that the acutely troublesome symptoms are generally self-limited. Anti-pruritic medications may be of benefit to some.

The approach to evaluation for chronic conditions associated with mineral fiber exposure is similar to the assessment of these conditions where there is no occupational exposure. A careful medical history, including a history of occupational and environmental exposures, forms the basis for care. Chest imaging to exclude other acute or reversible disease processes is indicated. Spirometry and possibly other measures of pulmonary function provide diagnostic and prognostic information.

There are no specific interventions uniquely beneficial for individuals with cancers that may be associated with mineral fiber exposure. Chronic bronchitis and airways obstruction should be approached in the usual fashion. Management should include reduction or elimination of adverse pulmonary exposures, including workplace dusts and tobacco smoke. Symptomatic treatment, reversal of reversible or intermittent airways obstruction, and infection control are also important. In the case of moderate-to-severe disease, referral to patient and family support and education programs may be helpful.

Disease prevention

Primary prevention

Given the classification of MMMF as potential human carcinogens by IARC, mineral fiber exposure should be limited to the extent feasible by technology. This can be done by several standard techniques. Where possible, substitutes should be used in place of the MMMF. This is often difficult since these products were, in many cases, replacements for asbestos. Lacking alternative materials, engineering controls to contain the source of exposure become the next best approach. When the process cannot be fully controlled, the worker must be isolated from the process generating the dust. Finally, the worker may be isolated by use of respiratory protection equipment. For uncontrolled exposures to RCF, as with asbestos, the appropriate type of respirator could be an air purifying or self-contained breathing apparatus (SCBA) with a full face-piece, operated in a pressure demand or other positive pressure mode. Respirators should be used with a complete respiratory protection plan. Administrative controls can also be used to reduce exposures by limiting the amount of time a worker spends in a contaminated environment. Administrative controls need to be coupled with personal samplers on the workers to closely monitor exposures and assure the maximum level of exposure is not surpassed.

Secondary prevention

There is no consensus approach to screening or surveillance of MMMF-exposed workers. However, in light of concern about asbestos-like effects, it would be prudent to closely monitor these workers for pulmonary health effects. The level of health risk from MMMF exposure most likely varies depending on the intensity and duration of exposure as well as with the specific physical and chemical characteristics of the fiber. Until the specific risks are better defined, a generic approach to surveillance of 'fiber-exposed' workers is reasonable. Baseline and periodic respiratory symptom questionnaires, spirometry, and chest radiographs should be offered. Since the diseases of concern have long latency, the frequency of observation should increase in each decade following first exposure. Careful collection and retention of exposure data should make future screening more productive as new knowledge from ongoing systematic observation of occupational cohorts becomes available.

References

1. Virta RL. Asbestos: geology, mineralogy, mining, and uses. US Department of Interior, US Geological Survey, Open-File Report 02-149 Version 1.0, URL: pubs.usgs.gov/of/2002/of02-149/index.html.
2. Virta RL. Worldwide asbestos supply and consumption trends from 1900 to 2000. US Department of Interior, US Geological Survey, Open-File Report 03-83, URL: pubs.usgs.gov/of/2003/of03-083/of03-083.pdf.
3. Mlynarski KW. US Geological Survey Minerals Yearbook. Washington, DC: Government Printing Office; 1998.
4. Environmental Protection Agency (EPA). EPA's asbestos and vermiculite home page. www.epa.gov/opptintr/asbestos/index.html. Accessed July 14, 2003.
5. Occupational Safety and Health Administration (OSHA). Preamble to final Rule: Occupational Exposure to Asbestos, Section 4-IV. Final regulatory impact and regulatory Flexibility Analysis. Federal Register 59: 40964-41162. Washington, DC: Government Printing Office; 1994.
6. McCrone WC. Asbestos identification. Chicago: The McCrone Research Institute; 1987.
7. Cassinelli ME, O'Connor PF, eds. NIOSH manual of analytical methods (NMAM), 4th edn. Methods nos. 7400, 7402, 9000, and 9002. Washington, DC: Government Printing Office; DHHS (NIOSH) Publication No. 94-113; 1994.
8. Kipen HM, Lilis R, Suzuki Y, et al. Pulmonary fibrosis in asbestos insulation workers with lung cancer: a radiological and histopathological evaluation. Br J Ind Med 1987; 44:96-100.
9. Oliver LC, Eisen EA, Green R, Sprince NL. Asbestos-related pleural plaques and lung function. Am J Ind Med 1988; 14:649-56.
10. Brodkin CA, Barnhart S, Checkoway H, Balmes J, Omenn GS, Rosenstock L. Longitudinal pattern of reported symptoms and accelerated ventilatory loss in asbestos-exposed workers. Chest 1996; 109:120-6.
11. Miller A, Lilis R, Godbold J, Chan E, Selikoff IJ. Relationship of pulmonary function to radiographic interstitial fibrosis in 2,611 long-term asbestos insulators. An assessment of the International Labour Office profusion score. Am Rev Respir Dis 1992; 145:263-70.
12. Wilkinson P, Hansell DM, Janssens J, et al. Is lung cancer associated with asbestos exposure when there are no small opacities on the chest radiograph? Lancet 1995; 345:1074-8.
13. Wagner GR. Screening and surveillance of workers exposed to mineral dusts. Geneva: World Health Organization; 1996.
14. Henschke CI, McCauley DI, Yankelevitz DF, et al. Early Lung Cancer Action Project: overall design and findings from baseline screening. Lancet 1999; 354:99-105.
15. Anonymous. Asbestos, asbestosis, and cancer: the Helsinki criteria for diagnosis and attribution. Scand J Work Environ Health 1997; 23:311-16.
16. US Department of Labor (DOL). Title 29 Code of Federal Regulations, Part 1910.1001. Occupational Safety and Health Administration, Asbestos Standard for General Industry, June 20, 1986 (as amended 1988, 1989, 1990, 1992, 1994, 1995, 1996, and 1998).
17. National Institute for Occupational Safety and Health (NIOSH). NIOSH hazard review: health effects of occupational exposure to respirable crystalline silica. Washington, DC: Government Printing Office; DHHS (NIOSH) Publication No. 2002-129; 2002.
18. IARC Working Group on the Evaluation of Carcinogenic Risks to Humans. Silica, some silicates, coal dust and para-aramid fibrils. Lyon, 15-22 October 1996. IARC Monogr Eval Carcinog Risks Hum 1997; 68:41-242.
19. Linch KD, Miller WE, Althouse RB, Groce DW, Hale JM. Surveillance of respirable crystalline silica dust using OSHA compliance data (1979-1995). Am J Ind Med 1998; 34:547-58.
20. Cassinelli ME, O'Connor PF, eds. NIOSH manual of analytical methods (NMAM), 4th edn. Methods nos. 7500, 7501, 7602,

and 7603. Washington, DC: Government Printing Office; DHHS (NIOSH) Publication No. 94-113; 1994.

21. American Thoracic Society. Adverse effects of crystalline silica exposure. Am J Respir Crit Care Med 1997; 155:761-5.

22. US Department of Labor, Occupational Safety and Health Administration. Title 29 Code of Federal Regulations, Part 1910.1000, Table Z-3. Mineral Dusts. Published at 39 FR 23502, June 27, 1974.

23. National Institute for Occupational Safety and Health (NIOSH). Criteria for a recommended standard. Occupational exposure to crystalline silica. Washington, DC: Government Printing Office; DHEW Publication No. (NIOSH) 75-120; 1974.

24. American Conference of Governmental Industrial Hygienists (ACGIH). 2003 TLVs® and BEIs®: based on the documentation of the threshold limit values for chemical substances and physical agents & biologic exposure Indices. Cincinnati: ACGIH Worldwide; 2003.

25. Federal Mine Safety & Health Act of 1977, Public Law 91-173, as amended by Public Law 95-164, Section 101.

26. Wagner GR, Attfield MD, Parker JE. Chest radiography in dust-exposed miners: promise and problems, potential and imperfections. Occup Med 1993; 8:127-41.

27. Marine WM, Gurr D, Jacobsen M. Clinically important respiratory effects of dust exposure and smoking in British coal miners. Am Rev Respir Dis 1988; 137:106-12.

28. Kissell FN. Handbook for dust control in mining. Washington, DC: Government Printing Office; DHHS (NIOSH) Publication No. 2003-147; 2003.

29. National Institute for Occupational Safety and Health (NIOSH). Criteria for a recommended standard. Occupational exposure to respirable coal mine dust. Washington, DC: Government Printing Office; DHHS (NIOSH) Publication No. 95-106; 1995.

30. International Agency for Research on Cancer. Man-made mineral fibres and radon. IARC Monogr Eval Carcinog Risks Hum 1988; 43.

31. National Toxicology Program on Carcinogens, tenth edition: carcinogen profiles 2002. Research Triangle Park, NC: NIEHS; 2002: III-46-47.

32. Lockey J, Lemasters G, Rice C, et al. Refractory ceramic fiber exposure and pleural plaques. Am J Respir Crit Care Med 1996; 154:1405-10.

Chapter 47
Toxic Gases

Akshay Sood

GENERAL CONSIDERATIONS

Specific toxic gases are discussed here. The clinical effects and management of acute-inhalation injury are discussed further in Chapter 19.5, and the effects of outdoor air pollutants in Chapter 51.

The circumstances of exposure to toxic gases and knowledge of their properties are useful in estimating the dose of exposure and anticipating the severity of injury.[1] Gases with potent odors or sensory irritant properties (e.g., hydrogen sulfide or sulfur dioxide) will motivate the exposed individual to flee the area, thus limiting the duration of exposure; whereas exposure to gases without these properties (e.g., carbon monoxide or phosgene) may be more prolonged and, thus, more deadly.

Any gas may act as an asphyxiant by physically displacing oxygen from the inhaled ambient air and subsequently lowering the alveolar oxygen tension. Some gases, such as carbon monoxide, cyanide, and hydrogen sulfide, may act as chemical asphyxiants by interfering with the oxygen transport system. Irritant gases, on the other hand, may directly injure the respiratory system, which may compromise the gas-exchanging function of the lung.

The dose of an inorganic gas delivered to the respiratory system is determined by several factors outlined in Table 47.1. The most important physicochemical determinant of the dose delivered is the solubility of the gas in water.[2] Because the respiratory system is lined with mucus in a watery solution, a more soluble gas (for example sulfur dioxide, ammonia and acid mists) will be predominantly taken up by the mucous lining of the nose and upper airway; and the smaller airways and alveoli are relatively spared. This is more likely to result in upper airway irritation and asthma-like symptomatology. However, under conditions of high concentrations of exposure, even highly soluble gases will penetrate the alveoli to cause acute alveolar lung injury. On the other hand, less soluble gases (for example, oxides of nitrogen, ozone, phosgene) are more likely to penetrate to these more distal airways even in conditions of exposure at relatively lower concentrations, and are thus more likely to produce a clinical picture of bronchiolitis or acute alveolar injury (see Chapter 19.5). Chlorine and hydrogen sulfide have intermediate solubility and can produce a full spectrum of pulmonary irritant effects involving both upper and lower airways. The solubility of a gas in the liquid lining of the respiratory system is described by Henry's law, and quantified by the Henry's law coefficient of the gas. US Standards for selected irritant and asphyxiant gases are listed in Table 47.2.

CARBON MONOXIDE

Carbon monoxide is a colorless, odorless, and non-irritant gas and is believed to be one of the most frequent causes of acute fatal poisoning in the United States, with an estimated 40,000 emergency department visits annually.[3] Normal non-smoking adults will have approximately 0.5% saturation with carboxyhemoglobin in the absence of any environmental exposure, and American adults commonly have about 1% carboxyhemoglobinemia with typical environmental exposures.

Exposure setting

Carbon monoxide is a product of the incomplete combustion of hydrocarbons. Tobacco smoke is the most important source. The concentration of carbon monoxide in mainstream cigarette smoke, though variable, averages approximately 400 ppm (0.04%), or eight times the current Occupational Safety and Health Administration (OSHA) permissible exposure limit (PEL). Among regular cigarette smokers, carboxyhemoglobin levels usually range from 3% to 8%, with levels up to and higher than 15% occurring in some very heavy smokers.

After cigarette smoke, the most common source of exposure to carbon monoxide is faulty or inadequately ventilated combustion sources. Automobile engine exhaust is the most important source of such exposure for American non-smokers and also accounts for the majority of deaths from carbon monoxide poisoning in the United States. Lethal concentrations of carboxyhemoglobin can be achieved within 10 minutes in the confines of a closed garage. Carbon monoxide toxicity can also occur in semi-enclosed spaces, working or living quarters adjacent to garages, and structural fires.

Improperly functioning or poorly ventilated home combustion appliances (such as gas clothes dryers with kinked exhaust hoses, heating furnaces, stoves, and ovens with continuously burning pilot lights) may produce carbon monoxide air concentrations exceeding 100 ppm, which may lead to levels of carboxyhemoglobin in the blood of 10% after 8 hours of exposure. An often overlooked source of carbon monoxide is methylene chloride, a common component of solvents like paint removers and furniture strippers. Once absorbed, methylene chloride is metabolized in the liver to carbon monoxide.

Environmental measurement

Colorimetric devices are available that can estimate individual exposure over a prolonged period. Instantaneous point

Physical and chemical characteristics of the gas
Inhaled concentration of gas
Duration of exposure
Minute ventilation (tidal volume × respiratory rate)
Physical and chemical characteristics of the gas

Table 47.1 Factors affecting the dose of an inorganic gas delivered to the respiratory system

air measurements may also be made with real-time instruments. When investigating homes for sources of carbon monoxide, indoor measurements of carbon dioxide as an indicator of unventilated combustion products are commonly used.

Biologic monitoring

Coburn and Forster developed a dose–response relationship model, between the partial pressure of carbon monoxide inhaled and the percent of carboxyhemoglobin saturation in blood. At normal body temperature and pH, carbon monoxide has approximately 220 times the affinity for hemoglobin as oxygen. Thus, when the partial pressure of carbon monoxide is 1/220th that of oxygen (or 0.1% carbon monoxide in air or approximately 1000 ppm),

blood at equilibrium will be 50% saturated by carbon monoxide and 50% saturated with oxygen. At low concentrations under conditions of rest, the percent of carboxyhemoglobin rises gradually over a period of hours to a plateau or steady state.[4,5] For concentrations of inhaled carbon monoxide greater than 100 ppm, the percent of carboxyhemoglobin can be related to the inhaled carbon monoxide concentration, the duration of exposure, and minute ventilation by the following equation:

$$\%COHb = [CO]_{air} \times KT$$

where COHb is carboxyhemoglobin, [CO] is the air concentration of carbon monoxide in parts per million, K is a constant that varies with minute ventilation, and T is the time in hours.

In a patient who presents with carbon monoxide poisoning of unknown concentration and duration who has been removed from exposure for a known period of time, it is possible to estimate the exposure concentration or earlier peak carboxyhemoglobin levels using the known carboxyhemoglobin levels and the duration since exposure. The time for the half reduction of blood carboxyhemoglobin levels is 320 minutes while breathing room air.

Substance	Type of standard	Level
Carbon monoxide	OSHA Permissible exposure limit: 8 hr TWA	50 ppm
	NIOSH Recommended exposure limit: 10 hr TWA	35 ppm
	NIOSH Recommended exposure limit: Ceiling Value	200 ppm
	NIOSH Immediately dangerous to life and health level	1200 ppm
Sulfur dioxide	OSHA Permissible exposure limit: 8 hr TWA	5 ppm
	NIOSH Recommended exposure limit: 10 hr TWA	2 ppm
	NIOSH 15 min. Short term exposure limit	5 ppm
	NIOSH Immediately dangerous to life and health level	100 ppm
Chlorine	OSHA Permissible exposure limit: ceiling value	1 ppm
	NIOSH Recommended exposure limit: 15 min ceiling value	0.5 ppm
	NIOSH Immediately dangerous to life and health level	10 ppm
Nitrogen dioxide	OSHA Permissible exposure limit: ceiling value	5 ppm
	NIOSH 15 min. Short term exposure limit	1 ppm
	NIOSH Immediately dangerous to life and health level	20 ppm
Cyanide	OSHA Permissible exposure limit: 8 hr TWA	10 ppm
	NIOSH 15 min. Short term exposure limit	4.7 ppm
	NIOSH Immediately dangerous to life and health level	50 ppm
Hydrogen sulfide	OSHA Permissible exposure limit: ceiling concentration	20 ppm
	OSHA Permissible exposure limit: acceptable maximum peak above ceiling concentration for an 8 hr shift[*]	50 ppm
	NIOSH Recommended Exposure limit: 10 min ceiling value	10 ppm
	NIOSH Immediately dangerous to life and health level	100 ppm
Ozone	OSHA Permissible exposure limit: 8 hr TWA	0.1 ppm
	NIOSH Recommended exposure limit: ceiling value	0.1 ppm
	NIOSH Immediately dangerous to life and health level	5 ppm
Phosgene	OSHA Permissible exposure limit: 8 hr TWA	0.1 ppm
	NIOSH Recommended exposure limit: 10 hr TWA	0.1 ppm
	NIOSH Recommended exposure limit: 15 min ceiling value	0.2 ppm
Ammonia	OSHA Permissible exposure limit: 8 hr TWA	50 ppm
	NIOSH Recommended exposure limit: 10 hr TWA	25 ppm
	NIOSH 15 min. Short term exposure limit:	35 ppm
	NIOSH Immediately dangerous to life and health level	300 ppm

*Acceptable maximum peak above ceiling concentration for an 8-hour shift, maximum duration 10 minutes, once, only if no other measured exposure occurs
OSHA: Occupational Safety and Health Administration
NIOSH: National Institute for Occupational Safety and Health. These standards are recommended, not legally mandated.
TWA: Time weighted average
ppm: parts per million

Table 47.2 United States occupational safety standards for selected irritant gases

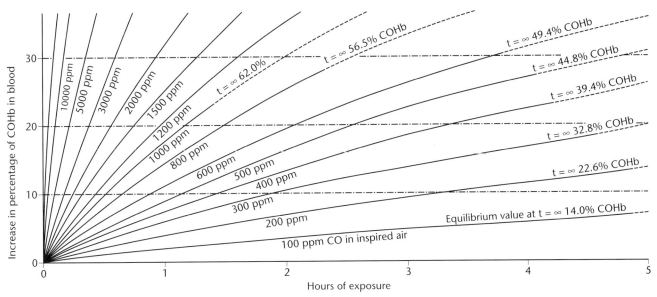

Figure 47.1: Increase in the percent of carboxyhemoglobin in the blood of resting subjects exposed by inhalation in relation to the concentration of carbon monoxide in the air and hours of exposure. Increasing the level of physical activity will increase the percent change in carboxyhemoglobin levels for a given air concentration and duration. (Adapted from Forbes W, Sargent F, Roughton F. The rate of carbon monoxide uptake by normal men. Am J Physiol 1945; 143:594–608.[5])

Therefore, for example, a patient brought to the emergency room with a carboxyhemoglobin level of 20%, 2 hours after rescue from a building in which the patient was found unconscious, may have had a peak carboxyhemoglobin level of about 25% (assuming that the interval elapsed is 0.375 half times of dissociation and that the current carboxyhemoglobin level is about 81% of the level 2 hours ago). A patient with a 50% carboxyhemoglobin level immediately on cessation of exposure has come into equilibrium with an inhaled carbon monoxide concentration of 0.1% in air or may have been exposed to an even higher concentration for a short duration, insufficient to reach steady-state equilibrium. The relationship among air concentration of carbon monoxide, hours of exposure, and the increase in the percent of carboxyhemoglobin is shown in Figure 47.1.

Pathophysiology

The major effect of carbon monoxide is to reduce the oxygen-carrying capacity of hemoglobin in the blood; hemoglobin bound to carbon monoxide is unavailable for binding with oxygen. In addition, carbon monoxide alters the relationship between arterial oxygen tension and hemoglobin saturation, making hemoglobin more avid for oxygen (a left shift of the oxygen–hemoglobin saturation curve) and making less oxygen available for release from hemoglobin in the vascular periphery (Fig. 47.2). The result is that the amount of available oxygen for tissues with a 60% carboxyhemoglobin level is substantially less than with a 60% loss of hemoglobin in cases of severe anemia. Other heme-containing enzyme systems like cytochrome a_3 may also be poisoned by carbon monoxide. These alterations result in cellular hypoxia.

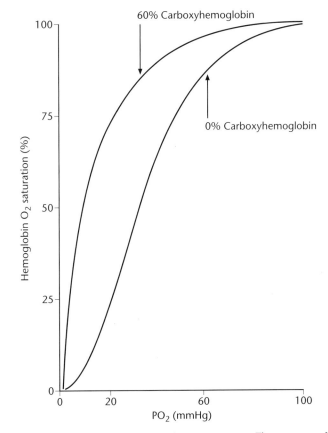

Figure 47.2: Oxygen–hemoglobin dissociation curve. The presence of carboxyhemoglobin shifts the curve to the left and changes it to a more hyperbolic shape. This results in a decrease in the oxygen-carrying capacity and impaired release of oxygen at the tissue level. (From: Ernst A, Zibrak JZ. Carbon monoxide poisoning. N Engl J Med 1998; 339: 1603–8.© 1998 Massachusetts Medical Society. All rights reserved.[9])

Recent investigations suggest other mechanisms of carbon monoxide-mediated toxicity. These include reoxygenation injury to the central nervous system by oxygen radicals[6] and lipid peroxygenation resulting in demyelination of lipids in the central nervous system.[7] These mechanisms are believed to be responsible for the delayed neuropsychiatric sequelae described with carbon monoxide. The toxic effects of carbon monoxide are manifest earlier in those with diseases or circumstances associated with limited or impaired oxygen delivery such as hemoglobin abnormalities (including anemia), high altitude, heavy cigarette smoking, critical degree of vascular stenosis, and heart and lung disease. Carbon monoxide exposure has an especially deleterious effect on the fetus in pregnant women.[8]

Acute clinical effects

The clinical symptoms of carbon monoxide poisoning are non-specific and often mistaken for a viral illness. These symptoms include headache, weakness, nausea, and dizziness.[4,9] Subtle alterations in visual perception and other central nervous system functions can be detected at carboxyhemoglobin levels above 5%. As the percent of carboxyhemoglobin in the blood rises, aortic and carotid oxygen chemoreceptors, which respond primarily to PaO_2 and not to oxygen saturation, will not increase the rate of firing, and hypoxia-driven hyperventilation and the accompanying symptom of dyspnea may not occur. Above 5% carboxyhemoglobinemia, a compensatory vasodilation to supply more blood to hypoxic tissues may occur with a resultant increase in cardiac output. If the ability to increase cardiac output in relation to vasodilation is exceeded, syncope may occur. Hyperventilation will finally occur when lactic acidosis develops. When the tissue hypoxia becomes more severe, seizures, coma, cardiac arrhythmias, myocardial infarction, or sudden death may supervene.[10]

The classic findings of cherry-red lips, cyanosis and retinal hemorrhages occur rarely.[11] Erythematous lesions with bullae over bony prominences have been described but are non-specific for carbon monoxide poisoning.[9] Necrosis of sweat glands is a characteristic histologic feature.

It is important to recognize that carboxyhemoglobin levels often do not correspond well to severity of symptoms, and the duration of exposure is an important factor mediating toxicity.[9] Further, the oxygen tension in plasma (measured as the PaO_2 on blood gas measurements) may be unaffected in carbon monoxide toxicity. Pulse oximetry cannot distinguish between oxyhemoglobin and carboxyhemoglobin at the commonly employed wavelengths and may therefore give a falsely normal reading of oxygen saturation. The percent of carboxyhemoglobin can be measured by co-oximetry (available on most blood gas machines used in hospitals).

Delayed effects

Of patients surviving acute carbon monoxide poisoning, 10–30% may have delayed neuropsychiatric sequelae that appear only after an interval (2–40 days) after an apparent complete recovery from the initial intoxication.[12] These include symptoms of mental deterioration, mood disorders, unusual behavior, irrational speech content, gait and other movement disturbances, parkinsonian deficits, and other focal neurologic signs. Abnormalities were seen on computed tomographic brain scans in about 50% in one series, commonly involving the globus pallidus. With prolonged follow-up, many but not all of the patients had complete resolution of these delayed sequelae.[12]

Chronic effects

Relatively little is known about chronic adaptation to low levels of carbon monoxide, other than that some heavy cigarette smokers have a secondary erythrocytosis, at least in part as a result of chronically elevated carboxyhemoglobin levels. In carefully controlled chamber-exposure studies, patients with ischemic heart disease experienced a decrease in time to the onset of angina during exercise following carbon monoxide exposure. However, the available evidence fails to support a causal relationship between exposure to carbon monoxide and atherosclerosis.[13] Current evidence on an arrhythmogenic effect is inconclusive.

Clinical evaluation strategy

A high index of clinical suspicion is essential for making the diagnosis of carbon monoxide toxicity. Measurement of blood carboxyhemoglobin levels is mandatory but alone may be insufficient to rule out the diagnosis. Since serum levels of carboxyhemoglobin may have already fallen by the time the patient reaches the emergency room, measurements of carbon monoxide levels in the exhaled air of patients, or measurement of carbon monoxide levels in the ambient air, or measurement of carboxyhemoglobin levels in the blood drawn at the scene of the event by the fire department or the paramedics may be helpful in confirming the diagnosis. Application of the half-time of dissociation of carbon monoxide can be used to extrapolate back to the carboxyhemoglobin levels that may have been present before the patient's arrival at the hospital.

Attention to clinical indicators, particularly a detailed neurologic examination and neuropsychologic testing, is important. Patients with current known overexposure, as indicated by carboxyhemoglobin levels of 25% or more, or a consistent clinical picture should be observed closely for rapidly evolving or delayed sequelae.

Management

The carbon monoxide-intoxicated patient should be first removed from the source of exposure. In addition to close monitoring and general supportive measures, increasing the arterial oxygen tension by administering 100% oxygen will improve tissue oxygenation, while increasing the rate of excretion of hemoglobin-bound carbon monoxide. The time for the half reduction of blood carboxyhemoglobin levels is 320 minutes breathing room air at 1 atmosphere, 80 minutes for 100% oxygen at 1 atmosphere, and 23 minutes using hyperbaric oxygen at 3 atmospheres. Increase in mechanical ventilation can also increase the

Coma
Any period of unconsciousness
Any abnormal score on the Carbon Monoxide
Neuropsychologic Screening Battery
Carboxyhemoglobin level > 40%
Pregnancy and carboxyhemoglobin level > 15% or evidence of
fetal distress
Signs of cardiac ischemia and arrhythmia
History of ischemic heart disease and carboxyhemoglobin
level ≥ 20%
Recurrent symptoms for up to 3 weeks after the original
treatment
Symptoms that do not resolve with normobaric oxygen after
4–6 hours

Data from Meyers RAM, Thom SR. Carbon monoxide and cyanide
poisoning. In: Kindwall EP, ed. Hyperbaric medicine practice. Flagstaff,
Arizona: Best Publishing, 1994, 357.[16]

Table 47.3 Suggested indications for hyperbaric oxygen therapy in patients with carbon monoxide poisoning.

excretion rate of carbon monoxide. Isocapnic hyperpnea in mechanically ventilated patients by providing very high minute ventilation while adding carbon dioxide to the respiratory circuit has been described to accelerate the elimination of carbon monoxide.[14]

The delivery of 100% oxygen at pressures greater than atmospheric in a high-pressure chamber (hyperbaric oxygen therapy) hastens the resolution of symptoms. However, it is unclear whether hyperbaric oxygen therapy influences the late sequelae and mortality.[15] The commonly suggested indications for hyperbaric oxygen therapy are summarized in Table 47.3.[16] Other than coma, there is disagreement about the absolute indications for instituting this therapy. Hyperbaric oxygen may carry the potential risk for central nervous system oxygen toxicity. In most cases, the therapy is unavailable within the critical first few hours after recognition of carbon monoxide poisoning.

Prevention
Most cases can be prevented by routine attention to proper function and ventilation of combustion sources. Heating oil or gas companies will often perform safety inspections and environmental measurements when a faulty furnace is suspected. Catalytic converters reduce the carbon monoxide content of car exhaust fumes. In evaluating indoor sources of combustion, measurements of carbon monoxide itself (or sometimes carbon dioxide as an index of unvented combustion products) are made during operation of the combustion source with maximal draft applied to the indoor area of interest. Electronic carbon monoxide alarms, designed like residential smoke detectors, are being increasingly used in residential and commercial buildings.

SULFUR DIOXIDE

Exposure settings
Sulfur dioxide gas is generated by the combustion of fossil fuels, as occurs in coal- and oil-fired power plants and in industrial processes such as petroleum refining, and smelt-ing of metal ores. It is also used as a bleaching agent in the textile, paper pulp, wool and fresh produce industries and as a fumigant for grain. Exposure at lower concentration occurs as an ambient outdoor air pollutant (see Chapter 51).

Environmental measurement
Commercially available sampling devices can continuously measure the ambient sulfur dioxide concentrations with a rapid response time to change in concentration. These devices provide early warning of rising levels of sulfur dioxide. They are therefore very useful in environmental air-monitoring stations and can also be adapted to industrial settings. Current occupational safety standards in the US are listed in Table 47.2.

Acute clinical effects
Being both soluble and a potent mucous membrane irritant, sulfur dioxide predominantly causes immediate symptoms of eye, nasal and upper airway irritation. Those acutely exposed to this irritant gas seek immediate escape. Those chronically exposed may develop sensory tolerance to its irritant properties and may be less aware of its presence.

Studies have shown impaired small airways mucosal clearance after exposure to aerosolized sulfuric acid. Asthmatic patients are more sensitive to the broncho-constricting action of sulfur dioxide. Cases of single, acute, high-level exposures followed by development of reactive airways dysfunction (RADS) have been reported (see Chapter 19.2). Severe inhalation cases are often complicated by acute lung injury and secondary bacterial pneumonia.

Chronic clinical effects.
After adjustment for levels of particulate matter less than 10 microns in aerodynamic diameter (PM_{10}) and ozone, there is little evidence that ambient environmental sulfur dioxide levels have a significant effect on mortality.[17-20] SO_2 levels may be associated with the frequency of respiratory symptoms,[21] though the association is stronger with particulate exposure.[22]

Clinical evaluation strategy
In the acutely exposed and symptomatic worker, management should be directed to detect and treat acute bronchospasm. Acute parenchymal lung injury is infrequent and occurs with heavy exposure. Lung examination, spirometry and pulse oximetry may be more useful than chest X-ray studies in detecting the airway abnormalities. Patients who appear stable after acute exposure should undergo follow-up evaluations of symptoms and pulmonary function testing.

Management
Treatment of inhalation injury due to sulfur dioxide is supportive. Early institution of bronchodilators with or without steroids is recommended, further discussed in Chapter 19.5.

Prevention

The education of those at risk in appropriate evacuation measures when a leak of sulfur dioxide is detected by odor may reduce subsequent higher-dose exposures. Continuous air monitoring in high-risk areas is available, using commercially available devices. Containment vessels of the gas should be properly stored, in well-ventilated areas, away from workers.

CHLORINE

Exposure settings

Molecular chlorine is a yellowish green gas used widely in many industrial processes such as making paper. Many occupational groups have a potential for exposure to chlorine in manufacture, transport, and utilization processes. The generation of chlorine gas by the inadvertent mixing of bleach (sodium hypochlorite) and phosphoric acid containing cleaning powders used for janitorial cleaning tasks has become a frequent cause of domestic and industrial exposure to chlorine.[23] Common settings for chlorine exposure include transportation or industrial accidents or spills, and accidents at swimming pools and sewage treatment facilities. Chlorine and phosgene gases were also used during World War I as chemical weapons.

Environmental measurement

Determination of exposure to airborne chlorine is made using a glass bubbler containing sulfamic acid, followed by analysis using an ion-specific electrode. Another method for determining exposure to airborne chlorine involves analysis using ion-chromatography. The current occupational safety standards in the US are listed in Table 47.2.

Acute clinical effects

Chlorine has strong odor, and sensory irritant properties. Slight irritation can be noted at 1–3 ppm, and easily noticeable irritation becomes evident with even brief exposure to 3–6 ppm. Chlorine inhalation may manifest any of the full spectrum of pulmonary irritant effects, from minor mucosal responses of the eyes, nose, throat, upper airway, nausea and vomiting to acute chemical tracheobronchitis, bronchospasm and non-cardiogenic pulmonary edema (see Chapter 19.5).[24,25]

Chronic clinical effects

Some survivors of short-term, uncontrolled, high-level chlorine exposures may develop RADS. Studies on residual effects of acute chlorine exposure on pulp mill workers also demonstrate a greater prevalence of respiratory symptoms and airflow obstruction.[26] However, data on the effect of chronic low-level chlorine exposures are inconclusive.[25,27,28]

Clinical evaluation strategy

Recently exposed patients should be observed for progressive airway and lung injury. Initial indicators of the severity of response include spirometry, arterial blood gas levels, and chest roentgenographic studies.

Management

Treatment is primarily supportive and can include use of antitussive agents, aerosolized bronchodilators, oxygen, maintenance of a patent airway, and (if necessary) intubation with positive pressure ventilation. The role of inhaled sodium bicarbonate and systemic corticosteroids remains unproven.

Prevention

Where chlorine gas is manufactured, transported, or used, good industrial hygiene practices and worker education regarding handling chlorine gas should prevent most acute high-level exposures. Rapid evacuation plans and the availability of emergency self-contained breathing devices can be life saving in the event of accidental release of the gas.

NITROGEN OXIDES

During high temperature combustion, oxygen reacts with nitrogen to generate oxides of nitrogen. Nitrogen dioxide is the major oxide of nitrogen causing inhalation respiratory disease in the workplace. The toxicity of nitrogen dioxide is attributed to its oxidative capabilities.

Exposure settings

Common sources of occupational exposure are the fermentation of freshly stored hay or corn in silos (causing silo filler's disease), pickling or etching of metal with nitric acid, cutting and burning flames or welding arcs, fuel combustion (for example, from ice skating rink resurfacing machines), the exposure of miners to products of underground blasting, and firefighters' exposure to the combustion of nitrogen-containing materials (as in the tragic results of the burning of nitrocellulose x-ray films during the Cleveland Clinic fire of 1929). The principal source of lower level environmental exposures is outdoor air pollution from motor vehicle emissions, and indoor air pollution from gas cooking ranges and kerosene space heaters (see Chapter 50 and 51).

Environmental measurement

A variety of methods are available for measuring nitrogen oxides. These include continuous sampling devices accurate at concentrations below the occupational standard. Current US occupational safety standards are listed in Table 47.2.

Acute clinical effects

Because of the relatively mild odor, minimal mucous membrane irritant properties and relatively low tissue solubility, these gases lack warning properties and have potential for causing damage to the small airways and alveoli. The onset of effects is characteristically delayed 1–30 hours after the acute exposure and may include reversible bronchitis, acute, and sometimes irreversible, bronchiolitis obliterans alone or with organizing pneumonia (BOOP), and non-cardiogenic pulmonary edema. Toxicity of oxides of nitrogen may be complicated by systemic absorption of nitrates and nitrites, producing hypotension or methemoglobinemia.

Survivors of massive acute exposures may experience the onset of chronic pulmonary disease up to 1 month following exposure, with progressive worsening of lung function, usually attributed to bronchiolitis obliterans.

Chronic clinical effects

While individual epidemiologic studies of ambient environmental exposures have shown inconsistent results,[29,30] a meta-analysis in 1992 showed a slightly increased risk for respiratory tract infections in children with indoor nitrogen dioxide exposures.[31] Studies involving controlled exposures of asthmatic volunteers to nitrogen dioxide have also yielded conflicting results.[29,30] There is little evidence that ambient nitrogen dioxide levels have a significant effect on mortality.[17]

Evaluation strategy

Because of the possibility of severe delayed respiratory toxicity following high acute exposures, careful serial examination is essential. Close inpatient monitoring during the first 24–48 hours after exposure may be warranted. After the initial period, regular follow-up evaluation during the first month is warranted.

Management

Systemic corticosteroid therapy may be useful in modulating the sequelae of acute exposure, and should be considered early in the course after a known massive exposure and in patients with spirometric abnormalities. Supportive treatment includes supplemental oxygen and ventilatory support.

Prevention

Engineering controls, including limitations on production, use of closed systems, and local ventilation, can avert exposure under routine workplace conditions. Welders working in enclosed spaces require appropriate respiratory protection in addition to local exhaust ventilation. Before entry, filled silos should be thoroughly vented with fresh air. When effective flushing of nitrogen dioxide cannot be verified, farmers should enter silos with self-containing breathing apparatus or clean air-supplied respirators under direct observation of a companion similarly equipped.

CYANIDE (HYDROGEN CYANIDE)

Exposure setting

Prussic acid (hydrogen cyanide) and cyanide salts are used as fumigating agents for killing insects and rodents in agricultural buildings and ships, in electroplating and metal cleaning,[32] and in the manufacture of nylon. Exposure may occur through inhalation of dust, combustion products of some plastics, by skin absorption (when liquid) or ingestion. Clinically relevant cyanide toxicity may also be present in smoke-exposed firefighters and other smoke inhalation victims (see Chapter 41).[33]

Environmental measurement

Cyanide compounds can be unstable in collection media, and often several forms must be assayed to develop an accurate profile of exposure. In workplace air, cyanide is commonly collected in an impinger containing sodium hydroxide. Biologic monitoring or exposure may be accomplished by measuring thiocyanate levels in the urine or blood (although care must be taken not to misinterpret low blood levels because toxicity is more closely related to levels in tissue than in blood). US current occupational safety standards for cyanide are listed in Table 47.2.

Acute clinical effects

Cyanide rapidly causes asphyxia in the mitochondria by binding to the enzyme cytochrome oxidase, preventing the utilization of oxygen in affected cells, and halting aerobic metabolism. Symptoms of toxicity may be non-specific. In cases of mild poisoning, these may include a bitter almond taste, irritation of mucous membranes, dyspnea, headache, dizziness, nausea or vomiting, and agitation. In more severe cases, hypotension, arrhythmias, cardiogenic and non-cardiogenic pulmonary edema, lactic acidosis, seizures and coma may also occur. The cardiovascular collapse is associated with a characteristic cherry-red skin color and a relatively normal heart rate. Acute cyanide exposure directly affects aortic and carotid chemoreceptors, causing hyperpnea, and respiratory arrest, resulting from the direct effects on the central nervous respiratory control system, soon follows. Death may occur within minutes. A delayed cyanide leukoencephalopathy, similar to that seen in survivors of carbon monoxide intoxication, occurs in a minority of those who recover from an acute episode of severe cyanide intoxication.

Chronic clinical effects

Cyanide salts are skin and mucous membrane irritants. Strong cyanide solution may produce skin ulcerations after direct contact with skin. Chronic cyanide exposure, particularly when dietary iodide levels are low, has also been reported to cause thyroid gland enlargement in workers. Goiter has also been associated with dietary intake of cassavas, which contain cyanide precursors. In those who have had chronic workplace exposure to cyanide at levels sufficient to produce symptoms without overt intoxication, residual symptoms of rash, bitter or almond taste, and headache have been reported as chronic sequelae up to 7 months after cessation of exposure.

Similar to acute cyanide intoxication, several neurologic deficits have been proposed following chronic cyanide exposure from cigarette smoke or from a diet rich in unprocessed cassava. These include a neuro-ophthalmologic syndrome, smoker's amblyopia, reportedly responsive to hydroxycobalamin, and a chronic demyelinating neurotoxic syndrome.

Sodium nitrite	10 ml of 3% solution (300 mg) IV over 5–20 minutes
Amyl nitrite	0.3 ml ampoule crushed every minute, via inhalation
Sodium thiosulfate	50 ml of 25% solution (12.5 g) IV over 10 min
Hydroxycobalamin	10 ml of 40% solution (4 g) IV over 20 min

*Recommended initial doses may be higher for children

Table 47.4 Recommended cyanide antidote dosage* regimens

Clinical evaluation strategy

In acute exposure, including smoke inhalation victims, little time is available for diagnostic efforts; the diagnosis should be made on clinical grounds and the antidote administered immediately,[33,34] further described below. In suspected subacute or chronic toxicity, the measurement of elevated blood or urine thiocyanate levels (commonly available in clinical laboratories in the monitoring of nitroprusside therapy) may confirm cyanide exposure. A blood level of cyanide greater than 0.2 µg/ml may indicate a toxic exposure, although adverse effects may occur at lower blood levels.

Management

Current treatment of cyanide poisoning consists of initiating basic support measures (removal from exposure, skin decontamination, and the administration of 100% normobaric oxygen) followed by the administration of antidotes outlined in Table 47.4. The objective is to bind and convert cyanide before it has saturated tissue cytochrome oxidase. Because irreversible poisoning and death may occur within minutes of exposure, antidotes must be administered without delay, usually available as a cyanide antidote kit, containing sodium nitrite, sodium thiosulfate, and amyl nitrite. The first step is rapid administration of nitrates. If the victim is breathing, amyl nitrite may be administered by inhalation until the intravenous infusion is started and intravenous sodium nitrite is administered to generate methemoglobin from hemoglobin, which is more avid for cyanide than is cytochrome oxidase. Next, sodium thiosulfate is administered, which stimulates the conversion of cyanmethemoglobin to thiocyanate, a less toxic product that is rapidly excreted in urine. If concomitant carboxyhemoglobinemia is also present, the induction of methemoglobinemia may be harmful. In such a case, thiosulfate can be given alone or additional nitrites can be given cautiously, aiming to keep the sum of methemoglobin and carboxyhemoglobin below 40%.

Intravenous administration of a preparation of hydroxycobalamin (vitamin B$_{12a}$) to form a renally excreted cyanocobalamin complex is a safe and effective alternative therapy used in Europe but not available in the United States in the necessary concentration.

Prevention

A high index of suspicion is needed to detect symptomatic exposure before a fatal event occurs. Because the symptoms of intoxication are non-specific, the removal of workers from the exposure area and measurement of blood or urine thiocyanate levels while engineering controls are re-evaluated may be life saving. Where a risk of skin exposure occurs, protective gloves, aprons, face shields, and other gear are indicated. The availability of eye-wash and emergency shower facilities is mandatory.

HYDROGEN SULFIDE

In addition to its irritant properties, hydrogen sulfide is an asphyxiant at the cellular level, acting in much the same way as cyanide, binding to and inactivating cytochrome c oxidase.[35] Hydrogen sulfide has a strong smell of sulfur or rotten eggs, with an odor threshold at about 5 parts per billion, well below the irritant threshold (>10 ppm) but at high concentrations (>100 ppm) the gas can inactivate the sense of smell by a toxic effect on the olfactory nerve. In cases of acute exposures, would-be rescuers without proper protective equipment may themselves become victims.

Exposure settings

Hydrogen sulfide is formed naturally from the decay of organic sulfur-containing material and may thus be encountered as an unwanted byproduct in human and animal waste water disposal systems (and hence the name sewer gas), farm manure containment areas, in processes using animal products (such as glue factories, tanneries, and felt-making operations), or from the decomposition of fish (such as in the holds of fishing vessels). It may also be formed in mineral deposits of sulfur and encountered in mining and blasting operations, particularly in the recovery and processing of petroleum containing high sulfur content. Hydrogen sulfide is denser than air and accumulates in low-lying areas.

Environmental measurement

Hydrogen sulfide may be measured in air by monitoring instruments using several techniques. Current US occupational safety standards are outlined in Table 47.2.

Acute clinical effects

The presenting symptoms relate to the inability of metabolizing cells to utilize oxygen, with central nervous system abnormalities which may include rapid loss of consciousness (termed as 'knockdown' in oil and natural gas workers) and respiratory paralysis.[35,36] Initial tachycardia and hyperpnea can lead to cardiovascular collapse and death. Hydrogen sulfide also has acute irritant effects ranging from mucosal irritation to pulmonary edema. The survivors of acute intoxication may have persistent central nervous system deficits.

Chronic clinical effects

Exposures to prolonged periods of low concentrations of hydrogen sulfide may cause conjunctival irritation, reduction in threshold for odor detection or complete anosmia. The latter may leave the worker less able to detect the warning properties of subsequent exposures. Chronic CNS effects may be cumulative over several 'knockdowns' and may be associated with changes in cognitive function, affect and personality.

Clinical evaluation strategy

Awareness of the circumstances or industries of exposure may help to identify hydrogen sulfide gas exposure. A smell of rotten eggs from a patient's breath, clothing or freshly drawn blood may be helpful. Time does not usually permit a more definitive assessment of the cause of a severe toxic event. Other than air monitoring instruments, urinary thiosulfate determination is the only practical test to monitor hydrogen sulfide exposure in workers.[35] However, ingestion of sulfur-rich food or water can dramatically influence these results. Increased lactic acid and anion gap acidosis suggest chemical asphyxia but there is no specific test to confirm hydrogen sulfide intoxication.

Management

In addition to the administration of 100% oxygen, the use of only the first step of the cyanide antidote listed in Table 47.4 – sodium nitrite – may be helpful. The rationale is to generate methemoglobin, which can successfully compete for hydrogen sulfide by forming sulfhemoglobin, thus freeing and reactivating cytochrome oxidase. Animal studies indicate a beneficial effect, although human efficacy is not well established. A potential toxicity of this therapy is a reduction in the oxygen-carrying capacity of the blood with the formation of sulfhemoglobin.

Prevention

The great potency and potential for irreversible and fatal outcomes of hydrogen sulfide mandate rigorous control technology and air monitoring wherever this gas is known to occur as a product of industrial processes. Education concerning risks and the need for evacuation and the availability of escape equipment (self-contained breathing devices) may be life saving in circumstances in which the gas may be encountered suddenly and without warning.

OZONE

Based on concentration per volume of air, ozone is one of the more toxic gases to the respiratory system. Because it is relatively insoluble, its effect is greatest at the level of distal airways and alveoli. The cytotoxicity of ozone is largely due to generation of free radicals and peroxygenation of unsaturated lipids. The toxicity of ozone, as discussed here, refers to the effects of low altitude or tropospheric ozone. At higher altitudes (stratospheric) ozone is in fact beneficial, as it blocks the harmful effects of cosmic waves.

Exposure setting

Ozone is generated intentionally as a bactericidal gas for purification of drinking water and for hot tubs and also as an unintentional byproduct of ultraviolet light within a certain range of wavelengths. Toxic concentrations of ozone have been described to occur in poorly ventilated areas from arc welding (particularly tungsten-inert gas shielded welding) operations[37] and from malfunctioning coronas of photocopy machines.

Automobiles are major environmental contributors of the compounds which produce ozone, one of the air pollutants regulated by the EPA.[38] Widespread environmental exposure to low concentrations of ozone occurs during air pollution episodes (see Chapter 51). Concentrations of ozone sufficient to cause symptoms and reversible respiratory effects have been described in the past within high-altitude commercial aircraft flying certain routes during certain seasons. However, in more modern aircraft, removal of ozone from cabin air by conditioning is readily accomplished.

Environmental measurement

The concentration of ozone in the air may drop off rapidly within inches from a point source. The measurement of ozone in air is most reliably accomplished with the use of real-time instruments with photochemical cells. The expense of these instruments and their requirement for recalibration make constant workplace monitoring uncommon. US occupational safety standards are listed in Table 47.2.

Acute clinical effects

Ozone has a characteristic odor reminiscent of chlorine bleach (hypochlorous acid), but olfactory adaptation occurs within minutes. There is a striking individual gradient in the threshold to respiratory system response. The more sensitive subjects in the normal population will demonstrate symptoms (cough or chest tightness on deep inspiration) and reversible obstructive pulmonary function effects with sustained aerobic exercise within minutes of exposure to ozone levels of 0.2 ppm. As the concentration rises, a greater proportion of the healthy population will experience acute symptoms. Higher acute concentrations may result in respiratory distress from airway narrowing and from acute lung injury or non-cardiogenic pulmonary edema. Systemic toxicity other than that secondary to acute lung injury has not been described.

Chronic clinical effects

Experimental exposures to ozone cause reversible decrements in lung function.[39] Several epidemiologic studies also suggest that ambient ozone exposure of asthmatics is associated with increased hospitalizations and emergency room visits. Whether repeated low level ozone exposures cause irreversible pulmonary changes remains unclear.[19] The mortality rate from all causes and from cardiovascular and respiratory illnesses is only weakly associated with increases in ozone levels.[17]

Clinical evaluation strategy

The clinician must try to determine whether the exposure was sufficient to require close monitoring and support. Similar to other potent pulmonary irritants, the presence of adventitious lung sounds, abnormalities on chest roentgenographs, arterial hypoxemia or oxygen desaturation may indicate an early or evolving acute pneumonitis requiring close monitoring.

Management

Although there is no specific therapy for ozone toxicity, the symptomatic worker may need supportive treatment, which may involve cough suppression and bronchodilator use. Acute lung injury may require supplementary oxygen and ventilatory support.

Prevention

When ozone production is anticipated, control technology is relatively straightforward. The gas is reactive with most surfaces (exceptions include glass, stainless steel, and Teflon) and can be largely converted back to molecular oxygen while piping it to the outdoors through local exhaust ventilation ducts. Real-time monitoring of the air concentration is easily achieved with commercially available instruments. Awareness of the potential for generating ozone when ultraviolet light of certain frequencies passes through oxygen can, in most instances, prevent generation of harmful concentrations of ozone in the air.

PHOSGENE

Also known by the synonyms carbonic acid dichloride, carbonyl chloride, chloroformyl chloride, and carbon oxychloride, phosgene is a colorless, oxidant gas, with low solubility, and odor of new-mown hay or rotting vegetable material. It is one of the most acutely toxic of all gases used in industry. Part of its extreme danger lies in its potency and lack of warning properties. The pathogenesis of phosgene poisoning is not clearly understood.[40]

Exposure setting

It is used as a synthesizing agent for manufacture of industrial chemicals such as isocyanates, urea, coal tar, dyes, pharmaceuticals and insecticides. Clinically significant acute inhalation exposure may also occur when chlorinated hydrocarbons are heated by flame or contact with a hot metal. The best described industrial instances of this type have been the welding of metals 'degreased' with solvents (trichloroethylene and 1,1,1,-trichloroethane),[41,42] and the use of carbon tetrachloride as a fire-fighting agent in poorly ventilated areas. Phosgene was also used as a rapidly fatal gas on the battlefields of World War I (Fig. 47.3).

Environmental measurement

For continuous air monitoring of phosgene, infrared spectrophotometry, gas chromatography, and a paper-tape method have been proposed.[43] Exposed workers should be encouraged to wear phosgene indicator badges, which act as dose-dependent colorimeters. The current occupational safety standards in the US are listed in Table 47.2.

Acute clinical effects

Initial symptoms and signs relate to irritation of eyes and upper airway. The severity of these early irritant effects is no guide to the severity of poisoning. Further, because of its relatively low solubility, a lethal dose may be inhaled without the victim's knowledge. This may result in direct alveolar injury, leading to acute pneumonitis and non-cardiogenic pulmonary edema, which may be fatal. Similar to nitrogen dioxide, the onset of non-cardiogenic pulmonary edema may be delayed for several hours (up to 12 or more) after the acute exposure.

Chronic clinical effects

Persisting pulmonary function abnormalities have been noted with long-term follow-up of those who survived acute phosgene lung injury. The nature of the chronic injury has not been well characterized.[44]

Clinical evaluation strategy

Any patient with phosgene exposure should be admitted for observation for at least 24 hours.[40] Immediately following exposure, patients with life-threatening exposure may be clinically indistinguishable from those with relatively mild exposure. Knowledge of the potential concentrations and the circumstances of the exposure may be one guide to determining risk. The presence of eye, nasal, or tracheal irritation may indicate the potential for life-threatening sequelae. Acute pneumonitis and pulmonary edema can progress to adult respiratory distress syndrome (ARDS).

Management

The treatment is primarily supportive, including maintenance of a patent airway and support of arterial oxygenation, if necessary, by positive pressure ventilation. Close observation of the asymptomatic or mildly symptomatic patient is the key to recognizing the delayed onset of ARDS. There is no known antidote to phosgene. However, particularly when administered early after a heavy exposure, systemic corticosteroids may have some benefit.[45] Intravenous theophylline and beta-adrenergic agonists have potential utility in reducing the development of pulmonary edema, based on animal models.[46]

Prevention

Use of phosgene requires the most thorough precautions against acute exposures. Industrial practices are needed to minimize the possibility of exposure, including isolation of the material, education of workers, use of phosgene indicator badges, the development of evacuation plans, and the availability of self-contained breathing devices for rapid escape.

AMMONIA

Ammonia is a soluble, colorless, irritant gas with a well-recognized pungent odor. High atmospheric concentration of this gas usually forces the exposed individual to attempt escape before significant pulmonary injury occurs. Ammonia reacts with water present in moist mucosal surfaces to form ammonium hydroxide, a potent alkali. This causes liquefactive necrosis of the mucosal surface, which in turn exposes more ammonia to the watery surface and results in further necrosis.

Exposure settings

Common exposure settings involve release of 'fumes' from a variety of household cleaning agents at home. Accidents involving the commercial use of refrigeration equipment and in the plastics, explosives and fertilizer industries are other exposure settings. Ammonia is also present in swine confinement buildings and is used as a soil fertilizer on farms.

Environmental monitoring

Ammonia levels in air can be monitored by collecting air through a glass tube containing sulfuric acid-impregnated carbon beads followed by analysis with ion chromatography. The current US occupational safety standards for ammonia are listed in Table 47.2.

Acute clinical effects

Ammonia is markedly irritating to the eyes, skin and mucous membranes of upper respiratory tracts and may cause severe edema of the larynx, resulting in upper airway obstruction. Higher exposures may result in the sloughing of the upper airway mucosa with extensive edema. Chemical bronchitis, bronchospasm, and non-cardiogenic pulmonary edema are also described. Furthermore, while the strong odor of the gas would tend to drive an individual away from the scene, blindness resulting from burn injuries to the eyes may trap the worker in the area, resulting in more severe respiratory injury. Complete recovery is usual with lesser exposures. Persistent effects following high exposures include reactive airways dysfunction syndrome (RADS), bronchopneumonia due to bacterial super-infection, bronchiectasis, airway stenosis, and bronchiolitis obliterans.

Chronic clinical effects

Chronic exposures are associated with reversible eye, nose and throat irritation.

Clinical evaluation strategy

Individuals with orofacial lesions may be at higher risk of developing acute laryngeal obstruction; however, this early complication can develop even in patients without visible injury. Patients with postexposure abnormalities clinically or on chest radiograph, pulmonary function test or increased arterial alveolar gradient on blood gas analysis should be observed in the hospital for at least 24 hours.

Management

Treatment is primarily supportive and aimed at maintenance of airway patency. Oxygen, bronchodilators, and assisted ventilation should be implemented as needed. Steroids and antibiotics are usually not effective.

Prevention

In addition to engineering controls, workers involved in handling of ammonia gas should be instructed to follow proper procedures, use personal protective equipment and have access to plenty of clean water for first aid.

References

1. Lee DHK, Falk HL, Murphy SL. Reactions to environmental agents. In: Geiger SR, ed. Handbook of physiology. Bethesda, MD: American Physiological Society, 1977.
2. Klocke RA. Pulmonary excretion of absorbed gases. In: Lee DHF, ed. Handbook of physiology. Reactions to environmental agents. Bethesda, MD: American Physiological Society, 1977: 555–62.
3. Hampson NB. Emergency department visits for carbon monoxide poisoning in the Pacific Northwest. J Emerg Med 1998; 16:695–8.
4. Coburn RF, ed. Biological effects of carbon monoxide. Ann NY Acad Sci 1970; 174:1–40.
5. Forbes W, Sargent F, Roughton F. The rate of carbon monoxide uptake by normal men. Am J Physiol 1945; 143:594–608.
6. Zhang J, Piantadosi CA. Mitochondrial oxidative stress after carbon monoxide hypoxia in the rat brain. J Clin Invest 1992; 90:1193–9.
7. Thom SR. Carbon monoxide-mediated brain lipid peroxidation in the rat. J Appl Physiol 1990; 68:997–1003.
8. Aubard Y, Magne I. Carbon monoxide poisoning in pregnancy. Br J Obstet Gynaecol 2000; 107:833–8.
9. Ernst A, Zibrak JD. Carbon monoxide poisoning. N Engl J Med 1998; 339:1603–8.
10. Turner M, Hamilton-Farrell M, Clark R. Carbon monoxide poisoning: an update. J Accid Emerg Med 1999; 16:92–6.
11. Hardy KR, Thom SR. Pathophysiology and treatment of carbon monoxide poisoning. J Toxicol Clin Toxicol 1994; 32:613–29.
12. Choi IS. Delayed neurologic sequelae in carbon monoxide intoxication. Arch Neurol 1983; 40:433–5.
13. Smith CJ, Steichen TJ. The atherogenic potential of carbon monoxide. Atherosclerosis 1993; 99:137–49.
14. Fisher JA, Rucker J, Sommer LZ, et al. Isocapnic hyperpnea accelerates carbon monoxide elimination. Am J Respir Crit Care Med 1999; 159:1289–92.
15. Juurlink D, Stanbrook M, McGuigan M. Hyperbaric oxygen for carbon monoxide poisoning (Cochrane Review). The Cochrane Library. Oxford: Update Software, 2000.
16. Meyers RAM, Thom SR. Carbon monoxide and cyanide poisoning. In: Kindwall EP, ed. Hyperbaric medicine practice. Flagstaff, Arizona: Best Publishing, 1994: 344–72.
17. Samet JM, Dominici F, Curriero FC, Coursac I, Zeger SL. Fine particulate air pollution and mortality in 20 US cities, 1987–1994. N Engl J Med 2000; 343:1742–9.
18. Schwartz J, Dockery DW. Increased mortality in Philadelphia associated with daily air pollution concentrations. Am Rev Respir Dis 1992; 145:600–4.
19. Committee of the Environmental and Occupational Health Assembly of the American Thoracic Society. Health effects of outdoor air pollution, Part 1. Am J Respir Crit Care Med 1996; 153:3–50.
20. Committee of the Environmental and Occupational Health Assembly of the American Thoracic Society. Health effects of outdoor air pollution, Part 2. Am J Respir Crit Care Med 1996; 153:477–98.
21. Chapman RS, Calafiore DC, Hasselblad V. Prevalence of persistent cough and phlegm in young adults in relation to long term ambient sulfur oxide exposure. Am Rev Respir Dis 1985; 132:261–4.
22. Euler GL, Abbey DE, Magie AR, Hodgkin JE. Chronic obstructive pulmonary disease symptom effects of long-term cumulative exposure to ambient levels of total suspended particulates and sulfur dioxide in California Seventh-Day Adventist residents. Arch Environ Health 1987; 42:213–22.
23. Hattis RP, Greer JR, Dietrich S, et al. Chlorine gas toxicity from mixture of bleach with other cleaning products in California. MMWR 1991;40:619–29.
24. Sexton JD, Pronchik DJ. Chlorine inhalation: the big picture. J Toxicol Clin Toxicol 1998; 36:87–93.
25. Das R, Blanc PD. Chlorine gas exposure and the lung: a review. Toxicol Ind Health 1993; 9:439–55.

26. Salisbury DA, Enarson DA, Chan-Yeung M, Kennedy SM. First-aid reports of acute chlorine gassing among pulpmill workers as predictors of lung health consequences. Am J Ind Med 1991; 20:71–81.

27. Kennedy SM, Enarson DA, Janssen RG, Chan-Yeung M. Lung health consequences of reported accidental chlorine gas exposures among pulpmill workers. Am Rev Respir Dis 1991; 143:74–9.

28. Patil LR, Smith RG, Vorwald AJ, Mooney TF Jr. The health of diaphragm cell workers exposed to chlorine. Am Ind Hyg Assoc J 1970; 31:678–86.

29. Samet JM, Marbury MC, Spengler JD. Health effects and sources of indoor air pollution. Part I. Am Rev Respir Dis 1987; 136:1486–508.

30. Chauhan AJ, Krishna MT, Frew AJ, Holgate ST. Exposure to nitrogen dioxide (NO_2) and respiratory disease risk. Rev Environ Health 1998; 13:73–90.

31. Hasselblad V, Eddy DM, Kotchmar DJ. Synthesis of environmental evidence: nitrogen dioxide epidemiology studies. J Air Waste Manage Assoc 1992; 42:662–71.

32. Blanc P, Hogan M, Mallin K, et al. Cyanide intoxication among silver reclaiming workers. JAMA 1985; 253:367–71.

33. Baud FJ, Barriot P, Toffis V, et al. Elevated blood cyanide concentrations in victims of smoke inhalation. N Engl J Med 1991; 325:1761–6.

34. Kulig K. Cyanide antidotes and fire toxicology. N Engl J Med 1991; 325:1801–2.

35. Milby TH, Baselt RC. Hydrogen sulfide poisoning: clarification of some controversial issues. Am J Ind Med 1999; 35:192–5.

36. Guidotti TL. Hydrogen sulphide. Occup Med (Lond) 1996; 46:367–71.

37. Lunau FW. Ozone in arc welding. Ann Occup Hyg 1967; 10:175–88.

38. U.S. Environmental Protection Agency. National air quality and emissions trends report. Research Triangle Park, NC: Office of Air Quality Planning and Standards, 1991.

39. McDonnell WF, Horstman DH, Hazucha MJ, et al. Pulmonary effects of ozone during exercise: dose–response characteristics. J Appl Physiol 1983; 54:1345–52.

40. Wyatt JP, Allister CA. Occupational phosgene poisoning: a case report and review. J Accid Emerg Med 1995; 12:212–3.

41. Dahlberg JA, Myrin LH. The formation of dichloracetyl chloride and phosgene from trichloroethylene in the atmosphere of the welding shop. Ann Occup Hyg 1971; 14:269–74.

42. Doig AT, Challen PJR. Respiratory hazards of welding. Ann Occup Hyg 1964; 7:223–9.

43. Tuggle RM, Esposito GG, Guinivan TL, et al. Field evaluation of selected monitoring methods for phosgene in air. Am Ind Hyg Assoc J 1979; 40:387–94.

44. Diller WF. Late sequelae after phosgene poisoning: a literature review. Toxicol Ind Health 1985; 1:129–36.

45. Diller WF, Zante R. A literature review: therapy for phosgene poisoning. Toxicol Ind Health 1985; 1:117–28.

46. Kennedy TP, Michael JR, Hoidal JR, et al. Dibutyryl cAMP, aminophylline, and beta adrenergic agonists protect against pulmonary edema caused by phosgene. J Appl Physiol 1981; 67:2542–52.

Chapter 48
Pesticides and Related Compounds

Matthew C Keifer, Catharina Wesseling, Rob McConnell

Pesticides are defined broadly in the United States under the Food, Insecticide, Fungicide, and Rodenticide Act (FIFRA) as substances intended for preventing, destroying, repelling, or mitigating a pest (e.g., insect, rodent, nematode, fungus, weed) or substances intended for use as plant regulators, defoliants, or desiccants. This definition includes materials such as hypochlorites, alcohols, aldehydes, hexachlorphene, and pinene-containing substances used as disinfectants. This chapter will focus principally on chemicals more commonly understood as pesticides, such as insecticides, herbicides, fungicides, and fumigants. Pesticides include a large group of diverse chemical substances with different functions and toxicities. The single characteristic in common is that of being dispersed purposefully into the environment with the intention of adversely affecting the health or behavior of a pest species.

HISTORIC AND CURRENT USE

Pesticides have a rich, though poorly documented history, with an intimate overlap between materials used to destroy or mitigate pests and those used as agents to poison humans. Some of the history of man's early use of chemicals to battle 'pests' survives in documentation in the ancient writings of the Egyptians and Chinese. Chinese writings refer to the use of sulfur as a fumigant. Odysseus, after slaying his wife's suitors, used sulfur to purify 'hall, house and courtyard'. Achilles in the *Iliad* also used sulfur in the cleansing of a chalice before offering a libation to Zeus during the siege of Troy. Leonardo da Vinci (1500) described the injection of arsenic into apple trees, not to control insect pests but as a means of assassination.

While many potions and other mixtures were recommended in an attempt to control pests prior to the 19th century, few were carefully tested, and most proved ineffective in larger scale agricultural use. One of the first pesticides to find broad use, and the first successful arsenical compound, was Paris green (copper acetoarsenate). Originally used as a paint pigment, Paris green was discovered to be insecticidal, and in 1867 found its first wide use in the control of the Colorado potato beetle. It was later used to control many other insect pests. Paris green was supplemented by several other arsenic-containing materials, such as London purple, which was a toxic waste product of the English dye industry. While easier to apply due to its higher water solubility, and having the advantage of visibility once applied, it proved nearly as damaging to the plants it protected as the insects it controlled. The most important product in the latter half of the 19th and early 20th century was lead arsenate. This was first introduced to replace Paris green, to which the gypsy moth was resistant. Lead arsenate became one of the most important and widely used pesticides and found use in many aspects of agriculture. Relatively safer for the applicator, due to its low volatility and skin absorption, it resulted in lead poisoning among fruit consumers, and even led to protests in England against use on imported apples. Despite objections to its use, lead arsenate remained the major insecticidal tool for the control of apple pests until the mid 1940s. It should be noted that despite their virtual replacement by synthetic organic pesticides, arsenical pesticides remained a source of poisoning even as late as the 1970s, when a national study of hospitalized pesticide poisonings estimated that 23 out of 770 poisonings were due to arsenic.[1]

Pyrethrum was an early effective botanic insecticide. The insecticidal qualities of chrysanthemums, from which pyrethrum derives, had been a secret closely guarded by merchants in the Caucasus, where pyrethrum flowers were grown, dried, and powdered. The secret was discovered and marketed widely in the Middle East in the early 1800s, making its way to US markets by the 1850s. An attempt to establish pyrethrum cultivation in the US by the Department of Agriculture failed in the early 1880s, and even in California, where the cultivation was successful, it did not prove economic for agricultural production.[2]

Historically, fungicide development paralleled that of insecticides, and at times overlapped, as many products were both insecticidal and fungicidal. Sulfur was the first effective fungicide, and it remains useful today. The use of copper sulfate to control bunt, a fungal disease, dates to 1761. The combination of copper sulfate and lime was initially used to deter pedestrians from disturbing grapes along vineyard paths. Its fungicidal value was recognized by an astute botanist, Alexis Millardet, when *Plasmopara viticola*, the fungus responsible for downy mildew, swept across the French countryside. Millardet noticed that only the roadside plants appeared resistant. After testing the mixture, Millardet promoted the use of copper sulfate and lime, which became known as Bordeaux mixture. In doing so, he helped save the French wine crop from devastation. Organic mercurial agents, initially used by Erlich in the treatment of syphilis, were introduced in the early 1910s and remained an important mainstay of seed treatment until recent times.

Modern organic chemistry led to the development of new pesticidal products in great abundance in the mid 1930s. The modern era of synthetic organic chemical control of pests dates to the discoveries of the fungicidal effects of the dithiocarbamates in 1934, the insecticidal effects of the organophosphates in 1936, and 1,1-bis-(*p*-chlorophenyl)-2,2,2-trichloroethane (DDT) in 1939.

Dithiocarbamates found use both as fungicides and as rubber polymerization accelerators. They were first patented as fungicides by chemists in 1934, but were little used or publicized until the introduction of thiram in 1949. At that time two other dithiocarbamates, the iron-containing ferbam and the zinc-containing ziram, were introduced. These were eventually joined by an expanding array of other effective organic fungicides.

Organophosphates were observed to have potent insecticidal qualities by a German scientist, Gerhard Shrader, who between 1935 and 1937 developed hundreds of compounds in search of new pesticidal chemicals. He developed several insecticides, including parathion, TEPP, and shraden. He also developed tabun, also known as GA, and along with his lab assistant was the first person in history to suffer an acute intoxication with a nerve agent. His work on insecticides led to development of several other war gases under the Nazi regime, though his original work appears to have been directed towards insecticides.

While looking for potential insecticides among thousands of chemical products, Paul Mueller discovered the insecticidal qualities of a long known but seemingly inert compound, dichloro-diphenyl trichloroethane (DDT), originally synthesized by Othmar Zeidler in 1873. Mueller, then working at the Ciba-Geigy facilities in Switzerland, discovered its remarkable potency, revolutionizing insect control. Its persistence, effectiveness, broad spectrum, and relative low acute mammalian toxicity made it appear to be a virtually perfect insecticide. DDT, used in the control of louse-born typhus, malaria, yellow fever and dengue fever, also revolutionized warfare. Due to the control of these diseases for the first time in history, fewer combatants died of infection than inflicted wounds. Mueller was subsequently awarded the Nobel Prize in Medicine for this discovery and its benefits in controlling vector-borne infectious diseases.[3]

Many other new insecticides, herbicides, fungicides, and fumigants were discovered during the decade surrounding World War I. Lindane's insecticidal activity was described by Van Linden, and applied as both a general use insecticide and a scabicide. After the war, surplus tear gas (chloropicrin) was adapted as a soil fumigant, but was eventually replaced by products such as dibromo-chloro-propane, 1,2 dibromo-propane, and methyl bromide.

DDT and other insecticides in the organochlorine family began to lose effectiveness due to insect resistance, and were restricted in the 1970s because of their environmental persistence and related ecologic damage. This resulted in increased use of the organophosphate and N-methyl carbamate insecticides. The use of these compounds in the agricultural workplace in the early 1950s resulted in frequent intoxications among workers more familiar with the less toxic DDT and lead arsenate. Recently the organophosphates have come under stricter scrutiny, due to their very high toxicity and frequent human intoxications. Several organophosphates have been removed from registration or have had significant restrictions included in their registered uses, including phosdrin, ethyl-parathion, chlorpyrifos and diazinon. An important class of insecticides included synthetic analogs of the natural pyrethrum molecule, leading to the many variants of synthetic pyrethroids, which today are widely used in both agriculture and non-agricultural insect control activities. However, the pyrethroids have encountered increasing resistance among target pests, reducing their usefulness and economic viability.

As organophosphates are increasingly more restricted, pyrethroids are encountering greater resistance and organochlorines are quickly vanishing, with new compounds being developed to fill their place. The mechanisms of action in many are sufficiently pest specific that toxicity in humans is less likely. Chitin inhibitors and insect pheromones are examples of these. The toxicity of these compounds for humans is likely to be low, except when dosed in large quantities, when allergic or idiopathic responses may be encountered, or if they are carcinogenic.

In the United States, with few exceptions, data are not available by state or region on the amounts of specific pesticides used in applications. California is the primary exception, where pesticide application information is reported and centrally available. New York also recently began to require that commercial applicators file application records annually. The amount of pesticides used worldwide exceeded 5.6 billion pounds in 1998 and 1999, of which 1.2 billion were used in the US. California alone reported 184,000,000 pounds of pesticides applied to agricultural crops in 2000.[4] Information for most other states can only be estimated by use of national surveys such as the National Agricultural Survey Service database.

While pesticides have contributed to a substantial increase in agricultural productivity worldwide, the associated environmental costs are less well documented. Pest control with insecticides has also played an important role in the control of malaria and other vector-borne diseases in most of the developed world. However, this advantage in developing countries has been ephemeral. In some endemic areas, the incidence of malaria has increased in recent years, partly as a result of insect resistance to DDT and other insecticides. The overuse of insecticides in agriculture has facilitated the development of resistance in insect vectors and made their control even more difficult.[3]

There are approximately 900 active ingredients currently registered for use in the United States. This number is in constant flux as pesticides lose registration or new agents are added. These chemicals are mixed with many other compounds, termed 'inert ingredients,' without pesticidal properties but not necessarily without health effects that can be found in more than 35,000 commercial products.

Pesticides are classified by function according to the class of pest they are active against, chemical class, and by toxicity (e.g., World Health Organization and US EPA). As demonstrated in Table 48.1, the EPA toxicity categories correspond to acute effects.

	Category			
Parameter	I	II	III	IV
Oral LD$_{50}$	50 mg/kg	50–500 mg/kg	500–5000 mg/kg	> 5000 mg/kg
Inhalation LD$_{50}$	0.2 mg/l	0.2–2 mg/l	2–20 mg/l	> 20 mg/l
Dermal LD$_{50}$	200 mg/kg	200–2000 mg/kg	2000–20,000 mg/kg	> 20,000 mg/kg
Eye effects	Corrosive; corneal opacity not reversible within 7 days	Corneal opacity reversible within 7 days; irritation persisting for 7 days	No corneal opacity; irritation reversible within 7 days	No irritation
Skin effects	Corrosive	Severe irritation at 72 hours	Moderate irritation at 72 hours	Mild or slight irritation at 72 hours
Signal word	Danger	Warning	Caution	Caution

LD$_{50}$, lethal dose for 50% of animals tested.

Table 48.1 Environmental Protection Agency toxicity categories for pesticides

EXPOSURE

In occupational settings, dermal exposure is commonly the primary source of overexposure; however, exposure by inhalation, ingestion, or a combination of routes may be important. The conjunctival membranes of the eye and other mucous membranes are sometimes included as a distinct route of systemic exposure. Many fumigants, which are often released as gases into enclosed spaces, are easily and efficiently absorbed by inhalation. Aerosols, fine mists, and powders may have particle sizes small enough to be inhaled deep into the lungs and absorbed. Larger particle fractions often deposit on upper and lower airway surfaces, where they are readily absorbed, and even coarse mists may deposit in the oropharynx and be swallowed. Many sprays and granules have particle sizes larger than 30 microns and do not reach the lungs effectively through inhalation.

While most pesticides have low odor thresholds and are often identifiable at low concentrations, many pesticides are of relatively low volatility, with dermal exposure being more significant than the inhalation route. It is important to emphasize that exposure to even low-volatility pesticides in enclosed spaces over significant durations, or exposure to highly volatile pesticides, including fumigants, may result in substantial exposure by the inhalation route. Though rarely of occupational import, many pesticides are efficiently absorbed from the gastrointestinal tract. Accidental splashes with pesticides expose mucous membranes of the eye, nose, and gut, and so represent an efficient route of absorption. Exposure route should be discerned and described clearly in the process of making the diagnosis of pesticide-related illness, and reporting overexposures.

Acute toxicity from dermal exposure depends on both the toxicity of the pesticide and on the ease with which it is absorbed (bioavailability). Absorption of pesticides, like absorption of medications through the skin, depends on the concentration and lipid solubility of the active ingredient, the absorptive potential of the solvent in which the product is formulated, the frequency and promptness with which skin is washed after contact. The integrity of the skin barrier can also influence the rate of absorption; abraded or highly vascularized inflamed skin surfaces enhance absorption. The part of the body exposed is also

very important in the ease of absorption.[5,6] Experiments with volunteers, for example, have shown that little as 8.6% of applied parathion may be absorbed through skin of the forearm, but as much as 100% may be absorbed through scrotal skin. Important in the first aid of overexposed victims is prompt decontamination. One study demonstrated that as much as 92% of applied parathion could be washed free 30 minutes after application, but as much as 70% could still be washed free after 300 minutes.

Some organophosphate agents can have potent interactions with other pesticides or with chemical contaminants within the same preparation. Malathion, for example, is much more toxic if administered with ethyl-p-nitrophenyl thionobenzenephosphorate (EPN). Isomalathion, present as a contaminant to malathion, resulted in epidemic poisoning among vector control spray operators in Pakistan.[7] Paraoxon and malaoxon, which are the principal toxic metabolites of parathion and malathion, have been reported to cause epidemic poisoning. Hot, dry conditions, perhaps in combination with contaminants in air pollution, enhance the environmental formation and persistence of paraoxon from parathion.[8] Alteration in toxicity through contaminants and storage conditions is not well characterized for most pesticides, and is generally not part of the toxicity studies required for pesticide registration.[9] The clinician should thus consider the possibility of toxicity enhancement through mixed applications, through more highly toxic contaminants, or through environmental activation, when the presenting toxicity is not fully explained by the estimated dose based on known pesticide characteristics.

Occupational exposure to pesticides occurs among manufacturers and formulators; during transport and storage; among mixers, loaders, and applicators working in fields, greenhouses, parks, and residential buildings (Fig. 48.1); among vector control and structural (especially termite control) applicators; and among farm workers entering fields or greenhouse workers handling foliage previously sprayed by pesticides (Table 48.2). Crop duster aviation mechanics have been reported to be at high risk for pesticide poisoning.[10] Other groups occasionally exposed include emergency crews or sewer workers involved in cleanup procedures. Perhaps the largest exposed group in developed countries is building maintenance workers, who apply household insecticides and disinfectants. Non-occupational environmental

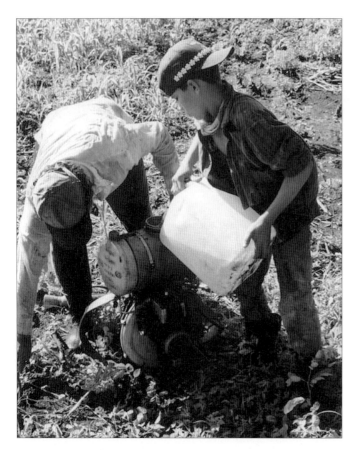

Figure 48.1: Nicaraguan child pouring pesticide. (Courtesy of Aurora Aragon MD, National University of Nicaragua, Leon)

Occupational exposure	Non-occupational exposure
Research chemistry	Residues from household and lawn applications
Manufacturing active ingredient	Termite control
Formulating end product	Accidental or intentional ingestion
Transportation	Food residues
Storage/warehouse work	Water residues
Mixing and loading	Hazardous waste sites
Agricultural application	Traffic accidents
Flaggers	Industrial spills
Structural application	
Building maintenance work	
Crop duster maintenance	
Farm work	
Greenhouse, nursery, mushroom house workers	
Livestock dippers	
Veterinarians	
Landscapers	
Park workers	
Forestry workers	
Entomologists	
Work on highways, railroads or rights of way	
Wood treatment workers	
Vector control workers	
Emergency workers	
Firefighters	
Sewer workers	
Hazardous waste workers	
Medical personnel	
Treating contaminated workers	

Table 48.2 Workplace and non-workplace exposures to pesticides

exposure occurs from drift,[11,12] contaminated water, residues in indoor air or food, or from exposure to hazardous waste that is improperly disposed of. Although non-occupational exposure is often low level, there have been numerous episodes of acute illness resulting from drift from nearby fields or from consumption of contaminated food. In the United States, an epidemic of more than 1300 poisonings (and possibly eight deaths) was associated with the consumption of California watermelons contaminated with aldicarb.[13] Intentional ingestion of pesticides is a frequent means of suicide, particularly in developing countries.[14]

EPIDEMIOLOGY
United States

No single surveillance system tracks pesticide poisonings in the US. In 1976, a national study of hospital admissions for pesticide poisonings noted that there was no system for recording pesticide poisonings in the United States. More than a quarter of a century later this remains the case. The majority of pesticide poisonings go unreported to any specific registry. Several states, including California, Washington, and New York (Table 48.3), have reporting systems that specifically identify pesticide poisonings. Other states require occupational intoxications to be reported, but many states have no reporting requirements.

The Environmental Protection Agency has estimated that some 10,000–20,000 medically treated pesticide poisonings occur annually in the US.[15] The mortality rate from unintentional acute pesticide poisoning in the United States in 1983 was estimated to be 2.7 per 10 million men (compared with 0.5 per 10 million women). The rate was three times higher among blacks than among whites. The mortality rate of pesticide poisoning related to suicide was 2.3 per 10 million for blacks and 2.6 per 10 million for whites. In California, which accounts for about one-third of the United States agricultural work force, 2001 registry data indicate that there were 979 reports of poisoning, 626 (63%) of which were judged after investigation to be potentially related to pesticides; 66% of poisonings were occupational. The largest group affected in agricultural settings was residue-exposed field workers (57 cases). Forty-two percent of these were identified as handlers, meaning that they were involved in some portion of the application process.

A significant drop in reports of pesticide-related illness has occurred in the past 10 years. In 1987, there were 2897 reported poisonings in California, 1754 (61%) of which were judged after investigation to be potentially related to pesticides. More than 80% of these were occupational poisonings. While some of this change may be related to reporting patterns, some is undoubtedly due to the elimination of several very toxic pesticides, such as phosdrin and ethyl parathion. The management of acute poisoning presented in this chapter will focus primarily on those pesticides that account for the most common and severe poisonings.

Arizona	Arizona Department of Health Services Pesticide Poisoning Surveillance and Reporting Program	Phone: 602-230-5830* Arizona Department of Health Services http://www.hs.state.az.us/edc/oeh/pestcide.htm
California	Multiple agencies involved in surveillance and investigation. County health officer should receive initial notification	Reporting form to be faxed to the county health officer http://www.oehha.org/pesticides/pdf/PIR_99.pdf
Florida	Florida Pesticide Exposure Surveillance Program Florida Department of Health	Reporting hotline: 1-800-282-3171 (within Florida) http://www9.myflorida.com/environment/hsee/pesticides/index.html
Louisiana	Louisiana Department of Health and Hospitals Office of Public Health Section of Environmental Epidemiology and Toxicology	Phone: 1-888-293-7020
Michigan	Michigan Department of Consumer and Industry Services Division of Occupational Health	Phone: 1-800-446-7805 (within Michigan) Downloadable reporting form in Portable Document File (PDF) format see: http://web2.chm.msu.edu/oem/resources.htm
New Mexico	Surveillance of pesticide related illness or injury Department of Health Office of Epidemiology	Phone: 505-827-0006 or 1-800-432-4404 (New Mexico only) Website link for reporting rule: http://www.health.state.nm.us/ Office of Epidemiology
New York	New York State Pesticide Poisoning Registry New York State Department of Health Center for Environmental Health Oregon Health Division	Environmental Helpline Phone: 1-800-458-1158 Reporting Regulation (Part 22, State Sanitary Code) – www.health.state.ny.us/nysdoh/environ/pest/appenda.htm
Oregon	Pesticide Poisoning Prevention Program Environmental and Occupational Epidemiology	Phone: (503) 73-4025 Fax: (503) 73-4798 http://www.ohd.hr.state.or.us/eoe/pest/
Texas	Pesticide Exposure Surveillance in Texas Texas Department of Health	Phone: 1-800-588-1248 (In Texas only) / 512-458-7269 Fax: 512-458-7699 http://www.tdh.state.tx.us/epitox/pesticides.htm
Washington	Office of Environmental Health & Safety Pesticide Program Washington State Department of Health	Washington Poison Center at 1-800-732-6985 General public and symptomatic individuals: 1-360-236-3361 http://www.doh.wa.gov/ehp/ts/PEST.HTM

*Contact information at the time of publication.

Table 48.3 States with established pesticide-related illness and injury surveillance systems

Under-reporting of pesticide poisonings, even in locations where reporting is mandatory, is likely to be a significant problem.[16] A study from Nicaragua, with results consistently observed for most of Central America (see also section on Developing Countries below) found reporting percentages as high as 30% in some regions[9] but as low as 2% in others.[17] Reporting is probably even less accurate for non-occupational compared to occupational poisonings. In one study, less than 1% of poison center referrals (most of which were non-occupational) were actually reported. Approximately 4% of poison control center consultations in the United States involve pesticide exposure (34% of consultations for children under 6 years of age).

Developing countries

While consumption of pesticides in developed countries has tended to decrease or remain stable, pesticide use has increased, and indeed been promoted, in developing countries. In Latin America, a high proportion of farmers use pesticides heavily, approaching 100% in some groups such as subsistence farmers. Recently, the widespread production of ornamental plants, tropical fruits, and vegetables for export has relied heavily on pesticide application.

In the early 1980s, based on data from Asian countries, it was projected that 90% of the estimated 3 million annual pesticide poisonings worldwide, and more than 99% of the 220,000 pesticide-related deaths, occurred in developing countries.[18] It was also estimated, based on extrapolation of interviews of several thousand agricultural workers in Asian countries, that 25 million occupational poisonings have occurred among agricultural workers in developing countries worldwide. These figures have not been updated and no new global estimates have been produced since their publication. In Costa Rica, it has been estimated that at least 4.5% of agricultural workers experience a pesticide-related illness each year.[19] In surveys of agricultural workers in several Asian countries, and of cotton workers in Mexico, 3–7% and 13–15%, respectively, reported poisoning in the previous year. In addition, pesticide poisoning may be more likely to be underdiagnosed than in the developed countries. In one ecologic study of mortality trends in the Philippines, a dramatic increase in diagnosed medical conditions that might be confused with pesticide poisoning was observed among men of working age in rural areas. The increase was not seen among those less likely to be exposed to pesticides, namely women or older or younger men. The increased mortality rate among men corresponded to the introduction of organochlorine pesticides into common agricultural practice in the 1970s, and was seen in a seasonal pattern that corresponded to the use of pesticides.[20] In Nicaragua, in 2000 it was estimated that among those persons with either domestic or occupational exposure to pesticides, 5% suffered a symptomatic poisoning episode.[21]

In general, large volumes of highly toxic pesticides are applied in the United States by relatively few workers loading crop dusters or tractor-drawn booms for application to large areas of land. Engineering controls, such as closed-system mixing and loading units, personal protective equipment, and medical supervision, are often available. By contrast, the small farmer in a developing country is likely to mix and load a backpack sprayer that may be poorly maintained, and to apply highly toxic insecticides without gloves, coveralls, or shoes.[22–24] Of concern, some 30% of the pesticide exports to other countries from the United States are of pesticides prohibited or restricted in the United States. Warning labels are often not in the language of the receiving country, with limited literacy among many farmers. In one epidemic, hungry victims washed seed grain treated with alkyl-mercury before eating it, in the mistaken belief that this would remove the toxin, with resulting widespread intoxication (see below). Severe malnutrition, especially protein deficiency, may markedly potentiate the toxicity of certain pesticides, such as captan and several acutely toxic organophosphates and carbamates.

Many of the most serious epidemics of pesticide poisoning have occurred in the developing world. Methyl mercury seed treatment has lead to poisoning epidemics in Latin America and the Middle East. An estimated 60,000 illnesses and 2000–2500 deaths from exposure to methyl isocyanate, used as an intermediary in insecticide manufacture, occurred in Bhopal, India during an uncontrolled release. More recently, in 1999, 24 children died in the Anduvian village of Taucamarca in Peru, after the milk supply at school was accidentally contaminated with methylparathion.

Increasingly, suicides have become an important pesticide-related health problem in developing countries.[25] While responsibility for this has been attributed to the person committing suicide,[26] suicides in agricultural workers can be viewed as an occupational disease (defined by WHO as "type IV") due to easy availability of the poisoning agent.[27] In Costa Rica, non-occupational accidental and suicidal pesticide poisonings were 11 times more frequent among agricultural workers than among the general population.[19] In Surinam, the incidence of paraquat suicides correlated closely with amounts of paraquat imported and distributed for agricultural use.[28] It is important to recognize that exposure to organophosphate pesticides may in itself cause psychiatric disorders including depression, leading to increased risk of suicides among farming populations.[29] In Serra Gaucha, Brazil, a high proportion of farm workers presented with minor psychiatric disorders,[30] which were strongly associated with pesticide exposures. In Ecuador, the suicide rate with pesticides was extremely high in a potato farming population;[31] suicidal ideation was four times more frequent among previously poisoned banana plantation workers than among workers who had never been poisoned.

GENERAL APPROACH TO THE PATIENT EXPOSED TO PESTICIDES

A pesticide-exposed patient, like a patient with a severely contagious disease, presents a risk for healthcare workers. Given the potential toxicity of some agricultural chemicals, management of a poisoning includes careful attention to the safety of the receiving healthcare professionals. Contaminated clothing, gastric, or bowel contents and secretions should be carefully handled and disposed of with great caution.

After (and sometimes during) support of respiration and circulation, decontamination is essential to curtail further dosing of the affected subject from skin or gut contamination. Among the first tasks of a healthcare worker presented with a patient overexposed to pesticides is to determine the chemical involved. In many countries, if the label on the container is available, it will list the active ingredients and their acute toxicity. In the United States, the label must list the EPA registration number and the EPA signal word, which indicates the relative acute toxicity (Table 48.1). The *Farm Chemicals Handbook*[32] is an index of most of the brand names available in the United States, and indicates the common chemical name of each active ingredient and the manufacturer. After the chemical name is known, useful resources for identifying the hazards of individual or groups of pesticides, and the management of related acute (and chronic) effects are listed in Table 48.4. In the United States, other resources include local poison control centers for the treatment of acute poisoning. An excellent resource, *Recognition and Management of Pesticide Poisoning*,[33] that is periodically updated and available through the EPA, is a detailed guide to treating acute poisoning.

Prompt induction of vomiting (or gastric lavage through a large-bore orogastric tube) is indicated to treat poisoning by ingestion. If consciousness is impaired or a petroleum distillate or corrosive was swallowed, gastric lavage should be performed. Caution must be exercised to avoid aspiration of petroleum distillates (producing a chemical pneumonitis), and use of a cuffed endotracheal tube in place before the stomach undergoes lavage should be considered. A chest x-ray study is indicated within a few hours after gastric lavage if aspiration of petroleum distillates is a possibility. Lavage should be followed by activated charcoal (50–100 g in 300 to 800 ml of water) to slow absorption and by a cathartic (e.g., sorbitol 1–2 g/kg of body weight to a maximum of 250 g per dose) to hasten transit time. Diazepam (Valium) 5–10 mg given slowly intravenously (not faster than 2 mg/minute) may be useful in controlling seizures.

If there is dermal exposure, the skin, hair, and nails should be bathed thoroughly with a mild detergent (or soap) and abundant water. The skin should not be scrubbed vigorously because damage to the superficial layers may enhance absorption. Further bathing with 70% alcohol may be helpful in removing additional residue. Skin, secretions, and clothing contaminated with pesticides should be

Useful references

- Farm Chemicals Handbook:[32] Useful for obtaining chemical names, if only a brand name is available; updated yearly.
- Handbook of Pesticide Toxicology:[95] After the chemical name is known (available from Farm Chemicals Handbook), a review of the toxicologic and human literature on a particular chemical can usually be found.
- Recognition and Management of Pesticide Poisonings:[33] Reviews the diagnosis and treatment of acute poisoning by the different groups of pesticides.
- Guidelines for Physicians: Medical Supervision of Pesticide Workers:[96] Reviews practical aspects of cholinesterase monitoring.
- Occupational Dermatitis from Pesticides: Patch Testing Procedures:[97] Describes dilutions for patch testing for specific pesticides.
- The Effects of Pesticides on Human Health:[98] Reviews chronic effects of pesticide exposure.
- Regulating Pesticides in Food:[99] Reviews carcinogenic effects of pesticides in food.
- EPA registration standards on individual pesticides: Reviews many unpublished studies, in addition to published literature.

Other resources (United States)

- National Pesticide Telecommunications Network: A 24-hour number for information on the acute or chronic effects of pesticides.
- Chemtrec 24-hour emergency number for information on handling spills.
- Centers for Disease Control (for outbreak or health hazard evaluations): National Institute for Occupational Safety and Health, Cincinnati, Ohio: for evaluation of workplace health hazards and outbreaks of illness. Center for Environmental Health and Injury Control, Atlanta, Georgia: for evaluation of environmental health hazards and outbreaks of illness.
- State and local health departments and the EPA-mandated state agency that is responsible for pesticide regulation.
- National Coalition Against the Misuse of Pesticides, Washington, DC: a non-governmental resource of local and national organizations providing information of alternatives to pesticides.

Table 48.4 Selected resources on pesticides

handled with gloves and bagged with impervious bags to prevent poisoning of health personnel. Contaminated clothing should be preserved, as testing of clothing may add to the characterization of exposure and medical management. If food contamination is suspected, food should be saved for future analysis, along with secretions (gastric contents, feces, and urine), blood, and serum. Deep freezing (at least –20 to –70 degrees C) of clothing, urine, feces, gastric contents, and blood samples is advisable to prevent degradation of the active ingredients.

INSECTICIDES

Cholinesterase inhibitors

1. Organophosphates
   Acephate (3*)
   Chlorpyrifos (2)
   Diazinon (2 or 3)
   Dichlorvos (1)
   Ethyl parathion (1)
   Ethion (2)
   Malathion (3)
   Methamidophos (1)
   Methyl parathion (1)
   Propetamphos (3)
   Trichlorfon (2)
2. Carbamates
   Aldicarb (1)
   Bendiocarb (2)
   Carbofuran (1 or 2)
   Carbaryl (1, 2 or 3)
   Methomyl (1 or 4)
   Promecarb (2)
   Propoxur (2)

*Throughout this chapter, the numbers in parentheses after the names of insecticides and other chemicals are the EPA toxicity category (described in Table 48.1).

Acute clinical effects

Although there are important differences in the treatment of acute poisoning with the organophosphate and N-methyl carbamate insecticides, their clinical presentations are similar. Acute poisoning with these two classes of pesticides accounts for the majority of systemic poisoning cases seen by clinicians in the United States. Both inhibit neuronal acetylcholinesterase, as shown schematically in Figure 48.2. Normal function of the cholinergic nervous system is modulated by this enzyme, which cleaves the principal neurotransmitter, acetylcholine, into choline and acetic acid. The inhibition of acetylcholinesterase results in an increase in acetylcholine and in overstimulation of the postsynaptic receptors in the cholinergic nervous system. These effects can be differentiated toxicologically into stimulation of the central nervous system, of the nicotinic receptors (skeletal muscle and autonomic ganglia) and the muscarinic receptors (secretory glands and postganglionic fibers in the parasympathetic nervous system) (Table 48.5). The nicotinic effects generally appear later, and usually in moderate to severe poisoning cases. Headache, anxiety, and sleep disturbance, often accompanied by salivation and anorexia, are common early symptoms of mild overexposure to cholinesterase inhibitors. Chest tightness is a symptom of moderately severe poisoning after dermal exposure, but it can be an early symptom if there is significant exposure to the respiratory tract. Seizures and impaired consciousness occur in more severe poisoning cases. Other reported acute effects include myopathy (including myocardiopathy), hypothermia, liver dysfunction, brady- or tachyarrhythmias, leukocytosis, and acute psychosis. Clinical findings may be variable, with postganglionic sympathetic stimulation dominating over parasympathetic findings. For example, varying degrees of miosis or even mydriasis may be observed following organophosphate poisoning.

Delayed or chronic effects of exposure to organophosphates

Chronic low-level exposure to organophosphates may result in weakness and malaise, often accompanied by headache and light-headedness, but without other specific symptoms. The etiologic relationship to pesticides of such non-specific symptoms may pose a clinical challenge (see section on Evaluation).

Several complications may occur in patients poisoned with organophosphates as follows.

1. There have been case reports of acute and persistent psychotic illness associated with poisoning by organophosphates.[34]
2. QT prolongation and torsade de pointes, a life-threatening ventricular tachycardia, have been reported to occur for up to several days after severe poisoning.[35]
3. The so-called intermediate syndrome, characterized by the paralysis of the proximal musculature and muscles of respiration and of cranial motor nerves, occurs 1–4 days after poisoning (after recovery from the life-threatening manifestations of acute poisoning). Supportive mechanical ventilation for up to 2 weeks typically results in recovery without specific treatment. The mechanism of the intermediate syndrome is not fully known, but may be related to either involution of acetylcholine receptors or continued severe cholinesterase inhibition.[36]
4. Organophosphate-induced delayed polyneuropathy (OPIDP), a distal dying-back axonopathy, is characterized clinically by cramping muscle pain in the legs, often followed by paresthesias and motor weakness. The onset occurs 10 days to 3 weeks following a severe poisoning episode. There may be marked foot drop and weakness of the distal upper extremities. In some patients pyramidal signs may develop. The best example of this problem was the epidemic of "Jake Leg", which resulted from widespread ingestion of tri-ortho-cresyl-pyrophosphate (TOCP) in adulterated ginger extract. TOCP is an organophosphate that is not an acetylcholinesterase inhibitor, and is used principally as a plasticizer and in hydraulic lubricants. The prognosis for complete recovery of victims with long tract signs is poor. Although objective evidence of sensory loss is often lacking, decreased vibration sense has been reported on examination almost 50 years after the onset of disease.[37] Neurophysiologic studies in humans and animals have demonstrated relatively normal nerve conduction velocities, with markedly decreased sensory amplitudes and muscle action potentials. The pathophysiology of the disease appears to involve the inhibition and subsequent aging of a poorly characterized esterase known as neuropathy target esterase (NTE), which is distinct from acetylcholinesterase. Although the assay for NTE activity is not available clinically, high levels of inhibition and aging of NTE activity in human lymphocytes have been shown to predict the onset of OPIDP in a patient poisoned with chlorpyrifos.[38] Most reported cases occurring after insecticide poisoning have involved methamidophos. In humans, OPIDP also has been reported to occur after poisoning with merphos, mipafox, leptophos, trichlorphon, trichloronat, chlorpyrifos, and fenthion.

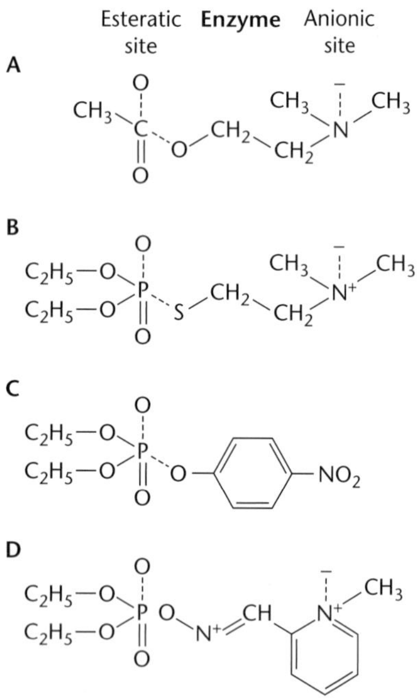

Figure 48.2: Reaction of acetylcholine (A), ecothiophate (B), and paraoxon (C) with acetylcholinesterase and positioning of 2-PAM for reactivation inhibited by diethoxy phosphate (D) derived from either of the two inhibitors. (Reprinted from Gallo M, et al. Organic phosphorus pesticides. In: Hayes W, Laws E, eds. Handbook of pesticide toxicology. © 1991, with permission from Elsevier.)

Muscarinic	Nicotinic	Central nervous system
Anorexia	Muscle twitching	Anxiety
Nausea and vomiting	Fasciculations	Irritability
Abdominal cramps	Weakness	Altered sleep
Diarrhea	Hypertension	Headache
Chest tightness (bronchoconstriction and increased secretions)	Hyperglycemia	Tremor
Increased salivation and lacrimation	Tachycardia (if severe)	Impaired cognition
Miosis and blurred vision (may be asymmetric and variable)		Seizures and coma (if severe)
Sweating		
Bradycardia		
Involuntary defecation and urination (if severe)		
From: Rosenstock L, Cullen M. Clinical occupational medicine. Philadelphia: WB Saunders Company, 1986.		

Table 48.5 Symptoms and signs of poisoning with anticholinesterases

5. In addition, persistent visual disturbances, difficulty concentrating, impaired memory, irritability, fatigue, and headache have been reported by individuals following poisoning with organophosphates. In large case series in the developed world, between 4% and 9% of poisoned individuals were reported to have clinically significant chronic neuropsychologic sequelae. In epidemiologic studies, even single episodes of severe organophosphate poisoning were associated with a persistent decrement in neuropsychologic function, including auditory attention, visual memory, visuomotor speed, sequencing and problem solving, motor steadiness, reaction time, and dexterity. Differences in the range of normal function, depending on cultural and, perhaps, socioeconomic factors are a challenge in clinical assessment; few tests are standardized for worker populations. In addition, there is large interindividual variability within the range of normal. An individual may have significant deterioration in neuropsychologic function and still remain within the interindividual normal range, if their premorbid function was high. Neuropsychologic evaluation should include an assessment of premorbid functioning, though previous neuropsychologic testing is rarely available. Chronic electroencephalographic disturbances, especially an increase in beta activity, have been reported among previously poisoned individuals.[39–41]

Evaluation

Although not always present, especially in mild poisoning, fasciculations with miosis are virtually diagnostic of poisoning with these agents. In cases of mild acute poisoning, a cautious diagnostic trial of atropine sulfate (0.4–1 mg intravenously slowly) will usually result in a prompt improvement of symptoms. In poisoning resulting from dermal exposure, the onset of symptoms is rarely delayed longer than 12 hours and almost never longer than 24 hours after the exposure ends. The symptoms usually occur within 2–3 hours of ingestion and more rapidly after exposure by inhalation. Although considerable variability exists, if the onset of symptoms is delayed longer, the clinician must reconsider the diagnosis or consider the possibility of continued occult exposure (to contaminated clothing, for example).[42,43] Although the results often are not available immediately, the measurement of cholinesterase levels in erythrocytes or in plasma is a useful confirmatory test.

Baseline cholinesterase levels are essential in interpreting values. Even mild depression of cholinesterase activity may result in symptoms, especially if the depression is sudden. Because there is a wide interindividual variation in normal cholinesterase activity, a low level is useful diagnostically, but a low normal level in an individual with symptoms of mild poisoning does not exclude the diagnosis. Rising cholinesterase for weeks to months after exposure may be useful in confirming the diagnosis. Most important is a comparison with baseline values, when available. Removal from exposure and serial measurements of cholinesterase activity are helpful diagnostic exercises in the setting of subtle non-specific symptoms (e.g., headache, malaise, and fatigue) and chronic low-level exposure to organophosphates. Cholinesterase inhibition in blood samples may rapidly reverse in the case of carbamate poisoning. Samples collected for cholinesterase testing should be chilled and tested as soon as possible after venepuncture. The use and interpretation of cholinesterase results are discussed further in a later section on monitoring pesticide-exposed workers. The evaluation of persistent neuropsychologic complaints after overexposure to organophosphates includes neurologic and neurobehavioral testing.[11,12,39]

Treatment

In addition to measures taken for all pesticide-intoxicated patients, the specific initial treatment of poisoning is the same for N-methyl carbamates and for organophosphates. The mainstay of treatment is atropine sulfate, which may be administered intravenously or intramuscularly. In mild to moderately severe poisoning, 1 mg is often enough to control symptoms, but may require further doses. The patient should be re-evaluated before each administration. Atropine toxicity (flushed, hot and dry skin, fever, and delirium) is a complication of overzealous treatment of mild cases of poisoning with cholinesterase inhibitors. In general, patients who are ill enough to require pharmacologic treatment (either with atropine or cholinesterase reactivators) should be observed for 12–24 hours after treatment.

Treatment temporarily may mask the symptoms as further absorption occurs or as insecticides are mobilized from temporary deposition in the fat stores.[44] In more severe poisoning, an initial dose of atropine sulfate (2.0 mg in adults or 0.05 mg/kg in children younger than 12 years old) should be administered. Treatment may be repeated at 10–15-minute intervals or titrated by an intravenous drip to achieve adequate atropinization (pulse 140/minute, mydriasis, and dry axillae).[33,45] A decreasing level of rales in the pulmonary fields is reported to be a useful crude guide to the efficacy of treatment. If necessary, tachycardia may be controlled with small doses of propranolol (Inderal). In one severely poisoned patient, 31 g of atropine sulfate were administered (during a 5-week period).

The pulmonary system fails first in fatal poisonings. Respiratory failure is multifactorial due to bronchorrhea resulting in airway compromise; stimulation of smooth muscle resulting in bronchospasm; cholinergic blockade of skeletal muscle resulting in diaphragmatic paralysis; and depression of respiratory centers. In patients requiring mechanical ventilation, frequent suctioning of copious pulmonary secretions is fundamental for effective treatment.

Atropine sulfate acts by blocking the postsynaptic receptors for acetylcholine. Another important treatment modality for organophosphate insecticide poisoning (but not for N-methyl carbamate poisoning) is the reactivation of acetylcholinesterase, for example, with pralidoxime (Protopam, 2-PAM; Fig. 48.2). Because atropine does not antagonize the nicotinic effects of acetylcholine on skeletal muscle, cholinesterase reactivation is critical in the treatment of respiratory muscle paralysis. In addition, oxime reactivators and atropine may each potentiate synergistically the therapeutic effect of the other. Treatment with 1 g of 2-PAM intravenously (in 5% glucose over several minutes; 20–50 mg/kg in children younger than age 12 years) can be repeated in 1 hour, if necessary. The half-life of pralidoxime is 0.9 hours in humans. Administration should be discontinued in cases of dangerous increases in blood pressure. Administration at a rate greater than 500 mg/minute can cause weakness, visual blurring, diplopia, dizziness, headache, tachycardia, and nausea. In one severe poisoning, 92 g was given over 23 days. However, because the acetylcholinesterase-phosphoryl bond strengthens (ages) with the loss of an additional alkyl group with time, treatment with 2-PAM is more effective the earlier it is given and, in some cases, becomes ineffective after 36–48 hours from the onset of poisoning. Blood should be drawn for the assay of cholinesterase activity before treatment with cholinesterase reactivators. Diazepam or barbiturates may be useful, but should be used with caution to manage seizures caused by cholinesterase inhibitors. The cause of seizures is often anoxia, and the delivery of oxygen to tissues should be a priority in treatment. Drugs that are contraindicated in the treatment of cholinesterase inhibitors include morphine, phenothiazines, reserpine, and theophylline.

Glycopyrolate, a potential substitute for atropine, has been under study in organophosphate pesticide poisonings. There may be some advantages such as reduced respiratory infections, but relatively little information is presently available in peer-reviewed journals.[33]

Because mild or subclinical cases of OPIDP following severe cholinergic poisoning may be much more common than previously suspected, patients poisoned with these or structurally similar organophosphates (Fig. 48.3) deserve a careful clinical evaluation of symptoms, motor strength, and vibration threshold. Electrophysiologic study of sensory amplitudes and muscle action potentials is indicated if the symptoms or examination suggest neuropathy. Rehabilitative treatment may be helpful, but there is no specific antidotal treatment to OPIDP.

Treatment of poisoning with N-methyl carbamates

Carbamate insecticides are reversible inhibitors of cholinesterase, and aggressive treatment with atropine will support life as the N-methyl carbamate is gradually metabolized and excreted. Even life-threatening cases generally recover within 12 hours. Cholinesterase reactivators, such as 2-PAM, generally are ineffective or only marginally effective in the treatment of N-methyl carbamate-poisoned patients. In animals, oxime reactivators have been shown to potentiate the toxicity of one N-methyl carbamate, carbaryl. Therefore, 2-PAM is not indicated in the treatment of N-methyl carbamate poisoning. However, if an organophosphate may also have been involved in a severe poisoning or if doubt exists as to whether an organophosphate or N-methyl carbamate caused the poisoning, 2-PAM should be administered, with the primary objective being to avoid respiratory paralysis from organophosphate poisoning.

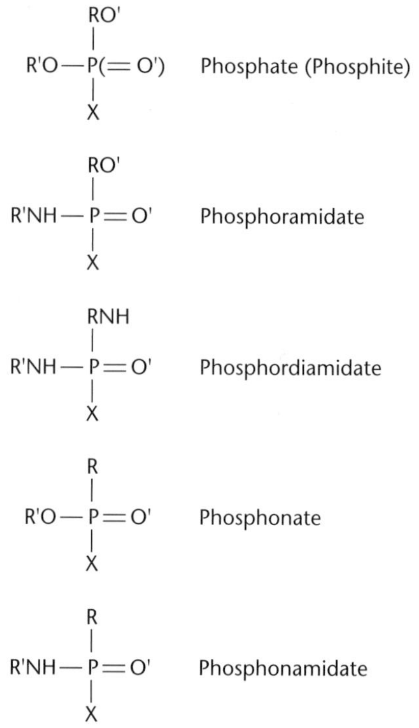

Figure 48.3: Organophosphates that have been associated with neurotoxicity. (From: Raffle P, Lee W, McCallum R, Murray R, eds. Hunter's diseases of occupations. Boston: Little, Brown, and Company, 1988.)

Pyrethrum and pyrethroids

Cismethrin (3)
Cypermethrin (2)
Cyfluthrin (2)
Deltamethrin (4)
Fenvalerate (2)
Flucythrinate (1)
Fluvalinate (2)
Pyrethrin (3)
Resmethrin (3)

In the mid-1800s, pyrethrum extracts of chrysanthemum flowers (containing pyrethrin and other active ingredients) were found to be effective insecticides. Although they are absorbed across the gut and through the lungs, they are minimally absorbed across intact skin, and they are relatively less toxic than other commonly used insecticides. Pyrethrum may cause asthma or allergic rhinitis, and contact dermatitis is frequent through allergic mechanisms. The mainstay of treatment for these conditions is avoidance of exposure. Acute allergic rhinitis may be treated with antihistamines, and severe asthmatic reactions should be treated similarly to asthma of other causes, and through strict avoidance of further exposures.

The many synthetic pyrethroid insecticides, which are closely related chemically to the naturally occurring pyrethrins, are more stable in the natural environment and are used in agriculture and in household pest control, although toxicity to non-target aquatic and terrestrial invertebrates is high. Ingestion of large doses of pyrethroids causes salivation, nausea, vomiting, diarrhea, irritability, tremor, inco-ordination, seizures, and death. Toxicity is thought to be mediated through functional changes in sodium channels. Treatment of acute poisoning is non-specific and supportive, including administration of activated charcoal and a cathartic following gastric aspiration and lavage.

Allergic responses to synthetic pyrethroids are uncommon. However, a high proportion of exposed workers report annoying itching and tingling of exposed skin, especially of the face, without visible inflammatory response. Symptoms resolve slowly (within 1 day) after exposure is discontinued. The mechanism of this seemingly local neurotoxic effect is not well understood, but application of vitamin E oil prior to exposure may be preventive. Caution should be taken to avoid eye contact, especially with fluvalinate, which is corrosive as formulated. Prolonged flushing of contaminated eyes with water or saline should be followed by referral to an ophthalmologist.

Organochlorine insecticides

Cyclodienes
Aldrin (1)
Chlordane (2)
Dieldrin (1)
Endosulfan (1)
Endrin (1)
Heptachlor (2)
Chlordecone (4)
DDT (2)
Lindane (Kwell) (2)
Toxaphene (1 or 2)

Many of these chemically diverse insecticides have been banned or restricted in the developed world because they persist in the environment and concentrate in the food chain, damaging wildlife. Fat levels of DDT in human surveys have decreased markedly since DDT was banned in the United States in 1973. In the developing world, DDT (for vector control in malaria-endemic areas) and toxaphene (in cotton cultivation) are still used, though movements to restrict the use of these persistent organic pollutants have had some effect at limiting their use in some countries (see Chapter 45). High concentrations of DDT in the fat and milk from humans and cows continue to be found in developing countries. Chlordane was, until recently, the agent of choice for termite control in most of the United States, and lindane still is used widely as an ectoparasiticide. Endosulfan is still registered and used in the US. Interestingly, the new pesticide fipronil has a similar but much more potent effect on the GABA receptor than do lindane, dieldrin, and endosulfan. The relative safety of the chemical appears to be due to its greater specificity for insect GABA A receptors than for those in mammals.[46,47]

Acute effects

Dermal absorption of the cyclodienes, chlordecone, and lindane is good. Because acute toxicity is high for chlorde-

cone, endrin, aldrin, and dieldrin, these account for most occupational poisonings. Most other acute poisonings result from ingestion. Acute toxicity reflects influence on neuronal membrane stability through interaction with either sodium channels or GABA receptors, resulting in hyperactivity in the central nervous system. Sudden seizures (especially from aldrin, dieldrin, endrin, lindane, and toxaphene) may occur up to 48 hours after exposure, and may be relatively intractable. Headache, nausea, dizziness, inco-ordination, confusion, tremor, and paresthesias are common. Tremor is characteristic of poisoning with DDT and chlordecone. Abnormal liver enzyme levels and renal tubular abnormalities may be seen.

Chronic effects

A very important historic event related to pesticide overexposure was epidemic occupational chlordecone (Kepone) poisoning in a manufacturing facility, characterized by anxiety, tremor, opsoclonus, personality changes, pleuritic and joint pains, weight loss, liver disease, and oligospermia. Indirect exposure was an important factor, with two family members of workers also poisoned by contaminated work clothes. A portion of the Chesapeake Bay in the United States was polluted by discharge from the plant. Almost all organochlorine insecticides have been found to be carcinogenic in at least one species of rodent. Idiosyncratic cases of aplastic anemia have been reported anecdotally in association with exposure to organochlorines, especially to chlordane and lindane.

Evaluation and treatment

The diagnosis of acute poisoning is made by a history of exposure in the appropriate clinical setting. Although the tests are not routinely available, organochlorines and their metabolites may be found in the blood or in fat. Treatment is supportive. Diazepam 5–10 mg by slow intravenous injection may be repeated at 10–15-minute intervals up to a total dose of 30 mg for the control of intractable seizures. Pentobarbital (100 mg by slow intravenous administration) is useful, not only for controlling seizures but also because it induces hepatic enzymes that may accelerate the metabolism of organochlorines. Additional doses may be given up to 500 mg. In studies of animals poisoned by aldrin and dieldrin, doses of pentobarbital that would otherwise cause anesthesia (20 mg/kg in dogs followed by 5 mg/kg twice daily) were required for periods of more than 2 weeks to control intractable seizures. Atropine and adrenergic amines are contraindicated because the organochlorines may potentiate myocardial irritability. Cholestyramine (Questran) was found to be effective in increasing elimination and ameliorating hepatic effects in chlordecone-poisoned patients. It has been recommended for treatment of poisoning by other organochlorines.

ANTICOAGULANT RODENTICIDES

Brodifacoum (1)
Diphacinone (1)
Warfarin (1, 2, or 3)

Since the synthesis of dicumarol in 1940, non-intentional ingestion of related anticoagulant baits has been common among children. Occupational poisoning by dermally absorbed warfarin has been reported. Some coumarin derivatives are used in medicine for the treatment of thrombo-embolic disease.

Acute effects

Increased capillary permeability and the antagonism of hepatic synthesis of vitamin K-dependent clotting factors II, VII, IX, and X produce bleeding gums and nose, ecchymoses, hematuria, and melena. Some, but not all, anticoagulant rodenticides produce diarrhea, small intestinal necrosis, urticaria, dermatitis, leukopenia, alopecia, and abnormal liver enzymes.

Evaluation and treatment

Diagnosis in the appropriate clinical setting is confirmed by an increased prothrombin time, which reaches a maximum 36–72 hours after ingestion. Treatment with the naturally occurring form of vitamin K_1 (phytonadione [aquamephyton]) is preferred. If ingestion is doubtful, the treatment may be oral, i.e., 15–25 mg (5–10 mg in children younger than 12 years old). If more than 1 mg/kg of coumarin or its related anticoagulant is ingested, vomiting should be induced with syrup of ipecac (within the first few hours, as bleeding may later become a complication of vomiting), or the stomach should undergo lavage. Treatment with vitamin K_1 5–10 mg intramuscularly (1–5 mg if younger than 12 years) is provided and repeated after 24 hours if the prothrombin time remains increased. If there is evidence of bleeding, phytonadione (in dextrose or saline) may be administered intravenously over 20 minutes (up to 10 mg; 5 mg if younger than 12 years old). If the bleeding is severe, treatment with fresh blood may be required. Prothrombin time and hemoglobin level should be monitored every 6–12 hours. Patients receiving intravenous vitamin K_1 should be monitored carefully, and treatment discontinued in the case of dyspnea, dizziness, flushing, decreased blood pressure, or cyanosis. Poisonings with diphacinone and brodifacoum may require larger doses of vitamin K_1 for more prolonged periods.

HERBICIDES

Alachlor (3)
Atrazine (3)
2,4-D (1 or 3)
2,4,5-T (3)
Butylate (3)
Cyanazine (2 or 3)
Glyphosate (2)
Metolachlor (3)
Metribuzin (3)
Paraquat (diquat) (2)
Trifluralin (3 or 4)

A broad and extensively used group of chemicals, herbicides include some chemicals with well-understood mechanisms of toxicity and others about which little is known. With some exceptions, most herbicides are generally of low acute toxicity. Herbicides make up the largest portion of the pesticidal chemicals used in the US. Some herbicides are important ground water contaminants and are animal carcinogens, including, for example, alachlor and atrazine.

Bipyridils (diquat and paraquat)

Among the most acutely toxic of the herbicidal chemicals is the bipyridil herbicide paraquat (Fig. 48.4). This extremely effective contact herbicide is widely used in both developing and developed countries. It is a restricted-use pesticide in the US. As a non-selective herbicide, paraquat is a desiccant and defoliant, and is widely used for control of broadleaf weeds and grasses. It is generally distributed as a liquid (e.g., 20% concentrate), and can be applied by aerial, tractor-based or backpack applications. Paraquat is sold under many trade names, sometimes combined with another bipyridil, diquat.

Paraquat has extremely low volatility with a slight amine-like odor. It is very soluble in water and poorly soluble in lipids. It is quickly destroyed by ultraviolet light. It does not generally leach from soil into ground water, as it binds quickly to or reacts with soil constituents.

The minimum lethal dose for human beings is thought to be approximately 35 mg/kg for paraquat. It has been involved in occupational and, more commonly, non-occupational self-induced deaths.[18,48] In Japan, where intentional ingestion is common, there are 2000 deaths each year attributable to paraquat. Occupational systemic poisoning in the United States is uncommon, but data from the Agricultural Health Study indicate that paraquat may be among several pesticides contributing to respiratory symptoms in farmers.[49] Severe occupational poisonings are rare in the US, but have been reported in Central America.[48] Dermal contact is an important exposure route.

Acute effects

Skin and ocular burns from splashes of the concentrate are among the most common consequences of overexposure to paraquat. A somewhat unique outcome among workers is loss of fingernails. Epistaxis is also reported among workers using the chemical. Painful burns and bleeding of the

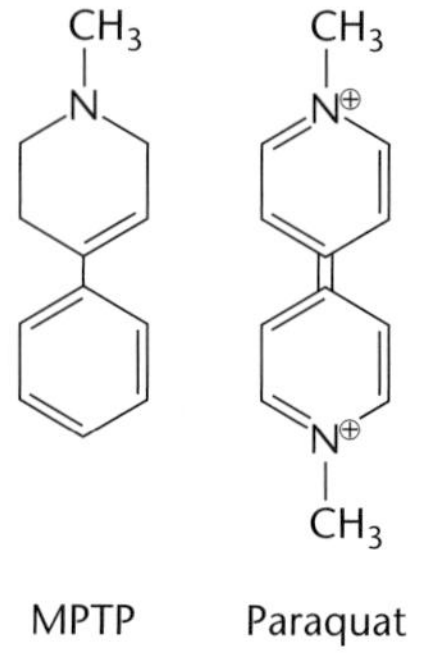

MPTP   Paraquat

Figure 48.4: Chemical structures of MPTP and paraquat.

gastrointestinal tract are common with ingestion. Approximately 20% of ingested paraquat is absorbed systemically, where it may cause acute hepatic necrosis and renal failure. Paraquat is concentrated from the systemic circulation into the lungs, where prominent pulmonary injury may occur; pulmonary edema may develop 2–4 days following ingestion, leading to pulmonary fibrosis in survivors.[50] Pneumothorax and pneumomediastinum are also common in the acute exposure setting.[51] Damage to muscle, including myocardium, and to the central nervous system have been reported. The mortality rate is greater than 50% in most case series of suicidal ingestion.

Paraquat is not well absorbed from intact skin; however, damaged skin is much more permeable to paraquat.[52] There are several reports of fatal paraquat poisoning caused by dermal absorption.[27] The lethal dose in 50% of rabbits repeatedly dermally dosed is only 4.5 mg/kg/day under occlusion. Occupational poisoning resulting from dermal absorption is more likely to occur in developing countries, where applicators may carry and mix concentrated paraquat in leaky backpack sprayers.

Chronic effects

Pulmonary fibrosis has been reported among survivors of paraquat poisoning.[53] Paraquat is structurally similar to 1-methyl-4-phenyl-1,2,3,6-tetrahydropyridine (MPTP), an illicit drug that caused an outbreak of acute-onset Parkinson's disease. Although it has been argued that paraquat does not cross the blood–brain barrier, ecologic studies and one case-control study suggest an association between herbicide exposure and Parkinson's disease.[54] In contrast, animal studies have failed to demonstrate a connection between paraquat and parkinsonism.

Evaluation and treatment

Contaminated skin should be washed thoroughly. Subsequent avoidance of exposure will usually result in resolution of rash and damage to the nails. If paraquat is splashed on to the eyes, they should be irrigated thoroughly with clean water, with referral to an ophthalmologist.

Paraquat absorption may be confirmed at the bedside by observing the colorimetric urinary reaction with sodium dithionite, performed by mixing the urine 2:1 with freshly prepared 1% sodium hydrosulfate in 1 N sodium hydroxide. Development of a blue color over a 60-second period indicates paraquat in excess of 0.5 mg/liter. The diagnosis should be confirmed by measuring plasma paraquat levels, which have been found to be useful prognostically in identifying those individuals likely to survive after ingestion. Those with plasma concentrations at 4, 6, 10, 16, and 24 hours after ingestion that are less than 2, 6, 0.3, 0.16, and 0.1 mg/liter, respectively, were likely to survive.

Unfortunately, there is no adequate specific antidote for paraquat poisoning. If paraquat ingestion is suspected, the stomach should be lavaged immediately with a slurry of Fuller's earth (100–150 g in 30% suspension; 2 g/kg in children). Lavage should be repeated every 2–4 hours until the slurry appears in the stool. A cathartic should be administered, unless intestinal ileus (a common complication of

poisoning) is present. Diuresis with isotonic saline, Ringer's solution, and 5% glucose in water is indicated to promote the excretion of paraquat and to correct dehydration and electrolyte imbalances, as long as the urinary output is adequate. Because paraquat-induced pulmonary toxicity is thought to arise from the generation of free radicals, which is enhanced by high oxygen concentrations, oxygen use should be minimized to the amount necessary to correct hypoxemia. One case report describes complete recovery from a combined paraquat-diquat ingestion with therapy including forced diuresis, hemofiltration with n-acetylcysteine, methylprednisolone, cyclophosphamide, vitamin E, cholchicine, and delayed continuous nitric oxide inhalation.[55]

Diquat

Poisoning with diquat is less common and generally less lethal than paraquat. The clinical presentation is similar to that of paraquat poisoning, except that central nervous system symptoms are more likely, including disorientation, psychotic behavior, and seizures. Renal failure is more prominent, as diquat does not concentrate in the lungs, with less severe pulmonary injury. Management is similar to that for paraquat poisoning.

Chlorophenoxy herbicides

2,4-D
2,4-DP,
2,4-DB,
2,4,5-T,
MCPA
Polychlorinated dibenzo-dioxins (PCDD) contaminants

Chlorophenoxy herbicides have been used widely in the United States and elsewhere against broad-leaved plants. During the American involvement in the Vietnam War, 2,4-D and 2,4,5-T were applied together for deforestation in a formulation known as Agent Orange. Chlorophenoxy herbicides are absorbed dermally, by inhalation, and by ingestion. Symptoms of irritant effects on the skin and mucous membranes are common. While acute systemic toxicity is generally low, after ingestion of large doses multiple organ systems may be affected, with resulting nausea, vomiting, diarrhea, myotonia, fever, confusion, leukocytosis, abnormal liver enzyme levels, elevated creatinine phosphokinase concentrations, myoglobinuria, T-wave flattening and inversion, and coma in severe poisonings. Treatment includes decontamination and forced alkaline diuresis with intravenous saline and dextrose with 44–88 mEq of sodium bicarbonate per liter, to maintain the urine pH at 7.6–8.8. Renal function and fluid balance should be carefully monitored. Heavy exposure to 2,4-D has been reported to cause peripheral neuropathy. In case-control studies, a history of exposure to 2,4-D has been associated epidemiologically with non-Hodgkin's lymphoma.

The chemical 2,4,5-T, which is no longer marketed in many of the industrialized countries, is contaminated with PCDD, of which the most toxic is 2,3,7,8-tetrachloro-dibenzodioxin (TCDD). TCDD bioaccumulates, and most of the low-level body burden for the general population comes from food, especially, fish, meat, and dairy products. In workers chronically and heavily exposed to TCDD, an increased overall incidence of cancer has been observed. The largest published cohort study of heavily exposed workers demonstrated an association between 2,4,5-T exposures and non-Hodgkin's lymphoma and soft tissue sarcoma – associations previously seen in some case-control studies. In animals, there are great differences in the interspecies toxicity of TCDD. In some animals, TCDD is an exceedingly potent carcinogen and teratogen, with acute hepatotoxic, immunotoxic, peripheral neuropathic, hematopoietic, and dermal effects. In accidents in which people have been highly exposed, TCDD has been reported in clinical series to be associated with chloracne, porphyria cutanea tarda, hepatic and renal disease, peripheral neuropathy, increased lipid levels, and possible accelerated atherosclerosis and neuropsychiatric disease.

The hallmark of TCDD exposure is the pale, small cyst characteristic of chloracne. However, among populations with environmental exposure to TCDD, such as veterans of the Vietnam War, individuals exposed to industrial waste in Seveso (Italy), Niagara Falls (New York), and Newark (New Jersey) or to TCDD-contaminated waste oil applied for dust control at Times Beach and other sites in Missouri, chloracne has been relatively uncommon. In epidemiologic studies of environmentally and occupationally exposed populations, subclinical depression of cell-mediated immunity, elevation of liver enzyme levels, and subclinical evidence for peripheral neuropathy have been observed variably.

Current or previous exposure to TCDD should be considered in the differential diagnosis of lesions compatible with chloracne, non-Hodgkin's lymphoma, and soft tissue sarcoma. If there is reason to suspect exposure to TCDD in these clinical settings, serum or adipose TCDD levels, although expensive, may be useful in helping to establish prior exposure. The mean half-life of TCDD in adipose tissue is approximately 7 years, and generally does not to exceed 15–20 parts per trillion in the general population.

The Veterans Administration has adopted regulations to compensate veterans exposed to Agent Orange during the Vietnam War for soft tissue sarcoma, non-Hodgkin's lymphoma, Hodgkin's disease, respiratory cancers, chloracne, peripheral neuropathy, and Type 2 diabetes.

Nitroaromatic herbicides

This group includes nitrophenolic and nitrocresol chemicals. These agents are used as herbicides, nematocides, insecticides, and fungicides. Now rarely used in the US, these chemicals are still used internationally and continue to contaminate surface water wells in agricultural areas. They are absorbed efficiently dermally, through the lung (if droplets are inhaled), or orally. A unique yellow discoloration to contaminated skin and fingernails may result from contact with these chemicals. With LD_{50s} in the 25–50 mg/kg range, they are highly toxic. These chemicals uncouple oxidative phosphorylation resulting in hyperthermia, tachycardia, fatigue, and, if sufficiently severe, death. Tissues with high metabolic needs such as liver, kidneys, nervous and reproductive systems are the most susceptible tissues. These chemicals are detectable in urine and serum by gas chromatographic methods. The fat solubility of these chemicals may assist in the diagnosis, as their elimination half-life is as long as 14 days. Treatment is directed at reducing hyperthermia and providing supportive care. Use of salicylates may paradoxically worsen hyperthermia, as they too uncouple oxidative phosphorylation. Atropine can worsen tachycardia. Decontamination is very important, and as with other highly toxic chemicals, caution should be exercised to avoid healthcare provider bystander exposure.[33]

Other herbicides

Dormex is a herbicide that contains hydrogen cyanide. Overexposure has lead to skin manifestations that include pruritic, erythematous, macular, or papular rashes. Skin burns have been reported. Other symptoms are related to systemic metabolic effects and include tachycardia, weakness, palpitations, headache, dizziness, vomiting and/or nausea, dyspnea, and hypotension.[56]

FUNGICIDES

Ferbam (4)
Hexachlorobenzene (4)
Mancozeb (4)
Maneb (4)
Methyl mercury
Pentachlorophenol (2)
Thiram (3)
Zineb (4)
Ziram (3)

Fungicides applied to seeds, crops, and gardens encompass a wide variety of chemical classes, including copper, cadmium, organomercury and organotin compounds, substituted benzenes, dithiocarbamates, thiophthalimides, and others. Acute toxicity is related to dose. In general, there is no specific antidotes for poisoning with these compounds. Supportive measures are described in the section on the general approach to the pesticide-exposed patient.

The dimethyldithiocarbamates ziram, ferbam, and thiram inhibit acetaldehyde dehydrogenase and have a disulfiram (Antabuse) effect. There have been reports of illness consistent with disulfiram reactions (nausea, vomiting, headache, diaphoresis, thirst, chest pain, and vertigo) among thiram-exposed workers who subsequently consumed alcohol-containing beverages. Ziram and ferbam are irritants; hemolysis has been reported in one case of ziram poisoning. All dithiocarbamates are metabolized to carbon disulfide, which may explain similarities in the symptoms of poisoning. Following ingestion, poisoning by thiram has been reported to cause nausea, headache, tremor, encephalopathy, hepatic and renal injury, and peripheral neuropathy. Treatment is supportive. Syrup of ipecac is contraindicated in the treatment of dithiocarbamate poisoning as it may contain ethanol.

The ethylene-bis-dithiocarbamates (maneb, mancozeb, and zineb) are metabolized to ethylene thiourea, a potent animal carcinogen. This metabolite may also account for the antithyroid effects that occur in animals exposed to these compounds. Ethylene thiourea may concentrate on cooked food previously treated with ethylene-bis-dithiocarbamates. Maneb is of interest because it contains manganese, which can produce a condition similar to Parkinson's disease. In one study of maneb-exposed workers in Brazil, movement disorders were reported suggestive of preclinical Parkinson's disease. Hemolytic anemia was reported in a worker with glucose-6-phosphate dehydrogenase deficiency exposed to zineb. Treatment includes decontamination and supportive care.

Although little used currently in the United States, alkyl mercury has resulted in occupational poisoning in seed treating facilities, and in epidemics of catastrophic fetotoxicity among peasants who consumed treated seed grain or meat from animals that had consumed this grain. Alkyl mercury compounds are absorbed from the gut and skin. Methyl mercury is volatile, and may be inhaled. Acute poisoning is manifested by headache, metallic taste, paresthesias, tremor, inco-ordination, slurred speech, constricted visual fields, hearing loss, loss of position sense, and spasticity. Among survivors, permanent neurologic effects are common. Decontamination is essential, and treatment of acute poisoning with D-penicillamine (Cuprimine, 0.5 g every 6 hours before meals and at bedtime for 5 days) may reduce the biologic half-life.

Consumption of hexachlorobenzene-treated seed grain in Turkey in the 1950s resulted in an epidemic of thousands of cases of poisoning that resembled porphyria cutanea tarda. Hexachlorobenzene is a potent inhibitor of uroporphyrinogen decarboxylase, resulting in increases in photosensitive porphyrins. Chronic bullous dermatitis, liver damage, hypertrichosis, and arthritis occurred in many exposed individuals. Acutely, hexachlorobenzene levels can be measured in blood, and metabolites can be measured in urine. Significantly elevated 24-hour urine concentrations of uro- and coproporphyrins in the appropriate clinical setting are diagnostic of porphyria cutanea tarda. Cholestyramine (3–8 g before each meal and at bedtime) has been recommended to accelerate elimination by interrupting the enterohepatic circulation of porphyrin metabolites in individuals with high levels in their tissues. Exposure to sunlight should be avoided in individuals with porphyria cutanea tarda.

Pentachlorophenol, used as a wood preservative, is well absorbed through the skin, and numerous occupational deaths have occurred from hyperthermia resulting from uncoupling of oxidative phosphorylation (similar to the nitroaromatics described above). Clinical features include fever, thirst, sweating, weakness, tachycardia and other arrhythmias, and tachypnea. Restlessness, anxiety, and dizziness reflect injury to the central nervous system. Albuminuria, glycosuria, azotemia, hepatomegaly, and elevated transaminase and alkaline phosphatase levels may be seen. Diagnosis is based on consistent clinical findings in the setting of exposure. Symptoms typically do not occur if the pentachlorophenol level in the serum or urine is less than 1 ppm. Treatment is directed toward reducing the body temperature, e.g., cooling blankets, cooling baths, and cold fluids by mouth. Salicylates are contraindicated, and other antipyretics are ineffective. Benzodiazepines may be used to control agitation. Fluid replacement is an important aspect of therapy given substantial insensible volume loss. Pentachlorophenol is contaminated with TCDD and other PCDDs; the chronic effects of pentachlorophenol exposure may result from PCDDs, especially hexachlorinated dioxin contaminants (see above, and Chapter 45). Aplastic anemia has been reported anecdotally in association with pentachlorophenol exposure. Elevated serum and urinary pentachlorophenol levels have been found in residents of log homes built with logs dipped in the pesticide.

FUMIGANTS AND NEMATOCIDES

Acrolein
Chloropicrin (2*, 0.1)
Dibromochloropropane (DBCP) (2, 0.01)
Dichlorobenzene (2, 75)
Dichloropropane (3, 75)
Dichloropropene (3, 1)
Ethylene dibromide (2, A2)
Ethylene oxide
Formaldehyde (0.1†, A2)
Methyl bromide (2,5)
Para-phostoxin (1, 0.3‡)
Sulfuryl fluoride (1,5)

Among the most acutely toxic of the pesticides are the chemicals used for fumigation. This application involves a chemical designed to permeate into otherwise unreachable spaces. Fumigants are generally non-specific toxicants selected to sterilize a space, object, or substance of a wide array of potential pests. The very non-specific nature of the biologic effects contributes to the collective hazard of these chemicals. Many chemicals have been used in the past as fumigants including oxides of sulfur, cyanides, chlorinated and other volatile solvents. The health effects of these chemicals are covered elsewhere in this book. Chemicals used widely as fumigants such as phosphine gas, methyl-bromide, dibromochloropropene, and 1,3-dichloropropene will be addressed in this section. Exposure is usually through inhalation, though exposure to liquid preparations during mixing and handling also occurs; ingestion of certain fumigant chemicals (particularly aluminum phosphide) is common in suicides in certain developing countries.

Grain may be fumigated by mixing with granulated fumigant compounds such as aluminum phosphide. The chemical reacts with the moisture in the grain, causing release of phosphine gas. A building may be fumigated by releasing or pumping fumigant into interior spaces after

---

*EPA toxicity category (described in Table 48.1) followed by threshold limit value (in parts per million); A2 indicates suspected human carcinogen.
†Threshold limit value.
‡Threshold limit value for phosphine.

sealing the entire structure in plastic or a tarp. Overexposure may occur during the venting or opening of buildings (e.g., grain storage facilities). Diffusion of residual fumigant from closed wall spaces has resulted in overexposure within fumigated living structures. Fumigants have caused problems by diffusing through previously unrecognized conduits into inhabited spaces distant from the fumigated area. Several halogenated hydrocarbon fumigants are suspected or proven animal carcinogens.

Aluminum phosphide ($AlPO_4$) is a fumigant that breaks down into phosphine and aluminum salts when combined with water. Phosphine is volatile and represents the fumigant moiety. $AlPO_4$ is either directly exposed to water by the user, or left in closed spaces to react with ambient moisture, gradually off-gassing phosphine. An example of this is the use of $AlPO_4$ in stored grain fumigation. $AlPO_4$ is also used for rodent control in the west, where it is inserted into rodent or mole burrows which are then sealed closed. Exposure to $AlPO_4$ generally occurs through inhalation. The odor threshold is between 0.02 and 3 ppm, with an odor described as that of rotten fish.

Methyl bromide is a fumigant gas that occurs naturally at very low levels, particularly near salt water, and in high concentrations is an effective soil sterilant. It is still used widely in California for nematode control in strawberry production. In California alone, some 16 million pounds of the gas were applied to the soil in 1997. The compound is also used for structural fumigation and has resulted in intoxications among people residing in fumigated buildings.

Acrolein is a colorless gas at room temperature. It has a pungent odor and is used as an algicide and aquatic herbicide. It reacts with sulfhydryl groups on enzymes interfering with enzymatic function. It is a prominent respiratory irritant and recognized asthmagen, and has an oral LD_{50} of 29 mg/kg in rodents.

Chloropicrin, developed as a lacrimating 'tear gas' agent in World War I, has found use as an insecticide and nematocide; the potent irritant qualities also act as a warning agent for less irritating, but more toxic, agents. It is thus often mixed with other fumigants to increase warning characteristics. It finds some use in the control of wood fungi.

Dibromochloropropane is a nematocide that is no longer registered in the US. It was formerly widely used in pineapple and banana production where it was applied through direct injection into the soil or through irrigated routes. It is a potent reproductive toxin causing direct damage to testicular tissues and has been associated with male infertility in many developing countries.

Acute effects

Mucous membrane and respiratory tract irritation are common with exposure to many of the fumigants. Chloropicrin and other irritants or odorants may be added to fumigants as warning agents. Several fumigants may be toxic at levels below odor threshold concentrations, resulting in overexposure without recognition of the chemical by those exposed.

The acute symptoms of occupational overexposure to phosphine are generally respiratory, and include acute chest discomfort with substernal burning, shortness of breath, chest tightness, as well as palpitations. Gastrointestinal symptoms are not uncommon, with diarrhea, nausea, abdominal pain, and vomiting. Central nervous system symptoms include headache, dizziness, and unstable gait. No specific diagnostic tests are available, and aluminum levels are not elevated in phosphine gas exposure. Abnormalities in liver enzymes and renal function parameters are reported. Phosphine is a poorly soluble gas and is thereby able to penetrate deeply into the lung without reacting with moisture in upper respiratory tract mucous membranes. This results in the potential for late-onset pulmonary edema and thus warrants close observation with hospitalization or prompt follow-up visit (including chest radiograph) within 24–48 hours of exposure.

Methyl bromide has a slightly sweet but barely noticeable odor, and is only moderately irritating, which makes it particularly dangerous. Overexposure causes respiratory irritation, pulmonary edema, anorexia, nausea, vomiting, headache, visual disturbances, agitation, dizziness, tremor, inco-ordination, myoclonus, and muscle weakness. Liquid methyl bromide can cause severe skin burns with substantial systemic absorption. Chloropicrin, which is intensely irritating, is added to methyl bromide formulations to warn applicators of overexposure. Due to its use as a structural fumigant in poorly ventilated indoor spaces, and its physical property of being heavier than air, it has been the cause of death and injury to people entering such structures, and from seepage through sewer systems into adjacent structures. In one case, accumulation of methyl bromide resulted in death and illness among infants.[57,58] Intoxication has also been reported during untarping of fumigated soil, a common activity in areas where soil fumigation is performed with methyl bromide.[59]

Aluminum phosphide (phostoxin), magnesium phosphide, and zinc phosphide slowly release phosphine gas; the release is more rapid in a moist environment. Phosphine is a mucous membrane and respiratory irritant that produces nausea, vomiting, diarrhea, headache, vertigo, fatigue, paresthesias, cough, dyspnea, chest tightness, and pulmonary edema. Renal, hepatic, cardiac, and central nervous system toxicity are common. Patients may smell of rotten fish or garlic. Deaths have occurred among individuals living near recently fumigated granaries or as a result of early re-entry into fumigated structures.

DBCP is irritating to skin and mucous membranes, and if absorbed in sufficient quantities can cause renal and liver damage. Acute high-level exposure may present with headache, nausea and vomiting, ataxia and slurred speech.

The nematocide dichloropropene (DCP) has an odor threshold between 1 and 4 ppm and an LC_{50} of between 855 and 1035 ppm in animal studies. Acute high-level overexposure results in liver, kidney, and lung injury in rats. A human fatality with DCP has been reported. DCP is both irritating and sensitizing to the skin and mucous membranes. Respiratory and mucous membrane irritation, headache, malaise, abdominal pain, and elevated hepatic transaminase levels were reported among persons who inhaled dichloropropene spilled in a highway accident.

Follow-up of exposed individuals documented altered personality, persistent headache and chest pain 2 years after the incident. Studies of dichloropropene have been inadequate to evaluate its carcinogenic effects, and it appears not to have the spermatotoxic effects of DBCP.

Chronic effects

Survivors of acute poisoning with methyl bromide may be left with residual organic brain damage, seizures, and personality changes. Ethylene dibromide is a potent animal carcinogen and a human spermatotoxin, and is no longer used in the United States. As early as 1961, published studies of rodents showed that DBCP caused diminished sperm counts and testicular atrophy. In 1977, almost half of a group of poorly protected production workers exposed to DBCP were demonstrated to be azospermic or oligospermic. Recovery was better among initially oligo- than among azospermic workers. DBCP is an animal carcinogen, and it has been removed from the continental United States market. However, biopersistence in ground water has been a problem, and in some parts of southern California, wells were found to be contaminated with residues as high as 39 parts per billion in 1979, years after the use of DBCP was banned.

Evaluation and treatment

Diagnosis of acute fumigant poisoning is made by consistent history and clinical findings in the setting of exposure to the responsible fumigant. Bromide ion may be elevated in blood and urine in poisonings with methyl bromide. With sulfuryl fluoride poisoning, fluoride may be measurable in blood. In general, treatment of poisoning includes decontamination of the eyes, skin, and gastrointestinal tract; respiratory support, including appropriate treatment of pulmonary edema with severe respiratory injury; and supportive care. Intravenous glucose may help reduce risk for hepatic injury. Dimercaprol (3–5 mg/kg every 6 hours in vegetable oil intramuscularly for four to six doses) has been used to treat poisoning with methyl bromide, although there is little evidence of efficacy.

OTHER REPELLANTS AND PESTICIDES

In the United States, N,N-diethyltoluamide (DEET) is the most commonly used insect repellent. Unlike other pesticides, repellents are purposely applied topically or to clothing by the general public. Severe irritation of the eyes and mucous membranes, and exacerbation of pre-existing skin disease have been reported. Application of formulations with high concentrations (more than 75% active ingredient) in tropical climates has resulted in severe dermatitis in antecubital and popliteal fossae (consistent with atopic reactions). It is rapidly absorbed dermally and by ingestion. Behavioral effects have been demonstrated in chronic feeding studies in rats, and several idiosyncratic cases of encephalopathy and death have been reported among children heavily treated with DEET. In one study of exposed workers, there was an increased prevalence of symptoms associated with impaired cognitive function and sleep disturbances, and a trend toward poorer objectively measured neurobehavioral performance among highly exposed workers. Low-concentration active ingredient formulations of DEET are recommended and should be applied primarily to clothing and boots. Skin application should be kept to a minimum, especially in individuals with pre-existing skin conditions and in children. Quantitative measurements of DEET are only available in specialized laboratories, where absorbed DEET or its metabolites may be measured in the blood or urine. Treatment of acute poisoning includes decontamination and supportive care.

Boric acid has been promoted as an alternative to synthetic organic insecticides (organophosphates, carbamates, and pyrethroids) for cockroach and other insect control. Although the acute toxicity is low with some irritant effects, there have been numerous instances of poisoning from ingestion of boric acid and borates, especially in children. Though poorly absorbed across normal skin, boric acid and borates are well absorbed across damaged or abraded skin. Injury to the gastrointestinal tract, vascular system, and brain has been observed. Nausea, vomiting, diarrhea, tremors, stiff neck, seizures, metabolic acidosis, elevated blood urea nitrogen level, and jaundice have been reported. A beefy red rash with a boiled lobster appearance is characteristic of poisoning. Treatment includes decontamination. Activated charcoal is not helpful in the management of ingestion. Occupational poisoning has not been reported, and no chronic effects have been reported among exposed workers or survivors of acute poisoning.

New pesticides

There has been a new expansion of pesticidal chemicals, that present new challenges to clinicians responsible for caring for exposed subjects. Chemicals affecting biologic systems specific to the pest, such as chitin production in insects, are less likely to produce acute effects in humans. Others, such as the neonicotinoids (e.g., imidacloprid), have direct toxicologic mechanisms relevant to humans. Spinosins, spinosoids, and indoxacarb may activate nicotinic receptors and interact with GABA receptors, but to a lesser degree in mammalian tissues. Chlorfenapyr appears to uncouple oxidative phosphorylation, though human toxicity has not been reported. Fipronil, an insecticide, appears to act through blocking of GABA receptors, similar to but more specifically than lindane and endosulfan. No human intoxications have yet been published. Amitraz is a central α-(2)-agonist, and some human toxicity has been reported with overdoses, with the initial signs and symptoms being altered consciousness, disorientation, vomiting, variable miosis or mydriasis, hypotension, bradycardia, tachypnea, hypothermia, and generalized seizures. Hyperglycemia, glycosuria, and minimal increase in transaminase levels have been observed. CNS depression resolved spontaneously within 4–28 hours in all, with generally a good clinical outcome.[60]

Given that many new chemicals are aimed at physiologic targets with homology in humans, it is likely that reports of human toxicity will emerge, as experience with these agents increases.

INERT INGREDIENTS

Pesticidal active ingredients are only a proportion of most pesticide formulations. In most countries, the rest of the formulation is listed on the label as inert ingredients, i.e., solvents, emulsifiers, spreaders, stickers, penetrants, anticaking agents, and other chemicals used in formulating the pesticide product. Volatile mixtures of aliphatic and aromatic hydrocarbons are the most common inert ingredients. Solvents and anticaking agents added to granulated formulations to prevent clumping, including some methyl naphthalenes, may be skin irritants and photosensitizers. Some hydrocarbon agents used to facilitate the penetration of active ingredients to the interior of plants (penetrants) may be skin and eye irritants. The identity of these ingredients, some of which have acute and chronic (carcinogenic, neurotoxic, or reproductive) systemic toxicities of their own, or may enhance absorption and bioavailability of the active pesticide, is frequently not provided. Many consumer groups have argued that inert ingredients should be identified to the public. Pesticide manufacturers maintain that such information is proprietary. A treating physician can request such information if it is necessary for the care of an exposed patient. The California Department of Food and Agriculture, unlike EPA, registers approximately 100 adjuvant chemicals as pesticides. In the treatment of acute pesticide poisoning, the potential effects of these components should be considered. In particular, tachypnea, cyanosis, tachycardia, hypoxia, and fever may indicate a lipoid pneumonitis from aspiration of petroleum distillates.

DERMATOLOGIC EFFECTS OF PESTICIDES

Dermatitis accounts for approximately one-third of reported pesticide-related illness, although for many more cases (for example, dermatitis in a golfer on a thiram-sprayed green), the cause may go unrecognized. One-half of all skin disease caused by pesticides in California is associated with the following six compounds: propargite, sulfur, glyphosate, methyl bromide, benomyl, and captan (Table 48.6). Many fungicides are skin irritants or sensitizers, especially chlorothalonil, thiram, maneb, zineb, captofol, copper compounds, tributyl, and triphenyl tin compounds, and benomyl. Irritant and allergic dermatoses are common among fungicide-exposed individuals. Although allergic dermatitis is more likely to have a delayed onset following exposure, the clinical features are similar to irritant dermatitis and include erythema, blistering, fissuring, cracking, and lichenification. Patch testing is often necessary to identify allergic dermatitis and to distinguish it from the many other causes of dermatitis in agricultural workers. Because contaminants or inert ingredients may be responsible for dermatitis, it is sometimes useful to test the commercial product in addition to the specific analytic-grade active ingredients. Treatment of contact dermatitis involves protection from exposure, including removal in cases of allergic or recalcitrant contact dermatitis (see Chapter 29.1), and may require moisturizing creams and topical steroids.

Phototoxic dermatitis has been caused by phenothiazine insecticides and by glyphosate. Chloracne and porphyria cutanea tarda associated with PCDDs and hexachlorobenzene are described above.

CARCINOGENIC EFFECTS OF PESTICIDES

Cohort studies of commercial pesticide applicators, who were exposed previously primarily to organochlorines, have

Pesticide	cases	Percent of total	cumulative
Propargite	241	18.7	18.7
Sulfur	195	15.1	33.9
Glyphosate	53	4.1	38.0
Propargite/sulfur	51	4.0	41.9
Methyl bromide	43	3.3	45.3
Benomyl	30	2.3	47.6
Captan	26	2.0	49.6
Petroleum products	24	1.9	51.5
Cyhexatin	21	1.6	53.1
Captan/sulfur	18	1.4	54.5
Dinitrophenol	18	1.4	55.9
Ethylene dibromide	15	1.2	57.1
Paraquat	15	1.2	58.2
Methomyl	13	1.0	59.2
Diazinon	12	0.9	60.2
Ziram	12	0.9	61.1
Captafol	11	0.9	62.0
DD mixture	11	0.9	62.8
Chlorothalonil	10	0.8	63.6
Dicofol	10	0.8	64.4
Captan/DCNA/sulfur	9	0.7	65.1
Acephate	8	0.6	65.7
Carbaryl	8	0.6	66.3
Dichloronitroanaline (DCNA)	8	0.6	66.9
Malathion	8	0.6	67.5
Naled	8	0.6	68.2
Dienochlor	8	0.6	68.8
Triadimefon	8	0.6	69.4
Dimethoate	6	0.5	69.9
Fenbutatin oxide	6	0.5	70.3
Anilazine	5	0.4	70.7
Benomyl/captan	5	0.4	71.1
Maneb	5	0.4	71.5
Simazine	5	0.4	71.9
Metam-sodium	5	0.4	72.3
Zineb	5	0.4	72.7
Other	168	13.0	85.7
Unknown	184	14.3	100.0
Total	1288	100.0	100.0

Reprinted with permission from: O'Malley MA, Mathias CG, Coye MJ. Epidemiology of pesticide related skin disease in California agriculture: 1978–83. In: Dosman J, Cockroft D, eds. Principles of health and safety in agriculture. © 1989 CRC Press, Inc., Boca Raton, FL.

Table 48.6 Pesticides associated with skin disease in agriculture as reported through the California Pesticide Illness Surveillance Program

Exposure	Cancer	Reference
Arsenic	Lung, liver, skin	IARC, 1980[100]
4-Chloro-*o*-toluidine (a metabolite of the pesticide chlordimeform)	Bladder	Stasik, 1988[101]
β-Naphthylamine (a contaminant of the pesticide 1-(1-naphthyl 1)-2-thiourea	Bladder	Hayes and Laws, 1991[95]
2,4-Dichlorophenoxy acetic acid	Non-Hodgkin's lymphoma	Hoar et al, 1986[102]
Paternal pesticide exposure	Acute lymphocytic leukemia	Lowengart et al., 1987[103]
Exposure	**Malformation**	Reference
Warfarin	Nasal hypoplasia	Hayes and Laws, 1991[95]
2,4,5-Trichlorophenoxyacetic acid	Various	Summarized in Lillienfeld and Gallo, 1989[104]
Herbicides	Neural tube defects, cleft palate	Balarajan and McDowell, 1983[105]
Residence in county with heavy use of pesticide	Congenital limb reduction defect	Scwartz and LoGerfo, 1988[106]
Multiple pesticides used in flower cultivation	Hemangioma	Restrepo et al, 1990[107]
Paternal pesticide exposure	Anencephaly	Brender and Suarez, 1990[108]

Table 48.7 Selected studies in which an association has been reported between cancer or congenital malformation and pesticide exposure

demonstrated a small increased risk of lung, bladder, brain, lymphatic, and hematopoietic cancers. In a few case-control studies, exposure to organochlorine insecticides (especially DDT, chlordane, and lindane) has been associated with soft tissue sarcoma, leukemia, and non-Hodgkin's lymphoma, although some workers may have had concomitant exposure to dioxin-contaminated herbicides. Among farm workers there are significant increases in risk for leukemia, stomach cancer, cervical cancer, and uterine cancer.[61] A proportional mortality study of farm workers also observed increases in buccal cavity, larynx, esophagus, stomach, skin, and cervical cancers.[62,63] Because most groups studied are exposed to multiple pesticides, it is difficult to identify specific carcinogenic agents, such as arsenic, which is a known cause of lung cancer, basal cell carcinoma of the skin, and hemangiosarcoma of the liver. In several case-control studies of childhood leukemia, parental use of pesticides in the home or garden was associated with a several-fold increase in risk. A few other selected pesticide exposures that are expected to cause human cancer are shown in Table 48.7. The relationships between chlorphenoxy acid herbicide exposures (including dioxin contaminants) and soft tissue sarcoma and non-Hodgkin's lymphoma have been discussed above. A list of pesticide agents associated with cancer is provided in Table 48.8. Toxicologic (usually rodent) studies are necessary to assess the risk of cancer from pesticides for which adequate epidemiologic data are not available.

In the United States, EPA generally sets legally established maximum limits (known as tolerances) for food residues, based on risk estimates from animal studies, which would allow no more than one additional cancer in 100,000 to 1 million persons exposed. Using EPA's risk estimates, one study estimating cumulative excess risk of cancer from food-borne residues to tolerances for 28 pesticides over a 70-year lifetime was 6 in 1000. Because children consume larger quantities of fruits and juices per kilogram of body weight than do adults, they may have a greater exposure to carcinogenic pesticide residues than is estimated by EPA for adults. This exposure occurs at a time when there exists the greatest potential latency for the subsequent development of cancer. Workers are another high-risk group because allow-

able exposures often are orders of magnitude greater than for consumers. The animal carcinogen alachlor, the most widely used herbicide in the United States, has been found to contaminate ground water, and has been banned for use in Massachusetts and Canada. Although most organophosphates have not been found to be carcinogenic in animals, dichlorvos is a probable human carcinogen. It has been estimated that there is a substantially increased risk of cancer from lifetime exposure to common household dichlorvos-impregnated insecticide strips. Many pesticides may be converted to carcinogenic nitroso compounds in the gastrointestinal tract; these include carbaryl, propoxur, fenuron, benzthiazuron, morpholine, atrazine, simazine, ziram, thiram, and ferbam.

REPRODUCTIVE EFFECTS OF PESTICIDES

Nasal hypoplasia is a well-recognized result of coumarin exposure among children of medically treated pregnant women. There are few other specific associations between a pesticide and congenital malformations, in part, because it is difficult to characterize exposure to a specific pesticide among pregnant women to allow assessment of teratogenicity. Unfortunately, exposure to mixtures of different pesticides is more frequent. The effects of exposure to herbicides, including those potentially contaminated with TCDD, have been most thoroughly investigated. More than 30 epidemiologic studies have looked at the relationship between birth defects, stillbirth, spontaneous abortion, and infertility, with chlorphenoxy acid herbicide exposure, yielding inconclusive results. Nevertheless, avoidance of exposure yielding to certain pesticides is important for pregnant women, especially during the first trimester, in view of the demonstrable animal teratogenicity of certain pesticides and some suggestive associations observed in epidemiologic studies, listed in Table 48.9.

The highest risk of adverse reproductive effect has been seen among male production workers heavily exposed to the nematocide DBCP. Production workers exposed to chlordecone also are reported to have developed oligospermia. An

Acetochlor
Acifluorfen
Alachlor
Amitrole
Aramite
Azobenzene
Benzene
β-Butyrolactone (solvent)
Chlorothalonil
Chromium (hexavalent compounds)
Creosotes
Cyclophosphamide
Daminozide
1,2-Dibromo-3-chloropropane
Dichlorophenyldichloroethane
Dichlorodiphenyldichloroethylene
Dichlorodiphenyltrichloroethane
p-Dichlorobenzene
1,1-Dichloroethane
1,2-Dichloropropane
1,3-Dichloropropene
Dieldrin
Epichlorohydrin
Ethylene dibromide
Ethylene dichloride (1,2-dichloroethane)
Ethylene oxide
Ethylene thiourea
Folpet
Formaldehyde (gas)
Furmecyclox
Griseofulvin
Heptachlor
Hexachlorobenzene
Hexachlorobenzodioxin (contaminant)
Lactofen
Lindane
Mancozeb
Maneb
Mestranol
Metiram
Mirex
Nitrofen (technical grade)
Pentachlorophenol
o-Phenylphenate sodium
Sulfallate
2,3,7,8-Tetrachlorodibenzo-para-dioxin (contaminant)
Toxaphene (polychorinated camphenes)
Tetrachloroethylene (perchloroethylene)
Trichloroethylene
Vinyl trichloride (1,1,2-trichloroethane)
Zineb

Adapted from California Department of Health Services. The Implementation of Proposition 65: A Progress Report, October 1, 1990.

Table 48.8 Pesticides associated with carcinogenicity

Developmental toxicity
Bromoxynil
Carbon disulfide
Chlordecone
Cyanazine
Cycloheximide
Cyclophosphamide
Cyhexatin
Dinocap
Dinoseb
Hexachlorobenzene
Mercury and mercury compounds
Methyl mercury
Nicotine
Warfarin
Female reproductive toxicity
Carbon disulfide
Cyclophosphamide (anhydrous)
Ethylene oxide
Male reproductive toxicity
Carbon disulfide
Cyclophosphamide
1,2-Dibromo-3-chloropropane
Dinitrobenzene
Dinoseb

Adapted from California Department of Health Services. The Implementation of Proposition 65: A Progress Report, October 1, 1990.

Table 48.9 Pesticides causing reproductive toxicity

cation, skin permeability, and use of personal protective equipment, must be assessed.

MONITORING POPULATIONS EXPOSED TO PESTICIDES

Well-established parameters for monitoring workers for overexposure to most pesticides do not exist. In contrast, pesticide parent compounds or metabolites can be measured for a large number of pesticides to confirm exposure. Among the best characterized metabolite profiles are those of the organophosphates. Metabolites of many organophosphate pesticides in urine can be identified, and increasingly the specificity of the metabolite profiles is allowing for the identification of specific pesticides from urine samples. Table 48.10 presents the metabolite tests presently available through the Centers for Disease Control Division of Laboratory Sciences.

Monitoring of workers for pesticide overexposure requires more than the ability to measure a parent compound or metabolite. An effective monitoring program should include a well thought out and efficient plan for obtaining samples, interpreting data, and acting upon the results. Although true cholinesterase activity in the nervous tissue is not accessible, cholinesterase activity may be measured effectively in the plasma and in erythrocytes. Cholinesterase depression is often a preclinical indicator of overexposure to these compounds. At least one preexposure baseline measurement should be obtained but an average of two or three measurements is preferable due to the variability in many laboratories. The need for a

epidemiologic study of workers exposed to ethylene dibromide, a fumigant that previously had been shown to be spermatotoxic in rodents, observed diminished sperm count with an increase in dysmorphic sperm compared to an unexposed referent group. Other spermatotoxins include carbaryl, nitroaromatic compounds, triphenyl tin, ordram, chlorbenzilate, and fenchlorphos, based primarily on toxicologic studies.

Estimating the reproductive risk to the individual worker depends on the teratogenic or spermatotoxic effect of a pesticide, which usually must be based on animal studies (Table 48.9). In addition, factors determining exposure, including the type of formulation, method of appli-

Pesticide(s)	Metabolite
Chlorpyrifos Chlorpyrifos methyl	3,5,6-trichloropyridinol
Diazinon	2-isopropyl-4-methyl-6-hydroxypyrimidine
Methyl parathion Parathion EPN	4-nitrophenol
Malathion	malathion diacid, malathion monoacid (and isomers)
Azinphosphos methyl	3-hydroxymethyl-1,2,3-benzotriazin-4 -one/ol
Isazaphos methyl	5-chloro-1,2-dihydro-1-isopropyl-[3H]- 1,2,4-triazol-3-one/ol
Pirimiphos methyl	2-diethylamino-6-methyl-4(1H)- pyrimidone/ol
Coumaphos	3-chloro-4-methyl-7-hydroxy coumarin
Acephate	acephate, methamidophos
Methamidophos	methamidophos

Web resources: http://www.inchem.org/
National Pesticide Information Center at Oregon State University: 1-800-858-7378; npic@ace.orst.edu

Table 48.10 Pesticides and the 'specific' metabolites that are measured at CDC

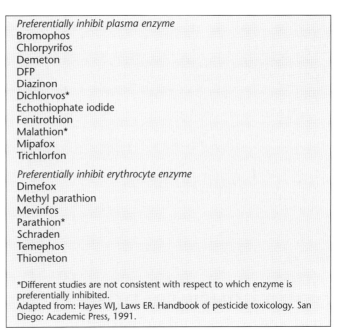

Preferentially inhibit plasma enzyme
Bromophos
Chlorpyrifos
Demeton
DFP
Diazinon
Dichlorvos*
Echothiophate iodide
Fenitrothion
Malathion*
Mipafox
Trichlorfon

Preferentially inhibit erythrocyte enzyme
Dimefox
Methyl parathion
Mevinfos
Parathion*
Schraden
Temephos
Thiometon

*Different studies are not consistent with respect to which enzyme is preferentially inhibited.
Adapted from: Hayes WJ, Laws ER. Handbook of pesticide toxicology. San Diego: Academic Press, 1991.

Table 48.11 Selected pesticides preferentially inhibiting erythrocyte or plasma cholinesterase

pre-exposure baseline is due to the fact that interindividual variability is large (observed 23% in one study).[64] The present standards in California recommend that if a worker's level falls below 80% of baseline, a workplace investigation should take place to ascertain the source of overexposure. Removal from exposure is required in California if erythrocyte cholinesterase activity falls to 70% or less of baseline or plasma cholinesterase falls to 60% of baseline value.

Workers removed from exposure should not return to work with pesticides until the cholinesterase activity returns to greater than 80% of baseline, and the reasons for the initial overexposure have been identified and corrected. Inter- and intra-laboratory variability over time may be considerable. Therefore, baseline and follow-up measurements of cholinesterase activity should be made by the same laboratory. Where feasible, in the setting of clinical screening or in epidemiologic studies, blood from the same unexposed individual (or individuals) may be included with samples of monitored workers to identify any major artifactual drift in laboratory results over time. The average range of variability of the activity of erythrocyte cholinesterase in unexposed individuals has been reported to be 8–12% (24–25% for plasma) over a 1-year period.

Where available, both erythrocyte and plasma cholinesterase measurements may be of value in the diagnosis and monitoring of exposed populations. There is some evidence that the plasma cholinesterase level may be a more sensitive indicator of low-level organophosphate exposure than is the erythrocyte cholinesterase concentration. The resolution of symptoms of acute poisoning also corresponds more closely to the early return of the plasma cholinesterase level to baseline. However, there are a few organophosphates (e.g., temephos and methyl parathion) that are reported preferentially to depress erythrocyte cholinesterase activity (Table 48.11). In addition, a variety of other conditions (including hepatic disease; many chronic diseases; acute infections; myxedema; pregnancy; and treatment with estrogens, β-blockers, steroids, and isoniazid) may depress plasma cholinesterase activity. Plasma cholinesterase levels also may be genetically low in a small proportion (3%) of the general population (of clinical importance because of the prolonged paralysis that follows administration of succinylcholine [Anectine]).

With the exception of anemia, there are few clinical conditions that will artifactually depress erythrocyte cholinesterase. Erythrocyte cholinesterase once inhibited by an organophosphate often remains depressed for the life of the erythrocyte (and thus better reflects accumulated effects of exposure over weeks or months). Some guidelines for the interpretation of cholinesterase activity are presented in Table 48.12. Cholinesterase measurements may be of limited utility for screening *n*-methyl carbamate insecticide exposed workers, because carbamate-induced inhibition of cholinesterase is rapidly reversible, particularly with the dilution used in many cholinesterase testing methods. Specialized isotope-based techniques can be applied, but these are not routinely available for most laboratories.[65]

Other monitoring tests for organophosphate exposure include urinary alkyl phosphates, which may be a more sensitive indicator of exposure to organophosphates than cholinesterase; however, these are not specific to individual agents. Measurement of urinary para-nitrophenol concentration has been used to monitor workers exposed to parathion. Although techniques are available for monitoring workers exposed to pesticides other than organophosphates (e.g., pentachlorophenol, DDT, synthetic anticoagulant rodenticides, and paraquat), these tests are not reliably predictive of clinical toxicity on an individual basis, and most are available only from specialized laboratories.

Clinical setting	Cholinesterase activity	
	Erythrocyte	Plasma
Acute, severe, organophosphate poisoning	Decreased	Decreased
Early recovery from poisoning (days to weeks)	Usually decreased	Decreased or normal
Late recovery from poisoning (weeks to 3 months)	Decreased or normal	Normal
Falsely normal activity:		
Mild poisoning (no baseline)	Often normal	Often normal
Carbamate poisoning	Often normal	Often normal
Early recovery of activity	Sometimes decreased	Often normal
Falsely decreased activity:		
Anemia	Often decreased	Normal
Liver disease	Normal	Decreased
Genetic plasma cholinesterase deficiency	Normal	Decreased
Pregnancy	Usually normal	Decreased

Table 48.12 Common clinical settings and relationship to cholinesterase activity

OTHER CONSIDERATIONS
Food and water contamination

The general public is routinely exposed to several pesticides. The National Health Assessment studies and other population studies have demonstrated that the vast majority of the US population have detectable levels of pesticide metabolites in urine. In a recent sampling of the US population (NHANES study) 2,5-dichlorophenol and n-naphthalene (constituents of moth repellents), TCP (the unique metabolite of chlorpyrifos), and pentachlorophenol (a wood preservative) were found in 94%, 86%, 82%, and 64%, respectively, of individuals sampled.[66] A study of a small sample of non-occupationally exposed individuals in Germany yielded similar findings.[67] In the United States, monitoring of pesticide residues in food by the Food and Drug Administration (FDA) routinely identifies 2–3% of samples with residues exceeding the EPA's tolerances, including 6% of samples of imported food. The FDA's testing methods can routinely test for only 163 of 316 pesticides for which legal maximum residue levels have been set. In addition, agricultural chemicals frequently impact on water quality. Although residues are generally low level, the EPA has found 74 pesticides in drinking water in 38 states. Forty-six of these pesticides are believed to have contaminated drinking water due to normal agricultural use. Although there are few epidemiologic studies, one investigation demonstrated subclinical abnormalities of immune function, including increased numbers of T8 lymphocytes and a decreased ratio of T4:T8 lymphocytes, among a cohort of women in Wisconsin drinking ground water contaminated with low levels of aldicarb (< 61 parts per billion). The impact of ground water contamination may be substantial, as over 75% of US cities and over 95% of rural populations in the US rely on ground water for drinking.

Domestic exposure to pesticides

Although for many workers pesticide use is associated with agriculture, the most intensive applications per acre occur in cities, where insecticides are applied for cockroach and termite control, and insecticides, fungicides, and herbicides are applied to gardens and lawns. In one study, the estimated infant exposure to chlorpyrifos after a routine treatment for fleas was 1.2–5.2 times the No Observable Adverse Effect Level (NOAEL).[66a] Although no systematic surveys have been conducted, in one study of chlordane-treated homes, more than 5% had persistent air-borne residues at levels above the National Academy of Sciences interim recommended limit of 5 micrograms/m³. Chlordane, which was until recently the treatment of choice for termite control, has been withdrawn by the manufacturer from the United States market; however, it continues to be marketed overseas. In Australia, increased breast milk organochlorine concentrations have correlated with applications for termite control.

A study of farm worker families from Washington State demonstrated a significant correlation between organophosphate pesticides in dust from homes and vehicles, with urinary metabolites in members of the household. This suggests an important contribution of indirect exposure to organophosphates among household contacts of farm workers.[68] A study of urban children demonstrated detectable levels of OP metabolites in nearly all participants studied, correlating with garden pesticide use.[69] A single study has pointed to food as the main source of organophosphate exposure in children; urban children eating an organic diet showed dramatically lower levels of organophosphate urinary metabolites than children eating a conventional diet.[70]

ISSUES IN DEVELOPING COUNTRIES
Central America: A case study of pesticides in the developing world

Pesticide use

Pesticide use in Central America continues to increase, with annual consumption as high as 2 kg per inhabitant and 20 kg per agricultural worker. Many of the most heavily used pesticides have high acute and chronic toxicity, including paraquat, mancozeb, terbufos, methamidophos, methyl bromide, carbofuran, methyl parathion, endosulfan, atrazine, copper arsenate, and aldicarb.[24] Additionally, the environmentally persistent organochlorine agents DDT, heptachlor, lindane, mirex, and pentachlorophenol are still registered in one or more Central American countries.[71]

Occupational exposures

Many toxic substances are frequently used in unsafe conditions, without adequate personal protective equipment, defective application equipment, and inappropriately high application rates. This results not only in risk to the applicator, but in contamination of the environment through runoff into waterways, and indirect exposure to living quarters. While there is evidence of increasing awareness of the dangers of pesticides, exposure assessment studies among small producers and plantation workers in Nicaragua and Costa Rica have observed significant ongoing problems in the handling of pesticides, despite training.[21,23] Production factors (manual applications, open mixing and loading systems) and application technologies (knapsack and aerial spraying) result in risk for high exposure levels, with frequent accidents. Personal protective devices, even when used properly, may not provide sufficient protection under tropical conditions. In hot and humid conditions, clothing saturated by perspiration or by contact with wet plants allows pesticides to penetrate the skin. Paradoxically, occlusion of pesticides under improperly fitting protective clothing may result in increased dermal uptake.[72]

Even when programs for safe pesticide use are fully implemented, protection of workers from pesticide-related illness remains limited as can be seen among pesticide poisonings on banana plantations in the Atlantic region of Costa Rica. Improvements in working conditions for applicators of toxic nematocides, including elimination of the extremely toxic aldicarb, resulted in a substantial decline in pesticide poisonings from 50 per 1000 in 1987 to 8 per 1000 banana workers in 1992. However, no further decrease could be achieved under the existing production techniques, with the incidence remaining about 7 per 1000 total banana workers between 1993 and 1996.[14]

Environmental exposure

Pesticide exposures extend to all sectors of the population. While less attention has been given to environmental than occupational health issues, non-occupational pesticide exposures in agricultural areas with intensive pesticide use may be considerable and complex. In Nicaragua, a population living in proximity to cotton fields with aerial spraying had significantly lower cholinesterase levels than a referent population in a non-adjacent field. These lowered levels were also associated with more acute and chronic health symptoms.[9] Organophosphate residues were detected in the urine of about 30% of children in El Salvador whose fathers sprayed methyl parathion.[73] In Costa Rica, a number of studies have analyzed pesticides in environmental samples in banana production areas. Surface waters, including rivers and creeks in national parks located downstream from banana plantations, have evidence of contamination by multiple pesticides.[74] Environmental samples taken near and inside houses and schools next to banana plantations demonstrated residues of the fungicide propiconazole in surface water and soil, and the insecticide chlorpyrifos in air samples.[75] Residues of multiple pesticides have been found in wells used for drinking water, in soil around the houses, in house and school dust, and in dust from mattresses of children (e.g., the fungicide chlorothalonil, the insecticide chlorpyrifos, and the nematocide ethoprophos).[76]

Health effects of pesticides in Central America

Investigating health effects of pesticide exposures is often a difficult task in developing countries, due to financial and technical constraint, limited infrastructure, and insufficient expertise in occupational and environmental hygiene and epidemiology. Research on acute poisonings has been carried out in all seven Central American countries, but research on chronic and delayed health effects has occurred primarily in Nicaragua and Costa Rica.

Acute poisonings

As early as in the 1980s, a well-organized pesticide poisoning surveillance system was established in a cotton-growing area in Nicaragua. Its existence facilitated a series of studies on pesticide health effects in the region. These included a study describing trends of poisonings in the area and an outbreak with carbofuran,[77] and several studies of depression of cholinesterase levels among mechanics of fumigation airplanes,[10] workers using closed pesticide mixing and loading systems, and among children living close to a fumigation airport.[78] A study assessing the degree of under-reporting concluded that despite education of physicians in the reporting area, only one-third of acute medically treated pesticide poisoning cases were reported to the registry. During the last half of the 1990s, surveillance systems of acute health effects from pesticides were established in all Central American countries, with 6934 acute pesticide poisonings reported during 2000. However, under-reporting and under-registration are estimated to be in excess of 95% in most countries.[79] Based on the degree of under-reporting in six of the seven countries, there are an estimated 400,000 symptomatic poisoning episodes annually.[17]

Skin injuries

Today, skin injuries are probably more widespread than systemic poisonings. Increasing rates of dermal lesions have been observed, particularly among female agricultural workers, with annual rates as high as 7.5 per 100 women employed in the banana and ornamental plant industries in Costa Rica.[80] Among men, the herbicide paraquat is the most frequently reported pesticide associated with skin and eye injuries in Costa Rica.[48] In 1993 and 1996, 40 and 25 per 100 herbicide sprayers on banana plantations, respectively, filed a claim for an occupational pesticide-related accident requiring medical attention – the majority due to paraquat.[48] The fungicide chlorothalonil has been identified as a risk factor for dermatitis among banana plantation workers in Panama.[81] On Panamanian banana plantations, pesticide applicators are at risk for allergic and contact dermatitis.[82] At least 16% of the workers were sensitized to one or more pesticides in use, including carbaryl, benomyl, ethoprophos, chlorothalonil, imazalil, glyphosate, thiabendazole, chlorpyrifos, oxyfluorfen, propiconazole, and tridemorph.

Chronic and delayed health effects

Cancer risk in populations of rural counties of Costa Rica with high pesticide use tends to be higher than in rural counties with low pesticide use. This ecologic association was evident for both the overall cancer risk, and the risk for a number of specific cancer sites, in particular female reproductive cancers in women, and lung cancer; in men and women.[83] Male banana workers in Costa Rica had excess risk for penile cancer, melanoma, and lung cancer; and female banana workers had increased risk for cervical cancer and leukemia.[84] The lung cancer excess was evident also among a subset of DBCP-exposed workers.[85]

The most striking reproductive effects have been related to sterility occurring in thousands of male banana workers exposed to DBCP during the 1970s throughout Central America and other countries.[86] In Costa Rica, wives of congenitally DBCP-exposed men have also claimed reproductive effects, such as sterility and congenital malformations, but no formal studies have been carried out. Genotoxic effects were observed among banana workers who had been exposed to the nematocide dibromochloropropane (DBCP) in the 1970s, more evident in those with specific polymorphisms.[87] Among female packing plant workers employed at banana plantations, with exposure to the fungicides thiabendazole and imazalile, an increased prevalence of genotoxic changes was observed.[88]

Persistent damage to the central and peripheral nervous systems has also been observed in workers previously poisoned with cholinesterase-inhibiting pesticides in both Nicaragua and Costa Rica.[39,77,85,89–91] Neurobehavioral deficits were found among male vector control sprayers in Costa Rica who had been previously exposed to DDT.[92] An association between long-term paraquat exposure and respiratory symptoms was observed in Nicaragua, but no alterations were found in tests of pulmonary function.[93]

Pesticide policies

For decades, 'safe use' approaches have been espoused by the pesticide industry to reduce risks in Central America and developing countries in general, presuming that pesticides are indispensable and, if properly handled, will not cause unreasonable harm.[94] Environmental contamination related to pesticide use has been attributed to insufficient regulation and unawareness among pesticide users, and it has been assumed that strengthening of regulations and education of users would lead to an acceptable level of pesticide safety. However, the major international 'safe use' initiatives have been limited in scope. Adherence to Food and Agriculture

Organization International Code of Conduct (the most important initiative to prevent undesirable effects of pesticides in developing countries by strengthening pesticide regulation) is voluntary. The Prior Informed Consent (PIC) list of the Rotterdam Convention contains only a few dozen pesticides, and does not include some pesticides causing unique problems in developing countries.

The 'Safe Use Initiative' of the Global Crop Protection Federation (today, Croplife International), aimed at widespread training in collaboration with governments, has not produced evidence of substantial improvements. In fact, many industry-based training materials promote pesticide use in developing countries, and a number of industrialized countries continue to manufacture domestically prohibited pesticides for export to developing countries. The WHO International Program for Chemical Safety (IPCS), with guidelines for pesticide registration and control in developing countries, emphasizes the prevention of acute health effects. Pesticides classified as 'nonhazardous' but with acknowledged chronic and delayed effects are ubiquitous, such as mancozeb, maneb, and chlorothalonil in Central America. Thus, 'safe use' programs have yet to achieve pesticide safety in agriculture in developing countries.

A major limitation experienced by many developing countries is lack of human and technical resources. Often the risk assessment performed by regulatory authorities in registering pesticides in these countries is no more than the copying of international guidelines or decisions by major regulatory agencies. There is often incomplete comprehension of this information. No resources exist to carry out systematic, continuous monitoring of hazards, exposure, or adverse health or ecologic effects. Preventive approaches, based on available technology, training and regulation, is generally absent in developing countries. Additionally, 'safe use' efforts often promote the use of pesticides, and may subtly encourage countries to desist from investing in sustainable agriculture, with alternative pest control approaches.

A reduction in pesticide use has been achieved in some developing countries. Many select examples do exist of successful Integrated Pest Management (IPM) programs, with drastically reduced pesticide use, in Southeast Asia and Central America, for important crops such as sugar cane, coffee, corn, citrus, and potato. Beyond IPM, organic agriculture integrates other principles of sustainable land use. Studies are increasingly showing that organic agriculture can produce compatible yields with traditional pesticide-dependent production systems, and may be more profitable in the longer term. However, profound changes in international and national agricultural policies, steering towards sustainable agriculture based on non-chemical pest management, are needed to effectively address pesticide-related health risks in developing countries.

PREVENTION AND REGULATION

Until recently, the most important legislation concerning pesticides in the United States has been the Food,

Insecticide, Fungicide, and Rodenticide Act (FIFRA) of 1947. First enforced by the FDA, EPA became the lead agency in its implementation in 1970. For a new pesticide to be registered for sale, the registrant must submit acute and subchronic toxicity studies, as well as chronic studies of neurotoxic, reproductive, mutagenic, and carcinogenic effects. Based on these data, food tolerances are set. Labeling requirements specifying permitted uses are designated, including general use (for sale to the general public) or restricted use (only for use under the supervision of trained licensed operators). Unfortunately, there was a large backlog of old pesticides that were registered without appropriate toxicologic studies under a "grandfather" clause in FIFRA. Many of these pesticides still have not been adequately evaluated.

In addition, the credibility of the registration process was undermined in the early 1980s, when it became known that the largest private contract testing laboratory in the United States had conducted 200 scientifically invalid or fraudulent studies that were relied on to support registration of 140 pesticides. A recent Federal survey found that the data required by EPA for chronic toxicity were incomplete for all 50 widely used agricultural pesticides reviewed. In the United States, regulations may vary from state to state, with some states having more stringent registration standards and re-entry intervals (Table 48.13). Because the EPA was primarily concerned with environmental and food contamination, there existed no standard requirement for data to be collected on worker exposure or worker health effects. As a result, relatively little was known or available about the health effects of pesticides among workers exposed to levels occurring in the agricultural workplace.

A new act, the Food Quality Protection Act (FQPA; FFDCA P.L. 104-170), amended the FIFRA and Federal Food, Drug, and Cosmetic Act in 1996. Under the amended Federal Insecticide, Fungicide, and Rodenticide Act (FIFRA) the EPA registers pesticides for use in the United States and prescribes labeling and other regulatory requirements to prevent unreasonable adverse effects on health or the environment. EPA also establishes food tolerances (maximum legally permissible levels) for individual pesticides in food. The FQPA facilitates a more consistent, scientifically-based, and protective approach to regulating pesticide use. The FQPA requires that EPA control, through registration, the amount of pesticides to which one is exposed through all possible routes of exposure. Pesticides are grouped according to mechanisms of action. For example, all cholinesterase inhibitors are considered and regulated as a whole. Reasonable certainty of no harm is a criterion for regulation, and accounts for vulnerable populations such as infants and children. Safer pesticides receive expedited handling and are thus encouraged.

Among pesticide laws, only the 1992 Worker Protection Standard (WPS) is designed to safeguard the health of agricultural workers and pesticide handlers. Other US pesticide regulations address primarily the risks posed by pesticides to the purchaser of the product, the environment, and the consumer. The WPS covers several important groups (e.g., handlers and field workers), regulating certain

| Pesticide | California | | | | | | EPA |
	Apples	Citrus	Corn	Grapes	Peaches	Other	All crops
All toxicity category I pesticides[a]	1	1	1	1	1	1	–
Aldicarb (Ternik)	1	1	1	1	1	1	1
Anilazine (Dyrene)	2	2	2	2	2	2	–
Carbofuran	–	–	14	–	–	–	2
Chlorpyrifos (Lorsban)	–	2	–	–	–	–	4
Diazinon	–	5	–	5	5	–	–
Dioxathion	–	30	–	30	30	–	1
Disulfoton	2	2	2	2	2	2	1
Endosulfan	2	2	2	2	2	2	2
Ethion	2	30	2	14	14	2	1
Guthion	14	30	–	21	14	14	1
Methidathion	2	30, 40[b]	2	2	2	2	1
Methomyl (Lannate)	2	2	2	7	2	–	2
Methyl parathion	14	14	14	14	21	14	1
Mevinphos (Phosdrin)	2	4	2	4	4	2	2
Monitor	2	2	2	2	2	2	1
Monocrotophos	2	2	2	2	2	2	1
Parathion (ethyl)	14	30, 45, 50, 90[c]	14	21	21	14	2
Phorate (Thimet)	2	2	7	2	2	2	1
Phosalone (Zoione)	–	7	–	35[d]	1	1	1
Propargite (Omite)	–	14	–	14	–	–	7
Propargite (Omite CR)	–	42[e]	–	–	–	–	–

[a]In California, all toxicity category I pesticides have a 1-day re-entry interval.
[b]Depending on the concentration used.
[c]Depending on the concentration used and the time of year applied.
[d]No longer registered for use on grapes in California because of several re-entry poisonings.
[e]No longer registered for use on citrus in California because of severe re-entry poisonings.
With permission from Moses M. Pesticides. In: Last J, Wallace RB, eds. Public health and preventive medicine, 13th edn. East Norwalk, Connecticut: Appleton & Lange, 1992.

Table 48.13 Field re-entry intervals in days or hours for selected pesticides (California and Environmental Protection Agency [EPA] Regulations)

application activities and stipulating several safety practices. Components of the regulation include training, re-entry, decontamination, personal protective equipment, and referral to medical providers. Workers are excluded from entering a pesticide-treated area during the restricted entry interval, which must be stated on the pesticide label. Personal protective equipment (PPE) must be provided to the handlers, and anyone entering the area before the restricted entry interval expires. PPE must be maintained by the employer. Notification must be posted clearly in areas of application to prevent early entry; water, soap, and towels for routine washing and emergency decontamination must be available to handlers.

The employer is responsible for assuring emergency transportation and information on the pesticide to a medical care facility, in the event that a worker or handler is made ill by exposure. Training is required for all workers and handlers, and a pesticide safety poster must be displayed. Handlers and workers must be informed of pesticide label requirements. Unlike standards developed by OSHA, no exposure measurements or biologic monitoring are required under WPS, despite the high toxicity of many of the chemicals involved. The effectiveness of the rule rests on the assumption that personal protective equipment will be effective for handlers, and that field workers will be adequately protected by restrictions from entering treated fields.

Exposure control

Engineering controls (for example, enclosed cabs with filtered air on tractor-pulled sprayers) have been demonstrated to reduce exposure markedly. Closed-system mixing and loading units, which are required for EPA category 1 pesticides in California, are reported to decrease exposure to these high-risk workers by as much as 10-fold. Correctly engineered mixing equipment will prevent the backflow of pesticides into water sources, and pastes may reduce exposure compared with liquids. Some inert solvent ingredients may reduce or increase toxicity. For example, parathion formulated with xylene is less toxic than an equivalent dose of parathion alone. Granules result in less respiratory exposure and perhaps less dermal exposure than powders, and powders in water-soluble bags may eliminate the need for human contact with the product during mixing and loading. Unfortunately, despite the fact that engineering controls are most effective in preventing overexposure, the WPS puts little emphasis on them. In California, engineering controls are required for all Category 1 pesticide loading operations.

Workers should be trained in the use of engineering controls, in appropriate personal hygiene (washing before eating, bathing on finishing work, and no smoking on the job), in the appropriate use of personal protective equipment, and in first aid measures in case of an accident. Gloves and coveralls are important measures of protection, although few data exist on the penetration of rubber or neoprene materials by the liquid formulations of many pesticides. Work clothes should be laundered separately

from regular clothing. In a study of clothing contaminated with dilute methyl parathion (1.25% active ingredient), a significant reduction in residues was seen with each of the first three washings, whereas clothing contaminated with methyl parathion concentrate continued to have significant residues after 10 washings. In general, clothing contaminated with pesticide concentrate should be discarded, and disposable coveralls should be considered for workers who are exposed to concentrates of hazardous pesticides.

References

1. Keefe TJ, Savage EP, Wheeler HW. Third national study of hospitalized pesticide poisonings in the United States, 1977–1982. Fort Collins, CO: Colorado State University, Epidemiologic Studies Center, 1990.
2. Whorton J. Before Silent Spring: pesticides and public health in pre-DDT America. Princeton, NJ: Princeton University Press, 1975.
3. Gladwell M. The mosquito killer. The New Yorker July 2, 2001.
4. California Pesticide Use Summaries (web based data base). http://www.ipm.ucdavis.edu/PUSE/2000/
5. Wolfe HR, Durham WF, Armstrong JF, et al. Exposure of workers to pesticides. Arch Environ Health 1967; 14:622–33.
6. Wester RC, Maibach HI. In vivo percutaneous absorption and decontamination of pesticides in humans. J Toxicol Environ Health 1985; 16:25–37.
7. Baker EL, Zack M, Miles JM, et al. Epidemic malathion poisoning in Pakistan malaria workers. Lancet 1978; i:31–34.
8. Woodrow JE, Seiber JN, Crosby DG, Moilanen KW, Soderquist CJ, Mourer C. Air-borne and surface residues of parathion and its conversion products in a treated plum orchard environment. Arch Environ Contam Toxicol 1977; 6:175–91.
9. Keifer M, McConnell R, Pacheco AF, Daniel W, Rosenstock L. Estimating underreported pesticide poisonings in Nicaragua. Am J Ind Med 1996; 30:195–201.
10. McConnell R, Pacheco Anton AF, Magnotti R. Crop duster aviation mechanics: high risk for pesticide poisoning. Am J Public Health 1990; 80:1236–9.
11. Keifer MC, Arne KH. Toxicity testing of pesticides sold in the United States. Occup Med 1997; 12:365–70.
12. Keifer MC, Mahurin RK. Chronic neurologic effects of pesticide overexposure. Occup Med 1997; 12:291–304.
13. Goldman LR, Smith DF, Neutra RR, et al. Pesticide food poisoning from contaminated watermelons in California, 1985. Arch Environ Health 1990; 45:229–36.
14. Wesseling C, van Wendel de Joode B, Monge P. Pesticide-related illness and injuries among banana workers in Costa Rica: a comparison between 1993 and 1996. Int J Occup Environ Health 2001; 7:90–7.
15. Blondell J. Epidemiology of pesticide poisonings in the United States, with special reference to occupational cases. Occup Med 1997; 12:209–20.
16. Kahn E. Pesticide related illness in California farm workers. J Occup Med 1976; 18:693–6.
17. Murray D, Wesseling C, Keifer M, Corriols M, Henao S. Surveillance of pesticide-related illness in the developing world: putting the data to work. Int J Occup Environ Health 2002; 8:243–8.
18. Jeyaratnam J. Acute pesticide poisoning: a major global health problem. World Health Stat Q 1990; 43:139–44.
19. Wesseling C, Castillo L, Elinder G. Pesticide poisonings in Costa Rica. Scand J Work Environ Health 1993; 19:227–35.
20. Loevinsohn ME. Insecticide use and increased mortality in rural central Luzon, Philippines. Lancet 1987; i: 1359–62.
21. Corriols M, Silva D, Marín J, Berroterán J, Lozano LM, Martínez J. Incidencia de intoxicaciones agudas por plaguicidas y estimación del subregistro en Nicaragua

(Incidence of acute pesticide intoxications and underregistration estimates in Nicaragua). Managua: OPS/OMS, 2002.

22. Kishi M. Farmers' perceptions of pesticides, and resultant health problems from exposures. Int J Occup Environ Health 2002; 8:175–81.

23. Aragón A, Aragón C, Thorn A. Pests, peasants, and pesticides on the Northern Nicaraguan Pacific Plain. Int J Occup Environ Health 2001; 7:295–302.

24. Wesseling C, Aragon A, Castillo L, et al. Hazardous pesticides in Central America. Int J Occup Environ Health 2001; 7:287–94.

25. Eddleston M, Karalliedde L, Buckley N, et al. Pesticide poisoning in the developing world – a minimum pesticides list. Lancet 2002; 360:1163–7.

26. Wilks MF. Paraquat poisoning. Lancet 1999; 353:321–2.

27. Wesseling C, McConnell R, Partanen T, Hogstedt C. Pesticides in developing countries: a review of occupational health impact and research needs. Int J Health Services 1997; 27:273–308.

28. Perriens J, Van Der Stuyft P, Chee H, Benimadho S. The epidemiology of paraquat intoxications in Surinam. Trop Geogr Med 1989; 41:266–9.

29. Stephens R, Spurgeon A, Calvert IA, et al. Neuropsychological effects of long-term exposure to organophosphates in sheep dip. Lancet 1995; 345:1135–9.

30. Faria NM, Facchini LA, Fassa AG, Tomasi E. A cross-sectional study about mental health of farm-workers from Serra Gaucha (Brazil). Rev Saude Publica 1999; 33:391–400.

31. Cole DC, Carpio F, Leon N. Economic burden of illness from pesticide poisonings in highland Ecuador. Rev Panam Salud Publica 2000; 8:196–201.

32. Farm chemicals handbook '90. Willoughby, OH: Meister Publishing, 1990.

33. Reigert R, Roberts J. Recognition and management of pesticide poisonings, 5th edn. EPA 735-R-98-003. Washington, DC: Environmental Protection Agency, 1999. http://www.epa.gov/pesticides/safety/healthcare/handbook/handbook.htm

34. Gershon S, Shaw FH. Psychiatric sequelae of chronic exposure to organosphosphorus insecticides. Lancet 1961; i: 1371–4.

35. Ludomirsky A, Klein HO, Sarelli P, et al. Q-T prolongation and polymorphous ('torsade de pointes') ventricular arrhythmias associated with organophosphorus insecticide poisoning. Am J Cardiol 1982; 49:1654–8.

36. Senanayake N, Karalliedde L. Neurotoxic effects of organophosphorus insecticides. N Engl J Med 1987; 316:761–3.

37. Morgan JP, Penovich P. Jamaica ginger paralysis. Forty-seven-year follow-up. Arch Neurol 1978; 35:530–2.

38. Lotti M, Moretto A, Zoppellari, et al. Inhibition of lymphocytic neuropathy target esterase predicts the development of organophosphate-induced delayed polyneuropathy. Arch Toxicol 1986; 59:176–9.

39. Rosenstock L, Keifer M, Daniell W, et al. Chronic central nervous system effects of acute organophosphate pesticide intoxication. Lancet 1991; 338:223–7.

40. Savage EP, Keefe TJ, Mounce LM, et al. Chronic neurologic sequelae of acute organophosphate pesticide poisoning. Arch Environ Health 1988; 43:38–45.

41. Wesseling C, Keifer M, Ahlbom A, et al. Long-term neurobehavioral effects of mild poisonings with organophosphate and n-methyl carbamate pesticides among banana workers. Int J Occup Environ Health 2002; 8:27–34.

42. Namba T, Nolte CT, Jackre J, et al. Poisoning due to organophosphate insecticides. Am J Med 1971; 50:475–92.

43. Midtling JE, Barnett PG, Coye MJ, et al. Clinical management of field worker organosphosphate poisoning. West J Med 1985; 142:414–8.

44. Metcalf RL, Branch CE, Swift TR, et al. Neurologic findings among workers exposed to fenthion in a veterinary hospital in Georgia. MMWR 1985; 34:402–3.

45. LeBlanc FN, Benson BE, Glig AD. A severe organophosphate poisoning requiring the use of an atropine drip. Clin Toxicol 1986; 24:69–76.

46. Narahashi T. Neuronal ion channels as the target sites of insecticides. Pharmacol Toxicol 1996; 79:1–14.

47. Zhao X, Salgado VL, Yeh JZ, Narahashi T. Differential actions of fipronil and dieldrin insecticides on GABA-gated chloride channels in cockroach neurons. J Pharmacol Exp Ther 2003; 306:914–24.

48. Wesseling C, van Wendel de Joode B, Ruepert C, et al. Paraquat in developing countries. Int J Occup Environ Health 2001; 7:275–86.

49. Hoppin JA, Umbach DM, London SJ, Alavanja MC, Sandler DP. Chemical predictors of wheeze among farmer pesticide applicators in the Agricultural Health Study. Am J Respir Crit Care Med 2002; 165:683–9.

50. Parkinson C. The changing pattern of paraquat poisoning in man. Histopathology 1980; 4:171–83.

51. Im JG, Lee KS, Han MC, Kim SJ, Kim IO. Paraquat poisoning: findings on chest radiography and CT in 42 patients. Am J Roentgenol 1991; 157:697–701.

52. Smith JG. Paraquat poisoning by skin absorption: a review. Hum Toxicol 1988; 7:15–9.

53. Yamashita M, Yamashita M, Ando Y. A long-term follow-up of lung function in survivors of paraquat poisoning. Hum Exp Toxicol 2000; 19:99–103.

54. Hertzman C, Wisen M, Bowering D, et al. Parkinson's disease: a case-control study of occupational and environmental risk factors. Am J Ind Med 1990; 17:349–55.

55. Eisenman A, Armali Z, Raikhlin-Eisenkraft B, et al. Nitric oxide inhalation for paraquat-induced lung injury. J Toxicol Clin Toxicol 1998; 36:575–84.

56. Pesticide-related illnesses associated with the use of a plant growth regulator – Italy, 2001. MMWR 2001; 50:845.

57. Langard S, Rognum T, Flotterod O, Skaug V. Fatal accident resulting from methyl bromide poisoning after fumigation of a neighbouring house; leakage through sewage pipes. J Appl Toxicol 1996; 16:445–8.

58. Horowitz BZ, Albertson TE, O'Malley M, Swenson EJ. An unusual exposure to methyl bromide leading to fatality. J Toxicol Clin Toxicol 1998; 36:353–7.

59. Herzstein J, Cullen MR. Methyl bromide intoxication in four field-workers during removal of soil fumigation sheets. Am J Ind Med 1990; 17:321–6.

60. Yilmaz HL, Yildizdas DR. Amitraz poisoning, an emerging problem: epidemiology, clinical features, management, and preventive strategies. Arch Dis Child 2003; 88:130–4.

61. Mills PK, Kwong S. Cancer incidence in the United Farmworkers of America (UFW), 1987–1997. Am J Ind Med 2001; 40:596–603.

62. Colt JS, Stallones L, Cameron LL, Dosemeci M, Zahm SH. Proportionate mortality among US migrant and seasonal farmworkers in twenty-four states. Am J Ind Med 2001; 40:604–11.

63. Colt JS, Engel LS, Keifer MC, Thompson ML, Zahm SH. Comparability of data obtained from migrant farmworkers and their spouses on occupational history. Am J Ind Med 2001; 40:523–30.

64. Fillmore CM, Lessenger JE. A cholinesterase testing program for pesticide applicators. J Occup Med 1993; 35:61–70.

65. Thomsen T, Kewitz H, Pleul O. A suitable method to monitor inhibition of cholinesterase activities in tissues as induced by reversible enzyme inhibitors. Enzyme 1989; 42:219–24.

66. Hill RH Jr, Head SL, Baker S, et al. Pesticide residues in urine of adults living in the United States: reference range concentrations. Environ Res 1995; 71:99–108.

66a. Fenske RA, Black KG, Elkner KP, et al. Potential exposure and health risks of infants following indoor residential pesticide applications. Am J Public Health 1990; 80: 689–93.

67. Koch HM, Hardt J, Angerer J. Biologic monitoring of exposure of the general population to the organophosphorus pesticides chlorpyrifos and chlorpyrifos-methyl by

determination of their specific metabolite 3,5,6-trichloro-2-pyridinol. Int J Hyg Environ Health 2001; 204:175–80.

68. Curl CL, Fenske RA, Kissel JC, et al. Evaluation of take-home organophosphorus pesticide exposure among agricultural workers and their children. Environ Health Perspect 2002; 110:A765.

69. Lu C, Knutson DE, Fisker-Andersen J, Fenske RA. Biologic monitoring survey of organophosphorus pesticide exposure among pre-school children in the Seattle metropolitan area. Environ Health Perspect 2001; 109:299–303.

70. Curl CL, Fenske RA, Elgethun K.Organophosphorus pesticide exposure of urban and suburban preschool children with organic and conventional diets. Environ Health Perspect 2003; 111:377–82.

71. UNEP Chemicals. Regionally based assessment of persistent toxic substances. Central American and the Caribbean regional report, 2002, Geneva.

72. Brouwer DH, De Vreede JAF, Meuling WJA, et al. Determination of the efficiency for pesticide exposure reduction with protective clothing: a field study using biologic monitoring. In: Honeycutt HC, ed. Worker exposure to agrichemicals. Baton Rouge, FL: Lewis Publishers, 2000;65–86.

73. Azaroff LS. Biomarkers of exposure to organophosphorous insecticides among farmers' families in rural El Salvador: factors associated with exposure. Environ Res 1999; 80:138–47.

74. Castillo LE. Pesticide impact of intensive banana production on aquatic ecosystems in Costa Rica. PhD thesis. Stockholm, Sweden: Stockholm University, 2000.

75. Smits N, Snippe R, de Vries J. Exposure to pesticides due to living next to a banana plantation. A pilot study. Internal report No. 312. Wageningen, The Netherlands: Wageningen Agricultural University, Environmental and Occupational Health Group, 1999.

76. Zuurbier M, Solano K, Arias D, Wesseling C, Ruepert C. Pesticide residues in the domestic environment, Limón, Costa Rica. 16th EPICOH Congress on Epidemiology in Occupational Health. Barcelona, September 11–14, 2002. Med Lav 2002; 93:P048.

77. McConnell R, Hruska A. An epidemic of pesticide poisoning in Nicaragua: implications for prevention in developing countries. Am J Public Health 1993; 83:1559–62.

78. McConnell R, Cedillo L, Keifer M, et al. Monitoring organophosphate insecticide exposed workers for cholinesterase depression: new technology for office or field use. J Occup Med 1992; 34:34–7.

79. Henao S, Arbelaez MP. Epidemiological situation of acute pesticide poisoning in the Central American Isthmus, 1992–2000. Epidemiol Bull 2002; 23:5–9.

80. Vergara AE, Fuortes L. Surveillance and epidemiology of occupational pesticide poisonings in banana plantations in Costa Rica. Int J Occup Environ Health 1998; 4: 199–201.

81. Penagos H, Jimenez V, Fallas V, O'Malley M, Maibach H. Chlorothalonil, a possible cause of erythema dyschromicum perstans (ashy dermatitis). Contact Derm 1996; 35:124–8.

82. Penagos H. Contact dermatitis caused by pesticides among banana plantation workers in Panama. Int J Occup Environ Health 2002; 8:14–18.

83. Wesseling C, Antich D, Hogstedt C, Rodriguez AC, Ahlbom A. Related articles, links geographical differences of cancer incidence in Costa Rica in relation to environmental and occupational pesticide exposure. Int J Epidemiol 1999; 28:365–74.

84. Wesseling C, Ahlbom A, Antich D, Rodríguez AC, Castro R. Cancer in banana plantation workers in Costa Rica. Int J Epidemiol 1996; 25:1125–31.

85. Wesseling C, Monge P, Partanen T, Guardado J. Banana workers in Costa Rica and cancer risk, an update. 16th EPICOH Congress on Epidemiology in Occupational Health. Barcelona, September 11–14, 2002. Med Lav 2002; 93:P107.

86. Slutsky M, Levin JL, Levy BS. Azoospermia and oligospermia among a large cohort of DBCP applicators in 12 countries. Int J Occup Environ Health 1999; 5:116–22.

87. Au WW, Sierra-Torres CH, Cajas-Salazar N, Shipp BK, Legator MS. Cytogenetic effects from exposure to mixed pesticides and the influence from genetic susceptibility. Environ Health Perspect 1999; 107:501–5.

88. Cuenca P, Ramírez V. Daño del ADN en trabajadoras bananeras expuestas a plaguicidas en Limón, Costa Rica. Revista Biología Tropical 2002; 50:507–18.

89. McConnell R, Delgado-Tellez E, Cuadra R, et al. Organophosphate neuropathy due to methamidophos: biochemical and neurophysiological markers. Arch Toxicol 1999; 73:296–300.

90. Miranda J, Lundberg I, McConnell R, et al. Onset of grip- and pinch-strength impairment after acute poisonings with organophosphate insecticides. Int J Occup Environ Health 2002; 8:19-26.

91. Miranda J, McConnell R, Delgado E, et al. Tactile vibration thresholds after acute poisonings with organophosphate insecticides. Int J Occup Environ Health 2002; 8:212–9.

92. van Wendel de Joode B, Wesseling C, Kromhout H, Monge P, García M, Mergler D. Chronic nervous system effects of long-term occupational exposure to DDT. Lancet 2001; 357:1014–6.

93. Castro-Gutiérrez N, McConnell R, Andersson K, Pacheco-Antón F, Hogstedt C. Respiratory symptoms, spirometry and chronic occupational paraquat exposure. Scand J Work Environ Health 1997; 23:421–7.

94. Wesseling C, Ruepert C, Chaverri F. Safe use of pesticides: a developing country point of view. In: Pimentel D, ed. Encyclopaedia of pest management. New York: Marcel Dekker, 2003.

95. Hayes WJ, Laws ER. Handbook of pesticide toxicology. San Diego, CA: Academic Press, 1991.

96. California Department of Health Services (CDHS). Guidelines for physicians. Medical supervision of pesticide workers. Berkeley, CA: CDHS, 1988.

97. Fisher AA. Occupational dermatitis from pesticides: patch testing procedures. Cutis 1983; 31:483–508.

98. Baker SR, Williamson CF, eds. The effects of pesticides on human health. Advances in modern environmental toxicology, vol. 18. Princeton, NJ: Princeton Scientific Co, 1990.

99. National Research Council. Regulating pesticides in food. Washington, DC: National Academy Press, 1987.

100. International Agency for Research on Cancer. IARC monographs on the evaluation of the carcinogenic risk of chemicals to humans, vol. 23. Lyon: IARC, 1980;39–141.

101. Stasik MJ. Carcinomas of the urinary bladder in a 4-chloro-o-toluidine cohort. Int Arch Occup Environ Health 1988; 60:21–24.

102. Hoar SK, Blair A, Holmes FF, et al. Agricultural herbicide use and risk of lymphoma and soft-tissue sarcoma. JAMA 1986; 256(9):1141–7. Erratum in: JAMA 1986; 256(24):3351.

103. Lowengart RA, Peters JM, Cicioni C, et al. Childhood leukemia and parents' occupational and home exposures. J Natl Cancer Inst 1987; 79:39–45.

104. Lillienfeld DE, Gallo MA. 2,4-D, 2,4,5-T and 2,3,7,8-TCDD: an overview. Epidemiol Rev 1989; 11:28–58.

105. Balarajan R, McDowall M. Congenital malformations and agricultural workers. Lancet 1983; 1(8333):1112–3.

106. Schwartz DA, LoGerfo JP. Congenital limb reduction defects in the agricultural setting. Am J Public Health 1988; 78(6):654–8.

107. Restrepo M, Munoz N, Day N, et al. Birth defects among children born to a population occupationally exposed to pesticides in Columbia. Scand J Work Environ Health 1990; 16:239–46.

108. Brender JD, Suarez L. Paternal occupation and anencephaly. Am J Epidemiol 1990; 131:517–21.

Chapter 49
Low-Level Environmental Exposures

Mark R Cullen

One of the cardinal rules of toxicology is that the biologic response to a physical or chemical hazard is a definable function of the exposure dose. Although this relationship may take one of several forms, depending on the toxin and the response, the general principle is that health effects from higher levels of exposure will be more frequent and/or more severe than those associated with lower levels. This is one of the guiding principles of occupational and environmental medicine (OEM) diagnosis and management.

Fortunately, extremely high levels of exposure to hazards, although risky, are generally uncommon. For any given substance, only a relatively small number of people, if any, are likely to be exposed to doses in the lethal or highly toxic range (e.g., accidental or uncontrolled exposure), although proportionally more may have moderate exposures (e.g., controlled occupational exposures). Many more people may encounter low-level exposures in the general environment (e.g., from air, water, or food contaminated by industrial wastes). A sizable number may have exposure to small doses of potential hazards such as may occur when ambient air is recycled indoors without dilution by fresh air. Finally, almost everybody is exposed to the extremely low levels of contaminants that are the background of modern society. This generic, inverse relationship between the level of hazardous exposure and the numbers of individuals exposed is depicted schematically in Figure 49.1.

Because so many more people are exposed to low levels than high ones, a substantial number of people with symptoms that are attributed to environmental factors are, in fact, only minimally exposed. Such patients are common in clinical practice, even though the proportion of all comparably exposed people who have complaints may be low.

For obvious reasons, patients with environmental complaints associated with small levels of exposure are much more difficult to evaluate than their more extensively exposed counterparts. Using the principles and approach enunciated in the Introduction and throughout this text, establishing a cause-and-effect relationship is difficult because the a priori likelihood for getting sick from such exposures is low; even rare diseases of other causes may strike as commonly. The exposures themselves, often many orders of magnitude lower than presently accepted threshold limit values (TLVs) or health guidelines, may be difficult or impossible to measure. The natural clinical response is to be skeptical, and many OEM experts have taken the view that such cases are so unlikely to have environmental origins that they should be quickly dismissed and shunted to the care of other specialists. This approach may be reinforced by the impression that complaints by these patients are being driven or amplified by considerations of financial gain, job alienation, or other non-health-related factors.

However, there are compelling scientific and empiric reasons why such cases cannot be trivially dismissed without careful individual consideration of each one.

1. For all mechanisms of toxicity other than direct action, there is no supportable evidence of a clear threshold dose below which the effects cannot occur. This is especially important for idiosyncratic (e.g., allergic) effects, which may occur at very low levels in sensitized individuals. Even assuming that the likelihood of the effects is a function of the dose, the sheer numbers exposed to low doses would predict that the effects would occasionally occur.

2. For direct-acting toxins, the existence of a threshold does not imply that the threshold is the same in all hosts. Again, theoretically assuming that certain variable host factors determine the threshold level, the large number exposed to low doses would favor occasional very low level reactors.

3. In some situations that have been well studied, such as the non-specific building-related illness (NSBRI, see Chapter 50), the epidemiologic pattern of responses strongly supports a toxic response to some environmental factor or factors, even though the mechanism for this remains obscure.

4. Certain recently described patterns of clinical responses to environmental agents are occurring too pervasively and recognizably to dismiss them out of hand, despite the absence of coherent toxicologic or epidemiologic explanation at this time.

Given these foundations, it is the premise of this chapter that individuals with complaints apparently related to an environmental factor or factors at low level merit OEM evaluation. In the sections that follow, we shall discuss the differential diagnosis of health problems associated with low-dose exposures, describe the approaches to the workup and management of these challenging cases, and delineate what is known about these patterns of illness not discussed elsewhere in this text.

DIFFERENTIAL DIAGNOSIS

Some patients or their physicians may come to believe, for whatever reasons, that a chronic or persistent symptom

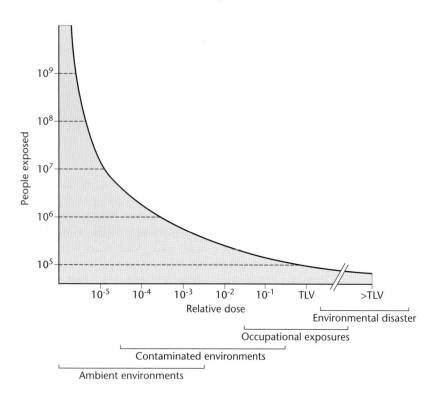

Figure 49.1: Exponential curve describing approximate relation between dose of any hazard, as an order of magnitude relative to a threshold limit value (TLV), and the number of persons likely to be exposed regularly at that level. In society as a whole, heavy disaster or occupational exposures affect relatively few persons, whereas millions experience low levels of exposure in contaminated food, air, and water

pattern or an established clinical abnormality or diagnosis is caused by a low-level environmental exposure. An example is the widespread attribution of various clinical syndromes to mercury exposure from amalgam in dental fillings (see Chapter 39.9). Similarly, an abnormality of liver function might be attributed to exposure to chemicals in a toxic waste site near the patient's home or a cancer might be attributed to an agent encountered occasionally or at very low levels at work. In such cases, the task of differential diagnosis is straightforward, if technically challenging. The approach is the one outlined in Chapter 3, i.e., the specific exposure is elucidated, the dose is quantified as best possible, data sets (toxicologic, epidemiologic, and clinical) are explored to determine the possibility and likelihood of relevant health effects, and the probability of the purported versus other possible causes is then calculated. The one caveat is to remember the possibility that the patient may be more susceptible than average, so that any significant possibility, even if not highly probable, must be taken seriously.

There are, however, a different subgroup of patients for whom this approach will not work. These are patients whose primary problem is that they react in some predictable way when exposed to certain environments or agents. Although they may differ greatly in the nature and scope of their symptoms, the circumstances that appear to induce them, and the severity of the complaints, they share certain features that are recognizable to the experienced practitioner as follows.

1. Symptoms, typically dermal, cardiorespiratory, gastrointestinal, neurologic, or musculoskeletal, occur episodically after exposure to some environment(s) or environmental agent(s).

2. Chronic fatigue, diffuse musculoskeletal pains or other non-specific complaints may prevail between episodes.
3. Constitutional signs of health, as measured by physical examination and routine laboratory studies, are preserved.

With such patients it is difficult either to confirm or exclude a toxicologic basis for the symptoms. Often, it is difficult to establish even the physiologic nature of the reactions, which may range from short-lived episodes of apparent autonomic discharge, e.g., tachycardia, tachypnea, and sweating, to protracted episodes of symptoms unassociated with measurable physiologic change. Nonetheless, the perceived temporal association between exposure and effect begs consideration of the following possibilities.

1. *Classic allergy to an environmental agent.* Many substances, especially certain small molecules, like formaldehyde, or certain biologic antigens, like those on mold, are ubiquitous in air, food, and water. For patients who are atopic or others whose complaint pattern could be explained by classic immunoglobulin or cell-mediated and related allergic responses, this possibility should never be overlooked. This otherwise straightforward diagnosis may be especially challenging because severely atopic patients often react to non-specific stimuli, such as irritants, and symptoms may persist between attacks, despite the absence of any stimulus, for unclear reasons.

2. *Chemically induced stimulation of a vascular or secretory disorder.* Migraine syndromes, hereditary diseases (such as porphyria), and endocrine tumors (such as pheochromocytoma) have been described that respond to specific chemical or physical stimuli, although almost always the stimulus has been a high-level exposure, such as a drug, alcohol, or other ingestion. Thus, although this possibility

is remote, it should be considered when highly stereotyped responses are described and other features consistent with such a diagnosis are noted.

3. *Classic anxiety disorder.* Phobias, especially claustrophobia and agoraphobia, may present as multisymptom reactions to specific environments; the environmental factor is presumably misinterpreted by the patient. Similarly, panic disorder, by definition attacks unprovoked by a defined stimulus, may be construed by the patient as being caused by the presence of a chemical or other contaminant. Obsessive-compulsive disorder may also present as reactions to environmental chemicals. Somatization disorder is characterized by a constellation of complaints referable to many organs that defy explanation. Typically the pattern is lifelong, and the symptoms do not cycle in any predictable fashion related to environmental exposure. These diagnostic considerations are important because the disorders are common and treatable. However, they are not diagnoses of exclusion (as is often presumed) but are, in fact, well-characterized, affirmatively diagnosable conditions that should be assessed by a specialist (see Chapter 28.3).

4. *Non-specific building-related illness (NSBRI).* As noted previously and described in detail in Chapter 50, an epidemiologically defined disorder caused by poor ventilation has emerged, which is characterized by fatigue, respiratory, dermal, and central nervous system complaints associated with a specific environment. The hallmarks are the concurrence of illness in coworkers and the isolation of difficulties to a single environment with improvement in others.

5. *Multiple chemical sensitivities (MCS).* This syndrome of unknown pathogenesis applies to the subgroup of these patients whose symptoms are referable to multiple systems and occur in multiple, unrelated environments in which low levels of chemicals are perceived. Common stimulants are perfumes and fragrances, petroleum derivatives, and smoke. The syndrome often, but not always, starts after a well-defined environmental event, such as a reaction to a more demonstrably toxic dose of an organic solvent, pesticide, or respiratory irritant, or after an episode of apparent NSBRI. Although manifestations of anxiety and/or depression are evident in many severely affected individuals, not all meet established criteria for primary anxiety. More importantly, neither the peculiar pattern of symptoms nor responses to therapy directed at these associated disorders suggest that MCS – whatever it is – is merely a misdiagnosis for anxiety or depression.

DIAGNOSTIC APPROACH TO PATIENTS WITH EPISODIC SYMPTOMS

Because the management and environmental ramifications differ greatly among these alternatives, it is crucial to differentiate them. However, usually these patients are referred to an OEM physician relatively late, after extensive workup and treatment has already been attempted, frustrating the patient, physicians (often many), and employ-

ers. For this reason, it is important to proceed efficiently and, to the extent possible, avoid extensive use of the laboratory and/or consultants to endlessly explore 'one last possibility' before providing a diagnosis and associated management plan.

Fortunately, although the stakes are high, the problem of differential diagnosis is not insurmountable, or even difficult, on close scrutiny. A detailed illness and exposure history, repeated and reviewed as often as is necessary, is the most important differential tool; the physical examination and laboratory results play an ancillary role. The following five historic features can provide considerable diagnostic insight.

1. *The spectrum of symptoms.* Classic allergies, secretory or vasospastic disorders, and panic disorder are characterized by fairly discrete and specific attacks. Usually, the manifestations of each attack are similar; between the attacks, there is recovery. Anxiety disorders (except pure panic) and MCS, on the other hand, share a more pleomorphic clinical character, often with diverse and changing patterns of symptoms and frequent persistence of symptoms between the exposures that precipitate the acute reactions.

2. *The diversity of environmental circumstances in which reactions are reported to occur.* NSBRI is characterized by reactions to a single, usually work, environment, in which the patient spends a large portion of time. An occurrence after only a brief exposure or in multiple settings rules this diagnosis out or suggests that NSBRI has been complicated by another problem, such as MCS. Similarly, although allergic reactions or stimulation of a secretory or vasospastic event could occur in several different settings, such reactions occurring ubiquitously or to dozens of apparently unrelated precipitants is biologically implausible.

3. *The nature of the environments that are associated with reactions.* Tolerance to an offending agent in one situation, e.g., at work, but not in another, e.g., outdoors, suggests that some characteristic of these environments other than the suspect agent is central; one must consider the possibilities of claustrophobia and agoraphobia. Such circumstantial factors also strongly militate against the classic allergy and secretory and vasospastic stimulation. Likewise, tolerance to tobacco smoke, which contains substantial doses of numerous chemicals at impressive levels, usually excludes MCS, although severe, dysfunctional addiction may rarely persist even after MCS is acquired.

4. *The predictability of environmental response.* The frequent occurrence of reactions in the absence of any environmental factor evident to the patient suggests the likelihood of panic, other anxiety disorder, or an endogenous precipitant of a secretory problem. Although unprovoked attacks occur in classic allergy or MCS, such episodes rule out NSBRI entirely or suggest it has become complicated.

5. *The onset of illness.* The patient's description of the earliest manifestations of illness, coupled with a detailed review of all prior medical conditions, can be helpful. NSBRI typically begins insidiously some time after beginning work in a specific building or after a building is renovated or otherwise physically altered. Classic allergies and MCS may occur after some period or episode of a demonstrably toxic

Syndrome	Spectrum of symptoms	Number of precipitating environments	Types of environments	Symptoms occur in unpredictable environment	Symptom onset
Classic allergy	Limited	Few	Specific	Occasionally	May be discrete
Secretory syndrome	Limited	Few	May appear diverse	Often	May be discrete
Panic disorder	Limited	Many	Diverse	Often	May be discrete
Anxiety disorders	Diverse	Many	May be recognizable	Often	Insidious
NSBRI*	Diverse	One	Single indoor environment	Never	Insidious or discrete
MCS	Diverse	Many	Diverse	Occasionally	Usually discrete

*NSBRI: Non-Specific Building Related Illness; MCS, Multiple Chemical Sensitivities.

Table 49.1 Differential features of disorders attributed to low-level environmental exposures

exposure associated with severe symptoms, whereas the anxiety disorders rarely have a clear beginning. The history in such patients typically reveals prior unexplained illness, often dating back to childhood. Although such a history does not exclude other possibilities, it should flag the need for a thorough investigation of these treatable disorders.

These historic features are summarized in Table 49.1. Collectively, they should allow the clinician to focus on the most likely entity or entities and reduce the need for exhaustive laboratory testing or referrals in all but the most difficult cases. Further evaluation and testing should follow the basic principles of the most likely candidates. Classic allergic disorders resulting from environmental agents are discussed in Chapters 19.2 and 50. NSBRI is discussed, along with specific building-related illnesses, in Chapter 50. The anxiety disorders are discussed in context in Chapter 28.3. The workup of migraine syndromes and secretory disorders, the rarest but possibly most serious consideration here, is beyond the scope of this text.

What remains is a discussion of the single most common diagnostic category for these patients, i.e., multiple chemical sensitivities (MCS). The remainder of the chapter is devoted to this controversial topic.

MULTIPLE CHEMICAL SENSITIVITIES (MCS)

This label was introduced in the mid 1980s to describe a group of patients who have symptoms in response to multiple low-level environmental exposures.[1] Gradually, the term MCS has emerged as the single most commonly used, but not exclusive designation for those who meet the following case definition.

1. The syndrome is acquired, usually after the occurrence of a more clearly evident (although not necessarily serious) health event caused by environmental exposure, such as solvent intoxication, respiratory tract irritation, pesticide poisoning, or NSBRI.
2. The patient experiences multiple symptoms referable to several organ systems, almost always including the central nervous system.
3. Although there may be persistent complaints between exposures, the symptoms are characteristically and predictably precipitated by a perceived environmental exposure.

4. The agents that may precipitate the symptoms are multiple and chemically diverse.
5. The doses of these agents that precipitate symptoms are at least two orders of magnitude lower than the established thresholds for acute health effects.
6. No test of physiologic function can explain the symptoms. Although there may be clinical abnormalities, such as mild bronchospasm or neuropsychologic dysfunction, these are typically non-specific and insufficient to explain the full scope of the illness pattern.
7. No other organic disorder is present that can better explain the pattern of symptoms.

Similar to other clinical case definitions of disorders of unknown cause that have no specific pathologic finding or test, problems exist with the MCS definition. Most obviously, many clinicians have used and continue to use other less well-defined terms to designate the disorders in these patients, causing confusion in the literature. A new designation[2] – idiopathic environmental intolerance – has some heuristic appeal but its introduction has only made matters worse. Furthermore, many patients whose syndrome fulfills part but not all of this case definition have had their condition diagnosed clinically as MCS anyway; this avoids having to deal with patients meeting the criteria for no known disorder but creates blurry margins for MCS. Finally, because many clinicians and investigators question whether MCS designates a unique disorder or a new presentation of another disease, which is toxic or psychologic (see subsequent discussion), many refuse to apply it under any circumstance.

These caveats notwithstanding, the MCS designation has allowed at least the beginning of some uniformity in the approach to the study and management of these curious cases. As long as the clinician recognizes that labeling a patient with MCS neither explains the basis of the illness – which remains unknown – nor ensures its successful resolution, a narrow use of this term applied to syndromes meeting the criteria above is probably clinically and scientifically reasonable at this time.

Epidemiology

Since the first edition of this book there has been substantial progress in our understanding of the epidemiology of MCS, despite the absence of a uniform definition or clear disease marker. Although no evidence has appeared to contradict the perception that clinically manifest MCS is uncommon,[3] population surveys in North Carolina and California[4,5] have demonstrated that as much as 6% of the population may have symptoms compatible with the diagnosis, sufficient to alter their lives in some ways to accommodate them. In the most comprehensive study of veterans of the Persian Gulf conflict of 1990–91, conducted among present and former military personnel in Iowa,[6] over 5% of military who returned from the war complained of symptoms which met the study criteria for MCS. Perhaps more alarmingly, military personnel *not* in the conflict, presumably a young healthy control population, had a rate of over 2.5% using the questionnaire instrument; two out of three in each group carried a physician diagnosis of MCS or equivalent designation. Another important contribution has been recent evidence of a strong overlap in symptom patterns between clinical patients with MCS and those with both chronic fatigue syndrome and fibromyalgia, better characterized syndromes which themselves lack pathogenic mechanisms or biologic disease markers.

The newly available data have lent further support to the idea that women are more frequently affected than men, by perhaps 2–4-fold,[3-6] but the disease is not unheard of in men, who constitute the majority of those with symptoms acquired after the war. Middle age is still the most commonly affected age group, but cases have been described from school age through retirement. Contrary to earlier speculation, risk for the disorder appears relatively evenly distributed by social class and race.[5,6]

Pathogenesis

As noted, the cause of MCS remains obscure. Broadly speaking, there are two schools of thought, i.e., the biologic and the psychologic. The former likens MCS to other allergic disorders and has postulated immune, epithelial, or central nervous system dysfunction as the basis for MCS. There were early data to support abnormal chemosensory responses in affected subjects, such as altered olfaction or trigeminal function, which could be related to such a proposed mechanism, but there are more comprehensive recent data which suggest the alteration is in conscious perception, not sensory function per se.[7,8] Data on immunologic defects and abnormal regional central nervous system metabolism have been reported but not confirmed by blinded and well-controlled studies.[9,10] Whether any such lesions, even if confirmed, are predisposing or represent the manifestation of disease also remains to be determined.

The psychologic view of the illness is based on the well-documented high rate of anxiety and affective symptoms evident in patients compared with other populations.[11-13] A model using classic constructs from behavioral theory has elegantly explained some cases, and therapy based on behavioral approaches has been anecdotally successful.[14] One investigator has reported a high rate of childhood abuse among patients with MCS, along with anecdotal

data on effective therapy focused on this issue.[15] Others have attempted to demonstrate that patient responses to environmental agents that purportedly cause symptoms do not do so predictably when blinded placebo challenges are interspersed among the offending agents, implying that suggestion or other psychologic factors are important. Acute reactions to chemicals in these patients bear some clinical resemblance to panic attacks, another feature suggesting a possible psychologic mechanism.[16]

Unfortunately, neither view has been subjected to adequate scrutiny. One randomized, double-blind controlled therapeutic trial of a selective serotonin uptake inhibitor with excellent activity against known anxiety disorders and depression found, surprisingly, that patients with MCS had no reactions to the placebo yet a marked increase in their apparent reactivity while receiving the active medication; none improved, as had been anticipated by the investigators.[17] All other existing studies have been cross-sectional and suffer from either inadequate control or unsatisfactory classification of patients using a standard set of criteria.

Given these inconsistencies, many suggest that both organic and psychologic factors may be operating. Meanwhile, it is probably prudent to avoid any dogmatic view that is likely to be incorrect when a fuller appreciation of MCS becomes available.

Clinical course

Uncertainties about its pathogenesis notwithstanding, much experience has been gained with MCS and its natural history. Two distinctive illness patterns are discernible among these patients. Some have striking attacks after exposure, followed by recovery to normal or near normal; they remain well as long as the offending agents are avoided. Others have persistent and often disabling symptoms, which are made worse by exposure but never entirely relieved. Contrary to the perception of many patients that the illness runs an inexorable downhill course, current experience suggests that MCS tends to run a naturally cyclic pattern after initial onset. Irrespective of the therapies the patient or clinician may try, the illness is punctuated by periods of greater and lesser discomfort associated with exposure to environmental agents and constitutional complaints. While it may be tempting to ascribe these changes to environmental or therapeutic factors, observations over longer periods suggest an unrelated rhythmicity.

The observation of the cyclic nature of the illness has two important clinical corollaries. First, no established, measurable physiologic consequences or complications over long-term follow-up have been documented. Limited data on psychotherapy to the contrary, there is no convincing evidence that patients with MCS ever revert to their premorbid state. This is not to say that major functional and symptomatic improvements are not achievable but that the goal of cure, i.e., return to prior health, does not occur spontaneously and is not generally achievable with present therapeutic modalities.

Treatment

As these considerations would suggest, there remain no established specific therapies for MCS. Almost every patient needs the following four things.

1. *Education.* A careful explanation of MCS, including what is and is not known about its cause and natural history, is required for the patient, their family, and often the employer. It is crucial that the patient understand that the disorder is neither lethal nor curable.

2. *Support.* This may include self-help groups, counselors, social workers, or more formal clinical care to manage the inevitable psychologic and social issues that the patient with MCS will have to confront. The goal should be return to the highest level of social, personal and occupational function of which the patient is capable. Problematically, patients who believe fervently that their disorder is purely physical in nature often resist such efforts, or view them as merely 'tactical'. Evidence suggests it is worthwhile trying to convince them otherwise.

3. *Environmental modification.* Although removing the patient from all contact with modern life is both highly counterproductive and unlikely to succeed, some changes are important, especially removal or reduction in the heaviest exposures that were associated with the onset of illness. Often, this entails a work modification and changes in the home environment to make it comfortable and safe. Unfortunately, clinicians inclined to the view that MCS is purely psychological often resist this aspect, wishing to avoid 'reinforcing' the patient's sometimes intractable view that the problem is purely physical. However, with or without the clinician's support, most patients make the changes anyway; withholding approval breeds distrust and undermines the possibility for a therapeutic relationship.

4. *Economic support.* If MCS results in profound levels of disability or a marked reduction in income because of job modification, it is necessary to use available entitlement and benefit programs to guarantee that severe hardship does not undermine treatment and rehabilitation. Rehabilitation to promote new occupational possibilities within limitations is highly desirable. The same comments as above with regard to the views of the clinician are also germane in this regard.

Beyond these measures, little else has been helpful for more than an occasional patient. Radical therapies, including isolation from all chemicals (e.g., moving to the desert or mountains), megavitamins, antioxidants, desensitization regimens, and fat purification are expensive and of unproved value. Behavioral therapy has been successful in a few widely reported cases[18] but has not been studied in a larger population, so efficacy currently remains unproven. Similarly, although psychiatric treatment, including either pharmacologic and/or psychotherapeutic modalities, is always indicated to manage depressive features or troubling anxiety when present, current evidence does not suggest that such therapy is particularly successful for modifying the manifestations of MCS, nor is it clinically indicated for that purpose.

References

1. Cullen MR. Workers with multiple sensitivities. Occup Med State Art Rev 1987; 2:655–62.
2. International Program on Chemical Safety. Conclusion and recommendations of a workshop on multiple chemical sensitivities. Reg Toxicol Pharmacol 1996; 24:S188–9.
3. Cullen MR, Pace PE, Redlich CA. The experience of the Yale Occupational and Environmental Medicine Clinic with multiple chemical sensitivities. Toxicol Ind Health 1992; 8:15–19.
4. Meggs WJ, Dunn KA, Bloch RM, et al. Prevalence and nature of allergy and chemical sensitivity in a general population. Arch Environ Health 1996; 51:275–82.
5. Kreutzer R, Neutra RR, Lashvay W. Prevalence of people reporting sensitivities to chemicals in a population-based survey. Am J Epidemiol 1999; 150:1–12.
6. Black DW, Doebbeling BN, Voelker MD, et al. Multiple chemical sensitivity syndrome. Symptom prevalence and risk factors in a military population. Arch Intern Med 2000; 160:1169–76.
7. Doty RL, Deems DA, Frye RE, et al. Olfactory sensitivity, nasal resistance and autonomic function in patients with multiple chemical sensitivities. Arch Otolaryngol Head Neck Surg 1988; 114:1422–7.
8. Dalton P, Hummel T. Chemosurgery function and response in idiopathic environmental intolerance. Occup Med State Art Rev 2000; 15:539–56.
9. Mitchell LS, Donnay A, Hoover D, et al. Immunologic parameters of multiple chemical sensitivity. Occup Med State Art Rev 2000;15:647–65.
10. Waxman AD. Functional brain assessment of multiple chemical sensitivities. Occup Med State Art Rev 2000; 15:611–6.
11. Simon GE, Katon WJ, Sparks PJ. Allergic to life: psychological factors in environmental illness. Am J Psychiatry 1990; 147:901–6.
12. Black DW, Rath A, Goldstein RB. Environmental illness: a controlled study of 26 subjects with 20th century disease. JAMA 1990; 264:3166–70.
13. Fiedler N, Kipen HM, Deluca J, et al. A controlled comparison of multiple chemical sensitivities and chronic fatigue syndrome. Psychosom Med 1996; 58:38–49.
14. Shusterman D, Balmes J, Cone J. Behavioral sensitization to irritants/odorants after acute overexposures. J Occup Med 1988; 30:565–7.
15. Selner JC, Standenmayer H. Psychologic factors complicating the diagnosis of work-related chemical illness. Immunol Allergy Clin North Am 1992; 12:909–19.
16. Leznoff A, Binkley KE. Idiopathic environmental intolerances: Results of challenge studies. Occup Med State Art Rev 2000; 15:529–38.
17. Cullen MR. Multiple chemical sensitivities: is there evidence of extreme vulnerability of the brain to environmental chemicals? In: Isaacson RL, Jensen KF, eds. The vulnerable brain and environmental risks, Vol. 3, Special hazards from air and water. New York: Plenum Press, 1994;65–75.
18. Gugliemi RS, Cid DJ, Spyker DA. Behavioral treatment of phobic avoidance in multiple chemical sensitivity. J Behav Ther Exp Psychiatry 1994; 25:197–209

Chapter 50
Exposures in Indoor Environments

Michael J Hodgson, Michelle R Addorisio

In industrialized societies individuals may spend up to 90% of their time indoors. Therefore, it is essential for the clinical practitioner to have an understanding of the indoor environment and its contribution to health. Providing adequate air quality, or ambient conditions, serves two separate and distinct, although overlapping, purposes – to provide comfort and protect health. Depending on the definition used, these two may not result from similar conditions. For example, benzene or asbestos concentrations may be imperceptible and yet pose at least a measurable risk. Yet, discomfort from offensive odors may not pose a health risk in the traditional sense. Nevertheless, such discomfort may lead to decreased productivity, increased concern, and social and organizational dysfunction. Since this discomfort may have a substantially greater influence on the overall performance of a workforce than more clearly measurable or estimable health risks, both health and comfort must be considered.

Indoor air quality presents a challenge to occupational and environmental health professionals that differs from traditional industrial worksites. First, it involves exposures that cross the divide between occupational and non-occupational settings. Second, little formal regulation exists. Although recommended exposure levels have been established by several organizations these may not be enforceable and serve as professional guidelines with an inadequately defined scientific basis.[1] Third, exposures usually are better characterized by assessment of processes and exposure determinants, rather than quantitative measurements of specific pollutants. Buildings and indoor environments in general must be examined as to whether they function as they are supposed to, i.e., whether they provide acceptable working or living conditions.[2,3]

This chapter addresses several approaches to indoor air quality in occupational settings. It presents an overview of the three standard approaches to buildings: occupant complaints, building systems, and pollutants. It summarizes current thinking about indoor exposures in the home. Finally, it makes recommendations on the prevention of building problems.

APPROACHES TO BUILDING PROBLEMS IN THE OCCUPATIONAL ENVIRONMENT

Three basic approaches are available to the investigation of building complaints or problems. The first focuses on health problems among building occupants and helps classify syndromes and identify diseases. Yet, it may not identify specific sources within buildings because the same pollutant may result from different building components. A typical example is the association of legionnaire's disease with both cooling towers and potable water systems. Therefore, although this approach may narrow the potential scope of the problem, it generally does not implicate a specific source.

The second approach focuses on environmental control, identifying deviations from good design, operations, and maintenance procedures. Deficiencies may be present and recognizable and still not be associated with the complaint or illness. This approach is therefore independent of medical evaluations and may not predict actual exposures or disease at any given time.[4]

The third approach focuses on specific pollutants and exposures. Frequently, the likely pollutants can be identified during a careful walk-through. Focusing on specific pollutants in problem-solving situations may utilize valuable resources on extensive quantitative air sampling measurements and actually delay identification and resolution of problems. This can lead to unnecessary turmoil, lost productivity, and progressive adverse health effects. A pollutant-oriented quantitative approach may be necessary from a research and regulatory standpoint, but frequently is not useful for solving practical indoor air clinical problems.

In the following sections, these three approaches are summarized separately and focus on disease identification, analysis of design deficiencies, and recognition and measurement of pollutant sources.

PARADIGM 1: DISORDERS ASSOCIATED WITH INDOOR POLLUTANTS

Health effects attributable to indoor pollutants have been recognized for centuries and began with the identification of adverse health effects from wood smoke in closed rooms in the 18th century. Max von Pettenkofer, in the mid 19th century, measured indoor CO_2 levels in an attempt to define health requirements. In the late 19th century, decreased ventilation was recognized as a contributing factor to the transmission of tuberculosis.

Building-related illness

During the last 20 years, complaints attributed to buildings have generally been classified as one of two broad groups:

Selected diseases	Selected agents
Rhinitis, sinusitis	Allergens, molds, spores Irritants – chemicals, cleaning agents, VOCs
Asthma	Irritant exposures, including cleaning agents, VOCs Allergens, molds, chemicals
Hypersensitivity pneumonitis	Wood dust, MDI, chemicals, thermotolerant bacteria related to moisture
Organic dust toxic syndrome (inhalation fevers)	Gram-negative bacteria, molds
Infectious diseases	
Legionnaire's disease	*Legionella pneumophila*
Tuberculosis	*Mycobacterium tuberculosis*
Upper respiratory tract infection	Viral infections
Allergic contact dermatitis	Molds, chemicals, photoactive copy paper, formaldehyde; molds; laser toners
Irritant contact dermatitis	Fiberglass, VOCs, low humidity, office products
Lung cancer	Radon, environmental tobacco smoke, asbestos

Table 50.1 Specific building-related illness agents

Mucus membrane irritation	Eye irritation, throat irritation, cough
Neurotoxic effects	Headaches, fatigue, lack of concentration, memory loss
Respiratory symptoms	Shortness of breath, cough, wheeze
Skin symptoms	Rash, pruritus, dryness
Chemosensory changes	Enhanced or abnormal odor perception; visual disturbances

Table 50.2 Typical symptoms in SBS

specific building-related illnesses and sick building syndrome (SBS). Building-related illnesses (BRI), which are listed in Table 50.1, are diseases that have multiple etiologies, one of which is a specific factor in an indoor environment.[5] They are summarized here but readers are referred to the appropriate chapters for a more detailed discussion. Some, such as eosinophilic fungal sinusitis, remain controversial. BRI are generally distinguished from the non-specific symptoms that make up sick building syndrome (SBS) (Table 50.2).[6] Although the distinction between specific building-related illnesses and SBS is widely used, outbreaks of specific diseases have often been associated with excess rates of non-specific symptoms in individuals that do not meet formal case definitions. This has been used as one argument to suggest that SBS may be an early stage of a BRI, which if left unchecked may progress to a recognizable pathophysiologic entity.[7,8]

Respiratory tract disease

Respiratory tract diseases such as rhinitis and asthma are the most common building-related illnesses. Diseases have been described at all levels of the respiratory system and are attributed to a variety of mechanisms but most often to

bioaerosols and irritants.[9,10] Diagnostic workups usually do not implicate any specific organism or single irritant. Disorders associated with bioaerosols are seen in settings with inadequate moisture control and poor housekeeping leading to bioaerosols growth. This growth is usually evident on visual inspection and through the sense of smell.[11]

Rhinitis and sinusitis

Complaints consistent with allergic and irritant rhinitis and sinusitis are commonly encountered in buildings and overlap with SBS (see also Chapter 20.3). The diagnosis is often based on the clinical history but may be embellished by tests, including nasal swabs, immunologic testing (skin and blood testing), rhinometry, and rhinomanometry. Recently, nasal lavage has documented abnormalities related to bioaerosols exposures.[12-14] Cases have been attributed to inadequate maintenance of ventilation units (see subsequent discussion). Even when preventive maintenance on central units is done, frequently no similar attempts are made to remove housings from window units for routine cleaning, perhaps because of cost or because of inadequate foresight. Accumulation of biologic materials supporting microbial growth is common as a consequence and may lead to odor complaints and allergic disease.

Asthma

Reversible airway dysfunction may be related to indoor air in buildings. Difficulties exist with defining whether cases are exacerbated by working in the building or whether some specific etiologic agent is present (i.e., occupational asthma).[13] Exposures may be present either at work/school or home, or in both settings concurrently. This makes the etiology of disease difficult to establish. Since substance-specific challenges are not practical and generally unavailable, alternative approaches are usually used. These include: spirometry before and after work and on a control day, peak flow tracings during the day, and sequential methacholine challenges[15] (see Chapter 19.2). It has been suggested that asthma exacerbations may be attributed to general growth of microbial agents on carpets or bedding, microbial contamination of ventilation systems, humidifiers, and to office products.

Management strategies for all three of these disorders may be frustrating, since the work environment may continue to exacerbate symptoms. Reassignment of a patient to other sites within the building may be attempted and is frequently met with success. Reduced exposures through improved ventilation and reduction of indoor sources can be effective with some patients. Removal from the environment may be necessary.[12] Following the patient's status with peak flow measurements or forced expiratory volumes will provide a reasonable indication of whether or not the patient's disease is reasonably controlled.

Humidifier fever

Humidifier fever, an acute inhalation syndrome similar to organic dust toxic syndrome related to malfunctioning air conditioning units, was one of the first diseases attributed to indoor spaces, initially in a carpentry shop. The symptoms include both systemic (headaches, feverishness, myalgias, and chills) and chest (chest tightness, cough, and wheezing) complaints, although the former are generally more prominent. The etiology is believed to be related to endotoxin and micro-organisms. The diagnosis is based largely on the clinical presentation and ruling out asthma and hypersensitivity pneumonitis.

Hypersensitivity pneumonitis

The syndrome of hypersensitivity pneumonitis may occur acutely, chronically, or in an intermediate form, with both chest and constitutional complaints (see Chapter 19.6). Symptoms include cough, chest tightness, fever, chills, and myalgias. In several outbreaks, wheezing was also reported.[12] The diagnosis is based on the clinical picture and confirmed by several or all of the following: lung function tests, chest x-ray studies, high resolution CAT scan, bronchoalveolar lavage, and biopsy. Serum antibodies can document exposure and an immune response. As awareness has increased, outbreaks have been documented with few clinical signs or physiologic abnormalities. Documentation of changes in lung function related to a specific site is generally possible and indicates the need for remedial action.

Outbreaks have usually been attributed to the contamination of ventilation systems. The primary sites have included: mold at the air intake, water pump contamination, sources for water incursion, contamination of duct liners and filters, and, rarely, sources such as those contaminated by residual sawdust, plumbing leaks, and standing water sources. The occurrence of this serious disease requires that the specific source be identified so that further cases may be prevented and the identified cases do not progress.[16]

Other non-infectious interstitial lung diseases

Several forms of non-allergic disease of the respiratory tract have been described. Asbestosis has been demonstrated in occupational groups with exposure to asbestos in indoor environments.[1] For example, maintenance plumbers and custodians in buildings and building tradespersons in general have been shown to be at increased risk for asbestos-related pleural disease. This occurs not because of work in buildings with exposure to ambient concentrations of asbestos fibers but because their job activities generate asbestos dust similar to that generated in industrial or construction environments.

Another form of interstitial lung disease may be associated with exposure to mycotoxin-producing fungi. Animal models document that mature rats develop pulmonary disease after exposure to spores of either *Aspergillus versicolor* or *Stachybotrys chartarum*. This effect is related to the methanol extractable fraction of the spores.[17] Case control studies suggest an association with industries, occupations, or exposures to bioaerosols. Case reports and clusters of interstitial disease suggest that moisture, dirt, and bioaerosols indoors are not as harmless as previously assumed.[18]

Infections

More important are the viral and bacterial infections attributed to building sources. Evidence exists that mechanical ventilation is associated with up to a 50% increase in respiratory tract infections and an estimated 500,000 lost work days.[19] Whether this is related to the recirculation of air, inadequate filtration, increased concentrations of air-borne droplet nuclei, relative humidity changes, or to increased infection susceptibility is a matter of dispute and scientific uncertainty. Several outbreaks of other viral illnesses, including measles and varicella, have been attributed to the dissemination of infectious particles after entrainment into the airstream. Tuberculosis and Q fever transmission can occur in a similar fashion. A single outbreak of pneumococcal pneumonia remains controversial, as it may have occurred from crowding alone rather than through airstream dissemination.[20]

The most frequently discussed bacterial infectious disease attributed to indoor spaces is caused by *Legionella* sp., including both legionnaire's disease and Pontiac fever.[17] The case fatality rate of 15% has not changed markedly, despite introduction of appropriate antibiotics. Two modes of transmission are recognized: (1) inhalation of droplet nuclei and (2) aspiration of Legionellaceae that colonizes the oropharynx in susceptible hosts (smokers, asthmatic patients, individuals with chronic obstructive pulmonary disease and immune suppression). Although most outbreaks in the first 15 years were attributed to cooling towers and to the drift of infected plumes, more recently an alternative hypothesis has been proposed. Most outbreaks reported since 1982 have been attributed to potable water systems. Although there are outbreaks clearly attributable to cooling towers and plume drift, potable water sources, including showers and home water heaters, are now a major concern.[21]

Since *Legionella* strains appear to be in more than one-half of water bodies in the United States, it is unclear why the disease is not more prevalent. The risk factors for transmission likely depend on the concentration of Legionellaceae in the water and host risk factors. In addition, electric water heaters, blind pipe ends, sluggish water flow, kinking in pipes, and leaks in water cooling systems may also contribute to disease transmission. Controversy exists as to whether cultures should be performed to keep Legionellaceae counts below a specific threshold or whether maintenance per se affects the rate of legionnaire's disease. In some settings, such as healthcare, this is standard practice.[22,23]

Work-related outbreaks have been documented in a broad range of settings, including cooling tower operations, steam turbine cleaners, plastic press cooling water leaks, and oil mists. Criteria for work-relatedness include growth of the agent from a specific source, serologic evidence for the presence of the same strain in victim and source, and adequate evidence of legionnaire's disease. Home sources should also be cultured since transmission from potable residential water is equally likely.

Dermatitis

Skin complaints have been described frequently in buildings and are also an integral component of the SBS. Although irritant, allergic, and photodermatitis have been documented, there is a question about the frequency and importance of each in indoor environments.

Irritant dermatitis

Irritant dermatitis has been attributed to chemical, physical, or a combination of both causes (see Chapter 29.1). The most easily recognized is induced by fiberglass fibers, classically described as itching without an obvious cause that is relieved by showering. The glass fibers may also be demonstrated in horizontal surface wipe samples. Itching occurring more frequently during the winter months may be associated with the lower relative humidity in indoor spaces, frequently below 20%. Such complaints have been attributed to the combination of low relative humidity and volatile organic compounds (VOC). Finally, some compounds, such as formaldehyde and phthalates in carbonless paper, are irritating on their own.

Allergic dermatitis

Cases of allergic skin disease have been described in buildings and are usually attributed to a specific source.[15]

Photodermatitis

Several reports have described erythema associated with video display terminal use, which has been localized to both the face and hands. The mechanism postulated was the relatively high intensity of the monochromatic light in such terminals compared with the broader range of frequencies from other sources. However, it is still difficult to prove an association since one of the cases listed was convincing but subsequently proved to be factitious.[24]

Lung cancer

Lung cancer is widely discussed as a chronic disease resulting from exposure to multiple risk factors. These include agents present in indoor environments, such as asbestos, radon, and environmental tobacco smoke (ETS).[25] Risk assessment for each of these does not suggest that work in the modern office is a significant risk factor. Individuals with traditional occupational exposures, such as plumbers and other building tradespersons, may be at risk for asbestos-related disease.

Sick building syndrome (SBS)

The term 'sick building syndrome' refers to problems related to indoor air quality in non-industrial buildings. Three very different approaches to its understanding have evolved and no operational criteria exist for its documentation. These three paradigms are: (1) building occupants and their symptoms, disease, or discomfort, (2) the environmental design and control of the building, and (3) specific pollutants and exposure assessment. It is clear that symptom prevalence varies from building to building, often without a recognized problem or an identified cause. Similarly, a substantial number of building systems do not meet professional design criteria or are operated in substandard ways. Finally, specific pollutants have been identified with reasonable measurement methods, physiologic markers of exposure, and predictable dose–response relationships.[19,26] Therefore, it is possible that many of the 'non-specific' symptoms of SBS may have a clear etiology.[7] The etiologic factors that are believed to contribute to SBS are defined in Table 50.3.

Building occupants

In the 1980s and 1990s numerous cross-sectional questionnaire investigations were published from several countries which suggested that complaint frequencies are associated with a series of environmental risk factors (Table 50.4). The most prominent risk factor was mechanical ventilation, which was consistently associated with a 50% increase in symptoms. Panel evaluations of office buildings in Denmark suggested that approximately 40% of the complaints could

Air contaminants	
Indoor sources	Building materials
	Moisture
	Office cleaning products
Outdoor sources	Automobile exhaust
	Industrial plants
	Moisture
HVAC system	Ventilation
	Heating/air conditioning
	Humidification
Work organization	Job satisfaction
	Stress
	Social structures
Host factors	Sex
	Atopy
	Airway hyper-reactivity
	Pre-existing disease

Table 50.3 Determinants of indoor air quality and symptoms

Volatile organic compounds	Formaldehyde; paints and resins; solvents; printed materials; printer and photocopier emissions
Dust/fibers	Asbestos; man-made mineral fibers (fiberglass); dirt, construction, and paper dust
Bioaerosols	Bacteria; fungi; molds; dust mites; viruses; pollen; animal danders and excreta
Entrapped outdoor sources	Vehicle exhaust; industrial exhaust
Physical factors	Temperature; humidity; noise; lighting
Contaminants generated by human activity	Carbon dioxide; perfume
Other	Fuel combustion products; radon; pesticides; cleaning agents; environmental tobacco smoke (ETS); building materials

Table 50.4 Common contaminants in indoor air

be attributed to ventilation systems, although it could not be determined if the pollutants were generated elsewhere and recirculated or if they were generated directly within the system. ETS, office machines, and human off-gassing contributed 25%, 20%, and 15% respectively to the remaining 60%.[27]

Over the last 15 years our understanding of the indoor environment and related health issues has increased significantly. While some symptoms, such as headaches, fatigue, and difficulty concentrating, are considered 'non-specific', others have better defined pathophysiologic mechanisms and markers.[28] In addition, it appears that personal characteristics modify the likelihood of symptoms. Atopic individuals describe higher symptom frequencies, have been shown to respond to irritants at lower levels, and have lower irritant thresholds than non-atopics.[29,30] Individuals with decreased tear-film break-up time and less protection for the ocular mucosa have higher rates of symptoms. Therefore, some of the symptom variability may result from defined, recognizable differences.

One of the better studied symptoms is mucosal irritation. Itching, irritation, tearing, and redness of the eyes, nasal mucosa, and throat mimic symptoms attributed to stimulating the irritant receptor, or the common chemical sense.[31] Physiologic techniques to measure these are well defined. Although headaches are widely recognized as a symptom of a poor indoor environment, there are no studies that examine them using standard diagnostic classifications. Data on headache treatment effectiveness in the office exist.[32] Dermal complaints have been reported to be associated with personality traits, dermal sensitivity to irritants, a history of eczema, and specific hormonal profiles.[15] Work stress is also associated with symptoms. Of some interest is the recent recognition that some mucosal symptoms appear related to specific fungal exposures in office buildings.

It is more difficult to address fatigue, headaches, lethargy, and other 'non-specific' symptoms.[32] Some data suggest they may in fact be related to endotoxin exposure and associated with moisture or humidity. Even though there appears to be a relationship between ventilation rates, moisture, infections, and symptoms, much still needs to be done to establish these associations. Stress and certain organizational factors at work may be risk factors.

PARADIGM 2: ENVIRONMENTAL DESIGN AND CONTROL

The first use of mechanical ventilation indoors occurred in 18th-century England when the new House of Parliament was fitted with blowers to distribute warmth from the furnaces. In 1860, Max von Pettenkofer calculated that indoor air was likely to be acceptable as long as the levels of carbon dioxide did not exceed 1000 ppm. Since 1892, the recommended indoor ventilation rates have ranged between 4 and 60 cubic feet of outdoor air per occupant per minute. The latter was recommended for tuberculosis prevention in the 1890s and to decrease tobacco irritation

in the 1970s; the former to keep miners alive in the early 19th century and during the energy crisis. The current standard recommends approximately 20.

At present, buildings in the US must be ventilated according to the local building code. Required outdoor air rates differ substantially between the building code and professional design recommendations. The most widely recognized standard, 'Ventilation for Acceptable Indoor Air Quality', promulgated by the American Society of Heating, Refrigerating, and Air-conditioning Engineers (ASHRAE), recommends approximately 20 cubic feet of outside air per occupant per minute for most commercial applications. Additional specific standards recommend boundaries and guidelines for thermal, acoustic, and lighting comfort. None were developed explicitly to protect completely against health effects.[1] Careful scrutiny of the scientific basis for each of these standards, therefore, suggests major gaps and assumptions. Health scientists must therefore remain aware that even when buildings 'meet all professional standards', a substantial proportion of occupants may be dissatisfied or even become ill from exposures.[11]

An ASHRAE commissioning guide provides detailed procedures to ensure that buildings 'work' at the beginning of their occupancy, but such guidelines are often not followed. Reviews of building systems suggest that the majority of buildings in the US simply do not meet professional design standards and therefore contribute to health concerns and occupant discomfort.

A review of structural and functional issues in problem buildings serves to identify specific sources. This may be done without necessarily linking the problem sources to concomitant medical problems or complaints, or even implicating specific pollutants. Nevertheless, the identification of engineering or architectural deficiencies by themselves should lead to remediation strategies.[4,29] Even if specific deficiencies have not caused the problem under investigation, they could do so in the future.

Newer building designs focus more on control of the microenvironment, such as: control of lighting, thermal parameters, and acoustics in the specific work zone.[2] In the long run, such systems may serve the occupants better, support higher productivity, and lead to greater occupant satisfaction.

Heating, ventilating, and air-conditioning systems

The first system usually examined closely in a problem building is the heating, ventilating, and air-conditioning (HVAC) system. HVAC systems were initially designed for pollutant removal and filter, but during the last 50 years they have served primarily to provide comfort. Ideally, ventilation systems distribute outside fresh air, condition (heat or cool) the air, control the humidity, and remove pollutants. Figure 50.1 provides a schematic of the design of a generic HVAC system.

Return and outside air are mixed in a plenum. The first basic assumption is that the outside air is clean. However, ambient air may not meet air quality guidelines

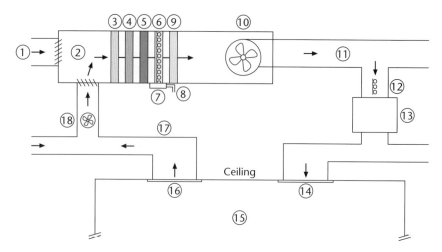

Figure 50.1: Schema of a basic ventilation system (HVAC). Arrows represent airflow; slashes represent dampers. (1) Outdoor air supply air intake, (2) mixing plenum, (3) prefilter, (4) filter, (5) heating coil, (6) cooling coil, (7) condensate/drip pan, (8) drain, (9) steam humidification, (10) supply fan, (11) supply duct, (12) reheat coil, (13) variable air volume box, (14) supply diffuser, (15) occupied space, (16) return air louver, (17) return air duct, (18) booster fan.

(Environmental Protection Agency guidelines and Clean Air Act) and therefore, the outdoor environment must be considered in evaluating systems. For example, placement of air intakes may lead to circadian changes in pollutant loads (intake at freeway level leading to carbon monoxide intake).

Air then passes through a filter bank to filter out the dust. All filters are rated for two specific factors. Arrestance refers to the ability to remove coarse dust. Dust spot efficiency refers to the ability to remove fine particulates of specific sizes, defined by mass median aerodynamic diameters. Various kinds of filters are frequently used to decrease cost, and most commercially available filters will not remove the particulate phase of ETS. Specific filters may remove gases and volatile organic compounds, but large banks are needed with frequent replacement for any useful filtration.

Next, air passes through a heat exchanger and is either heated with electricity or hot water or cooled by cold water, halocarbons, ammonia, or glycol ethers. As the air is cooled, water will condense on the cooling coils when the cooling coil surface is below the dew point temperature of the air (based on the water content). Although the temperature of the air leaving the coil is no different from air in which less latent cooling has occurred, the water content is substantially lower. The condensed water collects in drain pans. Adequate drainage is of paramount importance to prevent the growth of microbial agents and their dissemination in the airstream. Supply fans then carry the air to ducts. Air is distributed to occupied spaces through supply air louvers, whose design ensures that air is brought to the breathing zone of occupants, and thus, the microenvironment.

Air is returned to the central system through collecting ducts, open plenums, or open spaces. Some availability of relief pressurization must be provided otherwise the outside air may not be able to be distributed against the local pressure.[27]

A major concern in all systems is the integrity of the lining of ducts and plenums. If unsealed fiberglass, spray insulation, or other porous material becomes wet after attracting dust, ideal conditions are present for the growth of micro-organisms. Inadequate latent cooling may leave more water in the distributed air and lead to microbial overgrowth.

Two basic forms of air conditioning are currently in use: variable air volume (VAV) and constant flow (CF) systems. VAV systems mix air of different temperatures to achieve a desired temperature in occupied spaces. That is, when the temperature in the occupied space has reached a pre-set level, no further air flow may occur until the temperature has exceeded the thermostat trigger. CV systems, on the other hand, regulate temperature by varying the amount of initial conditioning and mixing, ensuring air flow at all times. Some VAV systems do have provisions for minimal air flow even when temperatures are in a desired range. Nevertheless, the balancing and maintenance of VAV systems require substantially more expertise than that of CV systems.[33]

Space design

Placement of distribution louvers, furniture, and partitions may influence the distribution of air flow and the adequacy of microenvironmental circulation. Retrofitting of walls in spaces without regard for the placement of louvers may lead to air quality complaints.

Office materials

A growing recognition that mucosal irritation is associated not only with inadequate ventilation but also with the accumulation of specific pollutant groups, i.e., VOC, has led architects, designers, and building owners to scrutinize the emissions from newer office products. A four-step process has been suggested to evaluate materials properly. Identification of target products allows the user or designer to identify potential sources of concern.[6,21] Screening for such products occurs based on information from existing databases and manufacturers' data. If no prior information is available on a product of interest, data may be collected on emissions rates, duration, and health effects. Finally, these three factors are reviewed, and manufacturers may be contacted for help in the modification of products before or after installation.

Products may be a primary or secondary problem source, e.g., materials with high surface areas, such as carpets, drapes, and upholstery, may actually serve as secondary sinks. These sinks absorb emitted agents at one point in time and contribute to the delayed decrease in concentrations of those agents by re-releasing the agent later on and therefore potentially contributing to adverse health effects.

PARADIGM 3: SPECIFIC POLLUTANTS – EXPOSURE ASSESSMENT

A discussion of specific pollutants ideally encompasses standard measurement techniques, exposure–effect relationships, and the pertinent standards. Providing this information for all the pollutants found in indoor environments is not possible here. Therefore, only a short discussion on seven of the more prominent pollutants will be given. These are also listed in Table 50.4, which compiles some of the common contaminants in indoor air. In an environmental evaluation, any consideration of pollutants must first address the representative pollutant and the multiple contaminant problems.

First, indoor environments involve multiple exposures. Sources of these contaminants include the outdoor environment, materials and products within the building, and the building occupants. Outdoor contaminants such as vehicle exhaust fumes can become trapped indoors. Individual agents are often present in concentration ranges of 1 to 100 parts per billion, which may be orders of magnitude below the recognized occupational criteria. Nevertheless, the best way of estimating their collective effects is currently uncertain. Most have both an odor and an irritant component to be considered.[34] Specific pollutant effects may be modified through additional exposures, such as noise and vibration, lighting factors, and thermal parameters.[21] It is therefore generally agreed that the use of environmental criteria alone, such as is commonly done in applied industrial hygiene, is unsuitable for evaluation of the non-industrial workplace.

Second, pollutants rarely are generated alone. Many sources emit multiple agents, leading to the search for a representative pollutant. For example, ETS consists of thousands of different compounds. Nicotine, or its metabolite cotinine, may be a reasonable indicator of recent exposure. Measurement difficulties and decay in the smoke question whether these are the ideal sentinel compounds.

Third, the shape of dose–response curves, effects thresholds, and susceptibility variability suggest that focusing on single levels for specific pollutants will not lead to effects on indoor environmental regulation.[35] Although a pollutant-oriented paradigm is useful for scientific discussions, measurement, and analysis, it is less useful for problem solving in regard to indoor air or for regulatory approaches to indoor environments.

Microbial agents

Evidence exists that microbial agents lead to allergic respiratory tract disease in public access buildings and residential environments. Symptoms appear more frequently in buildings with higher endotoxin levels or moisture problems, and in atopic individuals. Microbial agents proliferate wherever dirt, water, air, and heat coincide. To break the cycle of replication, the reservoir must be eradicated. This is best done through moisture prevention and cleaning.[28,36] Measurement of air-borne levels is of great scientific interest but typically of little practical use in individual cases. Speciation of the organisms demonstrates the presence of agents with the potential to form mycotoxins, and may provide useful scientific information. Also, immunologic testing, i.e., substance-specific challenge or documentation of antibodies, may be part of the evaluation.[37] Usually, in practice, sources can be identified by visual inspection or smell, and remediated without such testing.

Although a guideline was suggested of 1000 colony-forming units per m^3 of micro-organisms for indoor environments, many practitioners have interpreted this as a standard distinguishing safety from hazard, which was not the intent of the initial guideline. Currently, levels in the range of 1000 to 10,000 colony-forming units with clear gradients from outdoor concentrations are viewed with concern, although there are no specific standard guidelines.

Volatile organic compounds

Chamber studies of volatile organic compounds (VOCs) have suggested that many of the complaints induced by indoor environments may result from exposure to low levels of VOCs. Systematic assessment has, over the last 10 years, identified irritant and odor thresholds for several homologous series of agents (aliphatic aldehydes, ketones, alcohols). There are many sources of VOCs in the indoor environment; these include, but are not limited to, paints, adhesives, cleaners, plastics, and fabric protectors.[38]

VOCs can be skin and mucous membrane irritants. These health symptoms appear to be related to the difference in VOC concentrations on entering and leaving a room, to screening measures of VOC quantities, and to pollutants grouped by exposure sources (carpets, paints, etc.). It has been postulated that VOCs may trigger migraines; however, this is not established and most indoor headaches are not labeled as such. Central nervous system toxicity of solvents has only been described after substantially high exposures. Usually, specific total VOC levels can be measured in indoor environments but are typically very low and not felt to pose a permanent health risk.[39]

Environmental tobacco smoke

Recently, research has been establishing a link between environmental tobacco smoke (ETS) and adverse health effects. Some component of non-specific complaints can result from this exposure. The primary cause of the irritation and health effects is believed to reside in the gaseous rather than the particulate phase.[10]

A broader issue is raised by epidemiologic literature that suggests a variety of chronic diseases are attributable to ETS. Although the literature is somewhat limited, the chronic conditions linked to ETS include: lung cancer, heart disease, asthma, and chronic obstructive pulmonary disease.[25,40] This evidence is based on ETS as a risk factor for intense household contacts (spouses or parents) and the proportion of chronic disease attributable to levels typically found in the office or other workplaces appears exceedingly small.

A third issue is that of irritation and odor discomfort and required ventilation. The gas phase of ETS carries potent irritants, including sulfur dioxide, ammonia, and formaldehyde.[40] Ventilation rates required to ventilate ETS adequately in rooms and buildings may need to be three-fold higher than those recommended by ASHRAE in the 62 standard. The ventilation rate required to address typical smoking in smoking environments leads to conditions described by some as 'a tornado on your desk'.

Asbestos

Asbestos products were used in a broad range of applications in buildings. With inadequate maintenance these materials decay, leading to some degree of exposure. The intensity of this exposure varies considerably, depending on the activities of the individuals under scrutiny. Office workers, in general, are considered at very low risk for asbestos-related disease. Air sampling has generally not indicated fiber exposures above background levels. The risk from asbestos exposure in public access buildings can reasonably be considered negligible in most environments.

Radon

Radon in indoor environments as a cause of lung cancer has come under considerable scrutiny. Although it is clearly important in certain parts of the world, in the United States the risk is primarily in residences and not the workplace. The Environmental Protection Agency has recommended remediation when levels in living space exceed 4 pcu/l, as measured over a 3-month period. The risk of lung cancer at these low doses remains a focus of study. A substantial portion of its risk arises from the potentiation of smoking risk, so that smoking cessation efforts may have substantially greater beneficial effects.[41]

Biomass and fossil fuels

In public access buildings, the entrainment of vehicle exhaust sometimes leads to carbon monoxide and irritant (NO_x/SO_2) exposures. Usually exposure is because of poorly designed and located air intakes.[23] It is important to monitor the source of these exposures because these reactive agents can form reaction products with unsaturated hydrocarbons

indoors, therefore generating two additional moles of products generally more reactive than the original agents.

Carbon dioxide

CO_2 has been the subject of great interest in indoor air and is frequently (mis)named a pollutant. It is widely used as an indicator of adequate ventilation based on considerations in the ASHRAE 62-89 standard. Because humans are the primary source of CO_2, many consider it a reasonable indicator of ventilation adequacy.[42] In fact, data generally support its use not just as an indicator of ventilation but also as a reasonable predictor of symptoms. However, CO_2 levels may not accurately reflect the ventilation. In relatively low occupant/density rooms (less than seven persons per 1000 ft^2) and in spaces that have not reached steady state due to unstable numbers of occupants or too short a time to equilibrate, measured CO_2 levels may be a poor indicator of overall ventilation and ventilation efficiency. Second, if there are unexpected, strong sources that far exceed the usually expected pollutant load, specific exposures may remain uncontrolled. Nevertheless, reviewing CO_2 levels is appropriate in many situations. Levels above 1000 ppm (0.1%) indicate that a specific environment does not meet basic ventilation requirements.[23] However, this is not an absolute level. In the presence of definable building system problems a level in the range of 500 ppm can be present.[43]

RESIDENTIAL EXPOSURES

Homes remain a major source of exposures, with no organized lobby to support problem prevention. As in commercial space, construction is regulated through the building code, which does not address ventilation rates, moisture control, or physical safety hazards.

Moisture and disease

Since the late 1980s, data have suggested an association between childhood airways disease and moisture in the home. Moisture is associated with dust mite and cockroach exposures, and careful intervention has been shown to reduce dust mite antigen levels.[44] More controversial is the relationship between fungi, moisture, and asthma in adults and children. Although rare, case reports identify fungi as a possible cause of asthma. Recent studies suggest an association of fungi and also endotoxin, which may serve as a reasonable marker of biomass or direct pulmonary effects.

A controversial issue regarding mold in the home is that of 'idiopathic pulmonary hemorrhage' associated with *Stachybotrys chartarum*. After an initial case-control study of 10 such cases in Cleveland, additional cases have been reported. An animal model was developed in rat pups, identifying capillary fragility as a consequence of controlled exposure to *Stachybotrys chartarum* toxins likely to cause protein synthesis inhibition. This can be measured with assays standardized to other well-known carcinogenic toxins such as fumonisin.[45,46] As for adult interstitial pneumonitis, the combination of an animal model with suggested mechanism, an exposure trail, a formal case-control study, and case reports suggest the possibility of a causal association. However, it should be noted that the data from these studies are inconclusive and are reviewed in detail in *Clinical Microbiology Reviews*.[47]

The question of moisture sources in the home remains of great interest and concern. This refers to any moisture incursion, leaks through roofs and wall penetrations, windows and doors, most of which represent straightforward construction defects. Additional moisture sources differ by geographic area. In the northern US, below-grade moisture seepage remains a very common problem. In humid areas, inadequate enthalpy control (high indoor moisture content, often exacerbated by improper air conditioning sizing) represent a more common problem. Often it is a combination of below-grade moisture incursion, enthalpy design problems, and bulk moisture incursion that leads to negative health effects.

Fossil fuel combustion

Also of concern is domestic exposure to indoor combustion of wood, grass, dung (biomass fuels), coal, or petroleum derivatives, such as kerosene (fossil fuels) for cooking and heating. Combustion products include gaseous irritants (NO_x/SO_2), asphyxiants (CO), and complex hydrocarbons in particulate (e.g., polycyclic aromatic hydrocarbons).[10] Levels of these pollutants in unvented houses may reach industrial doses, especially in the Third World; the levels may be lower in developed countries but are still worrisome.[25]

Given overall health patterns, the biggest concerns in developing countries have focused on epidemic childhood acute respiratory illness. Evidence suggests stove exposures enhance the risk of this multifactorial killer, and may increase the risk of low birth weight, lung cancer, and possibly obstructive airways disease.[25]

In developed countries, stove and heater exposures are considered a possible contributor to childhood respiratory infection and diminished lung function. Exposures may be a risk factor for the development of asthma or for more severe asthma in established cases. Long-term sequelae remain inadequately investigated. In addition, an association between indoor CO exposures and adverse cardiovascular and central nervous system effects has been suggested. Unusual point sources, entrainment of exhaust from portable grills, entrainment of exhaust from garages, and furnace air supply interruption are associated with mortality and morbidity.[10]

DIAGNOSTIC STRATEGIES AND PREVENTION

Separate diagnostic strategies should be pursued for individual patients and the workplace. If the patient's complaints fit a specific pattern (i.e., a specific building-related illness), the likely source should be identified and remediated. Where no prior reports of an exposure–effect relationship exist, a diagnostic trial may be necessary. Identification of the likely pathophysiologic outcome allows the investigator to focus on a specific target organ under conditions that are measurable and reproducible. If an effect is identified, this may provide adequate evidence for intervention. If no change is identified, at least no disease severe enough to lead to pathophysiologic changes is present.

At the same time, the building should be evaluated, preferably by someone with ventilation expertise. Walk-throughs generally involve a review of the building's plans, inspection of various components of the HVAC system, and a review of other building systems and sources, such as may be present in mixed-use buildings. Occupant interviews or a questionnaire survey may be useful to characterize complaints, although they may not be helpful unless some specific disease is under investigation.[39] Likely causes may be identified during the initial review, and a hypothesis should be formulated. Additional evidence may then be collected and some intervention undertaken. Buildings must frequently be examined under different environmental conditions (e.g., temperatures and seasons) because many problems become evident when the conditions change.[48] If necessary, targeted sampling to document the presence of specific exposures may be useful to persuade the responsible parties of the appropriateness of or need for intervention. In general, extensive sampling is not helpful early in building investigations.

There is growing recognition of the importance of preventive maintenance and careful planning in renovation work. The former includes regular servicing of induction units, cleaning systems, and the like.[49] None of these have been subjected to scientific scrutiny as the new industry has arisen. The latter requires considerations of timing and design in renovation. Renovation during continued occupancy without isolation of the renovated space or isolation of the HVAC system serving the construction sites leads to avoidable mistakes and occupant exposure.[50]

A widely discussed approach to indoor air is to focus on prevention of sick buildings, called the healthy building movement. This has led to several changes in design and construction practices including: closer co-ordination between architects and engineers, the use of outside peer reviewers for overall project evaluation, the rigorous evaluation and commissioning of newly constructed buildings, the selection of low-emitting materials, and the contracting of designers and builders for a period after the completion to oversee the maintenance.[6]

Finally, careful scrutiny of the workplace organizational function may prevent the development of problems. Several studies have suggested that, in addition to specific environmental contaminants, various work stress parameters may influence building-related complaints. The development of crisis buildings is generally caused by poor labor–management communication. The failure to act appropriately early in the course of building complaints and to take occupant concerns seriously may contribute to many of the health complaints that are clearly preventable.

As the Occupational Safety and Health Administration has withdrawn its proposed standard, no regulatory approach appears imminent. Other occupational environments, such as healthcare with the Joint Commission on Accreditation of HealthCare Organizations, have developed effective self-regulation. Office buildings are a large enough class of buildings, with enough hazards, to warrant some similar approach.

References

1. Bracker A, Storey E. Assessing occupational and environmental exposures that cause lung disease. Clin Chest Med 2002; 23:695–705.
2. Bolle R. Indoor climate and health. Int J Circumpolar Health 2000; 59:228–39.
3. Hoppe P, Martinac I. Indoor climate and air quality. Review of current and future topics in the field of ISB study group 10. Int J Biometeorol 1998; 42:1–7.
4. Schneider T. Measuring strategies and monitoring of the indoor environment. J Environ Monit 1999; 1:427–34.
5. Kipen HM, Fiedler N. Environmental factors in medically unexplained symptoms and related syndromes: the evidence and the challenge. Environ Health Perspect 2002; 110(Suppl 4):597–9.
6. Samet JM, Spengler JD. Indoor environments and health: moving into the 21st century. Am J Public Health 2003; 93:1489–93.
7. Hodgson M. Sick building syndrome. Occup Med 2000; 15:571–85.
8. Hodgson M. The sick-building syndrome. Occup Med 1995; 10:167–75.
9. Chang CC, Ruhl RA, Halpern GM, Gershwin ME. The sick building syndrome. I. Definition and epidemiological considerations. J Asthma 1993; 30:285–95.
10. Harrison P. Lifestyle and indoor air pollution: irritative agents. Eur Respir Monogr 2002; 7:117–32.
11. Franco G. New trends in occupational and environmental diseases: the role of the occupational hygienist in recognizing lung diseases. Monaldi Arch Chest Dis 1994; 49:239–42.
12. Welch LS. Severity of health effects associated with building-related illness. Environ Health Perspect 1991; 95:67–9.
13. Meggs WJ. RADS and RUDS – the toxic induction of asthma and rhinitis. J Toxicol Clin Toxicol 1994; 32:487–501.
14. Meggs WJ. Hypothesis for induction and propagation of chemical sensitivity based on biopsy studies. Environ Health Perspect 1997; 105(Suppl 2):473–8.
15. Brooks SM. Host susceptibility to indoor air pollution. J Allergy Clin Immunol 1994; 94:344–51.
16. Weltermann BM, Hodgson M, Storey E, et al. Hypersensitivity pneumonitis: a sentinel event investigation in a wet building. Am J Ind Med 1998; 34:499–505.
17. Mahmoudi M, Gershwin ME. Sick building syndrome. III. Stachybotrys chartarum. J Asthma 2000; 37:191–8.
18. Hodgson MJ, Morey P, Leung WY, et al. Building-associated pulmonary disease from exposure to Stachybotrys chartarum and Aspergillus versicolor. J Occup Environ Med 1998; 40:241–9.
19. Thorn A. The sick building syndrome: a diagnostic dilemma. Soc Sci Med 1998; 47:1307–12.
20. Hoge CW, Reichler MR, Dominguez EA, et al. An epidemic of pneumococcal disease in an overcrowded, inadequately ventilated jail. N Engl J Med 1994; 331:643–8.
21. Oliver LC, Shackleton BW. The indoor air we breathe. Public Health Rep 1998; 113:398–409.
22. Gold DR. Indoor air pollution. Clin Chest Med 1992; 13:215–29.
23. Sabir M, Shashikiran U, Kochar SK. Building related illnesses and indoor air pollution. J Assoc Physicians India 1999; 47:426–30.
24. Berg M, Arnetz BB, Liden S, Eneroth P, Kallner A. Technostress. A psychophysiological study of employees with VDU-associated skin complaints. J Occup Med 1992; 34:698–701.
25. Blanc PD. The role of household exposures in lung disease in women. Eur Respir Monogr 2003; 8:118–30.
26. Tsai YJ, Gershwin ME. The sick building syndrome: what is it when it is? Compr Ther 2002; 28:140–4.
27. Wargocki P, Sundell J, Bischof W, et al. Ventilation and health in non-industrial indoor environments: report from a European multidisciplinary scientific consensus meeting (EUROVEN). Indoor Air 2002; 12:113–28.
28. Adverse Human Health Effects Associated with Molds in the Indoor Environment. Arlington Heights, IL: American College of Occupational and Environmental Medicine, 2002;1–10.
29. Letz GA. Sick building syndrome: acute illness among office workers – the role of building ventilation, air-borne contaminants and work stress. Allergy Proc 1990; 11:109–16.
30. Bascom R, Kesavanathan J, Swift DL. Human susceptibility to indoor contaminants. Occup Med 1995; 10:119–32.
31. Bascom R. The upper respiratory tract: mucous membrane irritation. Environ Health Perspect 1991; 95:39–44.
32. Schwartz BS, Stewart WF, Lipton RB. Lost workdays and decreased work effectiveness associated with headache in the workplace. J Occup Environ Med 1997; 39:320–7.
33. Seppanen O, Fisk WJ. Association of ventilation system type with SBS symptoms in office workers. Indoor Air 2002; 12:98–112.
34. Chester AC. Sick-building syndrome fatigue as a possible predation defense. Integr Physiol Behav Sci 1995; 30:68–83.
35. Pasanen AL. A review: fungal exposure assessment in indoor environments. Indoor Air 2001; 11:87–98.
36. Gravesen S. Microbiology on indoor air '99 – what is new and interesting? An overview of selected papers presented in Edinburgh, August, 1999. Indoor Air 2000; 10:74–80.
37. Malkin R, Martinez K, Marinkovich V, Wilcox T, Wall D, Biagini R. The relationship between symptoms and IgG and IgE antibodies in an office environment. Environ Res 1998; 76:85–93.
38. Hodgson M, Levin H, Wolkoff P. Volatile organic compounds and indoor air. J Allergy Clin Immunol 1994; 94:296–303.
39. Hodgson M. Field studies on the sick building syndrome. Ann NY Acad Sci 1992; 641:21–36.
40. Eisner MD. Environmental tobacco smoke and adult asthma. Clin Chest Med 2002; 23:749–61.
41. Samet JM, Marbury MC, Spengler JD. Health effects and sources of indoor air pollution. Part I. Am Rev Respir Dis 1987; 136:1486–508.
42. Apte MG, Fisk WJ, Daisey JM. Associations between indoor CO_2 concentrations and sick building syndrome symptoms in US office buildings: an analysis of the 1994-1996 BASE study data. Indoor Air 2000; 10:246–57.
43. Seppanen OA, Fisk WJ, Mendell MJ. Association of ventilation rates and CO_2 concentrations with health and other responses in commercial and institutional buildings. Indoor Air 1999; 9:226–52.
44. Robbins CA, Swenson LJ, Nealley ML, Gots RE, Kelman BJ. Health effects of mycotoxins in indoor air: a critical review. Appl Occup Environ Hyg 2000; 15:773–84.
45. Rao CY, Burge HA, Brain JD. The time course of responses to intratracheally instilled toxic Stachybotrys chartarum spores in rats. Mycopathologia 2000; 149:27–34.
46. Rao CY, Brain JD, Burge HA. Reduction of pulmonary toxicity of Stachybotrys chartarum spores by methanol extraction of mycotoxins. Appl Environ Microbiol 2000; 66:2817–21.
47. Kuhn DM, Ghannoum MA. Indoor mold, toxigenic fungi, and Stachybotrys chartarum: infectious disease perspective. Clin Microbiol Rev 2003; 16:144–72.
48. Samet JM, Marbury MC, Spengler JD. Health effects and sources of indoor air pollution. Part II. Am Rev Respir Dis 1988; 137:221–42.
49. Crawford JO, Bolas SM. Sick building syndrome, work factors and occupational stress. Scand J Work Environ Health 1996; 22:243–50.
50. Kreiss K. The epidemiology of building-related complaints and illness. Occup Med 1989; 4:575–92.

Chapter 51

Exposures in Outdoor Air

Mark W Frampton, Jonathan M Samet, Mark J Utell

Outdoor air pollution has numerous man-made and natural sources. In the US, approximately one-half of the population is exposed to pollutants at levels exceeding the current federal air quality standards. Concern for adverse health effects may be raised by persistent pollution with sustained exposure, as occurs in regions with photochemical pollution or smog; by dramatic releases of toxic chemicals, such as in the tragic release of methylisocyanate in the Bhopal incident and the subsequent release of aldicarboxime in Institute, West Virginia; by the presence of visible sources of community pollution such as smelters, power plants, or refineries; and by outbreaks of symptoms or illnesses possibly caused by air pollution. But even without visible or dramatic emissions, air pollution may harm public health.[1,2]

Assessment of the adverse effects of outdoor air pollution typically requires toxicologic and epidemiologic investigations.[3] Addressing these adverse effects may require reduction of emissions through engineering controls or changes in source operations, or even elimination of some sources. Legislation or prolonged litigation may be involved. While control of air pollution is a societal matter, physicians and other healthcare practitioners need to understand the effects of outdoor air pollution as they relate to the care of individual patients, and to potential community concerns. Patients often turn to their physicians for advice concerning possible harmful consequences of air pollution. For example, high levels of photochemical oxidants (i.e., smog) may prompt persons with asthma or chronic obstructive pulmonary disease (COPD) to ask about the safety of being outside; healthy persons may ask about the consequences of exercising.

Physicians also may be viewed as the community's experts on the consequences of air pollution or other forms of environmental contamination.[4] They may serve as sources of information and expertise for environmental groups, voluntary health agencies, municipal boards or other governmental bodies. Thus, the range of physician involvement with outdoor air pollution is potentially broad, spanning from the care of individual patients to issues of local, regional, or even national scope.

This chapter provides a broad perspective for clinicians on the adverse effects of outdoor air pollution. It reviews the principal forms of outdoor air pollution and associated health effects and considers approaches at the levels of the community and the individual patient for reducing morbidity and mortality resulting from exposure. Emphasis is placed on the problems likely to be found in the developed world; the situation in many developing countries is, regrettably, far worse.

SOURCES AND TYPES OF OUTDOOR AIR POLLUTION

Pollutant types	Sources
Particulate matter, sulfur oxides	Fossil fuel combustion, motor vehicles, power plants, combustion of coal for heating
Photochemical oxidant	Fossil fuel combustion, motor vehicles, oil refineries, power plants, other hydrocarbon sources
Carbon monoxide	Fossil fuel combustion, motor vehicles, industry
Toxic air pollutants	Fossil fuel combustion, industry, other

Table 51.1 Principal types and sources of pollutants

Outdoor air pollution has myriad natural and man-made sources. From the perspective of concern about adverse health effects, outdoor air pollutants can be classified into four broad groups (Table 51.1). Combustion of sulfur-containing fossil fuels, primarily coal and crude petroleum products, produces sulfur oxide and particulate pollution. The combustion gases, sulfur oxides and nitrogen oxides, are precursors of acid pollution and contribute to the formation of small particles. The use of tall stacks promotes the formation of acidic sulfate and nitrate species by spewing precursor pollutants high into the atmosphere, where the prolonged residence time facilitates the occurrence of chemical reactions that form acid particles.

Photochemical pollution or smog results from the action of sunlight on a precursor mixture of hydrocarbons, nitrogen oxides, and carbon monoxide (CO). This type of pollution tends to occur in areas with a high density of motor vehicles and warm, sunny climates. Although smog was first found in the Los Angeles air basin, it is now a regional problem in many parts of the US, including the East Coast. Smog is a complex mixture containing diverse oxidant pollutants; acidic species may also be present. The concentration of ozone is used to index the severity of photochemical pollution.

CO is also produced by combustion sources, both stationary and non-stationary. The toxic pollutants have diverse sources, including both small and large industries, and vehicles.

PERSONAL EXPOSURE TO AIR POLLUTION

Patterns of time-use and activity place children and adults in diverse indoor and outdoor environments throughout the day, each environment having its own unique set of air contaminants. Perhaps because of the distinct sources contaminating outdoor air and indoor air and the separate regulatory mechanisms for outdoor air, the workplace, and the home, the health effects of air pollution have often been addressed separately for outdoor and indoor air.

However, the concept of total personal exposure is more relevant for health; personal exposure to air pollution represents the time-weighted average of pollutant concentrations in microenvironments, which are environments having relatively homogeneous air quality (Fig. 51.1). Thus, for an office worker, relevant microenvironments might include home, office, car, outdoors at home, outdoors at work, and a movie theater. For some pollutants, such as ozone or acid aerosols, outdoor environments make the predominant contribution to total personal exposure; for others, such as

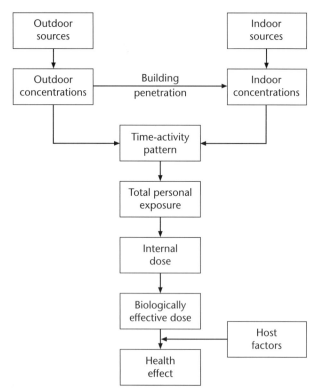

Figure 51.1: Framework for considering exposure, dose, and development of health effects. (Modified from Committee on the Epidemiology of Air Pollutants, Board on Toxicology and Environmental Health Hazards, Commission on Life Sciences, National Research Council. Epidemiology and air pollution. Washington, DC: National Academy Press; 1985.)

radon and formaldehyde, indoor locations are most important. In considering the health consequences of air pollution, the physician should recognize that outdoor air is only one potential vector for pollution exposure.

PRINCIPLES OF INHALATION INJURY (see Chapters 19.5 and 47)

Atmospheric pollutants exist in both gaseous and particulate forms. In relating clinical diseases to specific exposures, the clinician should recognize that penetration and retention of toxic gases in the respiratory tract can vary widely, depending on the physical properties of the gas (e.g., solubility), the concentration of the gas in the inspired air, the rate and depth of ventilation, and the extent to which the material is reactive. Gases that are highly water soluble, such as sulfur dioxide (SO_2), are almost completely extracted by the nose and pharynx of resting healthy subjects during brief exposures. In contrast, the removal of less water-soluble gases, such as nitrogen dioxide (NO_2) or ozone, is much less complete, and thus, these gases penetrate deeper into the respiratory tract. CO is poorly soluble in water and is not removed in the upper airways. On reaching the lung, CO diffuses across the alveolar–capillary membrane and binds avidly to hemoglobin in the blood.

Penetration of gases into the deep lung, and thus the total dose to the lung, can be greatly enhanced by exercise. Not only does exercise increase the dose directly by increasing minute ventilation but also, because many people switch from nasal to oral breathing during moderate to heavy exercise, the more efficient removal by the nasal passages is bypassed.

Pollutants in particulate form are usually found in nature as aerosols. These small liquid droplets or solid particles are dispersed in the atmosphere with sufficient stability to remain in suspension. Examples of common aerosols are sulfuric acid mists, sulfate salts, and nitrate salts. Although deposition of inhaled particles depends on multiple factors, including the aerodynamic properties of the particle (primarily its size), airway anatomy, and breathing pattern, several generalizations can be made. Inhaled particles larger than 10 μm are effectively filtered out of the respiratory tract by the nose and nasopharynx. These relatively large particles tend to deposit rapidly because of impaction against surfaces and gravitational forces. Particles trapped in the nose and nasopharynx are cleared in nasal secretions, coughed out, or swallowed. Particles less than 10 μm in aerodynamic diameter may be deposited in the tracheobronchial tree; deposition in the lung's alveoli is maximal for particles of 1 to 2 μm diameter. Particles smaller than 0.5 μm are carried by diffusion to the alveolar level, where they collide with gas molecules by brownian movement and come into contact with alveolar surfaces. Removal of particles from the upper airways is efficient and occurs within hours; this rapid clearance contrasts with clearance from the deep lung by alveolar macrophages, which may require days to months.

Population	Potential mechanism	Consequences
Infants	Immature defense mechanisms of the lung	Increased risk for respiratory infection
Elderly	Impaired respiratory defenses; reduced functional reserve	Increased risk for respiratory infection; increased risk for clinically significant effects on function
Asthmatics	Increased airways responsiveness	Increased risk for exacerbation and respiratory symptoms
Persons with COPD	Reduced level of lung function	Increased risk for clinically significant effects on function
Persons with CHD	Impaired myocardial oxygenation	Increased risk for myocardial ischemia
Cigarette smokers	Impaired defense and clearance; lung injury	Increased damage through synergism

CHD, coronary heart disease; COPD, chronic obstructive pulmonary disease.

Table 51.2 Populations considered most susceptible to air pollution

The mechanisms by which inhaled gases and particles injure the lung are diverse and not yet fully understood. The respiratory epithelium is the first point of contact with inhaled pollutants. Oxidant gases and reactive components of inhaled particles may injure respiratory epithelium via generation of reactive oxygen species. Airway epithelial cells and alveolar macrophages may respond with release of pro-inflammatory cytokines and chemokines, initiating a cascade of events, leading to airway inflammation, edema, and increased airways responsiveness. Inhalation of particulate matter is also associated with adverse cardiovascular events. The mechanisms remain unclear, but hypotheses include neurogenic reflexes influencing cardiac function, or translocation of particles to the heart. Organic materials on particles may also act as initiators or promoters of cancer.

DETERMINANTS OF RESPONSE

The likelihood of an adverse response to an inhaled pollutant depends on the degree of exposure to the pollutant and individual characteristics that determine the susceptibility of the exposed person. The relation between exposure and response may have different forms, depending on the mechanism by which the pollutant causes disease. If some minimum degree of exposure is required to produce disease, then a threshold is present. Alternatively, the risk of effect may increase with any exposure; the relationship may be linear or take a curvilinear or other form. For most inhaled pollutants, the evidence indicates increasing risk with increasing exposure. Most often, a linear relationship without a threshold is assumed, although the relevant data may be compatible with alternative exposure–response relationships. The assumption that a threshold does not exist implies that any exposure carries some risk. The shape of the dose–response relationship is relevant to the setting of regulations to protect public health.

The concept of susceptibility is highly relevant to the care of individual patients.[5] Physicians inherently consider susceptibility in the diagnosis and management of disease. Does family history increase the probability of disease? Does age increase the chance of an adverse drug reaction? Susceptibility refers to an altered degree of responsiveness, whether increased or decreased. Epidemiologists use mathematical approaches to describe the degree of altered susceptibility associated with having a particular characteristic. In considering the combined effects of two factors, synergism is considered present if the combined effect exceeds that predicted by the sum of the risks produced by the two factors acting independently. For some risk factors and diseases, the synergism is multiplicative; the combined risk equals the product of the two independent risks, such as lung cancer, asbestos, and smoking. For others, the interaction may be less than or greater than multiplicative, depending on the mechanism of interaction.

Factors determining susceptibility may include inherent individual characteristics (e.g., sex, age, degree of airways responsiveness, or presence of $alpha_1$-antitrypsin deficiency) and exposure to other agents that also have adverse effects on the same target organ (e.g., cigarette smoke or asbestos). Thus, many segments of the population have been considered at increased risk from air pollution (Table 51.2). An array of epidemiologic and laboratory evidence as well as clinical judgment support the determination that these and other groups are susceptible. For example, during the dramatic London Fog of 1952, infants, the elderly, and persons with cardiorespiratory diseases experienced a particularly high rate of mortality. Laboratory exposure studies suggest that persons with asthma or with coronary artery disease may experience adverse effects from exposure to SO_2 and CO, at lower concentrations than healthy persons, and these exposure levels often occur in the US. Patients with chronic respiratory conditions are frequently aware of their own susceptibility and report being affected adversely by exposures that might seem trivial to healthy persons.

Aspects of lifestyle may also increase the risk of an adverse effect from inhaled pollutants. Cigarette smoking impairs defense mechanisms and induces chronic inflammation and permanent structural damage in the lung. The combined effects of smoking and air pollutants may be additive or synergistic. Exercise may increase the likelihood of an adverse effect by increasing the dose of pollutants delivered to target sites in the lung as ventilation increases to meet metabolic demands. The choice of microenvironments may also influence exposure; the decision to spend time outside during a period of higher pollution concentrations may markedly increase personal exposure.

SOURCES OF INFORMATION ON AMBIENT AIR QUALITY

Achieving full understanding of the health effects of any air pollutant is a daunting task. The relevant literature includes information on sources and concentrations, and complementary data from toxicologic investigations, human exposures, and epidemiologic studies. Each approach has specific strengths and weaknesses in evaluating the impact of pollutants on human health.[6]

Epidemiologic studies involve examining the relation between exposure and health effects in the community setting and typically in large populations. Respiratory effects are usually assessed by questionnaire and by tests of pulmonary function that can be used in the field setting, most often spirometry. Inherent methodologic problems may limit the results of epidemiologic studies. Accurate estimation of exposure to a pollutant is typically difficult, and many outdoor pollutants of concern are components of complex mixtures. Confounding factors including environmental agents other than the pollutant of concern and factors determining the susceptibility of subjects may further limit interpretation of epidemiologic studies.

Controlled human exposures, involving short-term inhalation of pollutants by small groups of subjects, allow strict control of the experimental subject and the environment. They often include more invasive measurements of effects than is possible in the population setting; some protocols even include bronchoscopy and lung biopsy, for example. The limitations of using environmental exposure chambers rest on ethical and practical considerations. The safety of volunteer subjects is a primary concern, so that chronic exposures cannot be performed and the investigator is limited to examining mild, acute, and reversible effects. Exposures to pollutants are usually for short durations, such as a few hours, and at low concentrations. The results of controlled human exposures cannot be extrapolated to chronic effects. Clinical studies have proved quite effective, however, in determining threshold concentrations of individual pollutants that may cause specific health effects; susceptible populations, particularly persons with asthma, have often been the focus of clinical studies.

Animal studies provide the opportunity to evaluate pathogenic mechanisms of injury by pollutants. Carefully performed exposure–response data can be collected using a wide array of biologic parameters in multiple species. The difficulty in interpreting data from animal exposures lies in extrapolation from an animal model to human health effects. Differences in respiratory tract morphology, regional deposition of pollutants within the lung, and interspecies differences in biologic and physiologic sensitivity to given concentrations of pollutants contribute to the uncertainty of this extrapolation. Additionally, we lack animal models that are closely comparable to the chronic human diseases associated with susceptibility to air pollution.

Information on air pollution from these investigative approaches is published in a broad array of journals and technical reports. Criteria documents prepared by the Environmental Protection Agency (EPA) for its regulatory process offer lengthy reviews that are periodically updated and available at the EPA website, but these summary reports are potentially overwhelming in size and scope. The American Thoracic Society periodically has prepared summary statements for health professionals on the health effects of ambient air pollution.

HEALTH EFFECTS OF SPECIFIC OUTDOOR POLLUTANTS

About 121 million people in the US lived in counties that exceeded at least one air quality standard during 2000.[7] By pollutant, the number of people affected include 81.5 million by ozone, 9.7 million by CO, and 75.0 million by particulate matter. Although the pollutants are considered on an individual basis in the following section, it should be re-emphasized that exposure is often difficult to characterize because a mixture of pollutants is usually involved, and risk attributed to any particular pollutant may reflect the toxicity of the air pollution mixture more generally. The following discussion refers to health effects at levels of exposure encountered in outdoor environments in the US at present. A fuller discussion of health effects of exposure to agents at high concentrations is provided in Chapters 19.5 and 47. This chapter does not address the health effects of the 'hazardous pollutants', because of the large number of agents of concern.

Particulate matter, acid aerosols, and sulfur oxides

Sulfur oxides are produced by combustion of fuels containing sulfur, such as coal from the Eastern United States and crude petroleum.[8] In the past, scientific research and regulatory concern in relation to the sulfur oxides were directed primarily at the health effects of SO_2, an oxidant gas. Particulate matter was considered separately. Particles in the air have numerous natural and human-made sources, including the same combustion processes that also produce SO_2 and another group of oxidant gases, the nitrogen oxides. These gases, through transformations, may make a substantial contribution to the mass of small particles in many parts of the US. The chemical composition of particles is complex and highly variable, but along with the size of the particle, the composition is a major determinant of toxicity in the respiratory tract.

Individuals with asthma are particularly susceptible to SO_2, responding to exposures in controlled experiments with increased airways resistance and reduced lung function. With hyperventilation, which increases the dose delivered to the respiratory tract, some asthmatics are adversely affected at levels common in ambient air and well below those that might occur transiently with direct exposure to the plume from a power plant or factory. From a clinical perspective, SO_2 might worsen asthma for persons living in communities with point sources, such as smelters.

The adverse effects of particles are thought to depend on their chemical composition, such as the presence of trace metals and hydrocarbons, and on size, which determines the site of deposition within the respiratory tract. Inflammation with symptoms and reduction of lung function in healthy persons, those with asthma, and persons with COPD are of concern, as is carcinogenesis. Diesel exhaust, for example, is mutagenic and causes lung cancer in toxicologic studies involving exposure of rodents to high concentrations. Epidemiologic data provide supporting evidence that diesel exhaust is a human carcinogen. In experimental animal models, diesel particles enhance allergic sensitization.

A now substantial body of epidemiologic evidence has raised concern that even current concentrations of particulate matter in cities of the US (and other developed countries) may be adversely affecting the public's health. Studies in many cities show small increments in numbers of deaths, particularly from cardiopulmonary causes, on days with higher particulate matter levels compared to days with lower levels. The National Morbidity, Mortality, and Air Pollution Study (NMMAPS), conducted in 90 US cities, found that for each 10 $\mu g/m^3$ increase in PM10 (particles smaller than 10 microns) daily deaths increased 0.5%.[9] There also appear to be adverse effects over the longer term. Mortality among persons with underlying cardiopulmonary disease is increased in more polluted cities compared with less polluted cities. There are supporting findings on particulate matter and measures of morbidity: particulate air pollution shows associations with rates of hospitalization and emergency room visits among children and adults with asthma, and among adults with heart disease. Analyses suggest particular risk associated with the most highly respirable fraction, those less than 2.5 microns in diameter (PM2.5).

The evidence was considered sufficiently compelling by the US EPA in 1997 to warrant a new standard for fine particulate matter (see Table 51.3). Many questions remain and are under active investigation; research is in progress on mechanisms and also on the toxicity-determining characteristics of particles.[10] From a clinical perspective, the new findings on particulate matter reinforce the need for clinicians to consider air pollution as a factor that may adversely affect the status of their patients with heart and lung disease.

Ozone

Photochemical pollution is a complex oxidant mixture produced by the action of sunlight on vehicle exhaust. Through a series of photochemical reactions involving hydrocarbons and nitrogen oxides, various oxidant pollutants are produced, including ozone, which serves as an index for this type of pollution. Photochemical pollution was first recognized about 40 years ago in southern California, where the combination of sunlight and heavy vehicle travel promotes its formation. Ozone has now

Pollutant	Standard	Averaging time
SO_2	0.03 ppm	Annual mean
	0.14 ppm	24-hour average
PM10	50 $\mu g/m^3$	Annual mean
	150 $\mu g/m^3$	24-hour average
PM2.5	15 $\mu g/m^3$	Annual mean
	65 $\mu g/m^3$	24-hour average
Ozone	0.08 ppm	8-hour average
NO_2	0.053 ppm	Annual mean
CO	9 ppm	8-hour average
	35 ppm	1-hour average

Table 51.3 National ambient air quality standards: criteria pollutants.

become a problem in many other locations including other western cities in the US with similar sprawling growth, in the eastern US during the summertime, and in many other densely urban locations throughout the world, such as Mexico City.

The toxicology of ozone has been extensively investigated.[11,12] Low-level exposures cause damage to the small airways of experimental animals; the demonstration of subtle fibrosis in one animal model raises concern for permanent structural alteration. Volunteers exposed to ozone at concentrations in the range of the present standard, often present during pollution episodes, have transient reductions of lung function; healthy subjects have a range of responsiveness that is broad but repeatable for individuals. More recently, evidence of an inflammatory response and biochemical changes in bronchoalveolar lavage fluid has been detected 18 hours after an exposure to ozone at a level below the current standard. Taken together, the progressive decrements in pulmonary mechanics during exposure coupled with the persistent biochemical changes many hours after cessation of exposure indicate the potential for chronic effects from repeated inhalation. Increased susceptibility to ozone in asthmatics has recently been demonstrated for the first time.[13] The evidence for short-term effects of ozone exposure on the lung function of healthy volunteers has raised concern about possible long-term effects of living in southern California and other locations with sustained photochemical pollution. Relevant epidemiologic data are suggestive of chronic effects of ozone, but these data are not definitive.

Nitrogen oxides

Nitrogen oxides, like sulfur oxides, are produced by combustion processes, and contribute to the formation of ozone and secondary particles.[14] NO_2 is regulated by the EPA as a criteria pollutant. Exposure also occurs indoors from unvented combustion sources such as kerosene heaters and gas stoves. NO_2 is an oxidant gas that can penetrate to the small airways and alveoli of the lung. The toxicologic evidence suggests that NO_2 exposure can impair lung defenses against respiratory pathogens and cause airways inflammation, with associated effects on lung function and respiratory symptoms. The epidemiologic evidence remains inconclusive, largely because of methodologic problems arising in attempting to separate the effects of NO_2 from those of other pollutants, especially fine particles. Similarly, controlled clinical studies provide inconsistent findings on the effects of low-level NO_2 exposure on the lung function of asthmatics. The conflicting results are probably related to differences in subject selection and exposure protocols. Individuals with COPD may represent a group with increased susceptibility to short-term NO_2 exposure, but further study of this issue is needed.

Carbon monoxide

CO, another criteria pollutant, binds to hemoglobin to form carboxyhemoglobin (COHb) and reduces the capacity of the blood to deliver oxygen to the tissues. At high levels, CO can cause severe neurologic damage and even death in otherwise healthy persons. At low levels, individuals may have reduced oxygen uptake during exercise. Evidence indicates that controlled CO exposure of patients with stable coronary artery disease can induce earlier subjective and objective evidence of myocardial ischemia at venous COHb levels as low as 2% to 4%.[15] Such data are relevant to the urban environment, where individuals may be exposed to sufficient air pollution to have blood COHb levels elevated to this range. Furthermore, moderate exercise results in even greater CO loading. Thus, for patients with coronary disease, exposure to CO can exacerbate myocardial ischemia. In addition, at a COHb level of 6%, patients with coronary artery disease have an increased frequency of arrhythmias. On a practical level, physicians should advise patients with exertional myocardial ischemia that personal exposure to CO is potentially modifiable. The unborn fetus as well as patients with COPD may be particularly susceptible to effects of CO.

Lead (see Chapter 39.8)

The population may be exposed to lead through multiple environmental media, including ambient air. Fortunately in the US, the importance of ambient air as a source of population exposure to lead has diminished with the removal of lead from gasoline, although point sources (e.g., smelters) may still be important in some communities. Children are particularly vulnerable to lead exposure, and for US children, lead paint in older, urban housing remains a significant source of exposure. Even levels previously considered safe have been associated with adverse effects on neural cognitive development. As the scientific evidence on lead and child health has developed, the Center for Disease Control has progressively reduced the blood level of lead considered acceptable, to the present value of 10 µg/dl. In some countries, leaded gasoline continues to be a significant source of environmental pollution.

CLINICALLY RELEVANT HEALTH EFFECTS OF OUTDOOR AIR POLLUTION

Our knowledge of the adverse consequences of outdoor air pollution, reviewed earlier, is largely based on investigative efforts directed at characterizing adverse effects in populations. Epidemiologic studies provide estimates of the average effect and the range of effects on groups. Studies involving controlled human exposures offer more relevant information for clinicians; however, the most susceptible subjects typically are not included in these studies.

Nevertheless, the available evidence suggests that even the relatively low outdoor levels of pollution found in the US and in other developed countries cause adverse effects of consequence in clinical practice (Table 51.4). Persons made susceptible by underlying heart or lung disease are most likely to present to clinicians with adverse effects

Pollutant types	Health effects
Particulate pollution, sulfur oxides	Increased mortality/morbidity from respiratory and cardiac disease; exacerbations of asthma and COPD; respiratory symptoms, particularly in children
Photochemical pollution	Acute respiratory symptoms; reduced lung function in exercising persons
Carbon monoxide	Ischemic symptoms in persons with coronary heart disease and possibly with peripheral vascular disease

COPD, chronic obstructive pulmonary disease.

Table 51.4 Some clinically relevant health effects of outdoor air pollution

related to exposure to outdoor air pollution. In the evaluation of persons with difficult-to-control asthma or COPD, personal exposures to inhaled agents both indoors and outdoors should be considered as potential factors. Similarly, CO exposures should be considered in patients with ischemic heart disease having persistent angina or arrhythmias.

Even healthy persons may have acute respiratory symptoms or eye irritation from exposure to photochemical oxidant pollution. With exercise during smog episodes, lung function may also be substantially, although transiently, reduced.

Outdoor air pollution may also contribute to the development of chronic diseases and respiratory cancer. However, in an individual patient, there are currently no markers that distinguish the causative role of air pollution separate from other factors, such as smoking. Short-term excursions to places with higher levels of both oxidant pollution as well as sulfur oxide and particulate pollution may also increase the occurrence of respiratory infections, particularly those involving the lower respiratory tract.

CONTROL STRATEGIES
Regulation of outdoor air quality

The principal US federal statute addressing outdoor air quality is the Clean Air Act, which was last amended in 1990. The Act's structure and authorities are complex; it addresses mobile (automobiles and trucks) and stationary sources of pollution (power plants and industry), and requires that air quality standards be established for two sets of pollutants, so-called criteria pollutants (Table 51.3) and hazardous pollutants. These two groups of pollutants are regulated through different mechanisms. For the criteria pollutants, National Primary Ambient Air Quality Standards are set after extensive review of all relevant evidence; the standards must afford protection to the entire population, including those with heightened susceptibility, and offer an adequate margin of safety. The hazardous pollutants are predominantly carcinogens, such as asbestos and radionuclides, and standards for maximum concentrations are also intended to provide a margin of safety. The most recent amendments listed 189 toxic agents for regulation at a prescribed and rapid pace. The Act includes mechanisms for achieving compliance with the standards and for enforcement. In spite of having federal standards in place for ambient air quality, excess levels of exposure are common in many areas of the country, particularly for ozone.

The goal of achieving a minimum level of air quality should afford protection to most persons. However, in some persons, particular combinations of susceptibility and exposure might still produce clinically relevant effects of individual pollutants at concentrations below the regulatory limits.

Patient-oriented control

Approaches for limiting the health risks of breathing polluted ambient air have received little investigation. Present understanding of the determinants of exposure suggests that modifying time-activity patterns to limit time outside during episodes of outdoor pollution represents the most effective strategy. The potentially limited efficacy of this approach in settings of high indoor air pollution needs to be recognized (see Chapter 50). The levels of some reactive pollutants tend to be lower indoors than outdoors. Ozone levels in buildings are lower than outdoor levels but can be driven upward by increasing the rate of exchange of indoor with outdoor air. Fine particles can also penetrate indoors. Nevertheless, healthcare providers can reasonably advise patients to stay indoors during pollution episodes. Vigorous exercise outdoors, which increases the dose of pollution delivered to the respiratory tract, also should be avoided at such times.

Susceptible patients should be counseled concerning the nature and degree of their susceptibility. The use of medication should follow the usual clinical indications, and therapeutic regimens should not be adjusted because of the occurrence of a pollution episode without evidence of worsening of symptoms or function. In the laboratory, inhalation of cromolyn sodium and bronchodilating agents may block the response to some pollutants, but use of these drugs solely because of exposure to air pollution cannot be advised.

Respiratory protective equipment has been developed for use in the workplace in order to minimize exposure to toxic gases and particles. Many of these devices, particularly those likely to be most effective, add to the work of breathing and cannot be tolerated by persons with respiratory disease. Under most circumstances, healthcare providers should not suggest respiratory protection as a method for reducing the risks of ambient air pollution. Similarly, air cleaners have not been proved to have health benefits, whether directed at pollutants generated by indoor sources or at indoor pollutants brought in with outside air.

Community-oriented control

Frequently, communities become concerned about the impact of particular local sources, perhaps a power plant, manufacturing facility, or a truck or bus depot. Disadvantaged communities and populations are aware that they may have greater exposure to air pollutants and other environmental contaminants than more well-to-do communities. The term 'environmental justice' is used for efforts to address these inequities. Concern about the health risks may quickly lead to controversy and litigation. Thus, understanding the health risks posed by local sources may be difficult and requires skills in community health as well as in epidemiology and toxicology. Local physicians may become involved through concerns

AQI value	Descriptor	PM2.5, 24 hr (µg/m³)	PM10, 24 hr (µg/m³)	PM2.5	PM10
0-50	Good	15	50	None	None
51-100	Moderate	40	150	None	None
101-150	Unhealthy for sensitive groups	65	250	People with respiratory or heart disease, the elderly, and children should limit prolonged exertion	People with respiratory disease, such as asthma, should limit outdoor exertion
151-200	Unhealthy	150	350	People with respiratory or heart disease, the elderly, and children should avoid prolonged exertion; everyone else should limit prolonged exertion	People with respiratory disease, such as asthma, should avoid outdoor exertion; everyone else, especially the elderly and children, should limit prolonged outdoor exertion
201-300	Very unhealthy	250	420	People with respiratory or heart disease, the elderly, and children should avoid any outdoor activity; everyone else should avoid prolonged exertion	People with respiratory disease, such as asthma, should avoid any outdoor activity; everyone else, especially the elderly and children, should limit outdoor exertion
301-400	Hazardous	350	500	Everyone should avoid any outdoor exertion; people with respiratory or heart disease, the elderly, and children should remain indoors	Everyone should avoid any outdoor exertion; people with respiratory disease, such as asthma, should remain indoors
401-500	Hazardous	500	600	Same as above	Same as above

Table 51.5 The Air Quality Index (AQI) for particulate matter

about the health of their patients or as advocates for the community's environment or for the polluting facility. Most often, the dimensions of such complex problems exceed the skills of local physicians. Nevertheless, involvement may be appropriate but guidance should be obtained from appropriate public health and environmental agencies.

The interplay of factors that must be manipulated to prevent environmentally induced disease is complex, but standards are considered to be objective indicators of successful preventive measures or strategies. In 1976, the EPA proposed cautionary statements for public reporting of outdoor air quality, the Pollutant Standards Index (PSI) for criteria pollutants. In the 1999 revision,[16] the name was changed to the Air Quality Index (AQI). The actions taken when 'Alert Levels' are reached or are expected to be reached include the issuance of health advisories or cautionary statements to the public. As an example, Table 51.5 shows the AQI, pollutant levels, and cautionary statements for particulate matter. The EPA's advice is intended to be applied by local air pollution agencies in preparing daily air quality summaries, which are disseminated to the media. The AQI provides useful guidelines for physicians and public health officials.

References

1. Bascom R, Bromberg PA, Costa DA, et al. State of the art review: health effects of outdoor air pollution. Part 1. Am J Respir Crit Care Med 1996; 153:3-50.
2. Dickey JH. Part VII. Air pollution: overview of sources and health effects. Dis Mon 2000; 46:566-89.
3. Lippmann M, Schlesinger RB. Toxicological bases for the setting of health-related air pollution standards. Annu Rev Public Health 2000; 21:309-33.
4. Modrak JE, Frampton MW, Utell MJ. Community air pollution: what a pulmonologist should know. Clin Pulm Med 1997; 4:266-72.
5. Brain JD, Beck BD, Warren AJ, et al, eds. Variations in susceptibility to inhaled pollutants: identification, mechanisms, and policy implications. Baltimore: The Johns Hopkins University Press; 1988.
6. Utell MJ, Frampton MW. Toxicologic methods: controlled human exposures. Environ Health Perspect 2000; 108(Suppl 4):605-13.
7. Office of Air Quality Planning and Standards. National air quality status and trends, 2000. Web page (2002) located at www.epa.gov/oar/aqtrnd00/sixpoll.html.
8. Utell MJ, Frampton MW. Sulfur dioxide and sulfuric acid aerosols. In: Rom WM, ed. Environmental and occupational medicine, 3rd edn. Boston: Little, Brown & Co; 1998: 631–9.
9. Samet JM, Zeger SI, Dominici F, et al. The national morbidity, mortality, and air pollution study. Part II: Morbidity and mortality from air pollution in the United States. Health Effects Institute Research Report Number 94; 2000.
10. Frampton MW, Utell MJ, Samet JM. Cardiopulmonary consequences of particle inhalation. In: Gehr P, Heyder J, eds. Particle–lung interactions. New York: Marcel Dekker; 2000:653-70.
11. Devlin RB, Raub JA, Folinsbee LJ. Health effects of ozone. Sci Med 1997; 4:8-17.
12. Mudway IS, Kelly FJ. Ozone and the lung: a sensitive issue. Mol Aspects Med 2000; 30:21:1-48.
13. Gent JF, Triche EW, Holford TR, et al. Association of low-level ozone and fine particles with respiratory symptoms in children with asthma. JAMA 2003; 290:1859–67.
14. Bascom R, Bromberg PA, Costa DL, et al. Health effects of outdoor air pollution. Part 2. Am J Respir Crit Care Med 1996; 153:477-98.
15. Allred EN, Bleecker ER, Chaitman BR, et al. Short-term effects of carbon monoxide exposure on the exercise performance of subjects with coronary artery disease. N Engl J Med 1989; 321:1426-32.
16. Anonymous. AQI reporting: final rule. Federal Register 1999 Aug 4; 64.

Chapter 52
Hazardous Waste

52.1 Hazardous Waste Workers
Michael Gochfeld

A hazardous waste includes any hazardous substance that is or has been treated, stored or discarded, as well as any uncontrolled release of such a material.[1] Knowledge regarding health risks of hazardous waste has increased substantially in the years since the Phillips and Silbergeld,[2] and Andelman and Underhill[3] reviews. Many new environmental epidemiologic studies have appeared which warrant treating community exposure in a separate chapter (52.2). While substantial progress has been made at many sites in the previous decade, Barry Johnson, former head of the Agency for Toxic Substances and Disease Registry, emphasized, 'the high percentage of sites with completed exposure pathways and the toxicity potential of substances in these pathways show that uncontrolled hazardous-waste sites are a major environmental threat to human health'.[4]

During the 1990s many US Department of Energy and Department of Defense hazardous waste programs were recognized as inadequate, with many hazardous waste sites and facilities in close proximity to populated areas. This has prompted a significant investment in environmental remediation. Also during the 1990s, whole new toxicologic problems such as endocrine disruptors were recognized, focusing attention on sublethal and non-cancer effects. Risk assessment procedures continued to evolve in terms of both mathematical and social complexity, and the field of risk communication to workers and communities has expanded.

Hazardous waste is a universal problem and the 1990s saw the recognition of hazardous waste as well as trade in hazardous materials and industries as a major problem particularly in Eastern Europe and in developing nations. The disproportionate exposure of poor people, both at home and abroad, to hazardous waste has made 'environmental justice' an important policy area. Partly for this reason, the international trade in hazardous waste poses serious ethical as well as environmental and economic problems. Altered processes to improve efficiency and reduce waste generation, coupled with recycling, offer the promise of minimizing many adverse impacts of solid and liquid forms of chemical, biologic, and radioactive wastes on people and the environment.

BACKGROUND

Well-publicized descriptions of events such as Love Canal (New York 1978), the Chemical Control fire (New Jersey 1980), and Samuel Epstein's 1982 book on *Hazardous Waste in America*[5] brought hazardous waste to public attention. As the number of recognized hazardous waste sites has grown, communities have come to realize that they live in close proximity to such sites, with increasing public concern. Until the 1960s, toxic and radioactive waste was considered a challenge for solid waste systems.[6] It was then recognized that disposal of toxic substances in landfills posed hazards, and attention focused on incinerator technologies. In the 1970s major laws governing toxic substances were implemented including the Toxic Substances Control Act 1976[7] and the Resource Conservation and Recovery Act 1976.[8] In the 1980s governmental agencies focused attention on the magnitude of hazardous waste generation and disposal[9,10] and on the hazards facing workers.[11]

Initially it was proposed that hazardous waste management be assigned to governmental agencies, e.g. the Army Corps of Engineers, rather than the private sector.[12] In the 1970s, New Jersey developed a state initiative to clean up contaminated sites and taxed chemical and petrochemical industries to support a 'Spill Fund' allowing immediate cleanup. This successful program became a model for the nationwide 'Superfund' program. In the ensuing decades it became apparent that hazardous waste is a social as well as a technologic problem. Recycling and pollution prevention joined cleanup and incineration on the waste management agenda. Now many different federal agencies play a role in some aspect of hazardous materials management.[12]

Hazardous waste poses a threat to workers with occupational exposures (this chapter) and to the public potentially exposed in their homes, schools, or communities (Chapter 52.2). Exposure may occur at or near the sites of generation, along transportation routes, and near sites of ultimate disposal (i.e. hazardous waste sites). Indeed, in many communities, hazardous waste has emerged as a major public health concern. Hazardous waste management is often divided into two areas: the management of abandoned hazardous waste sites and the control of hazardous waste that continues to be produced, each governed by different federal laws.[13] Source reduction of waste ('pollution prevention') is an important component of the latter. The modern emphasis on brownfields redevelopment offers the opportunity to utilize partially remediated sites, with economic and social benefits, and low risk to future site occupants.

This and the next chapter cover individual workers and community exposures, respectively, and how such exposures can be evaluated and prevented. For most purposes, the clinician need not distinguish between a worker who manages currently generated hazardous waste on a factory site and one who manages formerly generated waste on an abandoned site. Although the two settings are subject to different regulations governing waste management, worker protection on both is covered by the same OSHA regulation.[14] Worker and community exposure are intertwined, because much of the hazardous waste remediation work is undertaken for the purpose of averting community exposure. Recent studies have attempted to balance the risk to workers from remediation against the community risks averted.

DEFINITION OF HAZARDOUS WASTE

Under RCRA[8] solid waste is determined to be hazardous if its 'quantity, concentration, or physical, chemical or infectious characteristic' leads to mortality or serious illness or otherwise poses a 'substantial present or potential hazard to human health or the environment, when improperly treated, stored, transported, or disposed of, or otherwise mismanaged'. The definition is very broad, and under the Toxic Substances Control Act of 1976[7] more than 55,000 chemicals are listed as falling under this definition. In reality most hazardous waste involves mixtures of several or many of these chemicals.

Procedures to identify hazardous waste

The Environmental Protection Agency developed tests to determine whether materials and soils qualified as hazardous. The Extraction Procedure (EP) designed to measure the extractability of inorganic materials from municipal solid waste has been supplanted by the Toxicity Characterization Leaching Procedure (TCLP). This uses a variety of solvents, including organic acids, to quantify how much organic and inorganic hazardous substances can be leached out of a waste or soil under controled conditions. Both tests determine the mobility of toxic constituents of wastes. In tests, a physical process is used to reduce the particle size, followed by the application of extraction solvents. The resulting leachate fluid is then analyzed for the presence of 39 designated contaminants to determine if they are present at levels of regulatory concern.

REGULATORY FRAMEWORK

The US Environmental Protection Agency (EPA) and many of the states regulate hazardous waste generation, transportation, and disposal. The Occupational Safety and Health Administration (OSHA) regulates worker exposure. The Agency for Toxic Substances and Disease Registry (ATSDR), a component of the Centers for Disease Control and Prevention (CDC), and the EPA are the federal agencies most likely to become involved in evaluating the community health impact of, and actual or potential exposure to hazardous waste. The Nuclear Regulatory Commission with the EPA are involved in regulations related to radioactive waste.

Two pieces of legislation are of primary importance in regulating hazardous waste. The Resource Conservation and Recovery Act of 1976[8] set requirements for the management of hazardous wastes that are currently being generated. The Comprehensive Environmental Response, Compensation and Liability Act of 1980 (CERCLA; often referred to as the 'Superfund Act') focused on abandoned hazardous waste sites, and developed a trust fund, through a tax on the chemical and petroleum industries, to provide for hazardous waste cleanups or remediation at these uncontroled or abandoned sites. This came to be known as Superfund, which is administered by EPA and modeled after the New Jersey Spill Response Act established to clean up chemical and oil spills. Both RCRA and CERCLA have been reauthorized with additional amendments, particularly the Superfund Amendment and Reauthorization Act (SARA 1988) which established a community infrastructure for managing toxic wastes and responding to hazardous chemical emergencies. Other relevant laws include the Water Pollution Control Act (1952), Clean Air Act (1963), Solid Waste Disposal Act (1965), Safe Drinking Water Act (1974), and Toxic Substances Control Act (1976).

EPA is authorized to perform short-term removal actions or longer-term remedial actions, and to force parties responsible for producing waste to conduct cleanups or reimburse EPA cleanups. Mitigation ranges from total cleanup to on-site containment, destruction or treatment, as well as cleaning up contaminated soil and ground water. Responsible parties can enter into administrative consent agreements with either EPA or a state, and undertake the site survey and mitigation under government supervision. If a responsible party refuses to participate, the government can undertake mitigation and assess triple damages. While regulations offer a framework for protecting workers, good planning and appropriate expertise in safety engineering, industrial hygiene, worker training, and occupational nursing and medicine are essential for implementation.[12]

EXPOSURE TO HAZARDOUS WASTES

Exposure to hazardous waste can be divided into occupational exposures (this chapter) and community exposures (Chapter 52.2).

Exposed workers

Employees who handle waste material directly are termed 'generator' workers. These employees may be exposed during storage procedures (e.g., loading into drums), pumping, inspection, maintenance of equipment, treating waste water, or preparing waste for shipment. Waste site employees may operate bulldozers, or crush waste drums for distribution. Transporter employees include truck, train, and barge loaders and operators. Environmental consultants, scientists, technicians, hydrologists, ecologists, geologists may inspect, sample, and analyze waste sites or perform ecologic risk assessments. Other specialized workers include well drillers who drill sampling wells on sites, remediation workers including laborers, building trades, and equipment operators, laboratory analysts who process wastes, public safety officials (e.g., security and firefighters) and workers from governmental agencies (e.g., inspectors and contract auditors).

Subcontract workers

Although responsible parties or public agencies will usually identify one or more prime contractors to conduct various phases of hazardous waste site investigation and remediation, much of the actual day-to-day work on site is likely to be done by subcontractors. Examples of subcontractors include those involved with infrastructure (road building and paving, fencing, electricians), site security, well drilling, construction/demolition, environmental monitoring and industrial hygiene, and medical monitoring. Much of the construction/demolition work on a site will be done by construction trades (e.g., laborers, equipment operators, painters, metal workers, masons) usually hired as subcontractors. Even if the prime contractor specializes in hazardous waste work, they will frequently use local contractors for many hazardous waste operations. These subcontractors rarely have safety and industrial hygiene resources, and provision for these services may be inadequate. Moreover, since subcontractor workers may not identify themselves as hazardous waste workers, they may not recognize the need for training, protection, or monitoring. Throughout this chapter, particular hazards facing subcontract workers will be identified.

Infrastructure

Many trades may become involved in building infrastructure on hazardous waste sites. Their exposure to hazardous substances will depend on their contact with contaminated media (e.g., soil or water), or concurrent remediation activities, or unanticipated exposure from explosions, fires, or spills. Hazardous waste work is usually a small part of their overall employment, and training and experience with hazardous waste are often scant.

Well drillers

Well drilling has become an important part of both site investigation and monitoring, with an estimated 37,000 new wells drilled annually for assessment of ground water quality and contamination. Well drillers experience mechanical safety hazards and noise, and their risk may be augmented by the protective equipment they are required to wear. Heat stress and exposure to toxic materials in soil and ground water are potential problems. Inadequately protected workers may be exposed to air-borne contaminants from the site, particularly if there is concurrent remediation or other sources of disturbance.[15] Vapor extraction systems and appropriate fans may be needed to reduce exposure.

Field workers

Many outdoor workers may be called on to assess resources or damages at hazardous waste sites (e.g., during ecologic assessments). Since they may not consider themselves or

be recognized as hazardous waste workers, there is a high likelihood that they will not have the training or protection or monitoring provided to other hazardous waste site workers.[16]

Worker injuries and exposures

Although potential exposure-related health risks facing hazardous waste workers have been reported frequently, documentation of exposure events is often minimized. In a study of an Ohio-based remediation company, 1607 illness/injury incident reports over a six-year period revealed that 75% involved mechanical trauma, 10% chemical exposure, 5% poisonous plants or insect bites, 2% temperature extremes, 1% cumulative trauma, with 7% unidentified.[17]

Community residents

Community residents may be exposed if their homes or workplace are in proximity to hazardous waste or contaminated industrial sites, resulting in soil contamination, because they walk or play on or near the site, or because their drinking water or air is contaminated by chemicals from the site (see Chapter 52.2).

Community vs worker risks

There are interactions between community and worker exposures. For example, strong environmental regulations regarding lead pollution of wetlands require bridge maintenance workers to work in enclosed 'tents' to contain lead dust. This, however, greatly increases the potential for worker exposure, and elevated blood lead levels are regularly encountered, even with aggressive use of personal protection.

Recently controversy has arisen over whether the risks to workers from hazardous waste remediation are warranted when weighed against the slight risk reduction to the public that remediation achieves,[18,19] which has encouraged focusing attention on cleanups where there are well characterized exposure pathways to the public.

With the practice of 'hazardous waste days', community exposure is reduced by the opportunity to bring household hazardous waste to centralized collection centers (usually on a county-wide basis). There the chemicals are classified, bulked, and shipped to permanent secure disposal sites. Workers (usually public works employees) involved in bulking activities are potentially exposed to hazardous materials, particularly in winter when such activities are likely to be conducted indoors in inadequately ventilated spaces.[20]

HAZARDOUS MATERIAL RELEASES: SPILLS, FIRES, EXPLOSIONS

Although the concept of 'hazardous waste' connotes landfills and drum dumps, the most serious health hazards are frequently posed by the sudden and accidental releases of chemicals during spills (tanks, pipelines, vehicles), fires, and explosions. This was highlighted by the tragic release of methyl isocyanate at Bhopal, India, which encouraged other countries to develop systems for preventing and responding to such emergencies. The train spills at Mississauga, Canada (chlorine, butane, toluene), and the metamsodium spill near Sacramento, California, highlighted transportation risks. The SARA Title III legislation emphasizes the need for local emergency planning groups, and the need to obtain information from chemical facilities located in each community, so that emergency responses can be anticipated. Such programs should involve community physicians, including emergency room and public health physicians, in the emergency planning; local hospitals need to have information on potential releases.

HAZARDOUS WASTE SITES AND NATIONAL PRIORITIES LIST

There is no single definition for a hazardous waste site, nor is the number of existing sites known with certainty. Estimates have ranged from 40,000[21] to 50,000 for the United States alone.[4] Only about 1500 sites have been listed on the National Priorities List (NPL), termed 'Superfund' sites. The NPL is EPA's list of uncontroled or abandoned sites identified for possible long-term remedial action under Superfund. The list is dynamic; once a site is successfully remediated according to EPA state agency criteria, it is removed from the list. The Department of Defense has developed an analogous Priority Model to rank the potential threat of contaminated sites to health and the environment, addressing the hazard, exposure pathway, and populations at risk.[22] The Department of Energy has developed an Environmental Restoration Priority System, which it uses to document its budget requirements.[22]

Although NPL sites are generally considered the most hazardous, many highly hazardous sites are not on the NPL. States have the option of seeking NPL listing for a site, or may choose not to do so if a responsible party is willing to undertake the investigation. Remediation of Superfund sites has been slowed by insurance and regulatory issues, which made it attractive to undertake cleanups under state auspices. EPA provides a website (http://www.epa.gov/superfund/sites/npl/npl.htm), which is the entry point for information on all NPL sites (Superfund sites).

At more than half of NPL sites, exposure pathways to human populations have been identified, indicating that they pose a health hazard. The sites are compared based on a hazard ranking system (HRS). Community involvement is included in the designation of a Superfund site, and a public comment period follows entry in the Federal Register that proposes listing a site on the NPL.

The first stage in the Superfund process is identification of the hazardous waste site. Once a site is identified, the state agency or EPA conducts a preliminary site assessment, including an inventory of known wastes on the site, to determine if there is a potential hazard. If a hazard exists, this may require emergency remediation or, more often, a

remedial investigation/feasibility study (RI/FS) is conducted, usually by private contractors.[23] The RI/FS serves as the mechanism for collecting data to:
1. characterize site conditions;
2. determine the nature of the waste;
3. assess risk to human health and the environment; and
4. conduct treatability testing to evaluate the potential performance and cost of treatment technologies.

The latter provides the mechanism for the potential development, screening, and detailed evaluation of alternative remedial actions.

Remediation may range from simple enclosure and warning signs to complete removal of waste, treatment of soil and ground water, and capping. The Superfund Trust monies can only be used for sites that meet the HRS criteria for inclusion on the National Priority List. Details on the HRS criteria and process are provided at: http://www.epa.gov/superfund/programs/npl_hrs/hrsint.htm

Hazard ranking system

The Hazard Ranking System (HRS) is the principal mechanism EPA uses to place uncontroled waste sites on the NPL. It is a numerically based screening system that uses initial site inspections and preliminary investigations to assess the potential of the site to pose a hazard to human health. The HRS yields three scores. The first evaluates the possibility that hazardous chemicals can migrate offsite. This depends on their likelihood of becoming air-borne (a function of soil dustiness and chemical volatility) or of moving through ground or surface water. These depend on geologic hydrologic features (slope, streams, aquifers), soil characteristics (organic content, colloidal nature, percolation), as well as on the chemicals' solubility characteristics. The second evaluates the likelihood that humans (often referred to as human 'receptors') or 'sensitive environments' will come in contact with the contaminated air, water, soil, or organisms. This depends on proximity, population density, prevailing winds, recreational activities, sources of drinking water and food, and the local topography. Some hazardous waste sites adjacent to residential areas are favored for recreational purposes, increasing the likelihood of human exposure. The third score is determined by the quantity and toxicity of the waste and its explosive or fire hazard properties.

The public is often confused by the designation Superfund site. This does not necessarily mean that a site will be cleaned up or even that it poses a real hazard. The listing designates the need for investigation of the site, and determination of how the site will be handled. Many Superfund sites remain today, unchanged from when they were listed nearly two decades ago. Posted public warnings at sites are variable. Occasionally Superfund sites, such as the Frontera Creek site in Puerto Rico, are found to pose little public health or ecologic threat.[24]

Under the law, responsibility for cleaning up or otherwise 'mitigating' a site lies with the responsible parties that generated the waste. Often the responsible parties cannot be identified, or may no longer represent a financially viable entity. Even when the original generator still exists, or when a legally responsible corporate heir is identified, years of legal action may ensue. In the interim, Superfund monies can be employed for mitigation, and the government will subsequently attempt to assess damages and seek reimbursement of the Fund.

CHEMICALS IN HAZARDOUS WASTE SITES

Discussion of chemical agents can be organized along structural (organic vs inorganic) or functional parameters (e.g., pesticides, solvents, etc). In order to characterize complex chemical mixtures it is essential to organize agents into groups that can be described generically. Fortunately, many chemicals are used only in research or in small quantities by very few industries, so that approximately 2000 are of widescale concern, and only about 300 are commonly used in large quantities. Indeed, since analytical laboratories normally provide information on only a few hundred chemicals, we are effectively limited to discussing those on which we have data. The US EPA has narrowed attention to about 150 chemicals, the so-called Hazardous Substance List or HSLs, which include the most toxic, widely encountered, or most useful surrogates (chemicals that may indicate that certain other chemicals or pollutants in general are present). This list includes 129 chemicals termed 'priority pollutants', plus some additional compounds. The priority pollutants are further broken down into groups based on analytical protocols: volatiles, semivolatiles, base neutrals, acid extractables, and heavy metals. Evaluations of hazardous waste sites or other contaminated sites often begin by measuring the priority pollutants in soil or water samples. Table 52.1.1 indicates the ten chemicals most commonly identified on Superfund sites. Thirty substances (18 of which are carcinogens) are present in 6% or more of the NPL sites.

The common solvents found in large amounts at hazardous waste sites are the aromatics (benzene, toluene, ethylbenzene, and xylene, abbreviated BTEX) and chlorinated alkanes and alkenes, particularly 1,1,1-trichloroethane, trichloroethylene (TCE), and tetrachloroethylene (perchlorethylene). These highly volatile compounds, vaporizing both into the atmosphere and into soil pores, are highly mobile, readily forming underground plumes, which can travel great distances, contaminating both ground and surface water. Heavy metals such as arsenic, lead, cadmium, mercury, and chromium are frequently present, although many compounds have low mobility and bioavailability. Polyaromatic hydrocarbons are also present at many waste sites and are the main contaminants of concern at gas plants and refineries.

Worker exposure occurs mainly at the source site during production, or during the onsite storage or shipping of the wastes. Occupational exposures also occur during transportation and at the final repository. However, most occupational health concerns focus on the hazardous waste remediation workers, who must be trained and protected to minimize exposure. Many hazardous organic chemicals break down quickly in the environment, but some are stable for years. In contrast, metal compounds persist indefinitely.

Chemical compatibility

Although many hazardous waste sites are drum dumps, tanks, or pits, there are also hazardous laboratory and industrial wastes that require sorting for proper disposal. Such sorting is conducted indoors and can be quite hazardous. These operations are conducted at generator sites to assure that waste streams are properly handled and that incompatible chemicals are not mixed. Incompatibilities can result in fires, explosions, splashes, or release of toxic gases. Oxidizers and reducers mixed together can cause serious reactions. The mixing of acids and bases can accomplish neutralization, but certain acid-base reactions can generate deadly hydrogen sulfide or cyanide compounds.[25] Such determinations often require working with open containers, and must be done under optimal ventilation with appropriate protective equipment.

RADIOACTIVE AND MIXED WASTES

Radioactive wastes have been generated in research laboratories, medical facilities, nuclear power plants, and in the development, manufacture, and testing of nuclear weapons. Although the latter activity was curtailed in 1989, the legacy of long-lived radionuclide wastes still exists on sites managed by the Department of Energy (DOE) and related contractors. The waste exists in tanks, drums, or containers of liquids and solids, both indoors and outdoors and above or below ground. Contamination occurs in soil, water, sediment, debris, and buildings. Radioactive sources, both sealed and unsealed, occur on DOE sites. Decommissioning, 'cocooning', and safe storage of cores of numerous reactors pose a particular challenge. In addition, numerous radiation targets and warheads await dismantling and disposal.

Radioactive waste exposure occurs at source sites, during transportation, and at repositories. Some short-lived isotopes decay very rapidly, releasing high energy over a short period of time, but many isotopes – particularly those generated

Chemical	Number of sites
Tricholoroethylene	129
Toluene	95
Benzene	94
Lead	93
Chloroform	68
PCBs	58
Tetrachloroethylene	57
Phenol	55
1,1,1-Trichloroethane	54
Chromium	53

*Data from Mitre Corp. 1983, after McDiarmid & Strickland 1990[64]

Table 52.1.1 Top ten chemicals reported in first 546 Superfund sites*

during the nuclear fuel cycle – have half-lives exceeding 100,000 years. Storage repositories must be secure to prevent leakage, theft, or disruption by geologic processes. The workers at greatest risk are those remediating the large scale Department of Energy sites, contaminated by nuclear waste from fuel and weapons production. Remediation activities are regulated by the DOE and contractors performing the work are responsible for meeting training, monitoring, and radiation protection requirements. Imposing and overseeing the regulations for lower-level subcontractors is a challenge for the DOE, which must have teams of industrial hygienists and radiation technicians to oversee subcontractors' performance.

High-level waste from nuclear reactors and nuclear weapons production is now in short-term storage at many nuclear facilities. Waste results in part from reprocessing spent fuel and fuel targets. Much is in liquid form and is potentially explosive. Although the federal government has sought to provide a permanent repository for such waste, and levied a tax on nuclear utilities to develop such a site, this has not been accomplished to date. In February 2002, President Bush approved the development of the Yucca Mountain facility as a permanent repository. This site in arid, sparsely populated country, with seismic stability, has faced opposition from state government and whether it will actually begin receiving such wastes by 2010 is uncertain. The safe and secure disposal of radioactive waste from nuclear power plants represents a severe challenge in the future development of nuclear energy.

Transuranic waste containing elements with higher atomic mass than uranium were formed during production of enriched uranium and plutonium for nuclear weapons. This contains more than 100 nanocuries per gram of α-emitters with half-lives greater than 20 years. This waste has been stored on Department of Energy facilities in several states. Volume reduction is the first step toward remediation followed by encapsulation and transportation to the Waste Isolation Pilot Plant (WIPP) in New Mexico. WIPP began development in the 1980s, but was only opened to receive wastes in 2001.

Low-level waste – a special case of hazardous waste is represented by low-level radioactive waste. In 1980 Congress shifted responsibility for the disposal of low-level radioactive wastes (LLRW) to the states. LLRW is defined as 'any radioactive material that is not high-level waste, transuranic waste (containing more than 100 nanocuries of alpha emitting isotopes with half life greater than 20 years), spent nuclear fuel, or by-product nuclear material', and is thus classified by the US Nuclear Regulatory Commission (NRC) by what it is not. LLRW is considered by many regulators to be relatively benign, including, for example, equipment and gloves used in manufacturing smoke detectors. However, it is difficult for the public to differentiate the hazards of HLRW from those of LLRW, and this hampers efforts to develop an effective disposal strategy. Moreover, some materials classified as LLRW may actually have high radioactivity.

About half the LLRW is generated from commercial nuclear reactors. The other half is from industrial and medical byproducts (including diagnostic and therapeutic materials). Examples include watch dials, radiographic equipment, and radiopharmaceuticals.[26] By definition, LLRW does not pose a substantial or lasting environmental threat to the biosphere or to humans. Compounds in this category require only marginal shielding and will decay rapidly. NRC[27] concluded that the threat to public health would be low and only shallow burial at closely monitored sites is required for safe disposal of LLRW.

Mixed wastes contain both toxic chemicals and radionuclides. These range from radiolabeled chemicals used in laboratory research and medical practice, to reactor cooling water containing chromium as a slimicide. They may vary from a few milliliters of a radiolabeled solvent to drums of inadequately characterized material. The safe handling, cleanup, and disposal of these wastes are largely under the jurisdiction of the NRC; however, some may be under mixed jurisdiction, complicating disposal.

BIOLOGIC WASTES

In the past decade, medical waste emerged as a significant public health hazard requiring its own regulations and management systems. Mismanagement of such waste, resulting in syringes, containers of blood, and contaminated medical waste washing up on New Jersey and New York beaches, captured extensive media attention and caused great economic losses to beachfront communities. The public outcry focused attention on this pervasive problem.

Waste from medical facilities is classified as infectious or non-infectious (mainly office and food wastes, or clinical supplies that have not come in contact with blood or other biologic materials). Infectious medical waste is generally defined as any solid waste that is generated in the diagnosis, treatment, or immunization of human beings or animals, in research, or in the production or testing of biologic agents, including but not limited to: soiled or blood-soaked bandages, culture dishes and other glassware, discarded surgical gloves or instruments, syringes and needles used to give shots or draw blood, lancets, cultures and swabs to inoculate cultures, and biologic material, and specimens. Sharps (needles, lancets, etc) are disposed of directly into specially designed and labeled rigid plastic containers. Other infectious waste is disposed of as 'red bag' waste in heavy gauge, red plastic bags.

Medical waste generators include private practitioners, clinics, hospitals and other healthcare facilities. Transporters, handlers and disposal facilities are also covered by regulation. Individual patients who generate medical wastes such as bandages and syringes at home are not covered. Most exposure takes place at the source site to clinical staff, housekeepers, and janitorial workers involved in the generation, collection and disposal of waste. Prior to the 1990s, many hospitals operated their own incinerators and disposed of infectious waste on site. Air quality and odor complaints coupled with stricter federal regulations governing emissions encouraged many hospitals to close down these local incinerators, and ship their wastes offsite to commercial medical waste treatment and disposal facilities.

The opportunity for exposure is greatest in those directly exposed to an infected patient (nurses, doctors, and other healthcare providers) and in those who collect the waste (housekeeping), particularly when sharps or broken glassware are disposed of improperly. Blood-borne pathogens such as the viral agents of AIDS and hepatitis are the main concerns, and the OSHA Blood-borne Pathogen Standard describes procedures for minimizing exposure. The risks vary with the frequency of the infections in the patient population, the infectiousness of the source blood, the nature of the object involved in the injury, and the characteristics of the injury itself. Needlestick events raise prominent health concerns due to risk of HIV, HBV, and HCV infection. Immunization against hepatitis B is required for personnel who may contact biologic waste, and a needlestick protocol including access to prophylaxis is necessary to prevent transmission of HIV.

The management of medical wastes includes grinding and chlorination, autoclaving, and incineration, which allow the material to enter the solid waste stream. In most cases medical wastes are collected in rigid red containers for sharps, and in red bags for other infectious medical wastes; these are shipped to companies that specialize in their destruction. Regulated medical waste haulers are used to transport the material to their destination. Medical waste disposal is regulated at the state level, but the emissions from medical waste incinerators are regulated by the US EPA. Other federal agencies regulate the transport of wastes (US Department of Transportation and US Postal Service), workplace exposures and blood-borne pathogens (US Department of Labor's Occupational Safety and Health Administration), and radioactive constituents in medical waste (Nuclear Regulatory Commission).

BIOLOGIC TARGETS OF HAZARDOUS CHEMICALS

Toxic chemicals damage living organisms in many ways; toxicologic research has revealed molecular mechanisms underlying genotoxicity, biochemical reactions, affecting organelles, and cells, organs and tissues. In some cases specific physiologic functions are inhibited. These may include diverse effects involving hematopoiesis, renal function, immune function, neurobehavioral performance, and reproduction. Exposure may occur to adults in general or to especially sensitive groups such as small children, pregnant women, or the elderly. Despite the great expansion of toxicologic knowledge, it is usually difficult to predict the effects of a particular exposure to hazardous waste, often involving complex mixtures, on an individual; assessing risk of adverse reproductive outcome or of developing cancer are particular challenges, which are the two greatest concerns voiced by exposed populations.

HAZARDS ASSOCIATED WITH SOLID WASTE MANAGEMENT

Workers who collect, sort, compact, or incinerate waste can be exposed to hazardous materials. Sanitation workers have died from noxious materials thrown out in trash. The more common hazards are organic dusts containing micro-organisms and endotoxins, as well as various chemicals. Landfill workers in New York reported more respiratory, dermatologic, and neurologic symptoms than other sanitation workers.[28] Garbage incinerators may emit toxic substances. Knox[29] found high rates of childhood cancer within 5 km of garbage incinerators, although the confounding effect of other industrial exposures could not be separated. Men living close to a Montreal landfill had elevated rates of several cancers.[30]

EXPOSURE PATHWAYS FOR WORKERS

Workers regularly exposed to hazardous waste are required to have training and protection to minimize exposure. Nonetheless exposure can occur when containers are breached, when there are leaks, spills, fires, explosions, or transportation accidents, or where safety measures are not followed.

Occupational exposure is often through inhalation of air-borne vapors or aerosols, but may also be through dermal contact. Inadvertent ingestion may occur if workers eat near the source of exposure or if their food and water are contaminated by aerial deposition. The importance of dermal absorption is probably underestimated in most exposure scenarios.

THE TIME COURSE OF EXPOSURE AND EFFECTS

The temporal features of exposure and effect are critical aspects of hazardous waste (or indeed any toxic) exposure. People may be exposed once to very high amounts (e.g., fire or explosion), or intermittently or continually to low levels. Similarly, effects may be manifest as acute, subacute, or chronic illness. Most troublesome is the long latent period between exposure and many effects. The consequences of some exposures are manifest immediately, while we have learned that the outcome of other exposures, particularly to carcinogens, may not appear for decades. For example, the latent period for mesothelioma from asbestos exposure may exceed 40 years. The long latency for cancer associated with environmental exposures poses challenges in establishing and attributing causality.

The practice of averaging exposure over time may be convenient for managing exposures in industry or for performing risk assessment, but is not biologically sound. Peak exposures may cause much greater damage than the same total amount distributed over time.

HAZARDOUS WASTE REMEDIATION

Remediation options vary greatly in scope and cost from fencing off a contaminated area to excavation and removal of contaminated soil, and pumping and treating the ground water. Research into methods for reducing the volume or toxicity of waste is extremely active. Chemical, physical, and biologic treatments, as well as administrative controls, can be utilized.[13,23]

There are a number of specialized treatments that can be used to diminish toxicity of hazardous wastes, including bio- and phytoremediation. Bioremediation employing bacteria to metabolically alter organic materials is widely used. An industry has developed around the 'invention' and patenting of new organisms designed to destroy particular substances, and includes the introduction and maintenance of the organisms on contaminated sites. Phytoremediation can be effective since roots and their accompanying microbial fauna can reduce the quantity of PAHs present.[31] Various plants have the propensity to extract particular substances (especially cations) from soil, and the plant material can be harvested and disposed of as solid hazardous waste.

Immobilization of radioactive wastes involves a variety of new technologies, including vitrification, which entails mixing the waste with borosilicate and heating it until it flows and then hardens as a glass that is then encased in steel canisters.

Remediation of waste often generates secondary waste. Excavation of dirt is the crudest method, and results in no volume reduction. Such dirt is hazardous waste, although it is sometimes mixed with much larger amounts of clean dirt (dilution) until the concentration of contaminants is 'acceptably low', and the soil can then be re-used, e.g., in road construction.

Pump and treat activities produce a water stream that must be processed in some way (for example, with charcoal columns) to remove the main contaminant(s) of concern. The resulting waste water is by no means pure and must be disposed of. Recharging into the ground or even an aquifer may be feasible if the removal efficiency has been high; different classes of compounds are removed with different efficiencies.[32]

High temperature treatments and incineration

Incineration remains a standby for destroying organics, although very high temperatures are required for polyhalogenated aromatic compounds such as PCBs and dioxins. It leaves behind an ash, mainly carbon and heavy metals. It requires either the construction of an onsite incinerator or the transport of wastes to a certified incinerator. Incinerator emissions can contain unwanted toxic chemicals as well. Recent studies exploiting advanced gas-phase thermal chemistry have identified how dioxins, furans, and other polyclic compounds are formed in incinerators, confirming earlier concerns about the gener-

ation of highly toxic air emissions during incineration. A variety of catalysts, including copper ions, play key roles in this transformation.[33] Workers at incinerators are responsible for receiving wastes, completing manifests, sorting wastes, feeding wastes into the incinerator, and maintaining operating conditions. They may be exposed to airborne emissions from the stacks, or during maintenance and cleaning operations. Fires and explosions occur occasionally, such as the Rollins fire in 1977 and the Chemical Control fire in 1980. Improved control methods and the training and monitoring of subcontractors who enter these sites have reduced the frequency of these events.

High temperature can also be applied in the field. In-situ thermal destruction applies a vacuum to subsurface or surface soil to pull air heated to 800°C through the soil. This can be highly efficient at destroying organics such as PCBs and PAHs with a high boiling point, and can greatly reduce the worker exposure involved in dig and carry operations. However, reducing PCB levels to the cleanup standard of 1 ppm may still require soil excavation.

CONCENTRATION, EXPOSURE, BIOAVAILABILITY, AND DOSE

Once an exposure pathway for workers or community has been established, it becomes necessary to estimate the degree of exposure. Usually the concentration in the environmental medium can be measured, and often exposure can be inferred. Bioavailability may be measured with laboratory simulations[34] or inferred from biomarkers.

Concentration

Concentration determines how much of a toxic material is present in environmental media, including the air (mg/m^3), water (mg/l), and soil or food (mg/kg). Laboratories that analyze these media provide information on the concentrations of dozens of toxic substances in the medium, which is the first step toward estimating hazard. In practice, the laboratories analyze for approximately 129 different substances that EPA has designated as Priority Pollutants.

Exposure

Exposure refers to how and how much of a substance enters the body. The movement of hazardous chemicals is very complex, and has challenged attempts to estimate exposure through modeling. Analytic procedures do allow some measurement of soil concentrations, air levels, and ground water plumes (an underground 'river' of hazardous material that moves slowly from its origin). This must be linked with behavioral data – how much time does an individual spend in proximity to the site, how might they be exposed to soil or dust or water, what level of protection do they use and how consistently? Such exposure data are frequently limited in environmental and occupational epidemiologic studies.

Exposure	Air	Soil/dust/fomites	Water	Food
Dermal	Generally not applicable	Some compounds absorbed from muds or slurries	Some substances absorbed from water or slurries	Not applicable
Inhalation	Primary route	Fine dusts, construction, road traffic	Aerosols during showering and cooking	Not applicable
Ingestion	Airborne deposition on food, crops	Toddlers ingest soil	Primary route	Primary route
Injection	Not applicable	'Sharps' for healthcare facilities	Not applicable	Not applicable

After Gochfeld 1991.[65]

Table 52.1.2 Exposure matrix for human exposure to environmental pollutants

Combining the four environmental media (air, water, soil/dust, and food) and the routes of exposure (dermal absorption, inhalation, ingestion, and occasionally injection) into an exposure matrix (Table 52.1.2) focuses attention on specific pathways.

Bioavailability

A critical factor in exposure analysis is bioavailability. The presence of a toxic material in soil does not establish that it can be taken up by plants or by people. For example, a soil with a high organic content may bind certain pollutants such that they cannot be released even when the soil is swallowed. For example, in rodent feeding studies Gallo and associates showed that dioxin-contaminated soil from Newark, New Jersey, yielded a much smaller proportion of its dioxin content than the sandier soil from Times Beach, Missouri.[35] Many risk assessments assume a bioavailability of 100%, a conservative assumption to maximize safety.

Dose and internal dose

Dose refers to how much of a substance reaches a target site in the body. A fundamental principle of toxicology is embodied in the dose–response concept. Simply stated, larger amounts of many chemicals typically produce larger effects. However, the dose–response relationship may be complex. In medicine, dose is measured by the amount that enters the body or gets absorbed into the blood stream, usually measured in mg of substance per kg of body weight per day. Of greater interest, but harder to quantify, is the internal dose delivered to the target tissue, which can sometimes be estimated using physiologically based pharmacokinetic models or by measuring biomarkers.

Thresholds

The first feature of the dose–response relationship that must be determined is whether there is a threshold, some level of exposure below which no effect (and no risk) occurs (see also Chapter 5). The antithesis of the threshold, the so-called no-threshold relationship, is exemplified by ionizing radiation and many other chemical carcinogens. Thus even very low exposures to ionizing radiation produce a finite risk of damage, without a threshold for radiation carcinogenesis.[36]

Determining a potential threshold in such circumstances is hampered by the practical challenges of directly studying the biologic effects of extremely low concentrations at which a threshold would exist. The current resolution, in keeping with the two-step model of carcinogenesis, is to treat initiators or genotoxic carcinogens (those which directly alter DNA) as if they have no threshold, and to treat promoters as if they have a threshold.

A second challenge to interpreting dose–response is illustrated in Figure 52.1.1, which compares two chemicals, both of which are shown with a threshold. If one uses the relative thresholds to compare toxicity, B appears to be more toxic than A, with an effect at a lower dosage. However, the midpoint of the curves show that B produces 50% of its effect (response dose or RD-50) at a very similar level to A. At higher doses, chemical A actually has greater toxicity than B, as indicated by the response rate. Hence, even the task of ranking chemicals by relative toxicity can become a difficult process.

CHEMICALS AND MIXTURES

Each individual chemical may exert one or more toxic effects on different target cells, tissues, or organs. For example, benzene, along with many other organic solvents, has general anesthetic properties when people are exposed acutely to high concentrations of vapors. Of greater concern, however, are the myelotoxic properties of

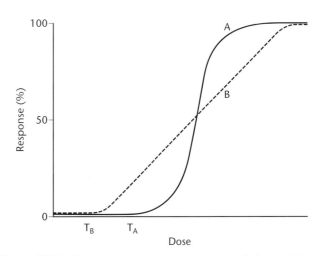

Figure 52.1.1: Dose–response curves showing the relative toxicity of two chemicals. If thresholds are compared, B is more toxic than A, but if the RD-50 is compared, then B appears to have similar toxicity to A. At higher doses, A has greater toxicity than B. (T-threshold dose).

benzene which result in aplastic anemia and leukemia. These effects occur in individuals with long-term exposure to much lower levels of benzene, levels below the odor threshold and below the threshold for neurotoxic effects.

One of the most troublesome features of hazardous waste sites is that the chemicals are present in mixtures, and that the actual composition of the mixtures is seldom fully known. Even when known, there is relatively little experience on how the toxicity of one compound is modified by simultaneous exposure to others. Three types of interaction occur: additive, where the effects of the two compounds together is equal to the cumulative effects both might have if they were administered separately; synergistic, where the two compounds together produce an effect greater than the sum of their individual effects (or at a lower combined dose); or protective, when one compound reduces the effect of the other. Synergistic actions pose the greatest threat, but are particularly difficult to estimate. One of the reasons to adopt an overprotective approach in environmental health is the uncertainty regarding the possibility of synergistic interactions where mixtures occur.

Explosive wastes and ordinance

The specialized task of dealing with ordinance and explosive wastes (OEW) and unexploded bombs, mines, and weapons (unexploded ordinance or UXO) is a specialized area of hazardous waste management. When such materials are identified they are usually dealt with by bomb squads on site, or in some cases transported to US Army facilities for detonation.[37]

CASE EXAMPLE OF A HAZARDOUS WASTE PROBLEM

On Earth Day 1980, the Chemical Control site in Elizabeth, New Jersey, exploded and burned. The fire raged for days, and many of the more than 40,000 55-gallon drums of chemical waste were damaged and their leaking contents were washed into the adjacent rivers by millions of gallons of fire-fighting water. The smoky plume blew for hours over surrounding neighborhoods. A study conducted by the National Institute for Occupational Safety and Health revealed that many firefighters had suffered measurable respiratory damage, since there was not adequate protective equipment for all of the personnel on site, and in some the damage was still evident five years later. No detailed study was made of the surrounding community (for descriptions and illustrations of the Chemical Control site see USEPA 1980[38] and Gochfeld & Burger 1990[24]).

The Chemical Control Company had operated for more than a decade, receiving waste from diverse chemical companies. In many cases the drums bore little or no labeling information, though many indicated the name of the generator company. Although the company was paid to dispose of the waste in a legal fashion, it merely stored the material on site. Its incinerator was never licensed, and

except for reports of some illegal nocturnal burning, waste continued to accumulate until the State of New Jersey closed the site in 1979 and took it over to begin the cleanup process.

The Chemical Control site was one of the nation's first Superfund sites. Despite the potentially disastrous prospect of a large hazardous waste site in close proximity to residential areas, the cleanup proceeded slowly, and provided insight into the problems that were to confound and retard cleanup and mitigation for the ensuing decade. Despite the fact that there was a hazardous waste incinerator already on site that could have been upgraded to safely dispose of much of the waste, the decision was made not to use it, but rather to ship all material offsite. This required opening every drum, sampling and identifying its contents, relabeling, and manifesting (or cataloging) it.

The process was accelerated when many of the generator companies were ordered to reclaim their identifiable wastes. It was, however, retarded by the difficulties in locating a suitable disposal site in another state and arranging safe transportation. Many of the drums (lab-packs) contained small vials of unlabelled wastes from research laboratories, and months were spent trying to identify and re-pack them. In the year that passed, only a small proportion of the material was moved offsite, prior to the fire and explosion.

The subsequent cleanup, complicated by the fire and rusted drums, required about five years and cost about $5,000,000 US. The period saw the emergence of companies specializing in hazardous waste cleanup, and one of the first medical surveillance programs instituted specifically for hazardous waste workers. Many of the lessons learned from the Chemical Control experience have shaped subsequent hazardous waste remediation approaches. In 2001 the site was a paved area surrounded by a high chain-link fence, awaiting 'brownfield' re-development.

EVALUATING AND PROTECTING THE HAZARDOUS WASTE WORKER

Protecting hazardous waste workers involves extensive training, determining their fitness to use respirators, careful selection of appropriate protective equipment, establishment of a standard operating procedures manual which includes appropriate safety planning, and medical surveillance. Whereas most of these procedures, including site monitoring by industrial hygienists, represent primary prevention, medical surveillance is secondary prevention (see Chapter 4.2). In addition to assessing early health effects in workers, it serves a quality assurance role, by being able to detect exposures that occur when there is a breakdown or inadequacy of the primary preventive strategies.

Health and Safety Plans

Hazardous waste investigations and remediation operations require a Health and Safety Plan (HASP) which includes both generic and site-specific components. This is the first step in worker and community protection. A typical HASP includes the following components: site description and layout of zones, hazards present, applicable standards and regulations, public safety, work site safety, site safety officer, chain of responsibility for subcontractors, hazard assessment including substances and amounts likely to be encountered, personnel protection and respiratory protection program, routine decontamination procedures for personnel and equipment, environmental monitoring procedures and equipment.

The HASP must also include provisions for emergency medical care for the site, and must designate employees with first aid and emergency response training. The HASP also identifies the necessary first aid equipment and procedures for emergency decontamination and evacuation, summoning emergency care, ambulance transport and notification of local emergency rooms regarding site hazards and work in progress.

Record keeping is an important part of the HASP. It includes names of all prime and subcontractor employees and visitors to a site, dates of deployment, training and equipment, as well as any exposure and medical monitoring data. The plan should include regular (preferably daily) safety briefings including all contractor, subcontractor, and regulatory personnel, with documentation of attendance and topics.[12] Some components of a HASP are discussed below.

Exclusion zone

Careful layout of a hazardous waste site will facilitate cost-effective operations and afford appropriate levels of protection. The HASP will identify the site zones including a exclusion or hot zone, a contamination reduction zone, and a support or clean zone. Appropriate layout of a hazardous waste site affords the opportunity to allow only adequately trained and protected workers into the most hazardous areas of the site. Other workers are allowed access to certain parts of the sites, i.e., command posts, while being excluded from the center. Staging areas for supplies and equipment, for the shipment of contained wastes, as well as decontamination areas and facilities need to be established and posted appropriately.[25]

Personal protective equipment

Personal protective equipment (PPE) plays a central role in protecting hazardous waste workers, because of the often unpredictable nature of their exposures. Nonetheless, engineering and administrative controls as well as good work practices remain important. PPE must be selected to be appropriate to possible exposure scenarios and hazards that may be encountered, yet must be sufficiently comfortable that it can and will be worn for the required period. Selection, training, and maintenance of the PPE are an integral part of the HASP. The goal is to provide the appropriate amount of protection. PPE may subject workers to heat stress, requiring adjustment of work practices.[39]

Respirator fit and fitness

Unlike industrial workers, the use of personal protective equipment plays a prominent role in protecting hazardous waste workers. Respiratory protection must be appropriate to the hazards that may be encountered. Wearers must be tested with their respirator to assure that there is a good fit (no leakage) (see also Chapter 4.1). They must have adequate training, not only in respirator selection, use, and maintenance, but also in hazard recognition and avoidance, i.e., exposure prevention.

There are four levels of protective equipment (Table 52.1.3) determined by the type and degree of contamination that may be encountered. Level D corresponds to requirements imposed on many industrial workers. Level C protection is encountered in industrial settings under special circumstances. In industry, Level B is likely to be used in confined space operations, and Level A primarily under emergency conditions. In hazardous waste activities Level B is not uncommon.

The OSHA Respirator Standard (CFR 1910.134) requires a medical evaluation to determine that there are no medical contraindications to using a respirator or wearing protective equipment. However, the criteria for making this determination are not absolute. Moreover, demographically, individuals applying for hazardous waste work tend to be young and healthy, such that cardiorespiratory contraindications to respirator use are likely to have low prevalence. With the 1998 Revision of the Standard, clearance can be provided simply by completing a questionnaire which can be reviewed by a licensed health provider.

In general, people with significant cardiorespiratory impairment (such as angina or recent myocardial infarction, uncontroled hypertension, arrhythmias or significant respiratory impairment from lung disease) should not do work that requires respiratory protection. Wearing respirators increases the work of breathing, increases physical workload, and can exacerbate heat stress (leading to peripheral vasodilatation). Rarely, individuals develop anxiety when wearing respirators and other protective equipment, and they should not be placed in locations where regular respirator use is required.

Significantly, the OSHA Standard does not require either chest radiographic studies or spirometry for determining respirator fitness. While it has been argued convincingly that in the absence of a history of cardiovascular or pulmonary disease these tests do not aid the clinician,[40] workers may be in a medical surveillance program where spirometry is required. Individuals with respiratory symptoms and a moderate decrease in function (e.g., FEU, or FVC 50-65% of predicted) require careful consideration. Such individuals might be cleared for level C, but not for level A or B protection. In jobs where the individual can pace their work, such a restriction may not be essential.

Additional conditions that must be considered, but are not currently regarded as an absolute contraindication for use of respirators, include pneumothorax, ruptured tympanic membrane, and use of contact lenses. While the need for increasing the intrapleural pressure to overcome

Level	Respirator	Body protection
Level D No measurable concentration. No exposure by inhalation or splashes.	None or dust mask.	Work coveralls. Dust mask as needed. Safety goggles. Hard hat/steel-toed shoes as designated.
Level C Known air concentration acceptable for air-purifying respirator. IDLH will not be reached. No skin damage or permeation. No unidentified vapors present.	Air-purifying respirator. Full face-piece.	Light, impermeable outer garment over work clothes.
Level B Air level may exceed capacity of air-purifying system. Unidentified vapor(s) likely to be present. Oxygen <19.5%. Dermal absorption possible, skin contact with head or neck not likely.	SCBA or other air-supplied system.	Full-body, impermeable garment, not encapsulated.
Level A Chemical concentration known to be above safe level or IDLH. Extremely hazardous or unidentified substance likely to be present. High splash potential. Likelihood of dermal absorption.	SCBA or other air-supplied system.	Full-body, encapsulating chemical suit.

Table 52.1.3 Levels of protective equipment for working on hazardous waste sites (IDLH = Immediately Dangerous to Life and Health)

increased dead space raises concern for pneumothorax, there is no evidence that respirator use poses a significant risk. Unless there is a history of a very recent or recurrent pneumothorax, this is not currently considered a contraindication. A ruptured tympanic membrane has been considered a possible route of exposure; however, remains a largely theoretical concern. The use of contact lenses has often been discouraged or forbidden for hazardous chemical work. The rationale is that chemicals might be absorbed under the lens by capillarity, that a soft lens might absorb chemicals, or that the lens might suddenly dislocate, causing the worker to remove their face mask. However, the improved visual acuity and visual field afforded by contact lenses may more than compensate for the risk, and it is reasonable that a person wearing contact lenses have the same eye protection as a person wearing no corrective lenses.

Respiratory protective equipment (RPE) plays an important role in protecting hazardous waste workers, but is not used uniformly. Mandatory fit-testing and training programs can play an important role in motivating workers to use RPE, while concerns about comfort and communication undermine RPE use.[41]

Preventing heat stress

A particular problem confronting workers who must exert themselves in chemically impervious protective clothing is heat stress (see Chapter 34). Outdoor work reduces risk for accumulation of hazardous vapors and fumes, but increases exposure to solar radiation. As heat load exceeds dissipation, body core temperature increases, performance declines, accident rates increase, and heat events (heat exhaustion, heat stroke) increase.[42] Ambient air temperature, radiant temperature, humidity, air motion, and metabolic heat production all contribute to increased heat load.

Acclimatization, work-site canopies, adequate hydration, and scheduling of work are among the approaches to reducing heat stress. Most important is an appropriate rest–work alternation schedule. In sunny areas this may require workers to spend more than 50% of their time at rest. Medical screening, other than a prior history of heat-related events, is of limited use in detecting individuals susceptible to heat stress. Certain equipment, including air-cooled suits, can be very beneficial. Small work sites can be covered by a canopy to exclude solar radiation, fans can be installed to increase air movement.

Decontamination

Decontamination procedures require planning to assure that workers practice the required 'decon' protocols when they move from zone 1 (hot zone) to zone 3. This requires proper removal and disposal of contaminated clothing and equipment, and the washing of non-disposable equipment (e.g., boots), such that contaminants are not tracked into clean areas or carried outside the hot zone. Details for appropriate design of a decon facility and program are provided by Lippitt and Prothero.[43] The selection of solvent (usually water), detergent, acid or base (if needed), and the proper drumming and disposal of the waste water are essential.

Training

Appropriate training ensures that workers know the hazards they will encounter and provides knowledge and skills for safe performance of work and protection. Training covers hazard recognition, exposure reduction (including PPE selection, use, and limitations), emergency escape procedures, emergency protocols including decontamination, and site-specific topics.[44] The OSHA Standard[14] requires a 40-hour training course with 8-hour annual refreshers, and additional training for supervisors. Actual 'hands-on' performance, including material handling while wearing protective gear, greatly enhances the learning experience, compared to passive classroom lectures.

Environmental monitoring

An important part of a Health and Safety Plan is environmental monitoring, which is a basic industrial hygiene procedure for worker protection. This is necessary to determine the level of protection required for particular tasks or particular parts of the site. In the absence of monitoring, a higher level of protection is required, which may increase the risk of heat stress, impose unnecessary discomfort on the wearer, and increase costs unnecessarily. A variety of monitoring devices are available, including real-time monitors with alarms to indicate the presence of excessive concentrations of volatile chemicals.[45] Monitoring for combustible gases, carbon monoxide, and for oxygen concentrations in confined space tasks is also essential.

Real-time field monitors have varying sensitivity and specificity. A chemical sensor for volatile organic compounds (VOC) can document underground plumes or air-borne emissions. They can be used as alarm systems. Real-time equipment includes portable gas chromatographs, flame ionization detectors (FID), or photoionization detectors (PIDs). Some are designed to read a particular substance or class of substances. Detector tubes, often used in factory settings, are often less suitable for hazardous waste sites. FIDs indicate total combustibles present, and are not very sensitive to temperature or humidity changes; they are not suitable for chlorinated hydrocarbons. PIDs are durable general purpose detectors that are non-specific and sensitive to humidity. The more expensive Fourier-transform infrared detectors (FTIR) can be tuned to specific substances (when there is a single substance of concern). These monitors do not require oxygen, in comparison with FIDs, and may be used in oxygen-deficient environments.[46] Confined spaces including buildings, tanks, and trenches represent particularly dangerous environments and require special protocols.[47] The level of air-borne contaminants present or potentially present determines the level of personal protective equipment required.

Employee job task analysis

A refinement of Health and Safety Plans is the Employee Job Task Analysis (EJTA) which requires supervisors to analyze the tasks required of each worker during every phase of a site investigation and remediation. This involves identifying and documenting critical functions and potential hazards, and links each worker with the appropriate level of training, protection, and medical clearance. The EJTA predicts, characterizes and helps prevent hazardous exposures. It has been initiated at Department of Energy remediation sites, and should extend to all hazardous waste operations.[48]

Medical monitoring for hazardous waste workers

Medical monitoring involves the longitudinal monitoring of workers with actual or potential exposure to workplace hazards (see also Chapter 59). The OSHA published the Hazardous Waste Standard or HAZWOPER,[14,49,50] which sets forth the requirements for 'medical surveillance' of hazardous waste workers (Paragraph F). There are some important limitations to the Standard. First, it emphasizes fitness rather than needs for surveillance. Second, it sets a threshold of 30 days of exposure above the permissible exposure limit for mandatory surveillance, which does not address individuals with briefer or intermittent high exposure levels and might include those with inadequate training or protection. Fortunately EPA contract specifications usually include comprehensive medical surveillance for all site workers. Finally, while the OSHA Standard leaves the content and interpretation of the surveillance program to the discretion of the physician, it does not stipulate a specific level of medical training or certification.

Medical monitoring of hazardous waste workers has posed many challenges.[51,52] Since hazardous waste workers with the greatest opportunity for exposure should have a high level of training and protective equipment, few actually experience significant unprotected exposure. This is reflected by studies showing relatively few abnormalities detected among hazardous waste workers.[53] On the other hand, workers with a lower level of exposures, but inadequate protection, may be at greater risk, and are less likely to be included in medical programs. Further, white collar hazardous waste workers were 67% more likely than blue collar workers to be in a surveillance program, even though they were less likely to be injured.[54]

Recommendations for medical monitoring programs

The medical monitoring program begins with a preliminary screening examination,[55] which can determine fitness and provide baseline data for comparison with subsequent evaluations. This is followed by periodic (usually annual) surveillance examinations. The extent, content, and frequency of examination depend on the type of work being performed. Annual examinations are common, but not required. The OSHA Standard gives the examining physician discretion over frequency of follow-up.

The examiner must have a clear picture of each worker's responsibilities and potential exposures; this requires more than a cursory understanding of the specific hazardous waste work. The anticipated task and job requirements should be developed for the EJTA (see above) and provided to the medical examiner in writing. The examiner should review these with each worker to verify the potential exposures.

Workers should complete a general health history form, including an occupational history, supplemented by specific information on past, current, and anticipated exposures. The past and current use of protective equipment should be reviewed, and the examiner should verify their appropriateness. The questionnaire and/or history should identify the frequency of work in the field, the kinds of sites visited, the substances encountered, the protective gear used, and the problems encountered on the site (including breakdown of operating procedures, explosions, exposures, or acute illness). Each worker should be asked specifically whether they have had mandated hazardous waste training, fit testing and training on their required protective equipment, and understanding of the Health and Safety Plan.

Each new employee should undergo a thorough baseline examination, including a detailed physical examination and blood tests (complete blood count and clinical chemistry profile with liver function testing). Workers who may require frequent exposure to heavy metals or pesticides may have baseline biomonitoring (e.g., blood lead or serum and red cell cholinesterase, respectively). Biologic monitoring was formerly a widespread and expensive component of the examinations, but in most cases has not proven fruitful and has been abandoned by many companies and providers. In some cases, baseline blood samples are archived for future analysis in the event of an exposure. Spirometry is usually performed as part of a respirator fitness examination, but is not required. Electrocardiograms are warranted for workers older than age 40 years or who have a history indicative of an increased risk of heart disease (e.g., family history, chest pain, hypercholesterolemia, hypertension). Stress tests are warranted only if clinically indicated. Audiometry is warranted for heavy equipment operators and others exposed to significant noise.

The periodic examination should include an interim history and targeted physical examination. Further test components depend on the history and exposure. No routine laboratory tests are required, but most examination batteries include spirometry and blood tests. Incident-related examinations are performed when there has been a spill or other exposure, or when a person has become sick as a result of work on a site. This examination depends on reports by the industrial hygienist or site safety officer, who should be able to identify the substance(s) to which the worker was exposed.

Positive results warrant appropriate follow-up, and findings that are believed to indicate chemical exposure must be reported to the health and safety officer as well as the employees, so that additional investigations and protection can be instituted. Usually such exposure occurs only when there is an accident or a breakdown in procedures. Under normal operating conditions, hazardous waste workers should be able to function with no appreciable chemical exposure and no increased health risk. Where health problems are detected, workers should be informed of procedures for filing worker's compensation claims.

Turnover and surveillance

Effective medical surveillance requires longitudinal tracking of the employee, so that current medical findings can be compared to past results. However, hazardous waste work is an industry with high worker turnover, and because each company uses different medical providers, it is

frequently the case that the current examiner has no prior medical record on a particular employee. Accordingly, each hazardous waste worker should receive a complete copy of test results and medical findings. The OSHA Standard requires that they also receive a written explanation of any significant findings. Providing workers with their medical records to take to future providers greatly enhances the value of the medical program.

Quality assurance for medical monitoring

Virtually all medical monitoring of hazardous waste workers is contracted out to physicians. Settings include academic or industrial medicine clinics or private practitioners. Some of these providers are very experienced, while others are unfamiliar with regulations, requirements, and risks. Likewise, some remediation companies lack expertise in identifying required medical services and receive little specific guidance from the OSHA HAZWOPER standard. Some medical companies specialize in providing medical monitoring services, and purchasers of such services must ascertain the experience and credentials of providers, as well as the appropriateness of the services offered. Some hazardous waste remediation firms operate in many states, using local providers for their medical monitoring. Therefore it is essential that the hazardous waste companies institute some form of quality assurance to ascertain that their employees are receiving the appropriate level of monitoring.[56]

Protecting subcontractor workers

As hazardous waste management has developed into an industry requiring increasing specialization, the work-force involved has become more diverse. Many employees are transient, spending only a few days at each site without considering themselves hazardous waste workers. For example, fencing contractors erect fences around sites, road-builders construct access roads and pave pads to support trailers and equipment, and electricians bring power lines to sites. Work on hazardous waste sites may thus represent only a small part of their work activities. Since these workers often do not have to wear respiratory protection for 30 days in a year, most of the subcontractors do not participate in any medical monitoring programs. Nonetheless, where respiratory protection is required, such workforces are required to meet the PPE provisions of the Hazardous Waste Standard as well as the training, fit testing, and fitness provisions of the OSHA Respirator Standard. Unfortunately, such programs are frequently not in place. The evaluation[57] and auditing[56] of hazardous waste workers protection should be an ongoing feature of any HASP.

INTERNATIONAL HAZARDOUS WASTE

Although hazardous waste and other environmental and public health issues are addressed in most industrialized nations, they frequently 'take a back seat' to economic development in developing nations. Traditionally, developing nations have been characterized by numerous small companies, employing few workers, with few resources or staff devoted to occupational or environmental safety and health. Even in countries with environmental regulations, enforcement is limited, due to the decentralized nature of waste generation. El-Fadel et al[58] demonstrated this with a case study in Lebanon, and warn that the impact of globalization is to superimpose large-scale industrialization on an infrastructure inadequate to deal with current hazardous waste generation. Wastes are disposed of on land and in water with little regard to containment, in a manner reminiscent of the mid-1900s in industrialized nations, without consideration for the much greater costs involved in cleaning up wastes decades in the future.

Assessing hazards at waste disposal sites is an international challenge, and methods have to be generalized to take into account different record keeping practices and cultural exposure patterns.[59] In some countries large populations live adjacent to or on landfills, and make their living by gleaning recoverable items from the dump. The sale of scrap metal, some of which has had radioactive contamination, has resulted in large-scale radiation exposure in countries such as Mexico, Taiwan, and Brazil. In the future, growing population pressures may require retrieving contaminated sites.

International trade in hazardous waste

Disposing of hazardous waste in compliance with laws has become an expensive process. On the one hand, high cost should be an incentive for pollution prevention and source reduction, including substituting less hazardous materials wherever possible. On the other hand, companies and countries look for less expensive disposal methods that increasingly involve shipping wastes to developing countries with economic incentives. Global environmental treaties are being developed, but are difficult to implement, particularly when hazardous waste is viewed as a commodity protected by world trade agreements.[60]

SOURCES OF INFORMATION

There are many volumes and compendia which provide information on specific hazardous substances. In addition, an increasing number of websites contain such information. The US EPA's Integrated Risk Information System (IRIS) has a web page that documents the scientific literature on which reference doses for non-carcinogens or slope factors for carcinogens are based. The Agency for Toxic Substance and Disease Registry (ATSDR) publishes and periodically updates monographs on specific chemicals commonly found in NPL sites. Fortunately this information is now available on the web at http://www.atsdr.cdc.gov/toxpro2.html (verified March 2004), or as CD or hardcopy free from ATSDR.

WASTE MINIMIZATION

A generation ago, Garrett Hardin[61] pointed out that our approach to regulation promoted rather than penalized the profligate disposal of waste materials, spreading the cost over society as a whole, rather than charging it to the polluters themselves. State and federal efforts to discover and control hazardous waste sites were already well under way by 1982, when Epstein and co-authors published their popular book,[5] and when medical evaluation approaches for populations exposed to hazardous waste were described.[62]

The increased cost and regulation of hazardous waste disposal have made waste minimization more attractive, and ultimately an economic necessity.[63] In 1984 the Hazardous and Solid Waste Amendments to RCRA stated that 'it is to be a national policy of the United States that, where feasible, the generation of hazardous waste is to be reduced or eliminated'. The Office of Technology Assessment[10] concluded that industry had been slow in achieving waste minimization, even though this may actually reduce costs. Unfortunately, in the ensuing years, progress towards waste minimization has been slow. Nonetheless, there are bright spots, such as a variety of efforts to minimize mercury in the waste stream through elimination of mercury batteries, exchange of mercury thermometers, and removal of mercury switches from automobiles.

References

1. Webb PJ. Information gathering, site characterization and information resources. In: Martin WF, Gochfeld M, eds. Protecting personnel at hazardous waste sites, 3rd edn. Boston: Butterworth-Heineman, 2000;23–50.
2. Phillips AM, Silbergeld EK. Health effects studies of exposure from hazardous waste sites – where are we today? Am J Ind Med 1985; 8:1.
3. Andelman JB, Underhill DW. Health effects from hazardous waste sites. Chelsea: Lewis, 1987.
4. Johnson BL, DeRosa C. The toxicologic hazard of superfund hazardous-waste sites. Rev Environ Health 1997; 12:235–51.
5. Epstein SS, Brown LO, Pope C. Hazardous waste in America. San Francisco: Sierra Club Books, 1982.
6. Skitt J. Disposal of refuse and other waste. New York: Halsted Press (John Wiley & Sons), 1972.
7. TSCA. The Toxic Substances Control. Act. PL 94-469, 90 Stat 2003, 1976.
8. RCRA. The Resource Conservation and Recovery Act, PL 94-580, 90 Stat 2795, 1976.
9. Wilkes A, Kiefer I, Levine B. Everybody's problem: hazardous waste. Office of Solid Waste SW-826. Washington DC: US EPA, 1980.
10. OTA. Serious reduction of hazardous waste. OTA-ITE-317. Washington DC: US Congress Office of Technology Assessment, 1986.
11. NIOSH. Occupational safety and health guidance manual for hazardous waste site activities. NIOSH 85-115. Washington DC: DHHS, National Institute for Occupational Safety and Health, 1985.
12. Martin WF, Gochfeld M. Introduction and federal programs. In: Martin WF, Gochfeld M, eds. Protecting personnel at hazardous waste sites, 3rd edn Boston: Butterworth-Heineman, 2000;1–22.
13. Blackman WC Jr. Basic hazardous waste management, 3rd edn. Boca Raton: Lewis, 2001.
14. OSHA (Occupational Safety and Health Administration). Standard on Hazardous Waste Operations and Emergency Responses, Final rule. CFR 1910.120. Fed Reg March 6, 1989: 54.
15. Sweet HR, Goldman D. Monitoring well health and safety. In: Martin WF, Gochfeld M, eds. Protecting personnel at

hazardous waste sites, 3rd edn. Boston: Butterworth-Heineman, 2000;483–97.

16. Burger J, Gochfeld M. Protecting ecological workers at hazardous waste sites. In: Martin WF, Gochfeld M, eds. Protecting personnel at hazardous waste sites, 3rd edn. Boston: Butterworth-Heineman, 2000;625–38.

17. Akbar-Khanzadeh F, Rejent GM. Incident trends for a hazardous waste cleanup company. Am Ind Hyg Assoc J 1999; 60:666–72.

18. Cohen JT, Becj, Rudel R. Life years lost at hazardous waste sites: remediation worker fatalities vs. cancer deaths to nearby residents. Risk Analysis 1997; 17:419–25.

19. Gochfeld M. Risk balancing for hazardous waste workers: alternative work, traffic fatalities, and unemployment. Risk Analysis 2004, in press.

20. Betsinger G, Brosseau LM, Golden J. Occupational health and safety in household hazardous waste management facilities. Am Ind Hyg Assoc J 2000; 61:575–83.

21. Hart FC. Preliminary assessment of cleanup costs of National Hazardous Waste Problems. Report to the US EPA, Feb 23, 1979.

22. National Research Council. Ranking hazardous waste sites. Washington DC: National Academy Press, 1994.

23. O'Brien & Gere Engineers. Hazardous waste site remediation: the engineer's perspective. New York: Van Nostrand Reinhold, 1988.

24. Gochfeld, M, Burger J. Investigations and activities at Superfund Sites. In: Gochfeld M, Favata EA, eds. Hazardous waste workers. Philadelphia: Hanley & Belfus, 1990.

25. Priester LE III, Wallace L. Engineering controls: site layout. In: Martin WF, Gochfeld M, eds. Protecting personnel at hazardous waste sites, 3rd edn. Boston: Butterworth-Heineman, 2000; 228–50.

26. Burns ME. Low level radioactive waste regulation. Chelsea: Lewis, 1988.

27. NRC. Managing low-level radioactive waste: a proposed approach. Washington DC: Nuclear Regulatory Commission, 1980.

28. Gelberg KH. Health study of New York City Department of Sanitation landfill employees. J Occup Environ Med 1997; 39:1103–10.

29. Knox E. Childhood cancers, birthplaces, incinerators and landfill sites. Int J Epidemiol 2000; 29:391–7.

30. Goldberg MS, Siemiatyck J, DeWar R, Desy M, Riberdy H. Risks of developing cancer relative to living near a municipal solid waste landfill site in Montreal. Arch Environ Health 1999; 54:291–6.

31. Olson PE, Flechter JS, Philp PR. Natural attenuation/phytoremediation in the vadose zone of a former industrial sludge basin. Environ Sci Pollut Res Int 2001; 8:243–9.

32. Leenheer JA, Hsu J, Barber LB. Transport and fate of organic wastes in ground water at the Stringfellow hazardous waste disposal site, southern California. J Contam Hydrol 2001; 51:163–78.

33. Taylor PH, Lenoir D. Chloroaromatic formation in incineration processes. Sci Total Environ 2001; 269:1–24.

34. Ellickson KM, Meeker RJ, Gallow MA, Buckley BT, Lioy PJ. Oral bioavailability of lead and arsenic from a NIST standard reference soil material. Arch Environ Contam Toxicol 2001; 40:128–35.

35. Umbreit TH, Hesse EJ, Gallo MA. Bioavailability and cytochrome P-450 induction from 2,3,7,8 tetrachlorodibenzo-P-dioxin contaminated soils from Times Beach, Missouri, and Newark, New Jersey. Drug Chem Toxicol 1988; 11:405–18.

36. Upton AC. Radiation hormesis: data and interpretation. Crit Rev Toxicol 2001; 31:581–95.

37. Pastorick JP. Ordnance, explosive waste, and unexploded ordnance. In: Martin WF, Gochfeld M, eds. Protecting personnel at hazardous waste sites, 3rd edn. Boston: Butterworth-Heineman, 2000;459–82.

38. Schwope AD, Janssen LL. Personal protective equipment. In: Martin WF, Gochfeld M, eds. Protecting personnel at hazardous waste sites, 3rd edn. Boston: Butterworth-Heineman, 2000; 251–94.

39. USEPA. Report of the scientific data collected in connection with the Chemical Control Operation Incident. Washington DC: US Environmental Protection Agency, 1980.

40. Hodous TK. Screening prospective workers for the ability to use respirators. J Occup Med 1986; 28:1074–80.

41. Salazar MK, Connon C, Takaro TK, Beaudet N, Barnhart S. An evaluation of factors affecting hazardous waste workers' use of respiratory protective equipment. AIHAJ 2001; 62:236–45.

42. Goldman RF. Heat stress in industrial protective encapsulating garments. In: Martin WF, Gochfeld M, eds. Protecting personnel at hazardous waste sites, 3rd edn. Boston: Butterworth-Heineman, 2000;295–355.

43. Lippitt JM, Prothero TG. Decontamination. In: Martin WF, Gochfeld M, eds. Protecting personnel at hazardous waste sites, 3rd edn. Boston: Butterworth-Heineman, 2000; 356–386.

44. Martin WF, Montgomery RC. Training. In: Martin WF, Gochfeld M, eds. Protecting personnel at hazardous waste sites, 3rd edn. Boston: Butterworth-Heineman, 2000; 387–419.

45. Levine SP. The role of air monitoring techniques in hazardous waste site personnel protection and surveillance strategies. In: Gochfeld M, Favata EA, eds. Hazardous waste workers. Philadelphia, Hanley & Belfus, 1990;109–16.

46. Levine SP. Air monitoring. In: Martin WF, Gochfeld M, eds. Protecting personnel at hazardous waste sites, 2nd edn. Boston: Butterworth-Heineman, 1994.

47. Bishop E. Air monitoring at hazardous waste sites. In: Martin WF, Gochfeld M, eds. Protecting personnel at hazardous waste sites, 3rd edn. Boston: Butterworth-Heineman, 2000; 137–81.

48. Takaro TK, Ertell K, Salazar MK, et al. Barriers and solutions in implementing occupational health and safety services at a large nuclear weapons facility. J Healthcare Qual 2000; 22:29–37.

49. Bingham E. Standards, regulation and public health. Med Clin North Am 1990; 74:527–36.

50. Melius JM. OSHA standard for medical surveillance of hazardous waste workers. In: Gochfeld M, Favata EA, eds. Hazardous waste workers. Philadelphia: Hanley & Belfus, 1990;143–50.

51. Melius JM. Medical surveillance for hazardous waste workers. J Occup Med 1986; 28:679–83.

52. Gochfeld M, Favata EA, eds. Hazardous waste workers. State-of-the-art reviews in occupational medicine, vol 5. Philadelphia: Hanley & Belfus, 1990.

53. Favata, E, Gochfeld, M. Medical surveillance of hazardous waste workers; ability of laboratory tests to discriminate exposure. Am J Ind Med 1988; 15:255–65.

54. Abatemarco DJ, Delnevo CD, Rosen M, Weidner BL, Gotsch AR. Medical surveillance practices of blue collar and white collar hazardous waste workers. J Occup Environ Med 1995; 37:578–82.

55. Gochfeld M. Medical surveillance and screening in the workplace: complementary preventive strategies. Environ Res 1992; 59:67–80.

56. Udasin I, Buckler G, Gochfeld M. Quality assurance audits of medical surveillance programs for hazardous waste workers. J Occup Med 1991; 33:1170–4.

57. Melius JM, Gochfeld M. Medical surveillance for hazardous waste workers. In: Martin WF, Gochfeld M, eds. Protecting personnel at hazardous waste sites, 3rd edn. Boston: Butterworth-Heineman, 2000; 207–27.

58. El-Fadel M, Zeinati M, el-Jisr K, Jamali D. Industrial-waste management in developing countries: the case of Lebanon. J Environ Manage 2001; 61:281–300.

59. World Health Organization. Methods of assessing risk to health from exposure to hazards released from waste landfills. Report from a WHO meeting, Lodz, Poland, 10–12 April 2000. Bilthoven, Netherlands: WHO Regional Office for Europe, European Centre for Environment and Health, 2001.

60. Asante-Duah K, Nagy IV. A paradigm of international environmental law: the case for controlling the transboundary movements of hazardous wastes. Environ Manage 2001; 27:779–86.

61. Hardin G. Tragedy of the commons. Science 1968; 162:1253–48.
62. Gochfeld M. Assessment of clinical toxicity in populations exposed to hazardous wastes. Proceedings of the international congress on industrial hazardous waste. Newark, New Jersey: Institute of Technology, 1982;352–65.
63. Higgins T. Hazardous waste minimization handbook. Chelsea: Lewis, 1989.
64. McDiarmid MA, Strickland PT. DNA adducts as markers of exposure in hazardous waste workers. In: Gochfeld M, Favata EA, eds. Hazardous waste workers. Philadelphia: Hanley & Belfus, 1990;49–58.
65. Gochfeld M. An exposure matrix for human exposure to environmental pollutants. Piscataway, New Jersey: Environmental and Occupational Health Sciences Institute, 1991.

52.2 Community Hazardous Waste Exposures

Michael Gochfeld

Many of the facts and principles regarding hazardous waste reviewed in Chapter 52.1 apply to community exposures as well. The impetus for the Resource Conservation and Recovery Act 1976 (RCRA) and the Comprehensive Environmental Response, Compensation and Liability Act 1980 (CERCLA), the statutes that govern hazardous waste management, was protection of public health by preventing community exposure. Residential and community exposure can occur from a variety of sources, including proximity to operating or abandoned industrial sites or landfills, from air-borne or water-borne contamination, from leaking pipelines or underground storage tanks, from transportation accidents, as well as uncontrolled releases such as fires and explosions. Several exposures, such as to medical and composted waste discussed in the previous chapter, can also affect community residents. Evaluating long-term, low-level exposures, including complex mixtures, poses a challenge to physicians practicing environmental medicine.[1]

HAZARDOUS WASTE VS HAZARDOUS MATERIALS EVENTS AND RELEASES

This chapter focuses on community exposure to hazardous waste. Communities can also be exposed to hazardous chemical and radioactive substances through uncontroled industrial releases, transportation spills, fires, and explosions. For the most part these events are beyond the scope of this chapter. In the state of Washington alone, between 1993 and 1995, an estimated 1269 such events were recorded, of which 294 involved human victims.[2] Title III of the Superfund Amendments and Reauthorization Act of 1986 (SARA Title III) established a new approach to managing chemical hazards, requiring industries to report the identity and amount of hazardous chemicals. SARA Title III also established local governmental boards to receive such data and evaluate hazards to the community, developing local emergency response plans where needed. However, implementation has been variable and often incomplete, in terms of both obtaining and processing data.[3]

EXPOSURE PATHWAYS

While the proximity to hazardous substances in waste sites is certainly a potential risk to health, there are two critical intervening factors: exposure pathway and biologically available dose. In order for people to become ill there must be a completed pathway of exposure involving contamination of air, water, food, soil, or dust, and entry into the body through inhalation, ingestion, or dermal routes. Proximity to a site is a major, though not essential aspect of this pathway. In general, air-borne contaminant concentration declines as the inverse square of distances from the source, although stack height, wind direction and velocity, physiognomic features (terrain, buildings), and physical properties of the contaminant (e.g., density compared to air) greatly influence this pathway. Ground water contamination can operate over relatively long distances when an entire aquifer is contaminated. About a third of the sites on the National Priorities List have documented complete pathways of exposure.[4]

The Agency for Toxic Substances and Disease Registry (ATSDR), a branch of the CDC, has the responsibility for evaluating health risks to communities with actual or potential exposure to hazardous wastes. This agency can perform public health assessments (Table 52.2.1), a primary purpose of which is to characterize pathways from contaminated environmental medium to human receptors. Community studies by ATSDR focus attention initially on the existence of a completed exposure pathway, from source, to environmental medium, to absorption route, to target organ. When such a pathway is documented, it is important to estimate the dose that can be transmitted, and how such a dose compares with known dose–response data for that substance. Seldom is there complete information on all components, and many uncertainties exist in estimating risk.

Marshall and colleagues[5] considered four pathways of exposure: air vapor, air particulates, ground water ingestion, and ground water inhalation (e.g., soil ingestion by toddlers). In studies of community exposure to industrial or hazardous waste sites, arbitrary cutoff distances have been used to distinguish an exposed from a non-exposed population. Areas were classified within one mile of each site according to (1) the probability of exposure to solvents, metals, and pesticides, and, if available, (2) the relative concentration of contaminants. The probability of exposure (low, medium, or high) for air vapor and particulates depends on the evaporation and soil retention potential of the contaminants, degree of containment, predominant wind direction, size of the contaminated area and amount of contaminant at the source, as well as any remediation or interventions. The probability of exposure for ground water ingestion and inhalation depends on whether there are water supply wells or affected basements within one mile, solubility of the contaminants, direction of ground water flow, and ground water sampling results. Relative concentration is based on sampling results for the appropriate environmental media.

EVALUATING COMMUNITY EXPOSURE TO HAZARDOUS WASTES

Inadequacy of exposure data (mainly retrospective) often represents a challenge in assessing the public health significance of hazardous waste. Such data are essential (1) to support epidemiologic studies of workplace and community exposure, (2) to conduct risk assessments, (3) to determine the utility of medical monitoring,[6] (4) to guide

Table 52.2.1. Outline of an ATSDR public health assessment

remediation and risk management activity,[7] and (5) to support litigation, remedial investigations, and cleanup. Many studies rely on proximity or distance to a source, but in order to make this a meaningful surrogate for exposure, the spatial resolution must be improved, requiring smaller areas with better characterized sampling strategies.[8]

Although many hazardous waste sites are former industrial properties, or landfills, and may be in rural areas away from densely populated areas, there are many sites that have residences within close proximity. In many cases, residential housing has been built on former industrial facilities, abandoned waste sites, or former manufactured gas plants, and many other sites have residential properties immediately abutting the property line. In some cases direct soil contamination of backyards has occurred due to runoff from the industrial sites, while in other cases concern may arise in a community downwind from a site. Other communities have had private or municipal wells contaminated by industrial waste.

The basic principles of exposure apply to community residents as well as to workers. Materials can move off-site through air, soil, water, and the food chain. People can be exposed through inhalation (air, dust), through dermal contact (soil, water), and through ingestion (soil, water, food). The picture is complicated frequently when communities have used abandoned waste sites for recreation.

Environmental media of concern and routes of exposure

Table 52.2.2 is an exposure matrix illustrating how material can move from the environment into the body. Air, soil, water, and food are the primary environmental media that can be contaminated. In addition to toxic vapors, airborne dusts or smoke from waste incinerators carry toxic particulate matter. Surface runoff or leachate through the soils may lead to contamination of surface or ground waters. In many cases, people actually enter the sites, experiencing direct contact with contaminated soil. This is particularly true in the case of children, who may ingest soil from their fingers after play. The problem is compounded by recreational use of abandoned sites. For example, dirt-bikes generate dust that can be inhaled or ingested. Once the soil and water are contaminated, there is opportunity for certain chemicals to be taken up by plants or plankton and thereby enter the food chain, with exposure to humans who may consume contaminated fish or wildlife.

The matrix (Table 52.2.2) has proven useful for demonstrating these relationships to policy makers and the public. It identifies the components that must be included in a risk assessment and those that are subject to remediation. For example, 'fallout' or air-borne deposition on the skin may not be important at a hazardous waste site, but may be significant in evaluating a proposed incinerator. Secondary interactions can also be incorporated in the matrix (e.g., air-borne deposition on edible portions of plants). The routes of exposure include ingestion, inhalation, and dermal absorption (injection is rarely applicable). In general, air-borne materials are inhaled, while contaminated water and food are typically ingested. Contaminants may become bioavailable through a combination of these routes.

Site	Air	Soil	Water	Food
Skin	Fallout and airborne deposition +	Direct contact + +	Direct contact + +	0
Lungs	Vapors and respirable particles + + + +	Airborne dust + +	Aerosols +	0
GI tract	Negligible swallowing of air +	Ingestion + +	Ingestion + + + +	Air deposition on leaves, soil on roots, toxic substances in leaves and fruits.* Superficial and systemic food chain biologic amplification + + + +

* Plants can be contaminated by airborne deposition on edible portions or by systemic uptake of material from soil or water.
From Gochfeld M. *An exposure matrix for human exposure to environmental pollutants.* Piscataway, NJ: Environmental and Occupational Health Sciences Institute, 1991.

Table 52.2.2 Exposure matrix for human exposure to environmental pollutants (Strength of pathway: + = Weak; ++ = moderate; ++++ = prominent)

Soil contamination with hazardous materials is widespread. Some contaminants are taken up from soil by garden plants. The contaminants in soil may leach into ground water, contaminating drinking water supplies. However, the main pathway of concern is the direct ingestion of soil by toddlers. The bioavailability of contaminants in soil is highly variable. They may be bound tightly to organic compounds, may exist in insoluble forms, or may be freely accessible when ingested. Various approaches have been used to estimate bioavailability, including the use of simulated gastric juice to extract lead and chromium compounds from soil. The bioavailability varied for lead from 39% to 70%, 41–66% for arsenic, and 34% for chromium.[9]

Community vs individual exposure

Most exposure investigations consider the community as a whole, particularly where air or ground water contamination is involved. This is sufficient to determine whether remediation is required or whether medical monitoring will be beneficial. It may also be the basis for litigation. However, for epidemiologic studies or where single households are affected, it may be important to determine exposure for individual families or even specific family members. This will also be essential in the screening phase of a medical monitoring program (see below).

Ongoing vs historic exposure

If exposure is ongoing or current, it is relatively easy to sample the relevant environmental media (e.g., drinking water, or indoor air in basement, showers, and bedrooms), ascertain behavioral patterns for family members, conduct 'market basket' analyses of food, and measure biomarkers of exposure in individuals. It is useful to narrow the assessment to one or a few agents that are suspected to have reached a family. Whereas the initial investigation (see Chapter 52.1) may seek to identify dozens of compounds, usually only about ten are found to be present in large quantities in a waste site; often only one or two of these are suspected of being significant for a household. For example, with leaking underground storage tanks from an adjacent gas station, the exposure evaluation may focus on petroleum hydrocarbons and benzene. Proximity to a chromium dump will focus attention on trivalent and hexavalent chromium.

It is often the case that exposure to hazardous materials ceased years previously and exposure can only be inferred by historical analytic data (air, soil, ground water), and by reconstruction of places and years of residences. In a New Jersey community where municipal wells were contaminated by a chemical company, several communities drank contaminated water for 10–20 years, but their exposure ceased in 1985. Medical monitoring, however, did not begin until 2002, by which time only residential information could be used to stratify the group by historical exposure probabilities.

Behavioral aspects

Often overlooked is the importance of individual behavior in determining or modifying exposure. The number of hours an individual spends at home, the amount of tap water consumed, the apportionment of time between different rooms, the amount of time and frequency of showering, the reliance on homegrown foods compared with commercial foods, the amount of fish consumed, are important variables. For children, especially toddlers, the amount of time spent at home compared with school, indoors compared with outdoors, crawling on floors and engaging in hand-to-mouth behavior are extremely important. Where soil is contaminated, the cover of playing areas (bare soil vs grass or pavement) and the activities on the soil are important.

Biomarkers

Some hazardous wastes such as heavy metals or polychlorinated organics persist in the body for long periods of time, stored in organs or fat, with slow excretion. These can be measured relatively non-invasively in blood or urine, and less effectively in the case of metals with hair and nails. Some exposures may be detected months or even years after exposure has ceased. Many small organic compounds, however, are quickly metabolized, and they or their contaminants can only be measured in the body if exposure is ongoing or relatively recent (days or weeks).

HIERARCHY OF EXPOSURE DATA AND SURROGATES

The National Research Council[10] identified a variety of exposure metrics and ranked them from best to poorest. This hierarchy of exposure-related data is presented in Table 52.2.3.

Quantified personal measurements
Quantified area or ambient measurements in the vicinity of residence or other sites of activity
Quantified surrogates of exposure (e.g., estimates of drinking water use)
Distance from site and duration of residence
Distance from site or duration of residence
Residence or employment in reasonable proximity to site where exposure can be assumed
Residence or employment in defined geographic area (e.g., county) of the site

Table 52.2.3 Exposure metrics as ranked by the National Research Council from best (top) to poorest (bottom)

Quantified personal measurements are virtually never available, even with recent or current exposures. Area measurements may have been obtained as part of surveys or compliance investigations. Surrogates of exposure such as distance and/or duration of residence are frequently used. The last measure, namely co-occurrence of site and receptor in the same geographic area, is also frequently used and is usually referred to as 'an ecologic study'. The NRC list is consistent with use of biomarkers as a quantified personal measurement. Kharrazi et al[11] successfully used odor complaints as a marker of exposure.

There have been several epidemiologic studies based on approximate distance between residence and source. Different authors used different distance criteria, based either on data constraints or on a priori judgments about significant distances. In an Australian study, distances of 300 m and 1000 m were used.[12] A 1994 study by Sosniak and colleagues[13] used one mile, measuring distance from the center of the zip code region to the center of the nearest site; such an approach may result in substantial misclassification of distance, requiring large numbers to assess an effect (see below). A very large study comparing adverse birth outcomes among populations within 2 km of British landfills, compared with reference populations showed very small, but statistically significant increases of all congenital anomalies, neural tube defects, hypospadias/epispadias, and low birthweight. The relative risks were all less than 1.1 except for gastroschisis (1.19). Conversely, heart defects were slightly but significantly lower among the exposed. No mechanism was identified to account for these findings.[14]

Many authors have concluded that enhanced availability and use of biomarkers to document exposure will advance environmental epidemiology. One common way to sample various biomarkers is through blood tests for a pollutant or its metabolites. However, exposure levels and the timing of exposure may not produce detectable signals of any biomarker in blood. ATSDR studied various analytes in blood in people living near to and far from an industrial complex, and found little difference in commonly encountered industrial volatile chemicals. The authors concluded that blood volatile organic compound (VOC) 'testing should be limited to populations living near sites where environmental testing has shown recent, elevated VOC exposure, or where unusual circumstances of illness may be attributed to VOC exposure'.[15]

HEALTH SURVEYS

When a community learns about a significant exposure to hazardous wastes, it is likely to request a health survey. In contrast, public health agencies may voice reluctance about such surveys, and are often not able to conduct a formal epidemiologic study. Such studies could include surveys and questionnaires, but might also include studies of birth or death certificates, data from birth defects or cancer registries, emergency room visits or hospitalizations, or comparisons of disease incidence or mortality in the affected community with that for a comparable community or the state. Unfortunately, in the absence of more detailed exposure data, one can rarely determine the exposure status of the individuals who become ill, and such studies are very likely to be inconclusive.

The importance of accurately determining exposure is that it will reduce the likelihood of misclassification errors (see Chapter 6). If an exposed person has a health problem, but is erroneously misclassified as an unexposed referent, or if a referent with no health problem is erroneously classified as exposed, the likelihood of detecting a difference in health status is compromised. Thus misclassification errors bias a study towards the null, reducing the likelihood of identifying an effect, even when an effect exists.

The ATSDR is charged to develop large-scale community health surveys. Surveys may involve little more than questionnaires or may involve extensive medical examinations and testing. In some cases, laboratory testing may be done as an exposure screening tool, as in urine testing for chromium, or breast milk screening for organochlorine compounds.

Health surveys may be aimed at estimating exposure, or may actually focus on the prevalence of particular disease endpoints. Careful attention must be given to designing such studies, particularly to the manner in which either negative or positive outcomes will be explained to the community, to government, and to responsible parties. Inadequately planned surveys may fail to uncover significant exposure, may provide spurious results that later undermine the community's efforts, and may discourage community and public health officials alike. However, since in many cases future exposure is terminated, a health survey, if it is to be conducted, should be undertaken in a timely manner, before evidence of exposure becomes diminished or lost.

One of the major difficulties with such health surveys and epidemiologic studies is the potential for bias and the difficulty of obtaining appropriate reference groups. By the time the study gets initiated, community members frequently have concerns regarding adverse health effects. Participants in health studies may be self-selected, introducing sources of bias and complicating interpretation of findings. However, it is essential to remember that the potential for selection bias does not mean that people have not been exposed or affected.

Self-reported exposures

Epidemiologists are divided over whether self-reported exposure can be relied on for hazardous waste studies. Dunne et al[12] found that people who believed that they had been exposed showed more symptoms than those who believed they had not. They attributed the difference to the effect of belief as advanced by Roht et al.[16] Ozonoff et al[17] likewise found an association between belief and self-reported findings. Since many aspects of exposure, visual and olfactory, are readily detectable by the exposed persons, it is likely that those who believed they were exposed actually had higher exposure than those who did not believe they had exposure. Indeed, Kharrazi et al[11] found that lower birth weights were associated with higher levels of odor reports.

Pets as sentinels

In some cases a sickness or death of a pet that has recently swallowed or drank from a mud puddle has called attention to local soil contamination. A study of pet dogs living near Superfund sites showed a higher frequency of micronuclei than in control dogs, suggesting actual exposure.[18] The rate of sinonasal cancer in pet dogs was more highly correlated with exposure to carcinogens in indoor air rather than outdoor pollution.[19]

NATIONAL EXPOSURE REGISTRY

ATSDR has established a National Exposure Registry (NER) as mandated by Superfund legislation. The purpose of the Registry is to assess and evaluate the potential relationship between adverse health effects and exposure to hazardous wastes, particularly the relationship between chronic health effects and long-term, low-level chemical exposures. The NER's trichloroethylene (TCE) subregistry has been used to demonstrate increased rates of hearing impairment and other conditions associated with historical exposure to TCE,[20] and offers one approach to identifying exposed individuals.

EPIDEMIOLOGIC STUDIES OF COMMUNITIES

There have been many attempts to identify or estimate the health impacts of community exposure to hazardous wastes, often by studying people in proximity to hazardous waste sites. Like many aspects of environmental epidemiology, the health risks of hazardous waste are often subtle and invariably complex. For some cancers there is a long latency between exposure and outcome. Even with events such as the Minamata disease outbreak (methylmercury poisoning in Minamata, Japan), where the health impacts were widespread and catastrophic, years elapsed before the causal agent was identified. Occupational health consequences lend themselves more readily to epidemiology, because populations are more circumscribed and exposures more quantifiable. However, the industrial hygiene literature indicates that substantial, and at times monumental, efforts of historic dose reconstruction may be required.

There are classic studies of communities exposed to hazardous waste; these include reproductive and developmental effects near the Love Canal (Niagara Falls, New York[21]) and leukemia (Woburn, Massachusetts[22]).

The importance of exposure estimates, misclassification bias, and power

Investigations of community exposure present problems of defining populations at risk, establishing reasonable refer-

ence populations, documenting pathways, and estimating concentrations and dose. The increasing mobility of society complicates the task of identifying populations at risk. The identification of suitable biomarkers of exposure and effect has greatly facilitated epidemiologic studies; improved exposure monitoring, spatial mapping, and statistical methods are also valuable. Nonetheless, many studies may yield wide confidence intervals due to small sample sizes; elevated risk ratios for disease may thus be difficult to interpret.

Although epidemiologic studies are often population based, the units of measurements are typically based on individuals and their disease outcomes. Thus it is necessary to have individualized exposure estimates that, as indicated above, may be challenging to ascertain. Most epidemiologic studies rely on surrogates of exposure or membership in a class. The inherent danger of such reliance is misclassification bias. If individuals with low or negligible exposure are included among those with high exposure (i.e., misclassification), the possibility of detecting an exposure is compromised. Once the potentially exposed population has been identified, usually based on some a priori distance assumption, a reference population is chosen. Sometimes the reference population is contiguous to the exposed one, and sometimes at a greater distance, including use of national reference populations. However, members of the reference population may also have been exposed to the same or similar hazards.

Within the exposed population, some individuals are more highly exposed than others, and these are presumably the ones likely to manifest the adverse health effect. However, by pooling these people with less exposed individuals, there is dilution of the effect being sought. This *invariably* reduces the power of any study to detect an adverse health effect. Yet, if a study attempts to stratify by exposure, the result may yield few people in an arbitrary 'high exposure' category, reducing power to detect effects.

Statistical power and hypothesis testing

The tradition of hypothesis testing and statistical significance arose in other disciplines and has been transferred directly to epidemiology, usually without critical consideration of its limitations (see Chapter 6). While setting an α (or 'P-value') of 0.05 may make sense in the context of many scientific investigations, it may be an unrealistic criterion for community-based epidemilogic studies, particularly since people do not need to be 95% confident when making health decisions or avoiding exposures. Studies of community exposure are limited by the size of the community, often in the hundreds, so that most studies begin with low power and can only detect as 'significant' a dramatic increase in the rate of disease.

Reference populations and confounders

Defining an appropriate reference population is a challenging aspect of designing studies in environmental settings. The reference population should be similar to the exposed population with regard to age, gender, ethnic, socioeconomic, and occupational characteristics, all of which are important risk factors for disease in general. Occupational exposures to hazardous materials would be especially confounding in a community study of the same hazards. Such matching represents a challenge that may not be achievable. Neighborhoods are often subtly structured, particularly with regard to socioeconomic factors. Even in a highly mobile society, people living close to an industrial facility are more likely to be employed there than those further away. People living close to a hazardous site are also more likely to be poor than those living further away, even within the same town.

Published studies appropriately identify the possibility of confounding. However, just because confounding may exist does not mean that it explains the findings. If a study has been undertaken to detect adverse health effects associated with a hazard, and observes a statistically significant positive association, it is important to strongly consider that that association is likely, even when the possibility of confounding is real. Only if the confounder can be shown to be a more likely cause of the outcome than the exposure should confounding be adduced as the primary explanation, and even then the exposure should not be disregarded. Interactions between confounders and the exposure (e.g., smoking and asbestos) may also represent an important causal factor.

Small area statistics

There are many challenges in performing environmental epidemiologic studies to evaluate exposure, risks, and health effects attributable to hazardous waste. These have been identified by many authors.[23] Small area statistics are a widespread problem in trying to study a single workplace or community. Characterizing populations living in proximity to (and at varying distances from) hazardous waste sites requires special statistical techniques. A general weakness is the lack of direct exposure measurement. An increased prevalence of self-reported health symptoms such as fatigue, sleepiness, and headaches among residents near waste sites has been reported in numerous studies. It is difficult to conclude whether these symptoms are an effect of direct toxicologic action of chemicals present in waste sites, an effect of stress and fears related to the waste site, or an effect of selection, recall, or reporting bias.

Although a substantial number of studies have been conducted, risks to health from landfill sites are challenging to quantify. There is often insufficient exposure information, and effects of low-level environmental exposure in the general population are by their nature difficult to establish. More interdisciplinary research can improve understanding of risks to human health related to hazardous waste disposal sites. As Vrijheid and colleagues emphasize, research needs to include 'epidemiologic and toxicologic studies on individual chemicals and chemical mixtures, well-designed single- and multisite landfill studies, development of biomarkers, and research on risk perception and sociologic determinants of ill health'.[23]

From cluster to waste site

Although most studies of health effects of hazardous wastes have examined populations living in proximity to known waste sites, some studies exemplify the reverse approach, beginning with an occurrence of similar disease among individuals. Best known, perhaps, is the investigation of a cluster of leukemia cases eventually attributed to drinking water contamination in Woburn, Massachusetts. A cluster of childhood brain cancer cases in Monmouth County, New Jersey, reported to the State Health Department by the local community, resulted in intensive environmental and epidemiologic study. The cluster has been linked to drinking water contamination, apparently by a novel and hitherto unrecognized contaminant from a nearby chemical plant.[24] Although controversy may continue to surround the current explanation or understanding of causation of these clusters, they remain important examples.

Detection of a cluster (an occurrence in time and space considerably above background levels) is not trivial. What seems like a cluster to a community may be coincidence when examined statistically,[25] yet actual clusters are important potential clues to environmental hazards.[26] A survey in 1990 indicated that about 1500 'clusters' are reported each year to state health departments. Some are followed up in detail, while some respondents emphasize the coincidental nature of apparent clusters.[27] Media coverage of clusters is uneven, but can both stimulate and interfere with subsequent investigations.[28] Some public health officials doggedly investigate reported clusters while others prefer to provide reassurance to the community that they are artifacts or coincidences.

Non-responders

Environmental epidemiologic studies often have a high rate of non-responders. Some of these are people who refuse to be interviewed ('refusers') while others are people who could not be contacted ('movers'). A study comparing these two types of non-responders to responders around a hazardous waste site showed no demographic difference between responders and refusers. Concern that refusers might be those who are healthy or unconcerned was refuted by the finding that refusers actually had somewhat higher levels of concern. By contrast, movers differed demographically, particularly in shorter residence and renting rather than owning,[29] that presumably allowed them to be more mobile and leave the area of hazardous exposure. People in this group, who may leave based on health-related symptoms, represent an important bias towards the null. (i.e., not detecting an effect that actually exists).

SPECIFIC HEALTH OUTCOMES

A variety of health effects are associated with hazardous material exposure. Communities are most concerned about long-term cancer risk or adverse reproductive outcomes. Some exposures may induce cytogenetic, neurobehavioral, hepatic, renal, pulmonary, endocrine, or dermal changes. In many instances however, non-specific symptoms are increased. Self-reported cases of disease, even physician-diagnosed events, are not always reliable. A cluster of 'ovarian cysts' reported in a contaminated university building included mostly cases of Bartholin cysts.[30] A study of medical records versus self-reported cancers showed a 15% over-reporting by participants living in a community with a hazardous waste processing facility.[31]

Cancer

Although cancer is one of the greatest concerns of communities near hazardous waste sites, few studies have directly investigated cancer, usually because of the long latency. The Knox study[32] did show an approximate doubling of childhood cancer risk for children living within 5 km of incinerators, with no relationship to landfills. In an Australian study, no relationship was found between exposure to mining wastes and cancer rates.[12]

Controversy has surrounded the reported cluster of childhood cancers, particularly leukemias and lymphomas, at Seascale, in the vicinity of the Sellafield nuclear reprocessing plant in the United Kingdom. However, one study found that the cancer cluster did not appear to be temporally related to the period of intense nuclear activity at Sellafield,[33] with population mixing potentially contributing to the observed lymphomas.[34]

Adverse reproductive outcomes

A variety of reproductive endpoints have been examined in populations with known or suspected hazardous waste exposure, and studies have been conducted on both local and national scales. Several occupational studies have shown that maternal exposure to certain chemicals is associated with lowered birth weight. A data linkage study between EPA's NPL and the National Maternal and Infant Health Survey found no excess of low birth weight, prematurity, infant mortality, or congenital malformations to mothers living within approximately a mile of hazardous waste sites.[13] About 80% of the British population lives within 2 km of a landfill. A study of populations around all 9565 landfills yielded 43,000 stillbirths and 124,000 congenital anomalies. There was a small excess of congenital anomalies and low (< 2500 g) or very low (< 1500 g) birthweight infants close to landfills, although no mechanism was demonstrated.[14] The confounding issue of whether populations at increased risk for low birthweight infants are more likely to reside close to landfills is an important one. Environmental justice studies (see below) indicate a higher proportion of minority and low income families living in proximity to environmental hazards.

Studies in New York[35] and California[36] also showed some excesses in specific congenital abnormalities associated with hazardous waste sites. A higher miscarriage rate was reported among people living close to old mining waste sites in Australia.[12] Thus there are some studies reporting miscarriages, low birth weight, and congenital

anomalies around hazardous waste sites. Interpretation is limited because the type of anomalies are not the same from study to study, nor are the specific exposures.

Families living near New Jersey's Lipari landfill (the highest priority on the Superfund list) had higher rates of low birthweight babies during the 1971–1975 period, than those more than 1 km from the site, and this excess was mainly due to a fivefold increase of low birthweight in homes immediately adjacent to the site.[37] This finding provided evidence that direct runoff and contamination was more likely a problem than air-borne contamination; the 1971–1975 period was temporally associated with the period of greatest runoff, and birthweights rose slowly after that time.

Elaborate study designs and detailed protocols have been developed for evaluating male and female reproductive function in exposed populations.[38,39] Depending on the magnitude of exposure, a tiered approach of (1) questionnaires, diaries, and review of parent and infant medical records; (2) cross-sectional biologic sampling for hormone levels, and (3) extensive prospective sampling linked to diaries has been proposed.[39] Five adverse outcomes, namely, structural anomalies, mutations, mortality, functional deficits, and impaired prenatal and postnatal growth, are amenable to investigation, beginning with questionnaires and medical records, and proceeding to neurodevelopmental testing and karyotyping. The highest level of investigation would include DNA adducts.[40]

Spatial mapping of birthweight data on a large sample initially posed computing challenges requiring novel approaches (e.g., Wartenberg et al[41]), which can be greatly facilitated by use of Geographic Information Systems (GIS).[42] However, selection of scale and sample size still pose problems, and despite increased availability of GIS, little progress has been made in incorporating it into environmental epidemiology.

Symptom prevalence studies

Many studies and reports indicate that people living in proximity to hazardous waste sites or other Locally Unwanted Land Uses (LULUs) have more symptoms than reference populations. Since such symptoms can be generated by events surrounding the site, by media coverage, lawsuits, controversies, and stress, symptom prevalence studies are potentially subject to bias and/or confounding. Lipscomb et al[43] attempted to provide a general estimate of background symptom prevalence in communities that could serve as an additional reference rate for future studies. A study of two Louisiana communities identified both hypochondriasis and respondent opinions as important contributors to reported symptoms.[16] Not surprisingly, they note that respondents who held a negative opinion of the site were two to three times more likely to identify symptoms. However, the converse interpretation – people with symptoms are more likely to form negative opinions – must also be taken seriously.

Based on a study of communities around five California waste sites, Neutra et al[44] concluded that neither classic exposure pathways and toxicology nor mass psychogenic illness accounted for increased symptom reporting. They suggested that 'environmental anxiety' be taken seriously as a stressor producing physiologic changes manifest as symptoms. Studies usually seek to compare rates in the target (putatively exposed population) with rates in some unexposed reference population. Rarely is it documented that the reference population is free of some other exposure sources.

A study of the BKK landfill (Los Angeles, CA) showed that the frequency of odor complaints statistically predicted lower birth weight.[11] Those reporting high odors had babies about two days earlier and 59 grams lighter than the reference population. The study cannot distinguish whether this observed effect is because odor produced anxiety and stress, or because odor was a good surrogate for exposure.

Mine, mill, and smelter waste

Children exposed to lead mining waste exhibited elevated blood levels, while rates of miscarriages were also higher near mine waste sites.[12]

ENVIRONMENTAL RISK ASSESSMENT

Public health assessments are often only qualitative in nature. When it comes to prioritizing risks or comparing hazards, more quantitative approaches such as 'risk assessment' have become popular. Although engineers have long been familiar with risk assessment in the design of structures, the concept was adopted in environmental health in the mid-20th century, and became prominent in the 1980s. The importance of improved information on hazardous waste sites was highlighted by the National Research Council, which recommended improvements in the system for setting remediation priorities – reducing expenditures on sites which posed minimal hazards and improving the identification and cleanup of highly hazardous sites.[10] The study noted the lack of toxicologic data on many hazardous waste components and the need to clarify the significance of long-term low-level exposures.

The risk assessment paradigm

The original approach to risk assessment included four phases that have been given various names.

Hazard identification involves identifying the specific hazard and its biologic effects. For a hazardous waste site this may involve characterizing the waste and identifying dozens of chemicals that may potentially contaminate surrounding communities. For each of these compounds, one or more endpoints are selected based on significance. At hazardous waste sites this is accomplished during the initial site discovery and the remedial investigation.

Dose–response assessment requires a review of the epidemiologic and toxicologic data base concerning the identified

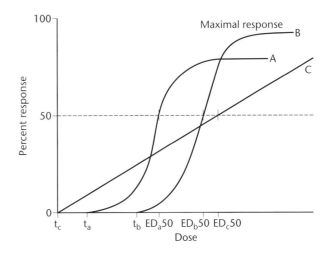

Figure 52.2.1: A typical dose–response curve showing the sigmoid curve typical (or assumed typical) of two toxic chemicals A and B with different toxicities. The linear no-threshold curve, which represents the dose–response relationship for a carcinogen, is represented by Line C.

hazards in order to determine at what levels exposed populations may experience adverse health outcomes. A typical dose response curve is 'S-shaped' with a flat subthreshold component, a steep effect component, and a plateau where maximum response is reached (Fig. 52.2.1). For cancer, however, a linear 'no threshold' dose–response curve is usually assumed (e.g., line C).

Exposure assessment involves a determination of how much, how long, and by what routes individuals may be exposed. Each potential exposure pathway must be examined and the quantities of material measured or estimated.

Risk characterization is the process of combining the above information to determine a 'safe' or 'de minimus' exposure level, above which an unacceptable public health risk may exist, and below which continued exposure is believed to have no significant health consequences. Various mathematical models have been employed to extrapolate downward from the high doses used in toxicologic experiments or encountered in occupational epidemiologic studies, to the much lower doses anticipated in residential or community exposure scenarios.

Over the past 20 years there has been an evolution in risk assessment. In the early 1980s the main debate was over which mathematical model was most appropriate for the various biologic processes involved in carcinogenesis. In the late 1980s it became apparent that exposure assessment data were notoriously lacking, and this scientific discipline enjoyed a renaissance. In the 1990s the toxicologic basis of risk assessment came under scrutiny, as analysis of epidemiologic data was refined. Subsequent attention focused on the 'uncertainty' in risk assessment. The mathematical results given to several decimal places and compared to a 'one in a million' (10^6) risk level convey an impression of mathematical precision which may not be justified by the data and assumptions employed. Often, errors in the dose–response analysis may be multiplied by errors in the exposure analysis, such that the resulting risk estimate may differ from the unknown reality by orders of magnitude. Default assumptions used in risk assessment have also come under scrutiny. Attempts to individualize exposure and risk are being investigated.

Risk assessment has engendered substantial controversy regarding all of these phases, particularly since the outcome of a single risk assessment may impose major cost burdens on polluters; conversely a low risk estimate may allow a community to be exposed to hazards that the residents find unacceptable. Risk assessment has become a common method for prioritizing hazardous waste exposure problems, and determining levels of exposure where intervention is necessary.[45] Given the uncertainties inherent in risk assessment, coupled with broad assumptions and sometimes conflicting data, the process is certainly vulnerable to controversy.

Risk assessment is currently used to determine whether a population exposed or potentially exposed to a hazard has sufficient risk of adverse outcomes to require intervention. Risk assessment provides information that risk managers can use to prioritize interventions. Originally it was considered critical that the estimations of risk be independent of the influence of cost or political considerations, which enter the risk management decision process. However, more recent approaches integrate the scientific/toxicologic risk assessment into a broader context that includes input from a large variety of stakeholders.[46]

Exposure scenarios for risk assessment

If a risk assessment is to be performed, one must develop a series of scenarios regarding potential exposure. These are sometimes labeled 'realistic' or 'worst-case' scenarios. One can consider this a sensitivity analysis; if the worst case scenario estimates a lifetime risk that is acceptable, then it is likely that few, if any, individuals in the community will have an unacceptable risk. Problems arise when the realistic scenario produces acceptable risk, but the worst case produces unacceptable risks. Controversy arises when a risk acceptable to the government may not be acceptable to the community or individuals. Regulatory agencies may use risk assessment to refuse or justify permits, or determine whether a cleanup is required. Since the decision over what scenarios to use is a policy decision rather than a scientific decision, and since scientists argue vehemently on both sides of the issue, the role of science in influencing policy is often clouded. Clinicians should be aware of these considerations when discussing policies and risks with patients, regardless of whether they are providing warnings or reassurance.

Some of the assumptions that are made in evaluating potential risk to a community are indicated below with some extreme examples.

House occupancy component:
- A newborn baby who will live in a house for 70 years, sitting on the front porch without ever leaving.
- A 5-year-old who will live in a house 16 hours a day until age 17, then leave and never return.

- An adult who will live in a house 16 hours a day, for 45 years.

Dietary component:
- People will obtain 100% of their food from locally caught fish or locally grown milk, meat, and produce.
- A realistic estimate of the contribution of locally grown produce and fish to overall diet is about 10%.

Childhood soil ingestion:
- An average child consumes about 50–100 mg of soil per day (for 4–6 months/year).
- In the South, where children might play outdoors all year, a malnourished child with pica might consume 1000 mg soil/day for 12 months/year.

Vulnerability of the population:
- A maximally exposed individual (MEI) is one who spends all their life at the point of maximum impact of air-borne and water-borne contamination, eating contaminated food. Specially susceptible groups include small children, the elderly, and the infirm.

Stealth farmer scenario:
- In planning for the indefinite storage of radioactive wastes on sites which are fenced, assume that a family climbs the fence and lives on top of the waste storage site, drinking well water, and growing crops and livestock in contaminated soil.

As described above, the role of risk assessment is currently debated, but the EPA at present accepts the formalized process of risk assessment as a basis for setting policy and making site-specific decisions. Environmental risk assessments are not designed to be predictive for individuals, but are intended to protect virtually all individuals. Risk assessments are limited by considering mainly cancer as an endpoint; by ignoring ecologic, aesthetic, and convenience values; and by making major, sometimes untestable, assumptions.

The Presidential/Congressional Commission on Risk Assessment and Risk Management

Throughout the 1990s, there was an increasing involvement of stakeholders in the risk assessment process. In addition to people who are exposed to hazardous waste, the term 'stakeholder' also refers to the generators, regulators, and local governments. Rather than endorsing the rigid separation of risk assessment and risk management, the Commission set risk assessment in a much larger risk management context, with stakeholder involvement at the center (Fig. 52.2.2). Stakeholders are to be involved in the decision of whether, when, and how to conduct a risk assessment, including what factors to consider and what assumptions to use. They are involved in discussions of how to interpret risk estimates, which remediation options (including the null option) to choose, and in the evaluation

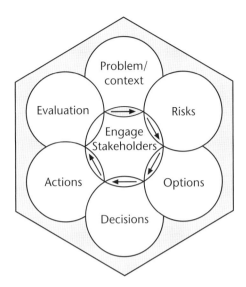

Figure 52.2.2: The model of a comprehensive risk management process as developed by the Presidential/Congressional Committee on Risk Assessment and Risk Management.

of interventions (i.e., whether risk has been reduced to an acceptable level).

Cancer risk assessment

Most of the attention in risk assessment has focused on carcinogens. The EPA has developed cancer slope factors that provide an estimate of the number of increased cancer cases per unit increase in lifetime dose. After selecting appropriate toxicologic studies, the linearized multistage model is applied to back extrapolate from the observed data to the dose that would correspond to one excess cancer death per million people exposed. To add an additional conservative step, the slope factor is designated as the 95th percent confidence limit around the point estimate of that dose. This represents a conservative estimate, not generally subject to verification epidemiologically. Since the average rate of cancer mortality is about 20% or 200,000 per million people, the one in a million excess corresponds to 200,001 cancer deaths per million (or one person dying of cancer who would otherwise have died of some other cause). Since even 10% increases in incidence are hard to detect in epidemiologic studies, the 1 in a million or ('10^6') excess mortality is only a theoretical construct.

Armed with the EPA slope factor, a risk assessor needs to estimate the lifetime exposure for the population and apply the slope factor to estimate the excess cancer mortality. Although the 10^6 'one in a million' risk is considered the de minimus risk, many decisions are made using the less protective 10^5 level; for occupational exposures the 10^4 level is frequently used. Estimates of the lung cancer risk for radon conclude that the 4 pCi/l remediation standard corresponds to an excess cancer mortality risk that may exceed 10^3. This would be unacceptably high if it were not for the fact that the radon occurs naturally and cannot be eliminated, although exposure can be interdicted.

Non-cancer risk assessment

In contrast to cancer endpoints, a threshold for risk is assumed for non-cancer endpoints. Using risk assessment approaches, the EPA sets reference doses (RfDs) for inhalation or ingestion, by selecting appropriate studies and identifying a no observed adverse effect level (NOAEL). Unfortunately, this level depends on the doses that were originally chosen for studies, most of which aimed at identifying the 50% effect (or 'ED-50') level rather than the NOAEL. In many studies, the only dose with no effect is the control or zero dose. In that case, the lowest observed adverse effect level (LOAEL) is selected. Since the threshold must be somewhere below the LOAEL, it is usually assumed to be one-tenth of the LOAEL, consistent with a safety or uncertainty factor (UF) of 10. If the base study is in animals, a tenfold UF is used to account for interspecies extrapolation. This is not always appropriate, since in some cases humans turn out to be less sensitive than the experimental animal.

Since risk assessment is concerned with lifetime risk, it is desirable to base the RfD on an animal study with lifetime exposure. In some cases, only shorter term studies are available, in which case another tenfold UF is incorporated to extrapolate from short-term to lifetime dose. This extrapolation accounts for accumulation in the body, and a longer opportunity for the endpoint to occur.

Whereas experimental animals are inbred to reduce individual variability, humans vary considerably, both genetically and in health status. Therefore a tenfold factor is introduced to protect the most sensitive individuals of a population. In some cases a threefold factor is used, but often even a tenfold factor may be inadequate to protect outliers.

Additional uncertainty factors may be used to account for multigenerational effects or for inadequacies in the underlying studies. The reference dose (RfD) is then calculated as follows:

$$RfD = NOAEL/(UF1 \times UF2 \times UF3)$$

or if there is no NOAEL:

$$RfD = LOAEL/(UF1 \times UF2 \times UF3 \times UF4)$$

The RfD is typically reported as micrograms (µg) intake per kg body weight per day. The exposure assessment then calculates the actual intake for an individual (usually averaged over a long period) and compares this to the RfD to achieve a hazard quotient (HQ).

$$HQ = daily\ intake/RfD.$$

An HQ less than 1 is considered acceptable, since the RfD itself has built in uncertainty factors. Where there are mixed exposures and several components can be analyzed at once, the HQ is calculated for each substance individually, and the HQs are summed to give an overall hazard index (HI). If the HI exceeds one, the exposure is considered unacceptable. This can be used as a basis for eliminating the hazard through cleanup, changing the water supply, or evacuation to a safer location.

Susceptibility

A major advancement in the 1990s was been the recognition of the importance of variation in susceptibility of human populations to various hazards. Whereas laboratory animals are inbred to reduce genetic variation and variance in response to an exposure, human populations have no such constraint. There is, however, no general rule to determine by what factor the most susceptible individuals differ from the population mean. Generally a tenfold correction factor is assumed to cover this difference. Much of the variation is presumed to have a genetic basis; in the 1990s there was a focus on genetic polymorphisms, particularly in metabolic enzymes such as the P450 group. A particular genotype may result in the underactivity or absence of an enzyme that normally speeds up the metabolism of a toxic compound, thereby increasing susceptibility. Conversely, if that enzymic conversion changes a parent compound into a more toxic metabolite, absence of the enzyme may favor direct excretion or an alternative pathway that reduces cancer risk.

This focus on genetic polymorphism research has been very fruitful; however, it is likely that many of the variations in susceptibility are polygenetic, involving the interaction of numerous gene loci. Moreover, genetic variation may interact with diet or other health conditions to modify the body's response to a particular toxicant.[47] Understanding the complexity of susceptibility is still in its infancy.

Precautionary principle

School children learn that in our legal system a suspect is considered innocent of a crime until proven guilty by a jury of peers. Unfortunately, in many countries chemicals are also considered 'innocent' of hazard until 'proven' hazardous, and skeptics set a very high barrier for proving hazard. An opposing view, now articulated as the Precautionary Principle, has been stated in various ways and contexts. Fundamentally, it recognizes that where there are threats of serious or irreversible damage, lack of full scientific certainty shall not be used as a reason for postponing measures to prevent environmental degradation. In other words, public health officials must not wait for every last bit of evidence before taking steps to reduce population exposure to potentially hazardous materials or situations. Even skeptics recognize the value of this principle, while arguing that it should be applied selectively.

The Precautionary Principle seems particularly applicable to hazardous waste, because of the difficulties in performing epidemiologic studies and conflicting published results. The National Research Council's Committee on Environmental Epidemiology concluded:

'Whether Superfund and other hazardous-waste programs actually protect human health is a critical question with respect to federal and state efforts to clean up hazardous wastes. To answer this question requires information on the scope of potential and actual human exposures to hazardous wastes and about the health effects that could be associated with these exposures. Based on its review of the published literature on the subject, the committee finds that the question cannot be answered. Although billions of dollars have been spent during the past decade to study and manage hazardous-waste sites in the US an insignificant amount has been devoted to evaluate the attendant health risks. This has resulted in an inadequate amount of information about the connections between exposure and effect.'[10]

BALANCING RISK: WORKERS VS COMMUNITIES

For nearly two decades, environmental remediation proceeded on the widespread assumption that any reduction in risk was good, and that reducing risk as close to zero as possible was desirable, if not feasible. The assumptions in many of the risk assessment scenarios were worst-case exposures, involving maximally exposed individuals. In such analyses, the countervailing risks to workers (or to communities exposed at a distance due to transportation accidents or exposures at the waste-receiving site) were conveniently ignored. It must be emphasized that reducing risks to workers is essential, particularly since such risks are usually more predictable than those hypothesized for the community.

Faced by the large sums of money expended on hazardous waste site remediation, to avert a relatively few resident deaths predicted by risk assessments, several researchers have called attention to the fact that the workers involved in remediation are at risk of death, and that such deaths are real (rather than theoretical) and may offset the number the cancer deaths averted. One study has shown that the years of life lost through injury or illness among hazardous waste remediation workers match or exceed the hypothetical cancer deaths to exposed residents if the site were not remediated.[48] A hypothetical example of "Years of Potential Life Lost" among 500 hazardous waste workers exceeded the years saved for the residential population of 5000 exposed to the site. Hoskin et al[49] quantified the mortality risk to workers using Bureau of Labor Statistics data for three different occupations often utilized in hazardous waste operations. These studies demonstrate that traumatic and traffic deaths, rather than chemical exposures, are the main problem for workers.

RISK COMMUNICATION AND RISK PERCEPTION

The important topic of risk communication is covered in Chapter 59 (see also Slovic[50] and Tinker[51]). Individuals vary greatly in their willingness to accept risks. Radiation and chemical workers tend to be more tolerant of these hazards than clerical employees in the same industries. Familiar and voluntary risks, or those carrying a perceived benefit, are frequently tolerated. In contrast, risks of similar magnitude that are unfamiliar and involuntary are rarely perceived as acceptable. The media often emphasize hazards without attempting to communicate levels of risk.[52,53]

Risk communication involves interpreting the nature and magnitude of health risks to communities and providing information on how to reduce further risks. Unfortunately, to some, risk communication involves reassuring the public that hazardous wastes will not hurt them, but in reality the task is very complex. Too often professionals assume that the public is not sophisticated enough to understand risk, but since risk decisions are a common occurrence in life, such condescension is unwarranted. If the risk communicator has enough information to present a clear picture of alternative risks, then individuals are likely to make informed choices. The choices, however, may not always appeal to health professionals or the risk manager.

Some communications resort to risk comparisons, comparing the lifetime cancer risk from a hazardous waste site to smoking so many packs of cigarettes a day, or to the probability of an asteroid striking earth.[54] Although seemingly sensible, such comparisons do not always have their desired effect since smoking, for example, is viewed as voluntary. An asteroid strike (high impact/low probability) differs categorically from waste exposure that is viewed as ongoing (therefore high probability).

Goldstein et al[55] extended the risk comparison approach by calculating that the lifetime risk of an individual on the ground being killed by an airplane was 4 in a million, and emphasized that people don't change their mode of living in response to such a small risk. People living near airports may well be less reassured than those living far away, particularly if there has been a recent air crash with community fatalities.[56]

Another approach is to convert a lifetime risk into an estimate of how many lifetimes it would take to experience one toxic-related cancer in a population of a given size. Weinstein et al[57] provide examples where cases would occur at intervals of centuries, and suggest that some audiences may find this informative or reassuring.

Patients and community residents can superimpose their own knowledge and belief systems on the messages imparted to them, allowing them to come up with their own, often unique interpretations. Faced with uncertainties in the data and various underlying values of audiences, physicians must develop a repertoire of approaches to communicating risk to the public and to other stakeholders.[58]

Risk perception and 'popular epidemiology'

It has long been apparent that professionals and lay persons have different perceptions of risk. Many papers have explored how people perceive risk. One reason for the different perceptions is in the kinds of data that communities utilize in conducting cursory epidemiologic assessments, often on an informal basis. They differ from professionals in how they gather and evaluate data, how

they weigh possible confounders, and how they interpret results, thereby leading to different perceptions.[59]

REDUCING COMMUNITY EXPOSURE

In the case where a risk assessment identifies an elevated or unacceptable risk, or where there is frank contamination, intervention is required. In extreme cases where an emergency exists, residents may be required or encouraged to evacuate. This will be a severe stress in itself, particularly if the exposure has been ongoing for a long time. A household or community may be warned or ordered to discontinue using water for drinking, cooking, and even for bathing or showering. Communities with well water may have emergency hook-up to municipal water, but when municipal water is contaminated, an alternative source for the water must be obtained. If the water is contaminated with non-volatile substances, then residents may continue to shower, but must obtain or be provided with bottled water for drinking and cooking. Long-term remediation may involve actual pumping out of aquifers, some form of chemical treatment, and replenishment. This is notoriously slow, inefficient, and costly. Point-of-entry treatment systems using ion exchange and filters may be used for some contaminated well water. When food is contaminated, advisories are issued banning fishing (or the consumption of fish) from certain bodies of water, ordering people not to consume certain garden crops, or even condemning certain sources of food.

Air-borne contamination that jeopardizes health is more likely to occur from incinerators or ongoing industrial activities. In the case of volatiles or dust blowing from a hazardous waste site, emergency containment or capping is called for.

Soil contamination poses more vexing, longer term challenges for reducing risk. Different agencies have different guidelines for identifying contaminated soil. Low-level contamination may be remediated in situ by some form of capping. Certain plastic geotextiles covered with clean fill may prevent people from contacting the contaminated soil. In some cases paving or planting of grass may be deemed sufficient.

When soil is contaminated above a certain level, it must be treated (either by chemical treatment in situ or by removal) to lower the level to a certain set standard (which is not always the same level that is considered hazardous). In many cases, companies must completely remove the top layer of soil (anywhere from 18 to 36 inches or more, depending on depth of contamination) from nearby residential communities, and replace it with clean topsoil, followed by extensive re-landscaping.

Household hazardous waste

Many households have hazardous wastes of their own half-used paint and solvent containers, pesticides, and cleansers. In some cases these may release volatiles into the home. In other cases they are a fire hazard, or a source of environmental contamination if disposed of improperly. Although the amount in a single home is small, the total amount in a community can be substantial. Many communities or counties have introduced household hazardous waste days or collection sites to facilitate the safe disposal of such wastes. Wastes are collected, chemicals are poured into bulk containers, and solid wastes are channeled either to special incinerators or landfills. However, occupational exposures at such sites can be significant, particularly to benzene and to mercury in broken fluorescent bulbs.[60]

BROWNFIELDS REDEVELOPMENT

A brownfield is an abandoned, idled, or under-used industrial or commercial facility where expansion or redevelopment is complicated by real or perceived environmental contamination. Residential risk is particularly problematic, and drives more extensive cleanup than redevelopment for industrial or commercial purposes. Development of industrial sites is not new. Many former manufactured gas plants were subsequently developed for housing; the school and adjacent properties at Love Canal represent another example of a brownfield. The costs of complete cleanup can sometimes be averted, or even amortized by new industrial development. Failure to develop such lands has become a national urban blight, while developing compatible remediation/redevelopment plans remains challenging.[61] New technologies for inactivating certain types of waste offer one possibility.[62] It has even been proposed that some hazardous waste sites be developed as museums to demonstrate how contamination occurs and its actual and potential impacts.[63]

THE ROLE OF MEDICAL SURVEILLANCE FOR THE COMMUNITY

A medical surveillance program must be predicated on the early detection of the effects of an exposure, at a point where intervention can prevent disease or disability. Where significant exposure to one or more toxic agents has occurred, medical evaluation can detect pathophysiologic changes. Where exposure is deemed not to be significant, appropriate reassurance may have greater benefit than the prolonged uncertainty associated with recurrent medical examinations. ATSDR has concluded: 'medical monitoring should be directed towards a target community identified as being "at significant increased risk for disease" on the basis of exposure. Significant increased risk will vary for particular sites depending upon such factors as the underlying risk of the outcome of concern, the risk attributable to the exposure, and the presence of sensitive subpopulations.'[64]

The decision regarding medical surveillance would be easier to make if risk assessments offered better precision, or if medical surveillance had better sensitivity and specificity. Legal action taken on behalf of communities or individuals exposed to hazardous waste often includes claims for ongoing medical surveillance as part of the damages sought. This places a unique burden on the medical community. Where exposure is likely to be negligible and the prevalence of toxic effects thereby low, the predictive value of even a sensitive screening test might be low.

Although medical surveillance is warranted in appropriate cases, it is certainly prudent to develop a registry of all residents in a community, including information such as dates and location of residence, data on soil and water contamination, age, time spent in home, and current health status. Maintaining a registry allows for the identification of potentially exposed residents at a future date, when more is known about the hazard, or when individuals show signs of illness. In the case of significant exposure to a toxic agent, baseline medical testing is often valuable. If the agent is one that can produce disease at a later date (e.g., carcinogens, reproductive toxins), follow-up examination may be warranted. However, where these conditions have a very low prevalence (i.e., where the risk is low), the predictive value of even a positive test may be low.

Criteria for inclusion in a medical surveillance program

The efficacy of any medical surveillance or screening program depends on the underlying prevalence of the endpoint being sought. Where this endpoint lies in the future, its prevalence can only be estimated. Therefore medical surveillance programs in industry or for communities depend on some assessment of the underlying prevalence of significant exposure, such that risk of adverse health effects in the future is increased.

Various approaches used to assess individual exposure (see above) can provide information for determining which individuals will benefit from medical surveillance and which will not. Ongoing medical surveillance can be justified where (1) there is or has been significant exposure to a hazard with documented exposure pathways, (2) when serious health consequences may occur, (3) when there is a substantial benefit from early diagnosis (or reassurance), and (4) when the onset of disease may be long delayed after exposure ceases. Where there is substantial anxiety, a one-time cross-sectional screening program may be appropriate, the results of which can serve to reassure the community or individuals, or can serve as the baseline for follow-up surveillance activities.

Screening versus surveillance

A medical monitoring program should include two phases: the initial or screening phase and the long-term surveillance phase. In the screening phase, the clinician obtains information on the past (or ongoing) exposures, and determines whether the participant is in a low, medium, or high exposure group. The former can be given reassurance that their risk of long-term health consequences is not appreciably increased, and that periodic follow-up examinations (surveillance phase) are not required. For individuals with high exposures, a close follow-up or surveillance (perhaps with annual examinations) is required. For individuals in the medium category, examinations can be performed less frequently (e.g., every 3–5 years).

The appropriate duration of the surveillance phase should address practical issues of latency. Since the longest latencies for cancer are of the order of decades, it may be reasonable to plan long term surveillance following termination of exposure.

COMMUNITY HAZARDOUS WASTE SOURCES

Household hazardous waste

Many households contain waste materials that are potentially hazardous, particularly flammable and volatile materials. Household hazardous waste is exempt from RCRA and CERCLA. This includes material collected, transported, stored, treated, disposed, recovered, or reused (RCRA 40 CFR 261.4). Such materials represent sources of exposure for the households in which they occur, as well as those who collect, process and dispose of them. Many communities have established household waste days to collect paints and stains, paint thinners, automotive wastes, antifreeze, cleaning agents, batteries, and pesticides. Medical wastes (bandages, syringes) are usually not collected in this manner. In a community survey, most householders try to use up materials where possible, but much is brought to the hazardous waste collection sites. However, because there may be few days a year when the sites are open, and because they are not conveniently located for everyone, much of this waste is disposed of as garbage, particularly when a house is being vacated for sale.

Solid waste incineration

The National Research Council estimates that the US has more than 100 municipal solid waste incinerators, 1600 medical waste incinerators, and 200 hazardous waste incinerators. Emissions of concern include particulates, metals, dioxins, and furans. The development of continuous emission monitors would allow incinerator operators to shut down or alter conditions when emissions are high. The Committee on Health Effects of Waste Incineration concluded that there were few studies effectively assessing health effects of incinerator emissions, particularly delayed effects.[65] The Committee made recommendations about improving future epidemiologic studies and exposure measurements.

ISSUES OF ENVIRONMENTAL JUSTICE

In the early 1990s, environmental justice emerged as a major ethical and public health issue (see Chapter 58), spearheaded by Robert Bullard's 'Dumping on Dixie'. Bullard and others have demonstrated that minority and poor communities are disproportionately exposed to hazardous waste sites, as well as industrial facilities and other locally unwanted land uses.[66,67] Whether this situation arises because the communities have little political influence or representation, making it easier to site such facilities, or because property values and rents are likely to be lower in such 'undesirable' neighborhoods does not change the fundamental relationship between poverty and exposure risk. Even in non-urban areas, minority populations may be at risk. In rural South Carolina, black fishermen consume substantially more fish than white fishermen, and are at higher risk from pollutants in the fish tissue,[68] while in the vicinity of a nuclear research laboratory (Los Alamos, NM), Hispanic populations had higher exposure from recreational activities than whites.[69]

Minority and poor families disproportionately live in communities with landfills, hazardous waste facilities, incinerators, industrial plants, and old housing with poor indoor air quality and lead-based paint, and children in these families are at risk of becoming the 'unwitting target of environmental injustices'.[70]

Environmental justice is a US governmental remedy that requires the application of fair strategies and processes in the resolution of inequality related to environmental contamination. The US response resulted in the establishment of offices of environmental justice within the EPA and ATSDR, and passage of important legislation and policies such as the Community Planning and Right-to-Know Act of 1986, Executive Order 12898 (Federal Actions to Address Environmental Justice in Minority Populations), and Executive Order 13045, a parallel order to protect low-income and minority children from actual and potential environmental hazards.

INTERNATIONAL TRADE IN HAZARDOUS WASTE

Closely linked to the issue of environmental justice is the international trade in hazardous waste. Developing nations concerned with balance of payment and international monetary debt generally pay more attention to short-term cash flow than to long-term environmental consequences.[71] Many countries have expressed a willingness to accept transboundary shipments of hazardous waste as a source of income, arguing, in some cases persuasively, that if short-term economic support is given to basic public health needs, this will have a salutary effect on health that offsets the long-term risks from the waste itself. Waste shipped from Taiwan to Cambodia was reported to have had short-term health consequences to people who reside near the site where the waste was dumped.[72] Highly industrialized countries that have been economically disadvantaged also have a serious hazardous waste legacy, as exemplified by a number of countries in Eastern Europe (e.g., Zejda et al[73]).

ECOLOGIC RISKS FROM CONTAMINATED SITES

Ecosystems and other natural resources of biologic, economic, recreational, or aesthetic value to humans can also be contaminated by hazardous wastes. Ecologic risk assessment has developed as a separate discipline,[74] emphasizing new methods to assess the effects of chemicals on ecosystems.[75] Runoff and leachate from landfills into adjacent ground or surface water of surrounding ecosystems is one means of contamination. Many habitats that have been used for disposal continue to maintain viable ecosystems that may develop some degree of tolerance for contamination. Although beyond the scope of this chapter, ecologic risk assessment has important parallels with human health risk assessment,[76] and it also influences how agencies responsible for hazardous waste, such as the US Department of Energy, provide for the long-term stewardship of sites that cannot be completely remediated with current technology.[77]

References

1. Goldstein, BD, Gochfeld M. Role of the physician in environmental medicine. Med Clin North Am 1990; 74:246–62.
2. Burgess JL, Kovalchick DF, Harter L, Kyes KB, Thompson JN. Hazardous materials events: an industrial comparison. J Occup Environ Med 2000; 42:546–53.
3. Lindell MK, Perry RW. Community innovation in hazardous materials management: progress in implementing SARA Title III in the United States. Superfund Amendments and Reauthorization Act. J Hazard Mater 2001; 88:169–94.
4. Johnson BL, DeRosa C. The toxicologic hazard of superfund hazardous-waste sites. Rev Environ Health 1997; 12:235–51.
5. Marshall EG, Geary NS, Cayo MR, Lauridsen PA. Residential exposure summary methodology for a reproductive health study of multiple hazardous waste sites. J Expo Anal Environ Epidemiol 1993; 3(Suppl 1):87–98.
6. Gochfeld M. Medical surveillance and screening in the workplace: complementary preventive strategies. Environ Res 1992; 59:67–80.
7. Georgopoulos PG, Lioy PJ. Exposure measurement needs for hazardous waste sites: two case studies. Toxicol Ind Health 1996; 12:651–5.
8. Krautheim KR, Aldrich TE. Geographic information system (GIS) studies of cancer around NPL sites. Toxicol Ind Health 1997; 13:357–62.
9. Hamel SC, Ellickson KM, Lioy PJ. The estimation of the bioaccessibility of heavy metals in soils using artificial biofluids by two novel methods: mass-balance and soil recapture. Parts I and II. Sci Total Environ 1999; 15:243–4,273–83.
10. NRC. Environmental epidemiology: public health and hazardous wastes. Washington DC: National Research Council, National Academy Press, 1991.
11. Kharrazi M, von Behren J, Smith M, et al. A community-based study of adverse pregnancy outcomes near a large hazardous waste landfill in California. Toxicol Ind Health 1997; 13:299–310.
12. Dunne MP, Burnett P, Lawton J, Raphael. B. The health effects of chemical waste in an urban community. Med J Aust 1990; 152:592–7.
13. Sosniak WA, Kaye WE, Gomez TM. Data linkage to explore the risk of low birthweight associate with maternal proximity to hazardous waste sites from the National Priorities List. Arch Environ Health 1994; 49:251–6.

14. Elliott P, Briggs D, Morris S, et al. Risk of adverse birth outcomes in populations living near landfill sites. Br Med J 2001; 323:363–8.
15. Hamar GB, McGeehin MA, Phifer BL, Ashley DL. Volatile organic compound testing of a population living near a hazardous waste site. J Expo Anal Environ Epidemiol 1996; 6:247–55.
16. Roht LH, Vernon SW, Weir FW, Pier SM, Sullivan P, Reed LJ. Community exposure to hazardous waste disposal sites: assessing reporting bias. Am J Epidemiol 1985; 122:418–33.
17. Ozonoff D, Colten ME, Cupples A, et al. Health problems reported by residents of a neighborhood contaminated by a hazardous waste facility. Am J Ind Med 1987; 11:581–97.
18. Backer LC, Grindem CB, Corbett WT, Cullens L, Hunter JL. Pet dogs as sentinels for environmental contamination. Sci Total Environ 2001; 274:161–9.
19. Bukowski JA, Wartenberg D, Goldschmidt M. Environmental causes for sinonasal cancers in pet dogs, and their usefulness as sentinels of indoor cancer risk. J Toxicol Environ Health A 1998; 54:579–91.
20. Burg JR, Gist GL. The National Exposure Registry: procedures for establishing a registry of persons environmentally exposed to hazardous substances. Toxicol Ind Health 1995; 11:231–48.
21. Paigen B, Goldman LR, Magnant MM, et al. Growth of children living near the hazardous waste site, Love Canal. Human Biol 1987; 59:489–508.
22. Lagokos SW, Wessen BJ, Zelen M. An analysis of contaminated well water and health effects in Woburn, Massachusetts. J Am Stat Assoc 1986; 81:583–96.
23. Vrijheid M, Dolk H, Stone D, Abramsky L, Alberman E, Scott JE. Socioeconomic inequalities in risk of congenital anomaly. Arch Dis Child 2000; 82:349–52.
24. Blumenstock J, Fagliano J, Bresnitz E. The Dover Township childhood cancer investigation. New Jersey Med 2000; December:25–30.
25. Waller LA. A civil action and statistical assessments of the spatial pattern of disease: do we have a cluster? Reg Toxicol Pharmacol 2000; 32:174–83.
26. Wartenberg D, Greenberg M. Solving the cluster puzzle: clues to follow and pitfalls to avoid. Stat Med 1993; 12:1763–70.
27. Greenberg M, Wartenberg D. Communicating to an alarmed community about cancer clusters: a fifty state survey. J Commun Health 1991; 16:71–82.
28. Greenberg M, Wartenberg D. Newspaper coverage of cancer clusters. Health Educ Q 1991; 18:363–74.
29. Whiteman DC, Dunne MP, Burnett PC. Psychological and social correlates of attrition in a longitudinal study of hazardous waste exposure. Arch Environ Health 1995; 50:281–6.
30. Gochfeld M. Investigation of a lymphoma cluster in a university building. Report to New Jersey Department of Health. Piscataway, NJ: Environmental and Occupational Health Sciences Institute, 1986.
31. Kaye WE, Hall HI, Lybarger JA. Recall bias in disease status associated with perceived exposure to hazardous substances. Ann Epidemiol 1994; 4:393–7.
32. Knox E. Childhood cancers, birthplaces, incinerators and landfill sites. Int J Epidemiol 2000; 29:391–7.
33. Cartwright RA, Dovey GJ, Kane EV, Gilman EA. Onset of the excess of childhood cancer in Seascale, Cumbria. J Public Health Med 2001; 23:314–22.
34. Dickinson HO, Parker L. Quantifying the effect of population mixing on childhood leukaemia risk: the Seascale cluster. Br J Cancer 1999; 81:144–51.
35. Geschwind SA, Stolwijk JA, Bracken M, et al. Risk of congenital malformations associated with proximity to hazardous waste sites. Am J Epidemiol 1992; 135:1197–207.
36. Shaw GM, Schulman J, Frisch JD, Cummins SK, Harris JA. Congenital malformations and birthweight in areas with potential environmental contamination. Arch Environ Health 1992; 47:147–54.

37. Berry M, Bove F. Birth weight reduction associated with residence near a hazardous waste landfill. Environ Health Perspect 1997; 105:856–61.

38. Wyrobek AJ, Schrader SM, Perreault SD, et al. Assessment of reproductive disorders and birth defects in communities near hazardous chemical sites. III. Guidelines for field studies of male reproductive disorders. Reprod Toxicol 1997; 11:243–59.

39. Scialli AR, Swan SH, Amler RW, et al. Assessment of reproductive disorders and birth defects in communities near hazardous chemical sites. II. Female reproductive disorders. Reprod Toxicol 1997; 11:231–42.

40. Savitz DA, Bornschein RL, Amler RW, et al. Assessment of reproductive disorders and birth defects in communities near hazardous chemical sites. I. Birth defects and developmental disorders. Reprod Toxicol 1997; 11:223–30.

41. Wartenberg D, Agamennone VJ, Ozonoff D, Berry RJ. A microcomputer-based vital records data base with interactive graphic assessment for states and localities. Am J Public Health 1989; 79:1531–6.

42. Stallones L, Nuckols JR, Berry JK. Surveillance around hazardous waste sites: geographic information systems and reproductive outcomes. Environ Res 1992; 59:81–92.

43. Lipscomb JA, Satin KP, Neutra RR. Reported symptom prevalence rates from comparison populations in community-based environmental studies. Arch Environ Health 1992; 47:263–9.

44. Neutra R, Lipscomb J, Satin K, Shusterman D. Hypotheses to explain the higher symptom rates observed around hazardous waste sites. Environ Health Perspect 1991; 94:31–8.

45. Gochfeld M. Hazardous waste. In: Rosenstock L, Cullen MR, eds. Textbook of clinical occupational and environmental medicine, 1st edn. Philadelphia: WB Saunders, 1994;876–88.

46. PCCRARM. Risk assessment and risk management. Washington, DC: Presidential/Congressional Committee on Risk Assessment and Risk Management, National Academy of Sciences, 1997.

47. Gochfeld M. Susceptibility biomarkers in the workplace: historical perspective. In: Mendelsohn ML, Mohr LC, Peeters JP, eds. Biomarkers: medical and workplace applications. Washington, DC: Joseph Henry Press, 1998;3–22.

48. Cohen JT, Beck BD, Rudel R. Life years lost at hazardous waste sites: remediation worker fatalities vs. cancer deaths to nearby residents. Risk Analysis 1997; 17:419–25.

49. Hoskin AF, Leigh JP, Planek TW. Estimated risk of occupational fatalities associated with hazardous waste site remediation. Risk Analysis 1994; 14:1011–7.

50. Slovic P. The perception of risk. Sterling, VA: Earthscan Press, 2000.

51. Tinker TL, Pavlova MT, Gotsch AR, Arkin EB. Communicating risk in a changing world. Solomon's Island, MD: OEM Press, 1998.

52. Sandman PM, Sachsman DB, Greenberg MR, Gochfeld. M. Environmental risk and the press. New Brunswick: Transactions Press, 1987.

53. Flynn J, Slovic P, Kunreuther H. Risk, media, and stigma: understanding public challenges to modern science and technology. Sterling, VA: Earthscan Press, 2001.

54. Gerrard MB. Risks of hazardous waste sites versus asteroid and comet impacts: accounting for the discrepancies in US resource allocation. Risk Analysis 2000; 20:895–904.

55. Goldstein BD, Demak M, Northridge M, Wartenberg D. Risk to groundlings of death due to airplane accidents: a risk communication tool. Risk Analysis 1992; 12:339–41.

56. Thompson KM, Rabouw RF, Cooke RM. The risk of groundling fatalities from unintentional airplane crashes. Risk Analysis 2001; 21:1025–10.

57. Weinstein ND, Kolb K, Goldstein BD. Using time intervals between expected events to communicate risk magnitudes. Risk Analysis 1996; 16:305–8.

58. Gochfeld M, Goldstein BD. Lessons in environmental health in the twentieth century. Annu Rev Public Health 1999; 20:35–53.

59. Brown P. Popular epidemiology and toxic waste contamination: lay and professional ways of knowing. J Health Soc Behav 1992; 33:267–81.

60. Betsinger G, Brosseau LM, Golden J. Occupational health and safety in household hazardous waste management facilities. AIHAJ 2000; 61:575–83.

61. Powers C. State brownfields policy and practice. Boston, MA: Institute for Responsible Management, Inc., 1995.

62. EPA. Road map to understanding innovative technology options for brownfields investigation and cleanup. USEPA 542-N-97-002. Washington, DC: US Environmental Protection Agency, 1997.

63. New Jersey Department of Environmental Protection. Report of the Mercury Task Force. Trenton, NJ: New Jersey Department of Environmental Protection, 2002.

64. ATSDR. Final criteria for determining the appropriateness of a medical monitoring program under CERCLA. Agency for Toxic Substances and Disease Registry. Fed Reg 1995; 60(145):36840–4.

65. NRC. Waste incineration and public health. Washington, DC: National Academy Press, 2000.

66. Popper FJ. Siting LULUs. Planning 1981; 47:12–18.

67. Bullard RD. Dumping in Dixie: race, class, and environmental quality. Boulder, CO: Westview, 1990.

68. Burger J, Gaines KF, Gochfeld M. Ethnic differences in risk from mercury among Savannah River fishermen. Risk Analysis 2001; 21:533–44.

69. Burger J. Recreation and risk around Los Alamos: are Hispanics more at risk? J Toxicol Environ Health A 2000; 61:265–80.

70. Powell DL, Stewart V. Children. The unwitting target of environmental injustices. Pediatr Clin North Am 2001; 48:1291–305.

71. Asante-Duah K, Nagy IV. A paradigm of international environmental law: the case for controlling the transboundary movements of hazardous wastes. Environ Manage 2001; 27:779–86.

72. Hess J, Frumkin H. The international trade in toxic waste: the case of Sihanoukville, Cambodia. Int J Occup Environ Health 2000; 6:331–44

73. Zejda JE, Jarosinska D, Biesiada M, et al. Results of the health survey of a population living in a vicinity of a large waste site. Eur J Public Health 2000; 8:238–44.

74. Suter GW II, Efroymson RA, Sample BE, Jones DS. Ecological risk assessment for contaminated sites. Boca Raton, FL: Lewis, 2000

75. Linthurst RA, Bourdeau P, Tardiff RG. Methods to assess the effects of chemicals on ecosystem. Scientific Group on Methods for Safety Evaluation of Chemicals Monograph No. 10. New York: John Wiley Sons, 1995.

76. Burger J, Gochfeld M. Ecological and human health risk assessment: a comparison. In: Di Giulio R, Monosson E, eds. Interconnections between human and ecosystem health. London: Chapman & Hall, 1996;127–48.

77. Burger J, Gochfeld M. Stewardship and the US Department of Energy: encompassing ecosystem protection. J Environ Planning Manage 2001; 44:437–54.

Chapter 53
Environmental Aspects of Food Safety

Mark R Cullen

INTRODUCTION

The major importance of food to health relates to nutrition. In developing countries, many of the common causes of morbidity and mortality relate to inadequacy of caloric or protein intake, deficiency in dietary components, or inadequacy of sanitation. In developed countries, and an increasing number of regions crossing through health 'transition', chronic diseases owe much of their origin to maldistribution of dietary elements and, increasingly, overconsumption and obesity. The fraction of all cardiovascular disease and cancer attributable to diet suggests it is on a par with, or possibly exceeds, tobacco as the major preventable cause of premature death in such societies.[1] These issues fall into the province of nutrition, crucial in the practice of general preventive medicine as well as virtually every clinical discipline, but beyond the scope of this text. Similarly beyond the scope of this chapter are the clinical problems of traditional food allergy and food intolerance, such as those to milk and lactose, and infectious enteropathies.

The past few decades, however, have witnessed changes in society and in the food supply which have thrust certain aspects of food safety directly into the purview of environmental medicine. Such matters as the contamination of the food chain with industrial chemicals such as mercury or polychlorinated biphenyls (PCBs); the intentional use of food additives (colorants, preservatives) and nutritional supplements; the unintended residues of pesticides, hormones, and antibiotics used in growing animal and vegetable products; and the dramatic incursions of new chemical and biologic products of biotechnology into the food chain (e.g., genetically modified [GM] organisms) have heightened concerns about the healthfulness of many foods above and beyond the traditional nutritional medicine or infectious disease concerns. These issues have been further thrust into the spotlight by the increasing recognition of food-borne infections associated not with poor sanitation per se but with modern food processing, such as 'mad cow disease' (also beyond the scope of this chapter). This is not to suggest that any of these environmental factors – even including the infectious risks – compete in importance with nutritional matters, nor that any major contribution to the risk for cardiovascular disease or cancer attributable to dietary behaviors is best explained by these environmental factors. But sufficient evidence of harm has been demonstrated to awaken unprecedented political and regulatory efforts around the world to re-evaluate food from an environmental perspective.

The goal of this chapter is to outline the major categories of environmental risk and/or concern associated with food (other than infectious and nutritional aspects), and provide a framework for clinical evaluation of patients with food-related exposures or concerns.

CHANGES IN SOCIETY, FOOD PRODUCTION, AND THE ENVIRONMENT WHICH MAY CONTRIBUTE TO RISK AND PERCEIVED RISK OF ADVERSE HEALTH

A complex constellation of societal changes has contributed to heightened environmental concern about the food we eat.

- Compared with earlier eras, most people eat a far higher fraction of their meals away from home. In the US, this fraction is approaching 50%, a reflection of modern worklife and lifestyle, enhanced by developments in food processing and service allowing unprecedented variety and convenience to support the cultural shift. As such, individuals and families have increasingly less control over the actual source of food and handling than previously.

- Because of changes in technology, single locations can process food for wide distribution. Once local, the food processing industry has become regional, national, and, increasingly, international business, providing more opportunities for environmental contamination and greater opportunity for a single mistake to affect large numbers of people.

- At the same time, the marketplace for raw and other minimally processed foods has markedly expanded. The increased demand for fresh food year round, concomitant with the technology for food distribution systems to satisfy this demand, has fostered increased importation of foods from regions of the world with less well regulated food-handling practices.

- Changing dietary and social eating patterns have lead to the introduction of new waves of food additives – such as non-absorbable fats and artificial sweeteners – as well as inclusion of natural nutrients (e.g., vitamins and herbals) as supplements at concentrations not previously in foods per se, some of which have never been tested at concentrations that could be consumed unwittingly and over long periods of time.

- Although many of the worst persistent polluting chemicals in the environment, such as PCBs and organochlorine pesticides, have now been banned from sale in many parts of the world, these have nonetheless persisted in the food chain and even spread to areas where they were never used. Other contaminants, such as mercury, are biologically magnified in the food chain, resulting in contamination covering the entire globe in unprecedented and unanticipated patterns, potentially causing risk remote from the original sources of contamination.

- In order to enhance production, agriculture (including for the purposes of this chapter both plant and animal production) has become increasingly mechanized and reliant on agrochemicals such as pesticides, hormones, and antibiotics. The wide variations in dietary behaviors present the possibility that exposure dose to some agents by some individuals could be substantial.

- The effectiveness of modern medicine in increasing the lifespan, allowing individuals with various immunologic and other biologic impairments to live for long periods, raises new questions about subsets of the population that may be at enhanced risk for food-borne illnesses and contamination.

- To meet the rising demand for fresh and nutritionally satisfactory foodstuffs, a panoply of GM vegetables – and, possibly in the near future, animal products – are entering into the marketplace, often without label or notice. Strategies for assuring the safety of these products have lagged behind the staggering pace of their development, currently the source of considerable political furore, especially in Europe.

- Emerging patterns of health and disease in highly developed societies have refocused concern on the possibility for a contribution of diet to such disorders as attention-deficit disorder, asthma, breast and prostate cancers, and endocrine disruption.

In the sections that follow, we shall review the following major areas of concern to environmental medicine practice.

I. Chemical contamination of foodstuffs
  - Accidental chemical contamination
  - Residues of agricultural products – pesticides, hormones, and antibiotics
  - Biopersistent or biomagnified contaminants
II. Food additives in processing
III. Contamination of food from packaging, cooking, and serving
IV. GM foods and related 'technologies'

CHEMICAL CONTAMINATION OF FOOD
Accidental contamination

Many of the most spectacular outbreaks of human exposure to hazardous chemicals have involved food. Most episodes have occurred when fresh staple foods, such as oil, rice, or other grains, have been contaminated during their growth or processing by industrial materials or waste. The best studied include the following.

Epping jaundice

In 1965, a small community near London experienced an epidemic of acute-onset jaundice following contamination of flour in a bakery with methylene dianiline (MDA or diaminodiphenylmethane). Victims developed gastrointestinal symptoms and fever over several days, with high levels of alkaline phosphatase in blood and milder rises in hepatic transaminases. Most recovered; long-term follow-up of 84 persons who were traced revealed no evidence of long-term sequelae, although the sample size was small.[2]

Minimata

In the late 1950s, an epidemic of a central nervous system (CNS) disease appeared in the region of Minimata Bay in Japan. Some adults were affected with tremor, ataxia, dysarthria, and visual disturbances – despite relatively well preserved cognition and memory. The impact on newborns was more profound, with motor disturbance and major developmental anomalies.[3] The cause was eventually attributed to consumption of large sea fish contaminated by mercury dumped in the bay from a factory manufacturing vinyl chloride; the mercury was biotransformed in the aquatic food chain to the highly neurotoxic methyl mercury. Interestingly, none of the systemic signs seen in inorganic merculialism, such as dermal, salivary, or renal changes (see Chapter 39.8), were noted. A similar outbreak occurred 15 years later in Iraq, where imported grain seeds that had been fumigated by organic mercurials were consumed rather than planted, with similar consequences.[4] These two outbreaks have formed the foundation for concern about the increased contamination by methyl mercury in fish throughout the world (see below).

Yusho

About a decade after the Minimata disaster, the Yusho prefecture in the western part of the Japanese archipelago was blighted by another – contamination of rice oil by PCBs, a now-banned class of industrial oils (see also Chapter 45). Up to 1800 people were affected by a syndrome initially recognized by ungainly skin and nail discoloration, cheesy ocular secretions, and chloracne.[5] Extensive evaluation as part of the so-called Yusho study revealed that peripheral nerve complaints and dysfunction were common, as were intractable headaches and lipid disturbances. Newborns were demonstrably affected to a greater degree than their mothers. Signs and symptoms persisted for years after resolution of the exposure, consonant with knowledge of the biopersistence of the causal agents; to date there has been no confirmation of increased cancer risks in the population.

An almost identical outbreak occurred in 1979 in Taiwan, dubbed Yucheng.[6]

Itai-itai

Long-term contamination of rice by cadmium in yet another part of Japan was recognized in 1971; the source was ground water carrying the metal from a mine tailing. Although renal dysfunction characteristic of poisoning with this metal was universal among heavily exposed subjects (see Chapter 39.4), the most common presenting clinical feature was pathologic fracture and extreme bone pain (which gave the outbreak its name – 'ouch-ouch'), primarily in middle-aged and elderly women, as a consequence of urinary calcium depletion. Much of our current knowledge of the consequence of industrial poisoning with this metal has resulted from extensive clinical and epidemiologic studies conducted on this population.[7]

Toxic oil syndrome

A spectacular epidemic of pneumonia with eosinophilia occurred in Madrid in May 1981. Thousands were affected; hundreds died while others went on to manifest chronic signs, including neuromuscular and visceral organ involvement. Investigations by local authorities, with the assistance of the Centers for Disease Control and Prevention (CDC), traced the outbreak to contamination of rapeseed oil (canola) by an aniline derivative – whose precise identity remains obscure after 20 years of research – hence the designation toxic oil syndrome (see Chapter 44). These oils had been sold via an informal market network over a several week period preceding the epidemic, which immediately petered out when the source was contained.[8,9] The clinical picture bears a strong resemblance to the eosinophilia–myalgia syndrome which occurred in epidemic form several years later in the US, and was eventually attributed to contamination of L-tryptophan sold as a herbal medicine for sleep in health food stores; studies revealed traces of aniline derivative in that outbreak as well, although again, the precise chemical structure of the causal agent remains obscure.[9]

Pesticides

Over the past 60 years there have been dozens of similar outbreaks caused by gross inadvertent application of agrochemicals to food. Virtually every class of pesticide has been implicated, and virtually every region of the world, developed and developing, has been affected. These episodes are cogently reviewed by Ferrer and Cabral.[4]

Residues of agricultural products in food (see Table 53.1)

Increasing use of chemicals to produce foodstuffs results in inevitable residues in products that come to market, only some of which can be 'washed off' or 'cooked away'. Although there has been an increasing pressure in developed countries to limit use of the most toxic agents, concern about long-term health consequences of residues persists for several reasons.

- Testing of many agricultural chemicals remains incomplete, especially as regards newer health concerns such as immunotoxicity or endocrine disruption.
- Agrochemicals are typically regulated individually, but multiple agents are present simultaneously in the typical food basket, with overlapping, possibly additive or synergistic, toxicities.
- Even for compounds regulated with established endpoints (such as cancer) taken into account, safety factors may not consider the impressive heterogeneity

Residue	Health concern	Most affected food(s)
Pesticides	Direct toxicity (especially in infants and children) Cancer Endocrine disruption Immunologic effects	Fruits, vegetables
Antibiotics	Drug-resistant flora Allergy Superinfection	Poultry
Hormones	Cancer Endocrine disruption	Dairy products, meat

Table 53.1 Residues of agricultural chemicals in human food

of dietary choices, especially among young children whose behavior may defy 'normative' assumptions used in establishing limits.[10] Recent evidence, for example, suggests that total organophosphate pesticide exposure of most children exceeds the current US recommended dietary levels, and a non-negligible fraction exceed even decade-old guidelines.

Despite these concerns, the following must be borne in mind. Ecologic studies comparing populations over time and from country to country[1] have not suggested the likelihood that residues in food explain much of the link between diet and cancer. For the pesticides in particular, best evidence suggests that overall, consumption of diets highest in raw fruits and vegetables confers protection from cancer despite possible contamination. Moreover, despite the theoretical concern, few empiric data have been generated to suggest that additive effects among related pesticides have contributed to measurable health effect, clinically or in populations.[11] Nonetheless, interest in this issue remains high, and the final verdict is still awaited.

There is growing evidence that the very widespread use of antimicrobial agents, especially for raising poultry, beef, and pork, has been responsible for emergence of resistant bacterial strains in the environment, and consequent human infection.[12,13] Consumers of treated meat are not necessarily at greater risk than others, since the spread of resistance through the ecosystem is complex; this is more a public health issue than individual health concern at the present time. A possible exception may be workers in the industry, who may be heavily colonized with such organisms (Silbergeld E, unpublished communication). Notably, neither allergic reactions nor other untoward side effects have been reported as a consequence of food ingestion per se, likely owing to the relatively trivial doses remaining in the final marketed products.

Likewise, although there remain substantial theoretical concerns about the use of hormones (see Chapter 27.1), the most widely used agent, supplemental bovine growth hormone in cow's milk, is essentially inert for humans.[14] Growth hormone-induced growth factors, which *are* biologically active for humans, are not secreted in the milk. The theoretical possibility that some fragments of these hormones would induce other endocrine responses remains unproven.

Finally, although there may be many reasons for consumer preference for so-called organic foods – grown or raised without the use of any of these chemicals – there remains no empiric evidence that they confer any better measure of health than comparable commercially grown products. Part of the problem has been wide variability in the interpretation of the designation 'organic', hence heterogeneity in the products.[15] However, because of widespread interest in these food alternatives, and the commercial pressures to expand their production, it is likely that further regulation of the industry will occur, as well as further scientific study attempting to delineate potential differences in health risk associated with their consumption.

Biopersistent contaminants in food (see Table 53.2)

Biopersistent organic chemicals, primarily polyhalogenated heterocyclic compounds like DDT and PCBs, and biomagnified metals, primarily methyl mercury, have created a hazard not previously envisioned. Unlike the residues discussed above, these agents have entered the food chain not primarily by virtue of the way food is raised or processed, but because of more profound contamination of the biosphere. An exception might be farmed salmon, in which PCBs have been attributed recently to feeding methods. As such, there are no 'organic' swordfish to be found, nor animals raised without trace dioxin content. Moreover, the dispersal of these contaminants throughout the world due to movements of air and water, and their persistence both in nature and biota, has extended the threat to much of the globe, even areas extremely remote from the original sources, such as the polar ice caps. Although the risk of acute effects or outbreaks from such contamination is slight, the public health consequences are potentially vast – in view of the magnitude and underlying health status of populations potentially at risk – and intractable, since the hazards are already widely disseminated and irremediable in the short term. The hazards of greatest concern are briefly discussed below, and in relevant exposure chapters elsewhere in the text.

Methyl mercury

As noted above, metallic or other forms of inorganic mercury are metabolized in the aquatic food chain to methyl mercury, which in turn is stored in muscle tissue of fish and not further excreted. Since this process continues for the lifespan of the fish, concentrations in the animals increase with their age, rendering large (old) catch a far greater potential risk to human health than crustaceans or fish consumed early in their lifespan. As discussed in Chapter 39.8, the greatest concern in populations with obligatory fish consumption (e.g., islanders) or individuals who consume large quantities by dietary preference is risk for in-utero absorption, since fetal brain is far more susceptible to injury than adult. For this reason, consumption of swordfish, tuna, and other similar species is recommended in modest quantities during pregnancy, although the extent of risk at currently extant levels worldwide is hotly disputed: some investigators believe the risk has been proven to be effectively nil[16] while others dispute this.[17]

PCBs

Although worldwide production of these oils has ceased, their persistence in the environment is such that levels are easily detected in the fatty tissue of mammals and many fish throughout the world. Recent studies from the Great Lakes and elsewhere suggest the possibility that small increments above the lowest background levels may induce measurable developmental effects in children, from either in-utero exposure or postpartum exposure in breast milk.[18] Study of the problem has been confounded by coexistence in fish of mercury, and methodologic difficulties teasing out relatively subtle differences in CNS performance of children, given the number of relevant covariates.

Dioxins

These cyclic organochlorines result from a range of industrial processes and from high-temperature oxidation of organic material such as fuels, plastics, and waste in the presence of chlorine. As discussed in Chapters 45 and 48, dioxins are the most potent synthetic toxins known, with carcinogenic, immune, and other systemic toxicities at picogram-per-kilogram (i.e., very low) doses. The human impact of background contamination in the food chain is the subject of intense speculation.[19] High-level environmental exposure is already suspected to cause diabetes mellitus, based on studies in Seveso, Italy, where a large community exposure occurred after an accident in 1976, and from Vietnam, where dioxins contaminated Agent Orange and other defoliants used in war.[20,21] Occupational exposures have been deemed carcinogenic.

FOOD ADDITIVES IN PROCESSING

An extraordinary array of synthetic chemicals is used by the food processing industry for various purposes, including sweetening (saccharine, aspartame), flavoring (nitrites, glutamates, papain, amylase, casein), preservation (BHT and BHA, sulfites), adding bulk and texture (polydextrose), packaging (polyglycerol), and coloring (tartrazine, azo dyes). In general, these compounds have been subjected to substantial toxicologic scrutiny because of the greater legal and regulatory requirements for food safety compared to other industrial uses. Nonetheless,

Chemical	Effects	Most affected foods
Polychlorinated biphenyls (PCBs)	Cancer Endocrine disruption Developmental toxicity	Fish (fresh water)
Organic mercury	Neurotoxicity Developmental toxicity	Fish (especially large game fish)
Organochlorine pesticides, dioxins, and related compounds	Cancer Endocrine disruption	Dairy products, meat

Table 53.2 Biopersistant contaminants in food

because exposure is so widespread and the possibility of idiosyncrasy so difficult to establish by traditional laboratory testing strategies, there has been substantial speculation and investigation regarding health effects. Current best evidence regarding these major additive groups is summarized below; detailed discussion of this extensive subject is beyond the scope of this chapter.

Overt clinical manifestations ascribable to dietary additives are uncommon, with estimates between three and 15 per 10,000 persons; the rates in children are higher, possibly approaching 1%–2%.[22] Far and away the best characterized reactions are allergic in nature, including asthma (with *sulfites* and *protein additives*), urticaria, and dermatitis, primarily in atopics. It is estimated that as many as 5% of asthmatics are sensitive to *sulfites*, though the reactions are typically mild when challenge tested.[23] Because of the occasional role of macronutrients in seizure disorders and migraine syndromes, it has been speculated that additives such as *tartrazine* might also be important triggers in some cases; blinded challenge studies have yielded at most equivocal evidence to support this.[24,25] *Nitrites* and *monosodium glutamate* (*MSG*) have each been implicated in the syndromes of flushing and headache, often related to consumption of Chinese food, but double-blind studies tend to refute the association.[26] More troublesome are data regarding attention-deficit disorder and behavioral disturbances in children, such as aggressive behavior in adolescents. Although the mechanisms remain highly conjectural, evidence does support an important role for dietary additives in a small minority of cases.[27] Strategies for identifying and documenting the relationship between these additives and clinical manifestations are discussed at the end of the chapter.

In addition to rare clinically recognizable consequences, carcinogenesis and endocrine disruption have been concerns, since some of these agents demonstrate adverse activity in in-vitro or whole-animal models. For example, *nitrites*, in theory, may be converted by flora in the gastrointestinal tract to the highly potent carcinogen group nitrosamines. Likewise, the preservative *potassium bromate* has proven positive for renal carcinoma in various assays, as, of course, has *saccharine*. Best evidence, however, suggests any effects due to these additives are dwarfed by effects – some harmful, some beneficial – of the foodstuffs to which these chemicals are added. It is worth mentioning, in this regard, that the most widely used preservatives, the phenolic antioxidants *BHT* and *BHA*, are likely anti-carcinogenic in practice, based on large populational studies.[1]

CONTAMINATION OF FOOD FROM IRRADIATION, PACKAGING, COOKING, AND SERVING

Beyond the factors that food might be exposed to during growth and production, there remains concern about irradiation and chemicals leached from packaging, cooking or serving materials.

Irradiation of fresh foods, especially poultry and meat, has become an increasingly common practice in response to concerns about bacterial pathogens such as salmonella. Unlike the complex and controversial subjects discussed above, there is neither a theoretical nor empiric basis for the belief that this practice may be harmful. Levels of radiation are too low to induce even trivial contamination by radionuclides and the energy transferred too low to modify substituents chemically. It is most likely that popular worry about this practice represents fallout from legitimate concerns about ionizing radiation exposures in other contexts.

The issue of chemical leaching is far less trivial. Canned and wrapped foods often accumulate higher levels of the material in which they are packed, and cooking adds still further to that burden. *Aluminum*, used for both purposes, has been prominent among concerns in this regard, especially since aluminum is an established neurotoxin in animal models, and in the setting of renal failure in humans, i.e., dialysis dementia which occurred when aluminum was added to dialysis solutions (see Chapter 39.1). Although there is speculation implicating this ubiquitous metal in degenerative disorders of the CNS, the evidence for such an effect remains weak; avoidance of such cookware or packaging for healthy individuals is without foundation at present. It might be argued theoretically that patients with renal failure should avoid aluminum exposures when possible, but there are no data to inform such a position.

Phthalates in plastic containers and wrapping can also leach into some foods. In vitro, these plasticizers have been shown to have a small estrogen-like effects only at doses exceeding those present in plastic-stored food.[28] Nonetheless, consideration is being given to substitutions based on risk assessment models.

More worrisome is the possibility of leaching from cookware made in regions of the world where environmental controls are limited. Most notorious in this regard is *lead*, used in glazes for pottery and crockware throughout the developing world because it is cheap and available. Heavy body burdens and even overt lead poisoning have been described from this route of exposure, rendering this an important component of history taking when lead poisoning is a consideration (see Chapter 39.7).

Finally, there is the issue of contamination of food by the products of combustion of fuel in cooking. The greatest concern is accumulation of *polyaromatic hydrocarbons* (*PAHs*) (see Chapter 44) on foods that are smoked or charcoal grilled. Exposure to these potent carcinogens in this setting has been documented;[29,30] excess risk due to consumption of these foods has not, although dermal and respiratory exposures to the same compounds industrially are associated with cancers of the lung and bladder. At present, the best dietary advice is to limit the fraction of overall consumption of food prepared by this route, but refinements in nutritional epidemiology may lead to strengthening or relaxation of such guidance in the near future.

GENETICALLY MODIFIED VEGETABLE AND ANIMAL PRODUCTS

The newest and most rapidly emerging environmental concern about food relates to GM plants and animals (see also Chapter 18.1). A number of such plant products have been introduced over the past decade. Consequently, substantial proportions of potatoes, corn, soy, and certain fruits are now produced from seeds into which genes from other species have been transfected and selected out, for purposes including pest resistance, climatologic hardiness, prolonged shelf-life, improved appearance or palatability, higher crop yields, and nutritional augmentation.

Most of the new products involve the insertion of vegetable or bacterial genes that produce well-characterized – and, generally, well-studied – structural proteins or enzymes. However, based on the pace of the technology, there will be countless variations in the near future, foreseeably including foods of animal origin as well.

There is evident concern in the community about the implications of this for the economy of agriculture as well as the control of the food chain in the hands of a few manufacturers implicit in the approach. Also, reasonable and as yet not fully addressed ecologic and environmental health concerns have surfaced, including:

- unforeseen selection pressures on ecosystems when large fields of plants with altered genes intrude;
- the possibility that genes could be transfected by natural vectors or otherwise recombine with plants in neighboring fields or even other species;
- the possible increased use of some herbicides for selection of genetically altered species over wild types, since, in order to select the new variants, genes are typically linked to genes for tolerance to herbicides, which are then sprayed on the fields to kill the wild types.

There are legitimate occupational issues raised for both the laboratory and field workers exposed to the GM products and their production (see Chapter 18).[1] The focus of this discussion, however, is the risk associated with consuming GM food.

Despite the vituperations and claims of some opponents of GM foods, the risk from consumption of these products appears modest. No outbreak or even case of systemic poisoning from consumption has been documented. Nonetheless, there are some credible concerns. An early one was the use of antibiotic-resistance genes to aid in the process of distinguishing the successful transgenic seeds from wild type.[5] Typically, kanamycin- and neosporin-resistance genes are employed for this purpose, most likely with no adverse human consequence of serious risk for emergence of polyresistant bacterial strains.[31] The best-founded concern relates to the possibility of increased allergy associated with altered or newly introduced proteins. Although theoretical information can be cited to exclude proteins that are *likely* to be antigenic – i.e., glycosylated proteins; those stable to temperature, pH, and protease degradation; and homologues of known antigens

– the possibility remains that post-transcriptional or other molecular modifications in the whole plant could render toxicologic predictions too imprecise to prevent allergic reactions from occurring.[32]

Another possibility is that a transgenic product could be toxic, especially if expressed in very large quantities in the edible portions of the plant as would be necessary for the new protein to change the taste/appearance/stability of the marketable product.[33] In general, these intentionally introduced proteins can be tested like any other potential chemical considered as a food additive. More problematic are the so-called *pleiotropic* effects of new genes. This refers to alteration of the expression of *other* plant genes or metabolism as an unanticipated consequence of the genetic modification, hence the overall composition of the food. For example, expression of a novel gene in potatoes was shown to enhance expression of certain potent plant alkaloids that caused an outbreak of food poisoning after conventional breeding experiments.[34] Another possibility is alteration in the distribution of native gene products by the new gene, such as expression in the fruit of cucubitracin, a bitter cucumber protein normally expressed only in stems and leaves. This problem is particularly vexing because meaningful toxicity testing would require testing the whole plant, not just the gene product itself, since the possibilities are limitless and unpredictable. To achieve this would require identifying some test animal species capable of consuming sufficient doses of the plant. The most obvious choice would be the livestock that normally consume such plants, but practical issues aside, such animals digest quite differently from humans, rendering such an approach very problematic, especially for conduct of long-term testing for chronic effects.

FOOD SAFETY IN CLINICAL ENVIRONMENTAL MEDICINE PRACTICE

As a matter of public health practice, the issue of diet concerns all practitioners. However, the possibility that contaminants in the food we generally eat, like the air we generally breathe and the water we generally drink, may contribute to background risks for chronic disease is not, in or of itself, an issue for clinical practice, except possibly in the management of those with unusual disorders or sensitivities. There are, however, four distinctive settings in which the issue of environmental food contamination might arise in clinical practice:

- in the workup of a patient with a cryptogenic illness – acute, episodic, or progressive – suspected possibly to have an environmental basis, such as urticaria, asthma, encephalopathy, migraine syndrome, or behavioral change;
- in the search for a 'source' when a patient – symptomatic or asymptomatic – is discovered to have a high body burden of a potentially toxic chemical, e.g., a metal or pesticide;
- in the evaluation of patients with multiple chemical sensitivities or other related conditions in which

gastrointestinal and systemic symptoms are perceived to be occurring in temporal relation to exposure to dietary constituents;

- in the evaluation and management of asymptomatic patients concerned about risk from exogenous exposures or classes of exposures, e.g., in a pregnant patient or a resident in a community in which a known source of contamination exists.

The approach to history taking, exposure assessment, and management in these settings and in general environmental medicine practice is briefly outlined below.

The dietary history in environmental medicine practice

It has not been routine in most occupational and environmental medicine practices to take detailed dietary histories. However, given the range of exposures that may be relevant to clinical evaluation, at least some information about diet should be included in every clinical assessment, along with work history, and home and ambient environments. Unless there is particular reason for concern based on the clinical issues listed above, however, this should be limited, and should not be confused with the dietary history that forms the foundation for nutritional medicine practice, general prevention-oriented primary healthcare, or the management of patients with chronic diseases to which diet has been proven to contribute – e.g., obesity, diabetes, lipid disorders, hypertension, etc. In those settings, the purpose of the dietary history is to establish a basis for nutritional modification, and considerable detail about food preferences and consumption is obligatory. In routine environmental medicine practice (excluding the specific settings listed above), on the other hand, the focus of the basic history is to discern whether *any aspect of dietary behavior might place an individual at unusual risk for an unsuspected environmental exposure or risk*. The elements of concern are:

- whether any food or class of foods is eaten in unusual proportion compared to normative behaviors; for example, does the patient consume fish at every meal, or extraordinary quantities of particular processed foods?
- whether 'unusual' foods are consumed which are known to have specific additives, such as herbs or supplements (a good context to inquire about any directly consumed in pill or other forms); and
- whether any foods are obtained from non-traditional sources, e.g., imported by family members, purchased from catalogues or other non-local suppliers, home-grown or processed, which could be locally contaminated, etc.

Negative responses to queries are probably sufficient as a screening procedure unless subsequent suspicions warrant greater detail.

The search for the 'source' for an elevated level of a potential toxin requires a more extensive evaluation. Overwhelmingly, the first matter is to confirm the evidence that the toxin has, in fact, accumulated in the body to excessive amount. Unfortunately, the proliferation of available laboratory assays and laboratories, combined

with substantial ignorance on the part of some practitioners who may order tests without appreciating the subtleties of their interpretation (see Chapter 3), has resulted in many 'false positives'. This situation is compounded in some areas by non-traditional practitioners, espousing unproven theories, who may order poorly standardized tests or large batteries such as hair analysis for metals and organic chemicals. Suspicion that a test result may not represent meaningful or conclusive evidence of an intoxication confers a crucial clinical obligation to resolve the issue clearly for the patient. Extensive investigation for a 'source' of the suspect toxin should *follow*, not precede, confirmation of the evidence at hand. However, once the evidence for an excessive burden of a toxin has been confirmed, then a careful exploration for possible sources must be conducted, and ingestion becomes an integral part of that search. In this regard, information must be sought regarding such matters as food preparation (e.g., cookware, utensils, or dishes from which metals could theoretically leach, sources of water used for cooking, seasonings or other materials used in food preparation), providers of food outside the home, foods consumed during travel, and even the remote possibility of foul play – surreptitious or intentional poisonings.

In the workup of acute, episodic or progressive symptoms, the temporal relationship between dietary behaviors and sources and the clinical problem is most important, as in the occupational history when workplace exposures are suspect. For example, in a progressive neuropathy, the onset in relation to change in diet would be noteworthy; for migraine, the nature of ingestions preceding headaches compared to other times. The task is most straightforward in presentations of acute disease, in which the approach to history taking parallels that for suspect food poisonings of any kind, with emphasis on most recently consumed meals and the pattern of symptoms among those who may have consumed the same items.

Patients with suspect multiple chemical sensitivities often complain about reactions to certain foods (see Chapter 49). In some cases, the reactions are limited to abdominal discomfort, and may mimic irritable bowel syndrome, a commonly associated illness. In others, however, foods are perceived as triggering diverse systemic, CNS, dermal, or other symptoms, similar to reported responses to air-borne exposures to irritants and odors. Recognizing that detailed knowledge of such patterns rarely contributes to elucidation of the underlying problem nor simplifies decision making, review of foods which trigger symptoms is preferable to frustratingly exhaustive searches or elimination diets that such patients often undertake by themselves under the misapprehension that the effort will reveal the unique 'cause' of their symptoms, if only they are diligent enough.

Finally, for the patient at special risk for exposure, or especially concerned – for example, regarding organic mercurials during pregnancy – the history should focus on known sources of such contaminants. This may require specific knowledge about local food sources, such as whether fish or game in the area are known to be contaminated (see below), coupled with a more detailed profile of what the patient consumes, at least semi-quantitatively, and where it comes from.

Establishing food-borne exposures

To a greater degree than in other aspects of occupational and environmental medicine practice, confirmation of exposure relies on use of biologic markers in the patient, most often direct levels in blood, urine, or hair; rarely, other body tissues. Although this does not pinpoint the source, it is often the only way to meaningfully estimate the amount of exposure that has occurred. Sometimes this is not possible, especially in situations where the chemical identity remains unknown, as in the case of toxic oil syndrome for example. In such cases, the pattern of symptoms among family members or others consuming the same foods is the best tool for clinical investigation.

Pinpointing the specific food-borne source of the contaminant may be substantially more challenging than confirming the presence of the toxin. Although in theory it might be possible to measure the suspect toxin in a food, this is rarely feasible – either the food is no longer present, the chemical is present in too low a concentration to easily measure, or the chemical identity is not adequately characterized. Even if measurable, normative values for comparison are generally lacking. As an alternative, the source may be identified by combining a dietary history with available data on food constituency or contamination. For example, an elevated blood mercury level might be 'confirmed' by combining a history of consumption of a given quantity of swordfish per week with data on average levels of mercury in swordfish in the community. Likewise, the presence of a food additive, such as MSG, or an herbal ingredient could be confirmed by food suppliers or preparers.

Another approach is to assess exposure levels and/or effects among other individuals with the same diet. For example, a working adult with an unexplained elevation of blood lead might be evaluated by checking lead levels of his or her spouse or children. Likewise, in suspect acute contamination, one would generally expect others who have consumed the same item(s) to be similarly affected, albeit not necessarily to comparable degree because of differences in the amount eaten or host variability.

Diagnostic evaluation: associating symptoms with foods

For the subset of cases where the possibility is raised that acute or recurrent symptoms might be induced by specific ingestions, elimination and/or challenge diets can have an important diagnostic role. The fundamental concept is straightforward, and similar to removal and rechallenge for workplace exposures (see Chapter 3). However, unlike the workplace, where few comparable exposures are likely to confound such 'trials', successful conduct of dietary challenges requires thoughtful guidance, especially if the suspect culprit is a food additive or contaminant that

could be present in a high fraction of items typically consumed. Rarely, a biologic marker may be helpful, such as skin or radioallergosorbent testing (RAST), most typically in pursuit of classic allergenic effects.

Managing environmental exposures/effects from food-borne sources

Once there is evidence that exposure has occurred, and reasonable knowledge about its source, there are two components to management. First, the toxic effects themselves need to be managed, depending on what they are. For example, organophosphate or lead poisoning from a food source would be treated as a similar poisoning from any source.

Second, the exposure should be eliminated. Fortunately, this is generally easier than in other occupational or environmental poisoning situations as long as dietary alternatives and the resources to utilize them exist. Food substitution is, in every case, the best solution. The major problems occur when there is no access to uncontaminated food; for example, in parts of the world where mercury-contaminated fish constitute the only source of protein, or when cultural or religious reasons make food substitution difficult. Even where confirmation is less certain – for example, in childhood behavioral disturbances or allergies arguably related to food additives – substitution can generally be undertaken by elimination diets without adverse social, economic, or other health consequences.

CONCLUSION

Far more testing is performed on the food supply, and far more attention paid to it, than either the ambient or workplace environment. Despite this, and despite centuries of experience, environmental aspects of food continue to cause risk to human health. The rapid intensification of agricultural production methods has necessitated larger, not smaller, reliance on chemicals and biologic products such as hormones and antibiotics. Moreover, the application of new genetic techniques to foodstuff, still in its developmental infancy, guarantees continued and novel challenges in the decades ahead.

References

1. Doll R, Peto R. The cause of cancer: quantitative estimates of avoidable risks of cancer in the United States today. J Natl Cancer Inst 1981; 66:1193-308.
2. Hall AJ, Harrington JM, Waterhouse JA. The Epping jaundice outbreak: a 24 year follow-up. J Epidemiol Commun Health 1992; 46:327-8.
3. McAlpine D, Araki S. Minimata disease: an unusual neurologic disorder caused by contaminated fish. Lancet 1958; ii:629-31.
4. Ferrer A, Cabral R. Toxic epidemics caused by alimentary exposure to pesticides: a review. Food Addit Contam 1991; 8:755-76.
5. Kuratsuma M, Yoshimura T, Matsuzaka J, Yamaguchi A. Epidemiologic study on Yusho, a poisoning caused by ingestion of rice oil contaminated with a commercial brand of

polychlorinated biphenyls. Environ Health Perspect 1972; 1:119-28.

6. Hsu S, Ma C, Hsu SK, Wu S, Hsu NH, Yeh C. Discovery and epidemiology of PCB poisoning in Taiwan. Am J Ind Med 1984; 5:71-9.

7. Friberg L, Piscator M, Norberg GF, Kjellstrom T. Cadmium in the environment, 2nd edn. Cleveland: CRC Press; 1974:128.

8. Aldridge WN. The toxic oil syndrome: from the disease towards a toxicologic understanding of its chemical aetiology and mechanism. Toxicol Lett 1992; 64-65(Spec No):59-70.

9. Philen RM, Posada M. Toxic oil syndrome and eosinophila-myalgia syndrome: May 8-10, 1991, WHO meeting report. Semin Arthritis Rheum 1993; 23:104-24.

10. Commission on Life Science. Pesticides in diets of infants and children. Washington, DC: National Academy Press; 1993

11. Carpy SA, Kobel W, Doe J. Health risk of low-dose pesticide mixtures: a review of 1985-1998 literature on combination toxicology and health risk assessment. J Toxicol Environ Health B Crit Rev 2000; 3:1-25.

12. O'Brien T. Emergence, spread and environmental effect of antimicrobial resistance: how use of an antimicrobial anywhere can increase resistance to any antimicrobial anywhere else. Clin Infect Dis 2002; 34(Suppl):S78-S84.

13. Barza M, Travers K. Excess infections due to antimicrobial resistance: the attributable fraction. Clin Infect Dis 2002; 34(Suppl):S126-30.

14. Juskevich JC, Guyer CG. Bovine growth hormone: human food safety evaluation. Science 1990; 249:875-84.

15. Anonymous. Organic foods: are they better? J Am Dietetic Assoc 1990; 90:920-2.

16. Davidson PW, Kost J, Myers GJ, Cox C, Clarkson TW, Shamlage CF. Methylmercury and neurodevelopment: reanalysis of the Seychelles Child Development Study outcome of 66 months of age. JAMA 2001; 285:1291-3.

17. Granjean P, Weihe P, White RF, et al. Cognitive deficit in 7-year-old children with prenatal exposure to methylmercury. Neurotoxicol Teratol 1997; 19:417-28.

18. Boersma ER, Lanting CI. Environmental exposure to PCBs and dioxins. Consequences for longterm neurological and cognitive development of the child and lactation. Adv Exp Med Biol 2000; 478:271-87.

19. Buchert A, Cederberg T, Dyke P, et al. Dioxin contamination in food. Environ Sci Pollut Res Int 2001; 8:84-8.

20. Pesatori AC, Zocchetti C, Guercilena S, Consonni D, Turrini D, Bertazzi PA. Dioxin exposure and nonmalignant health effects: a mortality study. Occup Environ Med 1998; 55:126-31.

21. Michalek JE, Akhter FZ, Kiel JL. Serum dioxin, insulin, fasting glucose and sex hormone-binding globulin in veterans of Operation Ranch Hand. J Clin Endocrinol Metab 1999; 84:1540-3.

22. Madsen C. Prevalence of food additive intolerance. Hum Exp Toxicol 1994; 13:393-9.

23. Weber RW. Food additives and allergy. Ann Allergy 1993; 70:183-90.

24. Camfield PR, Camfield CS, Dooley JM, Gordon K, Jollymare S, Weaver DF. Aspartame exacerbates EEG spike-wave discharge in children with generalized absence epilepsy: a double-blind controlled study. Neurology 1992; 42:1000-3.

25. Shaywitz BA, Anderson GM, Novotny EJ, Ebersole JS, Sullivan CM, Gillespie SM. Aspartame has no effect on seizures or epileptiform discharge in epileptic children. Ann Neurol 1994; 35;98-103.

26. Geha RS, Berser A, Ren C, et al. Review of alleged reaction to monosodium glutamate and outcome of a multicenter double-blind placebo-controlled study. J Nutr 2000; 130:1058S-62S.

27. Breakey J. The role of diet and behavior in children. J Paediatr Child Health 1997; 33:190-4.

28. Picard K, Lhuguenot JC, Lavier-Caniverc MC, Chagnon MC. Estrogenic activity and metabolism of n-butyl benzylphthalate in vitro: identification of the active molecule(s). Toxicol Appl Pharmacol 2001; 172:108-18.

29. Rothman N, Poirier MC, Haas RA, et al. Association of PAH-DNA adducts in peripheral white blood cells with dietary exposure to polyaromatic hydrocarbons. Environ Health Perspect 1993; 99:265-7.

30. Fritz W, Soos K. Smoked food and cancer. Bibl Nutr Dieta 1980; 29:57-64.

31. Nap JP, Bijvoet J, Stiekema WJ. Biosafety of kanamycin resistant plants. Transgenic Res 1992; 1:239-49.

32. Nordlee JA, Taylor SL, Townsend JA, Thomas LA, Bush RK. Identification of a brazil-nut allergen in transgenic soybeans. N Engl J Med 1996; 334:688-92.

33. Ewen SWB, Pusztai A. Effects of diets containing genetically modified potatoes expressing Galanthus nivalis lectin on rat small intestine. Lancet 1999; 354:1353-4.

34. Sinden SL, Webb RE. Effects of variety and location on the glycoalkaloid content of potatoes. Am Potato J 1972; 49:334-8.

Chapter 54

Occupational and Environmental Exposures to Waterborne Microbial Diseases

Mansour Samadpour, Peter S Evans, Karin D E Everett, Prajakta Ghatpande, Gregory J Ma, Robert R Miksch

INTRODUCTION

Diseases caused by waterborne microbial agents continue to be a leading environmental concern, and are responsible for human morbidity and mortality throughout the world. Freshwater microbes annually are responsible for four billion cases of diarrhea (2.2 million deaths), according to the World Health Organization (WHO). Poor hygiene that is associated with use of unclean water has resulted in an estimated 200 million schistosomiasis infections, with six million cases of blindness worldwide.[1] Freshwater sources, historically, have been associated with epidemics: during the 1800s in the United States there were eight major cholera outbreaks (caused by *Vibrio cholerae*) and three typhoid outbreaks (caused by *Salmonella typhosa*).

The fear of historically important waterborne infectious diseases like cholera and typhoid fever has been eliminated or substantially reduced in developed countries today, mostly due to sewage treatment and implementation of water treatment and delivery systems. However, even chlorinated drinking water is not sterile, and many people work in occupations with considerable exposure to water containing wastes. In addition, molecular diagnostic methods and DNA-based biodiversity studies are revealing that old pathogens are causing new problems, and novel microbes are being discovered in every setting. Epidemiologic reports have led to the recognition of emerging waterborne pathogens. As part of its regulatory role, the Environment Protection Agency (EPA) Office of Drinking Water prepares a list of 25 priority pollutants for scrutiny and research. In March of 1998, the agency published its Drinking Water Contaminant Candidate List in the Federal Register.[2] It was notable that ten of the 25 pollutants of concern were micro-organisms: *Acanthamoeba*, Adenoviruses, *Aeromonas hydrophila*, Caliciviruses (Norwalk and Norwalk-like viruses), Coxsackieviruses, *Cyanobacteria* (blue-green algae), Echoviruses, *Helicobacter pylori*, Microsporidia (e.g., *Cyclospora cayetanensis*), *Mycobacterium avium* and *Mycobacterium intracellulare*.

Humans and animals are exposed to microbes throughout their lives in work, home, and recreational environments. To be responsible for disease in humans or other animals, any one of these agents must be present in sufficient concentration to produce disease (infectious dose) and a susceptible host must come into contact with contaminated water.[3] Those that are waterborne are transmitted by drinking/eating, dermal/mucosal contact, or aerosol inhalation. Waterborne pathogens can also become foodborne when food is grown or prepared using water containing pathogenic microbes. Foodborne disease organisms are tracked by the Centers for Disease Control (CDC) Foodborne and Diarrheal Branch.[4] Eleven of the 16 foodborne diseases under surveillance by the CDC are also waterborne microbes.

Waterborne microbial pathogens belong to three major groups: bacterial, viral, and eukaryotic. These microbes cause a wide variety of diseases, including acute gastrointestinal, upper and lower respiratory, meningitis, myocarditis, dermatitis, cirrhosis, bacteremia, hemolytic uremic syndrome, and thrombotic thrombocytopenic purpura (see also Chapter 22). Because diseases vary greatly in severity, the US characterizes pathogens as Notifiable, Select, or Foreign Animal Disease (FAD) agents. Notifiable agents require notification of state public health physicians; the specific agents reported may vary from state to state. Waterborne Notifiable disease agents include *Cryptosporidium parvum*, enterohemorrhagic *Escherichia coli*, *Giardia intestinalis*, *Legionella pneumophila*, *Vibrio cholerae*, Poliovirus, and agents such as *Shigella sonnei*, which causes dysentery.[5]

GENERAL US POPULATIONS AT RISK
Outbreaks of waterborne illness in the USA

The US EPA and the CDC conduct surveillance for waterborne outbreaks in the USA.[6] In the distant past, waterborne outbreaks were caused by agents associated with disease in developing nations such as *Vibrio cholerae* (cholera), *Entamoeba* (amebiasis), *Shigella* (dysentery), and *Salmonella* (typhoid fever). In more recent years, outbreaks

Etiologic agent	Community outbreaks	Cases	Non-community outbreaks	Cases	Individual outbreaks	Cases	Cumulative outbreaks	Cases
AGI	11	10,162	36	4717	11	246	58	15,125
C. jejuni	1	172	3	66	1	102	5	340
C. parvum	5	404,642	1	27	2	39	8	404,708
Cryptosporidium spp.	2	3000	1	551	0	0	3	3551
E. coli O157:H7	3	208	2	37	3	12	8	257
E. coli O157:H7/C. jejuni	0	0	1	781	0	0	1	781
G. intestinalis	8	1891	3	139	6	25	17	2055
Giardia spp.	2	95	2	28	0	0	4	123
Hepatitis A	0	0	0	0	1	10	1	10
Non-O1 Vibrio cholerae	1	11	0	0	0	0	1	11
Norwalk-like virus	0	0	3	356	0	0	3	356
P. shigelloides	0	0	1	60	0	0	1	60
S. flexneri	0	0	0	0	1	33	1	33
S. sonnei	1	83	4	473	0	0	5	556
S. typhimurium	1	625	0	0	0	0	1	625
Salmonella spp.	1	124	0	0	1	84	2	208
Aichi virus	1	148	1	70	0	0	2	218
Cumulative microbial	37	421,161	58	7305	26	551	121	429,017

Data from MMWR Surveillance Summaries 1993, 1996, 1998, 2000, and 2002.

Table 54.1 United States outbreaks by etiologic agent in drinking water, 1991–2000 by water system type

have been linked to newly identified pathogens such as *Campylobacter, Cryptosporidium, E. coli* O157, *Giardia,* hepatitis A, *Legionella, Naegleria,* Acanthamoeba, Norwalk virus, *Pleisiomonas shigelloides, Pseudomonas,* and *Schistosoma spindale.* Improvements in sanitary infrastructure, including waste water treatment and drinking water protection, have drastically reduced the burden of waterborne disease, as well as the number of outbreaks. However, massive waterborne disease outbreaks continue to occur. The largest recent waterborne outbreak involved more than 400,000 cases of cryptosporidiosis in Milwaukee, Wisconsin, in 1993.[7] Another waterborne outbreak in Washington County, New York, in 1999[8] resulted in 148 cases of *E. coli* O157:H7 and *Campylobacter jejuni* infections. Outbreaks of waterborne illness have been associated with drinking water as well as recreational exposure to swimming pools, and natural water (bodies containing fresh and salt water).

Agents posing the greatest waterborne disease potential are transmitted through the fecal–oral route (Table 54.1). Consequently, prevention from diseases associated with these organisms is accomplished by protecting drinking water sources and recreational waters from contamination with human or animal waste. On the other hand, a limited number of waterborne pathogens (e.g., *Legionella* spp., *Vibrio* spp., *Aeromonas hydrophila,* and *Pseudomonas aeruginosa*) are indigenous to the water environment. Control of these agents and their potential infections is dependent on controlling exposure to water containing these organisms or by treating the water to remove or inactivate the infectious agents.

Drinking water

During the period 1991–1998, there were 81 outbreaks of waterborne disease associated with drinking water.[6] Of these, 41 were described as 'acute gastrointestinal illness' (AGI) of unknown etiology. The flagellated protozoan

parasite *Giardia* was the leading causative agent for 15 of the remaining 40 outbreaks. *Giardia* was the leading cause of waterborne outbreak in the preceding ten-year period as well. Another eukaryotic parasite, *Cryptosporidium parvum,* was the next leading cause (Table 54.2), accounting for ten of the 40 outbreaks. However, *C. parvum* accounted for the largest number of cases due to waterborne pathogens, mainly due to the Milwaukee outbreak that involved more than 400,000 cases. *Shigella sonnei* and *E. coli* O157:H7 each was responsible for four outbreaks. Two outbreaks were attributed to *Shigella flexneri* and the remaining five outbreaks were attributed one each to: *Salmonella typhimurium, Pleisiomonas shigelloides,* non-O1 *Vibrio cholerae,* hepatitis A, and a 'small round structured virus'. The low number of waterborne outbreaks of infectious disease is a tribute to the success of water treatment processes, especially the final disinfection and maintenance of residual disinfectant in the distribution systems. It is to be mentioned that while bacterial and viral pathogens are controlled effectively by the current disinfection processes, a successful control regimen for pathogens such as *Giardia* and *Cryptosporidium* involves the use of alternative disinfection technologies, such as ozonation and ultraviolet treatment, prolonged contact time with chlorine, and efforts to protect the source waters from resistant pathogens.

Recreational waters

The larger list of agents associated with recreational water outbreaks reflects the higher diversity of organisms present in untreated, natural waters (Table 54.3). In the period 1990–1998, 14,962 cases of disease associated with recreational water exposure were reported to the CDC.[9–12] *Pseudomonas* spp. were consistently reported every year during this period as a causative agent in 607 cases. However, the largest number of cases, 10,269, were

Recreational facility	Location	Disinfectant	Cases estimated/confirmed	Year
Pool	Doncaster, UK	Chlorine	NA/79	1988
Pool	Los Angeles County	Chlorine	44/5	1988
Pool	British Columbia	Chlorine	66/23	1990
Pool	Gloucestershire, UK	Ozone/chlorine	NA/13	1992
Water slide	Idaho	Chlorine	500/NA	1992
Pool (wave)	Oregon	Chlorine	NA/52	1992
Pool (motel)	Wisconsin	Chlorine	51/22	1993
Pool (motel)	Wisconsin	Chlorine	64/NA	1993
Pool	Wisconsin	Chlorine	5/NA	1993
Pool	Wisconsin	Chlorine	54/NA	1993
Pool (motel)	Missouri	Chlorine	101/26	1994
Lake	New Jersey	None	2070/46	1994
Pool	Sutherland, New South Wales	Chlorine	NA/70	1994
Pool	Kansas	NA	101/26	1995
Water park	Georgia	Chlorine	2470/62	1995
Water park	Nebraska	NA	NA/14	1995
Pool	Florida	NA	22/16	1996
Water park	California	Chlorine	3000/29	1996
Pool	Andover, UK	Chlorine	8/NA	1996
Lake	Indiana	None	3/NA	1996
River	NW England & Wales	None	27/7	1997
Pool	SW England & Wales	Ozone & chlorine	NA/9	1997
Fountain	Minnesota	Sand filter	369/73	1997
Three pools	Canberra, Australia	NA	NA/210	1998
Pool	Oregon	NA	51/8	1998
Pools	Queensland	NA	129/NA	1997
Pools	New South Wales	NA	370/NA	1998
Pools	Hutt Valley, New Zealand	NA	NA/171	1998

NA: not applicable

Table 54.2 Cryptosporidiosis outbreaks associated with recreational waters[21]

Etiologic agent	Lake/pond outbreaks	Cases	Pool outbreaks	Cases	Hot tub outbreaks	Cases	Other outbreaks	Cases	Cumulative outbreaks	Cases
Adenovirus 3	1	595							1	595
AGI	9	1046	3	132			3	80	15	1258
Campylobacter jejuni			1	6					1	6
Cryptosporidium							2	526	2	526
Cryptosporidium parvum	4	649	29	4632			2	526	35	5807
E. coli O157:H7	8	317	3	51			3	4	14	372
Giardia	1	4	3	30					4	34
Giardia intestinalis	3	73	2	157			1	6	6	236
Legionella					2	10	2	51	4	61
Legionella pneumophila							1	20	1	20
Leptospira	2	381							2	381
Leptospira interrogans	1	21							1	21
Naegleria	5	5					5	5	10	10
Naegleria fowleri	3	3						2	3	5
Norwalk	1	18					1	55	2	73
Norwalk-like virus	2	198	1	9			2	619	5	826
Pseudomonas			2	64	5	34	2	34	9	132
c/w *Pseudomonas*					3	10	1	45	4	55
Pseudomonas aeruginosa			11	335	19	157	1	50	31	542
c/w *P. aeruginosa*					3	24	1	15	4	39
Schistosoma spp.	6	173							6	173
c/w *Schistosoma* spp.	2	10					1	30	3	40
Schistosoma spindale	1	2							1	2
Shigella flexneri	1	35	1	6					2	41
Shigella sonnei	10	851	1	9			1	300	12	1160
Shigella sonnei and *C. parvum*							1	38	1	38
Unknown					1	12	1	33	2	45
Cumulative microbial	60	4381	57	5431	33	247	31	2439	181	12,498

Data from MMWR Surveillance Summaries 1993, 1996, 1998, 2000, and 2002.

Table 54.3 United States outbreaks by etiologic agent, for the period of 1991–2000 in recreational waters

attributed to *Cryptosporidium parvum* in seven of these eight years. *Shigella sonnei* was also reported in seven out of eight years as an etiologic agent in 1190 cases. Acute gastrointestinal illness (AGI) of unknown etiology and *E. coli* O157:H7 were both reported in five out of the eight years, for 253 and 257 cases respectively. *Giardia* and *Naegleria* were both reported in four of the eight years for 252 and 17 cases respectively. Three organisms, *Leptospira*, Norwalk virus and *Legionella*, were reported in three of the eight years for 375, 48, and 45 cases respectively. The following six causes were mentioned in one year each out of the eight-year period: adenovirus 3 (595 cases), *E. coli* O157:H7 and *Shigella sonnei* mixture (80 cases), *Shigella flexneri* (35 cases), unknown etiology (33 cases), chemical (26 cases), and *Salmonella* serotype Java (3 cases). The primary settings for recreational water associated outbreaks are swimming pools, lakes or ponds, and hot tubs[9–13] (Table 54.3). Microbial hazards associated with marine and estuarine environments are discussed in the next section.

The risk associated with recreational exposure to pathogens has been assessed in epidemiologic studies by comparing disease or symptom incidence rates for swimmers versus non-swimmers, or swimmers exposed to recreational waters with varying levels of microbial pollution. Pruss[14] reviewed 22 published epidemiology studies and concluded that there was agreement in a strong association of gastrointestinal (GI) symptoms and exposure to waters containing enterococci, fecal streptococci, thermotolerant coliforms, and *E. coli*. Pruss' conclusion, based on evaluating epidemiologic designs, was that enterococci and fecal streptococci were the most reliable indicator organisms for GI symptoms associated with exposure to marine and fresh waters; and that *E. coli* was a reliable indicator organism in fresh water and nearly as reliable as enterococci in marine waters. The observed illness threshold values described in the studies evaluated by Pruss were low for the enterococci and fecal streptococci and higher for the thermotolerant coliforms.[14–16] As a practical matter, the methodologies for recovery of these indicator organisms are not precise when applied to environmental water samples. Consequently, the higher threshold values for the *E. coli* and thermotolerant coliforms[17–19] are a more pragmatic yardstick for predicting the causal relationship between swimming and illness.

Swimming pools are frequently the setting for infectious disease outbreaks. Factors determining microbiologic water quality of swimming pools include the free chlorine concentration and pH, as well as the rate of water filtration and recirculation. Wading pools used by infants and other children prior to toilet training are often the site of disease transmission. The shallow depth and relatively low water volume in these pools leads to faster disinfectant depletion rates (due to the effects of ultraviolet light) and a higher concentration of organic matter following accidental bowel movements.[20]

A variety of eukaryotic, viral and bacterial pathogens are transmitted through swimming pools. *Cryptosporidium*, one of the most important waterborne pathogens of the past decade,[9–13] is a frequent cause of recreational water-

borne outbreaks[21] (Table 54.2). The persistence of *Cryptosporidium* oocysts in swimming pools is due to the extreme resistance to inactivation by chlorine and inadequate filtration by conventional pool filters.[22] Outbreaks of conjunctivitis due to a variety of Adenovirus serotypes, gastroenteritis due to exposure to Norovirus, Enterovirus, or enterobacteria such as *Shigella* spp. and *Escherichia coli* are often linked to inadequately chlorinated pools.

Marine waters

Exposure to a diverse group of micro-organisms, including diatoms, dinoflagellates, microalgae, as well as blue-green algae (a bacterial species), has been linked to mild to severe neurologic and gastrointestinal complaints in coastal and estuarine environments throughout the world. Marine micro-organisms may be free-living, or associated with a variety of fish and shellfish species. Clearly, foodborne transmission for these agents is an important means of exposure, but the role of recreational or occupational exposure to these micro-organisms has been suspected and is being evaluated.

Scromboid, amnesic shellfish poisoning (ASP), diarrhetic shellfish poisoning (DSP), paralytic shellfish poisoning (PSP), and ciguatera fish poisoning (CFP) follow the ingestion of fish or shellfish contaminated with marine micro-organisms. In these diseases, microbial contamination leads to the accumulation of toxic compounds producing a variety of neurologic and gastrointestinal symptoms. The diseases are encountered throughout the world, at a low rate. The CDC estimates 30 cases per year and one fatality per four years in the USA.[4] Diagnosis is usually based upon symptoms and history of shellfish consumption. In most cases, treatment is limited to supportive care; however, specific therapies are available for scromboid and CFP.

Individuals exposed to coastal waters risk contact to marine micro-organisms through recreational or occupational exposure to the environment. Marine micro-organisms or their toxins may be ingested or contact skin and mucous membranes. Air-borne transmission of aerosolized microbes or toxins is also possible. Environmental exposure may play a role in the transmission of neurotoxic shellfish poisoning (NSP) as well as possible estuary associated syndrome (PEAS).

NSP is primarily thought of as a foodborne illness associated with the consumption of shellfish caught during red tides, which are blooms of a marine dinoflagellate, *Karenia brevis* (formerly *Gymnodinium breve*), that regularly occur along the Gulf of Mexico and Atlantic coasts of the USA. A *K. brevis* toxin, brevetoxin, is responsible for NSP symptoms, which include altered sensations in the mouth and extremities, dizziness, loss of co-ordination, muscle aches, and gastrointestinal symptoms. Brevitoxin may also be aerosolized when it is released from cells by lysis or excretion and incorporated into marine aerosol by wind and breaking surf along the coast.[23] Air samples taken during red tide conditions along the Atlantic and Gulf coasts of Florida, as well as the Atlantic coast of North Carolina, were measured at 160–180 ng/mm^2.[23] The CDC is currently conducting a study to assess the health effects of exposure to aerosolized red tide agent.[5]

Another disease in which recreational or occupational exposure is thought to be potentially involved is PEAS, which is associated with two species of marine dinoflagellate, *Pfiesteria piscicida* and *P. shumwayae*. *Pfiesteria* has been implicated in massive fish kills occurring in estuaries along the southeastern Atlantic coast of the USA. Fish and shellfish located at the site of *Pfiesteria* blooms are lethargic, disoriented, and contain ulcers.[24] Although water-soluble *Pfiesteria* toxins are hypothesized to exist, none have been isolated and characterized in the laboratory, or detected in the environment, and a recent report challenged the notion that *P. shumwayae* even has the capacity to produce dinoflagellate-like toxin.[25] Studies documenting the effects of *Pfiesteria* species on humans originated with observations of respiratory, gastrointestinal, optical, and neurologic symptoms following exposure to aerosol in a laboratory.[26] Subsequent retrospective epidemiologic investigations have compared the health status of symptomatic individuals in contact with *Pfiesteria* blooms to controls.[27,28]

Mild flu-like illness as well as learning and memory difficulties were reported to be associated with exposure, but exposure assessments other than self-report were not possible. A large prospective study was unable to identify health issues in a cohort of individuals with recreational or occupational exposure,[29] and a cross-sectional study comparing the health of watermen working either in estuaries (site of *Pfiesteria*-associated fish kills) or the ocean failed to find significant differences upon medical, neurologic, neuropsychologic, or neurobehavioral evaluation system 2 (NES-2) evaluation, but did note a significantly reduced visual contrast sensitivity among the estuarian watermen.[30] Further studies, especially those that specifically measure exposure to *Pfiesteria* or its toxins, are needed to establish PEAS as a human disease.[31]

OCCUPATIONAL POPULATIONS AT RISK

Individuals are exposed to pathogens by virtue of their occupational responsibilities. A good example is exposure of physicians and allied healthcare professionals to viruses (e.g., hepatitis B, C, D, and human immunodeficiency virus) present in blood and other clinical specimens. Likewise, some workers are routinely exposed to waterborne pathogens present in natural waters, as well as sewage and aerosols.

Workers exposed to cooling towers, industrial water conditioning, and water supplies

Closed water management systems, such as those used for water cooling, conditioning, and supply, are difficult to maintain, and often accumulate biofilms. These biofilms provide a protective niche for many waterborne protozoa and bacteria. From a medical perspective, an important inhabitant of biofilms is *Legionella* spp., the causative agent of legionnaire's disease. This bacterial pathogen may be associated with single-celled protozoa; when growing inside the protozoan, it is unaffected by relatively high levels of biocides.[32] Aerosols containing *Legionella* bacteria are created when the bacteria are shed into water, which is then sprayed or splashed. In this way, *Legionella* gains access to the respiratory systems by inhalation. Free-living *Legionella* spp. have also been isolated directly from waters and soils. *Legionella* bacteria have been recovered from water samples taken from cooling towers,[33] cooling systems,[34] and hospital water supplies,[35,36] and inhabit water fittings, pipework, and materials in hospital hot-water systems.[37] Large outbreaks have been associated with these water supplies.[38–40]

Waste water workers

Waste water is a complex mixture of potentially hazardous organisms and chemicals in water, and workers may be exposed to pathogens through ingestion, contact with the skin or mucosal surfaces, or by aerosol inhalation. The purpose of waste water treatment is to protect public health by collecting, transporting, and treating waste water. This treatment has greatly reduced the frequency of water-associated disease in the United States, but continues to have an enormous worldwide impact on populations.

Despite the seemingly high potential for hazardous exposures to waste water treatment workers, many reports suggest that the risk of infection, as measured by pathogen loads or seroprevalence, is similar to other segments of the working population.[41–44] Questionnaire-based prevalence studies have documented illness rates in waste water treatment workers. For example, Thorn and colleagues found an elevated risk of non-specific respiratory, gastrointestinal, and central nervous system symptoms among 1394 Swedish municipal sewage workers, compared to controls that were unexposed, or partially exposed to sewage.[45] Using factor analysis, Douwes and colleagues defined four symptom clusters reported by 147 Dutch sewage workers.[46] Two clusters ('flu-like illness' and 'neurological symptoms') were statistically significantly associated with exposure to sewage. Other studies[47,48] did not find significantly higher illness rates among sewage workers, although Pahren and Jakubowski did find that the rate of gastrointestinal illness in inexperienced waste water workers was 2–4 times higher than in experienced workers or the control group.

Although the results of epidemiologic studies are mixed, the potential for exposure to disease agents cannot be discounted. Samples taken from municipal sewage treatment plants or conveyance systems can potentially contain any or all of the pathogenic micro-organisms from the community served by the plant. Waterborne microbial pathogens relevant for sewage treatment workers can be divided into those causing respiratory tract, cutaneous, and enteric diseases. The etiologic agents may be bacteria, viruses, protozoans, or helminths. These organisms typically enter human hosts by ingestion, inhalation, or direct contact with dermal or mucosal surfaces.

Respiratory tract pathogens

Aerosolized waste water can transmit viral and bacterial microbes to the lungs of workers. Aerosols may also be deposited on food or the surfaces of objects (fomites). The microbes described below may become etiologic agents of respiratory disease. *Legionella* species can be found in waste water, but there is little published information about waste water workers' potential risk of infection. One reported outbreak of Pontiac fever (non-pneumonic legionellosis) demonstrates that treated industrial waste water from a food manufacturer may have contributed to their common infections with *Legionella* based on their antibody titers.[49] Notably, the *Legionella* serotype isolated from five workers matched that isolated from sewage sludge during the same time period, and a sludge centrifugation process was identified as a potential source of the aerosol.

Mycobacterium spp., bacteria which cause tuberculosis and skin ulcerations, have been identified from waters and waste water treatment plants, and aerosols created in those environments may offer a previously unexpected source of infection.[50,51] Additional waste waterborne organisms cause respiratory disease in other countries. One of these, *Burkholderia (Pseudomonas) pseudomallei*, causes a pneumonia known as meliodosis in sub-tropical Australia and tropical southeast Asia.[52] As waste water treatment plants modernize and become more enclosed for odor control, aerosols become a more important exposure route.

Cutaneous pathogens

Gram-negative bacilli constitute the largest group of aquatic pathogens causing skin infections.[53] Skin infections and rashes have been reported for a variety of organisms not typically considered to be associated with waste water, but these reports underscore the importance of the combination of exposure, agent, and susceptible host. *Staphylococcus*, *Enterococcus*, *Streptococcus*, and *Clostridium* have a clinical history of causing cutaneous infections, and in some instances, serious tissue necrosis. *Mycobacterium ulcerans* has been epidemiologically linked to skin ulcerations through contact with waste water.[54] *Pseudomonas* spp., *Aeromonas hydrophila*, and *Flavobacter* are other bacteria causing non-enteric diseases, typically rashes, but sometimes associated with toxin production and secondary sequelae.[52]

Enteric pathogens

Enteric bacteria are the predominant, pathogenic infectious agents in waste water, and a large variety of pathogenic and opportunistic bacteria can be detected (Table 54.4). Enteric bacteria commonly cause gastrointestinal disorders, but some cause health effects beyond the gastrointestinal tract. Over the last 20 years in the USA, pathogenic forms of *E. coli* (enterotoxigenic, enteropathogenic, enterohemorrhagic, and enteroaggregative) have been found in waste water.[55–57] Enterohemorrhagic *E. coli*

O157:H7 causes not only bloody diarrhea, but also hemolytic-uremic syndrome in children, which is characterized by renal failure and a high case fatality rate. In the USA, *Salmonella* and *Shigella* bacteria are responsible for infection associated with foods that have been irrigated with waste water.[58] However, the most severe form of salmonellosis, typhoid fever, is rarely seen in the US.

Pathogenic species of *Leptospira* can be acquired from water contaminated with the urine of infected animals, causing vomiting, high fever, severe headache, chills, and muscle aches, and may include abdominal pain, diarrhea, jaundice (yellow discoloration of skin and sclerae), red eyes, or a rash. Severe infections result in liver and kidney dysfunction and a high mortality rate.[59] Rodents, particularly rats, are common hosts of infection, but a variety of wild and domestic mammals can be infected. The organisms can survive for months in water, and isolation from waste water is not uncommon, particularly in tropical and semi-tropical climates.[60] Fewer than 100 cases of leptospirosis are reported each year in the United States.[8] Other bacteria causing gastrointestinal ailments include *Campylobacter*, *Helicobacter*, and *Arcobacter*.[61]

The most commonly detected viruses in waste water belong to the *Enterovirus* group of the Picornaviruses, which consists of small single-stranded RNA viruses and includes *Poliovirus*, *Echovirus*, and *Coxsackievirus*. Other viruses associated with waste water and fecal contamination include *Adenovirus*, *Aichi virus*, *Astrovirus*, hepatitis A and E, *Calicivirus*, and *Reovirus*. *Rotavirus* (a member of the Reoviridae) is the most infectious of all the enteric viruses and should be considered a high risk in waste water.[62]

Protozoan parasites such as *Entamoeba histolytica*, *Giardia intestinalis*, and *Cryptosporidium parvum* are recovered from waste water more frequently than from other environmental sources. These parasites are also recovered from natural fresh and estuarine waters in the USA and worldwide.[63–67] *Toxoplasma gondii* and *Cyclospora* are also frequently recovered from waste water. *Entamoeba histolytica* causes amebiasis (amebic dysentery), and more serious extraintestinal disease affecting the liver. *Giardia intestinalis (lamblia)* and *Cryptosporidium parvum* have been implicated in waterborne cases of diarrhea, with flatulence and greasy stools, primarily from drinking surface water and inadequate treatment systems. Non-human animals serve as secondary or carrier hosts. The recurring contamination of water and cycling of these organisms to humans creates an almost endless source of infection. Helminth parasites (worms) found in waste waters include *Ascaris lumbricoides* (roundworm), *Necator americanus* (hookworm), *Trichuris trichiuria* (whipworm), *Toxocara canis* (canine roundworms), and *Strongyloides stercoralis* (the agent of strongyloidiasis). These worms all have life cycles that are dependent on a host during part of the reproductive cycle, and produce infective cysts, the form likely to be encountered in waste water. Helminthic eggs/cysts that make it past the waste water treatment process may survive in soils and sludges for up to ten years.[68]

Type	Disease or syndrome caused	Amount in waste water	Infectious dose
Bacteria		Med to High	High
Aeromonas hydrophila	Enteritis (inflammation of the intestine)		High
Burkholderia pseudomallei	Meliodosis		High
Campylobacter	Enteritis, diarrhea		High
Clostridium perfringens	Enteritis (indicator)		High
Escherichia coli, pathogenic	Enteritis, diarrhea		High
Francisella tularensis	Tularemia		High
Leptospira	Jaundice, meningitis, Weil's disease		High
Listeria monocytogenes	Listeriosis		High
Mycobacterium	Tuberculosis, skin ulcers		High
Pseudomonas	Skin, ear infections		High
Salmonella (1700 types)	Enteritis, typhoid		High
Shigella (4 species)	Enteritis, diarrhea		Low*
Staphylococcus aureus	Skin infections		High
Vibrio cholerae and *V. parahaemolyticus*	Cholera, skin infections		High
Yersinia enterocolitica and *Y. pseudotuberculosis*	Enteritis		High
Helminths		Low	Low
Ascaris lumbricoides	Ascariasis		Low
Ancylostoma duodenale	Hookworm infections		Low
Trichuris trichiura	Trichiuriasis		Low
Taenia (tapeworm)	Taeniasis		Low
Toxocara	Abdominal pains		Low
Strongyloides	Abdominal pains		low
Protozoa		Low to Med	Low
Entamoeba histolytica and *Entamoeba coli*	Enteritis, chronic diarrhea, dysentery, liver abscess		Low
Giardia intestinalis	Giardiasis, enteritis		Low
Cryptosporidium parvum	Enteritis, diarrhea		Low
Ballantidium coli	Enteritis, diarrhea		Low
Naegleria fowleri	Meningoencephalitis		Low
Acanthamoeba spp.	Meningoencephalitis		Low
Viruses		Med to High	Low
Poliovirus (3 types)	Paralysis, meningitis		Low
Echovirus (34 types)	Meningitis, diarrhea		Low
Coxsackievirus A and *B* (30 types)	Meningitis, conjunctivitis, chronic fatigue syndrome, myocardia, diabetes		Low
Hepatitis A and E viruses	Epidemic 'infectious' hepatitis		Low
Enterovirus 68–71	Meningitis, conjunctivitis		Low
Rotavirus (+4 types)	Enteritis		Low
Reovirus (3 types)	Enteritis, respiratory		Low
Adenovirus (+40 types)	Enteritis, eye and respiratory		Low
Norwalk and Norwalk-like viruses	Gastroenteritis		Low
Calicivirus and *Astrovirus*	Enteritis		Low
Coronavirus	Enteritis		Low
Parvovirus (2 types)	Enteritis, respiratory in children		Low

* Low infectious dose means only a few viral particles/cells/cysts/eggs are required to cause infection; high indicates many are required to cause an infection.
Data from Feachem et al. 1983[256] and Payment 1991.[50]

Table 54.4 Diseases associated worldwide with pathogens in waste water and their relative loading

Agricultural workers

In 2002, people working in agriculture, forestry, fishing, hunting, and mining accounted for 1.8% of the US workforce.[69] These individuals may be exposed to disease sources having natural reservoirs in animals (zoonoses), may be specific for humans, may produce toxins, or may be commensals that have acquired genetic elements that express pathogenic traits. The risk posed by transmission of waterborne disease from the agriculture watershed to the population is substantial.[70] Virulent bacteria and parasites can remain viable in the watershed environment, become amplified by agricultural practices, or contaminate the food supply with toxin (as in the case of algal blooms) or pathogens. Surveillance of farm workers has demonstrated that water quality is a serious occupational

hazard.[71,72] Drinking water may be contaminated in the farm environment with pesticides, other agricultural chemicals, and microbes. Agricultural waste containing pathogens such as *Salmonella* spp., *E. coli* O157:H7, *Campylobacter*, *Cryptosporidium parvum*, and many others, can contaminate surface and ground water that is used as sources for drinking water, or for recreational contacts.

Manure and agricultural waste water

Agricultural workers are exposed to many waterborne organisms through their contact with animals, animal feces, and fecally contaminated soil and water. The principal fecal sources are livestock and poultry, followed by wildlife and companion animals.[70] Manure from cattle, horses, pigs, and poultry is routinely processed and used as farm and commercial fertilizer. An additional source of agricultural exposure to infectious agents is the use of biosolids (sludge) from municipal waste water treatment plants,[73] where pathogens surviving sewage treatment are a potential health threat. Protozoan cysts can survive in water as long as 180 days; helminth (worm) ova can survive in soil seven years; bacteria and viruses may live up to a year.[74,75] Additionally, fecally contaminated water from animal feeding operations may leach into surface or ground water. On-farm recycling can also release pathogens into the environment. Manure contains numerous eukaryotes (protozoa), as well as anaerobic, aerobic, and facultatively aerobic bacteria that contribute to the decomposition of manure.[76] For this reason, manure is stored and decomposed as an aerated liquid slurry concentrate. Sludge and lagoon water are removed periodically and applied to farmland. Unprocessed sewage may be carried from lagoons and storage ponds into overland flow or subsurface water. Obviously, the occupational hazards of waste water workers would also be applicable in these situations.

Waterborne hazards in the agricultural watershed include protozoa, bacteria, viruses, and helminths. *Cryptosporidium parvum* and *Giardia* spp. are the protozoal pathogens of primary concern. Of lesser concern are *Entamoeba histolytica*, *Toxoplasma gondii*, and *Balantidium coli*.[9–13,70] Anaerobic and facultatively anaerobic bacteria make up the bulk of the feces. In a study of bacteria obtained from chicken intestines, 70% of the contents of the ileum were related to the *Lactobacillus* genus, and the rest were related to *Clostridia*, *Streptococcus*, and *Enterococcus*.[77] In the cecum, clostridial relatives comprised 65%, and the remainder were related to *Fusobacterium*, *Lactobacillus*, and *Bacteroides*. Facultatively aerobic organisms belonging to genera *Escherichia*, *Klebsiella*, *Enterobacter*, and *Citrobacter*, among others (fecal coliforms), are used as measures of fecal contamination in the environment because they are easily cultured and nearly always present in fecal matter.

Pathogenic bacteria are also transmitted in the feces, and these include *Escherichia coli* O157:H7, *Streptococcus* spp., *Enterococcus* spp., *Campylobacter* spp., *Salmonella* spp., *Yersinia enterocolitica*, *Brucella* spp., and *Leptospira*.[9–13] Parasitic worms transmitted by feces include platyhelminths and *Ascaris* spp.[70] Human viruses present in human sewage include *Adenovirus*, *Astrovirus*, *Hepatitis*, *Noroviruses*, *Rotavirus*, and *Coxsackievirus*.[78] However, most viruses, unlike many bacteria, parasites and helminths, are host specific. Viruses present in animal feces having zoonotic potential include hepatitis E, and influenza virus.

Contamination of crops
One of the major causes of water- or food-borne outbreaks associated with the agricultural sector is the use of contaminated irrigation water. The use of partially treated or untreated waste water introduces waterborne pathogens into the irrigation system.[79–81] Additionally, pathogens may enter the watershed through the application of manure or other biosolids to the land.[70,82,83] In the USA, use of these biosolids is regulated by the EPA Part 503 Biosolids Rule. However, these regulations may not be stringent enough to remove thermally tolerant viruses.[84,85]

After waste water or biosolids are applied to land, waterborne pathogens may persist and contaminate vegetation and crops. The life cycle of waterborne parasites may be supported by intermediate hosts found in irrigation canals.[86] Pathogens may contaminate crops by adhering to leaf or root surfaces.[87,88] Additionally, recent studies have shown that *E. coli* O157:H7 can migrate to internal edible parts of the plant tissue and become inaccessible to disinfectants and surface cleaning.[82,83]

Other occupational hazards

Stojek and Dutkiewicz[89] investigated the possibility of *Legionella* infection among outdoor gardeners in eastern Poland. They found that potting soil as well as the aerosolized water from the sprinklers was contaminated with *Legionella*, and could pose a threat.

In healthcare settings *Legionella* bacteria were found in the water of dental units sampled from 28 dental facilities in six US states.[90] The *Legionella* spp. levels observed in the dental unit waters was 1000/ml or more in 36% of the samples collected, and 10,000/ml or more in 19% of the samples. In an investigation of *Legionella* infection in a dental office, Atlas and colleagues identified high levels of *Legionella* spp., *L. pneumophila* and *L. longbeachae* in the dentist's operating area, suggesting that aerosols from dental units were the source of the *Legionella* infection.

WATERBORNE BACTERIAL PATHOGENS

Bacteria represent a diverse group of microbes that live in a wide variety of environments. Depending on the taxonomic subgroup, they may produce spores, survive in distilled water, remain alive for centuries in salt deposits, live endosymbiotically in protozoa, fungi, or insects, or synthesize toxins that in tiny amounts can cause substantial human illness or death.

Aeromonas

Introduction
Aeromonas species are free-living, facultatively anaerobic, gram-negative rods found in fresh water and sewage. *Aeromonas hydrophila* causes illness in fish, reptiles, amphibians, ducks and other water birds, and mammals, including humans.[91,92] Some *A. hydrophila* strains may produce a toxin that can cause diarrheal symptoms in patients.[93] *A. hydrophila* cultured from stool specimens grows readily on the differential media used to culture enteric gram-negative rods, and can easily be confused with the enteric bacteria.[94]

Clinical symptoms
Two distinct types of gastroenteritis have been associated with *A. hydrophila*: a cholera-like illness with watery diarrhea, and a dysenteric illness characterized by loose stools containing blood and mucus.[91] It also causes cellulitis and

other primary or nosocomial infections.[91,94] *A. hydrophila* can be found in blood of individuals with seriously impaired host defenses or endocarditis. It is occasionally isolated from the feces of patients with diarrhea.[94]

Mode of transmission

Aeromonas hydrophila is a motile rod commonly isolated from water, soil, or food, and occasionally from the human intestinal tract. It can cause freshwater wound infections.[94] Transmission may be via water, food or, more rarely, person to person.

Control measures

Most *Aeromonas* strains are susceptible to tetracyclines, aminoglycosides, and cephalosporins that can be used for the treatment.[94]

Escherichia coli

Introduction

Escherichia coli belongs to a large bacterial family, the Enterobacteriaceae, which lives in the intestinal tracts of animals. *E. coli* is a facultatively anaerobic gram-negative rod that adheres to mucus overlying the inside of the large intestine. It is acquired orally shortly after birth from other individuals, foods, or water. Many strains are sensitive to antibiotics. *E. coli* is a consistent inhabitant of the human intestinal tract and so its presence in nature is used as an indicator of fecal pollution and water contamination. Despite its role as a commensal organism in humans, *E. coli* is sometimes responsible for three types of infections: intestinal diseases (gastroenteritis), urinary tract infections (UTI), and neonatal meningitis.

The serotype O157:H7 of *Escherichia coli* has emerged as a significant pathogen from the enterohemorrhagic *Escherichia coli* (EHEC) group. Though commonly associated with foodborne illnesses, waterborne occurrence is also observed. Two potent toxins involved in the clinical complications of EHEC infection are Shiga-like toxins I and II. Shiga-like toxin I is identical to the cytotoxin produced by *Shigella dysenteriae*.[95] Antibiotic resistance genes are also frequently present in pathogenic strains. Drinking unchlorinated well water or accidental swallowing of water while engaging in recreational activities has been responsible for hundreds of cases.[96,97] Cattle are the primary reservoirs of EHEC. Humans can also act as a reservoir in the cases of human-to-human transmission. The pathogen can be shed for a week or less in adults, though three weeks is the common excretion period observed. A prolonged carriage is comparatively infrequent.[95]

Clinical symptoms

Pathogenic *E. coli* strains are classified as localized, diffuse, or aggregative, and typically cause fever, abdominal cramps, nausea, vomiting, and diarrhea. Diarrhea is often bloody. The incubation period for the illness ranges from one to ten days, with a median of 3–4 days. The pathogen is typically shed for a week or less in adults, but may be

found for up to three weeks. Clinical complications of the illness include hemolytic-uremic syndrome and thrombotic thrombocytopenic purpura. Uropathogenic *E. coli* colonize from the feces or perineal region and ascend the urinary tract to the bladder, causing typical urinary tract infection symptoms of dysuria, urgency, and frequency; the urine may be cloudy, foul smelling, and bloody.

Mode of transmission

Cattle are a primary reservoir of EHEC. Consumption of insufficiently cooked meat previously contaminated with *E. coli* O157:H7 during slaughter is one of the major causes of *E. coli* O157:H7 outbreaks. Humans can act as reservoirs in human-to-human transmission. A fecal–oral route of transmission is observed, with transmission from the diarrheal stools of an infected person to others, if inadequate personal hygiene is followed. Other common sources of infection include contaminated sprouts, lettuce, salami, unpasteurized milk, juice, sewage-contaminated water, and swimming in water contaminated with *E. coli* O157:H7.

Susceptibility and resistance

The infective dose of *E. coli* O157:H7 appears to be less than ten organisms. *E. coli* O157:H7 is susceptible to heat. Thus cooking meat or boiling water will help prevent transmission. Strains that have acquired pathogenicity factors may be resistant to tetracycline, ampicillin, erythromycin, trimethoprim-sulfamethoxazole, and amoxicillin/clavulanate.

Control measures

Drinking pasteurized milk, juice, or cider will help prevent the transmission of the pathogen. Chlorine or other commercially used disinfectants can kill *E. coli* O157:H7.

Helicobacter pylori

Introduction

Helicobacter pylori (formerly *Campylobacter pylori*) is a spiral-shaped bacterium found in the gastric mucous layer or adherent to the epithelial lining of the stomach. *H. pylori* causes more than 90% of duodenal ulcers and up to 80% of gastric ulcers. It is estimated that over half of the world's population may be infected with *H. pylori*. In the United States, *H. pylori* is most prevalent among older adults, African-Americans, Hispanics, and lower socioeconomic groups.[98]

Clinical symptoms

H. pylori causes chronic active, persistent, atrophic gastritis, as well as duodenal and gastric ulcers in adults and children. Infected persons have a 2–6-fold increased risk of developing gastric cancer and mucosal-associated lymphoid-type lymphoma compared with uninfected counterparts. The most common ulcer symptom is gnawing or burning pain in the epigastrium, most severe when the stomach is empty, between meals, and in the early morning hours. Other ulcer symptoms may include nausea, vomiting, loss of appetite, and bleeding; prolonged bleeding may cause anemia, weakness, and fatigue. Bleeding may be associated with hematemesis, hematochezia, or melena.[99]

Mode of transmission

It is not clearly understood how *H. pylori* is transmitted or why some patients become symptomatic while others do not. The bacteria are most likely spread from person to person through fecal–oral or oral–oral routes.[100] Possible environmental reservoirs include contaminated water sources.[101] Iatrogenic spread through contaminated endoscopes has been documented, but can be prevented by proper cleaning of equipment.[102]

Control measures

Therapy for *H. pylori* infection consists of ten days to two weeks of a regimen of effective antibiotics, such as amoxicillin, tetracycline (not to be used for children <12 years), metronidazole, or clarithromycin, plus either ranitidine bismuth citrate, bismuth subsalicylate, or a proton pump inhibitor.[103] Acid suppression by the H2 blocker or proton pump inhibitor therapy in conjunction with the antibiotics helps alleviate abdominal pain and nausea, heal gastric mucosal inflammation, and enhance antibiotic efficacy against *H. pylori* at the gastric mucosal surface.

Legionella pneumophila

Introduction

The research so far has identified more than 30 species and at least 14 serogroups of *Legionella pneumophila*. The most common strain responsible for more than 90% of known infections is the Pontiac sub-type (MAb2).[104] The *Legionella* species have often been observed to inhabit soil, rivers, and lakes. These organisms can colonize man-made water handling and storage systems. *Legionella* are often observed to inhabit cooling towers, evaporative condensers, showers, water storage, distribution systems, and other aquatic systems such as whirlpool spa baths.[104] *L. pneumophila* was shown to grow intracellularly in amebae, like *Acanthamoeba, Hartmannella, Valkampfia*, and *Naegleria* spp., and in other protozoa, like ciliates of the *Tetrahymena pyriformis* group.[105–110] Not only do these hosts provide nutrients for *Legionella* organisms, they also protect them from adverse environmental conditions.[111] Legionellosis has two distinct presentations: legionnaire's disease, the more severe form of infection, which includes severe pneumonia; and Pontiac fever, a flu-like illness without associated pneumonia.[111]

Clinical symptoms

Common symptoms include pneumonia with fever, chills, cough with variable sputum, prominent myalgias, headache, tiredness, loss of appetite, and diarrhea.[94,103] Persons with Pontiac fever experience fever and myalgias, but do not have pneumonia. They generally recover in 2–5 days without treatment. Incubation periods for legionnaire's disease and for Pontiac fever are 2–10 days, and 5–66 hours, respectively.[103]

Mode of transmission

Legionella spp. have often been observed to be associated with cold and hot water distribution systems, heaters, pools, and spas.[111] Persons may be exposed to these mists in homes, workplaces, hospitals, or public places. Legionellosis is not passed from person to person,[103] and there is no evidence of persons becoming infected from auto air conditioners or household window air-conditioning units.

Control measures

High dose erythromycin is the antibiotic currently recommended for treating persons with legionnaire's disease. In severe cases, a second drug, rifampin, may be added. Other drugs such as newer macrolides, clarithromycin, and azithromycin are also found to be effective.[103] Pontiac fever typically has a self-limited course, even without treatment. Improved design and maintenance of cooling towers and plumbing systems to limit the growth and spread of *Legionella* organisms are the foundations of legionellosis prevention.

Leptospira

Introduction

Leptospires are obligate aerobes that may be stained using carbol fuchsin counterstain. They produce both catalase and oxidase and have an optimum growth temperature of 28–30 degrees C. These tightly coiled, thin, flexible spirochetes are 5–15 μm long with very fine spirals 0.1–0.2 μm wide.[94] One end of the microbe is often bent into a distinctive hook and there are two internally located flagellar bundles for translational motility. Leptospirosis is a zoonosis of ubiquitous distribution, caused by infection with pathogenic *Leptospira* species passed in animal urine. The complex taxonomy of leptospires, previously based on serology, has been modified by genotypic classification.[112]

Clinical symptoms

Leptospirosis is particularly common in tropical regions. The spectrum of human leptospirosis ranges from subclinical infection to a severe syndrome of multi-organ infection with high mortality (Weil's disease). The incubation period ranges from four to 19 days.[95] Disease can develop in two phases: the first acute phase lasts about a week and includes fever, chills, headache, myalgias, vomiting, diarrhea, and occasionally skin rash. The second or immune phase produces antibody response and shedding of Leptospira.[113] Other symptoms may include aseptic meningitis, with intense headache, stiff neck, and pleocytosis in the cerebrospinal fluid.[114] Uveitis is a well-known late complication of systemic leptospirosis.

Mode of transmission

Rats, mice, wild rodents, dogs, swine, and cattle have been identified as the primary sources of zoonotic *Leptospira* infection, passing it through urine. *Leptospira* is ingested with contaminated food or water or can enter through skin lesions and mucous membranes.[114] Transmission can occur through contact with contaminated water, moist soil, vegetation, animals, or urine.[103] US military personnel serving in tropical regions are at risk for infection.[112]

Control measures

The epidemiology of leptospirosis is influenced by changes in animal husbandry, climate, and human behavior.[112] Once contracted by a person, the treatment of choice is antibiotic therapy (doxycycline, penicillin or tetracycline).[94] Control consists of preventing exposure to potentially contaminated water and reducing contamination by rodent control.

Plesiomonas shigelloides

Introduction

Plesiomonas shigelloides is a ubiquitous, facultatively anaerobic gram-negative rod with a polar flagellum. It is found in wells and unfiltered, untreated surface water. *P. shigelloides* is most common in tropical and subtropical areas. Most isolates from humans have been from stool cultures of patients with diarrhea. *P. shigelloides* grows on the differential media used to isolate *Salmonella* and *Shigella* from stool specimens. Some *Plesiomonas* strains share antigens with *Shigella sonnei*, so cross-reactions with *Shigella* A and C antisera do occur.[94]

Clinical symptoms

Symptoms usually occur within 48 hours of exposure. *P. shigelloides* produces self-limited diarrhea with blood or mucus, abdominal cramps, and vomiting or fever.[115]

Mode of transmission

Plesiomonas shigelloides is transmitted by drinking or preparing food with untreated water, eating uncooked shellfish, or traveling to developing countries.[116–118] It has been isolated from freshwater fish and this has been postulated as a source of transmission as well.[119]

Control measures

Routine testing for total fecal coliform bacteria, turbidity, and chlorine residual may enable early detection of fecal contamination and rapid decontamination. Disinfection with chlorine and filtration of potable water systems have substantially reduced waterborne outbreaks and subsequent morbidity and mortality. Agricultural runoff should not be used for drinking or food preparation.

Pseudomonas aeruginosa

Introduction

Pseudomonads are gram-negative, motile, aerobic rods, some of which produce water-soluble pigments. They are ubiquitous in soil, water, plants, animals, and moist environments such as hospitals.[94] Of the two million nosocomial infections in the US each year, 10% are caused by *P. aeruginosa*.[120] It is a common cause of pneumonia in inten-

sive care unit (ICU) settings. *Pseudomonas* infections can be spread within hospitals by healthcare workers, medical equipment, sinks, disinfectant solutions, and food.[120] Multidrug-resistant (MDR) *Pseudomonas aeruginosa* infection has been widely described in cystic fibrosis patients; some hospital units have MDR *P. aeruginosa* rates as high as 40%.[121] MDR *P. aeruginosa* occurs in isolated outbreaks in intensive care units, hematologic units, and among immunocompromised patients, including oncology and HIV patients.[121] *Pseudomonas aeruginosa* is both a frank pathogen and an opportunist, dependent almost entirely on the host susceptibility.

Clinical symptoms

P. aeruginosa infects skin, soft tissues, urinary tracts, eyes, ear, central nervous system, bones, joints, heart, and lung. Infection causes a similarly large range of symptoms, consistent with bacteremia: fever, inflammation, rash, myalgias, swelling, and other organ-specific symptoms (e.g., respiratory symptoms of dyspnea and cough). Wounds and burns can give rise to meningitis through hematogenous spread. *P. aeruginosa* invasion of the blood stream can lead to fatal sepsis. Hemorrhagic necrosis of skin (ecthyma gangrenosum) occurs often in sepsis due to *P. aeruginosa*. *P. aeruginosa* exotoxin A causes tissue necrosis that can be lethal.[94]

Mode of transmission

Pseudomonas is primarily a nosocomial pathogen, and it may be passed person to person or environmentally. The organism thrives in moist environments, including sinks, water baths, showers, hot tubs, and other wet areas.[94] It may be indigenous to water supplies or distribution systems if chlorine residuals are inadequate, or if water in long runs of distribution pipe is inadequately circulated.

Susceptibility and resistance

The most active antimicrobial agent against *P. aeruginosa* isolates is amikacin, in a study of 10,361 isolates at centers in the United States during 1995–2000.[122] It is important to assess sensitivities given the toxicity of aminoglycoside therapy. MDR *P. aeruginosa* and some other pseudomonads may be non-responsive to ciprofloxacin, ceftazidime, imipenem, gentamicin, and piperacillin.[121] Three-drug combinations are sometimes the only effective treatment.

Control measures

Pseudomonas infections should not be treated with single-drug therapy, as the bacteriocidal response rate is low with such therapy, and organisms can rapidly develop resistance for a single drug.

Shigella sonnei

Introduction

Shigella are gram-negative, non-motile, non-spore forming rod-shaped bacteria. Approximately 18,000 cases of shigellosis are reported in the United States every year.[123] *Shigella sonnei* (serogroup D) accounts for two-thirds of these. *Shigella sonnei* may be differentiated from the other *Shigellae*; however, the other species cannot be separated without serotyping, including *Shigella dysenteriae* (serogroup A), *Shigella flexneri* (B), and *Shigella boydii* (C).[124] In the CDC surveillance period 1991–2000, approximately 1700 people in the US developed shigellosis infection; one-third of these were due to contaminated drinking water and the remainder were associated with recreational water sources. Shigellosis accounts for less than 10% of the reported outbreaks of foodborne illness in the USA, and is frequently found in water polluted with human feces.

Clinical symptoms

Shigellosis involves the large and distal small intestine, and is characterized by diarrhea, fever, vomiting, stomach cramps, occasional toxemia, and tenesmus. Illness can be self-limited, and in some cases only a watery diarrhea occurs. More frequently, stools contain blood and mucus (dysentery) as a result of mucosal ulceration and confluent colonic crypt microabscesses. The incubation period ranges between 12 hours to one week, and lasts for about 4–7 days. Convulsions are an important complication in young children.[95]

Mode of transmission

Direct or indirect fecal–oral transfer is the primary route of transmission. Flies can facilitate transmission of the pathogen from feces to food. Drinking or swimming in contaminated water is another form of transmission.[95]

Susceptibility and resistance

A recent retrospective study found that most *Shigella* isolates are susceptible to ceftriaxone, ciprofloxacin, and gentamicin, but resistant to ampicillin and trimethoprim-sulfamethoxazole.[125]

Control measures

Improved hygiene in food handling, bathing in hot springs, and chlorine disinfection of potable water systems will reduce person-to-person transmission, outbreaks, and subsequent morbidity and mortality.

Salmonella typhimurium

Introduction

There are numerous pathogenic serotypes of *Salmonella*, although *Salmonella typhimurium* and *salmonella enteritidis* are the most common serotypes in the United States.[123] The vast majority of the more than 2500 serovars belong to one species: *S. enterica* (formerly *cholerasuis*[124]). *Salmonella* infections are common throughout the world. The incidence rate is highest in infants and young children. About 60–80% of cases are sporadic, though large outbreaks can be associated with hospitals, restaurants, and institutional settings, including nursing homes and orphanages. The common reservoirs of salmonellosis are domestic and wild animals, including poultry and fowl (including eggs), swine, cattle, rodents, and pets such as iguanas, tortoises, turtles, terrapins, chicks, dogs, and cats. Mild and asymptomatic human cases can also act as a carrier.[126]

Clinical symptoms

The typical clinical symptoms include frequent fever, headache, abdominal pain, diarrhea, nausea, and vomiting. Severe dehydration frequently occurs in elderly and infant cases. Anorexia and diarrhea may be experienced for several days. Septicemia and focal infection can develop as the illness progresses beyond the phase of acute enterocolitis,[95] including septic arthritis, cholecystitis, endocarditis, meningitis, pericarditis, pneumonia, pyoderma, pyelonephritis, and tissue abscesses. The incubation period ranges from six to 72 hours, with a median of 12–36 hours. An exposure dose of 100–1000 organisms is generally required, although for some highly virulent strains the infectious dose (ID) is thought to be as few as ten organisms.[95] A temporary carrier state is often observed for months in infants.

Mode of transmission

Salmonella inhabit the intestinal tracts of humans, animals, and birds, therefore the fecal–oral route is the most common. This is often mediated by water and food.

Susceptibility and resistance

HIV infected persons are at a higher risk of non-typhoidal *Salmonella* septicemia.

Control measures

Measures that will help reduce the risk of *Salmonella* transmission include pasteurization of milk, treatment of municipal water supplies, improvements in farm and animal hygiene, and wider use of egg pasteurization.[123]

Campylobacter jejuni

Introduction

Campylobacter jejuni belongs to the group of spiral shaped bacteria. Ninety-nine percent of the human illnesses of campylobacteriosis are caused by *Campylobacter jejuni*.[127] The common reservoirs for the pathogen are poultry, cattle, puppies, kittens, other pets, swine, sheep, rodents, and birds.[128] *Campylobacter* grows best at the body temperature of birds (40–42 degrees C), but some important species (e.g., *C. jejuni var.* doyle) will not grow at 42 degrees C, but rather at 37 degrees C.[129]

Foodborne campylobacteriosis is more common than waterborne campylobacteriosis. A waterborne outbreak at the Washington County Fair in New York in 1999 is one of the significant outbreaks of *Camplyobacter jejuni*, where a total of 781 cases were identified in conjunction with *E. coli* O157:H7.[130]

Over the period of 1991–2000, a total of five outbreaks affecting 340 people, and one outbreak affecting six people, were reported in association with drinking water and recreational water, respectively.[9–13]

Clinical symptoms

Campylobacteriosis is characterized by diarrhea, cramps, abdominal pain, and fever. The stools may be bloody, with mucus and WBCs in diarrheal stools. Occult blood can also be observed in the stools. A typhoid-like syndrome, with reactive arthritis, febrile convulsions, Guillain–Barré syndrome, and meningitis can also occur.[127] Severe gastroenteritis may mimic acute appendicitis. The onset of illness is usually observed between 2–5 days after exposure, though it can range between 1–10 days. Clinical illness usually lasts 2–5 days but in prolonged cases may last up to ten days.[131]

Mode of transmission

Birds, especially chicken flocks, are the most common reservoir of the pathogen. The organism is easily spread from bird to bird through a common water source or contact with the infected feces.[131] Primarily transmission can occur by handling raw poultry, or eating raw or undercooked poultry meat. Previous studies have reported that larger outbreaks are associated with drinking unpasteurized milk or contaminated water.[127] Infection can also be facilitated by contact with stools of an infected animal.

Susceptibility and resistance

The organism cannot survive drying, and tolerates poorly an oxygen-rich environment.

Control measures

Simple prevention measures can help control *Campylobacter jejuni* transmission, including avoiding consumption of uncooked meat or consumption of unpasteurized milk and untreated surface water.

Mycobacteria

Introduction

Mycobacteria are rod-shaped, non-spore forming, aerobic bacilli with thick, multi-layered lipid-rich walls. Mycobacteria are fastidious extracellular bacteria requiring special culture conditions, supplemented media, and prolonged incubation time. Nonetheless, they cause disease in a wide variety of vertebrates, including humans, livestock, birds, and fish. A number of *Mycobacterium* species are waterborne, including but not limited to *Mycobacterium avium*, *Mycobacterium intracellulare*, *Mycobacterium scrofulaceum*, *Mycobacterium marinum*, and *Mycobacterium chelonae*. *Mycobacterium avium* and *Mycobacterium intracellulare* grow in natural water sources and drinking water over a temperature range of 10–45 degrees C.[132] Mycobacteria species may be both saprophytic and pathogenic. Their growth rates are much slower than those of most other bacteria.

Clinical symptoms

Symptoms depend on the route of infection. In respiratory infection, symptoms include those associated with pneumonia as well as wheeze, bronchitis, and asthma.[133] Cutaneous infection results in granulomatous lesions of the skin.[53]

Mode of transmission

Cell surface hydrophobicity permits adherence to solid substrates (e.g., pipes or leaves) in aquatic environments, which results in Mycobacteria's persistence and resistance to being washed away.[133] Mycobacteria can colonize dental units and drinking water sources. Pulmonary illness and infection have been a consequence of exposure to aerosols generated by hot tubs, spas, and coolant baths, including hypersensitivity pneumonitis in occupants of water-damaged buildings, swimming pool attendants, and workers exposed to metal working fluid.

Susceptibility and resistance

Immunocompromised individuals and the elderly are particularly susceptible to mycobacterial infection.

Control measures

Mycobacterium are very resistant to the disinfectants used in water treatment, including chlorine and ozone.[133] Water filtration removes particulates that carry Mycobacteria; their numbers can be reduced using UV light or high temperatures (e.g., 40 degrees C), surfactants, or detergent-like disinfectants.

Vibrio cholerae

Introduction

Vibrio species are among the most common bacteria in surface waters worldwide. They are curved, gram-negative, aerobic rods, and are motile, possessing a polar flagellum. They do not form spores. *Vibrio cholerae* serogroup O1 and related Vibrio species cause cholera in humans, while other Vibrio species may cause sepsis or enteritis. Vibrio species are members of the family Enterobacteriaceae, including the medically important species *V. cholerae* serogroup O1, *V. cholerae* serogroup non-O1, *V. parahaemolyticus*, *V. mimicus*, *V. vulnificus*, *V. hofisae*, *V. fluvialis*, *V. damsela*, *V. alginolyticus*, and *V. metschnikovii*.[94]

Clinical symptoms

After an incubation period of less than a day to five days, depending on size of the inoculum,[134] there is a sudden onset of nausea and vomiting accompanied by profuse diarrhea with abdominal cramps. The stools resemble 'rice water' and contain mucus, epithelial cells, and large numbers of Vibrio bacteria. There is rapid loss of fluid and electrolytes, which leads to profound volume depletion that can lead to circulatory collapse, and anuria. The mortality rate without treatment is 25–50% in some epidemics.[135,136]

Mode of transmission

Worldwide epidemics of cholera occurred in the 1800s and early 1900s. The 'classic' biotype was prevalent through the early 1960s; the El Tor biotype, discovered in 1905, became prevalent in the late 1960s and has caused pandemic disease in Asia, the Middle East, and Africa.[94] The disease has been rare in North America since the mid-1800s, but an endemic focus may exist on the Gulf Coast of Louisiana and Texas.[94] From the endemic areas, the disease can be carried along shipping lanes, trade routes, and migration routes, and spread by individuals with mild or early illness and by water, food, flies, and person-to-person contact. The carrier state seldom exceeds 3–4 weeks, and true chronic carriers are rare. Vibrio species survive in water for up to three weeks.[94]

Therapy

The most important part of therapy consists of water and electrolyte replacement to correct the severe volume and electrolyte depletion. Many antimicrobial agents are effective against *V. cholerae*. Oral tetracycline tends to reduce stool output in cholera and shortens the period of excretion of bacteria.[94]

WATERBORNE VIRAL PATHOGENS

Waterborne viruses are present in large numbers in a variety of marine environments.[137,138] Exposure to waterborne viruses may occur by drinking or recreational use of contaminated water, or following the consumption of improperly cooked marine or freshwater molluscs, which capture and concentrate viruses and other pathogens. Additionally, contaminated natural water or inadequately treated human or animal sewage can be put to agricultural use, exposing workers, crops and, potentially, consumers to waterborne viral pathogens. The diseases associated with waterborne viruses include acute gastroenteritis, hepatitis, conjunctivitis, acute respiratory disease, and meningitis.

Since viruses are at least an order of magnitude smaller than bacteria or protozoa and many are structurally and biochemically distinct, methods that rely on bacterial indicators, such as the coliform count, do not detect or enumerate viruses in samples of treated water accurately.[139] Newer methods, such as the use of bacteriophage indicators, quantitative PCR, and outgrowth on mammalian cell culture, are considered to be more reliable.

Waterborne viruses have properties that determine their distribution and stability in the environment, as well as the methods required to detect, enumerate, and purify them from contaminated water. First, waterborne viruses possess a capsid consisting primarily of protein subunits fitting together to form a structure with higher order symmetry. The capsid makes these viruses extremely resistant to non-ionic detergents, compared to enveloped viruses, which derive their outer layer from a biologic membrane of their host cell. Second, the genetic material of waterborne viruses, unlike bacteria or protozoa, may consist of single- or double-stranded forms of DNA or RNA. Molecular methods used to detect the presence of viruses in water samples commonly rely on PCR, which utilizes a thermostable DNA polymerase. Because this enzyme amplifies DNA, but not RNA molecules, viruses with RNA genomes must first be converted to a DNA copy. This is often accomplished with an RNA-dependent DNA polymerase (reverse transcriptase), although a new polymerase capable of both activities is available commercially.

This section will focus on six virus families that pose health hazards to humans, and are known to be present in untreated and treated waters. The virology, clinical, and epidemiologic manifestations of the diseases and methods of detection in water are discussed below.

Adenovirus

Introduction

The Adenovirus (Ad) family includes more than 50 distinct types producing respiratory, ophthalmic, and enteric syndromes in humans. The Ad DNA genome is complex, encoding numerous polypeptides, and variation in gene content may explain the tissue tropism and biologic character distinguishing these Ad types.

Clinical symptoms

Waterborne adenoviruses of medical and public health importance lead to cases of conjunctivitis and gastroenteritis. Human adenovirus of types 3, 4, and 7 are commonly responsible for adenoviral hemorrhagic conjunctivitis (AHC), identified by the presence of small subconjunctival hemorrhages, inflammation of the corneal epithelium and upper respiratory disease. AHC appears 4–12 days (average eight days) following exposure. Infections with Ad types 8, 19, or 37 can lead to epidemic keratoconjunctivitis (EKC) 5–12 days following exposure. Other Ad types have also been linked to both AHC and EKC. Enteric Ads of types 40 and 41 are associated with cases of acute gastrointestinal disease, typically in children less than four years old and immunocompromised individuals. Symptoms typically appear in 8–10 days, and may last 1–2 weeks. Outbreaks are commonly set in daycare centers, hospitals, and nursing homes, and particularly affect immunocompromised individuals.[140]

Transmission

Although Ad conjunctivitis is often due to direct or indirect contact with eye discharge, outbreaks have been linked to inadequately chlorinated swimming pools or inadequate disinfection of eye washing stations in work settings, and ophthalmic solutions in physician offices. Enteric Ad infections are typically transmitted via the fecal–oral route. Enteric Ads are often found in natural and treated water samples, and the presence of Ad is not correlated with bacterial indicator organisms.[141–143]

Detection

A variety of diagnostic methods are typically used to detect and type adenovirus infections, including direct visualization by electron microscopy, serum neutralization, immunologic methods (immune fluorescence, enzyme linked immunoassay, and hemagglutination inhibition assay), virus isolation on permissive cell lines and PCR-restriction fragment length polymorphism. The latter two methods are useful for detection of Ads in environmental samples.

Control and prevention
Outbreaks of AHC and EKC can be prevented by assuring the sterility of instruments and hands contacting the conjunctiva (with systemic sterilization or the use of disposable equipment and gloves). Maintaining the proper concentration of free chlorine in swimming pools will prevent transmission of adenovirus in swimming pools. Adenoviral vaccines are not available in the US.

Calicivirus

Introduction
The Calicivirus family consists of encapsidated RNA viruses that were once described as 'small, round structured viruses', because of their uniform size and shape when viewed by electron microscopy. Two Calicivirus subgroups are currently believed to infect humans: Sapovirus (formerly 'Sapporo-like virus') and Norovirus (formerly 'Norwalk-like virus').

Clinical symptoms
Noroviruses are a very common cause of acute non-bacterial gastroenteritis in the developed world. Symptoms, which include acute-onset nausea and vomiting, watery non-bloody diarrhea with abdominal cramps, fever, myalgias, appear 24–48 hours following exposure and last 24–60 hours.

Mode of transmission
Outbreaks often occur when large groups are exposed to a common source of infection, which could be contact with an infected individual, contaminated food, or water. Fecal–oral transmission is undoubtedly important, but other routes, such as inhalation of aerosolized virus[144] or ingestion of virus attached to objects or surfaces, are likely. Water plays an important role in the transmission of viruses during outbreaks, as well as sporadic cases. Although few studies have definitively demonstrated the presence of Calicivirus in natural and treated waters, exposure to water has been independently associated with infection during outbreaks,[145–148] and virus, often having a nucleic acid sequence identical to virus shed by cases, has been isolated from water sources implicated in some outbreaks.[145,149,150] The settings for Calicivirus outbreaks have been restaurants, hospitals, cruise ships, vacation resorts, schools, concerts, and nursing homes.[149,151–153] Unlike many other gastroenteritis viruses, Calicivirus infects individuals of all ages, and adults are often associated with outbreaks. This suggests that virus-specific immunity is short-lived or unable to cross-neutralize viral variants.[44]

Detection
The use of electron microscopy and serology to diagnose Calicivirus infections is being replaced by tests using RT-

PCR amplification of viral genomes extracted from stool or environmental samples. The nucleic acid sequence of genes amplified using these tests can be determined and compared to sequences obtained from environmental specimens to link cases and potential sources or vectors.

Prevention and control
Fastidious hygienic measures, including frequent hand washing, will prevent many cases. However, because virus may be present in aerosol and is stable in the environment, outbreak sites should be thoroughly cleaned to prevent further transmission. Shellfish, which often contains Caliciviruses, should be thoroughly cooked

Picornaviruses

Introduction
The Picornavirus family includes waterborne pathogens of medical and public health importance, including Enteroviruses (including the viruses that cause poliomyelitis), as well as hepatitis A virus. Picornaviruses are characterized by a small proteinaceous capsid enclosing a positive-sense RNA genome. The genetic organization of the picornaviral genome is similar, but nucleic acid sequences can be quite diverse.

Clinical symptoms
Important waterborne enteroviruses include coxsackieviruses and poliovirus. Multiple *Coxsackievirus* serotypes are responsible for transient cases of pharyngitis and myalgia as well as diseases with long-lasting sequelae including myocarditis, meningitis, and perhaps insulin-dependent diabetes. Rare cases of acute flaccid paralysis (AFP) are still caused by *Poliovirus*, although this virus is a target for worldwide eradication. Incubation periods for enterovirus infection range from 3–5 days for *Coxsackievirus* pharyngitis, to 3–31 days for poliovirus AFP. Enteroviruses may persist in the stool for several weeks following infection. Hepatitis A virus (HAV) causes significant food- or waterborne outbreaks throughout the world. The disease is characterized by symptoms, including jaundice, dark urine, fever, anorexia, abdominal pain, and malaise, that appear 15–50 days after exposure. Symptoms can last from 1–2 weeks to several months, and virus is shed to the stool for 1–3 weeks after exposure, often before the onset of illness. The HAV mortality rate is very low, but infection can be lethal, especially in the elderly and individuals with chronic liver disease.

Mode of transmission
Waterborne picornaviruses are commonly identified in samples of natural waters as well as waste water samples,[154–160] and exposure to recreational water or marine molluscs has been epidemiologically linked to some outbreaks,[161,162] especially in the case of hepatitis A.[163,164] Fecal–oral transmission is commonly observed with HAV, and common source outbreaks are often associated with contaminated food or water, or through an infected food handler. Because of the extraordinary heat and pH stability

demonstrated by the virus, even cooked items may be a source of infection. For example, HAV infectivity is partially retained in shellfish heated to 60 degrees C for one hour.[165] Other transmission routes may be epidemiologically important, including direct contact (via hands or fomites), sexual contact, and blood transfusion.

Detection
Picornaviruses may be detected by isolation in permissive cell culture and suckling mice. Serologic methods (virus neutralization, IgG and IgM ELISA) may be used to diagnose polio or HAV infection in unvaccinated individuals. RT-PCR and sequence analysis of amplified genes may be used to detect virus in the environment and among cases, and is an invaluable tool for tracing outbreaks

Control and prevention
Good personal hygiene practices are necessary to prevent fecal–oral transmission, as is access to clean water in developing nations. Food- and waterborne HAV can be destroyed by thorough cooking. Shellfish should be heated to 85–90 degrees C (185–194 degrees F) for four minutes, or steamed for 90 seconds prior to eating. Inactivated and attenuated (oral) poliovirus vaccines form the basis of a worldwide campaign to eradicate this virus. An inactivated HAV vaccine is available and highly effective even after a single dose, but is not routinely recommended for children less than two years of age, or for older children and adults in low-risk populations. HAV immunoglobulin (Ig) can prevent clinical symptoms if given within two weeks of exposure.

The presence of oral poliovirus vaccine (OPV) in water samples is an important issue in nations that are using OPV to eradicate AFP because OPV is capable of reverting to virulence and, in some documented instances, causing outbreaks.[166,167]

Hepatitis E

Introduction
Hepatitis E virus (HEV) is not assigned to a family, but these viruses, which consist of a positive-sense RNA genome enclosed within a compact, proteinaceous capsid, share genetic and morphologic characteristics with Caliciviruses and the Rubella virus family.

Clinical symptoms
Infection leads to a clinical disease similar to that caused by HAV, including a long (15–60 days) incubation period, and the presence of infectious virus in blood and stool prior to the appearance of symptoms. During outbreaks, symptoms are more common among older individuals. Mortality is generally low, except among women in their third trimester of pregnancy, where the case-fatality rate is about 20%.

Mode of transmission
The disease is endemic and outbreaks are common in developing countries in South Asia, North Africa, the Middle East, and Mexico, and especially in regions with poor sanitation infrastructure. HEV outbreaks are primarily linked to fecally contaminated water, although other transmission routes including food or infected food handlers have been observed. Household-based secondary transmission is rare.[168] In the industrialized nations, infection is usually confined to individuals traveling in endemic regions. Exposure estimates based on serologic surveys may be confounded by cross-reaction,[169] with related virus circulating in swine and other animals. The capacity of these viruses to cause human disease is currently under investigation, but they have not been linked to large disease outbreaks. Fecally contaminated water has been identified as an important HEV transmission route in epidemiologic investigations.[170–172] This predilection to waterborne transmission is underscored by surveys identifying HEV nucleic acid in samples of sewage, as well as natural and treated water collected throughout the world.[159,173,174] The public health significance of sewageborne HEV-like viruses remains to be determined.

Detection
HEV infection is usually confirmed by serologic identification of circulating IgM and IgG, or the presence of viral RNA in blood or stool by RT-PCR, tests which are not routinely available in the USA.

Prevention and control
Travelers to endemic areas of the world should be educated about precautions to prevent the acquisition of food and waterborne diseases, including HEV. This is especially true for women in the third trimester of pregnancy. Proper sanitation infrastructure is needed to control outbreaks in developing nations. HEV-specific therapy and vaccination are not available.

Rotavirus

Introduction
Rotavirus, an encapsidated, multisegmented double-stranded RNA virus belonging to the Reovirus family, is a common cause of severe gastroenteritis in children throughout the world. Rotavirus isolates are serologically distinguished into six groups, three (groups A, B, and C) of which appear to cause human disease. Rotaviruses have been isolated from animals, but zoonotic transmission does not occur.

Clinical symptoms
The virus induces a typical gastroenteritis, characterized by vomiting, watery diarrhea, and fever, 1–3 days after exposure. Symptoms may last 4–6 days, during which the patient excretes virus into stool. In most cases, prolonged excretion is not observed.

Mode of transmission
Rotavirus transmission is primarily through fecally contaminated food and water or contact with contaminated

surfaces, although the presence of virus in respiratory secretions may allow air-borne transmission. Most cases of symptomatic disease are found among children less than five years old. However, a large serogroup B rotavirus outbreak on mainland China affected mostly adults,[175] and there is evidence that adult Rotavirus gastroenteritis, caused by genotype G2 variant of a serogroup A virus, is the cause of some outbreaks in the USA.[176] The presence and stability of Rotavirus in a variety of natural and treated water[177–179] accounts for the epidemiologic importance of waterborne virus transmission.[160,180] However, it was not detected in two recent surveys of ground water in the USA.[181,182]

Detection

Infected individuals are usually identified by the demonstration of viral antigen in stool using an enzyme-linked immunoassay (ELISA), and may be confirmed with additional tests, including RT-PCR amplification of viral nucleic acid from stool.

Prevention and control

Since virus can survive for long periods on contaminated surfaces and in water, hygienic measures designed to prevent fecal–oral transmission may not be effective. Breastfeeding does not prevent infection, but significantly reduces the severity of diarrhea. A Rotavirus vaccine is currently not available in the USA.

Astrovirus

Introduction

Astrovirus are encapsidated, single-stranded, positive-sense RNA viruses that were first identified in 1975.[183] They have a star-like appearance when viewed by electron microscopy.

Clinical symptoms

Acute gastroenteritis caused by Astrovirus infection has a typical presentation, and is usually found in children throughout the world.[184–186] Adult infection is rarely observed, although outbreaks have occurred among the elderly residents of nursing homes. The importance of Astrovirus infection is probably under-recognized in the USA due to the lack of diagnostic capacity.

Mode of transmission

The primary mode of transmission is probably fecal–oral, although the stability of the virus may allow it to survive on and be transmitted by inanimate objects.[187]

Detection

The potential detection methodologies employed include EIA and RT-PCR.[184,186,187]

Prevention and control

Like Rotavirus, hygienic measures designed to prevent fecal–oral transmission may not be effective.

Other/emerging waterborne viruses

Other viruses linked to human disease and present in natural or treated waters include Circovirus, Torovirus, Picobirnavirus, and the Aichi virus, a newly identified member of the Picornavirus family.[188] Additionally, Caliciviruses associated with marine mammals are believed to be the source of land-based zoonoses.[189] The epidemiologic strength and public health importance of these associations remain to be determined.

WATERBORNE EUKARYOTIC PATHOGENS

Eukaryotes are living cells with organelles, including nuclei that contain the genetic material. They are generally large enough to be easily seen with a light microscope, and include protozoans, helminths, and fungi. The protozoans *Cryptosporidium parvum* and *Giardia intestinalis* are notifiable disease agents, requiring the notification of state public health physicians when they are found in patients.

Single-celled protozoan parasites typically have complex life cycles with specific intermediate host requirements. Most have at least two developmental forms: the vegetative 'trophozoite' and the cyst that can survive under adverse environmental conditions. Humans are host to nearly 300 species of parasitic worm and over 70 species of protozoa.[190] Protozoa come in all sizes; those that are best understood are much larger than bacteria, some even visible without a microscope. Protozoa often live freely in water, although parasites may prefer a host organism or may even be unable to reproduce in the environment.

Acanthamoeba

Introduction

Acanthamoeba is one of the protozoan Amebae parasites. It is found in most water, including fresh, brackish, sea, tap, bottled mineral, sewage, gastrointestinal washings, contact lens solution, and eyewash station water; it is also found in hot tubs, soil, dust, and air, and in heating, air-conditioning, ventilation, humidifiers, dialysis, and dental units.[191–194] *Acanthamoeba* has been cultured from the upper airways of apparently healthy people and may be part of the normal flora. It is one of several ameboid eukaryotic lineages that undergoes slow gliding movements (others include *Hartmannella*, *Valkampfia*, and *Naegleria*).[111] *Acanthamoeba* may be free-living, parasitic, or opportunistic. In response to dry or cold environmental conditions, the motile trophozoite transforms into the cyst, protected and easily distributed throughout the environment. Cysts survive in water, soil, and dust for a year, unaffected by freezing, many chemicals, and some medications used to treat the vegetative forms.

Keratitis and pneumonitis are the principal water-related syndromes caused by *Acanthamoeba* spp.[192,195–199]

Swimmers and diving activities in natural waters may offer an exposure route. In immunocompromised hosts, *Acanthamoeba* species also produce granulomatous amebic encephalitis, a chronic central nervous system disease.[200] Some sources cite the lower respiratory tract as one possible route of invasion, through the inhalation of cysts from air, aerosols, or dust. Another route may be via skin infections.[192,196,199,201]

Acanthamoeba may serve as a vector for pathogenic bacteria because it is host to *Legionella pneumophila*, *Vibrio cholerae*, *Mycobacterium avium*, and emerging pathogens, such as *Parachlamydia* and *Simkania*.[202,203] These endosymbionts can enhance *Acanthamoeba* virulence or behave as pathogens on their own. The *Parachlamydia* strain Hall's coccus, for example, is transmitted by these amebae and was associated with fever in patients who used humidifiers in Vermont.[204,205] *Acanthamoeba* hosts *L. pneumophila* and carries it in the cysts; *Mycobacterium avium* grows saprozoically on products secreted by *Acanthamoeba* and is found in the outer walls of the double-walled cysts.[206] Cysts may provide a reservoir for the bacteria when environmental conditions become unfavorable.

Clinical symptoms

Wearers of contact lenses (hard, soft, or extended wear lenses) may develop keratitis, which is a sensation of a foreign body in the eye, tearing, blurred vision, photophobia, blepharospasm, and swelling of the upper eyelid. Keratitis can progress to corneal abscess; severe pain may imply a deep, long-standing infection, chronic ulceration of the corneal epithelium, and eventual loss of vision. Non-specific symptoms may be falsely diagnosed as herpes simplex keratitis, herpes zoster, fungal, and bacterial infection.[207]

Mode of transmission

Acanthamoeba has been found in the upper respiratory tract of healthy people as well as people with compromised immune systems. Most episodes of keratitis follow water exposure, such as a history of swimming in lakes and ponds while wearing contact lenses.[196,199] *Acanthamoeba* infections are also linked to non-sterile home-made saline solutions for contact lenses.[199] *Acanthamoeba* enters skin or membranes through a cut or wound, or through the nostrils. Once inside the body, it can travel to the lungs and through the blood stream to other parts of the body, especially the central nervous system.

Susceptibility and resistance

Acanthamoeba is resistant to most commonly used antibacterial, antifungal, antiprotozoal, and antiviral agents. Some patients have been successfully treated using ketoconazole, miconazole, and propamidine isethionate.

Control measures

Inhalation of cysts in dust or water can be limited by using a respirator or breathing mask. Eye infection can be limited by adhering to strict contact lens hygiene and cleaning regimens and not wearing lenses in pools, hot tubs, lakes,

rivers, or oceans. *Acanthamoeba* is on the Candidate Contaminant List published by USEPA, and is undergoing consideration for regulation.

Entamoeba histolytica

Introduction

Entamoeba histolytica is one of the intestinal Amebae parasites. In the US, those at risk for amebiasis due to *E. histolytica* include travelers, immigrants, migrant workers, immunocompromised individuals, institutionalized individuals, and sexually active homosexual males.[208]

Clinical symptoms

The incubation period varies from one to four months. Four major intestinal syndromes are caused by infection: (1) asymptomatic colonization; (2) acute amebic colitis, presenting with lower abdominal pain, bloody stools, and fever; (3) fulminant colitis in children presenting with diffuse abdominal pain, profuse bloody diarrhea, and fever; and (4) ameboma, an asymptomatic lesion or a tender mass accompanied by symptomatic dysentery.[209] Parasites can become disseminated and cause fatal disease.

Mode of transmission

E. histolytica infects people worldwide. Transmission in water is common in developing countries, where human feces is sometimes used for fertilizer.[208]

Susceptibility and resistance

Metronidazole, chloroquine, and dehydroemetine are effective in the treatment of invasive amebiasis.[209,210]

Control measures

E. histolytica is controlled by improving hygiene, adequately disposing of fecal waste, and adequately washing fruits and vegetables.

Cryptosporidium parvum

Introduction

Cryptosporidium is a coccidian parasite that is present in large numbers in surface waters and that also lives in the intestines of animals and humans. Its outer shell helps it survive outside the body for long periods of time and makes it highly resistant to chlorine disinfection.[211] *Cryptosporidium parvum* is a common cause of drinking or recreational waterborne disease outbreaks in humans in the United States.[211]

Clinical symptoms

Diarrhea, loose or watery stool, and stomach upset caused by *Cryptosporidium parvum* persists for about two weeks. Illness can be accompanied by fever, and the severity of symptoms may increase or subside in cycles. Asymptomatic cases have also been observed.[211]

Mode of transmission

Cryptosporidium is transmitted by the fecal–oral route. It is found in soil, food, water, or surfaces contaminated with feces of infected humans or animals. It is acquired by accidental swallowing of water from swimming pools, hot tubs, jacuzzis, fountains, lakes, rivers, springs, ponds, or streams contaminated with feces from infected humans or animals.

Susceptibility and resistance

Cryptosporidium is highly resistant to chlorine and requires high levels and increased contact time for inactivation. *Cryptosporidium* can be viable for days in a swimming pool with public health mandated levels of chlorine.[13]

Control measures

Physical removal of the parasite from water by filtration has become an important component of municipal water treatment systems.[212] Filters must be capable of removing particles <1 μm to control *Cryptosporidium*.[212] *Cryptosporidium* is killed by boiling for one minute.[212]

Cyclospora cayetanensis

Introduction

Cyclospora cayetanensis is a Coccidia parasite previously known as a 'cyanobacterium-like' or 'coccidia-like' body (CLB). Cyclosporiasis is most common in tropical and subtropical areas. There are many life-cycle variations in the genus *Cyclospora*, so the complete life cycle of *C. cayetanensis* has not been fully described. Infected persons excrete the oocyst stage of *Cyclospora* in their feces. When excreted, oocysts are not infectious and require 5–13 days to sporulate and become infectious.[211,213] Parasites may be found in the jejunal enterocytes.

Clinical symptoms

Cyclosporiasis onset begins with one day of malaise and low-grade fever, followed by rapid onset of diarrhea.[213] Infection is characterized by nausea, anorexia, abdominal cramping, watery diarrhea, constipation, and weight loss.[214] Symptoms last an average of seven weeks.[215–217] In AIDS patients, infections tend to last up to four months.[218]

Mode of transmission

Transmission of *Cyclospora* directly from an infected person to someone else is unlikely. Indirect transmission occurs when an infected person contaminates the environment and oocysts have sufficient time in water or food to become infectious.[211]

Susceptibility and resistance

Trimethoprim-sulfamethoxazole is an effective treatment for *Cyclospora* infection.[211]

Control measures

Avoiding food or water that may be contaminated with stool is the best way to prevent infection. Reinfection can occur.

Giardia intestinalis

Introduction

Giardia is a flagellate parasite that lives in the intestine of infected humans or animals. Giardiasis is the most prevalent waterborne disease in the United States.[219] The causative agent, *Giardia intestinalis*, was at one time called *Giardia lamblia*. *Giardia* is the most commonly diagnosed intestinal parasite in US public health laboratories.[12] From 1976 to 1994 it was found to be the etiologic agent most frequently associated with drinking water in the US.[197] The cyst is the stage found most commonly in non-diarrheal feces. Cysts are hardy, surviving several months in cold water. Animals may serve as a reservoir in the wild.

Clinical symptoms

A wide range of clinical symptoms are observed with *Giardia* infection, including diarrhea, flatulence, bloating, weight loss, abdominal cramps, nausea, malabsorption, foul smelling stools, steatorrhea, fatigue, anorexia, and chills.[12] The incubation period for giardiasis is 3–25 days.[12] Asymptomatic infections can also be observed.[211] Most children under the age of five have been infected with *Giardia* at least once.[75]

Mode of transmission

The organism is transmitted by a fecal–oral route from person to person. *Giardia* cysts ingested with contaminated food or water develop into trophozoites that attach to the small intestine.[12,75] Encystation occurs as parasites transit toward the colon.

Susceptibility and resistance

Giardia is sensitive to metronidazole (Flagyl), quinacrine hydrochloride, and furazolidone. High temperatures decrease the viability of *Giardia* in the environment. *Giardia* survives a month at 21 degrees C, but cysts are killed in ten minutes at 54 degrees C.[27]

Control measures

Improved hygiene, with adequate disposal of fecal waste and washing of fruits and vegetables is the most effective control method. Use of granular filters and coagulation are effective against *Giardia*. Commonly used water disinfectants achieve adequate *Giardia* inactivation. Boiling water for one minute kills *Giardia* cysts.[75]

Isospora belli

Introduction

Isospora belli is a Coccidia parasite related to *Cryptosporidium* spp., *Cyclospora* spp., and *Toxoplasma* spp.[220] Humans are the only known host.[213] Intestinal involvement and symptoms are usually transient, unless the patient is immunocompromised.[220] *I. belli* has been associated with outbreaks of diarrhea in institutional settings, daycare centers, World War II veterans from the Pacific, immigrants, and individuals with HIV infection.

Clinical symptoms

Symptoms develop a week after *I. belli* oocyst ingestion, including diarrhea, weight loss, abdominal pain, cramping, and low-grade fever.[210,221] The disease is usually self-limiting; however, oocyst shedding may persist for 2–3 weeks after the patient recovers.[210,221,222] Chronic illness occurs occasionally in infants or in otherwise healthy adults.[223] Disseminated infection may result from ingestion of large numbers of oocysts.[220,224]

Mode of transmission

Infective *I. belli* sporulated oocysts are spread through ingestion of food and water contaminated with feces.[213,225]

Susceptibility and resistance

Several drugs will effectively treat *I. belli*: trimethoprim-sulfamethoxazole, co-trimoxazole, pyrimethamine-sulfadiazine, primaquine phosphate-nitrofurantoin, and primaquine phosphate-chloroquine-phosphate.[213]

Control measures

Prevention of disease can be accomplished with improved personal hygiene and sanitation to eliminate possible fecal–oral transmission from food, water, or environmental surfaces.[213]

Microsporidia

Introduction

Intestinal Microsporidia includes over 100 genera and 1000 species. They are obligate intracellular parasites found in both vertebrates and invertebrates.[213] At least four genera are implicated in human disease: *Encephalitozoon*, *Enterocytozoon*, *Pleistophora*, and *Vittaforma*.[226,227] *Enterocytozoon bieneusi* is known to have tissue specificity for the human intestinal tract.[228–230]

Clinical symptoms

Because the route of human infection has not been fully characterized, the incubation period for microsporidial disease is unknown. Most infections are found in association with HIV infection. Microsporidia can cause chronic diarrhea without blood, dehydration, weight loss greater than 10% of body weight, keratitis, conjunctivitis, hepatitis, peritonitis, myositis, central nervous system infection, renal disease, sinusitis, and disseminated disease.[229,213–235] It has been speculated that Microsporidia may be present at low levels in human populations, becoming activated if an individual's immune system is compromised.[228,236–240]

Mode of transmission

E. bieneusi appears to be a zoonotic pathogen.[241] Common environmental sources of Microsporidia include surface water and runoff. It is possible that Microsporidia may undergo human-to-human fecal–oral, urinary–oral, ocular inoculation, sexual, or transplacental transmission.[242–244] Respiratory transmission occurs by inhalation, aspiration of gastrointestinal contents, or hematogenous dissemina-

tion.[228] *E. bieneusi* can survive in 4 degrees C water for more than one year.

Susceptibility and resistance

Topical fumagillin appears to be successful against microsporidial keratoconjunctivitis.[245,246] *E. intestinalis* responds to albendazole therapy, but *E. bieneusi* does not. No other treatment success has been achieved.[230,239,247,248]

Control measures

Control can be facilitated with improved hygiene, adequate disposal of fecal waste, and washing of contaminated fruits and vegetables.

Naegleria

Introduction

Naegleria is one of the Amebae parasites, commonly found in soil and warm fresh water (lakes, rivers, and hot springs, unchlorinated swimming pools, and in warm water discharge pools from industrial plants).[213] In the United States, the disease is generally acquired while swimming and diving in freshwater lakes and ponds. Only *Naegleria fowleri* has been found to infect humans, causing primary amebic meningoencephalitis, a rapidly progressing meningoencephalitis that is almost always fatal. Significant numbers of *N. fowleri* are found in water with high concentrations of iron and manganese and in water layers containing filamentous cyanobacteria and eubacteria, which serve as food sources.

Clinical symptoms

Naegleria fowleri infection is accompanied by headache, fever, nausea and vomiting, stiff neck, encephalopathic symptoms of confusion, apathy, loss of balance and bodily control, seizures, and hallucinations. Infection often results in death within 7–10 days. The incubation period is 2–7 days. Other symptoms include abnormalities of taste and smell, seizures, cerebellar ataxia, nuchal rigidity, photophobia, palsies of the third, fourth, and sixth cranial nerves, and increased intracranial pressure and coma. Cardiac abnormalities may also develop. Subclinical infections are possible in healthy people when *N. fowleri* colonizes the nose and throat.[191,199,249,250] Eye infections may lead to blindness.[91]

Mode of transmission

Naegleria fowleri enters the body through the nose and travels to the brain and spinal cord while the person is swimming underwater or diving. Infection is most common during the dry, hot summer months, when the temperature is above 27 degrees C. The preferred environment for *N. fowleri* is the soil; however, heavy rains and runoff introduce this organism into lakes, ponds, and surface waters.[251,252] *N. fowleri* can also be associated with household washing and bathing.[252]

Susceptibility and resistance

Amphotericin B, an antifungal drug, is the only agent with established clinical efficacy in the treatment of *N. fowleri*, although therapy with this drug is not always effective and has been associated with adverse effects on the kidneys and other organs.

Control measures

Avoidance is the best control measure, achieved by not swimming in warm, fresh water, such as ponds or warm water discharge pools, or unchlorinated swimming pools or polluted waters.

Schistosomiasis

Introduction

Schistosoma are flukes (worms/helminths) belonging to the class Trematode. Flukes in infected humans are found in the liver and blood. Schistosomiasis occurs among people living in tropical and subtropical zones, with water-borne transmission from freshwater snails. In the US, schistosomiasis is principally found only in immigrants from endemic areas or Americans returning from endemic areas.[253] It is an occupational disease in people who are unable to avoid contact with untreated water.[254] Adult worms can live 20–30 years in the veins of the human abdominal cavity, with hundreds of eggs each day excreted in feces or urine. Affected occupations include agriculture, fishing, washing and bathing.

Clinical symptoms

Schistosoma symptoms vary with the species of worm and the phase of infection. Initial invasion of skin may cause itching and rash, heavy infestation may cause fever, chills, lymph node enlargement, and liver and spleen enlargement. Urinary symptoms include frequency, dysuria, and hematuria. Intestinal symptoms include abdominal pain and diarrhea (which may be bloody).

Mode of transmission

Transmission of the parasites does not occur in the United States because of lack of suitable snail hosts, although dermatitis due to avian schistosomes occurs in the Great Lakes region. There the typical hosts are migratory water birds, including shorebirds, ducks, and geese.[255]

Susceptibility and resistance

Schistosoma infection can be treated with praziquantel.

Control measures

Infection with *Schistosoma* can be avoided by eradication of snails and by avoiding swimming or bathing in untreated water from endemic areas.

References

1. World Health Organization. Global water supply and sanitation assessment 2000 report. Geneva: WHO, 2000. http://www.who.int/docstore/water_sanitation_health/ Globassessment/Global1.htm
2. US EPA. Ground water & drinking water drinking water contaminant candidate list. March 2, 1998, 63 FR 10273. United States Environmental Protection Agency. http://www.epa.gov/safewater/ccl/cclfs.html
3. Cooper RC. Disease risk among sewage plant operators: a review. Sanitary Engineering and Environmental Health Research Laboratory, Report 91-1. Berkeley: University of California, 1991.
4. CDC. Food-borne and Diarrheal Branch, Division of Bacterial and Mycotic Diseases. Atlanta: Centers for Disease Control, 2003. http://www.cdc.gov/ncidod/dbmd/food-borne/index.htm
5. CDC. Nationally Notifiable Infectious Diseases, United States 2003. Atlanta: Centers for Disease Control, 2003. http://www.cdc.gov/epo/dphsi/phs/infdis2003.htm
6. Levine WC, Stephenson WT, Craun GF. MMWR CDC Surveillance Summaries 1990; 39:1–13.
7. MacKenzie WR, Hoxie NJ, Proctor ME, et al. A massive outbreak in Milwaukee of *Cryptosporidium* infection tansmitted through the public water supply. N Engl J Med 1994; 331:161–7.
8. CDC. Summary of notifiable diseases, United States, 1998. MMWR 1999; 47.
9. CDC/MMWR. Surveillance for waterborne disease outbreaks, United States, 1991–1992. MMWR Surveillance Summaries November 19, 1993; 42(SS-05):1–22.
10. CDC. Surveillance for waterborne disease outbreaks, United States, 1993–1994. MMWR Surveillance Summaries April 12, 1996; 45(SS-1):1–33.
11. CDC/MMWR. Surveillance for waterborne disease outbreaks, United States, 1995–1996. MMWR Surveillance Summaries December 11, 1998; 47(SS-5):1–34.
12. CDC/MMWR.. Surveillance for waterborne disease outbreaks, United States, 1997–1998. MMWR Surveillance Summaries May 26, 2000; 49(SS04):1–35.
13. CDC/MMWR. Surveillance for waterborne disease outbreaks, United States, 1999–2000. Surveillance Summaries November 22, 2002; 51(SS08);1–28.
14. Pruss A. Review of epidemiological studies on health effects from exposure to recreational water. Int J Epidemiol 1998; 27:1–9.
15. Cabelli VJ, Dufour AP, McCabe LJ, Levin MA. Swimming-associated gastroenteritis and water quality. Am J Epidemiol 1982; 115(4):606–16.
16. Zmirou D, Ferley JP, Balducci F, et al. Evaluation of microbial indicators of health risk related to river swimming places. Rev Epidemiol Sante Publique 1990; 38:101–10.
17. Cheung WH, Chang KC, Hung RP. Variations in microbial indicator densities in beach waters and health-related assessment of bathing water quality. Epidemiol Infect 1991; 106(2):329–44.
18. Seyfried PL, Tobin RS, Brown NE, Ness PF. A prospective study of swimming-related illness. II. Morbidity and the microbiological quality of water. Am J Public Health 1985; 75:1071–5.
19. Van Asperen IA, Medema G, Borgdorff MW, Sprenger MJW, Havelaar AH. Risk of gastroenteritis among triathletes in relation to faecal pollution of fresh waters. Int J Epidemiol 1998; 27:309–15.
20. CDC. Surveillance data from swimming pool inspections – selected states and counties, United States, May–September 2002. MMWR 2003; 52(22):513–6.
21. Carpenter C, Fayer R, Trout J, Beach MJ. Chlorine disinfection of recreational water for Cryptosporidium parvum. Emerg Infect Dis 1999; 5:579–84.
22. CDC. Protracted outbreaks of Cryptosporidiosis associated with swimming pool use – Ohio and Nebraska, 2000. MMWR 2001; 50(20):406–10.
23. Pierce RH, Henry MS, Blum PC, et al. Brevetoxin concentrations in marine aerosol: human exposure levels during a Karenia brevis harmful algal bloom. Bull Environ Contam Toxicol 2003; 70:161–5.
24. Swinker M, Tester P, Koltai Attix D, Schmechel D. Human health effects of exposure to *Pfiesteria piscicida*: a review. Microbes Infect 2002; 4:751–62.

25. Berry JP, Reece KS, Rein KS, et al. Are Pfiesteria species toxicogenic? Evidence against production of ichthyotoxins by *Pfiesteria shumwayae*. Proc Natl Acad Sci USA 2002; 99:10970.

26. Glasgow HB Jr, Burkholder JM, Schmechel DE, Tester PA, Rublee PA. Insidious effects of a toxic estuarine dinoflagellate on fish survival and human health. J Toxicol Environ Health 1995; 46:501–22.

27. Grattan LM, Oldach D, Perl TM, et al. Learning and memory difficulties after environmental exposure to waterways containing toxin-producing Pfiesteria or Pfiesteria-like dinoflagellates. Lancet 1998; 352(9127):532–9.

28. Haselow DT, Brown E, Tracy JK, et al. Gastrointestinal and respiratory tract symptoms following brief environmental exposure to aerosols during a pfiesteria-related fish kill. J Toxicol Environ Health A 2001; 63:553–64.

29. Moe CL, Turf E, Oldach D, et al. Cohort studies of health effects among people exposed to estuarine waters: North Carolina, Virginia, and Maryland. Environ Health Perspect 2001; 109(Suppl 5):781–6.

30. Swinker M, Koltai D, Wilkins J, et al. Estuary-associated syndrome in North Carolina: an occupational prevalence study. Environ Health Perspect 2001; 109:21–6.

31. Samet J, Bignami GS, Feldman R, Hawkins W, Neff J, Smayda T. Pfiesteria: review of the science and identification of research gaps. Report for the National Center for Environmental Health, Centers for Disease Control and Prevention. Environ Health Perspect 2001; 109(Suppl 5):639–59.

32. Fields BS, Benson RF, Besser RE. Legionella and Legionnaires' disease: 25 years of investigation. Clin Microbiol Rev 2002; 15:506–26.

33. Tobin RS, Ewan P, Walsh K, Dutka B. A survey of Legionella pneumophila in water in 12 Canadian cities. Water Res 1986; 20:495–501.

34. Kusnetsov JM, Martikainen PJ, Jousimies-Somer HR, et al. Physical, chemical and microbiological water characteristics associated with the occurrence of Legionella in cooling tower systems. Water Res 1993; 27:85–90.

35. Best M, Yu VL, Stout J, Goetz A, Muder RR, Taylor F. Legionellaceae in the hospital water-supply. Epidemiological link with disease and evaluation of a method for control of nosocomial legionnaires' disease and Pittsburgh pneumonia. Lancet 1983; 2(8345):307–10.

36. Sabria M, Garcia-Nunez M, Pedro-Botet ML, et al. Presence and chromosomal subtyping of Legionella species in potable water systems in 20 hospitals of Catalonia, Spain. Infect Control Hosp Epidemiol 2001; 22:673–6.

37. Emmerson AM. Emerging waterborne infections in health-care settings. Emerg Infect Dis 2001; 7:272–6.

38. Fraser DW, Tsai TR, Orenstein W, et al. Legionnaires' disease: description of an epidemic of pneumonia. N Engl J Med 1977; 297:1189–97.

39. Formica N, Tallis G, Zwolak B, et al. Legionnaires' disease outbreak: Victoria's largest identified outbreak. Commun Dis Intell 2000; 24:199–202.

40. Garcia-Fulgueiras A, Navarro C, Fenoll D, et al. Legionnaires' disease outbreak in Murcia, Spain. Emerg Infect Dis 2003; 9:915–21.

41. Clark CS, Linnemann CC, Clark JG, Gartside PS. Enteric parasites in workers occupationally exposed to sewage. J Occup Med 1984; 26:273–4.

42. Clark CS, Linnemann CC Jr, Gartside PS, Phair JP, Blacklow N, Zeiss CR. Serologic survey of rotavirus, Norwalk agent and *Prototheca wickerhamii* in waste water workers. Am J Public Health 1985; 75:83–5.

43. Clark CS, Linneman CC. The use of serum antibody as a means to determine infections from exposure to waste waters and refuse. CRC Crit Rev Environ Control 1986; 16:305–26.

44. Glas C, Hotz P, Steffen R. Hepatitis A in workers exposed to sewage: a systematic review. Occup Environ Med 2001; 58:762–8.

45. Thorn J, Beijer L, Rylander R. Work related symptoms among sewage workers: a nationwide survey in Sweden. Occup Environ Med 2002; 59:562–6.

46. Douwes J, Mannetje A, Heederik D. Work-related symptoms in sewage treatment workers. Ann Agric Environ Med 2001; 8:39–45.

47. Friis L, Agreus L, Edling C. Abdominal symptoms among sewage workers. Occup Med (Lond) 1998; 48:251–3.

48. Pahren H, Jakubowski W, eds. Waste water aerosols and disease. Proceedings of a symposium. US Environmental Protection Agency publication No. EPA-600/9-80-028. Washington DC: EPA, 1980.

49. Gregersen P, Grunnet K, Uldum SA, Andersen BH, Madsen H. Pontiac fever at a sewage treatment plant in the food industry. Scand J Work Environ Health 1999; 25:291–5.

50. Payment P. Waste water chlorination from a public health microbiology perspective. Ottawa: Health and Welfare Canada, 1991.

51. Szabo I, Kiss KK, Varnai I. Epidemic pulmonary infection associated with *Mycobacterium xenopi* indigenous in sewage-sludge. Acta Microbiol Acad Sci Hung 1982; 29:263–6.

52. Ashbolt NJ, Ball A, Dorsch M, et al. The identification and human health significance of environmental aeromonads. Water Sci Technol 1995; 31:263–70.

53. Elko L, Rosenbach K, Sinnott J. Cutaneous manifestations of waterborne infections. Curr Infect Dis Rep 2003; 5:398–406.

54. Johnson PDR, Veitch MGK, Leslie DE, Flood PE, Hayman JA. The emergence of *Mycobacterium ulcerans* infection near Melbourne. Med J Aust 1996; 165:76–8.

55. Muniesa M, Jofre J. Occurrence of phages infecting *Escherichia coli* O157:H7 carrying the Stx 2 gene in sewage from different countries. FEMS Microbiol Lett 2000; 183:197–200.

56. Tanji Y, Mizoguchi M, Yoichi M, et al. Seasonal change and fate of coliphages infected to *Escherichia coli* O157:H7 in a waste water treatment plant. Water Res 2003; 37:1136–42.

57. Grant SB, Pendroy CP, Bellin CL, Mayer JK, Palmer CJ. Prevalence of enterohemorrhagic *Escherichia coli* in raw and treated municipal sewage. Appl Environ Microbiol 1996; 62:3466–9.

58. Bryan FL. Diseases transmitted by foods contaminated by waste water. J Food Protect 1977; 40:45–59.

59. Speelman, P. Leptospirosis. In: Fauci AS, Braunwald E, Isselbacher KJ, et al, eds. Harrison's principles of internal medicine, 14th edn. New York: McGraw-Hill, 1998.

60. Wilson R, Fujioka R. Development of a method to selectively isolate pathogenic leptospira from environmental samples. Water Sci Technol 1995; 31:275–82.

61. Wesley IV. Helicobacter and Arcobacter species – risks for foods and beverages. J Food Protect 1996; 59:1127–32.

62. Gerba CP, Rose JB, Haas CN. Sensitive populations: who is at the greatest risk? Int J Food Microbiol 1996; 30:113–23.

63. Ferguson CM, Coote BG, Ashbolt NJ, Stevenson IM. Relationships between indicators, pathogens and water quality in an estuarine system. Water Res 1996; 30:2045–54.

64. Haas CN, Rose JB. Distribution of Cryptosporidium oocysts in a water supply. Water Res 1996; 30:2251–4.

65. Ho BSW, Tam TY, Hutton P, Yam WC. Detection and enumeration of Giardia cysts in river waters of Hong Kong by flocculation-percoll/sucrose gradient-immunofluorescence method. Water Science and Technology 1995; 31:431–434.

66. Ongerth JE, Hunter GD, DeWalle FB. Watershed use and Giardia cyst presence. Water Res 1995; 29:1295–9.

67. Wallis PM, Erlandsen SL, Isaac-Renton JL, Olson ME, Robertson WJ, van Keulen H. Prevalence of Giardia cysts and Cryptosporidium oocysts and characterization of Giardia spp. isolated from drinking water in Canada. Appl Environ Microbiol 1996; 62:2789–97.

68. Khuroo MS. Ascariasis. Gastroenterol Clin North Am 1996; 25:553–77.

69. US Census Bureau 2000. United States Department of Commerce. http://www.census.gov/acs/www/Products/Profiles/Chg/2002/0102/Tabular/010/01000US3.htm

70. Rosen BH. Waterborne pathogens in agricultural watersheds. Technical note. Raleigh: Watershed Science Institute, 2000.

71. National Occupational Research Agenda. Surveillance of hired farm worker health and occupational safety. Atlanta: NIOSH, 1998.

72. Vela-Acosta MS, Bigelow P, Buchan R. Assessment of occupational health and safety risks of farmworkers in Colorado. Am J Ind Med 2002; 2:19–27.

73. Page AL, Gleason TL III, Smith JE Jr, Iskander JK, Sommers LE. Utilization of municipal wasterwater and sludge on land. Riverside: University of California,1983.

74. Kelly WR. Animal and human health hazards associated with the utilization of animal effluents. In: A workshop in the EEC: programme of coordination of research on effluents, November 21–23. Dublin, Ireland: Commission of the European Communities, 1978.

75. EPA. Giardia: drinking water fact sheet. Office of Water, 4304. Washington DC: United States Environmental Protection Agency, 2000. http://www.epa.gov/waterscience/humanhealth/microbial/giardiafs.pdf

76. Chastain JP, Henry S. Manure management. Florence: Agricultural Research & Extension in the Pee Dee Region of South Carolina, Clemson University, 2003. http://www.clemson.edu/peedeerec/

77. Lu J, Idris U, Harmon B, et al. Diversity and succession of the intestinal bacterial community of the maturing broiler chicken. Appl Environ Microbiol. 2003; 69(11):6816–24.

78. Awwa Research Foundation. Workshop on emerging pathogens. Denver: Awwa RF, 1999.

79. Fasciolo GE, Meca MI, Gabriel E, Morabito J. Effects on crops of irrigation with treated municipal waste waters. Water Sci Technol 2002; 45:133–8.

80. Okafo CN, Veronica JU, Musa G. Occurrence of pathogens on vegetables harvested from soils irrigated with contaminated streams. Sci Total Environ 2003; 311:49–56.

81. Shuval HJ. Waste water irrigation in developing countries: health effects and technical solutions. Technical paper 51. Washington DC: World Bank, 1990;35–38.

82. Solomon EB, Yaron S, Matthews KR. Transmission of *Escherichia coli* O157:H7 from contaminated manure and irrigation water to lettuce plant tissue and its subsequent internalization. Appl Environ Microbiol 2002; 68:397–400.

83. Solomon EB, Potenski CJ, Matthews KR. Effect of irrigation method on transmission to and persistence of *Escherichia coli* O157:H7 on lettuce. J Food Protect 2002; 65:673–6.

84. Gerba CP, Pepper IL, Whitehead LF 3rd. A risk assessment of emerging pathogens of concern in the land application of biosolids. Water Sci Technol 2002; 46:225–30.

85. Committee on Toxicants and Pathogens in Biosolids Applied to Land. Biosolids applied to land. Washington DC: National Academy of Sciences, 2002.

86. Bizuneh A, Birrie H, Debele K. Colonization of irrigation canals by *Bulinus abyssinicus* and upsurge of urinary schistosomiasis in the middle Awash Valley of Ethiopia. Ethiopian Med J 1995; 33:259–63.

87. Amahmid O, Asmama S, Bouhoum K. The effect of waste water reuse in irrigation on the contamination level of food crops by Giardia cysts and Ascaris eggs. Int J Food Microbiol 1999; 49:19–26.

88. Armon R, Gold D, Brodsky M, Oron G. Surface and subsurface irrigation with effluents of different qualities and presence of Cryptosporidium oocysts in soil and on crops. Water Sci Technol 2002; 46:115–22.

89. Stojek NM, Dutkiewicz J. Legionella in sprinkling water as a potential occupational risk factor for gardeners. Ann Agric Environ Med 2002; 9:261–4.

90. Atlas RM, Williams JF, Huntington MK. Legionella contamination of dental-unit waters. Appl Environ Microbiol 1995; 61:1208–13.

91. FDA. Bad Bugs Book. Food-borne pathogenic micro-organisms and natural toxins handbook. Washington DC: Center for Food Safety & Applied Nutrition, US Food & Drug Administration, 2003. http://www.cfsan.fda.gov/~mow/chap17.html

92. WILDPro 2003. *Aeromonas hydrophila*. The Electronic Library. http://212.187.155.84/pass_06june/Lists_Diseases/Disease.htm

93. Haque QM, Sugiyama A, Iwade Y, et al. Characterization of *Aeromonas hydrophila*: a comparative study of strains isolated from diarrheal feces and the environment. Southeast Asian J Trop Med Public Health 1996; 27:132–8.

94. Jawetz E, Melnick JL, Adelberg EA. Pseudomonas, acinetobacter, aeromonas and plesiomonas. In: Review of medical microbiology, 17th edn. Norwalk: Appleton & Lange, 1987.

95. APHA. In: Chin J, ed. Control of communicable diseases manual, 17th edn. Washington DC: American Public Health Association, 2000;155–8.

96. New York State Department of Health. Novello AC, MD, MPH, Commissioner. 2000. The Washington County Fair outbreak report.

97. Public Health Dispatch: Outbreak of *Escherichia coli* 0157:H7 and *Campylobacter* among attendees of the Washington County Fair–New York, 1999. MMWR Weekly 1999; 48:803–5.

98. Taylor DN, Parsonnet J. Epidemiology and natural history of *H. pylori* infections. In: Blaser MJ, Smith PF, Ravdin J, Greenberg H, Guerrant RL, eds. Infections of the gastrointestinal tract. New York: Raven Press, 1995;551–64.

99. CDC. *Helicobacter pylori* and peptic ulcer disease. Division of Bacterial and Mycotic Diseases. http://www.cdc.gov/ulcer/history.htm

100. Thomas JE, Gibson GR, Darboe MK, Dale A, Weaver LT. Isolation of *Helicobacter pylori* from human feces. Lancet 1992; 340:1194–5.

101. Klein PD, Graham DY, Gaillour A, Opekun AR, Smith EO. Water source as risk factor for *Helicobacter pylori* infection in Peruvian children. Lancet 1991; 337:1503–6.

102. Tytgat GN. Endoscopic transmission of *Helicobacter pylori*. Aliment Pharmacol Ther 1995; 9(suppl 2):105–10.

103. Chin J. Control of communicable diseases manual, 17th edn. Washington DC: American Public Health Association, 2000.

104. Healthy Buildings International Pty Ltd. Legionella in building water systems: risk assessment and proactive monitoring. Data sheet. Pymble, NSW, Australia, HBI: 2001. http://www.hbi.com.au/contents.html

105. Barker J, Brown MRW, Collier PJ, Farrell I, Gilbert P. Relationship between *Legionella pneumophila* and *Acanthamoeba polyphaga*: physiologic status and susceptibility to chemical inactivation. Appl Environ Microbiol 1992; 58:2420–5.

106. Fields BS. Legionella and protozoa: interaction of a pathogen and its natural host. In: Barbaree JM, Breiman RF, Dufour AP, eds. Legionella: current status and emerging perspectives. Washington, DC: American Society for Microbiology, 1993;129–30.

107. Fields BS, Sanden GN, Barbaree JM, Morrill WE, Wadowsky RM. Intracellular multiplication of *Legionella pneumophila* in amoebae isolated from hospital hot water tanks. Curr Microbiol 1989; 18:131–37.

108. Newsome AL, Baker RL, Miller RD, Arnold RR. Interactions between *Naegleria fowleri* and *Legionella pneumophila*. Infect Immun 1985; 50:449–52.

109. Rowbotham TJ. Current views on the relationships between amoebae, Legionellae and man. Isr J Med Sci 1986; 22:678–89.

110. Wadowsky RM, Fleisher A, Kapp NJ, et al. Multiplication of virulent and avirulent strains of *Legionella pneumophila* in cultures of *Hartmannella vermiformis*. In: Barbaree JM, Breiman RF, Dufour AP, eds. Legionella: current status and emerging perspectives. Washington, DC: American Society for Microbiology, 1993;145–47.

111. Szewzyk U, Szewzyk R, Manz W, Schleifer KH. Microbiological safety of drinking water. Ann Rev Microbiol 2000; 54:81–127.

112. Levett PN. Leptospirosis. Clin Microbiol Rev 2001; 14:296–326.

113. Edwards GA, Domm DM. Human leptospirosis. Medicine 1960; 39:117–56.

114. Kelley PW. Leptospirosis. In: Gorbach SL, Bartlett JG, Blacklow NR, eds. Infectious diseases, 2nd edn. Philadelphia: WB Saunders, 1998;1580–7.

115. Holmberg SD, Wachsmuth IK, Hickman-Brenner FW, et al. Plesiomonas enteric infections in the United States. Ann Intern Med 1986; 105(5):690–4.

116. Soweid AM, Clarkston WK. Plesiomonas shigelloides: An unusual cause of diarrhea. Am J Gastroenterol 1995; 90:2235–6.

117. Jeppesen C. Media for Aeromonas spp., Plesiomonas shigelloides and Pseudomonas spp. food and environment. Int J Food Microbiol 1995; 26:25–41.

118. San Joaquin VH. Aeromonas, Yersinia, and miscellaneous bacterial enteropathogens. Pediatr Ann 1994; 23:544–8.

119. Van Damme LR, Vandepitte J. Frequent isolation of *Edwardsiella tarda* and *Pleisiomonas shigelloides* from healthy Zairese freshwater fish: a possible source of sporadic diarrhea in the tropics. Appl Environ Microbiol 1980; 39:475–9.

120. The Gale Encyclopedia of Medicine. 2002, *as cited by* Rowland B, 2002. Health A to Z. Your family health site. http://www.healthatoz.com/healthatoz/Atoz/ency/pseudomonas_infections.html

121. Tacconelli E, Tumbarello M, Bertagnolio S, et al. Multidrug resistant pseudomonas aeruginosa bloodstream infections: analysis of trends in prevalence and epidemiology. Emerg Infect Dis 2002; 8(2):220–1

122. Friedland I, Stinson L, Ikaiddi M, et al. Phenotypic antimicrobial resistance patterns in Pseudomonas aeruginosa and Acinetobacter: results of a Multicenter Intensive Care Unit Surveillance Study, 1995–2000. Diagn Microbiol Infect Dis 2003; 45(4):245–50.

123. CDC. 2003c. Shigellosis. Internet article. http://www.cdc.gov/ncidod/dbmd/diseaseinfo/shigellosis_g.htm

124. Holt JG, Krieg NR, Sneath PHA, Staley JT, Williams ST, eds. Bergey's manual of determinative bacteriology, 9th edn. Philadelphia: Williams and Wilkins, 1994.

125. Greenberg D, Marcu S, Melamed R, Lifshitz M. Shigella bacteremia: a retrospective study. Clin Pediatr (Phila) 2003; 42(5):411–5.

126. Refsum T, Hier E, Kapperud G, Vardund T, Holstad G. Molecular epidemiology of *Salmonella enterica* serovar Typhimurium isolates determined by pulse-field gel electrophoresis: comparison of isolates from avian wildlife, domestic animals and the environment in Norway. Appl Environ Microbiol 2002; 68:5600–6.

127. Tauxe RV. Epidemiology of *Campylobacter jejuni* infections in the US and other industrialized nations. In: Nachamkin I, Blaser MJ, Tomkins LS, eds. *Campylobacter jejuni*: current status and future trends. Washington DC: American Society for Microbiology, 1992;9–19.

128. Stern NJ. Reservoirs for *Campylobacter jejuni* and approaches for intervention in poultry. In: Nachamkin I, Blaser MJ, Tomkins LS, eds. *Campylobacter jejuni*: current status and future trends. Washington DC: American Society for Microbiology, 1992;49–60.

129. Goossens H, Butzler J-P. Isolation and identification of Campylobacter spp. In: Nachamkin I, Blaser MJ, Tomkins LS, eds. *Campylobacter jejuni*: current status and future trends. Washington DC: American Society for Microbiology, 1992;93–109

130. Novello AC. 2000. The Washington County Fair outbreak report. New York State Department of Health.

131. Skirrow MB, Blaser MJ. Clinical and epidemiological considerations. In: Nachamkin I, Blaser MJ, Tomkins LS, eds. *Campylobacter jejuni*: current status and future trends. Washington DC: American Society for Microbiology, 1992;3–8.

132. Jones JJ, Falkinham JO 3rd. Decolorization of malachite green and crystal violet by waterborne pathogenic mycobacteria. Antimicrob Agents Chemother 2003; 47:2323–6.

133. Falkinham JO, 3rd. Mycobacterial aerosols and respiratory disease. Emerg Infect Dis 2003; 9(7):763–767.

134. Levine MM, Black RE, Clements ML, Nalin DR, Cisneros L, Finkelstein RA. Volunteer studies in development of vaccines against cholera and enterotoxigenic *Escherichia coli*: a review. In: Holme T, Holmgren J, Merson MH, Mollby R, eds. Acute enteric infections in children. New prospects for treatment and prevention. Amsterdam: Elsevier, North-Holland Biomedical Press, 1981;443–59.

135. Morris JG Jr, Black RE. Cholera and other vibrioses in the United States. N Engl J Med 1985; 312:343–50.

136. Pierce NF, Mondol A. Clinical features of cholera. In: Barua D, Burrows W, eds. Cholera. Philadelphia: WB Saunders, 1974;202–20.

137. Culley AI, Lang AS, Suttle CA. High diversity of unknown picorna-like viruses in the sea. Nature 2003; 424(6952): 1054–7.

138. Griffin DW, Donaldson KA, Paul JH, Rose JB. Pathogenic human viruses in coastal waters. Clin Microbiol Rev 2003; 16:129–43.

139. Baggi F, Demarta A, Peduzzi R. Persistence of viral pathogens and bacteriophages during sewage treatment: lack of correlation with indicator bacteria. Res Microbiol 2001; 152:743–51.

140. Van R, Wun CC, O'Ryan ML, Matson DO, Jackson L, Pickering LK. Outbreaks of human enteric adenovirus types 40 and 41 in Houston day care centers. J Pediatr 1992; 120:516–21.

141. Van Heerden J, Ehlers MM, Van Zyl WB, Grabow WO. Incidence of adenoviruses in raw and treated water. Water Res 2003; 37:3704–8.

142. Jiang S, Noble R, Chu W. Human adenoviruses and coliphages in urban runoff-impacted coastal waters of Southern California. Appl Environ Microbiol 2001; 67:179–84.

143. Pina S, Puig M, Lucena F, Jofre J, Girones R. Viral pollution in the environment and in shellfish: human adenovirus detection by PCR as an index of human viruses. Appl Environ Microbiol 1998; 64:3376–82.

144. Marks PJ, Vipond IB, Regan FM, Wedgwood K, Fey RE, Caul EO. A school outbreak of Norwalk-like virus: evidence for air-borne transmission. Epidemiol Infect 2003; 131:727–36.

145. Kukkula M, Maunula L, Silvennoinen E, von Bonsdorff CH. Outbreak of viral gastroenteritis due to drinking water contaminated by Norwalk-like viruses. J Infect Dis 1999; 180:1771–6.

146. Boccia D, Tozzi AE, Cotter B, et al. Waterborne outbreak of Norwalk-like virus gastroenteritis at a tourist resort, Italy. Emerg Infect Dis 2002; 8:563–8.

147. Kaplan JE, Goodman RA, Schonberger LB, Lippy EC, Gary GW. Gastroenteritis due to Norwalk virus: an outbreak associated with a municipal water system. J Infect Dis 1982; 146:190–7.

148. Anderson AD, Heyford AG, Sarisky JP, et al. A waterborne outbreak of Norwalk-like virus among snowmobilers–Wyoming, 2001. J Infect Dis 2003; 187(2):303–6.

149. Brown CM, Cann JW, Simons G, et al. Outbreak of Norwalk virus in a Caribbean island resort: application of molecular diagnostics to ascertain the vehicle of infection. Epidemiol Infect 2001; 126:425–32.

150. Hafliger D, Hubner P, Luthy J. Outbreak of viral gastroenteritis due to sewage-contaminated drinking water. Int J Food Microbiol 2000; 54(1–2):123–6.

151. Moe CL, Christmas WA, Echols LJ, Miller SE. Outbreaks of acute gastroenteritis associated with Norwalk-like viruses in campus settings. J Am Coll Health 2001; 50:57–66.

152. Evans MR, Meldrum R, Lane W, et al. An outbreak of viral gastroenteritis following environmental contamination at a concert hall. Epidemiol Infect 2002; 129:355–60.

153. Fankhauser RL, Monroe SS, Noel JS, et al. Epidemiologic and molecular trends of "Norwalk-like viruses" associated with outbreaks of gastroenteritis in the United States. J Infect Dis 2002; 186(1):1–7.

154. Ali MA, Abdel-Dayem TM. Myocarditis: an expected health hazard associated with water resources contaminated with Coxsackie viruses type B. Int J Environ Health Res 2003; 13(3):261–70.

155. Griffin DW, Gibson CJ 3rd, Lipp EK, Riley K, Paul JH 3rd, Rose JB. Detection of viral pathogens by reverse transcriptase PCR and of microbial indicators by standard methods in the canals of the Florida Keys. Appl Environ Microbiol 1999; 65:4118–25. Erratum in: Appl Environ Microbiol 2000; 66:876.

156. Kueh CS, Grohmann GS. Recovery of viruses and bacteria in waters off Bondi beach: a pilot study. Med J Aust 1989; 151:632–8.

157. Keswick BH, Gerba CP, Goyal SM. Occurrence of enteroviruses in community swimming pools. Am J Public Health 1981; 71:1026–30.

158. Schvoerer E, Ventura M, Dubos O, et al. Qualitative and quantitative molecular detection of enteroviruses in water from bathing areas and from a sewage treatment plant. Res Microbiol 2001; 152:179–86.

159. Viadya SR, Chitambar SD, Arankalle VA. Polymerase chain reaction-based prevalence of *hepatitis A*, hepatitis E and TT viruses in sewage from an endemic area. J Hepatol 2002; 37(1):131–6.

160. Kittigul L, Raengsakulrach B, Siritantikorn S, et al. Detection of poliovirus, hepatitis A virus and rotavirus from sewage and water samples. Southeast Asian J Trop Med Public Health 2000; 31:41–6.

161. Lenaway DD, Brockmann R, Dolan GJ, Cruz-Uribe F. An outbreak of an enterovirus-like illness at a community wading pool: implications for public health inspection programs. Am J Public Health 1989; 79:889–90.

162. D'Alessio D, Minor TE, Allen CI et al. A study of the proportions of swimmers among well controls and children with enterovirus-like illness shedding or not shedding an enterovirus. Am J Epidemiol 1981; 113(5):533–41.

163. DeSerres G, Cromeans TL, Levesque B, et al. Molecular confirmation of hepatitis A virus from well water: epidemiology and public health implications. J Infect Dis 1999; 179(1):37–43.

164. Bloch AB, Stramer SL, Smith JD, et al. Recovery of hepatitis A virus from a water supply responsible for a common source outbreak of hepatitis A. Am J Public Health 1990; 80:428–30.

165. Nelson KE, Thomas DL. Viral Hepatitis. In KE Nelson, CM Williams, NMH Graham (eds). Infectious Disease Epidemiology. Theory and Practice. (pp.567–610). Gaithersburg, MDI, 2001. Aspen Publishers.

166. Kew O, Morris-Glasgow V, Landaverde M, et al. Outbreak of poliomyelitis in Hispaniola associated with circulating type 1 vaccine-derived poliovirus. Science 2002; 296(5566):356–9.

167. Yang CF, Naguib T, Yang SJ, et al. Circulation of endemic type 2 vaccine-derived poliovirus in Egypt from 1983 to 1993. J Virol 2003; 77:8366–77.

168. Arankalle VA, Chadha MS, Mehendale SM, Tungatkar SP. Epidemic hepatitis E: serological evidence for lack of intrafamilial spread. Indian J Gastroenterol 2000; 19:24–8.

169. Quiroga JA, Cotonat T, Castillo I, Carreno V. Hepatitis E virus seroprevalence in acute viral hepatitis in a developed country confirmed by a supplemental assay. J Med Virol 1996; 50:16–9.

170. Rab MA, Bile MK, Mubarik MM, et al. Water-borne hepatitis E virus epidemic in Islamabad, Pakistan: a common source outbreak traced to the malfunction of a modern water treatment plant. Am J Trop Med Hyg 1997; 57:151–7.

171. Benjelloun S, Bahbouhi B, Bouchrit N, et al. Seroepidemiological study of an acute hepatitis E outbreak in Morocco. Res Virol 1997; 148:279–87.

172. Corwin AL, Tien NT, Bounlu K, et al. The unique riverine ecology of hepatitis E virus transmission in South-East Asia. Trans R Soc Trop Med Hyg 1999; 93:255–60.

173. Clemente-Casares P, Pina S, Buti M, et al. Hepatitis E virus epidemiology in industrialized countries. Emerg Infect Dis 2003; 9:448–54.

174. Jothikumar N, Aparna K, Kaamatchiammal S, Paulmurugan R, Saravanadevi S, Khanna P. Detection of hepatitis E virus in raw and treated waste water with the polymerase chain reaction. Appl Environ Microbiol 1993; 59:2558–62.

175. Su CQ, Wu YL, Shen HK, et al. An outbreak of epidemic diarrhoea in adults caused by a new rotavirus in Anhui Province of China in the summer of 1983. J Med Virol 1986; 19(2):167–73.

176. Griffin DD, Fletcher M, Levy ME, et al. Outbreaks of adult gastroenteritis traced to a single genotype of rotavirus. J Infect Dis 2002; 185:1502–5.

177. Hurst CJ, Gerba CP. Stability of simian rotavirus in fresh and estuarine water. Appl Environ Microbiol 1980; 39:1–5.

178. Raphael RA, Sattar SA, Springthorpe VS. Long-term survival of human rotavirus in raw and treated river water. Can J Microbiol 1985; 31:124–8.

179. Pancorbo OC, Evanshen BG, Campbell WF, Lambert S, Curtis SK, Woolley TW. Infectivity and antigenicity reduction rates of human rotavirus strain Wa in fresh waters. Appl Environ Microbiol 1987; 53:1803–11.

180. Aulicino FA, Orsini P, Carere M, Mastrantonio A. Bacteriological and virological quality of seawater bathing areas along the Tyrrhenian coast. Int J Environ Health Res 2001; 11(1):5–11.

181. Fout GS, Martinson BC, Moyer MW, Dahling DR. A multiplex reverse transcription-PCR method for detection of human enteric viruses in ground water. Appl Environ Microbiol 2003; 69:3158–64.

182. Borchardt MA, Bertz PD, Spencer SK, Battigelli DA. Incidence of enteric viruses in ground water from household wells in Wisconsin. Appl Environ Microbiol 2003; 69:1172–80.

183. Kurtz JB, Lee TW. Astroviruses: human and animal. Ciba Found Symp 1987; 128:92–107.

184. Herrmann JE, Taylor DN, Echeverria P, Blacklow NR. Astroviruses as a cause of gastroenteritis in children. N Engl J Med 1991; 324(25): 1757–60.

185. Dalton RM, Roman ER, Negredo AA, Wilhelmi ID, Glass RI, Sanchez-Fauquier A. Astrovirus acute gastroenteritis among children in Madrid, Spain. Pediatr Infect Dis J 2002; 21:1038–41.

186. Cunliffe NA, Dove W, Gondwe JS, et al. Detection and characterisation of human astroviruses in children with acute gastroenteritis in Blantyre, Malawi. J Med Virol 2002; 67:563–6.

187. Abad FX, Villena C, Guix S, et al. Potential role of fomites in the vehicular transmission of human astroviruses. Appl Environ Microbiol 2001; 67(9):3904–7.

188. Glass RI, Bresee J, Jiang B, et al. Gastroenteritis viruses: an overview. Novartis Found Symp 2001; 238:5–19; discussion 19–25.

189. Smith AW, Skilling DE, Cherry N, Mead JH, Matson DO. Calicivirus emergence from ocean reservoirs: zoonotic and interspecies movements. Emerg Infect Dis 1998; 4:13–20.

190. Cox FEG. History of Human Parasitology. Clin Microbiol Rev 2002; 15(4):595–612.

191. Martinez AJ. Free-living amebas: infection of the central nervous system. Mt Sinai J Med 1993; 60:271–8.

192. Martinez AJ, Visvesvara GS. Laboratory diagnosis of pathogenic free-living amoebas: Naegleria, Acanthamoeba, and Leptomyxid. Clin Lab Med 1991; 11:861–72.

193. Pankhurst CL, Johnson NW, Woods RG. Microbial contamination of dental unit waterlines: the scientific argument. Int Dent J 1998; 48(4):359–68.

194. Seal D, Stapleton F, Dart J. Possible environmental sources of Acanthamoeba spp in contact lens wearers. Br J Ophthalmol 1992; 76(7):424–7.

195. Anderlini P, Przepiorka D, Luna M, et al. Acanthamoeba meningo-encephalitis after bone marrow transplantation. Bone Marrow Transplant 1994;14(3):459–61.

196. Bottone EJ. Free-living amebas of the genera Acanthamoeba and Naegleria: an overview and basic microbiologic correlates. Mt Sinai J Med 1993; 60:260–70.

197. CDC MMWR. Acanthamoeba keratitis associated with contact lenses – United States, 1986. 1986; 35(25):405–8.

198. Marrie TJ, Raoult D, La Scola B, Birtles RJ, de Carolis E and Canadian Community-Acquired Pneumonia Study Group. Legionella-like and other amoebal pathogens as agents of community-acquired pneumonia. Emerg Infect Dis 2001; 7:1026–9.

199. Visvesvara GS. Epidemiology of infections with free-living amebas and laboratory diagnosis of microsporidiosis. Mt Sinai J Med 1993; 60:283–8.

200. Marciano-Cabral F, Puffenbarger R, Cabral GA. The increasing importance of Acanthamoeba infections. J Eukaryot Microbiol 2000; 47(1):29–36.

201. Gardner HA, Martinez AJ, Visvesvara GS, Sotrel A. Granulomatous amebic encephalitis in an AIDS patient. Neurology 1991; 41(12):1993–5.

202. Dvoskin B, Friedman MG, Kahane S, Mathias M. Infection of Acanthamoeba polyphaga with Simkania negevensis and S. negevensis survival within amoebal cysts. Appl Environ Microbiol 2001; 67:4789–95.

203. Nwachuku N, Gerba CP. Health effects of Acanthamoeba spp. and its potential for waterborne transmission. Rev Environ Contam Toxicol 2004; 180:93–131.

204. Birtles RJ, Rowbotham TJ, Storey C, Marrie TJ, Raoult D. Chlamydia-like obligate parasite of free-living amoebae. Lancet 1997; 349:925–6.

205. Maurin M, Bryskier A, Raoult D. Antibiotic susceptibilities of Parachlamydia acanthamoeba in amoebae. Antimicrob Agents Chemother 2002; 46:3065–7.

206. Steinert M, Birkness K, White E, Fields B, Quinn F. Mycobacterium avium bacilli grow saprozoically in coculture with Acanthamoeba polyphaga and survive within cyst walls. Appl Environ Microbiol 1998; 64:2256–61.

207. Divers Alert Network. DAN safety tips. Alert Diver 2002; 4th quarter. https://www.daneurope.org/eng/ad8pag3.htm

208. Bruckner DA. Amebiasis. Clin Microbiol Rev 1992; 5:356–69.

209. Reed SL. Amebiasis: an update. Clin Infect Dis 1992; 14:385–93.

210. Garcia LS, Bruckner DA. Diagnostic medical parasitology. Washington DC: American Society for Microbiology, 1993.

211. CDC, Division of Parasitic Diseases. 2001. Cryptosporidiosis fact sheet.

212. CDC, MMWR. Assessing the public health threat associated with water borne cryptosporidiosis: Report of a workshop, Recommendations and reports. June 1995.

213. Garcia LS. Practical Guide to Diagnostic Parasitology. Washington DC, 1999. ASM Press.

214. Pape JW, Verdier RI, Boncy M, et al. Cyclospora infection in adults infected with HIV. Ann Intern Med 1994; 121:654–7.

215. Casemore DP. Cyclospora: another 'new' pathogen. J Med Microbiol 1994; 41:217–9.

216. Hoge CW, Shlim DR, Rajah R, et al. Epidemiology of diarrhoeal illness associated with coccidian-like organism among travelers and foreign residents in Nepal. Lancet 1993; 341:1175–9.

217. Smith PM. Traveler's diarrhoea associated with a cyanobacterium like body. Med J Aust 1993; 158:724.

218. Hart AS, Mark TR, Ramesh S, Caryn SP, Andrea SL, Frank KE. Novel organism associated with chronic diarrhoea in AIDS. Lancet 1990; 335:169–70.

219. National Park Service. Public Health Program. Washington DC: US Department of the Interior, 2003. http://www.nps.gov/public_health/inter/info/factsheets/fs_giardia.htm

220. Mannheimer SB, Soave R. Protozoal infections in patients with AIDS: cryptosporidiosis, isosporiasis, cyclosporiasis, and microsporidiosis. Infect Dis Clin North Am 1994; 8:483–98.

221. Wittner M, Tanowitz HB, Weiss LM. Parasitic infections in AIDS patients. Cryptosporidiosis, isosporiasis, microsporidiosis, cyclosporiasis. Infect Dis Clin North Am 1993; 7:569–86.

222. La Via WV. Parasitic gastroenteritis. Pediatr Ann 1994; 23(10):556–60.

223. Benator DA, French AL, Beaudet LM, et al. Isospora belli infection associated with acalculous cholecystitis in a patient with AIDS. Ann Intern Med 1994; 121:663–664.

224. Markus MB. Origin of extra-intestinal stages of Isospora belli in the acquired immune deficiency syndrome (AIDS). Med Hypotheses 1991; 35: 278.

225. Comin CE, Santucci M. 1994. Submicroscopic profile of Isospora belli enteritis in a patient with acquired immune deficiency syndrome. Ultrastruct Pathol 1994; 18:473–82.

226. Butcher PD, Cevallos AM, Carnaby S, Alstead EM, Swarbrick ET, Farthing MJ. Phenotypic and genotypic variation in Giardia lamblia isolates during chronic infection. Gut 1994; 35:51–4.

227. Harskeeri RA, Van Gool T, Schuitema AR, Didier ES, Terpstra WJ. Reclassification of the microsporidian Septata intestinalis to Encephalitozoon intestinalis on the basis of genetic and immunological characterization. Parasitology 1995; 110:277–85.

228. Bryan RT. Microsporidia. In: Mandel G, Bennett JE, Dolin R, eds. Principles and practices of infectious diseases. New York: Churchill Livingstone, Inc., 1995; 2513–24.

229. Canning EU, Hollister WS. New intestinal protozoa-coccidia and microsporidia. Trans R Soc Trop Med Hyg 1990; 84:181–6.

230. Lom J. Introductory remarks on microsporidia in the AIDS era. Folia Parasitol (Prague) 1993; 40:255–6.

231. Cali A, Meisler D, Lowder C, et al. Corneal microsporidiosis: characterization and identification. J Protozool 1991; 38:215S–217S.

232. Modigliani R. Occurrence of new microsporidian found in intestines of AIDS patients. J Protozool 1985; 32:250–4.

233. Pol S, Romana C, Richard S, et al. Enterocytozoon bieneusi infection in acquired immunodeficiency syndrome-related sclerosing cholangitis. Gastroenterology 1992; 102:1778–81.

234. Rabeneck L, Gyorkey F, Genta RM, Gyorkey P, Foote LW, Risser JM. The role of microsporidia in the pathogenesis of HIV-related chronic diarrhea. Ann Intern Med 1993; 119:895–9.

235. Schattenkerk J, Van Gool T, Van Ketel R, et al. Clinical significance of small intestinal microsporidiosis in HIV-1-infected individuals. Lancet 1991; 337:895–8.

236. Blaser MJ, Smith PD, Ravdin JI, Greenberg HB, Guerrant RL. Infections of the gastrointestinal tract. New York: Raven Press, 1995.

237. McDougall RJ, Tandy MW, Boreham RE, Stenzel DJ, O'Donoghue PJ. Incidental finding of a microsporidian parasite from an AIDS patient. J Clin Microbiol 1993; 31:436–9.

238. Michiels JF, Hofman P, Saint Paul MC, Loubiere R, Bernard E, LeFichoux Y. Pathological features of intestinal microsporidiosis in HIV positive patients. A report of 13 new cases. Pathol Res Pract 1993; 189:377–83.

239. Neafie RC, Marty AM. Unusual infections in humans. Clin Microbiol Rev 1993; 6:35–49.

240. Weber R, Sauer B, Luthy R, Nadal D. Intestinal coinfection with Enterocytozoon bieneusi and Cryptosporidium in a human immunodeficiency virus-infected child with chronic diarrhea. Clin Infect Dis 1993; 17:480–3.

241. Dengjel B, Zahler M, Hermanns W, et al. Zoonotic potential of Enterocytozoon bieneusi. J Clin Microbiol 2001; 4495–4499.

242. Glaser CA, Angulo FJ, Rooney JA. Animal-associated opportunistic infections among persons infected with the human immunodeficiency virus. Clin Infect Dis 1994; 18:14–24.

243. Muscat I. Human microsporidiosis. J Infect 1990; 21:125–9.

244. Vavra J, Nohynkova E, Machala L, Spala J. An extremely rapid method for detection of microsporidia in biopsy materials from AIDS patients. Folia Parasitol 1993; 40:273–4.

245. Rosenberger D. Successful treatment of microsporidial keratoconjunctivitis with topical fumagillin in a patient with AIDS. Cornea 1993; 12:261–5.

246. Yee R. Resolution of microsporidial epithelial keratopathy in a patient with AIDS. Ophthalmology 1990; 98:196–201.

247. Asmuth DM, DeGirolami PC, Federman M, et al. Clinical features of microsporidiosis in patients with AIDS. Clin Infect Dis 1994; 18:819–25.

248. Lumb R, Swift J, James C, Papanaoum K, Mukherjee T. Identification of the microsporidian parasite, *Enterocytozoon bieneusi* in faecal samples and intestinal biopsies from an AIDS patient. Int J Parasitol 1993; 23:793–801.

249. Kilvington S, Beeching J. Development of PCR for identification of *Naegleria fowleri* from the environment. Appl Environ Microbiol 1995; 61:3764–7.

250. Ma P, Visvesvara GS, Martinez AJ, et al. Naegleria and Acanthamoeba infections: review. Rev Infect Dis 1990; 12(3): 490–513.

251. Elder MJ, Kilvington S, Dart JK. A clinicopathologic study of in vitro sensitivity testing and *Acanthamoeba keratitis*. Invest Ophthalmol Vis Sci 1994; 35:1059–64.

252. Marciano-Cabral F. Biology of Naegleria spp. Microbiol Rev 1988; 52:114–33.

253. CDC. Schistosomiasis. The Yellow Book, Health Information for International Travel. Washington DC: National Center for Infectious Diseases, 2003–04. http://www.cdc.gov/travel/diseases/schisto.htm

254. World Health Organization. Public health importance: schistosomiasis. Geneva: WHO, 1997.

255. CDC-MMWR. 1992. Cercarial dermatitis outbreak at a state park Delaware, 1991; 41(14); 225–8.

256. Feachem DG, Bradley DJ, Garelick H, Mara DD. Sanitation and disease: health aspects of excreta and waste water management. New York: John Wiley and Sons, 1983.

Section 5
Policy, Regulation and Control

Chapter 55
Ethics in Occupational Medicine

Anne Krantz, Linda S Forst

The practice of medicine often occurs at the interface between clinical science and social relationships; in occupational medicine, this is almost always true. In occupational medicine, these social relationships are frequently economic and societal forces that distort the traditional relationship between physician and patient. The conflicts that arise from these forces, and their ethical implications, must be recognized and overcome by the occupational medicine physician in order to practice in this field with the highest professional standards. This chapter reviews the basis for the ethical practice of medicine, some of the ethical challenges encountered in the practice of occupational medicine, and the role of codes of ethics in this field.

ETHICS IN GENERAL MEDICAL PRACTICE

The primacy of the relationship between doctor and patient is the nucleus around which principles of ethical medical practice are formulated. Four principles central to biomedical ethics have been elucidated by Beauchamp and Childress.[1] *Non-maleficence* is the duty to not intentionally cause harm to the patient, expressed by the familiar dictum, *Primum non nocere*. *Beneficence* is the duty to act in the best interest of the patient, and to promote his or her welfare. *Respect for autonomy* is the duty to safeguard the decision-making capacity of patients, and is the basis for the principle of informed consent. Finally, there are considerations of *justice*, which relate to the fair allocation of healthcare resources.[1]

The American College of Physicians gives guidance to the practicing physician in the application of these principles to the clinical context.[2] To serve a patient's best interest, the physician must understand the patient's complaints, goals, and expectations. The provision of care requires informed consent. The physician must respect the privacy of the patient, and afford maximum confidentiality. Disclosure of relevant medical information must be done in a way that the patient understands. The physician must be professionally competent. Finally, the practicing physician must be aware of the social, organizational, and financial conflicts of interest that might influence the provision of care, and base his or her actions only on what is appropriate medical care.[2]

CONFLICTS OF INTEREST IN OCCUPATIONAL MEDICINE

A conflict of interest is 'a set of conditions in which professional judgment concerning a primary interest (such as a patient's welfare or the validity of research) tends to be unduly influenced by a secondary interest (such as financial gain)'.[3] In occupational medicine, financial conflicts of interest arise when the physician has a dual relationship: one with a patient (who is an employee), and at the same time, one with an employer, insurer, or other entity that employs or pays the physician for the patient's care. These entities are likely to have their own financial interest in the patient's (employee's) diagnosis, treatment, and ability to return to work. Thus, there may be undue pressure, real or perceived, on the physician to provide care or opinions that are not in the patient's best interest, or do not reflect the doctor's best professional judgment. Examples of potential conflicts of interest include the following.

- A company physician decides on the timing of returning an employee to work after an injury; the physician is explicitly or implicitly aware of the employer's concern for the costs of the employee's lost workdays.
- A physician performs an independent medical examination and renders an opinion regarding the work-relatedness of an illness; the patient was referred by a workers' compensation insurance carrier, which provides the physician with many such referrals.
- A physician in a hospital-based occupational health program plans to refer a patient with a work-related injury to the most qualified neurosurgeon; the physician is well aware that the hospital expects the occupational health program will generate referrals for its own sub-specialist physicians and ancillary services.

Conflicts of interest also pertain to the work of occupational health-related professions outside medicine, including nursing, industrial hygiene, and other sciences. For example:

- an occupational health scientist employed by the manufacturer of a persistent organic pollutant is a member of a panel which will advise the government of the extent of environmental contamination and health effects from the pollutant, and the optimal strategy for abatement; the scientist knows that the costs of abatement will be borne by the manufacturer.

Several features of financial conflicts of interest have been discussed by Thompson.[3] Firstly, it is incorrect to dismiss financial conflict of interest as just one among the many competing interests which must always be weighed in the complicated practice of medicine. Physicians (occupational or otherwise) have a primary responsibility for the wellbeing of the patient, which takes precedence over financial or corporate interests. On the other hand, the mere presence of financial conflicts of interest does not mean that the physician necessarily does not act in the patient's best interest, or uses other than his or her best professional judgment. Nor is it necessarily an attack on the integrity of a physician to note that a conflict of interest exists. However, it is usually the case that many elements go into the process of medical decision making, and the influence of dual relationships may be subtle. The avoidance of conflicts of interest not only protects the professionalism of the physician, but also contributes to public confidence in the integrity of the profession.[3] Thus, it is critical for physicians to recognize conflicts of interest and develop structural precautions to prevent them or minimize their influence.

An example of an important structural precaution that can minimize conflicts of interest is the freedom of an employee to choose his or her own physician for the care of a work-related injury or illness. This arrangement exists in some states. Thus, for example, if an employer knows that a worker can seek care outside, there will be less pressure on the company physician, or the contracted occupational health program, to provide substandard care, or return an injured employee to work prematurely. Another safeguard for workers would be a contractual right for a union to veto the selection of a company physician. For the physician, a practice structured so that it is not unduly dependent upon a single referral source will minimize the perceived pressure which that referral source exerts, and, in the event that the referral source has expectations that the physician believes are unethical, make it easier to decline the business. For the health scientist in the example above, a structural policy that avoids a conflict of interest would be one that prevents scientific panels having, as participants, those with a financial interest in the outcome of the question being studied.

What role does disclosure play in the management of conflicts of interest? While disclosure of a financial conflict of interest is important in the ethical care of the patient, it does not, by itself, alter the potential influence which that conflict may exert. For example, a patient may independently seek care for an illness from a primary care physician who also provides occupational health services for the patient's employer. If the patient has no other choice, perhaps due to geographic or financial limitations, of pursuing care elsewhere, then disclosure does not change the potential effect that the conflict may exert in the patient's care. Importantly, as noted by Rodwin,[4] a physician's obligation to act in the best interests of the patient is not limited by disclosing a conflict of interest. In the case of the occupational health scientist above, the mere disclosure of the relationship with the manufacturer does not prevent the conflict.

The current practice of occupational medicine often does occur in settings where financial conflicts of interest are unavoidable, for example, when clinical judgments are made by a company physician. In addition to the structural safeguards that may be developed for the worker/patient, the physician's individual ability to maintain an approach that uniformly puts the patient/worker's best interest above corporate interests is paramount. The best circumstance is when the company physician is allowed to practice with no interference from management, and is successful in convincing the employer that its long-term interests are best served by protecting workers from hazardous exposures. When there is conflict, however, the physician's position can be bolstered by the presence of a professional code of ethics (see below).

PATIENT CONFIDENTIALITY

Occupational medicine may be considered a subset of forensic medicine in that many, if not the majority, of work-related injury and illness claims are adjudicated within the workers' compensation system. As such, these cases are reviewed by many different groups of professionals. If the worker's compensation claim is immediately accepted by employers or insurance companies, they still may require that a copy of the medical record be sent for evaluation by a claims analyst before payment is made. If the claim is contested, attorneys may be called in and claims may go before an arbitrator at the state industrial commission; review of medical records is essential to adjudication of the case. The patient's primary provider and the designated 'company physician' may gain access to each other's records in order to deliver optimal care or to render an opinion regarding fitness for work. Case managers, human resources personnel, and owners/supervisors may all have the opportunity to scrutinize an injured worker's records, particularly in small companies where one or a few managers fill those roles. On rare occasions, enforcement agencies like the Occupational Safety and Health Administration (OSHA) or the health department may gain access to medical records.

There are both ethical and legal considerations that apply to patient confidentiality in the occupational medicine setting. In the US, the patient's right to privacy and confidentiality is implicit in the doctor–patient relationship. Injured workers, who typically have more experience with general healthcare than occupational healthcare, may expect that all provider–patient relationships are the same. The occupational physician has the obligation to inform the patient of the difference.

Even if the patient is made aware of the role of the occupational physician, 'fidelity' to the patient requires that the physician obtain consent to release medical information to a third party. To protect this right, healthcare institutions have developed medical release forms that require the patient's signature, and protocols for releasing medical information. Occupational clinics have adapted these

I have authorized _____ Medical Center to render treatment of my work-related injury/illness and to release any or all medical information, both written and verbal, regarding my work-related injury/illness (including, but not limited to, medical records, billing information, and x-rays) to my employer and its representatives, insurance carriers, and physicians for the duration of the injury.

I further give consent to _____ Medical Center for the performance of drug testing, either urine, blood or breath, in accordance with my employer's drug testing policy. I also authorize the release of such results to my employer.

This consent remains in effect until revoked in writing by me.

Signed _____   Date _____

Witness _____

Figure 55.1: Sample occupational medicine consent form.

documents to inform the patient of the role of the provider in this case and to gain consent for release of medical information to all interested parties (Fig. 55.1). Although this protocol may interfere with the injured worker's comfort and openness with the provider, it is essential to the principle of non-maleficence.

A series of statutes and court decisions define the boundaries of patient confidentiality in occupational medicine. An implied contract between patient and physician in all clinical interactions is recognized in most of the 50 states in the US and there is much case law that upholds this understanding. Because of the changes in healthcare delivery and payment over the past several decades, the National Conference of Commissioners on Uniform State Laws approved and recommended enactment of the Universal HealthCare Information Act in 1985.[5] The Act cites:

- 'the emergence of third party payment plans';
- 'the growing involvement of government agencies in virtually all aspects of healthcare';
- 'the exponential increase in the use of computers and automated information systems for healthcare record information as conditions that have challenged confidentiality protections';
- 'the sheer amount of personal data kept in healthcare records'; and
- 'the [increased] number of individuals who monitor those records'.

This model rule requires that a medical release be signed and dated by the patient, that it identify the nature of the information that will be disclosed, and that it identify who will receive the information. The permission lasts no more than 30 months without renewal. There are situations where patient consent is not required. Those that apply to occupational health include:

- healthcare providers who need it to render healthcare to the patient;
- for quality assurance peer review;
- for administrative or legal purposes;
- for prevention of danger to the patient or others;
- for research;
- when required by the public health system; or
- in compliance with compulsory processes.

In addition, there have been many court decisions whereby physicians hired by a party other than the patient (e.g., the employer) were exempt.[6] When medical information regarding an employee is released to the company physician, there is an implicit obligation that this information is not re-disclosed to other parties in the company.[6]

Under workers' compensation statutes, records describing a work-related injury or illness may be disclosed to the insurer, the employer, or the state workers' compensation fund in most states. Independent medical examinations are considered the property of the payer – usually the employer.

Under the Health Insurance Portability and Accountability Act of 1996 (HIPAA),[7] the US Department of Health and Human Services developed a standard regarding access to medical records. This law went into effect in 2002. Under the standard, providers and insurance companies must provide patients with a document describing how their health information may be used and disclosed. Patients have a right to see their records, request amendments, know of any disclosures made, and request that specific non-routine disclosures not be made. Explicit authorization is required to release the information for non-routine purposes, and then the minimal amount of information should be released. Providers and insurers must train their employees regarding HIPAA requirements, write privacy procedures, identify a 'privacy officer', and develop a procedure for accepting complaints from individuals regarding violation of their rights. Criminal and civil penalties have been established for breaching confidentiality. This will clearly affect the management of occupational medicine records.

Patients' trust in the occupational physician and their willingness to supply information regarding their health status make confidentiality a critical assurance in the occupational healthcare setting. While HIPAA goes a long way to defining appropriate disclosure of medical information, respect for privacy and autonomy of the employee/patient is the ethical goal of the occupational provider.

OCCUPATIONAL HEALTH RESEARCH

The protocol for protection of human subjects in medical research was established by the US Department of Health and Human Services,[8] and based on the Belmont Report.[9] Here, the ethical principles central to clinical practice are applied to the research setting:
- 'autonomy'– respect for individuals and informed consent;
- 'beneficence'– concern about the common good and reducing risk to the individual; and
- 'justice' – apportioning benefits and burdens of research fairly.

A key difference between clinical principles and research principles is the omission of maleficence in the latter: it is recognized that in research, harm may in fact be done, and the goal is to minimize its risk. Although federal law applies only to projects that are funded by the government, most research institutions have adopted this protocol for all research.

There are two major activities in occupational health that are regarded as research. One is use of data collected routinely for the purpose of medical or exposure monitoring and surveillance. The second is de novo collection of data from workers or their environment to address a scientific hypothesis. The former falls in the category of review of secondary data and, if confidentiality can be maintained, does not require informed consent. The latter entails enrollment of workers and is thus guided by rules related to human subjects research.

Some would consider workers a 'vulnerable population', because job security could be jeopardized by their willingness or unwillingness to participate, and also because confidentiality may be difficult to maintain in the closed environment of the workplace. For this reason, Rothstein states that workers should be afforded 'additional protections beyond those normally provided to research participants'.[10] Drawing from laws relating to research on other populations, research involving workers would be permitted only if it:
- evaluates issues related to the subjects' workplace and involves minimal risk;
- evaluates conditions that affect workers as a group; and
- is likely to improve the health of the individual enrolled worker.

There should be no connection between enrolling in the research and benefits unrelated to the research. For example, the worker should not get (or be denied) special treatment regarding payment or desirable job tasks based on his or her willingness to participate.

Emanuel proposes that workers be considered a 'community', rather than a 'vulnerable population', since they are targeted *because of* their work, rather than as a convenience sample.[11] In this scheme, workers are considered partners in the research; they or their representatives are then contributors to all aspects of study execution. They would be involved with protocol development, consent processes, research conduct, data access, and dissemination of results. This would allow for direct oversight by the subjects themselves, and afford a greater level of protection from research risks.

Although not common, carrying out one's duty to safeguard the health of workers and the public can have dire professional consequences. In 1994, Dr David Kern was a faculty member at a university medical school, the director of the university's occupational medicine program, and the director of an occupational and environmental health service which provided clinical services at a hospital affiliated with the university.[12] After seeing a patient at the affiliated hospital with suspected occupational lung disease, Dr Kern arranged a site visit at the patient's workplace, which manufactured finely cut nylon (flock) and flocked fabric. The site visit would serve a dual purpose: to investigate possible etiologies for the illness, and to educate students and trainees. At the start of the site visit, Dr Kern signed a confidentiality agreement regarding the limits of disclosure of information and trade secrets at the plant.

Some time later, Dr Kern saw a second patient with interstitial lung disease from the same plant. He contacted a public health agency (NIOSH) about his concern for a suspected outbreak of an occupational lung disease, and arranged a consulting agreement with the company to undertake an investigation of the suspected outbreak. During the course of the investigation, Dr Kern identified other cases, and eventually sought to present his clinical findings to the scientific public. He was asked by the company to refrain from submitting a planned abstract of his findings for presentation at an international scientific meeting. He was then asked by the affiliated hospital (of which the company was a benefactor) to withdraw his submitted abstract. The hospital also sought to delay Dr Kern's communication with workers participating in the study about clinical recommendations based on Dr Kern's understanding of the disease. Eventually, the hospital terminated the occupational and environmental health service, despite later learning that his academic freedom had been violated. Dr Kern maintained that the confidentiality agreement had little if anything to do with the outbreak investigation, and, in any case, 'it should not be allowed to deter us from our professional responsibilities'.[12]

Dr Kern's actions were in keeping with the highest standards of public health practice: he notified a public health agency when he suspected an outbreak; he sought permission to undertake an outbreak investigation; he sought to keep all relevant parties informed of the results; and, importantly, he sought to inform other scientists of the results in a timely manner, so that other workers might be protected. Unfortunately, his story 'illustrates the conflict-prone nature of the practice of occupational medicine'.[13]

The workplace 'outbreak investigation' is an intermediate form of research, in that it is designed to address a hazard that may affect the immediate health of the workforce. Outbreak investigations are conducted expeditiously, sometimes not allowing time to adequately plan and communicate pertinent issues to the employee-subjects, or to cultivate a partnership. They generally proceed in a single workplace with a small number of employees, limiting statistical power and limiting the ability to generalize results. They may be performed or mandated by an enforcement agency such as OSHA or a public health department, bypassing institutional review procedures required of other types of research. Still, results of outbreak investigations in the workplace fall in the domain of research, and should be published, particularly when results are relevant to occupational and public health.

CODES OF ETHICS IN OCCUPATIONAL MEDICINE

Many professional organizations of physicians and other biomedical scientists have adopted codes of ethics or conduct. In general, these codes articulate core values and principles of their respective professions, establish behavioral norms expected by members of the profession, and provide moral guidance for practitioners faced with conflict or uncertainty. Ethical codes can help establish an 'ethics standard of care' for the profession and, through their development and ratification by a professional group, contribute to the 'ethics education' of the members of that group.[14]

Criticisms of codes of ethics include that they may simply represent an effort by professionals to police themselves, in order to avoid outside scrutiny. They are voluntary, and professional organizations have no way of enforcing them. Their content may be non-specific, so that while they outline expected values, they may not sufficiently delineate expected or proscribed behaviors necessary to achieve those values. These limitations notwithstanding, the establishment of codes of ethics for physicians and other health professionals is increasingly common and generally considered desirable.

Numerous codes of ethics for occupational medicine and related public health professions have been adopted or proposed.[2,15-20] In the process of selecting a code of conduct for the Association of Occupational and Environmental Clinics (AOEC), Brodkin et al. suggested seven principles most relevant to the ethical practice of occupational medicine, and therefore desirable as elements of any such code. These principles are:

- an obligation to promote a safe and healthy workplace and environment;
- an obligation to maintain professional competence;
- an obligation to advise and report;
- avoidance of conflict of interest;
- avoidance of discrimination;
- an obligation to maintain ethical standards; and
- an obligation to maintain patient confidentiality.[21]

Another code stresses the importance of transparency, with an obligation to declare conflicts of interest.[19] Because the practice of occupational health is multidisciplinary, it is also relevant that all health and safety professionals have equivalent ethical standards.[22]

The 1996 AOEC review found that the most robust code of those reviewed was that of the International Commission on Occupational Health. It was the most detailed, applied to the full range of occupational health practitioners, and addressed both clinical and public health dimensions.[21] This code is reproduced below. The American College of Occupational and Environmental Medicine adopted a code in 1993,[2] which has been supplemented by subsequent discussions of confidentiality[23] and research on workers.[10] A code of conduct that includes an explicit declaration of conflict of interest has also been proposed.[19]

Efforts to protect workers and the public from occupational and environmental hazards occur in a setting fraught with powerful and competing social and economic forces. Amid these forces, the occupational health professional's first priority is to the health of the worker and public. The health and safety professional must be ever mindful of the interests that conflict with that priority, and of the expectation, from patients, colleagues, and society, that one will practice according to the highest standards of ethical practice. Codes that recognize this priority remind practitioners of the ethical standards of their profession, and strengthen their ability to work effectively. These codes must remain living documents, their contents and implications being periodically reviewed and debated, to maintain a high level of attention to the ethical practice of occupational and environmental health.

Acknowledgment
The authors thank Dr Peter Orris for his insights and guidance.

References

1. Beauchamp TL, Childress JF. Principles of biomedical ethics, 4th edn. New York: Oxford University Press; 1994.
2. American College of Physicians. Ethics manual. Fourth edition. Ann Intern Med 1998; 128:576-94.
3. Thompson DF. Understanding financial conflicts of interest. N Engl J Med 1993; 329:573-6.
4. Rodwin MA. Physicians' conflicts of interest. The limitations of disclosure. N Engl J Med 1989; 320:1405-8.
5. Uniform HealthCare Information Act, 1985. www.law.upenn.edu/bll/ulc/fnact99/1980s/uhcia85.pdf. Accessed 7-27-02.
6. Tilton SH. Right to privacy and confidentiality of medical records. Occup Med 1996; 11:17-28.
7. Health Insurance Portability and Accountability Act of 1996 (HIPAA), P.L. 104-91. aspe.hhs.gov/admnsimp/pl104191.htm. Accessed 7-27-02.
8. Federal Register, 1999. CFR 46.101-46.409.
9. National Commission for the Protection of Human Subjects of Biomedical and Behavioral Research. The Belmont Report. Washington DC: US Government Printing Office; 1979.
10. Rothstein MA. Ethical guidelines for medical research on workers. J Occup Environ Med 2000; 42:1166-71.
11. Emanuel E. Introduction to occupational medical ethics. Occup Med 2001; 17:549-58.

12. Kern DG. The unexpected result of an investigation of an outbreak of occupational lung disease. Int J Occup Environ Health 1998; 4:19-32.

13. Nemery B. The conflict-prone nature of occupational health research and practice. Int J Occup Environ Health 1998; 4:35-7.

14. Goodman KW. Codes of ethics in occupational and environmental health. J Occup Environ Med 1996; 38:882-3.

15. AAOHN. AAOHN code of ethics and interpretive statements. Atlanta, GA: American Association of Occupational Health Nurses; 1991.

16. American Board of Industrial Hygiene. Code of ethics for the practice of industrial hygiene. ABIH 1994. www.abih.org/Docs/Code-of-Ethics.htm. Accessed 6-27-02.

17. American College of Occupational and Environmental Medicine. Code of ethical conduct. J Occup Med 1994; 29:28.

18. American Occupational Medicine Association. Code of ethical conduct for physicians providing occupational medical services. J Occup Med 1976; 18:703.

19. Anonymous. International code of conduct (ethics) for occupational health and safety professionals. Int J Occup Environ Health 2001; 7:230-2.

20. International Commission of Occupational Health. International code of ethics for occupational health professionals. Singapore: ICOH; 1992.

21. Brodkin AC, Frumkin H, Kirkland KH, Orris P, Schenk M. AOEC position paper on the organizational code for ethical conduct. J Occup Environ Med 1996; 38:869-81.

22. Ladou J, Tennenhouse DJ, Feitshans IL. Codes of ethics (conduct). Occup Med 2002; 17:559-85.

23. Rischitelli DG. The confidentiality of medical information in the workplace. J Occup Environ Med 1995; 37:583-93.

Appendix

International Code of Ethics for Occupational Health Professionals

International Commission on Occupational Health

Introduction

1. The aim of occupational health practice is to protect and promote workers' health, to sustain and improve their working capacity and ability, to contribute to the establishment and maintenance of a safe and healthy working environment for all, as well as to promote the adaptation of work to the capabilities of workers, taking into account their state of health.

2. The field of occupational health is broad and covers the prevention of all impairments arising out of employment, work injuries and work-related disorders, including occupational diseases and all aspects relating to the interactions between work and health. Occupational health professionals should be involved, whenever possible, in the design and choice of health and safety equipment, appropriate methods and procedures and safe work practices and they should encourage workers' participation in this field as well as feedback from experience.

3. On the basis of the principle of equity, occupational health professionals should assist workers in obtaining and maintaining employment notwithstanding their health deficiencies or their handicap. It should be duly recognised that there are particular occupational health needs of workers as determined by factors such as gender, age, physiologic condition, social aspects, communication barriers or other factors. Such needs should be met on an individual basis with due concern to protection of health in relation to work and without leaving any possibility for discrimination.

4. For the purpose of this Code, the expression "occupational health professionals" is meant to include all those who, in a professional capacity, carry out occupational safety and health tasks, provide occupational health services or are involved in an occupational health practice. A wide range of disciplines are concerned with occupational health since it is at an interface between technology and health involving technical, medical, social and legal aspects. Occupational health professionals include occupational health physicians and nurses, factory inspectors, occupational hygienists and occupational psychologists, specialists involved in ergonomics, in rehabilitation therapy, in accident prevention and in the improvement of the working environment as well as in occupational health and safety research. The trend is to mobilise the competence of these occupational health professionals within the framework of a multidisciplinary team approach.

5. Many other professionals from a variety of disciplines such as chemistry, toxicology, engineering, radiation health, epidemiology, environmental health, applied sociology, insurance personnel and health education may also be involved, to some extent, in occupational health practice. Furthermore, public health and labour authorities, employers, workers and their representatives and first aid workers have an essential role and even a direct responsibility in the implementation of occupational health policies and programmes, although they are not occupational health specialists by profession. Finally, many other professions such as lawyers, architects, manufacturers, designers, work analysts, work organisation specialists, teachers in technical schools, universities and other institutions as well as the media personnel have an important role to play in relation to the improvement of the working environment and of working conditions.

6. The term "employers" means persons with recognised responsibility, commitment and duties towards workers in their employment by virtue of a mutually agreed relationship (a self-employed person is regarded as being both an employer and a worker). The term "workers" applies to any persons who work, whether full time, part time or temporarily for an employer; this term is used here in a broad sense covering all employees, including management staff and the self-employed (a self-employed person is regarded as having the duties of both an employer and a worker). The expression "competent authority" means a minister, government department or other public authority having the power to issue regulations, orders or other instruction having the force of law, and who is in charge of supervising and enforcing their implementation.

7. There is a wide range of duties, obligations and responsibilities as well as complex relationships among those concerned and involved in occupational safety and health matters. In general, obligations and responsibilities are defined by statutory regulations. Each employer has the responsibility for the health and safety of the workers in his or her employment. Each profession has its responsibilities which are related to the nature of its duties. It is important to define the role of occupational health professionals and their relationships with other professionals, with the competent authority and with social partners in the purview of economic, social, environmental and health policies. This calls for a clear view about the ethics of

occupational health professionals and standards in their professional conduct. When specialists of several professions are working together within a multidisciplinary approach, they should endeavour to base their action on shared sets of values and have an understanding of each other's duties, obligations, responsibilities and professional standards.

8. Some of the conditions of execution of the functions of occupational health professionals and the conditions of operation of occupational health services are often defined in statutory regulations, such as regular planning and reviewing of activities and continuous consultation with workers and management. Basic requirements for a sound occupational practice include a full professional independence, i.e. that occupational health professionals must enjoy an independence in the exercise of their functions which should enable them to make judgements and give advice for the protection of the workers' health and for their safety within the undertaking in accordance with their knowledge and conscience. Occupational health professionals should make sure that the necessary conditions are met to enable them to carry out their activities according to good practice and to the highest professional standards. This should include adequate staffing, training and retraining, support and access to an appropriate level of senior management.

9. Further basic requirements for acceptable occupational health practice, often specified by national regulations, include free access to the workplace, the possibility of taking samples and assessing the working environment, making job analyses and participating in enquiries and consulting the competent authority on the implementation of occupational safety and health standards in the undertaking. Special attention should be given to ethical dilemmas which may arise from pursuing simultaneously objectives which may be competing such as the protection of employment and the protection of health, the right to information and confidentiality, and the conflicts between individual and collective interests.

10. The occupational health practice should meet the aims of occupational health which have been defined by the ILO and WHO in 1950 and updated as follows by the ILO/WHO Joint Committee on Occupational Health in 1995:

Occupational health should aim at: the promotion and maintenance of the highest degree of physical, mental and social well-being of workers in all occupations; the prevention amongst workers of departures from health caused by their working conditions; the protection of workers in their employment from risks resulting from factors adverse to health; the placing and maintenance of the workers in an occupational environment adapted to their physiologic and psychological capabilities; and, to summarise, the adaptation of work to man and of each man to his job. The main focus in occupational health is on three different objectives: (i) the maintenance and promotion of workers' health and working capacity; (ii) the improvement of working environment and

work to become conducive to safety and health; and (iii) development of work organisations and working cultures in a direction which supports health and safety at work and in doing so also promotes a positive social climate and smooth operation and may enhance productivity of the undertakings. The concept of working culture is intended in this context to mean a reflection of the essential value systems adopted by the undertaking concerned. Such a culture is reflected in practice in the managerial systems, personnel policy, principles for participation, training policies and quality management of the undertaking.

11. It cannot be overemphasised that the central purpose of any occupational health practice is the primary prevention of occupational and work-related diseases and injuries. Such practice should take place under controlled conditions and within an organised framework – preferably involving professional occupational health services – in order to ensure that it is relevant, knowledge-based, sound from a scientific, ethical and technical point of view, and appropriate to the occupational risks in the enterprise and to the occupational health needs of the working population concerned.

12. It is increasingly understood that the purpose of a sound occupational health practice is not merely to perform assessments and to provide services but implies caring for workers' health and their working capacity with a view to protect, maintain and promote them. This approach of occupational healthcare and occupational health promotion addresses workers' health and their human and social needs in a comprehensive and coherent manner which includes preventive healthcare, health promotion, curative healthcare, first-aid rehabilitation and compensation where appropriate, as well as strategies for recovery and reintegration into the working environment. Similarly, the importance of considering the links between occupational health, environmental health, quality management, product safety and stewardship, public and community health and security is increasingly understood. This strategy is conducive to the development of occupational safety and health management systems, an emphasis on the choice of clean technologies and alliances with those who produce and those who protect in order to make development sustainable, equitable, socially useful and responsive to human needs.

BASIC PRINCIPLES

The following three paragraphs summarise the principles of ethics and values on which is based the International Code of Ethics for Occupational Health Professionals.

The purpose of occupational health is to serve the health and social well-being of the workers individually and collectively. Occupational health practice must be performed according to the highest professional standards and ethical principles. Occupational health professionals must contribute to environmental and community health.

The duties of occupational health professionals include protecting the life and the health of the worker, respecting human dignity and promoting the highest ethical principles in occupational health policies and programmes. Integrity in professional conduct, impartiality and the protection of the confidentiality of health data and of the privacy of workers are part of these duties.

Occupational health professionals are experts who must enjoy full professional independence in the execution of their functions. They must acquire and maintain the competence necessary for their duties and require conditions which allow them to carry out their tasks according to good practice and professional ethics.

DUTIES AND OBLIGATIONS OF OCCUPATIONAL HEALTH PROFESSIONALS

Aims and advisory role

1. The primary aim of occupational health practice is to safeguard and promote the health of workers, to promote a safe and healthy working environment, to protect the working capacity of workers and their access to employment. In pursuing this aim, occupational health professionals must use validated methods of risk evaluation, propose effective preventive measures and follow up their implementation. The occupational health professionals must provide competent and honest advice to the employers on fulfilling their responsibility in the field of occupational safety and health as well as to the workers on the protection and promotion of their health in relation to work. The occupational health professionals should maintain direct contact with safety and health committees, where they exist.

Knowledge and expertise

2. Occupational health professionals must continuously strive to be familiar with the work and the working environment as well as to develop their competence and to remain well informed in scientific and technical knowledge, occupational hazards and the most efficient means to eliminate or to minimise the relevant risks. As the emphasis must be on primary prevention defined in terms of policies, design, choice of clean technologies, engineering control measures and adapting work organisation and workplaces to workers, occupational health professionals must regularly and routinely, whenever possible, visit the workplaces and consult the workers and the management on the work that is performed.

Development of a policy and a programme

3. The occupational health professionals must advise the management and the workers on factors at work which may affect workers' health. The risk assessment of occupational hazards must lead to the establishment of an occupational safety and health policy and of a programme of prevention adapted to the needs of undertakings and workplaces. The occupational health professionals must propose such a policy and programme on the basis of scientific and technical knowledge currently available as well as of their knowledge of the work organisation and environment. Occupational health professionals must ensure that they possess the required skill or secure the necessary expertise in order to provide advice on programmes of prevention which should include, as appropriate, measures for monitoring and management of occupational safety and health hazards and, in case of failure, for minimising consequences.

Emphasis on prevention and on a prompt action

4. Special consideration should be given to the rapid application of simple preventive measures which are technically sound and easily implemented. Further evaluation must check whether these measures are effective or if a more complete solution must be sought. When doubts exist about the severity of an occupational hazard, prudent precautionary action must be considered immediately and taken as appropriate. When there are uncertainties or differing opinions concerning nature of the hazards or the risks involved, occupational health professionals must be transparent in their assessment with respect to all concerned, avoid ambiguity in communicating their opinion and consult other professionals as necessary.

Follow-up of remedial actions

5. In the case of refusal or of unwillingness to take adequate steps to remove an undue risk or to remedy a situation which presents evidence of danger to health or safety, the occupational health professionals must make, as rapidly as possible, their concern clear, in writing, to the appropriate senior management executive, stressing the need for taking into account scientific knowledge and for applying relevant health protection standards, including exposure limits, and recalling the obligation of the employer to apply laws and regulations and to protect the health of workers in their employment. The workers concerned and their representatives in the enterprise should be informed and the competent authority should be contacted, whenever necessary.

Safety and health information

6. Occupational health professionals must contribute to the information for workers on occupational hazards to which they may be exposed in an objective and understandable manner which does not conceal any fact and emphasises the preventive measures. The occupational health professionals must co-operate with the employer, the workers and their representatives to ensure adequate information and training on health and safety to the management personnel and workers. Occupational health professionals must provide appropriate information to the employers, workers and their representatives about the level of scientific certainty or uncertainty of known and suspected occupational hazards at the workplace.

Commercial secrets

7. Occupational health professionals are obliged not to reveal industrial or commercial secrets of which they may become aware in the exercise of their activities. However, they must not withhold information which is necessary to protect the safety and health of workers or of the community. When needed, the occupational health professionals must consult the competent authority in charge of supervising the implementation of the relevant legislation.

Health surveillance

8. The occupational health objectives, methods and procedures of health surveillance must be clearly defined with priority given to adaptation of workplaces to workers who must receive information in this respect. The relevance and validity of these methods and procedures must be assessed. The surveillance must be carried out with the informed consent of the workers. The potentially positive and negative consequences of participation in screening and health surveillance programmes should be discussed as part of the consent process. The health surveillance must be performed by an occupational health professional approved by the competent authority.

Information to the worker

9. The results of examinations carried out within the framework of health surveillance must be explained to the worker concerned. The determination of fitness for a given job, when required, must be based on a good knowledge of the job demands and of the work-site and on the assessment of the health of the worker. The workers must be informed of the opportunity to challenge the conclusions concerning their fitness in relation to work that they feel contrary to their interest. An appeals procedure must be established in this respect.

Information to the employer

10. The results of the examinations prescribed by national laws or regulations must only be conveyed to management in terms of fitness for the envisaged work or of limitations necessary from a medical point of view in the assignment of tasks or in the exposure to occupational hazards, with the emphasis put on proposals to adapt the tasks and working conditions to the abilities of the worker. General information on work fitness or in relation to health or the potential or probable health effects of work hazards, may be provided with the informed consent of the worker concerned, in so far as this is necessary to guarantee the protection of the worker's health.

Danger to a third party

11. Where the health condition of the worker and the nature of the tasks performed are such as to be likely to endanger the safety of others, the worker must be clearly informed of the situation. In the case of a particularly hazardous situation, the management and, if so required by national regulations, the competent authority must also be informed of the measures necessary to safeguard other persons. In his advice, the occupational health professional must try to reconcile employment of the worker concerned with the safety or health of others that may be endangered.

Biologic monitoring and investigations

12. Biologic tests and other investigations must be chosen for their validity and relevance for protection of the health of the worker concerned, with due regard to their sensitivity, their specificity and their predictive value. Occupational health professionals must not use screening tests or investigations which are not reliable or which do not have a sufficient predictive value in relation to the requirements of the work assignment. Where a choice is possible and appropriate, preference must always be given to non-invasive methods and to examinations, which do not involve any danger to the health of the worker concerned. An invasive investigation or an examination which involves a risk to the health of the worker concerned may only be advised after an evaluation of the benefits to the worker and the risks involved. Such an investigation is subject to the worker's informed consent and must be performed according to the highest professional standards. It cannot be justified for insurance purposes or in relation to insurance claims.

Health promotion

13. When engaging in health education, health promotion, health screening and public health programmes, occupational health professionals must seek the participation of both employers and workers in their design and in their implementation. They must also protect the confidentiality of personal health data of the workers, and prevent their misuse.

Protection of community and environment

14. Occupational health professionals must be aware of their role in relation to the protection of the community and of the environment. With a view to contributing to environmental health and public health, occupational health professionals must initiate and participate, as appropriate, in identifying, assessing, advertising and advising for the purpose of prevention on occupational and environmental hazards arising or which may result from operations or processes in the enterprise.

Contribution to scientific knowledge

15. Occupational health professionals must report objectively to the scientific community as well as to the public health and labour authorities on new or suspected occupational hazards. They must also report on new and relevant preventive methods. Occupational health professionals involved in research must design and carry out their activities on a sound scientific basis with full professional independence and follow the ethical principles attached to research work and to medical research, including an evaluation by an independent committee on ethics, as appropriate.

CONDITIONS OF EXECUTION OF THE FUNCTIONS OF OCCUPATIONAL HEALTH PROFESSIONALS

Competence, integrity and impartiality

16. Occupational health professionals must always act, as a matter of prime concern, in the interest of the health and safety of the workers. Occupational health professionals must base their judgements on scientific knowledge and technical competence and call upon specialised expert advice as necessary. Occupational health professionals must refrain from any judgement, advice or activity which may endanger the trust in their integrity and impartiality.

Professional independence

17. Occupational health professionals must seek and maintain full professional independence and observe the rules of confidentiality in the execution of their functions. Occupational health professionals must under no circumstances allow their judgement and statements to be influenced by any conflict of interest, in particular when advising the employer, the workers or their representatives in the undertaking on occupational hazards and situations which present evidence of danger to health or safety.

Equity, non-discrimination and communication

18. The occupational health professionals must build a relationship of trust, confidence and equity with the people to whom they provide occupational health services. All workers should be treated in an equitable manner, without any form of discrimination as regards their condition, their convictions or the reason which led to the consultation of the occupational health professionals. Occupational health professionals must establish and maintain clear channels of communication among themselves, the senior management responsible for decisions at the highest level about the conditions and the organisation of work and the working environment in the undertaking, and with the workers' representatives.

Clause on ethics in contracts of employment

19. Occupational health professionals must request that a clause on ethics be incorporated in their contract of employment. This clause on ethics should include, in particular, their right to apply professional standards, guidelines and codes of ethics. Occupational health professionals must not accept conditions of occupational health practice which do not allow for performance of their functions according to the desired professional standards and principles of ethics. Contracts of employment should contain guidance on the legal, contractual and ethical aspects and on management of conflict, access to records and confidentiality in particular. Occupational health professionals must ensure that their contract of employment or service does not contain provisions which could

limit their professional independence. In case of doubt about the terms of the contract legal advice must be sought and the competent authority must be consulted as appropriate.

Records

20. Occupational health professionals must keep good records with the appropriate degree of confidentiality for the purpose of identifying occupational health problems in the enterprise. Such records include data relating to the surveillance of the working environment, personal data such as the employment history and occupational health data such as the history of occupational exposure, results of personal monitoring of exposure to occupational hazards and fitness certificates. Workers must be given access to the data relating to the surveillance of the working environment and to their own occupational health records.

Medical confidentiality

21. Individual medical data and the results of medical investigations must be recorded in confidential medical files which must be kept secured under the responsibility of the occupational health physician or the occupational health nurse. Access to medical files, their transmission and their release are governed by national laws or regulations on medical data where they exist and relevant national codes of ethics for health professionals and medical practitioners. The information contained in these files must only be used for occupational health purposes.

Collective health data

22. When there is no possibility of individual identification, information on aggregate health data on groups of workers may be disclosed to management and workers' representatives in the undertaking or to safety and health committees, where they exist, in order to help them in their duties to protect the health and safety of exposed groups of workers. Occupational injuries and work-related diseases must be reported to the competent authority according to national laws and regulations.

Relationships with health professionals

23. Occupational health professionals must not seek personal information which is not relevant to the protection, maintenance or promotion of workers' health in relation to work or to the overall health of the workforce. Occupational health physicians may seek further medical information or data from the worker's personal physician or hospital medical staff, with the worker's informed consent, but only for the purpose of protecting, maintaining or promoting the health of the worker concerned. In so doing, the occupational health physician must inform the worker's personal physician or hospital medical staff of his or her role and of the purpose for which the medical information or data is required. With the agreement of the worker, the occupational health physician or the occupational health nurse may, if necessary, inform the worker's personal physician of relevant health data as well as of

hazards, occupational exposures and constraints at work which represent a particular risk in view of the worker's state of health.

Combating abuses

24. Occupational health professionals must co-operate with other health professionals in the protection of the confidentiality of the health and medical data concerning workers. Occupational health professionals must identify, assess and point out to those concerned procedures or practices which are, in their opinion, contrary to the principles of ethics embodied in this Code and inform the competent authority when necessary. This concerns in particular instances of misuse or abuse of occupational health data, concealing or withholding findings, violating medical confidentiality or of inadequate protection of records in particular as regards information placed on computers.

Relationships with social partners

25. Occupational health professionals must increase the awareness of employers, workers and their representatives of the need for full professional independence and commitment to protect medical confidentiality in order to respect human dignity and to enhance the acceptability and effectiveness of occupational health practice.

Promoting ethics and professional audit

26. Occupational health professionals must seek the support and co-operation of employers, workers and their organisations, as well as of the competent authorities, for implementing the highest standards of ethics in occupational health practice. Occupational health professionals must institute a programme of professional audit of their activities to ensure that appropriate standards have been set, that they are being met and that deficiencies, if any, are detected and corrected and that steps are taken to ensure continuous improvement of professional performance.

This Code has been reproduced with the permission of International Commission on Occupational Health © ICOH 2002.

Chapter 56

Occupational and Environmental Legislation, Regulation, and Litigation in the United States

Gina Solomon, Adrianna Quintero, Amanda Hawes, Ellen Widess

INTRODUCTION

Physicians working in occupational and environmental medicine (OEM) often become involved in legal issues whether or not they seek such involvement. Understanding the legal and regulatory framework of OEM can be important in numerous clinical situations. Finding information about chemical exposure or toxicity requires knowledge of the governmental resources available. Physicians must be aware of legally mandated disease reporting requirements. Regulatory agencies can be important resources but it is important to know where their jurisdictions begin and end. Providing good information and advice to patients may require knowledge of available legal and regulatory options. Finally, patients may choose to bring legal action against a party that they presume responsible for their disease or injury, and the treating physician's medical record and testimony take on enormous importance in such a case.

The field of occupational and environmental law is relatively new. Most of the legislation in the field was passed since 1970, and most of the important litigation has taken place in the past two decades. Although the legislative framework of occupational law (other than labor relations and workers' compensation) is primarily centralized in the Occupational Safety and Health Act (OSHAct), environmental law is more diffuse. Environmental law is a confusing field with many governing laws, overlapping jurisdictions, and inconsistencies, making it difficult to understand, and resulting in some surprising gaps and omissions. The general public often assumes that the government would not allow dangerous chemicals to be used in the workplace, used in consumer products, or released into the air or water of their community. The assumption that the government has the authority to prevent hazardous chemical exposures is not legally correct, although there are some hazards that have been effectively addressed through law and regulation.

This chapter is designed to give the clinician an overview of the laws, regulatory agencies, and litigation relevant to the practice of occupational and environmental medicine. Workers compensation law is covered in Chapter 57.1. There are agencies with legal responsibility for investigating certain environmental or occupational hazards. There are also legal and regulatory resources for clinicians, including sources of information relevant to

chemical toxicity and to exposure. The clinician in turn has some legal obligations. Tort law is an area of ongoing development. Physicians have an important role in gathering information that may be helpful in a tort framework, and medical professionals should understand what is expected both of the treating physician and of the expert witness.

OCCUPATIONAL HEALTH LAWS AND REGULATORY AGENCIES

The Occupational Safety and Health Act, OSHA, and NIOSH

In 1970 President Richard Nixon signed the Occupational Safety and Health Act (OSHAct). This law was the first comprehensive attempt in the US to regulate occupational health and safety. The law created two government agencies, the Occupational Safety and Health Administration (OSHA) within the Department of Labor, and the National Institute for Occupational Safety and Health (NIOSH) within the Centers for Disease Control and Prevention (CDC) in the Department of Health and Human Services.

The OSHAct created important health and safety provisions for most workers. However, state and federal employees are exempt from protection under this law. The law creates a general duty for the employer 'to furnish to each of his employees employment and a place of employment which are free from recognized hazards that are causing or are likely to cause death or serious harm to his employees' (Section 5(a)(1)). OSHA sometimes uses this 'general duty clause' to cite employers for violations of the law even when the employer has not violated any specific workplace standard.

The OSHAct also requires OSHA to set standards governing health and safety in the work environment. The agency must 'set the standard which most adequately assures, to the extent feasible, on the basis of the best available evidence, that no employee will suffer material impairment of health or functional capacity even if such employee has regular exposure to the hazard dealt with by such standard for the period of his working life' (Section 6(b)(5)). Thus the language of the law appears to be highly protective of the health and safety of the worker. Unfortunately, subsequent court interpretations of the legislation, and decades of actual implementation have shown serious deficiencies. Due to the cumbersome process of collecting the scientific evidence and moving forward with rulemakings, OSHA has succeeded in only adopting interim standards from industry organizations and setting a small handful of specific standards of its own.

The OSHA effort to promulgate an ergonomics standard to address musculoskeletal disorders in the workplace, for example, began in 1992. After a cumbersome 8-year process, more than 8000 written comments, and more than 700 witnesses testifying at numerous public hearings, the agency issued a standard in November of 2000. In March of 2001, the new ergonomics standard was repealed due to a change in political administration in Washington DC. In the first 16 years of its history, OSHA promulgated only 24 standards. Observers have noted that the history of OSHA standard setting has been a process 'characterized by frustration, delay and missed opportunity'.[1] The courts have placed a heavy burden of proof on OSHA to demonstrate a 'significant risk of harm' and to show that a given standard is 'reasonably necessary and appropriate to remedy a significant risk of material health impairment'.[2] The definition of 'significant risk' has been a longstanding cause of contention. OSHA generally considers a cancer risk of one-in-a-thousand to be a significant risk. This contrasts sharply with the Environmental Protection Agency's one-in-a-million significant risk level.

The OSHAct has given OSHA some police powers to enforce the law. The law originally gave inspectors the right to enter any workplace covered by the law without prior notification. The Supreme Court held that this right is in violation of the Fourth Amendment and OSHA inspectors are now required to obtain search warrants. Inspectors are allowed to speak privately with any employee. When violations are identified, the agency may issue citations that must be posted in the workplace, and may assess fines. The fine for a serious violation may not exceed $1000, whereas the fine for a willful violation that results in the death of an employee or a repeated violation may be up to $10,000 per violation. Because OSHA has been chronically short-staffed, employers can expect rarely (if ever) to see an OSHA inspector at their door. The infrequent nature of the inspections and the relatively small fines are often not a sufficient incentive to make employers address workplace health and safety problems. Because OSHA citations must be posted, employees know if their workplace was inspected and if violations were found. The presence of OSHA does not necessarily mean hazardous health and safety conditions were found at the facility, since violations of record keeping are common. Conversely an OSHA inspection that fails to identify any violations does not necessarily mean the workplace is safe – only that no OSHA standards were violated. OSHA will sometimes inspect workplaces in response to complaints from unions or groups of workers. Physicians can also contact OSHA if they have information to suggest unsafe

or unhealthy workplace conditions. OSHA frequently follows up on tips from physicians.

OSHA does require that employers keep records of some important health and safety-related items. Workplaces must maintain on 'OSHA Log' with information about workplace injuries and illnesses. An injury is recordable if it involves medical treatment, loss of consciousness, work restrictions, or job transfer. Several OSHA standards require monitoring of exposure either through industrial hygiene sampling or biologic monitoring. The employer must maintain accurate records of these employees' exposures, and keep the records for at least 30 years. Employers must also file reports of work injuries and illnesses to OSHA for statistical purposes. OSHA compiles annual statistics on work injuries and illnesses, and on results of OSHA inspections. These reports are available to the public from OSHA. Although these reporting requirements have provided useful statistics on workplace injuries, they are much less useful for work-related disease. The diseases may not be diagnosed as work related, or may occur after an individual has left the job. Thus there is likely under-reporting of work-related illness.

Individual states are legally allowed to create their own versions of OSHA, as long as the state OSHA protections are at least as stringent as the federal protections. Now more than half of the states have their own state OSHA agencies, with standards and penalties that are generally significantly more stringent than those of federal OSHA. In some states coverage has been extended to state government workers. States with their own OSHA may have somewhat different reporting requirements and standards. In addition, workplace inspections are done by state rather than federal inspectors. Physicians should know if their state has an OSHA agency, and should know whom to contact if they identify potentially unsafe workplace conditions.

NIOSH is the research and educational arm of the federal workplace health and safety program. NIOSH researches occupational illness and injuries, recommends criteria for occupational health and safety standards to OSHA, and educates the public and the medical community about occupational health and safety issues. NIOSH also conducts health hazard evaluations (HHEs) of workplaces.[3] An HHE must be requested by an employer, a union representative, or by a group of workers. These investigations are most useful when a new or unusual work-related illness is suspected or when no specific OSHA standard applies. The requestor of an HHE may request confidentiality. NIOSH will triage requests and responds to some by sending teams of investigators to the workplace to conduct an in-depth investigation. If necessary, NIOSH teams can obtain a judicial warrant to perform an HHE even in the face of employer hostility. NIOSH also compiles a list of known toxic substances, known as RTECS (Registry of Toxic Effects of Chemical Substances) and writes summaries of the toxic effects of various chemicals.[4] Information is readily available from NIOSH either via the internet or via telephone at 1-800-35-NIOSH.

In 1987, NIOSH initiated the Sentinel Event Notification System for Occupational Risks (SENSOR), a project conducted in collaboration with the health departments of 10 states and designed to improve the reporting and surveillance of work-related health conditions. SENSOR states include California, Connecticut, Massachusetts, Michigan, Minnesota, New Jersey, New York, Oregon, Washington, and Wisconsin. States vary with regard to the health conditions tracked, but several states track traumatic injuries, occupational asthma, carpal tunnel syndrome, lead poisoning, noise-induced hearing loss, silicosis, dermatitis, injuries among teen workers, and other work-related disorders. In many of these states, physicians are legally required to report occupational diseases or injuries, and this information is critical to accurate tracking of work-related disorders by state and federal agencies.

The Mine Safety and Health Act and the Mine Safety and Health Administration (MSHA)

Passed in 1977 as a revision to the Federal Coal Mine Health and Safety Act of 1969, this statute created a federally administered compensation scheme for coal dust pneumoconiosis, known as the 'Black Lung Program'. The legislation also created the Mine Safety and Health Administration (MSHA) in the Department of Labor. MSHA is charged with addressing health and safety risks to all surface and underground miners. MSHA has set numerous health and safety standards and has established an inspection strategy that is quite different from the OSHA model. Each mine operator must provide routine sampling data for regulatory purposes to the agency. MSHA also does some inspection and sampling to confirm the submitted data. This approach guarantees that some data are available to the government on a routine and ongoing basis, irrespective of the actual frequency of government inspections. MSHA has attempted to control pneumoconiosis by establishing requirements for routine medical monitoring of miners, economic protection for workers transferred because of findings on medical monitoring, and a national surveillance program in coal mines administered by NIOSH.

Child Labor and the Fair Labor Standards Act

The Fair Labor Standards Act (FLSA) of 1938 includes several basic requirements relevant to occupational health. The FLSA requires payment of a minimum wage, overtime pay for work weeks longer than 40 hours, and restrictions on child labor. The child labor provisions include some restrictions on hours of work by youth under age 16, and a list of jobs considered too dangerous for workers under age 18 to perform. The restrictions on work hours do not apply to children working at family farms or family businesses, and the restrictions on hazardous work apply more narrowly to workers under age 16 in agricultural settings. In 1998, the Institute of Medicine released a report on child labor in the United States.[5] The report recommended several changes in FLSA to better protect youth at work.

Suggestions included limitations on working hours for children between the ages of 16 and 18, updating of the list of hazardous jobs to reflect hazardous exposures in modern workplaces, applying the same protections to children working in agriculture that apply to children in other job settings, updating OSHA standards to make sure they protect children, and increasing enforcement of the FLSA to reduce widespread violations. To date, there has been little progress on updating and amending child labor laws and regulations. Physicians should be aware that many children do work, and may be exposed to workplace hazards. An occupational history and reporting of work-related illnesses and injuries is particularly important in this population.

Agricultural workers

Jurisdiction over the agricultural work environment is divided between OSHA, the Environmental Protection Agency (EPA), and states. OSHA oversees Field Sanitation Regulations, which require employers to provide workers with drinking water, toilets, and hand washing facilities. Agriculture is specifically exempt from many OSHA standards, such as those regulating electrical hazards, unguarded machinery, confined spaces, heat stress, carcinogens, and access to medical and exposure records. Farms with fewer than 10 employees and that do not have farm labor camps are completely exempt from OSHA oversight, meaning that only an estimated 5% of farms in the US fall under OSHA's jurisdiction at all. Several states, including Washington and California, have more stringent agricultural worker protection laws.

The EPA's Office of Pesticide Programs (OPP) oversees worker protection from pesticides, and promulgated the Worker Protection Standard (WPS); 'designed to reduce the risks of illness or injury resulting from workers' and handlers' occupational exposures to pesticides used in the production of agricultural plants on farms or in nurseries, greenhouses, and forests and also from the accidental exposure of workers and other persons to such pesticides'.[6] Under the WPS, when an exposure occurs, employers must transport workers from the job site to a medical care facility and provide information about the pesticide to which the worker may have been exposed. EPA also sets restricted entry intervals (REIs) for pesticides, specifying how long employers must wait after a pesticide application before allowing workers to re-enter the area. OPP publishes an important resource for clinicians describing the signs and symptoms of pesticide poisoning, treatment for, and toxicology of, over 1500 pesticide products.[7] OPP has also worked in collaboration with other agencies to develop an initiative aimed at instructing healthcare providers about pesticide toxicology.[8]

Environmental health laws and regulatory agencies

In the United States, the laws and regulations designed to protect human health from environmental hazards are numerous and complex, including components at the federal and state level. It may be difficult for the clinician to determine who is responsible for what and where to turn for information. The Environmental Protection Agency (EPA) is the federal agency charged with administering the bulk of environmental regulations. The agency, created by President Nixon in 1970, brought together a patchwork of existing federal programs and laws concerned with environmental protection. EPA is administratively divided into 10 regions across the country. Each region addresses local and national issues. There are also numerous offices within the EPA with regulatory authority over specific classes of chemicals or environmental media. The EPA's mission includes protection of the natural environment and protection of human health. Despite the latter focus, there are few physicians, health professionals, or epidemiologists at the agency.

The EPA houses a wealth of information that may be useful to health professionals, some collected from outside parties, some developed by the EPA's Office of Research and Development. This information is available through EPA websites such as Envirofacts, a website that provides access to information about environmental issues including information on toxic chemical releases, hazardous waste, superfund, air and water releases and others.[9] One of the more valuable sources of information is the Integrated Risk Information System (IRIS). Developed for EPA staff to address the need for information on substances for use in risk assessments and regulatory activities, IRIS is a collection of data files with information on health effects of numerous chemicals.[10]

Information that is not readily available on government websites can generally be obtained by filing a Freedom of Information Act (FOIA) request.[11] The FOIA allows anyone to request any government information (other than confidential business information, classified materials, and draft documents).[12] The requestor is charged a fee for copying the documents, and must also pay for the time staff spend searching for documents. The requestor can ask for a fee waiver if the documents will be used in the public interest and the information will be made available to the public.

Even with the information the EPA makes available, healthcare professionals are left to unravel this information for themselves and their patients. Doctors are often called upon not only to diagnose environmental illness but also to help their patients understand scientific data, sift through government records, even provoke regulatory action. Physicians should understand the legal framework, so that they may treat patients with complaints linked to environmental or occupational exposures with this regulatory structure in mind. This may be especially important when a patient presents with a condition that does, or may at some future time, warrant further action either through the filing of a complaint with the agency or by initiating legal action. While a full understanding of the laws and regulations and an assessment of any claims should be left to an attorney with knowledge of environmental law, the following summary presents an overview of the laws with which treating physicians should be familiar.

Pesticide law: FIFRA and FFDCA

Two laws deal with the impacts on human health resulting from the use of pesticides: the Federal Insecticide, Fungicide, and Rodenticide Act (FIFRA),[13] and the Federal Food, Drug, and Cosmetic Act (FFDCA).[14] Under FIFRA, a pesticide cannot be sold or distributed in the United States until it is registered by the EPA. Registration of a pesticide means that it has been approved for sale and use. The EPA must make a determination that the pesticide, when considered with any restrictions imposed regarding its use, will perform its intended function and will not generally cause unreasonable adverse effects on the environment when used in accordance with widespread and commonly recognized practices. This determination is based on a balancing of the economic, social, and environmental costs against the benefit the pesticide provides. FIFRA also gives the EPA the authority to request any data necessary from the manufacturer to ensure that the product will not likely cause unreasonable adverse effects.

FIFRA has been amended several times to account for increasing public concern about the adverse effects of pesticides, and the advancement of scientific knowledge. In 1988, Congress amended FIFRA to require the re-registration of over 600 pesticides using the science reflected in the EPA's updated practices.[15] As part of this process, EPA produces Re-registration Eligibility Decision documents (REDs) and risk assessments. Both the risk assessments and the REDs are published documents that contain valuable summaries of the health effects, ecologic and occupational risks of individual pesticides.[16]

The Federal Food, Drug, and Cosmetic Act (FFDCA) is the nation's major law regulating contaminants in food, including pesticides. While the Food and Drug Administration (FDA) implements most of the FFDCA, the EPA carries out its pesticide standard setting provisions. Under the FFCDA, the EPA establishes tolerances (maximum legally permissible levels) for pesticide residues in food. Any pesticide chemical residue in or on a food is considered unsafe unless a tolerance or an exemption is in effect, and the residue is in compliance with that tolerance or exemption.

The Food Quality Protection Act of 1996 (FQPA) amended both the FIFRA and the FFDCA, setting a tougher standard for pesticide use on food. This law fundamentally changed the way the EPA regulates pesticides by mandating a health-based standard aimed at protecting infants and children. Under the FQPA, the EPA is required to reassess the safety of all existing tolerances by August 2006. The EPA must now consider the public's total exposure to pesticides (through food, water and home environments) when setting tolerances for pesticide levels on food. These decisions must protect infants and children whose developing systems may be more sensitive to pesticide exposure. The law also requires the EPA to determine whether a pesticide has a common mechanism of toxicity with any other pesticides.

FQPA also requires the EPA to establish and implement the Endocrine Disruptor Screening Program to test chemicals for endocrine effects. Congress specifically addressed the issue of endocrine disruption in the Food Quality Protection Act (FQPA) and Safe Drinking Water Act amendments of 1996. The Endocrine Disruptor Screening Program focuses on providing methods and procedures to detect and characterize endocrine activity of pesticides, commercial chemicals, and environmental contaminants. This information will be available to members of the public, and will help guide regulatory action.

Toxic chemicals: TSCA

In 1976, Congress enacted the Toxic Substances and Control Act (TSCA)[17] fueled by public concern over polychlorinated biphenyls (PCBs) and their persistence in the environment. TSCA, administered by the EPA's Office of Toxic Substances, authorizes the agency to regulate the manufacture, distribution, import and processing of industrial chemicals and heavy metals and require their testing. TSCA directs the EPA to conduct a risk–benefit analysis in determining the least burdensome manner in which to reduce the risk a chemical poses while considering the benefits provided by the chemical or chemical process.

Perhaps the most valuable aspects of TSCA to physicians are the data-gathering provisions. Under TSCA, the EPA has the authority to gather exposure and health data on a broad spectrum of chemicals. Data submissions required from industry, and other databases with information on approved chemicals, provide a valuable body of information, though often not in a user-friendly form. The EPA can require manufacturers, importers and processors of chemical substances to maintain records and report such data as the EPA may reasonably require, including chemical or mixture identity, use, health and environmental effects. Under TSCA, companies can be required to record, retain and in some cases report 'allegations of significant adverse reactions' – reactions that may indicate a substantial impairment of function or long-lasting or irreversible damage to health or the environment. Information on unpublished studies pertaining to the effects of chemicals submitted by industry to the EPA is available in the Toxic Substances Control Act Test Submissions (TSCATS) database.[18]

TSCA's intent was to give the EPA the authority to monitor the more than 75,000 chemicals currently produced or imported into the US. Unfortunately the law has failed to fulfill its original intent, in part because courts have generally placed a heavy burden of proof on the EPA in regulating under TSCA. The EPA cannot even require testing of a chemical until the compound is shown to present an 'unreasonable risk' or may pose a substantial or significant environmental or human health hazard. The interpretation of the term 'unreasonable risk' has generally been very strict, and the EPA has acted only rarely to regulate toxic chemicals using its authority under TSCA.[19]

Toxic waste: Superfund and RCRA

In 1980, Congress enacted the Comprehensive Environmental Response, Compensation and Liability Act (CERCLA), commonly known as 'Superfund', to require the clean-up of sites contaminated with toxic waste. The EPA's Office of Emergency and Remedial Response (OERR) has the authority to respond to releases or threatened releases of hazardous substances that may endanger public health or the environment. CERCLA is retroactive, allowing the EPA to hold liable those responsible for disposal of hazardous wastes before the law was enacted in 1980. CERCLA also established a trust fund to provide for clean-up when no responsible party can be identified.

CERCLA was amended in 1986 by the Superfund Amendments and Reauthorization Act (SARA).[20] The amendments strengthened the focus on human health risks from hazardous waste sites and encouraged greater citizen participation in making decisions on clean-up. Title III of SARA is an important source of public information, and is also known as the Emergency Planning and Community Right-to-Know Act (EPCRA). EPCRA requires the EPA to develop and maintain a toxic chemical database known as the Toxics Release Inventory (TRI).[21] This publicly available database contains information regarding toxic chemicals that are manufactured, treated, transported, or released into the environment. Manufacturers and facilities that use hazardous chemicals are required to report information on their discharges to air, water, land, and their transport for off-site disposal. There are over 600 chemicals that are subject to reporting on the TRI. TRI information is publicly available and accessible electronically. EPCRA also requires that emergency responders, including healthcare personnel, must have immediate access to information on what chemicals are released at any manufacturing facility in the event of an emergency.

CERCLA also created the Agency for Toxic Substances and Disease Registry (ATSDR). ATSDR, an agency of the US Department of Health and Human Services, is the principal federal public health agency involved with hazardous waste sites and emergencies resulting from releases of hazardous substances into the environment. ATSDR conducts health assessments at waste sites, health consultations concerning hazardous substances, health surveillance and registries, information development and dissemination, and education and training. ATSDR evaluates communities in proximity to hazardous waste sites to identify priority sites for remediation.

ATSDR also prepares toxicologic profiles of common chemicals, and ToxFAQs, a series of summaries about hazardous substances.[22] ATSDR maintains HazDat, a central database developed to provide access to information on the release of hazardous substances from Superfund sites, impacts on the general population and health information. ATSDR administers a National Exposure Registry (NER) to track the health status of individuals in communities that have been heavily exposed to specific contaminants. There are currently four active subregistries: trichloroethylene (TCE), 1,1,1-trichloroethane (TCA), benzene, and dioxin. An additional service provided by ATSDR is a referral network to occupational and environmental health clinics, including clinics with a pediatric focus (e.g., Association of Occupational and Environmental Clinics (AOEC) and Pediatric Environmental Health Specialty Units (PEHSU)).

The Resource Conservation and Recovery Act (RCRA) controls the transport, storage, and disposal of hazardous wastes onto land. RCRA was enacted in 1976 to address the management and disposal of municipal and industrial waste. RCRA is administered by the EPA's Office of Solid Waste. RCRA sets standards for the transport, labeling, and disposal of waste and includes provisions for clean-up of existing contaminated sites. The EPA and the states enforce these standards through a monitoring program using inspections, reviews, and sampling to determine a waste handler's compliance with the RCRA requirements. Under RCRA, citizens are authorized to bring direct enforcement actions against violators, known as a 'private right of action' under the law.

Air and water: the Clean Air Act, Clean Water Act, and Safe Drinking Water Act

The EPA regulates the risk posed by air pollutants to human health and the environment through the Clean Air Act (CAA), which regulates air emissions from area, stationary, and mobile sources by setting limits on how much of a pollutant can be in the air anywhere in the United States.[23] The law allows individual states to have stronger pollution controls, but prohibits weaker pollution controls than those set nationwide. The CAA established two types of national air quality standards: primary standards set limits to protect public health; and secondary standards protect public welfare, visibility and damage to animals, crops, and structures.

The CAA requires the EPA to promulgate National Ambient Air Quality Standards (NAAQS) for pollutants which the EPA has determined pose a risk to public health. These standards must be set at levels that protect the most sensitive members of the population, such as asthmatics, with a margin of safety. The EPA may require facilities emitting pollutants to conduct air quality monitoring, the results of which are made public.[24]

Each state must devise a State Implementation Plan (SIP), a collection of the regulations a state will use to clean up the air in polluted areas, which the EPA must approve. Standards are then administered by the states. The EPA assists the states by providing scientific research, engineering designs and money to support clean air programs. The goal of the Clean Air Act was to set and achieve NAAQS for every state by 1975; however, many areas of the country failed to meet the deadlines. In 1990 the Act was again amended to address previously overlooked problems such as acid rain, ground-level ozone, stratospheric ozone depletion, and air toxics. In 1997, the EPA set more stringent health-based standards for ozone and particulate air pollution. According to the American Lung Association, in the period between 1999 and 2001, approximately 137 million people in the US were living in areas that do not meet the new NAAQS.[25] The 1990 CAA established a permitting program for major air pollution sources such as power plants, enabled the EPA to fine violators, and included provisions to reduce interstate air pollution. The CAA was also important in setting the stage for the federal

citizen suit. This provision, now contained in many environmental laws, allows any person to bring a civil action against any other entity, including the EPA, to enforce the law.

The Clean Water Act (CWA) is a 1977 amendment to the Federal Water Pollution Control Act of 1972.[26] The CWA sets the goal of making all the nation's waters fishable and swimmable, and gives the EPA the authority to set national water quality standards for contaminants in surface waters. The CWA makes it unlawful for any person to discharge any pollutant from a point source into navigable waters unless a permit is obtained.[27] Permits control the amount and concentration of pollutants discharged into lakes, rivers, or the ocean. The EPA is charged with the duty of monitoring which dischargers are violating their permits. Unfortunately, this basic information is not available to the public through the EPA's Office of Water website.[28] The US Geological Survey also provides a wealth of information on the nation's water.[29]

The Safe Drinking Water Act (SDWA) was established to protect the quality of drinking water. Originally passed in 1974 and amended in 1986 and 1996, the SDWA does not regulate private wells serving less than 25 people. The law focuses on surface water and ground water actually or potentially designated for drinking. The Act authorizes the EPA to establish national primary drinking water standards (NPDWS) for drinking water. NPDWS set enforceable maximum contaminant levels for physical, chemical, biologic, or radiologic substances in drinking water sources. The EPA sets these standards by identifying contaminants that may adversely affect public health and that occur at a level and with a frequency that pose a threat to public health. The EPA determines an unenforceable maximum contaminant level goal (MCLG) at a level below which there is no expected health risk. Finally, the agency sets a maximum contaminant level (MCL), the maximum legally permissible level of a contaminant in treated drinking water. The MCL may be significantly higher than the MCLG, because it takes into account the maximum contaminant level goal, and the cost of achieving the level. The SDWA also contains a provision permitting citizens to file lawsuits in federal court in response to violations of drinking water standards by water suppliers or in response to the actions of the EPA.

Some of the more important features in the SDWA are its right-to-know components. The Consumer Confidence Report is the centerpiece of the right-to-know provisions in the SDWA Amendments of 1996. Water suppliers must produce annual drinking water quality reports for their customers. These reports enable the public to make informed decisions about their health and their environment by providing information about the source of local drinking water; the level of any contaminant found and the MCL for comparison; the likely source of any contaminant detected, and the potential health effects of any contaminants detected in violation of an EPA health standard. Physicians should familiarize themselves with these reports as they can be confusing, and patients may require assistance interpreting the reports. The EPA maintains drinking water data in several databases. The Safe Drinking Water Information System (SDWIS) is the EPA's national regulatory compliance database for the drinking water program. It includes information on the nation's 170,000 public water systems. The National Contaminant Occurrence Database (NCOD) tracks contaminants in drinking water to support the EPA's decisions regarding which contaminants to regulate.[30]

TORT LAW

With few exceptions, 'no-fault' workers' compensation is an injured worker's exclusive remedy against an employer. Nevertheless, tort litigation is increasingly common in occupational and environmental health. In some states, for example, a worker may sue an employer whose conduct is egregious and malicious, or if the conduct results in death; worker lawsuits are also sometimes directed against manufacturers and suppliers of chemical products, tools, or devices used in the workplace, or against other involved parties (e.g., a ventilation contractor). Individuals and communities in environmental exposure situations may also rely on tort law as a way of seeking compensation for their alleged injuries. A common public misperception of tort law is that juries typically award undeserving plaintiffs millions for minimal injuries. In fact, most tort cases are settled prior to trial and many that go to a jury for decision end up with a verdict for the defendant. Jury awards in tort cases are designed to compensate a person who has been wronged and who has suffered wage loss, medical expenses or other 'special damages' and who has also endured pain and suffering. When a jury finds the conduct of a defendant to be malicious, fraudulent or otherwise grossly appalling, punitive damages may be awarded to teach the wrongdoer a lesson and to try to deter similar conduct in the future. As a result, a small proportion of highly publicized lawsuits do end with large jury awards for the plaintiff.

The role of the treating physician in tort cases

When a patient brings a legal claim for compensation and asserts that a third party (the 'defendant') is legally responsible for an injury or illness, the records of treatment for that injury or illness may be subpoenaed and entered into evidence as part of the legal process. Subpoenas may also request records of a patient's prior medical history. Disputes over the relevance of old medical records may arise, along with debates about a patient's privacy and what is a legitimate scope of inquiry. Besides producing records of treatment when obliged to do so, the treating physician may be asked to testify as to the nature and extent of injury and the patient's prognosis. This process starts with a deposition, an out-of-court question and answer session, under oath, before a court reporter. Treating physicians may also be required to give testimony in court if the case proceeds to trial. Sometimes the treating physician will be asked about recognized risk factors for the patient's injury or condition,

and for an opinion on likely contributing causes in the individual case.

In cases of occupational or environmental exposure and disease, specialties in science and medicine that are germane to issues of causation generally include toxicology, epidemiology, occupational medicine, and industrial hygiene. A treating physician with knowledge and experience in such a field can be an effective witness whose opinion on causation will be given great weight. Conversely, a physician who does not customarily address issues of causation of occupational or environmental injury or disease in his/her regular medical practice may choose to defer to a physician or scientist who does specialize in such issues. Witnesses who are paid by litigants to express their opinions in the legal process are potentially vulnerable to charges of bias. At the same time, judges and jurors are sorely in need of expert assistance and interpretation in working their way through the complex medical and scientific issues raised in occupational and environmental health cases.

Admissibility of expert opinions

In 1923, a federal court held that an expert opinion should only be admitted at trial if the proponent of the opinion could demonstrate that the expert's views and opinion had been 'generally accepted' in the relevant scientific community.[31] In the 70 years following the so-called Frye decision, both the federal courts, as well as virtually every state court in the United States, relied upon the Kelly/Frye rule for admissibility of expert opinion. The California Supreme Court clarified that courts often refer to the narrow, 'common sense' purpose of the Kelly/Frye rule: to protect the jury from techniques which, though 'new' or 'experimental', convey a 'misleading aura of certainty'. The California court has specified that 'Kelly/Frye only applies to that limited class of expert testimony which is based in whole or part, on a technique, process, or theory which is *new* to science and, even more so, the law'.[32] Many would argue that expert opinions about the likely causal factors in disease are not appropriate for Kelly/Frye evaluation for the reason that the generally accepted methodology for evaluating causation is a weight-of-the evidence approach as outlined by Bradford Hill many decades ago, and is not a new or untried technique at all.

In 1993, the United States Supreme Court ruled, in *Daubert v. Merrell Dow Pharmaceuticals Inc.*, that in jurisdictions which follow federal rules of evidence, the Kelly/Frye rule for admissibility of expert scientific testimony has been pre-empted by a subsequently enacted federal rule of evidence, the Federal Rule of Evidence 702.[33] Some jurisdictions continue to use the Kelly/Frye rule, others use the test of admissibility outlined in Daubert.

Under Daubert, a trial judge deciding whether to admit expert scientific testimony at trial should specifically determine whether the expert's testimony: (1) reflects 'scientific knowledge' and (2) will assist the judge and jury in understanding or determining a material fact at issue. These determinations, in turn, require a specific assessment as to whether the reasoning or methodology underlying the testimony is 'scientifically valid' and whether that reasoning or methodology can properly be applied to the facts at issue.

The Court explained that many factors will bear on these assessments, including whether the scientific hypothesis can be (and has been) tested, whether it has been subjected to peer review and publication, its error rate, and whether the theory or technique has attracted widespread acceptance within a relevant scientific community. The Court indicated that the judge's analysis should be flexible, and no one factor should be considered determinative. The Court further emphasized that, *for purposes of determining admissibility of testimony, the focus must be on the principles and methodology underlying an expert's testimony, rather than on the expert's conclusions.*

In theory, this approach appears comparable to the Kelly/Frye rule still used in many state court jurisdictions. In practice, Daubert has given judges greater latitude in deciding whether to admit or bar experts from testimony in tort litigation. Despite the apparently reasonable standards laid out by the Supreme Court in Daubert, lower courts have taken divergent approaches to implementing the decision. Some federal courts have indicated that scientific opinions are admissible when they are based on methods reasonably or traditionally relied on by other experts in the same field, and the fact that such an opinion does not conclusively establish a cause–effect relationship will not render the opinion inadmissible under Daubert.[34]

In a key federal district court case, however, the judge barred the plaintiff's witnesses from testimony, reasoning that they did not engage in activities in a relevant field of expertise. The question at hand related to the potential teratogenic effects of a medication, and the plaintiff witnesses were experts in clinical medicine, pharmacology, and toxicology. The judge ruled that the only relevant and admissible field of expertise would be teratology.[35] Other courts have barred experts from presenting testimony based on case reports or case studies, or even based on animal studies, saying that these cannot reasonably be relied upon to support causation.[36] One court excluded expert testimony on the association between ethylene dioxide and brain tumors because the expert was relying on animal studies rather than human epidemiologic studies, even though the substance is classified as a carcinogen by regulatory agencies.[37]

Scientific uncertainty and the standard of proof

In tort cases, judges and juries are expected to decide whether, in light of the available evidence and data, it is more likely than not, to a reasonable degree of scientific and medical certainty, that a given exposure was a substantial contributing factor in the production of a specific disease or condition. It is not unusual for the state of evidence to be incomplete or subjected to the degree of scientific rigor that physicians are taught to expect of

scientific data. In law, the relevant question is whether the exposure, activity or conduct in question was a substantial contributing cause to the outcome. It need not be the sole cause. The degree of confidence that it was a contributing cause is sometimes expressed in probabilities – that it is more likely than not that it was a contributing cause (a 51% probability) or the 'preponderance of the evidence' indicates that it is a contributing cause. This is a different concept than 'beyond a reasonable doubt', the standard in criminal cases. The standard in tort cases is also different from the concept that an association can be considered to be causal only if it satisfies a test of statistical significance. In the courtroom, questions of causation generally draw on the disciplines of epidemiology, toxicology, industrial hygiene, occupational medicine, and clinical medicine, as interpreted and explained to the judge or jury by appropriately trained, qualified and experienced practitioners from these disciplines.

Physicians and scientists routinely use guidelines based on those proposed by Bradford Hill for assessing causation when they express opinions about causation in legal proceedings.[38] Because the Bradford Hill guidelines are well recognized and widely used in the scientific and medical community, their use as a methodologic approach for assessing causation is generally accepted in the courtroom. Consistency, specificity and strength of the association, the existence of an animal model, biologic plausibility of the putative association, temporality, and reasoning by analogy are all relevant considerations. None is a sine qua non. Further, diagnostic conclusions should be based on a consideration of differential diagnostic possibilities.

Challenges in tort litigation

Despite the lowered standard of proof compared to the 'beyond a reasonable doubt' standard in criminal cases, it can still be quite challenging to prove causation in a toxic tort context. In many cases of potential association between an occupational or environmental exposure and disease, there is likely to be less scientific research to draw on for determining causation than in situations such as those involving pharmaceutical drugs, where medical records of dosage and pre-market testing data are generally available. Many occupational and environmental diseases have long latency periods, making it a challenge to associate current illnesses with exposure that may (or may not) have occurred many years in the past. The requirement of the federal Hazard Communication Standard of 1986, that employers maintain exposure records for a 30-year minimum, is a helpful start in uncovering the nature and extent of potentially contributory exposures on the job. Biologic monitoring and medical surveillance data can be of particular use in documenting past exposures. At the same time, it is well recognized that people live complicated lives with numerous potential exposures in their homes, communities and workplaces. The identification of a substantial contributing cause can become very confusing when there are numerous potential causal factors. Studies on the health outcomes of persons engaged in similar work as the litigant and/or with similar exposures can shed useful light on causal factors, especially when the studies report consistent patterns, can detect dose–response trends, and are consistent with what is generally understood about the biology of the disease in question.

Establishing a causal connection in an individual case can be challenging for a variety of reasons. First, the sciences of toxicology and epidemiology have inherent limitations that narrow the interpretations one may draw from the available data; thus different evaluators may draw very different conclusions from the same overall body of literature. Animal data can provide a framework for evaluating the potential of a chemical to cause or contribute to effects in humans, but extrapolation from animal data to human risk requires consideration of inter-species differences, dosage, route of exposure, and whether mechanistic studies indicate likely relevance of the animal finding in humans. Completely controlled human studies are often out of the question due to ethical concerns about intentionally dosing humans with a toxic chemical to monitor its effects. In the real world, workers exposed to toxic materials are much more likely to be exposed to a mix of chemical compounds than to a single chemical, as would be the case in an animal toxicology experiment.

Epidemiologic studies may also be of limited application standing alone because of small or unrepresentative population sizes, inability to control for all confounding variables, difficulties in measuring historic exposure, and risks of recall bias. Judges have often been unfriendly to conclusions based on in-vitro studies, toxicology studies, and case reports, often demanding several positive, statistically significant epidemiologic studies prior to allowing evidence to come before a jury.[39] In this regard, under a 'weight-of-the-evidence' approach, a series of studies which consistently report positive associations between a given exposure and a disease endpoint may provide a compelling case for causation, even if none standing alone 'proves' the association. This observation is well to keep in mind given the struggle that some courts have had with epidemiologic data – sometimes according it much more and sometimes much less weight than the epidemiologic community itself would.

Several courts have narrowed the admissibility of epidemiologic studies since Daubert. Courts have ruled, for example, that it is unreasonable for experts to rely on studies with a relative risk less than 2.0 to support causation,[40] or that experts cannot present or rely on data from epidemiologic studies if the studies are not statistically significant with a P value less than 0.05, or with a confidence interval that includes one. These rulings appear to many to unduly narrow the scope of admissible evidence in tort cases, to accord less weight to epidemiologic data than scientists do, and to exclude studies that could be scientifically relevant to the understanding of causation.

The sciences of epidemiology and toxicology, as well as the structure of the laws and the rules by which regulatory agencies operate, make it possible to deal with some issues such as risk assessment and the consideration of precautionary principles on a population level. These same scientific tools and disciplines may also be useful and relevant in the situation that a clinician is most likely to be addressing – an individual instance of disease in a given patient. In this individual context, a concerned clinician has an opportunity to become involved in a constructive way, usually in conjunction with the input of specialists in such disciplines as occupational medicine, toxicology, industrial hygiene, and epidemiology.

Clinicians can contribute to a better societal understanding of the role of occupational and environmental exposures in the development of disease and thus assist in preventing future instances. These same efforts help individuals to document the prevalence of disease among similarly exposed persons. For example, the treating physician should make a patient's work history and exposure information a routine and readily abstractable part of the chart, along with standard social history and life style information. Patients often assume that their treating physicians know if a job or environmental exposure is a risk factor for disease and will not necessarily volunteer information if the treater does not show interest in eliciting it. The treating physician should also participate in coordinated efforts to report and track exposures and disease. The observations of astute clinicians have played a significant role in the discovery of many exposure/disease connections.

Regulators, legislators, judges, and juries with no scientific background must often weigh scientific information to make necessary legal decisions – some involving individuals who are already sick, some affecting populations at risk for future disease. Often these decision makers must call on physicians or other scientists to help interpret the science and guide appropriate health-protective decisions. The clinician should be aware of the resources available through government agencies, and should be able to direct a patient to these resources as appropriate.

References

1. Ashford NA, Caldart CC. Technology, law, and the working environment. New York: Van Nostrand Reinhold, 1991;100.
2. Industrial Union Department v. American Petroleum Institute 448 US 607 (1980).
3. http://www.cdc.gov/niosh/hhe.html
4. http://www.cdc.gov/niosh/rtecs.html
5. Committee on the Health and Safety Implications of Child Labor, National Research Council and Institute of Medicine. Protecting youth at work: health, safety, and development of working children and adolescents in the United States. Washington DC: National Academy Press, 1998.
6. 40 CFR § 170.1, et seq.
7. Reigart R, Roberts J. Recognition and management of pesticide poisonings, 5th edn. EPA 735-R-98-003. Washington DC: US Environmental Protection Agency, 1999.
8. http://www.neetf.org/Health/providers/index.shtm
9. http://www.epa.gov/enviro/index_java.html
10. http://www.epa.gov/iris/intro.htm
11. 5 U.S.C § 552.
12. http://www.epa.gov/foia/
13. 7 U.S.C § 136 et seq.
14. 21 U.S.C § et seq.
15. FIFRA § 4(a), 7 U.S.C § 136a-1.
16. http://www.epa.gov/pesticides/
17. 15 U.S.C § 2601 et seq.

18. http://esc.syrres.com/efdb/TSCATS.htm
19. Environmental Defense Fund v. Environmental Protection Agency 636 F.2d 1267 (D.C. Cir. 1980).
20. 42 U.S.C § 9601 et seq (1986).
21. http://www.epa.gov/tri/
22. http://www.atsdr.cdc.gov/
23. 42 U.S.C § 7401 et seq (1970).
24. http://www.epa.gov/airnow/
25. American Lung Association> State of the air, 2003. Washington DC: American Lung Association, 2003. http://www.lungaction.org/reports/sota03_full.html
26. 33 U.S.C § 1251 et seq.
27. 33 U.S.C § 1362(6).
28. http://www.epa.gov/watrhome/
29. http://water.usgs.gov/
30. http://www.epa.gov/safewater/databases.html
31. Frye v. United States, 293 F. 1013 (1923).
32. People v. Stoll, 49 Cal. 3d 1136, 1156, 265 Cal. Rptr 111 (1989).
33. Daubert v. Merrell Dow Pharmaceuticals, Inc. 509 U.S. 579 (1993).
34. See, e.g., Zuchowicz v. United States, 140 F. 3d 381, 387 (2d Cir. 1998); Ambrosini v. Labarraque, 101 F.3d 129, 139 (D.C. Cir. 1996); Upjohn Co. v. Ambrosini, 520 U.S. 1205 (1997); Kennedy v. Collagen Corporation, 161 F.3d 1226 (D.C. Cir. 1998).
35. Wade-Greaux v. Whitehall Laboratories, Inc. 974 F. Supp.1441 (D. Virgin Islands), 1994.
36. Bryant AH, Reinert A. Epidemiology in the legal arena and the search for truth. Am J Epidemiol 2001; 154:S27–S35.
37. Allen v. Pennsylvania Engineering Corp. 102 F.3d 194 (5th Cir.) 1996.
38. Bradford Hill A. The environment and disease: association or causation? Proc Roy Soc Med 1965; 58:295–300.
39. Brock v. Merrell Dow Pharmaceuticals, Inc. 874 F.2d 307 (5th Cir.), 1989.
40. See Kelley v. American Heyer-Schulte Corp. 957 F. Supp. 873 (W.D. Tex) 1997 and Merrell Dow Pharmaceuticals, Inc. v. Havner 953 S.W.2d 706 (Tex.), 1997.

Chapter 57

Legal and Regulatory Issues in the Workplace

57.1 Government Agencies/Statutes/Legislation
Mark A Rothstein

PHYSICIAN–PATIENT RELATIONSHIP IN THE OCCUPATIONAL SETTING
When does the relationship exist?

Traditionally, the physician–patient relationship has been based on the contract created when an individual selects a physician and the physician agrees to perform certain medical services. The contract model does not seem appropriate, however, when the physician is selected and paid by a third party rather than the individual recipient of the medical services. This third-party relationship, which applies in many employer-required medical examinations, is not unique to the occupational setting. Insurance, Social Security, workers' compensation, and other third-party medical examinations involve similar relationships.

Historically, the law has provided that there is no physician–patient relationship between an individual and a third-party physician, including in the occupational setting.[1] There is some evidence, however, that this view is changing, and the current state of the law is unclear. Courts that adhere to the dichotomy between employer-provided and traditional, patient-obtained medical care look to whether the physician is treating or merely examining the individual or for whose benefit the physician is performing the service. When the physician is merely examining the individual to determine employability or performing services for the benefit of the employer, no physician–patient relationship has generally been found. If the physician renders treatment[2] or is providing services for the benefit of the employee,[3] then a physician–patient relationship may be found.

These distinctions between employer-provided and patient-obtained medical care are probably too simplistic and artificial when applied to contemporary practice. Today, physicians employed by corporations examine *and* treat; their services may benefit *both* employer and employee. Similarly, patient-chosen physicians may increasingly assume roles in recommending and promoting changes in the workplace environment. However, independent medical examinations to determine the presence or extent of disability continue to stand outside the realm of the doctor–patient relationship.

Legal consequences of relationship or absence of relationship

If a physician–patient relationship is established, a physician is required to use 'that degree of care, skill and proficiency which is commonly exercised by the. . . careful and prudent physician engaged in similar practice under the same or similar circumstances'.[4] The standard of care required of a specialist is higher. It is the degree of care, skill, and proficiency commonly exercised by a specialist in good standing.

In the context of an occupational medical examination, the physician–patient relationship would establish a number of duties on the part of the physician. These include the duty:

- to inform the patient of his or her conditions and of all medical facts of which the patient reasonably should know;
- to notify the patient of the results of tests and of the physician's diagnosis, including issues of work-relatedness and impairment;
- to inform the patient of the need for treatment;
- to refer the patient to a specialist;
- to give the patient proper instructions for self-care;
- to advise the patient of the conditions that could aggravate the illness; and
- to preserve the confidentiality of the patient's medical information.

When there is no physician–patient relationship, most, if not all, of these duties are inapplicable. Some courts hold that the physician has no duty except to avoid injuring the individual during the course of the examination. Other courts hold that the physician owes the individual some degree of reasonable care or, if the physician undertakes to give some medical advice during the course of the examination, to exercise the same degree of care as one who renders services gratuitously.

Liability issues

Employer-salaried and, to a lesser extent, employer-retained independent contractor physicians are generally immune from employee lawsuits for two reasons. First, the existence of a legal duty to act with reasonable care usually depends on a physician–patient relationship. Second, co-employees (including a co-employee physician) may not be legally responsible for harms sustained by the employee because of workers' compensation laws, which limit liability of an employer and all co-employees to that which can be recovered under workers' compensation.[5] Nevertheless, there are exceptions.

As in more traditional medical malpractice cases, an injury caused during the course of an employer-mandated medical examination could establish liability on the part of the examining physician as well as that of the employer.[6] Not surprisingly, these situations are rare. A more common allegation is that in conducting a medical examination, the physician failed to diagnose a serious illness and the delay in treatment aggravated the individual's condition or reduced the likelihood of successful treatment. Even though an employer may be under no duty to conduct an examination, once the duty is assumed, any negligence in performing the examination may be actionable. For example, in *Green v. Walker,*[7] the defendant physician contracted with an employer to perform an annual physical examination of an offshore cook. The physician then allegedly negligently failed to diagnose the early stages of lung cancer, and the employee subsequently died. In a medical malpractice action brought by the man's widow, the United States District Court for the Eastern District of Louisiana granted summary judgment to the defendant on the ground that there was no physician–patient relationship. The United States Court of Appeals for the Fifth Circuit reversed this ruling. According to the court, even in the absence of a traditional physician–patient relationship, a physician owes a duty of reasonable care to an employee undergoing an employer-mandated medical examination.

Another theory on which plaintiffs have sued is that a negligent medical assessment resulted in an improper job placement.[8] Actions against employer-salaried physicians and employers for improper job placement normally are found to be barred by workers' compensation, but actions against independent contractor physicians are more likely to be successful.

Besides providing medical examinations, some company physicians become involved, to varying degrees, in the actual treatment of employees, from first aid to ongoing care. A number of lawsuits have alleged malpractice in treatment. Again, although most personal injury actions have been barred by workers' compensation,[9] in some cases of alleged negligent treatment, the courts have held that the plaintiffs have stated a legally cognizable claim.[10]

MEDICAL EVALUATION UNDER THE AMERICANS WITH DISABILITIES ACT
Coverage

The Americans with Disabilities Act (ADA) of 1990[11] is the first comprehensive federal law to prohibit discrimination in employment against an estimated 43 million Americans

with physical or mental disabilities. The ADA covers most private employers and state and local government employers. Federal employers are covered under comparable provisions of the Rehabilitation Act.[12] The ADA does not pre-empt state discrimination laws (such as a state law that covers small employers). The enforcement procedures and remedies are the same as exist under Title VII of the Civil Rights Act of 1964, which prohibits discrimination based on race, color, religion, sex, or national origin, and is enforced by the Equal Employment Opportunity Commission (EEOC).

Medical examinations

The ADA limits the way companies and physicians may assess the health status of applicants and employees (Table 57.1.1). Section 102(d)(2) of the ADA prohibits pre-employment examinations and questionnaires. An employer may not 'conduct a medical examination or make inquiries of a job applicant as to whether such applicant is an individual with a disability or as to the nature or severity of such disability'. The only permissible inquiries are about the ability of the applicant to perform job related functions. For example, an employer could ask if an applicant had a driver's license or could climb telephone poles, if these tasks were part of the job, but could not ask about specific medical conditions.

After a conditional offer of employment, an employer may require an 'employment entrance examination' (pre-placement examination) pursuant to Section 102(d)(3). These examinations, however, must be given to all conditional offerees, regardless of disability. Certainly, the examinations need not be identical for each individual and may vary based on the job requirements; the age, sex, and medical history of the individual; and other factors.

Pre-placement examinations need not be job related, although only job-related medical criteria may be used to screen out qualified individuals with disabilities.[13] Thus, many physicians limit pre-placement examinations to assessing medical conditions that bear directly on the individual's ability to perform the job. Among other things, this means that physicians:

- tailor each examination to the specific demands of the job;
- only use medical screening procedures with a high positive predictive value (thus precluding, for example, the use of low-back X-ray studies for screening out asymptomatic individuals); and

Timing	Legality
Pre-employment examinations	Impermissible
Pre-placement examinations (after conditional offer of employment)	Permissible
Current employee examinations	Permissible if job related or voluntary

Table 57.1.1 Medical examinations under the ADA

- use less comprehensive examinations for less physically demanding jobs.

The limited scope of pre-placement examinations under the ADA suggests two necessary responses by examining physicians. First, individuals undergoing an examination should be informed of the limited nature of the medical assessment and advised that it is not designed to substitute for a comprehensive examination by their personal physician. Although legal, broad release forms authorizing access to all private medical records of an individual result in employers obtaining more medical information than may be lawfully used. Thus, physicians and employers should consider more limited releases.

Records, disclosures, and accommodations

Section 102(d)(3) of the ADA regulates medical records. '[I]nformation obtained regarding the medical conditions or history of the applicant [must be] collected and maintained on separate forms and in separate medical files and [must be] treated as a confidential medical record. . .' For most companies with on-site medical facilities, this is standard procedure already. Most problems arise at facilities without on-site medical departments that use contract physicians to perform pre-placement examinations. These contract physicians frequently do not want to maintain huge files of non-patients who were examined only once. Although EEOC regulations to implement the ADA do not address this issue, it would appear that an employer would be in compliance if contractor-generated medical records were stored at the worksite separate from other files, and with controlled access.

The ADA also limits the disclosures that physicians can make to non-medical personnel. Section 102(d)(3) provides that 'supervisors and managers may be informed regarding necessary restrictions on the work or duties of the employee and necessary accommodations'. They may not be given any other medical information, such as specific diagnoses. This provision is consistent with principles of confidentiality addressed in Chapter 55, and mandated under the Health Insurance Portability and Accountability Act (HIPAA), 1996, which went into effect in 2002. Releases authorizing wider disclosure of medical information raise substantial legal concerns. Significantly, because Section 104(d) provides that a drug test is not a 'medical examination', disclosing the results of a pre-placement drug test to management would be legally permissible (although arguably in contravention of appropriate ethical principles).

Section 103(d) of the ADA, dealing with infectious and communicable diseases, permits the exclusion of individuals from food-handling jobs if they have an infectious or communicable disease (such as hepatitis A) that the Secretary of Health and Human Services determines may be transmitted through food handling. Although the ADA does not contain any express provisions concerning HIV, it is clear that HIV testing, isolation, or other discrimination against people who are seropositive for HIV or who have AIDS is unlawful under the ADA, if the individuals with or without reasonable accommodation are otherwise qualified and capable of performing job-related duties.

The ADA provisions applicable to periodic medical examinations of employees are more explicit than those applicable to pre-placement examinations. Pursuant to Sections 102(b)(6) and 102(d)(4), all medical examinations and inquiries must be 'job-related and consistent with business necessity'. Employers may offer medical examinations of a non-job-related nature, such as comprehensive medical examinations and wellness programs, but employee participation must be voluntary.

The responsibility of occupational physicians may encompass determining what 'reasonable accommodation' will permit an otherwise qualified individual with disabilities to perform the job. According to Section 101(9) of the ADA, reasonable accommodation may include making facilities accessible; job restructuring; part-time or modified work schedules; reassignment to a vacant position; modification of equipment; appropriate adjustment of examinations, training materials, or policies; and the provision of qualified readers or interpreters. Reasonable accommodation is not required, however, if it would impose an 'undue hardship' on the employer based on the nature and cost of the accommodation, the size and financial resources of the facility or company, and the nature of the workforce.

One of the many reasons an individual with disabilities may be considered medically unqualified for a particular job is the employer's concern that the individual may pose a safety or health threat to the individual, coworkers, customers, or the public. Section 103(b) provides that 'the term "qualification standards" may include a requirement that an individual shall not pose a direct threat to the health or safety of other individuals in the workplace.'[14] Although this language is narrow and does not include harm to the individual employee with a disability, the interpretive regulation of the EEOC is broader. It defines 'direct threat' to include the affected individual, requires these determinations to be made on the basis of reasonable medical judgment, and lists four factors to consider. These factors are the duration of the risk, the nature and severity of the potential harm, the likelihood that the potential harm will occur, and the imminence of the potential harm. The legislative history and the EEOC regulations make it clear that a 'direct threat' claim of an employer is difficult to prove. Patronizing assumptions, generalized fears, and speculative or remote risks are insufficient.

In *Chevron USA Inc v Echazabal*,[15] an individual who had worked for independent contractors at a Chevron Oil refinery was denied a position with Chevron because he had a history of hepatitis C. Although he had worked at the facility for 20 years without any health problems, Chevron said that chemicals at the refinery could damage his liver. The Supreme Court held it was lawful for the employer to consider the individual's risk to 'self' as well as 'others'. Another case finding a direct threat involved an individual with uncontrolled epilepsy who worked with hazardous machinery.[16]

OCCUPATIONAL SAFETY AND HEALTH ADMINISTRATION (OSHA)-REQUIRED AND OTHER MANDATORY PRACTICES

Mandatory examinations

Generally speaking, there is no legal duty for an employer to perform pre-placement or other medical examinations. There are, however, some governmentally mandated employee medical examinations. These medical examinations are conducted for two main purposes:

- to protect the health and safety of the employee; and
- to protect the health and safety of the public.

Perhaps the best example of a medical examination designed to protect the health of employees is an OSHA-mandated examination. These examinations, however, only pertain to employees with exposure to about two dozen specific toxic substances[17] (see Chapter 59). In general, physicians must furnish employers with a statement of suitability for employment in the regulated area; the employer must offer employees periodic (usually annual) examinations; and, in some instances, employers also must provide examinations at termination of employment. The failure to offer these required medical examinations may lead to the issuance of OSHA citations and the assessment of penalties.

Three of the most common questions regarding OSHA-mandated medical examinations are:

1. Is the medical examination mandatory?
2. Who selects the physician?
3. Who pays for the examination?

First, Section 6(b)(7) of the Occupational Safety and Health Act provides that medical examinations shall 'be made available' to exposed employees. OSHA has interpreted this language to mean that the employer must offer the examination; however, the employee may refuse to take the examination. Nevertheless, OSHA does not protect a refusal to participate. Unless the issue is covered by the terms of a collective bargaining agreement, an employer may make cooperation with medical examinations a valid condition of employment.

Second, the Act does not specifically indicate whether the employer or employee has the right to select a physician to perform medical examinations. Early on, OSHA determined that the employer should have the option of choosing the physician and should have access to the results of the examination. This policy has been followed in all of the health standards.

Third, Section 6(b)(7) of the Act makes it clear that medical examinations shall be made available 'by the employer or at his cost'. OSHA's health standards have included language indicating that all costs for medical examinations must be borne by the employer. The employer also may be required to compensate employees for time spent taking the examination (outside normal working hours) and for extra transportation expenses.

Although physicians should be familiar with OSHA's medical examination provisions (see Chapter 59), these regulations may be of limited value for the following four reasons.

1. The provisions only apply to specific occupational exposures and, therefore, are of limited scope.
2. The provisions list required procedures but often give little guidance as to the significance of specific clinical or laboratory findings.
3. The provisions do not indicate what procedures or tests may or may not be performed.
4. With a few exceptions, there is no mention about what personnel actions are required, permitted, or prohibited on the basis of test or examination results.

Another law requiring medical examinations to protect employee health is the Mine Safety and Health Act.[18] Section 203(a) of the Act requires that all miners working in a coal mine be given a chest X-ray study within 6 months after commencement of employment, a second X-ray study 3 years later, and a third X-ray study 2 years after that if the second X-ray study showed evidence of pneumoconiosis.

There are a number of federal laws mandating employee medical screening to protect the health and safety of the public. Two of the most important of these laws prescribe medical certification for over-the-road truckers and airline pilots. The Department of Transportation's (DOT) Bureau of Motor Carrier Safety has issued detailed regulations for the physical examination of drivers operating motor vehicles in interstate commerce.[19] Successful completion of the examination is a prerequisite for driver certification. Physicians are provided with a form and instructions about specific conditions to evaluate. Similar regulations have been promulgated by the Federal Aviation Administration (FAA) for airline flight crews.[20] Unlike the motor carrier examinations, which may be performed by any licensed physician, aviation medical examinations may be performed only by physicians designated by the FAA under the auspices of the Federal Air Surgeon.

The DOT and FAA examinations contemplate a role for the physician different from that in other examinations. Because of concern for public safety, detailed procedures and standards have been adopted that remove a great deal of the discretion from the physician. If the standards are excessively stringent and serve to disqualify individuals who would normally be considered fit, it may be viewed as an acceptable price to pay for protecting the public.

A number of state laws also require pre-placement medical examinations to protect public health and safety. Among the occupations for which a medical examination may be mandated are teachers, school bus drivers, police, firefighters, divers, transportation, and maritime workers. Laws in many states also mandate the reporting of various occupational diseases.[21]

Access to exposure and medical records

The primary purpose of OSHA's rule on access to exposure and medical records is 'to enable workers to play a meaningful role in their own health management'.[22] The regulation applies to all covered general industry, maritime, and construction employers. It is, however, limited to employers having employees exposed to toxic substances or harmful physical agents. Unlike other OSHA record-keeping requirements, the access regulation does *not* require that certain documents be prepared but only that existing records be maintained and made available to employees and other parties designated in the regulation.

Any current or former employee being assigned or transferred to work where there will be exposure to toxic substances or harmful physical agents has a right of access to four kinds of exposure records:
- environmental monitoring records;
- biologic monitoring results;
- material safety data sheets; and
- any other record disclosing the identity of a toxic substance or harmful physical agent.

Any worker who has a right of access to exposure records may designate a representative to exercise access rights. Recognized or certified collective bargaining agents (i.e., labor unions) are automatically considered 'designated representatives' and have a right of access to employee exposure records without individual employee consent. OSHA also has a right of access to exposure records.

Access to employee medical records is more restricted (Table 57.1.2). Employees have a right of access to their entire medical files regardless of how the information was generated or is maintained. Excluded from the definition of 'employee medical record' are certain physical specimens, certain records concerning health insurance claims, and certain records concerning voluntary employee medical assistance programs. A limited discretion is also given physicians to deny access in cases in which there is a specific diagnosis of a terminal illness or psychiatric condition. Collective bargaining agents must obtain specific written consent before gaining access to employee medical records. OSHA has a right of access to employee medical records, but those records in a personally identifiable form are subject to detailed procedures and protections. The Occupational Safety and Health Review Commission has held that OSHA has a right of access to employee medical records as part of its enforcement process and in discovery before a Commission hearing.[23] The Commission also has held that a release referring only

to medical records does not require the disclosure of employee exposure records.[24]

With a few exceptions, employers must preserve exposure records for at least 30 years and must preserve medical records for the duration of employment plus 30 years. With the exception of X-ray studies, employers may keep the records in any form, such as microfilm, microfiche, or computer disk. On receipt of a request, access must be provided in a reasonable time, place, and manner within 15 days. In responding to an initial request, an employer may provide a copy without cost, provide copying facilities at no cost, or may loan the record for a reasonable time. Administrative costs may be charged for subsequent copying requests.

Although identities of substances, exposure levels, and health status data may not be withheld, the employer may delete any other trade secret data that disclose manufacturing processes or disclose the percentage of a chemical substance in a mixture, so long as the employee or designated representative is notified of the deletion. Access to other trade secrets may be on written agreement not to misuse this information.

The access regulation also includes an exemption from record retention requirements for medical and exposure records for short-term employees (the short-term employee may be handed the records), permission for employers to store medical records on microfilm, protections for employer trade secrets, and a requirement that unions must have need before they may see an employee's exposure records without the employee's consent, thereby allowing employers to deny blanket requests.

Hazard communication

OSHA's original Hazard Communication Standard[25] covered an estimated 14 million employees in 300,000 manufacturing establishments. Among other things, it required chemical manufacturers and importers to assess the hazards of chemicals they produce or import, and all employers engaged in manufacturing to provide information to their employees concerning hazardous chemicals by means of hazard communication programs including labels, material safety data sheets, training, and access to written records. One of the purposes of the standard was to pre-empt state right-to-know laws.

The standard originally applied only to chemical manufacturers and importers (SIC Codes 20 to 39), applied only to 600 substances, and excluded hazardous wastes, foods, drugs, and pesticides. By contrast, many state right-to-know laws cover more classes of employers and many more substances.

An amendment to the Hazard Communication Standard expanded coverage beyond the manufacturing sector to cover all workers. The revised standard contains three new provisions:
- a requirement that at multi-employer worksites, employers exchange their material safety data sheets, either individually or through a central location;
- an exemption from labeling requirements for consumer products used in the same manner and quantities as intended for consumer use; and

---

1. Applies to employers with employees exposed to toxic substances or harmful physical agents
2. Employees have a right of access to their entire medical files, except for health insurance claims and employee assistance program records
3. Unions must obtain written consent before gaining access
4. OSHA has a right of access, with specific provisions to protect confidentiality
5. Records must be retained for at least 30 years
6. Upon receipt of an employee request, access must be provided within 15 days

Table 57.1.2 Key provisions of OSHA's access to employee medical records regulation

- an exemption from labeling requirements for drugs regulated by the Food and Drug Administration.

WORKERS' COMPENSATION
General provisions

The workers' compensation system consists of a series of state and federal laws designed to provide income replacement, medical expenses, and rehabilitation services to individuals disabled by work-related injury or illness. Each state has its own workers' compensation law, and federal laws provide additional coverage for federal civilian employees, longshoring and harbor workers, seamen, railroad workers, and coal miners.

Workers' compensation is essentially a form of employer-provided life and disability insurance for work-related injury, illness, and death. With only a few exceptions, such as domestic household employees, all private sector employees are covered. For commercially purchased or state-administered plans, premiums are paid by the employer into an insurance fund, which pays worker claims. For self-funded employers, claims are paid directly by the employer. Work-related injuries are compensable without regard to who was at fault. Common law defenses, such as contributory negligence, assumption of the risk by the employee, and claiming the injury was caused by a co-employee, are inapplicable.

Workers' compensation law generally precludes an employee from suing or otherwise being reimbursed for injury or harm by the employer. Only third parties, such as suppliers of hazardous materials or equipment, can be sued (see Chapter 56). Further, the compensation laws do not preclude other types of defenses by an employer, such as that work did not cause the injury or illness. As in other legal actions, the burden remains on the employee who has been hurt or become ill to prove that an injury or illness is compensable.

Although each state law sets its own eligibility requirements, benefit levels, and claims procedures, most state laws are similar. An employee is usually required to notify the employer of an injury or illness, and to file a timely claim with the state agency that administers the workers' compensation system. All states have waiting periods before a claimant is eligible for benefits. In virtually all jurisdictions, contested workers' compensation cases are adjudicated by an administrative agency. This procedure is less formal than a court proceeding, and generally faster and less expensive. Denial of claims frequently results in lengthy appeal processes, especially in occupational disease cases. Further, the administrative determination is invariably subject to judicial review.

Eligibility for benefits

The claimant has the burden of demonstrating eligibility for workers' compensation, and this usually requires medical documentation of the claimant's injury or illness. In many states, the administrator of the workers'

compensation system has the authority to order the claimant to undergo a medical examination by an examiner selected and paid by the state agency. Refusal to submit to a medical examination will bar the recovery of benefits, but claimants usually need not submit to potentially dangerous or painful procedures.

Virtually all workers' compensation laws use a four-way classification of disabilities:
- temporary partial;
- temporary total;
- permanent partial; and
- permanent total.

Temporary claims are relatively easy to determine. Temporary partial disability is applicable when it is determined that the claimant is unable to perform at his or her regular job but is able to engage in some other gainful employment. Temporary compensation is based on wage loss and includes medical and hospital expenses. Temporary total disability exists when the claimant is unable to work at all for a limited period of time. All states have waiting periods (from 3 to 7 days) before a claimant is eligible for wage replacement benefits. There are usually no waiting periods, however, for medical benefits.

From a medical standpoint, it may be difficult to determine when the period of temporary total disability has ended or, if a degree of impairment remains, when the temporary total disability becomes a permanent partial disability. The dates most frequently used for deciding that a temporary total disability has become a permanent partial disability are the date the claimant has reached maximum medical improvement (i.e., no further improvement in medical status is anticipated), the date the impairment has become stationary, or the date the claimant is able to return to work.

Awards for permanent partial disability may be scheduled or unscheduled. Scheduled benefits are legislatively set and involve total or partial loss of use of specific body members, in cases in which wage loss is presumed. These scheduled benefits may be given in addition to benefits received for temporary total disability; in such cases the claimant is entitled to a scheduled payment, regardless of the economic consequences of the impairment. In other words, the basis of the award is medical impairment rather than wage loss.

For unscheduled permanent partial disability cases, the wage loss principle is generally used. Degree of disability is calculated by comparing the individual's earnings before the injury or illness with his or her earning capacity after the injury or illness. This later estimate, of course, depends on the medical determination of impairment as well as other non-medical factors relative to the claimant's employment opportunities.

Many workers' compensation laws and regulations are vague about the method to be used by examining physicians in calculating the claimant's level of impairment (see Chapter 8). Some states use the American Medical Association's Guide to the Evaluation of Physical Impairment (currently in the fifth edition); other states have their own systems. Commonly, the physician will initially determine the degree of impairment caused by an injury or illness to a specific organ system or body part, and subsequently calculate the degree of impairment to the body as a whole.

Medical opinions

The examining or treating physician has two major responsibilities to the patient in workers' compensation matters. First, and most crucial, is determination of whether an illness or injury is, in fact, work related, the sine qua non of eligibility for this benefit as compared with others. For sudden injuries and acute diseases, this connection may be obvious; for chronic or delayed effects of work, determination of causation may be more challenging. The standard used in most compensation systems is 'more probably than not', or more than 50% likely to be work related. Although strategies for arriving at this opinion are beyond the scope of this chapter, the physician must recognize that the clinical continuum becomes a categorical 'all or nothing' as far as eligibility for this benefit is concerned.

The second obligation of the physician is determination of disability status. Part of this determination is entailed in the assessment of physical impairment, discussed in Chapter 8. However, the physician also must translate this clinical information into a decision about whether and what work the patient can do, because this factor is vital to the compensation system's decision about the assignment of benefits. This task requires knowledge not only of the illness or injury and the patient, but also of the job tasks, exposure, and physical demand requirements.

In workers' compensation cases, it is not unusual for there to be conflicting medical evidence concerning the work-relatedness or level of the claimant's disability. There is some disagreement among the states on how conflicting medical evidence should be resolved. The industrial commission or workers' compensation board is charged with determining which conflicting medical testimony is to be accepted. Deference usually is given to the opinions of the treating physician. The theory behind giving greater weight to the testimony of treating physicians is that a treating physician is likely more experienced than an examining physician with the specific health status of an individual patient. Although it could be argued that the testimony of some treating physicians may be affected by advocacy for their regular patients, the countering argument is that some third-party examining physicians may have biases, including financial interests, related to the third parties who have retained their services.

DRUG TESTING
Overview

Perhaps the most ubiquitous procedure performed in company medical departments is drug testing. Although pre-placement drug testing is most common, some companies also test 'for cause', post-rehabilitation, periodically, or randomly. Some companies limit testing to employees in safety-sensitive positions; others test all applicants or employees.

Pursuant to an Executive Order issued by President Reagan in 1986,[26] about half of all federal government employees are subject to drug testing. Some comparable state laws also mandate the testing of state employees. In the private sector, certain employees in safety-sensitive jobs, such as transportation and nuclear workers, are subject to federally mandated drug testing. The Drug Free Workplace Act,[27] applicable to recipients of federal grants, requires grantees to have a written substance abuse policy but does not require drug testing. Therefore, most private sector drug testing has been voluntarily adopted by employers.

Drug testing is a forensic procedure rather than a medical test. Nevertheless, physicians are often assigned a major role in the process. For example, under the Department of Health and Human Services' guidelines for federal drug-testing programs, a 'Medical Review Officer' (termed 'MRO') is responsible for interviewing tested individuals about prescription drug use and reviewing and interpreting drug test results.[28]

Legal issues

The legality, morality, and efficacy of drug testing remain subjects of great controversy. Whether drug testing is legal depends on many factors, including the following: whether the employment is in the public or private sector, whether the drug testing is government mandated, whether the employees are represented by a union, whether there is an applicable state drug-testing law, and whether the testing involves employees in safety-sensitive jobs (Table 57.1.3). In general, private sector employers are given great leeway in drug testing.

About half the states have enacted their own laws to regulate drug testing. The laws vary widely, and deal with issues such as whether probable cause is needed to test, which job classifications may be subject to testing, the permissible time for testing, sample collection methods, confidentiality, analytic methodology, and laboratory certification.[29]

Because of the large number of potential legal issues involving drug testing, legal counsel should be consulted about these matters. Nevertheless, some general advice will help avoid problems. First, occupational health personnel must be particularly careful about maintaining the confidentiality of drug test results. Second, all drug-screening tests should be confirmed using gas chromatography, mass spectrometry, or comparable technology. Third, observed

1. Private or public sector?
2. Government mandated?
3. State drug-testing law?
4. Collective bargaining agreement?
5. Confirmatory testing used?
6. Pre-employment, pre-placement, periodic, for cause, or random?
7. Safety-sensitive position?

Table 57.1.3 Factors determining the legality of drug testing

urination is likely to be challenged as an invasion of privacy. Fourth, random testing is the most likely form of testing to be invalidated by the courts, and it is often considered unlawful except in cases of clear-cut public safety considerations.

References

1. See, for example, Murphy v. Blum, 554 N.Y.S.2d 640 (App. Div. 1990) (annual employment physical); Lee v. City of New York, 560 N.Y.S.2d 700 (App. Div. 1990) (pre-employment physical); Elia v. Erie Ins. Exch., 581 A.2d 209 (Pa. Super. Ct. 1990) (insurance physical); Beaman v. Helton, 573 So. 2d 776 (Miss. 1990) (Social Security examination). For a further discussion, see Rothstein MA. Legal issues in the medical assessment of physical impairment by third-party physicians. J Legal Med 1984; 5:503-48.
2. Hendy v. Losse, 274 Cal. Rptr. 31 (1990).
3. Hickey v. Travelers Ins. Co., 558 N.Y.S.2d 554 (App. Div. 1990).
4. Brown v. United States, 419 F.2d 337, 341 (8th Cir. 1969).
5. Kerr v. Olson, 798 P.2d 819 (Wash. Ct. App. 1990).
6. Hagan v. Antonio, 397 S.E.2d 810 (Va. 1990) (malpractice based on fondling applicant during pre-employment examination).
7. 910 F.2d 291 (5th Cir. 1990).
8. Mahfouz v. J.A.C.E. Oilfield Sales & Serv., Inc., 569 So. 2d 1074 (La. Ct. App. 1990).
9. Panaro v. Electrolux Corp., 545 A.2d 1086 (Conn. 1988); Deller v. Naymick, 342 5.E.2d 73 (W. Va. 1985).
10. Nolan v. Jefferson Down's, Inc., 592 So.2d 831 (La. Ct. App. 1991), writ denied, 596 50.2d 558 (La. 1992).
11. 42 U.S.C. §§12101-12213.
12. 29 U.S.C. §791.
13. 29 C.F.R. Part 1630.
14. 42 U.S.C. §12113(b).
15. Echazabal v. Chevron USA, Inc., 536 US 73(2002).
16. Moses v. American Nonwovens, Inc., 97 F.3d 446 (11th Cir. 1996), cert. denied, 519 U.S. 1118 (1997).
17. 29 C.F.R. §§1910.1001-1910.1048.
18. 30 U.S.C. §§801-962.
19. 49 C.F.R. §§391.41-391.49.
20. 14 C.F.R. §§67.1-67.31.
21. Freund E, Seligman PJ, Chorba TL, et al. Mandatory reporting of occupational diseases by clinicians. JAMA 1989; 262:3041-4.
22. 45 Fed. Reg. 35,212 (1980), codified at 29 C.F.R. § 1910.20.
23. General Motors Corp., 9 OSHC 1879, 1981 OSHD ¶25,341 (ALJ), petition for review dismissed Nos. 81-1919, 81-3323 (2d Cir. 1982); West Pt. Pepperell, Inc., 9 OSHC 1784, 1981 OSHD ¶25,356 (1981).
24. Johnson & Johnson Prods., Inc., 11 OSHC 2097, 1984 OSHD ¶26,988 (1984), petition for review withdrawn No. 84-2588 (7th Cir. 1984).
25. 29 C.F.R. §1910.1200.
26. Executive Order 12,564, 52 Fed. Reg. 23,889 (1986).
27. 41 U.S.C. §§701-707.
28. 52 Fed. Reg. 30,638,30,643 (1987).
29. Rothstein MA, et al. Employment law, 2nd edn. Volume 1, § 1.26. St Paul, Minnesota: West Group; 1999.

57.2 **Environmental Justice**

Rachel Rubin, Linda Rae Murray

INTRODUCTION

Environmental and occupational hazards and the resultant illnesses, diseases and injuries caused by exposure to these hazards frequently go unrecognized. Modern industrial production generates pollutants that may contaminate surroundings and quality of life, and sometimes threaten human health.

The Environmental Justice movement is a global phenomenon, and reflects a challenge to the present distribution of rewards and burdens of our industrial world. In the US, the Environmental Justice movement reflects the confluence of several major social movements. In general terms, this movement reflects the blending of the civil rights movement, the broad movement for social and economic justice, and concerns for the environment. Some critics have attempted to interpret the Environmental Justice movement more narrowly as a debate about siting of toxic landfills and disproportionate burden of environmental hazards. In particular, the Environmental Protection Agency (EPA) defines Environmental Justice as 'the fair treatment and meaningful involvement of all people regardless of race, color, national origin, or income with respect to the development, implementation, and enforcement of environmental laws, regulations, and policies'.[1] This definition neglects the relationship between environmental protection through promulgating and enforcing laws equitably, and ensuring environmental health and wellbeing. The struggle for environmental health inherently coexists with other social needs, including fair wages, safe jobs, access to quality healthcare, good schools and recreation facilities, adequate housing, and communities free of violence, drugs and poverty.[2]

The Environmental Justice movement at its core is concerned with challenging the status quo and with the equitable distributions of society's burdens and resources.

HISTORICAL OVERVIEW

The environmental movement in the US traces its history from early conservation and preservationist movements of the late 1800s and early 1900s. In 1969, the National Environmental Policy Act was passed and signed by President Nixon. This policy act was the most comprehensive legislation concerning environmental health in US history. During the 1970s, this movement reached the mainstream of American political discussion and concentrated on the passage of legislation addressing the environment. The 1969 Act created a council on environmental quality that published an annual report on the state of the environment. Its 1971 report acknowledged that environmental quality is affected by race and class status of communities.[3] The Clean Air Act of 1970 was a major revision to the 1963 Act and set much more demanding standards for control of air pollution. Similarly, the Federal Water Pollution Control Act, more commonly known as

the Clean Water Act, was passed in 1971. The establishment of the EPA in 1970 moved beyond established federal agencies that had not effectively addressed environmental issues, independent of other socioeconomic interests.[4,5]

There is a broader context in which the history of mainstream environmental movements can be understood. Schlosberg argues that it is more useful to see the first wave of the American environmental movement as a synthesis of early preservationist/conservationist concerns and the urban public health issues of the Progressive era in the early 20th century. This approach allows some understanding of race, class, and gender issues. This history includes the work of individuals such as Alice Hamilton in criticizing the impact of occupational hazards on the health of workers and the communities in which they lived. Social activism, publicizing the effects of industrialization and the dangers of the urban environment (e.g., poor housing, overcrowding, sewage, and water quality), and the settlement movements can then be understood in a broader context of contributing to today's environmental justice movement. In addition to foreign immigrant communities affected by urban industrial environments, the early decades of the last century saw the beginning of the historic internal migration of African-Americans from the rural south to urban industrial centers. This period saw a widening of the disparities in morbidity and mortality for African-Americans compared to the white population. The dominant theory of the day proposed that these disparities were due to racial differences; this theory was directly challenged by 'environmentalism' which maintained that differences of housing, working conditions, diet, availability of medical care, and other environmental factors, not genetics, explained the disparity between the health status of the races. In black communities across the nation, community-based organizations joined with African-American public health and medical professionals to attack and eliminate these health disparities. These early movements foreshadowed today's modern Environmental Justice movement.[6–9]

During the 1960s and 1970s, a number of 'environmental' issues were again taken up by community groups. Struggles against lead poisoning and poor housing conditions, while ignored by mainstream environmental groups, were important issues for organizations representing people of color. Occupational health and safety struggles among workers of color have informed the Environmental Justice movement. In the 1970s, interaction between labor unions, environmental groups, and minority organizations focused on issues of the urban environment; by the mid-1970s a number of efforts were formalized. A number of unions played an important role in educating their rank-and-file workers about health and safety issues; the United Auto Workers (UAW) and the Oil, Chemical, and Atomic Workers (OCAW) are notable examples. The UAW held a conference on the urban environment that included church groups, unions, and organizations devoted to social and economic justice. The Urban League began a project directed at addressing environmental concerns of the inner city. In 1977, the Urban Environmental Conference (UEC) began holding nationwide conferences attempting to build coalitions between occupational health and safety activists, communities of color, and environmentalists. In 1979, the National Urban League, the UEC, and the Sierra Club held a national conference, 'City Care: A Conference on the Urban Environment', attended by 700 participants. A few years later, the UEC held a national conference, 'Taking Back Our Health – An Institute on Surviving the Toxic Threat to Minority Communities'. This conference emphasized the connections between minority occupational health and safety labor activists and their communities. However, these early efforts had little impact on the mainstream environmental movement.[10]

In 1982, over 500 African-Americans were arrested attempting to stop construction of a polychlorinated biphenyl (PCB) landfill near Afton in Warren County, North Carolina. Many writers consider this protest to be a formative event of the modern Environmental Justice movement. Civil rights and environmental activists came together to plan and stage numerous demonstrations in Warren County. Among the arrested were Dr Benjamin Chavez Junior, then executive director of the United Church of Christ Commission for Racial Justice, Dr Joseph Lowery of the Southern Christian Leadership Conference, and Congressman Walter Faunteroy.[10,11]

Following the protests in Warren County, Congressman Faunteroy requested a congressional study of hazardous waste sites and race. In 1983, the General Accounting Office (GAO) reported that three out of four hazardous waste sites in EPA's Region 4 (eight southern states) were located near communities composed mainly of minorities.[12] In 1985, the Council of Energy Resource Tribes commissioned by the EPA conducted a survey revealing as many as 1200 hazardous waste sites on or near 25 Indian reservations.[13]

In 1987, the Commission for Racial Justice of the United Church of Christ (UCC) published its seminal report, 'Toxic Wastes and Race in the United States'. This report showed that race was the most significant factor, more so than income, in determining the placement of hazardous waste facilities in communities. Three out of every five African-Americans or Hispanics live in a community with unregulated commercial hazardous waste facilities.[14] Despite some methodologic problems with the UCC study, it placed the question of disproportionate exposure to environmental hazards in the public arena. The Reverend Benjamin Chavez coined the term 'environmental racism' while presenting the UCC report, and the debate took an even more controversial tone.

Since the late 1980s, hundreds of community organizations not tied to national mainstream environmental groups have protested local environmental issues. Many of these local struggles have been well documented. They include work around 'Cancer Alley' in the Mississippi delta, Chicanas in east LA who protested against the building of a toxic waste incinerator, residents of public housing projects in south-east Chicago, and many others.[13,15–17]

In 1990, as an outgrowth of its own struggles against corporate polluters, the Southwest Organizing Project (SWOP) brought together African-Americans, Asian-Americans, Latino-Americans, and Native Americans from the southwestern states to organize issues around environmental health from the perspective of peoples of color. Activists and SWOP wrote an open letter to major mainstream environmental organizations criticizing their failure to address minority issues and particularly for their discriminatory hiring practices of environmental organization staff.[10,18]

During the Fall of 1991, more than 650 people attended the First National People of Color Environmental Leadership Summit from almost all states of the union, many American-Indian nations, Puerto Rico, Canada, Latin America, and the Marshall Islands. Attendees adopted a document entitled 'Principles of Environmental Justice', which provided a framework for the Environmental Justice movement. The 17-point document addresses the need for public policy free from discrimination or bias, a right to participate as equal partners in decision making, for producers to be strictly responsible for detoxification and containment of their products, the right of all workers to a safe and healthy work environment, and the need for urban and rural ecologic policies to clean up and rebuild communities. The principles also address more general social issues, including the fundamental right to self-determination of all peoples, and fair access for all to resources. While these principles make explicit the connections between the right to a clean toxin-free workplace, home, and community, they extend to more general sociopolitical issues, as well as quite controversial issues such as ceasing production of 'all toxins, hazardous wastes, and radioactive materials'.[19]

GOVERNMENTAL RESPONSE TO ENVIRONMENTAL JUSTICE

In 1990, the EPA established the Environmental Equity Workgroup to evaluate the available evidence of environmental injustices. The Group confirmed the widespread existence of major environmental inequities, and recommended the formation of the Office of Environmental Justice. The Office has been responsible for addressing issues of environmental justice into all EPA policies and activities. Many have criticized the EPA's formulation of environmental equity as a narrowing of the principles of environmental justice.[20] However, the establishment of the Office of Environmental Justice and EPA administrator Carol Browner's declaration of environmental justice as one of its seven main priorities in 1993 was a major step forward in acknowledging and addressing environmental injustices.

In 1994, President Bill Clinton signed Executive Order 12898 entitled 'Federal Actions to Address Environmental Justice in Minority Populations and Low-Income Populations'. This Order called for all federal agencies to make environmental justice part of their mission, where applicable.

Agencies were charged with 'identifying and addressing any or all disproportionately high and adverse human health or environmental effects in its policies, programs and activities'. The Order established the Interagency Working Group on Environmental Justice, which provides guidance to federal agencies in identifying environmental injustices in their policies, programs, and activities, and acts as a clearing-house for federal agencies to develop environmental justice strategies, help coordinate environmental justice-related data collection, research activities between agencies, examine existing data, and hold public meetings for fact-finding and addressing community concerns. In addition, the Order calls for each federal agency to develop an environmental justice strategy. Federal environmental health research, where practical and appropriate, should include diverse segments of the population, especially those at high risk from environmental hazards, such as minority and low-income populations.[21]

Since the issuance of Executive Order 12898, the various federal agencies (i.e., Health and Human Services, Housing and Urban Development, Defense, Labor, EPA, Commerce, Transportation, Energy, amongst others) have developed environmental justice strategies with varying degrees of implementation. Various rollbacks in environmental protections have been attempted, but grassroots activism and various committed government officials have continued to struggle for environmental justice and sound environmental policies.

EVIDENCE FOR DISPROPORTIONATE EXPOSURE AND HEALTH EFFECTS RELATED TO DEMOGRAPHIC AND SOCIOECONOMIC FACTORS

There is evidence to suggest that low-income and minority communities and workers may be exposed disproportionately to environmental hazards. Numerous hazardous waste sites, legal and illegal, have been placed in communities of color and low-income neighborhoods. These sites can leak contaminants into water and soil of the surrounding community. Factory emissions can contaminate the air of surrounding communities. Multiple exposure routes with complex mixtures of toxicants may produce synergistic effects on human health that are difficult to quantify.

Research has centered around three types of problems: health-based problems; land-use and space-based problems; and structural/economic problems.[22] With regard to health-based problems of environmental justice, a series of classic case studies in occupational health document differential exposure of workers of color, and the often resultant disparities in occupational disease and injuries. Perhaps the most devastating industrial disaster in US history occurred at Gauley Bridge, West Virginia. This project of dry tunneling through a mountain of silica rock resulted in the deaths of hundreds of workers from acute silicosis and the development of chronic lung disease in

thousands of others.[23] These workers were disproportionately African-American. (See excerpt from the paper by Ashley Lucas and Ariadne Paxton[24] overleaf.)

Asian immigrants are exposed to dangerous solvents in the dry-cleaning industry, where they work in disproportionate numbers. The classic studies of steelworkers showed that the higher rates of lung cancer among African-American steelworkers resulted not from genetic differences, but from occupational segregation to work duties on the tops of the coke ovens. Investigators have described many examples that demonstrate segregated patterns of employment. Even after correction for length of employment and educational status, workers of color are often disproportionately exposed to greater occupational hazards compared with their counterparts.[25-34] In addition to occupational exposures and diseases are numerous health impacts on communities, such as childhood lead poisoning. The age and quality of housing and geographic proximity to lead-based industries and highways are among the factors that help to explain the higher blood lead levels among African-American and Mexican-American children.[35-37] The increasing disparity in asthma in African-American and Latino children in urban areas compared to whites is also well documented, with concern for environmental risk factors.[38-40]

RESEARCH ADDRESSING ENVIRONMENTAL JUSTICE

A number of researchers have reviewed the evidence for disproportionate exposure to environmental hazards by race, ethnicity, and class. The overall picture is contradictory, and plagued with numerous methodologic challenges. A number of studies have used zip code and smaller geographic areas to look at the location of industrial sources of pollution and toxic waste sites. The early UCC study used 1980 census data to assess toxic waste sites and correlations with community demographics.[14] The study showed that race and, secondarily, income were particularly important predictors of geographic proximity to hazardous waste facilities. However, the 26 million people of color living near closed and abandoned waste sites in the UCC study were not significantly greater than the percentage of whites living near these sites. A number of investigators have chosen to define environmental injustice using an ecologic approach. In this approach, a differential siting of CERCLA toxic waste sites according to race is emphasized. This rather simplistic model ignores the rich literature and research on race-related effects, and reduces this complicated issue to a single ecologic variable, namely the location of certain types of toxic waste dumps.

Many investigators looking at the demographic characteristics of populations residing around toxic waste sites appropriately emphasize that income is an important variable. Some of these investigators also argue that race is not a factor – rather, income level is the major variable – and dismiss the interactions between race and income. There are also methodologic problems with the unit of analysis used in these studies. Geographic areas such as counties and zip

The Hawk's Nest Incident

The Gauley Bridge Disaster

Preparation for Disaster

In 1927, construction of a hydroelectric plant on the New River in Gauley Bridge, West Virginia, began under the Union Carbide and Carbon Corporation. Union Carbide then formed the New Kanahwa Power Company and the Rinehart and Dennis Company of Charlottesville, Virginia, was contracted to begin construction. Workers came from all over the Southeast. The majority of these new employees were African-American. One procedure used to build the tunnel was called 'mucking'. This was the process by which the broken rock was removed from the tunnel. The removal of the broken rock aided the dispersal of dust that might have been contaminated with silica dust. This dust might have infected several hundred men. The rock was then carried out of the tunnel via 'dinkeys' (or small locomotives).

Working in the Tunnel

The work schedule was a 6-day workweek with two 10-hour shifts per day. The workforce was composed unevenly of African-Americans and Caucasians, with more African-Americans employed by Union Carbide to work in the tunnels than white workers. As a result, more African-Americans died from silicosis. The company provided its workers with housing. The housing was scarcely better than living in a shack, but the white workers were charged less rent for their accommodations than their African-American counterparts. There were not even close to enough beds for all the workers and their families. The cost of living in the villages, much like the rent, was determined by race. Working in the tunnel consisted of two 3-hour shifts. Holes were drilled in the rock for several feet and then dynamite was inserted in the holes to blast out the remainder of the rock. The clearing out of debris involved a lot of contact with dust that contained silica. In addition to the dusty conditions, the use of gasoline-powered equipment also polluted the already contaminated air. It has been reported that mainly black workers were forced to clean out the tunnel after the blast and that was by far the most dangerous part of the job. Length of employment rarely lasted over a year as a result of the dangerous working conditions. The records of medical services rendered to the workmen have never been fully recovered. Physicians of the time were not very familiar with silicosis as a disease. It resembled tuberculosis and was often misdiagnosed as such. It also appears that Union Carbide never took any steps to assess the risk of the workers being exposed to silica dust. There are accounts from workers saying that they emerged daily from the tunnels coated in dust from head to toe, and members of the community said that the workers were often so dust covered that they left footprints as they walked away from the tunnels back to their houses. The officials of Union Carbide and Rinehart and Dennis said that if there was any dust coverage on the workers, it was minimal.

Recognition of Disaster

In 1932, several lawsuits began to be filed on behalf of some of the afflicted workers. By the mid-1930s, the courts had ruled in favor of compensating the plaintiffs. The allocation of money was based on race and marital status, just as wages and housing had been earlier. A single black man would receive $400, while a married white man received $1000. The families of deceased workers received an extra $600. In 1935, the West Virginia House of Delegates passed a new state workers' compensation law which would compensate workers who were infected with silicosis. Despite this giant step forward in compensating workers for illness contracted on the job, there were many loopholes. These loopholes cleared the employer of responsibility for the disease and made eligibility for this law almost impossible for workers. The hearings that existed at this time did not do enough to relieve or compensate the victims and their families, despite the new legislation.

How Many Died?

An actual number of how many people died as a result of silicosis in Gauley Bridge has never been determined; however, the estimate has been set at around 700 deaths and several thousand diagnosed with lung disease. The victims, for the most part, remain anonymous. There were no headstones for the graves that have been found. The one consistent factor is that proportionally more blacks than whites died in this great disaster. Black deaths were also under-reported, thus skewing the number of deaths even further.

Epilogue

The prospects for local men to work in the mines after working at Hawk's Nest were slim to none when the operators discovered that these men had been exposed to silica dust, which could be killing them. After the afflicted were compensated, Rinehart and Dennis never again competed for a major project. Union Carbide claimed no responsibility for silicosis. Up until at least 1940, silicosis remained absent from the list of diseases that could be claimed under the workman's compensation laws. There is no longer any indication of where the camps once stood on the construction site.

---

codes may be too large to provide a meaningful assessment of exposure and demographics. The studies do not address the issue of whether people of color settled in these polluted areas because they were not welcome in more desirable neighborhoods or communities, or whether impoverished and disenfranchised communities were systematically chosen for toxic waste disposal facilities.[14,41–47]

A number of studies have examined ambient concentrations of air pollutants in various community locations. The evidence is contradictory, with some investigators finding differences based on race, or income, or both. These studies have also been limited by exposure assessment, as the movement of air pollutants is dependent on meteorologic conditions, which may be poorly characterized.[22,48,49]

Societal racism and class distinction are seen by many in the Environmental Justice movement as the most proximal causes for the disproportionate burden of environmental exposures. These ideologic philosophies are delineated by the resultant lack of political and economic power in poor communities and communities of color. The fact that poor people, and especially workers of color, labor in jobs that are often more hazardous and live in communities more likely to be located near hazardous industries or waste sites contributes to their increased exposure to environmental toxins. Patterns of discrimination in areas of housing and education, for example, can result in large numbers of minority populations being exposed to environmental toxins.[28,50] Race- and ethnicity-specific data should be collected to characterize more completely the extent of this problem. Caution should be exercised, however, when categorizing populations into specific racial or ethnic groupings. Racial and ethnic groupings are not biologic or genetic categories, nor do they correlate systematically with socioeconomic status, occupational categories, or other relevant variables.

In addition to challenges in exposure characterization and frequent exposure to a complex mixture of toxicants, a major problem with many current epidemiologic studies related to environmental injustices is that most populations studied are relatively small in size. A statistically significant and robust association between an exposure and a disease cannot be observed when the population studied is too small to document an effect. In addition, few studies have attempted to determine the role socioeconomic or race factors play in the development of potential disease clusters in workplaces or communities. Socioeconomic factors are treated as confounders as opposed to variables of interest to investigate with respect to disease development.[44] The 1999 Institute of Medicine Report entitled 'Toward Environmental Justice' supports three principles for public research to address environmental justice issues, namely:

- improvement of scientific methodologies;
- involvement of affected populations; and
- communication of findings to all stakeholders.[44]

This will require greater resources and improvements in research methodologies, including development of participatory research approaches.

PUBLIC HEALTH MODEL

The Environmental Justice movement emphasizes that environmental health be addressed in terms of public health principles and policy.

Interventions are thus inherently connected to other civil rights and social justice issues. Community empowerment has the potential for the greatest impact. Governmental actions, such as the Executive Order issued by Clinton, that facilitate consideration of environmental justice issues when designing programs can profoundly change the actions of environmental agencies. These broader conceptual approaches challenge the thinking of governmental agencies and the mainstream environmental movement. Whether or not such broad approaches increase our understanding of environmental health, or cloud it with irrelevant issues, is at the heart of the debate around environmental justice.

Currently, Executive Order 12898 is the basis for federal policies regarding environmental justice. The Order directed all federal agencies to develop environmental justice policies and strategies specific to their areas of responsibility. In particular, the US EPA strategies focus on five major areas:

- public participation and accountability, partnerships, outreach and communication with stakeholders, including minority populations and/or low-income populations;
- health and environmental research, including minority and/or low-income populations;
- data collection, analysis and stakeholder access to public information;
- Native American and indigenous environmental protection; and
- enforcement, compliance, assurance, and regulatory reviews.[1]

All of these areas need attention and development to appropriately address and prevent environmental injustices. Public participation must be collaborative. Government, community, and industry partnerships are essential for effective hazard and illness identification through data collection, as well as research, risk communication, and remediation and prevention efforts. Placing the burden of providing definitive evidence linking adverse health outcomes to specific environmental exposures on community residents is not appropriate. Effective intervention will require an understanding that these communities, generally minority and poor, do not necessarily have the resources or expertise to gather the needed data and information.[44] Risk communication approaches should be grounded in a clear understanding of the cultural contexts involved. It is imperative to train and utilize community residents, as a matter of policy, to aid in development and implementation of educational programs. The National Environmental Justice Advisory Council in 1996 proposed a 'public participation checklist for government agencies'[51] to facilitate this approach, including identification of stakeholders and providing opportunities to offer input into decisions that may impact their health, property values, and lifestyles. Such an approach is based on participatory research, involving 'the affected communities in the planning, implementation, evaluation and dissemination of results'.[44,52] Soliciting community input before beginning the project, using community residents to gather data where appropriate, and continual feedback on the progress of the research will likely minimize distrust and maximize needed community cooperation and participation.[53]

ROLE OF THE HEALTHCARE WORKER

Physicians, nurses, and other healthcare workers, particularly occupational and environmental medicine specialists, have a critical role addressing environmental injustices. When patients present to their primary care providers with concerns regarding workplace or community environmental exposures, most medical practitioners do not have the appropriate knowledge to fully address the concerns. Rarely is a public health approach taken to determine whether an entire community is at risk.

Primary care practitioners need to be aware of occupational and environmental resources in their community. Many local health departments, university hospitals or schools of public health have environmental health experts who know of occupational and environmental medicine clinicians in the area.

Unfortunately, poor and rural communities, which include many communities of color, may not have access to quality primary healthcare, much less to trained specialists. One useful resource is the Association of Occupational and Environmental Clinics (AOEC), which is a network of clinics in the US and Canada that specialize in the evaluation of occupational and environmental diseases and injuries.[54] There are over 60 full-service occupational and environmental clinics, 12 pediatric environmental health specialty units, and 250 individual members in the network.

Finally, it is important to recognize that the physician's role goes beyond the individual doctor–patient relationship and should enter the arena of public involvement with communities in need. Any public health intervention needs to be developed as a partnership between community members, the primary healthcare providers for the community, and the occupational and environmental research and educational experts.

CONCLUSION

In summary, the Environmental Justice movement views race and social class as two fundamental issues impeding environmental equity. Ongoing disparities devalue the lives of those from lower socioeconomic strata and peoples of color, resulting in disproportionate exposure to environmental toxins, and concomitant health risks.

The lack of political and economic power among people of color and the poor frequently means that environmental health concerns in these communities receive inadequate attention or are ignored completely. It also means that the range of options open to these communities is much narrower. For example, one frequent argument for siting a toxic waste facility or an incinerator in impoverished communities is that such enterprises will result in badly needed jobs. This inappropriate emphasis on economic issues must be viewed skeptically in the overall context of public health and social justice.

The Environmental Justice movement has not been characterized by a large national infrastructure, but is rather organized as a network of local and regional organizations.[9] Dana Alston's summation speech at the First National People of Color Environmental Leadership Summit emphasizes the social, spiritual, and political nature of this movement:

'The environment affords us the platform to address the critical issues of our time: questions of militarism and defense policy; religious freedom; cultural survival; energy and sustainable development; the future of our cities; transportation; housing; land and sovereignty rights; self-determination; and employment. We can go on and on. For us, the issues of the environment do not stand alone by themselves. They are not narrowly defined. Our vision of the environment is woven into an overall framework of social, racial and economic justice. It is deeply rooted in our cultures and our spirituality. It is based on a long tradition of understanding and respect for the natural world. The environment, for us, is where we live, where we work and where we play.'[19]

The Environmental Justice movement has been criticized for focusing on things not accomplished, and links to causation not proven, and an overly broad approach to the issues of occupational and environmental health. However, in its relatively short history it has challenged the approach to 'environmentalism' as a merely regulatory function. The movement has caused the US EPA and other government agencies to rethink their approach to community participation. It has broadened the concept of environmental issues to include social and economic justice, and has embraced a public health model for its approach to issues.[9]

References

1. US Environmental Protection Agency. Environmental Justice website: es.epa.gov/oeca/main/ej/ 2002.
2. Bryant B, ed. Environmental justice: issues, policies, and solutions. Washington, DC: Island Press; 1995.
3. Bryant B. Domestic chronology of environmental justice. University of Michigan personal webpage: www.personal.umich.edu/~bbryant/ejtimeline.html
4. Sale K. The green revolution: the American environmental movement 1962-1992. New York: Hill and Wang; 1993.
5. Shabecoff P. A fierce green fire: the American environmental movement. New York: Hill and Wang; 1993.
6. Byrd WM, Clayton LA. An American health dilemma volume I: a medical history of African-Americans and the problem of race: beginnings to 1900. New York: Routledge; 2000.
7. Byrd WM, Clayton LA. An American health dilemma volume II: race, medicine, healthcare in the United States. New York: Routledge; 2001.
8. McBride D. From TB to AIDS: epidemics among urban Blacks since 1900. New York: State University of New York Press; 1991.
9. Schlosberg D. Environmental justice and new pluralism: the challenge of difference of environmentalism. Oxford: Oxford University Press; 1999.
10. Tingling-Clemmons M. From one Earth day to the next: twenty years of action by people of color. In: Alston D, ed. We speak for ourselves: social justice, race and environment. Washington, DC: The Panos Institute; 1990.
11. A brief history of environmental justice. Thurgood Marshall School of Law, Environmental Justice Clinic webpage. Texas Southern University, Houston. www.tsulaw.edu/environ/environ.htm
12. US General Accounting Office. Siting of hazardous waste landfills and their correlation with racial and economic status of surrounding communities. GAO/RCED-83-168, B-211461. Washington, DC: Government Printing Office; 1983.
13. Bullard RD, ed. Unequal protection: environmental justice & communities of color. San Francisco: Sierra Club Books; 1994.
14. United Church of Christ Commission for Racial Justice. Toxic wastes and race in the United States: a national report on the racial and socio-economic characteristics of communities surrounding hazardous waste sites. New York: United Church of Christ; 1987.
15. Alston D, ed. We speak for ourselves: social justice, race and environment. Washington DC: The Panos Institute; 1990.
16. Bullard RD. Race, class and the politics of place. In: Dumping in Dixie: race, class and environmental quality. Boulder, CO: Westview; 1990.
17. Cole LW, Foster SR. From the ground up: environmental racism and the rise of the environmental justice movement. New York: New York University Press; 2001.
18. Moore R, Head L. Building a net that works: SWOP. In: Bullard RD, ed. Unequal protection: environmental justice & communities of color. San Francisco: Sierra Club Books; 1994.
19. Lee C, ed. Proceedings of the First National People of Color Environmental Leadership Summit. New York, United Church of Christ Commission for Racial Justice. 1992.
20. U.S. Environmental Protection Agency. Environmental equity: reducing risk for all communities. EPA230-R-92-008. Washington, DC: US Environmental Protection Agency, 1992.
21. Clinton WJ. Federal Actions to Address Environmental Justice in Minority Populations and Low-income Populations.

Presidential Executive Order No 12898. Federal Register Vol 59, No 32, February 16, 1994.

22. Gelobter M. The meaning of urban environmental justice. Fordham Urban Law J 1994; 21:841-56.

23. Cherniack M. The Hawk's Nest incident: America's worst industrial accident. New Haven, CT: Yale University Press; 1986.

24. Lucas A, Paxton A. About the Hawk's Nest incident – background for Muriel Rukeyser's *The Book of the Dead*. In: Nelson C, ed. Modern American poetry. Department of English, University of Illinois at Urbana-Champaign, website: www.english.uiuc.edu/maps/poets/m_r/rukeyser/hawksnest.htm, 1999.

25. Davis ME. The impact of workplace health and safety on black workers: assessment and prognosis. Labor Law J 1980; 31:723-32.

26. Friedman-Jimenez G. Occupational disease among minority workers: a common and preventable public health problem. Am Assoc Occup Health Nurs J 1989; 37:64-70.

27. Friedman-Jimenez G. Achieving environmental justice: the role of occupational health. Fordham Urban Law J 1994; 21:605-29.

28. Friedman-Jimenez G, Ortiz JS. Occupational health. In: Molina CW, Aguirre-Molina M, eds. Latino health in the US : a growing challenge. Washington, DC: American Public Health Association; 1994:341-89.

29. Frumkin H, Walker ED. Minority workers and communities. In: Wallace RB, ed. Maxcy-Rosenau-Last public health and preventive medicine, 14th edn. Stamford, CT: Appleton and Lange; 1998:682.

30. Frumkin H, Walker ED, Friedman-Jimenez G. Minority workers and communities. Occup Med 1999; 14:495-517.

31. Kidd-Taylor A, Murray LR. Minority workers. In: Levy BS, Wegman DH, eds. Occupational health: recognizing and preventing work-related disease and injury, 4th edn. New York: Lippincott, Williams & Wilkins; 2000.

32. Robinson JC. Trends in racial inequality and exposure to work-related hazards, 1968-1986. Am Assoc Occup Health Nurs J 1989; 37:56-63.

33. Robinson JC. Exposure to occupational hazards among Hispanics, blacks and non-Hispanic whites in California. Am J Public Health 1989; 79:629-30.

34. Robinson JC. Racial inequality and the probability of occupation-related injury or illness. Health and Society 1984; 62:567-90.

35. Lanphear BP, Weitzman M, Eberly S. Racial differences in urban children's environmental exposure to lead. Am J Public Health 1996; 86:1460-3.

36. Mahaffey KR, Annest JL, Roberts J, Murphy RS. National estimates of blood lead levels, United States, 1976-1980: association with selected demographic and socio-economic factors. N Engl J Med 1982; 307:573-9.

37. Sargent JD, Brown MJ, Freeman JL, Bailey A, Goodman D, Freeman DH. Childhood lead poisoning in Massachusetts communities: its association with sociodemographic and housing characteristics. Am J Public Health 1995; 85:528-34.

38. Marder D, Targonski P, Orris P, Persky V, Addington W. Effect of racial and socio-economic factors on asthma mortality in Chicago. Chest (Suppl) 1992; 101:426S-92S.

39. Weiss KB, Wagener DK. Changing patterns of asthma mortality: identifying target populations at high risk. JAMA 1990; 264:1683-7.

40. Weitzman M, Gortmaker S, Sobol A. Racial, social, and environmental risks for childhood asthma. Am J Dis Child 1990; 144:1189-94.

41. Been V. What has fairness got to do with it? Environmental justice and the siting of locally undesirable land uses. Cornell Law Review, September 1993.

42. Goldman B. Not just prosperity: achieving sustainability with environmental justice. Vienna, VA; National Wildlife Federation; 1993.

43. Gould JM. Quality of life in American neighborhoods, levels of affluence, toxic waste, and cancer mortality in residential zip code areas. Boulder, CO: Westview; 1986.

44. Institute of Medicine, Committee on Environmental Justice. Toward environmental justice: research, education and health policy needs. Washington, DC: National Academy Press; 1999.

45. Mohai P, Bryant B. Environmental racism: reviewing the evidence. In: Race and the incidence of environmental hazards: a time for discourse. Boulder, CO: Westview; 1992.

46. White H. Race, class, and environmental hazards. In: Camacho D, ed. Environmental injustices, political struggles: race, class and the environment. Durham, NC: Duke University Press; 1998.

47. Zimmerman R. Social equity and environmental risk. Risk Anal 1993; 13:649-66.

48. Perlin S, Setzer RW, Creason J, Sexton K. Distribution of industrial air emissions by income and race in the United States: an approach to the Toxic Release Inventory. Environ Sci Technol 1995; 29:69-80.

49. Wernette DR, Nieves LA. Breathing polluted air: minorities are disproportionately exposed. EPA J 1992; March/April:16-17.

50. Lopez R. Segregation and black/white differences in exposure to air toxics in 1990. Environ Health Perspect 2002; 110(Suppl 2):289-95.

51. US Environmental Protection Agency, National Environmental Justice Advisory Council, Accountability Subcommittee. The model plan for public participation. Washington, DC: US EPA, Office of Environmental Justice; 1996.

52. Drevdahl D. Coming to voice: the power of emancipatory community interventions. Adv Nurs Sci 1995; 18:13-24.

53. O'Fallon LR, Dearry A. Community-based participatory research as a tool to advance environmental health sciences. Environ Health Perspect 2002; 110(Suppl 2):155-9.

54. The Association of Occupational and Environmental Clinics. Washington, DC. www.aoec.org.

Chapter 58

Integrating Clinical Care with Prevention of Occupational Illness and Injury

Robin Herbert, Jaime Szeinuk

INTRODUCTION

Occupational medicine is a unique clinical specialty that links the direct clinical care of individuals with occupational illnesses or injuries to workplace preventive efforts.[1] Thus, the occupational medicine physician has an opportunity not only to impact the identified patient, but also to prevent disease or injury in similarly exposed coworkers.[1]

As in other medical specialties, prevention efforts in occupational medicine can be categorized as primary, secondary, or tertiary.[2] The goal of primary prevention is to prevent injuries or the onset of disease, either by preventing exposure to workplace hazards or by preventing health effects due to exposure. Secondary prevention seeks to identify and treat asymptomatic individuals in whom preclinical disease has developed, before the condition becomes clinically apparent. Tertiary prevention seeks to prevent disability, disease progression, or death due to clinically apparent illness or injury.[3]

Occupational and environmental medicine practitioners can contribute to the prevention of occupational diseases and injuries in a number of ways. Examples of primary interventions that healthcare providers can initiate in individual clinical encounters include immunizations against occupational infectious diseases and provision of patient education about the effects of exposures sustained in the workplace and about ways to minimize those exposures. Examples of provider-based secondary prevention include blood lead monitoring and screening for asbestos-related malignancies. Examples of tertiary prevention initiatives that can be conducted in the clinical setting include treatment of occupational cancers or occupational asthma. In the workplace, primary preventive efforts include the substitution of less toxic chemicals and processes and ventilation systems to reduce exposure. Examples of secondary disease preventive efforts include workplace-based screening for occupational disease. Examples of workplace-based tertiary modifications include job modifications to prevent reinjury and facilitate return to work.

This chapter will describe approaches in the clinical setting to the primary, secondary, and tertiary prevention of occupational disease and injury, and will also provide an overview of Occupational Safety and Health Administration (OSHA)-mandated examinations for targeted populations, which provide the opportunity for secondary disease prevention.

PRIMARY PREVENTION OF OCCUPATIONAL ILLNESS AND INJURY

Primary prevention of occupational illness and injury is largely based on minimizing exposure to workplace hazards. While the healthcare provider may have limited ability to effect reductions of hazardous workplace exposures, there are a number of ways in which he or she can work towards primary prevention of occupational disease and injury in the clinical setting. These are described below.

1. Identification of occupational hazards by taking an occupational history, with follow-up to employers regarding hazard abatement

By taking a careful occupational history, the healthcare provider can identify possible occupational hazards and can play an important role in prevention by communicating with employers about reduction of hazardous exposures that are identified in the occupational history. Ultimately, the employer has responsibility for, and control over, whether or not appropriate preventive measures are employed in the workplace. However, the healthcare provider can function as an advocate for workplace safety in a way that individual workers cannot. For example, a study of predictors of employer-based risk reduction efforts for workers with upper extremity work-related diseases found that a physician recommending specific workplace exposure modifications increased the likelihood of their implementation.[4] However, despite the potential effectiveness of healthcare provider communication with employers regarding workplace interventions, the healthcare provider should never communicate with an employer or other party without explicit permission from the patient, as such activities can result in severe consequences for some workers, particularly those in vulnerable populations.

2. Use of the sentinel health event approach

When an occupational disease or injury is identified in an individual patient, it should be treated as an index case, or sentinel health event, whenever feasible. As defined by Rutstein et al., an occupational sentinel health event 'is a disease, disability or ultimately death which is occupationally related and which occurrence may 1) provide the impetus for epidemiologic or industrial hygiene studies; or 2) serve as a warning signal that materials substitution, engineering continuation, personal protection or medical care may be required'.[5] This approach thus relies upon public health-based follow-up of index cases of occupational injury or illness with the goal of decreasing exposure, as well as preventing disease or injury in similarly exposed coworkers. In the sentinel health event approach, following identification of an index case, similarly exposed coworkers should be screened for disease and/or exposure (e.g., blood lead levels). Reduction of the inciting exposure should be initiated. Healthcare providers can play an important role in recognition and follow-up of sentinel health events. Follow-up can potentially result in both primary prevention (hazard identification followed by exposure reduction) and secondary disease prevention (screening of similarly exposed workers). However, again, the healthcare provider should never communicate with employers or unions without explicit permission from the patient.

3. Patient/worker education about minimizing hazardous workplace exposures, and about modifying non-occupational risk factors that may potentiate the effects of occupational exposures

Healthcare providers can contribute to the primary prevention of occupational injury and illness by providing patient/worker education about the health effects of exposures sustained by the patient, and about ways in which the worker might minimize exposures to workplace hazards. For example, because motor vehicle fatalities are the leading cause of fatal occupational injuries in the US, healthcare providers should inquire about and encourage seatbelt use in patients whose jobs involve driving.[3,6] Similarly, healthcare providers should ask lead-exposed patients about availability and use of handwashing facilities, and patients should be instructed not to eat in work areas where there is the potential for contamination of food with lead.[7] Reviewing proper use of respirators is another example of a strategy for primary prevention.

Additionally, the healthcare provider should counsel the patient about individual, modifiable behaviors which may increase the risk of occupational diseases. For example, cigarette smoking, in addition to being an independent risk factor for a larger number of diseases, acts in synergy with asbestos to increase the risk of lung cancer. Therefore, primary preventive efforts in an asbestos-exposed worker who also smokes cigarettes would include both providing education and communicating with the employer about minimizing exposure to asbestos and adhering to OSHA standards, but also working on smoking cessation with the individual patient.

4. Use of the US Preventive Services Task Force recommendations on periodic health examinations

Healthcare providers can contribute to primary prevention of some occupational diseases by utilizing appropriate components of the *Guide to Clinical Preventive Services*, a report of the US Preventive Services Task Force.[3] The guide recommends specific components of periodic health examinations for various high-risk populations, including certain working groups. For example, the guide recommends that healthcare workers receive hepatitis A and B vaccine, influenza vaccine, and regular purified protein derivatives.[3]

SECONDARY PREVENTION OF OCCUPATIONAL ILLNESS

The goal of secondary disease prevention is to detect disease at a stage when cure or control is possible. Secondary prevention relies primarily on screening. The general principles of screening are that:

- a test or series of tests will identify asymptomatic persons at risk for a specific disease;
- persons with a positive result on a screening can be further evaluated to determine whether they have the disease;
- ideally, once the disease is established, early intervention can change the course of disease, resulting in decreased morbidity and mortality.[3,8]

In the clinical setting, secondary prevention of occupational illness can occur in the milieu of mandated screening examinations (e.g., OSHA, Department of Transportation [DOT]) or as part of routine clinical care provision.

SCREENING FOR OCCUPATIONAL DISEASE UNDER THE OSHA STANDARDS

In the US, OSHA has promulgated a series of federal regulations, the OSHA Standards, which deal with various aspects of biologic monitoring and medical surveillance for some hazardous workplace exposures.[9] OSHA requires employers to provide mandated periodic screening examinations for workers with certain exposures (e.g., asbestos) or job titles (e.g., hazardous waste workers). The occupational medicine professional should be familiar with the requirements of periodic screening examinations under the OSHA law. Regulations can be obtained by logging into the OSHA website at www.osha-slc.gov/OshStd_toc/OSHA_Std_toc. html. Because many of the OSHA standards were written 10 to 20 years ago, provisions of the law need to be supplemented by review of newer scientific criteria about the potential health effects of the exposures for which the workers are being evaluated, and appropriate screening modalities for the health effects of interest. The occupational medicine provider should review the known toxicity of exposures for which he or she is conducting examinations, and be familiar with both the use of biomarkers of exposure to the substance(s) under consideration, as well as the best screening methods for health conditions associated with the exposure(s). Finally, when planning or conducting a medical screening program, the occupational medicine practitioner should be certain to refer all laboratory and ancillary tests to well-known, respected and certified laboratories and diagnostic facilities, as there can be significant variation in techniques and laboratory procedures that sometimes may render false or equivocal results.

OSHA has strict regulations regarding patient confidentiality and record keeping for OSHA-mandated examinations. The healthcare provider must be aware of the regulations when planning to conduct an OSHA-mandated screening program (see Chapter 57.1). OSHA usually only permits the healthcare provider to inform the employer of issues related to the specific hazard for which the worker is being screened, in order to protect patient confidentiality. The provider is generally obligated to maintain medical records and test results for long periods of time, which vary according to the exposure.

Table 58.1 summarizes both the requirements of the OSHA Standards on medical screening for workers with specific exposures, and other OSHA regulations regarding medical screening of workers in specific trades, such as hazardous waste workers. For each exposure, the table presents the toxicant in consideration together with the number of the OSHA Rule that covers this specific substance. Next is a review of target occupation and industries where exposure to this substance is most commonly encountered. A list of the target organs that have been found to have susceptibility to organ damage by the specific substance, and the carcinogenic potential of the substance, follow. Finally, a summary of the recommendations under the OSHA Standard and a succinct review of a series of tests recommended for periodic monitoring of workers exposed to these specific toxicants is provided. For Standards in which the OSHA recommendations for medical surveillance are sparse or vague, the table has been supplemented with additional recommendations about appropriate surveillance techniques for particular exposures.

One of the purposes of the medical examinations under the OSHA Standards is to establish a baseline for future health monitoring of workers exposed to occupational toxins. Baseline evaluation is important in providing a basis for subsequent assessment and changes in the health of the individual and in evaluating her or his risk factors to exposure to toxins. Baseline examinations can also provide the opportunity to provide education to the patient/worker about the potential deleterious health effects of the agents to which he or she may be exposed, and to assess the presence or absence of co-morbid conditions that may affect risk of developing an occupational disease. Thus, when performing the required periodic medical and laboratory examinations, the occupational medicine professional should take time to compare current with previous results in order to detect early, subclinical changes in test results. Although these may not yet be 'clinically significant', such changes and trends may be the first sign of early tissue damage that, when detected in a timely manner, should lead to avoidance or control of exposure to prevent development of clinically apparent disease.

In addition to the routinely recommended tests and evaluations for workers with particular exposures, it is important for the occupational medicine professional to be aware that some workers may have greater susceptibility to the effects of some substances, or may have other medical conditions that make it difficult to use particular protective equipment. Consequently, it is recommended that in certain cases the healthcare provider should be prepared to evaluate situations not directly related to the specific toxicant in question, to the extent that they may affect occupational safety and health. For example, workers with skin diseases may be unable to tolerate wearing protective clothing or particular gloves. Some workers with chronic respiratory diseases may not tolerate wearing negative pressure (air-purifying) respirators. Additional tests and procedures may be required to help the healthcare provider determine which workers are medically unable to be exposed to certain toxicants or to wear specific work protection equipment. Supplemental testing may include, for example, evaluation of cardiovascular function, baseline and repeated chest X-ray, pulmonary function test (spirometry), periodic monitoring of blood-forming organs (i.e., complete blood count), liver and kidney function tests, or early markers of kidney damage such as low-molecular-weight proteins in the urine (e.g., beta-2 microglobulin). However, medical surveillance should not be used for employment purposes such as hiring and firing.[10] Furthermore, the healthcare provider should be aware of the Americans with Disabilities Act (ADA) provisions of federal law (see Chapter 57.1).

Screening at-risk workers who are not covered by OSHA-mandated examinations

There are many workers who sustain exposures known to be associated with increased risk of occupational cancers and other occupational illnesses whose employers are not required to provide OSHA-mandated screening examinations, but who might benefit from periodic screening examinations. They include, for example, workers exposed to known carcinogens such as chromium, radiation, nickel, and coal tar pitch, and workers in industries that have been associated with significant health hazards and/or cancer risk, such as the rubber industry, furniture workers (wood dust), and steel foundries.

In general, screening for either occupational exposure resulting in detectable internal dose (utilizing biomarkers) or for asymptomatic occupational disease should be considered in the following settings in addition to those mandated by OSHA:

- when a sentinel health event is identified, as described earlier in this chapter;
- when an occupational history reveals that a patient's work involves exposure to a given agent such as lead, for which a screening device is available;

Exposure[9] OSHA Rule #	Workers at risk/uses	Target organs[12]	Medical screening and surveillance
2-Acetylaminofluorene (13-carcinogens) 1910.1014	Chemical research, experimental carcinogen	Liver, bladder, kidney, pancreas, skin	*Trigger:* Working in a regulated area *Examinations:* 1; 2*; 5 *Exam components:* PE focusing on increased risk for cancer such as reduced immunologic competence, treatment with steroids or cytotoxics, pregnancy and cigarette smoking; work and medical history; genetic and environmental factors *Tests:* Urinalysis, urine cytology and cystoscopy * Annually
Acrylonitrile 1910.1045	Manufacture of acrylic fibers for the apparel, carpeting, and home furnishing industries; in plastic pipes and pipefitting; in automotive parts, appliances, and building components; in the petrochemical industry; to make acrylamide; prior to World War II, used in the production of oil-resistant rubbers	Eyes, skin, cardiovascular system, liver, kidney, CNS Cancer: brain, lung, bowel	*Trigger:* Exposure at or above the AL (2 ppm) *Examinations:* 1; 2; 3; 4; 5 *Exam components:* PE with special attention to CNS dysfunction symptoms such as headaches, dizziness or weakness, respiratory system, GI system, thyroid and skin; work and medical history. Persons unusually susceptible to effects of anoxia or those with anemia would be expected to be at increased risk *Tests:* **CXR; FOB (for workers >40);** blood cyanide, blood plasma, urinalysis; urinary level of acrylonitrile and urinary excretion of thiocyanate over a TWA; additional tests as needed
Alpha-Naphthylamine (13-carcinogens) 1910.1004	Dyes, prints	Bladder, skin	*See 2-acetylaminofluorene* *Tests:* Urinalysis, urine cytology and cystoscopy
4-Aminodiphenyl (13-carcinogens) 1910.1011	Rubber, byproduct of aniline dye manufacturing, used in cancer research	Bladder, skin Cancer: bladder	*See 2-acetylaminofluorene* *Tests:* Urinalysis, urine cytology and cystoscopy
Arsenic 1910.1018	For hardening lead in battery grids, bearings, and cable sheets; in the manufacture of calcium, copper, and lead arsenate pesticides (arsenic trioxide and pentoxide); as pigment and refining agent in glass and as preservative in tanning and taxidermy; copper acetoarsenite and chromated copper arsenate (CCA) as a wood preservative; also used as herbicide and desiccant for cotton harvesting; in veterinary pharmaceuticals and feed additives; arsine gas in the microelectronics industry	Liver, kidney, skin, lungs, lymphatic system, nose, nervous system, reproductive system Cancer: lung, skin, liver (angiosarcoma)	*Trigger:* (1) Exposure at or above the AL (5 mg/m³) for at least 30 days/year; (2) Exposure for 10 or more years above the AL, though worker may no longer be exposed above the level; (3) Assignment to areas in which exposure will probably exceed action level *Examinations:* 1; 2*; 3; 4; 5 *Exam components:* PE; nasal and skin; work and medical history, including smoking history, respiratory symptoms Tests: **CXR;** CBC; reticulocyte count; LFT; PFT; urinalysis; total urine arsenic levels (measurement of dimethylarsinic acid and monomethylarsonic acid eliminates confusion with dietary sources); additional tests as needed * Annually for employees 45 years of age or younger with less than 10 years of exposure, and every 6 months for all other employees
Asbestos 1910.1001 (General Industry) 1926.1101 (Construction)	Asbestos is present in over 3000 manufactured products, which include: building, construction, cement work, insulation, fireproofing, textiles, pipes and ducts for water, air, and chemicals, automobile brake pads and linings (friction products), in construction work involving demolition or salvage, alteration, repair, maintenance, renovation or installation of products; in removal or encapsulation of old asbestos-containing materials	Respiratory system, GI system, eyes Cancer: lung, pleura and peritoneum, colon, ?kidney	*Trigger:* (1) Exposure at or above the PEL (0.1 fiber per cm³ of air) for a combined period of 30 or more days/year; (2) Requirement to wear respiratory protective equipment because of asbestos jobs *Examinations:* 1; 2*; 4; 5 *Exam components:* PE; work and medical history with emphasis directed to symptoms of the respiratory system, cardiovascular system, and digestive tract; completion of the standard respiratory disease questionnaire at the initial exam, and of the follow-up questionnaire yearly *Tests:* **CXR (B-reading); PFT (FVC, FEV₁);** FOB, colonoscopy, low-dose spiral CT scan of the chest; additional tests as needed. * Within 10 days following the 13th day of exposure and at least annually thereafter
Benzene 1910.1028	For extraction in chemical analyses and as a specialty solvent; in the production of ethyl benzene for the production of styrene; in gasoline	Blood, bone marrow, CNS, eyes, respiratory system, skin, liver, kidney Cancer: leukemia	*Trigger:* (1) Exposure at or above the AL (0.5 ppm) for at least 30 days/year; (2) Exposure at or above the PEL (1 ppm) for at least 10 days/year; (3) Assignment to areas in which exposure will probably exceed action level

Table 58.1 Requirements of the OSHA Standards on medical screening for workers with specific exposures, and other OSHA regulations regarding medical screening of workers in specific trades

Exposure[9] OSHA Rule #	Workers at risk/uses	Target organs[12]	Medical screening and surveillance
			Examinations: 1; 2; 3; 5 *Exam components:* PE; work and medical history, including smoking history, hematologic symptoms, and family history of blood dyscrasia *Tests:* **CBC (including red blood cell indices, reticulocyte count)**; LFT; PFT for workers required to use respirators; urinalysis; additional tests as needed. **MRP**
Benzidine (13-carcinogens) 1910.1010	Dyes, detection of blood, reagent for metals	Bladder, skin, kidney, liver, blood Cancer: bladder	*See 2-Acetylaminofluorene* *Tests:* PFT; urinalysis; occult blood in urine (recommended each month); urine cytology (recommended every 6 months); cystoscopy
Beta-Naphthylamine (13-carcinogens) 1910.1009	Dyes	Bladder, skin Cancer: bladder	*See 2-Acetylaminofluorene* *Tests:* Urinalysis; urine cytology; cystoscopy
Beta-Propiolactone (13-carcinogens) 1910.1013	Disinfectant, organic synthesis	Kidney, skin, lungs, eye	*See 2-Acetylaminofluorene* *Tests:* PFT
Bis-chloromethyl ether (13-carcinogens) 1910.1008	Ion-exchange resins, bactericide, pesticide, dispersing agent, water repellant, solvent for polymerization, flameproofing agents	Eye, skin, respiratory system Cancer: lung	*See 2-Acetylaminofluorene* *Tests:* PFT
Blood-borne pathogens 1910.1030	This term refers to pathogenic micro-organisms that are present in human blood and can cause disease in humans. These pathogens include, but are not limited to, hepatitis B virus (HBV) and human immunodeficiency virus (HIV). Healthcare workers with direct patient contact, but also workers at laboratory facilities, and housekeeping and laundry workers in healthcare facilities, are at risk	Liver, immune system	*Trigger:* Reasonably anticipated skin, eye, mucous membrane, or parenteral contact with blood or other potentially infectious materials* *Examinations:* 1†; 3‡ *Exam components:* Evaluations and procedures including hepatitis B vaccination series and post-exposure evaluation and follow-up, including prophylaxis, provided in a timely fashion, at no cost to the employee and under the supervision of a licensed physician * Other potentially infectious materials include: 1) human body fluids: semen, vaginal secretions, cerebrospinal fluid, synovial fluid, pleural fluid, pericardial fluid, peritoneal fluid, amniotic fluid, saliva in dental procedures, any body fluid that is visibly contaminated with blood, and all body fluids in situations where it is difficult or impossible to differentiate between body fluids; 2) unfixed tissue or organ (other than intact skin) from a human (living or dead); and 3) HIV-containing cell or tissue cultures, organ cultures, and HIV- or HBV-containing culture medium or other solutions; and blood, organs, or other tissues from experimental animals infected with HIV or HBV † Hepatitis B vaccination within 10 working days of initial assignment, unless already immune or vaccine contraindicated ‡ Post-exposure monitoring: following a report of an exposure incident, the employer shall make immediately available to the exposed employee a confidential medical evaluation and follow-up, including at least the following elements. 1. Documentation of the route(s) of exposure, and the circumstances under which the exposure incident occurred. 2. Identification and documentation of the source individual, unless the employer can establish that identification is unfeasible or prohibited by state or local law. 3. The source individual's blood shall be tested as soon as feasible and after consent is obtained in order to determine HBV and HIV infectivity. If consent is not obtained, the employer shall establish that legally required consent cannot be obtained. When the source individual's consent is not required by law, the source individual's blood, if available, shall be tested and the results documented. When the source individual is already known to be infected with HBV or HIV, testing for the source individual's known HBV or HIV status need not be repeated. 4. Results of the source individual's testing shall be made available to the exposed employee, and the employee shall be informed of applicable laws and regulations concerning disclosure of the identity and infectious status of the source individual. 5. Collection and testing of blood for HBV and HIV serologic status if consented by the employee. 6. Post-exposure prophylaxis, when medically indicated, as recommended by the US Public Health Service, counseling, and evaluation of reported illness.

Table 58.1 (Cont'd) Requirements of the OSHA Standards on medical screening for workers with specific exposures, and other OSHA regulations regarding medical screening of workers in specific trades

Exposure[9] OSHA Rule #	Workers at risk/uses	Target organs[12]	Medical screening and surveillance
1,3 Butadiene 1910.1051	Manufacture of acrylic fibers for apparel, carpeting, home furnishing, plastic pipes and pipefitting, automotive parts, appliances, and building components; exposure occurs in the petrochemical industry	Eyes, respiratory system, CNS, reproductive system; Cancer: hematopoietic cancer	*Trigger:* (1) Exposure at or above the AL (0.5 ppm) on 30 or more days; (2) Exposure at or above the PEL (1 ppm TWA) on 10 or more days a year *Examinations:* 1; 2; 3*; 4; 5 *Exam components:* PE emphasis directed on the hematopoietic and reticuloendothelial systems and skin; work and medical history; environmental history; standardized medical questionnaire *Tests:* **CBC with differential and platelet count every year** * Include CBC within 48 hours of exposure and monthly for 3 months; and PE if employee reports irritation of eyes, nose, throat, lungs, or skin, blurred vision, coughing, drowsiness, nausea, or headache
Cadmium 1910.1027 1926.1127	Smelting and refining of zinc, lead, and copper; recovery and refining of cadmium products; manufacture of batteries, paints, and plastics; welding and brazing, and electroplating operations	Respiratory system, prostate, blood; Cancer: lungs and prostate	*Trigger:* (1) Exposure at or above the AL (2.5 mg/m³) for at least 30 days/year; (2) Exposure for 10 or more years above the AL though they may no longer be exposed above the level; (3) Assignment to areas in which exposure to cadmium will be encountered *Examinations:* 1; 2*; 3; 4; 5 *Exam components:* PE; prostate palpation in men >40 years of age; work and medical history, including smoking history, respiratory symptoms *Tests†:* Biologic monitoring including: **cadmium in blood, cadmium in urine and beta-2-microglobulin in urine, serum creatinine; CBC; BUN; CXR; PFT (FVC, FEV₁);** urinalysis for proteinuria; pulmonary diffusion capacity; prostate-specific antigen; additional tests as needed. **MRP** * Semi-annually † Biologic monitoring should be conducted quarterly
Coke oven emissions (COE) 1910.1029(j)	COE are the benzene-soluble fraction of total particulate matter present during the destructive distillation or carbonization of coal for the production of coke. Work-titles included under this Standard are: lidman, tar chaser, larry-car operator, luterman, machine operator and benchman on the coke side, benchman on the pusher side, heater, quenching car operator, pusher machine operator, screening station operator, wharfman, oven patcher, oven repairman, spellman, and maintenance personnel	Skin, respiratory system, urinary tract; Cancer: skin, lungs, kidney, and bladder	*Trigger:* Working in a regulated area for at least 30 days per year *Examinations:* 1; 2*; 4; 5 *Exam components:* PE including weight and skin examination; work and medical history, including smoking history and respiratory symptoms *Tests:* **CXR; PFT (FVC, FEV₁);** urinalysis for sugar, **albumin, hematuria; urine cytology examination;** additional tests as needed * Semi-annual for employees 45 years of age or older or with 5 or more years of employment, and annual examinations for all other employees
Compressed air spaces 1926.803	Tunnel operators, caisson operator, deep-sea divers, air personnel at high altitudes	Central and peripheral nervous system, joints, bones	*Trigger:* Working in a regulated area *Examinations:* 1; 2; 3 *Exam components:* Medical examination directed to assure that employee is in good physical condition for working in compressed air spaces.* Special attention given to: weight, vascular system, coagulation mechanisms, respiratory system, osseous system * The physician must be familiar with and experienced in the physical requirements and the medical aspects of compressed air work and treatment of decompression illness. S/he shall be available at all times while work is in progress. S/he shall be physically qualified and be willing to enter a pressurized environment

Table 58.1 (Cont'd) Requirements of the OSHA Standards on medical screening for workers with specific exposures, and other OSHA regulations regarding medical screening of workers in specific trades

Exposure[9] OSHA Rule #	Workers at risk/uses	Target organs[12]	Medical screening and surveillance
Cotton dust 1910.1043	Yarn manufacturing, slashing and weaving, waste house textile operations. Workers are NOT exposed in woven or knitted materials, harvesting or ginning of cotton	Respiratory system, cardiovascular system, byssinosis	*Trigger:* Exposure at or above the following AL: yarn manufacture and cotton washing – 100 μg/m³; textile operations – 250 μg/m³; slashing and weaving – 375 μg/m³ *Examinations:* 1; 2*; 5 *Exam components:* Work and medical history; standardized questionnaire; Schilling grading system *Tests:* **PFT (FVC, FEV₁, FEV₁, FEV₁/FVC)[†]** **MRP** * Annually for workers exposed above the AL. Every 2 years for workers exposed at or below the AL. Every 6 months for workers whose initial FEV₁ is above 80% but decreases by 5% or 200 ml on the first day of work, of for those employees whose initial FEV₁ is below 80%. Exam should include all the elements of the initial examination and comparison with previous test results [†] Before worker enters the workplace on the first day of the working week preceded by at least 35 hours of no exposure to cotton dust (PFT must be repeated during the shift not less than 4 hours and no more than 10 hours after beginning the work shift, and in any case no more than 1 hour after cessation of exposure)
1,2-Dibromo-3-chloropropane (DBCP) 1910.1044	Nematocide used on citrus fruits, grapes, peaches, pineapples, soybeans, and tomatoes. Its use has been banned in the US since 1979	Eyes, skin, respiratory system, CNS, liver, kidney, spleen, reproductive system, digestive system. Cancer: in animals; nasal cavity, tongue, pharynx, lungs, stomach, adrenal and mammary glands	*Trigger:* Working in a regulated area *Examinations:* 1; 2; 3; 5 *Exam components:* PE including examination of the genitourinary tract, testicle size and body habitus; reproductive history *Tests:* **Serum specimen for RIA determinations of FSH, LH and total estrogen (females), and sperm count in males**
3,3'-Dichlorobenzidine and its salts (13-carcinogens) 1910.1007	Dyes (azo dyes), pigments	Bladder, liver, lung, skin, GI	*See 2-Acetylaminofluorene* *Tests:* PFT
4-Dimethylaminoazo-benzene (13-carcinogens) 1910.1015	pH indicator, test for identification of peroxidized fats, for determination of free chlorhydric acid in gastric juice	Skin, respiratory system, liver, kidney, bladder	*See 2-Acetylaminofluorene*
Ethylene oxide (EtO) 1910.1047 1926.1147	In the manufacture of ethylene glycol (antifreeze and an intermediate for polyester fibers, films, and bottles), non-ionic surface-active agents (used for home laundry detergents and dishwashing liquids), glycol ethers (used for surface coatings), and ethanolamines (for soaps, detergents, and textile chemicals). Used as a pesticide fumigant and as sterilant in hospitals, medical products manufacture, libraries, museums, beekeeping, spice and seasoning fumigation, animal and plant quarantine, transportation vehicle fumigation, and dairy packaging	Eyes, skin, respiratory system, liver, CNS, blood, kidney, and reproductive system. Cancer: peritoneal cancer, leukemia	*Trigger:* Exposure at or above the AL (0.5 ppm) for at least 30 days/year without regard to respirator use *Examinations:* 1; 2; 3; 4; 5 *Exam components:* PE with emphasis directed on symptoms related to the pulmonary, hematologic, neurologic, and reproductive systems and to the eyes and skin; work and medical history *Tests:* **CBC to include at least a white cell count (including differential cell count), red cell count, hematocrit, and hemoglobin; additional tests as needed*** * If requested by the worker, pregnancy testing or laboratory evaluation of fertility will be provided, as deemed appropriate by the physician
Ethyleneimine (13-carcinogens) 1910.1012	Textile finishing agent, insect sterilant, antineoplastic, manufacture of resinous products	Eye, skin, respiratory system, liver, kidney	*See 2-Acetylaminofluorene* *Tests:* CXR; PFT

Table 58.1 (Cont'd) Requirements of the OSHA Standards on medical screening for workers with specific exposures, and other OSHA regulations regarding medical screening of workers in specific trades

Exposure[9] OSHA Rule #	Workers at risk/uses	Target organs[12]	Medical screening and surveillance
Formaldehyde 1910.1048	In the manufacture of urea-formaldehyde foam and resins used as adhesives in particle board, fiberboard and plywood. Used as tissue fixative and embalming agent and as preservative in cosmetics, glues and shampoos	Eyes, respiratory system, skin Cancer: nasal cavity, nasopharynx	*Trigger:* Exposure at or above the AL (0.75 ppm) *Examinations:* 1; 2; 3; 5 *Exam components:* PE with special emphasis directed to symptoms and signs related to the pulmonary system and to the eyes and skin; work and medical history *Tests:* **PFT (FVC, FEV$_1$, FEF)**; blood and urine; additional tests as needed **MRP**
Hazardous waste 1910.120 1926.65	More common potential exposures: aromatic hydrocarbons, asbestos, dioxin, halogenated aliphatic hydrocarbons, heavy metals, herbicides, organochlorine insecticides, organophosphate and carbamate insecticides, polychlorinated byphenyls, other toxic chemicals, safety hazards, radiation, heat or cold stress, explosions and fires	Lungs, kidneys, central nervous system, blood, skin, eyes, stress, cancer. Additional target organs as per exposures	*Trigger:* Working in a regulated area *Examinations:* 1*; 2; 3; 4; 5 *Exam components:* PE including vision and audiometric tests, determination of fitness to work wearing protective equipment and baseline monitoring for specific exposures; work and medical history; relevant lifestyle habits *Tests:* LFT; kidney function; urinalysis; CBC; CXR. Baseline and periodic tests for specific toxicants should be tailored to exposure, such as: serum PCB testing, lead and zinc protoporphyrin (ZPP), cadmium, arsenic and organophosphate pesticides. PFT and electrocardiogram if necessary to assess worker's capacity to perform while wearing protective equipment * Freezing pre-employment serum specimen for later testing is suggested
Lead 1910.1025 1926.62	Manufacture of storage batteries; as an alloy in pipes, cable sheathing, solder; in paints and plastics as pigments and stabilizers; as glazes for ceramics; in construction for attenuation of sound and vibration and for the shielding of radioactivity; in ammunition, bronze and brass, cosmetics and jewelry; organic lead (tetramethyl lead) used as antiknock agent in gasoline	Eyes, GI tract, CNS, kidney, blood, gingival tissue	*Trigger:* (1) Exposure at or above the AL (50 μg/m^3) at any time calls for biologic monitoring of blood lead levels (BLL) and ZPP levels; (2) Exposure above 30 μg/m^3 TWA for more than 30 days/year; (3) Employees whose BLL exceed 40 μg/dl *Examinations:* 1*; 2†;3‡; 5 *Exam components:* PE with emphasis on neurologic, GI, and cardiovascular systems, teeth, gums, and renal system; work and medical history *Tests:* **BLL**; ZPP††; hemoglobin; hematocrit; BUN; serum creatinine; red cell indices; examination of the peripheral blood smear to evaluate red blood cell morphology; routine urinalysis with microscopic examination; X-ray fluorescence of the bone; additional tests as needed MRP‡‡**

* All workers assigned to work in an area in which air-borne lead concentrations reach or exceed the 30 μg/m^3 TWA for more than 30 days/year

† Annually for workers exposed above 30 μg/m^3 for more than 30 days/year, or whose BLL conducted at any time during the preceding 12 months resulted in level of 40 μg/dl or higher

‡ Medical examination must be provided as soon as possible after notification by the worker that s/he has developed signs or symptoms commonly associated with lead intoxication, that s/he desires medical advice regarding lead exposure and the ability to procreate a healthy child, or that s/he has demonstrated difficulty in breathing during a respirator fitting test or during respirator use. Examination is also to be made available to each worker removed from exposure to lead due to risk of sustaining material impairment to health, or otherwise limited or specially protected pursuant to medical recommendations

** Workers exposed above 30 μg/m^3 for more than 30 days/year or whose BLL is above 40 μg/dl but exposed for no more than 30 days/year, should have BLL determined at least every 2 months for the first 6 months of exposure and every 6 months thereafter. Frequency is increased to every 2 months for workers whose last BLL was 40 μg/dl or above. For workers who are removed from exposure to lead due to an elevated blood lead, a new BLL must be measured monthly

†† Recommended on each occasion a BLL measurement is made

‡‡ When the BLL reaches 50 μg/dl, confirmed by a follow-up BLL performed within 2 weeks after the employer receives the results of the first BLL. Return of the employee to his or her job status depends on a worker's BLL declining to 40 μg/dl. In addition to the above BLL criterion, temporary worker removal may also take place as a result of medical determinations and recommendations

Table 58.1 (Cont'd) Requirements of the OSHA Standards on medical screening for workers with specific exposures, and other OSHA regulations regarding medical screening of workers in specific trades

Exposure[9] OSHA Rule #	Workers at risk/uses	Target organs[12]	Medical screening and surveillance
Methylene chloride (MC) 1910.1052	Paint stripping, polyurethane foam manufacturing, and cleaning and degreasing	Eyes, skin, cardiovascular system, liver, CNS Cancer: in animals; lung, liver, salivary and mammary glands	*Trigger:* (1) Exposure at or above the AL (12.5 ppm) on 30 or more days per year, or above the 8-hour TWA PEL (25 ppm) or the STEL (125 ppm) on 10 or more days per year; (2) Exposure above the PEL or STEL for any time period where an employee has been identified as being at risk from cardiac disease or from some other serious MC-related health condition *Examinations:* 1; 2*; 3; 4; 5 *Exam components:* PE with emphasis on lungs, cardiovascular, liver, nervous, skin, hematologic; work and medical history *Tests:* **Carboxyhemoglobin (before- and after-shift); resting ECG; hematocrit; LFT; cholesterol levels;** additional tests as needed **MRP** *For employees 45 years of age or older, within 12 months, and for employees younger than 45 years of age, within 36 months of the initial surveillance
Methyl chloromethyl ether (13-carcinogens) 1910.1006	*See Bis-chloromethyl ether*	Eye, skin, respiratory system	*See Bis-chloromethyl ether*
Methylene-dianiline (MDA) 1910.1050 1926.60	Production of rigid polyurethane foams, as a curing agent and as epoxy resin hardener	Eyes, liver, cardiovascular system, spleen Cancer: bladder	*Trigger:* (1) Exposure at or above the AL (5 ppb) for 30 or more days per year; (2) Dermal exposure to MDA for 15 or more days per year; (3) Exposure in an emergency situation and for employees who show signs or symptoms of MDA exposure *Examinations:* 1; 2; 3; 5 *Exam components:* PE with emphasis directed on skin and liver; work and medical history with emphasis on past work exposure to MDA or any other toxic substance, history of drugs, alcohol, tobacco, or medication routinely taken, and history of dermatitis, chemical skin sensitization, or previous hepatic disease *Tests:* **LFT, urinalysis repeated annually** **MRP**
4-Nitrobiphenyl (13-carcinogens) 1910.1003 1915.1003 1926.1103	Rubber industry	Bladder, blood	*See 2-Acetylaminofluorene* *Tests:* Urinalysis; urine cytology; cystoscopy
N-nitroso-dimethyl amine (13-carcinogens) 1910.1016	Used as antioxidant for lubricants, softener of copolymers; formerly used in rocket fluids; present in cigarette smoke	Liver, kidney, lungs	*See 2-Acetylaminofluorene* *Tests:* LFT; PFT
Noise 1910.95 1926.52	Construction, manufacturing, military, mining, production, and transportation industries	Ears	*Trigger:* Exposure to sound levels in excess of those shown in the following table, when measured on the acoustic scale of a standard sound level meter at slow response: PERMISSIBLE NOISE EXPOSURES* Duration per day, hours — Sound level dBA, slow response 8 — 90 6 — 92 4 — 95 3 — 97 2 — 100 1 1/2 — 102 1 — 105 1/2 — 110 1/4 or less — 115 *Examinations:* 1; 2; 4

Table 58.1 (Cont'd) Requirements of the OSHA Standards on medical screening for workers with specific exposures, and other OSHA regulations regarding medical screening of workers in specific trades

Exposure[9] OSHA Rule #	Workers at risk/uses	Target organs[12]	Medical screening and surveillance
Noise continued			Exam components: Hearing conservation program whenever employee noise exposures equal or exceed an 8-hour TWA sound level of 85 decibels measured on the A scale (slow response). Program consists of obtaining valid audiograms as follows: a baseline study, within 6 months of an employee's first exposure at or above the AL, annual new audiograms for each eligible employee, which should be compared with the baseline audiogram, and an audiogram at termination of employment. If the annual audiogram shows that an employee has suffered a standard threshold shift, the employer may obtain a retest within 30 days and consider the results of the retest as the annual audiogram, and the audiologist, otolaryngologist, or physician in charge of the program shall determine whether there is a need for further evaluation.
			* When the daily noise exposure is composed of two or more periods of noise exposure of different levels, their combined effect should be considered, rather than the individual effect of each. If the sum of the following fractions: $C(1)/T(1) + C(2)/T(2) + C(n)/T(n)$ exceeds unity, then the mixed exposure should be considered to exceed the limit value. Cn indicates the total time of exposure at a specified noise level, and Tn indicates the total time of exposure permitted at that level. Exposure to impulsive or impact noise should not exceed 140 dB peak sound pressure level
Respirator use[13] 1910.134	Used to prevent inhalation of harmful substances and to provide a source of respirable air when breathing in oxygen-deficient atmospheres	Respiratory system, skin, senses, musculo-skeletal system, cardiovascular, psychologic effects	Trigger: Use of respiratory protective equipment Examinations: 1; 2; 5 Exam components: Work and medical history; standard medical questionnaire; follow-up evaluation (interview) required if answering 'yes' to questions 1–8 or 10–15 of the standard questionnaire; if evaluation finds a significant clinical problem, clinical examination and special tests as recommended by healthcare professional; re-evaluations determined by individual's health status, medical recommendation, changes in working conditions or observations from the respiratory protection program or at the time of annual fit-testing; additional tests as needed
Vinyl chloride 1910.1017	Production of polyvinyl chloride resins for plastic piping and conduit, floor coverings, home furnishing, electrical applications, records, toys, packaging, and transportation industry (auto tops, upholstery, and mats). Standard does NOT apply to handling or use of fabricated products made of polyvinyl chloride	Liver, CNS, blood, respiratory system, lymphatic system, skin Cancer: hepatic angiosarcoma	Trigger: Exposure in excess of the AL (0.5 ppm) Examinations: 1; 2*; 5 Exam components: PE focusing on enlargement of the liver, spleen, or kidneys, or dysfunction in these organs, skin, connective tissue, and pulmonary abnormalities; work and medical history including alcohol intake, past history of hepatitis, past exposure to potential hepatotoxic agents including drugs and chemicals, past history of blood transfusions, and past history of hospitalizations Tests: **Serum determination of total bilirubin, alkaline phosphatase, aminotransferases and gamma-glutamyl transpeptidase, urinary coproporphyrins**, ultrasonography of the liver * Examinations should be performed at least every 6 months for each employee who has been employed in vinyl chloride manufacturing for 10 years or longer, and annually for all other employees

Examinations are provided as 1=pre-placement examination; 2=periodic examination; 3=emergency/exposure examination and tests; 4=termination examination; 5=evaluation of ability to wear a respirator. OSHA-mandated medical tests and procedures are in **bold**.

AL, action level; BUN, blood urea nitrogen; CBC, complete blood count; CNS, central nervous system; CXR, chest X-ray; EKG, electrocardiogram; FOB, fecal occult blood; FVC, forced vital capacity; FEV, forced expiratory flow; FEV₁, forced expiratory volume in 1 second; GI, gastrointestinal; LFT, liver function tests; MRP, medical removal plan; PE, physical examination; PFT, spirometry; RIA, radioimmunoassay; TWA, time-weighted average; ?, = possible association.

Table 58.1 (Cont'd) Requirements of the OSHA Standards on medical screening for workers with specific exposures, and other OSHA regulations regarding medical screening of workers in specific trades

- when the patient has had significant exposure to an agent or agents known to be associated with a disease for which screening tools exist and there is evidence that early detection may improve outcomes; or
- when the US Preventive Services Task Force recommends screening, e.g., the Task Force recommendation that patients with potential tuberculosis contact receive regular PPD skin testing; PPD testing should be performed in settings with recognized high potential for exposure to tuberculosis, such as prisons.

Screening programs for occupational diseases should be based on the standard principles of screening previously described. Unfortunately, there is limited information available for the occupational healthcare provider on the efficacy of screening for disease in occupationally exposed populations. The American College of Occupational and Environmental Medicine (ACOEM) has developed protocols for the detection of various occupational conditions, based on target organ, disease type, and exposure; the National Institute for Occupational Safety and Health (NIOSH) website also provides guidance.[11]

An important and often overlooked barrier to secondary prevention of occupational diseases is access to follow-up diagnostic testing and treatment. In some states, the worker's compensation system may unfortunately pose barriers to prompt care. Additionally, healthcare providers need to recognize that the treatment of any occupational diseases that are identified should include attempting to decrease occupational exposure to the causal agent. Ideally, this should be accomplished both for the identified patient and for similarly exposed coworkers.

TERTIARY PREVENTION OF OCCUPATIONAL ILLNESS AND INJURY

Tertiary prevention of illness and injury is focused on minimizing morbidity, disability, and mortality due to occupational diseases and injuries. Examples of tertiary occupational disease prevention include surgery for the treatment of lung cancer in an asbestos-exposed worker or carpal tunnel release in a worker with work-related carpal tunnel syndrome. In addition to medical treatment, tertiary preventive services include disability prevention. Disability prevention may be facilitated by:

- providing appropriate therapeutic medical care;
- coordinating with the employer regarding return-to-work issues such as modified duty, in which work tasks or schedules may be changed to allow return to work; and
- in those situations in which the worker cannot return to the previous job, facilitating vocational rehabilitation. An example of a situation in which return to work at the previous job might not be feasible would be in a worker with isocyanate-induced asthma – in that situation, the affected worker should be referred to appropriate vocational rehabilitation programs.

Managing return to work for patients with occupational health problems requires intensive coordination between the healthcare provider, the employer, and, where it exists, the union. As is true with requests to modify exposure for primary disease prevention, healthcare providers should explicitly request the patient's permission prior to communicating with the union or the employer about return to work. An example of how the healthcare provider can assist in return to work efforts is provided by that of a reporter who has undergone carpal tunnel surgery for work-related carpal tunnel syndrome and is now ready to return to work. Often, after receiving surgery, the patient will receive hand therapy to minimize his or her chance of reinjury. In the interim, the healthcare provider can work with the employer to initiate ergonomic changes designed to prevent both exacerbation of the carpal tunnel syndrome and development of new musculoskeletal disorders. Appropriate changes might include improvements in the computer workstation by provision of an adjustable keyboard, an adjustable chair, and voice-recognition software, and introduction of a modified schedule, in which the patient progressively increases repetitive work activities and is provided with alternative tasks to minimize hand-intensive work.

CONCLUSION

In conclusion, primary, secondary, and tertiary prevention of occupational health problems should be an integral part of the practice of occupational medicine. Successful prevention endeavors often require time-intensive efforts by healthcare providers coupled with management cooperation. Finally, healthcare providers should familiarize themselves with exposures that trigger OSHA-mandated screening examinations.

References

1. Herbert R, London M, Nagin D, Beckett W. The diagnosis and treatment of occupational diseases: integrating clinical practice with prevention. Am J Ind Med 2000; 37:1-5.
2. Rudolph L, Deitchman S, Dervin K. Integrating occupational health services and occupational prevention services. Am J Ind Med 2001; 40:307-18.
3. US Preventive Services Task Force. Guide to clinical preventive services, 2nd ed. Baltimore: Williams & Wilkins; 1996. Available at www.ahrq.gov/clinic/cpsix.htm. Last accessed August 15, 2001.
4. Keogh J, Gucer P, Gordon J, Nuwayhid I. Patterns and predictors of employer risk-reduction activities (ERRAs) in response to a work-related upper extremity cumulative trauma disorder (UECTD): reports from workers' compensations claimants. Am J Ind Med 2000; 38:489-97.
5. Rutstein D, Mullan R, Frazier T, Halperin W, Melius J, Sestito J. Sentinel health events (occupational): a basis for physician recognition and public health surveillance. Am J Public Health 1983; 73:1054-62.
6. Herbert R, Landrigan PJ. Work-related death: a continuing epidemic. Am J Public Health 2000; 90:541-5.
7. Levin S, Goldberg M. Clinical evaluation and management of lead-exposed construction workers. Am J Ind Med 2000; 37:23-43.
8. Patz EF, Goodman PC, Bepler G. Screening for lung cancer. N Engl J Med 2000; 343;1627-33.
9. Occupational Safety and Health Administration, US Department of Labor. OSHA Regulations (Standards – 29 CFR).

Available at www.osha-slc.gov/OshStd_toc/OSHA_Std_toc.html. Last accessed August 15, 2001.

10. American College of Occupational and Environmental Medicine (ACOEM). Medical surveillance in the workplace. Position statement. Available at: www.acoem.org/paprguid/papers/msurv.htm. Reprinted from the September 1989 ACOEM Report, web page last updated 4/21/97. Last accessed June 15, 2001.

11. NIOSH. Specific medical tests published in the literature for OSHA regulated substances. Available at: www.cdc.gov/niosh/nmed/medstart.html. Last accessed August 15, 2001.

12. National Institute for Occupational Safety and Health, US Department of Health and Human Services, Public Health Service, Centers for Disease Control and Prevention. NIOSH Pocket Guide to Chemical Hazards. DHHS (NIOSH) Publication No. 2000-130, July 2000.

13. National Institute for Occupational Safety and Health, Occupational Safety and Health Administration (OSHA), US Coast Guard, US Environmental Protection Agency. Occupational safety and health guidance manual for hazardous waste site activities. Washington, DC: US Department of Health and Human Services, Public Health Service, Centers for Disease Control, National Institute for Occupational Safety and Health, October 1985.

Chapter 59
Communication and Assessment of Risk

Bernard D Goldstein, Audrey R Gotsch

INTRODUCTION

The success of a physician's practice must always be judged in terms of the outcome of health and wellbeing of the patients. This reflects not only the correctness of the physician's diagnosis and actions but also the physician's ability to communicate recommendations to the patient. Communication is thus a central skill in the practice of medicine and risk communication is, in a sense, a subset of patient communication. Since before the time of Hippocrates, communicating risk to patients has been an important tool used by physicians. In recent years, however, the concept of risk communication has been extended to the health and wellbeing of the community.[1-3]

Modern medicine has two competing trends in terms of the need for physicians to communicate effectively. The move toward superspecialization places many physicians in positions where there is little or no opportunity to explain anything to a patient, e.g., pathologists and radiologists. Conversely, the increased desire of patients to be involved in medical decisions that affect them in this era of holistic medicine places more demands on the communication skills of those physicians who do have patient contact. This is further complicated by the increasing complexity of modern medicine and by the rapid movement from a passive to an active information era. Coverage by mass media may lead to the patient learning about the significance of a study outcome published in the latest issue of the *New England Journal of Medicine* before the physician's own copy of the journal arrives in the mail. The blossoming of the internet as a communications medium is providing patients with new information sources, many of which are not subject to even a modest amount of peer review.

The risk communication focus in this chapter will be on those aspects of risk communication that are pertinent to physicians involved in occupational and environmental medicine on a full- or part-time basis. We describe some of the basic behavioral theories that provide the foundation for sound risk communication, and generalize from single patient issues familiar to the general physician to special problems involved in the workplace, to the often more difficult problems encountered in environmental medicine when communicating with groups of individuals, communities, or representatives of different interested parties, regulatory agencies, and the media.

Risk communication will be addressed broadly in this chapter to include the one-on-one activities of physicians dealing with individuals, and the issues faced by the public such as the risk assessments of chemical and physical agents. It is the latter application of the risk communication concept that has gained widespread use among governmental agencies and various interest groups who are exploring means to improve their ability to communicate about risks.

Concern about health risks of chemical and physical agents in the environment has led physicians to become more involved in responding to the public about controversial issues related to the levels of risk to human health. If appropriate societal balance is to be maintained between the risks and benefits posed by environmental agents, it is crucial that physicians increase their understanding and communication skills regarding these issues. The next section provides an overview of the risk assessment paradigm at a level that is useful for a physician to understand and to translate to the public. The ensuing section addresses the basic concepts that provide the foundation for effective communication. These are followed by a consideration of a number of issues pertinent to the communication of risks.

RISK ASSESSMENT PARADIGM

The risk assessment paradigm consists of four major steps: hazard identification; dose–response evaluation; exposure assessment; and risk characterization. It is derived from standard engineering approaches, such as those that attempt to determine the likelihood that a bridge will fall based upon knowledge of the strengths of the structural components, the weight that will be carried and external forces such as wind speed. It is also derived from the three 'laws' of toxicology: the dose makes the poison, the specificity of the biologic hazards posed by chemical and physical agents, and the unity of the animal kingdom, including humans.

The first law of toxicology, the dose makes the poison, is attributed to Paracelsus. It is central to all toxicology and is equivalent to the dose–response evaluation step of risk assessment. Basically, everything causes risk, even water – it is all a matter of dose. The second law of toxicology, recently attributed to Pare, is that the inherent structure of a chemical and the biologic niche in which it reacts confer a very high level of specificity to the type of effects, i.e., the hazard, caused by a chemical. As examples, radioactive iodine preferentially causes thyroid cancer because of the specific iodine uptake mechanisms of the thyroid gland, and carbon monoxide interferes with oxygen delivery because of its propensity to bind to the oxygen-combining site of hemoglobin. Note that risk is conferred only by the combination of hazard and exposure – no matter how intrinsically hazardous a chemical is, there is no risk unless there is some exposure to it leading to the internal dose at the organ of concern.

The third law of toxicology, that humans are animals, is the basis for using laboratory animals for the extrapolation of hazard identification and dose–response information to humans. There are certainly differences between humans and laboratory animals, but these are relatively minor compared to the broad degree of similarity in structure and function of organelles, cells, tissues and organs. Understanding the relevant differences permits extrapolation from animals to humans. Where ethically possible, human data are of value because they avoid the pitfalls inherent in extrapolation. But human data usually have been obtained from relatively high-level exposure situations, often in the workplace. Accordingly, extrapolation from such data to lower levels and to the general population also is necessary.

Exposure assessment, the third step of risk assessment, is the measurement of internal dose, often indirectly. Physicians are most comfortable with the situation of drugs in which dose is usually obvious because it is prescribed. In the workplace it is often industrial hygienists who evaluate the extent of exposure of individual workers, sometimes through the use of area-wide measurements or, ideally, of personal monitors. Exposure assessment for members of the general population, for example to the effluent of a factory, often requires simplifying assumptions which are best made by taking into account worst case situations for the most sensitive members of the general population.

Translation of external dose to internal dose to the target tissue often depends upon the availability of biologic markers. In the two examples above, one can use radioactive scanning of the thyroid gland to determine radioactive iodine uptake, and carboxy hemoglobin levels to provide an accurate marker of the extent of carbon monoxide exposure over the past 4–6 hours, as well as a predictor of its adverse effects. But there are very few such internal indicators. In many cases, increased susceptibility to chemical exposures will represent changes in the internal pathways that lead to the formation or detoxification of toxic intermediates at a target tissue. In other words, genetic polymorphisms that alter human susceptibility to chemicals often act to alter the extent to which external exposure is converted to internal dose to target tissue.

Risk characterization, the last step of a risk assessment, is the interface between the risk assessor and the risk manager.[4] Too often risk is characterized in terms of an abstruse and poorly understood mathematical formulation. The aim of risk characterization should be to serve as the basis for the communication of risk information. The risk should be characterized in such a way that it is readily translatable into who is at risk, for what diseases, and under what circumstances.[2] The parameter should include the duration of time for adverse outcomes to develop, which is often better understood than the usual numerical statement of chances per million.[5] The key

uncertainties underlying the risk assessment should be included as part of the characterization, but a mathematical formulation of the extent of uncertainty is usually unnecessary and can further obscure the goal of the risk assessment.[6]

RISK COMMUNICATION AND MAJOR HEALTH EDUCATION CONCEPTS

A basis for effective risk communication exists in the body of theoretical concepts and research knowledge underpinning the practice of health education. Of the major health education concepts, perhaps the most important for risk communication is the health belief model, which explains behavioral change on the basis of patients' belief in their own susceptibility to a disease or condition, its severity, the effectiveness of techniques for its prevention or treatment, and their own capacity for making use of those techniques. This section summarizes the health belief model as well as other major health education concepts, such as empowerment, locus of control, social learning theory, social support, and diffusion of innovations.

The health belief model

The health belief model developed in the 1950s from stimulus–response and cognitive theories of behavior.[7] The model was conceptualized by Hochbaum[8] and his colleagues in the US Public Health Service who examined the motivating factors for individuals to participate in free tuberculosis screening programs sponsored by the US Public Health Service. Their work identified three critical motivational factors: people's perception of themselves as personally susceptible to tuberculosis, even in the absence of symptoms; their belief in the effectiveness of chest radiographs as a detection technique; and their belief that early detection and treatment would benefit them. The single most important variable in moving individuals to take action was the belief in their own susceptibility to tuberculosis.

Since this initial study, the health belief model has been refined through further research and is now applied to the full spectrum of behaviors that affect health. Training in the application of the model can greatly enhance physicians' ability to perform risk communication in environmental and occupational medicine settings.

Components of the health belief model

The health belief model, as it is now generally formulated, holds that individuals will take action to prevent damage to their health, to screen for disease, or to control disease, if they: (1) regard themselves as personally susceptible to a given condition; (2) believe the condition to have serious consequences; (3) believe that the action will either reduce their susceptibility or reduce the severity of the condition; and (4) believe that the anticipated barriers to (or costs of) taking action are outweighed by the benefits.[7] The combination of perceived susceptibility and perceived severity is often referred to as 'perceived threat'. In most formulations of the model, educational level and other demographic factors are taken into account as influencing perceptions of susceptibility, severity, benefits, and barriers.

A refinement of the health belief model has involved the introduction of Bandura's concept of self-efficacy.[9] This concept relates to the individual's belief that he or she can effectively perform a given action believed to be protective of health; self-efficacy amplifies the model's reliance on the perception of benefits. For example, if workers are to use protective equipment during exposure to an occupational hazard, they must believe not only that the equipment will protect them but also that they are capable of using the equipment consistently and effectively. Studies point to the significance of self-efficacy as a critical factor in behavior change.[10,11]

Implications of the health belief model for risk communication

The health belief model underscores the importance of risk communication and provides an important framework for physicians to use in conducting it. The model points to the fact that risk communication must be a part of a comprehensive strategy for communicating about health beliefs if it is to be effective in producing behavior change.[12] For example, providing information about an occupational hazard may not cause workers to modify their actions if it is not also accompanied by information that stresses the workers' self-efficacy.

The evidence is strong that attention to the variables outlined in the model can lead to sustained changes in behavior, whether one is dealing with an individual patient, a group of patients, or a community. Such changes can be accomplished if communication is designed to underline the susceptibility of an individual or group to a particular risk, the severity of the risk, the effectiveness of a course of action in protecting health, the capacity of the individual or group to perform the action, and the relative weight of the benefits of the action as opposed to its costs.

Interventions can be more effectively planned if data are available on the health beliefs of the target population. For example, if workers in a particular industry accept their susceptibility to occupational asthma and understand that appropriate clean-up and ventilation procedures can help prevent it,[13] but do not regard asthma as a severe enough condition to warrant the inconvenience of utilizing the procedures, an intervention could be designed that would emphasize the severity of the disease (while at the same time giving appropriate weight to the other variables identified in the model). In another population, however, it might be more important to emphasize susceptibility or in another setting self-efficacy, depending on the baseline health beliefs of the target group.

Empowerment and locus of control

Closely related to the idea of self-efficacy are the concepts of empowerment and locus of control. The latter has to do

with an individual's conception of the ability to control threats to health. If control is perceived as external, such as controllable only by an employer or by civil authorities, the individual is unlikely to have any motivation for behavior change that could protect his or her health.[14,15] Motivation for action is far more likely when patients believe themselves to have some control over risks to health. The locus of control may be at the individual level (in quitting smoking or in taking appropriate safety precautions on the job) or it may be at the level of the community, for example, in persuading industries to properly discharge their hazardous wastes.

Empowerment is a process through which individuals or communities take control over risks and over their environment, acting to protect their health.[16,17] It is often viewed as a process whereby problem-solving ability is increased. In the patient–provider relationship, the provider who empowers patients enables them to take an active role in protecting their health, rather than encouraging them to take the passive role of sick people who wait to be cured. As Lewis explains, the provider's role is not so much to 'intervene' as to enable patients to 'modify their interpersonal environment in ways that foster positive health behavior. In the process, personal levels of power and control, including self-efficacy, are enhanced'.[18]

Empowerment plays an important role in approaches to improving health through community organization, where the physician can also have a critical enabling role. Communication about risk at the community level means empowering both the community as a whole and individuals within it. Community action to restore areas of contamination, frequently cited as brownfields, is an example of community empowerment. Involvement with community efforts, with its resulting increase in social support, has been shown to increase the individual's sense of control and to produce significant physical and emotional health benefits.[10,19] As communities become empowered they are better able to engage in collective problem solving and to reduce risks. Research indicates that community empowerment may be statistically reflected in declines of alcoholism, suicide, and divorce rates.[20,21]

Social learning theory

Social learning theory explains health behavior change in terms of dynamic inter-relationships among behavior, personal factors, and environmental influences; the interaction of these three components is called reciprocal determinism. The theory identifies a variety of personal factors as critical, including the individual's ability to symbolize the meanings of behavior, to foresee the outcomes of behavior, to learn by observing others, to regulate behavior, and to reflect on and analyze experience.[10,22] Environmental factors extend to all external influences on a person's behavior, including both physical and social dimensions. Some proponents of social learning theory use a behaviorist framework, in that they consider health behavior in terms of positive and negative reinforcements. This branch of the theory places strong emphasis on the individual's locus of control – those with an internal locus of control being more likely to initiate change themselves, those with an external locus of control more likely to be influenced by others.[23]

The other important branch of social learning theory, developed in the early 1960s, emphasizes cognitive constructs, among them 'observational learning', which holds that behavior can be learned by observing the behavior of others and the rewards others receive, without the rewards having to be received directly by the observer.[24] Among other constructs that the theory identifies as critical in determining behavior, one of the most important is 'behavioral capability', which distinguishes two components of behavior – knowledge and skill. To make a behavior change a person needs to know not only what the behavior is, but also how to perform it. This concept points to the importance in risk communication not only of addressing the behaviors that can reduce risk, but also of providing training and practice in the skills involved in performing the relevant behaviors.

Social learning theory provides a foundation for risk communication by identifying both behaviorist and cognitive constructs in individual behavior; and by placing these within the framework that recognizes that behavior does not occur within a vacuum; that it is a continuous interaction between a person's behavior and the environment where the behavior takes place (reciprocal determinism). It provides an especially valuable theoretical foundation for the design of multilevel, multicomponent interventions, in which individual behavior change and change within the environment are addressed simultaneously.

Diffusion theory

Diffusion theory examines the process by which innovations – ideas, practices, and services – are communicated among members of a social system. It sees innovations as developing from a realm of expertise, known as the resource system, and ultimately being adopted by a given population, known as the user system. The theory identifies the central factors of successful diffusion efforts and points to potential system failure points. Among the attributes of innovations that are likely to meet with successful diffusion and adoption are cost-efficiency, simplicity, flexibility, a low degree of risk, and compatibility with the target population's economic, sociocultural, and philosophical value systems. Innovations are also more likely to be adopted if they show a relative advantage over existing methods and if they are reversible – allowing the individual or group adopting the innovation to return to earlier methods if need be.[25,26]

Classic diffusion theory saw the adoption process as a relatively straightforward movement from the source that provides the needed knowledge or expertise required to make the change to the agency or individual making the change. Modern formulations of the theory describe a reciprocal, multistep process that may extend well beyond adoption itself (taking into account the need to maintain changes in behavior). Rogers[26] identifies a six-step diffusion

process: (1) recognition of a problem or need; (2) basic and applied research; (3) development, in which an innovation is given a form intended to meet the needs of a particular population; (4) production, marketing, and distribution; (5) diffusion and adoption; and (6) consequences.

The constant interaction of the behavior, the individual and the environment involved in adoption of innovations is emphasized by a refinement of diffusion theory known as the linkage approach.[27,28] This approach identifies a linkage system involved in developing innovation and diffusion strategies; the linkage system includes members of both the resource system and the user system, whose collaboration is facilitated by 'change agents' (themselves often members of the other systems). The linkage approach draws on social marketing research to describe the collaboration between user and resource systems in developing and adopting innovations. The role of the resource system is seen as one of helping the user system determine its needs, expectations, and limitations. In this context, the theory emphasizes the collection of quantitative and qualitative data about a target population, segmentation of a population into subgroups, and tailoring of innovations to suit the needs and sociocultural characteristics of a particular group or subgroup.[25]

Risk communication can benefit from the use of diffusion theory to analyze how innovations in research knowledge can be effectively transmitted to practitioners and ultimately to the general population. Diffusion theory also offers a means for determining the most effective techniques for developing real-world applications of risk communication approaches that have been developed in demonstration settings.[3,25,26]

WHO IS INVOLVED IN RISK COMMUNICATION?
The risk communicator

The most important determinant for success in communicating risk is the perceived credibility of the individual engaged in the communication process.[29] While many other aspects of risk communication include technical skills that can be learned by the physician, credibility is not a skill that can be learned; it is a standing that needs to be earned.[30] Obviously, part of the physician's credibility will depend, at least initially, on his or her employment affiliation. For example, the physician employed by a company will have a different level of credibility if there is a difference of opinion concerning the extent of employee risk than a physician representing workers who is not employed by the same industry. Company physicians can and do build credibility with employees through activities on a one-to-one basis as part of their routine practice of occupational medicine, and this can be extremely helpful when the physician assumes the role of a risk communicator.

Corporations also differ among themselves in their inherent credibility on health issues. It is hard to imagine that a company that fights to obtain 'give-backs' on health insurance at the collective bargaining table will be very convincing when it attempts to communicate a concern about reducing risk for a worker or community. Perhaps the least credible industry will be one that is seen as inherently inimical to public health. For example, it is unlikely that anyone in the workforce or general community would believe any communication concerning the risk of a chemical hazard that emanated from a cigarette company, or an otherwise neutral industry that happened to be owned by a major tobacco corporation.

Similar to general clinical medicine, the basis for risk communication is a history that includes questions that will identify potential risks. Such a medical history allows the physician to understand the full range of risks facing the patient and facilitates the use of communication techniques appropriate for the individual's level of understanding and concern.[31] A careful history that identifies work, home, or recreational activities that could lead to chemical exposures is crucial (see Chapter 3). The work practice and its possible adverse consequences should be sufficiently understood so that alternative activities leading to protection can be stressed. As is clear from studies of cigarette smokers, the physician can be highly effective in reinforcing messages that may be present in the workplace or available through product labels. Conversely, the absence of such reinforcement, when the risk is or should be known to the physician, may be perceived by the patient as a form of acquiescence in the unsafe activity.

Physicians also need to consider that concern about risks expressed by an individual can actually mask other issues. For example, stress due to job dissatisfaction, problems with an employer, or even unstable home situations may result in non-specific symptoms which are attributed to a chemical or physical agent in the workplace. In community issues, concern about property values or changes in the ambience of a community may also be expressed as health issues.

Physicians have a responsibility not to abuse their position of trust in a community by allowing such ancillary factors as property values or community ambience to interfere with their judgments about health risk. A particularly egregious example of abusing this position occurred when a surgeon, active in local medical society affairs, predicted in a letter to the Mayor and the local media that dire health consequences from air pollution would be caused by the siting of a natural gas co-generation plant in the local industrial park. The community contained many senior citizens who were thus led by concern for their health to strongly oppose the development of the plant. This opposition occurred even though the community was experiencing frequent brownouts during the hottest days of the year which could have led to heat stress due to the lack of functioning air conditioning equipment, as well as to potential problems with medical assistance equipment which also required electricity. The physician later admitted to his colleagues that he had overstated the health problem because of his concern with the change in the character of his previously rural community.

Recipients of the risk message

Workers

Communicating the level of risk that may be present for a worker in a specific industry presents many of the same challenges that exist for communicating to an individual patient. Workers, as well as patients, are more likely to heed advice belatedly about preventive measures when they are suffering from a problem caused by their failure to take preventive action. A physician is derelict in responsibility if he or she simply conducts first aid after a workplace accident and allows the workers to return to the same setting where the injury occurred. Any injury in the workplace must lead to a full inquiry as to its cause. To the extent that the worker's actions, whether negligent or not, played any role, it is crucial that the physician actively communicate to the individual worker, to coworkers and to management the cause of the injury in order to avert a future problem, and to encourage the worker to seek appropriate training.[32]

Every physician encounter with a worker should be viewed as an opportunity for the prevention of occupational disease. The best way to reinforce safe work practice and to inform workers of potential hazards is for the physician to thoroughly understand the job tasks that are conducted within the workplace. Physicians with responsibility for a group of workers are obligated to familiarize themselves with the range of tasks that are performed in their setting. One of the best ways to evaluate the workplace is simply to ask workers what they believe to be the most dangerous part of their job, and to follow up on site by observing them on the job. This not only educates the physician, but it also establishes a link that will foster effective risk communication between the physician and the worker.

The obligation to understand the workplace also extends to the primary care practitioner who sees patients in his or her office independent of any formal relationship with the employer. All patients should be questioned regarding their workplace responsibilities. Again, questioning that goes beyond the patient's job title and approaches an understanding of the potential workplace hazards is itself a risk communication tool. Demonstration of concern by a physician is a highly effective way of letting a worker know that workplace hazards do exist, and reinforces health and safety messages that are provided at the workplace. How effective the physician may be in obtaining information from the patient will be determined by the physician's communication skills.

Peer group support can be a major determinant in how workers respond to job threats. Changing risky work behaviors frequently requires an understanding of the group dynamics that may lead a population of workers to fail to act in a safe manner. Sometimes long-standing traditions of work practice or 'macho' attitudes, particularly among young males, may interfere with safety at the workplace. In addition, certain preventive actions may be cumbersome or uncomfortable, such as wearing protective clothing, and therefore may not always be accepted by workers. Effective risk communication in such situations is facilitated by understanding the peer structure and using an approach that maximizes the likelihood that peer pressure will lead to the reinforcement of safe work practices. Change is possible; if 'macho' hockey players can be convinced to wear protective headgear, so can construction workers.

Physicians also have the opportunity to communicate the risks of personal health behaviors to workers that are not due to workplace hazards. Health promotion activities aimed at high blood pressure, obesity, high cholesterol levels and other risk factors have proven to be effective in decreasing adverse health consequences among workers and may be cost-effective for employers who develop these programs.

General public

While physicians are accustomed to discussing issues in terms of health, it must be emphasized that the residents in communities respond to environmental risks for many other reasons, stated and unstated. One potentially strong force in environmental issues is a sense of outrage of what *they* are doing to *me*. Whether or not health is the primary or actual concern, health will almost always be a stated issue.[30,33,34]

So, to whom does the public listen? Note that we have not asked the question 'Where do members of the public get their information?'. There have been a number of attempts to study the latter question, but there is an important distinction between where one obtains information and whether the information is believed. Despite the fact that at least in the US, the public rates doctors and universities as highly credible sources,[35] they are rarely accessed as a source for information. Perhaps the most important point is that the American public is highly skeptical about their usual sources of information regarding environmental matters; surveys have rated industry, government, and the press as very poor sources, with environmental groups rated only slightly better if at all.

An effective strategy is to include family members, also part of the general public, in discussions with employees about health roles and may facilitate discussion of dose–response. For example, a worker may be exposed to a chemical at levels that he or she can smell at the workplace with no concern about its health effects, but will be genuinely frightened by the exposure of family members to much smaller amounts if it becomes part of a community problem. Similarly, the worker's spouse, based on warnings about relatively small amounts in the general environment, realizes that there is reason to be concerned when a worker is exposed to higher levels.[36]

In every society risks to children are of particular concern, as has been demonstrated by the public alarm about alar in apples. Asbestos in schools has presented a particularly difficult problem in risk communication. Asbestos is dreaded as a carcinogen for very good reasons; however, depending upon its location and physical state, there may be less risk leaving the asbestos in place, or seal-ing it, than there is in dislodging the asbestos and removing it. The process of removing asbestos may be risky to the workers and tends to put asbestos into the air where it can be inhaled by children. Unfortunately, consultants hired by schools to give advice on asbestos removal may themselves be in the business of removing asbestos. We need to be at least as cautiously skeptical about so-called 'environmental experts' as we are with advice from medical consultants.

Decision makers

Physicians with expertise in environmental and occupational health are often asked by societal decision makers for advice on risk assessment and communication. In some ways community physicians and healthcare providers may be better able than academic scientists to empathize with the problems of decisionmakers. The latter are often facing time pressures caused by court, legislative, or political factors and, like physicians, may not have the luxury of obtaining all the needed data before a decision needs to be made.

Like a physician faced with a puzzling diagnostic problem, it is important to the decision maker to be able to cull significant information from a mass of data, to logically place a particular issue into a coherent framework, and to synthesize seemingly disparate information. When issues involve human health, the lay decision maker can be greatly assisted by a lucid explanation of the health risks and their implications by an even-handed physician.

Often the question is not so much whether an effect will occur, but how important it is to human health. For example, using sensitive modern techniques, researchers can accurately determine the level of an air pollutant capable of causing as little as 3% constriction of airways. Industry may tell a lay decision maker to ignore such minimal broncho-constriction, as it is well within the range of physiologic changes that occur when one goes from a warm room to a cold outdoor environment. On the other hand, clinicians are well aware of the morbidity due to asthma-induced bronchoconstriction; while small on a population basis, pollutants may have a marked effect in susceptible individuals.

Many occupational medicine physicians work for corporations and will become involved in interactions between the corporation and the community, particularly when issues affecting public health are raised. To function effectively in this situation the physician must understand the numerous cultural issues that profoundly affect the interface between a corporation and a community. Many of these represent the difference in the populations involved. Not uncommonly, industries with significant workplace hazards or emissions are located in economically disadvantaged communities whose predominant populations are often African-American or Hispanic, while the key corporate decision makers tend to be members of the relatively wealthy white population, who live in distant communities. The term 'environmental justice' is used to characterize the recognition that minority and disadvantaged

	Industry culture	Community culture
Secrecy	Good	Bad
Organizational clarity	Good	Rare
Redundancy	Bad	Good
Accountability	Good	Rare to non-existent
Initiative on community issues	Dangerous	Rewarded
Metric of success	Extrinsic: easily measurable as dollars	Intrinsic: difficult to measure

Table 59.1 Current issues inherent to risk communication by industrial organizations

communities bear a disproportionate burden of polluting and hazardous industries. The issues posed by environmental injustice are increasingly important and are not solvable without careful and respectful attention to the voice and involvement of the community (see Chapter 57.2).

It must be emphasized, however, that even without the issues considered under the sphere of environmental justice, there remain substantial differences between the culture of industries and the culture of communities (Table 59.1). Secrecy in the form of trade secrets is central to the continued competitive success of industries, while within a community secrecy is met with suspicion. The corporate world strives for organizational clarity, while communities tend to derive strength from a plethora of overlapping organizations that combine or go their own way depending upon the specific issue they are addressing. To a corporation redundancy is wasteful, while to a community it may be the only way to get the message across; success in the corporate world may be relatively easily measured in terms of dollars, while for a community member success is much more of an intrinsic metric that is not so readily gauged.

None of these cultural differences between corporations and communities is absolute but the physician must be aware of them when in the position of representing an industry to the community. In fact, there are really only two laws of interaction with the community for government or for industry. The first is if you have already irrevocably made a decision, do not approach the community as if there is a true dialogue in mind, as they will certainly see through the falseness of such an approach; and, second, there are no laws, each situation is different and each community is different. There are, however, reasonably obvious rules of engagement which include openness, transparency, honesty and respect.[33,34,37]

The press

Physicians have not been trained to communicate with the press, and are often astounded that what they say or do is transmitted so poorly by the press to the public.

The first task is to understand the press.[38] Five characteristics seem particularly pertinent.

1. Similar to physicians, members of the press consider themselves to be professionals performing a very important public service.

2. Members of the press are often highly suspicious cynics and iconoclasts; a desire to bring down idols and the successful may be part of their personal make-up and a key to success in their field.
3. In America the press is less subject to checks and balances than any major institution.
4. They may have minimal scientific or medical background.
5. Different professional subgroups of the press, e.g., daily newspaper reporters, magazine writers, or TV newscasters, have different needs in order to accomplish their jobs.

It is important to understand how members of the press handle a situation in which they may have very little background and may know little about the underlying technical concerns of specific issues. However, what an ethical journalist has been trained to do is to provide a balanced presentation of an issue. This leads to obtaining one quote from an industry representative and one quote from an environmental representative on a health issue or, more commonly, asking industry and environmental or labor groups for names of health experts for them to interview. This seemingly balanced and appropriate approach can, however, lead to the impression of greater uncertainty than otherwise would be present. There is almost always going to be some degree of disagreement among experts on any critical issue; however, most experts will usually have broad areas of agreement. The procedure used by journalists to obtain information tends to focus on areas of disagreement, or experts who are at one end or another of the usual spectrum of opinions. Involvement of attorneys may further polarize the discussion.

OTHER FACETS OF EFFECTIVE RISK COMMUNICATION
Understanding the issue

It is crucial for effective communication to understand the dimensions of the issue of concern.[39,40] As physicians we have all learned the importance of saying, 'I don't know', when we are in an area of medicine beyond our expertise. This certainly is also true when communicating to individuals or the public about risks. It is also crucial to appreciate the patient's or public's level of knowledge and empathize with their concerns in order to effectively communicate one's message.

Regarding the risks of chemical or physical agents, it is important to address toxicologic principles, including dose–response; the specificity of the effects of chemical and physical agents; and experience with animal testing as a controlled test for potential human response.

Many toxic compounds, namely direct-acting or intrinsic toxins, have thresholds below which there is no risk of an adverse effect. Others, such as mutagens and carcinogens for which it is assumed that any one molecule is capable of producing an effect, have very low-level risks at low concentrations. The relationship between dose and toxicity may be poorly understood by the public. In addition, surveys illustrate that the public frequently does not understand the association between the environment and public health.[41] The specificity of the effects of chemicals may also be poorly understood. The same person who readily understands that a knife, found near a person with a bullet wound in the heart, cannot be the murder weapon will readily assume that because asbestos can cause lung cancer it must also cause brain cancer.

A good analogy for physicians to use to communicate concepts of dose effects, and specificity of chemical and physical agents is to talk about medicines as chemicals. People understand that sufficiently high doses of aspirin can be lethal; conversely, an amount of aspirin can be so small that it will be of no value whatsoever in affecting pain. They also understand that aspirin is of no value for constipation and that a laxative will not decrease the pain of arthritis.

Tell the bad news

There is an obligation to report known or suspected health hazards (see Chapter 55). Not communicating such hazards when it is appropriate to do so is more than just loss of credibility or bad press; it is a major legal liability issue. Industry physicians who failed to inform workers about the information linking asbestos to lung cancer and mesothelioma have been subjected to law suits. An important corollary is that when industry finds out something has gone wrong, it should move to get the information out as quickly and openly as possible, preferably with a commitment to address and correct the issue.

An excellent example of the appropriate means to release information to the public is the issue of dioxins in paper products. The American paper industry became aware of the presence of varying amounts of dioxins in bleached paper products, which include such items as tampons, baby wipes, surgical gauze, food containers, and toilet paper. The industry organization, after an internal debate, elected to rapidly inform the public and the appropriate governmental agencies about the concern, along with a plan to investigate the causes and make any necessary process alterations. This issue received EPA acquiescence. Considering the personal intimacy of some of these paper items, the public response has been remarkably low key. Imagine, however, where the industry would be now if it had tried to hide the issue. Had such information 'leaked out' the EPA would have had enormous pressure to act confrontationally rather than co-operatively. Instead, there has been a constructive approach to obtain the scientific and technical information necessary to tackle this difficult problem.

Redundancy counts, and counts again

Communication to patients or the general public also requires reinforcement. The best time to tell people about a potential problem is before an adverse event occurs. Unfortunately, few people are listening or are interested enough at that stage to pay attention. However, that does not mean that no one is paying attention. What it does mean is there is value in being proactive and in recounting what is known, assuming that only a small percentage of individuals, or of a larger audience is going to receive any one message. There is rarely one audience only, but rather a multiplicity of individuals who are reached through a variety of media, starting with school children and extending through senior citizen groups.

Redundancy has a negative connotation to it, and should rather be viewed as a consistent message. This strategy has worked very well for public interest groups, including environmental groups that have specific issues that are of concern to them. Continually presenting an issue until the point is made is an approach that has characterized effective environmental organizations.

Do not condescend

The most important lesson that physicians and other experts have to learn when dealing with the public is not to be condescending. Empathic recognition of the problem perceived by the public is always the best approach. For instance, an approach that is bound to fail is to respond to a concern expressed by the public about a chemical in food by pointing out that foods are themselves chemicals, or that illness and death are a part of life.

References

1. National Research Council. Improving risk communication. Report of the Committee on Risk Perception and Communication. Washington, DC: National Academy Press, 1989.
2. National Research Council. Understanding risk. Informing decisions in a democratic society. Washington, DC: National Academy Press, 1996.
3. Gotsch AR, Goldstein BD, eds. Communicating environmental risk to the public. Health Educ Q 1991; 18:269–404.
4. Goldstein BD. The who, what, when, where, and why of risk characterization. Policy Stud J 1995; 23:70–75.
5. Weinstein MD, Kolb K, Goldstein BD. Using time intervals between expected events to communicate risk magnitudes. Risk Analysis 1996; 16:305–8.
6. Goldstein BD, Risk management will not be improved by mandating numerical uncertainty analysis for risk assessment. Univ Cincinnati Law Rev 1995; 63-4:1599–610.
7. Rosenstock IM. The health belief model. In: Glanz K, Lewis FM, Rimer BK, eds. Health behavior and health education. San Francisco, CA: Jossey-Bass, 1990.
8. Hochbaum GM. Public participation in medical screening programs: a sociopsychological study. Public Health Service Publication no. 572, 1958.
9. Bandura A. Social learning theory. Englewood Cliffs, NJ: Prentice-Hall, 1977.
10. Bandura A. Social foundations of thought and action. Englewood Cliffs, NJ: Prentice-Hall, 1986.
11. Marlatt GA, Gordon JR, eds. Relapse prevention. New York: Guilford Press, 1985.
12. Tinker TL, Pavlova MT, Gotsch AR, Bratic Arkin E. Communicating risk in a changing world. Solomons Island, MD: The Ramazzini Institute, 1998.
13. Bailey WC, Clark NM, Gotsch AR, Lemen RJ, Rosenstock IM. Asthma prevention. Chest 1992; 102:216S–31S.

14. Israel BA, Schurman SJ. Social support, control, and the stress process. In: Glanz K, Lewis FM, Rimer BK, eds. Health behavior and health education. San Francisco, CA: Jossey-Bass, 1990.

15. Lewis FM. The concept of control: a typology and health-related variables. Adv Health Educ Prom 1987; 2:277–309.

16. Minkler M. Improving health through community organization. In: Glanz K, Lewis FM, Rimer BK, eds. Health behavior and health education. San Francisco, CA: Jossey-Bass, 1990.

17. Rappaport J. Studies in empowerment: introduction to the issue. Prev Hum Serv 1984; 3:1–7.

18. Lewis FM. Perspectives on models of interpersonal health behavior. In: Glanz K, Lewis FM, Rimer BK, eds. Health behavior and health education. San Francisco, CA: Jossey-Bass, 1990.

19. Cohen S, Syme SL, eds. Social support and health. Orlando, FL: Academic Press, 1985.

20. Israel B. Social networks and social support: implications for natural helper and community level interventions. Health Educ Q 1985; 12:66–80.

21. Minkler M. Building supportive ties and sense of community among the inner-city elderly: the tenderloin senior outreach project. Health Educ Q 1985; 12:303–14.

22. Perry CL, Baranowski T, Parcel GS. How individuals, environments, and health behavior interact: social learning theory. In: Glanz K, Lewis FM, Rimer BK, eds. Health behavior and health education. San Francisco, CA: Jossey-Bass, 1990.

23. Rodin J. Personal control through the life course. In: Heise R, ed. Implications of the life-span perspective for social psychology. Hillsdale, NJ: Erlbaum, 1987.

24. Bandura A, Walters RH. Social learning and personality development. New York: Holt, Rinehart & Winston, 1963.

25. Orlandi MA, Landers KC, Weston R, Haley N. Diffusion of health promotion innovations. In: Glanz K, Lewis FM, Rimer BK, eds. Health behavior and health education. San Francisco, CA: Jossey-Bass, 1990.

26. Rogers EM. Diffusion of innovations, 3rd edn. New York: Free Press, 1962.

27. Orlandi MA. Promoting health and preventing disease in healthcare settings: an analysis of barriers. Prev Med 1987; 16:119–30.

28. Orlandi MA. The diffusion and adoption of worksite health promotion innovations: an analysis of the barriers. Prev Med 1986; 15:522–36.

29. Siegrist M, Cvetkovich G. Perception of hazards: the role of social trust and knowledge. Risk Analysis 2000; 20:713–19.

30. Sandman PM, Weinstein ND, Miller CK. High risk or low: how location on a 'risk ladder' affects perceived risks.' Risk Analysis 1994: 14:35.

31. Abatemarco D, Delnevo C, Rosen M, Weidner L, Gotsch AR. Medical surveillance practices of blue collar and white collar hazardous waste workers. J Occup Med 1995; 37:578–82.

32. Weidner BL, Gotsch AR, Delnevo CD, Newman JB, McDonald B. Worker health and safety training: assessing impact among emergency responders. Am J Ind Med 1998; 33:241–6.

33. Covello VT, Flamm WG, Rodricks JV, Tardiff RG. The analysis of actual versus perceived risks. New York: Plenum, 1983.

34. Fischoff B. Risk perception and communication unplugged: twenty years of process. Risk Analysis 1995; 15:137–45.

35. Goldstein BD, Gotsch AR, Lioy PJ. Environmental health in New Jersey. New Jersey Med 1988; 85:894–6.

36. Goldstein BD, Dickason OE, Morresey L, Tardiff R. Communication of risk due to community and workplace petroleum exposure. Indoor Environ 1994; 3:96–102.

37. Chess C. Evaluating environmental public participation: methodological questions. J Environ Planning Manage 2000; 43:769–84.

38. West B, Sandman PM, Greenberg MR. The reporter's environmental handbook. New Brunswick, NJ: Rutgers University Press, 1995.

39. Sjoberg L. Factors in risk perception. Risk Analysis 2000; 20:1–11.

40. Slovic P. Perception of risk. Science 1987; 236:280–5.

41. Gotsch AR. Surveys show nation is failing environmental health 101. Vital signs: perspectives of the President of APHA. The Nation's Health. Washington, DC: American Public Health Association, 1999.

Index